AF819775

Medico Achiever's Series

NEET

Objective

Physics

Volume 2

Medico Achiever's Series

NEET

Objective

Physics

Volume 2

DC Pandey
[B. Tech, M. Tech, Pantnagar, ID 15722]

arihant
SUCCESS AND NOTHING LESS

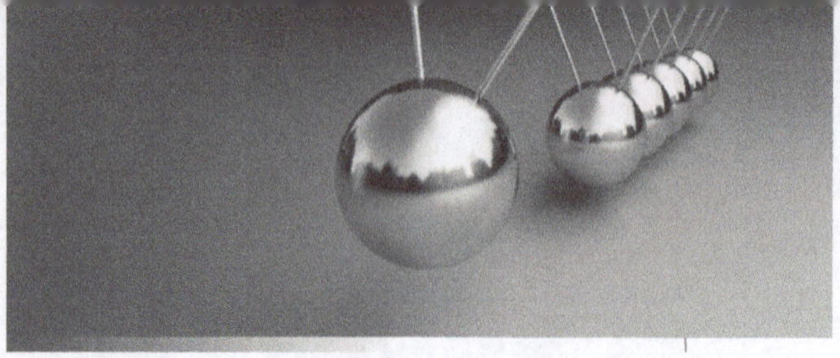

arihant
SUCCESS AND NOTHING LESS

Arihant Prakashan (Series), Meerut

Administrative & Production Offices

Regd. Office
'Ramchhaya' 4577/15, Agarwal Road, Darya Ganj, New Delhi -110002
Tele: 011- 47630600, 43518550

Head Office
Kalindi, TP Nagar, Meerut (UP) - 250002
Tel: 0121-7156203, 7156204

Sales & Support Offices

Agra, Ahmedabad, Bengaluru, Bareilly, Chennai, Delhi, Guwahati, Hyderabad, Jaipur, Jhansi, Kolkata, Lucknow, Nagpur & Pune.

PO No : TXT-XX-XXXXXXX-X-XX

Published by Arihant Publications (India) Ltd.

For further information about the books published by Arihant, log on to www.arihantbooks.com or e-mail at info@arihantbooks.com

Follow us on

PRODUCTION TEAM

Supported by **Dr. Manish Kumar Gupta**

Project Head	*Cover Designer*	*Inner Designer*
Yojna Sharma	Bilal Hashmi	Ankit Tyagi
Page Layouting	*Proof Readers*	*Figure Designer*
Rajbhaskar Rana	Princi Mittal, Mansi	Mohit

Preface

Mastery on Physics is important for students who are planning to make their career in medicine. The competition is no longer easy for a seat in a prestigious medical colleges today. Present changes in NEET exam Pattern have increased this challenge many a fold. To face this, they require an objective approach in their studies. A student can master the concepts and the skills required to tackle the questions asked in different entrances such as NEET (National Eligibility cum Entrance Test) through this approach.

NEET Objective Physics books of **Medico achiever's series** are borne out of my experience of teaching Physics to medical aspirants. The content of these books is framed to provide help in facing present day challenges by future medicos.

The exclusive features of our new magnified edition are

- The Chapter begins *via* **Overview with NEET connection.** This feature provides 4-way benefits as **Chapter Abstract, Insight of important topics, Suggestions to grip the chapter** and **NEET analytics** as video support.
- The whole chapter has been divided into smaller **modules**. Theory part of each module is elaborated with following unparallel features -
  - **Concept Ladder** Focused box matter with enhanced and important info
  - **Mentor's Tip** Specialised tips, Tricks and advice by the mentor
- Another speciality of modular theory is its syncing with PYQs through unique features like –
  - **NEET Snapshots** Facts from selected conceptual PYQs with proper elaborations
  - **NEET Close up** Simulators to sync Numerical PYQs with theory and having skill builders as additional practice tool.
  - **NEET Exclusive Extra Bytes** Important facts from past exams/ topics still important for NEET
- Assignments of the chapters have been divided into three parts:
  - **Step Up Practice** Scientifically designed modular Practice exercise, present just after the theory in each module.
  - **Gearing up for NEET** Mixed bag of assorted MCQs with all special format question types as asked in NEET.
  - **Final Check through PYQs** Last 10-years PYQs arranged in Modular format.

I am thankful to Dr. Manish Kumar Gupta, Academic Head and HOD Physics, Shivaji Career Institute for his support in finalizing this edition of Book.

Huge efforts have been made from my side to keep this book error free, inspite of that if any error or whatsoever is skipped in the book then that is purely incidental. Please write to me about that so that it can be corrected in the further edition of the book. Further, Suggestions from the respected Teachers & Students are also welcome as these are the foundation stones for the further improvement and success of our book.

DC Pandey

DEDICATION

This book is dedicated to my honourable grandfather

(Late) Sh. Pitamber Pandey

a Kumaoni poet, and a resident of village Dhaura (Almora), Uttarakhand

Key Features

Learning Objectives

Glimpse of Modular Distribution of Topics.

Learning Objectives

Module-I

- Electric Charge
- Conductors and Insulators
- Methods of Charging
- Coulomb's Law
- Forces between Multiple Charges (Superposition Principle)
- Applications of Electric Force (Coulomb's Law)

Module-II

- Electric Field
- Electric Field Lines
- Continuous Charge Distribution
- Electric Field of a Charged Ring
- Electric Dipole
- The Field of an Electric Dipole or Dipole Field
- Force on Dipole
- Torque on an Electric Dipole
- Work Done in Rotating a Dipole in a Uniform Electric Field

Electric Charges and Fields

Chapter Overview with NEET Connection

Electric charge is one of the fundamental concept of Physics. This chapter explains different properties of charge along with conceptualisation of their interactions with other charged as well as uncharged bodies. It also explains the measurement of strength and weakness of this interaction in terms of electric field.

Special format questions can be easily framed on the following topics of this chapter

- Methods of charging
- Coulomb's law
- Electric field lines
- Electric field due to dipole
- Gauss' law and its applications

For better understanding of this chapter

- Properties of vectors should be memorised.
- Strong grip over differentiation and integration is required.

Chapter overview with NEET connection

Present on the first page of every chapter and contain

- Chapter abstract
- Insight of Important Topics
- Suggestions to grip the chapter in a better way
- NEET analytics as video support

Concept Ladder

Focused Box matter with enhanced and important info to provide better grip over the concept.

(viii) The dimensional formula of charge is $[q] = [AT]$.

(ix) Frankline is the smallest unit of charge. It is also known as esu.

$$1 \text{ Frankline} = 1 \text{ esu} = \frac{1}{10} \text{ emu}$$

(x) Charge is always associated with mass.

Concept ladder

Mass of a body slightly changes while charging.

Mass $M-\Delta m$ ← Positive charging — Mass M — Negative charging → Mass $M+\Delta m$

Here, Δm = Number of electrons transferred during charging × Mass of electron.

$$\Delta m = Nm_e$$

Similarly, magnitude of force between q_1 and q_3,

$$|\mathbf{F}_2| = F_2 = \frac{1}{4\pi\varepsilon_0} \cdot \frac{q_1 q_3}{r^2}$$

where, $q_3 = 3\,\mu\text{C} = 3 \times 10^{-6}\,\text{C}$.

$$\Rightarrow \quad F_2 = \frac{(9.0\times 10^9)\,(1.0\times 10^{-6})\,(3.0\times 10^{-6})}{(1.0)^2}$$

$$= 2.7\times 10^{-2}\ \text{N}$$

Now, net force, $|\mathbf{F}_{net}| = \sqrt{F_1^2 + F_2^2 + 2F_1F_2\cos 120^\circ}$

$$= \left(\sqrt{(1.8)^2 + (2.7)^2 + 2\,(1.8)\,(2.7)\left(-\frac{1}{2}\right)}\right) \times 10^{-2}\ \text{N}$$

$$= 2.38\times 10^{-2}\ \text{N}$$

Mentor's Tip

Always use vector's parallelogram law of vector addition you learnt in class 11th Physics to solve resultant forces.

Mentor's Tips

Specialised Tips, Tricks and advices by the Mentor for performance enhancement in NEET.

Key Features

NEET Snapshot

When a sphere enclosed an electric dipole with charge $+q$C, then the total electric flux across the sphere is zero. ***[NEET 2019]***

When a sphere enclosed a charged dipole,

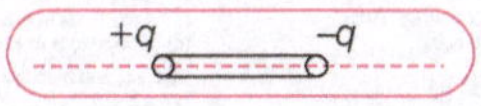

Here, $q = \pm qC$

Thus, according to the Gauss' law, the net electric flux across the closed surface is equal to the net charge enclosed by it, divided by ε_0, i.e.

$$\phi_E = \frac{q_{in}}{\varepsilon_0} = \frac{+q-q}{\varepsilon_0} = 0$$

NEET Snapshot

Unique element having facts with proper elaborations to sync selected conceptual questions of PYQs with the theory.

NEET Close-up

Example Similar to PYQ Asked in NEET 2023

An electric dipole is placed at an angle of 45° with an electric field of intensity 2×10^6 NC^{-1}. It experiences a torque equal to $2\sqrt{2}$ N-m. If the dipole length is 1 cm, then the magnitude of charge on the dipole is

(a) 3×10^{-3} C (b) 2×10^{-4} C (c) 4×10^{-2} C (d) 6×10^{-3} C

Sol. (*b*) Given, $\theta = 45°$,

$$E = 2\times10^6 \text{ NC}^{-1}$$

Dipole length, $2l = 1 \text{ cm} = 1\times10^{-2}$ m

Torque, $\tau = 2\sqrt{2}$ N-m

Skill Builder

An electric dipole is placed at an angle of 90° with an electric field of intensity 5×10^5 NC^{-1}. It experiences a torque equal to 15 N-m. If the dipole length is 3 cm, then the magnitude of charge on the dipole is

(a) 5 mC (b) 2 mC

(c) 1 mC (d) 3 mC

For more Practice Refer Q.Nos. 32, 36 of Gearing up for NEET.

NEET Close up

Unparallel concept elevation tool, helpful in syncing PYQs with theory and provide additional practice through skill builders.

NEET Exclusive EXTRA BYTES

- Ultimate test of charging is repulsion because attraction may also occur between one charged and another uncharged body.
- A normal charged particle [which is stable or moving with very low speed, then speed of light ($v << c$) has fixed specific mass, i.e. $\frac{q}{m} = 1.76\times10^{11}$ C/kg.
- Coulomb's law is used for two point charges. While using this for expanded and limited size bodies, one should take all the charge at the centre of the body and then even this, law will be valid only for points outside of that expanded body.
- Coulomb's force between two charges is independent of nearby existing other charged /uncharged bodies.
- Dielectric constant (K) of a medium is numerically equal to the ratio of the force on two point charges in free space to that in the medium.

$$K = \frac{F_{\text{Free space}}}{F_{\text{medium}}}$$

- A charged particle always experiences electric force in an electric field whether it is stable or moving .
- For any regular polygon containing same charges at all corners, electric field at centre is always zero.
- Electric lines of force start and end perpendicular at the surface of the conductor.
- Electric field inside a hollow sphere may or may not be zero, while it is always zero inside solid conductors.
- An electric dipole experiences only torque (not force) in an uniform electric field while it may experience force also in non-uniform electric field.
- Electric field and Coulomb force for different distributions.

Distribution	Point charge	Dipole	Quadrupole	Octupole
E or F is proportional to	$\frac{1}{r^2}$	$\frac{1}{r^3}$	$\frac{1}{r^4}$	$\frac{1}{r^5}$

NEET Exclusive Extra Bytes

Important facts from Past Exams/ Topics still expected in NEET.

Key Features

STEP UP Practice 1

1. One metallic sphere A is given positive charge whereas another identical metallic sphere B of exactly same mass as of A is given equal amount of negative charge. Then,
(a) mass of A and mass of B still remain equal
(b) mass of A increases
(c) mass of B decreases
(d) mass of B increases

2. When 10^{14} electrons are removed from a neutral metal sphere, then the charge on the sphere becomes
(a) 16 μC (b) −16 μC
(c) 32μC (d) −32μC

3. A conductor has 14.4×10^{-19}C positive charge. The conductor has (charge on electron = 1.6×10^{-19}C)
(a) 9 electrons in excess (b) 27 electrons in short
(c) 27 electrons in excess (d) 9 electrons in short

4. Charge on α-particle is
(a) 4.8×10^{-19} C (b) 1.6×10^{-19} C
(c) 3.2×10^{-19}C (d) 6.4×10^{-19} C

5. Two similarly charged bodies can
(a) only attract each other
(b) only repel each other
(c) may attract or repel each other
(d) neither attract nor repel each other

Step UP Practice

Scientifically designed first practice exercise to check modular learning.

GEARING UP FOR NEET

Single Option Correct

1 Charge q_2 of mass m revolves around a stationary charge q_1 in a circular orbit of radius r. The orbital periodic time of q_2 would be
(a) $\left[\frac{4\pi^2 mr^3}{kq_1q_2}\right]^{1/2}$ (b) $\left[\frac{kq_1q_2}{4\pi^2 mr^3}\right]^{1/2}$
(c) $\left[\frac{4\pi^2 mr^4}{kq_1q_2}\right]^{1/2}$ (d) $\left[\frac{4\pi^2 mr^2}{kq_1q_2}\right]^{1/2}$

2 Two identical charged spheres suspended from a common point by two massless strings of length l are initially a distance $d (d << l)$ apart because of their mutual repulsion. The charge begins to leak from both the spheres at a constant rate. As a result, the spheres approach each other with a velocity v. Then, v as a function of distance x between them is,
(a) $v \propto x^{-1/2}$ (b) $v \propto x^{-1}$
(c) $v \propto x^{1/2}$ (d) $v \propto x$

3 In the given figure, two tiny conducting balls of identical mass m and identical charge q hang from non-conducting threads of equal length L. Assume that θ is so small that $\tan\theta \simeq \sin\theta$, then for equilibrium, x is equal to

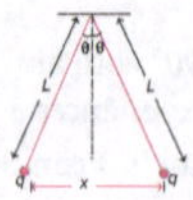

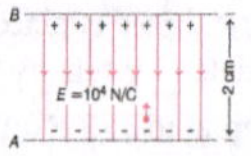

(a) 0.85×10^7 ms^{-1} (b) 1.0×10^7 ms^{-1}
(c) 1.25×10^7 ms^{-1} (d) 1.65×10^7 ms^{-1}

6 Four point positive charges of same magnitude (Q) are placed at four corners of a rigid square frame as shown in figure. The plane of the frame is perpendicular to Z-axis. If a negative point charge is placed at a distance z away from the frame ($z << L$), then

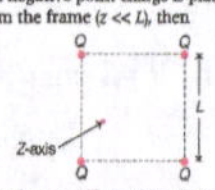

(a) negative charge oscillates along the Z-axis
(b) it moves away from the frame
(c) it moves slowly towards the frame and stays in the plane of the frame
(d) it passes through the frame only once

Gearing up for NEET

Mixed bag of assorted MCQs with all special format questions types asked in NEET.

Final Check Through PYQs

Module-I Electric Charges and Coulomb's Law

1 The acceleration of an electron due to the mutual attraction between the electron and a proton when they are 1.6 Å apart is, ($m_e \simeq 9 \times 10^{-31}$ kg, $e = 1.6 \times 10^{-19}$C)
$\left(\text{Take, } \frac{1}{4\pi\varepsilon_0} = 9 \times 10^9 \text{ Nm}^2\text{C}^{-2}\right)$
[NCERT (New) Pg. 8, NEET (Oct.) 2020]
(a) 10^{24} m/s^2
(b) 10^{23} m/s^2
(c) 10^{22} m/s^2
(d) 10^{25} m/s^2

2 Two point charges A and B, having charges $+Q$ and $-Q$ respectively, are placed at certain distance apart and force acting between them is F. If 25% charge of A is transferred to B, then force between the charges becomes *[NCERT (New) Pg. 8, NEET (National) 2019]*
(a) $\frac{9F}{16}$ (b) $\frac{16F}{9}$
(c) $\frac{4F}{3}$ (d) F

3 Suppose the charge of a proton and an electron differ slightly. One of them is $-e$ and the other is $(e + \Delta e)$. If the net of electrostatic force and gravitational force between two hydrogen atoms placed at a distance d (much greater than atomic size) apart is zero, then Δe is of the order [Given mass of hydrogen, $m_h = 1.67 \times 10^{-27}$ kg] *[NCERT (New) Pg. 8, NEET 2017]*
(a) 10^{-20} C (b) 10^{-23} C
(c) 10^{-37} C (d) 10^{-47} C

4 Two identical charged spheres suspended from a common point by two massless strings of lengths l, are initially at a distance d ($d << l$) apart because of their mutual repulsion. The charges begin to leak from both the spheres at a constant rate. As a result, the spheres approach each other with a velocity v. Then, v varies as a function of the distance x between the sphere, as
[NCERT (New) Pg. 8, NEET 2016]
(a) $v \propto x$ (b) $v \propto x^{-1/2}$
(c) $v \propto x^{-1}$ (d) $v \propto x^{1/2}$

Final Check through PYQs

Specialised PYQs section having last 10 years PYQs arranged in modular format to check the preparation levels and gain confidence to face NEET.

Syllabus

UNIT I Electrostatics

Electric charges: Conservation of charge. Coulomb's law forces between two point charges, forces between multiple charges: superposition principle and continuous charge distribution.

Electric field: Electric field due to a point charge, Electric field lines. Electric dipole, Electric field due to a dipole. Torque on a dipole in a uniform electric field.

Electric flux, Gauss's law and its applications to find field due to infinitely long uniformly charged straight wire, uniformly charged infinite plane sheet and uniformly charged thin spherical shell. Electric potential and its calculation for a point charge, electric dipole and system of charges; potential difference, Equipotential surfaces, Electrical potential energy of a system of two point charges and of electric dipole in an electrostatic field.

Conductors and insulators, Dielectrics and electric polarization, capacitors and capacitances, the combination of capacitors in series and parallel, capacitance of a parallel plate capacitor with and without dielectric medium between the plates. Energy stored in a capacitor.

UNIT II Current Electricity

Electric current, Drift velocity, mobility and their relation with electric current. Ohm,s law, Electrical resistance, V-I characteristics of Ohmic and non-ohmic conductors. Electrical energy and power, Electrical resistivity and conductivity. Series and parallel combinations of resistors; Temperature dependence of resistance.

Internal resistance, potential difference and emf of a cell, a combination of cells in series and parallel. Kirchhoff's laws and their applications. Wheatstone bridge, Metre Bridge.

UNIT III Magnetic Effects of Current and Magnetism

Biot - Savart law and its application to current carrying circular loop. Ampere's law and its applications to infinitely long current carrying straight wire and solenoid. Force on a moving charge in uniform magnetic and electric fields.

Force on a current-carrying conductor in a uniform magnetic field. The force between two parallel currents carrying conductors-definition of ampere. Torque experienced by a current loop in a uniform magnetic field: Moving coil galvanometer, its sensitivity and conversion to ammeter and voltmeter.

Current loop as a magnetic dipole and its magnetic dipole moment. Bar magnet as an equivalent solenoid. magnetic field lines; Magnetic field due to a magnetic dipole (bar magnet) along its axis and perpendicular to its axis. Torque on a magnetic dipole in a uniform magnetic field. Para, dia and ferromagnetic substances with examples, Effect of temperature on magnetic properties.

UNIT IV Electromagnetic Induction and Alternating Currents

Electromagnetic induction: Faraday's law, Induced emf and current: Lenz's law, Eddy currents, Self and mutual inductance. Alternating currents, peak and RMS value of alternating current/voltage : reactance and impedance: LCR series circuit, resonance : power in AC circuits, wattless current, AC generator and transformer.

UNIT V Electromagnetic Waves

Displacement current, Electromagnetic waves and their characteristics, Transverse nature of electromagnetic waves, Electromagnetic spectrum (radio waves, microwaves, infrared, visible, ultraviolet. X-rays. Gamma rays), Applications of e.m. waves.

UNIT VI Optics

Reflection of light, spherical mirrors, mirror formula. Refraction of light at plane and spherical surfaces, thin lens formula and lens maker formula. Total internal reflection and its applications.

Magnification, power of a lens, Combination of thin lenses in contact, Refraction of light through a prism. Microscope and astronomical telescope (reflecting and refracting) and their magnifying powers.

Wave optics: wavefront and Huygens' principle, Laws of reflection and refraction using Huygens principle,

Interference, Young's double-slit experiment and expression for fringe width, coherent sources, and sustained interference of light. Diffraction due to a single slit, width of central maximum.. Polarization, plane-polarized light: Brewster's law, uses of plane-polarized light and Polaroid.

UNIT VII Dual Nature of Matter and Radiation

Dual nature of radiation. Photoelectric effect. Hertz and Lenard's observations; Einstein's photoelectric equation: particle nature of light. Matter waves-wave nature of particle, de-Broglie relation.

UNIT VIII Atoms and Nuclei

Alpha-particle scattering experiment; Rutherford's model of atom; Bohr model, energy levels, hydrogen spectrum. Composition and size of nucleus, atomic masses, mass-energy relation, mass defect; binding energy per nucleon and its variation with mass number, nuclear fission, and fusion.

UNIT IX Electronic Devices

Semiconductors; semiconductor diode: I-V characteristics in forward and reverse bias; diode as a rectifier; I-V characteristics of LED. the photodiode, solar cell, and Zener diode; Zener diode as a voltage regulator. Logic gates (OR, AND, NOT, NAND and NOR).

UNIT X Experimental Skills

Familiarity with the basic approach and observations of the experiments and activities:

1. Varnier calipers-its use to measure the internal and external diameter and depth of a vessel.
2. Screw gauge-its use to determine thickness/diameter of thin sheet/wire.
3. Simple pendulum-dissipation of energy by plotting a graph between the square of amplitude and time.
4. Metre Scale - the mass of a given object by the principle of moments.
5. Young's modulus of elasticity of the material of a metallic wire.
6. Surface tension of water by capillary rise and effect of detergents,
7. Co-efficient of viscosity of a given viscous liquid by measuring terminal velocity of a given spherical body.
8. Speed of sound in air at room temperature using a resonance tube.
9. Specific heat capacity of a given (i) solid and (ii) liquid by method of mixtures.
10. The resistivity of the material of a given wire using a metre bridge.
11. The resistance of a given wire using Ohm's law.
12. Resistance and figure of merit of a galvanometer by half deflection method.
13. The focal length of;
    (i) Convex mirror
    (ii) Concave mirror and
    (iii) Convex lens, using the parallax method.
14. The plot of the angle of deviation vs angle of incidence for a triangular prism.
15. Refractive index of a glass slab using a travelling microscope.
16. Characteristic curves of a p-n junction diode in forward and reverse bias.
17. Characteristic curves of a Zener diode and finding reverse break down voltage.
18. Identification of Diode, LED,. Resistor. A capacitor from a mixed collection of such items.

Content

For deeper insight
Scan the QR Code

Chapter 1

Electric Charges and Fields

Learning Objectives

Module-I

- Electric Charge
- Conductors and Insulators
- Methods of Charging
- Coulomb's Law
- Forces between Multiple Charges (Superposition Principle)
- Applications of Electric Force (Coulomb's Law)

Module-II

- Electric Field
- Electric Field Lines
- Continuous Charge Distribution
- Electric Field of a Charged Ring
- Electric Dipole
- The Field of an Electric Dipole or Dipole Field
- Force on Dipole
- Torque on an Electric Dipole
- Work Done in Rotating a Dipole in a Uniform Electric Field

Module-III

- Electric Flux
- Area Vector
- Gauss' Law

Module-IV

- Applications of Gauss' Law

Chapter Overview with NEET Connection

Electric charge is one of the fundamental concept of Physics. This chapter explains different properties of charge along with conceptualisation of their interactions with other charged as well as uncharged bodies. It also explains the measurement of strength and weakness of this interaction in terms of electric field.

Special format questions can be easily framed on the following topics of this chapter

- Methods of charging
- Coulomb's law
- Electric field lines
- Electric field due to dipole
- Gauss' law and its applications

For better understanding of this chapter

- Properties of vectors should be memorised.
- Strong grip over differentiation and integration is required.

Introduction

Electric charges have unique properties of attraction, repulsion, conduction, induction, etc., which causes many specific effects associated with it. Study of these properties are done under static and dynamic behaviour of charge. In this chapter, we will study about properties of electric charges, Coulomb's law and its application, properties of electric dipole, electric flux, Gauss' law and its application to calculate electric field produced by complex distribution of charges.

Module 1

Electric Charges and Coulomb's Law

• Electric Charge • Conductors and Insulators • Methods of Charging • Coulomb's Law
• Forces between Multiple Charges (Superposition Principle) • Applications of Electric Force (Coulomb's Law)

Electric Charge

Electric charge can be defined as an intrinsic property of elementary particles of matter which give rise to electric force between various objects. It is represented by q. The SI unit of electric charge is coulomb (C). A proton has positive charge$(+e)$ and an electron has negative charge $(-e)$, where $e = 1.6 \times 10^{-19}$ C.

William Gilbert first observed two types of charges and their proper concept was given by **Benjamin Frankline.**

Important points regarding electric charge

The following points regarding electric charge are as follows

(i) Like charges repel each other and unlike charges attract each other.

(ii) The property which differentiates two kinds of charge is called the **polarity of charge.** If an object possesses an electric charge, then it is said to be **electrified** or **charged.** When its net charge is zero, then it is said to be **neutral (just like neutron).**

(iii) Charge is a scalar quantity as it has magnitude but no direction. It can be of two types as positive and negative. When some electrons are removed from the atom, it acquires a positive charge and when some electrons are added to the atom, it acquires a negative charge.

(iv) Charge can be transferred from one body to another.

(v) Charge is invariant, *i.e.* it does not depend on the velocity of charged particle.

(vi) A charged particle at rest produces electric field. A charged particle with unaccelerated motion produces both electric and magnetic fields but does not radiate energy. But an accelerated charged particle not only produces an electric and magnetic fields but also radiates energy in the form of electromagnetic waves.

(vii) 1 coulomb $= 3 \times 10^9$ esu $= \frac{1}{10}$ emu of charge, where esu is electrostatic unit of charge and emu is electromagnetic unit of charge. Its CGS unit is stat coulomb.

(viii) The dimensional formula of charge is $[q] = [\text{AT}]$.

(ix) Frankline is the smallest unit of charge. It is also known as esu.

$$1 \text{ Frankline} = 1 \text{ esu} = \frac{1}{3 \times 10^{10}} \text{ emu}$$

(x) Charge is always associated with mass.

Concept ladder

Mass of a body slightly changes while charging.

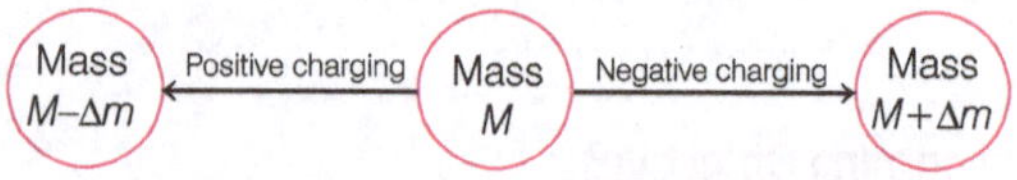

Here, Δm = Number of electrons transferred during charging × Mass of electron.

$$\boxed{\Delta m = Nm_e}$$

Properties of an Electric Charge

If the size of charged bodies is very small as compared to the distance between them, we treat them as **point charges.** In addition to being positive or negative, the charges have the following properties :

Charge is Additive

If a system contains n charges q_1, q_2, q_3 ...., q_n, then the total charge of the system is obtained simply by algebric (including their respective signs) sum of all charges.

$$q_{\text{net}} = q_1 + q_2 + q_3 + \ldots + q_n$$

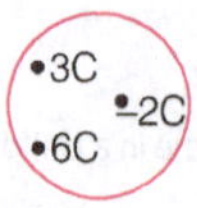

Here, net charge of this system is

$$q_{\text{net}} = 3\text{C} - 2\text{C} + 6\text{C} = 7\text{C}$$

Charge is Conserved

Total charge of an isolated system always remains constant. This property is known as **Law of Conservation of Charge.**

Conservation of charge holds good for all kinds of reactions.

Charge is Quantised

Charge cannot have any arbitrary value. Its value is always an integer multiplier of e [charge of electron]

In general, $q = \pm ne$ where, n = integer.

> **Concept ladder** Protons and neutrons are combination of other entities called **quarks**, which have charges of $\pm\frac{1}{3}e$ and $\pm\frac{2}{3}e$. However, isolated quarks have not been observed, hence quantum of charge is still e.

Example 1 *What is the total charge of a system containing five charges +1, + 2, −3, + 4 and −5 in some arbitrary unit?*

Sol. As charges are additive in nature, *i.e.* the total charge of a system is the algebraic sum of all the individual charges located at different points inside the system, *i.e.*

$$q_{net} = q_1 + q_2 + q_3 + q_4 + q_5$$

$\therefore$ Total charge = +1 + 2 − 3 + 4 − 5 = −1 in the same unit.

Example 2 *How many electrons are there in one coulomb of negative charge?*

Sol. The negative charge is due to the presence of excess electrons. An electron has a charge whose magnitude is $e = 1.6 \times 10^{-19}$ C, the number of electrons is equal to the charge q divided by the charge e on each electron.

Therefore, the number n of electrons is

$$n = \frac{q}{e} = \frac{1.0}{1.6 \times 10^{-19}} = 6.25 \times 10^{18} \text{ electrons}$$

Example 3 *A sphere of lead of mass 10 g has net charge -2.5×10^{-9} C.*

(i) Find the number of excess electrons on the sphere.

(ii) How many excess electrons are per lead atom? Atomic number of lead is 82 and its atomic mass is 207 g/mol.

Sol. (i) The charge on an electron $= -1.6 \times 10^{-19}$C

Net charge on sphere $= -2.5 \times 10^{-9}$C

So, the number of excess electrons $= \frac{-2.5 \times 10^{-9}\text{C}}{-1.6 \times 10^{-19}\text{C}}$

$= 1.56 \times 10^{10}$ electrons

(ii) Atomic number of lead is 82.

Atomic mass of lead is 207 g/mol.

$\therefore$ 10 g of lead will have $\frac{10 \text{ g}}{207 \text{ g/mol}} \times 6.02 \times 10^{23}$ atoms/mol

$= 2.91 \times 10^{22}$ atoms

$\therefore$ The number of excess electrons per lead atom

$= \frac{1.56 \times 10^{10}}{2.91 \times 10^{22}} = 5.36 \times 10^{-13}$ electrons

Conductors and Insulators

Now we understand that, the quantisation of electric charge is the property by virtue of which all free charges are integral multiple of a basic unit of charge represented by *e*.

Conductors The substances through which electric charges can flow easily are called conductors.

Metals, human body and animal bodies, graphite, acids, etc. are examples of conductors.

Insulators The substances through which electric charges cannot flow easily are called insulators.

Most of the non-metals like glass, diamond, porcelain, plastic, nylon, wood, mica, etc. are examples of insulators.

Methods of Charging

There are mainly three methods of charging a body, which are given below.

1. Charging by Rubbing or Friction

When two bodies are rubbed together, some electrons from one body gets transferred to the another body. The positive and negative charges appear on the bodies in equal amount simultaneously due to the transfer of electrons.

The body that donates the electrons becomes positively charged while that which receives electrons becomes negatively charged, *e.g.* when a glass rod is rubbed with a silk cloth, the glass rod acquires some positive charge by losing electrons and the silk cloth acquires negative charge of the same amount of gaining electrons.

Ebonite rod on rubbing with wool becomes positively charged making the wool negatively charged.

2. Charging by Contact or Conduction

Take two conductors, one is charged and other is uncharged. Bring the conductors in contact with each other. The charge (whether negative or positive) under its own repulsion will spread over both the conductors.

Thus, the conductors will be charged with the same sign. This is called as charging by conduction (through contact).

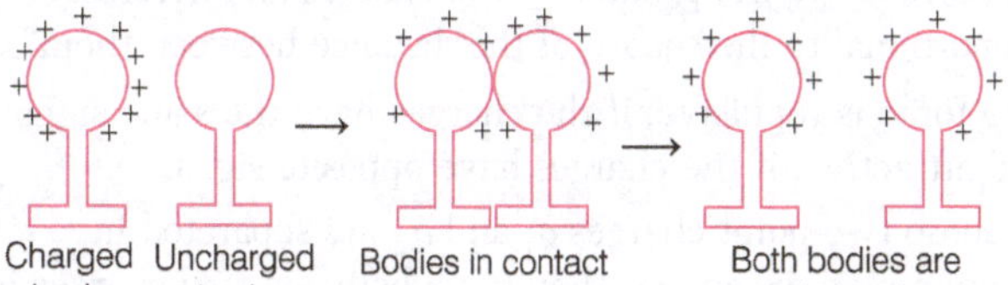

> **Mentor's Tip**
> If two conducting spheres of radii R_1 and R_2 and initial charges Q_1 and Q_2 respectively, then their final charges after conduction (Q_1' and Q_2' respectively) can be given by
>
> $$Q_1' = R_1\left[\frac{Q_{total}}{R_{total}}\right] \Rightarrow Q_2' = R_2\left[\frac{Q_{total}}{R_{total}}\right] \Rightarrow \frac{Q_1'}{Q_2'} = \frac{R_1}{R_2}$$

3. Charging by Induction

If a charged body is brought near an uncharged body, then one side of neutral body (closer to charged body) becomes oppositely charged while the other side becomes similarly charged as shown in figure.

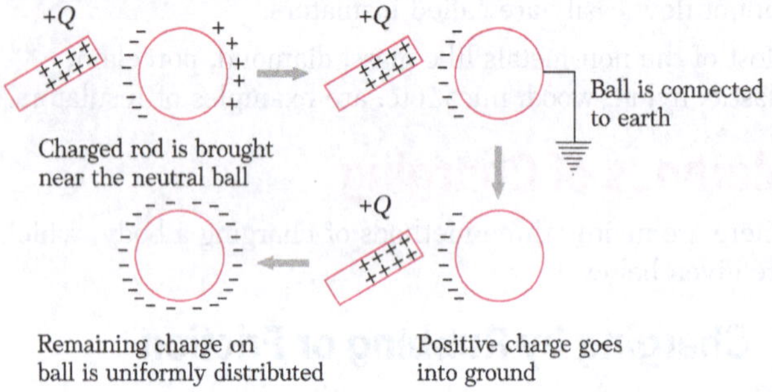

Charging by induction

In this process, charging is done without actual contact of bodies.

Concept ladder

Important points regarding induction

- In case of metals, induced charge is equal and opposite of inducing charge i.e. $q_{\text{induced}} = -q_{\text{inducing}}$
- For other bodies, $q_{\text{induced}} = -q_{\text{inducing}}\left[1 - \frac{1}{\varepsilon_r}\right]$
- Induction happens in bodies, not in point charges/masses.
- Net electrostatic force between inducing and induced bodies is always attractive.
- Since, attraction can happen in (a) opposite charges and (b) a charged body and uncharged body, **repulsion is the sure test of electrification.**

Coulomb's Law

Coulomb's law is a quantitative statement about the force between two point charges, which he derived using torsion balance experiment. It states that "the force of interaction between any two point charges is directly proportional to the product of the charges and inversely proportional to the square of the distance between them".

The force is repulsive, if the charges have the same signs and attractive, if the charges have opposite signs.

Suppose two point charges q_1 and q_2 are separated in vacuum by a distance r, then force between two charges is given by

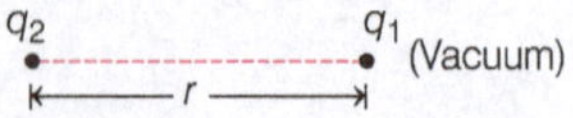

Two charges separated by distance r

$$F_e = \frac{kq_1q_2}{r^2}$$

The constant k is usually put as $k = \frac{1}{4\pi\varepsilon_0}$, where ε_0 is called the **permittivity of free space** and has the value $\varepsilon_0 = 8.854 \times 10^{-12} \text{C}^2/\text{N-m}^2$. For all practical purposes, we will take $\frac{1}{4\pi\varepsilon_0} \simeq 9 \times 10^9 \text{N-m}^2/\text{C}^2$.

NEET Close-up

Example Similar to PYQ Asked in NEET 2020

The acceleration of an electron due to the mutual attraction between the electron and a proton when they are 2.1 Å apart is ($m_e \approx 9.1 \times 10^{-31}$ kg, $e = 1.6 \times 10^{-19}$ C)

$\left[\text{Take, } \frac{1}{4\pi\varepsilon_0} = 9 \times 10^9 \text{ Nm}^2\text{C}^{-2}\right]$

(a) 0.58×10^{22} m/s^2 (b) 5.88×10^{22} m/s^2
(c) 5.22×10^{23} m/s^2 (d) 0.85×10^{22} m/s^2

Sol. (*a*) Force of mutual attraction between the electron and proton (where, $r = 2.1$ Å $= 2.1 \times 10^{-10}$ m) is given as

$$F = \frac{1}{4\pi\varepsilon_0} \times \frac{e^2}{r^2} = 9 \times 10^9 \times \frac{(1.6 \times 10^{-19})^2}{(2.1 \times 10^{-10})^2}$$

$$= \frac{23.04 \times 10^{-29}}{4.41 \times 10^{-20}} = 5.22 \times 10^{-9}$$

$$\therefore \text{Acceleration of electron} = \frac{F}{m_e} = \frac{5.22 \times 10^{-9}}{9 \times 10^{-31}}$$

$$= 0.58 \times 10^{22} \text{ m/s}^2$$

Skill Builder

The acceleration of an electron due to the mutual attraction between the electron and proton is 0.85×10^{22} m/s^2. The distance between them is ($e = 1.6 \times 10^{-19}$) C.

$\left[\text{Take, } \frac{1}{4\pi\varepsilon_0} = 9 \times 10^9 \text{ Nm}^2\text{C}^{-2}\right]$

(a) 5.2 Å (b) 5 Å (c) 4.4 Å (d) 1.73 Å

For more Practice Refer Q.No. 18 of Gearing up for NEET.

Coulomb's Law in Vector Form

Consider two point charges q_1 and q_2 placed in vacuum at a distance r from each other, repel each other.

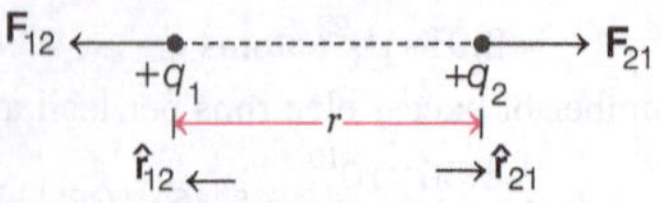

Repulsive Coulombian forces for $q_1q_2 > 0$

In vector form, Coulomb's law may be expressed as

$$\mathbf{F}_{12} = \text{Force on charge } q_1 \text{ due to } q_2$$

$$= \frac{1}{4\pi\varepsilon_0} \cdot \frac{q_1q_2}{r^2} \hat{\mathbf{r}}_{12}$$

where, $\hat{\mathbf{r}}_{12} = \dfrac{\mathbf{r}_{12}}{r}$ is a unit vector in the direction from q_1 to q_2.

Similarly, $\mathbf{F}_{21}$ = force on charge q_2 due to q_1

$$= \frac{1}{4\pi\varepsilon_0} \cdot \frac{q_1 q_2}{r^2} \hat{\mathbf{r}}_{21}$$

where, $\hat{\mathbf{r}}_{21} = \dfrac{\mathbf{r}_{21}}{r}$ is a unit vector in the direction from q_2 to q_1.

Similar case arises for attraction between two charges.

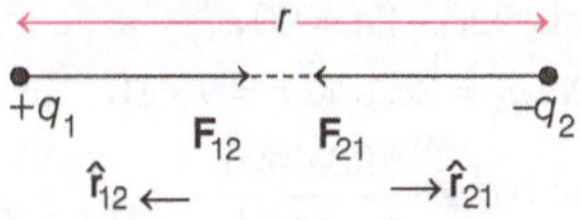

Attractive Coulombian forces for $q_1 q_2 < 0$

NEET Close-up

Example Similar to PYQ Asked in NEET 2019

Two point charges P and Q, having charges $+2Q$ and $-2Q$ respectively are placed at certain distance apart and force acting between them is F. If 20% charge of P is transferred to Q, then forces between the charges becomes

(a) $\dfrac{9}{16}F$ (b) $\dfrac{9}{25}F$

(c) $\dfrac{16}{25}F$ (d) $\dfrac{4}{5}F$

Sol. (c) The force between two point charges P and Q having charges $+2Q$ and $-2Q$ respectively is given by

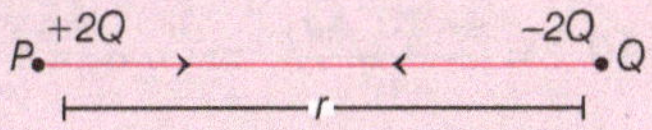

$$F = \frac{KQ_PQ_Q}{r^2} = \frac{K(2Q)(-2Q)}{r^2} = -\frac{4KQ^2}{r^2} \quad \text{...(i)}$$

When 20% charge of P is transferred to Q, then new amount of charge on P and Q respectively become

$$Q'_P = \frac{4}{5}(2Q)$$

$$Q'_Q = \left(\frac{20}{100}Q_P + Q_Q\right) = \left(\frac{1}{5}Q_P + Q_Q\right)$$

$$= \left(\frac{1}{5}(2Q) - 2Q\right) = \left(\frac{2}{5}Q - 2Q\right) = \frac{-8Q}{5}$$

So, the force between the two charges now becomes

$$F' = \frac{KQ'_P\,Q'_Q}{r^2} = \frac{K\left(\frac{8Q}{5}\right)\left(\frac{-8Q}{5}\right)}{r^2}$$

$$= \frac{-64KQ^2}{25r^2} = \frac{16}{25}F \quad \text{[From Eq. (i)]}$$

Thus, the new force between the charge is $\dfrac{16}{25}$ times the initial force between the charges.

Skill Builder

A force of 10 N is acting on two point charges L and M, having charges $\dfrac{+Q}{2}$ and $\dfrac{-Q}{2}$ respectively are placed at r cm apart. If 15% charge of L is transferred to M, then force between the charges becomes

(a) $\dfrac{17}{40}$ N (b) $\dfrac{289}{40}$ N (c) $\dfrac{17}{80}$ N (d) $\dfrac{289}{400}$ N

For more Practice Refer Q.No. 21 of Gearing up for NEET.

Important Points Related to Coulomb's Law

Important points related to Coulomb's law are given below

(i) The electric force is an action reaction pair, *i.e.* the two charges exert equal and opposite forces on each other. Thus, Coulomb's law obeys Newton's third law. $\mathbf{F}_{12} = -\mathbf{F}_{21}$

(ii) The electric force is conservative in nature.

(iii) Coulomb's law as we have stated above can be used for point charges in vacuum. When a dielectric medium is completely filled in between charges, rearrangement of the charges inside the dielectric medium takes place and the force between the same two charges decreases by a factor of K (dielectric constant).

$$F'_e = \frac{F_e}{K} = \frac{1}{4\pi\varepsilon_0 K} \cdot \frac{q_1 q_2}{r^2}$$

$$= \frac{1}{4\pi\varepsilon} \cdot \frac{q_1 q_2}{r^2} \quad \text{(in medium)}$$

Here, $\varepsilon = \varepsilon_0 K$ is called **permittivity of the medium.** For vacuum $K = 1$, for metal $K = \infty$.

(iv) The electric force is much stronger than gravitational force, $F_e >> F_g$.

As value of $\dfrac{1}{4\pi\varepsilon_0} = 9 \times 10^9$ N-m^2/C^2, which is much more than the value of gravitational constant,

$$G = 6.67 \times 10^{-11} \text{ N-m}^2 \text{ kg}^{-2}.$$

Concept ladder

- Coulomb's Force is a central force (and hence conservative too).
- Coulomb's force can be used for two point charges only. However, If sizes of charged bodies are very small as compared to distance between them, we can still apply this formula.
- Coulomb's force between two charges is independent of presence /absence of third charge.
- In the Coulomb's expression for finding force between two charges, do not use sign of charge because F is magnitude of force in the expression.

Example 4 Find the electrostatic force on q_2 in vector form for following diagram

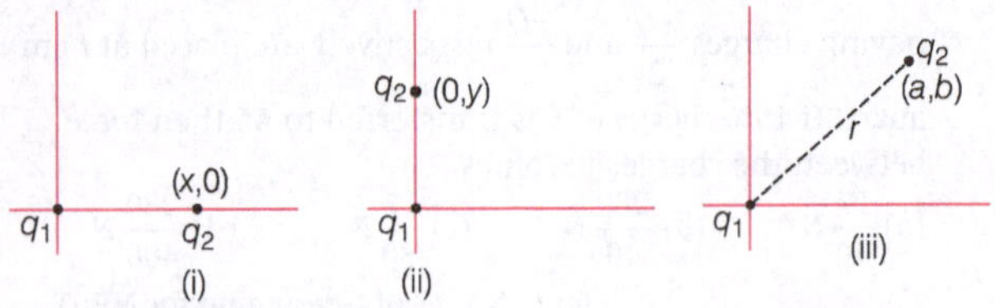

Sol. (i) $\mathbf{F}_{21} = \dfrac{Kq_1q_2}{x^2}\hat{\mathbf{i}}$ or $\dfrac{Kq_1q_2}{x^3}\mathbf{x}$

(ii) $\mathbf{F}_{21} = \dfrac{Kq_1q_2}{y^2}\hat{\mathbf{j}}$ or $\dfrac{Kq_1q_2}{y^3}\mathbf{y}$

(iii) $\mathbf{F}_{21} = \dfrac{Kq_1q_2}{r^2}\hat{\mathbf{r}} = \dfrac{Kq_1q_2}{(a^2+b^2)}\dfrac{a\hat{\mathbf{i}}+b\hat{\mathbf{j}}}{(a^2+b^2)^{\frac{1}{2}}} = \dfrac{Kq_1q_2}{(a^2+b^2)^{\frac{3}{2}}}(a\hat{\mathbf{i}}+b\hat{\mathbf{j}})$

Example 5 *A proton and an electron are placed 1.6 cm apart in free space. Find the magnitude and nature of electrostatic force between them.*

Sol. Charge on electron $= -1.6\times10^{-19}$ C

Charge on proton $= 1.6\times10^{-19}$ C

Using Coulomb's law,

$F = \dfrac{q_1q_2}{4\pi\varepsilon r^2}$, where r is the distance between proton and electron

$= \dfrac{9\times10^9\times(1.6\times10^{-19})(-1.6\times10^{-19})}{(1.6\times10^{-2})^2}$

$= -9\times10^{-25}$ N

Negative sign indicates that the force is attractive in nature.

Example 6 *The electrostatic force on a small sphere of charge 0.4 μC due to another small sphere of charge −0.8 μC in air is 0.2 N. (i) What is the distance between the two spheres? (ii) What is the force on the second sphere due to the first?*

Sol. (i) Using the relation, $F = \dfrac{1}{4\pi\varepsilon_0}\cdot\dfrac{q_1q_2}{r^2}$, we get

$$r^2 = \frac{1}{4\pi\varepsilon_0}\cdot\frac{q_1q_2}{F}$$

Here, $q_1 = 0.4\,\mu\text{C} = 0.4\times10^{-6}$ C,

$q_2 = 0.8\,\mu\text{C} = 0.8\times10^{-6}$ C

and $F = 0.2$ N

$\Rightarrow r^2 = 9\times10^9\times\dfrac{0.4\times10^{-6}\times0.8\times10^{-6}}{0.2}$

$= 144\times10^{-4}\,\text{m}^2$

Therefore, distance between the two spheres,

$r = 12\times10^{-2}\,\text{m} = 0.12$ m

(ii) Electrostatic forces always, appear in pairs and follows Newton's third law of motion.

$\therefore |\mathbf{F}_{21}|$ = Force on q_2 due to q_1 = 0.2 N and is attractive in nature.

Example 7 *Nucleus of ${}_{92}U^{238}$ emits α-particle (${}_2He^4$). α-particle has atomic number 2 and mass number 4. At any instant, α-particle is at a distance of 9×10^{-15} m from the centre of nucleus of uranium. What is the force on α-particle at this instant?*

$${}_{92}U^{238} \longrightarrow {}_2He^4 + {}_{90}Th^{234}$$

Sol. Force, $F = \dfrac{1}{4\pi\varepsilon_0}\dfrac{q_1q_2}{r^2}$

${}_{92}U^{238}$ has charge $92e$. When α-particle is emitted, charge on residual nucleus is $92e - 2e = 90e$.

$\therefore \quad q_1 = 90e,\ q_2 = 2e$, and $r = 9\times10^{-15}$ m

$\therefore \quad F = 9\times10^9\times\dfrac{(90e)(2e)}{(9\times10^{-15})^2}$

Force on α-particle,

$$F = \frac{9\times10^9\times90\times(1.6\times10^{-19})^2\times2}{(9\times10^{-15})^2} = 512\,\text{N}$$

Example 8 *Two identical spheres having positive charges are placed 3m apart repel each other with a force 8×10^{-3} N. Now, charges are connected by a metallic wire and they begin to repel each other with a force of 9×10^{-3} N. Find initial charges on the spheres.*

Sol. Let charges are q_1 and q_2 placed 3 m apart from each other.

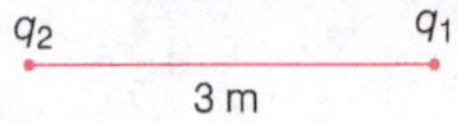

$\therefore \quad F = \dfrac{1}{4\pi\varepsilon_0}\dfrac{q_1q_2}{r^2}$ (Coulomb's law)

$\Rightarrow \quad 8\times10^{-3} = \dfrac{9\times10^9 q_1q_2}{(3)^2} \Rightarrow q_1q_2 = 8\times10^{-12}$

When the spheres are touched or connected by a metallic wire, charge on each sphere will be $\left(\dfrac{q_1+q_2}{2}\right)$.

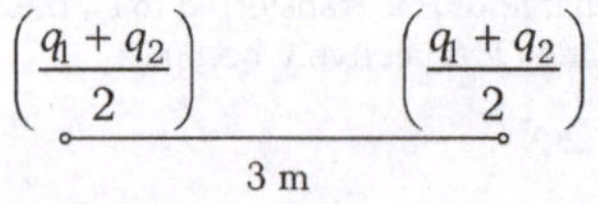

According to given condition in the question,

$\Rightarrow \quad 9\times10^{-3} = \dfrac{9\times10^9\left(\dfrac{q_1+q_2}{2}\right)^2}{(3)^2}$

$\Rightarrow \quad \left(\dfrac{q_1+q_2}{2}\right)^2 = 9\times10^{-12} \Rightarrow q_1+q_2 = 6\times10^{-6}$ ...(i)

Now, $(q_1-q_2)^2 = (q_1+q_2)^2 - 4q_1q_2$

$= (6\times10^{-6})^2 - 4\times8\times10^{-12} = 4\times10^{-12}$

$\Rightarrow \quad q_1 - q_2 = 2\times10^{-6}$ ...(ii)

Solving Eqs. (i) and (ii), we get

$q_1 = 4\times10^{-6}\,\text{C} = 4\,\mu\text{C},\ q_2 = 2\times10^{-6}\,\text{C} = 2\,\mu\text{C}$

Therefore, initial charges on the sphere are 4 μC and 2 μC.

Mentor's TIP

Identical spheres get equal charges when connected through a wire. The magnitude of this charge will always be equal to the average of both the charges.

Example 9 *Two protons are placed at some separation in vacuum. Find the ratio of electric and gravitational force acting between them.*

Sol. Let the distance between two protons having charge $+e$ and mass m is placed at a distance r from each other as shown in figure.

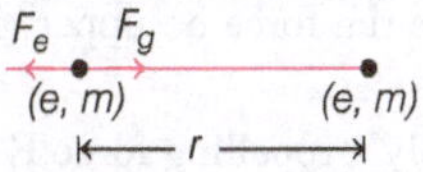

From Coulomb's law, $F_e = \frac{1}{4\pi\varepsilon_0}\frac{q_1 q_2}{r^2} = \frac{1}{4\pi\,\varepsilon_0}\frac{e \times e}{r^2}$

From gravitation law, $F_g = G\frac{m_1 m_2}{r^2} = G\frac{m \times m}{r^2}$

where, F_e and F_g are electric and gravitational forces respectively. On putting the values, we get

$$\frac{F_e}{F_g} = \frac{\frac{1}{4\pi\varepsilon_0}\frac{e^2}{r^2}}{\frac{Gm^2}{r^2}} = \frac{1}{4\pi\varepsilon_0}\frac{e^2}{m^2}\cdot\frac{1}{G}$$

$$= \frac{(9 \times 10^9)(1.6 \times 10^{-19})^2}{(1.67 \times 10^{-27})^2} \times \frac{1}{(6.67 \times 10^{-11})}$$

$$= 1.2 \times 10^{36} \simeq 10^{36}$$

Thus, $F_e >> F_g$

Example 10 *An electron revolves around a fixed charge of 9e in horizontal circle of radius r. Calculate its revolving speed.*

Sol. For circular motion,

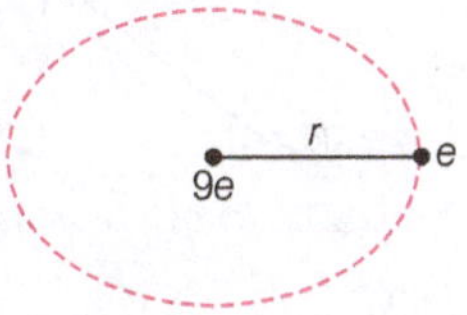

Centripetal force = Coulomb force

$$\Rightarrow \frac{m_e v^2}{r} = \frac{Ke(9e)}{r^2} \Rightarrow v = 3e\sqrt{\frac{K}{m_e r}}$$

Forces between Multiple Charges
(Superposition Principle)

According to the principle of superposition, "total force on a given charge due to number of charges is the vector sum of individual forces acting on that charge due to all the charges". The individual forces are unaffected due to the presence of other charges.

Suppose a system contains n point charges $q_1, q_2, \dots, q_n$. Then, by the principle of superposition, the force on q_1 due to all the other charges is given by

$$\mathbf{F}_1 = \mathbf{F}_{12} + \mathbf{F}_{13} + \dots\dots + \mathbf{F}_{1n}$$

$$\mathbf{F}_1 = \frac{q_1}{4\pi\varepsilon_0}\left[\frac{q_2\hat{\mathbf{r}}_{12}}{r_{12}^2} + \frac{q_3\hat{\mathbf{r}}_{13}}{r_{13}^2} + \dots\dots \frac{q_n\hat{\mathbf{r}}_{1n}}{r_{1n}^2}\right]$$

$$= \frac{q_1}{4\pi\varepsilon_0}\sum_{i=2}^{n}\frac{q_i\,\hat{\mathbf{r}}_{1i}}{r_{1i}^2}$$

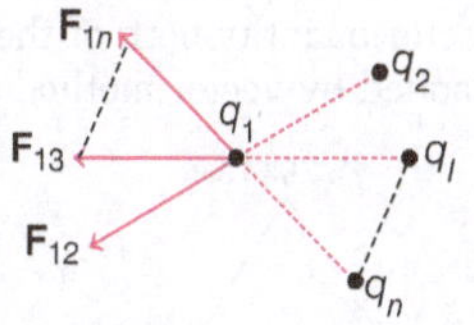

Force between the charges $q_1, q_2, q_3, \dots, q_n$

Example 11 *Equal charges each of 20 μC are placed at x = 0, 2, 4, 8, 16 cm on X-axis. Find the force experienced by the charge at x = 2 cm.*

Sol. Force on charge at $x = 2$ cm due to charge at $x = 0$ cm and $x = 4$ cm are equal and opposite, so they cancel each other.

Net force on charge at $x = 2$ cm is resultant of repulsive forces due to two charges at $x = 8$ cm and $x = 16$ cm.

$$\therefore\ F = \frac{q_1 \times q_2}{4\pi\varepsilon_0}\left[\frac{1}{(0.08 - 0.02)^2} + \frac{1}{(0.16 - 0.02)^2}\right]$$

$$= 9 \times 10^9 [20 \times 10^{-6}]^2\left[\frac{1}{(0.06)^2} + \frac{1}{(0.14)^2}\right] \cong 1.2 \times 10^3\ \text{N}$$

Example 12 *Five point charges each of value +q are placed on five vertices of a regular hexagon of side a metre. What is the magnitude of the force on a point charge of value −q coulomb placed at the centre of the hexagon?*

Sol. Let the centre of the hexagon be O. When the centre is joined with the vertices of a hexagon, then six triangles are formed. Consider ΔODE

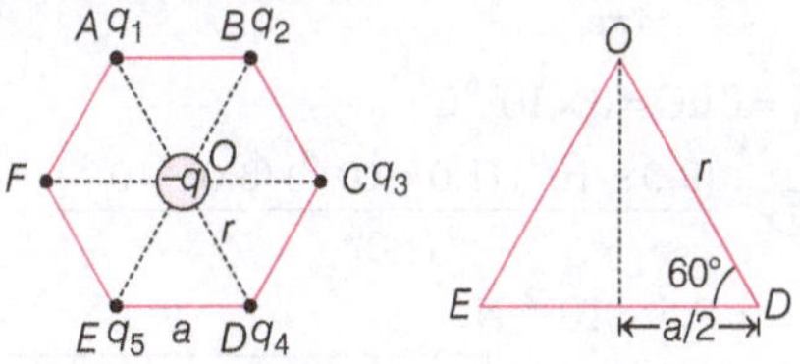

$$\frac{a/2}{r} = \cos 60° = \frac{1}{2}$$

$$\therefore \quad a = r$$

Given, $q_1 = q_2 = q_3 = q_4 = q_5 = q$

Net force on $-q$ is due to q_3 because forces due to q_1 and q_4 are equal and opposite, so cancel each other. Similarly, forces due to q_2 and q_5 also cancel each other. Hence, the net force on $-q$ is

$$F = \frac{1}{4\pi\,\varepsilon_0} \cdot \frac{(q)(q)}{r^2} \quad \text{(towards } q_3\text{)}$$

or $$F = \frac{1}{4\pi\,\varepsilon_0} \cdot \frac{q^2}{a^2}$$

Example 13 *Three charges $q_1 = 1\,\mu C$, $q_2 = -2\,\mu C$ and $q_3 = 3\,\mu C$ are placed on the vertices of an equilateral triangle of side 1.0 m. Find magnitude of electric force acting on charge q_1.*

Sol. Charge q_2 will attract charge q_1 (along the line joining them) and charge q_3 will repel charge q_1. Therefore, two forces will act on q_1, one due to q_2 and another due to q_3. Since, the force is a vector quantity both of these forces (say $\mathbf{F}_1$ and $\mathbf{F}_2$) will be added by vector method.

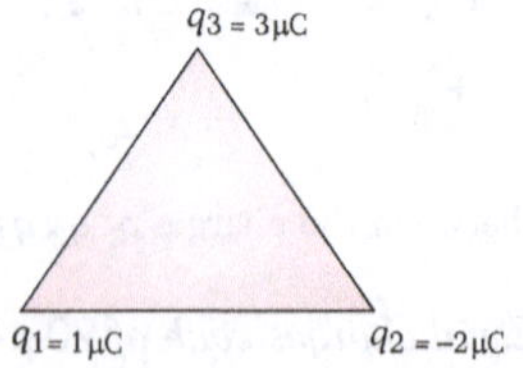

In the figure,

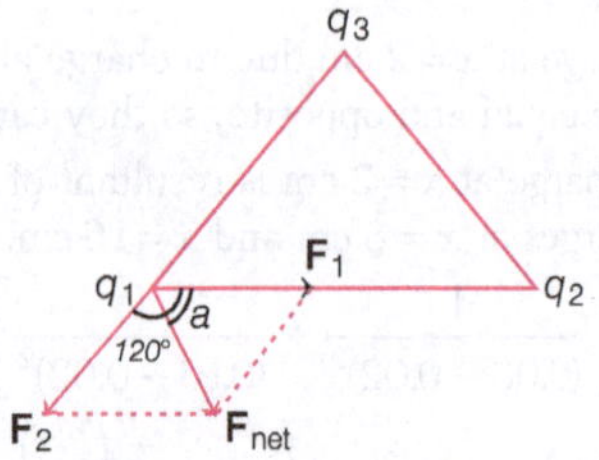

Magnitude of force between q_1 and q_2,

$$|\mathbf{F}_1| = F_1 = \frac{1}{4\pi\varepsilon_0} \cdot \frac{q_1 q_2}{r^2}$$

where, $q_1 = 1\,\mu C = 1 \times 10^{-6} C$ and $q_2 = 2\,\mu C = 2 \times 10^{-6} C$.

$$\Rightarrow \quad F_1 = \frac{(9.0 \times 10^9)(1.0 \times 10^{-6})(2.0 \times 10^{-6})}{(1.0)^2} = 1.8 \times 10^{-2}\ \text{N}$$

Similarly, magnitude of force between q_1 and q_3,

$$|\mathbf{F}_2| = F_2 = \frac{1}{4\pi\varepsilon_0} \cdot \frac{q_1 q_3}{r^2}$$

where, $q_3 = 3\,\mu C = 3 \times 10^{-6} C$.

$$\Rightarrow \quad F_2 = \frac{(9.0 \times 10^9)(1.0 \times 10^{-6})(3.0 \times 10^{-6})}{(1.0)^2}$$

$$= 2.7 \times 10^{-2}\ \text{N}$$

Now, net force, $|\mathbf{F}_{net}| = \sqrt{F_1^2 + F_2^2 + 2F_1 F_2 \cos 120^\circ}$

$$= \left(\sqrt{(1.8)^2 + (2.7)^2 + 2\,(1.8)\,(2.7)\left(-\frac{1}{2}\right)}\right) \times 10^{-2}\ \text{N}$$

$$= 2.38 \times 10^{-2}\ \text{N}$$

Mentor's TiP

Always use vector's parallelogram law of vector addition you learnt in class 11th Physics to solve resultant forces.

Example 14 *Four charges Q, q, Q and q are kept at the four corners of a square as shown below. What is the relation between Q and q, so that the net force on a charge q is zero?*

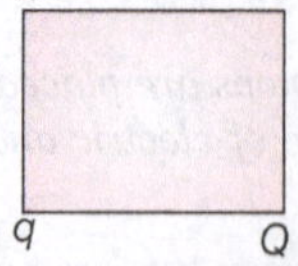

Sol. Here, both the charges q will have same sign either positive or negative. Similarly, both the charges Q will have same sign. Let us make the force on upper right corner q equal to zero.

Lower q will apply a repelling force $\mathbf{F}_1$ on upper q because both the charges have same sign. To balance this force both Q must apply attractive forces $\mathbf{F}_2$ and $\mathbf{F}_3$ of equal magnitude, hence Q and q will have opposite signs. Now, the resultant of $\mathbf{F}_2$ and $\mathbf{F}_3$ will be $F\sqrt{2}$ (Parallelogram law of vector addition), if $|\mathbf{F}_2| = |\mathbf{F}_3| = F$. Also note that $F\sqrt{2}$ will be exactly opposite to F_1.

So, $$F_1 = F\sqrt{2}$$

From Coulomb's law,

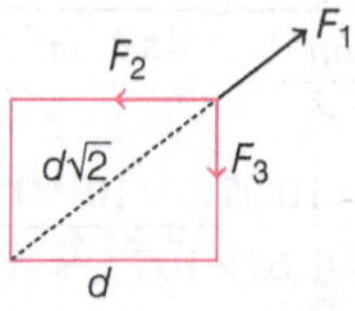

$$F_1 = \frac{kq^2}{(d\sqrt{2})^2} \quad \text{and} \quad F_2 = F_3 = \frac{kQq}{d^2}$$

Resultant of F_2 and F_3, $F_{23} = \sqrt{2}F$

From the diagram, $F_1 = \sqrt{2}F$

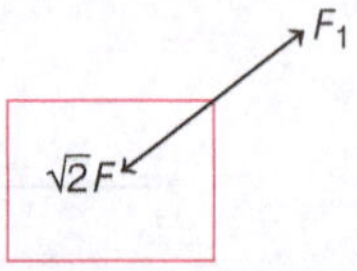

$$\therefore \quad \frac{q^2}{(d\sqrt{2})^2} = \frac{\sqrt{2}Qq}{d^2}$$

$$\therefore \quad Q = \frac{q}{2\sqrt{2}}$$

But as we said Q and q have opposite sign, so $q = -2\sqrt{2}Q$.

Applications of Electric Force (Coulomb's Law)

1. For Solving Problems Related to String

Let us consider two identical balls, having mass m and charge q. These are suspended from a common point by two insulating strings each of length L as shown in figure.

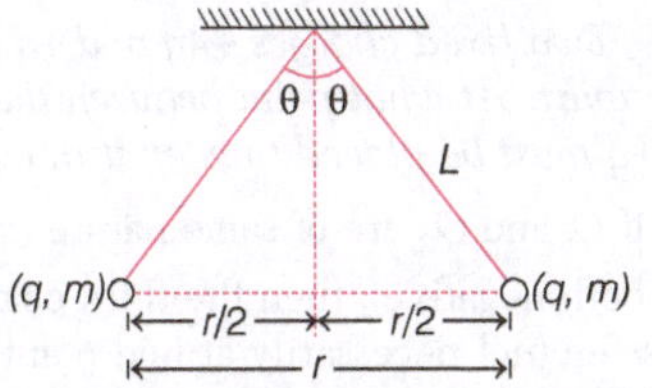

Two identical charged balls are suspended from same point

The balls repel and come into equilibrium at separation r. The ball is in equilibrium under the following forces :

(i) Weight of the ball, $w = mg$ and, (ii) Electric force,

$$F_e = \frac{1}{4\pi\varepsilon_0} \frac{q \cdot q}{r^2} = \frac{q^2}{4\pi\varepsilon_0 r^2} \quad \text{...(i)}$$

(iii) **Tension in the string** For this, let us draw FBD of a ball under consideration.

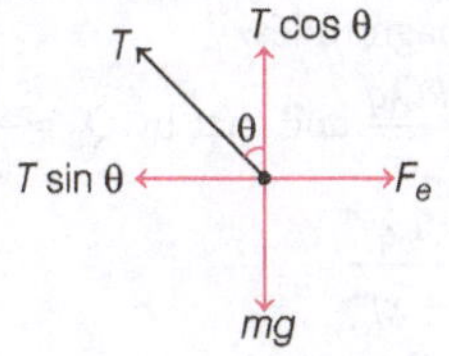

FBD of right ball

It is clear from FBD that,

$$T \sin\theta = F_e \quad \text{...(ii)}$$

$$T \cos\theta = mg \quad \text{...(iii)}$$

On dividing Eq. (ii) by Eq. (iii), we get

$$\Rightarrow \quad \tan\theta = \frac{F_e}{mg} \quad \text{...(iv)}$$

or $\quad T = \sqrt{(T \sin\theta)^2 + (T\cos\theta)^2}$

$$= \sqrt{F_e^2 + (mg)^2} \quad \text{...(v)}$$

From geometry of the figure,

$$\tan\theta = \frac{r/2}{\sqrt{L^2 - \frac{r^2}{4}}}$$

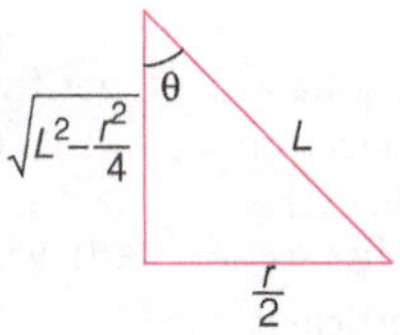

Formation of a triangle through $r/2$ and L

If θ is small, $\tan\theta \simeq \sin\theta = \dfrac{r/2}{L}$.

Now, let us solve some problems related to this to make our concepts more clear.

Example 15 *Two identical pith balls, each of mass m and charge q are suspended from a common point by two strings of equal length l. Find charge q in terms of given quantities, if angle between the strings is 2θ in equilibrium.*

Sol. Let x be the separation between balls in equilibrium. According to the question, following figure can be drawn

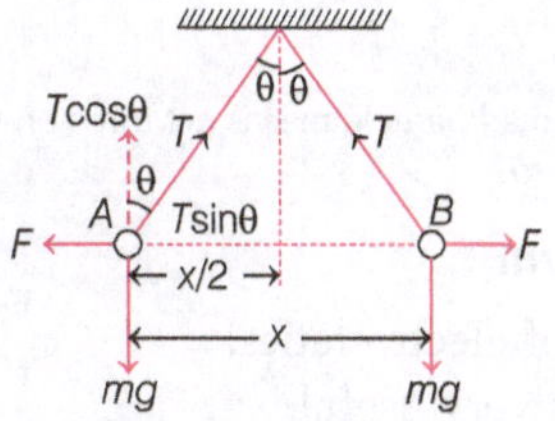

Each ball is in equilibrium under the action of the following forces

(a) Weight of the ball, mg

(b) Repulsive electric force,

$$F = \frac{1}{4\pi\,\varepsilon_0} \frac{q^2}{x^2}$$

(c) Tension in the string, T

Resolving T in the horizontal and vertical direction, since ball is in equilibrium,

$$T \sin\theta = F \quad \text{...(i)}$$

$$T \cos\theta = mg \quad \text{...(ii)}$$

By Eqs. (i) and (ii), we get

$$\tan\theta = \frac{F}{mg} = \frac{\frac{1}{4\pi\,\varepsilon_0} \frac{q^2}{x^2}}{mg} \quad \text{...(iii)}$$

Form figure, $\dfrac{x}{2} = l \sin\theta \Rightarrow x = 2l\sin\theta$

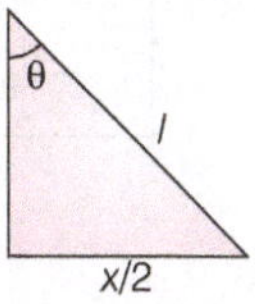

Put value of x in Eq. (iii), we get

$$q^2 = 4\pi\varepsilon_0 mgx^2 \tan\theta$$

$$= 4\pi\varepsilon_0 mg(2l\sin\theta)^2 \tan\theta$$

$$q = [16\pi\varepsilon_0\, mgl^2 \sin^2\theta \tan\theta]^{1/2}$$

Example 16 *A particle A having charge q and mass m is placed at the bottom of a smooth inclined plane of inclination θ. Where should a block B, having same charge and mass, be placed on the incline plane, so that it may remain in equilibrium?*

Sol. The following figure can be drawn in accordance with the question.

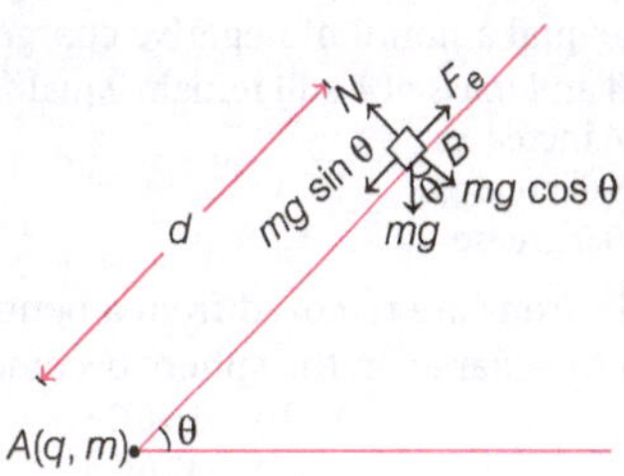

Let block B be placed at distance d. The block B is in equilibrium. So, $mg \cos\theta$ is balanced by normal reaction and $mg \sin\theta$ by repulsive electric force, *i.e.* $F_e = mg \sin\theta$

$$\Rightarrow \frac{1}{4\pi\varepsilon_0}\frac{q^2}{d^2} = mg\sin\theta \Rightarrow d = q\sqrt{\frac{1}{4\pi\varepsilon_0 mg\sin\theta}}$$

Mentor's TiP

Equilibrium of charged particle means net force on the charged particle must be zero.

2. Lami's Theorem

In few problems of electrostatics, Lami's theorem is very useful. According to this theorem, if three concurrent forces F_1, F_2 and F_3 as shown in figure are in equilibrium or if $F_1 + F_2 + F_3 = 0$, then

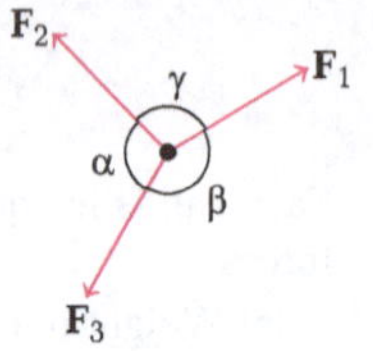

Three forces passing through a point

$$\frac{F_1}{\sin\alpha} = \frac{F_2}{\sin\beta} = \frac{F_3}{\sin\gamma}$$

Concept ladder

- When a point charge is placed linearly between two fixed charges of same polarity

$$x = \left(\frac{\sqrt{q_{small}}}{\sqrt{q_{small}} + \sqrt{q_{large}}}\right) r$$

- When a point charge is placed linearly aside of two fixed charges of opposite polarity.

$$x = \left(\frac{\sqrt{q_{small}}}{\sqrt{q_{large}} - \sqrt{q_{small}}}\right) r$$

Here, x is distance of point charge from smaller charge.

Example 17 *Two fixed charges $+4q$ and $+q$ are at a distance 3 m apart. At what point between the charges, a third charge $+q$ must be placed to keep it in equilibrium?*

Sol. Remember, if Q_1 and Q_2 are of same nature (means both positive or both negative), then the third charge should be placed between (not necessarily at mid-point) Q_1 and Q_2 on the straight line joining them. But, if Q_1 and Q_2 are of opposite nature, then the third charge will be put outside and close to that charge which is lesser in magnitude.

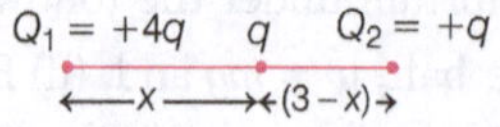

Here, Q_1 and Q_2 are of same nature that of third charge q, so it will be kept in between at a distance x from Q_1 (as shown in figure). Hence, q will be at a distance $(3 - x)$ from Q_2. Since, q is in equilibrium, so net force on it must be zero. The forces applied by Q_1 and Q_2 on q are in opposite direction, so as to just balance their magnitudes.

Force on q by $Q_1 = \frac{kQ_1 q}{x^2}$ and that by $Q_2 = \frac{kQ_2 q}{(3-x)^2}$

Now, $\frac{kQ_1 q}{x^2} = \frac{kQ_2 q}{(3-x)^2}$

or $\frac{Q_1}{x^2} = \frac{Q_2}{(3-x)^2}$

or $\frac{4}{x^2} = \frac{1}{(3-x)^2}$

Take the square root, $\frac{2}{x} = \frac{1}{(3-x)}$

or $6 - 2x = x$ (after cross multiplication) or $x = 2$ m. So, q will be placed at a distance 2 m from Q_1 and at 1m from Q_2.

STEP UP Practice 1

1. One metallic sphere A is given positive charge whereas another identical metallic sphere B of exactly same mass as of A is given equal amount of negative charge. Then,
   (a) mass of A and mass of B still remain equal
   (b) mass of A increases
   (c) mass of B decreases
   (d) mass of B increases

2. When 10^{14} electrons are removed from a neutral metal sphere, then the charge on the sphere becomes
   (a) 16 μC (b) −16 μC
   (c) 32μC (d) −32μC

3. A conductor has 14.4×10^{-19}C positive charge. The conductor has (charge on electron $= 1.6 \times 10^{-19}$C)
   (a) 9 electrons in excess (b) 27 electrons in short
   (c) 27 electrons in excess (d) 9 electrons in short

4. Charge on α-particle is
   (a) 4.8×10^{-19} C (b) 1.6×10^{-19} C
   (c) 3.2×10^{-19}C (d) 6.4×10^{-19} C

5. Two similarly charged bodies can
   (a) only attract each other
   (b) only repel each other
   (c) may attract or repel each other
   (d) neither attract nor repel each other

6. Consider a neutral conducting sphere. A positive point charge is placed outside the sphere. The net charge on the sphere is
(a) negative and distributed uniformly over the surface of the sphere
(b) negative and appears only at the point on the sphere closest to the point charge
(c) negative and distributed non-uniformly over the entire surface of the sphere
(d) zero

7. A metallic sphere having no net charge is placed near a finite metal plate carrying a positive charge. The electric force on the sphere will be
(a) towards the plate (b) away from the plate
(c) parallel to the plate (d) zero

8. There are two charges $+1\mu C$ and $+5\mu C$. The ratio of the forces acting on them will be
(a) 1 : 5 (b) 1 : 1
(c) 5 : 1 (d) 1 : 25

9. The force between two charges 0.06 m apart is 5 N. If each charge is moved towards the other, so that new distance becomes 0.04 m, then the force between them will become
(a) 7.20 N (b) 11.25 N (c) 22.50 N (d) 45.00 N

10. The charges on two spheres are $+7\mu C$ and $-5\,\mu C$, respectively. They experience a force F. If each of them is given an additional charge of $-2\mu C$, then the new force attraction will be
(a) F (b) $F/2$
(c) $F/\sqrt{3}$ (d) $2F$

11. Two charges of equal magnitudes and at a distance r exert a force F on each other. If the charges are halved and distance between them is doubled, then the new force acting on each charge is
(a) $F/8$ (c) $F/4$ (c) $4F$ (d) $F/16$

12. Two charges placed in air repel each other by a force of 10^{-4}N. When oil is introduced between the charges, then the force becomes 2.5×10^{-5}N.
The dielectric constant of oil is
(a) 2.5 (b) 0.25
(c) 2.0 (d) 4.0

13. Two point charges placed at a certain distance r in air exert a force F on each other. Then, the distance r' at which these charges will exert the same force in a medium of dielectric constant K is given by
(a) r (b) r/K
(c) $r/\sqrt{K}$ (d) $r\sqrt{K}$

14. F_g and F_e represent gravitational and electrostatic force respectively between electrons situated at a distance of 10 cm. The ratio of F_g/F_e is of the order of
(a) 10^{42} (b) 10^{-21}
(c) 10^{24} (d) 10^{-43}

15. Two particles of equal mass m and charge q are placed at a distance of 16 cm. They do not experience any force. The value of $\frac{q}{m}$ is
(a) l (b) $\sqrt{\frac{\pi\varepsilon_0}{G}}$
(c) $\sqrt{\frac{G}{4\pi\varepsilon_0}}$ (d) $\sqrt{4\pi\varepsilon_0 G}$

16. A charge q_1 exerts some force on a second charge q_2. If a third charge q_3 is brought near q_2, then the force exerted by q_1 on q_2
(a) decreases
(b) increases
(c) remains the same
(d) increases, if q_3 is of same sign as q_1 and decreases, if q_3 is of opposite sign as q_1

17. Electric charges of $1\mu C$, $-1\mu C$ and $2\mu C$ are placed in air at the corners A, B and C respectively of an equilateral triangle ABC having length of each side 10 cm. The resultant force on the charge at C is
(a) 0.9 N (b) 1.8 N (c) 2.7 N (d) 3.6 N

18. Two identical spheres A and B with charge Q are placed at a particular distance from each other and repel each other with force F. Anohter identical neutral sphere C is brought into contact with sphere A and then with B and finally removed from the system. Calculate new force between A and B.
(a) $\frac{F}{4}$ (b) $\frac{F}{2}$ (c) F (d) $\frac{3F}{8}$

19. Two point charges of $9Q$ and $-16Q$ are placed 1m apart from each other. Find equilibrium position for another charge of 1C from $9Q$ charge.
(a) 3m on left (b) 3m on right
(c) 4m on left (d) 4m on right

20. According to the given diagram charge $-q$ should be displaced such as it should oscillate. Find its direction of displacement.

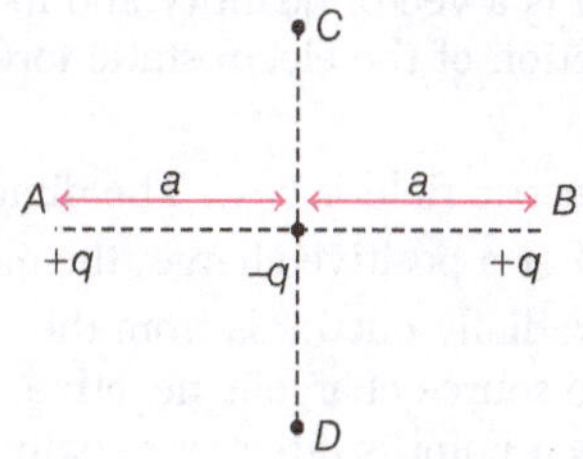

(a) Along A or C (b) Along B or D
(c) Along C or D (d) Along A or B

21. Match the columns

Column I	Column II
A. Discharging	I. Similar charged plates fixed from one ends
B. Earthing	II. A wire in domestic supply line
C. Attraction	III. Thunderstorm
D. Repulsion	IV. One charged and one neutral plate fixed from one ends.

Choose the correct answer from the options given below
(a) A→II, B→I, C→III, D→IV
(b) A→I, B→III, C→II, D→IV
(c) A→III, B→II, C→IV, D→I
(d) A→IV, B→III, C→I, D→II

Module 2

Electric Field and Electric Dipole

- Electric Field • Electric Field Lines • Continuous Charge Distribution • Electric Field of a Charged Ring
- Electric Dipole • The Field of an Electric Dipole or Dipole Field • Force on Dipole
- Torque on an Electric Dipole • Work Done in Rotating a Dipole in a Uniform Electric Field

Electric Field

The region surrounding a charge or distribution of charge in which its electrical effects can be observed or experienced is called the **electric field of the charge** or **distribution of charge.**

Electric field at a point can be defined in terms of a vector function **E** called **electric field strength.**

Electric Field Strength

The electric field strength (often called electric field) at a point is defined as the electrostatic force $\mathbf{F}_e$ per unit positive test charge. Thus, if the electrostatic force experienced by a small test charge q_0 is $\mathbf{F}_e$, then field strength at that point is defined as

$$\mathbf{E} = \lim_{q_0 \to 0} \frac{\mathbf{F}_e}{q_0}$$

The electric field is a vector quantity and its direction is same as the direction of the electrostatic force $\mathbf{F}_e$ on a positive charge.

The SI unit of electric field is N/C. The dimensions for **E** is $[MLT^{-3}A^{-1}]$. For a positive charge, the electric field will be directed radially outwards from the charge. On the other hand, if the source charge is negative, the electric field vector at each point is directed radially inwards.

Example 18 *An electric field of 10^5 N/C points due west at a certain spot. What are the magnitude and direction of the force that acts on a charge of + 2 μC and – 5 μC at this spot?*

Sol. Electrostatic force, $F = qE$

where, q = charge

and E = electric field.

Here, $q_1 = +2\mu C = 2\times10^{-6}$ C

and $q_2 = -5\mu C = -5\times10^{-6}$ C

∴ Force on charge q_1, $F_1 = (2\times10^{-6})(10^5) = 0.2$ N (due west)

and force on charge q_2, F_2

$= (-5\times10^{-6})(10^5) = 0.5$ N (due east)

Example 19 *Calculate the magnitude of an electric field which can just suspend a deuteron of mass 3.2×10^{-27} kg freely in air.*

Sol. Upward force (qE) on the deuteron due to electric field E is equal to weight mg of deuteron, $qE = mg$

$$\therefore \quad E = \frac{mg}{q} = \frac{3.2\times10^{-27}\times9.8}{1.6\times10^{-19}} = 19.6\times10^{-8}\ \text{NC}^{-1}$$

Example 20 *A pendulum of mass 60 mg carrying a charge of 3×10^{-6} C is at rest in a horizontal electric field of 2×10^2 V / m. Find the tension in the thread of the pendulum and the angle it makes with the vertical ($g = 10\ m/s^2$)*

Sol. Given, $m = 60$ mg $= 60\times10^{-6}$ kg

$q = 3\times10^{-6}$ C

$E = 2\times10^2$ V/m

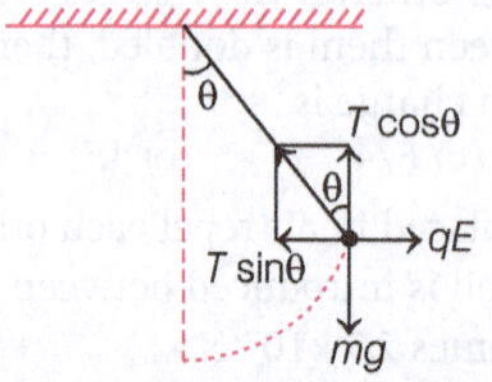

Let T be the tension in the thread and θ be the angle it makes with vertical, as shown in figure. When the bob is in equilibrium.

$$T\sin\theta = qE \quad \text{...(i)}$$

$$T\cos\theta = mg \quad \text{...(ii)}$$

Eq. (i) divided by Eq. (ii),

$$\tan\theta = \frac{q\cdot E}{m\cdot g}$$

$$\tan\theta = \frac{3\times10^{-6}\times2\times10^2}{60\times10^{-6}\times10}$$

$$\tan\theta = 1$$

$$\tan\theta = \tan 45^\circ \Rightarrow \theta = 45^\circ$$

So, from Eq. (i), tension in the thread $T\sin\theta = qE$

$$T\sin45^\circ = 3\times10^{-6}\times2\times10^2$$

$$T = 6\sqrt{2}\times10^{-4}\ \text{N}$$

Motion of a Charged Particle in a Uniform Electric Field

Case-I A charged particle initially at rest is placed in a uniform electric field.

Consider a charged particle of charge q, mass m situated in a uniform electric field E. Force on the particle is given by $\mathbf{F} = q\mathbf{E}$

$$\Rightarrow \quad \text{Acceleration } (\mathbf{a}) = \frac{\mathbf{F}}{m} = \frac{q\mathbf{E}}{m} = \text{constant}$$

(a) Velocity after time t

$$\mathbf{v} = \mathbf{u} + \mathbf{a}t = 0 + \frac{q\mathbf{E}}{m} \cdot t$$

$$\Rightarrow \quad \mathbf{v} = \frac{q\mathbf{E}}{m} \cdot t$$

$$\Rightarrow \quad \mathbf{v} \propto t$$

(b) Displacement of particle in time t

$$\mathbf{s} = \mathbf{u}t + \frac{1}{2}\mathbf{a}t^2$$

$$= 0(t) + \frac{1}{2} \cdot \frac{q\mathbf{E}}{m} \cdot t^2$$

$$\Rightarrow \quad \mathbf{s} = \frac{q\mathbf{E}}{2m} \cdot t^2$$

$$\Rightarrow \quad s \propto t^2$$

(c) Kinetic energy gained by the particle in time t

$$K = \frac{1}{2} mv^2 = \frac{1}{2} m \left(\frac{qE}{m} t\right)^2 = \frac{q^2E^2t^2}{2m}$$

$$\Rightarrow \quad K \propto t^2$$

Example 21 *An electron moves a distance of 8 cm. When accelerated from rest by an electric field of strength 9×10^5 N/C. Calculate the time of travel. [The mass and charge of electron are 9×10^{-31} kg and 1.6×10^{-19} C]*

Sol. Force exerted on the electron by the electric field,

$$F = e \cdot E$$

$$\therefore \text{ Acceleration, } \quad a = \frac{F}{m} = \frac{eE}{m}$$

$$a = \frac{1.6 \times 10^{-19} \times 9 \times 10^5}{9 \times 10^{-31}}$$

$$a = 0.16 \times 10^{16} \text{ m/s}^2$$

Now, $\quad u = 0,$

$$s = 8 \text{ cm} = 8 \times 10^{-2} \text{ m}$$

As $\quad s = ut + \frac{1}{2} at^2$

$$8 \times 10^{-2} = 0 + \frac{1}{2} \times 0.16 \times 10^{16} \times t^2$$

$$t^2 = \frac{16 \times 10^{-2}}{16 \times 10^{16}} \times 10^2$$

$$= 10^{-16}$$

$$t = 10^{-8} \text{ s}$$

Case II If charged particle is initially moving perpendicular to the uniform electric field.

(a) Resultant velocity after time t

Along X-axis

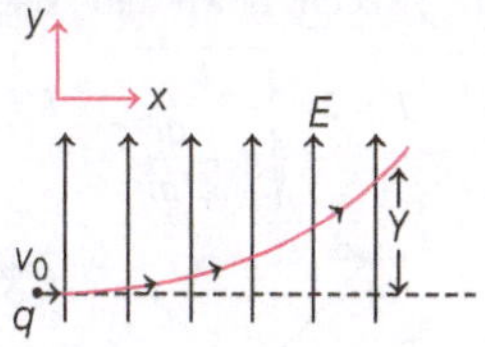

$$u_x = v_0, a_x = 0, v_x = u_x + a_x t$$

$$v_x = v_0 + 0$$

$$\Rightarrow v_x = v_0$$

Along Y-axis

$$u_y = 0, a_y = \frac{qE}{m}$$

$$\Rightarrow v_y = u_y + a_y t$$

$$v_y = 0 + \frac{qE}{m} t$$

$$\Rightarrow v_y = \frac{qE}{m} t$$

$$\therefore |\mathbf{v}| = \sqrt{v_x^2 + v_y^2} = \sqrt{v_0^2 + \frac{q^2E^2t^2}{m^2}}$$

(b) Equation of trajectory

Along X-axis,

$$u_x = v_0, a_x = 0, s_x = x$$

$$s = ut + \frac{1}{2} at^2 \Rightarrow x = v_0 t \quad \text{...(i)}$$

Along Y-axis,

$$u_y = 0, a_y = \frac{qE}{m}, s_y = y$$

$$s = ut + \frac{1}{2} at^2 \Rightarrow y = \frac{1}{2}\left(\frac{qE}{m}\right) t^2 \quad \text{...(ii)}$$

Value of t from Eq. (i) put in Eq. (ii)

$$y = \frac{1}{2}\left(\frac{qE}{m}\right)\left(\frac{x}{v_0}\right)^2$$

$$\Rightarrow \quad y = \frac{1}{2}\frac{qEx^2}{mv_0^2}$$

$\therefore y \propto x^2$, i.e., path is parabolic.

Concept ladder

Effect on time period of simple pendulum (T) due to uniform electric field

If only gravity is acting, $T = 2\pi\sqrt{\frac{l}{g}}$

If bob of pendulum has $+q$ charge and surrounding an electric field **E** applied, then

Case I E acting upward	Case II E acting downward	Case III E acting horizontally
$T = 2\pi\sqrt{\dfrac{l}{g - \dfrac{qE}{m}}}$	$T = 2\pi\sqrt{\dfrac{l}{g + \dfrac{qE}{m}}}$	$T = 2\pi\sqrt{\dfrac{l}{\sqrt{(g)^2 + \left(\dfrac{qE}{m}\right)^2}}}$

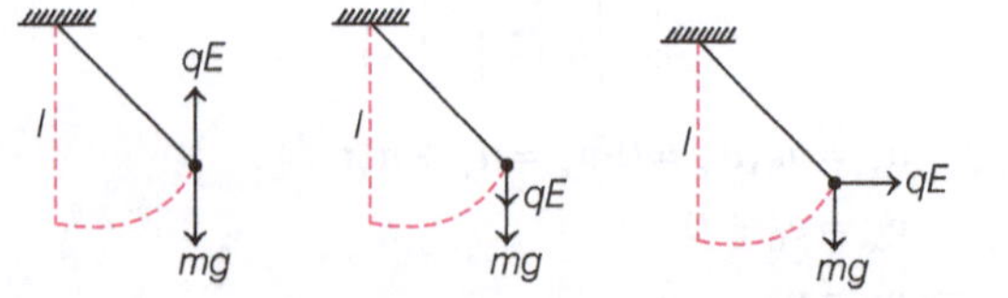

Electric Field due to a Point Charge

The electric field produced by a point charge q can be obtained in general terms from Coulomb's law. The magnitude of the force exerted by the charge q on a test charge q_0 is

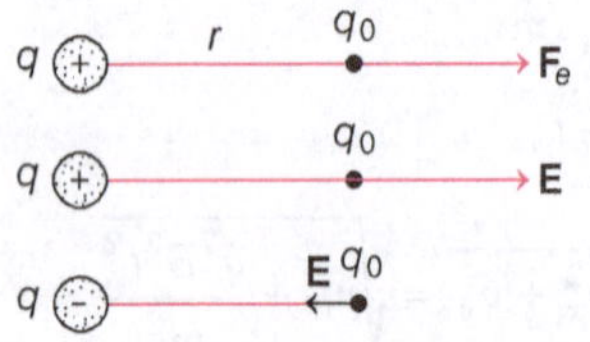

Direction of electric field due to positive and negative charges

$$F_e = \frac{1}{4\pi\varepsilon_0}\cdot\frac{qq_0}{r^2}$$

Therefore, the intensity of the electric field at this point is given by $E = \dfrac{F_e}{q_0}$

$$\boxed{E = \frac{1}{4\pi\varepsilon_0}\cdot\frac{q}{r^2}}$$

Vector form

- Let a point p at a distance of r from a charge Q, the electric field at that point will be

$$\mathbf{E}_p = \frac{1}{4\pi\varepsilon_0}\frac{Q}{r^2}\hat{\mathbf{r}}$$

$$\Rightarrow \quad \mathbf{E}_p = \frac{1}{4\pi\varepsilon_0}\frac{Q}{r^3}\mathbf{r}$$

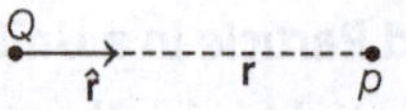

- Where $\hat{\mathbf{r}}$ is the position vector of point of observation (p) with respect to source point charge (Q).
- In vector form charge (Q) is used with sign.

Mentor's TiP

In electric field region, a point with zero resultant electric field is called neutral point.

Example 22 *A point charge Q is placed at point A(0, 0). Calculate the electric field at B(x, y) in vector form.*

Sol. $\mathbf{E} = \dfrac{KQ}{r^3}\mathbf{r}$ and $\mathbf{r} = \mathbf{r}_B - \mathbf{r}_A = x\hat{\mathbf{i}} + y\hat{\mathbf{j}}$

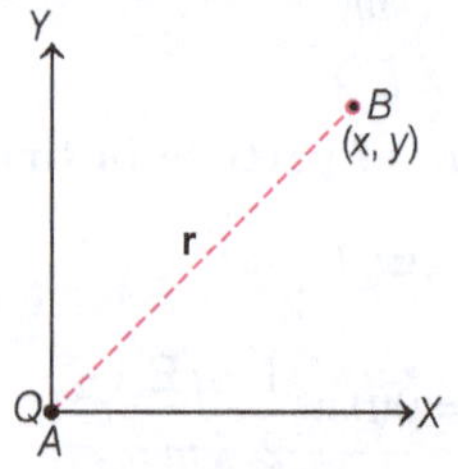

$$\mathbf{E} = \frac{kQ}{(x^2 + y^2)^{3/2}}(x\hat{\mathbf{i}} + y\hat{\mathbf{j}})$$

Example 23 *Two point charges $q_1 = 16\ \mu C$ and $q_2 = 4\ \mu C$, are separated in vacuum by a distance of 3.0 m. Find the point on the line between the charges, where the net electric field is zero.*

Sol. Between the charges, the two field contributions have opposite directions and the net electric field is zero at a point (say P), where the magnitudes of $\mathbf{E}_1$ and $\mathbf{E}_2$ are equal. However, since, $q_2 < q_1$, point P must be closer to q_2, in order that the field of the smaller charge can balance the field of the greater charge.

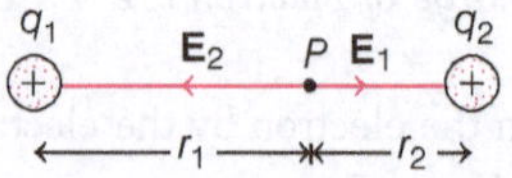

At P, $\quad E_1 = E_2$

or $\quad \dfrac{1}{4\pi\varepsilon_0}\cdot\dfrac{q_1}{r_1^2} = \dfrac{1}{4\pi\varepsilon_0}\cdot\dfrac{q_2}{r_2^2}$

$\therefore \quad \dfrac{r_1}{r_2} = \sqrt{\dfrac{q_1}{q_2}} = \sqrt{\dfrac{16}{4}} = 2$ ...(i)

Also, $\quad r_1 + r_2 = 3.0$ m ...(ii)

Solving these equations, we get

$r_1 = 2$ m

and $\quad r_2 = 1$ m

Thus, the point P is at a distance of 2 m from q_1 and 1 m from q_2.

Example 24 *A ball of mass m having a charge q is released from rest in a region where a horizontal electric field E exists.*
(i) Find the resultant force acting on the ball.
(ii) Find the trajectory followed by the ball.

Sol. The forces acting on the ball are weight of the ball in vertically downward direction and the electric force in the horizontal direction.

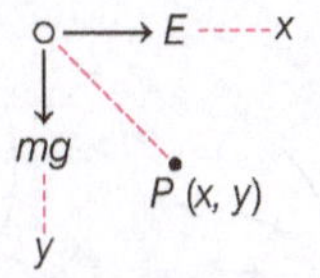

(i) Resultant force, $F = \sqrt{(mg)^2 + (qE)^2}$

(ii) Let the ball be at point P after time t.

As, $F = ma = qE$

$\therefore \quad a = \dfrac{qE}{m}$

$$\left.\begin{aligned} x\text{-direction}, \ x &= \frac{1}{2}\frac{qE}{m}t^2 \\ y\text{-direction}, \ y &= \frac{1}{2}gt^2 \end{aligned}\right\}$$

$$\frac{y}{x} = \frac{g}{qE/m}$$

$\Rightarrow \quad y = \dfrac{mgx}{qE}$

Hence, trajectory is a straight line.

Example 25 *A ball having charge q and mass m is suspended from a string of length L between two parallel plates, where a vertical electric field E is established. Find the time period of simple pendulum, if electric field is directed (i) downward and (ii) upward.*

Sol. (i) When electric field is downward

For simple pendulum,

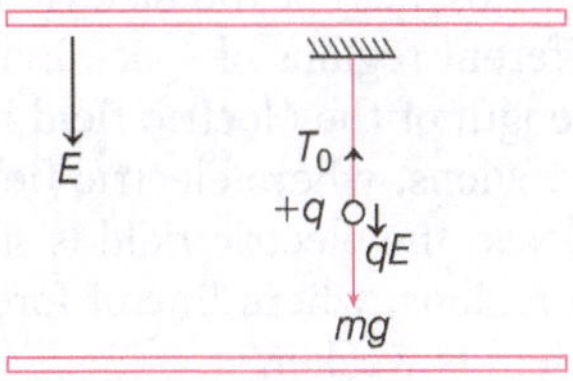

Time period, $T = 2\pi\sqrt{\dfrac{L}{a}}$

where, a is the effective acceleration.

$$a = \frac{\text{net external force on the ball}}{\text{mass of the ball}}$$

$\Rightarrow \quad a = \dfrac{mg + qE}{m} = g + \dfrac{qE}{m}$

$\therefore$ Time period, $T = 2\pi\sqrt{\dfrac{L}{g + \dfrac{qE}{m}}}$

(ii) When electric field is upward

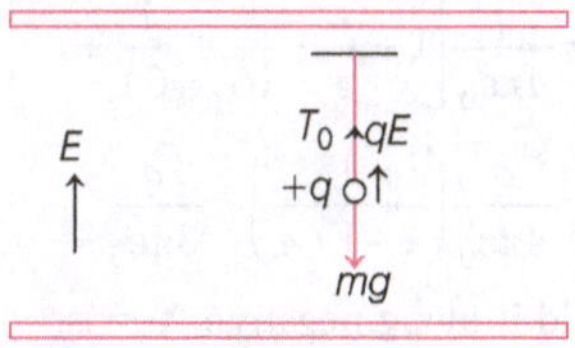

Effective acceleration,

$$a = \frac{mg - qE}{m} = g - \frac{qE}{m}$$

$\therefore$ Time period, $T = 2\pi\sqrt{\dfrac{L}{g - \dfrac{qE}{m}}}$

Example 26 *Find out electric field intensity at point A(0, 1 m, 2 m) due to a point charge −20 μC situated at point B($\sqrt{2}$ m, 0, 1 m).*

Sol. $$\mathbf{E} = \frac{KQ}{|\mathbf{r}|^3}\mathbf{r}$$

$\Rightarrow \quad \mathbf{r} = \mathbf{r}_A - \mathbf{r}_B = (\hat{\mathbf{j}} + 2\hat{\mathbf{k}}) - (\sqrt{2}\hat{\mathbf{i}} + \hat{\mathbf{k}})$

$= (-\sqrt{2}\hat{\mathbf{i}} + \hat{\mathbf{j}} + \hat{\mathbf{k}})$

$|\mathbf{r}| = \sqrt{(\sqrt{2})^2 + (1)^2 + (1)^2} = 2$

$$\mathbf{E} = \frac{9 \times 10^9 \times (-20 \times 10^{-6})}{8}(-\sqrt{2}\hat{\mathbf{i}} + \hat{\mathbf{j}} + \hat{\mathbf{k}})$$

$= 22.5 \times 10^3 \, (\sqrt{2}\hat{\mathbf{i}} - \hat{\mathbf{j}} - \hat{\mathbf{k}})$ N/C.

Example 27 *Three identical charges each of q are placed at three corners of an equilateral triangle of side length a. Find net electric field at centre of triangle.*

Sol.

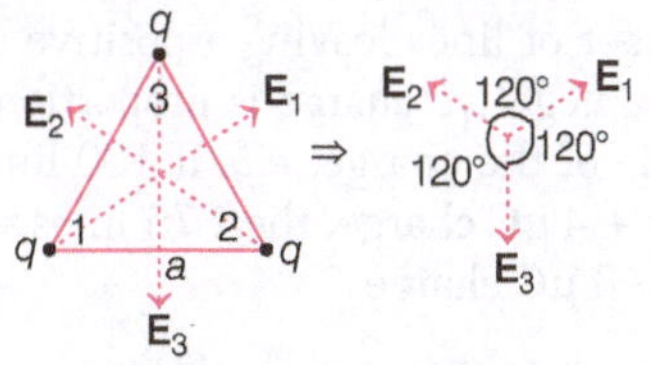

$$\mathbf{E}_{\text{net}} = \mathbf{E}_1 + \mathbf{E}_2 + \mathbf{E}_3 \Rightarrow \mathbf{E}_{\text{net}} = 0$$

Note If identical charges are placed at each corner of a regular polygon, then resultant electric field at centre of polygon is zero.

Example 28 *An infinite number of charges each equal to q are placed along X-axis at x = 1, x = 2, x = 4, x = 8 and so on. Find the electric field at the point x = 0 due to this set up of charges.*

Sol. At the point $x = 0$, the electric field due to all the charges are in the same negative x-direction and hence get added up.

$$E = \frac{1}{4\pi\varepsilon_0}\left[\frac{q}{1^2} + \frac{q}{2^2} + \frac{q}{4^2} + \frac{q}{8^2} + \dots\right]$$

$$= \frac{q}{4\pi\varepsilon_0}\left[1 + \frac{1}{4} + \frac{1}{16} + \frac{1}{64} + \dots\right]$$

$$= \frac{q}{4\pi\varepsilon_0}\left(\frac{1}{1 - 1/4}\right) = \frac{q}{3\pi\varepsilon_0}$$

This electric field is along negative X-axis.

Electric Field Lines

An electric field line is an imaginary line or curve drawn through a region of space, so that its tangent at any point is in the direction of the electric field vector at that point.

Electric field lines were introduced by Michael Faraday to visualise electric field.

The electric field lines have the following properties :

(i) The tangent to a field line at any point gives the direction of **E** at that point.

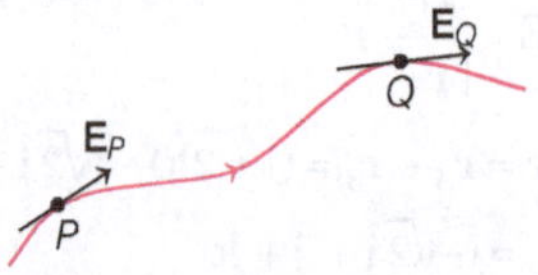

Electric field at points P and Q

In the given figure, electric field at points P and Q are along the tangents (E_P and E_Q). This is also the path on which a positive test charge will tend to move, if free to do so.

(ii) Electric field lines always begin from a positive charge and end on a negative charge and do not start or stop in mid-space.

(iii) The number of lines leaving a positive charge or entering a negative charge is proportional to the magnitude of the charge. *e.g.* if 100 lines are drawn leaving a + 4 μC charge, then 75 lines would have to end on a -3 μC charge.

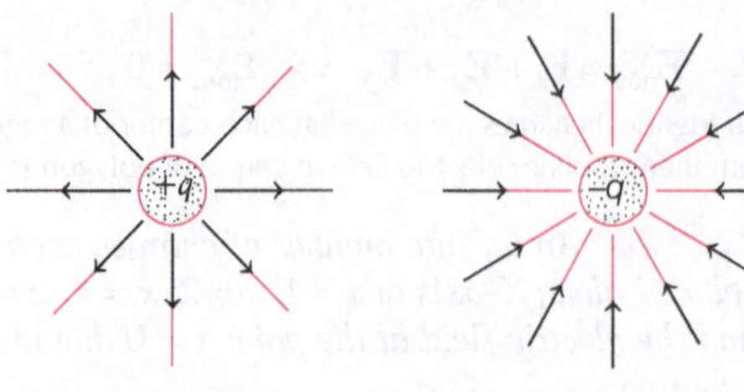

(a) (b)

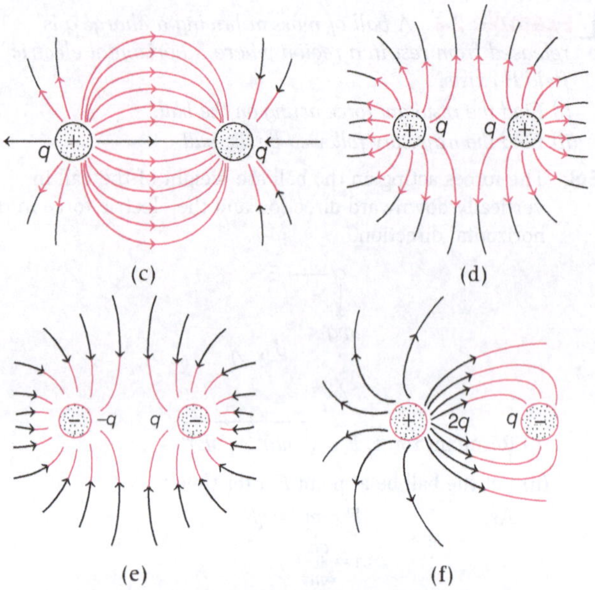

Electric field lines associated with a single as well as combination of charges

(iv) Two lines can never intersect. If it happens, then two tangents can be drawn at their point of intersection, *i.e.* intensity at that point will have two directions which is not possible.

(v) In a uniform field, the field lines are straight, parallel and uniformly spaced.

(vi) The electric field lines can never form closed loops as a field line can never start and end on the same charge.

(vii) In a region, where there is no electric field, electric field lines are absent. This is why inside a conductor (where, electric field is zero), no electric field lines exist.

(viii) Electric field lines of force ends or starts normally from the surface of a conductor.

(ix) The relative closeness of the electric field lines of force in different regions of space indicates the relative strength of the electric field in different regions. In regions, where electric field lines of force are closer, the electric field is stronger, whereas in regions, where line of force are farther apart, the field is weaker.

Therefore, in the given figure $|E_A| > |E_B|$.

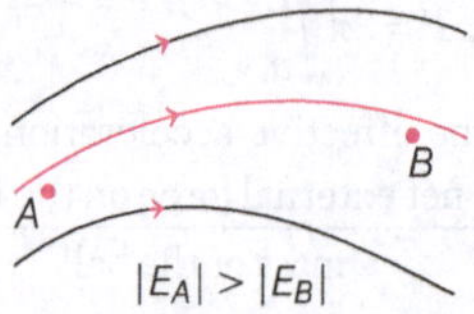

Electric field strength at points A and B

Continuous Charge Distribution

In most of the cases, we deal with charges having magnitude greater than the charge of an electron. For this, we can imagine that the charge is spread in a region in a continuous manner. Such a charge distribution is known as continuous charge distribution.

Consider a point charge q_0 lying near a region of continuous charge distribution which is made up of large number of small charges dq as shown in figure.

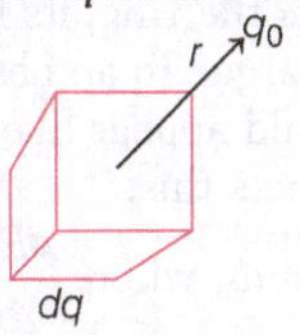

Force on a point charge q_0 due to a continuous charge distribution

According to Coulomb's law, the force on a point charge q_0 due to small charge dq is

$$\mathbf{F} = \frac{q_0}{4\pi\varepsilon_0}\int \frac{dq}{r^2}\hat{\mathbf{r}} \quad \text{...(i)}$$

where, $\hat{\mathbf{r}} = \frac{\mathbf{r}}{r}$

There are three types of continuous charge distribution

1. Line Charge Distribution (λ)

It is a charge distribution along a one-dimensional curve or line in space as shown in figure.

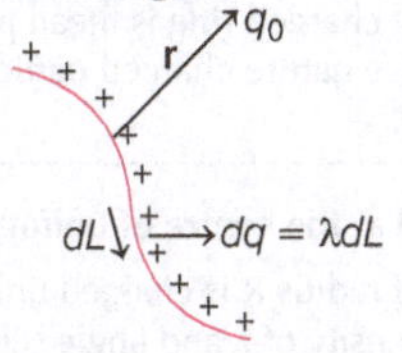

Line charge distribution

The charge contained per unit length of the line at any point is called **linear charge density**. It is denoted by λ.

i.e. $$\lambda = \frac{dq}{dL}$$

Its SI unit is Cm^{-1}.

Electric field due to the line charge distribution at the location of charge q_0 is

$$\mathbf{E}_L = \frac{1}{4\pi\varepsilon_0}\int_L \frac{\lambda}{r^2}dL\,\hat{\mathbf{r}}$$

2. Surface Charge Distribution (σ)

It is a charge distribution spread over a two-dimensional surface S in space as shown in figure.

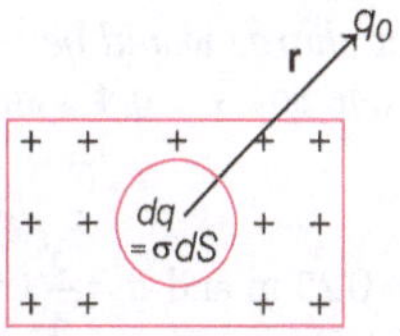

Surface charge distribution

The charge contained per unit area at any point is called surface charge density. It is denoted by σ.

i.e. $$\sigma = \frac{dq}{dS}$$

Its SI unit is Cm^{-2}.

Electric field due to the surface charge distribution at the location of charge q_0 is

$$\mathbf{E}_S = \frac{1}{4\pi\varepsilon_0}\int_S \frac{\sigma}{r^2}dS\,\hat{\mathbf{r}}$$

3. Volume Charge Distribution (ρ)

It is a charge distribution spread over a three-dimensional volume or region V of space as shown in figure.

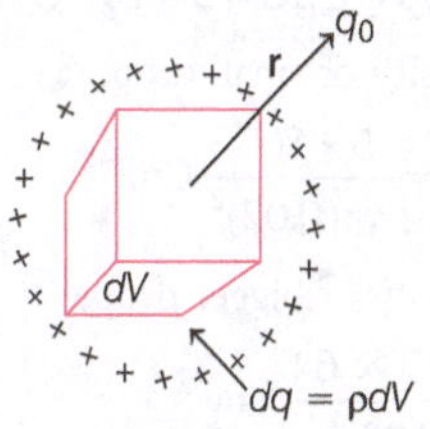

Volume charge distribution

The charge contained per unit volume at any point is called volume charge density. It is denoted by ρ.

i.e. $$\rho = \frac{dq}{dV}$$

Its SI unit is coulomb per cubic metre (Cm^{-3}).

Electric field due to the volume charge distribution at the location of charge q_0 is

$$\mathbf{E}_V = \frac{1}{4\pi\varepsilon_0}\int_V \frac{\rho}{r^2}dV\,\hat{\mathbf{r}}$$

Mentor's Tip

For three types of charge distribution Linear, surface and volume

$$dq = \lambda dL = \sigma dS = \rho dV$$

This formula is very similar to three types of mass distribution in mechanics.

Example 29 *What charge would be required to electrify a sphere of radius 25 cm, so as to get a surface charge density of $\frac{3}{\pi}$ Cm^{-2}?*

Sol. Given, $r = 25$ cm $= 0.25$ m and $\sigma = \frac{3}{\pi}\ Cm^{-2}$

As, $\sigma = \frac{q}{4\pi r^2}$

$\therefore\quad q = 4\pi r^2 \sigma = 4\pi \times (0.25)^2 \times \frac{3}{\pi} = 0.75\,C$

Example 30 *Sixty four drops of radius 0.02 m and each carrying a charge of 5μC are combined to form a bigger drop. Find how the surface charge density of electrification will change, if no charge is lost?*

Sol. Volume of each small drop $= \frac{4}{3}\pi(0.02)^3\ m^3$

Volume of 64 small drops $= \frac{4}{3}\pi(0.02)^3 \times 64\ m^3$

Let R be the radius of the bigger drop formed, then

$\frac{4}{3}\pi R^3 = \frac{4}{3}\pi(0.02)^3 \times 64$ or $R^3 = (0.02)^3 \times 4^3$

$\therefore\quad R = 0.02 \times 4 = 0.08$ m

Charge on small drop $= 5\mu C = 5 \times 10^{-6} C$

Surface charge density of small drop,

$$\sigma_1 = \frac{q}{4\pi r^2} = \frac{5 \times 10^{-6}}{4\pi(0.02)^2}\ Cm^{-2}$$

Surface charge density of bigger drop,

$$\sigma_2 = \frac{5 \times 10^{-6} \times 64}{4\pi(0.08)^2}\ Cm^{-2}$$

$$\therefore\quad \frac{\sigma_1}{\sigma_2} = \frac{5 \times 10^{-6}}{4\pi(0.02)^2} \times \frac{4\pi(0.08)^2}{5 \times 10^{-6} \times 64} = \frac{1}{4} = 1:4$$

Electric Field of a Charged Ring

Electric field at a distance x from the centre of uniformly charged ring of total charge q on its axis is given by

$$E_x = \left(\frac{1}{4\pi\varepsilon_0}\right)\frac{qx}{(x^2 + R^2)^{3/2}}$$

Direction of this electric field is along the axis and away from the ring in case of positively charged ring and towards the ring in case of negatively charged ring.

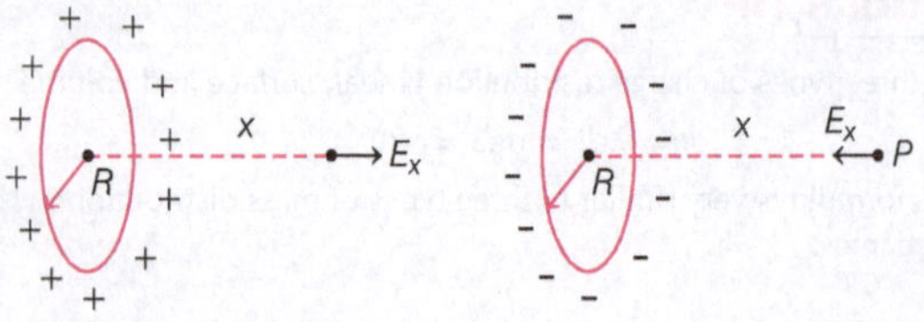

Electric field of positively and negatively charged rings

Special Cases

From the above expression, we can see that

(i) $E_x = 0$ at $x = 0$, *i.e.* field is zero at the centre of the ring. This would occur because charges on opposite sides of the ring would push a test charge at the centre, in the opposite directions with equal effort and so the forces would add to zero.

(ii) $E_x = \frac{1}{4\pi\varepsilon_0} \cdot \frac{q}{x^2}$ for $x \gg R$, *i.e.* when the point P is much farther from the ring, its field is the same as that of a point charge. To an observer far from the ring, the ring would appear like a point and the electric field reflects this.

(iii) E_x will be maximum, where $\frac{dE_x}{dx} = 0$. Differentiating E_x w.r.t. x and putting it equal to zero, we get $x = \pm \frac{R}{\sqrt{2}}$ and E_{max} comes out to be, $\frac{2}{3\sqrt{3}}\left(\frac{1}{4\pi\varepsilon_0} \cdot \frac{q}{R^2}\right)$.

Graph between Electric Field and Distance from Centre (x) for Uniformly Charged Ring

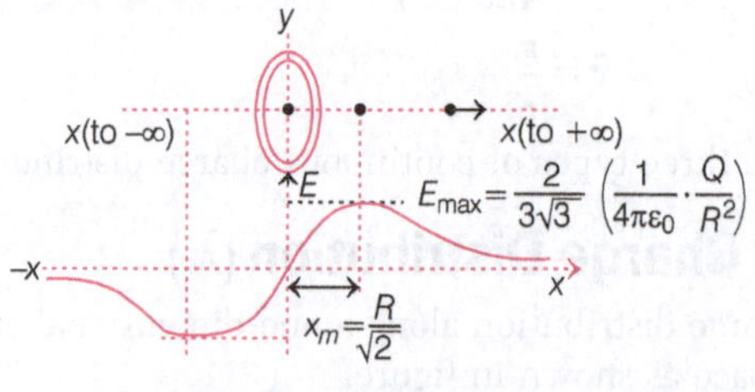

Note Centre of uniformly charged ring is mean position of stable equilibrium for unlike nature charged particle along axial displacement.

Concept ladder

Electric field at the centre of uniformly charged arc

An arc of radius R is charged uniformly with linear charge density of λ and angle subtended at centre is α.

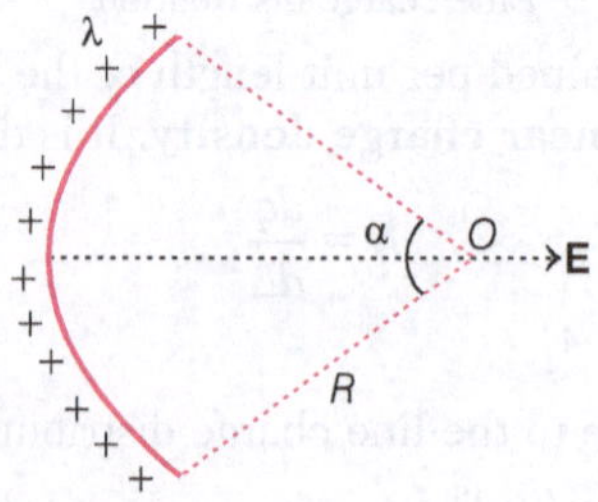

Electric field at centre of this arc is as

$$E = \frac{2k\lambda}{R}\left(\sin\frac{\alpha}{2}\right)$$

If charge on arc is Q, then $Q = \lambda R\alpha$

$\lambda = \frac{Q}{R\alpha}$ (α in radian) and $E = \frac{2kQ}{R^2\alpha}\left(\sin\frac{\alpha}{2}\right)$

Example 31 *A charge of 4×10^{-9} C is distributed uniformly over the circumference of a conducting ring of radius 0.3 m. Calculate the field intensity at a point on the axis of the ring at 0.4 m from its centre and also at the centre.*

Sol. Given, $q = 4\times10^{-9}$ C, $x = 0.4$ m and $R = 0.3$ m

Electric field intensity at 0.4 m from its centre,

$$E = \frac{qx}{4\pi\varepsilon_0 (R^2 + x^2)^{3/2}}$$

$$= \frac{9\times10^9 \times 4\times10^{-9}\times 0.4}{(0.3^2 + 0.4^2)^{3/2}}$$

$$E = \frac{14.4}{(0.5)^3}$$

$$= 115.2 \text{ N/C}$$

At the centre of the ring, $x = 0$

$\therefore$ Electric field intensity, $E = 0$

Electric Dipole

- A system of two equal and opposite charges separated by a small distance is called electric dipole, shown in figure. Every dipole has a characteristic property called dipole moment. It is defined as the product of magnitude of either charge and the separation between the charges, given as

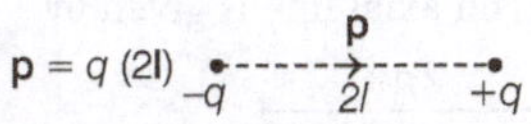

- In certain molecules, the centres of positive and negative charges do not coincide. This results in the formation of electric dipoles.
- Atom is non-polar because the centres of positive and negative charges in it coincide. Polarity can be induced in an atom by the application of electric field in that case. It is called as induced dipole.
- **Dipole Moment** Dipole moment $\mathbf{p} = q(2\mathbf{l})$
  1. It is a vector quantity directed from negative to positive charge of dipole.
  2. **Dimension** [LTA], SI unit : Coulomb × Metre (or C-m)

Example 32 *A system has two charges, $q_A = 2.5\times10^{-7}$ C and $q_B = -2.5\times10^{-7}$ C located at points A(0, 0, −15 cm) and B(0, 0, +15 cm) respectively. What is the electric dipole moment of the system?*

Sol. Electric dipole moment,

p = magnitude of either charge × dipole length

$= q_A \times AB = 2.5\times10^{-7}\times 0.30$

$= 7.5\times10^{-8}$ C-m

The electric dipole moment is directed from B to A, i.e. from negative charge to positive charge.

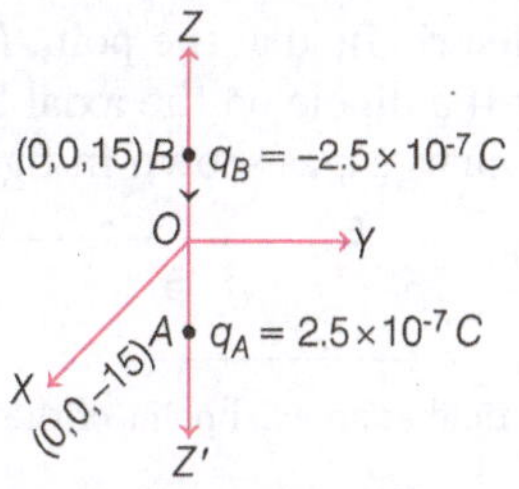

Example 33 *Three charges are placed as shown. Find dipole moment of the arrangements.*

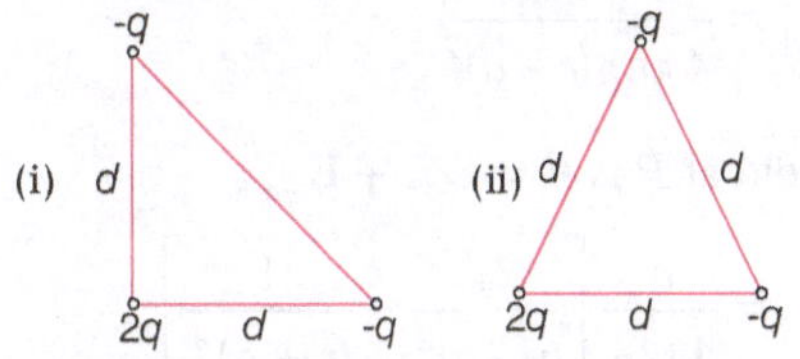

Sol. (i) Here, two dipoles are formed. These are shown in diagram below.

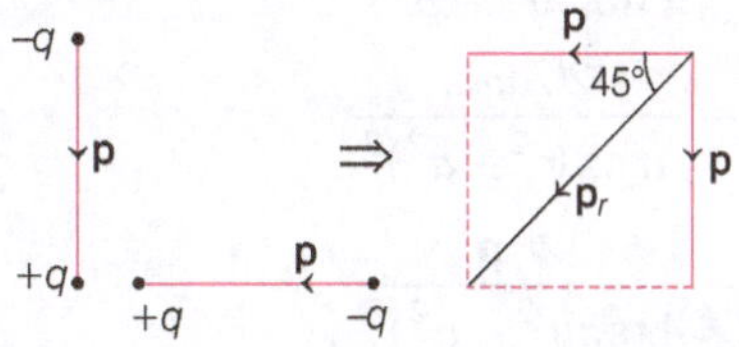

Resultant dipole moment, $p_r = 2p\cos 45° = \sqrt{2}p = \sqrt{2}qd$

and $\theta = 45°$

(ii) The two dipoles formed are as shown below.

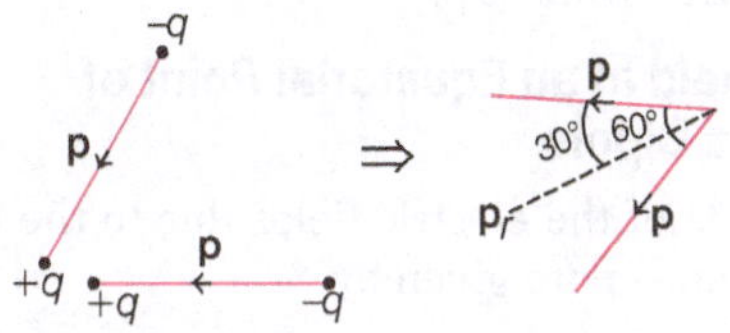

$\therefore$ The resultant dipole moment,

$p_r = 2p\cos 30° = \sqrt{3}p = \sqrt{3}\,qd$ and $\theta = 30°$

The Field of an Electric Dipole or Dipole Field

The electric field produced by an electric dipole is called a **dipole field**. The total charge of the electric dipole is zero but dipole field is not zero. It can be found using Coulomb's law and the superposition principle. We will find electric field of an electric dipole at two points as discussed below.

1. Electric Field at an Axial Point of an Electric Dipole

Let us calculate electric field at the point P at a distance r from the centre of the dipole on the axial line of the dipole on the side of the charge q as shown in figure.

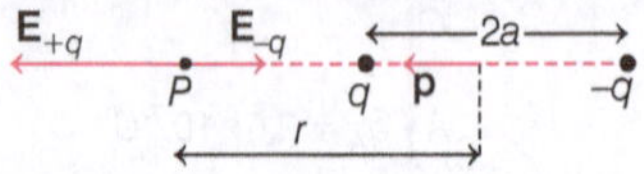

Electric field at an axial point of the dipole

$$\mathbf{E}_{-q} = \frac{-q}{4\pi\varepsilon_0 (r+a)^2}$$

$$\mathbf{E}_{+q} = \frac{q}{4\pi\varepsilon_0 (r-a)^2}$$

The total field at P is $\mathbf{E} = \mathbf{E}_{+q} + \mathbf{E}_{-q}$

$$= \frac{q}{4\pi\varepsilon_0}\left[\frac{1}{(r-a)^2} - \frac{1}{(r+a)^2}\right]$$

$$= \frac{q}{4\pi\varepsilon_0} \frac{4ar}{(r^2-a^2)^2} \qquad (\because 2aq = p)$$

$$\therefore \qquad \mathbf{E} = \frac{2(2aq)r}{4\pi\varepsilon_0 (r^2-a^2)^2}$$

$$= \frac{2r\,\mathbf{p}}{4\pi\varepsilon_0 (r^2-a^2)^2}$$

For short dipole, *i.e.* for $r >> a$, $\boxed{\mathbf{E} = \dfrac{2\mathbf{p}}{4\pi\varepsilon_0 r^3}}$

Direction of $\mathbf{E}$ is same as $\mathbf{p}$.

2. Electric Field at an Equatorial Point of an Electric Dipole

The magnitude of the electric fields due to the two charges $+q$ and $-q$ are given by

$E_{+q} = \dfrac{q}{4\pi\varepsilon_0 (r^2+a^2)}$ and $E_{-q} = \dfrac{q}{4\pi\varepsilon_0 (r^2+a^2)}$ and they are equal in magnitude. The directions of E_{+q} and E_{-q} are as shown in the figure.

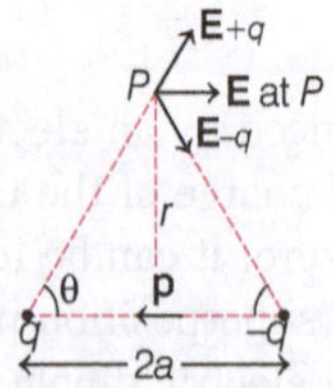

The components of electric field normal to the dipole axis cancel away. The components of electric field along the dipole axis add up. The total electric field $\mathbf{E}$ at P is opposite to dipole moment vector $\mathbf{p}$.

So, we have $\mathbf{E} = -[(E_{+q} + E_{-q})\cos\theta]$

$$= \frac{-2q}{4\pi\varepsilon_0 (r^2+a^2)} \cdot \frac{a}{(r^2+a^2)^{1/2}} \left(\because \cos\theta = \frac{a}{(r^2+a^2)^{\frac{1}{2}}}\right)$$

$$\Rightarrow \quad \mathbf{E} = \frac{-2aq}{4\pi\varepsilon_0 (r^2+a^2)^{3/2}} = \frac{-\mathbf{p}}{4\pi\varepsilon_0 (r^2+a^2)^{3/2}} \quad [\because 2aq = p]$$

For short dipole, $r >> a$

$$\therefore \qquad \boxed{\mathbf{E} = \frac{-\mathbf{p}}{4\pi\varepsilon_0 r^3}}$$

Concept ladder

- The electric field due to short dipole at large distance ($r >> a$) is proportional to $\frac{1}{r^3}$.
- If we take the limit, when the dipole size $2a$ approaches zero, the charge q approaches infinity in such a way that the product, $p = q \times 2a$ is finite. Such a dipole is referred to as a point dipole (ideal dipole).
- In the limit $r >> a$ for dipole size $2a$, the dipole is known as point dipole (on ideal dipole)

Example 34 *Two opposite charges each of magnitude $2\mu C$ are 1 cm apart. Find electric field at a distance of 5 cm from the mid-point on axial line of the dipole. Also, find the field on equatorial line at the same distance from mid-point.*

Sol. Electric field (E) on axial line is given by

$$\frac{2pr}{4\pi\varepsilon_0 (r^2-a^2)^2}$$

where, p is dipole moment = either charge × dipole length

Thus, $p = q \cdot 2a = (2\times10^{-6}) \times (0.01)$

Also, $r = 5\times10^{-2}$ m

$$\therefore \quad E_a = \frac{9\times10^9 \times 2(2\times10^{-6}\times10^{-2})\times 5\times10^{-2}}{[(5\times10^{-2})^2 - (0.5\times10^{-2})^2]^2}$$

$$= 2.93\times10^6 \text{ NC}^{-1}$$

Similarly, electric field (E) on equatorial line is given by

$$E_e = \frac{p}{4\pi\varepsilon_0 (r^2+a^2)^{3/2}}$$

The symbols have the same meaning as above,

$$E_e = \frac{9\times10^9 \times (2\times10^{-6}\times10^{-2})}{[(5\times10^{-2})^2 + (0.5\times10^{-2})^2]^{3/2}}$$

$$\therefore \quad E_e = 1.42\times10^6 \text{ NC}^{-1}$$

3. Electric Field at the Position (r, θ)

Due to the positive charge of the dipole, electric field at point P will be in radially outward direction and due to the negative charge it will be radially inward. Now, we have considered the radial component (E_r) and transverse component (E_θ) of the net electric field (E) as shown in figure.

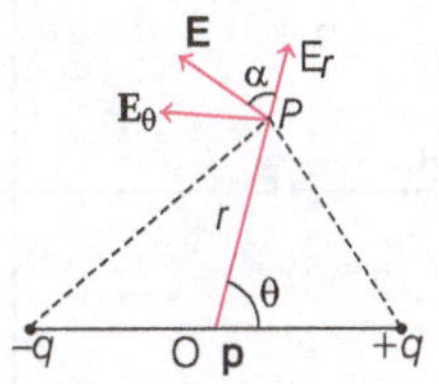

Radial and transverse component of the electric field E of the dipole at point $P(r, \theta)$

$$\therefore \quad E_r = \frac{1}{4\pi\varepsilon_0} \cdot \frac{2p\cos\theta}{r^3}$$

and $$E_\theta = \frac{1}{4\pi\varepsilon_0} \cdot \frac{p\sin\theta}{r^3}$$

$\therefore$ Net electric field at point P is $E = \sqrt{E_r^2 + E_\theta^2}$

$$\Rightarrow \quad E = \frac{1}{4\pi\varepsilon_0} \frac{p}{r^3} \sqrt{1+3\cos^2\theta}$$

Direction of the electric field, $\tan\alpha = \frac{E_\theta}{E_r} = \frac{1}{2}\tan\theta$

Example 35 *What is the magnitude of electric field intensity due to a dipole of moment 2×10^{-8} C-m at a point distance 1 m from the centre of dipole, when line joining the point to the centre of dipole makes an angle of 60° with dipole axis?*

Sol. Given, $p = 2\times10^{-8}$ C-m, $r = 1$ m and $\theta = 60°$

$\therefore$ Electric field intensity, $E = \frac{p}{4\pi\varepsilon_0 r^3}\sqrt{3\cos^2\theta + 1}$

$$= \frac{2\times10^{-8}\times9\times10^9}{(1)^3} \times \sqrt{3(\cos 60°)^2 + 1} = 238.1 \text{ N/C}$$

Force on Dipole

Suppose an electric dipole of dipole moment $|\mathbf{p}| = 2aq$ is placed in a uniform electric field **E** at an angle θ, where θ is the angle between **p** and **E**. A force $\mathbf{F}_1 = q\mathbf{E}$ will act on positive charge and $\mathbf{F}_2 = -q\mathbf{E}$ on negative charge.

Since, $\mathbf{F}_1$ and $\mathbf{F}_2$ are equal in magnitude but opposite in direction.

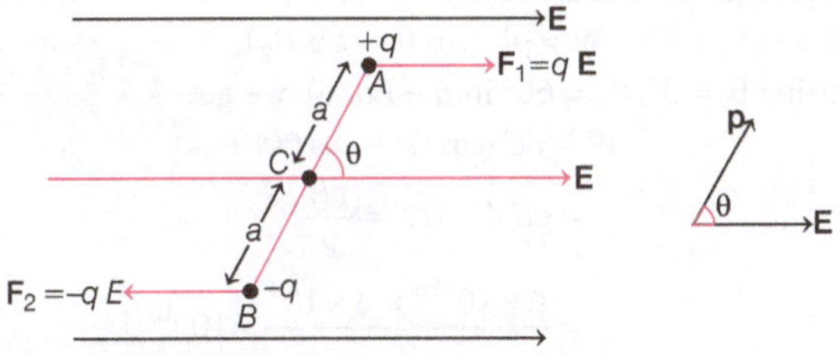

Electric dipole in a uniform electric field

Hence, $\mathbf{F}_1 + \mathbf{F}_2 = 0$

or $\mathbf{F}_{net} = 0$

Thus, net force on a dipole in uniform electric field is zero. While in a non-uniform electric field, it may or may not be zero.

Torque on an Electric Dipole

The two equal and opposite forces shown in the above diagram act at different points of the dipole. They form a couple which exerts a **torque**. This torque has a magnitude equal to the magnitude of either force multiplied by the arm of the couple, *i.e.* perpendicular distance between the two anti-parallel forces.

Magnitude of torque $= qE \times 2a\sin\theta = 2qaE\sin\theta$

$$\tau = pE\sin\theta \qquad [\because p = (2a)q]$$

or $$\boldsymbol{\tau} = \mathbf{p}\times\mathbf{E}$$

Thus, the magnitude of torque is $\tau = pE\sin\theta$. The direction of torque is perpendicular to the plane of paper inwards. Further this torque is zero at $\theta = 0°$ or $\theta = 180°$, *i.e.* when the dipole is parallel or anti-parallel to **E** and maximum at $\theta = 90°$.

Thus, variation of τ with θ is as shown in graph below.

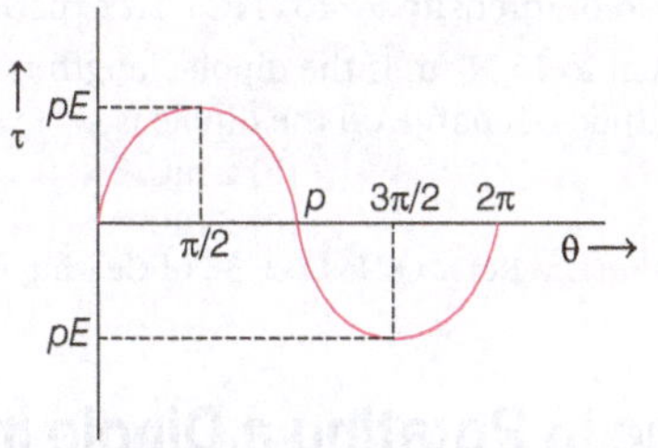

Variation of τ with θ

Example 36 *An electric dipole with dipole moment 4×10^{-9} C-m is aligned at 30° with the direction of a uniform electric field of magnitude 5×10^4 NC^{-1}. Calculate the magnitude of the torque acting on the dipole.*

Sol. Using the formula, $\tau = pE\sin\theta$ ...(i)

Here, dipole moment, $p = 4\times10^{-9}$ C-m

and $E = 5\times10^4$ NC^{-1}

Angle between E and p, $\theta = 30°$.

Substituting these values in Eq (i), we get

$$\tau = 4\times10^{-9}\times5\times10^4\times\sin 30°$$

$$= 20\times10^{-5}\times\frac{1}{2} = 10^{-4} \text{ N-m}$$

NEET Close-up

Example Similar to PYQ Asked in NEET 2023

An electric dipole is placed at an angle of 45° with an electric field of intensity 2×10^6 NC^{-1}. It experiences a torque equal to $2\sqrt{2}$ N-m. If the dipole length is 1 cm, then the magnitude of charge on the dipole is

(a) 3×10^{-3} C (b) 2×10^{-4} C (c) 4×10^{-2} C (d) 6×10^{-3} C

Sol. (b) Given, $\theta = 45°$,

$$E = 2 \times 10^6 \text{ NC}^{-1}$$

Dipole length, $2l = 1 \text{ cm} = 1 \times 10^{-2}$ m

Torque, $\tau = 2\sqrt{2}$ N-m

We know that, $\tau = pE \sin\theta$

$$\Rightarrow \quad p = \frac{\tau}{E \sin\theta} = \frac{2\sqrt{2}}{2 \times 10^6 \times \sin 45°}$$

$$\Rightarrow \quad p = 2 \times 10^{-6} \text{ C-m}$$

$$\Rightarrow \quad 2l \cdot q = 2 \times 10^{-6}$$

$$\Rightarrow \quad q = \frac{2 \times 10^{-6}}{2l} = \frac{2 \times 10^{-6}}{1 \times 10^{-2}} = 2 \times 10^{-4} \text{ C}$$

Skill Builder

An electric dipole is placed at an angle of 90° with an electric field of intensity 5×10^5 NC^{-1}. It experiences a torque equal to 15 N-m. If the dipole length is 3 cm, then the magnitude of charge on the dipole is

(a) 5 mC (b) 2 mC
(c) 1 mC (d) 3 mC

For more Practice Refer Q.Nos. 32, 36 of Gearing up for NEET.

Work Done in Rotating a Dipole in a Uniform Electric Field

When an electric dipole is placed in a uniform electric field **E**, [Fig. (a)] a torque, $\tau = \mathbf{p} \times \mathbf{E}$ acts on it. If we rotate the dipole through a small angle $d\theta$ as shown in Fig. (b), the work done by the torque is

$$dW = \tau d\theta \Rightarrow dW = -pE \sin\theta \, d\theta$$

The work is negative as the rotation $d\theta$ is opposite to the torque.

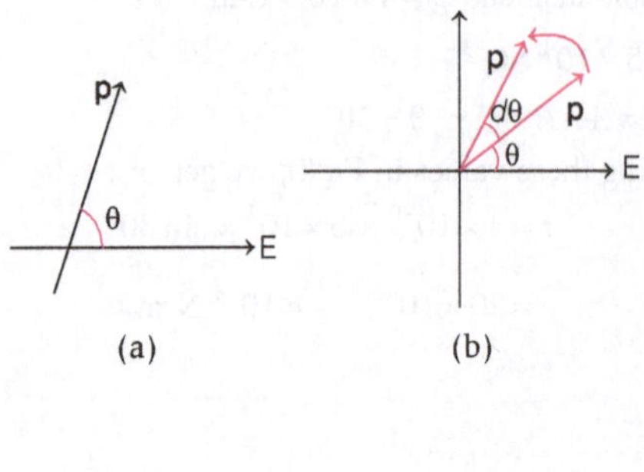

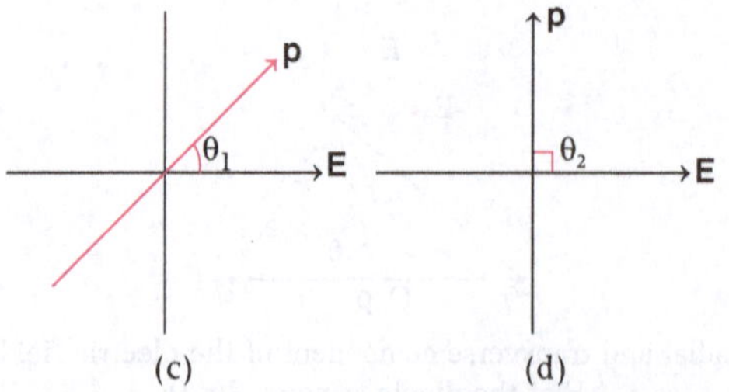

Dipole at different angles with electric field

Total work done by external forces in rotating a dipole from $\theta = \theta_1$ to $\theta = \theta_2$ [Figs. (c) and (d)] will be given by

$$W = \int_{\theta_1}^{\theta_2} pE \sin\theta d\theta$$

$$W_{\text{external force}} = pE (\cos\theta_1 - \cos\theta_2)$$

and work done by electric forces,

$$W_{\text{electric force}} = -W_{\text{external force}}$$
$$= pE (\cos\theta_2 - \cos\theta_1)$$

Taking $\theta_1 = \theta$ and $\theta_2 = 90°$, we have

$$W_{\text{electric dipole}} = p \cdot E (\cos 90° - \cos\theta)$$
$$= -pE \cos\theta$$
$$= -\mathbf{p} \cdot \mathbf{E}$$

Concept ladder If dipole is placed in non-uniform electric field, then magnitude and direction of electric field is different at every point and it will experience both net force and net torque.

Example 37 *An electric dipole of dipole moment $p = 5 \times 10^{-18}$ C-m lying along uniform electric field $E = 4 \times 10^4$ NC^{-1}. Calculate the work done is rotating the dipole by 60°.*

Sol. It is given that, electric dipole moment,

$$p = 5 \times 10^{-18} \text{ C-m}$$

Electric field strength, $E = 4 \times 10^4$ NC^{-1}

When the electric dipole is placed in an electric field **E**, a torque $\tau = \mathbf{p} \times \mathbf{E}$ acts on it. This torque tries to rotate the dipole through an angle θ.

If the dipole is rotated from an angle θ_1 to θ_2, then work done by external force is given by

$$W = pE (\cos\theta_1 - \cos\theta_2) \quad \text{...(i)}$$

Putting $\theta_1 = 0°$, $\theta_2 = 60°$ in the Eq. (i), we get

$$W = pE (\cos 0° - \cos 60°)$$
$$= pE (1 - 1/2) = \frac{pE}{2}$$
$$= \frac{5 \times 10^{-18} \times 4 \times 10^4}{2} = 10^{-13} \text{ J}$$

$$\Rightarrow \quad W = 0.1 \times 10^{-12} \text{ J} = 0.1 \text{ pJ}$$

STEP UP Practice 2

1. Electric field strength due to a point charge of 5 μC at a distance 80 cm from the charge is
(a) 8×10^4 NC^{-1} (b) 7×10^4 NC^{-1}
(c) 5×10^4 NC^{-1} (d) 4×10^4 NC^{-1}

2. **Statement I** The relative closeness of electric field lines does not indicate the relative strength of electric field.
Statement II Electrostatic field lines do not form closed loops.
In the light of the above statements, choose the most appropriate answer from the options given below.
(a) Both Statement I and Statement II are incorrect.
(b) Statement I is correct but Statement II is incorrect
(c) Statement I is incorrect but Statement II is correct
(d) Both Statement I and Statement II are correct

3. The electric field due to a charge at a distance of 3 m from it, is 500 NC^{-1}. The magnitude of the charge is
$\left[\text{Take, } \dfrac{1}{4\pi\varepsilon_0} = 9\times10^9 \text{ N-m}^2/\text{C}^2\right]$
(a) 2.5 μC (b) 2.0 μC (c) 1.0 μC (d) 0.5 μC

4. **Statement I** On going away from a point charge or a small electric dipole, electric field decreases at the same rate in both the cases.
Statement II Electric field is inversely proportional to square of distance from the charge of an electric dipole.
In the light of the above statements, choose the most appropriate answer from the options given below.
(a) Both Statement I and Statement II are incorrect.
(b) Statement I is correct but Statement II is incorrect
(c) Statement I is incorrect but Statement II is correct
(d) Both Statement I and Statement II are correct

5. Two charges + 5 μC and + 10 μC are placed 20 cm apart. The net electric field at the mid point between the two charges is
(a) 4.5×10^6 NC^{-1}, directed toward + 5 μC
(b) 4.5×10^6 NC^{-1}, directed toward + 10 μC
(c) 13.5×10^6 NC^{-1}, directed toward +5 μC
(d) 13.5×10^6 NC^{-1}, directed toward + 10 μC

6. Two point charges $+8q$ and $-2q$ are located at $X = 0$ and $x = L$, respectively. The location of a point on the X-axis at which the net electric field due to these two point charge is zero, is
(a) $8L$ (b) $4L$ (c) $2L$ (d) $\dfrac{L}{4}$

7. A cube of side b has a charge q at each of its vertices. The electric field due to this charge distribution at the centre of this cube will be $\dfrac{1}{4\pi\varepsilon_0}$ times
(a) $\dfrac{q}{b^2}$ (b) $\dfrac{q}{2b^2}$ (c) $\dfrac{32q}{b^2}$ (d) zero

8. Figures below show regular hexagons, with charges at the vertices. In which of the following cases the electric field at the centre is not zero?

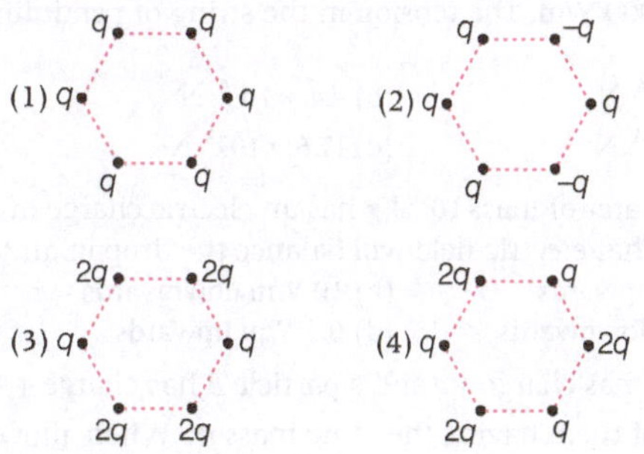

(a) 1 (b) 2
(c) 3 (d) 4

9. An electron is sent in an electric field of intensity 9.1×10^6 N/C. The acceleration produced is
(a) 1.6 m/s^2 (b) 1.6×10^{18} m/s^2
(c) 3.2×10^{18} m/s^2 (d) 0.8×10^{18} m/s^2

10. A charged particle of mass m and charge q is released from rest in a uniform electric field of constant magnitude E. The kinetic energy of the particle after time t is
(a) $\dfrac{2E^2t^2}{mq}$ (b) $\dfrac{Eq^2m}{2t^2}$
(c) $\dfrac{E^2q^2t^2}{2m}$ (d) $\dfrac{Eqm}{2t}$

11. A uniform electric field is along Y-axis in horizontal plane. An electron is projected towards X-axis in this electric field. The path of motion of electron is
(a) Circular (b) Elliptical
(c) Parabola (d) Straight line

12. An electron is placed in vacuum in uniform electric field E, then for balancing of electron, magnitude and direction of electric field will be ($g = 10$ m/s^2)
(a) 5.69×10^{-11} N/C, vertically upward
(b) 5.69×10^{-11} N/C, vertically downward
(c) 5.69×10^{-10} N/C, vertically upward
(d) 5.69×10^{-10} N/C, vertically downward

13. Two charges Q and $-q$, ($q > Q$) are placed at points A and B, then point where $E = 0$

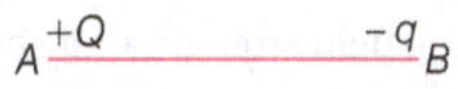

(a) In between A and B
(b) Left hand side of A
(c) Right hand side of B
(d) E will not be zero at any point

14. A charge Q is placed at the centre of a square. If electric field intensity at corner is E_1 and at the mid point of side is E_2 then ratio of $\frac{E_1}{E_2}$ is

(a) $\frac{1}{\sqrt{2}}$ (b) $\sqrt{2}$ (c) $\frac{1}{2}$ (d) 2

15. A simple pendulum of 80 mg-wt and carrying charge 2×10^{-8} C is in equilibrium in a horizontal uniform electric field of 20,000 V/m. The tension in the string of pendulum will be

(a) 22×10^{-4} N (b) 4.4×10^{-4} N
(c) 8.8×10^{-4} N (d) 17.6×10^{-4} N

16. A drop of water of mass 10^{-6} kg has an electric charge of 1000 nC. What electric field will balance the drop in air?

(a) 10 V/m upwards (b) 10 V/m downwards
(c) 0.1V/m downwards (d) 0.1 V/m upwards

17. A particle A has charge $+q$ and a particle B has charge $+4q$ with each of them having the same mass m. When allowed to move from rest in uniform electric field for same time interval, the ratio of their speed $\frac{v_A}{v_B}$ will become

(a) 2:1 (b) 1:2 (c) 1:4 (d) 4:1

18. A positively charged pendulum is oscillating in a uniform electric field pointing vertical upwards. Its time period as compared to that when it oscillates without electric field.

(a) is less (b) is more
(c) Remains unchanged (d) Starts fluctuating

19. The figure shows some of the electric field lines corresponding to an electric field. The figure suggests.

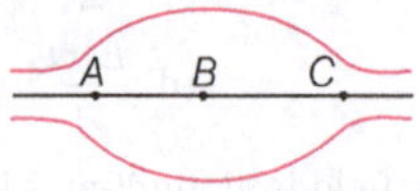

(a) $E_A > E_B > E_C$ (b) $E_A = E_B = E_C$
(c) $E_A = E_C > E_B$ (d) $E_A = E_C < E_B$

20. **Statement I** An electric dipole placed at an angle of 30° with an electric field intensity 2×10^5 N/C. It experiences a torque of 4 N-m, the charge on the dipole is 4 mC, if the dipole length is 2 cm.

Statement II Torque on an electric dipole in an electric field is equal to the cross product between dipole moment and electric field.

In the light of the above statements, choose the most appropriate answer from the options given below.

(a) Both Statement I and Statement II are incorrect.
(b) Statement I is correct but Statement II is incorrect
(c) Statement I is incorrect but Statement II is correct
(d) Both Statement I and Statement II are correct

21. If E_a be the electric field strength of a short dipole at a point on its axial line and E_e that on the equatorial line at the same distance, then

(a) $E_e = 2E_a$ (b) $E_a = 2E_e$
(c) $E_a = E_e$ (d) None of these

22. **Statement I** When a dipole is placed at an angle from the direction of uniform electric field it experiences torque.

Statement II When electric dipole is parallel or anti-parallel to electric field then net torque is non-zero.

(a) Both Statement I and Statement II are incorrect.
(b) Statement I is correct but Statement II is incorrect
(c) Statement I is incorrect but Statement II is correct
(d) Both Statement I and Statement II are correct

23. Electric field at a far away distance r on the axis of a dipole is E_0. What is the electric field at a distance $2r$ on perpendicular bisector?

(a) $\frac{E_0}{16}$ (b) $-\frac{E_0}{16}$ (c) $\frac{E_0}{8}$ (d) $-\frac{E_0}{8}$

24. The electric field due to an electric dipole at a distance r from its centre in axial position is E. If the dipole is rotated through an angle of 90° about its perpendicular axis, then the magnitude of electric field at the same point will be

(a) E (b) $\frac{E}{4}$ (c) $\frac{E}{2}$ (d) $2E$

25. **Statement I** The electric field due to dipole on its equatorial line at a distance is equal to half the electric field at axial line at same distance from mean point.

Statement II Electric field due to dipole varies inversely to the square of the distance.

In the light of the above statements, choose the most appropriate answer from the options given below.

(a) Both Statement I and Statement II are incorrect.
(b) Statement I is correct but Statement II is incorrect
(c) Statement I is incorrect but Statement II is correct
(d) Both Statement I and Statement II are correct

26. When an electric dipole **p** is placed in a uniform electric field **E**, then at what angle between **p** and **E** the value of torque will be maximum?

(a) 90° (b) 0° (c) 180° (d) 45°

27. An electric dipole of moment **p** is placed normal to the lines of force of electric intensity **E**, then the work done in deflecting it through an angle of 180° is

(a) pE (b) $+2pE$
(c) $-2pE$ (d) zero

28. A molecule with a dipole moment **p** is placed in an electric field of strength **E**. Initially, the dipole is aligned parallel to the field. If the dipole is to be rotated to anti-parallel to the field, then the work required to be done by an external agency is

(a) $-2pE$ (b) $-pE$ (c) pE (d) $2pE$

29. Two opposite and equal charges of 4×10^{-8}C are placed 2×10^{-2} cm away from each other. If this dipole is placed in an external electric field of 4×10^8 NC^{-1}, then the value of maximum torque and the work done in rotating it through 180° will be

(a) 64×10^{-4} N-m and 64×10^{-4} J
(b) 32×10^{-4} N-m and 32×10^{-4} J
(c) 64×10^{-4} N-m and 32×10^{-4} J
(d) 32×10^{-4} N-m and 64×10^{-4} J

30. Two electric dipoles of moment p and $64p$ are placed in opposite direction on a line at a distance of 25 cm. The electric field will be zero at point between the dipoles whose distance from the dipole of moment p is

(a) 5 cm (b) $\frac{25}{9}$ cm (c) 10 cm (d) $\frac{4}{13}$ cm

31. An electric dipole is situated in an electric field of uniform intensity E whose dipole moment is p and moment of inertia is I. If the dipole is displaced slightly from the equilibrium position, then the angular frequency of its oscillations is

(a) $\left(\frac{pE}{I}\right)^{1/2}$ (b) $\left(\frac{pE}{I}\right)^{3/2}$ (c) $\left(\frac{I}{pE}\right)^{1/2}$ (d) $\left(\frac{p}{IE}\right)^{1/2}$

32. An uncharged sphere of metal is placed in between two charged plates as shown. The lines of force look like

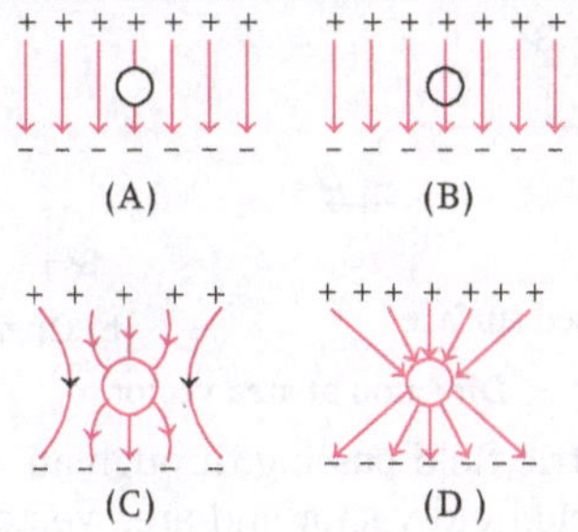

(a) A (b) B
(c) C (d) D

Module 3

Electric Flux and Gauss' Law

- Electric Flux
- Area Vector
- Gauss' Law

Strength of electric field crossing or emerging through a given area is defined in terms of flux of that electric field. Gauss' law represents dependency of this electric flux on the charged enclosed inside the closed surface. This session explains both of the phenomena and helps in solving conceptual as well as numerical problems on the basis of electric flux and Gauss' law.

Electric Flux

Electric flux over an area in an electric field is a measure of the number of field lines crossing a surface. It is denoted by ϕ_E. Let $\mathbf{E}$ be electric field at the location of the surface element $d\mathbf{S}$. The electric flux through the entire surface is given by

$$\phi_E = \int_S \mathbf{E} \cdot d\mathbf{S}$$

$$\Rightarrow \quad \phi_E = \int_S E\, dS \cos\theta$$

$$= E\cos\theta \int_S dS$$

Here, θ is smaller angle between $\mathbf{E}$ and $d\mathbf{S}$.

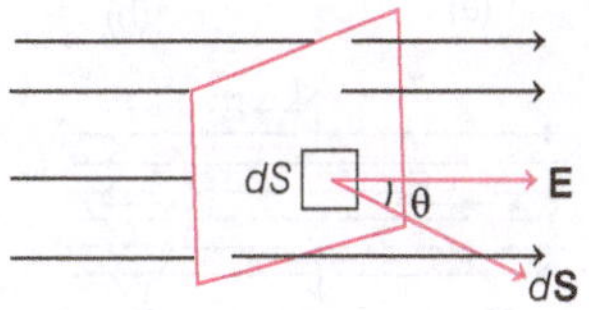

Electric flux over an area $d\mathbf{S}$

For a closed surface, θ is the angle between $\mathbf{E}$ and outward normal to the area element.

Electric flux is a scalar quantity having SI unit V-m or N-m^2 C^{-1}.

An electric flux can also be defined as the flow of the electric field lines through a surface. When field lines leave or flow out of a closed surface, ϕ_E is positive and when they enter or flow into the surface, ϕ_E is negative.

Area Vector

Area is a vector quantity. The direction of a planar area vector is specified by normal to the plane, *e.g.* in case of closed surface like cube, sphere, etc., direction of area vector $\mathbf{S}$ in outward direction is considered to be positive.

In case of open surface, any normal direction can be considered positive.

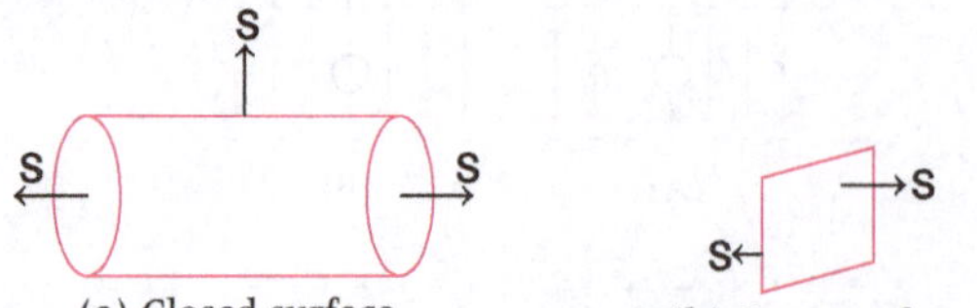

(a) Closed surface (b) Open surface

Direction of area vector

The flux of electric field passing through an area is the dot product of electric field vector and area vector.

i.e. $\phi = \mathbf{E} \cdot \mathbf{S} = ES\cos\theta$

It is real scalar physical quantity with units (volt × m) and dimensions

$$[\phi_E] = [\mathbf{E}d\mathbf{A}] = \left[\frac{\mathbf{F}}{q} d\mathbf{A}\right] = \left[\frac{\text{MLT}^{-2}}{\text{AT}} \text{L}^2\right] = [\text{ML}^3\text{T}^{-3}\text{A}^{-1}]$$

Concept ladder For a closed body outward flux is taken to be positive while inward negative.

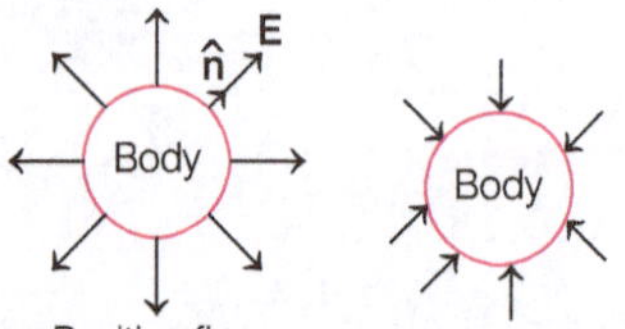

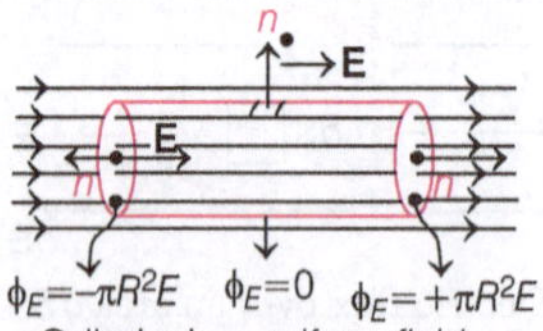

Cylinder in a uniform field

(c)

Example 38 *The electric field in a region is given by* $\mathbf{E} = a\hat{\mathbf{i}} + b\hat{\mathbf{j}}$, *here, a and b are constants. Find the net flux passing through a square area of side l parallel to YZ-plane.*

Sol. A square area of side l parallel to YZ-plane in vector form can be written as $\mathbf{S} = l^2\hat{\mathbf{i}}$

Given, $\mathbf{E} = a\hat{\mathbf{i}} + b\hat{\mathbf{j}}$

∴ Electric flux passing through the given area will be

$$\phi_E = \mathbf{E} \cdot \mathbf{S}$$
$$= (a\hat{\mathbf{i}} + b\hat{\mathbf{j}}) \cdot (l^2\hat{\mathbf{i}}) = al^2$$

Example 39 *Find the flux from the given area.*

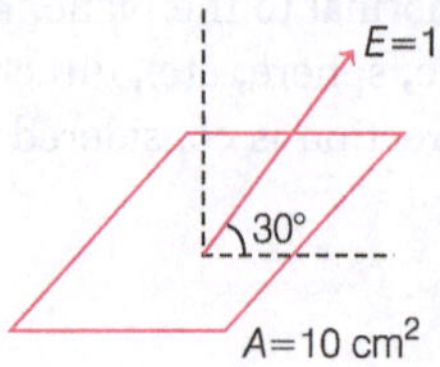

Sol. $\phi = EA\cos\theta = 10 \times 10 \times 10^{-4} \times \cos 60°$
$= 5 \times 10^{-3}$ V-m

Example 40 *The electric field in a region is given by* $\mathbf{E} = \frac{E_0}{a} x\hat{\mathbf{i}}$. *Find the electric flux passing through a cubical volume bounded by the surfaces* $x = 0$, $x = a$, $y = 0$, $y = a$, $z = 0$ *and* $z = a$.

Sol. The given situation is shown below

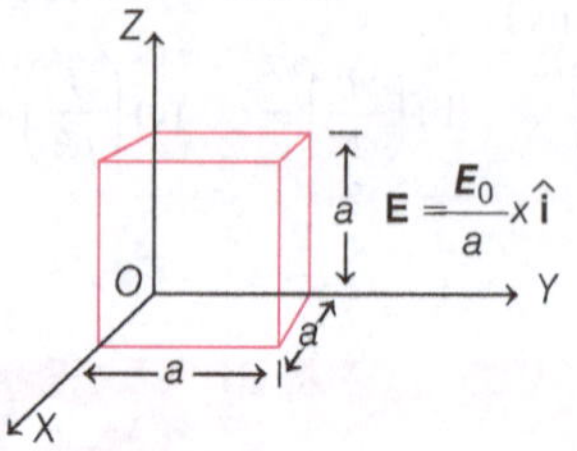

On four faces, electric field and area vector are perpendicular, hence there will be no flux. One face is at origin, *i.e.* $x = 0$ ⇒ $E = 0$, hence there will be no flux. On the sixth face, $x = a$

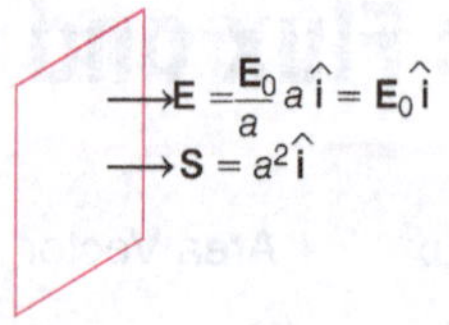

∴ Net electric flux, $\phi = \mathbf{E} \cdot \mathbf{S} = E_0\hat{\mathbf{i}} \cdot a^2\hat{\mathbf{i}} = E_0 a^2$

Example 41 *A cylinder is placed in a uniform electric field* **E** *with axis parallel to the field. Find the total electric flux through the cylinder.*

Sol. The dircetion of **E** and $d\mathbf{S}$ on different sections of cylinder are shown below

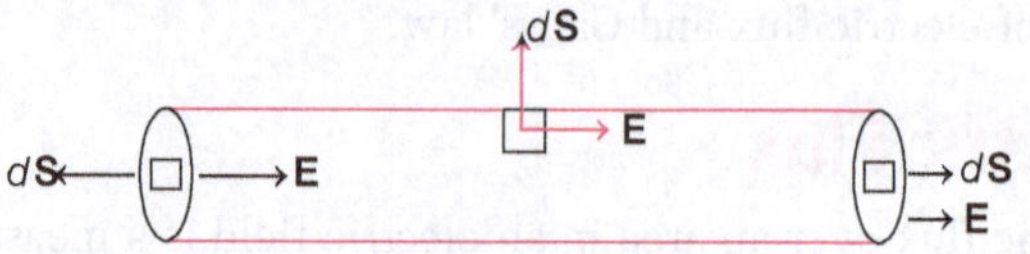

Flux through the entire cylinder,

$$\phi_E = \underbrace{\int \mathbf{E} \cdot d\mathbf{S}}_{\text{Right plane face}} + \underbrace{\int \mathbf{E} \cdot d\mathbf{S}}_{\text{Left plane face}} + \underbrace{\int \mathbf{E} \cdot d\mathbf{S}}_{\text{curved surface}}$$

$$\Rightarrow \phi_E = \int \mathbf{E} \cdot d\mathbf{S} \cos 180° + \int \mathbf{E} \cdot d\mathbf{S} \cos 0° + \int \mathbf{E} \cdot d\mathbf{S} \cos 90°$$
$$= -\mathbf{E}\int d\mathbf{S} + \mathbf{E}\int d\mathbf{S} + \mathbf{0}$$
$$= -\mathbf{E} \times \pi r^2 + \mathbf{E} \times \pi r^2 = 0$$

Gauss' Law

According to this law, the total flux linked with a closed surface is $\frac{1}{\varepsilon_0}$ times the charge enclosed by the surface (gaussian surface).

Mathematically $\phi_E = \oint \mathbf{E} \cdot d\mathbf{S} = \dfrac{q_{\text{enclosed}}}{\varepsilon_0}$

Important Points Regarding Gauss' Law

1. Flux through a shape is independent of its shape, size and position of charge inside it.
2. Electric field intensity at any gaussian surface depends on all charges in and around it.
3. If $E = 0$, then $\phi_E = 0$ but if $\phi = 0$, then E may or may not be zero.

NEET Snapshot

The number of flux line entering the surface must be equal to the number of flux lines leaving it, if $\oint \mathbf{E} \cdot d\mathbf{S} = 0$ over a surface. ***[NEET 2023]***

The electric flux is proportional to the number of electric field line and the term $\oint_s E \cdot dS$ represent electric flux over the closed surface. It means $\oint_s E \cdot dS$ represent the algebraic sum of the number of flux lines entering the surface and number of flux lines leaving the surface.

Scan for Video

Electric Flux Calculation of Some Specific Structures

Using $\phi_E = \int \mathbf{E} \cdot d\mathbf{S}$ and $\phi_E = \dfrac{q_{\text{enclosed}}}{\varepsilon_0}$

1. Cylinder in uniform **E**

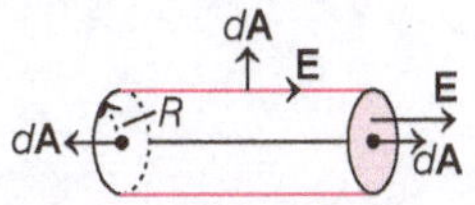

$\phi_{\text{in}} = -\pi R^2 E$ and $\phi_{\text{out}} = \pi R^2 E$
$\Rightarrow \phi_{\text{total}} = 0$

2. Hemisphere in uniform **E**

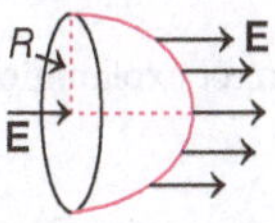

$\phi_{\text{in}} = \phi_{\text{circular}} = -\pi R^2 E$ and
$\phi_{\text{out}} = \phi_{\text{curved}} = \pi R^2 E$
$\Rightarrow \phi_{\text{total}} = 0$

3. Cube in uniform **E**

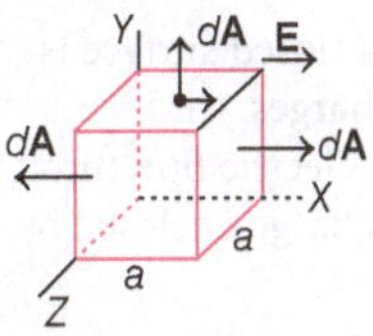

$\phi_{\text{in}} = -a^2 E$ and $\phi_{\text{out}} = a^2 E$
$\Rightarrow \phi_{\text{total}} = 0$

4. Charge q in a hemisphere

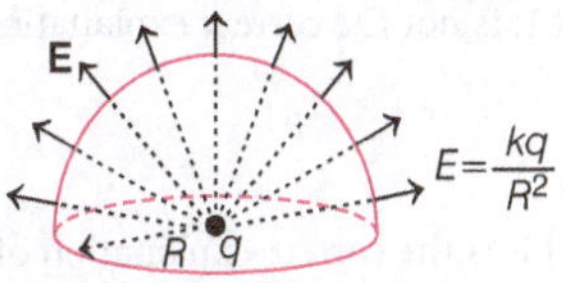

Electric field is radial

$\phi = 2\pi R^2 \times \dfrac{q}{4\pi\varepsilon_0 R^2} = \dfrac{q}{2\varepsilon_0}$

5. Charge q on circular surface of cylinder

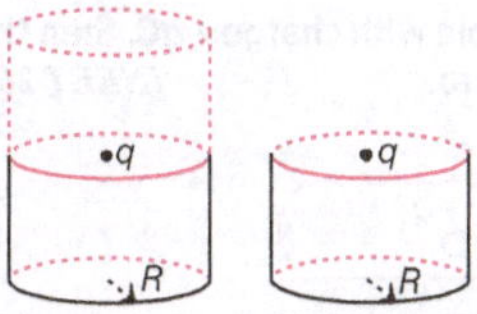

$\phi = \dfrac{q}{2\varepsilon_0}$

6. Charge q on an edge of cube

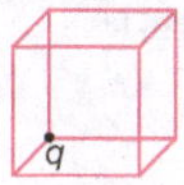

$\phi = \dfrac{q}{8\varepsilon_0}$

Mentor's TIP

- Gauss' law is valid only for closed surfaces (3D closed structures). for surfaces (2D), use basic formula of electric flux
$$\phi_E = \int \mathbf{E} \cdot d\mathbf{S}$$
- Gauss' law is valid for all vector fields obeying inverse square law.
- If a body contains q at its centre, then electric flux through each half of the surface will be $\dfrac{q}{2\varepsilon_0}$.
- If the same body have n identical faces, then flux through each face will be $\dfrac{q}{n\varepsilon_0}$.

Example 42 *An uniformly charged conducting sphere of 2.4 m diameter has a surface charge density of 80.0 $\mu C/m^2$. (i) Find the charge on the sphere. (ii) What is the total electric flux leaving the surface of the sphere?*

Sol. (i) Using the relation $\sigma = \dfrac{q}{4\pi R^2}$, we get

$$q = 4\pi R^2 \times \sigma = 4 \times \frac{22}{7} \times (1.2)^2 \times 80 \times 10^{-6}$$
$$= 1.45 \times 10^{-3}\ \text{C}$$

(ii) Using Gauss' theorem, we get

$$\phi = \frac{q}{\varepsilon_0} = \frac{1.45 \times 10^{-3}}{8.854 \times 10^{-12}} = 1.64 \times 10^8\ \text{N-m}^2\text{C}^{-1}$$

Example 43 *A point charge causes an electric flux of -1.0×10^3 $N\text{-}m^2C^{-1}$ to pass through a spherical Gaussian surface of 10.0 cm radius centred on the charge. (i) If the radius of the Gaussian surface is doubled, how much flux will pass through the surface? (ii) What is the value of the point charge?*

Sol. (i) According to Gauss' law, the electric flux through a Gaussian surface depends upon the charge enclosed inside the surface and not upon its size. Thus, the electric flux will remain unchanged,

i.e. -1.0×10^3 N-m^{2}C^{-1}.

(ii) Using the formula $\phi = \dfrac{q}{\varepsilon_0}$ (Gauss's theorem), we get

$$\Rightarrow \quad q = \varepsilon_0 \phi = 8.854 \times 10^{-12} \times (-1.0 \times 10^3)$$
$$= -8.854 \times 10^{-9}\text{C} = -8.8\,\text{nC}$$

NEET Snapshot

When a sphere enclosed an electric dipole with charge $+q$C, then the total electric flux across the sphere is zero. *[NEET 2019]*

When a sphere enclosed a charged dipole,

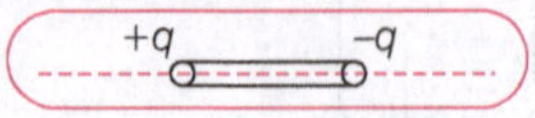

Here, $q = \pm qC$

Thus, according to the Gauss' law, the net electric flux across the closed surface is equal to the net charge enclosed by it, divided by ε_0, i.e.

$$\phi_E = \frac{q_{in}}{\varepsilon_0} = \frac{+q-q}{\varepsilon_0} = 0$$

Example 44 *A long string with charge per unit length λ on it passing through a cube of side a. Then, find maximum flux passing through the cube.*

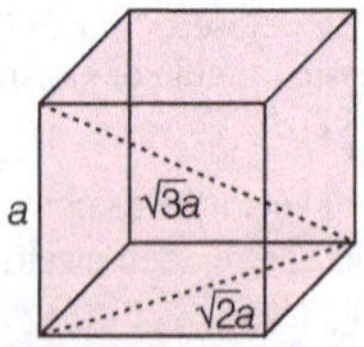

Sol. Maximum length of string through cube (when it is passing along body diagonal of cube) is $= \sqrt{3}a$

Maximum charge inside cube $= \sqrt{3}a\lambda \Rightarrow \phi_{max} = \dfrac{\sqrt{3}a\lambda}{\varepsilon_0}$

Example 45 *In a region of space, the electric field is in the x-direction and proportional to x, i.e., $\mathbf{E} = E_0 x\hat{\mathbf{i}}$.* Consider an imaginary cubical volume of edge a, with its edges parallel to the axes of coordinates. What is the charge enclosed by this volume?

Sol. The idea behind this question is that we have to calculate the total electric flux of the field $\mathbf{E} = E_0 \times \hat{\mathbf{i}}$ through this cube and have to make it equal to $\dfrac{q_{enc}}{\varepsilon_0}$. Then, q will be calculated.

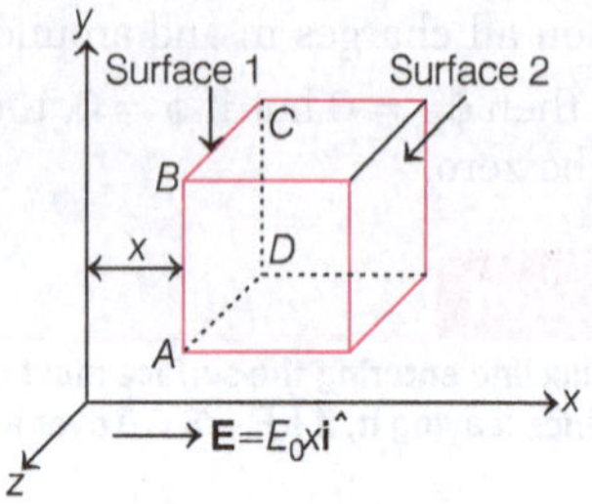

The electric flux on the surface 1 is incoming flux

$$\phi_1 = EA\cos 180° = E_0 x(a^2)(-1) = -E_0 xa^2$$

The electric flux on the surface 2 is outgoing flux

$$\phi_2 = EA\cos 0° = E_0(x+a)(a^2)(+1)$$
$$= E_0 xa^2 + E_0 a^3$$

Net flux through the cube is $\phi = \phi_1 + \phi_2$

$$= -E_0 xa^2 + E_0 xa^2 + E_0 a^3 = E_0 a^3$$

Using the Gauss' law, net flux

$$\phi = \frac{q_{enc}}{\varepsilon_0} = E_0 a^3 \Rightarrow q_{enc} = \varepsilon_0 E_0 a^3$$

STEP UP Practice 3

1. What is the value of electric flux in XY-plane of area of $10\ m^2$, if $\mathbf{E} = (5\hat{\mathbf{i}} + 10\hat{\mathbf{j}})$ N/C ?
   (a) 50 SI Unit (b) 100 SI Unit
   (c) $50\sqrt{5}$ SI Unit (d) zero

2. A charged wire of linear charge density k is placed along axis of cylinder of length a. Electric flux associated to cylinder is
   (a) $\dfrac{ka}{\varepsilon_0}$ (b) $\dfrac{2ka}{\varepsilon_0}$
   (c) $\dfrac{ka}{2\varepsilon_0}$ (d) None of these

3. **Assertion** (A) Electric flux through an open surface depends only on the electric field's magnitude.
   Reason (R) Electric flux is defined as the dot product of the electric field and the surface area vector.
   In the light of the above statements, choose the correct answer from the options given below.
   (a) Both A and R are true but R is not the correct explanation of A.
   (b) A is true but R is false.
   (c) A is false but R is true.
   (d) Both A and R are true and R is the correct explanation of A.

4. **Assertion** (A) Electric flux through a closed surface is affected by the presence of external charges.
   Reason (R) According to Gauss' law, electric flux through a closed surface depends only on the charge enclosed by the surface, not external charges.
   In the light of the above statements, choose the correct answer from the options given below.
   (a) Both A and R are true but R is not the correct explanation of A.
   (b) A is true but R is false.
   (c) A is false but R is true.
   (d) Both A and R are true and R is the correct explanation of A.

5. A point charge q is placed on one of the vertices of a cube of side l. What will be flux linked to the cube ?
(a) $\frac{q}{\varepsilon_0}$ (b) $\frac{q}{2\varepsilon_0}$ (c) $\frac{q}{4\varepsilon_0}$ (d) $\frac{q}{8\varepsilon_0}$

6. **Assertion** (A) Gauss' law is valid only for static electric fields.
Reason (R) The electric flux through a closed surface is proportional to the enclosed charge.
In the light of the above statements, choose the correct answer from the options given below.
(a) Both A and R are true but R is not the correct explanation of A.
(b) A is true but R is false.
(c) A is false but R is true.
(d) Both A and R are true and R is the correct explanation of A.

7. A charge q is placed in a metallic box as shown in figure.

Relation between electric field intensities at A and B is
(a) $E_A > E_B$ (b) $E_A = E_B$
(c) $E_A < E_B$ (d) None of these

8. A point charge inside an ellipsoid is displaced from one foci to another foci. Its linked electric flux
(a) will increase
(b) remains unchanged
(c) will decrease
(d) will become zero

9. A charge q is situated at one vertices of a cube. Electric flux linked with each surface of the cube will be
(a) $\frac{q}{8\varepsilon_0}$ (b) $\frac{q}{48\varepsilon_0}$
(c) $\frac{q}{24\varepsilon_0}$ (d) $\frac{q}{\varepsilon_0}$

10. **Assertion** (A) The electric field just inside a charged conducting surface is always zero.
Reason (R) The electric field lines emanating from the surface are normal to the surface due to the repulsion between like charges.
In the light of the above statements, choose the correct answer from the options given below.
(a) Both A and R are true but R is not the correct explanation of A.
(b) A is true but R is false.
(c) A is false but R is true.
(d) Both A and R are true and R is the correct explanation of A.

11. Which of the following is not correctly paired?
(a) Electrical field due to dipole $\longrightarrow E \propto \frac{1}{r^3}$
(b) Electric field due to point charge $\longrightarrow E \propto \frac{1}{r^2}$
(c) Electric flux through a closed surface $\longrightarrow \oint \mathbf{E} \cdot d\mathbf{A}$
(d) Electric flux through a closed surface if there is no Constant charge enclosed by surface $\longrightarrow \oint \mathbf{E} \cdot d\mathbf{A} = 0$

12. **Assertion** (A) Gauss' law applied to any shape of the closed surface.
Reason (R) Gauss' law is independent of the shape of the surface as long as it encloses the charge.
In the light of the above statements, choose the correct answer from the options given below.
(a) Both A and R are true but R is not the correct explanation of A.
(b) A is true but R is false.
(c) A is false but R is true.
(d) Both A and R are true and R is the correct explanation of A.

13. An imaginary cube of side a is in region of uniform electric field **E**.

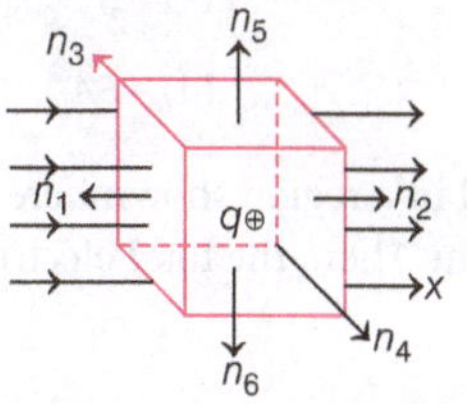

The cube is then turned by angle θ about a vertical axis.

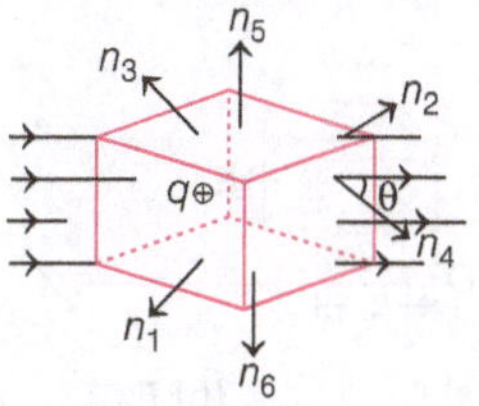

Which of the following is not correctly paired?
(a) Flux through surface 1, $\phi_{E_1} \longrightarrow -Ea^2 \cos\theta$
(b) Flux through surface 2, $\phi_{E_2} \longrightarrow Ea^2 \cos\theta$
(c) Flux through surface 3, $\phi_{E_3} \longrightarrow 0$
(d) Flux through surface 4, $\phi_{E_4} \longrightarrow Ea^2 \sin\theta$

14. A cube is placed in a electric field as shown in figure. Total flux related to it will be

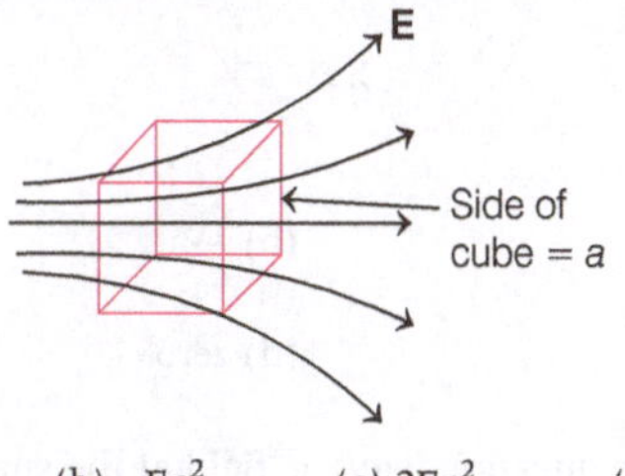

(a) Ea^2 (b) $-Ea^2$ (c) $2Ea^2$ (d) zero

15. A sheet of area A is rotated from perpendicular position to angle of θ with electric field **E**. Which of the following pair is not correctly paired according to θ and their corresponding electric field.
(a) $0° \longrightarrow$ (i) $-EA$ (b) $30° \longrightarrow$ (ii) EA
(c) $60° \longrightarrow$ (iii) $-0.134EA$ (d) $90° \longrightarrow$ (iv) 0

16. A charge q is placed at the centre of the open end of a cylindrical vessel. The flux of electric field through the surface of vessel is
(a) zero (b) $\frac{q}{\varepsilon_0}$ (c) $\frac{q}{2\varepsilon_0}$ (d) $\frac{2q}{\varepsilon_0}$

17. A sheet of area A is rotated from perpendicular position to angle of 30° with electric field $\mathbf{E}$ as shown in figure. Change in electric flux passing through the sheet will be

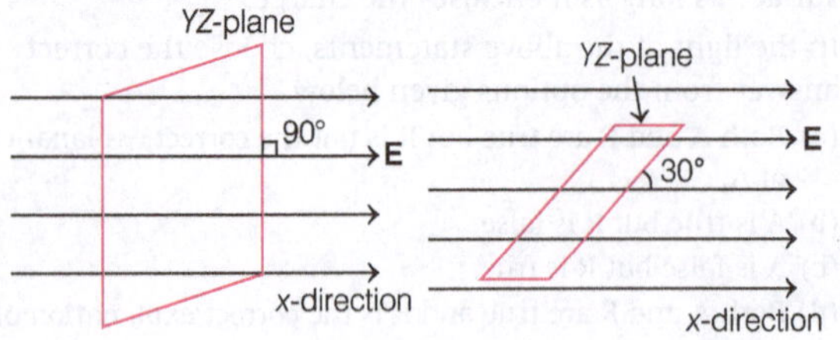

(a) EA
(b) $\frac{EA}{2}$
(c) $\frac{-EA}{2}$
(d) $-EA$

18. The electric field in a region shown here is given by $\mathbf{E} = E_0 x^{3/2}\hat{\mathbf{i}}$ volt/m. Then, the total electric flux through the cube of side a is

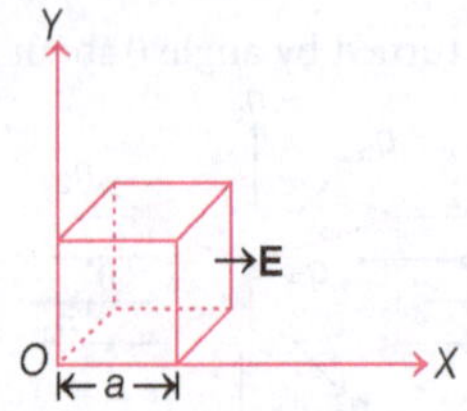

(a) zero
(b) E_0
(c) $E_0 a^{5/2}$
(d) $E_0 a^{7/2}$

19. Consider the charge configuration for a sphere given below. Electric flux linked with the sphere will be

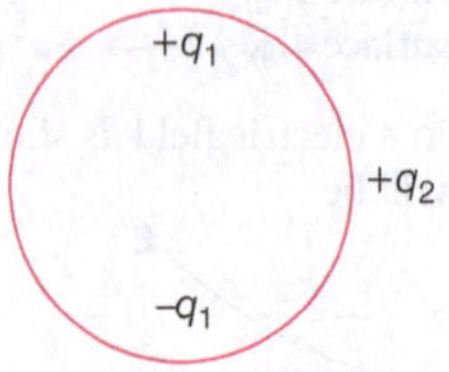

(a) $\frac{q_2}{\varepsilon_0}$
(b) $\frac{q_1}{\varepsilon_0}$
(c) $\frac{-q_1}{\varepsilon_0}$
(d) zero

20. In the above question, electric field at the surface of sphere coil be due to
(a) q_1 only
(b) q_1 and q_2 only
(c) zero
(d) All three charges

21. A charge q is surrounded by a closed surface consisting of an inverted cone of height h and base radius R, and a hemisphere of radius R as shown in the figure. The electrical flux through the conical surface is

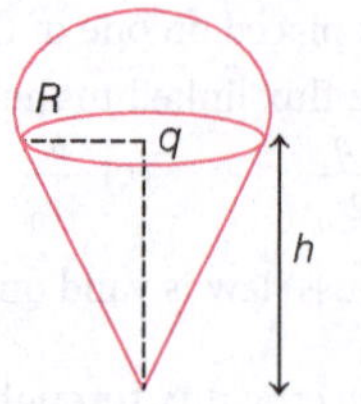

(a) $\frac{2q}{\varepsilon_0}$
(b) $\frac{q}{3\varepsilon_0}$
(c) $\frac{3q}{2\varepsilon_0}$
(d) $\frac{q}{2\varepsilon_0}$

22. If linear charge density of a wire as shown in the figure is λ, then

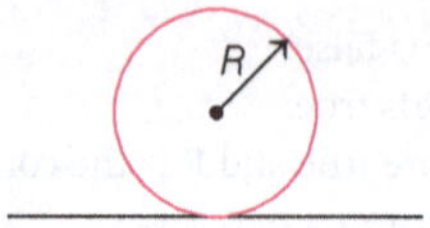

(a) electric field at the centre is $\frac{\lambda}{2\varepsilon_0}$
(b) electric field at the centre of the loop is $\frac{\lambda}{2\pi\varepsilon_0 R}$
(c) electric field at the centre of the loop is $\frac{\lambda}{2\pi\varepsilon_0 R} + \frac{\lambda}{2\varepsilon_0 R}$
(d) None of the above

23. Figure shown below is a distribution of charges. The flux of electric field due to these charges through the surface S is

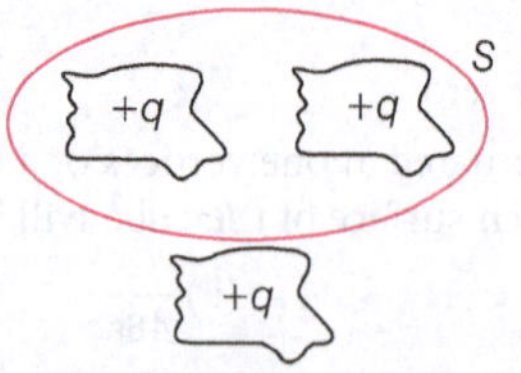

(a) $3q/\varepsilon_0$
(b) $2q/\varepsilon_0$
(c) q/ε_0
(d) zero

24. A cylinder of radius R and length L is placed in a uniform electric field E parallel to the cylinder axis. The total flux for the surface of the cylinder is given by
(a) $2\pi R^2 E$
(b) $\pi R^2/E$
(c) $(\pi R^2/\pi R)/E$
(d) zero

25. A square surface of side L metres is in the plane of the paper. A uniform electric field $\mathbf{E}$ (volt/m), also in the plane of the paper, is limited only to the lower half of the square surface, (see figure). The electric flux in SI units associated with the surface is

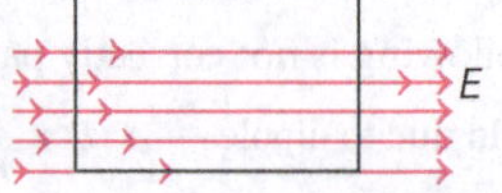

(a) zero
(b) EL^2
(c) $EL^2/(2\varepsilon_0)$
(d) $EL^2/2$

Module 4

Applications of Gauss' Law

- Applications of Gauss's Law

Applications of Gauss' Law

Gauss's law of electrostatics (refer Module-3) is very helpful in calculation of electric field at any given point due to various types of charge distributions. These calculations are otherwise difficult as well as lengthy with the help of standard formula of electric field (Module-2).

This session discusses about various shapes in charge distributions and calculation of electric field (s) at different points due to these charges.

To calculate electric field by using Gauss' law Gaussian surface is considered such that

1. It should be symmetrical in shape and size.
2. Point of observation should be located at Gaussian surface for symmetry of point of observation.
3. Distribution of charge inside Gaussian surface should be symmetric.

Gaussian Surface Consideration

- Consider cylindrical Gaussian surface for linear and cylindrical charge distribution.
- Spherical Gaussian surface consider for point charge and spherical charge distribution.
- **Concept** $\oint \mathbf{E} \cdot d\mathbf{A} = \dfrac{q_{enc}}{E_0}$

1. Electric Field Due to an Infinitely Long Straight Uniformly Charged Wire

Consider a long line charge with a linear charge density (charge per unit length), λ. To calculate the electric field at a distance r from the line charge, we construct a Gaussian surface, a cylinder of any arbitrary length l of radius r and its axis coinciding with the axis of the line charge. This cylinder have three surfaces. One is curved surface and the two plane parallel surfaces.

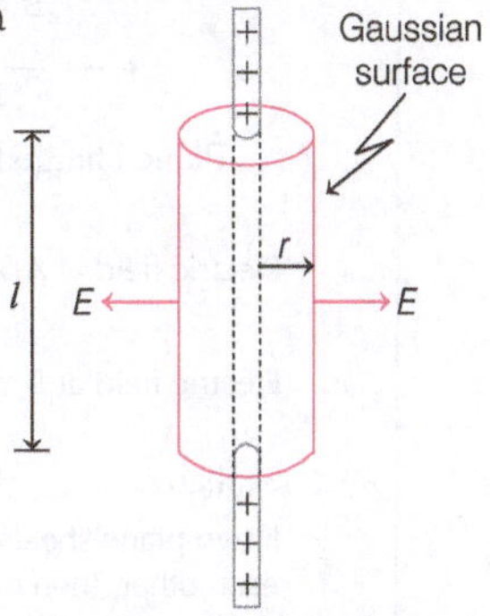

Cylindrical Gaussian surface around a line charge

Field lines at plane parallel surfaces are tangential, so flux passing through these surfaces is zero. The magnitude of electric field is having the same magnitude (say E) at curved surface and simultaneously the electric field is perpendicular at every point of this surface.

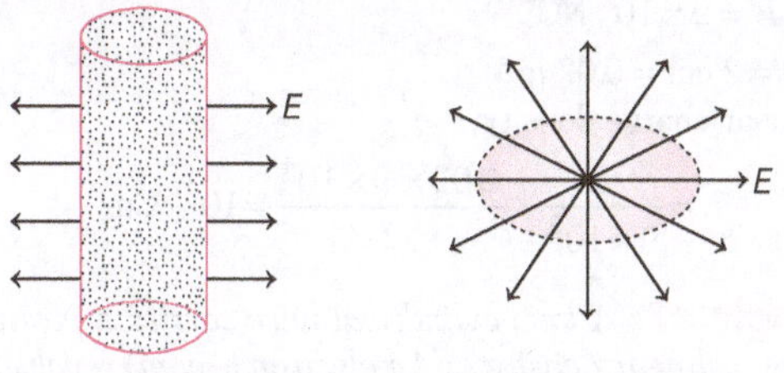

Electric flux through different surfaces

Hence, we can apply the Gauss' law as

$$E \cdot S = \frac{q_{in}}{\varepsilon_0}$$

Here, S = area of curved surface = $(2\pi rl)$

and q_{in} = net charge enclosing this cylinder = λl.

$$\therefore \quad E\,(2\pi rl) = \frac{\lambda l}{\varepsilon_0}$$

$$\therefore \quad \boxed{E = \frac{\lambda}{2\pi\varepsilon_0 r}}$$

i.e. $\quad E \propto \dfrac{1}{r}$

So, E-r graph is a rectangular hyperbola as shown in figure.

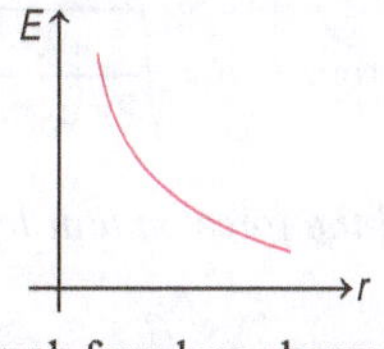

E-r graph for a long charged wire

Concept ladder

Electric field due to a finite length of straight charged wire,

$$E = \frac{1}{4\pi\varepsilon_0}\frac{\lambda}{r}(\sin\theta_1 + \sin\theta_2)$$

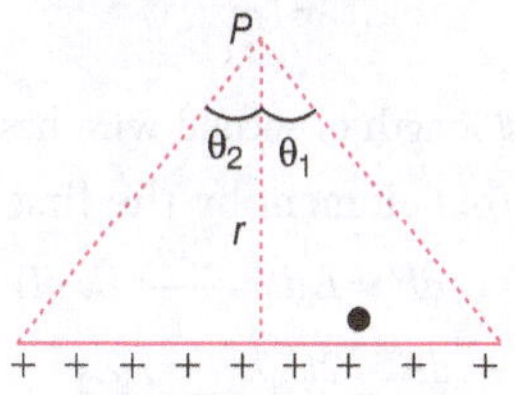

Example 46 *An infinite line charge produces a field of 9×10^4 NC^{-1} at a distance of 2 cm. Calculate the linear charge density.*

Sol. As we know that, electric field due to an infinite line charge is given by the relation,

$$E = \frac{1}{2\pi\varepsilon_0} \cdot \frac{\lambda}{r}$$

where, λ is linear charge density and r is the distance of a point where an electric field is produced from the line charge.

or $$\lambda = 2\pi\varepsilon_0 r E$$

Here, $E = 9 \times 10^4$ NC^{-1}

and $r = 2$ cm $= 0.02$ m

$\therefore$ Linear charge density,

$$\lambda = \frac{1}{9 \times 10^9} \times \frac{0.02 \times 9 \times 10^4}{2} = 10^{-7} \text{ Cm}^{-1}$$

Example 47 *A long cylindrical wire carries a positive charge of linear density λ. An electron $(-e, m)$ revolves around it in a circular path under the influence of the attractive electrostatic force. Find the speed of the electron.*

Sol. Electric field at perpendicular distance r,

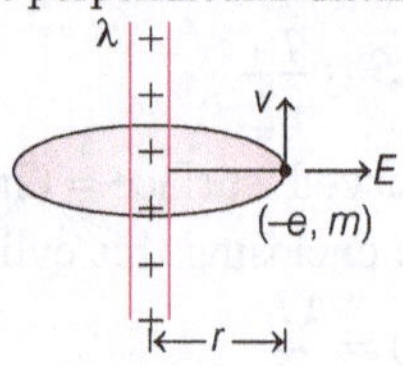

$$E = \frac{\lambda}{2\pi\varepsilon_0 r}$$

The electric force on electron, $F = eE$

To move in circular path, necessary centripetal force is provided by electric force.

$$F_c = \frac{mv^2}{r} \Rightarrow \frac{mv^2}{r} = eE = \frac{e\lambda}{2\pi\varepsilon_0 r} \Rightarrow v = \sqrt{\frac{e\lambda}{2\pi\varepsilon_0 m}}$$

$\therefore$ Speed of the electron, $$v = \sqrt{\frac{e\lambda}{2\pi\varepsilon_0 m}}$$

Example 48 *Find the force on unit length of one wire due to another wire.*

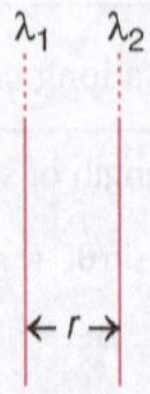

Sol. Suppose that dl length of second wire has charge dq, then the force on this element by the first wire is

$$dF = E_1 dq = \frac{2k\lambda_1}{r}(\lambda_2 dl)$$

$$\Rightarrow \quad \frac{dF}{dl} = \frac{2k\lambda_1\lambda_2}{r} = \frac{\lambda_1\lambda_2}{2\pi\varepsilon_0 r}$$

2. Electric Field due to a Plane Sheet of Charge

Consider a flat thin sheet, infinite in size with constant surface charge density σ (charge per unit area).

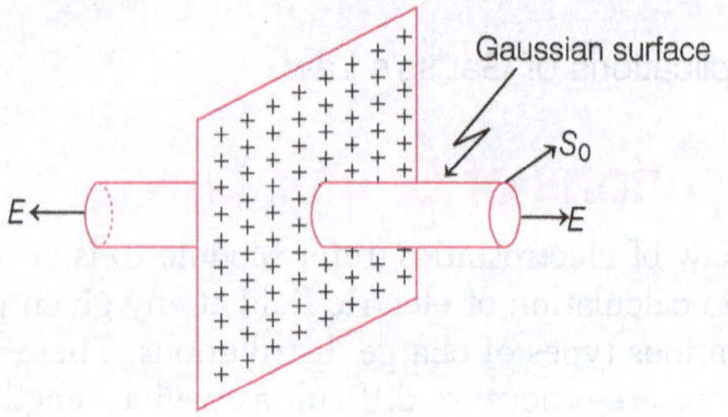

Cylindrical Gaussian surface for a plane charged sheet

Let us draw a Gaussian surface (a cylinder) with one end on one side and other end on the other side and of cross-sectional area S_0. Field lines will be tangential to the curved surface, so flux passing through this surface is zero. At plane surfaces, electric field has same magnitude and perpendicular to surface. Hence, using $E \cdot S = \frac{q_{in}}{\varepsilon_0}$

$$\therefore \quad E(2S_0) = \frac{(\sigma)(S_0)}{\varepsilon_0}$$

$$\therefore \quad \boxed{E = \frac{\sigma}{2\varepsilon_0}}$$

Thus, we see that the magnitude of the field due to plane sheet of charge is independent of the distance from the sheet.

Concept ladder Suppose two plane sheets having charge densities $+\sigma$ and $-\sigma$ are placed at some separation.

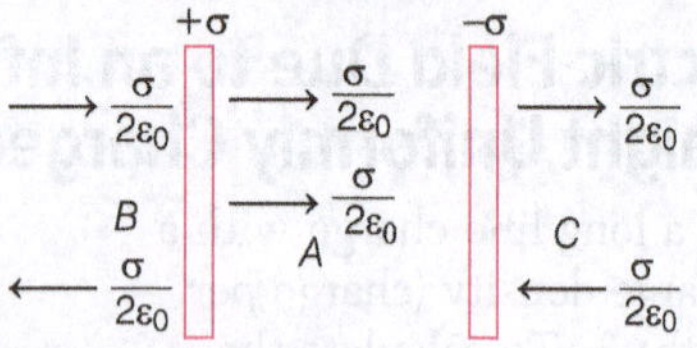

Plane charged sheets placed close to each other

Electric field at A, $E_A = \frac{\sigma}{2\varepsilon_0} + \frac{\sigma}{2\varepsilon_0} = \frac{\sigma}{\varepsilon_0}$

Electric field at B, $E_B = \frac{\sigma}{2\varepsilon_0} - \frac{\sigma}{2\varepsilon_0} \Rightarrow E_B = 0$

Similarly, $E_C = 0$

If two plane sheets having opposite charges are kept close to each other, then electric field exists only between them.

Example 49 *A large plane sheet of charge having surface charge density 5×10^{-6} Cm^{-2} lies in XY-plane. Find the electric flux through a circular area of radius*

0.1 *m, if the normal to the circular area makes an angle of* 60° *with the Z-axis.*

Sol. Given, $\sigma = 5 \times 10^{-6}\ \text{Cm}^{-2}$, $r = 0.1$ m and $\theta = 60°$

Flux, $\phi = E \cdot S \cos\theta = \left(\dfrac{\sigma}{2\varepsilon_0}\right)\pi r^2 \cos\theta$

$$= \frac{5 \times 10^{-6}}{2 \times 8.85 \times 10^{-12}} \times \frac{22}{7} \times (0.1)^2 \cos 60°$$

$\therefore \quad \phi = 4.44 \times 10^3\ \text{N-m}^2/\text{C}$

Example 50 *Two large, thin metal plates are placed parallel and close to each other. On their inner faces, the plates have surface charge densities of opposite signs and of magnitude* $1.77 \times 10^{-11}\ \text{C/m}^2$. *What is electric field ?*

(i) to the left of the plates, *(ii) to the right of the plates*

(iii) and in between the plates?

Sol. (i) Electric fields due to both the plates outside them, will be equal in magnitude and opposite in direction, so net field will be zero.

(ii) Electric field outside the plates will be equal in magnitude and opposite in direction, so net electric field will be zero.

(iii) In between the plates, the electric fields due to both the plates will be adding up, so net field will be

$\dfrac{\sigma}{2\varepsilon_0} + \dfrac{\sigma}{2\varepsilon_0} = \dfrac{\sigma}{\varepsilon_0}$ from positive to negative plate.

$$\therefore \quad E = \frac{\sigma}{\varepsilon_0} = \frac{1.77 \times 10^{-11}}{8.85 \times 10^{-12}} = 2\ \text{N/C}$$

3. Electric Field near a Charged Conducting Surface

When a charge is given to a conducting plate, it distributes, itself over the entire outer surface of the plate. The surface charge density σ is uniform and is the same on both surfaces, if plate is of uniform thickness and of infinite size. This is similar to the previous one, the only difference is that, this time charges are on both sides. Hence, applying $E \cdot S = \dfrac{q_{in}}{\varepsilon_0}$

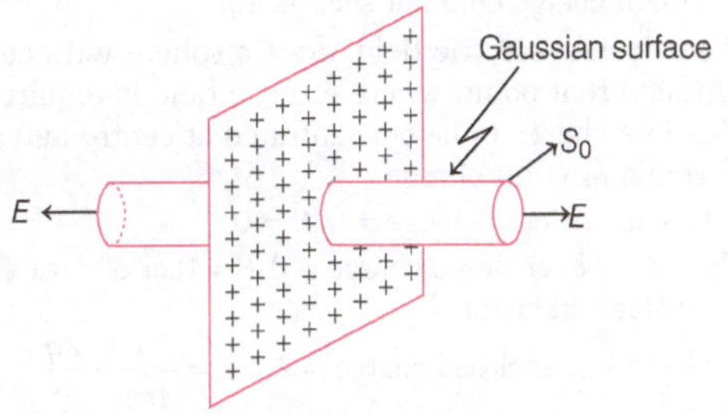

Cylindrical Gaussian surface for a conducting surface

Here, $\quad S = 2S_0$ and $q_{in} = (\sigma)(2S_0)$

$$\therefore \quad E(2S_0) = \frac{(\sigma)(2S_0)}{\varepsilon_0}$$

$$\therefore \quad \boxed{E = \frac{\sigma}{\varepsilon_0}}$$

The electric field near a charged conducting surface of any shape is σ/ε_0 and perpendicular to the surface.

4. Electric Field due to a Uniformly Charged Thin spherical Shell

Let O be the centre and R be the radius of a thin, isolated spherical shell or solid conducting sphere carrying a charge $+q$ which is uniformly distributed on the surface. We have to determine electric field intensity due to this shell at points outside the shell, on the surface of the shell and inside the shell.

At External Point

We can construct a Gaussian surface (a sphere) of radius $r > R$. At all points of this sphere, the magnitude of electric field is same and its direction is perpendicular to the surface. Thus, we can apply Gauss's theorem,

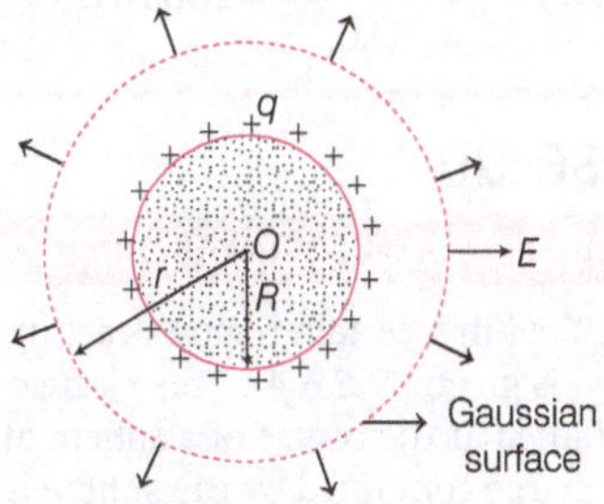

Spherical Gaussian surface around a spherical shell

$$E \cdot S = \frac{q_{in}}{\varepsilon_0} \quad \text{or} \quad E(4\pi r^2) = \frac{q}{\varepsilon_0}$$

$$\therefore \quad \boxed{E = \frac{1}{4\pi\varepsilon_0} \cdot \frac{q}{r^2}}$$

Hence, the electric field at any external point is the same as, if the total charge is concentrated at centre.

At the surface of sphere, $r = R$

$$\therefore \quad \boxed{E = \frac{1}{4\pi\varepsilon_0} \cdot \frac{q}{R^2}}$$

At an Internal Point

In this case, the Gaussian surface encloses no charge,

i.e. $\quad \phi = E(4\pi r^2) = 0, \ E_{inside} = 0$

The electric field intensity is zero everywhere inside the charged shell.

The variation of electric field (E) with the distance from the centre (r) is as shown in figure.

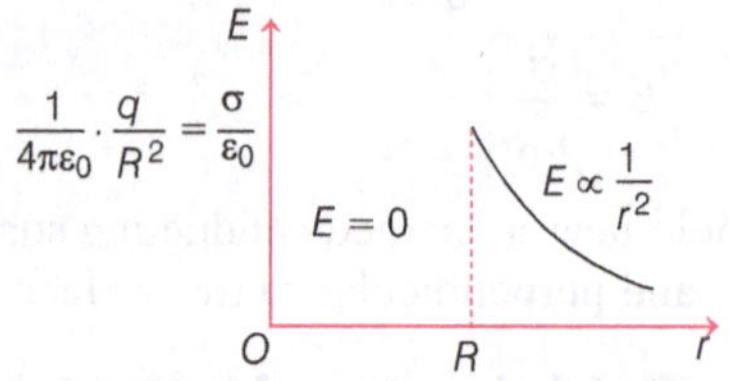

E-r graph for a spherical shell

(i) At the surface, graph is discontinuous.

(ii) $E_{\text{surface}}=\dfrac{1}{4\pi\varepsilon_0}\cdot\dfrac{q}{R^2}=\dfrac{q/4\pi R^2}{\varepsilon_0}=\dfrac{\sigma}{\varepsilon_0}$

Example 51 *A thin spherical shell of metal has a radius of 0.25 m and carries charge of 0.2 μC. Calculate the electric intensity at 3.0 m from the centre of the shell.*

Sol. The intensity at an external point at a distance r from the centre of the shell is given by $E=\dfrac{1}{4\pi\varepsilon_0}\cdot\dfrac{q}{r^2}$

Here, $r = 3.0$ m

$$\therefore\quad E=(9.0\times10^9)\times\frac{2\times10^{-7}}{(3.0)^2}=200\text{ N/C}$$

NEET Close-up

Example Similar to PYQ Asked in NEET 2015

The electric field in a certain region is acting radially outward and is given by $E = 4r$. This electric field is due to a charge contained at the centre of a sphere of radius b. The amount of charge contained by the sphere is

(a) $4\pi\varepsilon_0 b^2$ (b) $4\pi\varepsilon_0 b$ (c) $16\pi\varepsilon_0 b^3$ (d) $16\pi\varepsilon_0 b^2$

Sol. (c) The given electric field is,

$$E = 4r \quad\quad ...(i)$$

Electric field at the surface of the sphere is,

$$E=\frac{1}{4\pi\varepsilon_0}\frac{q}{b^2} \quad\quad ...(ii)$$

Eqs. (i) and (ii) are equal, if $r = b$.

$$\frac{1}{4\pi\varepsilon_0}\frac{q}{b^2}=4b$$

$$\Rightarrow\quad q=16\pi\varepsilon_0 b^3$$

Skill Builder

The electric field in a certain region is acting radially inward and is given by $E = 3r^2$. This electric field is due to a charge contained at the centre of a sphere of radius c. The amount of charge contained by the sphere is

(a) $3\pi\varepsilon_0 c^3$ (b) $6\pi\varepsilon_0 c$ (c) $12\pi\varepsilon_0 c^4$ (d) $8\pi\varepsilon_0 c^2$

For more Practice Refer Q.No. 9 of step up practice 4 and Q. No. 56, 65 of Gearing up for NEET.

Example 52 *An electric dipole is placed at the centre of a spherical shell. Find the electric field at an external point of the shell.*

Sol. Net charge inside the sphere, $q_{\text{in}} = 0$.

Therefore, according to Gauss' law, net flux passing through the sphere is zero. Therefore, electric field at an external point will be zero.

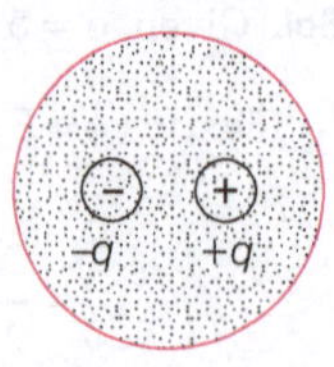

Example 53 *A small conducting spherical shell with inner radius a and outer radius b is concentric with a larger conducting spherical shell with inner radius c and outer radius d. The inner shell has total charge +2q and the outer shell has charge +4q.*

(i) What is the total charge on the (a) inner surface of the small shell, (b) outer surface of the small shell, (c) inner surface of the large shell (d) and outer surface of the large shell?

(ii) Calculate the electric field in terms of q and the distance r from the common centre of two shells for (a) r < a, (b) a < r < b, (c) b < r < c, (d) c < r < d (e) and r > d.

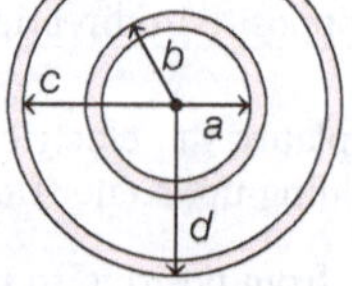

Sol. Charge distribution,

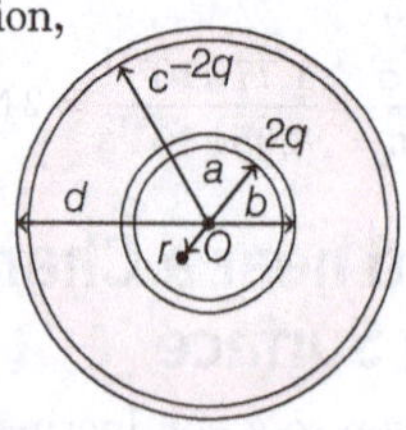

(i) Total charge on inner shell $= 2q$

Total charge on outer shell $= 4q$

Charge distribution

(a) Charge on inner surface of small shell = 0

(b) Charge on outer surface of small shell $= 2q$

(c) Charge on inner surface of large shell $= -2q$

(facing surface have equal and opposite charges)

(d) Charge on outer surface of large shell $= 6q$

(total charge on outer shell is $4q$)

(ii) To calculate electric field, draw a sphere with centre O through that point, where electric field is required. Assume charge to be concentrated at centre and apply formula of point charge.

(a) $r < a$, enclosed charge = 0, $E = 0$

(b) $a < r < b$, enclosed charge = 0, $E = 0$ or electric field inside conductor = 0

(c) $b < r < c$, enclosed charge $= 2q$, $E=\dfrac{1}{4\pi\varepsilon_0}\cdot\dfrac{2q}{r^2}$

(d) $c < r < d$, enclosed charge = 0, $E = 0$, or electric field inside conductor = 0

(e) $r > d$, enclosed charge $= 6q$, $E=\dfrac{1}{4\pi\varepsilon_0}\cdot\dfrac{6q}{r^2}$

5. Electric Field due to a non-Conducting Solid Sphere of Charge

Suppose positive charge q is uniformly distributed throughout the volume of a non-conducting solid sphere of radius R.

At an Internal Point

For finding the electric field at a distance r ($< R$) from the centre, let us choose our Gaussian surface a sphere of radius r, concentric with the charge distribution.

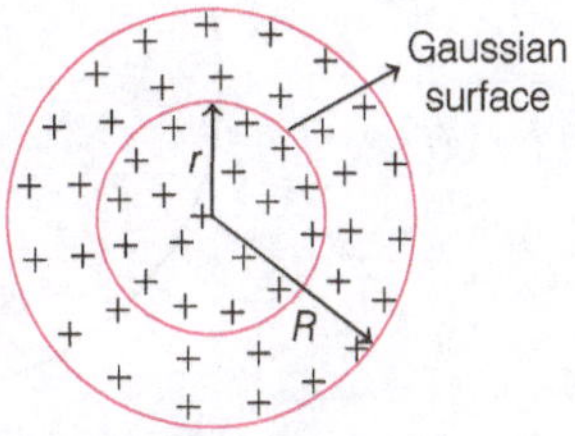

Spherical Gaussian surface inside a solid sphere

From symmetry, the magnitude of electric field E has the same value at every point on the Gaussian surface and the direction of **E** is radial at every point on the surface. So, applying Gauss' law, we have

$$ES = \frac{q_{in}}{\varepsilon_0} \quad \text{...(i)}$$

Here, $S = 4\pi r^2$ and $q_{in} = (\rho)\left(\frac{4}{3}\pi r^3\right)$

Here, ρ = charge per unit volume $= \frac{q}{(4/3)\pi R^3}$

Substituting these values in Eq. (i), we get

$$E = \frac{1}{4\pi\varepsilon_0} \cdot \frac{q}{R^3} \cdot r$$

or $E \propto r$

At the centre of sphere, $r = 0$, so $E = 0$

At the surface of sphere, $r = R$, so $E = \frac{1}{4\pi\varepsilon_0} \cdot \frac{q}{R^2}$

At an External Point

To find the electric field outside the charged sphere, we use a spherical Gaussian surface of radius r ($> R$). This surface encloses the entire charged sphere, so $q_{in} = q$ and

Gauss's law gives, $E(4\pi r^2) = \frac{q}{\varepsilon_0}$

or $E = \frac{1}{4\pi\varepsilon_0} \cdot \frac{q}{r^2}$ or $E \propto \frac{1}{r^2}$

Thus, for a uniformly charged solid sphere, we have the following formulae for magnitude of electric field.

$$E_{\text{inside}} = \frac{1}{4\pi\varepsilon_0} \cdot \frac{q}{R^3} \cdot r$$

$$E_{\text{surface}} = \frac{1}{4\pi\varepsilon_0} \cdot \frac{q}{R^2}$$

and $$E_{\text{outside}} = \frac{1}{4\pi\varepsilon_0} \cdot \frac{q}{r^2}$$

Thus, the electric field at any external point is the same as, if the total charge is concentrated at centre.

The variation of electric field (E) with the distance from the centre of the sphere (r) is shown in figure.

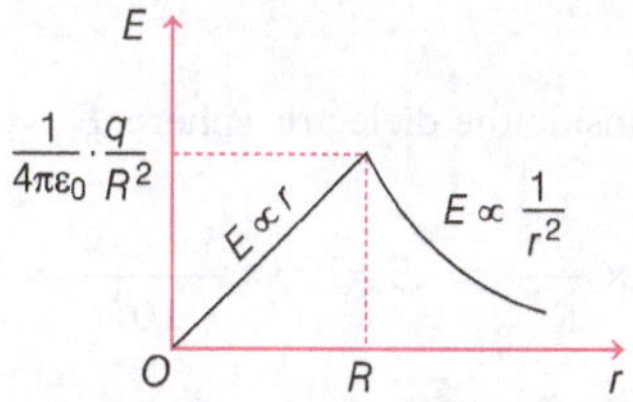

E-r graph for a soild non-conducting sphere

Mentor's TiP

If we set $r = R$ in either of the two expressions for E (outside and inside the sphere), we get the same result, $E = \frac{1}{4\pi\varepsilon_0} \cdot \frac{q}{R^2}$

this is because E is continuous function of r in this case. By contrast, for the charged conducting sphere, the magnitude of electric field is discontinuous at $r = R$ (it jumps from $E = 0$ to $E = \sigma/\varepsilon_0$).

NEET Close-up

Example Similar to PYQ Asked in NEET 2020

Radius of a spherical conductor is 20 cm. Conductor having charge of 2.8×10^{-9} C distributed uniformly. Then magnitude of electric field at a point 27 cm from the centre of the sphere is (in N/C)

(a) 2823×10^2 (b) 2286×10^3
(c) 3923×10^3 (d) 3457×10^2 N/C

Sol. (*d*) Given,

Radius, $r = 20 \text{ cm} = 20 \times 10^{-2}$ m

Charge, $q = 2.8 \times 10^{-9}$ C

Electric field at a point ($x = 27$ cm) from the centre of the sphere is $E = \frac{1}{4\pi\varepsilon_0} \frac{q}{x^2}$

$$= 9 \times 10^9 \times \frac{2.8 \times 10^{-9}}{(27 \times 10^{-2})^2}$$

$$= 3.457 \times 10^2 \text{ N/C}$$

Skill Builder

A spherical conductor has a charge of 1.6×10^{-6} C distributed uniformly. It has radius of 5 cm. The magnitude of electric field at point 10 cm from the centre of the conductor is

(a) 14.4×10^5 N/C (b) 12.3×10^4 N/C
(c) 16.2×10^5 N/C (d) 18.9×10^4 N/C

For more Practice Refer Q.No. 15, 18, 19 of step up exercise 4 and Q. No. 54, 55, 59 of Gearing up for NEET.

Example 54 *At a point 20 cm from the centre of a uniformly charged dielectric sphere of radius 10 cm, the electric field is 100 V/m. Find the electric field at 3 cm from the centre of the sphere.*

Sol. Electric field outside the dielectric sphere, $E_{out} = \frac{1}{4\pi\varepsilon_0} \cdot \frac{q}{r^2}$

Electric field inside the dielectric sphere, $E_{in} = \frac{1}{4\pi\varepsilon_0} \cdot \frac{q}{R^3} x$

$\therefore \quad E_{in} = E_{out} \times \frac{r^2 x}{R^3} \Rightarrow E = 100 \times \frac{3 \times (20)^2}{10^3} = 120 \text{ V/m}$

Example 55 *A non-conducting solid sphere of radius R is charged uniformly. Electric field at distance R / 2 from centre of sphere is E, then calculate electric field at distance 2R from centre of sphere.*

Sol. $E_{in} = \frac{kQr}{R^3} \Rightarrow \left[r = \frac{R}{2}\right]$

$\Rightarrow E = \frac{\frac{kQR}{2}}{R^3} = \frac{kQ}{2R^2};$

$E_{out} = \frac{kQ}{r^2} = \frac{kQ}{(2R)^2} = \frac{kQ}{4R^2}; E_{out} = \frac{E}{2}$

Example 56 *Two concentric conducting spherical shell of radii a and b (b > a) are charged with q and Q respectively.* Calculate electric field at distance r from their common centre in the following cases.

(i) $a > r > 0$ (ii) $r = a$

(iii) $b > r > a$ (iv) $r = b$

(v) $\infty > r > b$

Sol. (i) $E_1 = 0 + 0 = 0$

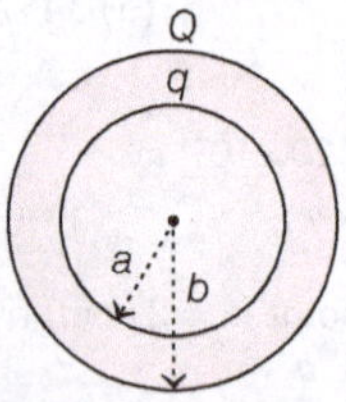

(ii) $E_2 = \frac{kq}{a^2} + 0 = \frac{kq}{a^2}$ (iii) $E_3 = \frac{kq}{r^2} + 0 = \frac{kq}{r^2}$

(iv) $E_4 = \frac{kq}{b^2} + \frac{kQ}{b^2} = \frac{k}{b^2}(q+Q)$ (v) $E_5 = \frac{kq}{r^2} + \frac{kQ}{r^2} = \frac{k}{r^2}(q+Q)$

Example 57 *A non conducting solid sphere is charged uniformly. A small spherical portion is removed from this solid sphere as shown. Then, electric field in the cavity is*

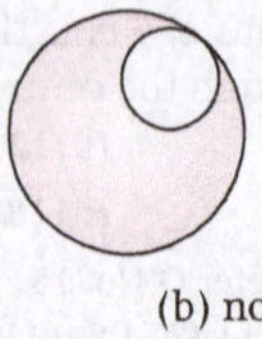

(a) zero (b) non-zero and uniform

(c) non-zero and non-uniform (d) None of these

Sol. (b) By principle of superposition

$\mathbf{E}_{entire} = \mathbf{E}_{Remaining} + \mathbf{E}_{removed}$

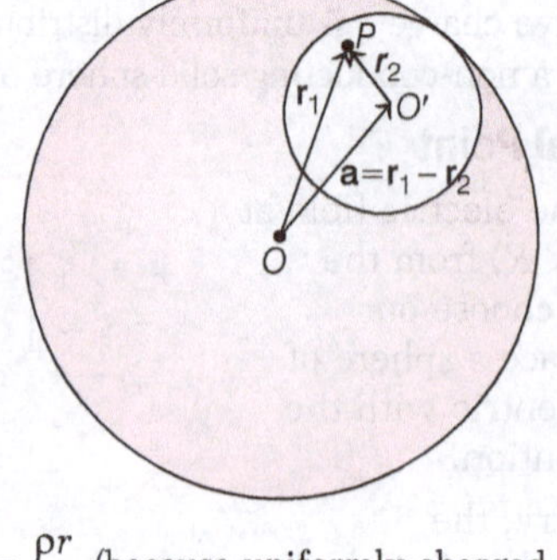

use $\mathbf{E}_{in} = \frac{\rho r}{3\varepsilon_0}$ (because uniformly charged sphere)

$\frac{\rho \mathbf{r}_1}{3\varepsilon_0} = \mathbf{E}_{remaining} + \frac{\rho \mathbf{r}_2}{3\varepsilon_0}$

$\Rightarrow \mathbf{E}_{remaining} = \frac{\rho \mathbf{r}_1}{3\varepsilon_0} - \frac{\rho \mathbf{r}_2}{3\varepsilon_0} = \frac{\rho}{3\varepsilon_0}(\mathbf{r}_1 - \mathbf{r}_2)$

$\mathbf{E}_{remaining} = \frac{\rho}{3\varepsilon_0}(\mathbf{a})$ where **a** is position vector of centre of cavity w.r.t. centre of entire sphere, which does not depend on location of point of observation inside the cavity.

Concept ladder Above expression of electric field concludes that electric field at all points inside the cavity is **non-zero** and **uniform.** Direction of this non-zero uniform electric field is along the line joining of centre of entire sphere and centre of cavity [Along $\mathbf{r}_1 - \mathbf{r}_2$ or **a**].

Example 58 *Two non-conducting spheres of radius R have charge Q uniformly distributed on them. The centres of spheres are at x = 0 and x = 3R. Find the magnitude and direction of the net electric field on the X-axis at*

(i) $x = 0$, *(ii)* $x = \frac{R}{2}$, *(iii)* $x = \frac{3R}{2}$ *(iv) and* $x = 4R$.

Sol. Electric field inside sphere at distance r from centre

$= \frac{1}{4\pi\varepsilon_0} \cdot \frac{Qr}{R^3}$

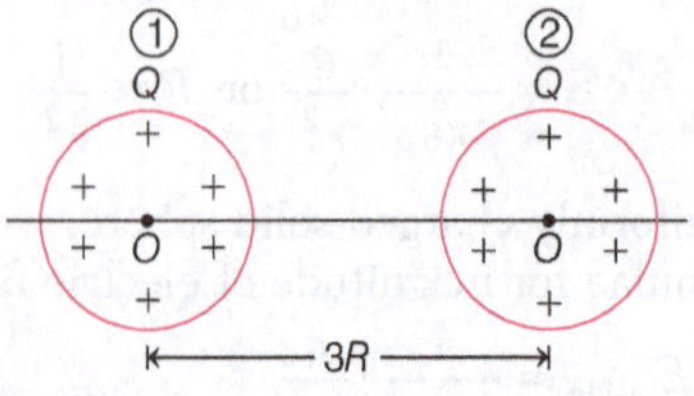

On the surface or outside, whole charge is assumed to be concentrated at centre.

(i) At $x = 0$, $E_1 = 0$, $E_2 = \frac{1}{4\pi\varepsilon_0} \frac{Q}{(3R)^2}$, towards left

$$E_{net} = E_2 = \frac{Q}{36\pi\,\varepsilon_0\,R^2}, \text{ along } -X\text{-axis}$$

(ii) At $x = R/2$,

$$E_1 = \frac{1}{4\pi\,\varepsilon_0}\cdot\frac{QR/2}{R^3} = \frac{Q}{8\pi\,\varepsilon_0\,R^2}, \text{ along } +X\text{-axis}$$

$$E_2 = \frac{1}{4\pi\,\varepsilon_0}\cdot\frac{Q}{(5R/2)^2} = \frac{Q}{25\pi\,\varepsilon_0\,R^2}, \text{ along } -X\text{-axis}$$

$$E_{net} = E_1 - E_2 = \frac{17Q}{200\pi\,\varepsilon_0\,R^2}, \text{ along } +X\text{-axis}$$

(iii) At $x = 3R/2$, $E_{net} = 0$ $\quad (\because E_1 = E_2)$

(iv) At $x = 4R$, $E_1 = \dfrac{1}{4\pi\varepsilon_0}\dfrac{Q}{(4R)^2}$, $E_2 = \dfrac{1}{4\pi\,\varepsilon_0}\dfrac{Q}{R^2}$

$$E_{net} = E_1 + E_2 = \frac{17Q}{64\pi\varepsilon_0 R^2}, \text{ along } +X\text{-axis}$$

Example 59 *Two large charged non-conducting parallel sheets are placed at a finite distance from each other as shown in figure. Find out electric field intensity at points B.*

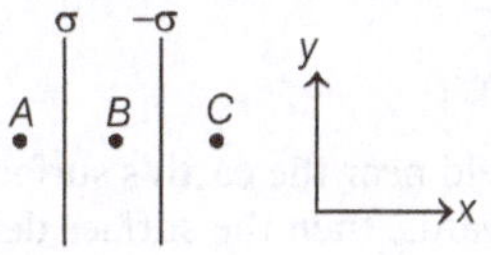

(a) $\dfrac{\sigma}{\varepsilon_0}\hat{\mathbf{i}}$ (b) $\dfrac{\sigma}{2\varepsilon_0}\hat{\mathbf{i}}$ (c) $\dfrac{\sigma}{\varepsilon_0}\hat{\mathbf{j}}$ (d) $\dfrac{\sigma}{2\varepsilon_0}\hat{\mathbf{j}}$

Sol. (a) $|\mathbf{E}_+| = |\mathbf{E}_-| = \dfrac{\sigma}{2\varepsilon_0}$

$$\mathbf{E}_A = \mathbf{E}_C = 0$$

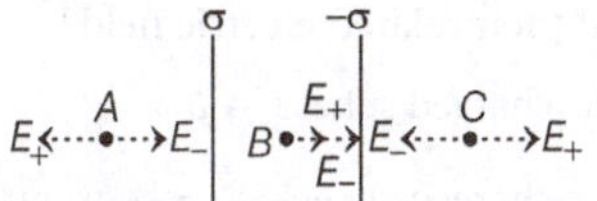

$$\mathbf{E}_E = \mathbf{E}_+ + \mathbf{E}_- = \frac{\sigma}{2\varepsilon_0}\hat{\mathbf{i}} + \frac{\sigma}{2\varepsilon_0}\hat{\mathbf{i}} = \frac{\sigma}{\varepsilon_0}\hat{\mathbf{i}}$$

Example 60 *Three large charged conducting parallel sheets are placed at a finite distance from each other as shown in figure. Find out electric field intensity at point C. (Area of each surface of sheet A)*

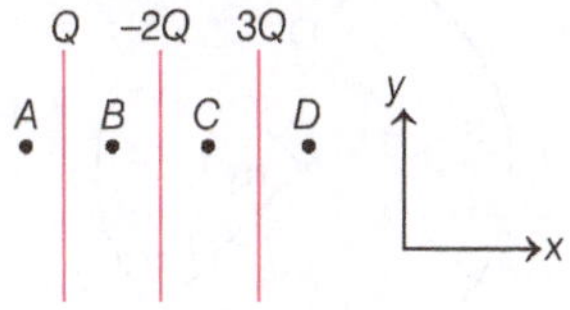

(a) $-\dfrac{Q}{\varepsilon_0 A}\hat{\mathbf{i}}$ (b) 0

(c) $-\dfrac{2Q}{\varepsilon_0 A}\hat{\mathbf{i}}$ (d) $\dfrac{Q}{\varepsilon_0 A}\hat{\mathbf{i}}$

Sol. (c) For point C

$$\mathbf{E}_{net} = \mathbf{E}_Q + \mathbf{E}_{-2Q} + \mathbf{E}_{3Q}$$

$$= +\frac{Q}{2A\varepsilon_0}\hat{\mathbf{i}} - \frac{2Q}{2A\varepsilon_0}\hat{\mathbf{i}} - \frac{3Q}{2A\varepsilon_0}\hat{\mathbf{i}}$$

$$= -\frac{2Q}{A\varepsilon_0}\hat{\mathbf{i}}$$

Example 61 *Two concentric uniformly charged spherical shells of radius R_1 and R_2 ($R_2 > R_1$) have total charges Q_1 and Q_2 respectively. Electric field for $r < R_1$ is.*

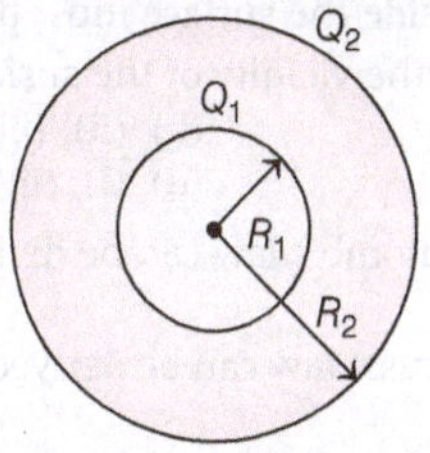

(a) $E = 0$ (b) E = constant

(c) $E \neq 0$ (d) None of these

Sol. (a) Inside the inner spherical shell, the electric field is zero due to symmetry and the fact that there is no enclosed charge within that region.

Example 62 *There are two non-conducting large sheet with surface charge densities $+\sigma$ and $-\sigma$ are placed parallel to each other at distance d as shown in figure. If a point charge (q, m) is released from the sheet A then calculate the velocity by which it will strike B (Neglect gravity).*

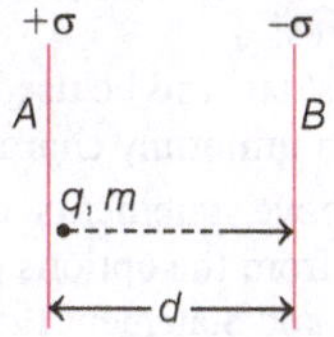

(a) $\sqrt{\dfrac{2\sigma d}{\varepsilon_0 m}}$ (b) $\sqrt{\dfrac{\sigma d}{\varepsilon_0 m}}$

(c) $\sqrt{\dfrac{2\sigma q d}{\varepsilon_0 m}}$ (d) zero

Sol. (c) Electric field between the plates $= \dfrac{\sigma}{\varepsilon_0}$

Force on charge q, $F = \dfrac{\sigma q}{\varepsilon_0}$

Acceleration, $a = \dfrac{\sigma q}{m\varepsilon_0}$

Velocity at plate B

$$v^2 - u^2 = 2as$$

$$v^2 - (0)^2 = 2\frac{\sigma q}{\varepsilon_0 m}d$$

$$v = \sqrt{\frac{2\sigma q d}{\varepsilon_0 m}}$$

STEP UP Practice 4

1. If the flux of the electric field through a closed surface is zero, then
   (i) the electric field must be zero everywhere on the surface
   (ii) the electric field may be zero everywhere on the surface
   (iii) the charge inside the surface must be zero
   (iv) the charge in the vicinity of the surfaces must be zero
   (a) (i), (ii) (b) (ii), (iii)
   (c) (ii), (iv) (d) (i), (iii)

2. **Statement I** Coulomb's law can be derived from Gauss' law.
   Statement II Gauss' law can be derived from Coulomb's law.
   In the light of the above statements, choose the most appropriate answer from the options given below.
   (a) Both Statement I and Statement II are incorrect.
   (b) Statement I is correct but Statement II is incorrect.
   (c) Statement I is incorrect but Statement II is correct.
   (d) Both Statement I and Statement II are correct.

3. An infinite line charge produces a field of 18×10^4 N/C at 0.02 m. The linear charge density is
   (a) 2×10^{-7} C/m (b) 10^{-8} C/ m
   (c) 10^7 C/m (d) 10^{-4} C/m

4. **Statement I** Gauss' law is applicable to open surfaces as well as closed surfaces.
   Statement II Gauss' law can be used to calculate the electric field due to a uniformly charged infinite line.
   In the light of the above statements, choose the most appropriate answer from the options given below.
   (a) Both Statement I and Statement II are incorrect.
   (b) Statement I is correct but Statement II is incorrect.
   (c) Statement I is incorrect but Statement II is correct.
   (d) Both Statement I and Statement II are correct.

5. A charge of 17.7×10^{-4} C is distributed uniformly over a large sheet of area 200 m^2. The electric field intensity at a distance 20 cm from it in air will be
   (a) 5×10^5 N/C
   (b) 6×10^5 N/C
   (c) 7×10^5 N/C
   (d) 8×10^5 N/C

6. **Statement I** Gauss' law is not applicable to find the electric field between two oppositely charged parallel plates.
   Statement II The electric field between the plates is uniform and can be easily calculated without Gauss' law.
   In the light of the above statements, choose the most appropriate answer from the options given below.
   (a) Both Statement I and Statement II are incorrect.
   (b) Statement I is correct but Statement II is incorrect.
   (c) Statement I is incorrect but Statement II is correct.
   (d) Both Statement I and Statement II are correct.

7. From what distance should a 100 eV electron be fired towards a large metal plate having a surface charge density of -2.0×10^{-6} Cm^{-2}, so that it just fails to strike the plate?
   (a) 0.50 mm (b) 0.44 mm
   (c) 0.60 mm (d) 0.77 mm

8. Which of the following is not correctly paired according to charge distribution and their Gaussian surface?
   (a) Line charge $\rightarrow$ Cylinder (co-axial)
   (b) Charged sheet $\rightarrow$ Cylinder (perpendicular)
   (c) Point charge $\rightarrow$ Circle
   (d) Charged sphere $\rightarrow$ sphere

9. A thin spherical shell of metal has a radius of 0.25 m and carries a charge of 0.2 μC. The electric field intensity at a point on the surface of the shell will be
   (a) 2.88×10^4 N/C
   (b) 3.4×10^4 N/C
   (c) 3.25×10^4 N/C
   (d) 3.88×10^4 N/C

10. If the electric field near the earth's surface be 300 V/m directed downwards, then the surface density of charge on earth's surface is
    (a) 3.0×10^{-9} C/m^2
    (b) 5.0×10^{-9} C/m^2
    (c) 2.6×10^{-9} C/m^2
    (d) 7.0×10^{-9} C/m^2

11. Which of the following is not correctly paired according to condition and their related electric field?
    (a) Outside the charged sphere $\rightarrow E \propto \frac{1}{r^2}$
    (b) Outside the charged sheet $\rightarrow E =$ constant
    (c) Inside the charged sphere $\rightarrow E = 0$
    (d) Near to the line charge $\rightarrow E \propto \frac{1}{r^2}$

12. Two concentric uniformly charged shells of radii R_1 and R_2 ($R_2 > R_1$) have total charges Q_1 and Q_2 respectively. Electric field for at point lies inside both the sphere is

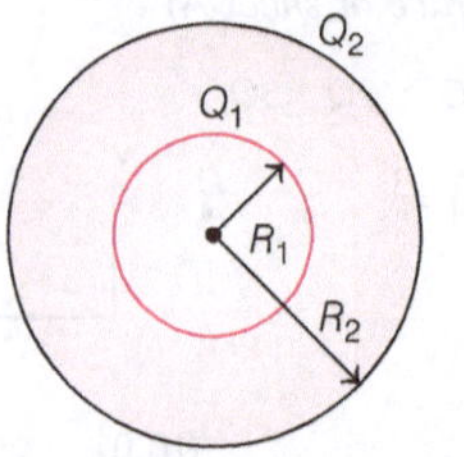

    (a) $E = 0$ (b) $E = \frac{KQ_1}{r^2}\hat{\mathbf{r}}$
    (c) $E = \frac{K(Q_1 + Q_2)}{r^2}\hat{\mathbf{r}}$ (d) None of these

13. A shell is made of conductor as shown in figure. It has inner radius a and outer radius b and carries charge Q. At its centre is a dipole $\mathbf{p}$ as shown. In this case,

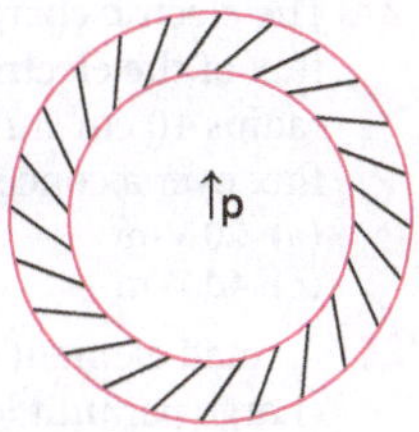

(a) surface charge density on the outer surface depends on $|\mathbf{p}|$.
(b) surface charge density on the inner surface of the shell is zero everywhere.
(c) electric field outside the shell is the same as that of a point charge at the centre of the shell.
(d) surface charge density on the inner surface is uniform and equal to $\frac{Q/2}{4\pi a^2}$

14. **Statement I** A metallic shield in the form of a hollow shell may be built to block an electric field.
Statement II The electric field inside a hollow spherical shield is zero at every point.
In the light of the above statements, choose the most appropriate answer from the options given below.
(a) Both Statement I and Statement II are incorrect.
(b) Statement I is correct but Statement II is incorrect.
(c) Statement I is incorrect but Statement II is correct.
(d) Both Statement I and Statement II are correct.

15. Find the electric field inside a non-conducting solid sphere which carries a charge density proportional to the distance from centre as $p = \alpha r$ (α is a constant)
(a) $\frac{\alpha r^2}{2\varepsilon_0}$ (b) $\frac{\alpha r^2}{4\varepsilon_0}$ (c) $\frac{\alpha r^2}{\varepsilon_0}$ (d) zero

16. **Statement I** The electric field outside a charged spherical shell depends on the amount of charge on the shell and its thickness.
Statement II The electric field inside a uniformally charged non-conducting solid sphere decrease with distance from the centre.
In the light of the above statements, choose the most appropriate answer from the options given below.
(a) Both Statement I and Statement II are incorrect.
(b) Statement I is correct but Statement II is incorrect.
(c) Statement I is incorrect but Statement II is correct.
(d) Both Statement I and Statement II are correct.

17. The angles of inclination of the suspended charged pendulum are 60° and 30° due to electric field of the surface charge densities σ_1 and σ_2 respectively. Then value of $\frac{\sigma_1}{\sigma_2}$ is

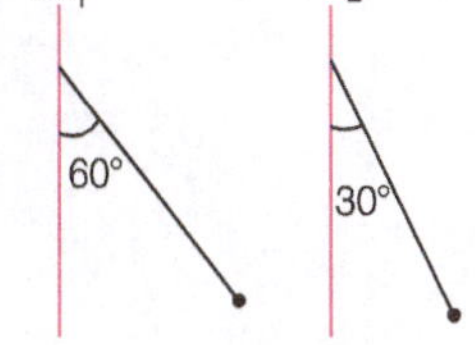

(a) $\sqrt{3}$ (b) 3
(c) $\frac{1}{\sqrt{3}}$ (d) $\frac{1}{3}$

18. The electric field at $2R$ from the centre of a uniformly charged non-conducting sphere of radius R is E. The electric field at a distance $\frac{R}{2}$ from the centre will be
(a) zero (b) $2E$ (c) $4E$ (d) $16E$

19. The electric field at a distance $\frac{3R}{2}$ from the centre of a charged conducting spherical shell of radius R is E. The electric field at a distance $\frac{R}{2}$ from the centre of the sphere is
(a) zero (b) E (c) $E/2$ (d) $E/3$

20. Electric field intensity at a point in between two parallel sheets with like charges of same surface charge densities (σ) is
(a) $\frac{\sigma}{2\varepsilon_0}$ (b) $\frac{\sigma}{\varepsilon_0}$ (c) zero (d) $\frac{2\sigma}{\varepsilon_0}$

21. Which of the following statement is correct?
(a) Electric field inside a conducting sphere is constant and non-zero.
(b) Electric field outside a conducting sphere is constant and non-zero
(c) Electric field inside a non-conducting sphere is constant and non-zero
(d) Electric field inside a non-conducting sphere is variable and non-zero

22. Which of the following is the incorrect statement
(a) Gaussian surfaces are imaginary surfaces.
(b) Electric field is always perpendicular at any point of Gaussian surface
(c) Cube can be chosen as Gaussian surface for a point charge
(d) Gaussian surfaces are symmetrical surfaces.

23. Two parallel metal plates having charges $+Q$ and $-Q$ face each other at a certain distance between them. If the plate are now dipped in kerosene oil tank, the electric field between the plates will
(a) becomes zero (b) increase
(c) decrease (d) remains same

24. A solid conducting sphere of radius a has a net positive charge $2Q$. A conducting spherical shell of inner radius b and outer radius c is concentric with the solid sphere and has a net charge $-Q$. The surface charge density on the inner and outer surfaces of the spherical shell will be

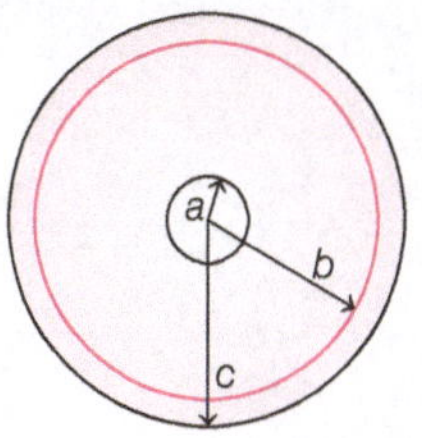

(a) $-\frac{2Q}{4\pi b^2}, \frac{Q}{4\pi c^2}$ (b) $-\frac{Q}{4\pi b^2}, \frac{Q}{4\pi c^2}$
(c) $0, \frac{Q}{4\pi c^2}$ (d) None of these

25. A mass $m = 20$ g has a charge $q = 3.0$ mC. It moves with a velocity of 20 ms^{-1} and enters a region of electric field of 80 NC^{-1} in the same direction as the velocity of the mass. The velocity of the mass after 3s in this region is
(a) 80 ms^{-1} (b) 56 ms^{-1}
(c) 44 ms^{-1} (d) 40 ms^{-1}

26. Three concentric metallic spherical shells of radii R, $2R$, $3R$ are given charges Q_1 Q_2 Q_3, respectively. It is found that the surface charge densities on the outer surfaces of the shells are equal. Then, the ratio of the charges given to the shells $Q_1 : Q_2 : Q_3$ is
(a) 1 : 2 : 3 (b) 1 : 3 : 5
(c) 1 : 4 : 9 (d) 1 : 8 : 18

27. The electric charges are distributed in a small volume. The flux of the electric field through a spherical surface of radius 10 cm surrounding the total charge is 20 V-m. The flux over a concentric sphere of radius 20 cm will be
(a) 20 V-m (b) 10 V-m
(c) 40 V-m (d) 5 V-m

28. A small element l is cut from a circular ring of radius a and charge per unit length λ. The net electric field at the centre of ring is
(a) zero (b) $\frac{-\lambda l}{4\pi\varepsilon_0 a^2}$
(c) infinity (d) $\frac{\lambda}{4\pi\varepsilon_0 l}$

NEET Exclusive EXTRA BYTES

- Ultimate test of charging is repulsion because attraction may also occur between one charged and another uncharged body.
- A normal charged particle [which is stable or moving with very low speed, then speed of light ($v << c$) has fixed specific mass, i.e. $\frac{q}{m} = 1.76 \times 10^{11}$ C/kg.
- Coulomb's law is used for two point charges. While using this for expanded and limited size bodies, one should take all the charge at the centre of the body and then even this, law will be valid only for points outside of that expanded body.
- Coulomb's force between two charges is independent of nearby existing other charged /uncharged bodies.
- Dielectric constant (K) of a medium is numerically equal to the ratio of the force on two point charges in free space to that in the medium.
$$K = \frac{F_{\text{Free space}}}{F_{\text{medium}}}$$
- A charged particle always experiences electric force in an electric field whether it is static or moving .
- For any regular polygon containing same charges at all corners, electric field at centre is always zero.
- Electric lines of force start and end perpendicular at the surface of the conductor.
- Electric field inside a hollow sphere may or may not be zero, while it is always zero inside solid conductors.
- An electric dipole experiences only torque (not force) in an uniform electric field while it may experience force also in non-uniform electric field.

GEARING UP FOR NEET

Single Option Correct

1 Charge q_2 of mass m revolves around a stationary charge q_1 in a circular orbit of radius r. The orbital periodic time of q_2 would be

(a) $\left[\dfrac{4\pi^2 mr^3}{kq_1q_2}\right]^{1/2}$ (b) $\left[\dfrac{kq_1q_2}{4\pi^2 mr^3}\right]^{1/2}$

(c) $\left[\dfrac{4\pi^2 mr^4}{kq_1q_2}\right]^{1/2}$ (d) $\left[\dfrac{4\pi^2 mr^2}{kq_1q_2}\right]^{1/2}$

2 Two identical charged spheres suspended from a common point by two massless strings of length l are initially a distance $d (d << l)$ apart because of their mutual repulsion. The charge begins to leak from both the spheres at a constant rate. As a result, the spheres approach each other with a velocity v. Then, v as a function of distance x between them is,

(a) $v \propto x^{-1/2}$ (b) $v \propto x^{-1}$

(c) $v \propto x^{1/2}$ (d) $v \propto x$

3 In the given figure, two tiny conducting balls of identical mass m and identical charge q hang from non-conducting threads of equal length L. Assume that θ is so small that $\tan\theta \simeq \sin\theta$, then for equilibrium, x is equal to

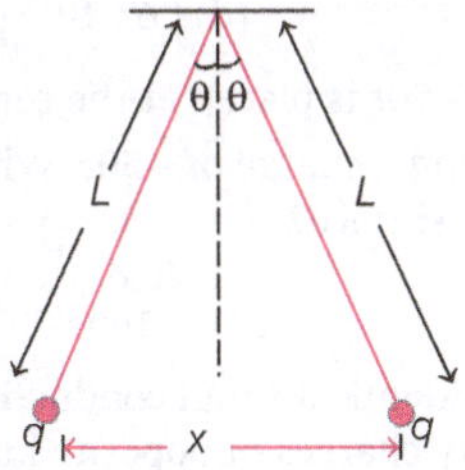

(a) $\left(\dfrac{q^2L}{2\pi\varepsilon_0 mg}\right)^{1/3}$ (b) $\left(\dfrac{qL^2}{2\pi\varepsilon_0 mg}\right)^{1/3}$

(c) $\left(\dfrac{q^2L^2}{4\pi\varepsilon_0 mg}\right)^{1/3}$ (d) $\left(\dfrac{q^2L}{4\pi\varepsilon_0 mg}\right)^{1/3}$

4 If a charge on the body is 1 nC, then how many electrons are present on the body?

(a) 1.6×10^{19} (b) 6.25×10^{9}

(c) 6.25×10^{27} (d) 6.25×10^{28}

5 An electron is released from the bottom plate A as shown in the figure ($E = 10^4$ N/C). The velocity of the electron when it reaches plate B will be nearly equal to

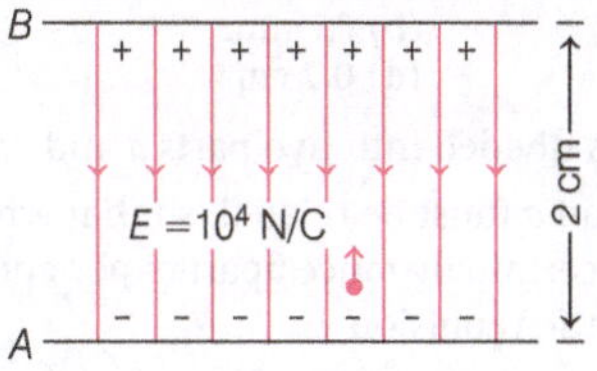

(a) 0.85×10^7 ms^{-1} (b) 1.0×10^7 ms^{-1}

(c) 1.25×10^7 ms^{-1} (d) 1.65×10^7 ms^{-1}

6 Four point positive charges of same magnitude (Q) are placed at four corners of a rigid square frame as shown in figure. The plane of the frame is perpendicular to Z-axis. If a negative point charge is placed at a distance z away from the frame ($z << L$), then

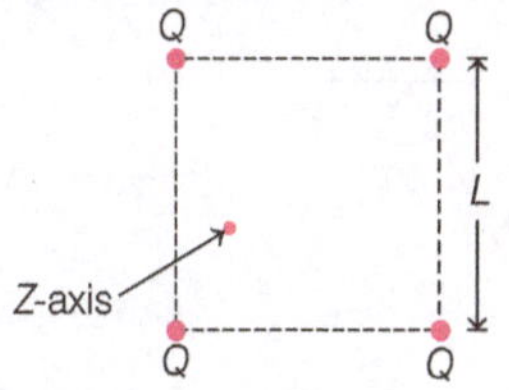

(a) negative charge oscillates along the Z-axis

(b) it moves away from the frame

(c) it moves slowly towards the frame and stays in the plane of the frame

(d) it passes through the frame only once

7 Two copper balls, each weighing 10 g, are kept in air 10 cm apart. If one electron from every 10^6 atoms is transferred from one ball to the other, then the coulomb force between them is (atomic weight of copper is 63.5)

(a) 2.0×10^{10} N (b) 2.0×10^{4} N

(c) 2.0×10^{8} N (d) 2.0×10^{6} N

8 Two equally charged, identical metal spheres A and B repel each other with a force F. The spheres are kept fixed with a distance r between them. A third identical, but uncharged sphere C is brought in contact with A and then placed at the mid-point of the line joining A and B. The magnitude of the net electric force on C is

(a) F (b) $F/4$

(c) $F/2$ (d) $4F$

9 Four charges equal to $-Q$ are placed at the four corners of a square and a charge q is at its centre. If the system is in equilibrium, the value of q is

(a) $\frac{-Q}{4}(1+2\sqrt{2})$ (b) $\frac{Q}{4}(1+2\sqrt{2})$
(c) $\frac{-Q}{2}(1+2\sqrt{2})$ (d) $\frac{Q}{2}(1+2\sqrt{2})$

10 An electron moving with the speed $5\times10^6 ms^{-1}$ is shooted parallel to the electric field of intensity 1×10^3 N/C. Field is responsible for the retardation of motion of electron. Now, evaluate the distance travelled by the electron before coming to rest for an instant. (Mass of electron $=9\times10^{-31}$ kg and charge $=1.6\times10^{-19}$ C)
(a) 7m (b) 0.7 mm
(c) 7 cm (d) 0.7 cm

11 A certain charge Q is divided into two parts q and $(Q-q)$. How the charge Q and q must be related, so that when q and $(Q-q)$ is placed at a certain distance apart experience maximum electrostatic repulsion ?
(a) $Q=2q$ (b) $Q=3q$
(c) $Q=4q$ (d) $Q=4q$

12 Two small spherical balls each carrying a charge $Q=10\,\mu C$ (10 micro-coulomb) are suspended by two insulating threads of equal lengths 1 m each, from a point fixed in the ceiling. It is found that in equilibrium threads are separated by an angle 60° between them, as shown in the figure. What is the tension in the threads ?
(Given, $\frac{1}{(4\pi\varepsilon_0)}=9\times10^9$ Nm/C²)

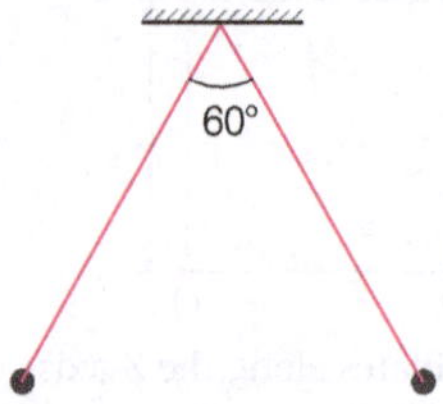

(a) 18 N
(b) 1.8 N
(c) 0.18 N
(d) None of the above

13 An infinite number of charges, each of charge $1\,\mu C$, are placed on the X-axis with coordinates $x=1, 2, 4, 8, \ldots, \infty$. If a charge of 1 C is kept at the origin, then what is the net force acting on 1C charge ?
(a) 9000 N (b) 12000 N
(c) 24000 N (d) 36000 N

14 Equal charges q are placed at the four corners A, B, C and D of a square of length a. The magnitude of the force on the charge at B will be
(a) $\frac{3q^2}{4\pi\varepsilon_0 a^2}$ (b) $\frac{q^2}{4\pi\varepsilon_0 a^2}$
(c) $\left(\frac{1+2\sqrt{2}}{2}\right)\frac{q^2}{4\pi\varepsilon_0 a^2}$ (d) $\left(2+\frac{1}{\sqrt{2}}\right)\frac{q^2}{4\pi\varepsilon_0 a^2}$

15 In figure two positive charges q_2 and q_3 fixed along the Y-axis, exert a net electric force in the + x-direction on a charge q_1 fixed along the X-axis. If a positive charge Q is added at $(x, 0)$, then the force on q_1 ***[NCERT Exemplar]***

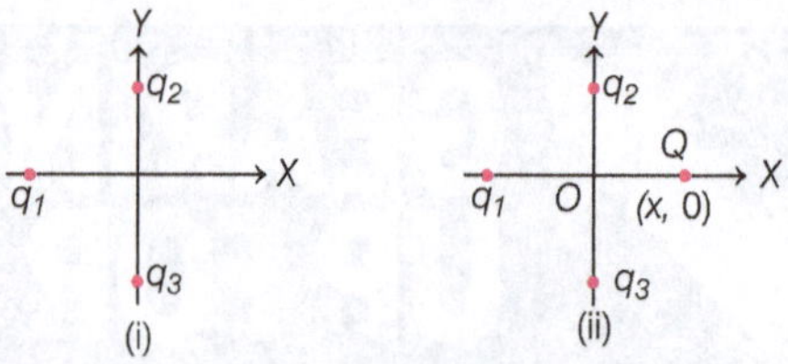

(a) shall increase along the positive X-axis.
(b) shall decrease along the positive X-axis.
(c) shall point along the negative X-axis.
(d) shall increase but the direction changes because of the intersection of Q with q_2 and q_3.

16 Two positive ions, each carrying a charge q, are separated by a distance d. If F is the force of repulsion between the ions, then the number of electrons missing from each ion will be (e being the charge on an electron)
(a) $\frac{4\pi\varepsilon_0 Fd^2}{e}$ (b) $\sqrt{\frac{4\pi\varepsilon_0 Fe^2}{d^2}}$
(c) $\sqrt{\frac{4\pi\varepsilon_0 Fd^2}{e^2}}$ (d) $\frac{4\pi\varepsilon_0 Fd^2}{e^2}$

17 Two spherical conductors B and C having equal radii and carrying equal charges on them repel each other with a force F, when kept apart at some distance. A third spherical conductor having same radius as that of B but uncharged is brought in contact with B, then brought in contact with C and finally removed away from both. The new force of repulsion between B and C is
(a) $F/4$ (b) $3F/4$
(c) $F/8$ (d) $3F/8$

18 Under the action of a given coulombic force, the acceleration of an electron is 2.5×10^{22} ms^{-2}. Then, the magnitude of the acceleration of a proton under the action of same force is nearly
(a) 1.6×10^{-19} ms^{-2} (b) 9.1×10^{31} ms^{-2}
(c) 1.4×10^{19} ms^{-2} (d) 1.6×10^{27} ms^{-2}

19 A ball with charge $-50e$ is placed at the centre of a hollow spherical shell having a charge of $-50e$. What is the charge on the shell's outer surface?
(a) $-50e$ (b) Zero
(c) $-100e$ (d) $+100e$

20 The centres of two identical small conducting spheres are 1 m apart. They carry charges of opposite kind and attract each other with a force F. When they are connected by a conducting thin wire they repel each other with a force $F/3$. What is the ratio of magnitude of charges carried by the spheres initially?
(a) 1 : 1 (b) 2 : 1
(c) 3 : 1 (d) 4 : 1

21 Two small conducting spheres of equal radius have charges $+10\,\mu C$ and $-20\,\mu C$ respectively and placed at a distance R from each other. They experience force F_1. If they are brought in contact and separated to the same distance, they experience force F_2. The ratio of F_1 to F_2 is
(a) 1 : 8 (b) −8 : 1
(c) 1 : 2 (d) −2 : 1

22 Two similar small spheres having $+q$ and $-q$ charge are kept at a certain distance. F force acts between the two. If in the middle of two spheres, another similar small sphere having $+q$ charge is kept, then it will experience a force in magnitude and direction as
(a) zero, having no direction
(b) $8F$, towards $+q$ charge
(c) $8F$, towards $-q$ charge
(d) $4F$, towards $+q$ charge

23 A conductor has been given a charge -3×10^{-7}C by transferring electron. Increase in mass (in kg) of the conductor and the number of electrons added to the conductor are respectively
(a) 2×10^{-16} and 2×10^{31} (b) 5×10^{-31} and 5×10^{19}
(c) 3×10^{-19} and 9×10^{16} (d) 2×10^{-18} and 2×10^{12}

24 Three equal charges are placed on the three corners of a square. If the force between q_1 and q_2 is F_{12} and that between q_1 and q_3 is F_{13}, then the ratio of magnitudes (F_{12}/F_{13}) is
(a) 1/2 (b) 2 (c) $1/\sqrt{2}$ (d) $\sqrt{2}$

25 Two point charges q and $2q$ are placed some distance apart. If the electric field at the location of q be E, then that at the location of $2q$ will be
(a) $3E$ (b) $E/2$
(c) E (d) None of these

26 A charge q is lying at mid-point of the line joining the two similar charges Q. The system will be in equilibrium, if the value of q is
(a) $Q/2$ (b) $-Q/2$ (c) $Q/4$ (d) $-Q/4$

27 Two small spheres of masses M_1 and M_2 are suspended by weightless insulating threads of lengths L_1 and L_2. The spheres carry charges Q_1 and Q_2, respectively. The spheres are suspended such that they are in level with one another and the threads are inclined to the vertical at angles of θ_1 and θ_2 as shown. Which one of the following conditions is essential, if $\theta_1=\theta_2$?

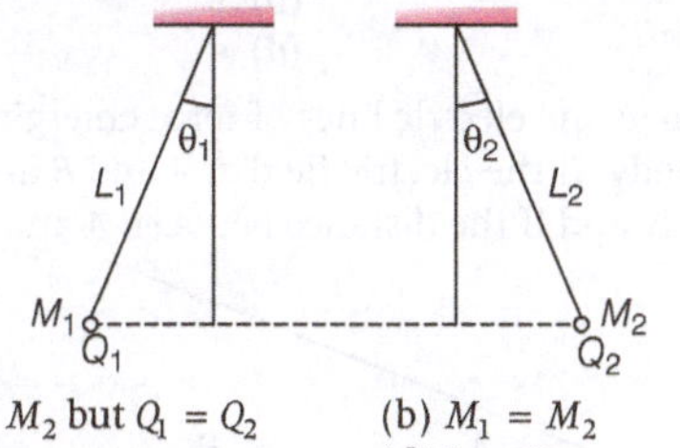

(a) $M_1\neq M_2$ but $Q_1=Q_2$ (b) $M_1=M_2$
(c) $Q_1=Q_2$ (d) $L_1=L_2$

28 Two point charges $+10^{-7}$C and -10^{-7}C are placed at A and B, 20 cm apart as shown in the figure. Calculate the electric field at C, 20 cm apart from both A and B.

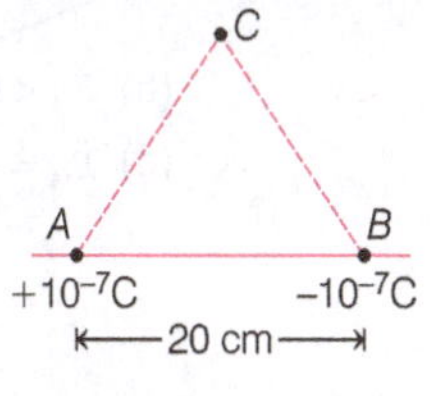

(a) 1.5×10^{-5} NC^{-1} (b) 2.2×10^{4} NC^{-1}
(c) 3.5×10^{6} NC^{-1} (d) 3.0×10^{5} NC^{-1}

29 Two point charges $q_1=2\mu$C and $q_2=1\,\mu$C are placed at distances $b=1$ cm and $a=2$ cm from the origin of the Y and X-axis as shown in figure. The electric field vector at point $P(a,b)$ will subtend an angle θ with the X-axis given by

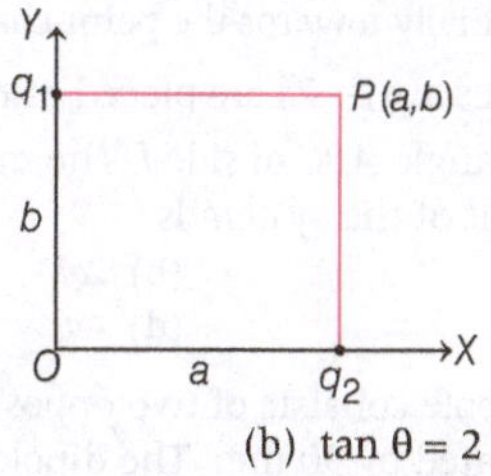

(a) $\tan\theta=1$ (b) $\tan\theta=2$
(c) $\tan\theta=3$ (d) $\tan\theta=4$

30 Three point charges as shown are placed at the vertices of an isosceles right-angled triangle. Which of the numbered vectors coincides in direction with the electric field at the mid-point M of the hypotenuse?

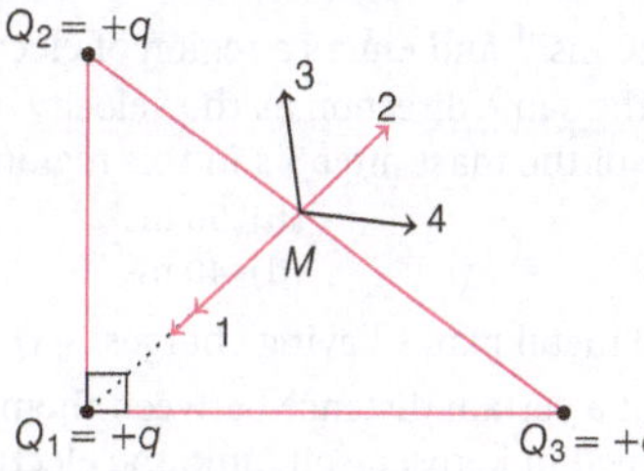

(a) 1 (b) 2
(c) 3 (d) 4

31 The figure shows the path of a positively charged particle 1 through a rectangular region of uniform electric field as shown in the figure. What is the direction of electric field and the direction of particles 2, 3 and 4?

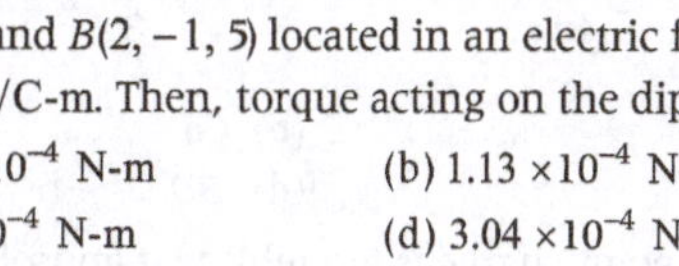

(a) Top, down, top, down
(b) Top, down, down, top
(c) Down, top, top, down
(d) Down, top, down, down

32 Two charges of $-4\,\mu$C and $+4\,\mu$C are placed at the points $A(1, 0, 4)$ and $B(2, -1, 5)$ located in an electric field $\mathbf{E}=20\hat{\mathbf{i}}$ V/C-m. Then, torque acting on the dipole will be
(a) 2.31×10^{-4} N-m (b) 1.13×10^{-4} N-m
(c) 8.0×10^{-4} N-m (d) 3.04×10^{-4} N-m

33 A drop of 10^{-6} kg water carries 10^{-6}C charge. What electric field should be applied to balance its weight? (assume, $g=10\text{ ms}^{-2}$)
(a) 10 V/m, upward (b) 10 V/m, downward
(c) 0.1 V/m, downward (d) 0.1 V/m, upward

34 A point charge $+q$ is placed at a distance d from an isolated conducting plane. The field at a point P on the other side of the plane is ***[NCERT Exemplar]***
(a) directed perpendicular to the plane and away from the plane.
(b) directed perpendicular to the plane but towards the plane.
(c) directed radially away from the point charge.
(d) directed radially towards the point charge.

35 Electric charges $q, q, -2q$ are placed at the corners of an equilateral triangle ABC of side l. The magnitude of electric dipole moment of the system is
(a) ql (b) $2ql$
(c) $\sqrt{3}ql$ (d) $4ql$

36 An electric dipole consists of two opposite charges each 0.05 μC separated by 30 mm. The dipole is placed in an uniform external electric field of 10^6 NC^{-1}. The maximum torque exerted by the field on the dipole is
(a) 6×10^{-3} Nm (b) 3×10^{-3} Nm
(c) 15×10^{-3} Nm (d) 1.5×10^{-3} Nm

37 A mass $m = 20$ g has a charge $q = 3.0$ mC. It moves with a velocity of 20 ms^{-1} and enters a region of electric field of 80 NC^{-1} in the same direction as the velocity of the mass. The velocity of the mass after 3 s in this region is
(a) 80 ms^{-1} (b) 56 ms^{-1}
(c) 44 ms^{-1} (d) 40 ms^{-1}

38 Two parallel metal plates having charges $+Q$ and $-Q$ face each other at a certain distance between them. If the plate are now dipped in kerosene oil tank, the electric field between the plates will
(a) become zero
(b) increase
(c) decrease
(d) remain same

39 q, $2q$, $3q$ and $4q$ charges are placed at the four corners A, B, C and D of a square. The field at the centre P of the square has the direction along

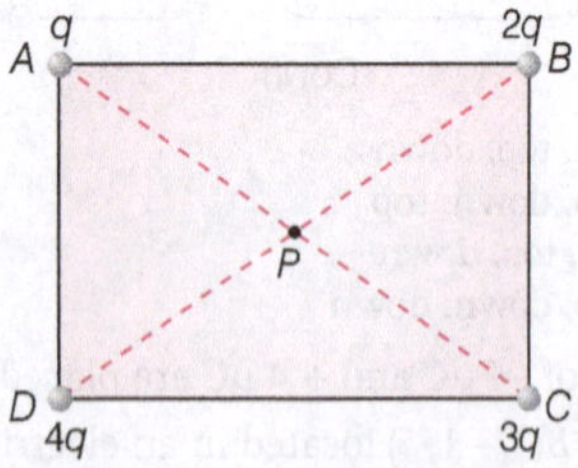

(a) AB (b) CB
(c) AC (d) BD

40 A positive point charge is brought near an isolated conducting sphere as shown in figure. The electric field is best given by ***[NCERT Exemplar]***

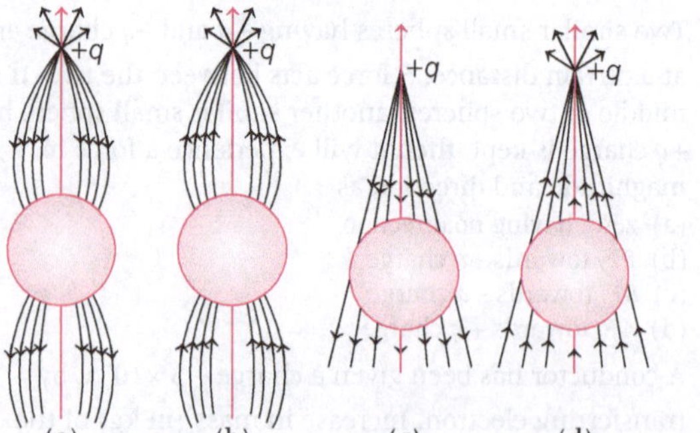

(a) (b) (c) (d)

41 What is the magnitude of a point charge due to which the electric field 30 cm away has the magnitude of 2 N/C? $[1/4\pi\varepsilon_0 = 9 \times 10^9 \text{N-m}^2/\text{C}^2]$
(a) 2×10^{-11} C (b) 3×10^{-11} C
(c) 5×10^{-11} C (d) 9×10^{-11} C

42 Two point charges of 20 μC and 80 μC are 10 cm apart. Where will the electric field strength be zero on the line joining the charges from 20 μC charge?
(a) 0.1 m (b) 0.04 m (c) 0.033 m (d) 0.33 m

43 The electric dipole of dipole moment p is placed in a uniform electric field E. Then, the
(a) torque experienced by the dipole is $E \times p$
(b) torque is zero, if p is perpendicular to E.
(c) torque is maximum, if p is perpendicular to E.
(d) potential energy is maximum, if p is parallel to E.

44 A metallic solid sphere is placed in a uniform electric field.The lines of force follow the path(s) shown in figure as

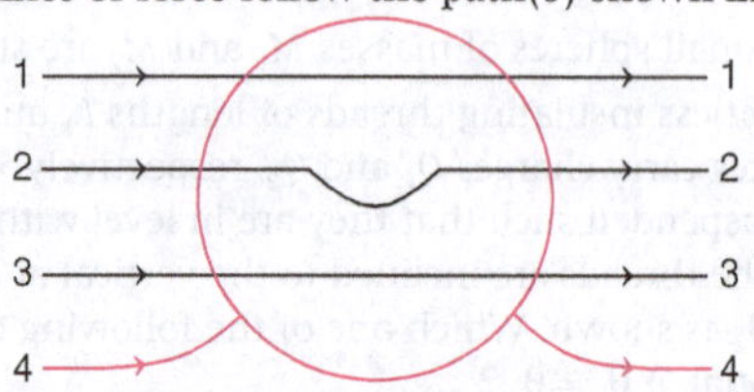

(a) 1 (b) 2
(c) 3 (d) 4

45 Figure shows the electric lines of force emerging from a charged body. If the electric field at A and B are E_A and E_B, respectively and if the distance between A and B is r, then

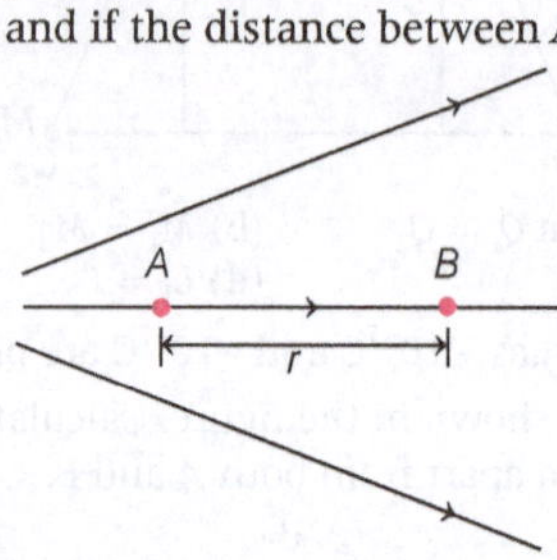

(a) $E_A > E_B$ (b) $E_A < E_B$
(c) $E_A = \dfrac{E_B}{r}$ (d) $E_A = \dfrac{E_B}{r^2}$

46 A hemisphere is uniformly charged positively. The electric field at a point on a diameter away from the centre is directed ***[NCERT Exemplar]***
(a) perpendicular to the diameter
(b) parallel to the diameter
(c) at an angle tilted towards the diameter
(d) at an angle tilted away from the diameter

47 Charge q is uniformly distributed over a thin half ring of radius R. The electric field at the centre of the ring is
(a) $\frac{q}{2\pi^2\varepsilon_0 R^2}$ (b) $\frac{q}{4\pi^2\varepsilon_0 R^2}$
(c) $\frac{q}{4\pi\varepsilon_0 R^2}$ (d) $\frac{q}{2\pi\varepsilon_0 R^2}$

48 A charge $10\,\mu C$ is placed at the centre of a hemisphere of radius $R = 10$ cm as shown. The electric flux through the hemisphere (in MKS units) is

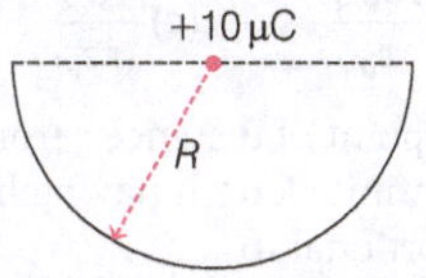

(a) 20×10^5 (b) 10×10^5 (c) 6×10^5 (d) 2×10^5

49 What is the nature of Gaussian surface involved in Gauss' law of electrostatics ?
(a) Scalar (b) Electrical
(c) Magnetic (d) Vector

50 The electric flux through the surface

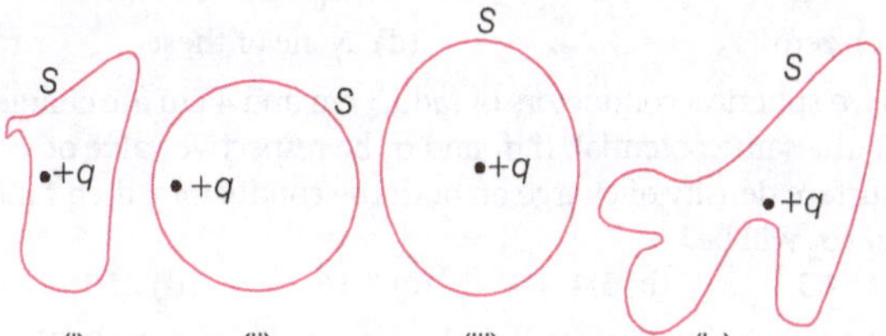

(i) (ii) (iii) (iv)

(a) in fig. (iv) is the largest.
(b) in fig. (iii) is the least.
(c) in fig. (ii) is same as fig. (iii) but is smaller than fig. (iv)
(d) is the same for all the figures.

51 If the electric field is given by $(5\hat{\mathbf{i}} + 4\hat{\mathbf{j}} + 9\hat{\mathbf{k}})$, then the electric flux through a surface of area 20 unit lying in the YZ-plane will be
(a) 100 unit (b) 80 unit
(c) 180 unit (d) 20 unit

52 The given figure shows a spherical Gaussian surface and a charge distribution. When calculating the flux of electric field through the Gaussian surface, then the electric field will be due to

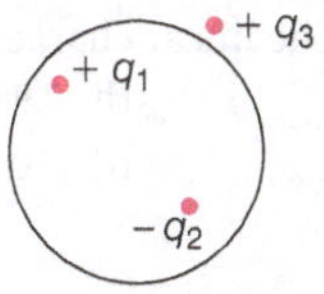

(a) $+q_3$ alone (b) $+q_1$ and $+q_3$
(c) $+q_1, +q_3$ and $-q_2$ (d) $+q_1$ and $-q_2$

53 The total electric flux emanating from a closed surface enclosing an α - particle is (e = electronic charge)
(a) $\frac{2e}{\varepsilon_0}$ (b) $\frac{e}{\varepsilon_0}$
(c) $\frac{4e}{\varepsilon_0}$ (d) $e\,\varepsilon_0$

54 A thin conducting ring of radius R is given a charge $+Q$. The electric field at the centre O of the ring due to the charge on the part AKB of the ring is E. The electric field at the centre due to the charge on the part $ACDB$ of the ring is

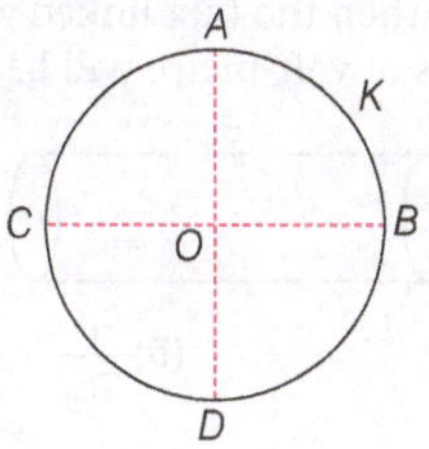

(a) E along KO
(b) $3E$ along OK
(c) $3E$ along KO
(d) E along OK

55 Two concentric conducting thin spherical shells A and B having radii r_A and r_B ($r_B > r_A$) are charged Q_A and $-Q_B$ ($|Q_B| > |Q_A|$). The electrical field along a line, (passing through the centre) is

(a)
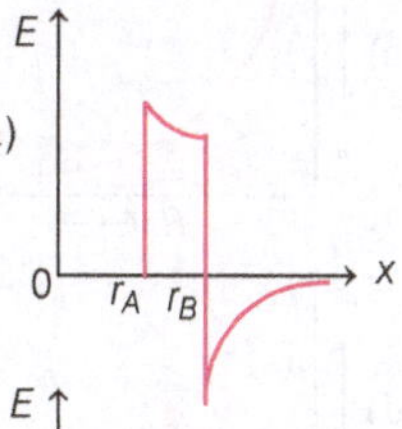

(b)
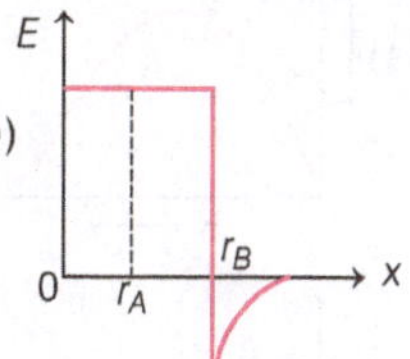

(c)
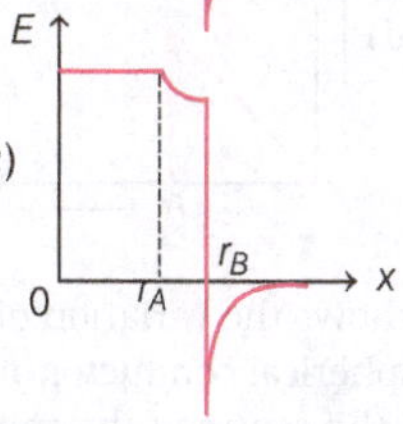

(d)
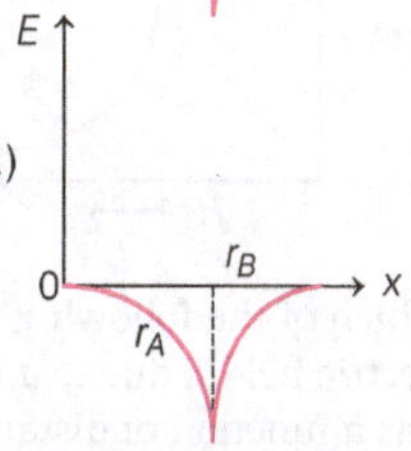

56 The adjacent diagram shows a charge $+Q$ held on an insulating support S and enclosed by a hollow spherical conductor. O represents the centre of the spherical conductor and P is a point such that $OP = x$ and $SP = r$. The electric field at point P will be

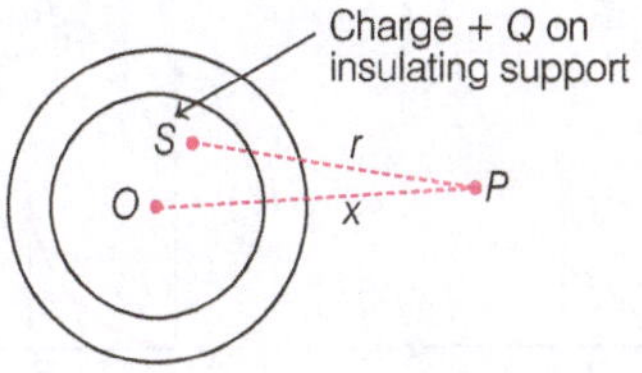

(a) $\frac{Q}{4\pi\varepsilon_0 x^2}$ (b) $\frac{Q}{4\pi\varepsilon_0 r^2}$
(c) 0 (d) None of these

57 If the electric field lines is flowing along axis of a cylinder, then the flux of this field through the cylindrical surface with the axis parallel to the field is [where r = radius of cylinder]

(a) $\frac{\sigma}{2\pi r\varepsilon_0}$ (b) $\frac{\sigma}{\varepsilon_0}$

(c) zero (d) $\frac{\sigma}{2\varepsilon_0}$

58 A hollow cylinder has a charge q coulomb within it. If ϕ is the electric flux in units of volt-metre associated with the curved surface B, then the flux linked with the plane surface A in units of volt-metre will be

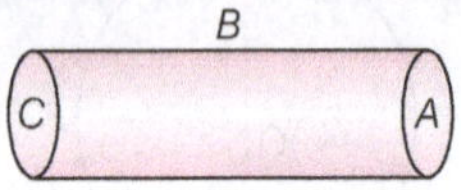

(a) $\frac{1}{2}\left(\frac{q}{\varepsilon_0}-\phi\right)$ (b) $\frac{q}{2\varepsilon_0}$

(c) $\frac{\phi}{3}$ (d) $\frac{q}{\varepsilon_0}-\phi$

59 In a uniformly charged non-conducting sphere of total charge Q and radius R, the electric field E is plotted as function of distance from the centre. The graph which would corresponds to the above will be

(a)
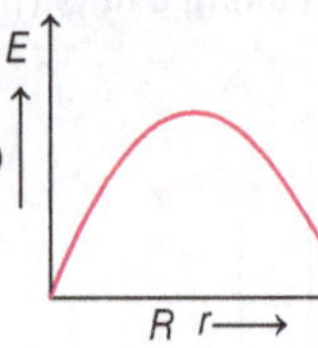

(b)
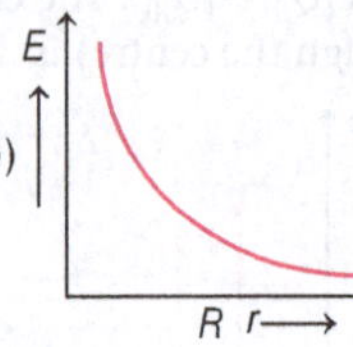

(c)
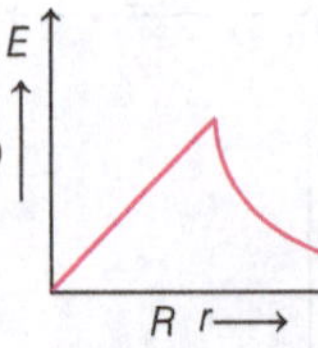

(d)
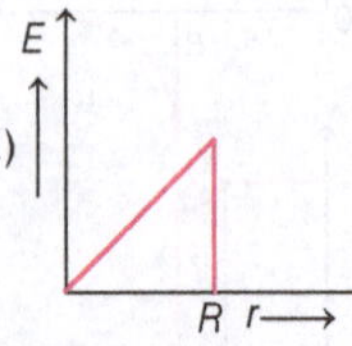

60 Which of the following graphs shows the variation of electric field E due to a hollow spherical conductor of radius R as a function of distance from the centre of the sphere?

(a)
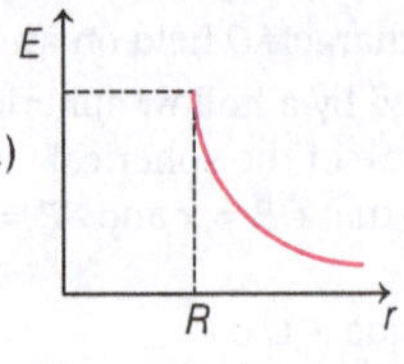

(b)
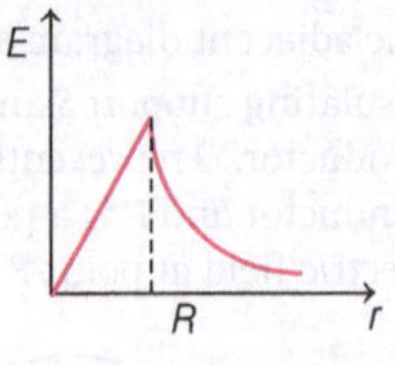

(c)
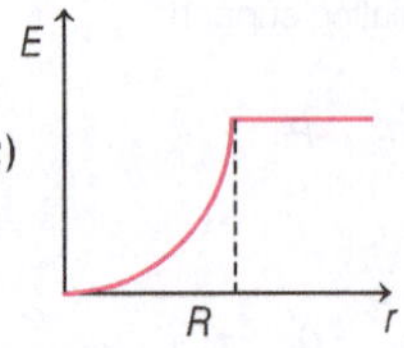

(d)
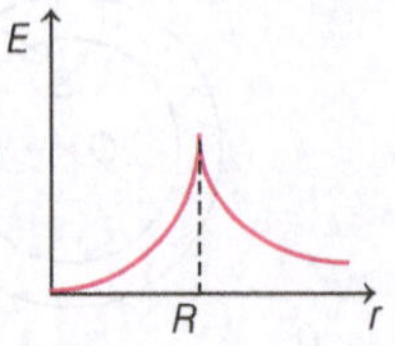

61 Electric charge is uniformly distributed along a long straight wire of radius 1 mm. The charge per centimetre length of the wire is Q coulomb. Another cylindrical surface of radius 50 cm and length 1 m symmetrically encloses the wire as shown in the figure. The total electric flux passing through the cylindrical surface is

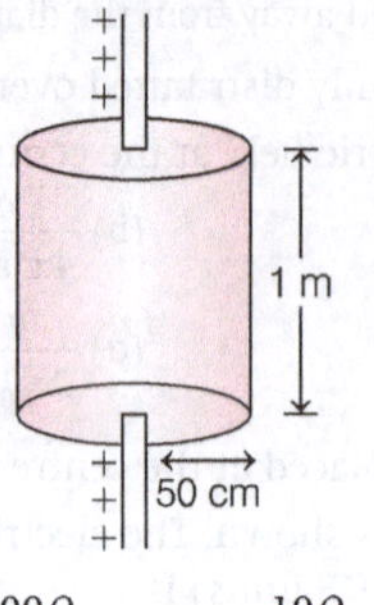

(a) $\frac{Q}{\varepsilon_0}$ (b) $\frac{100Q}{\varepsilon_0}$ (c) $\frac{10Q}{(\pi\varepsilon_0)}$ (d) $\frac{100Q}{(\pi\varepsilon_0)}$

62 Electric field at a point of distance r from a uniformly charged wire of infinite length having linear charge density λ is directly proportional to

(a) r^{-1} (b) r (c) r^2 (d) r^{-2}

63 A ring of radius R is uniformly charged. Linear charge density is λ. An imaginary sphere of radius R is drawn with its centre on circumference of ring. Total electric flux passing through the sphere would be

(a) $\frac{2\pi R\lambda}{\varepsilon_0}$ (b) $\frac{\pi R\lambda}{\varepsilon_0}$

(c) zero (d) None of these

64 Two spherical conductors of radii 3 cm and 4 cm are charged to the same potential. If σ_1 and σ_2 be respective value of surface density of charge on both the conductors, then ratio of σ_1/σ_2 will be

(a) 4/3 (b) 3/4 (c) 9/16 (d) 25/10

65 Three concentric metallic spherical shells of radii R, $2R$, $3R$ are given charges Q_1, Q_2, Q_3, respectively. It is found that the surface charge densities on the outer surfaces of the shells are equal. Then, the ratio of the charges given to the shells $Q_1 : Q_2 : Q_3$ is

(a) 1 : 2 : 3 (b) 1 : 3 : 5

(c) 1 : 4 : 9 (d) 1 : 8 : 18

66 The electric field at a distance $\frac{3R}{2}$ from the centre of a charged conducting spherical shell of radius R is E. The electric field at a distance $\frac{R}{2}$ from the centre of the sphere is

(a) zero (b) E (c) $E/2$ (d) $E/3$

67 An infinite line charge produces a field of 7.18×10^8 N/C at a distance of 2 cm. The linear charge density is

(a) 7.27×10^{-4} C/m (b) 7.98×10^{-4} C/m

(c) 7.11×10^{-4} C/m (d) 7.04×10^{-4} C/m

Assertion and Reason

Directions (Q. No. 1-8) *These questions consist of two statements each printed as Assertion (A) and Reason (R). While answering these questions you are required to choose anyone of the following four responses.*

(a) If both Assertion and Reason are true and Reason is the correct explanation of Assertion.

(b) If both Assertion and Reason are true but Reason is not the correct explanation of Assertion.

(c) If Assertion is true but Reason is false.

(d) If Assertion is false but Reason is true.

1 **Assertion** (A) Due to two point charges, electric field cannot be zero at two points.

Reason (R) Electric field is a vector quantity.

2 **Assertion** (A) Electric lines of forces cross each other.
Reason (R) Electric field at a point gives one direction.

3 **Assertion** (A) If a dipole is enclosed by a surface, then according to Gauss' law, electric flux linked with it will be zero.

Reason (R) The net charge enclosed by the surface is zero.

4 **Assertion** (A) A uniformly charged disc has a pin hole at its centre. The electric field at the centre of the disc is zero.

Reason (R) Disc can be supposed to be made up of many rings. Also, electric field at the centre of uniformly charged ring is zero.

5 **Assertion** (A) In a uniform electric field, electrons move in the opposite direction of electric field.
Reason (R) This is because of the negative charge of an electron.

6 **Assertion** (A) In a region, where uniform electric field exists, the net charge within volume of any size is zero.

Reason (R) The electric flux within any closed surface in region of uniform electric field is zero.

7 **Assertion** (A) Total flux through a closed surface is zero, if no charge is enclosed by the surface.

Reason (R) Gauss' law is true for any closed surface, no matter what its shape or size is.

8 **Assertion** (A) The surface charge densities of two spherical conductors of different radii are equal. Then, the electric field intensities near their surface are also equal.

Reason (R) Surface charge density is equal to charge per unit area.

Statement Type Questions

Directions (Q.No. 1-8) *In the following questions Statement I and Statement II are given. Read these statements and choose the most appropriate answer from the options given below.*

(a) Both Statement I and Statement II are incorrect.

(b) Statement I is correct but Statement II is incorrect.

(c) Statement I is incorrect but Statement II is correct.

(d) Both Statement I and Statement II are correct.

1 **Statement I** A system contains two point charges q_1 and q_2, the total charge of the system is obtained simply by adding algebraically q_1 and q_2.

Statement II All free charges are integral multiples of a basic unit charge.

2 **Statement I** When the medium between two charges is replaced by another medium with a higher dielectric constant, the electric force between them decreases.

Statement II Electric dipole moment varies inversely to the dielectric constant.

3 **Statement I** A point charge is brought in an electric field. The field at a nearby point is increase, whatever be the nature of the charge.
Statement II The electric field is independent of the nature of charge.

4 **Statement I** When a dipole is placed at an angle from the direction of a uniform electric field, then it experiences torque.

Statement II When electric dipole is parallel at anti-parallel to the electric field then net torque is non-zero.

5 **Statement I** Torque on a dipole in a field is maximum when they are perpendicular to each other.
Statement II Electric field of an infinite plane sheet of charge is directly proportional to surface charge density.

6 **Statement I** Electric lines of field cross each other.

Statement II Electric field at a point superimpose to give one resultant electric field.

7 **Statement I** Three point charges Q_1, Q_2 and Q_3 are shown in the figure . The flux over the Gaussian surface depends on only one charge point.

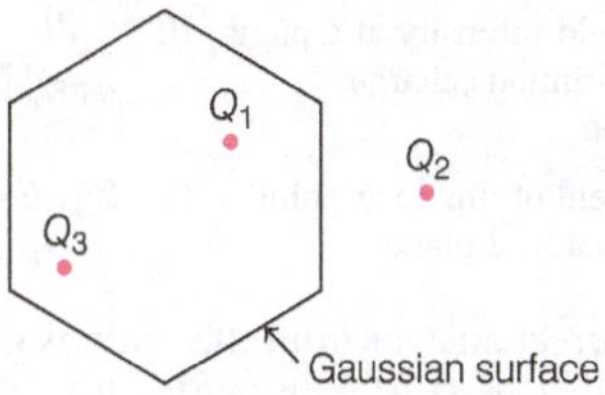

Statement II Electric flux depends on the all charge near by.

8 **Statement I** A point charge is lying at the centre of a cube of each side. The electric flux emanating from each surface of the cube is $\frac{1}{6}$th of the total flux.

Statement II According to Gauss' theorem, total electric flux through a closed surface enclosing a charge is equal to $\frac{1}{\varepsilon_0}$ times the magnitude of the charge enclosed.

Match the Columns

1 Match the field lines given in Column I with the charge configuration due to which field lines exist in Column II.

Column I	Column II
A. 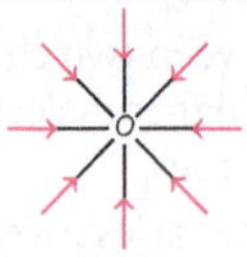	I A pair of equal and opposite charges
B. 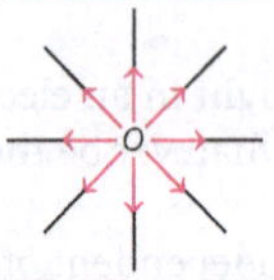	II A pair of positive charges
C. 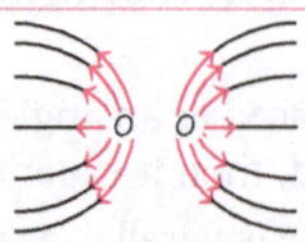	III A single positive charge
D. 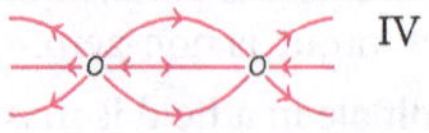	IV A single negative charge.

Choose the correct answer from the options given below.
(a) A-IV, B-II, C-III, D-I (b) A-I , B-II, C-III, D-IV
(c) A-IV, B-III, C-II, D-I (d) A-I, B-IV, C-III, D-II

2 Match the following in Column I with Column II.

Column I	Column II
A. Torque on a dipole in uniform electric field	I $\frac{1}{4\pi\varepsilon_0}\int\frac{dq}{r^2}$
B. Electric field of a dipole at a point on the dipole axis	II $\frac{p}{4\pi\varepsilon_0 r^3}$
C. Electric field intensity at a point due to continuous charge distribution	III $\frac{2p}{4\pi\varepsilon_0 r^3}$
D. Electric field of dipole at point on the equatorial plane	IV $2qaE\sin\theta$

Choose the correct answer from the options given below.
(a) A-IV , B-II, C-I, D-III (b) A-IV, B-I, C-II, D-III
(c) A-IV, B-III, C-I, D-II (d) A-II , B-II, C-III, D-IV

3 Match the following two columns and choose the option from codes given below.

Column I	Column II
A. Electric charge	I $[M^{-1}L^{-3}T^4A^2]$
B. Electric field strength	II $[MLT^{-3}A^{-1}]$
C. Absolute permittivity	III $[M^0LTA]$
D. Electric dipole	IV None

Choose the correct answer from the options given below.
(a) A-IV , B-II, C-I, D-III
(b) A-I , B-II, C-III, D-IV
(c) A-II, B-III, C-I, D-IV
(d) A-IV, B-II, C-III, D-IV

4 Match Column I with their respective formula in Column II.

Column I	Column II
A. Electric field outside the spherical shell	I $E\Delta S\cos\theta$
B. Quantity of heat	II 0
C. Electric flux through an area element	III $\frac{q}{4\pi\varepsilon_0 r^2}\hat{\mathbf{r}}$
D. Electric field inside the spherical shell	IV Charge

Choose the correct answer form the options given below.
(a) A-II, B-IV, C-I, D-III (b) A-III , B-IV, C-I, D-II
(c) A-I , B-IV, C-III, D-II (d) A-II , B-III, C-I, D-II

5 Match the following quantities in Column I with Column II

Column I	Column II
A. Infinite sheet of charge	I $E\propto\frac{1}{r^2}$
B. Infinite line charge	II $E\propto\frac{1}{r}$
C. Electric dipole	III $E=\text{constant}$
D. Point charge	IV $E\propto\frac{1}{r^3}$

Choose the correct answer form the options given below.
(a) A-II , B-III, C-I, D-IV (b) A-III , B-II, C-IV, D-I
(c) A-IV , B-I, C-III, D-II (d) A-II , B-I, C-IV, D-III

6 Four metallic plates are charged as shown in figure below, match the following two columns. Then, choose the option from codes given below.

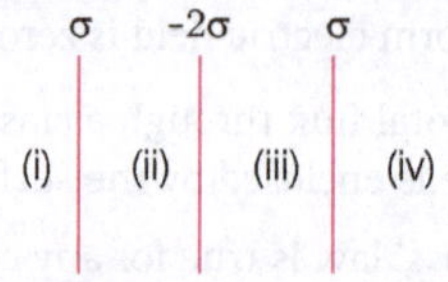

Column I	Column II
A. Electric field in region-I	I $\frac{\sigma}{\varepsilon_0}$
B. Electric field in region-II	II $\frac{-\sigma}{\varepsilon_0}$
C. Electric field in region - III	III $\frac{\sigma}{2\varepsilon_0}$
D. Electric field in region-IV	IV Zero

Choose the correct answer form the options given below.
(a) A-I , B-IV, C-II, D-III (b) A-IV , B-I, C-II, D-IV
(c) A-III , B-II, C-I, D-I (d) A-IV , B-IV, C-I, D-II

Final Check Through PYQs

Module-I Electric Charges and Coulomb's Law

1 The acceleration of an electron due to the mutual attraction between the electron and a proton when they are 1.6 Å apart is, $(m_e \simeq 9 \times 10^{-31}$ kg, $e = 1.6 \times 10^{-19}$C)

$$\left(\text{Take, } \frac{1}{4\pi\varepsilon_0} = 9 \times 10^9 \text{ Nm}^2\text{C}^{-2}\right)$$

[NCERT (New) Pg. 8, NEET (Oct.) 2020]

(a) 10^{24} m/s^2
(b) 10^{23} m/s^2
(c) 10^{22} m/s^2
(d) 10^{25} m/s^2

2 Two point charges A and B, having charges $+Q$ and $-Q$ respectively, are placed at certain distance apart and force acting between them is F. If 25% charge of A is transferred to B, then force between the charges becomes ***[NCERT (New) Pg. 8, NEET (National) 2019]***

(a) $\frac{9F}{16}$ (b) $\frac{16F}{9}$
(c) $\frac{4F}{3}$ (d) F

3 Suppose the charge of a proton and an electron differ slightly. One of them is $-e$ and the other is $(e + \Delta e)$. If the net of electrostatic force and gravitational force between two hydrogen atoms placed at a distance d (much greater than atomic size) apart is zero, then Δe is of the order [Given mass of hydrogen, $m_h = 1.67 \times 10^{-27}$ kg] ***[NCERT (New) Pg. 8, NEET 2017]***

(a) 10^{-20} C (b) 10^{-23} C
(c) 10^{-37} C (d) 10^{-47} C

4 Two identical charged spheres suspended from a common point by two massless strings of lengths l, are initially at a distance d $(d << l)$ apart because of their mutual repulsion. The charges begin to leak from both the spheres at a constant rate. As a result, the spheres approach each other with a velocity v. Then, v varies as a function of the distance x between the sphere, as ***[NCERT (New) Pg. 8, NEET 2016]***

(a) $v \propto x$ (b) $v \propto x^{-1/2}$
(c) $v \propto x^{-1}$ (d) $v \propto x^{1/2}$

Module-II Electric Field and Electric Dipole

5 An electric dipole is placed at an angle of 30° with an electric field of intensity 2×10^5 NC^{-1}. It experiences a torque equal to 4 N m. Calculate the magnitude of charge on the dipole, if the dipole length is 2 cm. ***[NCERT (New) Pg. 27, NEET 2023, 2016]***

(a) 6 mC (b) 4 mC (c) 2 mC (d) 8 mC

6 Two point charges $-q$ and $+q$ are placed at a distance of L, as shown in the figure.

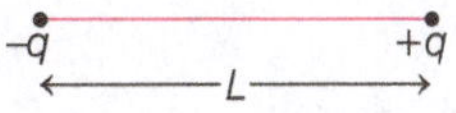

The magnitude of electric field intensity at a distance $R(R >> L)$ varies as ***[NCERT (New) Pg. 24, NEET 2022]***

(a) $\frac{1}{R^3}$ (b) $\frac{1}{R^4}$ (c) $\frac{1}{R^6}$ (d) $\frac{1}{R^2}$

7 A dipole is placed in an electric field as shown. In which direction will it move? ***[NNCERT (New) Pg. 23, NEET 2021]***

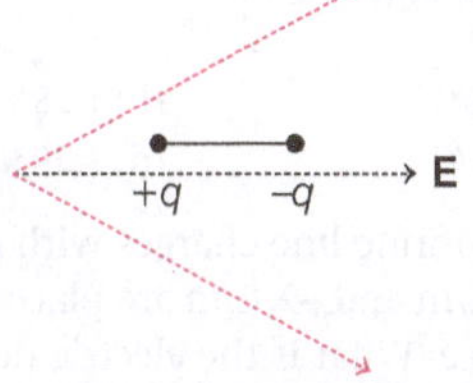

(a) Towards the left as its potential energy will increase
(b) Towards the right as its potential energy will decrease
(c) Towards the left as its potential energy will decrease
(d) Towards the right as its potential energy will increase

8 Polar molecules are the molecules ***[NCERT (New) Pg. 23, NEET 2021]***

(a) having zero dipole moment
(b) acquire a dipole moment only in the presence of electric field due to displacement of charges.
(c) acquire a dipole moment only when magnetic field is absent
(d) having a permanent electric dipole moment

9 The electric field at a point on the equatorial plane at a distance r from the centre of a dipole having dipole moment P is given by ($r >>$ separation of two charges forming the dipole, ε_0 = permittivity of free space)
[NCERT (New) Pg. 24, NEET (Oct.) 2020]

(a) $E = \frac{\mathbf{p}}{4\pi\varepsilon_0 r^3}$

(b) $E = \frac{2\mathbf{p}}{4\pi\varepsilon_0 r^3}$

(c) $E = -\frac{\mathbf{p}}{4\pi\varepsilon_0 r^2}$

(d) $E = -\frac{\mathbf{p}}{4\pi\varepsilon_0 r^3}$

10 An electron falls from rest through a vertical distance h in a uniform and vertically upward directed electric field E. The direction of electric field is now reversed, keeping its magnitude the same. A proton is allowed to fall from rest in it through the same vertical distance h. The time of fall of the electron, in comparison to the time of fall of the proton is
[NCERT (New) Pg. 14, NEET 2018]

(a) 10 times greater
(b) 5 times greater
(c) smaller
(d) equal

Module-III Electric Flux and Gauss's Law

11 If $\oint \mathbf{E} \cdot d\mathbf{S} = 0$ over a surface, then
[NCERT (New) Pg. 28, NEET 2023]

(a) the magnitude of electric field on the surface is constant.
(b) all the charges must necessarily be inside the surface.
(c) the electric field inside the surface is necessarily uniform.
(d) the number of flux lines entering the surface must be equal to the number of flux lines leaving it.

12 A sphere encloses an electric dipole with charge $\pm 3 \times 10^{-6}$ C. What is the total electric flux across the sphere? *[NCERT (New) Pg. 28, NEET (Odisha) 2019]*

(a) -3×10^{-6} N-m^2/C
(b) zero
(c) 3×10^{6} N-m^2/C
(d) 6×10^{-6} N-m^2/C

Module-IV Applications of Gauss' Law

13 A spherical conductor of radius 10 cm has a charge of 3.2×10^{-7} C distributed uniformly. What is the magnitude of electric field at a point 15 cm from the centre of the sphere?
[NCERT (New) Pg. 28, NEET (Sep.) 2020]

$\left(\frac{1}{4\pi\varepsilon_0} = 9 \times 10^9 \text{ Nm}^2/\text{C}^2\right)$

(a) 1.28×10^5 N/C
(b) 1.28×10^6 N/C
(c) 1.28×10^7 N/C
(d) 1.28×10^4 N/C

14 Two parallel infinite line charges with linear charge densities $+\lambda$ C/m and $-\lambda$ C/m are placed at a distance of $2R$ in free space. What is the electric field mid-way between the two line charges?
[NCERT (New) Pg. 28, NEET (National) 2019]

(a) $\frac{2\lambda}{\pi\varepsilon_0 R}$ N/C
(b) $\frac{\lambda}{\pi\varepsilon_0 R}$ N/C
(c) $\frac{\lambda}{2\pi\varepsilon_0 R}$ N/C
(d) Zero

15 A hollow metal sphere of radius R is uniformly charged.The electric field due to the sphere at a distance r from the centre
[NCERT (New) Pg. 28, NEET (National) 2019]

(a) zero as r increases for $r < R$, decreases as r increases for $r > R$
(b) zero as r increases for $r < R$, increases as r increases for $r > R$
(c) decreases as r increases for $r < R$ and for $r > R$
(d) increases as r increases for $r < R$ and for $r > R$

16 The electric field in a certain region is acting radially outward and is given by $E = Ar$. A charge contained in a sphere of radius a centred at the origin of the field will be given by *[NCERT (New) Pg. 28, AIPMT 2015]*

(a) $4\pi\varepsilon_0 Aa^2$
(b) $A\varepsilon_0 a^2$
(c) $4\pi\varepsilon_0 Aa^3$
(d) $\varepsilon_0 Aa^3$

Answers

Step up Practice 1

1 (d)	2 (a)	3 (d)	4 (c)	5 (c)	6 (d)	7 (a)	8 (b)	9 (b)	10 (a)
11 (d)	12 (d)	13 (c)	14 (d)	15 (d)	16 (c)	17 (b)	18 (d)	19 (a)	20 (c)
21 (c)									

Step up Practice 2

1 (b)	2 (c)	3 (d)	4 (a)	5 (a)	6 (c)	7 (d)	8 (b)	9 (b)	10 (c)
11 (c)	12 (a)	13 (b)	14 (c)	15 (c)	16 (a)	17 (c)	18 (b)	19 (c)	20 (c)
21 (b)	22 (b)	23 (b)	24 (c)	25 (b)	26 (a)	27 (d)	28 (d)	29 (d)	30 (a)
31 (a)	32 (c)								

Step up Practice 3

1 (d)	2 (a)	3 (d)	4 (c)	5 (d)	6 (a)	7 (a)	8 (b)	9 (c)	10 (a)
11 (d)	12 (d)	13 (c)	14 (d)	15 (b)	16 (c)	17 (c)	18 (d)	19 (d)	20 (d)
21 (d)	22 (d)	23 (b)	24 (d)	25 (a)					

Step up Practice 4

1 (b)	2 (b)	3 (a)	4 (c)	5 (a)	6 (a)	7 (b)	8 (c)	9 (a)	10 (c)
11 (d)	12 (a)	13 (c)	14 (d)	15 (b)	16 (a)	17 (b)	18 (b)	19 (a)	20 (c)
21 (d)	22 (c)	23 (c)	24 (a)	25 (b)	26 (b)	27 (a)	28 (b)		

Gearing up for NEET

1 (a)	2 (a)	3 (a)	4 (b)	5 (a)	6 (a)	7 (c)	8 (a)	9 (b)	10 (c)
11 (a)	12 (b)	13 (b)	14 (c)	15 (a)	16 (c)	17 (d)	18 (c)	19 (c)	20 (c)
21 (b)	22 (c)	23 (d)	24 (b)	25 (b)	26 (d)	27 (b)	28 (b)	29 (b)	30 (b)
31 (a)	32 (b)	33 (a)	34 (a)	35 (c)	36 (d)	37 (b)	38 (c)	39 (b)	40 (a)
41 (a)	42 (c)	43 (c)	44 (d)	45 (a)	46 (a)	47 (a)	48 (c)	49 (d)	50 (d)
51 (a)	52 (c)	53 (a)	54 (d)	55 (a)	56 (a)	57 (c)	58 (a)	59 (c)	60 (a)
61 (b)	62 (a)	63 (d)	64 (a)	65 (b)	66 (a)	67 (b)			

Assertion and Reason

1 (a)	2 (d)	3 (a)	4 (a)	5 (a)	6 (a)	7 (b)	8 (b)

Statement Type Questions

1 (d)	2 (b)	3 (a)	4 (b)	5 (d)	6 (a)	7 (a)	8 (d)

Match the Columns

1 (c)	2 (c)	3 (a)	4 (b)	5 (b)	6 (b)

Final Check Through PYQs Module I

1 (c)	2 (a)	3 (c)	4 (b)

Final Check Through PYQs Module II

5 (c)	6 (a)	7 (b)	8 (d)	9 (d)	10 (c)

Final Check Through PYQs Module III

11 (d)	12 (b)

Final Check Through PYQs Module IV

13 (a)	14 (b)	15 (a)	16 (c)

Hints and Solutions

Step up Practice 1

5. (*c*) Normally similar charges repel each other.

If one charge is much greater than another and both charged bodies are placed near to each other, then induced charge on body with smaller charge will have higher (and opposite) induced charge resulting attraction between both bodies.

18. (*d*) During process

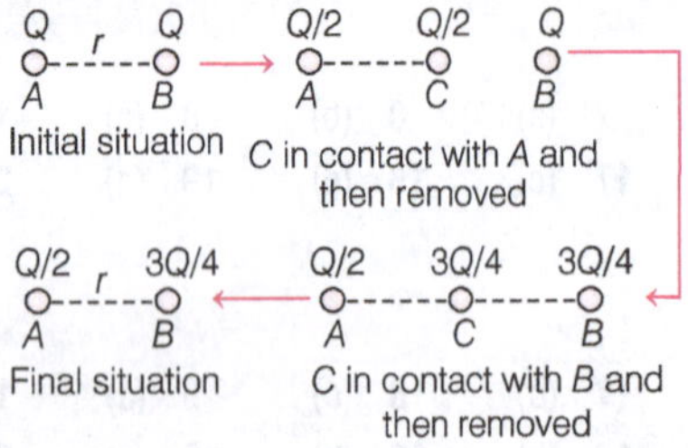

$$F_{\text{initial}} = F = \frac{KQ^2}{r^2}$$

$$F_{\text{new}} = \frac{K(Q/2)(3Q/4)}{r^2} = \frac{3}{8}\frac{KQ^2}{r^2} = \frac{3}{8}F$$

19. (*a*) For dissimilar charges

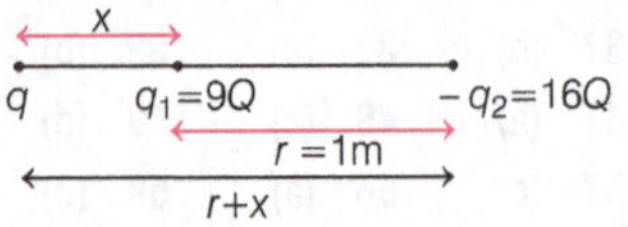

$$x = \left(\frac{\sqrt{q_1}}{\sqrt{q_2} - \sqrt{q_1}}\right) r = \left(\frac{\sqrt{9Q}}{\sqrt{16Q} - \sqrt{9Q}}\right) \times 1$$

$$= \frac{3}{4-3} \times 1 = 3 \text{ m leftwards from } 9Q \text{ charge.}$$

20. (*c*) Charge $-q$ is under equilibrium at given situation. This equilibrium is stable under displacement in vertical (*C-D*) direction as it will tend to reach again at its current position due to attraction of positive charges.

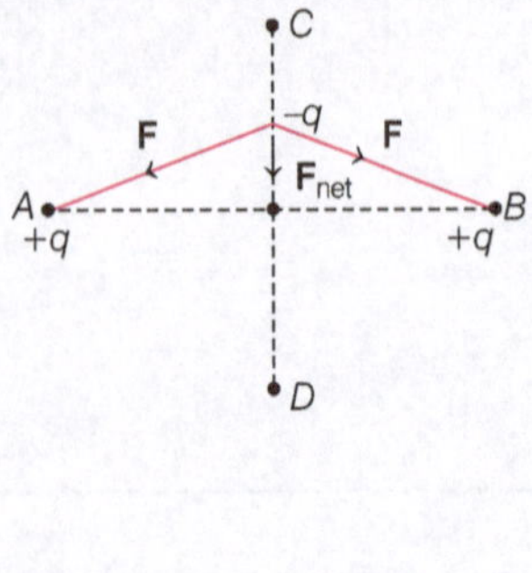

Hence, it should be displaced either towards *C* or towards *D*.

21. (*c*) A → III, B → II, C → IV, D → I

Step up Practice 2

1. (*b*) Given, charge $(Q) = 5\,\mu\text{C}$

Distance separation $(r) = 80 \times 10^{-2} = 8 \times 10^{-1}$ m

Electric field due to a point charge is given as

$$E = \frac{kQ}{r^2}$$

Thus, $E = \dfrac{9 \times 10^9 \times 5 \times 10^{-6}}{(8 \times 10^{-1})^2}$

$$= \frac{45 \times 10^3}{64 \times 10^{-2}} = 0.703 \times 10^5$$

$$E = 7 \times 10^4 \text{ NC}^{-1}$$

2. (*c*) The electric field strength is determined by the density of field lines, the more lines per unit area, stronger the electric field. Therefore, Statement I is incorrect but Statement II is correct.

3. (*d*) Here, $E = 500 \text{ NC}^{-1}$

distance $(r) = 3$ m

Thus, $E = 9 \times 10^9 \times \dfrac{Q}{r^2}$

$\Rightarrow \quad 500 = 9 \times 10^9 \times \dfrac{Q}{(3)^2}$

$\Rightarrow \quad Q = 0.5\,\mu\text{C}$

4. (*a*) For electric dipole, the field falls as cube of distance from the centre of dipole. But for point charge, it falls as square of distance. So, both Statement I and Statement II are incorrect.

5. (*a*) Given, $q_1 = 10\,\mu\text{C}$ and $q_2 = 5\,\mu\text{C}$

Let the electric field at point *P* due to q_1 is

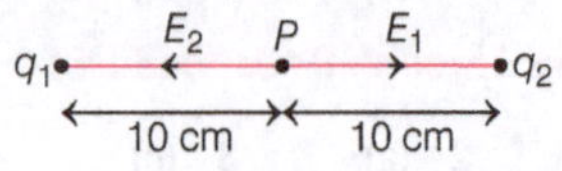

E_1 is due to q_1 and due to q_2 is E_2

$$E_P = \frac{9 \times 10^9}{(0.1)^2}(10 - 5) \times 10^{-6}$$

$$= 4.5 \times 10^6 \text{ N/C}$$

as $\quad E_1 > E_2$

Electric field is directed toward $+5\,\mu\text{C}$

6. (c) Here, resultant intensity = 0

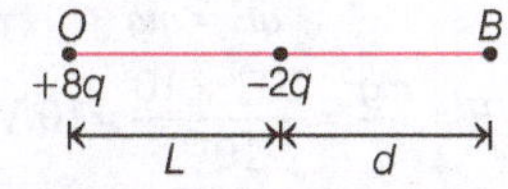

$$\because \quad \frac{1}{4\pi\varepsilon_0}\frac{8q}{(L+d)^2} - \frac{1}{4\pi\varepsilon_0}\frac{2q}{d^2} = 0$$

or $\quad (L+d)^2 = 4d^2$ or $d = L$

$\therefore$ Distance from origin = $2L$

7. (d) The electric field at the centre of the cube, due to the eight charges, gets cancelled. This is because the charges are distributed symmetrically with respect to the centre of the cube. Hence, the electric field is zero at the centre.

8. (b) In Figs. (1), (3) and (4), net electric field is zero because electric field at a point due to positive charge acts away from the charge and due to negative charge, it acts towards the charge so for Fig. (2), net electric field is not zero.

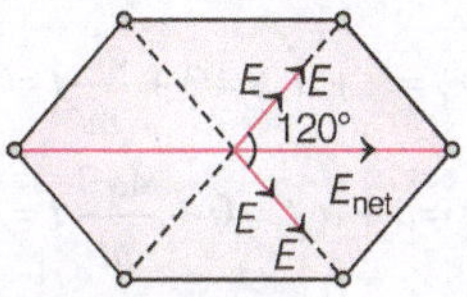

Here, net electric field in Fig. (2) is

$$= \sqrt{(2E)^2 + (2E)^2 + (2E)(2E)\cdot 2\cos 120^\circ} = 2E$$

which is not zero.

9. (b) Given,

Mass of electron, $m = 9.1\times 10^{-31}$ kg

Intensity of electric field, $E = 9.1\times 10^{6}$ N/C

From, Newton's second law of motion.

$$F = ma \quad \text{...(i)}$$

the force on a charge exerted by an electric field is given as

$$F = q_0 E \quad \text{...(ii)}$$

where, E is the intensity of the field and q_0 is the charge of the body

By modifying first equation,

$$a = \frac{F}{m} \quad \text{...(iii)}$$

Substituting the value of F in the Eq. (iii) from Eq. (ii), we get

$$a = \frac{q_e E}{m}$$

$$\Rightarrow \quad a = \frac{(9.1\times 10^{6})(1.6\times 10^{-19})}{9.1\times 10^{-31}}$$

[$\because$ charge of electron $= 1.6\times 10^{18}$ m/s^2]

$$\therefore \quad a = 1.6\times 10^{18} \text{ m/s}^2$$

10. (c) A force produced because of the electric field

$$F = qE$$

$$a = \frac{qE}{m}$$

Particle starts from rest and acceleration is constantly applying in the equation of motion

$$v = u + at$$

$$v = 0 + \frac{qEt}{m}$$

$$v = \frac{qEt}{m}$$

Now, $\quad \text{KE} = \frac{1}{2}mv^2 = \frac{1}{2}m\left(\frac{qEt}{m}\right)^2 = \frac{q^2E^2t^2}{2m}$

11. (c) When charge enters the electric field perpendicularly, it follow a parabolic path.

12. (a) Given, $g = 10$ m/s^2

Charge of an electron, $q = -1.6\times 10^{-19}$ C

mass of an electron, $m = 9.11\times 10^{-31}$ kg

As we know, $\quad E = \frac{(mg)}{q} = \frac{9.11\times 10^{-31}\times 10}{1.6\times 10^{-19}}$

$$E = 5.69\times 10^{-11} \text{ N/C}$$

So, the magnitude of the electric field is approximately 5.69×10^{-11} N/C.

Since the electric field oppose the gravitational force. Therefore, the direction of the electric field will be opposite to the direction of the gravitational field, which is upwards.

13. (b) Left hand side of A

(i) For the unlike charges, the electric field is zero outside of the smaller magnitude charge.

(ii) For like charge, the electric field will be zero closer to the smaller charge and will be along the line joining the two charges.

(iii) For opposite charges of equal magnitude, there will not be any zero electric fields.

14. (c) **Case I**

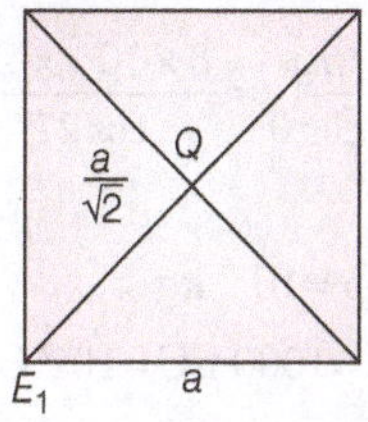

$$E_{\text{at corner}} = \frac{1}{4\pi\varepsilon_0}\frac{Q}{\left(\frac{a}{\sqrt{2}}\right)^2}$$

$$E_1 = \frac{1}{4\pi\varepsilon_0}\frac{2Q}{a^2}$$

Case II

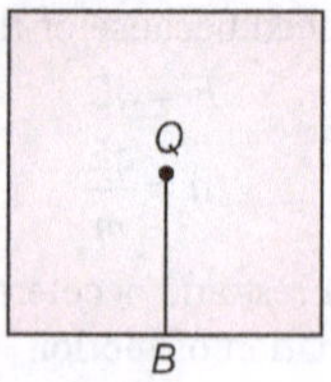

$$E_B = \frac{1}{4\pi\varepsilon_0} \frac{Q}{\left(\frac{a}{2}\right)^2}$$

$$\Rightarrow \quad E_2 = \frac{1}{4\pi\varepsilon_0} \frac{4Q}{a^2}$$

$$\therefore \quad \frac{E_1}{E_2} = \frac{\left(\frac{1}{4\pi\varepsilon_0} \frac{2Q}{a^2}\right)}{\left(\frac{1}{4\pi\varepsilon_0} \frac{4Q}{a^2}\right)} = \frac{1}{2}$$

15. (*c*) From the given data

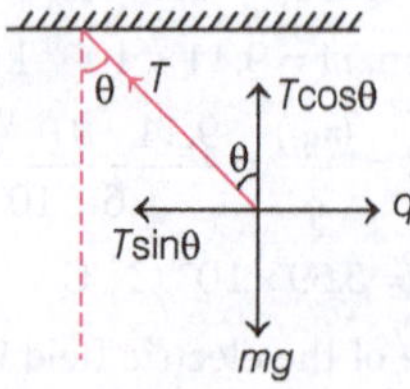

$$E = 20000 \text{ V/m} = 20 \times 10^3 \text{ V/m}$$

$$m = 80 \times 10^{-5} \text{ kg}$$

$$q = 2 \times 10^{-8} \text{ C}$$

$$\tan\theta = \left(\frac{qE}{mg}\right) \qquad [T\cos\theta = mg,\ T\sin\theta = qE]$$

$$\tan\theta = \frac{20 \times 10^3 \times 2 \times 10^{-8}}{8 \times 10^{-5} \times 9.8}$$

$$\tan\theta = \frac{40}{8 \times 9.8} = 0.51$$

$$\theta = 27^\circ$$

From equation,

$$T = \frac{mg}{\cos\theta} = \frac{8 \times 10^{-5} \times 9.8}{\cos 27^\circ} = 8.8 \times 10^{-4} \text{ N}$$

16. (*a*) Given,

mass of water drop $= 10^{-6}$ kg

electric charge $(q) = 1000 \text{ nC} = 10^{-6}$ C

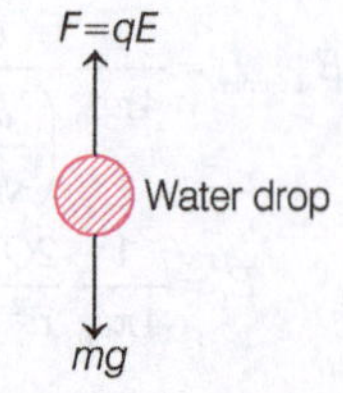

$$\because \quad F = mg$$

$$\Rightarrow \quad qE = mg$$

$$\Rightarrow \quad E = \frac{mg}{q} = \frac{10^{-6} \times 10}{10^{-6}} = 10 \text{ V/m},$$

upward because charge is positive.

17. (*c*)

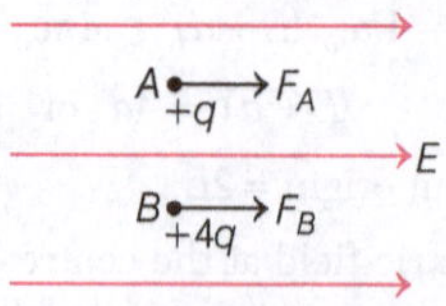

Electric force on a charge particle placed in electric field.

$$F = qE$$

$$\Rightarrow \quad F_A = qE$$

$$\Rightarrow \quad a_A = \frac{F_A}{m_A} = \frac{qE}{m}$$

$$\Rightarrow \quad F_B = 4qE$$

$$\Rightarrow \quad a_B = \frac{F_B}{m_B} = \frac{4qE}{m}$$

$$\Rightarrow \quad v_A = u + a_A t = 0 + \frac{qE}{m} t = \frac{qE}{m} t$$

$$\Rightarrow \quad v_B = u + a_B t = 0 + \frac{4qE}{m} t = \frac{4qE}{m} t$$

$$\therefore \quad \frac{v_A}{v_B} = \frac{1}{4} \text{ or } 1:4$$

18. (*b*) As we know,

Time period of the pendulum, $T = 2\pi\sqrt{\frac{l}{g_{\text{eff}}}}$

Since the pendulum is positively charged and the electric field is in the upward direction.

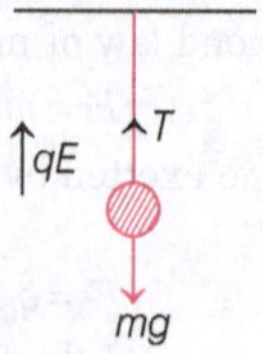

So, now in electric field

Time period of pendulum

$$T' = 2\pi\sqrt{\frac{l}{g\left(1 - \frac{qE}{mg}\right)}} \qquad \left[\because g_{\text{eff}} = \left(g - \frac{qE}{m}\right)\right]$$

Therefore, we can say that time period of pendulum is increase in presence of electric field.

19. (*c*) At points *A* and *C*, electric field lines are equally spaced and dense that's why $E_A = E_C > E_B$

20. (*c*) Torque on an electric dipole in an electric field,

$$\boldsymbol{\tau} = \mathbf{p} \times \mathbf{E}$$

$$\Rightarrow \quad |\tau| = pE\sin\theta$$

$$4 = p \times 2 \times 10^5 \sin 30^\circ$$

$$p = 4 \times 10^{-5} \text{ C-m}$$

$$q2l = 4 \times 10^{-5} \text{ C-m}$$

where, $2l = 2 \text{ cm} = 2 \times 10^{-2}$ m

$$q = \frac{4 \times 10^{-5}}{2 \times 10^{-2}} = 2 \times 10^{-3} \text{ C} = 2 \text{ mC}$$

21. (*b*) Electric field at axial point, at distance r from the centre is

$$E_a = \frac{2kp}{r^3}$$

Electric field at equatorial point, at distance r from the centre is

$$E_e = \frac{kp}{r^3}$$

Therefore, $E_a = 2E_e$

22. (*b*) Statement I is correct but Statement II is incorrect. In parallel and anti-parallel orientations, the angle (θ) between the dipole moment and the electric field is neither 0° and 180°. Leading to a sine (θ) term in the torque formula becoming zero, resulting in zero net torque.

23. (*b*) As we know electric field E along the axis of dipole

$$E_0 = \frac{2kp}{r^3} \quad \text{...(i)}$$

where, p is dipole moment

The electric field in the direction of perpendicular bisector of dipole at distance $2r$

$$E = \frac{kp}{(2r)^3} \quad \text{...(ii)}$$

From Eqs. (i) and (ii), we get

$$E = \frac{E_0}{16}$$

Hence, E is in the opposite direction of p

Hence, $E = -\frac{E_0}{16}$

24. (*c*)

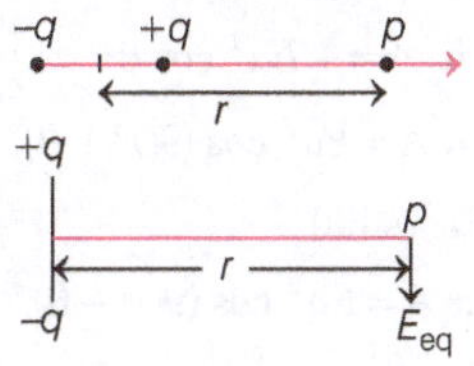

Given, $|\mathbf{E}_{ax}| = E$

$$|\mathbf{E}_{ax}| = \frac{2kp}{r^3}$$

$$|\mathbf{E}_{equ}| = \frac{kp}{r^3}$$

After 90° rotation, the point lies on the equatorial line of the given dipole.

$$\therefore \quad E_{eq} = \frac{E_{ax}}{2} = \frac{E}{2}$$

25. (*b*) Statement I is correct but Statement II is incorrect. Electric field due to dipole varies inversely to the cube of the distance

i.e., $E \propto \frac{1}{r^3}$.

26. (*a*) As we know,

Torque due to dipole and electric field, $\tau = p \times E \sin \theta$

And for maximum torque, $\sin \theta$ should be 1

So, $\sin \theta = 1$

$$\theta = 90°$$

27. (*d*) Work done, W = change in potential energy

$$= -pE[\cos \theta_2 - \cos \theta_1]$$

Initial angle of **p** with **E**; $\theta_1 = 90°$

Final angle, $\theta_2 = 90° + 180° = 270°$

$$= -pE[\cos 270° - \cos 90°] = 0$$

28. (*d*) Here, dipole moment is p and electric field strength is E.

Initially, the dipole is along the direction of electric field.

$\therefore$ Initial potential energy of dipole

$$U_i = -pE \cos \theta_1$$

$$\Rightarrow \quad U_i = -pE \cos 0° = -pE$$

Now, the dipole is rotated and kept in the direction anti-parallel to the direction of electric field.

Potential energy of dipole is $U_f = -pE \cos \theta_2$

$$\Rightarrow \quad U_f = -pE \cos 180° = +pE$$

Work done in rotating the electric dipole

$$W = pE - (-pE) = 2pE$$

29. (*d*) Dipole moment

$$= q \times 2a = 4 \times 10^{-8} \times 2 \times 10^{-2} \times 10^{-2}$$

$$= 8 \times 10^{-12} \text{C-m}$$

$$\tau_{max} = pE$$

$$\tau_{max} = 8 \times 10^{-12} \times 4 \times 10^{8} = 32 \times 10^{-4} \text{Nm}$$

Maximum work done in rotating through 180°

$$W_{max} = 2pE = 2 \times 32 \times 10^{-4} = 64 \times 10^{-4} \text{J}$$

30. (*a*) Suppose neutral point N lies at a distance x from dipole of moment p or at a distance $(25 - x)$ from dipole of moment 64 p.

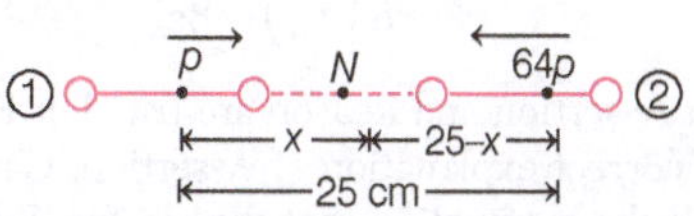

At point N electric field due to dipole 1 = Electric field due to dipole 2

$$\Rightarrow \quad \frac{1}{4\pi\varepsilon_0} \cdot \frac{2p}{x^3} = \frac{1}{4\pi\varepsilon_0} \cdot \frac{2(64p)}{(25 - x)^3}$$

$$\Rightarrow \quad \frac{1}{x^3} = \frac{64}{(25 - x)^3}$$

$$\Rightarrow \quad x = 5 \text{ cm}$$

31. (*a*) When dipole is given a small angular displacement θ about it's equilibrium position, then the restoring torque will be

$$\tau = -pE\sin\theta = -pE\theta \text{ (as } \sin\theta = \theta)$$

or
$$I\frac{d^2\theta}{dt^2} = -pE\theta \quad \left(\text{as } \tau = I\alpha = I\frac{d^2\theta}{dt^2}\right)$$

As,
$$\frac{d^2\theta}{dt^2} = -\omega^2\theta$$

$$\Rightarrow \quad \omega^2 = \frac{pE}{I}$$

$$\Rightarrow \quad \omega = \sqrt{\frac{pE}{I}}$$

32. (*c*) Electric field lines of force never intersect the conductor. They are perpendicular and slightly curved near the surface of conductor.

Step up Practice 3

1. (*d*) Electric flux in *XY*-plane of area of 10 m^2 is zero because the surface is lying in the *XY*-plane, its area vector will be along the *Z*-axis but in **E** there are only *x* and *y* components present.

2. (*a*) The linear charge density *k* gives the charge per unit length, so total charge *Q* on the wire is $k \cdot a$, where *a* is the length of the cylinder.
Therefore, the electric flux through the cylinder surface is $\phi = \frac{Q}{\varepsilon_0} = \frac{ka}{\varepsilon_0}$

3. (*d*) Both Assertion and Reason are true and Reason is the correct explanation of Assertion.

4. (*c*) Electric flux through a closed surface is not affected by the presence of external charges because Gauss's law states that the electric flux through a closed surface depends only on the net charge enclosed by the surface. Hence, Assertion is false but Reason is true.

5. (*d*) Assume eight identical hypothetical cube, so that the given charge *q* appears at the centre of the bigger cube.
Thus, the electric flux passing through the given cube is
$$\phi = \frac{1}{8}\left(\frac{q}{\varepsilon_0}\right) = \frac{q}{8\varepsilon_0}$$

6. (*a*) Both Assertion and Reason are true but Reason is not the correct explanation of Assertion. Gauss' law is based on the assumption that the electric field does not change with time and is proportional to the charge enclosed by the surface.

7. (*a*) The charge *q* is placed near to the point *A*. Hence, $E_A > E_B$

8. (*b*) Electric flux is remains unchanged because electric flux depends only on the amount of charge but not on the position of charge.

9. (*c*)

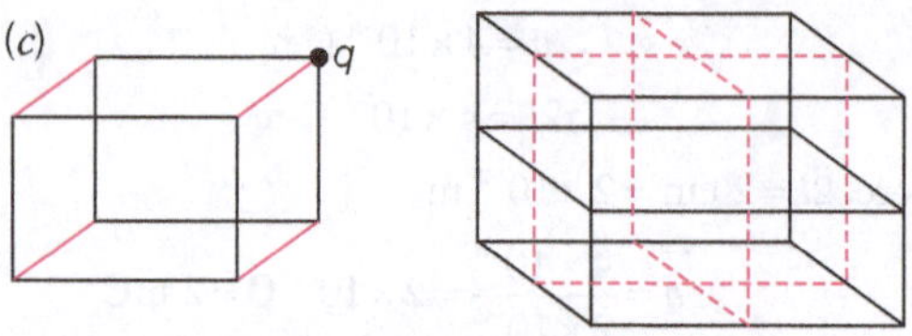

Eight identical cube are required so that the given charge *q* appear at the centre of the bigger cube. Since the flux is shared between 8 cubes the flux through each is $\left(\frac{1}{8}\right)\frac{q}{\varepsilon_0}$.
[entire surface]
Now flux $\left(\frac{1}{8}\text{th}\right)$ will pass through three of the faces of smaller cube and three face won't have any effect.
This $\frac{1}{8}$th will be divided into 3 parts again.
So, the total will be $\left(\frac{1}{24}\right)\frac{q}{\varepsilon_0}$ from each face.

10. (*a*) Both Assertion and Reason are true but Reason is not the correct explanation of Assertion.
Inside a conductor, charges redistribute themselves to cancel any electric field, resulting in zero electric field inside.

11. (*d*) Electric flux through a closed surface is zero if there is no charge enclosed by surface.

12. (*d*) Both Assertion and Reason are true and Reason is the correct explanation of Assertion.
Gauss' law holds for any closed surface, regardless of its shape, as long as it encloses the charge.

13. (*c*) The field **E** is directed into faces 1 and 3 so the fluxes through them are negative **E** is directed out of faces 2 and 4, so the fluxes through them are positive.
We find
$$\phi_{E_1} = \mathbf{E}_1 \cdot \hat{\mathbf{n}}_1 A = Ea^2\cos\theta\,(180° - \theta)$$
$$= -Ea^2\cos\theta$$
$$\phi_{E_2} = \mathbf{E}\cdot\hat{\mathbf{n}}_2 A = +Ea^2\cos\theta$$
$$\phi_{E_3} = \mathbf{E}\cdot\hat{\mathbf{n}}_3 A = Ea^2\cos(90° + \theta)$$
$$= -Ea^2\sin\theta$$
$$\phi_{E_4} = \mathbf{E}\cdot\hat{\mathbf{n}}_4 A = Ea^2\cos(90° - \theta)$$
$$= Ea^2\sin\theta$$

14. (*d*) Cube is placed in a uniform electric field, therefore electric field entering from one surface of cube is same as electric field coming out from opposite surface of the cube, due to this net electric flux becomes zero.

15. (*b*) Before rotation, $\phi_0 = \mathbf{E}\cdot\mathbf{A}$
After rotation
(A) When $\theta = 0°$
$$\phi_1 = EA\cos(90° - 0°)$$

$$\phi_1 = 0$$
$$\phi_{net} = \phi_1 - \phi_0 = -EA$$

(B) $\theta = 30°$

$$\phi_2 = EA\cos(90° - 30°)$$
$$\phi_2 = \frac{EA}{2}$$
$$\phi_{net} = \frac{EA}{2} - EA = -\frac{EA}{2}$$

(C) when $\theta = 60°$

$$d_{net} = \frac{\sqrt{3}}{2}EA - EA$$
$$= -0.134\,EA$$

(D) When $\theta = 90°$

$$\phi_{net} = EA - EA = 0$$

16. (*c*) To apply Gauss' theorem it is essential that charge should be placed inside a closed surface. So imagine on another similar cylindrical vessel above it. So, the flux through the surface will be half of the total flux.

$$\phi = \frac{q}{2\varepsilon_0}$$

17. (*c*) Before rotation

$$\phi_1 = \mathbf{E}\cdot\mathbf{A}$$

After rotation,

Angle between electric field vector and area vector of surface is $(90° - 30°)$

$$\phi_2 = \mathbf{E}\cdot\mathbf{A} = EA\cos 60°$$
$$\phi_2 = \frac{EA}{2}$$

So, change in electric flux passing through the sheet will be

$$= \phi_2 - \phi_1 = \frac{EA}{2} - EA$$
$$\phi_{net} = -\frac{EA}{2}$$

18. (*d*) Given, $E = E_0 x^{3/2}\hat{\mathbf{i}}$ V/m

$\therefore$ Electric field at $x = 0$

$$E = E_0(0)$$
$$E = 0$$

Again, Electric field at $x = a$

$$E = E_0 a^{3/2}\hat{\mathbf{i}} \text{ V/m}$$

If side of cube is a, then surface area of the face is a^2 therefore,

$\Rightarrow \quad \phi = \mathbf{E}\cdot d\mathbf{S}$

$\Rightarrow \quad \phi = E\cdot dS$

$\Rightarrow \quad \phi = E_0 a^{3/2} \times a^2$

$\Rightarrow \quad \phi = E_0 a^{7/2}$

19. (*d*) As we know from Gauss' theorem electric flux due to any charge, or a system of charges outside a Gaussian surface over its surface is zero.

Therefore, electric flux is only due to q_1 and $-q_1$

$$\phi_1 = \frac{q_1}{\varepsilon_0}, \text{ from charge } q_1$$
$$\phi_2 = \frac{-q_1}{\varepsilon_0}, \text{ from charge } -q_1$$
$$\phi_{net} = \frac{q_1}{\varepsilon_0} - \frac{q_1}{\varepsilon_0}$$
$$\phi_{net} = 0$$

20. (*d*) The electric field is due to all charges present whether inside or outside the given surface.

21. (*d*) Total flux from complete closed surface $= \dfrac{q}{\varepsilon_0}$

Half of the flux will pass through hemisphere.

$\therefore$ Flux through cone $= \dfrac{q}{2\varepsilon_0}$

22. (*d*) Electric field at centre due to circular portion is zero because electric field due to each charged element at centre will be cancel out by the electric field due the charged element of its just opposite side.

23. (*b*) Flux of electric field,

$$\phi = \frac{1}{\varepsilon_0} \times Q_{in} = \frac{1}{\varepsilon_0}(2q)$$

24. (*d*) Flux through surface A, $\phi_A = E \times \pi R^2$ and B, $\phi_B = -E \times \pi R^2$

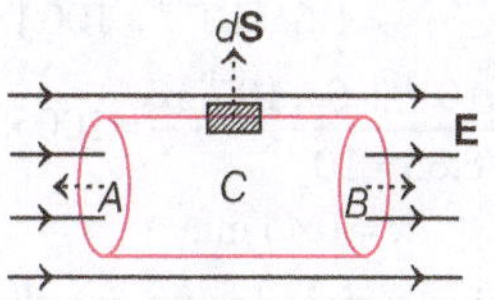

Flux through curved surface C,

$$\phi_C = \int \mathbf{E}\cdot d\mathbf{S} = \int EdS\cos 90° = 0$$

$\therefore$ Total flux through cylinder $= \phi_A + \phi_B + \phi_C = 0$

25. (*a*) Electric flux, $\phi_E = \int \mathbf{E}\cdot d\mathbf{S}$

$$= \int E\,dS\cos\theta = \int E\,dS\cos 90° = 0$$

Step up Practice 4

2. (*b*) Statement I is correct but Statement II is incorrect.

Coulomb's law can be derived from Gauss' law but *vice-versa* is not correct.

3. (*a*) Electric field,

$$E = \frac{\lambda}{2\pi\varepsilon_0 r} = \frac{2\lambda}{4\pi\varepsilon_0 r}$$

or $$\lambda = \frac{E \times 4\pi\varepsilon_0 r}{2}$$

$$= 18\times 10^4 \times \frac{1}{9\times 10^9} \times \frac{0.02}{2}$$
$$= 2\times 10^{-7} \text{ C/m}$$

4. (c) Statement I is incorrect but Statement II is correct. Gauss's law relates the flux of the electric field through a closed surface to the charge enclosed within that surface. Open surfaces do not enclose a volume. So, the concept of enclosed charge does not apply.

5. (a) Surface charge density, $\sigma = \frac{q}{A}$

$$= \frac{17.7 \times 10^{-4}}{200}$$

The electric field outside the sheet is given by

$$E = \frac{\sigma}{2\varepsilon_0} = \frac{17.7 \times 10^{-4}}{2 \times 8.85 \times 10^{-12} \times 200}$$
$$= 5 \times 10^5 \text{ N/C}$$

6. (a) Both Statement I and Statement II are incorrect. Gauss's law can be applied to find the electric field between two oppositely charged parallel plates by choosing a Gaussian surface that spans the region between them.

7. (b) Electric field, $E = \sigma/\varepsilon_0$

$$F = Ee = \frac{\sigma e}{\varepsilon_0} = \frac{(2.0 \times 10^{-6})(1.6 \times 10^{-19})}{8.85 \times 10^{-12}}$$

The work done by the electron against this force in travelling a distance x metre, $W = Fx$

Also, $W = K = 100$ eV

$$= 1.6 \times 10^{-19} \times 100 \text{ J}$$

$$\therefore \quad \frac{(2.0 \times 10^{-6})(1.6 \times 10^{-19})x}{8.85 \times 10^{-12}} = 100 \times (1.6 \times 10^{-19})$$

$$x = 0.44 \text{ mm}$$

8. (c) The Gaussian surface for a point charge and a charged sphere is a sphere of a particular radius around the charge.

9. (a) Electric field, $E = \frac{1}{4\pi\varepsilon_0} \cdot \frac{q}{R^2}$

$$= (9 \times 10^9) \times \frac{0.2 \times 10^{-6}}{(0.25)^2}$$
$$= 2.88 \times 10^4 \text{ N/C}$$

10. (c) We have, $E = \sigma/\varepsilon_0$

$$\Rightarrow \quad \sigma = E\varepsilon_0 = 300 \times (8.85 \times 10^{-12})$$
$$= 2.6 \times 10^{-9} \text{ C/m}^2$$

11. (d)

(a) Electric field outside the charged sphere is $\frac{kQ}{r^2}$

$$\therefore \quad E \propto \frac{1}{r^2}$$

(b) Electric field is constant outside a charged sheet because the field lines are perpendicular to the sheet by symmetry.

(c) Electric field inside the charged sphere is zero because for a closed Gaussian sphere, the net charge enclosed is zero.

(d) Electric field near to the line charge is $\frac{\lambda}{2\pi\varepsilon_0 r}$

$$\therefore \quad E \propto \frac{1}{r}$$

12. (a) Point lies inside both the sphere it mean, we find electric field at $r < R_1$

Therefore,

$$E_{net} = E_{inner} + E_{outer} = 0 + 0$$
$$E_{net} = 0$$

13. (c) Using Gauss's law, let charge on dipole is q,

$$\oint \mathbf{E} \cdot d\mathbf{A} = \frac{Q_{in}}{\varepsilon_0}$$
$$= \frac{Q + q - q}{\varepsilon_0} = \frac{Q}{\varepsilon_0}$$
$$E \times 4\pi r^2 = \frac{Q}{\varepsilon_0}$$
$$E = \frac{1}{4\pi\varepsilon_0} \times \frac{Q}{r^2} = \frac{kQ}{r^2} \text{ For } r \geq R$$

Hence, the electric field outside the shell is the same as that of a point charge inside the shell.

14. (d) Both Statement I and Statement II are correct. In a hollow spherical shield, the charge is present only on its surface and the intensity at every point inside the shell is zero. Hence, the metallic shield in the form of hollow shell may be used to block an electric field.

15. (b) According to Gauss' law,

Electric flux through a closed surface, $\phi = \frac{q_{enc}}{\varepsilon_0}$

Inside a sphere of radius R, we can consider a Gaussian surface in the form of a sphere with radius (r) where $(r < R)$

$$q_{enc} = \int_0^r \rho \cdot 4\pi r'^2 \, dr'$$
$$q_{enc} = \int_0^r \alpha r' \cdot 4\pi r'^2 \, dr' \qquad [\because \rho = \alpha r']$$
$$q_{enc} = \pi\alpha r^4$$
$$\therefore \quad \phi = \frac{\pi\alpha r^4}{\varepsilon_0}$$

By Gauss' law

$$\phi = E \cdot 4\pi r^2$$
$$\Rightarrow \quad \frac{\pi\alpha r^4}{\varepsilon_0} = E \cdot 4\pi r^2$$
$$\therefore \quad E = \frac{\alpha r^2}{4\varepsilon_0}$$

16. (*a*) The electric field outside a charged spherical shell depends only on the total charged enclosed, and it is independent of the shell's thickness.

The expression of the electric field inside the sphere when $(r < R)$, $E = \frac{1}{4\pi\varepsilon_0} \cdot \frac{Q}{R^3} \cdot r$

So, $E \propto r$

17. (*b*) The angle of inclination is related to the electric field (E) by $\tan\theta = \frac{qE}{mg}$

Since,
$$\frac{\tan 60°}{\tan 30°} = \frac{\frac{qE_1}{mg}}{\frac{qE_2}{mg}}$$

By simplifing the expression

$$\Rightarrow \quad \frac{E_1}{E_2} = \frac{\sqrt{3}}{\frac{1}{\sqrt{3}}}$$

$$\Rightarrow \quad \frac{E_1}{E_2} = \sqrt{3} \times \sqrt{3} = 3$$

As we know, electric field is related to surface charge density (σ) by

$$E = \frac{\sigma}{\varepsilon_0}$$

So, $\frac{\sigma_1}{\sigma_2} = \frac{E_1}{E_2}$

$\therefore$ $\frac{\sigma_1}{\sigma_2} = 3$

18. (*b*) Let volume charge density of sphere is ρ

$\Rightarrow$ charge on sphere $q = \frac{4}{3}\pi R^3 \rho$

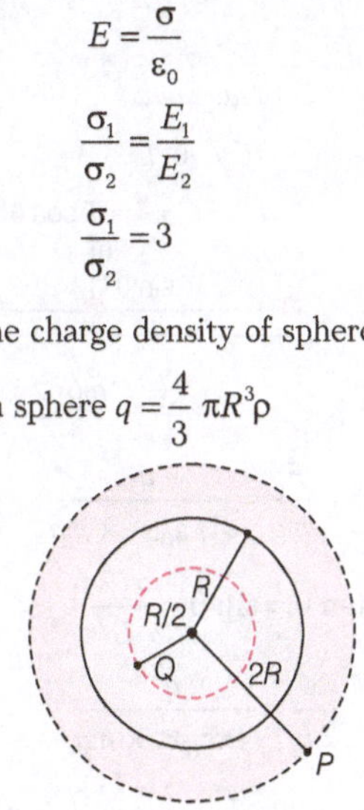

$$\Rightarrow \quad E_p = \frac{1}{4\pi\varepsilon_0}\frac{q}{(2R)^2} = \frac{1}{4\pi\varepsilon_0}\frac{\frac{4}{3}\pi R^3\rho}{4R^2} = E \quad \text{(given)}$$

$$\Rightarrow \quad E_Q = \frac{1}{4\pi\varepsilon_0}\frac{q}{\left(\frac{R}{2}\right)^2} = \frac{1}{4\pi\varepsilon_0}\frac{\frac{4}{3}\left(\frac{R}{2}\right)^3\rho}{\left(\frac{R}{2}\right)^2}$$

$$\Rightarrow \quad \frac{E_p}{E_Q} = \frac{\frac{1}{4}}{\frac{1}{2}} = \frac{1}{2}$$

$$\Rightarrow \quad \frac{E_p}{E_Q} = \frac{1}{2} \quad \Rightarrow \quad E_Q = 2E_P = 2E$$

19. (*a*) Electric field inside shell is zero.

20. (*c*) Situation is shown in the figure

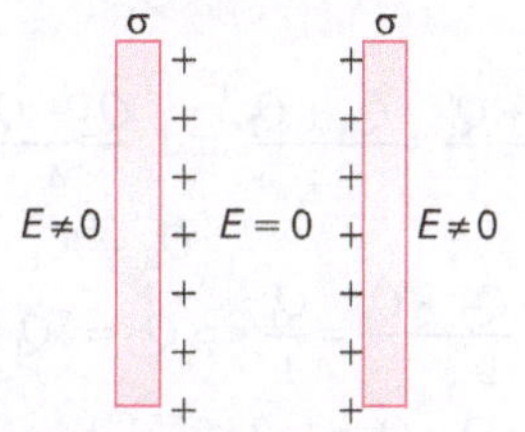

Electric field between two parallel sheets

$$= \frac{2}{2\varepsilon_0}(\sigma - \sigma) = 0$$

23. (*c*) Electric field in vacuum, $E_0 = \frac{\sigma}{\varepsilon_0}$

In medium, $E_2 = \frac{\sigma}{\varepsilon_0 K}$

If $K > 1$, then $E_2 < E_0$.

i.e. if the plates are dipped in kerosene oil tank, the electric field between the plates will decrease.

24. (*a*) Surface charge density $(\sigma) = \frac{\text{Charge}}{\text{Surface area}}$

So, surface charge density on the inner surface

$$\sigma_{\text{inner}} = \frac{-2Q}{4\pi b^2}$$

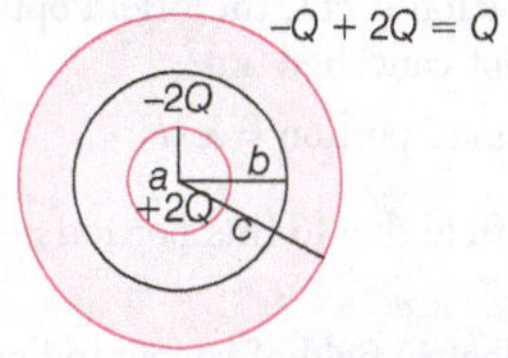

and surface charge density on the outer surface,

$$\sigma_{\text{outer}} = \frac{Q}{4\pi c^2}$$

25. (*b*) When charged particle enters in a uniform electric field, then force on charged particle, $F = qE$

Also, $F = ma$

$\therefore$ $ma = qE$

or acceleration, $a = \frac{qE}{m} = \frac{3 \times 10^{-3} \times 80}{20 \times 10^{-3}} = 12 \text{ ms}^{-2}$

So, from equations of motion

$$v = u + at = 20 + 12 \times 3 = 56 \text{ ms}^{-1}$$

26. (*b*) On the outer surfaces of the shell, surface charge densities are equal

$$\frac{Q_3 + Q_2 + Q_1}{4\pi(3R)^2} = \frac{Q_2 + Q_1}{4\pi(2R)^2} = \frac{Q_1}{4\pi R^2}$$

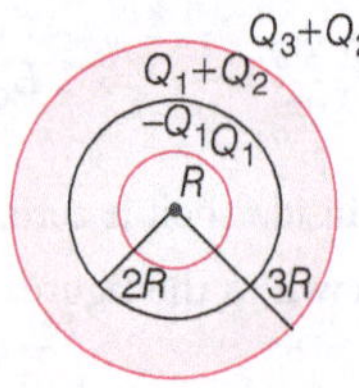

$$\frac{Q_3+Q_2+Q_1}{9}=\frac{Q_2+Q_1}{4} \text{ and } \frac{Q_2+Q_1}{4}=\frac{Q_1}{1}$$

$$\Rightarrow \qquad Q_2 = 3Q_1$$

$$\therefore \quad \frac{Q_3+Q_2+Q_1}{9}=\frac{Q_1}{1} \Rightarrow Q_3 = 5Q_1$$

Hence, $Q_1 : Q_2 : Q_3 = 1:3:5$

27. (*a*) According to Gauss's law, total flux coming out of a closed surface enclosing charge q is given by

$$\phi = \int \mathbf{E}\cdot d\mathbf{S} = \frac{q}{\varepsilon_0}.$$

From this expression, it is clear that total flux linked with a closed surface only depends on the enclosed charge and independent of the shape and size of the surface.

$$\phi = \int \mathbf{E}\cdot d\mathbf{S} = \frac{q}{\varepsilon_0} = 20 \text{ V-m} \qquad \text{[given]}$$

This $\frac{q}{\varepsilon_0}$ is constant as long as the enclosed charge is constant.

The flux over a concentric sphere of radius 20 cm = 20 V-m.

28. (*b*) If ring is complete, then net field at centre is zero. As small portion is cut, then field opposite to this portion is not cancelled out.

Charge of small portion $= \lambda \cdot l$

$\therefore$ Electric field due to this portion $= \frac{\lambda l}{4\pi\varepsilon_0 a^2}$

Let E_R is electric field of remaining portion.

$$\therefore \qquad E_R + \frac{\lambda l}{4\pi\varepsilon_0 a^2} = 0 \Rightarrow E_R = \frac{-\lambda l}{4\pi\varepsilon_0 a^2}$$

Gearing up For NEET

1. (*a*) $\frac{1}{4\pi\varepsilon_0}\frac{q_1 q_2}{r^2} = mr\omega^2 = \frac{4\pi^2 mr}{T^2} \qquad \left(\because \omega = \frac{2\pi}{T}\right)$

$$\Rightarrow \qquad T^2 = \frac{(4\pi\varepsilon_0)r^2(4\pi^2 mr)}{q_1 q_2}$$

$$\therefore \text{ Time period, } T = \left[\frac{4\pi^2 mr^3}{kq_1 q_2}\right]^{1/2}$$

2. (*a*) $\because T\sin\theta = F$

$$= \frac{q^2}{4\pi\varepsilon_0 x^2} \text{ and } T\cos\theta = mg$$

Dividing the two equations, we get

$$\therefore \quad \tan\theta = \frac{1}{4\pi\varepsilon_0}\frac{q^2}{x^2 mg}$$

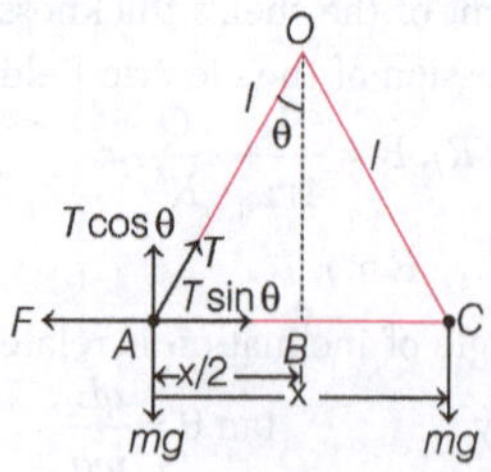

$$\text{or} \qquad \frac{x}{2l} = \frac{q^2}{4\pi\varepsilon_0 x^2 mg} \qquad \left(\because \tan\theta \approx \sin\theta = \frac{x}{2l}\right)$$

$$\text{or} \qquad \frac{x}{2l} \propto \frac{q^2}{x^2} \text{ or } q^2 \propto x^3$$

$$\Rightarrow \qquad q \propto x^{\frac{3}{2}} \Rightarrow \frac{dq}{dt} \propto \frac{3}{2}x^{\frac{1}{2}}\frac{dx}{dt} \qquad \left(\frac{dq}{dt} = \text{constant}\right)$$

$$\therefore \qquad v \propto x^{-\frac{1}{2}} \qquad \left(\because v = \frac{dx}{dt}\right)$$

3. (*a*) In equilibrium,

$$F_e = T\sin\theta \qquad \text{...(i)}$$

$$\text{and} \qquad mg = T\cos\theta \qquad \text{...(ii)}$$

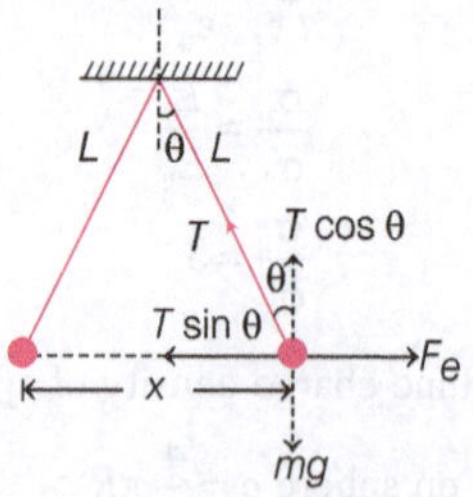

$$\tan\theta = \frac{F_e}{mg} = \frac{q^2}{4\pi\varepsilon_0 x^2 \times mg}$$

$$\text{Also,} \qquad \tan\theta \approx \sin\theta = \frac{x/2}{L}$$

$$\text{Hence,} \qquad \frac{x}{2L} = \frac{q^2}{4\pi\varepsilon_0 x^2 \times mg}$$

$$\Rightarrow \qquad x^3 = \frac{2q^2 L}{4\pi\varepsilon_0\, mg} \Rightarrow x = \left(\frac{q^2 L}{2\pi\varepsilon_0\, mg}\right)^{1/3}$$

4. (*b*) Given, charge on the body,

$$q = 1\text{ nC} = 1\times 1\times 10^{-9}\text{ C} \qquad (\because 1\text{ nC} = 10^{-9}\text{ C})$$

Charge on the electron, $e = 1.6\times 10^{-19}$ C

From the property of quantisation of charge, $q = ne$

$$\Rightarrow \text{Number of charges, } n = \frac{q}{e} = \frac{1\times 10^{-9}}{1.6\times 10^{-19}}$$

$$= 0.625\times 10^{-9}\times 10^{19}$$

$$= 6.25\times 10^{9}$$

5. (*a*) The force acting on the electron $= eE$

Acceleration of the electron $= \dfrac{eE}{m}$

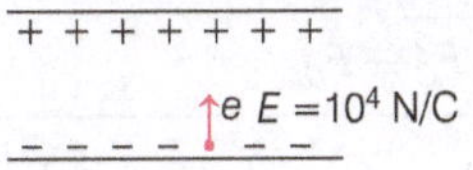

Here, $s = 2 \times 10^{-2}\text{m}, u = 0, v = ?$

$$\therefore \quad v^2 - u^2 = 2as$$

$$\Rightarrow \quad v^2 = 2\left(\frac{e}{m}\right)E \times 2 \times 10^{-2}\text{ m}$$

Also, $\dfrac{e}{m} = 1.76 \times 10^{11}$ C/kg

$$\therefore \quad v^2 = 2 \times 1.76 \times 10^{11} \times 10^4 \times 2 \times 10^{-2}$$
$$= 7.04 \times 10^{13}$$
$$= 70.4 \times 10^{12}$$

The velocity of the electron when it reaches plate *B*,

$$v \approx 0.85 \times 10^7 \text{ m/s}$$

6. (*a*) On negative charge, the resultant force acts as a restoring force and proportional to displacement. When it reaches in the *XY*-plane, the resultant force is zero and the mass moves down along *Z*-axis due to inertia. Thus, oscillation is set along *Z*-axis.

7. (*c*) Number of electrons,

$$n = \frac{6 \times 10^{23}}{63.5} \times 10 \times \frac{1}{10^6} = \frac{6 \times 10^{18}}{63.5}$$

As, $q = ne$

$$q = \frac{6 \times 10^{18} \times 1.6 \times 10^{-19}}{63.5}$$

or $q = 1.5 \times 10^{-2}$ C

$$\therefore \quad F = \frac{9 \times 10^9 \times 1.5 \times 10^{-2} \times 1.5 \times 10^{-2}}{\left(\dfrac{10}{100}\right)^2}$$

$$= 2.0 \times 10^8 \text{ N}$$

8. (*a*) **Case I**

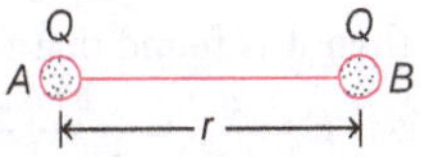

$$F = \frac{1}{4\pi\varepsilon_0} \cdot \frac{Q^2}{r^2}$$

Case II

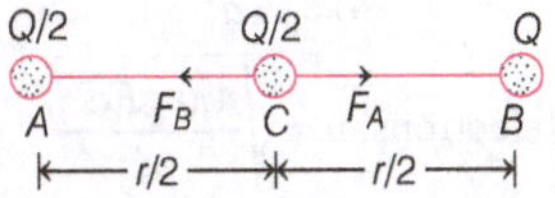

When sphere *C* is touched to *A*, then equal charge *Q*/2 distributes on *A* and *C*.

$$\therefore \quad F_A = \frac{1}{4\pi\varepsilon_0} \frac{(Q/2)^2}{(r/2)^2} = \frac{1}{4\pi\varepsilon_0} \cdot \frac{Q^2}{r^2}$$

$$F_B = \frac{1}{4\pi\varepsilon_0} \cdot \frac{(Q)(Q/2)}{(r/2)^2} = 2 \cdot \frac{1}{4\pi\varepsilon_0} \cdot \frac{Q^2}{r^2}$$

$\therefore$ Net force on *C*, $F_{\text{net}} = F_B - F_A$

$$= \frac{1}{4\pi\varepsilon_0} \cdot \frac{Q^2}{r^2} = F$$

9. (*b*) The system is in equilibrium means the force experienced by each charge is zero. It is clear that charge placed at centre would be in equilibrium for any value of *q*, so we are considering the equilibrium of charge placed at any corner.

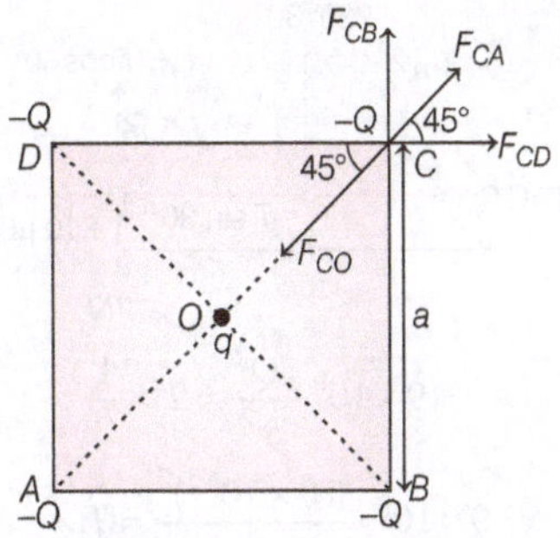

$$F_{CD} + F_{CA}\cos 45° + F_{CO}\cos 45° = 0$$

$$\Rightarrow \frac{1}{4\pi\varepsilon_0} \frac{(-Q)(-Q)}{a^2} + \frac{1}{4\pi\varepsilon_0} \frac{(-Q)(-Q)}{(\sqrt{2}a)^2} \times \frac{1}{\sqrt{2}}$$
$$+ \frac{1}{4\pi\varepsilon_0} \frac{(-Q)q}{(\sqrt{2}a/2)^2} \times \frac{1}{\sqrt{2}} = 0$$

$$\Rightarrow \frac{1}{4\pi\varepsilon_0} \cdot \frac{Q^2}{a^2} + \frac{1}{4\pi\varepsilon_0} \cdot \frac{Q^2}{2a^2} \cdot \frac{1}{\sqrt{2}}$$
$$- \frac{1}{4\pi\varepsilon_0} \cdot \frac{2Qq}{a^2} \cdot \frac{1}{\sqrt{2}} = 0$$

$$\Rightarrow Q + \frac{Q}{2\sqrt{2}} - \sqrt{2}q = 0 \Rightarrow 2\sqrt{2}Q + Q - 4q = 0$$

$$\Rightarrow \quad 4q = (2\sqrt{2} + 1)Q$$

Therefore, $q = \dfrac{Q}{4}(2\sqrt{2} + 1)$

10. (*c*) Electric force, $qE = ma \Rightarrow a = \dfrac{qE}{m}$

$$\therefore \quad a = \frac{1.6 \times 10^{-19} \times 1 \times 10^3}{9 \times 10^{-31}} = \frac{1.6}{9} \times 10^{15} \text{ m/s}^2$$

$\because \quad u = 5 \times 10^6 \text{ ms}^{-1}$ and $v = 0$

$\therefore$ From $v^2 = u^2 - 2as \Rightarrow s = \dfrac{u^2}{2a}$

$\therefore$ Distance, $s = \dfrac{(5 \times 10^6)^2 \times 9}{2 \times 1.6 \times 10^{15}} = 7$ cm (approx.)

11. (*a*) The electrostatic force of repulsion between the charge *q* and (*Q* − *q*) at separation *r* is given by

$$F = \frac{1}{4\pi\varepsilon_0} \cdot \frac{q(Q-q)}{r^2} = \frac{1}{4\pi\varepsilon_0} \cdot \frac{qQ - q^2}{r^2}$$

For maximum electrostatic force of repulsion, then $\frac{\partial f}{\partial q} = 0$

i.e. $\frac{1}{4\pi\varepsilon_0} \cdot \frac{(Q-2q)}{r^2} = 0$

As, $1/4\pi\varepsilon_0 r^2$ is constant, therefore $Q - 2q = 0$ or $Q = 2q$

12. (b) In the following figure, in equilibrium,

$F_e = T \sin 30°$ and $r = 1\text{ m}$

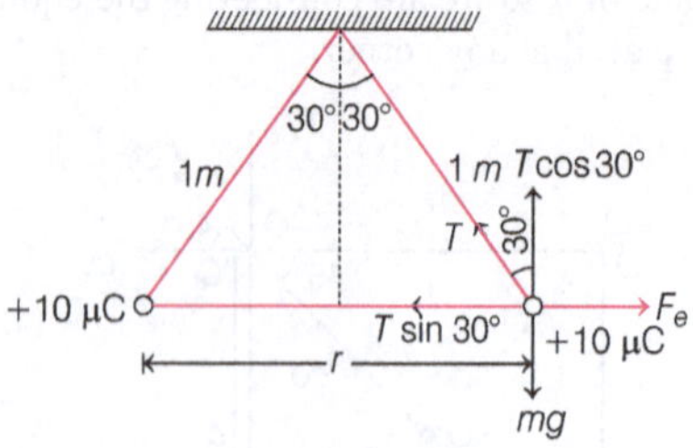

$$\Rightarrow \quad 9 \times 10^9 \cdot \frac{Q^2}{r^2} = T \times \frac{1}{2}$$

$$\Rightarrow \quad 9 \times 10^9 \cdot \frac{(10 \times 10^{-6})^2}{1^2} = T \times \frac{1}{2}$$

$\therefore$ Tension in the threads, $T = 1.8\text{ N}$

13. (b) The schematic diagram of distribution of charges on X-axis is shown in figure below.

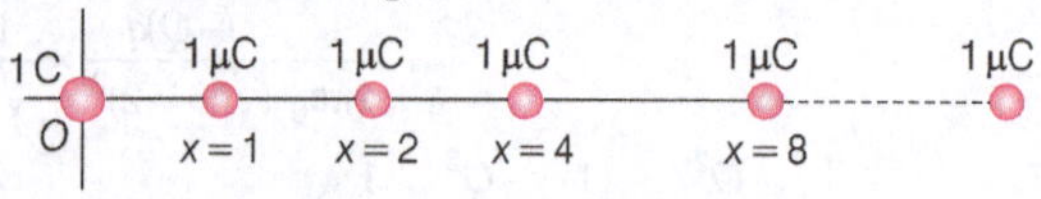

Total force acting on 1 C charge is given by

$$F = \frac{1}{4\pi\varepsilon_0}\left[\frac{1 \times 1 \times 10^{-6}}{(1)^2} + \frac{1 \times 1 \times 10^{-6}}{(2)^2} + \frac{1 \times 1 \times 10^{-6}}{(4)^2} + \frac{1 \times 1 \times 10^{-6}}{(8)^2} + \dots \infty\right]$$

$$= \frac{10^{-6}}{4\pi\varepsilon_0}\left(\frac{1}{1} + \frac{1}{4} + \frac{1}{16} + \frac{1}{64} + \dots \infty\right)$$

$$= 9 \times 10^9 \times 10^{-6}\left(\frac{1}{1 - (1/4)}\right)$$

$$= 9 \times 10^9 \times 10^{-6} \times \frac{4}{3} = 9 \times \frac{4}{3} \times 10^3 = 12000\text{ N}$$

14. (c) The given situation is shown below.

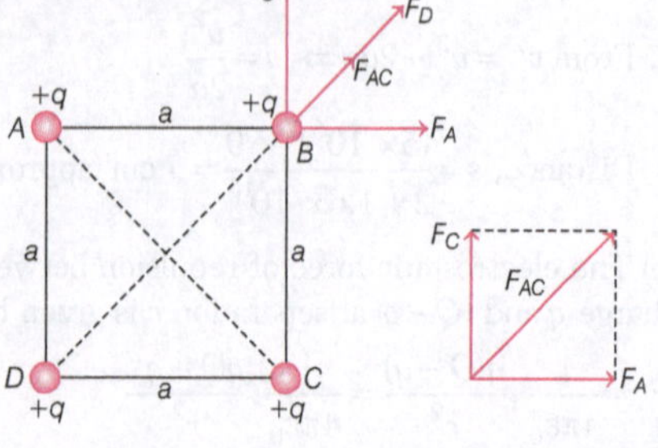

Here, $F_A = \frac{1}{4\pi\varepsilon_0} \cdot \frac{q^2}{a^2}$ and $F_C = \frac{1}{4\pi\varepsilon_0} \cdot \frac{q^2}{a^2}$

Net force on B, $F_{\text{net}} = F_{AC} + F_D$

$$= \sqrt{F_A^2 + F_C^2} + F_D$$

$$= \sqrt{\left\{\left(\frac{1}{4\pi\varepsilon_0} \frac{q^2}{a^2}\right)^2 + \left(\frac{1}{4\pi\varepsilon_0} \frac{q^2}{a^2}\right)^2\right\}} + \frac{1}{4\pi\varepsilon_0} \cdot \frac{q^2}{(a\sqrt{2})^2}$$

$$= \frac{1}{4\pi\varepsilon_0} \cdot \frac{q^2}{a^2}\left(\sqrt{2} + \frac{1}{2}\right)$$

$$= \frac{1}{4\pi\varepsilon_0} \cdot \frac{q^2}{a^2}\left(\frac{1 + 2\sqrt{2}}{2}\right)$$

15. (a) The net force on q_1 by q_2 and q_3 is along the $+x$-direction, so nature of force between q_1, q_2 and q_1, q_3 is attractive. This can be represent by the figure given below.

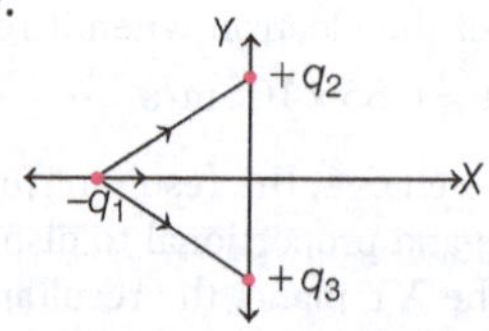

The attractive force between these charges states that q_1 is a negative charge (since, q_2 and q_3 are positive). Thus, nature of force between q_1 and newly introduced charge Q (positive) is attractive and net force on q_1 by q_2, q_3 and Q are along the same direction as given in the diagram below.

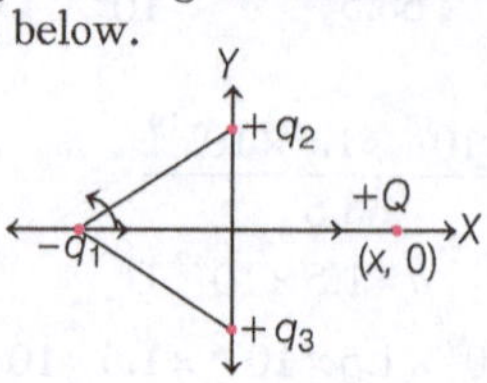

The figure given above clearly shows that the force on q_1 shall increase along the positive X-axis due to the positive charge Q.

16. (c) Two positive ions, each carrying a charge q are kept at a distance d, then it is found that force of repulsion between them is $F = \frac{kqq}{d^2} = \frac{1}{4\pi\varepsilon_0} \frac{qq}{d^2}$

where, $\quad q = ne$

$$\therefore \quad F = \frac{1}{4\pi\varepsilon_0} \frac{n^2 e^2}{d^2}$$

Number of electrons, $n = \sqrt{\frac{4\pi\varepsilon_0 F d^2}{e^2}}$

17. (d) Initially force, $F = k\frac{Q^2}{r^2}$

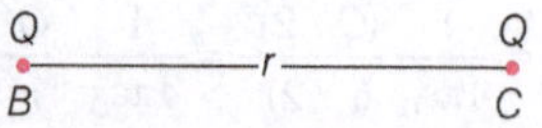

Finally, when a third spherical conductor comes in contact alternatively with B and C then removed, the charges on B and C become $Q/2$ and $3Q/4$, respectively.

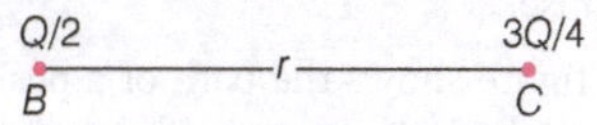

Now, force, $F' = k\dfrac{(Q/2)(3Q/4)}{r^2} = \dfrac{3}{8}F$

18. (c) The acceleration of the electron due to given coulombic force, F is $a_e = \dfrac{F}{m_e}$ ...(i)

where, m_e is the mass of the electron.

The acceleration of the proton due to same force F is

$$a_p = \frac{F}{m_p} \quad \text{...(ii)}$$

where, m_p is the mass of the proton.

On dividing Eq. (ii) by Eq. (i), we get $\dfrac{a_p}{a_e} = \dfrac{m_e}{m_p}$

$$a_p = \frac{a_e m_e}{m_p} = \frac{(2.5\times 10^{22}\ \text{ms}^{-2})(9.1\times 10^{-31}\ \text{kg})}{(1.67\times 10^{-27}\text{kg})}$$

$= 13.6\times 10^{18}\text{ms}^{-2}$

$\approx 1.4\times 10^{19}\text{ms}^{-2}$

19. (c) Let the induced charge on inner surface and outer surface be q_1 and q_2 respectively, then $q_1 + q_2 = -50e$.

Here, charge q_1 induced due to the ball is $+50e$.

So, $+50e + q_2 = -50e$

$\Rightarrow q_2 = -100e$

20. (c) From Coulomb's law,

$$q_1 q_2 \propto F \quad \text{...(i) } [\because r = 1\text{ m}]$$

$$\left(\frac{q_1 - q_2}{2}\right)\left(\frac{q_1 - q_2}{2}\right) \propto \frac{F}{3} \quad \text{...(ii)}$$

Dividing Eq. (i) by Eq (ii), we get

$$\frac{q_1}{q_2} = \frac{3}{1}$$

21. (b) We have, $q_1' = q_2' = \left(\dfrac{q_1 + q_2}{2}\right) = \left(\dfrac{10 - 20}{2}\right)$

$$q_1' = q_2' = -5\ \mu\text{C}$$

$$\therefore \frac{F_1}{F_2} = \frac{q_1 q_2}{q_1' q_2'} = \frac{(10)(-20)}{(-5)\times(-5)} = -\frac{8}{1} \quad (\because F \propto q)$$

22. (c) Situation is shown in figure below

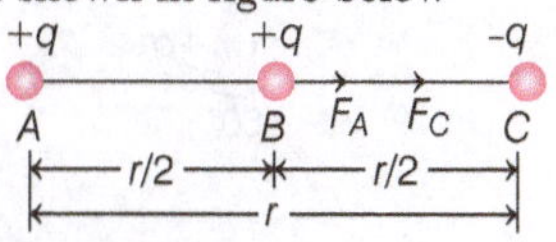

Force between A and C,

$$F = \frac{1}{4\pi\varepsilon_0}\cdot\frac{q^2}{r^2}$$

When sphere B is kept at the mid-point of line joining A and C, then net force on B is

$$F_{\text{net}} = F_A + F_C = \frac{1}{4\pi\varepsilon_0}\cdot\frac{q^2}{(r/2)^2} + \frac{1}{4\pi\varepsilon_0}\cdot\frac{q^2}{(r/2)^2}$$

$$= 8\cdot\frac{1}{4\pi\varepsilon_0}\cdot\frac{q^2}{r^2} = 8F$$

23. (d) Here, $q = -3\times 10^{-7}\text{C}$

Number of electrons transferred to the conductor is

$$n = \frac{q}{e} = \frac{-3\times 10^{-7}\text{C}}{-1.6\times 10^{-19}\text{C}} \approx 2\times 10^{12}$$

Mass of one electron, $m_e = 9.1\times 10^{-31}$ kg

Increase mass of the conductor $= m_e \times n$

$= 9.1\times 10^{-31}\times 2\times 10^{12}$

$= 18.2\times 10^{-19}\text{ kg} \approx 2\times 10^{-18}\text{ kg}$

24. (b) Force, $F_{12} = \dfrac{k(q^2)}{a^2}$

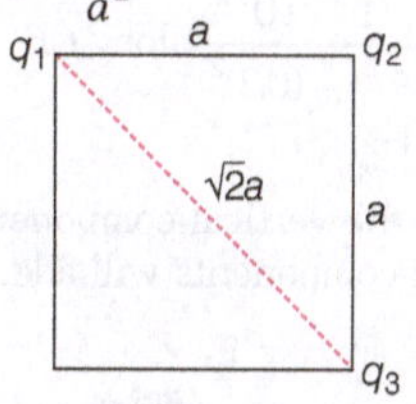

Force, $F_{13} = \dfrac{k(q^2)}{(\sqrt{2}a)^2}$

$\therefore$ Ratio, $\dfrac{F_{12}}{F_{13}} = \dfrac{2}{1}$

25. (b) As, electric field at q is E, so force on charge q,

$$F = qE \quad \text{...(i)}$$

Let the electric field at $2q$ be E', so force on $2q$ will be

$$F' = 2qE' \quad \text{...(ii)}$$

But, according to Coulomb's law, $F' = F$

$\Rightarrow 2qE' = qE$ [from Eqs. (i) and (ii)]

$\Rightarrow E' = E/2$

26. (d) For the system to be in equilibrium, net force on charge Q should be zero. So, Q and q should be unlike in nature.

$$\therefore \frac{k\cdot Qq}{r^2} + \frac{kQ\cdot Q}{(2r)^2} = 0 \text{ or charge, } q = \frac{-Q}{4}$$

27. (b) The three forces acting on each sphere are

(i) tension (ii) weight

(iii) electrostatic force of repulsion

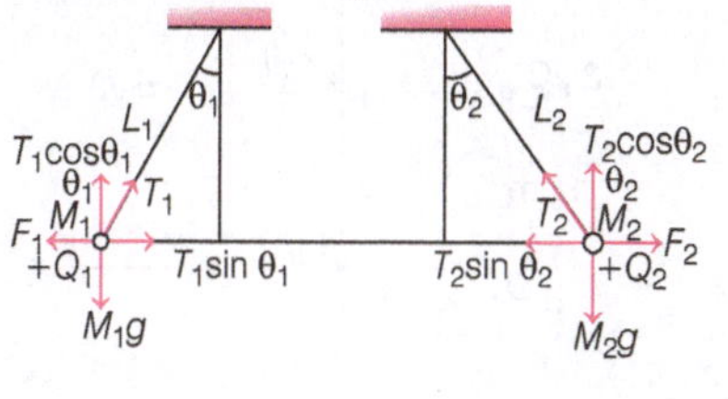

For sphere 1, in equilibrium, from figure,

$T_1 \cos\theta_1 = M_1 g$ and $T_1 \sin\theta_1 = F_1$

$\therefore \quad \tan\theta_1 = \dfrac{F_1}{M_1 g}$

For sphere 2, in equilibrium, from figure,

$T_2 \cos\theta_2 = M_2 g$ and $T_2 \sin\theta_2 = F_2$

$\therefore \quad \tan\theta_2 = \dfrac{F_2}{M_2 g}$

Force of repulsion between two charges are same.

$\therefore \quad F_1 = F_2$

Here, $\theta_1 = \theta_2$ only, if $\dfrac{F_1}{M_1 g} = \dfrac{F_2}{M_2 g} \Rightarrow M_1 = M_2$

28. (b) The electric field at C due to charge $+10^7$C at A is

$$\mathbf{E}_1 = \frac{1}{4\pi\varepsilon_0}\frac{10^{-7}}{(0.2)^2} \text{ along } AC$$

The electric field at C due to charge -10^{-7}C at B is

$$\mathbf{E}_2 = \frac{1}{4\pi\varepsilon_0}\frac{10^{-7}}{(0.2)^2} \text{ along } CB$$

As, $\quad |\mathbf{E}_1| = |\mathbf{E}_2|$

By symmetry, the vertical components will cancel out and horizontal components will add.

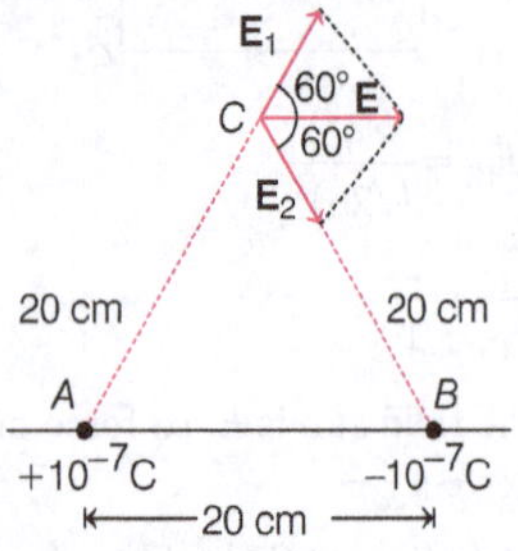

$\therefore$ The resultant electric field at C is

$$E = 2E_1 \cos 60° = 2 \times \frac{1}{4\pi\varepsilon_0}\frac{10^{-7}}{(0.2)^2} \times \frac{1}{2}$$

$$= \frac{9 \times 10^9 \times 10^{-7}}{(0.2)^2}$$

$$= 2.2 \times 10^4 \text{ N/C}$$

29. (b) $E \propto \dfrac{q}{r^2} \Rightarrow \tan\theta = \dfrac{E_0}{E_0/2} = 2$

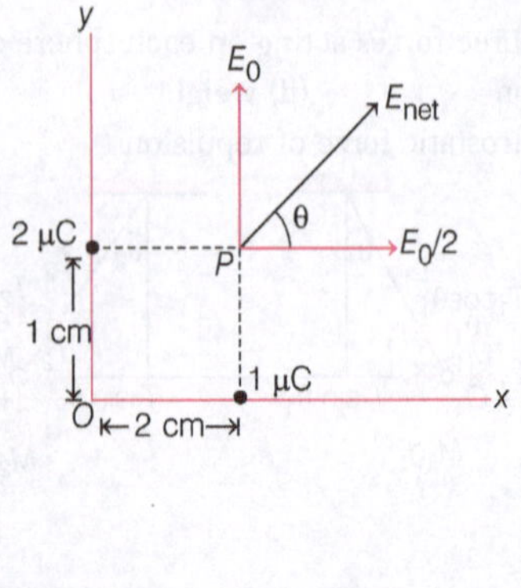

30. (b) Electric field due to Q_2 and Q_3 cancel each other. So, the vector numbered 2 coincides in direction with electric field due to Q_1 at mid-point M of the hypotenuse.

31. (a) The figure shows the path of a positive charged particle (1) through a rectangular region of uniform electric field.

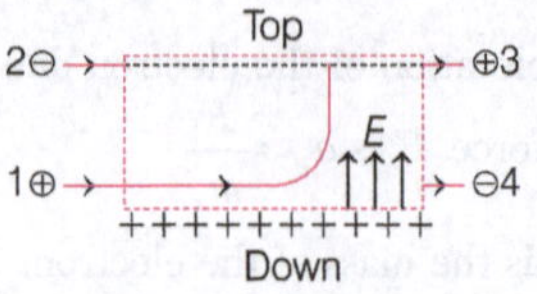

Since, positive charged particle moves in a parabolic path in electric field, it means the direction of electric field is upward. The direction of particle (2) which is negative is downward.

The direction of deflection of particle (3) which is positive is upward and direction of deflection of particle (4) is downward.

32. (b) Given, $A(1, 0, 4)$ and $B(2, -1, 5)$

$\therefore \quad \mathbf{AB} = [(2-1)\hat{\mathbf{i}} + (-1-0)\hat{\mathbf{j}} + (5-4)\hat{\mathbf{k}}]$

$\mathbf{AB} = [\hat{\mathbf{i}} - \hat{\mathbf{j}} + \hat{\mathbf{k}}]$

Torque, $\tau = \mathbf{p} \times \mathbf{E} = q\mathbf{AB} \times \mathbf{E}$

$\tau = 4 \times 10^{-6}(\hat{\mathbf{i}} - \hat{\mathbf{j}} + \hat{\mathbf{k}}) \times 20\hat{\mathbf{i}}$

$\tau = 8 \times 10^{-5}(\hat{\mathbf{k}} + \hat{\mathbf{j}})$

Magnitude of torque,

$\tau = 8 \times 10^{-5}\sqrt{1^2 + 1^2}$

$\tau = 1.13 \times 10^{-4}$ N-m

33. (a) By using, $QE = mg$

$E = \dfrac{mg}{Q} = \dfrac{10^{-6} \times 10}{10^{-6}} = 10$ V/m, upward because charge is positive.

34. (a) When a positive point charge brought near an isolated conducting plane, then some negative charge develops on the surface of the plane towards the charge and an equal positive charge develops on opposite side to the plane. So, the field at point P on other side is directed perpendicular to plane and away from it.

35. (c) The situation is shown below.

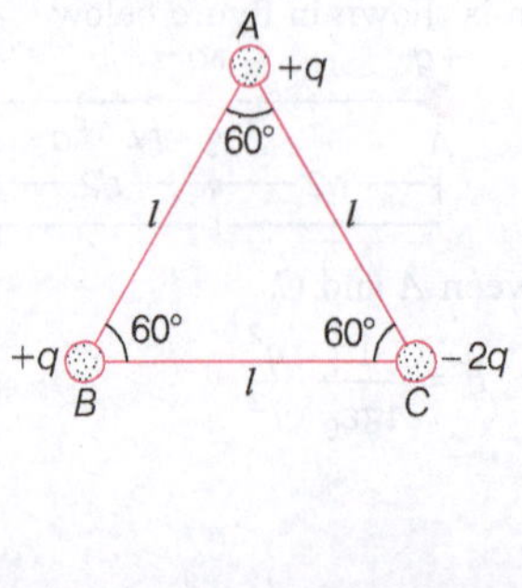

The direction of dipole moment is shown in figure.

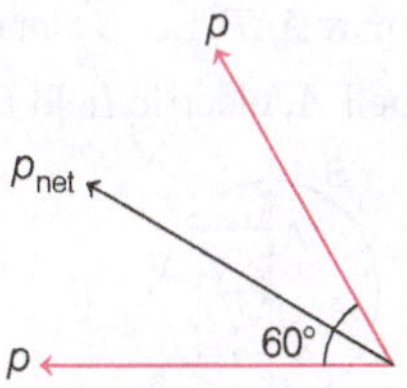

Net electric dipole moment,

$$p_{net} = \sqrt{p^2 + p^2 + 2pp\cos 60°} = \sqrt{3}p$$

$$= \sqrt{3}\,ql \qquad [\because p = ql]$$

36. (*d*) Given, $q = 0.05\,\mu C = 5 \times 10^{-8} C$

$2a = 30\text{ mm} = 0.03\text{ m}$ and $E = 10^6\text{ NC}^{-1}$

Torque acting on an electric dipole placed in an uniform electric field,

$$\tau = pE\sin\theta$$

For maximum torque, $\theta = 90°$

$$\therefore \quad \tau_{max} = pE = E(q \times 2a)$$

$$= 10^6 \times 5 \times 10^{-8} \times 0.03$$

$$= 1.5 \times 10^{-3}\text{ Nm}$$

37. (*b*) When charged particle enters in a uniform electric field, then force on charged particle, $F = qE$

Also, $F = ma$

$\therefore \quad ma = qE$

or acceleration, $a = \dfrac{qE}{m} = \dfrac{3 \times 10^{-3} \times 80}{20 \times 10^{-3}} = 12\text{ ms}^{-2}$

So, from equations of motion

$$v = u + at = 20 + 12 \times 3 = 56\text{ ms}^{-1}$$

38. (*c*) Electric field in vacuum, $E_0 = \dfrac{\sigma}{\varepsilon_0}$

In medium, $E_2 = \dfrac{\sigma}{\varepsilon_0 K}$

If $K > 1$, then $E_2 < E_0$.

i.e. if the plates are dipped in kerosene oil tank, the electric field between the plates will decrease.

39. (*b*) $\mathbf{E}_q + \mathbf{E}_{3q}$ is along PA

$\mathbf{E}_{2q} + \mathbf{E}_{4q}$ is along PB

$\therefore$ $\mathbf{E}_{net}$ is along CB.

40. (*a*) When a positive point charge is brought near an isolated conducting sphere without touching the sphere, the free electrons in the sphere are attracted towards the positive charge making left side negatively charged. This leaves an excess of positive charge on the rear (right) surface of sphere as shown below.

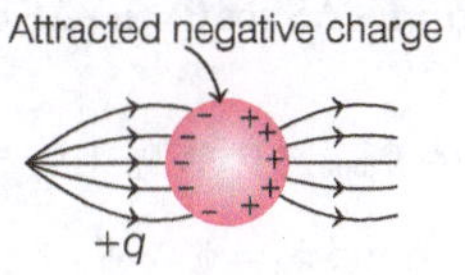

Electric field lines start from positive charge and end at negative charge (in this case from positive point charge to negative charge created inside the sphere).

Also, electric field line emerges from a positive charge, in case of single charge and ends at infinity.

Here, all these conditions are fulfilled in figure (a).

41. (*a*) Electric field due to a point charge, $E = \dfrac{q}{4\pi\varepsilon_0 r^2}$

$$\therefore \quad q = E \times 4\pi\varepsilon_0 r^2 = 2 \times \frac{1}{9 \times 10^9} \times \left(\frac{30}{100}\right)^2$$

$$= 2 \times 10^{-11}\text{ C}$$

42. (*c*) Let neutral point be obtained at a distance x from $20\,\mu C$ charge. Hence, at neutral point

$$\frac{1}{4\pi\varepsilon_0}\frac{20 \times 10^{-6}}{x^2} = \frac{1}{4\pi\varepsilon_0}\frac{80 \times 10^{-6}}{(0.10 - x)^2}$$

$$\frac{20}{x^2} = \frac{80}{(0.10 - x)^2}$$

$$x = +0.033\text{ m}$$

43. (*c*) Torque on dipole, $\tau = p \times E\sin\theta$. So, torque is maximum if p is perpendicular to E. Potential energy $U = -pE = -pE\cos\theta$

Hence, when $\theta = 180°$, i.e. p is anti-parallel to E, then potential energy will be maximum.

44. (*d*) Electric lines of force are perpendicular to the surface of a conductor. Inside the sphere, no lines are present.

Hence, options (d) is correct.

45. (*a*) Electric lines are closer at A. So, the strength of elctric field at A is more than at B, i.e. $E_A > E_B$.

46. (*a*) When the point is situated on a diameter away from the centre of a uniformly positive charged hemisphere, then the electric field is perpendicular to the diameter. The component of electric field intensity parallel to the diameter cancel out.

47. (*a*) From figure, $dl = R\,d\theta$,

Charge on dl, $dq = \lambda R\,d\theta$

Electric field at centre due to dl is $\left(\because \lambda = \dfrac{q}{\pi R}\right)$

$$dE = k\frac{\lambda R d\theta}{R^2}$$

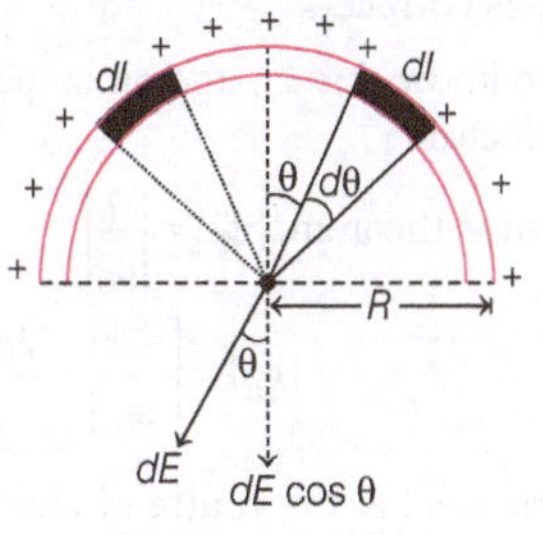

We need to consider only the component $dE \cos \theta$, as the component $dE \sin \theta$ will cancel out because of the field at C due to the symmetrical element dl'.

Total field at centre, $|E| = 2\int_0^{\pi/2} dE \cos \theta$

$$= \frac{2k\lambda}{R} \int_0^{\pi/2} \cos \theta \, d\theta$$

$$= \frac{2k\lambda}{R} = \frac{q}{2\pi^2 \varepsilon_0 R^2}$$

48. (c) According to Gauss' theorem, electric flux through the sphere $= \frac{q}{\varepsilon_0}$.

$\therefore$ Electric flux through the hemisphere $= \frac{1}{2}\frac{q}{\varepsilon_0}$

$$= \frac{10 \times 10^{-6}}{2 \times 8.854 \times 10^{-12}} = 0.56 \times 10^6 \text{ N-m}^2\text{C}^{-1}$$

$$\approx 0.6 \times 10^6 \text{ N-m}^2\text{C}^{-1}$$

$$= 6 \times 10^5 \text{ N-m}^2\text{C}^{-1}$$

49. (d) The Gauss's law of electrostatics gives a relation between electric flux through any closed hypothetical surface called a Gaussian surface and the charge enclosed by the surface. The Gaussian surface has a direction outwards the enclosed path. It obeys vector algebra rules.

So, the nature of Gaussian surface is vector.

50. (d) Gauss' law of electrostatic states that, the total electric flux through a closed surface is equal to the charge enclosed divided by the permittivity, *i.e.* $\phi = \frac{Q}{\varepsilon_0}$.

Thus, electric flux through a surface does not depend on the shape, size or area of a surface but it depends on the total charge enclosed by the surface.

So, here in this question, all the figures have same electric flux as all of them has single positive charge.

51. (a) Electric flux is equal to the scalar product of an area vector and electric field. **E**. As the suface is lying in YZ-plane,

$\therefore \quad \phi = \mathbf{E} \cdot d\mathbf{A} = (5\hat{\mathbf{i}} + 4\hat{\mathbf{j}} + 9\hat{\mathbf{k}})\,(20\hat{\mathbf{i}}) = 100$ unit

52. (c) The electric field is due to all charges present whether inside or outside of the given surface. So, option (c) is correct.

53. (a) As, we know that charge on α- particle is double to that on electron

$\because$ By Gauss' theorem, $|\phi_E| = \left|\frac{q}{\varepsilon_0}\right|$

$$|\phi_E| = \left|\frac{-2e}{\varepsilon_0}\right| = \frac{2e}{\varepsilon_0}$$

54. (d) Electric field at the centre of charged circular ring is zero. Hence, electric field at O due to the part $ACDB$ is equal in magnitude and opposite in direction that due to the part AKB, i.e. E along OK.

55. (a) Inside the shell A, electric field $E_{in} = 0$

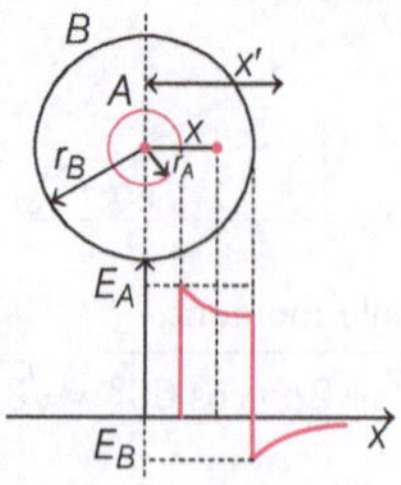

At the surface of shell A,

$$E_A = \frac{kQ_A}{r_A^2} \quad \text{[a fixed positive value]}$$

Between the shell A and B, at a distance x from the common centre,

$$E = \frac{k \cdot Q_A}{x^2} \quad \text{[as } x \text{ increases, } E \text{ decreases]}$$

At the surface of shell B,

$$E_B = \frac{k(Q_A - Q_B)}{r_B^2}$$

[a fixed negative value because $|Q_A| < |Q_B|$]

Outside the both shell, at a distance x' from the common centre,

$$E_{out} = \frac{k(Q_A - Q_B)}{x'^2}$$

[as x' increases negative value of E_{out} decrease and it becomes zero at $x = \infty$]

56. (a) According to Gauss' theorem,

$$\oint \mathbf{E} \cdot d\mathbf{S} = \frac{1}{\varepsilon_0} Q_{enclosed}$$

$$E \cdot 4\pi x^2 = \frac{Q}{\varepsilon_0}$$

Electric field at the point P, $E = \frac{Q}{4\pi\varepsilon_0 x^2}$

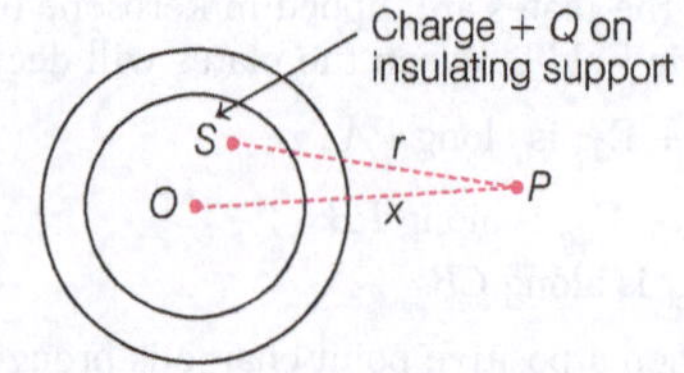

57. (c) Assuming there is a small area ΔS on the cylindrical surface. The normal to this area will be perpendicular to the axis of the cylinder, but the electric field parallel to axis.

Hence, $\quad \Delta\phi = E \cdot \Delta S \cos \theta = E \cdot \Delta S \cos \frac{\pi}{2} = 0$

58. (a) Total flux, $\phi_{total} = \phi_A + \phi_B + \phi_C = \frac{q}{\varepsilon_0}$

$\because \qquad \phi_B = \phi$ and $\phi_A = \phi_C = \phi'$ [assumed]

$\therefore 2\phi' + \phi = \frac{q}{\varepsilon_0}$

The flux through the plane surface A,

$$\phi' = \frac{1}{2}\left(\frac{q}{\varepsilon_0} - \phi\right)$$

59. (c) The field increases linearly from centre inside the sphere (from $r = 0$ to $r = R$) become maximum at the surface of the sphere and decrease rapidly with distance $\left(\propto \frac{1}{r^2}\right)$ outside the sphere. So, the graph will be as shown.

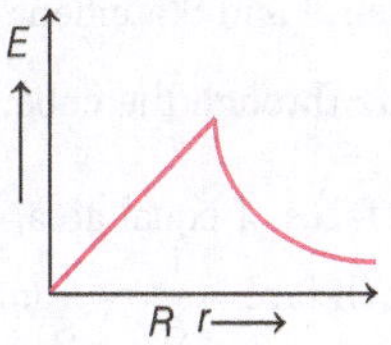

60. (a) Electric field due to a hollow spherical conductor is given by following equations $E = 0$, for

$r < R$ ...(i)

and $E = \frac{Q}{4\pi\varepsilon_0 r^2}$, for $r \geq R$ ...(ii)

i.e. inside the conductor, field will be zero and outside the conductor, will vary according to $E \propto \frac{1}{r^2}$.

61. (b) Charge enclosed by cylindrical surface (length 100 cm) is $Q_{\text{encl}} = 100Q$. By applying Gauss's law,

$$\phi = \frac{1}{\varepsilon_0}(Q_{\text{encl}}) = \frac{1}{\varepsilon_0}(100\,Q)$$

$\because$ The lines are parallel to the surface.

62. (a) We know that, electric field at distance r from an infinitely long linear charge is given by

$$E = \frac{\lambda}{2\pi\varepsilon_0 r}$$

$\Rightarrow \lambda = 2\pi\varepsilon_0 . rE$ or $E \propto r^{-1}$

63. (d) As imaginary sphere of radius R is drawn with its centre on circumference of ring.

So, $q_{\text{in}} < \pi R\lambda$.

where, λ is linear charge density.

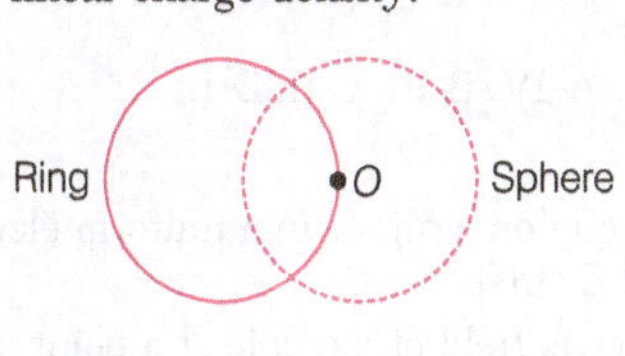

$\therefore \phi < \frac{\pi R\lambda}{\varepsilon_0}$

64. (a) $V \propto \frac{q}{R}$

$V \propto \sigma R$

$V_1 = V_2$

$\sigma_1 R_1 = \sigma_2 R_2$

$\frac{\sigma_1}{\sigma_2} = \frac{R_2}{R_1} = \frac{4}{3}$

65. (b) On the outer surfaces of the shell, surface charge densities are equal.

$$\frac{Q_3 + Q_2 + Q_1}{4\pi(3R)^2} = \frac{Q_2 + Q_1}{4\pi(2R)^2} = \frac{Q_1}{4\pi R^2}$$

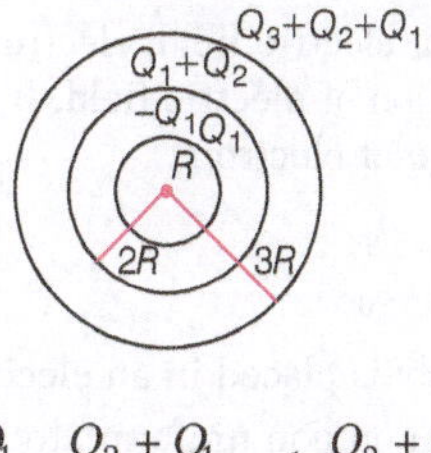

$$\frac{Q_3 + Q_2 + Q_1}{9} = \frac{Q_2 + Q_1}{4} \text{ and } \frac{Q_2 + Q_1}{4} = \frac{Q_1}{1}$$

$\Rightarrow Q_2 = 3Q_1$

$\therefore \frac{Q_3 + Q_2 + Q_1}{9} = \frac{Q_1}{1} \Rightarrow Q_3 = 5Q_1$

Hence, $Q_1 : Q_2 : Q_3 = 1 : 3 : 5$

66. (a) Electric field inside shell is zero.

67. (b) Given, $E = 7.18 \times 10^8$ N/C

and $r = 2 \text{ cm} = 2 \times 10^{-2}$ m

Electric field is given by $E = \frac{\lambda}{2\pi\varepsilon_0 r}$

$$\lambda = 2\pi\varepsilon_0 rE = \frac{4\pi\varepsilon_0 rE}{2} = \frac{2 \times 10^{-2} \times 7.18 \times 10^8}{2 \times 9 \times 10^9}$$

$= 7.98 \times 10^{-4}$ C/m

Assertion and Reason

1. (a) Electric field becomes zero when the sum of the electric field vectors with the same intensity acting in opposite direction cancel each other.

But electric field at a point is due to two point charges given by

$$\mathbf{E} = \mathbf{E}_1 + \mathbf{E}_2 = \frac{Kq_1\hat{\mathbf{r}}_1}{r_1^2} + \frac{Kq_2\hat{\mathbf{r}}_2}{r_2^2}$$

In case of electric field, it gives both magnitude and direction. So, it is a vector quantity.

2. (d) If electric lines of force cross each other, then the electric field at the point of interesection will have two directions simultaneously which is not possible physically.

3. (a) If a dipole is enclosed by a surface as shown in figure,

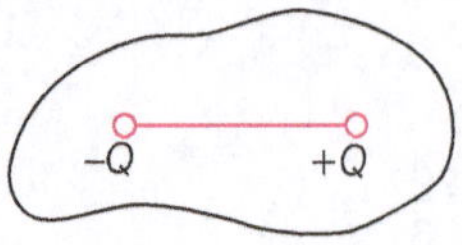

then $Q_{\text{enclosed}} = Q - Q = 0$

$\therefore$ $\phi = 0$ (from Gauss' law)

4. (a) The electric field due to disc is superposition of electric field due to its constituent ring as given in reason.

5. (a) In a uniform electric field, electrons move in the opposite direction of electric field. It is because of the negative charge of electron.

6. (a) Flux, $\phi_{\text{net}} = \frac{q_{\text{in}}}{\varepsilon_0}$

If a closed body is placed in an electric field (either uniform on non uniform), total flux linked with it will be zero,

i.e. $\phi_{\text{net}} = 0 \Rightarrow q_m = 0$

7. (b) Gauss' law implies that the total electric flux through a closed surface is zero if no charge is enclosed by the surface and it is true for any closed surface, independent of its shape and size.

8. (b) As, $\sigma_1 = \sigma_2$ (given)

$\therefore$ $\frac{q_1}{4\pi r_1^2} = \frac{q_2}{4\pi r_2^2}$, or $\frac{q_1}{q_2} = \frac{r_1^2}{r_2^2}$

[let r_1 and r_2 be two different radii]

Then, the ratio of electric field intensities near the surface of spherical conductor.

$$\frac{E_1}{E_2} = \frac{q_1}{4\pi\varepsilon_0 r_1^2} \times \frac{4\pi\varepsilon_0 r_2^2}{q_2} = \frac{q_1}{q_2} \times \frac{r_2^2}{r_1^2} = 1, \text{ i.e. } E_1 = E_2$$

Statement Type Questions

1. (d) Both Statement I and Statement II are correct.

2. (b) Statement I is correct but Statement II is incorrect.

In a medium, $F_m = \frac{F}{k}$

From above expression, it is quite clear that greater the value of k smaller is the force between the two charges. Also, electric dipole moment is directly proportional to dielectric constant.

3. (a) Electric field at the nearby point will be resultant of existing field and field due to the charge brought. It may increase or decrease if the charge is positive or negative depending on the position of the point with respect to the charge brought.

4. (b) In parallel and anti-parallel orientations, the angle (θ) between the dipole moment and electric field is either 0° and 180° leading to a sine (θ) term in the torque formula becoming zero, resulting in zero net torque, Therefore, Statement I is correct but Statement II is incorrect.

5. (d) Both Statement I and Statement II are correct.

6. (a) Two field lines never intersect.

7. (a) According to Gauss' law, electric flux depends on the enclosed charges only. Here, the enclosed charge are Q_1 and Q_3 only. Hence, both Statement I and Statement II are incorrect.

8. (d) Both Statement I and Statement II are correct .

The electric flux through the cube, $\phi = \frac{q}{\varepsilon_0}$

A cube has six faces of equal area. Therefore, electric flux through each face $= \frac{1}{6}\phi = \frac{1}{6}(q/\varepsilon_0)$.

Therefore, equal to $\frac{1}{6}$ th of the total flux.

Match the Columns

1. (c) Figures show the field lines around some simple charge configurations. The field lines of a single positive charge are radially outward while those of a single negative charge are radially inward. The field lines around a system of two positive charges (q, q) give a pictorial description of their mutual repulsion. While that of a pair of equal and opposite charges shows attraction.

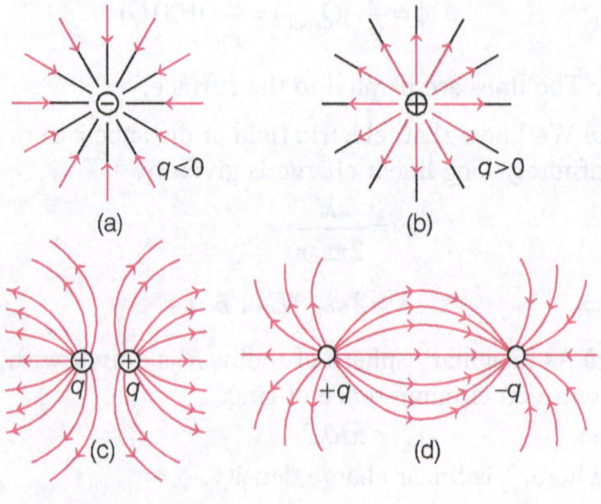

Hence, A-IV, B-III, C-II, D-I.

2. (c)

A. Torque on a dipole in a uniform electric field is $2qa\,E\sin\theta$.

B. Electric field of a dipole at a point on the dipole axis is $\frac{2p}{4\pi\varepsilon_0 r^3}$.

C. Electric field intensity at a point due to continuous charge distribution is $\frac{1}{4\pi\varepsilon_0}\int\frac{dq}{r^2}$.

D. Electric field of dipole at point on equitorial plane is $\frac{p}{4\pi\varepsilon_0 r^3}$.

$\therefore$ A-IV, B-III, C-I, D-II.

3. (*a*) Electric charge = [AT]

Electric field strength = $[MLT^{-3}A^{-1}]$

Absolute permittivity = $[M^{-1}L^{-3}T^{4}A^{2}]$

Electric dipole = $[M^{0}L^{1}T^{1}A^{1}]$

Hence, A-IV, B-II, C-I, D-III.

4. (*b*) A. Electric field outside the spherical shell is denotes as $E=\frac{q}{4\pi\varepsilon_0 r^2}\hat{\mathbf{r}}\ (r\geq R)$

where, r is the distance of the point from the centre of the shell and R is the radius of the shell, q is the total charge of the shell : $q=4\pi K^2\sigma$

B. The quantity of heat generated or absorbed in an electrical circuit can be expressed in terms of charge.

C. Electric flux $\Delta\phi$ through an area element ΔS is defined by $\Delta\phi=E\times\Delta S=E\Delta S\cos\theta$, which is proportional to the number of field lines cutting the area element.

D. Electric field inside the spherical shell is zero, this is due to the charge redistribution on the surface. canceling the field inside.

Hence, A-III, B-II, C-IV, D-I.

5. (*b*)

A. For infinite sheet of charge, E = constant.

B. For infinite line charge, $E\propto\frac{1}{r}$.

C. For electric dipole, $E\propto\frac{1}{r^3}$.

D. For a point charge, $E\propto\frac{1}{r^2}$.

Hence, A-III, B-II, C-IV, D-I.

6. (*b*) $E_{\text{I}}=\frac{(\sigma)+(-2\sigma+\sigma)}{2\varepsilon_0}=0$;

$$E_{\text{II}}=\frac{(\sigma)-(-2\sigma+\sigma)}{2\varepsilon_0}=\frac{\sigma}{\varepsilon_0}$$

$$E_{\text{III}}=\frac{(\sigma-2\sigma)-\sigma}{2\varepsilon_0}=-\frac{\sigma}{\varepsilon_0};$$

$$E_{\text{IV}}=\frac{(\sigma-2\sigma+\sigma)}{2\varepsilon_0}=0$$

Hence, A-IV, B-I, C-II, D-IV.

Final Check Through PYQs

1. (*c*) Force of mutual attraction between the electron and proton.

(when, $r=1.6\ \text{Å}=1.6\times10^{-10}$ m) is given as

$$F=9\times10^9\times\frac{e^2}{r^2}=9\times10^9\times\frac{(1.6\times10^{-19})^2}{(1.6\times10^{-10})^2}$$

$$=9\times10^{-9}\text{N}$$

$\therefore$ Acceleration of electron

$$=\frac{F}{m_e}=\frac{9\times10^{-9}}{9\times10^{-31}}=10^{22}\ \text{m/s}^2$$

2. (*a*) The force between two point charges A and B having charge $+Q$ and $-Q$ respectively is given by

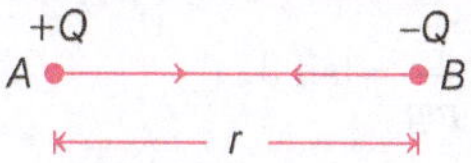

$$F=\frac{KQ_AQ_B}{r^2}=\frac{KQ(-Q)}{r^2}=-\frac{KQ^2}{r^2}\quad\text{...(i)}$$

When 25% charge of A is transferred to B, then new amount of charge on A and B respectively become

$$Q'_A=\frac{3}{4}Q$$

$$Q'_B=\left(\frac{25}{100}Q_A+Q_B\right)=\left(\frac{1}{4}Q-Q\right)=\frac{-3}{4}Q$$

So, the force between the two charges now becomes

$$F'=\frac{KQ'_AQ'_B}{r^2}=\frac{K\left(\frac{3Q}{4}\right)\left(-\frac{3}{4}Q\right)}{r^2}$$

$$=\frac{-9KQ^2}{16r^2}=\frac{9}{16}F\quad\text{[From Eq. (i)]}$$

Thus, the new force between the charges is 9/16 times the initial force between the charges.

3. (*c*) Net charge on one H-atom

$$q=-e+e+\Delta e=\Delta e$$

Net electrostatic repulsive force between two H-atoms

$$F_r=\frac{Kq^2}{d^2}=\frac{K(\Delta e)^2}{d^2}$$

Similarly, net gravitational attractive force between two H-atoms,

$$F_G=\frac{Gm_r^2}{d^2}$$

It is given that,

$$F_r-F_G=0$$

$$\Rightarrow\quad\frac{K(\Delta e)^2}{d^2}-\frac{Gm_r^2}{d^2}=0$$

$$\Rightarrow\quad(\Delta e)^2=\frac{Gm_r^2}{K}$$

$$(\Delta e)^2 = \frac{(6.67\times10^{-11})(1.67\times10^{-27})^2}{9\times10^9}$$

$\Rightarrow \quad \Delta e = 1.437\times10^{-37}$ C

4. (b) According to question, two identical charged spheres are suspended from a common point by two massless strings of length L.

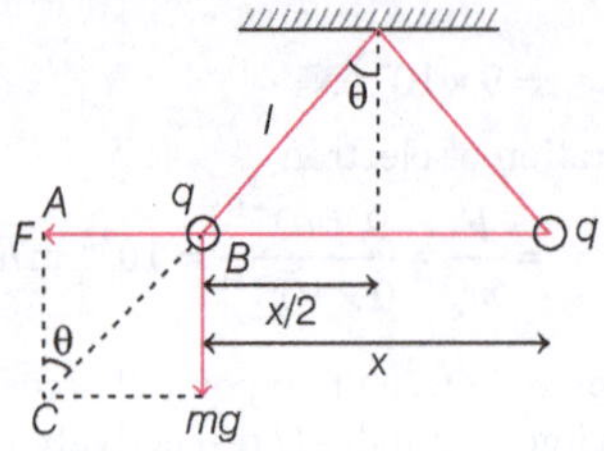

$\because$ In ΔABC, $\dfrac{F}{mg} = \tan\theta$ ...(i)

Since, the charges begins to leak from both the spheres at a constant rate. As a result, the spheres approach each other with velocity v.

Therefore, Eq. (i) can be rewritten as

$$\frac{Kq^2}{x^2 mg} = \frac{x/2}{\sqrt{l^2 - \frac{x^2}{4}}}$$

$$\Rightarrow \quad \frac{Kq^2}{x^2 mg} = \frac{x}{2l} \quad \text{or} \quad q^2 \propto x^3$$

$$\Rightarrow \quad q \propto x^{3/2}$$

$$\Rightarrow \quad \frac{dq}{dt} \propto \frac{d(x^{3/2})}{dx}\cdot\frac{dx}{dt}$$

$$\Rightarrow \quad \frac{dq}{dt} \propto x^{1/2}.v$$

$$\Rightarrow \quad v \propto \frac{1}{x^{1/2}} \quad \text{or} \quad v \propto x^{-1/2}$$

5. (c) Given, $\theta = 30°$

$E = 2\times10^5\ \text{NC}^{-1}$

Dipole length, $2l = 2$ cm $= 2\times10^{-2}$ m

Torque, $\tau = 4$ N-m

We know that, $\tau = pE\sin\theta$

$$\Rightarrow \quad p = \frac{\tau}{E\sin\theta} = \frac{4}{2\times10^5\times\sin30°}$$

$$\Rightarrow \quad p = 4\times10^{-5}\ \text{C-m}$$

$$\Rightarrow \quad 2l\cdot q = 4\times10^{-5}$$

$$\Rightarrow \quad q = \frac{4\times10^{-5}}{2l} = \frac{4\times10^{-5}}{2\times10^{-2}}$$

$$= 2\times10^{-3}\ \text{C} = 2\ \text{mC}$$

6. (a) The arrangement of charges shown in the figure is an electric dipole. Hence, electric field at point P at a distance $R(R >> L)$ from the dipole is equal to electric field due to electric dipole on axial position.

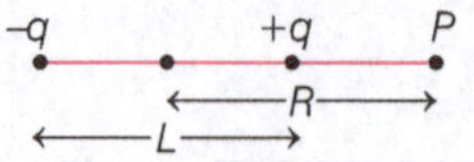

i.e., $$E = \frac{1}{4\pi\varepsilon_0}\cdot\frac{2p}{R^3}$$

where, $p = qL$ (Electric dipole moment)

$$\therefore \quad E \propto \frac{1}{R^3}$$

7. (b) We know that, the direction of electric dipole moment is from negative charge to positive charge.

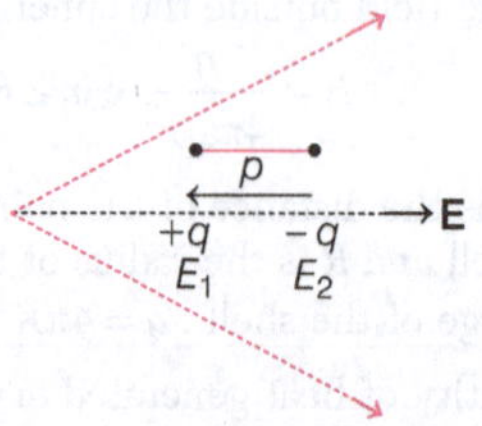

The strength of the electric field at $+q$ is greater than that of $-q$ charge, i.e. $|E_1| > |E_2|$.

So, the net force on the dipole act towards the right side.

We know that, a system always moves to decrease its potential energy.

So, the given dipole move towards right side as its potential energy will decrease.

8. (d) In polar molecules, the positive charge and negative charge do not overlap each other. So, the total charge on the polar molecule is zero. Thus, these types of molecules have permanent electric dipole moment. e.g. Water is polar molecule.

9. (d) Electric field due to electric dipole on equatorial plane at a distance r from the centre of dipole is given as

$$\mathbf{E} = -\frac{1}{4\pi\varepsilon_0}\frac{\mathbf{p}}{r^3}$$

10. (c) Force on a charged particle in the presence of an electric field is given as

$$F = qE \quad \text{...(i)}$$

From Newton's second law of motion, force on a particle with mass m is given as

$$F = ma \quad \text{...(ii)}$$

where, a is the acceleration.

From Eqs. (i) and (ii), we get

$$F = ma = qE$$

$$\Rightarrow \quad a = \frac{qE}{m} \quad \text{...(iii)}$$

Now, consider that a particle falls from rest through a vertical distance h. Therefore, $u = 0$ and the second equation of motion becomes

$$s = ut + \frac{1}{2}at^2$$

or $$h = 0 \times t + \frac{1}{2}at^2$$

$$= \frac{1}{2} \times \frac{qE}{m}t^2 \quad \text{[from Eq. (iii)]}$$

$\Rightarrow$ $$t^2 = \frac{2hm}{qE} \text{ or } t = \sqrt{\frac{2hm}{qE}}$$

Since, the particles given in the question is electron and proton; and the quantity $\sqrt{\frac{2h}{qE}}$ (here, $q_p = q_e = e$) for both of them is constant. Thus, we can write, $t = k\sqrt{m}$

where, $$k = \sqrt{\frac{2h}{qE}} \text{ or } t \propto \sqrt{m}$$

As, mass of proton (m_p) >> mass of electron (m_e).

Thus, the time of fall of an electrons would be smaller than the time of fall of a protons.

11. (*d*) According to Gauss' law, $\oint \mathbf{E} \cdot d\mathbf{S}$ represents total electric flux passing through a closed surface.

If $\oint \mathbf{E} \cdot d\mathbf{S} = 0$, then it signifies that the number of electric flux lines entering the surface must be equal to the number of flux lines leaving the surface.

12. (*b*) When a sphere encloses a charged dipole,

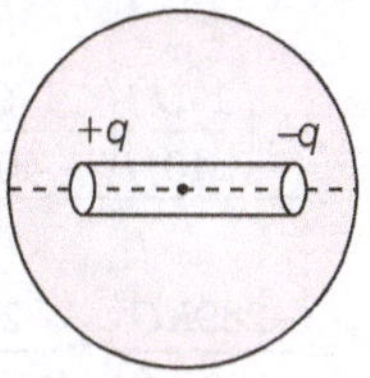

Here, $q = \pm 3 \times 10^{-6}$ C

Thus, according to Gauss's law, the net electric flux across the closed surface is equal to the net charge enclosed by it divided by ε_0, i.e.

$$\phi_E = \frac{q_{in}}{\varepsilon_0} = \frac{+3 \times 10^{-6} - 3 \times 10^{-6}}{\varepsilon_0} = 0$$

Hence, electric flux across the sphere is zero.

Note For a dipole or quadrupole, net electric flux will always be zero.

13. (*a*) Given, radius, $r = 10$ cm $= 10 \times 10^{-2}$ m

Charge, $q = 3.2 \times 10^{-7}$ C

Electric field at a point ($x = 15$ cm) from the centre of the sphere is

$$E = \frac{1}{4\pi\varepsilon_0} \cdot \frac{q}{x^2} = 9 \times 10^9 \times \frac{3.2 \times 10^{-7}}{(15 \times 10^{-2})^2}$$

$$= 1.28 \times 10^5 \text{ N/C}$$

Hence, correct option is (a).

14. (*b*) Consider two infinite line charges with linear charge densities $+\lambda$ C/m and $-\lambda$ C/m respectively, which are lying in y-direction as shown in the figure below.

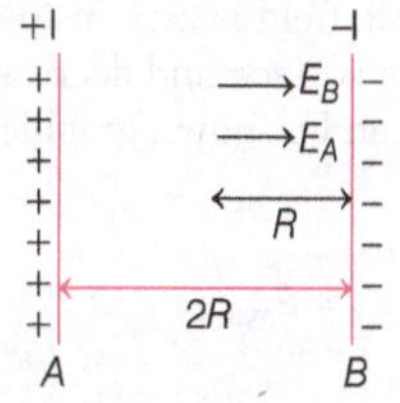

Then, the electric field due to line A at the mid way between the two line charges, i.e. at R is

$$|\mathbf{E}_A| = \frac{\lambda}{2\pi\varepsilon_0 R} \text{ N/C} \quad \text{... (i)}$$

which lies along +ve X-axis (outward), i.e. from A to B.

Similarly, the electric field due to line B at the mid way between the two line charges, i.e. at R is

$$|\mathbf{E}_B| = \frac{\lambda}{2\pi\varepsilon_0 R} \text{ N/C} \quad \text{... (ii)}$$

Due to negative charge on B, $\mathbf{E}_B$ also lies along +ve X-axis (inward), i.e. from A to B.

So, the resultant electric field at R is given as

$$|\mathbf{E}_R| = |\mathbf{E}_A| + |\mathbf{E}_B|$$

Substituting the values from Eqs. (i) and (ii) neq (iii) we get

$$|\mathbf{E}_R| = \frac{\lambda}{2\pi\varepsilon_0 R} + \frac{\lambda}{2\pi\varepsilon_0 R} = \frac{\lambda}{\pi\varepsilon_0 R} \text{ N/C}$$

Which also lies along the + ve X-axis, i.e. from A to B.

15. (*a*) As the hollow sphere is uniformly charged, so the net charge will appear on the surface of the sphere.

(i) The electric field at a point outside the hollow sphere is

$$\phi = \oint_S \mathbf{E} \cdot d\mathbf{S} = \frac{Q_{\text{enclosed}}}{\varepsilon_0} \quad \text{[from Gauss' law]}$$

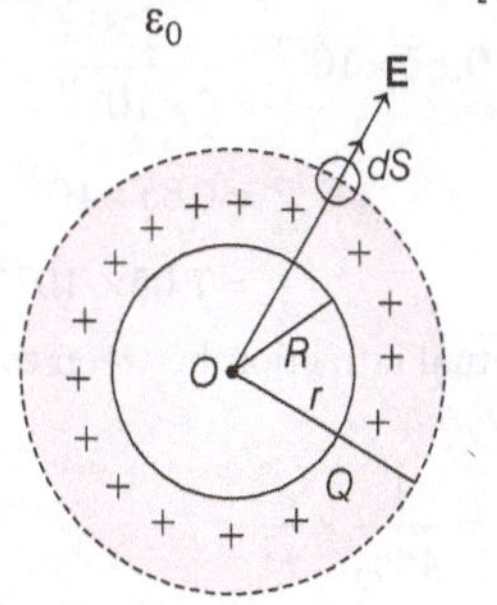

$\Rightarrow$ $$E(4\pi r^2) = \frac{Q}{\varepsilon_0}$$

$\Rightarrow$ $$E = \frac{Q}{4\pi\varepsilon_0 r^2} \Rightarrow E \propto \frac{1}{r^2}$$

(ii) The electric field at the surface ($r = R$),

$$E = \frac{Q}{4\pi\varepsilon_0 R}$$

(iii) The electric field inside hollow sphere is

$$E = \frac{Q}{4\pi\varepsilon_0 r} = 0 \qquad [\because Q_{inside} = 0]$$

Thus, the electric field is zero inside the hollow sphere maximum at the surface and decreases as r increases for $r > R$. This can be shown graphically as

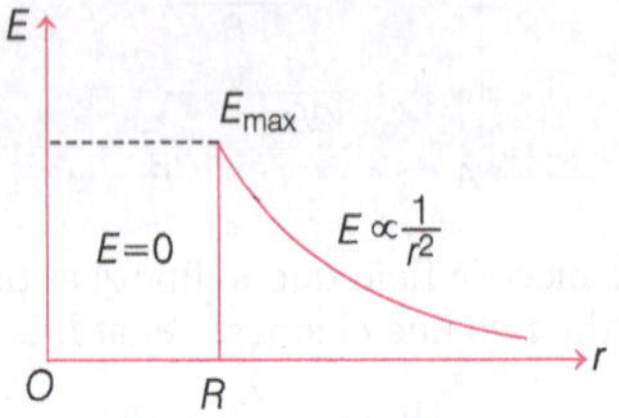

16. (c) Given, $E = Ar$ ...(i)

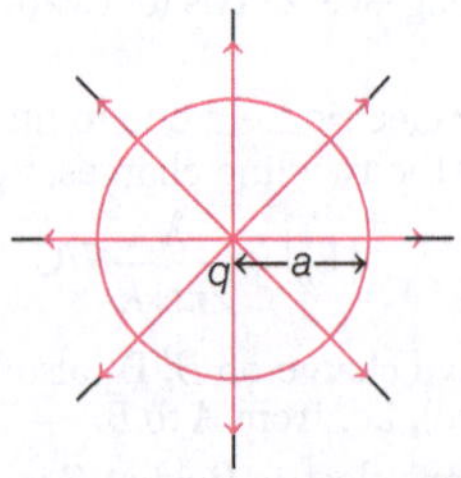

Here, $r = a \Rightarrow E = \frac{1}{4\pi\varepsilon_0} \cdot \frac{q}{a^2}$

From Eq. (i), we get

$$\frac{1}{4\pi\varepsilon_0} \cdot \frac{q}{a^2} = Aa \Rightarrow q = 4\pi\varepsilon_0 A a^3$$

Skill Builder

Sol. of Skill Builder on Pg. 04

(d) Acceleration of electron $= \frac{F}{m}$

$$0.85 \times 10^{22} = \frac{F}{9 \times 10^{-31}}$$

$$F = 0.85 \times 10^{22} \times 9 \times 10^{-31}$$

$$= 7.65 \times 10^{-9}$$

Force of mutual attraction between the electron and proton is given as

$$F = \frac{1}{4\pi\varepsilon_0} \times \frac{e^2}{r^2}$$

$$7.65 \times 10^{-9} = 9 \times 10^9 \times \frac{(1.6 \times 10^{-19})^2}{r^2}$$

$$r^2 = \frac{9 \times 10^9 \times (1.6 \times 10^{-19})^2}{7.65 \times 10^{-9}}$$

$$r^2 = 3.0117 \times 10^{-20}$$

$$r = \sqrt{3.0117 \times 10^{-20}}$$

$$= 1.73 \times 10^{-10} = 1.73 \text{ Å}$$

Sol. of Skill Builder on Pg. 05

(b) The force between two point charges L and M having charges $\frac{+Q}{2}$ and $\frac{-Q}{2}$ respectively is given by

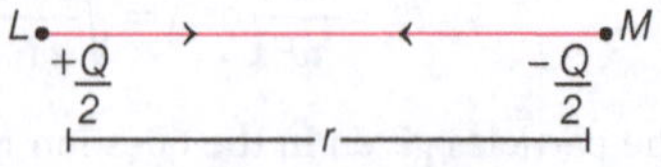

$$F = \frac{KQ_L Q_M}{r^2} = \frac{K\left(\frac{+Q}{2}\right)\left(\frac{-Q}{2}\right)}{r^2}$$

$$= \frac{-KQ^2}{4r^2} \qquad \text{...(i)}$$

When 15% charge of L is transferred to M, then new amount of charge on L and M respectively becomes

$$Q'_L = \frac{Q}{2} - \frac{Q}{2} \times \frac{15}{100} = \frac{Q}{2} - \frac{3Q}{40} = \frac{17Q}{40}$$

$$Q'_M = \left(\frac{15}{100} Q_L + Q_M\right)$$

$$= \left(\frac{3}{20} \cdot \frac{Q}{2} - \frac{Q}{2}\right) = \left(\frac{3Q}{40} - \frac{Q}{2}\right) = \frac{-17Q}{40}$$

So, the force between the two charges now becomes

$$F' = \frac{KQ'_L Q'_M}{r^2}$$

$$= \frac{K\left(\frac{17Q}{40}\right)\left(-\frac{17Q}{40}\right)}{r^2}$$

$$= \frac{-289KQ^2}{1600r^2} = \frac{+289}{400}\left(-\frac{KQ^2}{4r^2}\right)$$

$$= \frac{289}{400} F \qquad \text{[From Eq. (i)]}$$

$$= \frac{289}{400} \times 10 \qquad \text{[Given, } F = 10 \text{ N]}$$

$$= \frac{289}{40} \text{ N}$$

Thus, new force is $\frac{289}{40}$ N.

Sol. of Skill Builder on Pg. 22

(c) Given, $\theta = 90°$,

$$E = 5 \times 10^5 \text{ NC}^{-1}$$

Dipole length, $2l = 3 \text{ cm} = 3 \times 10^{-2}$ m

Torque, $\tau = 15$ N-m

We know that, $\tau = pE\sin\theta$

$$\Rightarrow \quad p = \frac{\tau}{E\sin\theta} = \frac{15}{5\times10^5\times\sin 90°}$$

$$\Rightarrow \quad p = 3\times10^{-5} \text{ C-m}$$

$$\Rightarrow \quad 2l\cdot q = 3\times10^{-5}$$

$$\Rightarrow \quad q = \frac{3\times10^{-5}}{3\times10^{-2}} = 1\times10^{-3}\text{ C} = 1\text{ mC}$$

■ Sol. of Skill Builder on Pg. 34

(*c*) The given electric field is,

$$E = 3r^2 \quad \text{...(i)}$$

Electric field at the surface of the sphere is,

$$E = \frac{1}{4\pi\varepsilon_0}\frac{q}{c^2} \quad \text{...(ii)}$$

Eq. (i) and Eq. (ii) are equal if $r = c$.

$$\frac{1}{4\pi\varepsilon_0}\frac{q}{c^2} = 3c^2$$

$$q = 12\pi\varepsilon_0 c^4$$

■ Sol. of Skill Builder on Pg. 35

(*a*) Given, radius, $r = 5$ cm

Charge, $q = 1.6\times10^{-6}$ C

Electric field at a point ($x = 10$ cm) from the centre of the sphere is

$$E = \frac{1}{4\pi\varepsilon_0}\cdot\frac{q}{x^2} = 9\times10^9\times\frac{1.6\times10^{-6}}{(10\times10^{-2})^2}$$

$$= 14.4\times10^5 \text{ N/C}$$

For deeper insight
Scan the QR Code

Chapter 2

Electrostatic Potential

Learning Objectives

Module-I

- Electric Potential
- Electrostatic Potential due to a Point Charge
- Electric Potential due to a Continuous Charge Distribution
- Electric Potential Due to Electric Dipole
- Relation between Electric Field and Electric Potential

Module-II

- Equipotential Surface
- Potential due to Charged Sphere
- Motion of Charged Particle in Electric Field
- Kinetic Energy of a Charged Particle
- Work Done by a Charged Particle

Module-III

- Electric Potential Energy
- Potential Energy of a System of Charges
- Potential Energy of a Dipole in a Uniform Electric Field

Chapter Overview with *NEET Connection*

- This chapter is base of many branches of Phyics and engineering like electronic devices and circuits. Without having good knowledge of this chapter, it will be difficult to understand other chapters like Moving Charges and Magnetism, Electromagnetic Induction, Alternating Current.

Special format questions can be easily framed on the following topics of this chapter

- Calculation of electric potential due to different charges arrangements.
- Relationship between electric field and electric potential.
- Calculation of work done required to move a charge inside electric field.
- Electric potential energy stored/exhausted in movement of charge in electric field.

For better understanding of this chapter

- Proper practice of differentiation and integration is required.
- Sign convention of work and energy should be revised from class 11th.

Introduction

When an external force does work on a body to move from one point to another, then potential energy get stored in the body. If the body does work against electric force, then the stored potential energy is known as electric potential energy.

In this chapter, we will study electric potential, electric potential due to electric dipole, equipotential surface, potential due to charged sphere and electric potential energy.

Module 1

Electric Potential

- Electric Potential
- Electrostatic Potential due to a Point Charge
- Electric Potential due to a Continuous Charge Distribution
- Electric Potential due to Electric Dipole
- Relation between Electric Field and Electric Potential

Electric Potential

The electric potential at any point in the region of electric field is defined as the amount of work done in bringing a unit positive test charge from infinity to that point along any arbitrary path. It is a scalar quantity and is denoted by V.

$$\text{Electric potential } (V) = \frac{\text{Work done } (W)}{\text{Charge } (q_0)}$$

Unit and Dimensional Formula of Electric Potential

Its SI unit is volt (V) and $1 \text{ volt} = \dfrac{1 \text{ joule}}{1 \text{ coulomb}}$

and CGS unit is stat volt (esu), where $1 \text{ volt} = \dfrac{1}{300}$ stat volt.

Its dimensional formula is $[ML^2T^{-3}A^{-1}]$.

- Electric potential is a relative term, it depends on reference point.

Concept ladder

This work is done against electric field (also known as external work done).

Also, there should not be any change in kinetic energy of the charge in this process. So, electric potential at point P,

$$V_P = \frac{W_{\infty \text{ to } P}}{q_0} \quad \text{(by external agent)}$$

or

$$V_P = -\frac{W_{\infty \text{ to } P}}{q_0} \quad \text{(by electric force)}$$

According to the nature of charge, electric potential can be positive (due to positive charge), negative (due to negative charge) or zero.

Example 1 *How much work will be done in bringing a charge of 400 μC from infinity to some point P in the region of electric field? Given that the electric potential at point P is 20 V.*

Sol. Electric potential at any point can be written as,

$$\text{Electric potential } (V) = \frac{\text{Work done } (W)}{\text{Charge } (q_0)}$$

Given, $V_P = 20 \text{ V}$ and $q_0 = 400\ \mu\text{C} = 400 \times 10^{-6} \text{ C}$

On putting the values in Eq. (i), we get

$$20 = \frac{W}{400 \times 10^{-6}}$$

$$\therefore \quad W = 20 \times 400 \times 10^{-6} = 8 \times 10^{-3} \text{ J}$$

Electric Potential Difference

The electric potential difference between two points A and B is equal to the work done by the external force in moving a unit positive charge against the electrostatic force from point B to A along any path between these two points.

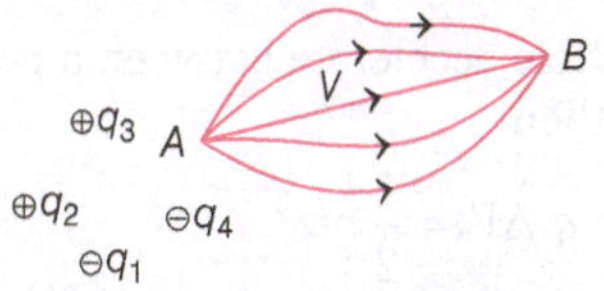

Electric potential between points A and B

If V_A and V_B be the electric potentials at points A and B respectively, then $\Delta V = V_A - V_B$

or $$\Delta V = \frac{W_{AB}}{q}$$

The SI unit of potential difference is volt (V).

The dimensional formula for electric potential difference is given by $[ML^2T^{-3}A^{-1}]$.

Mentor's TIP

- Following three formulae are very useful in the problems related to work done in electric field.

  $(W_{a-b})_{\text{electric force}} = q_0(V_a - V_b)$

  $(W_{a-b})_{\text{external force}} = q_0(V_b - V_a) = -(W_{a-b})_{\text{electric force}}$

  $(W_{a-b})_{\text{external force}} = -q_0(V_a - V_b)$

- Here, q_0, V_a and V_b are to be substituted with sign.

Example 2 *The electric potential at point A is 20 V and at B is −40 V. Find the work done by an external force and electrostatic force in moving an electron slowly from B to A.*

Sol. Here, the test charge is an electron, i.e.

$$q_0 = -1.6 \times 10^{-19} \text{ C}$$

$V_A = 20$ V and $V_B = -40$ V

Work done by external force,

$$(W_{B-A})_{\text{external force}} = q_0(V_A - V_B)$$
$$= (-1.6 \times 10^{-19})[(20) - (-40)]$$
$$= -9.6 \times 10^{-18} \text{ J}$$

Work done by electric force,

$$(W_{B-A})_{\text{electric force}} = -(W_{B-A})_{\text{external force}}$$
$$= -(-9.6 \times 10^{-18} \text{ J})$$
$$= 9.6 \times 10^{-18} \text{ J}$$

Mentor's TiP

Here, we can see that an electron (a negative charge) moves from B (lower potential) to A (higher potential) and the work done by electric force is positive. Therefore, we may conclude that whenever a negative charge moves from a lower potential to higher potential, work done by the electric force is positive or when a positive charge moves from lower potential to higher potential, the work done by the electric force is negative.

Accelerated Charge or Charge Under Electric Field

If a charge moves under only the effect of electric field, then Δ KE = Work done by electric force.

If a charged particle accelerate between a potential difference ΔV, then

$$q\,\Delta V = \frac{1}{2} mv^2$$

Example 3. *A bullet of mass 2 g having a charge of 2 μC. Then through what potential difference must it be accelerated starting from rest to acquire a speed of 10 m/s.*

Sol. Kinetic energy $K = \frac{1}{2} mv^2$

$$q\,\Delta V = \frac{1}{2} mv^2$$

$$\Rightarrow \quad \Delta V = \frac{mv^2}{2q}$$

$$\Delta V = \frac{(2 \times 10^{-3})(10)^2}{2(2 \times 10^{-6})}$$

$$\Delta V = 50 \times 10^3 \text{ V} = 50 \text{ kV}$$

Example 4. *When a charge Q is displaced from potential of 100 V to 600 V, then its kinetic energy increases 8×10^{-15} J. Calculate Q.*

Sol. Kinetic energy $K = Q\Delta V$

$$\Rightarrow \quad Q = \frac{K}{\Delta V} = \frac{8 \times 10^{-15}}{100 - 600}$$
$$= -1.6 \times 10^{-17}$$
$$Q = -1.6 \times 10^{-17} \text{ C}$$

Electrostatic Potential due to a Point Charge

Let, P be the point at a distance r from the origin O at which the electric potential due to point charge $+q$ is required.

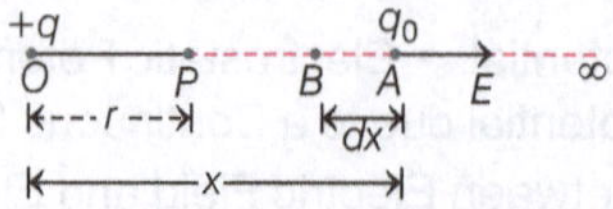

Electrostatic potential due to a point charge

The electric potential at a point P is the amount of work done in carrying a unit positive charge from ∞ to point P.

Suppose a test charge q_0 is placed at point A at distance x from O.

The electrostatic force acting on charge q_0 is given by

$$F = \frac{1}{4\pi\varepsilon_0} \frac{qq_0}{x^2}, \text{ along } OA \quad \text{...(i)}$$

Small work done in moving the charge through a small distance dx from A to B is given by

$$dW = \mathbf{F} \cdot \mathbf{dx}$$
$$= Fdx \cos 180° = -Fdx \quad (\because \cos 180° = -1)$$

Total work done in moving a positive test charge q_0 from ∞ to the point P is given by

$$W = \int_{\infty}^{r} -Fdx$$

$$= \int_{\infty}^{r} -\frac{1}{4\pi\varepsilon_0} \frac{qq_0}{x^2} dx$$

$$= -\frac{qq_0}{4\pi\varepsilon_0}\left[\frac{-1}{x}\right]_{\infty}^{r} \quad \left(\because \int x^{-2} dx = -\frac{1}{x}\right)$$

$$W = \frac{qq_0}{4\pi\varepsilon_0 r} \quad \text{...(iii)}$$

From the definition of electric potential,

$$\therefore \quad V = \frac{W}{q_0} = \frac{q}{4\pi\varepsilon_0 r} \quad \text{...(iv)}$$

A positively charged particle produces a positive electric potential. A negatively charged particle produces a negative electric potential.

Here, we assume that electrostatic potential is zero at infinity. Eq. (iv) shows that at equal distances from a point charge q, value of V is same.

Hence, electrostatic potential due to a single charge is spherically symmetric.

Figure given below shows the variation of electrostatic potential with distance, i.e. $V \propto \frac{1}{r}$.

For positive charge

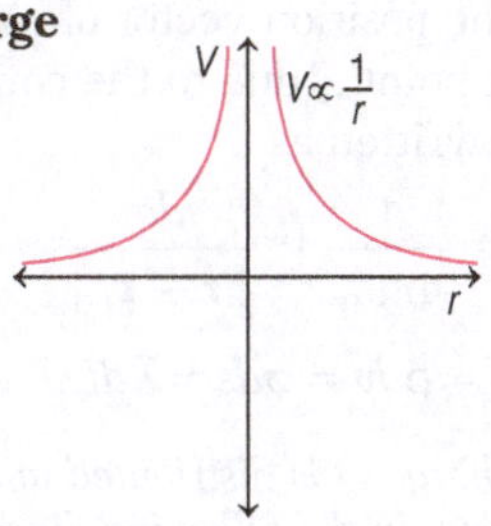

For negative charge

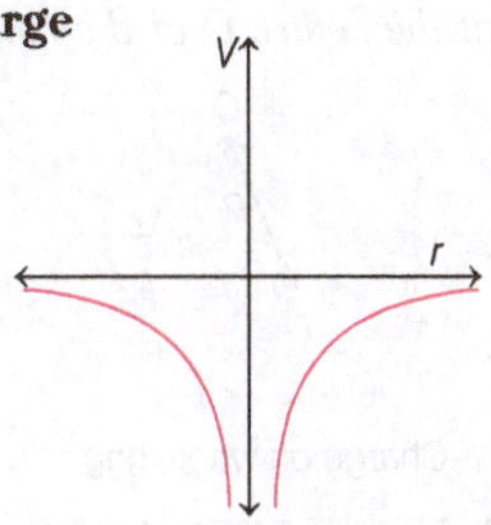

Example 5. *Determine the potential at a point 0.50 m*
(i) from a +20 μC point charge and
(ii) from a −20 μC point charge.

Sol. The potential due to a point charge is given by

$$V = \frac{kq}{r}$$

(i) Potential due to a positive 20 μC charge,

$$V = \frac{kq}{r} = (9.0 \times 10^9)\left(\frac{20 \times 10^{-6}}{0.50}\right)$$

$$= 3.6 \times 10^5 \text{ V}$$

(ii) Potential due to a negative −20 μC charge,

$$V = (9.0 \times 10^9)\left(\frac{-20 \times 10^{-6}}{0.50}\right)$$

$$= -3.6 \times 10^5 \text{ V}$$

Example 6. *What is the electrostatic potential at the surface of a silver nucleus of diameter 12.4 fermi? [Atomic number (Z) for silver is 47]*

Sol. Given, radius of silver nucleus,

$$r = \frac{12.4}{2} = 6.2 \text{ fm}$$

$$= 6.2 \times 10^{-15} \text{ m} \qquad (1 \text{ fermi} = 10^{-15} \text{ m})$$

and $Z = 47$

∴ Charge, $q = Ze = 47 \times 1.6 \times 10^{-19}$ C

∴ Electrostatic potential,

$$V = \frac{q}{4\pi\varepsilon_0 r}$$

$$= \frac{9 \times 10^9 \times 47 \times 1.6 \times 10^{-19}}{6.2 \times 10^{-15}}$$

$$= 1.09 \times 10^7 \text{ V}$$

Mentor's TiP

Potential due to system of charges at a given point is the algebraic sum of potentials due to all charges at that point.

Example 7. *Three point charges each of Q are placed at three corners of an equilateral triangle of side length a. Calculate electrical potential at centre of equilateral triangle.*

Sol. $V = \frac{kQ}{r} + \frac{kQ}{r} + \frac{kQ}{r} = \frac{3kQ}{r}$

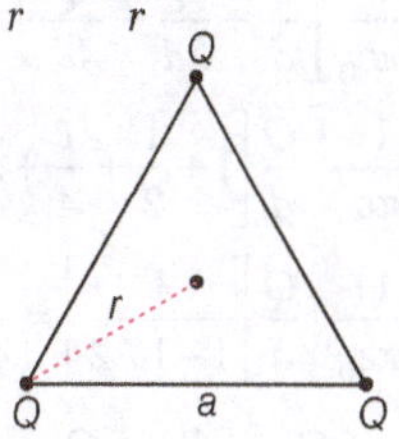

$$r = \frac{a}{\sqrt{3}}$$

$$\Rightarrow \qquad V = \frac{3kQ}{a}\sqrt{3} = \frac{3\sqrt{3}\,kQ}{a}$$

Example 8. *Two point charges of Q and 4Q are placed at distance r from each other. Calculate potential at the point on the line joining of the charges where resultant electric field is zero.*

Sol. Resultant electric field is zero at

$$x = \frac{\sqrt{Q}}{\sqrt{Q} + \sqrt{4Q}}\, r = \frac{\sqrt{Q}}{\sqrt{Q}\,(1+2)}\, r$$

$$\Rightarrow \qquad x = \frac{r}{3} \text{ (neutral point from } Q)$$

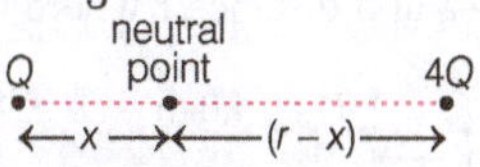

Potential at neutral point

$$V = \frac{kQ}{x} + \frac{k(4Q)}{(r-x)} = \frac{kQ}{r/3} + \frac{k4Q}{2r/3} = \frac{9kQ}{r}$$

Example 9. *Two point charges Q and −Q are placed at (a, 0) and (−a, 0) respectively. Charge q is transfered from origin to position of (2a, 0). Calculate required work done.*

Sol.

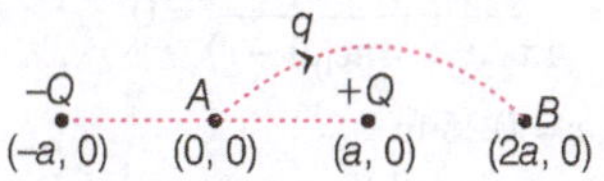

$$V_A = \frac{kQ}{a} - \frac{kQ}{a} = 0;$$

$$V_B = \frac{kQ}{a} - \frac{kQ}{3a} = \frac{2kQ}{3a}$$

$$W_{AB} = q(V_B - V_A)$$

$$= q\left(\frac{2kQ}{3a} - 0\right) = \frac{2kqQ}{3a} = \frac{Qq}{6\pi\varepsilon_0 a}$$

Example 10. *Find the electric potential at the origin O, if (i) Infinite charges each of Q are placed, at x = d, 2d, 4d.... ∞. (ii) A charge +Q is placed at each of the points x = d, x = 3d, x = 5d, ... ∞ on the X-axis, and a charge −Q is placed at each of the points, x = 2d, x = 4d, x = 6d, ..., ∞.*

Sol. (i)

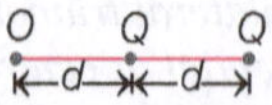

Electric potential,

$$V_O = \frac{1}{4\pi\varepsilon_0}\left[\frac{Q}{d}+\frac{Q}{2d}+\frac{Q}{4d}+\ldots\infty\right]$$

$$= \frac{1}{4\pi\varepsilon_0}\cdot\frac{Q}{d}\left[1+\frac{1}{2}+\frac{1}{4}+\ldots\infty\right]$$

$$= \frac{1}{4\pi\varepsilon_0}\cdot\frac{Q}{d}\left[\frac{1}{1-1/2}\right] = \frac{1}{4\pi\varepsilon_0}\cdot\frac{2Q}{d}$$

(ii)

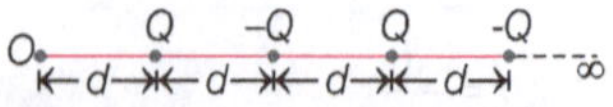

Electric potential,

$$V_O = \frac{1}{4\pi\varepsilon_0}\left[\frac{Q}{d}-\frac{Q}{2d}+\frac{Q}{3d}-\frac{Q}{4d}+\ldots\infty\right]$$

$$= \frac{1}{4\pi\varepsilon_0}\cdot\frac{Q}{d}\left[1-\frac{1}{2}+\frac{1}{3}-\frac{1}{4}+\ldots\infty\right]$$

$$= \frac{1}{4\pi\varepsilon_0}\cdot\frac{Q}{d}\log_e 2$$

Example 11. *Find out the points on the line joining two charges +q and −3q (kept at a distance of 1.0 m), where electric potential is zero.*

Sol. Let P be the point on the axis either to the left or to the right of charge $+q$ at a distance r where potential is zero.

Hence,

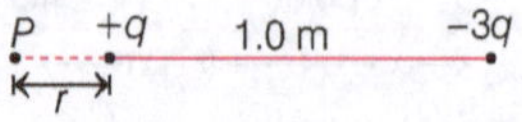

or

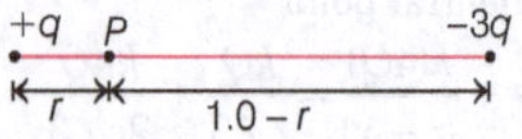

$$V_P = \frac{q}{4\pi\varepsilon_0 r} - \frac{3q}{4\pi\varepsilon_0(1+r)} = 0$$

Solving this, we get $r = 0.5$ m

Further, $V_P = \dfrac{q}{4\pi\varepsilon_0 r} - \dfrac{3q}{4\pi\varepsilon_0(1-r)} = 0$

which gives, $r = 0.25$ m

Thus, the potential will be zero at point P on the axis which is either 0.5 m to the left or 0.25 m to the right of charge $+q$.

Electric Potential due to a Continuous Charge Distribution

We can imagine that a continuous charge distribution consists of a number of small charge elements located at position $\mathbf{r}_i$. If $\mathbf{r}$ is the position vector of point P, then the electric potential at point P due to the continuous charge distribution can be written as

$$V = \frac{1}{4\pi\varepsilon_0}\int \frac{dq}{|\mathbf{r}-\mathbf{r}_i|}$$

Here, $dq = \rho dv = \sigma ds = \lambda dL$

Example 12. *A charge Q is distributed uniformly on a ring of radius R as shown in the following diagram. Find the electric potential at the centre O of the ring.*

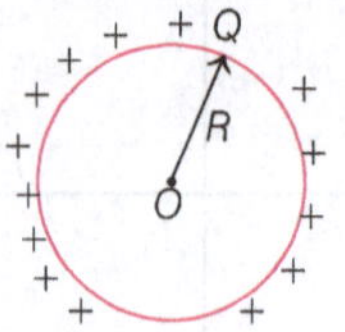

Charge on whole ring

Sol. Consider a small charge dq. Electric potential at O due to dq,

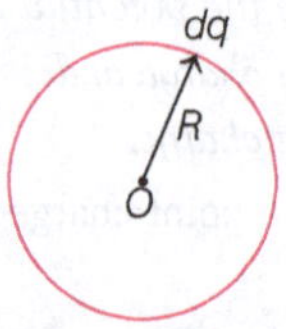

$$dV = \frac{1}{4\pi\varepsilon_0}\cdot\frac{dq}{R}$$

$$V_0 = \Sigma dV = \frac{1}{4\pi\varepsilon_0 R}\Sigma dq = \frac{1}{4\pi\varepsilon_0}\cdot\frac{Q}{R}$$

Electric Potential due to Electric Dipole

Let AB be an electric dipole of length $2a$ and let P be any point, where $OP = r$.

Let θ be the angle between r and the dipole axis.

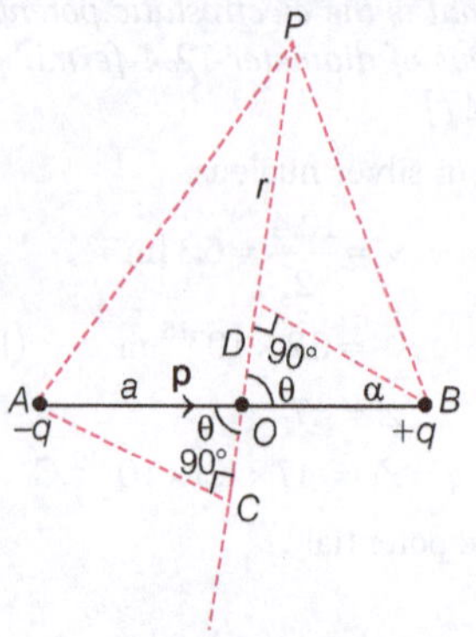

Electric dipole

Here, $AB = 2a$, $AO = OB = a$ and $OP = r$

In ΔOAC, $\cos\theta = \dfrac{OC}{OA} = \dfrac{OC}{a}$

$\therefore \quad OC = a\cos\theta$

Also, $OD = a\cos\theta$

If $r >> a, PA = PC$

$= OP + OC = r + a\cos\theta$

$PB = PD = OP - OD = r - a\cos\theta$

V is the potential due to electric dipole,

$$V = \left(\frac{1}{4\pi\varepsilon_0}\right)\left[\frac{q}{PB} - \frac{q}{PA}\right]$$

$$V = \left(\frac{1}{4\pi\varepsilon_0}\right)q\left[\frac{1}{(r - a\cos\theta)} - \frac{1}{(r + a\cos\theta)}\right]$$

$$V = \left(\frac{1}{4\pi\varepsilon_0}\right)\left[\frac{2aq\cos\theta}{r^2 - a^2\cos\theta}\right]$$

$$V = \left(\frac{1}{4\pi\varepsilon_0}\right)\frac{p\cos\theta}{(r^2 - a^2\cos^2\theta)} \quad (\because p = 2aq)$$

If $r >> a$, $a^2\cos^2\theta$ can be neglected in comparison to r^2, then the resultant potential at point P,

$$V = \frac{1}{4\pi\varepsilon_0}\frac{p\cos\theta}{r^2}$$

where, p is dipole moment.

Special Cases

(i) When the point P lies on the axial line of the dipole on the side of positive charge,

$\theta = 0° \Rightarrow \cos\theta = 1$

$$\therefore \quad V = \left(\frac{1}{4\pi\varepsilon_0}\right)\frac{p}{(r^2 - a^2)}$$

If r is very large as compared to $2a$, i.e. $r >> 2a$, then a^2 can be neglected in comparison to r^2, then potential at the point P,

$$V = \frac{1}{4\pi\varepsilon_0}\cdot\frac{p}{r^2}$$

(ii) When P lies on other side, $\theta = 180°$

$\Rightarrow \quad \cos\theta = -1$

$$\therefore \quad V = -\left(\frac{1}{4\pi\varepsilon_0}\right)\frac{p}{(r^2 - a^2)}$$

If $r >> a$, then $V = -\frac{1}{4\pi\varepsilon_0}\cdot\frac{p}{r^2}$

(iii) When the point P lies on equatorial line, $\theta = 90°$

$\Rightarrow \quad \cos\theta = 0$

$\therefore \quad V = 0$

(iv) In general, $V = \left(\frac{1}{4\pi\varepsilon_0}\right)\frac{\mathbf{p}\cdot\mathbf{r}}{r^3}$, for a short dipole, at a point whose position vector with respect to dipole is **r**.

NEET Close-up

Example Similar to PYQ Asked in NEET 2023

An electric dipole is placed as shown in the figure.

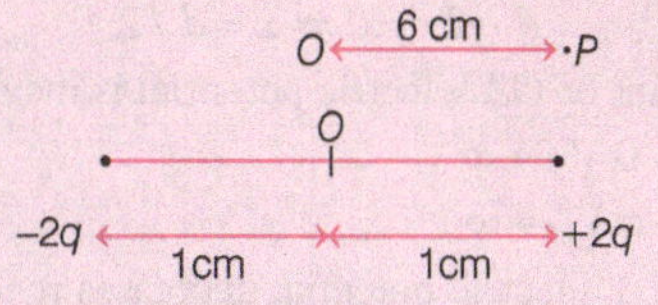

The electric potential (in 10^2 V) at point P due to the dipole is (ε_0 = permittivity of free space and $\frac{1}{4\pi\varepsilon_0} = K$)

(a) $\left(\frac{1}{9}\right)qK$ (b) $\left(\frac{1}{18}\right)qK$ (c) $\left(\frac{3}{8}\right)qK$ (d) $\left(\frac{2}{3}\right)qK$

Sol. (a) Electric potential at point P due to electric dipole,

$$V = \frac{1}{4\pi\varepsilon_0}\cdot\frac{p}{r^2} = K\frac{p}{r^2} = K\frac{2q \times 2a}{r^2}$$

Here, $r = 6\text{ cm} = 6 \times 10^{-2}$ m

$2a = (1 + 1)\text{ cm} = 2\text{ cm} = 2 \times 10^{-2}$ m

$$\therefore \quad V = \frac{K(2q)(2 \times 10^{-2})}{(6 \times 10^{-2})^2} = \left(\frac{1}{9}\right)Kq \times (10^2\text{ V})$$

Skill Builder

An electric dipole consists of two charges of equal magnitude and opposite sign separately by a distance $2a$ as shown in figure. The dipole is along the X-axis and is centred at the origin.

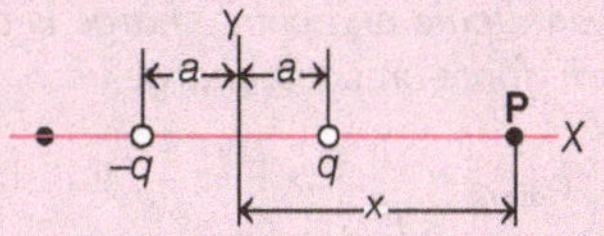

The electric potential at point P is

(a) $\frac{K_e qa}{x^2 - a^2}$ (b) $\frac{2K_e qa}{x^2 - a^2}$ (c) $\frac{2K_e qa}{x^2 + a^2}$ (d) $\frac{K_e qa}{(x - a)^2}$

For more Practice Refer Q. No. 12, 15 of step up practice 1 and Q.No. 3, 14, 26 of Gearing up for NEET.

Example 13. *Sketch the variation of electric potential on the X-axis with respect to x for $x = -\infty$ to $x = +\infty$ in the following case.*

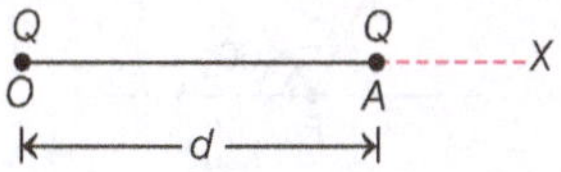

Sol.

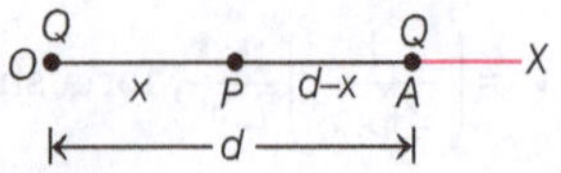

Electric potential at P,

$$V_P = \frac{1}{4\pi\varepsilon_0}\left[\frac{Q}{x} + \frac{Q}{d-x}\right] = \frac{Q}{4\pi\varepsilon_0} \cdot \frac{d}{x(d-x)}$$

V_P is minimum, if $x(d-x)$ is maximum.

$x(d-x)$ is maximum,

if $\frac{d}{dx} x(d-x) = 0$

$\Rightarrow \quad d - 2x = 0 \Rightarrow x = d/2$

At mid-point of OA, electric potential is maximum.

At $O: x \to 0, V \to \infty$

At $A: x \to d, V \to \infty$

From O to A, electric potential decreases reaching to minimum value and then increases.

Left of O: At distance x from O,

$$V = \frac{1}{4\pi\varepsilon_0}\left[\frac{Q}{x} + \frac{Q}{d+x}\right]$$

$x \to 0, V \to \infty, x \to -\infty, V \to 0$

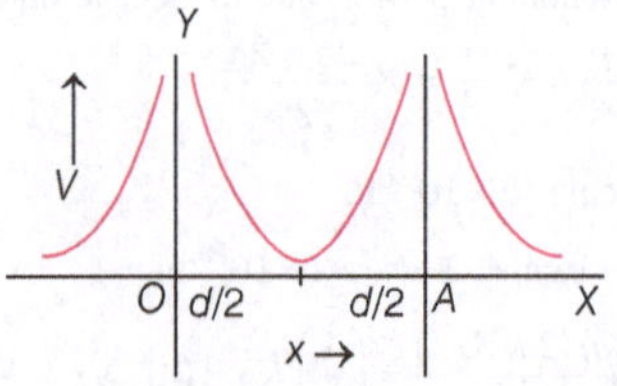

Right of A : At distance x from O,

$$V = \frac{1}{4\pi\varepsilon_0}\left[\frac{Q}{x} + \frac{Q}{x-d}\right]$$

$x \to d, V \to \infty, x \to \infty, V \to 0$

Example 14. *A point charge is placed in electric field of electric dipole. Electric force on point charge is F. If distance between dipole and point charge is doubled, then find new electric force on point charge?*

Sol. $F = qE_{\text{dipole}}; \left(E_{\text{dipole}} \propto \frac{1}{r^3}\right) \Rightarrow F \propto \frac{1}{r^3}$. If distance is doubled, then $\Rightarrow F_2 = \frac{F}{8}$

Example 15. *A small dipole of dipole moment p is placed at the origin along X-axis. A charge q is transfered from A(r, 120°) to B(r, 60°) in electric field of dipole. Calculate work done on the charge. (Assume gravity free space)*

Sol.

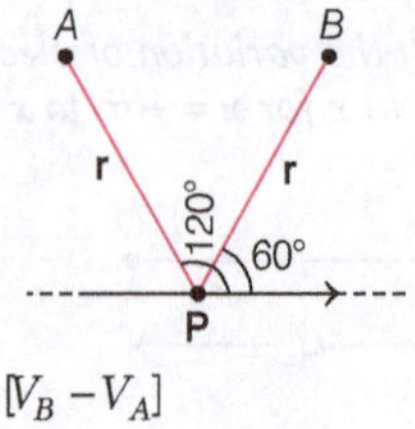

$$W_{AB} = q[V_B - V_A]$$

$$= q\left[\frac{kp\cos 60^\circ}{r^2} - \frac{kp\cos 120^\circ}{r^2}\right]$$

$$W_{AB} = \frac{qkp}{r^2}\left[\frac{1}{2} - \left(-\frac{1}{2}\right)\right] = \frac{kpq}{r^2} = \frac{pq}{4\pi\varepsilon_0 r^2}$$

Relation between Electric Field and Electric Potential

Let us first consider the case when electric potential V is shown and we want to calculate **E**. The relation is as under, in case of cartesian coordinates.

$$\mathbf{E} = E_x\hat{\mathbf{i}} + E_y\hat{\mathbf{j}} + E_z\hat{\mathbf{k}}$$

Here, $E_x = -\frac{\partial V}{\partial x} = -$ (partial derivative of V w.r.t. x)

$E_y = -\frac{\partial V}{\partial y} = -$ (partial derivative of V w.r.t. y)

$E_z = -\frac{\partial V}{\partial z} = -$ (partial derivative of V w.r.t. z)

$$\mathbf{E} = -\left[\frac{\partial V}{\partial x}\hat{\mathbf{i}} + \frac{\partial V}{\partial y}\hat{\mathbf{j}} + \frac{\partial V}{\partial z}\hat{\mathbf{k}}\right]$$

Sometimes it is also written as,

$$\mathbf{E} = -\text{gradient } V$$

$$= -\text{grad } V = -\nabla V = -\frac{dV}{dr}$$

$$\boxed{\mathbf{E} = -\frac{dV}{dr}}$$

Here, negative sign shows that the potential decreases in the direction of electric field.

Potential gradient is a vector quantity.

Concept ladder

- If electric field is variable

  $V_A - V_B = -\int_{r_B}^{r_A} \mathbf{E} \cdot d\mathbf{r}$

- If electric field is uniform, then in vector form,

  $V_A - V_B = -\mathbf{E} \cdot (\mathbf{r}_A - \mathbf{r}_B)$

  and in scalar form,

  $V_A - V_B = \pm E(d)$

  where, d is distance between points.

Example 16. *The electric potential in a region is represented as $V = 2x + 3y - z$*

Obtain expression for electric field strength.

Sol. As we know,

$$\mathbf{E} = -\left[\frac{\partial V}{\partial x}\hat{\mathbf{i}} + \frac{\partial V}{\partial y}\hat{\mathbf{j}} + \frac{\partial V}{\partial z}\hat{\mathbf{k}}\right]$$

So, $\frac{\partial V}{\partial x} = \frac{\partial}{\partial x}(2x + 3y - z) = 2$

$$\frac{\partial V}{\partial y} = \frac{\partial}{\partial y}(2x + 3y - z) = 3$$

$$\frac{\partial V}{\partial z} = \frac{\partial}{\partial z}(2x + 3y - z) = -1$$

Electric field, $\mathbf{E} = -2\hat{\mathbf{i}} - 3\hat{\mathbf{j}} + \hat{\mathbf{k}}$

Example 17. *In uniform electric field, $\mathbf{E} = 10\ \text{NC}^{-1}$, as shown in figure, find*

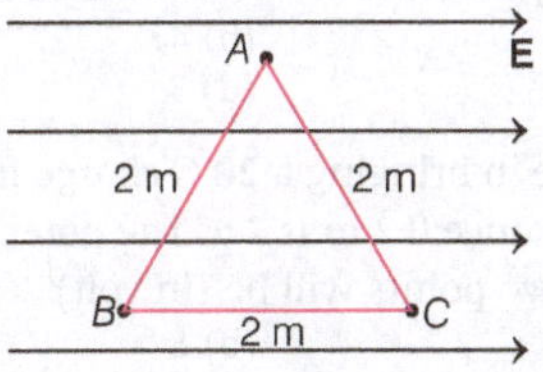

(i) $V_A - V_B$

(ii) $V_B - V_C$

Sol. (i) $V_B > V_A$, so $V_A - V_B$ will be negative.

Further, horizontal distance between A and B is

$$d_{AB} = 2\cos 60° = 1\ \text{m}$$

$$\therefore \quad V_A - V_B = -Ed_{AB} = (-10)(1) = -10\ \text{V}$$

(ii) $V_B > V_C$, so $V_B - V_C$ will be positive.

Further, $d_{BC} = 2.0$ m

$$\therefore \quad V_B - V_C = (10)(2) = 20\ \text{V}$$

Example 18. *A uniform electric field of $100\ \text{Vm}^{-1}$ is directed at $30°$ with the positive X-axis as shown in figure. Find the potential difference V_{BA}, if $OA = 2$ m and $OB = 4$ m.*

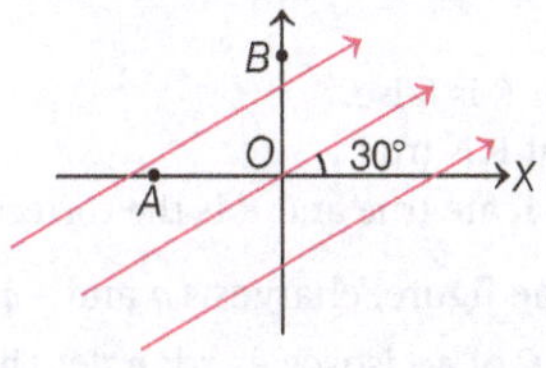

Sol. Electric field in vector form can be written as

$$\mathbf{E} = (100\cos 30°\ \hat{\mathbf{i}} + 100\sin 30°\ \hat{\mathbf{j}})\ \text{Vm}^{-1}$$

$$= (50\sqrt{3}\ \hat{\mathbf{i}} + 50\hat{\mathbf{j}})\ \text{Vm}^{-1}$$

$$A = (-2\ \text{m}, 0, 0)$$

and $\quad B = (0, 4\ \text{m}, 0)$

$$\therefore \quad V_{BA} = V_B - V_A = -\int_A^B \mathbf{E}\cdot d\mathbf{r}$$

$$= -\int_{(-2\,\text{m},0,0)}^{(0,4\,\text{m},0)} (50\sqrt{3}\ \hat{\mathbf{i}} + 50\hat{\mathbf{j}})\cdot(dx\,\hat{\mathbf{i}} + dy\,\hat{\mathbf{j}} + dz\,\hat{\mathbf{k}})$$

$$= -[50\sqrt{3}\ x + 50y]_{(-2\,\text{m},0,0)}^{(0,4\,\text{m},0)}$$

$$= -100(2 + \sqrt{3})\ \text{V}$$

Example 19. *Electric field is given by $E = \dfrac{100}{x^2}$ V/m. Find the potential difference between $x = 10$ m and $x = 20$ m.*

Sol. $V_1 - V_2 = -\int_{x_2}^{x_1} \mathbf{E}\cdot dx$

$$= -\int_{20}^{10} \frac{100}{x^2}\,dx = -100\left[-\frac{1}{x}\right]_{20}^{10} = 5\ \text{V}$$

Example 20. *There is a long linear charge distribution of linear charge density λ as shown. Calculate work done to transfer a charge q from point A to B.*

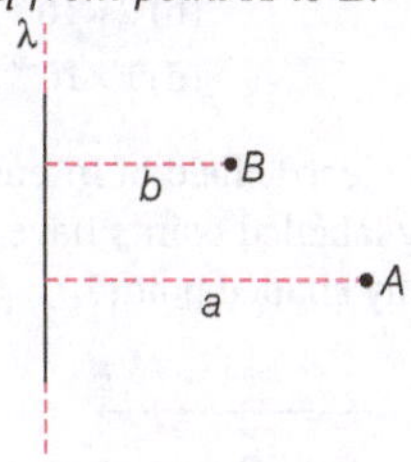

Sol. $W_{AB} = q(V_B - V_A)$ ...(i)

$$V_B - V_A = -\int_{r_A}^{r_B} \mathbf{E}\cdot d\mathbf{r};\ E = \frac{\lambda}{2\pi\varepsilon_0 r}$$

$$V_B - V_A = -\int_a^b \frac{\lambda}{2\pi\varepsilon_0 r}\,dr$$

$$= -\frac{\lambda}{2\pi\varepsilon_0}[\log_e r]_a^b = \frac{\lambda}{2\pi\varepsilon_0}[\log_e r]_b^a$$

$$= \frac{\lambda}{2\pi\varepsilon_0}\ln\frac{a}{b} \quad \text{...(ii)}$$

By Eqs. (i) and (ii)

$$\Rightarrow \quad W_{AB} = \frac{q\lambda}{2\pi\varepsilon_0}\ln\frac{a}{b}$$

Example 21. *Electric field in a region is $\mathbf{E} = 3\hat{\mathbf{i}} + 4\hat{\mathbf{j}}$ V/m. Calculate potential difference between points A(2, 3) and B(5, 7).*

Sol. $V_A - V_B = -\mathbf{E}\cdot(\mathbf{r}_A - \mathbf{r}_B) = -\mathbf{E}\cdot[(2\hat{\mathbf{i}} + 3\hat{\mathbf{j}}) - (5\hat{\mathbf{i}} + 7\hat{\mathbf{j}})]$

$$= (9 + 16)\ \text{volt} = 25\ \text{V}$$

Example 22. *An oil drop B has charge 1.6×10^{-19} C and mass 1.6×10^{-14} kg. If the drop is in equilibrium position, then what will be the potential difference between the plates. [The distance between the plates is 10 mm]*

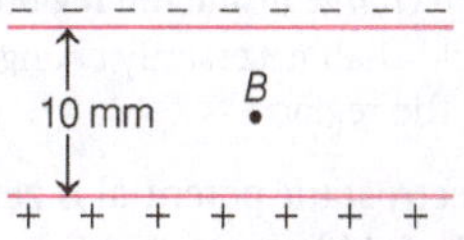

Sol. When a charged particle is in equilibrium in vertically directed electric field, the following formula is often used $qE = mg$

$$qE = mg \Rightarrow q\left(\frac{\Delta V}{d}\right) = mg$$

$$\Rightarrow \quad \Delta V = \frac{mgd}{q} = \frac{1.6\times10^{-14}\times 9.8\times10\times10^{-3}}{1.6\times10^{-19}}$$

$$\Rightarrow \quad \Delta V = 10^4\ \text{V}$$

STEP UP Practice 1

1. Find the work done by some external force in moving a charge $q = 4\ \mu C$ from infinity to a point, where electric potential is 10^4 V.
(a) 4×10^{-2} J (b) 2×10^{-2} J
(c) 8×10^{-2} J (d) 1×10^{-2} J

2. There is a uniform electric field of intensity E which is as shown. How many labelled points have the same electric potential as the fully shaded point?

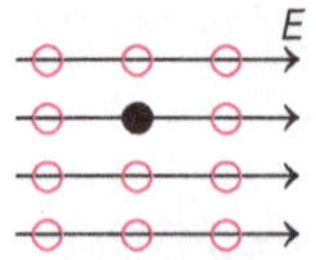

(a) 2 (b) 3
(c) 8 (d) 11

3. The electric potential at a point in free space due to a charge Q coulomb is $Q \times 10^{11}$ volts. The electric field at the point is
(a) $4\pi\varepsilon_0 Q \times 10^{20}$ Vm^{-1} (b) $12\pi\varepsilon_0 Q \times 10^{22}$ Vm^{-1}
(c) $4\pi\varepsilon_0 Q \times 10^{22}$ Vm^{-1} (d) $12\pi\varepsilon_0 Q \times 10^{20}$ Vm^{-1}

4. In an hydrogen atom, the electron revolves around the nucleus in an orbit of radius 0.53×10^{-10} m. Then, the electrical potential produced by the nucleus at the position of the electron is
(a) -13.6 V (b) -27.2 V
(c) 27.2 V (d) 13.6 V

5. Three charges $2q, -q, -q$ are located at the vertices of an equilateral triangle. At the centre of the triangle
(a) the field is zero but potential is non-zero
(b) the field is non-zero but potential is zero
(c) Both field and potential are zero
(d) Both field and potential are non-zero

6. In a region of constant potential
(a) the electric field is uniform
(b) the electric field is zero
(c) there can be no charge inside the region
(d) the electric field shall necessarily change if a charge is placed outside the region

7. **Statement I** Electrostatic potential is zero at a point, where the electric field is zero.
Statement II The electric potential is constant in a given region, the electric field in that region is zero.
In the light of the above statements, choose the most appropriate answer from the options given below.
(a) Both Statement I and Statement II are incorrect.
(b) Statement I is correct but Statement II is incorrect.
(c) Statement I is incorrect but Statement II is correct.
(d) Both Statement I and Statement II are correct.

8. A particle of mass 1.96×10^{-15} kg is kept in equilibrium between two horizontal metal plates having potential difference of 400 V separated apart by 0.02 m. Then, the charge on the particle is (e = electronic charge)
(a) $2e$ (b) $4e$
(c) $6e$ (d) $3e$

9. The work done in bringing a 20 C charge from point A to point B for distance 0.2 m is 2 J. The potential difference between the two points will be (in volt)
(a) 0.2 (b) 8
(c) 0.1 (d) 0.4

10. The electric field in a certain region is given by $E = (5\hat{\mathbf{i}} - 3\hat{\mathbf{j}})$ kV/m. The potential difference $V_B - V_A$ between points A and B, having coordinates (4, 0, 3) m and (10, 3, 0) m respectively, is equal to
(a) 21 kV (b) 23 kV
(c) -39 kV (d) 39 kV

11. **Assertion** (A) Electric potential on the axis of a charged ring is maximum at a point perpendicular to the centre of the ring.
Reason (R) At the point perpendicular to the centre of the ring, the distance from each point charge on the ring is maximum.
In the light of above statements, choose the most appropriate answer from the options given below
(a) Both A and R are true but R is not the correct explanation of A.
(b) A is true but R is false.
(c) A is false but R is true.
(d) Both A and R are true and R is the correct explanation of A.

12. As shown in the figure, charges $+q$ and $-q$ are placed at the vertices B and C of an isosceles triangle. The potential at the vertex A is

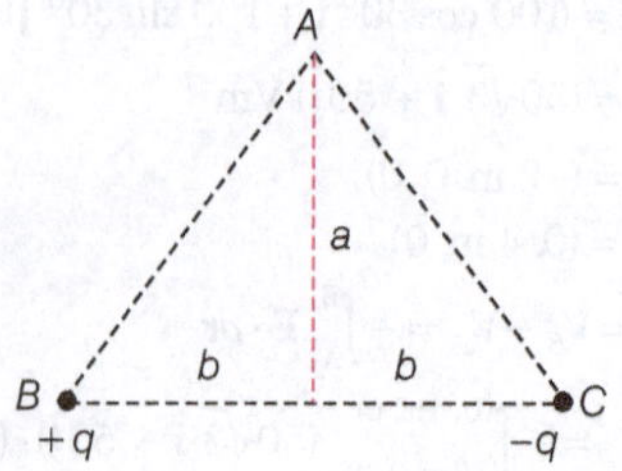

(a) $\frac{1}{4\pi\varepsilon_0} \cdot \frac{2q}{\sqrt{a^2 + b^2}}$
(b) zero
(c) $\frac{1}{4\pi\varepsilon_0} \cdot \frac{q}{\sqrt{a^2 + b^2}}$
(d) $\frac{1}{4\pi\varepsilon_0} \cdot \frac{(-q)}{\sqrt{a^2 + b^2}}$

13. In the rectangle shown below, the two corners have charges $q_1 = -5\,\mu C$ and $q_2 = 2.0\,\mu C$. The work done in moving a charge $+3.0\,\mu C$ from B to A is (take, $k = 10^{10}\ N\text{-}m^2/C^2$)

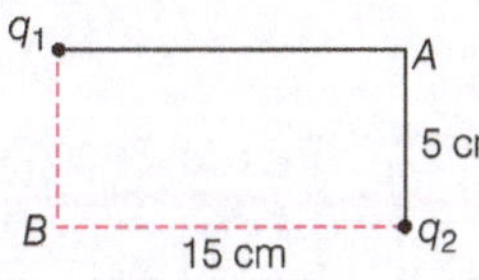

(a) 2.8 J (b) 3.5 J
(c) 4.5 J (d) 5.5 J

14. In an electric field $E = (3\hat{i} + 5\hat{j})$ N/C, electric potential at origin is 0 volt. Below the given options which one is not correct?
(a) Potential at (3, 0) is −9 V
(b) Potential at (−4, 0) is 12 V
(c) Potential at (0, 6) is −30 V
(d) Potential at (0, − 5) is 24 V

15. Two point charges $-q$ and $+q$ are located at points $(0, 0, -a)$ and $(0, 0, a)$ respectively. The potential at a point $(0, 0, z)$, where $z > a$ is
(a) $\frac{qa}{4\pi\varepsilon_0 z^2}$ (b) $\frac{qa}{4\pi\varepsilon_0 a}$
(c) $\frac{2qa}{4\pi\varepsilon_0 (z^2 - a^2)}$ (d) $\frac{2qa}{4\pi\varepsilon_0 (z^2 + a^2)}$

16. Two plates are 2 cm apart and a potential difference is 10 V is applied between them, then the electric field between the plates is
(a) 20 NC^{-1} (b) 500 NC^{-1}
(c) 5 NC^{-1} (d) 250 NC^{-1}

17. At a certain distance from a point charge the electric field is 500 Vm^{-1} and the potential is 3000 V. What is this distance?
(a) 6 m (b) 12 m
(c) 36 m (d) 144 m

18. Two charges of 4 μC each are placed at the corners A and B of an equilateral triangle ABC of side length 0.2 m in air. The electric potential at C is $\left[\frac{1}{4\pi\varepsilon_0} = 9 \times 10^9\ N\text{-}m^2C^{-2}\right]$
(a) 9×10^4 V (b) 18×10^4 V
(c) 36×10^4 V (d) 36×10^{-4} V

19. The electric potential V at any point $O(x, y, z$ all in metres) in space is given by $V = 4x^2$ V. The electric field at the point (1 m, 0, 2 m) in volt metre^{-1} is
(a) 8, along negative X-axis
(b) 8, along positive X-axis
(c) 16, along negative X-axis
(d) 16, along positive Z-axis

20. The electric potential V is given as a function of distance x (metre) by $V = (5x^2 + 10x - 9)$ V. Value of electric field at $x = 1$ is
(a) −20 Vm^{-1} (b) 6 Vm^{-1}
(c) 11 Vm^{-1} (d) −23 Vm^{-1}

21. **Statement I** Electric potential due to dipole $\propto \frac{1}{r^2}$.

Statement II Electric potential due to a point charge $\propto \frac{1}{r^2}$.

In the light of the above statements, choose the most appropriate answer from the options given below
(a) Both Statement I and Statement II are incorrect.
(b) Statement I is correct but Statement II is incorrect.
(c) Statement I is incorrect but Statement II is correct.
(d) Both Statement I and Statement II are correct.

22. In the following question condition of electric potential and proportionality of their r are given which of the following pair is not correctly paired.
(a) Point charge —$1/r$
(b) Electric dipole —$1/r^2$
(c) Quadrupole —$1/r^3$
(d) Octupole —$1/r^8$

23. Find correct statement
(a) Electric potential can't be calculated for variable electric field.
(b) Electric potential can't be calculated for constant electric field.
(c) Electric potential difference is absolute quantity.
(d) Electric potential difference can't be calculated for variable electric field.

Module 2

Applications of Electric Potential

- Equipotential Surface • Potential due to Charged Sphere • Motion of Charged Particle in Electric Field
- Kinetic Energy of a Charged Particle • Work Done by a Charged Particle

Equipotential Surface

Any surface over which the electric potential is same everywhere is called an **equipotential surface.** For a single charge q, the potential is given by $V = \frac{1}{4\pi\varepsilon_0} \frac{q}{r}$.

This shows that if r is constant, then V will be constant. Thus, equipotential surfaces of a single point charge are concentric spherical surfaces centred at the charge.

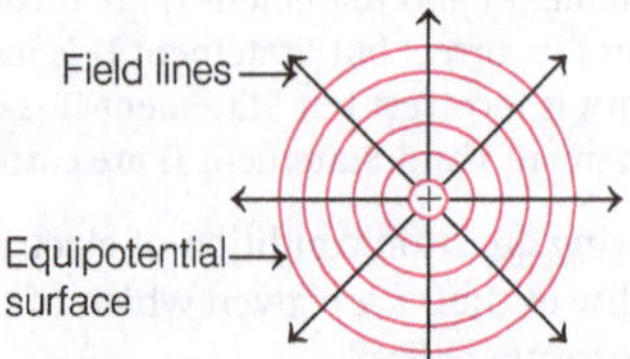

Concentric spherical surfaces having charge q at the centre

Properties of a Equipotential Surfaces

(i) Potential difference between any two points on an equipotential surface is zero.

(ii) Two equipotential surfaces can never intersect each other. If two equipotential surfaces intersect each other, then at the point of intersection of these, there will be two directions of electric field which is impossible.

(iii) As, the work done by electric force is zero when a test charge is moved along the equipotential surface, it follows that **E** must be perpendicular to the surface at every point, so that the electric force $q_0\mathbf{E}$ will always be perpendicular to the displacement of a charge moving on the surface. Thus, field lines and equipotential surfaces are always mutually perpendicular.

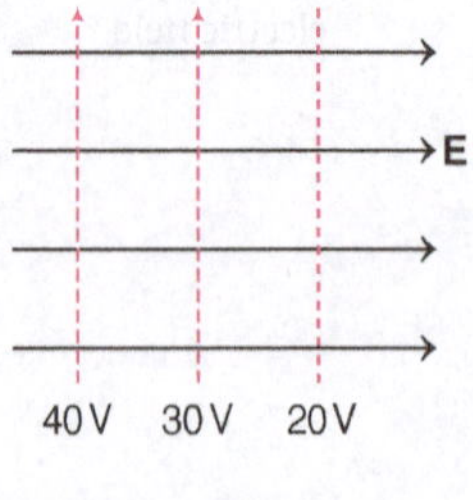

(iv) Equipotential surfaces are always perpendicular to electric line of force.

Equipotential Surface for Charge Distribution

(i) The equipotential surfaces are a family of concentric spheres for a point charge or a sphere of charge as shown in the following figures.

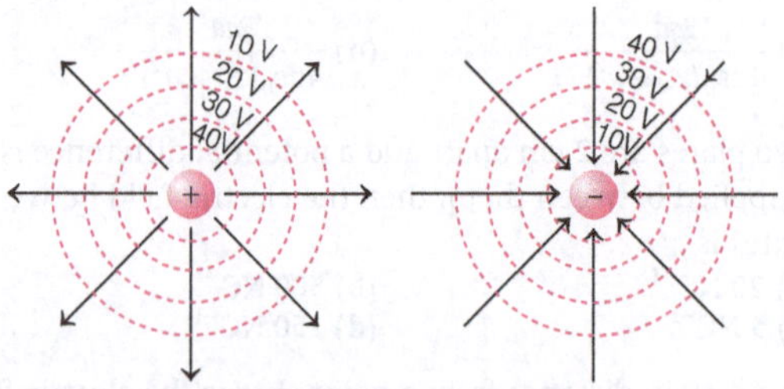

Equipotential surfaces

(ii) When potential is applied between two charged plates, electric field (**E**) is setup between them and this **E** is normal to the equipotential surface as shown below

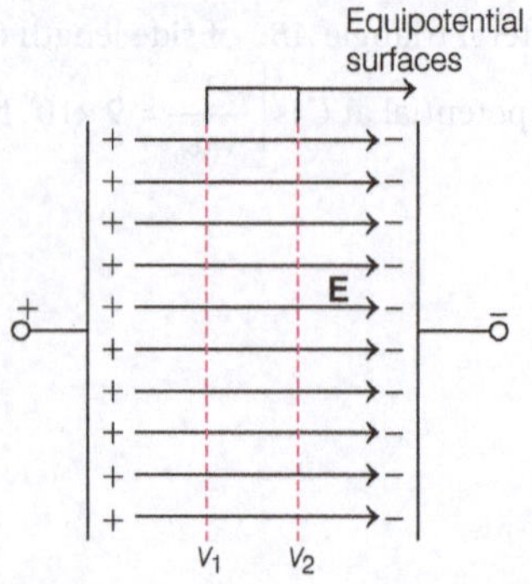

Equipotential surfaces between two charged plates

(iii) The equipotential surfaces are a family of concentric cylinders for a line of charge or cylinder of charge. Equipotential surface for line charge is shown below

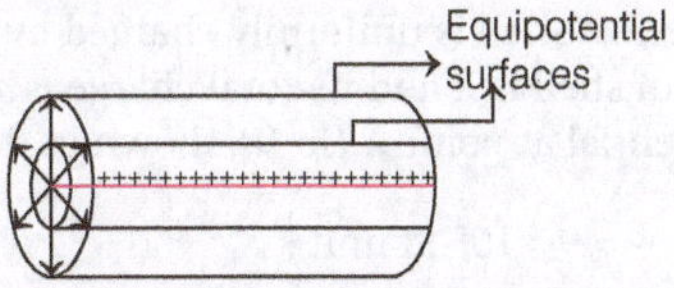

Equipotential surfaces for a line charge distribution

(iv) Equipotential surfaces for two positive charges of equal magnitude are shown below

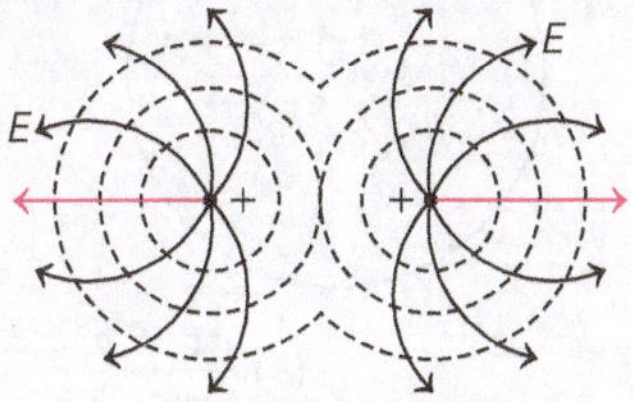

Equipotential surfaces for like charges

(v) Equipotential surfaces for two equal and opposite charges can be drawn as

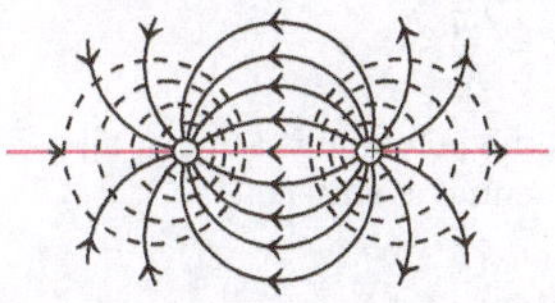

Equipotential surfaces for unlike charges

Mentor's TIP

While drawing the equipotential surfaces, we should keep in mind the two main points.

- These are perpendicular to electric field lines at all places.
- Electric field lines always flow from higher potential to lower potential.

Example 23 *A charge +Q is placed at the centre of a circle. What will be the amount of work done in carrying a charge q from B to C in the figure?*

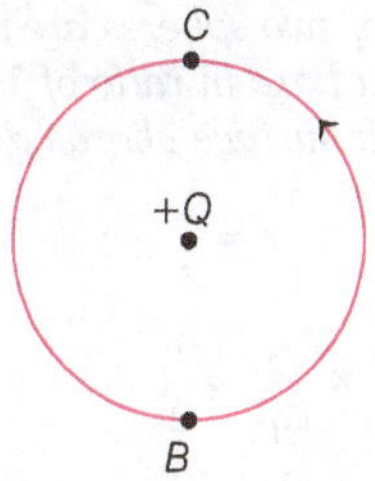

Sol. As circumference of circle in given figure is equipotential surface.

Hence, $V_C - V_B = 0 \Rightarrow W = q(V_C - V_B) = 0$

Example 24 *Some equipotential surfaces are shown in the figure below. Calculate electric field and direction of the electric field in this region.*

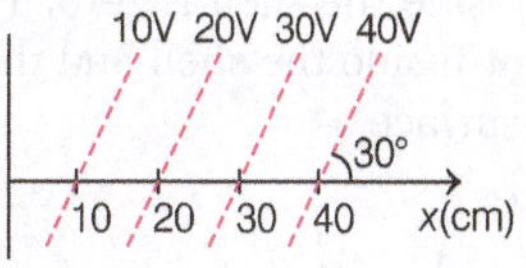

Sol. We know that, **E** is always perpendicular to the equipotential surfaces and points in that direction in which the potential is decreasing.

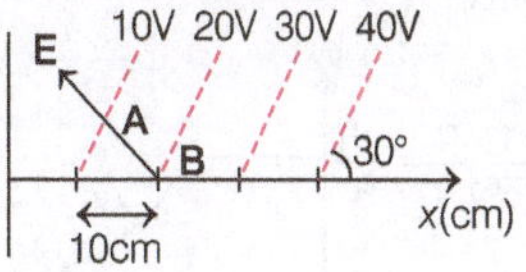

So it will be as shown below

Electric field in this region is uniform so potential difference $\Delta V = Ed$

$$E = \frac{\Delta V}{d}$$

(Here d is the length of $AB = 10 \sin 30°$ cm $= 5$ cm $= 5 \times 10^{-2}$ m)

$$E = \frac{10\text{ V}}{5 \times 10^{-2}\text{ m}} = 200\text{ V/m}$$

Hence, the electric field **E** has the value 200 V/m and makes 120° with positive X-axis.

Potential Due to Charged Sphere

Electric potential due to conducting and non-conducting charged sphere are given below

Electric Potential due to a Conducting Charged Sphere or Shell

Let us consider a uniformly charged spherical shell. The radius of shell is R and its total charge is q, which is uniformly distributed over the surface. We can construct a Gaussian surface (a sphere) of radius $r > R$.

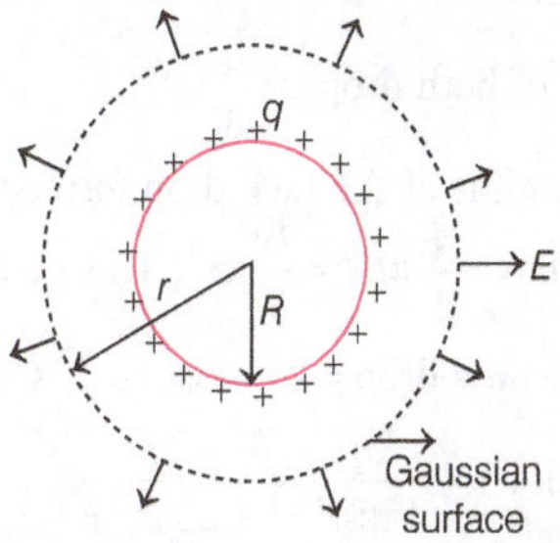

At external points, the potential at any point is the same when the whole charge is assumed to be concentrated at the centre. At the surface of the sphere, $r = R$

$\therefore$ Potential, $V = \dfrac{1}{4\pi\varepsilon_0} \cdot \dfrac{q}{R}$

The electric field inside the shell is zero. This implies that potential is constant inside the shell and therefore equals to its value at the surface.

Thus, we can write,

$$V_{\text{inside}} = V_{\text{surface}} = \frac{1}{4\pi\varepsilon_0} \cdot \frac{q}{R} \text{ and } V_{\text{outside}} = \frac{1}{4\pi\varepsilon_0} \cdot \frac{q}{r}$$

The potential (V) varies with the distance from the centre (r) as shown in figure.

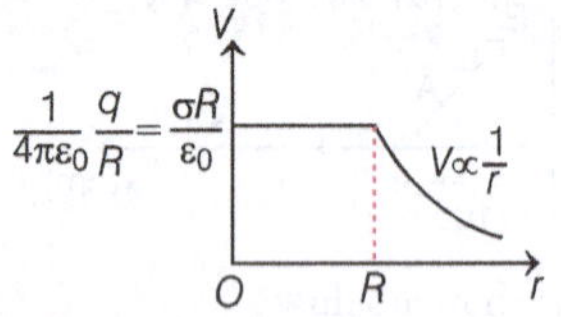

NEET Snapshot

If two spheres are charged with the same charge, then the potential on the smaller sphere is greater. ***[NEET 2022]***

Since, $V \propto \dfrac{1}{R}$, thus the sphere having smaller radius will have greater potential.

Scan for Video

Example 25 *A spherical drop of water carrying a charge of* 3×10^{-19} *C has a potential of 500 V at its surface. What is the radius of the drop? If two drops of the same charge and the same radius combine to form a single spherical drop, what is the potential at the surface of the new drop?*

Sol. The potential V is given by $V = \dfrac{q}{4\pi\varepsilon_0 r}$

Here, $q = 3 \times 10^{-19}$ C and $V = 500$ V

Hence, $r = \dfrac{q}{4\pi\varepsilon_0 V} = \dfrac{9 \times 10^9 \times 3 \times 10^{-19}}{500} = 5.4 \times 10^{-12}$ m

Volume of one drop is $\dfrac{4}{3}\pi r^3$.

Total volume of both drops is $\dfrac{8}{3}\pi r^3$.

Let r' be the radius of the new drop formed, equating the volumes, we have $\dfrac{4}{3}\pi r'^3 = \dfrac{8}{3}\pi r^3$. This gives, $r' = 2^{1/3} r$.

Charge on the new drop $= 2q = 6 \times 10^{-19}$ C

New potential, $V' = \dfrac{2q}{4\pi\varepsilon_0 r'} = \dfrac{2q}{4\pi\varepsilon_0 2^{1/3} r}$

Hence, by putting values, we get

$$V' = \frac{1000}{2^{1/3}} = 794 \text{ V}$$

NEET Close-up

Example Similar to PYQ Asked in NEET 2024

A thin spherical shell is uniformly charged by some source. The radius of shell is R and its total charge is q, then the electric potential at point A (in V) shown in the figure is

$\left(\text{Take, } \dfrac{1}{4\pi\varepsilon_0} = 9 \times 10^9 \text{ SI unit}\right)$

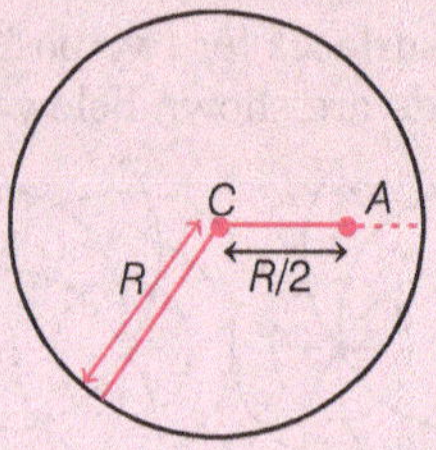

(a) $\dfrac{1}{4\pi\varepsilon_0} \cdot \dfrac{q}{R}$ (b) $\dfrac{1}{8\pi\varepsilon_0} \cdot \dfrac{q}{R}$

(c) $\dfrac{1}{4\pi\varepsilon_0} \cdot \dfrac{2q}{R}$ (d) $\dfrac{1}{2\pi\varepsilon_0} \cdot \dfrac{q}{R}$

Sol. (*a*) As we know, for a uniformly charged spherical shell,

$$V = \frac{Kq}{R}$$

Also, for $r \le R$, the potential is same at all points which is equal to the potential at surface.

Thus,

$$V_{\text{at } \frac{R}{2}} = \frac{1}{4\pi\varepsilon_0} \cdot \frac{q}{R}$$

Skill Builder

Electric potential on the surface of a charged spherical shell of radius 20 cm is 80 V, then the value of electric potential at a distance of 30 cm from the centre of spherical shell is

(a) 50.2 V
(b) 48.6 V
(c) 53.3 V
(d) 61.5 V

For more Practice Refer Q.No. 11 of step up practice 2 and Q.No. 31 of Gearing up for NEET.

Example 26 *Radii of two spheres are* r_1 *and* r_2 *respectively. Their electric potential are in ratio of 1 : 2 respectively. Find the ratio of their surface charge densities.*

Sol. Given, $\dfrac{V_1}{V_2} = \dfrac{1}{2}$

$$\Rightarrow \frac{kq_1}{r_1} \times \frac{r_2}{kq_2} = \frac{1}{2}$$

$$\Rightarrow \frac{r_1 q_1}{r_1^2} \times \frac{r_2^2}{r_2 q_2} = \frac{1}{2}$$

$$\frac{\sigma_1}{\sigma_2} = \frac{r_2}{2r_1}$$

Electric Potential due to Concentric Shells

1. Consider two concentric conducting shells of radii r_1 and r_2 $(r_2 > r_1)$ carrying uniformly distributed charges Q_1 and Q_2 respectively. Potential at the surface of each shell is

Potential on inner shell, $V_1 = \dfrac{Q_1}{4\pi\varepsilon_0 r_1} + \dfrac{Q_2}{4\pi\varepsilon_0 r_2}$

Potential on outer shell, $V_2 = \dfrac{Q_1}{4\pi\varepsilon_0 r_2} + \dfrac{Q_2}{4\pi\varepsilon_0 r_2}$

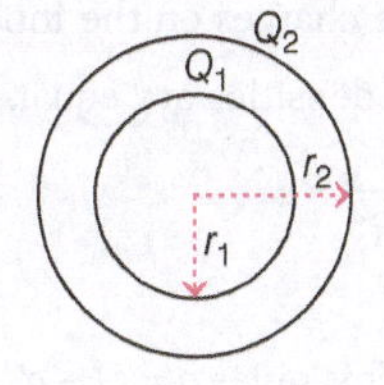

2. The figure shows three conducting concentric shells of radii a, b and c $(a < b < c)$ having charges Q_a, Q_b and Q_c respectively.

Potential at A,

$$V_A = \frac{1}{4\pi\varepsilon_0}\left[\frac{Q_a}{a} + \frac{Q_b}{b} + \frac{Q_c}{c}\right]$$

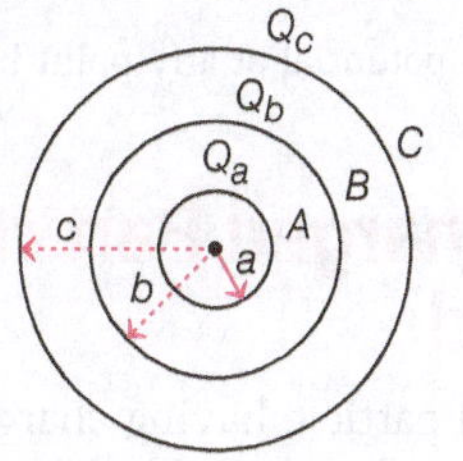

Potential at B,

$$V_B = \frac{1}{4\pi\varepsilon_0}\left[\frac{Q_a}{b} + \frac{Q_b}{b} + \frac{Q_c}{c}\right] = \frac{1}{4\pi\varepsilon_0}\left[\frac{Q_a + Q_b}{b} + \frac{Q_c}{c}\right]$$

Potential at C,

$$V_C = \frac{1}{4\pi\varepsilon_0}\left[\frac{Q_a}{c} + \frac{Q_b}{c} + \frac{Q_c}{c}\right] = \frac{1}{4\pi\varepsilon_0 c}[Q_a + Q_b + Q_c]$$

3. The figure shows two concentric spheres having radii r_1 and r_2 respectively $(r_2 > r_1)$. If charge on inner sphere is $+Q$ and outer sphere is earthed, then suppose that Q' appeared on outer sphere so

(i) Potential at the surface of outer sphere

$$V_C = \frac{Q}{4\pi\varepsilon_0 r_2} + \frac{Q'}{4\pi\varepsilon_0 r_2} = 0 \Rightarrow Q' = -Q$$

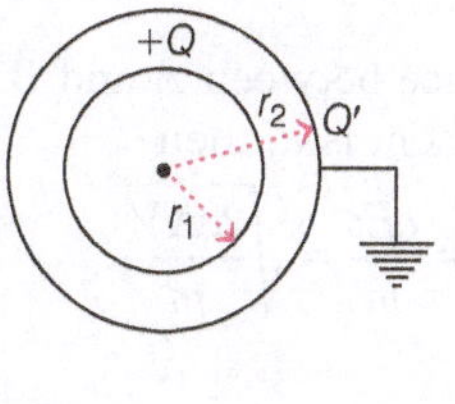

Mentor's TiP

When an object is grounded, then its potential considered zero. (Q' induced on inner surface of outer sphere because outer surface is earthed)

(ii) Potential of the inner sphere

$$V_1 = \frac{Q}{4\pi\varepsilon_0 r_1} + \frac{-Q}{4\pi\varepsilon_0 r_2}$$

$$= \frac{Q}{4\pi\varepsilon_0}\left[\frac{1}{r_1} - \frac{1}{r_2}\right]$$

4. In the above case if outer sphere is given a charge $+Q$ and inner sphere is earthed, then

(i) In this case potential at the surface of inner sphere is zero, so if Q' is appeared on inner sphere, then

$$V_1 = \frac{Q'}{4\pi\varepsilon_0 r_1} + \frac{Q}{4\pi\varepsilon_0 r_2} = 0$$

i.e. $Q' = -\dfrac{r_1}{r_2}Q$

(charge on inner sphere is less than that of the outer sphere).

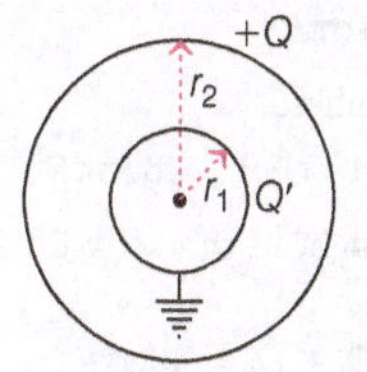

(ii) Potential at the surface of outer sphere

$$V_2 = \frac{Q}{4\pi\varepsilon_0 r_2} + \frac{Q'}{4\pi\varepsilon_0 r_2}$$

$$= \frac{1}{4\pi\varepsilon_0 r_2}\left[Q - Q\frac{r_1}{r_2}\right] = \frac{Q}{4\pi\varepsilon_0 r_2}\left[1 - \frac{r_1}{r_2}\right]$$

Example 27 *Two equipotential spheres are drawn round a point charge. As we move away from the charge, will the spacing between two spheres having a constant potential difference decrease, increase or remain constant.*

Sol. In the given figure, we have $V_1 > V_2$

$\therefore$ $V_1 = \dfrac{1}{4\pi\varepsilon_0}\cdot\dfrac{q}{r_1}$

and $V_2 = \dfrac{1}{4\pi\varepsilon_0}\cdot\dfrac{q}{r_2}$

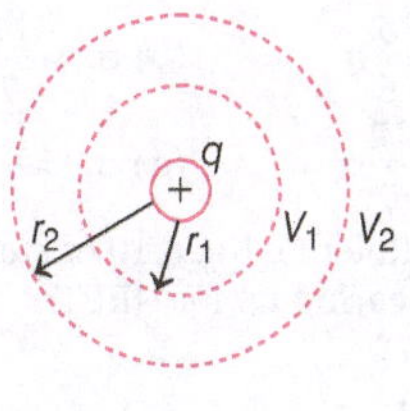

Now, $$V_1 - V_2 = \frac{q}{4\pi\varepsilon_0}\left(\frac{1}{r_1} - \frac{1}{r_2}\right)$$

$$= \frac{q}{4\pi\varepsilon_0}\left(\frac{r_2 - r_1}{r_1 r_2}\right)$$

$$\therefore \quad (r_2 - r_1) = \frac{(4\pi\varepsilon_0)(V_1 - V_2)}{q}(r_1 r_2)$$

For a constant potential difference $(V_1 - V_2)$, $r_2 - r_1 \propto r_1 r_2$ i.e. the spacing between two spheres $(r_2 - r_1)$ increases as we move away from the charge, because the product $r_1 r_2$ will increase.

NEET Close-up

Example Similar to PYQ Asked in NEET 2019

Two metal spheres, one of radius R and the other of $3R$ respectively have same surface charge density σ. They are brought in contact and then separated. The new surface charge densities are

(a) $\sigma_1 = \frac{5}{2}\sigma, \sigma_2 = 3\sigma$ (b) $\sigma_1 = \frac{5}{2}\sigma, \sigma_2 = \frac{5}{6}\sigma$

(c) $\sigma_1 = 5\sigma, \sigma_2 = \frac{5}{3}\sigma$ (d) $\sigma_1 = \frac{5}{3}\sigma, \sigma_2 = \frac{5}{6}\sigma$

Sol. (*a*) Charge on first sphere,

$$Q_1 = 4\sigma\pi R^2$$

Charge on second sphere,

$$Q_2 = 4\sigma\pi(3R)^2 = 36\sigma\pi R^2$$

When they are brought in contact with each other, the total charge will be

$$Q_t = Q_1 + Q_2 = 40\sigma\pi R^2$$

When two charge bodies are connected,

$$V_1 = V_2$$

$$\frac{Q_1'}{4\pi\varepsilon_0 R} = \frac{Q_2'}{4\pi\varepsilon_0 (3R)}$$

$$\Rightarrow \quad \frac{Q_1'}{Q_2'} = \frac{1}{3} \Rightarrow Q_1' = \frac{1}{4}Q_t \text{ and } Q_2' = \frac{3}{4}Q_t$$

After separation, new surface charge density will be

$$\sigma_1 = \frac{Q_1'}{4\pi R^2} = \frac{1}{16}\frac{Q_t}{\pi R^2} = \frac{40\sigma\pi R^2}{16\pi R^2} = \frac{5}{2}\sigma$$

$$\sigma_2 = \frac{Q_2'}{4\pi(3R)^2} = \frac{3}{4}\frac{Q_t}{9\pi R^2} = \frac{3}{4}\frac{36\sigma\pi R^2}{9\pi R^2} = 3\sigma$$

Skill Builder

Two metal sphere, one of radius $2R$ and the other of $4R$ respectively have same surface charge density 6. They are brought in contact and then seperated. The new surface charge densities are

(a) $\sigma_1 = \frac{10}{3}\sigma, \sigma_2 = \frac{5}{6}\sigma$ (b) $\sigma_1 = \frac{10}{7}\sigma, \sigma_2 = \frac{8}{3}\sigma$

(c) $\sigma_1 = \frac{15}{4}\sigma, \sigma_2 = \frac{12}{7}\sigma$ (d) $\sigma_1 = \frac{18}{4}\sigma, \sigma_2 = \frac{16}{3}\sigma$

For more Pratice Refer Q. No. 8,10 of step up practice 2 and Q. No. 34, 40, 47 of Gearing up for NEET.

Example 28 *A point charge of $-q$ is transferred from centre to surface on non-conducting solid sphere of radius R and charge Q. Calculate work done.*

Sol. $W_{cs} = q(V_s - V_c)$

$$= -q\left(\frac{KQ}{R} - \frac{3}{2}\frac{KQ}{R}\right) = \frac{KqQ}{2R}$$

Example 29 *A charge Q is distributed over two concentric hollow spheres of radii r and R (> r) such that the surface densities are equal. Find the potential at any point inside the smaller sphere.*

Sol. Let q and q' be the charges on the inner and outer sphere.

As surface charge densities are equal.

$$\therefore \quad \frac{q}{4\pi r^2} = \frac{q'}{4\pi R^2}$$

or $$qR^2 = q' r^2$$

Also, $q + q' = Q$. This gives $q = Q - q'$

Solving the two equations, we get

$$q = \frac{Qr^2}{R^2 + r^2}, q' = \frac{QR^2}{R^2 + r^2}$$

Now, potential at the centre is given by

$$V_C = \frac{q}{4\pi\varepsilon_0 r} + \frac{q'}{4\pi\varepsilon_0 R} = \frac{Q(r + R)}{4\pi\varepsilon_0(R^2 + r^2)}$$

This is equal to potential at any point inside the smaller sphere.

Motion of Charged Particle in Electric Field

Consider a charged particle having charge q and mass m is initially at rest in an electric field of strength E. The particle will experience an electric force which causes its motion. The force experienced by the charged particles is F, where

$$F = qE$$

$\therefore$ Acceleration produced by this force is

$$a = \frac{F}{m} = \frac{qE}{m} \quad \text{...(i)}$$

Suppose at point A particle is at rest and after some time t, it reaches the point B and attains velocity v.

$$\therefore \quad v = at$$

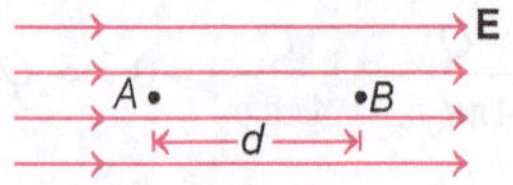

If potential difference between A and B be ΔV and the distance between them is d, then

$$v = \frac{qEt}{m} = \sqrt{\frac{2q\Delta V}{m}} \quad \text{...(ii)}$$

As, momentum, $p = mv$

$$p = m\left(\frac{qEt}{m}\right) = qEt \qquad \text{[from Eq. (ii)]}$$

or $$p = m \times \sqrt{\frac{2q\Delta V}{m}} = \sqrt{2mq\Delta V}$$

Kinetic Energy of a Charged Particle

Kinetic energy gained by the particle in time t,

$$K = \frac{1}{2}mv^2 = \frac{1}{2}m\left(\frac{qEt}{m}\right)^2 \qquad \text{[from Eq. (ii)]}$$

$$= \frac{q^2E^2t^2}{2m}$$

or $$K = \frac{1}{2}m \times \frac{2q\Delta V}{m} = q\Delta V$$

Example 30 *A bullet of mass 2 g is moving with a speed of 10 m/s. If the bullet has a charge of 2μC, through what potential it be accelerated starting from rest, to acquire the same speed?*

Sol. Use the relation, $qV = \frac{1}{2}mv^2$

Here, $q = 2 \times 10^{-6}$ C, $m = 2 \times 10^{-3}$ kg and $v = 10\ \text{ms}^{-1}$

Therefore, ptoential, $V = \frac{mv^2}{2q}$

$$= \frac{2 \times 10^{-3} \times (10)^2}{2 \times 2 \times 10^{-6}} = \frac{10^{-1}}{2 \times 10^{-6}} = 5 \times 10^4\ \text{V} = 50\ \text{kV}$$

Work Done by a Charged Particle

According to work energy theorem, gain in kinetic energy = work done in displacement of charge, i.e. $W = q\Delta V$

where, ΔV = potential difference between the two positions of charge q, i.e. $\Delta V = \mathbf{E} \cdot \Delta \mathbf{r} = E\Delta r \cos\theta$, where θ is the angle between direction of electric field and direction of motion of charge.

If charge q is given a displacement $\mathbf{r} = (x\hat{\mathbf{i}} + y\hat{\mathbf{j}} + z\hat{\mathbf{k}})$ in an electric field $\mathbf{E} = (E_x\hat{\mathbf{i}} + E_y\hat{\mathbf{j}} + E_z\hat{\mathbf{k}})$, then the work done is

$$W = q(\mathbf{E} \cdot \mathbf{r}) = q(E_x x + E_y y + E_z z)$$

Work done in displacing a charge in an electric field is path independent because electric force in field is conservative.

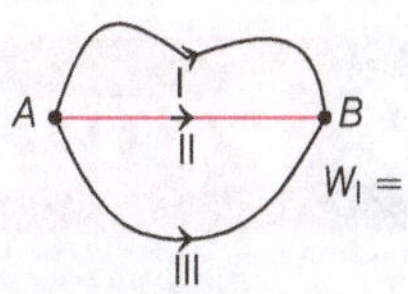

Different path followed by charged particle

When charged particle enters perpendicularly in an electric field, it describes a parabolic path as shown.

Example 31 *A block having charge q and mass m is resting on a smooth horizontal surface at a distance d from the wall is as shown. Discuss the motion of the block when a uniform electric field E is applied horizontally towards the wall assuming that collision of the block with the wall is completely elastic.*

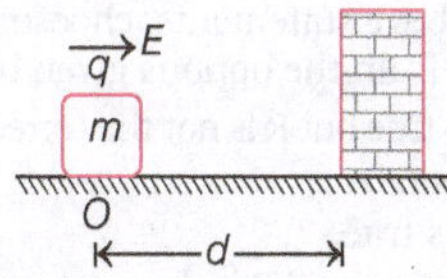

Sol. The figure can be shown as

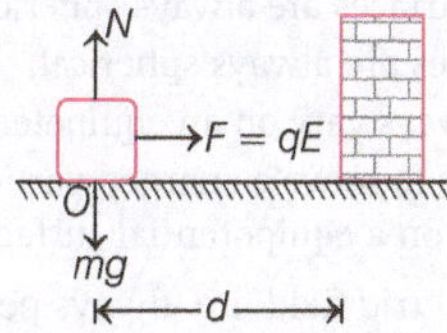

Acceleration of the block can be given as $a = \frac{qE}{m}$.

Time taken by the block to reach the wall at distance, $d = \left(\frac{1}{2}at^2\right)$ is

$$t = \sqrt{\frac{2d}{a}} = \sqrt{\frac{2d}{qE/m}} = \sqrt{\frac{2md}{qE}}$$

After completely elastic collision, the speed of the block is reversed and then it moves under retardation and comes to rest at O. Again it is accelerated towards the wall and so on. In fact, it is executing oscillatory motion of the time period

$$T = 2t = 2\sqrt{\frac{2md}{qE}}$$

As, force qE is constant, the motion of block is not simple harmonic.

STEP UP Practice 2

1. The work done to move a charge along an equipotential surface from A to b
(a) cannot be defined as $\int_A^B \mathbf{E}\cdot d\mathbf{l}$
(b) must be defined as $\frac{\mathbf{E}}{dl}$
(c) is zero
(d) can have a non-zero value

2. **Assertion** (A) Work done in moving a charge along an equipotential surface is zero.
Reason (R) Two equipotential surfaces can never intersect each other.
In the light of the above statements, choose the most appropriate answer from the options given below
(a) Both A and R are true but R is not the correct explanation of A.
(b) A is true but R is false.
(c) A is false but R is true.
(d) Both A and R are true and R is the correct explanation of A.

3. Find correct statement
(a) Equipotential surfaces are always spherical.
(b) Gaussian surfaces are always spherical.
(c) Electric field always vary on an equipotential surface.
(d) No work is done to move a charged particle from one point to another point on a equipotential surface.

4. **Assertion** (A) Electric field are always perpendicular to equipotential surface.
Reason (R) Electric potential decreases in the direction of electric field.
In the light of the above statements, choose the most appropriate answer from the options given below
(a) Both A and R are true but R is not the correct explanation of A.
(b) A is true but R is false.
(c) A is false but R is true.
(d) Both A and R are true and R is the correct explanation of A.

5. Which of the following statement is incorrect regarding equipotential surfaces?
(a) Equipotential surfaces are closer in regions of large electric fields compared to regions of lower electric field.
(b) Equipotential surfaces will be more crowded near sharp edge of a conductor.
(c) Equipotential surfaces will always be equally spaced.
(d) Equipotential surfaces will be more crowded near regions of large charge densities.

6. **Statement I** For any charge configuration, equipotential surface through a point is normal to the electric field.
Statement II Two equipotential surfaces intersect each other.
In the light of the above statements, choose the most appropriate answer from the options given below
(a) Both Statement I and Statement II are incorrect.
(b) Statement I is correct but Statement II is incorrect.
(c) Statement I is incorrect but Statement II is correct.
(d) Both Statement I and Statement II are correct.

7. A hollow metal sphere of radius 5 cm is charged, so that the potential on its surface is 10 V. The potential at the centre of the sphere is
(a) 0 V
(b) 10 V
(c) same as at point 5 cm away from the surface
(d) same as at point 25 cm away from the surface

8. Two charged spheres of radii R_1 and R_2 having equal surface charge density. The ratio of their potential is
(a) $\frac{R_1}{R_2}$ (b) $\frac{R_2}{R_1}$ (c) $\left(\frac{R_1}{R_2}\right)^2$ (d) $\left(\frac{R_2}{R_1}\right)^2$

9. If a charged spherical conductor of radius 10 cm has potential V at a point distant 5 from its centre, then the potential at a point distant 15 cm from the centre will be
(a) $\frac{1}{3}V$ (b) $\frac{2}{3}V$ (c) $\frac{3}{2}V$ (d) $3V$

10. A spherical conductor of radius 2 m is charged to a potential of 120 V. It is now placed inside another hollow spherical conductor of radius 6 m. Calculate the potential to which the bigger sphere would be raised.
(a) 20 V (b) 60 V
(c) 80 V (d) 40 V

11. The electrostatic potential of a uniformly charged thin spherical shell of charge Q and radius R at a distance r from the centre is
(a) $\frac{Q}{4\pi\varepsilon_0 r}$ for points outside that $\frac{Q}{4\pi\varepsilon_0 R}$ for points inside the shell
(b) $\frac{Q}{4\pi\varepsilon_0 r}$ for both points inside and outside the shell
(c) zero for points outside and $\frac{Q}{4\pi\varepsilon_0 r}$ for points inside the shell
(d) zero for both points inside and outside the shell

12. The diameter of a hollow metallic sphere is 60 cm and the sphere carries a charge of 500 μC. The potential at a distance of 100 cm from the centre of the sphere will be
(a) 6×10^7 V (b) 7×10^6 V
(c) 4.5×10^6 V (d) 5×10^6 V

13. **Statement I** The electric potential inside a conducting sphere remains constant from centre to surface.
Statement II It becomes possible to define potential at a point in an electric field because electric field is a non-conservative field.
In the light of the above statements, choose the most appropriate answer from the options given below
(a) Both Statement I and Statement II are incorrect.
(b) Statement I is correct but Statement II is incorrect.
(c) Statement I is incorrect but Statement II is correct.
(d) Both Statement I and Statement II are correct.

14. A hollow sphere of radius 0.1 m has a charge of 5×10^{-8}C. The potential at a distance of 5 cm from the centre of the sphere is $\left(\frac{1}{4\pi\varepsilon_0}=9\times10^9\text{Nm}^2\text{c}^{-2}\right)$

(a) 3000 V (b) 5000 V
(c) 4500 V (d) 6000 V

15. The electric potential at the surface of an atomic nucleus ($Z = 50$) of radius 9.0×10^{-15} cm

(a) 80 V (b) 8×10^6 V (c) 9 V (d) 9×10^5 V

16. **Assertion** (A) The electric potential outside a uniformly charged conducting sphere is inversely proportional to the distance from the surface of the sphere.

Reason (R) Outside the sphere, the electric field behaves as all the charge is concentrated at the centre.

In the light of above statements, choose the most appropriate answer from the options given below

(a) Both A and R are true but R is not the correct explanation of A.
(b) A is true but R is false.
(c) A is false but R is true.
(d) Both A and R are true and R is the correct explanation of A.

17. The radii of two concentric spherical conducting shells are r_1 and r_2 ($r_2 > r_1$). The charge on the outer shell is q. The charge on the inner shell which is connected to the earth is

(a) $q\left(\frac{r_2}{r_1}\right)$ (b) $q^2\left(\frac{r_1}{r_2}\right)$ (c) $-q\left(\frac{r_1}{r_2}\right)$ (d) $q^2\left(\frac{r_2}{r_1}\right)$

18. A hollow conducting sphere of radius R has a charge $(+q)$ on its surface. What is the electric potential within the sphere at a distance $r = R/3$ from its centre?

(a) Zero (b) $\frac{1}{4\pi\varepsilon_0}\frac{Q}{r}$ (c) $\frac{1}{4\pi\varepsilon_0}\frac{Q}{R}$ (d) $\frac{1}{4\pi\varepsilon_0}\frac{Q}{r^2}$

19. Three concentric spherical shells have radii a, b and c ($a < b < c$) and have surface charge densities σ, $-\sigma$ and σ, respectively. If V_A, V_B and V_C denote the potentials of the three shells, ... for $c = a + b$, we have

(a) $V_C = V_A \neq V_B$ (b) $V_C = V_B \neq V_A$
(c) $V_C \neq V_B \neq V_A$ (d) $V_C = V_B = V_A$

20. In the uniform electric field shown in the figure, potential difference between points C and D is

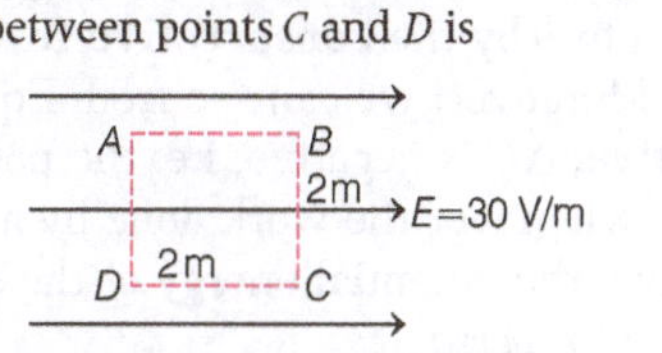

(a) –60 V (b) zero (c) +60 V (d) 30 V

21. Find correct statement

(a) For any concentric charged shells, charge is induced from outer shell to inner shell.
(b) Two concentric charged shells never induces charge.
(c) If outer shell is grounded, charge induced on outer surface is equal to charge of inner surface.
(d) If inner shell is grounded, charge induced on inner shell is equal to charge of outer shell.

22. **Statement I** Potential difference between the surfaces of two concentric spherical shells does not depend on the charge on the outer shell.

Statement II Two concentric spherical shell of different radii are at potentials V_A and V_B. If outer shell is earthed, then potential difference will not be changed.

In the light of the above statements, choose the most appropriate answer from the options given below.

(a) Both Statement I and Statement II are incorrect.
(b) Statement I is correct but Statement II is incorrect.
(c) Statement I is incorrect but Statement II is correct.
(d) Both Statement I and Statement II are correct.

23. A point charge of magnitude $+2\,\mu$C is fixed at (0, 0, 0). An isolated uncharged spherical conductor is fixed with its centre at (3 cm, 0, 0). The potential at the centre of the sphere is

(a) 0.30 MV (b) 0.25 MV
(c) 0.60 MV (d) 0.15 MV

24. A sphere of 4 cm radius is suspended within a hollow sphere of 6 cm radius. If the inner sphere is charged to a potential 3 esu while the outer sphere is earthed, then the charge on the inner sphere will be

(a) $\frac{1}{4}$ esu (b) 30 esu
(c) 36 esu (d) 54 esu

25. Below the given options which one is not correct?

(a) Electric potential inside conducting sphere $\rightarrow$ Variable
(b) Electric field inside conducting sphere $\rightarrow$ Zero
(c) Electric potential inside non-conducting sphere $\rightarrow$ Variable (non-linear)
(d) Electric field inside non-conducting $\rightarrow$ Variable (linear) sphere

26. Below the given options which one is not correct?

(a) Equipotential surface $\rightarrow W = 0$
(b) Non-conducting charged sphere $\rightarrow V_{\text{centre}}$ = Minimum
(c) Conducting charged sphere $\rightarrow V_{\text{in}}$ = constant
(d) Non-uniform electric potential $\rightarrow W = q\cdot\Delta V$

27. According to electric potential due to continuous charge distribution, which of the following option is not correct ?

(a) Potential due to an electric dipole varies as $\propto\frac{1}{r^2}$
(b) Potential difference between any two points on an equipotential surface is = 0
(c) Electric potential due to uniformly charged thin spherical shell ($r < R$) $\propto\frac{1}{r}$
(d) Potential due to a point charge varies as $\propto\frac{1}{r}$

28. Obtain the energy in joule acquired by an electron beam when accelerated through a potential difference of 2000 V. How much speed will the electron gain?

(a) $\frac{8}{3}\times10^7$ m/s (b) $\frac{7}{3}\times10^7$ m/s
(c) $\frac{5}{3}\times10^7$ m/s (d) $\frac{2}{3}\times10^7$ m/s

29. A particle A has charge $+16q$ and a particle B has charge $+4q$ with each of them having the same mass m. When allowed to fall from rest through the same electric potential difference, the ratio of their speed $\frac{v_A}{v_B}$ will becomes

(a) 2 : 1 (b) 1 : 2 (c) 1 : 4 (d) 4 : 1

30. What potential difference must be applied to produce an electric field that can accelerate an electron to one-tenth the velocity of light?

(a) 1352 V (b) 2511 V (c) 2531 V (d) 3521 V

31. An α particle is carried from a point at potential 70 volt to a point at 50 volt from the rest, then its kinetic energy will be

(a) 40 eV (b) 20 eV
(c) 20 MeV (d) 40 MeV

32. Proton, Deuteron and α-particles are in rest. If they are accelerated by a potential of V volt, then ratio of their kinetic energies is

(a) 1 : 2 : 4 (b) 1 : 1 : 2
(c) 1 : 2 : 2 (d) 1 : 1 : 1

33. When an electron is moved in an electric field, then it gains energy of 200 eV. Find out potential difference between two points.

(a) 200 V (b) 400 V
(c) 0 (d) 100 V

34. Assertion (A) Work done by an electric field on a charged particle depends on the path taken by the particle.

Reason (R) Force exerted by the field oppose the direction of motion of the particle.

In the light of the above statements, choose the most appropriate answer from the options given below

(a) Both A and R are true but R is not the correct explanation of A.

(b) A is true but R is false.

(c) A is false but R is true.

(d) Both A and R are true and R is the correct explanation of A.

Module 3

Electric Potential Energy

- Electric Potential Energy • Potential Energy of a System of Charges
- Potential Energy of a Dipole in a Uniform Electric Field

Electric Potential Energy

When a charged particle moves in an electric field, the field exerts a force (electric force) that can do work on the particle. This work can be expressed in terms of electric potential energy.

It is represented by U. Electric potential can be written as potential energy per unit charge, i.e. $V = \frac{W}{q} = \frac{U}{q}$

Electric potential energy is defined only in a conservative field.

Relation between Work and Energy

If the force **F** is conservative, the work done by **F** can always be expressed in terms of a **potential energy** U. When the charge particle moves from a point, where the potential energy is U_a to a point where it is U_b, the change in potential energy is, $\Delta U = U_b - U_a$.

This is related by the work $W_{a\to b}$ as

$$W_{a\to b} = U_a - U_b = -(U_b - U_a) = -\Delta U \quad \text{...(i)}$$

Here, $W_{a\to b}$ is the work done in displacing the charge particle from a to b by the **conservative force** (here electrostatic). Moreover, we can see from Eq. (i) that if $W_{a\to b}$ is positive, ΔU is negative, i.e. the potential energy decreases. So, whenever the work done by a conservative force is positive, the potential energy of the system decreases and *vice-versa.*

That's what happens when a charge particle is thrown upwards, the work done by gravity is negative, and the potential energy increases.

Concept ladder

If a charge moves from one position to another position in an electric field, its potential energy changes. In this process Work done by external force for this charge

$W_{\text{external}} = U_f - U_i$ and

Work done by field, $W_{\text{field}} = U_i - U_f$

Electron Volt

One electron volt (1 eV) is the energy equal to the work done in moving a single elementary charge particle, such as the electron or the proton through a potential difference of exactly one volt (1 V).

$$1 \text{ eV} = e\,(1 \text{ V})$$
$$= (1.6 \times 10^{-19} \text{ C})\,(1 \text{ J/C})$$
$$= 1.6 \times 10^{-19} \text{ J}$$

Example 32 *A spherical oil drop of radius 10^{-4} cm has a total charge equivalent to 40 electrons. Calculate the energy that would be required to place an additional electron on the drop.*

Sol. Initial charge on the oil drop,

$$q = 40 \times 1.6 \times 10^{-19}$$
$$= 64 \times 10^{-19} \text{ C}$$

Potential of the oil drop $= \dfrac{q}{4\pi\varepsilon_0 r} = \dfrac{9 \times 10^9 \times 64 \times 10^{-19}}{10^{-6}}$

$$= 576 \times 10^{-4} \text{ V}$$

Now, energy required = work done in bringing an electron from infinity to a point of potential.

As, potential $= \dfrac{\text{work}}{\text{charge}}$

$\therefore$ Work = Potential × Charge

$$= 576 \times 10^{-4} \times 1.6 \times 10^{-19}$$
$$= 921.6 \times 10^{-23} \text{ J}$$

Example 33 *A uniform electric field E_0 is directed along positive y-direction. Find the change in electric potential energy of a positive test charge q_0 when it is displaced in the field from $y_i = a$ to $y_f = 2a$ along the Y-axis.*

Sol. Electrostatic force on the test charge,

$F_e = q_0 E_0$ (along positive y-direction)

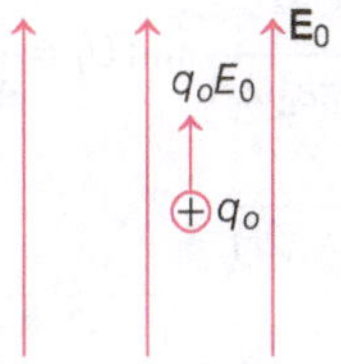

$\therefore$ $W_{i \to f} = -\Delta U$ or $\Delta U = -W_{i \to f}$

$$= -[q_0 E_0 (2a - a)] = -q_0 E_0 a$$

Note Here, work done by electrostatic force is positive. Hence, the potential energy is decreasing.

Example 34 *Find the change in electric potential energy, ΔU as a charge of 2.20×10^{-6} C, moves from a point A to point B, given that the change in electric potential between these points is $\Delta V = V_B - V_A = 24.0$ V.*

Sol. As, $\Delta V = \dfrac{\Delta U}{q_0}$, where ΔU is change in potential energy

$\therefore$ $\Delta U = q_0 \Delta V$

$$= (2.20 \times 10^{-6})\,(24.0)$$
$$= 5.28 \times 10^{-5} \text{ J}$$

Example 35 *A charge is moved in an electric field of a fixed charge distribution from point A to another point B slowly. The work done by external agent in doing so, is 100 J. What is the work done by the electric field of the charge distribution as the charge moves from A to B?*

Sol. Work done, $W_{\text{ext}} = \Delta U$

$$= U_B - U_A = 100 \text{ J}$$

As, $\mathbf{F}_{\text{ext}} = -\mathbf{F}_E$ for the charge to move slowly, so

$$W_E = -W_{\text{ext}} = -100 \text{ J}$$

Potential Energy of a System of Charges

The potential energy for a system of two point charges and for a collection of more than two charges are given below.

Potential Energy for a System of Two Point Charges

Potential energy of the system of two charges q_1 and q_2 will be the work done to bring them from infinity to point A and point B, respectively.

Work done to bring charge q_1 from infinity to point A,

$$W_1 = 0$$

Work done to bring charge q_2 from infinity to point B,

$$W_2 = q_2 (V_B - V_A)$$

As, $W_2 = q_2 \times \dfrac{1}{4\pi\varepsilon_0} \dfrac{q_1}{r}$

Now, potential energy of the system of charges q_1 and q_2,

$$U = W_1 + W_2$$
$$U = \frac{1}{4\pi\varepsilon_0} \cdot \frac{q_1 q_2}{r}$$

Concept ladder

Electrostatic potential energy of spherical shell and non-conducting solid sphere.

Shape	Electrostatic potential energy
Uniformly charged thin spherical shell	$U = \dfrac{KQ^2}{2R}$
Uniformly charged non-conducting solid sphere	$U = \dfrac{3}{5}\dfrac{KQ^2}{R}$

Example 36 *In a hydrogen atom, the electron and proton are bound together at a distance of about 0.53 Å. Estimate the potential energy of the system in eV, assuming zero potential energy at infinite separation between the electron and the proton.*

Sol. Charge on electron, $q_1 = -1.6\times10^{-19}$ C

Charge on proton, $q_2 = 1.6\times10^{-19}$ C

Separation between electron and proton,

$$r = 0.53\ \text{Å} = 0.53\times10^{-10}\ \text{m}$$

The change in energy when electron-proton system is formed is

$$\Delta U = \frac{1}{4\pi\varepsilon_0}\cdot\frac{q_1q_2}{r}$$

$$= (9\times10^9)\times\frac{(-1.6\times10^{-19})(1.6\times10^{-19})}{0.53\times10^{-10}}$$

$$= -4.35\times10^{-18}\ \text{J} = -\frac{4.35\times10^{-18}}{1.6\times10^{-19}} = -27.2\ \text{eV}$$

At infinite separation, the potential energy is zero, therefore the energy when the system is formed, is

$$U = 0 + \Delta U = -27.2\ \text{eV}$$

Example 37 *A point charge $q_1 = -5.8\ \mu C$ is held stationary at the origin. A second point charge $q_2 = +4.3\ \mu C$ moves from the point (0.26 m, 0, 0) to (0.38 m, 0, 0). How much work is done by the electric force on q_2?*

Sol. Work done by the electrostatic forces $= U_i - U_f$

$$= \frac{q_1q_2}{4\pi\varepsilon_0}\left(\frac{1}{r_i}-\frac{1}{r_f}\right) = \frac{q_1q_2}{4\pi\varepsilon_0}\left(\frac{r_f-r_i}{r_ir_f}\right)$$

$$= \frac{(-5.8\times10^{-6})(4.3\times10^{-6})(9\times10^{9})(0.38-0.26)}{(0.38)(0.26)}$$

$$= -0.272\ \text{J}$$

Example 38 *What minimum work must be done by an external force to bring a charge $q = 3.0\ \mu C$ from a great distance away (take, $r = \infty$) to a point 0.50 m from a charge $Q = 20.0\ \mu C$?*

Sol. The change in potential energy equal to the positive of the work required by an external force $W = \Delta U = q(V_B - V_A)$.

We get the potential V_B and V_A using $V = \frac{kQ}{r}$

The work required is equal to the change in potential energy,

$$W = q(V_B - V_A) = q\left(\frac{kQ}{r_B}-\frac{kQ}{r_A}\right)$$

where, $r_B = 0.500$ m and $r_A = \infty$.

$$\text{Work done, } W = \frac{(3.00\times10^{-6}\text{C})\times(9\times10^{+9})(2.00\times10^{-5})}{(0.50)}$$

$$= 1.08\ \text{J}$$

Example 39 *A point charge $q_1 = 9.1\ \mu C$ is held fixed at origin. A second point charge $q_2 = -0.42\ \mu C$ and a mass 3.2×10^{-4} kg is placed on the X-axis, 0.96 m from the origin. The second point charge is released at rest. What is its speed when it is 0.24 m from the origin?*

Sol. From conservation of mechanical energy, we have decrease in gravitational potential energy = increase in kinetic energy

$$\text{or}\quad \frac{1}{2}mv^2 = U_i - U_f$$

$$= \frac{q_1q_2}{4\pi\varepsilon_0}\left(\frac{1}{r_i}-\frac{1}{r_f}\right) = \frac{q_1q_2}{4\pi\varepsilon_0}\left(\frac{r_f-r_i}{r_ir_f}\right)$$

Speed of the second charge,

$$v = \sqrt{\frac{q_1q_2}{2\pi\varepsilon_0 m}\left(\frac{r_f-r_i}{r_ir_f}\right)}$$

$$= \sqrt{\frac{(9.1\times10^{-6})(-0.42\times10^{-6})\times2\times9\times10^9}{3.2\times10^{-4}}}\cdot\sqrt{\left(\frac{0.24-0.96}{(0.24)(0.96)}\right)}$$

$$= 26\ \text{ms}^{-1}$$

Example 40 *A proton is fixed at origin. Another proton is released from rest, from a point at a distance r from origin. Taking charge of origin as e and mass as m, find the speed of the proton (i) at a distance 2r from origin, (ii) at large distance from origin.*

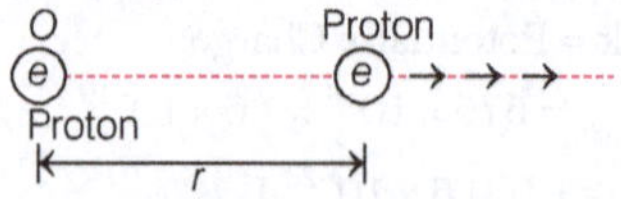

Sol. The proton moves away under electrostatic repulsion.

As there is no external force, $W_{ext} = 0$

$$\Rightarrow \quad \Delta KE + \Delta PE = 0$$

$$\Rightarrow \quad \left(\frac{1}{2}mv^2\right) + (U_f - U_i) = 0$$

(i) We have,

$$U_f = \frac{e^2}{4\pi\varepsilon_0(2r)} \text{ and } U_i = \frac{e^2}{4\pi\varepsilon_0(r)}$$

$$\therefore \quad \frac{1}{2}mv^2 = \frac{e^2}{4\pi\varepsilon_0(2r)}$$

or speed of the proton, $v = \sqrt{\frac{e^2}{4\pi\varepsilon_0 rm}}$

(ii) We have, $U_f = 0$, $U_i = \frac{e^2}{4\pi\varepsilon_0 r}$

$$\therefore \quad \frac{1}{2}mv^2 = \frac{e^2}{4\pi\varepsilon_0 r}$$

Speed of the proton, $\sqrt{\frac{2e^2}{4\pi\varepsilon_0 rm}}$

Potential Energy for a System of More than Two Charges

When more than two charged particles are there in a system. The potential energy of system is given by sum of potential energies of all pairs of charges.

For example if a system of three charges q_1, q_2 and q_3 given in the figure

$$\text{Potential energy of system } (U) = \frac{kq_1q_2}{r_{12}} + \frac{kq_2q_3}{r_{23}} + \frac{kq_1q_3}{r_{13}}$$

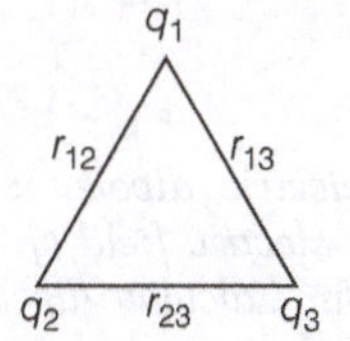

Note For potential energy of a particular charge only is the sum of potential energies of that charge with the others.

For example, for q_1

$$\Rightarrow \quad U_{q_1} = \frac{kq_1q_2}{r_{12}} + \frac{kq_1q_3}{r_{13}}$$

Example 41 *Three point charges of 0.1 C each are placed at the corners of an equilateral triangle with side 1 m. If this system is supplied energy at the rate of 1 kW, how much time will be required to move one of the charges to the mid-point of the line joining the two others?*

Sol.

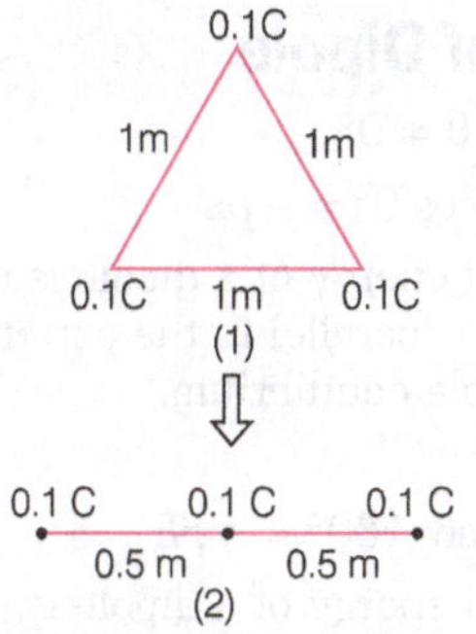

$$U_1 = \frac{1}{4\pi\varepsilon_0}\left[\frac{0.1 \times 0.1}{1} \times 3\right]$$

$$= 9 \times 10^9 \times 3 \times 10^{-2} = 27 \times 10^7 \text{ J}$$

$$U_2 = \frac{1}{4\pi\varepsilon_0}\left[\frac{0.1 \times 0.1}{0.5} \times 2 + \frac{0.1 \times 0.1}{1}\right]$$

$$= 9 \times 10^9 \times 0.05 = 45 \times 10^7 \text{ J}$$

$$W_{1 \to 2} = U_2 - U_1 = 18 \times 10^7 \text{ J}$$

Rate at which energy is supplied is given by

$$P = \frac{W}{t}$$

$$\therefore \quad t = \frac{W}{P} = \frac{18 \times 10^7}{10^3} = 18 \times 10^4 \text{ s} = 50 \text{ h}$$

Example 42 *Four charges $q_1 = 1\ \mu C$, $q_2 = 2\ \mu C$, $q_3 = -3\ \mu C$ and $q_1 = 4\ \mu C$ are kept on the vertices of a square of side 1 m. Find the electric potential energy of this system of charges.*

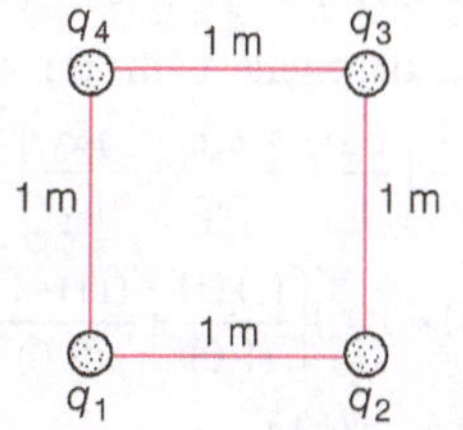

Sol. We have,

$$r_{41} = r_{43} = r_{32} = r_{21} = 1 \text{ m}$$

and
$$r_{42} = r_{31} = \sqrt{(1)^2 + (1)^2} = \sqrt{2} \text{ m}$$

Potential energy of a system of three charges,

$$U = \frac{1}{4\pi\varepsilon_0}\left[\frac{q_4q_3}{r_{43}} + \frac{q_4q_2}{r_{42}} + \frac{q_4q_1}{r_{41}} + \frac{q_3q_2}{r_{32}} + \frac{q_3q_1}{r_{31}} + \frac{q_2q_1}{r_{21}}\right]$$

$$U = (9.0 \times 10^9)(10^{-6})(10^{-6})$$

$$\left[\frac{(4)(-3)}{1} + \frac{(4)(2)}{\sqrt{2}} + \frac{(4)(1)}{1} + \frac{(-3)(2)}{1} + \frac{(-3)(1)}{\sqrt{2}} + \frac{(2)(1)}{1}\right]$$

$$= (9.0 \times 10^{-3})\left[-12 + \frac{5}{\sqrt{2}}\right] = -7.62 \times 10^{-2} \text{ J}$$

Mentor's TiP

Here, negative sign of U implies that positive work has been done by electrostatic forces in assembling these charges at respective distances from infinity.

Example 43 *Two point charges are located on the X-axis, $q_1 = -1\ \mu C$ at $x = 0$ and $q_2 = +1\ \mu C$ at $x = 1$ m.*

(i) Find the work that must be done by an external force to bring a third point charge $q_3 = +1\ \mu C$ from infinity at $x = 2$ m.

(ii) Find the total potential energy of the system of three charges.

Sol. (i) The work that must be done on q_3 by an external force is equal to the difference of potential energy ΔU when the charge is at $x = 2$ m and the potential energy when it is at infinity.

$$\therefore \quad W = \Delta U = U_f - U_i$$

$$= \frac{1}{4\pi\varepsilon_0}\left[\frac{q_3q_2}{(r_{32})_f} + \frac{q_3q_1}{(r_{31})_f} + \frac{q_2q_1}{(r_{21})_f}\right]$$

$$- \frac{1}{4\pi\varepsilon_0}\left[\frac{q_3q_2}{(r_{32})_i} + \frac{q_3q_1}{(r_{31})_i} + \frac{q_2q_1}{(r_{21})_i}\right]$$

Here, $(r_{21})_i = (r_{21})_f$ and $(r_{32})_i = (r_{31})_i = \infty$

$$\therefore \quad W = \frac{1}{4\pi\varepsilon_0}\left[\frac{q_3q_2}{(r_{32})_f} + \frac{q_3q_1}{(r_{31})_f}\right]$$

Substituting the values, we get

$$W = (9.0 \times 10^9)(10^{-12})\left[\frac{(1)(1)}{(1.0)} + \frac{(1)(-1)}{(2.0)}\right]$$

$$= 4.5 \times 10^{-3}\ \text{J}$$

(ii) The total potential energy of the three charges is given by

$$U = \frac{1}{4\pi\varepsilon_0}\left(\frac{q_3 q_2}{r_{32}} + \frac{q_3 q_1}{r_{31}} + \frac{q_2 q_1}{r_{21}}\right)$$

$$= (9.0 \times 10^9)\left[\frac{(1)(1)}{(1.0)} + \frac{(1)(-1)}{(2.0)} + \frac{(1)(-1)}{(1.0)}\right]10^{-12}$$

$$= -4.5 \times 10^{-3}\ \text{J}$$

Potential Energy of a Dipole in a Uniform Electric Field

Electrostatic potential energy of a dipole placed in a uniform electric field is defined as the work done in rotating a dipole from a direction perpendicular to the field to the given direction, i.e.

$$U = W_{90^\circ \to \theta} = \int_{90^\circ}^{\theta} pE \sin\theta \, d\theta$$

$$= pE\,[-\cos\theta]_{90^\circ}^{\theta}$$

$$U = -pE\cos\theta = -\mathbf{p}\cdot\mathbf{E}$$

When an electric dipole is placed in uniform electric field, then

(i) If $\theta = 0^\circ$ 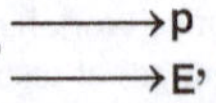

$F = 0, \tau = 0, U = -pE$ (minimum)

$\Rightarrow$ So dipole is in stable equilibrium.

(ii) If $\theta = 90^\circ$ 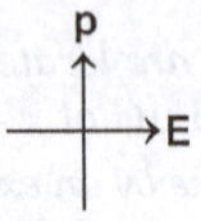

$F = 0, \tau = pE, U = 0$

(ii) If $\theta = 180^\circ$ 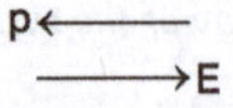

$F = 0, \tau = 0, U = pE$ (maximum)

$\Rightarrow$ So dipole is in unstable equilibrium.

Mentor's TIP

Keep following points in mind while solving electric dipole related problems.

- If electric dipole is placed in uniform electric field, then electric force act on dipole is zero while torque on dipole may be zero or non-zero.
- If electric dipole is placed in non-uniform electric field, then electric force act on dipole is non-zero while torque on dipole may be zero or non-zero.
- Electric dipole placed in electric field, tends to rotate such that its dipole moment become parallel to external electric field.

Force on an Electric Dipole in Non-uniform Electric Field

- When a short dipole is placed in a non-uniform electric field it will experience a force.
- The interaction energy of the dipole in electric field E is $U = -\mathbf{p}\cdot\mathbf{E}$.
- If $E = f(r) \Rightarrow U = f(r)$, so the force on dipole due to electric field is $F = -\dfrac{\Delta U}{\Delta r}$
- If the dipole is placed in the direction of electric field, then $\mathbf{F} = -\mathbf{p}\cdot\dfrac{d\mathbf{E}}{dr}$

Example 44 *An electric dipole, when held at 30° with respect to a uniform electric field of 10^4 N/C experiences a torque of 9×10^{-26} Nm. Calculate dipole moment of the dipole.*

Sol. Torque $\tau = pE\sin\theta$

$\Rightarrow 9 \times 10^{-26}\ \text{Nm} = p(10^4\ \text{N/C})(\sin 30^\circ)$

$\therefore \quad p = 1.8 \times 10^{-29}$ C-m

Example 45 *An electric dipole of dipole moment p is placed in uniform electric field E, then calculate work done to rotate it from orientation of stable equilibrium to unstable equilibrium.*

Sol. $W_{0 \to 180^\circ} = pE(\cos 0^\circ - \cos 180^\circ)$

$\because W_{0 \to 180^\circ} = pE(1 - (-1)) = 2pE$

Equilibrium of Dipole

Work done, when $\theta = 0^\circ$

$$U = -pE\cos 0^\circ = -pE$$

Thus, the potential energy of a dipole is minimum when its dipole moment is parallel to the external field. This is the position of stable equilibrium.

(ii) When $\theta = 180^\circ$

$$U = -pE\cos 180^\circ = +pE$$

Thus, the potential energy of a dipole is maximum when its dipole moment is antiparallel to the external field. This is the position of unstable equilibrium.

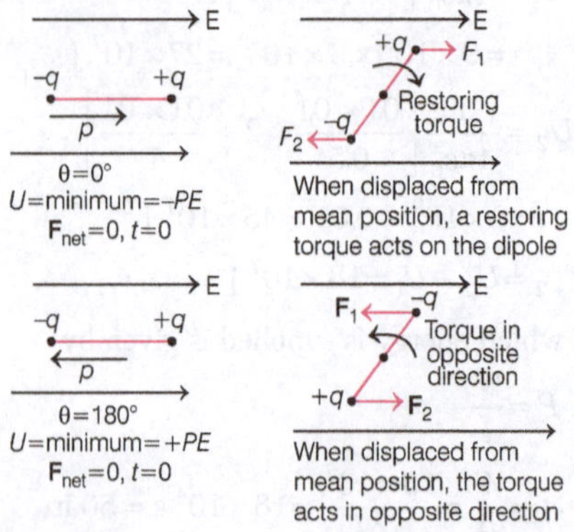

Example 46 *Two point charges +2e and −2e are situated at a distance of 2.4 Å from each other and constitute an electric dipole. This dipole is placed in a uniform electric field of* 4.0×10^5 Vm^{-1}. *Calculate*

(i) electric dipole moment

(ii) potential energy of the dipole in equilibrium position

(iii) and work done in rotating the dipole through 180° from the equilibrium position.

Sol. (i) The electric dipole moment is

$$p = q \times 2l$$

where, q is the charge of one end of the dipole and $2l$ is the distance between the two charges.

Here, $q = 2e = 3.2 \times 10^{-19}$ C and $2l = 2.4$ Å $= 2.4 \times 10^{-10}$ m

$$\because p = (3.2 \times 10^{-19}) \times (2.4 \times 10^{-10}) = 7.68 \times 10^{-29} \text{ C-m}$$

(ii) The potential energy of a dipole in an electric field E is

$$U = -pE \cos\theta$$

where, θ is the angle between the axis of the dipole and the field. In equilibrium position,

$$\theta = 0°, \text{ and so } U_0 = -pE$$

Here, $p = 7.68 \times 10^{-29}$ C-m and $E = 4.0 \times 10^5$ Vm^{-1}

$$\therefore U_0 = -(7.68 \times 10^{-29}) \times (4.0 \times 10^5) = -3.07 \times 10^{-23} \text{ J}$$

(iii) The work done (increase in energy) in rotating the dipole through angle θ from the direction of the electric field E is given by

$$W = pE(1 - \cos\theta)$$

If $\theta = 180°$ or $\cos\theta = -1$,

then, $W = 2pE = 2 \times (7.68 \times 10^{-29}) \times (4.0 \times 10^5)$

$$= 6.14 \times 10^{-23} \text{ J}$$

Concept ladder

- Electrostatic force between two point charges $\Rightarrow F \propto \frac{1}{r^2}$
- Electrostatic force between a point charge and a dipole $\Rightarrow F \propto \frac{1}{r^3}$
- Electrostatic force between two dipoles $\Rightarrow F \propto \frac{1}{r^4}$

STEP UP Practice 3

1. When a positive charge q is taken from lower potential point to a higher potential point, then its potential energy will
(a) decrease (b) increase
(c) remain unchanged (d) become zero

2. When one electron is taken towards the other electron, then the electric potential energy of the system
(a) decreases (b) increases
(c) remains unchanged (d) becomes zero

3. The charge and mass of particle are 2 times and 4000 times the charge and mass of an electron respectively. This particle is accelerated through a potential difference of 5 volt. If initially the particle was at rest, then its final kinetic energy will be
(a) 10 eV (b) 5 eV
(c) 100 eV (d) 2×10^3 eV

4. Two positive point charges of 12 μC and 8 μC are 10 cm apart. The work done in bringing them 4 cm is
(a) 5.8 J (b) 5.8 eV
(c) 13 J (d) 13 eV

5. Select the correct pair
(a) Electric potential energy — eV
(b) Electric potential — V/m
(c) Electric field — C-m
(d) Electric dipole moment — J/C

6. The electrostatic potential energy between proton and electron separated by a distance 1 Å is
(a) 13.6 eV (b) 27.2 eV
(c) −14.4 eV (d) 1.44 eV

7. **Assertion** (A) The expression of potential energy $U = \frac{1}{4\pi\varepsilon_0} \frac{q_1 q_2}{r_{12}}$, is unaltered whatever way the charges are brought to the specified locations.
Reason (R) Path-independence of work for electrostatic force.
In the light of the above statements, choose the correct answer from the options given below
(a) Both A and R are true but R is not the correct explanation of A.
(b) A is true but R is false.
(c) A is false but R is true.
(d) Both A and R are true and R is the correct explanation of A.

8. A proton moves a distance d in a uniform electric field **E** as shown in the figure. Does the electric field do a positive or negative work on the proton? Does the electric potential energy of the proton increase or decrease?

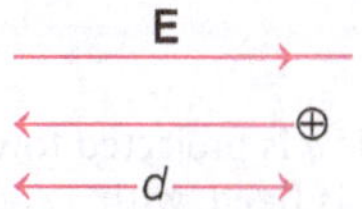

(a) Negative, increase (b) Positive, decrease
(c) Negative, decrease (d) Positive, increase

9. **Assertion** (A) If a charged particle is moved from one point to another point, the work done by electrostatic field is the change in potential energy.
Reason (R) Work done by external non-conservative force is always equal to the change in PE.
In the light of the above statements, choose the correct answer from the options given below

(a) Both A and R are true but R is not the correct explanation of A.
(b) A is true but R is false.
(c) A is false but R is true.
(d) Both A and R are true and R is the correct explanation of A.

10. Two positive point charges of 12 and 5 microcoulombs, are placed 10 cm apart in air. The work needed to bring them 6 cm closer is
(a) 2.4 J (b) 3.6 J (c) 4.8 J (d) 6.0 J

11. A charged sphere of diameter 4 cm has a charge density of 10^{-4} coulombs/cm^2. The work done in joules when a charge of 40 nano-coulombs is moved from infinity to a point which is at a distance of 2 cm from the surface of the sphere is
(a) 14.4π (b) 28.8π (c) 144π (d) 288π

12. Identify the wrong statement.
(a) The electrical potential energy of a system of two protons shall increase if the separation between the two is decreased.
(b) The electrical potential energy of a proton-electron system will increase if the separation between the two is decreased.
(c) The electrical potential energy of a proton-electron system will increase if the separation between the two is increased.
(d) The electrical potential energy of a system of two electrons shall increase if the separation between the two is decreased.

13. **Assertion** (A) Electric potential and electric potential energy are different quantities.
Reason (R) For a system of positive test charge and point charge, electric potential energy is equal to electric potential.
In the light of above statements, choose the correct answer from the options given below
(a) Both A and R are true but R is not the correct explanation of A.
(b) A is true but R is false.
(c) A is false but R is true.
(d) Both A and R are true and R is the correct explanation of A.

14. Two points P and Q are maintained at the potentials of 10 V and –4 V, respectively. The work done in moving 100 electrons from P to Q is
(a) -9.60×10^{-17} J
(b) 9.60×10^{-17} J
(c) -2.24×10^{-16} J
(d) 2.24×10^{-16} J

15. A charged particle q is projected towards another charged particle Q, which is fixed, with a speed v. It approaches Q upto a closest distance r and then returns. If q were given a speed of $2v$, the closest distances of approach would be

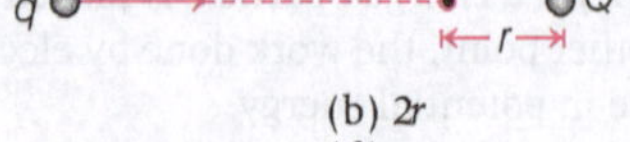

(a) $r/4$ (b) $2r$
(c) $r/2$ (d) r

16. Three identical charges each of $2\ \mu C$ are placed at the vertices of a triangle ABC as shown in the figure.

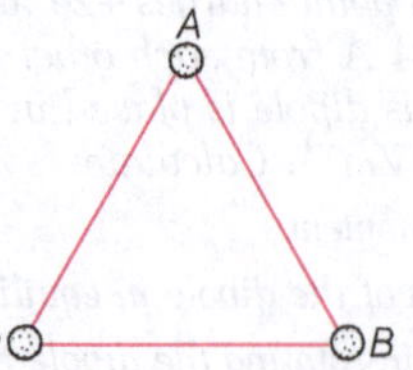

If $AB + AC = 12$ cm and $AB \cdot AC = 32\ cm^2$, the potential energy of the charge at A is
(a) 1.53 J (b) 5.31 J (c) 3.15 J (d) 1.35 J

17. If three charges are placed at the vertices of equilateral triangle of charge q each, what is the net potential energy, if the side of equilateral triangle is l cm?
(a) $\frac{1}{4\pi\varepsilon_0}\frac{q^2}{l}$ (b) $\frac{1}{4\pi\varepsilon_0}\frac{2q^2}{l}$
(c) $\frac{1}{4\pi\varepsilon_0}\frac{3q^2}{l}$ (d) $\frac{1}{4\pi\varepsilon_0}\frac{4q^2}{l}$

18. Three charges Q, $+q$ and $+q$ are placed at the vertices of an equilateral triangle of side l as shown in the figure. If the net electrostatic energy of the system is zero, then Q is equal to

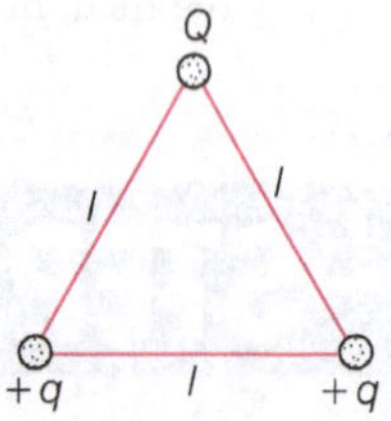

(a) $-\frac{q}{2}$ (b) $-q$
(c) $+q$ (d) zero

19. If identical charges $(-q)$ are placed at each corner of a cube of side b, then electric potential energy of charge $(+q)$ which is placed at centre of the cube will be
(a) $\frac{8\sqrt{2}q^2}{4\pi\varepsilon_0 b}$ (b) $\frac{-8\sqrt{2}q^2}{\pi\varepsilon_0 b}$ (c) $\frac{-4\sqrt{2}q^2}{\pi\varepsilon_0 b}$ (d) $\frac{-4q^2}{\sqrt{3}\pi\varepsilon_0 b}$

20. Two charges q_1 and q_2 are placed 30 cm apart as shown in the figure. A third charge q_3 is moved along the arc of a circle of radius 40 cm from C to D. The change in the potential energy of the system is $\frac{q_3}{4\pi\varepsilon_0}k$, where k is

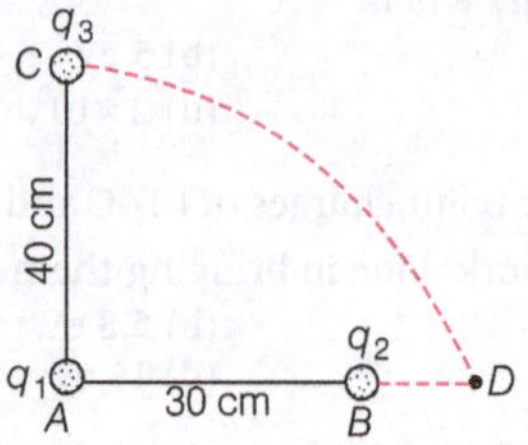

(a) $8q_2$ (b) $8q_1$
(c) $6q_2$ (d) $6q_1$

21. Three point charges of 1 C, 2 C and 3 C are placed at the corners of an equilateral triangle of side 100 cm. The work done to move these charges to the corners of a similar equilateral triangle of side 50 cm, will be
(a) 9.9×10^{10} J (b) 9.9×10^{9} J
(c) 5.2×10^{10} J (d) 5.9×10^{9} J

22. Figure shows an arrangement of three point charges. The total electropotential energy of the arrangement is zero. Find ratio q/Q.

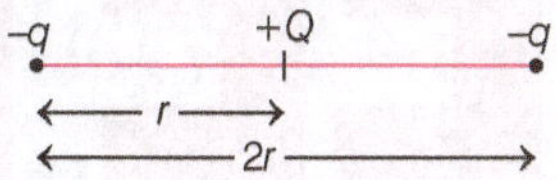

(a) 2 : 1 (b) 1 : 2
(c) 4 : 1 (d) 1 : 1

23. **Assertion** (A) At a point of given potential, PE of a positive charge is always positive.
Reason (R) At a point of given negative potential, PE of a negative charge is always positive.
In the light of above statements, choose the correct answer from the options given below
(a) Both A and R are true but R is not the correct explanation of A.
(b) A is true but R is false.
(c) A is false but R is true.
(d) Both A and R are true and R is the correct explanation of A.

24. For dipole $q = 2 \times 10^{-6}$ C and $d = 0.01$ m, calculate the maximum torque for this dipole if $E = 5 \times 10^{5}$ N/C.
(a) 1×10^{-3} N-m
(b) 10×10^{-2} N-m
(c) 10×10^{-3} N-m
(d) 1×10^{2} N-m

25. A molecule with a dipole moment p is placed in a electric field of strength E. Initially, the dipole is aligned parallel to the field. If the dipole is to be rotated to be anti-parallel to the field, then the work required to be done by an external agency is
(a) $-2pE$ (b) $-pE$
(c) pE (d) $2pE$

26. Select the incorrect pair for a dipole in electric field.
(a) $\theta = 0° \rightarrow U = -$ ve (max)
(b) $\theta = 90° \rightarrow U = 0$
(c) $\theta = 180° \rightarrow U = +$ ve (max)
(d) $0 < \theta < 90° \rightarrow U = +$ ve

27. Find correct statement
(a) Electric dipole moment is scalar quantity.
(b) Electric potential energy is zero when dipole is placed antiparallel to the electric field.
(c) Torque on a dipole is zero when dipole is placed antiparallel to the electric field.
(d) Torque on a dipole is zero when dipole is placed perpendicular to the electric field.

NEET Exclusive EXTRA BYTES

- If potential energy at infinite is zero, then
  (i) Work done to form a charge system, $W = U_f$.
  (ii) Work done to separate a charge system, $W = -U_i$.
- Electric potential of earth is assumed to zero.
- Direction of electric field is from high potential to low potential, irrespective of charge distribution.
- When we move in direction of **E**, electric potential reduces.
- Equipotential surface may or may not be real.
- Electric field inside equipotential volume is always zero.
- Electric potential at equatorial line of electric dipole is always zero.
- In any uniform electric field, force on dipole is always zero but torque may be present.
- Torque on a dipole in non-uniform electric field may be zero.
- **Electric potential due to**
  (i) point charge is inversely proportional to distance.
  (ii) electric dipole is inversely proportional to square of distance.
  (ii) electric quadruple is inversely proportional to cube of distance.

GEARING UP FOR NEET

Single Option Correct

1. From a point charge there is a fixed point A. At that point there is an electric field of 500 V/m and potential of 3000 V. Then, the distance of point A from the point charge is
(a) 6 m (b) 12 m (c) 36 m (d) 144 m

2. Which of the following is not true?
(a) For a point charge, the electrostatic potential varies as $1/r$
(b) For a dipole, the potential depends on the position vector and dipole moment vector
(c) The electric dipole potential varies as $1/r$ at large distance
(d) For a point charge, the electrostatic field varies as $1/r^2$

3. The potential at a point due to an electric dipole will be maximum and minimum when the angles between the axis of the dipole and the line joining the point to the dipole are respectively
(a) 90° and 180° (b) 0° and 90°
(c) 90° and 0° (d) 0° and 180°

4. The ionisation potential of mercury is 10.39 V. How far an electron must travel in an electric field of 1.5×10^6 V/m to gain sufficient energy to ionise mercury?
(a) $\frac{10.39}{1.6 \times 10^{-19}}$ m (b) $\frac{10.39}{2 \times 1.6 \times 10^{-19}}$ m
(c) $10.39 \times 1.6 \times 10^{-19}$ m (d) $\frac{10.39}{1.5 \times 10^6}$ m

5. The electric potential at any point x, y and z in metres is given by $V = 3x^2$. The electric field at a point (2, 0, 1) is
(a) 12 Vm^{-1} (b) -6 Vm^{-1} (c) 6 Vm^{-1} (d) -12 Vm^{-1}

6. A uniform electric field having a magnitude E_0 and direction along the positive X-axis exists. If the potential V is zero at $x = 0$, then its value at $X = +x$ will be
(a) $+xE_0$ (b) $-xE_0$
(c) $+x^2E_0$ (d) $-x^2E_0$

7. The electric potential at a point (x, y, z) is given by

$V = -x^2y - xz^3 + 4$

The electric field $\mathbf{E}$ at that point is
(a) $\mathbf{E} = \hat{\mathbf{i}}\,(2xy + z^3) + \hat{\mathbf{j}}\,x^2 + \hat{\mathbf{k}}\,3xz^2$
(b) $\mathbf{E} = \hat{\mathbf{i}}\,2xy + \hat{\mathbf{j}}\,(x^2 + y^2) + \hat{\mathbf{k}}\,(3xy - y^2)$
(c) $\mathbf{E} = \hat{\mathbf{i}}\,z^3 + \hat{\mathbf{j}}\,xyz + \hat{\mathbf{k}}\,z^2$
(d) $\mathbf{E} = \hat{\mathbf{i}}\,(2xy - z^3) + \hat{\mathbf{j}}\,xy^2 + \hat{\mathbf{k}}\,3z^2x$

8. Potential difference between two points $(V_A - V_B)$ in an electric field $\mathbf{E} = (2\hat{\mathbf{i}} - 4\hat{\mathbf{j}})$ N/C, where $A = (0, 0)$ and $B = (3\text{ m}, 4\text{ m})$ is
(a) 10 V (b) -10 V (c) 16 V (d) -16 V

9. Assume that an electric field $\mathbf{E} = 30x^2\hat{\mathbf{i}}$ exists in space. Then, the potential difference $V_A - V_o$, where V_o is the potential at the origin and V_A is the potential at $x = 2$ m, is
(a) 120 V (b) -120 V (c) -80 V (d) 80 V

10. The potential at a point x (measured in μm) due to some charges situated on the X-axis is given by $V(x) = \frac{20}{(x^2 - 4)}$ V. The electric field E at $x = 4$ μm is given by
(a) 5/3 V/μm and in the negative x-direction
(b) 5/3 V/μm and in the positive x-direction
(c) 10/9 V/μm and in the negative x-direction
(d) 10/9 V/μm and in the positive x-direction

11. Four point charges each $+q$ is placed on the circumference of a circle of diameter $2d$ in such a way that they form a square. The potential at the centre (in CGS unit) is
(a) zero (b) $\frac{4q}{d}$ (c) $\frac{4d}{q}$ (d) $\frac{q}{4d}$

12. If a charged spherical conductor of radius 5 cm has potential V at a point distant 5 cm from its centre, then the potential at a point distant 30 cm from the centre will be
(a) $\frac{1}{3}V$ (b) $\frac{1}{6}V$ c) $\frac{3}{2}V$ (d) $3V$

13. Four electric charges $+q$, $+q$, $-q$ and $-q$ are placed at the corners of a square of side $2L$. The electric potential at point A, midway between the two charges $+q$ and $+q$, is
(a) $\frac{1}{4\pi\varepsilon_0}\frac{2q}{L}\left(1 + \frac{1}{\sqrt{5}}\right)$ (b) $\frac{1}{4\pi\varepsilon_0}\frac{2q}{L}\left(1 - \frac{1}{\sqrt{5}}\right)$
(c) zero (d) $\frac{1}{4\pi\varepsilon_0}\frac{2q}{L}(1 + \sqrt{5})$

14. Two unlike charges of magnitude q are separated by a distance $2d$. The potential at a point midway between them is
(a) zero (b) $\frac{1}{4\pi\varepsilon_0}$
(c) $\frac{1}{4\pi\varepsilon_0}\cdot\frac{q}{d}$ (d) $\frac{1}{4\pi\varepsilon_0}\cdot\frac{2q}{d}$

15. In a uniform electric field a charge of 3 C experiences a force of 3000 N. The potential difference between two points 1 cm apart along the electric lines of force will be
(a) 10 V (b) 100 V
(c) 30 V (d) 300 V

16. An electron charge 10^{-3} μC is placed at the origin (0, 0) of *xy*-coordinate system. Two points *A* and *B* are situated at $(\sqrt{2}, \sqrt{2})$ and (2, 0), respectively. The potential difference between the points *A* and *B* will be
(a) 9 V (b) zero
(c) 2 V (d) 3.5 V

17. Electric potential at any point is $V = -5x + 3y + \sqrt{15}z$, then the magnitude of the electric field is
(a) $3\sqrt{2}$ (b) $4\sqrt{2}$
(c) $5\sqrt{2}$ (d) 7

18. Point charge $q_1 = 2\,\mu C$ and $q_2 = -1\,\mu C$ are kept at points $x = 0$ and $x = 6$, respectively. Electrical potential will be zero at points
(a) $x = 2$ and $x = 9$ (b) $x = 1$ and $x = 5$
(c) $x = 4$ and $x = 12$ (d) $x = -2$ and $x = 2$

19. Eight small drops, each of radius *r* and having same charge *q* are combined to form a big drop. The ratio between the potentials of the bigger drop and the smaller drop is
(a) 8 : 1 (b) 4 : 1 (c) 2 : 1 (d) 1 : 8

20. Eight oil drops of same size are charged to a potential of 50 V each. These oil drops are merged into one single large drop. What will be the potential of the large drop?
(a) 50 V (b) 100 V
(c) 200 V (d) 400 V

21. A spherical conductor of radius 2 m is charged to a potential of 120 V. It is now placed inside another hollow spherical conductor of radius 6 m. Calculate the potential of bigger sphere, if the smaller sphere is made to touch the bigger sphere.
(a) 120 V (b) 60 V
(c) 80 V (d) 40 V

22. In Millikan's oil drop experiment, an oil drop carrying a charge *Q* is held stationary by a potential difference 2400 V between the plates. To keep a drop of half the radius stationary, the potential difference had to be made 600 V. What is the charge on the second drop?
(a) $\frac{Q}{4}$ (b) $\frac{Q}{2}$ (c) Q (d) $\frac{3Q}{2}$

23. Two charges $+6\,\mu C$ and $-4\,\mu C$ are placed 15 cm apart as shown. At what distances from *A* to its right, the electrostatic potential is zero (distances in cm)?

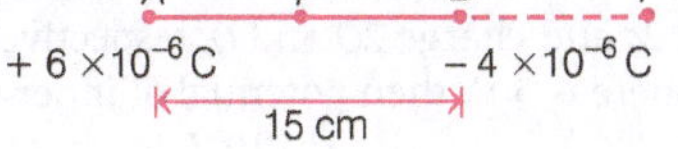

(a) 5, 9, 60 (b) 9, 45, infinity
(c) 20, 45, infinity (d) 9, 15, 45

24. An electron initially at rest falls a distance of 1.5 cm in a uniform electric field of magnitude 2×10^4 N/C. The time taken by the electron to fall this distance is
(a) 1.3×10^2 s (b) 2.1×10^{-2} s
(c) 1.6×10^{-10} s (d) 2.9×10^{-9} s

25. Charge *Q* is uniformly distributed on a dielectric rod *AB* of length $2l$. The potential at *P* shown in the figure is equal to

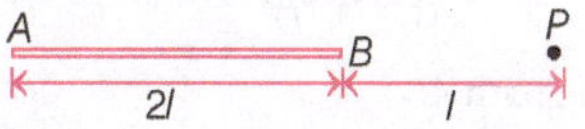

(a) $\frac{Q}{4\pi\varepsilon_0(2l)}$ (b) $\frac{Q}{4\pi\varepsilon_0(l)}\ln(2)$
(c) $\frac{Q}{4\pi\varepsilon_0(2l)}\ln(3)$ (d) None of these

26. In the figure given below, *O* is the centre of line joining *AB*. Two charges of opposite nature and same magnitude are placed at points *A* and *B*, respectively.

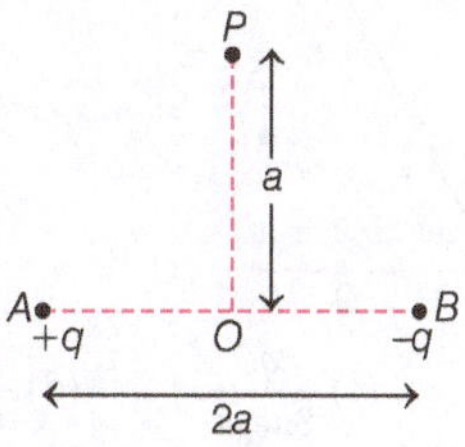

The potential at point *P* is
(a) $\frac{2kq}{a\sqrt{2}}$ (b) zero
(c) $\frac{kq}{a\sqrt{2}}$ (d) cannot be determined

27. An electron moving with the speed 5×10^6 m/s is shooted parallel to the electric field of intensity 1×10^3 N/C. Field is responsible for the retardation of motion of electron. Now evaluate the distance travelled by the electron before coming to rest for an instant (mass of $e = 9 \times 10^{-31}$ kg, charge $= 1.6 \times 10^{-19}$ C).
(a) 7 m (b) 0.7 mm (c) 7 cm (d) 0.7 cm

28. Angle between equipotential surface and lines of force is
(a) zero (b) 180° (c) 90° (d) 45°

29. A charge of 5 C is given a displacement of 0.5 m. The work done in the process is 10 J. The potential difference between the two points will be
(a) 2 V (b) 0.25 V (c) 1 V (d) 25 V

30. The work done in carrying a charge of 5 μC from a point *A* to a point *B* in an electric field is 10 mJ. Then, potential difference $(V_B - V_A)$ is
(a) +2 kV (b) –2 kV
(c) +200 kV (d) –200 kV

31. A hollow metal sphere of radius 10 cm is charged such that the potential on its surface becomes 80 V. The potential at the centre of the sphere is
(a) 80 V (b) 800 V
(c) 8 V (d) zero

32. In the electric field of a point charge q, a certain charge is carried from point A to B, C, D and E. Then, the work done

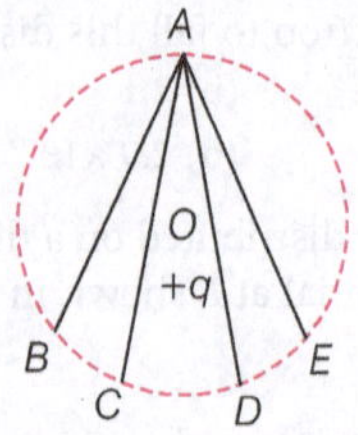

(a) is least along the path AB
(b) is least along the path AD
(c) is zero along all the paths AB, AC, AD and AE
(d) is least along AE

33. Three charges, each $+q$, are placed at the corners of an isosceles triangle ABC of sides BC and AC, $2a$. D and E are the mid-points of BC and CA. The work done in taking a charge Q from D to E is

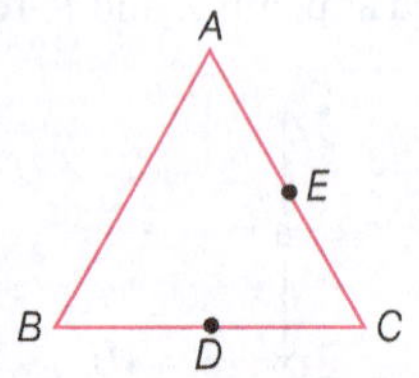

(a) zero (b) $\frac{3qQ}{4\pi\varepsilon_0 a}$ (c) $\frac{3qQ}{8\pi\varepsilon_0 a}$ (d) $\frac{qQ}{4\pi\varepsilon_0 a}$

34. A solid conducting sphere having a charge Q is surrounded by an uncharged concentric conducting hollow spherical shell. Let the potential difference between the surface of the solid sphere and that of the outer surface of the hollow shell be V.

If the shell is now given a charge of $-3Q$, then the new potential difference between the same two surface is

(a) V (b) $2V$
(c) $4V$ (d) $-2V$

35. Two spheres A and B of radius a and b respectively are at same electric potential. The ratio of the surface charge densities of A and B is

(a) $\frac{a}{b}$ (b) $\frac{b}{a}$ (c) $\frac{a^2}{b^2}$ (d) $\frac{b^2}{a^2}$

36. A particle A has charge $+q$ and a particle B has charge $+4q$ with each of them having the same mass m. When allowed to fall from rest through the same electric potential difference, the ratio of their speed $\frac{v_A}{v_B}$ will become

(a) $2:1$ (b) $1:2$
(c) $1:4$ (d) $4:1$

37. At a distance of 1 m from a fixed charge of 1 mC, a particle of mass 2 g and charge 1 μC is held stationary. Both the charges are placed on a smooth horizontal surface. If the particle is made free to move, then its speed at a distance of 10 m from the fixed charge will be

(a) 10 ms^{-1} (b) 20 ms^{-1}
(c) 60 sm^{-1} (d) 90 ms^{-1}

38. Two spherical conductors of radii 4 cm and 5 cm are charged to the same potential. If σ_1 and σ_2 be respective value of surface density of charge on both the conductors, then the ratio of σ_1 / σ_2 will be

(a) $\frac{16}{25}$ (b) $\frac{25}{10}$
(c) $\frac{4}{5}$ (d) $\frac{5}{4}$

39. A hollow charged metal sphere has radius r. If the potential difference between its surface and a point at a distance $3r$ from the centre is V, then electric field intensity at a distance $3r$ is

(a) $\frac{V}{2r}$ (b) $\frac{V}{3r}$ (c) $\frac{V}{6r}$ (d) $\frac{V}{4r}$

40. In the rectangle, shown below, the two corners have charges $q_1 = -5\ \mu C$ and $q_2 = +2.0\ \mu C$. The work done in moving a charge $+6.0\ \mu C$ from B to A is (take, $1/4\pi\varepsilon_0 = 10^{10}\ N\text{-}m^2/C^2$)

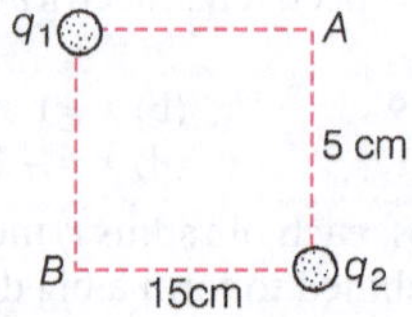

(a) 2.8 J (b) 3.5 J
(c) 4.5 J (d) 5.6 J

41. A thin spherical conducting shell of radius R has a charge q. Another charge Q is placed at the centre of the shell. The electrostatic potential at a point P, a distance $R/2$ from the centre of the cell is

(a) $\frac{(q+Q)}{4\pi\varepsilon_0}\frac{2}{R}$ (b) $\frac{2Q}{4\pi\varepsilon_0 R}$
(c) $\frac{2Q}{4\pi\varepsilon_0 R} - \frac{2q}{4\pi\varepsilon_0 R}$ (d) $\frac{2Q}{4\pi\varepsilon_0 R} + \frac{q}{4\pi\varepsilon_0 R}$

42. Consider a system composed of two metallic spheres of radii r_1 and r_2 connected by a thin wire and switch S as shown in the figure. Initially S is in open position, and the spheres carry charges q_1 and q_2, respectively. If the switch is closed, the potential of the system is

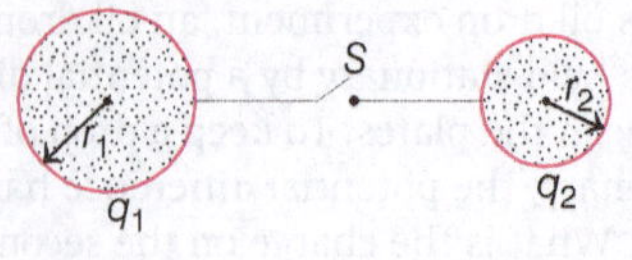

(a) $\frac{1}{4\pi\varepsilon_0}\frac{q_1 q_2}{r_1 r_2}$ (b) $\frac{1}{4\pi\varepsilon_0}\left(\frac{q_1+q_2}{r_1+r_2}\right)$
(c) $\frac{1}{4\pi\varepsilon_0}\left(\frac{q_1}{r_1}+\frac{q_2}{r_2}\right)$ (d) $\frac{1}{4\pi\varepsilon_0}\left(\frac{q_1+q_2}{\sqrt{r_1 r_2}}\right)$

43. A and B are two thin concentric hollow conductors having radii a and $2a$ and charge $2Q$ and Q, respectively. If potential of outer sphere is 5 V, then potential of inner sphere is

(a) 20 V (b) 10 V
(c) $\frac{25}{3}$ V (d) $\frac{50}{3}$ V

44. There are four concentric shells A, B, C and D of radii a, $2a$, $3a$ and $4a$, respectively. Shells B and D are given charges $+q$ and $-q$, respectively. Shell C is now earthed. The potential difference $V_A - V_C$ is $\left(\text{take, } K = \frac{1}{4\pi\varepsilon_0}\right)$

(a) $\frac{Kq}{2a}$ (b) $\frac{Kq}{3a}$

(c) $\frac{Kq}{4a}$ (d) $\frac{Kq}{6a}$

45. A point charge q is placed at a distance r from a centre O of an uncharged spherical shell of inner radius R and outer radius $2R$. The distance $r < R$. The electric potential at the centre of the shell will be

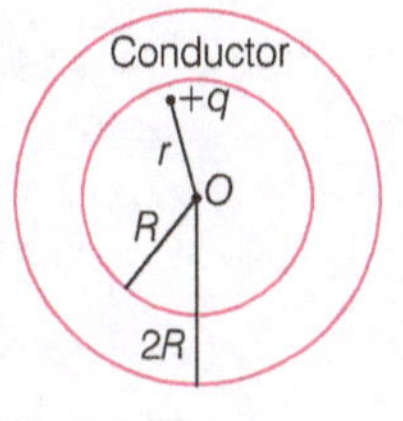

(a) $\frac{q}{4\pi\varepsilon_0}\left(\frac{1}{r} - \frac{1}{2R}\right)$ (b) $\frac{q}{4\pi\varepsilon_0 r}$

(c) $\frac{q}{4\pi\varepsilon_0}\left(\frac{1}{r} + \frac{1}{2R}\right)$ (d) $\frac{q}{4\pi\varepsilon_0}\left(\frac{1}{r} - \frac{1}{R}\right)$

46. A hollow sphere of radius r is put inside another hollow sphere of radius R. The charges on the two are $+Q$ and $-q$ as shown in the figure. A point P is located at a distance x from the common centre such that $r < x < R$. The potential at the point P is

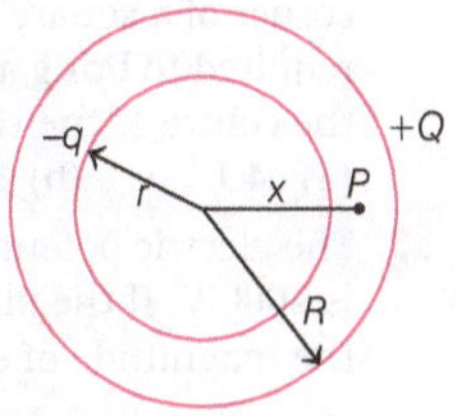

(a) $\frac{1}{4\pi\varepsilon_0}\left(\frac{Q-q}{x}\right)$ (b) $\frac{1}{4\pi\varepsilon_0}\left(\frac{Q}{R} - \frac{q}{r}\right)$

(c) $\frac{1}{4\pi\varepsilon_0}\left(\frac{Q}{R} - \frac{q}{x}\right)$ (d) $\frac{1}{4\pi\varepsilon_0}\left(\frac{q}{r} - \frac{Q}{x}\right)$

47. The arc AB with the centre C and the infinitely long wire having linear charge density λ are lying in the same plane. The minimum amount of work to be done to move a point charge q_0 from point A to B through a circular path AB of radius a is equal to

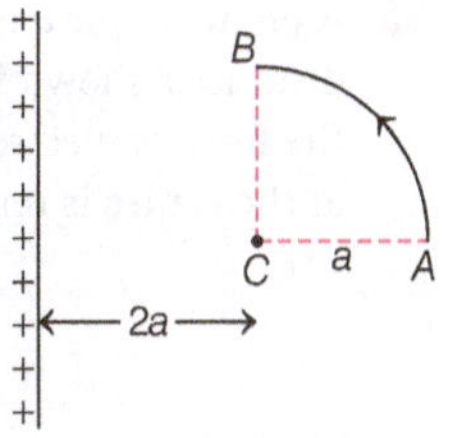

(a) $\frac{q_0\lambda}{4\pi\varepsilon_0}\ln\left(\frac{2}{3}\right)$ (b) $\frac{q_0\lambda}{2\pi\varepsilon_0}\ln\left(\frac{3}{2}\right)$

(c) $\frac{q_0\lambda}{2\pi\varepsilon_0}\ln\left(\frac{2}{3}\right)$ (d) None of these

48. Three identical metallic uncharged spheres A, B and C of radius a are kept on the corners of an equilateral triangle of side d ($d >> a$). A fourth sphere (radius a) which has charge Q touches A and is then removed to a position far away. B is earthed and then the earth connection is removed. Sphere C is then earthed, the charge on sphere C is

(a) $\frac{Qa}{2d}\left(\frac{2d-a}{2d}\right)$ (b) $\frac{Qa}{2d}\left(\frac{2d-a}{d}\right)$

(c) $\frac{Qa}{2d}\left(\frac{a-d}{d}\right)$ (d) $\frac{2Qa}{d}\left(\frac{d-a}{2d}\right)$

49. A solid conducting sphere of radius a having a charge q is surrounded by a concentric conducting spherical shell of inner radius $2a$ and outer radius $3a$ as shown in figure. The amount of heat produced when switch is closed.

$\left(\text{Take, } K = \frac{1}{4\pi\varepsilon_0}\right)$

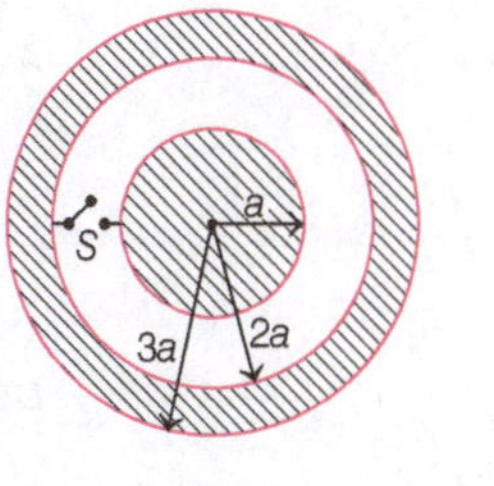

(a) $\frac{Kq^2}{2a}$ (b) $\frac{Kq^2}{3a}$ (c) $\frac{Kq^2}{4a}$ (d) $\frac{Kq^2}{6a}$

50. Two equal charges q are placed at a distance of $2a$ and a third charge $-2q$ is placed at the mid-point. The potential energy of the system is

(a) $\frac{q^2}{8\pi\varepsilon_0 a}$ (b) $\frac{6q^2}{8\pi\varepsilon_0 a}$ (c) $\frac{-7q^2}{8\pi\varepsilon_0 a}$ (d) $\frac{-9q^2}{8\pi\varepsilon_0 a}$

51. Two conducting spheres of radii 3 cm and 1 cm are separated by a distance of 10 cm in free space. If the spheres are charged to same potential of 10 V each, then the force of repulsion between them is

(a) $\left(\frac{1}{3}\right)\times 10^{-9}$ N (b) $\left(\frac{2}{9}\right)\times 10^{-9}$ N

(c) $\left(\frac{1}{9}\right)\times 10^{-9}$ N (d) $\left(\frac{4}{9}\right)\times 10^{-9}$ N

52. Two identical thin rings each of radius 10 cm carrying charges 10 C and 5 C are coaxially placed at a distance 10 cm apart. The work done in moving a charge q from the centre of the first ring to that of the second is

(a) $\frac{q}{8\pi\varepsilon_0}\left[\frac{\sqrt{2}+1}{\sqrt{2}}\right]$ (b) $\frac{q}{8\pi\varepsilon_0}\left[\frac{\sqrt{2}-1}{\sqrt{2}}\right]$

(c) $\frac{q}{4\pi\varepsilon_0}\left[\frac{\sqrt{2}+1}{\sqrt{2}}\right]$ (d) $\frac{q}{4\pi\varepsilon_0}\left[\frac{\sqrt{2}-1}{\sqrt{2}}\right]$

53. Figure shows three spherical and equipotential surfaces A, B and C around a point charge q. The potential difference $V_A - V_B = V_B - V_C$. If t_1 and t_2 be the distance between them, then

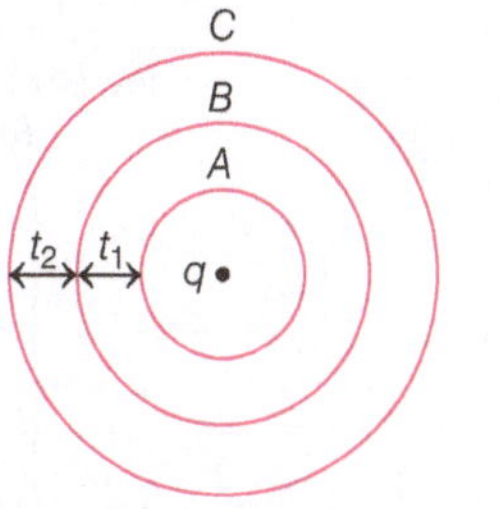

(a) $t_1 = t_2$ (b) $t_1 > t_2$

(c) $t_1 < t_2$ (d) $t_1 \le t_2$

54. A small conducting sphere of radius r is lying concentrically inside a bigger hollow conducting sphere of radius R. The bigger and smaller spheres are charged with Q and q ($Q > q$) and are insulated from each other. The potential difference between the spheres will be

(a) $\frac{1}{4\pi\varepsilon_0}\left(\frac{q}{r} - \frac{Q}{R}\right)$ (b) $\frac{1}{4\pi\varepsilon_0}\left(\frac{Q}{R} + \frac{q}{r}\right)$

(c) $\frac{1}{4\pi\varepsilon_0}\left(\frac{q}{r} - \frac{q}{R}\right)$ (d) $\frac{1}{4\pi\varepsilon_0}\left(\frac{q}{R} - \frac{Q}{r}\right)$

55. Four charges are arranged at the corners of a square $ABCD$ of side d, as shown in the figure. The work required to put together this arrangement is

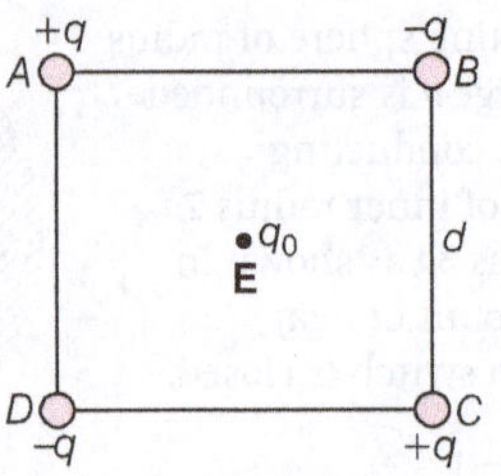

(a) $\frac{-q^2}{4\pi\varepsilon_0 d}(4-\sqrt{2})$ (b) $\frac{-q^3}{4\pi\varepsilon_0 d}(4-\sqrt{2})$

(c) $\frac{-q^4}{4\pi\varepsilon_0 d}(4-\sqrt{2})$ (d) $\frac{q^2}{4\pi\varepsilon_0 d}(4-\sqrt{2})$

56. An electric dipole when placed in a uniform electric field E will have minimum potential energy if the dipole moment makes the following angle with E

(a) π (b) $\pi/2$

(c) zero (d) $3\pi/2$

57. How much kinetic energy will be gained by an α-particle in going from a point at 70 V to another point at 50 V?

(a) 40 eV (b) 40 keV (c) 40 MeV (d) 0 eV

58. If 4×10^{20} eV energy is required to move a charge 0.25 C between two points, then what will be the potential difference between them?

(a) 178 V (b) 256 V

(c) 356 V (d) None of these

59. Figure shows some equipotential lines distributed in space. A charged object is moved from point A to point B.

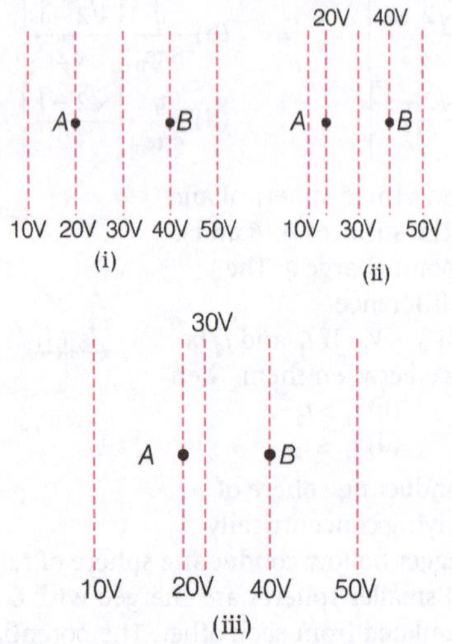

(a) The work done in Fig. (i) is the greatest

(b) The work done in Fig. (ii) is least

(c) The work done is the same in Fig. (i), Fig. (ii) and Fig. (iii)

(d) The work done in Fig. (iii) is greater than Fig. (ii) but equal to that in Fig. (i)

60. Two equal charges q of opposite sign separated by a distance $2a$ constitute an electric dipole of dipole moment p. If P is a point at a distance r from the centre of the dipole and the line joining the centre of the dipole to this point makes an angle θ with the axis of the dipole, then the potential at P is given by ($f >> 2a$) (where, $p = 2qa$).

(a) $V = \frac{p \sin\theta}{4\pi\varepsilon_0 r^2}$ (b) $V = \frac{p\cos\theta}{4\pi\varepsilon_0 r}$

(c) $V = \frac{p\sin\theta}{4\pi\varepsilon_0 r}$ (d) $V = \frac{p\cos\theta}{4\pi\varepsilon_0 r^2}$

61. Three charges Q, $+q$ and $+q$ are placed at the vertices of a right angled isosceles triangle as shown. The net electrostatic energy of the configuration is zero, if Q is equal to

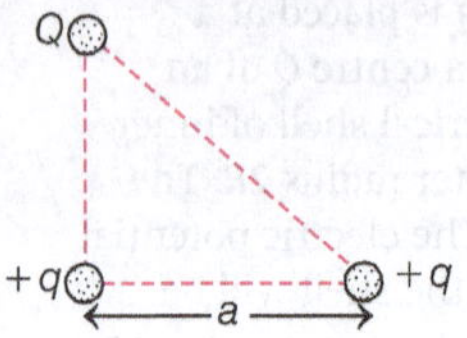

(a) $\frac{-q}{1+\sqrt{2}}$ (b) $\frac{-2q}{2+\sqrt{2}}$ (c) $-2q$ (d) $+q$

62. Four identical charges $+50\,\mu$C each are placed, one at each corner of a square of side 2 m. How much external energy is required to bring another charge of $+50\,\mu$C from infinity to the centre of the square?

(a) 64 J (b) 41 J (c) 16 J (d) 10 J

63. The electric potential difference between two parallel plates is 2000 V. If the plates are separated by 2 mm, then what is the magnitude of electrostatic force on a charge of 4×10^{-6} C located midway between the plates?

(a) 4 N (b) 6 N (c) 8 N (d) 1.5×10^{-6} N

64. Two positive charges $12\,\mu$C and $8\,\mu$C are 10 cm apart. The work done in bringing them 6 cm closer is

(a) 5.8 J (b) 5.8 eV (c) 13 J (d) 13 eV

65. A point charge q is surrounded by six identical charges at distance r shown in the figure. How much work is done by the force of electrostatic repulsion, when the point charge at the centre is removed to infinity?

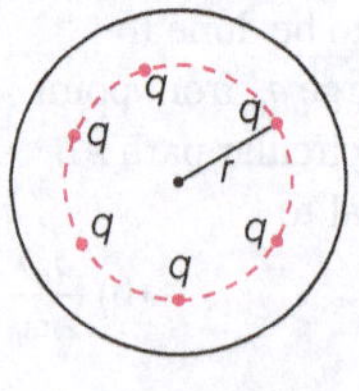

(a) $6q/4\pi\varepsilon_0 r$ (b) $6q^2/4\pi\varepsilon_0 r$

(c) $36q^2/4\pi\varepsilon_0 r$ (d) Zero

66. Three charges $-q$, $+Q$ and $-q$ are placed in a straight line as shown.

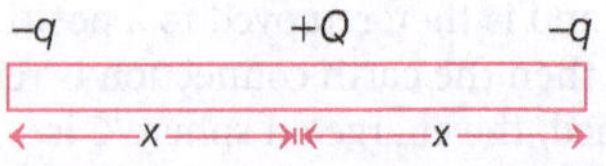

If the total potential energy of the system is zero, then the ratio $\frac{q}{Q}$ is

(a) 2 (b) 5.5 (c) 4 (d) 1.5

67. The mutual electrostatic potential energy between two protons which are at a distance of 9×10^{-15} m, in $_{92}U^{235}$ nucleus is
(a) 1.56×10^{-14} J (b) 5.5×10^{-14} J
(c) 2.56×10^{-14} J (d) 4.56×10^{-14} J

68. Three charges Q, $+q$ and $+q$ are placed at the vertices of an equilateral triangle. If the net electrostatic energy of the system is zero, then Q is equal to
(a) $(-q/2)$ (b) $-q$
(c) $+q$ (d) zero

69. Three particles, each having a charge of $10\,\mu C$ are placed at the corners of an equilateral triangle of side 10 cm. The electrostatic potential energy of the system is (given $\frac{1}{4\pi\varepsilon_0} = 9 \times 10^9\ N\text{-}m^2/C^2$)
(a) zero (b) infinite
(c) 27 J (d) 100 J

70. An electric dipole, made up of positive and negative charges each of $3.5\,\mu C$ and placed at a distance 4.2 cm apart is placed in an electric field of $5.87 \times 10^5\ NC^{-1}$. What will be the maximum torque which the field can exert on the dipole? Also, obtain the work that must be done to turn the dipole from 0° to 180°.
(a) $86.289 \times 10^{-3}\ Nm^{-1}, 1.70 \times 10^{-1}$ J
(b) $75.26 \times 10^{-3}\ Nm^{-1}, 1.70 \times 10^{-1}$ J
(c) $86.289 \times 10^{-3}\ Nm^{-1}, 3.70 \times 10^{-3}$ J
(d) $55.26 \times 10^{-3}\ Nm^{-1}, 1.70 \times 10^{-3}$ J

71. A molecule of a substance has a permanent electric dipole moment of magnitude 10^{-29} C-m. A mole of this substance is polarised (at low temperature) by applying a strong electrostatic field of magnitude $10^6\ Vm^{-1}$. The direction of the field is suddenly changed from an angle of 60° to 0°. Estimate the heat released from the substance in aligning its dipoles along the new direction of the field.
(a) −3 J (b) 3 J
(c) −6 J (d) 6 J

Assertion and Reason

Directions (Q. No. 1-5) *These questions consist of two statements each printed as Assertion (A) and Reason (R). While answering these questions you are required to choose anyone of the following four responses.*

(a) Both Assertion and Reason are true and Reason is the correct explanation of Assertion.
(b) Both Assertion and Reason are true but Reason is not the correct explanation of Assertion.
(c) Assertion is true but Reason is false.
(d) Assertion is false but Reason is true.

1. **Assertion** (A) Conductor having equal positive charge and volume, must also have same potential.
Reason (R) Potential depends on charge and geometry of conductor.

2. **Assertion** (A) When two positive point charges move away from each other, then their electrostatic potential energy decreases.
Reason (R) Change in potential energy between two points is equal to the work done by electrostatic forces.

3. **Assertion** (A) In the absence of an external electric field, the dipole moment per unit volume of a polar dielectric is zero.
Reason (R) The dipoles of a polar dielectric are randomly oriented.

4. **Assertion** (A) Polar molecules have permanent dipole moment.
Reason (R) In polar molecules, the centre of positive and negative charges coincides even when there is no external field.

5. **Assertion** (A) A point charge is placed in a uniform field pointing North. There is no change in potential energy of charge when it is moved along a line pointing East-West.
Reason (R) Electric field of a point charge is non-uniform.

Statement Type Questions

Direction (Q. Nos. 1-5) *These questions consist of two statements, choose the most appropriate answer from the options given below.*

(a) Both Statement I and Statement II are incorrect.
(b) Statement I is correct but Statement II is incorrect.
(c) Statement I is incorrect but Statement II is correct.
(d) Both Statement I and Statement II are correct.

1. **Statement I** Electric potential is scalar and electric intensity is vector quantity.
Statement II The value of electric potential and electric intensity at the middle point of the line joining an electron and proton is zero.

2. **Statement I** The two adjacent conductors carrying same charge can be at different potential.
Statement II The potential of a conductor depends on the charge on it as well as shape and size of its surrounding charged bodies and their separation from the body.

3. **Statement I** There can be a potential difference between two neighbouring conductors carrying equal positive charge.

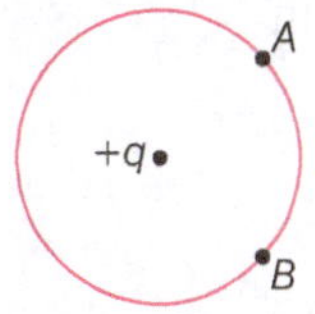

Statement II Work done is zero if a point charge $+q$, is taken from a point A to the point B on the circumference of a circle.

4. **Statement I** A small electric dipole is moved translationally from higher potential to lower potential in uniform electric field. Work done by electric field is positive.

Statement II When a positive charge is moved from higher potential to lower potential, work done by electric field is positive.

5. **Statement I** Potential energy of the system is equal to the total work done in assembling the configuration.

Statement II For a system of positive test charge electric potential is equal to electric potential energy.

Match the Columns

1. In an electric field $\mathbf{E} = (2\hat{\mathbf{i}} + 4\hat{\mathbf{j}})$ N/C, electric potential at origin is 0 V. Match the following Column I and Column II.

Column I	Column II
A. Potential at (4*m*, 0)	I. 8 V
B. Potential at (−4*m*, 0)	II. −8 V
C. Potential at (0, 4*m*)	III. 16 V
D. Potential at (0, − 4*m*)	IV. −16 V

Choose the correct answer from the options given below
(a) A-I, B-II, C-IV, D-III
(b) A-II, B-I, C-IV, D-III
(c) A-I, B-II, C-III, D-IV
(d) A-IV, B-II, C-I, D-III

2. Consider a dipole with dipole moment 4.8×10^{-30} cm. Let a point *P* lies 4.1×10^{-9} m away from centre of dipole. Match the values of potentials given in column II with column I.

Column I	Column II
A. Point is along axis of dipole nearer to positive charge	I. -18×10^{-3} V
B. Point is 45° above the axis but nearer to positive charge	II. 1.8×10^{-3} V
C. Point is 45° above the axis but nearer to negative charge	III. 2.6×10^{-3} V
D. Point is along of dipole nearer to negative charge	IV. -2.6×10^{-3} V

Choose the correct answer from options given below.
(a) A-II, B-III, C-I, D-IV
(b) A-III, B-II, C-I, D-IV
(c) A-IV, B-I, C-II, D-III
(d) D-II, B-IV, C-I, D-III

3. Consider four spherical metallic shells *A*, *B*, *C* and *D* of radii $\frac{3}{2}$ m, $\frac{5}{2}$ m, $\frac{7}{2}$ m and $\frac{9}{2}$ m, respectively with surface charge densities σ, − σ, σ and −σ, respectively. Now, match the following columns.

Column I	Column II
A. Potential of *A*	I. $(-15)\frac{\sigma}{\varepsilon_0}$
B. Potential of *B*	II. $\left(-\frac{13}{5}\right)\frac{\sigma}{\varepsilon_0}$
C. Potential of *C*	III. $(-2)\frac{\sigma}{\varepsilon_0}$
D. Potential of *D*	IV. $\left(-\frac{8}{3}\right)\frac{\sigma}{\varepsilon_0}$

Choose the correct answer from the options given below.
(a) A-IV, B-II, C-I, D-III
(b) A-III, B-II, C-I, D-IV
(c) A-II, B-I, C-III, D-IV
(d) A-I, B-III, C-II, D-IV

4. Match the Column I (potential) with Column II (value) for electric potential at different points P_1, P_2, P_3 and P_4 as shown in the figure with respect to an electric dipole.

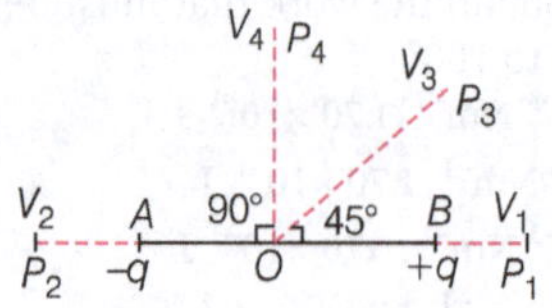

Each points P_1, P_2, P_3 and P_4 are equal distance *r* from mid-point *O* of dipole.

Column I	Column II
A. V_1	I. 0
B. V_2	II. $\frac{p}{4\sqrt{2}\pi\varepsilon_0 r^2}$
C. V_3	III. $\frac{-p}{4\pi\varepsilon_0 r^2}$
D. V_4	IV. $\frac{p}{4\pi\varepsilon_0 r^2}$

Choose the correct answer from the options given below.
(a) A-I, B-III, C-II, D-IV
(b) A-III, B-II, C-IV, D-I
(c) A-IV, B-II, C-I, D-III
(d) A-IV, B-III, C-II, D-I

Final Check Through PYQs

Module-I Electric Potential

1. Assertion (A) The potential (V) at any axial point, at 2 m distance (r) from the centre of the dipole of dipole moment vector **P** of magnitude, 4×10^{-6} C m, is $\pm 9 \times 10^{3}$ V. $\left(\text{Take, } \frac{1}{4\pi\varepsilon_0} = 9 \times 10^{9} \text{ SI units}\right)$

Reason (R) $V = \pm \frac{2P}{4\pi\varepsilon_0 r^2}$, where r is the distance of any axial point, situated at 2 m from the centre of the dipole.

In the light of the above statements, choose the correct answer from the options given below.

[NCERT (New) Pg. 49, NEET 2024]

(a) Both A and R are true but R is not the correct explanation of A.
(b) A is true but R is false.
(c) A is false but R is true.
(d) Both A and R are true and R is the correct explanation of A.

2. An electric dipole is placed as shown in the figure.

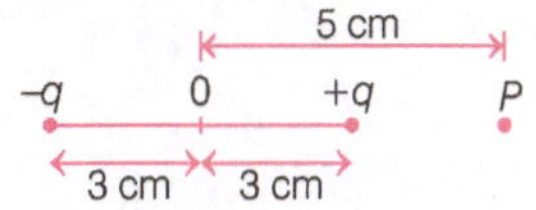

The electric potential (in 10^2 V) at point P due to the dipole is (ε_0 = permittivity of free space and $\frac{1}{4\pi\varepsilon_0} = K$)

[NCERT (New) Pg. 49, NEET 2023]

(a) $\left(\frac{5}{8}\right)qK$ (b) $\left(\frac{8}{5}\right)qK$ (c) $\left(\frac{8}{3}\right)qK$ (d) $\left(\frac{3}{8}\right)qK$

3. In a certain region of space with volume 0.2 m^3, the electric potential is found to be 5 V throughout. The magnitude of electric field in this region is

[NCERT (New) Pg. 55, NEET (Sep.) 2020]

(a) 0.5 N/C (b) 1 N/C (c) 5 N/C (d) zero

4. A short electric dipole has a dipole moment of 16×10^{-9} C-m. The electric potential due to the dipole at a point at a distance of 0.6 m from the centre of the dipole, situated on a line making an angle of 60° with the dipole axis is $\left(\frac{1}{4\pi\varepsilon_0} = 9 \times 10^{9} \text{ Nm}^2/\text{C}^2\right)$

[NCERT (New) Pg. 49, NEET (Sep.) 2020]

(a) 200 V (b) 400 V (c) zero (d) 50 V

5. If potential (in volts) in a region is expressed as $V(x, y, z) = 6xy - y + 2yz$, the electric field (in N/C) at point (1, 1, 0) is *[NCERT (New) Pg. 55, AIPMT 2015]*

(a) $-(3\hat{i} + 5\hat{j} + 3\hat{k})$ (b) $-(6\hat{i} + 5\hat{j} + 2\hat{k})$
(c) $-(2\hat{i} + 3\hat{j} + \hat{k})$ (d) $-(6\hat{i} + 9\hat{j} + \hat{k})$

Module-II Applications of Electric Potential

6. A thin spherical shell is charged by some source. The potential difference between the two points C and P (in V) shown in the figure is $\left(\text{Take, } \frac{1}{4\pi\varepsilon_0} = 9 \times 10^{9} \text{ SI units}\right)$

[NCERT (New) Pg. 51, NEET 2024]

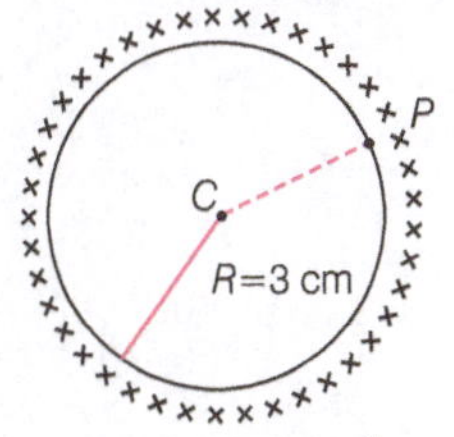

(a) 3×10^5 (b) 1×10^5
(c) 0.5×10^5 (d) zero

7. The angle between the electric lines of force and the equipotential surface is *[NCERT (New) Pg. 54, NEET 2022]*

(a) 45° (b) 90°
(c) 180° (d) 0°

8. Two hollow conducting spheres of radii R_1 and R_2 ($R_1 > R_2$) have equal charges. The potential would be

[NCERT (New) Pg. 51, NEET 2022]

(a) more on smaller sphere
(b) equal on both the spheres
(c) dependent on the material property of the sphere
(d) more on bigger sphere

9. Twenty seven drops of same size are charged at 220 V each. They combine to form a bigger drop. Calculate the potential of the bigger drop.

[NCERT (New) Pg. 51, NEET 2021]

(a) 660 V (b) 1320 V (c) 1520 V (d) 1980 V

10. Two charged spherical conductors of radii R_1 and R_2 are connected by a wire. Then, the ratio of surface charge densities of the spheres (σ_1 / σ_2) is

[NCERT (New) Pg. 51, NEET 2021]

(a) $\frac{R_1}{R_2}$ (b) $\frac{R_2}{R_1}$

(c) $\sqrt{\left(\frac{R_1}{R_2}\right)}$ (d) $\frac{R_1^2}{R_2^2}$

11. The variation of electrostatic potential with radial distance r from the centre of a positively charged metallic thin shell of radius R is given by the graph

[NCERT (New) Pg. 52, NEET (Oct.) 2020]

(a) 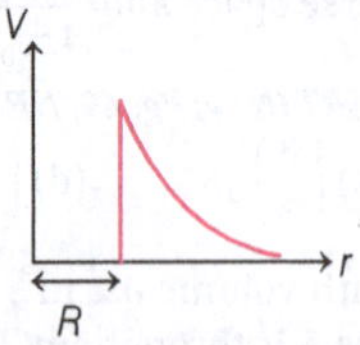

(b) 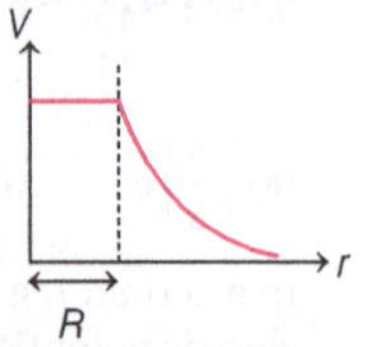

(c) 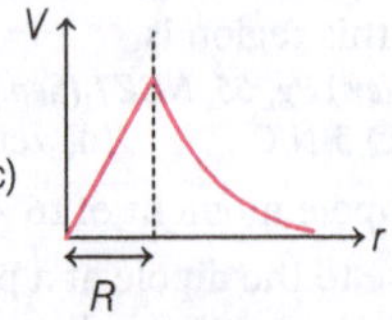

(d) 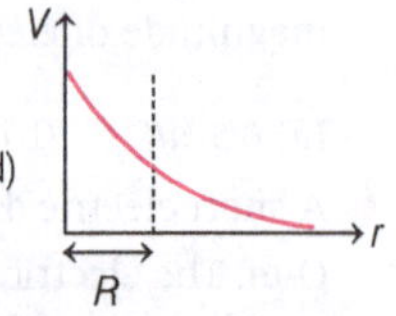

12. Two metal spheres, one of radius R and the other of radius $2R$ respectively have the same surface charge density σ. They are brought in contact and separated. What will be the new surface charge densities on them? ***[NCERT (New) Pg. 52, NEET (Odisha) 2019]***

(a) $\sigma_1 = \frac{5}{6}\sigma, \sigma_2 = \frac{5}{2}\sigma$

(b) $\sigma_1 = \frac{5}{2}\sigma, \sigma_2 = \frac{5}{6}\sigma$

(c) $\sigma_1 = \frac{5}{2}\sigma, \sigma_2 = \frac{5}{3}\sigma$

(d) $\sigma_1 = \frac{5}{3}\sigma, \sigma_2 = \frac{5}{6}\sigma$

13. The diagrams below show regions of equipotentials.

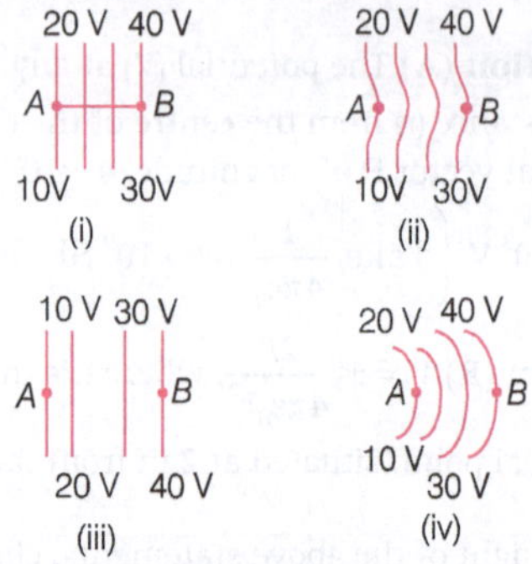

A positive charge is moved from A to B in each diagram. ***[NCERT (New) Pg. 54, NEET 2017]***

(a) Maximum work is required to move q in figure (iii)

(b) In all the four cases, the work done is the same

(c) Minimum work is required to move q in figure (i)

(d) Maximum work is required to move q in figure (ii)

Final Check

Answers

Step up Practice 1

1 (a)	2 (b)	3 (c)	4 (c)	5 (b)	6 (b)	7 (c)	8 (c)	9 (c)	10 (a)
11 (d)	12 (b)	13 (a)	14 (d)	15 (c)	16 (b)	17 (a)	18 (c)	19 (a)	20 (a)
21 (b)	22 (d)	23 (c)							

Step up Practice 2

1 (c)	2 (a)	3 (d)	4 (a)	5 (c)	6 (b)	7 (b)	8 (a)	9 (b)	10 (d)
11 (a)	12 (c)	13 (b)	14 (c)	15 (b)	16 (c)	17 (c)	18 (c)	19 (a)	20 (a)
21 (c)	22 (d)	23 (c)	24 (c)	25 (a)	26 (b)	27 (c)	28 (a)	29 (a)	30 (c)
31 (a)	32 (b)	33 (a)	34 (c)						

Step up Practice 3

1 (b)	2 (b)	3 (a)	4 (c)	5 (a)	6 (c)	7 (d)	8 (a)	9 (b)	10 (b)
11 (a)	12 (b)	13 (b)	14 (c)	15 (a)	16 (d)	17 (c)	18 (a)	19 (d)	20 (a)
21 (a)	22 (c)	23 (c)	24 (c)	25 (d)	26 (d)	27 (c)			

Gearing up for NEET

1 (a)	2 (c)	3 (d)	4 (d)	5 (d)	6 (b)	7 (a)	8 (b)	9 (c)	10 (d)
11 (b)	12 (b)	13 (b)	14 (a)	15 (a)	16 (b)	17 (d)	18 (c)	19 (b)	20 (c)
21 (d)	22 (b)	23 (b)	24 (d)	25 (c)	26 (b)	27 (c)	28 (c)	29 (a)	30 (a)
31 (a)	32 (c)	33 (a)	34 (a)	35 (b)	36 (b)	37 (d)	38 (d)	39 (c)	40 (d)
41 (d)	42 (b)	43 (c)	44 (d)	45 (a)	46 (c)	47 (b)	48 (c)	49 (c)	50 (c)
51 (a)	52 (b)	53 (c)	54 (c)	55 (a)	56 (c)	57 (a)	58 (b)	59 (c)	60 (d)
61 (b)	62 (a)	63 (a)	64 (a)	65 (b)	66 (c)	67 (c)	68 (a)	69 (c)	70 (a)
71 (b)									

Assertion and Reason

1 (d)	2 (b)	3 (a)	4 (c)	5 (b)

Statement Type Questions

1 (b)	2 (d)	3 (d)	4 (c)	5 (b)

Match the Columns

1 (b)	2 (b)	3 (b)	4 (d)

Final Check through PYQs : Module-I

1 (b)	2 (d)	3 (d)	4 (d)	5 (b)

Final Check through PYQs : Module-II

6 (d)	7 (b)	8 (a)	9 (d)	10 (b)	11 (b)	12 (d)	13 (b)

Hints and Solutions

Step up Practice 1

1. (a) Using the relation, $W = qV_a$
where, V_a is the electric potential at point A.
We have, $W = (4 \times 10^{-6})(10^4) = 4 \times 10^{-2}$ J

2. (b) Electric line of force always flow from higher potential to lower potential, so given figure in the question, if we move from labelled point to the right side, the potential will decrease. If we move from labelled point to the left side, the potential will increase. If we move perpendicular to these lines, the electric potential doesn't change. So, there are 3 more points other than labelled point which will be at the same potential.

3. (c) Electric potential at a distance r due to point charge Q is $V = \frac{kQ}{r}$ and electric field at same point is $E = \frac{kQ}{r^2}$

$$\Rightarrow E = \frac{kQ}{(kQ/V)^2} = \frac{V^2}{kQ}$$

$$= \frac{(Q \times 10^{11})^2}{kQ} = 4\pi\varepsilon_0 Q \times 10^{22} \text{ V/m} \quad \left(\because k = \frac{1}{4\pi\varepsilon_0}\right)$$

4. (c) The electrical potential produced by the nucleus at the position of the electron,

$$V = 9 \times 10^9 \times \frac{q}{r}$$

$$= 9 \times 10^9 \times \frac{(+1.6 \times 10^{-19})}{0.53 \times 10^{-10}} = 27.2 \text{ V}$$

5. (b) Obviously, from charge configuration, at the centre electric field is non-zero. Potential at the centre due to charge $2q$, $V_{2q} = \frac{2q}{r}$ and potential due to $-q$ charge,

$$V_{-q} = -\frac{q}{r}$$

(where, r = distance of centre point)

$\therefore$ Total potential, $V = V_{2q} + V_{-q} + V_{-q} = 0$

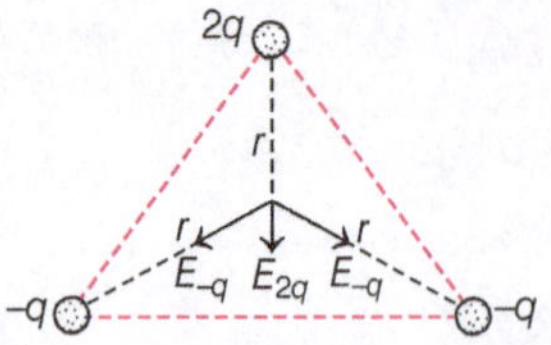

6. (b) The electric field intensity E and electric potential V are related as $E = -\frac{dV}{dr}$ and for V = constant. $\frac{dV}{dr} = 0$
This imply that electric field intensity, $E = 0$.

7. (c) Statement I is incorrect and Statement II is correct.
Electric field is equal to the negative of potential gradient

$$E = -\frac{dV}{dr}$$

This implies that even if the electric field at a point is zero, the potential may have some non-zero constant value at that point.

8. (c) We have, $mg = qE$

$$q = \frac{mg}{E} = \frac{mg}{V/d}$$

$$= \frac{1.96 \times 10^{-15} \times 10}{(400/0.02)}$$

$$= \frac{1.96 \times 10^{-14}}{2 \times 10^4} = 0.98 \times 10^{-18}$$

$$= 9.8 \times 10^{-19} \approx 6e$$

9. (c) Potential difference,

$$\Delta V = \frac{W}{q} = \frac{2}{20} = 0.1 \text{ V}$$

10. (a) The electric field,

$$\mathbf{E} = 5\hat{\mathbf{i}} - 3\hat{\mathbf{j}} \text{ kV/m}$$

$$\Delta\mathbf{r} = (10-4)\hat{\mathbf{i}} + (3-0)\hat{\mathbf{j}} + (0-3)\hat{\mathbf{k}} = 6\hat{\mathbf{i}} + 3\hat{\mathbf{j}} - 3\hat{\mathbf{k}}$$

$$V_{AB} = \mathbf{E} \cdot \Delta\mathbf{r} = (5\hat{\mathbf{i}} - 3\hat{\mathbf{j}}) \cdot (6\hat{\mathbf{i}} + 3\hat{\mathbf{j}} - 3\hat{\mathbf{k}}) \text{ kV}$$

$$= 21 \text{ kV}$$

11. (d) Both A and R are true and R is the correct explanation of A.

12. (b) Potential at A = Potential due to $(+q)$ charge + Potential due to $(-q)$ charge

$$V_A = \frac{1}{4\pi\varepsilon_0}\frac{q}{\sqrt{a^2+b^2}} + \frac{1}{4\pi\varepsilon_0}\frac{(-q)}{\sqrt{a^2+b^2}} = 0$$

13. (a) $V_A = 10^{10}\left[\frac{-5 \times 10^{-6}}{15 \times 10^{-2}} + \frac{2 \times 10^{-6}}{5 \times 10^{-2}}\right] = \frac{1}{15} \times 10^6$ V

$$V_B = 10^{10}\left[\frac{2 \times 10^{-6}}{15 \times 10^{-2}} - \frac{5 \times 10^{-6}}{5 \times 10^{-2}}\right]$$

$$= -\frac{13}{15} \times 10^6 \text{ V}$$

$$\therefore \quad W = q(V_A - V_B)$$

$$= 3 \times 10^{-6}\left[\frac{1}{15} \times 10^6 - \left(-\frac{13}{15} \times 10^6\right)\right] = 2.8 \text{ J}$$

14. (d) The electric potential between two points a and b is

$$V_B - V_A = -\int_a^b \mathbf{E} \cdot d\mathbf{r}$$

(a) $V_{(3,0)} - V_{(0,0)} = -\int_0^3 (3\hat{\mathbf{i}} + 5\hat{\mathbf{j}}) \cdot (dx\,\hat{\mathbf{i}} + dy\,\hat{\mathbf{j}})$

$= -\int_0^3 (3dx + 5dy)$

(As y is constant so $dy = 0$)

$= -3\,[x]_0^3$

$V_{(3,0)} = -9\text{ V}$

(b) Similar for

$V_{(-4,0)} - V_{(0,0)} = -3\int_0^{-4} dx$

$V_{(-4,0)} = 12\text{ V}$

(c) $V_{(0,6)} - V_{(0,0)} = -\int_0^6 (3\hat{\mathbf{i}} + 5\hat{\mathbf{j}}) \cdot (dx\,\hat{\mathbf{i}} + dy\,\hat{\mathbf{j}})$

$= -\int_0^6 (3dx + 5dy)$

(As x is constant so $dx = 0$)

$= -5\int_0^6 dy = -5\,[y]_0^6$

$V_{(0,6)} = -30\text{ V}$

(d) Similar for

$V_{(0,-5)} - V_{(0,0)} = -5\int_0^{-5} dy = -5\,[y]_0^{-5}$

$V_{(0,-5)} = +25\text{ V}$

15. (*c*) Potential at P due to $(+q)$ charge

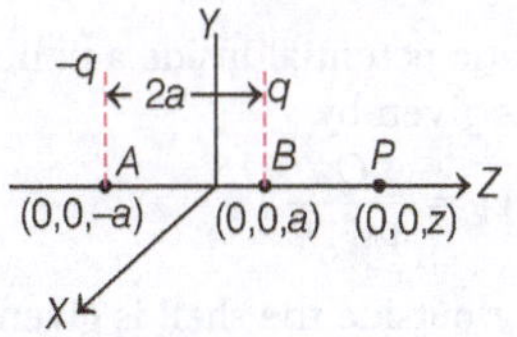

$$V_1 = \frac{1}{4\pi\varepsilon_0} \cdot \frac{q}{(z-a)}$$

Potential at P due to $(-q)$ charge,

$$V_2 = \frac{1}{4\pi\varepsilon_0} \cdot \frac{-q}{(z+a)}$$

Total potential at P due (AB) electric dipole,

$$V = V_1 + V_2 = \frac{1}{4\pi\varepsilon_0} \cdot \frac{q}{(z-a)} - \frac{1}{4\pi\varepsilon_0} \cdot \frac{q}{(z+a)}$$

$$= \frac{2qa}{4\pi\varepsilon_0 (z^2 - a^2)}$$

16. (*b*) Electric field, $E = \frac{V}{d} = \frac{10}{2 \times 10^{-2}} = 500\text{ N/C}$

17. (*a*) We have, $V = E \times d$

$\Rightarrow$ Distance, $d = \frac{V}{E} = \frac{3000}{500} = 6\text{ m}$

18. (*c*)

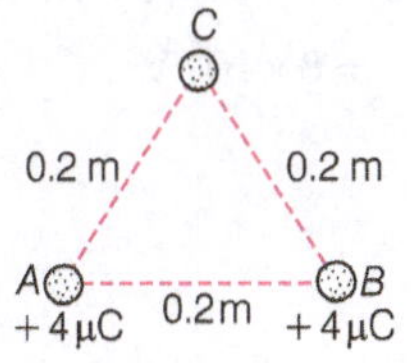

Potential at C,

$$V = 2\left(\frac{1}{4\pi\varepsilon_0} \cdot \frac{q}{r}\right)$$

$$= 2 \times \left(9 \times 10^9 \times \frac{4 \times 10^{-6}}{0.2}\right)$$

$$= 36 \times 10^4\text{ V}$$

19. (*a*) The electric potential

$V(x, y, z) = 4x^2\text{ V}$

Now, $\mathbf{E} = -\left(\hat{\mathbf{i}}\frac{\partial V}{\partial x} + \hat{\mathbf{j}}\frac{\partial V}{\partial y} + \hat{\mathbf{k}}\frac{\partial V}{\partial z}\right)$

Now, $\frac{\partial V}{\partial x} = 8x$, $\frac{\partial V}{\partial y} = 0$ and $\frac{\partial V}{\partial z} = 0$

Hence, $\mathbf{E} = -8x\hat{\mathbf{i}}$ V/m. So, at point (1 m, 0, 2 m)

$\mathbf{E} = -8\hat{\mathbf{i}}$ V/m or 8, along negative X-axis.

20. (*a*) We have, electric field,

$$E = -\frac{dV}{dx} = -\frac{d}{dx}(5x^2 + 10x - 9)$$

$$= -10x - 10$$

$$\therefore (E)_{x=1} = -10 \times 1 - 10$$

$$= -20\text{ V/m}$$

21. (*b*) Statement I is correct but Statement II is incorrect.
Electric potential due to a point charge q at a distance r from is given by, $V = \frac{1}{4\pi\varepsilon_0} \cdot \frac{q}{r}$.

22. (*d*) The octupole potential can be expressed as

$$V_{\text{oct}}(r) = \frac{1}{4\pi\varepsilon_0} \frac{1}{r^4} \Sigma_{i,j,k}\, Q_{ijk}\, \hat{\mathbf{r}}_i \hat{\mathbf{r}}_j \hat{\mathbf{r}}_k$$

$\therefore$ Potential due to octupole varies as $\frac{1}{r^4}$.

23. (*c*) Electric potential can be calculated for both variable and constant electric fields. In case of a constant electric field, the electric potential, $V = Ed$, where (E) is the magnitude of the electric field and (d) is the distance from the point to a reference. For a variable electric field, the potential is calculated by integrating the electric field over the path from the reference point to the point of interest.
Electric potential difference can also be calculated for variable electric field.
So, we can say that only statement (c) is correct.

Step up Practice 2

1. (*c*) Work done in displacing a charge particle is given by $W_{AB} = q(V_B - V_A)$ and the line integral of electric field from point A to B gives potential difference

$$V_B - V_A = -\int_A^B \mathbf{E} \cdot d\mathbf{l}$$

For equipotential surface, $V_B - V_A = 0$ and hence $W = 0$.

2. (*a*) Both A and R are true but R is not the correct explanation of A.

Work done in moving a charge along an equipotential surface is zero because electric potential is constant along an equipotential surface.

3. (*d*) Equipotential surfaces are not always spherical. They can take various shapes depending on the configuration of electric charges creating the electric field.

Gaussian surfaces can take various shapes depending on the symmetry of the charge distribution being analysed.

Electrical field always perpendicular to an equipotential surface.

So, only statement (d) is correct.

4. (*a*) Both A and R are true but R is not the correct explanation of A.

Electric field line are perpendicular to equipotential surfaces because the potential is constant along them not necessarily because potential decreases in the direction of the field.

5. (*c*) Equipotential surfaces will not always be equally spaced. These are closer in regions with high electric fields than in regions with low electric fields.

6. (*b*) Statement I is correct but Statement II is incorrect. If two equipotential surfaces intersect, there would be two values of electric potential at the point of intersection, which is not possible.

7. (*b*) Since, potential inside the hollow sphere is same as that on the surface.

8. (*a*) Let Q_1 and Q_2 are the charges on sphere of radii R_1 and R_2, respectively.

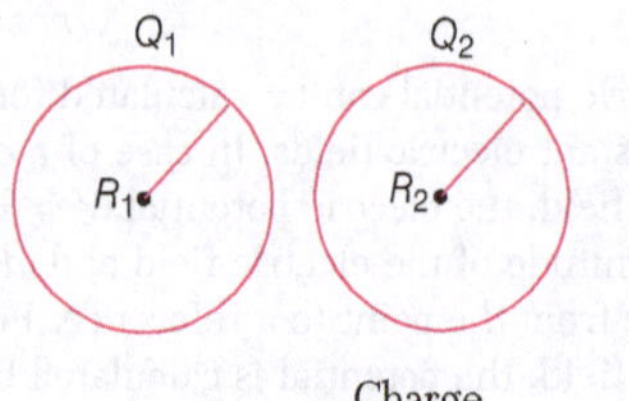

Surface charge density, $\sigma = \dfrac{\text{Charge}}{\text{area}}$

According to given problem, $\sigma_1 = \sigma_2$

$$\frac{Q_1}{4\pi R_1^2} = \frac{Q_2}{4\pi R_2^2}$$

$$\therefore \quad \frac{Q_1}{Q_2} = \frac{R_1^2}{R_2^2} \quad \text{...(i)}$$

In case of a charged sphere,

$$V_s = \frac{1}{4\pi\varepsilon_0}\frac{Q}{R}$$

$$\therefore \quad V_1 = \frac{1}{4\pi\varepsilon_0}\frac{Q_1}{R_1}, V_2 = \frac{1}{4\pi\varepsilon_0}\frac{Q_2}{R_2}$$

$$\Rightarrow \quad \frac{V_1}{V_2} = \frac{Q_1}{R_1} \times \frac{R_2}{Q_2} = \frac{Q_1}{Q_2} \times \frac{R_2}{R_1}$$

$$= \left(\frac{R_1}{R_2}\right)^2 \times \left(\frac{R_2}{R_1}\right) = \frac{R_1}{R_2} \text{ [using Eq. (i)]}$$

9. (*b*) Potential inside the sphere will be same as that on its surface, i.e. $V = V_{\text{surface}} = \dfrac{q}{10}$ stat volt,

$$V_{\text{out}} = \frac{q}{15} \text{ stat volt}$$

$$\therefore \quad \frac{V_{\text{out}}}{V} = \frac{2}{3} \Rightarrow V_{\text{out}} = \frac{2}{3}V$$

10. (*d*) If charge acquired by the smaller sphere is q, then its potential,

$$120 = \frac{kq}{2} \quad \text{...(i)}$$

Whole charge comes to outer sphere.

Also, potential of the outer sphere, $V = \dfrac{kq}{6}$ ...(ii)

From Eqs. (i) and (ii), we get

$$V = 40 \text{ V}$$

11. (*a*) Electrostatic potential inside a uniformly thin shell of radius R is given by

$$V_R = \frac{Q}{4\pi\varepsilon_0 R}$$

and at point r outside the shell is given by

$$V_r = \frac{Q}{4\pi\varepsilon_0 r}$$

12. (*c*) Potential, $V = \dfrac{1}{4\pi\varepsilon_0} \cdot \dfrac{q}{r} = 9 \times 10^9 \times \dfrac{500 \times 10^{-6}}{1.0}$

$$= 4.5 \times 10^6 \text{ V}$$

13. (*b*) Statement I is correct but Statement II is incorrect. It becomes possible to define potential at a point in an electric field because electric field is a conservative field.

14. (*c*) Potential, $V = \dfrac{1}{4\pi\varepsilon_0}\dfrac{q}{R} = \dfrac{(9 \times 10^9) \times (5 \times 10^{-8})}{0.1}$

$$= 4500 \text{V}$$

15. (*b*) Potential, $V = \dfrac{Kq}{r} = \dfrac{KZe}{r}$

$$= \frac{9 \times 10^9 \times 50 \times 1.6 \times 10^{-19}}{9 \times 10^{-15}}$$

$$= 8 \times 10^6 \text{ V}$$

16. (c) A is false but R is true.
The electric potential outside a uniformly charged conducting sphere is inversely proportional to the distance from the centre of the sphere.

17. (c) Let q' be the charge on the inner shell. Then, the potential of the inner is
V = potential due to its own q' + potential due to the outer charge

$$= \frac{1}{4\pi\varepsilon}\left(\frac{q'}{r_1} + \frac{q}{r_2}\right)$$

But $V = 0$, because the inner shell is earthed.

$$\therefore \quad \frac{q'}{r_1} + \frac{q}{r_2} = 0$$

$$q' = -q\left(\frac{r_1}{r_2}\right)$$

18. (c) Inside a conducting body, potential is same everywhere and equals to the potential at its surface.

19. (a) $V_A = \frac{\sigma}{\varepsilon_0}(a - b + c)$

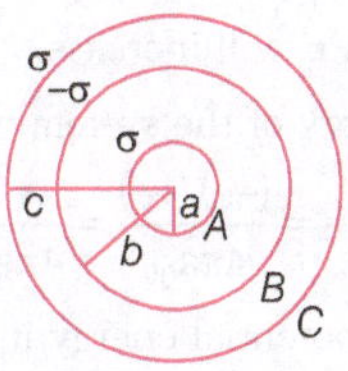

$$V_B = \frac{\sigma}{\varepsilon_0}\left(\frac{a^2}{c} - b + c\right)$$

$$\Rightarrow \quad V_C = \frac{\sigma}{\varepsilon_0}\left(\frac{a^2}{c} - \frac{b^2}{c} + c\right)$$

On putting $c = a + b$

$$\Rightarrow \quad V_A = V_C \neq V_B$$

20. (a) Using the relation, $V = Ed$
where, V = potential difference between the two points
E = magnitude of electric field (E)
d = projection of line along E

$$V_{CD} = V_C - V_D = (-30) \times (2) = -60 \text{ V}$$

21. (c) For any concentric charged shells, charge is not induced from outer shell to inner shell because the charge on the outer shell will redistribute themselves in a way that cancels out the electric field inside the inner shell, resulting is no net charge induced on the inner shell.
Two concentric charged shells can induces charge under certain condition i.e. outer shell grounded, Inner shell grounded. If outer shell is grounded, charge induced an outer surface is equal to charge of inner surface.
But if inner shell is grounded, charge induced on inner shell is not equal to charge of outer shell.

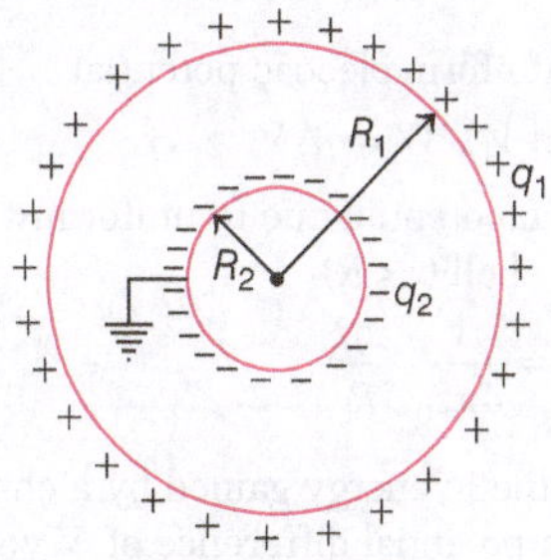

$$q_2 = -q_1\frac{R_2}{R_1}$$

Hence, only statement (c) is correct.

22. (d) Both Statement I and Statement II are correct.

23. (c) $q = 2\,\mu\text{C} = 2 \times 10^{-6}$ C

$$r = 3 \text{ cm} = 3 \times 10^{-2} \text{ m}$$

Induced charge will not produce/contribute to potential.

$$V = \frac{kq}{r}$$

$$V = \frac{9 \times 10^9 \times 2 \times 10^{-6}}{3 \times 10^{-2}}$$

$$V = 6 \times 10^5 \text{ V}$$

$$\Rightarrow \quad V = 0.60 \text{ MV}$$

24. (c) Let the charge on the inner sphere be Q, then the charge induced on the inner surface of the outer sphere is $-Q$.
∴ Electric potential V of the inner sphere is given by,

$$V = \frac{Q}{4} - \frac{Q}{6}$$

$$V = 3 \text{ esu}$$

$$\therefore \quad 3 = \frac{Q}{4} - \frac{Q}{6}$$

$$\Rightarrow \quad Q\left[\frac{1}{4} - \frac{1}{6}\right] = 3$$

$$\Rightarrow \quad \frac{Q}{12} = 3$$

∴ Charge on the inner sphere, $Q = 36$ esu

25. (a) The electric potential is constant for conducting charge sphere.

26. (b) No work is done to move a charged particle from one point to another point on a equipotential surface.
In non-conducting charged sphere, charge is uniformly distributed. Hence the electric potential at the centre is 1.5 times the electric potential at the surface of the sphere.

The potential is constant for conducting charged sphere because the electric field inside a conducting sphere is zero.

For non-uniform electric potential

$W = q(V_2 - V_1),\ W = q\Delta V$

27. (c) Electric potential due to uniformly charged thin spherical shell $(r < R)$

$$V = \frac{1}{4\pi\varepsilon_0} \cdot \frac{q}{R}$$

28. (a) The kinetic energy gained by a charge of q coulomb through a potential difference of V volt is

$$K = qV$$
$$K = (1.6 \times 10^{-19})(2000)$$
$$= 3.2 \times 10^{-16}\ \text{J}$$

We have, $K = \frac{1}{2} mv^2$

$$v = \sqrt{\frac{2K}{m}} = \sqrt{\frac{2 \times 3.2 \times 10^{-16}}{9 \times 10^{-31}}}$$
$$= \frac{8}{3} \times 10^7\ \text{m/s}$$

29. (a) Speed of the particle, $v = \sqrt{\frac{2QV}{m}}$

$$\Rightarrow \quad v \propto \sqrt{Q} \Rightarrow \frac{v_a}{v_B} = \sqrt{\frac{Q_A}{Q_B}}$$
$$= \sqrt{\frac{16q}{4q}} = \frac{2}{1}$$

30. (c) The kinetic energy of the electron,

$$K = eV = \frac{1}{2} mv^2$$
$$\Rightarrow \quad V = \frac{1}{2} \frac{mv^2}{e}$$

Here, $v = \frac{c}{10} = \frac{3 \times 10^8}{10}$

$$= 3 \times 10^7\ \text{m/s}$$
$$V = \frac{1}{2} \frac{(9.0 \times 10^{-31})(3.0 \times 10^{-7})^2}{(1.6 \times 10^{-19})}$$

Potential, $V = 2531$ V

31. (a) Kinetic energy, KE $= qV$

For α particle, KE $= (2e)[V_B - V_A] = 2e\,[20]$ volt

$$\text{KE} = 40\ \text{eV}$$

32. (b) The kinetic energy gained by a charged particle is

$$K = qV$$

Kinetic energy of a proton,

$$K_p = +1 \times V = V$$

Kinetic energy of a deuteron

$$K_d = +1 \times V = V$$

Kinetic energy of a α-particle

$K_\alpha = +2 \times V = 2V$

Hence, $K_p : K_d : K_\alpha = V : V : 2V$

$\Rightarrow K_p : K_d : K_\alpha = 1 : 1 : 2$

33. (a) Given,

Electron gain energy, $K = 200$ eV

$$K = qV$$
$$V = \frac{K}{q}$$
$$\therefore \quad V = \frac{200\ \text{eV}}{e}$$

Hence, $V = 200$ V

34. (c) A is false but R is true.

Electric force is a conservative force. So, the work done by a conservative force is independent of the path taken by the particle.

Step up Practice 3

1. (b) ΔPE = Work done by external agent

$$= (V_f q - V_i q),\ V_f > V_i$$

$\Rightarrow$ ΔPE > 0, i.e. PE will increase.

2. (b) Potential energy of the system will be given by

$$= \frac{(-e)(-e)}{4\pi\varepsilon_0 r} = \frac{e^2}{4\pi\varepsilon_0 r}$$

As, r decreases, potential energy increases.

3. (a) From work energy theorem,

Work done = Change in KE

$$qV = \text{KE}_f - \text{KE}_i \quad [\because \text{KE}_i = 0]$$
$$\Rightarrow \quad \text{KE}_f = V(2e)$$
$$\text{KE}_f = 5 \times 2 \times 1.6 \times 10^{-19}\ \text{J}$$
$$\text{KE}_f = 10\ \text{eV}$$

4. (c) Work done, $W = U_f - U_i$

$$= 9 \times 10^9 \times QQ_2 \left[\frac{1}{r_2} - \frac{1}{r_1}\right]$$
$$\Rightarrow \quad W = 9 \times 10^9 \times 12 \times 10^{-6} \times 8 \times 10^{-6} \left[\frac{1}{4 \times 10^{-2}} - \frac{1}{10 \times 10^{-2}}\right]$$
$$= 12.96\ \text{J} \approx 13\ \text{J}$$

6. (c) Electric potential energy,

$$U = \frac{1}{4\pi\varepsilon_0} \frac{q_1 q_2}{d}$$
$$\therefore \quad U = \frac{9 \times 10^9 \times 1.6 \times 10^{-19} \times (-1.6 \times 10^{-19})}{1 \times 10^{-10} \times 1.6 \times 10^{-19}}\ \text{eV}$$
$$= -9 \times 10^9 \times 1.6 \times 10^{-9}\ \text{eV}$$
$$= -14.4\ \text{eV}$$

7. (*d*) The potential energy, $U = \frac{1}{4\pi\varepsilon_0}\frac{q_1q_2}{r_{12}}$ is unaltered whatever way the charges are brought to the specified locations, because of path-independence of work for electrostatic force.

Therefore, both A and R are true and R is the correct explanation of A.

8. (*a*) Since, the proton is moving against the direction of electric field, so work is done by the proton against electric field. It implies that electric field does negative work on the proton. Again, proton is moving in electric field from low potential region to high potential region, hence its potential energy increases.

9. (*b*) A is true but R is false.

Non-conservative force depends on path. Hence, work done by non-conservative force is not equal to the change in PE.

10. (*b*) Potential energy of charges Q_1 and Q_2 at 10 cm apart,

$$U_i = \frac{1}{4\pi\varepsilon_0}\frac{12\times10^{-6}\times5\times10^{-6}}{0.1}$$

$$= \frac{9\times10^9\times60\times10^{-12}}{0.1}$$

$$= 54\times10^{-1} = 5.4\text{ J}$$

Potential energy of charge Q_1 and Q_2 at 6 cm apart,

$$U_2 = \frac{9\times10^9\times60\times10^{-12}}{0.06} = 9\text{ J}$$

$\therefore$ Work done = (9 − 5.4) J

= 3.6 J

11. (*a*) Radius $= 2\times10^{-2}$ m

Charge density $= 10^{-4}\text{ C/cm}^2 = 1\text{ C/m}^2$

$$q' = 4\times10^{-8}\text{ C}$$

Distance from the centre of sphere, $r = (2+2)\times10^{-2}$ m

$\Rightarrow$ Work done

$$W = \frac{Kqq'}{r} = \frac{K\sigma Aq'}{r}$$

$$\Rightarrow W = \frac{9\times10^9\times1\times4\pi\times4\times10^{-4}\times4\times10^{-8}}{4\times10^{-2}}$$

$$\Rightarrow W = 14.4\pi\text{ J}$$

12. (*b*) The potential energy is relative quantity, it depends on reference position, while comparing potential energy in two positions, consider negative sign.

(a) $U \propto \frac{e^2}{r}$, if r is decreased, U is increased.

(b) $U \propto -\frac{e^2}{r}$, if r is decreased, U is decreased.

(c) $U \propto -\frac{e^2}{r}$, if r is increased, U is increased.

(d) $U \propto \frac{e^2}{r}$, if r is decreased, U is increased.

So option (b) is wrong.

13. (*b*) A is true but R is false.

Electric potential and electric potential energy are different quantities.

If test charge $= Q$ and point charge q, the electric potential is $V = \frac{Kq}{r}$ and potential energy

$$W = QV = \frac{KqQ}{r}$$

Thus, $V \neq W$

14. (*c*) Potential difference

$$\Delta V = V_Q - V_P$$

$$= -4\text{ V} - 10\text{ V} = -14\text{ V}$$

Work done $\Delta W = q\Delta V$

$$= 1.6\times10^{-19}\times100\times(-14)$$

$$= -2.24\times10^{-16}\text{ J}$$

15. (*a*) At infinity PE = 0

Case I Applying energy conservation

$$0 + \frac{1}{2}mv^2 = \frac{KQq}{r} + 0$$

$$\Rightarrow \quad \frac{1}{2}mv^2 = \frac{KQq}{r} \quad \text{...(i)}$$

Case II Applying energy conservation

$$\frac{1}{2}m(2v)^2 = \frac{KQq}{r'} \quad \text{...(ii)}$$

From Eqs. (i) and (ii)

$$r' = \frac{r}{4}$$

16. (*d*) We have, $AB + AC = 12$ cm ...(i)

$$AB\cdot AC = 32\text{ cm}^2$$

$$\therefore\ AB - AC = \sqrt{(AB) + AC)^2 - 4AB\cdot AC}$$

$$AB - AC = 4\text{ cm}$$

From Eqs. (i) and (ii), we get

$$AB = 8\text{ cm}, AC = 4\text{ cm}$$

Potential energy at point A,

$$U_A = \frac{1}{4\pi\varepsilon_0}\left[\frac{q_Aq_B}{AB} + \frac{q_Aq_C}{AC}\right]$$

$$= \frac{9\times10^9\times4\times10^{-12}}{10^{-2}}\left(\frac{1}{8}+\frac{1}{4}\right) = 1.35\text{ J}$$

17. (*c*) Potential energy,

$$U = \frac{1}{4\pi\varepsilon_0}\left[\frac{Q_1Q_2}{r_1} + \frac{Q_2Q_3}{r_2} + \frac{Q_1Q_3}{r_3}\right]$$

Net potential energy, $U_{\text{net}} = \frac{3}{4\pi\varepsilon_0}\cdot\frac{q^2}{l}$

18. (*a*) Potential energy of the system,

$$U = K\frac{Qq}{l} + \frac{Kq^2}{l} + \frac{KqQ}{l} = 0$$

$$\Rightarrow \quad \frac{Kq}{l}(Q + q + Q) = 0$$

$$\Rightarrow \quad Q = -\frac{q}{2}$$

19. (*d*) Length of the diagonal of a cube having each side b is $\sqrt{3}b$. So, distance of centre of cube from each vertex is $\frac{\sqrt{3}}{2}b$.

Hence, potential energy of the given system of charge is

$$U = 8 \times \left[\frac{1}{4\pi\varepsilon_0} \cdot \frac{(-q)(q)}{\sqrt{3}b/2}\right] = \frac{-4q^2}{\sqrt{3}\,\pi\varepsilon_0 b}$$

20. (*a*) Change in potential energy

$$(\Delta U) = U_f - u_i$$

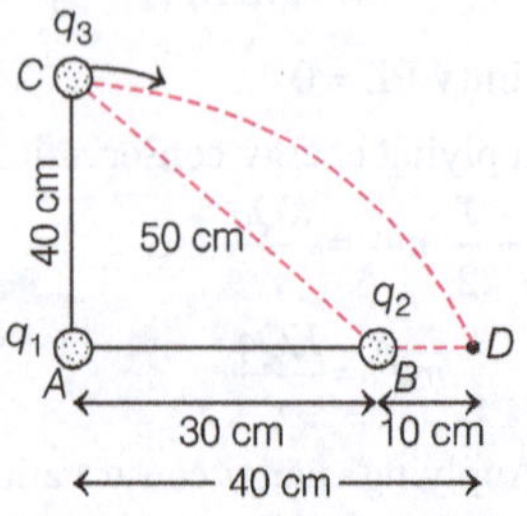

$\Rightarrow$ Potential energy,

$$\Delta U = \frac{1}{4\pi\varepsilon_0}\left[\left(\frac{q_1q_3}{0.4} + \frac{q_2q_3}{0.1}\right) - \left(\frac{q_1q_3}{0.4} + \frac{q_2q_3}{0.5}\right)\right]$$

$$\Rightarrow \quad \Delta U = \frac{1}{4\pi\varepsilon_0}[8q_2q_3]$$

$$= \frac{q_3}{4\pi\varepsilon_0}(8q_2)$$

$$\therefore \quad k = 8q_2$$

21. (*a*) Given, $q_1 = 1\text{ C}, q_2 = 2\text{ C}, q_3 = 3\text{ C}$ and $r_1 = 100\text{ cm} = 1\text{ m}$

Initial PE of system,

$$U_1 = \frac{1}{4\pi\varepsilon_0 r_1}(q_1q_2 + q_2q_3 + q_3q_1)$$

$$= \frac{9 \times 10^9}{1}(1 \times 2 + 2 \times 3 + 3 \times 1)$$

$$= 99 \times 10^9\text{ J}$$

When $r_2 = 50\text{ cm} = 0.5\text{ m}$

Initial PE of system,

$$U_2 = \frac{1}{4\pi\varepsilon_0 r_2}(q_1q_2 + q_2q_3 + q_3q_1)$$

$$= \frac{9 \times 10^9}{0.5}(1 \times 2 + 2 \times 3 + 3 \times 1)$$

$$= 2 \times 99 \times 10^9\text{ J}$$

Work done, $W = U_2 - U_1$

$$= 2 \times 99 \times 10^9 - 99 \times 10^9$$

$$= 99 \times 10^9\text{ J}$$

$$= 9.9 \times 10^{10}\text{ J}$$

22. (*c*) Total electropotential energy can be calculated by algebraic sum of all potential energies.

$$U_{\text{total}} = \frac{-KqQ}{r} + \frac{-KqQ}{r} + \frac{K(-q)(-q)}{2r}$$

$$= \left[-2Qq + \frac{q^2}{2}\right]\frac{K}{r}$$

Since $\quad U_{\text{total}} = 0$

$$\Rightarrow \quad -2Qq + \frac{q^2}{2} = 0$$

$$\Rightarrow \quad q = 4Q \text{ or } \frac{q}{Q} = \frac{4}{1}$$

23. (*c*) A is false but R is true.

24. (*c*) Torque, $\tau_{\max} = pE = q(2l)E$

$$= 2 \times 10^{-6} \times 0.01 \times 5 \times 10^5$$

$$= 10 \times 10^{-3}\text{ N-m}$$

25. (*d*) Work done, $W = pE(1 - \cos\theta)$

$$= pE(1 - \cos 180°)$$

$$W = pE[1 - (-1)] = 2pE$$

26. (*d*) When an electric dipole is placed in uniform electric field, then $U = -pE\cos\theta$.

Gearing up for NEET

1. (*a*) Potential, $V = E \cdot d$

$\therefore$ Distance from the point charge,

$$d = \frac{V}{E} = \frac{3000}{500} = 6\text{ m}$$

2. (*c*) The electric dipole potential varies $1/r$ at large distance, is not true, because $V = \frac{1}{4\pi\varepsilon_0} \cdot \frac{p}{r^2}$, i.e. $V \propto \frac{1}{r^2}$.

3. (*d*) Potential at a point due to electric dipole

$$V = \frac{p\cos\theta}{r^2}$$

If $\theta = 0°$, then V will be maximum and if $\theta = 180°$, then V will be minimum.

4. (*d*) The potential which is required to ionise the electron from outermost shell of mercury is called ionisation potential. The electric field strength is given by $E = \frac{V}{d}$.

where, d is distance between plates creating electric field.

Given, $V = 10.39$ V, $E = 1.5 \times 10^6$ V/m

Distance travelled by electron to gain ionisation energy,

$$\therefore d = \frac{V}{E} = \frac{10.39}{1.5 \times 10^6} \text{ m}$$

5. (*d*) Electric field, $E = -\frac{dV}{dr} = -\frac{d}{dx}(3x^2) = -6x$

At pont (2, 0, 1)

Electric field, $E = -12 \text{ Vm}^{-1}$

6. (*b*) We have, $E_0 = -\frac{dV}{dx}$ or $dV = -E_0 dx$

On integrating both sides, we get

$$\int_0^{V_x} dV = \int_0^x E_0 dx$$

$$\Rightarrow \quad V_x = -xE_0$$

7. (*a*) Potential gradient is related with electric field according to the following relation, $E = \frac{-dV}{dr}$.

$$\mathbf{E} = -\frac{\partial V_\mathbf{r}}{\partial r} = \left[-\frac{\partial V}{\partial x}\hat{\mathbf{i}} - \frac{\partial V}{\partial y}\hat{\mathbf{j}} - \frac{\partial V}{\partial z}\hat{\mathbf{k}}\right]$$

$$= [\hat{\mathbf{i}}\,(2xy + z^3) + \hat{\mathbf{j}}\,x^2 + \hat{\mathbf{k}}\,3xz^2]$$

8. (*b*) Potential difference between two points,

$$V_A - V_B = \int_A^B (2\hat{\mathbf{i}} - 4\hat{\mathbf{j}}) \cdot (dx\hat{\mathbf{i}} + dy\hat{\mathbf{j}})$$

$$= [2x - 4y]_{(0,0)}^{(3m,\,4m)} = -10 \text{ V}$$

9. (*c*) We have, potential difference,

$$V_A - V_o = -\int_o^A E_x dx$$

Potential difference,

$$V_A - V_o = -\int_0^2 30x^2 dx$$

$$= -30\left(\frac{2^3}{3}\right) = -80 \text{ V}$$

10. (*d*) We have, $V(x) = \frac{20}{x^2 - 4}$

Electric field at $x = 4\ \mu$m

$$E = \frac{-dV}{dx} = \frac{20}{(x^2 - 4)^2}(2x - 0)$$

$$= \frac{160}{144} = \frac{10}{9} \text{ V/}\mu\text{m}$$

Direction of electric field E will be along positive x-direction.

11. (*b*) Potential at centre due to all charges,

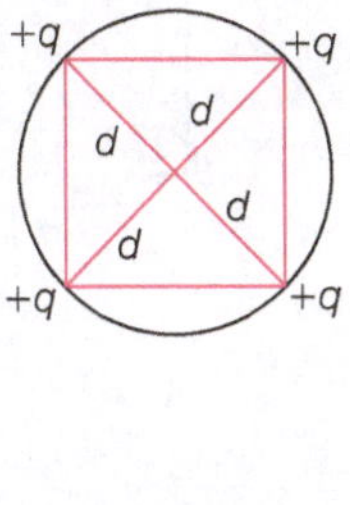

$$V = \frac{1}{4\pi\varepsilon_0}\left[\frac{q}{d} + \frac{q}{d} + \frac{q}{d} + \frac{q}{d}\right]$$

$$= \frac{1}{4\pi\varepsilon_0}\frac{4q}{d} \text{ in SI unit} = \frac{4q}{d} \text{ in CGS unit}$$

12. (*b*) Radius of spherical conductor,

$$R = 5 \text{ cm} = 5 \times 10^{-2} \text{ m}$$

According to given situation,

$$V = \frac{1}{4\pi\varepsilon_0} \cdot \frac{q}{R}$$

$$V = \frac{1}{4\pi\varepsilon_0} \cdot \frac{q}{5 \times 10^{-2}}$$

$$\Rightarrow \quad \frac{q}{4\pi\varepsilon_0} = 5 \times 10^{-2} V \quad \text{...(i)}$$

Again, electric potential at distance

$$r = 30 \text{ cm} = 30 \times 10^{-2} \text{ m}$$

From the centre,

$$V' = \frac{1}{4\pi\varepsilon_0} \cdot \frac{q}{30 \times 10^{-2}}$$

$$= \left(\frac{q}{4\pi\varepsilon_0}\right) \times \frac{1}{30 \times 10^{-2}} = \frac{5 \times 10^{-2}}{30 \times 10^{-2}} V$$

$$= \frac{V}{6} \quad \text{[from Eq. (i)]}$$

13. (*b*) Potential, $V = \frac{1}{4\pi\varepsilon_0}\frac{q}{r}$

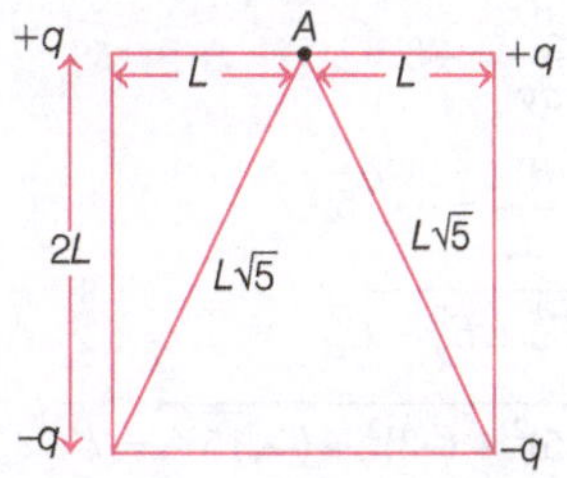

Here, $V = 2V_{+\text{ve}} + 2V_{-\text{ve}}$

$$V = \frac{1}{4\pi\varepsilon_0}\left[\frac{2q}{L} - \frac{2q}{L\sqrt{5}}\right]$$

The electric potential at mid-point A,

$$V = \frac{2q}{4\pi\varepsilon_0 L}\left(1 - \frac{1}{\sqrt{5}}\right)$$

14. (*a*) Potential at O due to charge at A,

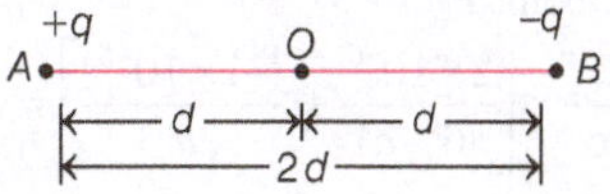

$$\therefore \quad V_1 = \frac{1}{4\pi\varepsilon_0} \cdot \frac{q}{d}$$

Potential at O due to charge at B,

$$V_2 = \frac{1}{4\pi\varepsilon_0}\frac{(-q)}{d}$$

∴Potential at mid-point O,

$$V = \frac{1}{4\pi\varepsilon_0}\frac{q}{d} + \frac{1}{4\pi\varepsilon_0}\cdot\frac{(-q)}{d} = 0$$

15. (a) Force, $F = qE = q\left(\frac{V}{d}\right)$

∴ Potential difference between two points,

$$V = \frac{F \cdot d}{q} = \frac{(3000)(10^{-2})}{3} = 10 \text{ V}$$

16. (b)

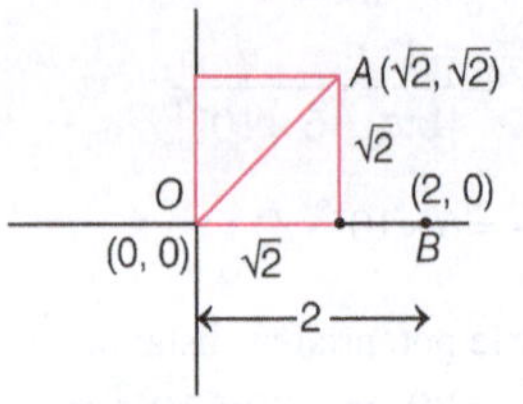

$$AO = \sqrt{(\sqrt{2})^2 + (\sqrt{2})^2}$$

$$AO = \sqrt{4} = 2 \text{ and } BO = 2$$

Potential difference between the points A and B

$$= V_A - V_B$$

$$= \frac{1}{4\pi\varepsilon_0}\cdot\frac{Q}{AO} - \frac{1}{4\pi\varepsilon_0}\cdot\frac{Q}{BO}$$

$$= 0 \qquad (\because AO = BO)$$

17. (d) $E_x = -\frac{dV}{dx} = -(-5) = 5,$

$$E_y = -\frac{dV}{dy} = -3$$

and $E_z = -\frac{dV}{dz} = -\sqrt{15}$

$$\therefore E_{\text{net}} = \sqrt{E_x^2 + E_y^2 + E_z^2}$$

$$= \sqrt{(5)^2 + (-3)^2 + (-\sqrt{15})^2} = 7$$

18. (c) Let, potential will be zero at two points P and Q, then

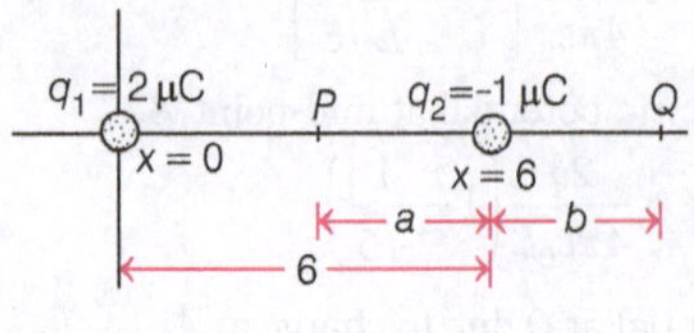

at internal point P

$$\frac{1}{4\pi\varepsilon_0}\times\left[\frac{2\times10^{-6}}{(6-a)} + \frac{(-1\times10^{-6})}{a}\right] = 0$$

$$\therefore \quad a = 2$$

So, distance of P from origin, $x = 6 - 2 = 4$

At external point Q,

$$\frac{1}{4\pi\varepsilon_0}\times\left[\frac{2\times10^{-6}}{(6+b)} + \frac{(-1\times10^{-6})}{b}\right] = 0$$

$$\therefore \quad b = 6$$

So, distance of Q from origin,

$$x = 6 + 6 = 12$$

19. (b) Let radius of big drop be R and radius of small drop be r,

∴Volume of big drop = 8 × volume of small drops

or $\frac{4}{3}\pi R^3 = 8 \times \frac{4}{3}\pi r^3$ or $R = 2r$

Potential of big drop,

$$V_{\text{big}} = \frac{KQ}{R} = \frac{K8q}{2r} \quad (q \text{ is charge on small drop})$$

$$\therefore \quad V_{\text{big}} = 4V_{\text{small}} \qquad \left(\because V_{\text{small}} = \frac{Kq}{r}\right)$$

$$\therefore \quad \frac{V_{\text{big}}}{V_{\text{small}}} = \frac{4}{1}$$

20. (c) We have, $8\left(\frac{4}{3}\pi r^3\right) = \frac{4}{3}\pi R^3$

$$\Rightarrow \quad R = 2r, Q = 8q$$

Further, $V = \frac{1}{4\pi\varepsilon_0}\cdot\frac{q}{r} = 50$ V

Potential of the large drop,

$$V' = \frac{1}{4\pi\varepsilon_0}\cdot\frac{Q}{R} = \frac{1}{4\pi\varepsilon_0}\cdot\frac{8q}{2r}$$

$$= 4 \times 50 = 200 \text{ V}$$

21. (d) We have, $V = \frac{KQ}{r}$

$$\Rightarrow \quad 120 = \frac{KQ}{2}$$

$$\therefore \quad KQ = 240 \text{ units}$$

When it is made to touch the bigger sphere, whole charge will transfer to bigger sphere.

∴Potential of bigger sphere,

$$V = \frac{KQ}{6} = \frac{240}{6} = 40 \text{ V}$$

22. (b) Let radius of drop is r. According to Millikan, for balance of drop,

$$QE = mg \text{ or } Q\frac{V}{d} = \left[\left(\frac{4}{3}\pi r^3\right)\rho\right]g$$

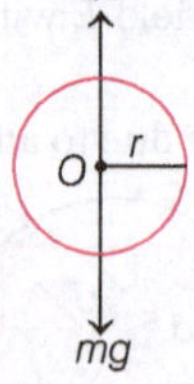

where, V is potential difference and ρ is density of drop.

$$\therefore \quad \frac{Q_1}{Q_2} = \left(\frac{r_1}{r_2}\right)^3 \times \frac{V_2}{V_1}$$

$$\Rightarrow \quad \frac{Q}{Q_2} = \left(\frac{r}{r/2}\right)^3 \times \frac{600}{2400} = 2$$

$$\Rightarrow \quad Q_2 = Q/2$$

23. (*b*)

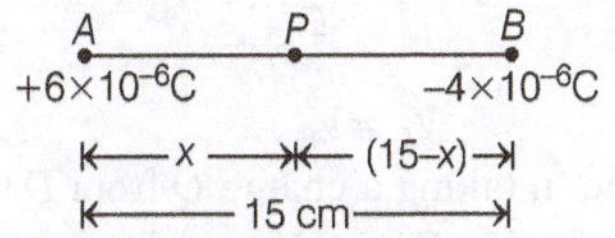

Let the potential be zero at point P at a distance x, from the charge $+6 \times 10^{-6}$ C at A as shown in the figure. Potential at P,

$$V = \frac{1}{4\pi\varepsilon_0}\left[\frac{6 \times 10^{-6}}{x} + \frac{(-4 \times 10^{-6})}{(15 - x)}\right]$$

$$0 = \frac{1}{4\pi\varepsilon_0}\left[\frac{6 \times 10^{-6}}{x} - \frac{4 \times 10^{-6}}{15 - x}\right]$$

$$0 = \frac{6 \times 10^{-6}}{x} - \frac{4 \times 10^{-6}}{15 - x}$$

$$\frac{6 \times 10^{-6}}{x} = \frac{4 \times 10^{-6}}{15 - x}$$

$$\Rightarrow \quad 6(15 - x) = 4x$$

$$90 - 6x = 4x \text{ or } 10x = 90$$

$$\Rightarrow \quad x = \frac{90}{10} = 9 \text{ cm}$$

The other possibility is that point of zero potential P may lie on AB produced at a distance x from the charge $+6 \times 10^{-6}$ C at A as shown in the figure.

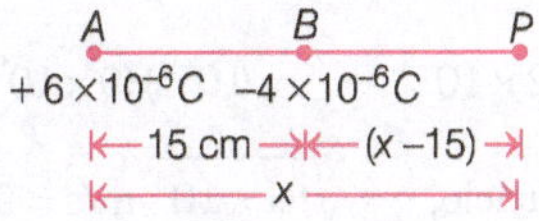

Potential at P,

$$V = \frac{1}{4\pi\varepsilon_0}\left[\frac{6 \times 10^{-6}}{x} + \frac{(-4 \times 10^{-6})}{(x - 15)}\right]$$

$$0 = \frac{1}{4\pi\varepsilon_0}\left[\frac{6 \times 10^{-6}}{x} - \frac{4 \times 10^{-6}}{x - 15}\right]$$

$$0 = \frac{6 \times 10^{-6}}{x} = \frac{4 \times 10^{-6}}{x - 15}$$

$$\Rightarrow \quad \frac{6}{x} = \frac{4}{x - 15}$$

$$6x - 90 = 4x$$

$$\Rightarrow \quad 2x = 90$$

$$\text{or} \quad x = \frac{90}{2} = 45 \text{ cm}$$

Thus, electrostatic potential is zero at 9 cm and 45 cm from the charge $+6 \times 10^{-6}$ C at A. Also, potential is zero at infinity.

24. (*d*) As the field is upward, so the negatively charged electron experiences a downward force of the magnitude of eE, where E is the magnitude of the electric field.

The acceleration of the electron is $a_e = \frac{eE}{m_e}$.

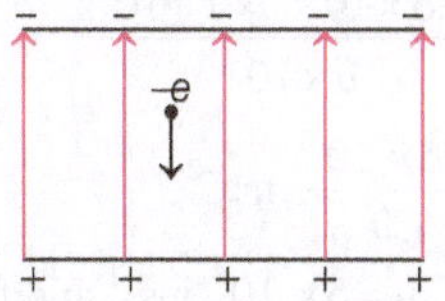

where, m_e is the mass of the electron.

Starting from rest, the time taken by the electron to fall through a distance h is given by

$$t_e = \sqrt{\frac{2h}{a_e}} = \sqrt{\frac{2hm_e}{eE}}$$

$$= \sqrt{\frac{2 \times 1.5 \times 10^{-2} \times 9.1 \times 10^{-31}}{1.6 \times 10^{-19} \times 2 \times 10^4}}$$

$$= 2.9 \times 10^{-9} \text{ s}$$

25. (*c*) We have, $dQ = \left(\frac{Q}{2l}\right) \cdot dx$

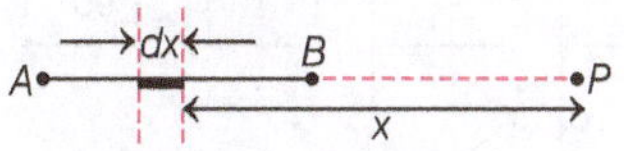

Potential of small part,

$$dV = \frac{1}{4\pi\varepsilon_0} \cdot \frac{dQ}{x}$$

$$= \frac{1}{4\pi\varepsilon_0} \cdot \frac{Q}{2l} \cdot \frac{dx}{x}$$

$\therefore$ Potential at P,

$$V = \int_{x=l}^{x=3l} dV$$

$$= \frac{1}{4\pi\varepsilon_0} \cdot \frac{Q}{2l} \ln(3)$$

26. (*b*) As O is the centre of line AB, so $AO = a$ and the distance of point P from A and B is

$$AP = BP = \sqrt{a^2 + a^2} = \sqrt{2}a$$

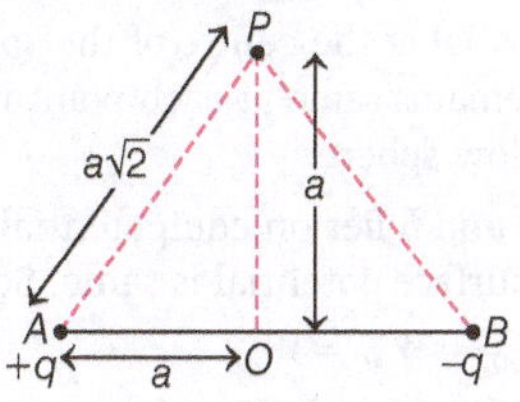

The potential at P due to charge $+q$ at A and $-q$ at B is

$$V_P = V_A + V_B = \frac{Kq}{AP} + \frac{K(-q)}{BP}$$

$$= \left(\frac{Kq}{a\sqrt{2}}\right) + \left(\frac{-Kq}{a\sqrt{2}}\right) = \text{zero}$$

27. (c) Electric force, $qE = ma$

$$\therefore \quad a = \frac{qE}{m}$$

$$\Rightarrow \quad a = \frac{1.6 \times 10^{-19} \times 1 \times 10^3}{9 \times 10^{-31}}$$

$$= \frac{1.6 \times 10^{15}}{9} \text{ ms}^{-2}$$

Initially speed, $u = 5 \times 10^6 \text{ ms}^{-1}$ and final speed, $v = 0$

$\therefore$ From $v^2 = u^2 - 2as$

$\Rightarrow$ Distance travelled by electron, $s = \dfrac{u^2}{2a}$

$$s = \frac{(5 \times 10^6)^2 \times 9}{2 \times 1.6 \times 10^{15}} = 7 \text{ cm}$$

28. (c) Angle between equipotential surface and line of force is 90°.

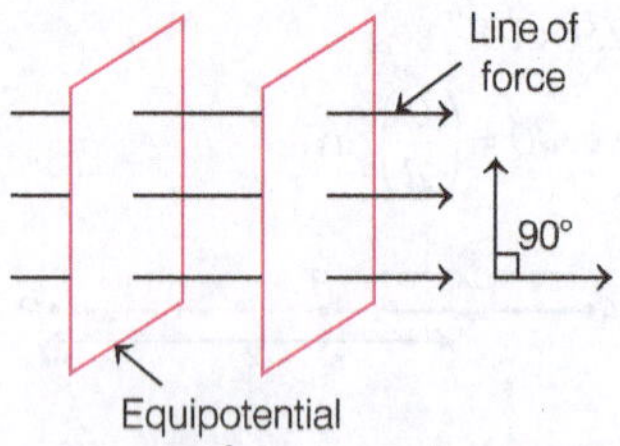

29. (a) $\because$ Potential difference $= \dfrac{\text{Work done}}{\text{Charge}}$

$$\therefore \quad W = qV$$

$$10 = 5 \times V$$

$$\therefore \quad V = 2 \text{ V}$$

30. (a) Work done,

$$W_{A \to B} = U_B - U_A = q(V_B - V_A)$$

Potential difference,

$$V_B - V_A = \frac{W_{A \to B}}{q}$$

$$= \frac{10 \times 10^{-3}}{5 \times 10^{-6}} = 2 \text{kV}$$

31. (a) The potential at the centre of the sphere is 80 V because it remains same at each point inside the metallic hollow sphere.

32. (c) A, B, C, D and E lies on equipotential surface. On sphere, the surface potential is same. So,

$$W_{AB} = W_{AC} = W_{AD}$$

$$= W_{AE} = q(V_f - V_i) = \text{zero}$$

33. (a) We have, $AC = BC$

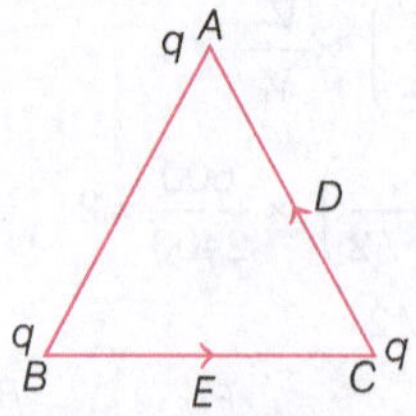

$$\therefore \quad V_D = V_E$$

Work done in taking a charge Q from D to E

$$W = Q(V_E - V_D)$$

$$W = 0$$

34. (a) Potential difference only depends upon the inner charge.

So, if the shell is given a charge of $-3Q$, the new potential difference between the same two surface is V.

35. (b) As electric potential of spheres are same, $V_A = V_B$

$$\Rightarrow \quad E_A \cdot a = E_B \cdot b$$

$$\therefore \quad \frac{\sigma_A a}{\varepsilon_0} = \frac{\sigma_B b}{\varepsilon_0} \text{ or } \frac{\sigma_A}{\sigma_B} = \frac{b}{a}$$

36. (b) When charge particle enters in a potential field, then

$$\frac{1}{2} mv^2 = qV$$

$$\therefore \quad v = \sqrt{\left(\frac{2qV}{m}\right)}$$

$$\therefore \quad \frac{v_A}{v_B} = \sqrt{\frac{q}{4q}} = \frac{1}{2}$$

37. (d) Here, $\dfrac{1}{2} mv^2 = \dfrac{q_1 q_2}{4\pi\varepsilon_0}\left(\dfrac{1}{r_i} - \dfrac{1}{r_f}\right)$

$$\frac{1}{2} \times 2 \times 10^{-3} \times v^2 = (10^{-9})(9 \times 10^9)(0.9)$$

Speed of particle, $v = \sqrt{8.1 \times 10^3}$ m/s = 90 m/s

38. (d) We have, $V \propto \dfrac{q}{R}$ $\quad \left(\because V = \dfrac{1}{4\pi\varepsilon_0} \cdot \dfrac{q}{R}\right)$

$$\because \quad \sigma = \frac{q}{4\pi R^2}$$

$$\therefore \quad q \propto \sigma R^2 \text{ or } V \propto \sigma R$$

Potential is same, i.e. $V_1 = V_2$

$$\therefore \quad \sigma_1 R_1 = \sigma_2 R_2$$

$$\Rightarrow \quad \text{Ratio of } \frac{\sigma_1}{\sigma_2} = \frac{R_2}{R_1} = \frac{5}{4}$$

39. (c) $V = \dfrac{q}{4\pi\varepsilon_0 r} - \dfrac{q}{4\pi\varepsilon_0 3r} = \dfrac{q}{6\pi\varepsilon_0 r}$

Electric field intensity at a distance $3r$ is given by

$$E = \frac{q}{4\pi\varepsilon_0 (3r)^2} = \frac{q}{4\pi\varepsilon_0 \cdot 9r^2}$$

Thus, $\frac{E}{V} = \frac{q(6\pi\varepsilon_0 r)}{4\pi\varepsilon_0 9r^2(q)} = \frac{1}{6r}$

$\Rightarrow \quad E = \frac{V}{6r}$

40. (*d*) Work done, $W = 6\times10^{-6}(V_A - V_B)$, where

$$V_A = 10^{10}\left[\frac{(-5\times10^{-6})}{15\times10^{-2}} + \frac{2\times10^{-6}}{5\times10^{-2}}\right] = \frac{1}{15}\times10^6\ \text{V}$$

and $$V_B = 10^{10}\left[\frac{(2\times10^{-6})}{15\times10^{-2}} - \frac{5\times10^{-6}}{5\times10^{-2}}\right] = -\frac{13}{15}\times10^6\ \text{V}$$

$$\therefore \quad W = 6\times10^{-6}\left[\frac{1}{15}\times10^6 - \left(-\frac{13}{15}\times10^6\right)\right] = 5.6\ \text{J}$$

41. (*d*) Electric potential at *P*,

$$V = \frac{kQ}{R/2} + \frac{kq}{R} = \frac{2Q}{4\pi\varepsilon_0 R} + \frac{q}{4\pi\varepsilon_0 R}$$

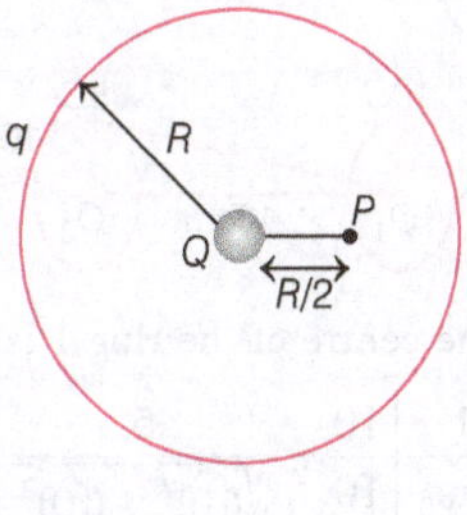

42. (*b*) Potential of the system,

$$V = \frac{\text{Net charge}}{\text{Net capacity}} = \frac{q_1 + q_2}{4\pi\varepsilon_0(r_1 + r_2)}$$

43. (*c*) $\frac{K(2Q)}{2a} + \frac{KQ}{2a} = 5$

or $\quad \frac{K(3Q)}{2a} = 5$

$\therefore \quad \frac{KQ}{a} = \frac{10}{3}$

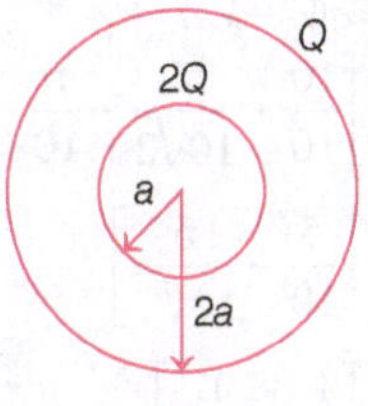

Now, potential of inner sphere,

$$V_m = \frac{K2Q}{a} + \frac{KQ}{2a} = \frac{5}{2}\frac{KQ}{a} = \frac{5}{2}\left(\frac{10}{3}\right) = \frac{25}{3}\ \text{V}$$

44. (*d*) Shell *C* is now earthed.

$\therefore \quad V_C = 0$

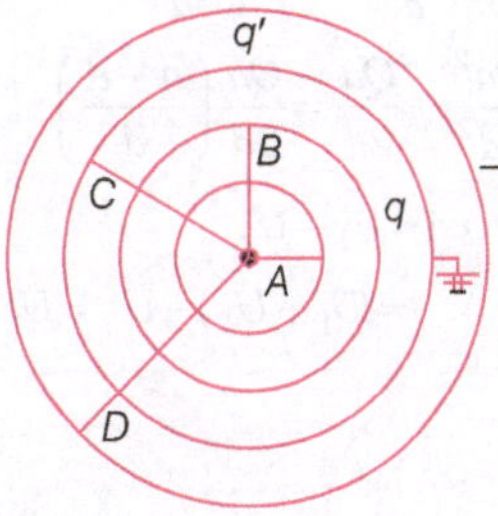

$\therefore \quad \frac{K(q+q')}{3a} - \frac{Kq}{4a} = 0$

$\therefore \quad q' = -\frac{q}{4}$

Now, potential difference,

$$V_A - V_C = \frac{Kq}{2a} - \frac{Kq/4}{3a} - \frac{Kq}{4a} - 0 = \frac{Kq}{6a}$$

45. (*a*) The induced charges will be as under.

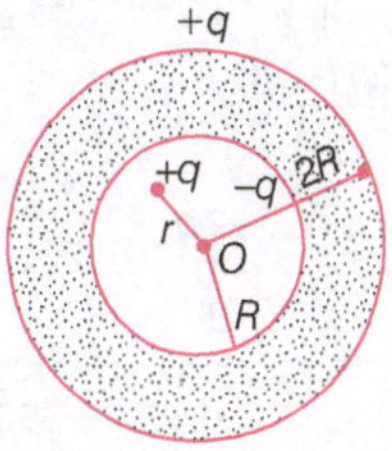

Potential at point *O* (the centre),

$$V_0 = \frac{1}{4\pi\varepsilon_0}\left[\frac{q}{r} - \frac{q}{R} + \frac{q}{2R}\right] = \frac{q}{4\pi\varepsilon_0}\left[\frac{1}{r} - \frac{1}{2R}\right]$$

46. (*c*) Potential at point *P*,

$$V = \frac{KQ}{R} - \frac{Kq}{x} = \frac{1}{4\pi\varepsilon_0}\left(\frac{Q}{R} - \frac{q}{x}\right)$$

47. (*b*) Work done, $W_{AB} - U_B - U_A = q_0(V_B - V_A)$

Potential, $V_B - V_A = -\int_A^B E\,dr$

$$= -\int_{3a}^{2a}\frac{\lambda}{2\pi\varepsilon_0 r} = \frac{\lambda}{2\pi\varepsilon_0}\ln\left(\frac{3}{2}\right)$$

$\therefore$ Work done, $W_{A\to B} = \frac{q_0\lambda}{2\pi\varepsilon_0}\ln\left(\frac{3}{2}\right)$

48. (*c*) $q_A = \frac{Q}{2}$

When *B* is earthed

$V_B = 0$

$\therefore \quad \frac{Kq_B}{a} + \frac{K(Q/2)}{d} = 0$

$\therefore \quad q_B = \frac{-Qa}{2d}$

When C is earthed

$$\therefore \quad \frac{Kq_C}{a} + \frac{K(Q/2)}{d} - \frac{K(Qa/2d)}{d} = 0$$

$$\therefore \quad q_C = \frac{Qa^2}{2d^2} - \frac{Qa}{2d} = \frac{Qa}{2d}\left(\frac{a-d}{d}\right)$$

49. (*c*) Heat produced $= U_i - U_f$

$$= (U_1 + U_2) - U_2 = U_1$$

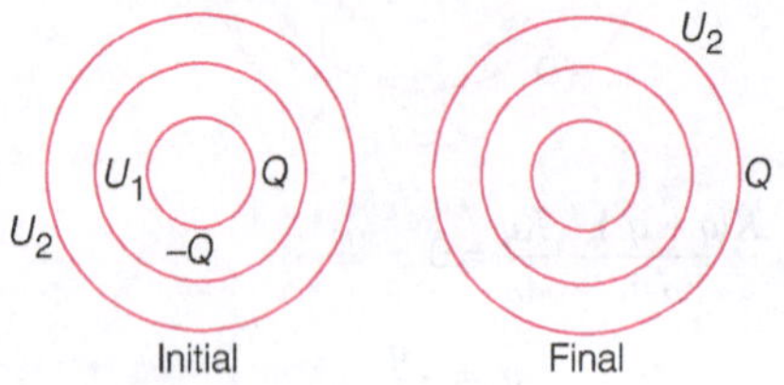

$$\text{Heat produced} = \frac{q^2}{2C}$$

$$= \frac{q^2}{2\left[4\pi\varepsilon_0\left\{\frac{a \times 2a}{2a - a}\right\}\right]} = \frac{Kq^2}{4a}$$

50. (*c*) $U_{AB} = \frac{1}{4\pi\varepsilon_0} \cdot \frac{(q)(-2q)}{a}$

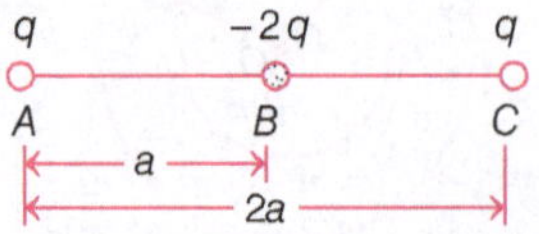

$$U_{BC} = \frac{1}{4\pi\varepsilon_0} \cdot \frac{(-2q)(q)}{a}$$

$$U_{CA} = \frac{1}{4\pi\varepsilon_0} \cdot \frac{(q)(q)}{2a}$$

Potential energy of the system,

$$U_{\text{system}} = \frac{1}{4\pi\varepsilon_0} \cdot \left[\frac{-2q^2}{a} - \frac{2q^2}{a} + \frac{q^2}{2a}\right]$$

$$U_{\text{system}} = \frac{-7q^2}{8\pi\varepsilon_0 a}$$

51. (*a*) Let Q_1 and Q_2 be the charge on the two conducting spheres of radii R_1 (= 3 cm) and R_2 (=1 cm), respectively.

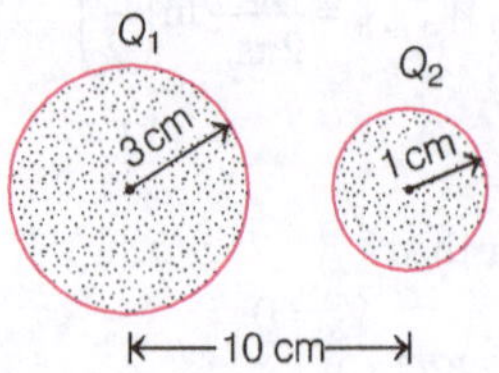

$$\therefore \quad \text{Potential, } V_1 = \frac{1}{4\pi\varepsilon_0} \frac{Q_1}{R_1}$$

$$\Rightarrow \quad 10 = \frac{9 \times 10^9 \times Q_1}{3 \times 10^{-2}}$$

$$\Rightarrow \text{Charge, } Q_1 = \frac{10 \times 3 \times 10^{-2}}{9 \times 10^9} \quad \text{...(i)}$$

and $$V_2 = \frac{1}{4\pi\varepsilon_0} \frac{Q_2}{R_2}$$

$$\Rightarrow \quad 10 = \frac{9 \times 10^9 \times Q_2}{1 \times 10^{-2}}$$

$$\Rightarrow \text{Charge, } Q_2 = \frac{10 \times 1 \times 10^{-2}}{9 \times 10^9} \quad \text{...(ii)}$$

According to Coulomb's law, force of repulsion between them is

$$F = \frac{1}{4\pi\varepsilon_0} \frac{Q_1 Q_2}{r^2}$$

$$= \frac{9 \times 10^9 \times 10 \times 3 \times 10^{-2} \times 10 \times 1 \times 10^{-2}}{9 \times 10^9 \times 9 \times 10^9 \times (10 \times 10^{-2})^2}$$

[using Eqs. (i) and (ii)]

$$= \left(\frac{1}{3}\right) \times 10^{-9} \text{ N}$$

52. (*b*)

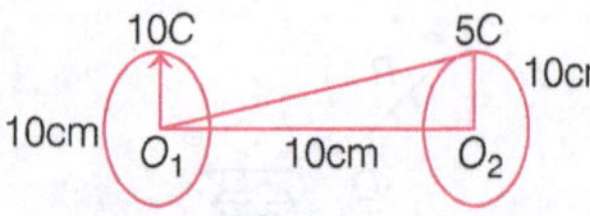

Potential at the centre of the ring 1 is

$$V_1 = \frac{1}{4\pi\varepsilon_0}\left[\frac{10}{10} + \frac{5}{\sqrt{(10)^2 + (10)^2}}\right]$$

$$= \frac{1}{4\pi\varepsilon_0}\left[\frac{10}{10} + \frac{5}{10\sqrt{2}}\right]$$

Potential at the centre of the ring 2 is

$$V_2 = \frac{1}{4\pi\varepsilon_0}\left[\frac{5}{10} + \frac{10}{\sqrt{(10)^2 + (10)^2}}\right]$$

$$= \frac{1}{4\pi\varepsilon_0}\left[\frac{5}{10} + \frac{10}{10\sqrt{2}}\right]$$

Work done, $W = q(V_1 - V_2)$

$$= \frac{q}{4\pi\varepsilon_0}\left[\frac{10}{10} + \frac{5}{10\sqrt{2}} - \frac{5}{10} - \frac{10}{10\sqrt{2}}\right]$$

$$= \frac{q}{4\pi\varepsilon_0}\left[\frac{5}{10} - \frac{5}{10\sqrt{2}}\right]$$

$$= \frac{q}{4\pi\varepsilon_0}\left[\frac{1}{2} - \frac{1}{2\sqrt{2}}\right]$$

$$= \frac{q}{8\pi\varepsilon_0}\left[\frac{\sqrt{2} - 1}{\sqrt{2}}\right]$$

53. (*c*) Potential difference between two equipotential surfaces *A* and *B*

$$V_A - V_B = kq\left(\frac{1}{r_A} - \frac{1}{r_B}\right)$$

$$= kq\left(\frac{r_B - r_A}{r_A r_B}\right) = \frac{kqt_1}{r_A r_B}$$

or $$t_1 = \frac{(V_A - V_B)\, r_A r_B}{kq} \text{ or } t_1 \propto r_A r_B$$

Similarly, $t_2 \propto r_B r_C$

Since, $r_A < r_B < r_C$, therefore $r_A r_B < r_B r_C$

$\therefore \quad t_1 < t_2$

54. (*c*) The potential of conducting sphere having charge *Q* at the surface, $A = \frac{1}{4\pi\varepsilon_0} \cdot \frac{Q}{R}$.

The potential of conducting sphere having charge *q* at the surface, $A = \frac{1}{4\pi\varepsilon_0} \cdot \frac{q}{R}$

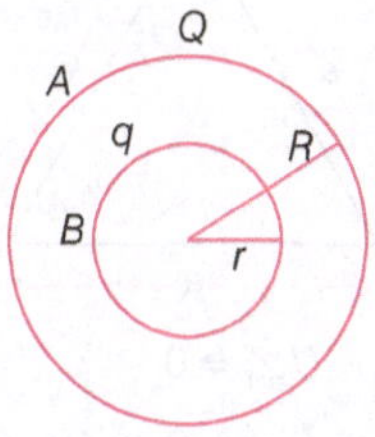

The potential at *B* is due to *Q* inside $= \frac{1}{4\pi\varepsilon_0} \cdot \frac{Q}{R}$

The potential at *B* due to $q = \frac{1}{4\pi\varepsilon_0} \cdot \frac{q}{r}$

$\therefore$ Potential at *A*,

$$V_A = \frac{1}{4\pi\varepsilon_0}\left(\frac{Q}{R} + \frac{q}{R}\right)$$

Potential at *B*,

$$V_B = \frac{1}{4\pi\varepsilon_0}\left(\frac{Q}{R} + \frac{q}{r}\right)$$

$$\therefore \quad V_B - V_A = \frac{1}{4\pi\varepsilon_0}\left(\frac{q}{r} - \frac{q}{R}\right)$$

55. (*a*) Suppose, first the charge $+q$ is brought to *A* and then the charges $-q$, $+q$ and $-q$ are brought to *B*, *C* and *D*, respectively. The total work needed can be calculated in steps

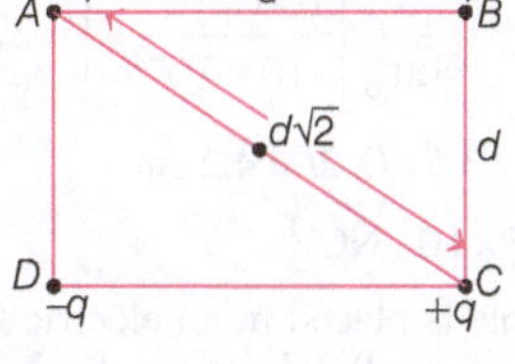

(i) Work needed to bring charge $+q$ to *A*, when no charge is present elsewhere is zero.

(ii) Work needed to bring $-q$ to *B* when $+q$ is at *A*. This is given by (charge at *B*) × (electrostatic potential at *B* due to charge $+q$ at *A*)

$$= -q \times \left(\frac{q}{4\pi\varepsilon_0 d}\right) = -\frac{q^2}{4\pi\varepsilon_0 d}$$

(iii) Work needed to bring charge $+q$ to *C* when $+q$ is at *A* and $-q$ is at *B*. This is given by (charge at *C*) × (potential at *C* due to charges at *A* and *B*)

$$= +q\left(\frac{+q}{4\pi\varepsilon_0 d\sqrt{2}} + \frac{-q}{4\pi\varepsilon_0 d}\right)$$

$$= \frac{-q^2}{4\pi\varepsilon_0 d}\left(1 - \frac{1}{\sqrt{2}}\right)$$

(iv) Work needed to bring $-q$ to *D* when $+q$ at *A*, $-q$ at *B* and $+q$ at *C*. This is given by (charge at *D*) × (potential at *D* due to charges at *A*, *B* and *C*)

$$= -q\left(\frac{+q}{4\pi\varepsilon_0 d} + \frac{-q}{4\pi\varepsilon_0 d\sqrt{2}} + \frac{q}{4\pi\varepsilon_0 d}\right)$$

$$= \frac{-q^2}{4\pi\varepsilon_0 d}\left(2 - \frac{1}{\sqrt{2}}\right)$$

Adding the work done in steps (i), (ii), (iii) and (iv), the total work required is

$$= \frac{-q^2}{4\pi\varepsilon_0 d}\left\{(0) + (1) + \left(1 - \frac{1}{\sqrt{2}}\right) + \left(2 - \frac{1}{\sqrt{2}}\right)\right\}$$

$$= \frac{-q^2}{4\pi\varepsilon_0 d}(4 - \sqrt{2})$$

56. (*c*) $U = -pE\cos\theta$, *U* is minimum at $\theta = 0°$.

57. (*a*) Kinetic energy gained by α-particle,

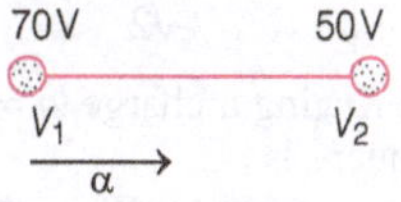

$$KE = q \cdot \Delta V = q(V_1 - V_2) = 2e(V_1 - V_2)$$

$$= 2 \times 1.6 \times 10^{-19}\,(70 - 50) = 40\text{ eV}$$

58. (*b*) By using, $KE = QV$

$$\Rightarrow \quad 4 \times 10^{20} \times 1.6 \times 10^{-19} = 0.25 \times V$$

Potential difference, $V = \frac{4 \times 10^{20} \times 1.6 \times 10^{-19}}{0.25} = 256\text{ V}$

59. (*c*) The work done by a electrostatic force is given by $W_{12} = q(V_2 - V_1)$. Here initial and final potentials are same in all three cases and same charge is moved, so work done is same in all three cases.

60. (*d*) As shown in figure, component of dipole moment along the line *OP* will be

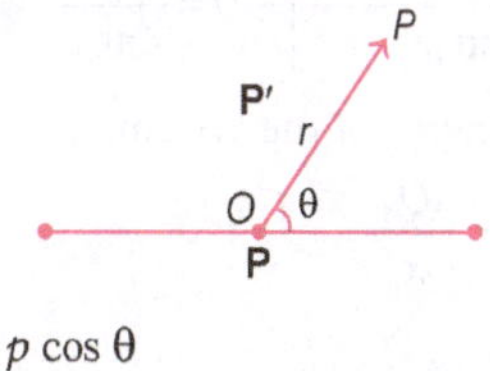

$$p' = p\cos\theta$$

Hence, electric potential at point P will be

$$V = \frac{1}{4\pi\varepsilon_0} \cdot \frac{p\cos\theta}{r^2}$$

61. (*b*) Net electrostatic energy,

$$U = \frac{kQq}{a} + \frac{kq^2}{a} + \frac{kQq}{a\sqrt{2}} = 0$$

$$\Rightarrow \quad \frac{kq}{a}\left(Q + q + \frac{Q}{\sqrt{2}}\right) = 0$$

$\therefore$ The value of $Q = -\dfrac{2q}{2+\sqrt{2}}$

62. (*a*)

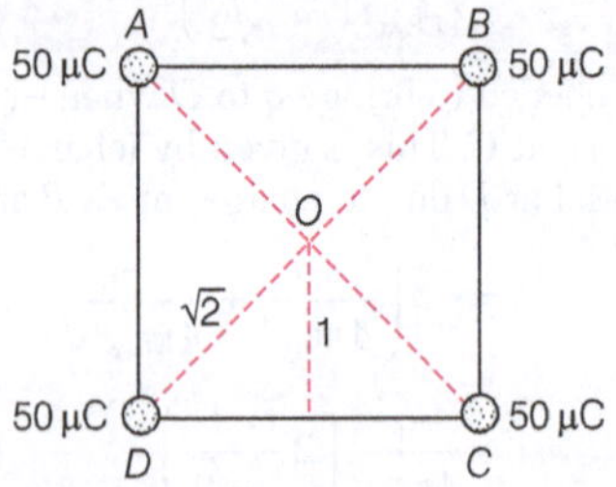

Potential at centre, $V_A = V_B = V_C = V_D = V$

$$= \frac{1}{4\pi\varepsilon_0} \cdot \frac{q}{r}$$

$$V = \frac{1}{4\pi\varepsilon_0} \cdot \frac{(50\times 10^{-6})}{(\sqrt{2})}$$

$\therefore$ Potential at the centre of square,

$$V_0 = 4\,\text{V}$$

$$V_0 = 4 \times \left[\frac{9\times 10^9 \times 50\times 10^{-6}}{\sqrt{2}}\right] = 90\sqrt{2}\times 10^4\ \text{V}$$

Work done in bringing a charge ($q = 50\ \mu$C) from ∞ to centre of the square is

$$\therefore \quad W = qV_0 = 50\times 10^{-6} \times 90\sqrt{2}\times 10^4$$

$$= 63.64\ \text{J} \simeq 64\ \text{J}$$

63. (*a*) Force, $F_e = qE = q\left(\dfrac{V}{d}\right) = (4\times 10^{-6})\left(\dfrac{2000}{2\times 10^{-3}}\right) = 4\ \text{N}$

64. (*a*) Work done, $W = U_f - U_i$

$$= \frac{q_1 q_2}{4\pi\varepsilon_0}\left[\frac{1}{r_f} - \frac{1}{r_i}\right]$$

$$= (9\times 10^9)(10^{-12})(12)(8)\left[\frac{1}{0.06} - \frac{1}{0.1}\right] = 5.8\ \text{J}$$

65. (*b*) Work done, $W = U_i - U_f$

$$= 6\left[\frac{1}{4\pi\varepsilon_0} \cdot \frac{q\cdot q}{r}\right] - 0 = \frac{6q^2}{4\pi\varepsilon_0 r}$$

66. (*c*) Potential energy of the system,

$$\frac{-kqQ}{x} - \frac{kQq}{x} + \frac{kq^2}{2x} = 0$$

$$\Rightarrow \quad \frac{-4kqQ + kq^2}{2x} = 0 \Rightarrow kq^2 = 4kQq$$

Ratio, $\dfrac{q}{Q} = 4$

67. (*c*) Electrostatic potential energy,

$$U = \frac{1}{4\pi\varepsilon_0} \cdot \frac{q_1 q_2}{r}$$

Here, $q_1 = q_2 = 1.6\times 10^{-19}$ C

and $r = 9\times 10^{-15}$ m

$$\therefore \quad U = \frac{9\times 10^9 \times 1.6\times 10^{-19} \times 1.6\times 10^{-19}}{9\times 10^{-15}}$$

$$= 2.56\times 10^{-14}\ \text{J}$$

68. (*a*) $U_{\text{net}} = \dfrac{1}{4\pi\varepsilon_0}\left[\dfrac{Qq}{a} + \dfrac{qq}{a} + \dfrac{Qq}{a}\right]$

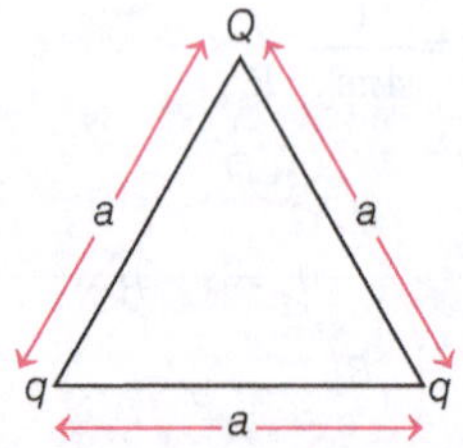

$$\because \quad U_{\text{net}} = 0$$

$$2Qq + q^2 = 0 \Rightarrow Q = -\frac{q}{2}$$

69. (*c*)

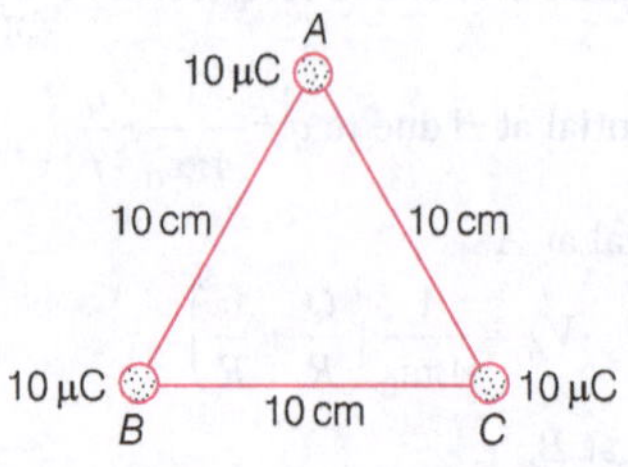

$$U_{AB} = \frac{1}{4\pi\varepsilon_0} \cdot \frac{(10)(10)\times 10^{-12}}{10\times 10^{-2}}$$

$$U_{BC} = \frac{1}{4\pi\varepsilon_0} \cdot \frac{(10)(10)\times 10^{-12}}{10\times 10^{-2}}$$

$$U_{AC} = \frac{1}{4\pi\varepsilon_0} \cdot \frac{(10)(10)\times 10^{-12}}{10\times 10^{-2}}$$

$$\therefore \quad U_{\text{total}} = U_{AB} + U_{BC} + U_{CA}$$

$$= \frac{3}{4\pi\varepsilon_0}\left[\frac{100\times 10^{-12}}{10\times 10^{-2}}\right] = 27\,\text{J}$$

70. (*a*) Given, $q = 3.5\ \mu$C, $2l = 4.2$ cm

and $E = 5.87\times 10^5\ \text{NC}^{-1}$

When a dipole is placed in an electric field **E**, torque exerted, $\tau = pE\sin\theta$, where p = dipole moment ($= q\times 2l$) and θ is the angle which dipole makes with the field.

For maximum torque, $\theta = 90°$

$$\tau_{max} = pE \sin 90°$$

i.e. $\tau_{max} = pE$

$\Rightarrow$ $\tau_{max} = q \times 2l \times E$

$$= (3.5 \times 10^{-6}) \times 4.2 \times 10^{-2} \times 5.87 \times 10^{5}$$

$$= 86.289 \times 10^{-3}\ \text{Nm}^{-1}$$

Work done in rotating the dipole from an angle θ_0 to θ,

$$W = \int_{\theta_0}^{\theta} pE \sin\theta\, d\theta$$

$$= pE[\cos\theta_0 - \cos\theta]$$

Here, $\theta_0 = 0°$ and $\theta = 180°$

$$W = pE(\cos 0° - \cos 180°)$$

$\Rightarrow$ $W = 2pE$

$$= 2 \times q \times 2l \times E$$

$$= 2 \times (3.5 \times 10^{-6}) \times (4.2 \times 10^{-2}) \times 5.8 \times 10^{5}$$

$$= 1.705 \times 10^{-1}\ \text{J} \simeq 1.70 \times 10^{-1}\ \text{J}$$

Hence, the maximum torque is 86.289×10^{-3} Nm^{-1} and work done is 1.70×10^{-1} J.

71. (*b*) Given, dipole moment of each molecule $= 10^{-29}$ C-m and number of molecules in 1 mole of the substance $= 6 \times 10^{23}$.

Therefore, total dipole moment of all molecules,

$$p = 6 \times 10^{23} \times 10^{-29}\ \text{C-m}$$

$$= 6 \times 10^{-6}\ \text{C-m}$$

Initial potential energy,

$$U_i = -pE\cos\theta$$

$$= -6 \times 10^{-6} \times 10^{6} \times \cos 60°$$

$$= -6 \times \frac{1}{2} = -3\ \text{J}$$

Final potential energy (when $\theta = 0°$),

[finally p and E are aligned in the same direction]

$$U_f = -6 \times 10^{-6} \times 10^{6} \times \cos 0° = -6\ \text{J}$$

Change in potential energy $= -6\ \text{J} - (-3\ \text{J}) = -3\ \text{J}$

So, there is a loss in potential energy. This must be the energy released by the substances in the form of heat in aligning its dipole.

$\therefore$ Heat energy $= -\text{PE} = -(-3\ \text{J}) = 3\ \text{J}$

Assertion and Reason

1. (*d*) Electric potential of a charged conductor depends not only on the amount of charge and volume but also on the shape of the conductor. Hence, if their shapes are different, they may have different electric potential.

2. (*b*) Potential energy of a system of two charges,

$$U = K\frac{q_1 q_2}{r}.$$

$\therefore$ When two positive point charges move away from each other, then their potential energy decreases and work done by electrostatic force can always be expressed in terms of a potential energy, when the particle moves from a point.

3. (*a*) Polar dielectric molecules are the one in which centres of positive and negative charges are separated even when there is no external field. It means, they have permanent dipoles.

So, in the absence of any external electric field, the different permanent dipoles are oriented randomly due to thermal agitation. So, the total dipole moment is zero.

4. (*c*) The molecules of a substance may be polar or non-polar. In a non-polar molecule, the centre of positive and negative charges coincides.

On the other hand, a polar molecule is one in which the centres of positive and negative charges are separated, even when there is no external field.

Such molecules have a permanent dipole moment.

5. (*b*) Line along East-West is an equipotential line.

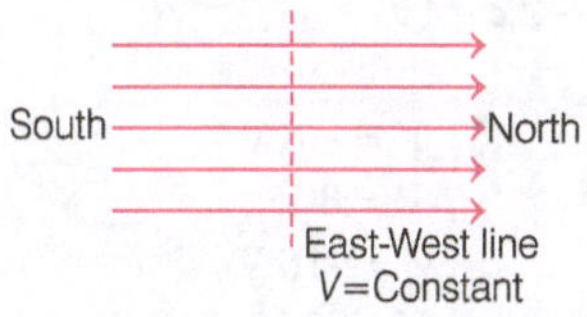

As V = constant along East-West line

qV or PE of charge remains constant along the line.

Also, field of a point charge is non-uniform.

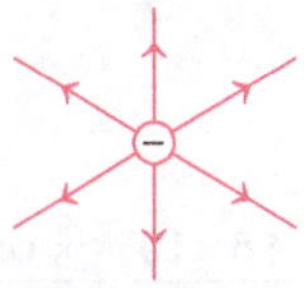

Statement Type Questions

1. (*b*) Statement I is correct but Statement II is incorrect.

Electric potential V is a scalar quantity. Therefore, electric potential at middle point will be the algebraic sum of potentials due to electron and proton, i.e.

$$V = \frac{K\,\Sigma q}{r} = 0$$

as $\Sigma q = -q + q = 0$

But if a unit positive charge held at the centre will be repelled by proton and attracted by electron with the same force, the net force on unit positive charge will not be zero. Therefore electric field intensity E, cannot be zero at the middle point.

2. (*d*) Both Statement I and Statement II are correct.

3. (*d*) Both Statement I and Statement II are correct.

4. (c) Statement I is incorrect but Statement II is correct.
In uniform electric field net force on an electric dipole is zero. Therefore no work is done in translational motion of the dipole.

5. (b) Statement I is correct but Statement II is incorrect.
Assume if test charge $= Q$ and point charge $= q$

The electric potential, $V = \dfrac{Kq}{r}$

and electric potential energy

$$W = QV$$

$$= \frac{KQq}{r}$$

Thus, V is not equal to W.

Match the Columns

1. (b) As, $\int dV = -\int \mathbf{E} \cdot d\mathbf{r}$

$\therefore \quad V_A - V_B = -\int_B^A \mathbf{E} \cdot d\mathbf{r}$

$\because \quad \mathbf{E} = (2\hat{\mathbf{i}} + 4\hat{\mathbf{j}})$ N/C

$V = -2x - 4y$

A. $(4m, 0)$ $\quad V = -8$ V
B. $(-4m, 0)$ $\quad V = 8$ V
C. $(0, 4m)$ $\quad V = -16$ V
D. $(0, -4m)$ $\quad V = 16$ V

Hence, A-II, B-I, C-IV, D-III.

2. (b) A.

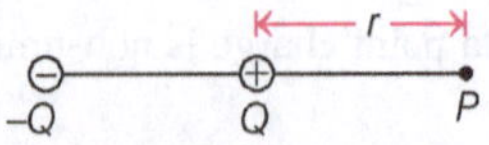

$$V = \frac{Kp\cos\theta}{r^2}$$

$$= \frac{9\times10^9 \times 4.8\times10^{-30} \times \cos 0°}{(4.1\times10^{-9})^2}$$

$$= 2.6\times10^{-3} \text{ V}$$

B. $V = \dfrac{Kp\cos\theta}{r^2} = 1.8\times10^{-3}$ V

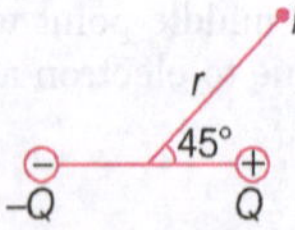

C. $V = \dfrac{1}{4\pi\varepsilon_0} \cdot \dfrac{p\cos\theta}{r^2}$

$$= \frac{9\times10^9 \times 4.8\times10^{-30} \times \cos 135°}{(4.1\times10^{-9})^2}$$

$$= -1.8\times10^{-3} \text{ V}$$

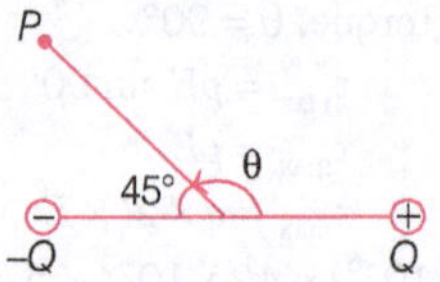

D.

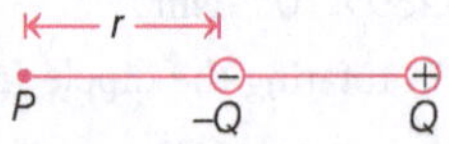

$$V = \frac{Kp\cos\theta}{r^2}$$

$$= \frac{9\times10^9 \times 4.8\times10^{-3} \times \cos 180°}{(4.1\times10^{-9})^2}$$

$$= -2.6\times10^{-3} \text{ V}$$

3. (b) $V_A =$ Potential due to charge q_A,

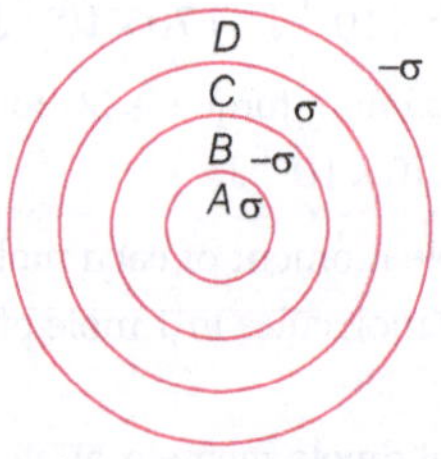

$$= K\left(\frac{q_A}{a} + \frac{q_B}{b} + \frac{q_C}{c} + \frac{q_D}{d}\right)$$

$$= K\left(\frac{4\pi a^2 \cdot \sigma}{a} + \frac{4\pi b^2 \cdot (-\sigma)}{b} + \frac{4\pi c^2 \cdot (\sigma)}{c} + \frac{4\pi D^2 \cdot (-\sigma)}{d}\right)$$

$$= \frac{1}{4\pi\varepsilon_0} \cdot 4\pi(\sigma a - \sigma b + \sigma c - \sigma d)$$

$$= \frac{\sigma}{\varepsilon_0}(a - b + c - d)$$

$$= \frac{\sigma}{\varepsilon_0}\left(\frac{3}{2} - \frac{5}{2} + \frac{7}{2} - \frac{9}{2}\right) = \frac{\sigma}{\varepsilon_0}(-2)$$

Also, $V_B = \dfrac{\sigma}{\varepsilon_0}\left[\dfrac{a^2}{b} - b + c - d\right]$

$$= -\frac{\sigma}{\varepsilon_0}\frac{13}{5}$$

$$V_C = \frac{\sigma}{\varepsilon_0}\left(\frac{a^2}{c} - \frac{b^2}{c} + c - d\right)$$

$$= \frac{\sigma}{\varepsilon_0}(-15)$$

$$V_D = \frac{\sigma}{\varepsilon_0}\left(\frac{a^2}{d} - \frac{b^2}{d} + \frac{c^2}{d} - d\right) = \frac{\sigma}{\varepsilon_0}\left(-\frac{8}{3}\right)$$

4. (*d*) Electric potential at any point due to electric dipole is given as

$$V = \frac{p\cos\theta}{4\pi\varepsilon_0 r^2}$$

A. At point P_1, $\theta = 0°$

$$\Rightarrow V_1 = \frac{1}{4\pi\varepsilon_0}\cdot\frac{p\cos 0°}{r^2} = \frac{p}{4\pi\varepsilon_0 r^2}$$

B. At point P_2, $\theta = 180°$

$$\Rightarrow V_1 = \frac{1}{4\pi\varepsilon_0}\cdot\frac{p\cos 180°}{r^2} = \frac{-p}{4\pi\varepsilon_0 r^2}$$

C. At point P_3, $\theta = 45°$

$$\Rightarrow V_3 = \frac{1}{4\pi\varepsilon_0}\cdot\frac{p\cos 45°}{r^2} = \frac{p}{4\sqrt{2}\pi\varepsilon_0 r^2}$$

D. At point P_4, $\theta = 90°$

$$\Rightarrow V_4 = \frac{1}{4\pi\varepsilon_0}\cdot\frac{p\cos 90°}{r^2} = 0$$

Hence, A-IV, B-III, C-II, D-I

Final Check Through PYQs

1. (*b*) The general expression of potential due to dipole is given by,

$$V = k\frac{P\cos\theta}{r^2}$$

where, P is magnitude of dipole moment and r is the distance.

For axial point where $\theta = 0°$,

$$V = k\frac{P}{r^2} = \frac{9\times10^9\times4\times10^{-6}}{(2)^2} = 9\times10^3\text{ V}$$

For axial point where $\theta = 180°$,

$$V = -k\frac{P}{r^2} = \frac{-9\times10^9\times4\times10^{-6}}{(2)^2} = -9\times10^3\text{ V}$$

2. (*d*)

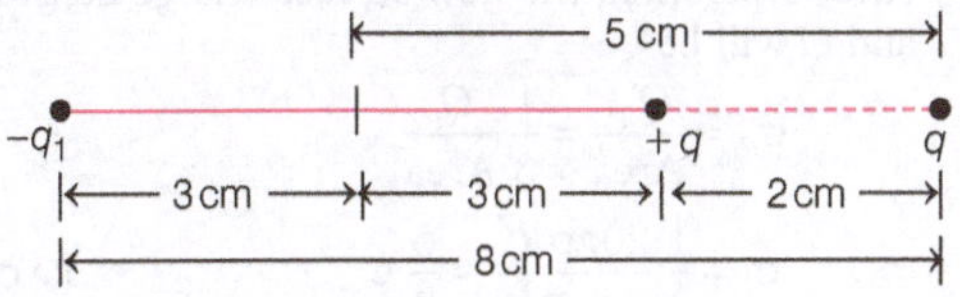

$$V = \frac{Kq}{2\times10^{-2}} - \frac{Kq}{8\times10^{-2}}$$

$$= Kq\left[\frac{3}{8}\right]\times10^2$$

3. (*d*) Given, volume, $V = 0.2\text{ m}^3$

Electric potential = 5 V = constant

$\because$ Electric field $E = \dfrac{-dV}{dr} = \dfrac{-d(5)}{dr} = 0$

4. (*a*) Given, electric dipole moment,

$$p = 16\times10^{-9}\text{ C-m}$$

Distance, $r = 0.6$ m

Angle, $\theta = 60° \Rightarrow \cos 60° = \frac{1}{2}$

Electric potential at a point which is at a distance r at some angle θ from electric dipole is

$$V = \frac{p\cos\theta}{4\pi\varepsilon_0 r^2}$$

$$= \frac{9\times10^9\times16\times10^{-9}\times\frac{1}{2}}{(0.6)^2}$$

$$= 2\times10^2 = 200\text{ V}$$

5. (*b*) Given, potential in a region,

$$V = 6xy - y + 2yz$$

Electric field in a region,

$$E = -\frac{\partial V}{\partial x}\hat{\mathbf{i}} - \frac{\partial V}{\partial y}\hat{\mathbf{j}} - \frac{\partial V}{\partial z}\hat{\mathbf{k}}$$

$$\Rightarrow E = -6y\hat{\mathbf{i}} - (6x - 1 + 2z)\hat{\mathbf{j}} - 2y\hat{\mathbf{k}}$$

At, (1, 1, 0), electric field can be expressed,

$$E = -(6\times1\hat{\mathbf{i}}) - (6\times1-1)\hat{\mathbf{j}} - 2\times1\hat{\mathbf{k}}$$

$$= -(6\hat{\mathbf{i}} + 5\hat{\mathbf{j}} + 2\hat{\mathbf{k}})\text{ N/C}$$

6. (*d*) Potential due to uniformly charged spherical shell is given by,

$$V = \frac{kq}{R} \quad (\text{For } r \le R)$$

$$\Rightarrow V_C = V_P$$

$$\Rightarrow V_C - V_P = 0$$

7. (*b*) Work done to move a charge (q) particle between any two points on equipotential surface is zero.

i.e. $W = q(V_2 - V_1)$

$\Rightarrow \mathbf{F}\cdot d\mathbf{s} = q(V - V)$ $\quad [\because V_1 = V_2 = V]$

$\Rightarrow q(\mathbf{E}\cdot d\mathbf{s}) = 0$ $\quad [\because \mathbf{F} = \mathbf{E}\cdot d\mathbf{s}]$

$\Rightarrow \mathbf{F}\cdot d\mathbf{s} = 0$

Therefore, $\mathbf{E} \perp d\mathbf{s}$

Since, $d\mathbf{s}$ lies in the plane of equipotential surface.

Thus, angle between the electric lines of force and the equipotential surface is 90°.

8. (*a*) Potential on the hollow conducting sphere of radius R due to charge Q is

$$V = \frac{1}{4\pi\varepsilon_0}\cdot\frac{Q}{R}$$

$\Rightarrow V \propto \dfrac{1}{R}$ $\quad$ [For same charge Q]

$$\Rightarrow \frac{V_1}{V_2} = \frac{R_2}{R_1}$$

Since, $R_1 > R_2$

$\therefore \dfrac{R_2}{R_1} < 1$

$$\therefore \quad \frac{V_1}{V_2} < 1$$

$$\therefore \quad V_1 < V_2$$

Hence, potential will more on smaller sphere.

9. (*d*) According to the question,

$$V_{\text{bigger}} = 27 \times V_{\text{small}}$$

$$\Rightarrow \quad \frac{4}{3}\pi R^3 = 27 \times \frac{4}{3}\pi r^3$$

$$\Rightarrow \quad R^3 = 27 \times r^3$$

$$\Rightarrow \quad R = 3r$$

Now, the potential of the small drop,

$$V = \frac{Kq}{r} \quad \text{...(i)}$$

The potential of the bigger drop,

$$V' = \frac{KQ}{R}$$

$$Q = 27q$$

So, the potential of the bigger drop,

$$V' = \frac{K \times 27q}{3r}$$

$$\Rightarrow \quad V' = 9\frac{Kq}{r}$$

$$V' = 9V \quad \text{[From Eq. (i)]}$$

$$= 9 \times 220 = 1980 \text{ V}$$

10. (*b*) When two charged spherical conductors are connected by a conducting wire, then the potential becomes same in both the spherical conductor, i.e.

$$V_1 = V_2$$

$$\Rightarrow \quad \frac{Kq_1}{R_1} = \frac{Kq_2}{R_2}$$

$$\Rightarrow \quad \frac{q_1}{q_2} = \frac{R_1}{R_2} \quad \text{...(i)}$$

$$\sigma = \frac{q_1}{4\pi R^2}$$

$$\therefore \quad \frac{\sigma_1}{\sigma_2} = \frac{\dfrac{q_1}{4\pi R_1^2}}{\dfrac{q_2}{4\pi R_2^2}}$$

$$\Rightarrow \quad \frac{\sigma_1}{\sigma_2} = \frac{q_1}{q_2}\frac{R_2^2}{R_1^2}$$

$$\Rightarrow \quad \frac{\sigma_1}{\sigma_2} = \frac{R_1}{R_2}\frac{R_2^2}{R_1^2} \quad \text{[From Eq. (i)]}$$

$$\Rightarrow \quad \frac{\sigma_1}{\sigma_2} = \frac{R_2}{R_1}$$

11. (*b*) For metallic spherical shell,

$$V_{\text{inside}} = V_{\text{surface}} = \frac{1}{4\pi\varepsilon_0} \cdot \frac{q}{R} = \text{constant}$$

Outside the spherical shell,

$$V \propto \frac{1}{r}$$

Hence, variation of potential (V) with distance r is given as

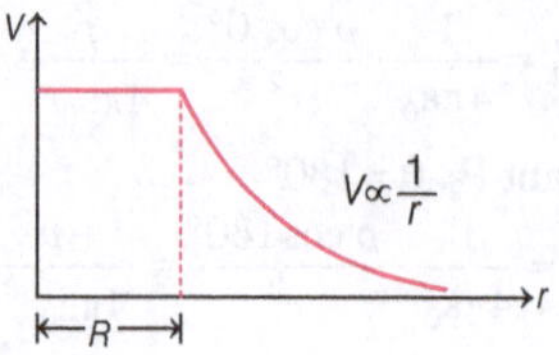

12. (*d*) Surface charge density,

$$\sigma = \frac{\text{Charge}}{\text{Area}} = \frac{Q}{A}$$

or $\quad Q = \sigma A$

$$Q_P = \sigma \times 4\pi R^2 = 4\pi\sigma R^2 \quad \text{...(i)}$$

and $Q_Q = \sigma \times 4\pi (2R)^2 = 16\pi\sigma R^2 \quad$ ...(ii)

When they are brought in contact with each other, the total charge will be

$$Q_t = Q_P + Q_Q$$

$$= 4\pi\sigma R^2 + 16\pi\sigma R^2 \quad \text{[From Eqs. (i) and (ii)]}$$

$$= 20\pi\sigma R^2 \quad \text{...(iii)}$$

When two charged bodies are connected

$$\therefore \quad V_1 = V_2$$

$$\frac{Q_P}{4\pi\varepsilon_0 R} = \frac{Q_Q}{4\pi\varepsilon_0 2R}$$

$$\Rightarrow \quad \frac{Q_P}{R} = \frac{Q_Q}{2R} \Rightarrow \frac{Q_P}{Q_Q} = \frac{1}{2}$$

$$\therefore \quad Q'_P = \frac{1}{3}Q_t \text{ and } Q'_Q = \frac{2}{3}Q_t$$

After separation, the new surface charge densities on P and Q will be

$$\sigma_P = \frac{Q'_P}{\text{Area}} = \frac{1}{3}\frac{Q_t}{\text{Area}}$$

$$\Rightarrow \quad \sigma_1 = \frac{1}{3}\frac{20\pi\sigma R^2}{4\pi R^2} = \frac{5}{3}\sigma \quad [\because \sigma_P = \sigma_1]$$

and $\quad \sigma_Q = \dfrac{Q'_Q}{\text{Area}} = \dfrac{2}{3}\dfrac{Q_t}{\text{Area}}$

$$\Rightarrow \quad \sigma_2 = \frac{2}{3} \times \frac{20\pi\sigma R^2}{4\pi (2R)^2} \quad [\because \sigma_Q = \sigma_2]$$

$$= \frac{2}{3} \times \frac{5}{4}\sigma = \frac{5}{6}\sigma$$

13. (*b*) We know that,

Work done (W) $= q\,\Delta V$

ΔV is same in all the cases. So, work done will be same in the all cases.

Skill Builder

Sol. of Skill Builder on Pg. 79

(*b*) For a point in figure,

$$V = K_e \Sigma \frac{q_i}{r_i} = K_e \left(\frac{q}{x-a} - \frac{q}{x+a} \right) = \frac{2K_e qa}{x^2 - a^2}$$

Sol. of Skill Builder on Pg. 86

(*c*) Potential at surface = 80 V

$$V = \frac{K \cdot Q}{R}$$

$$80 = \frac{K \cdot Q}{0.2}$$

$$K \cdot Q = 16$$

Potential at 30 cm from centre

$$V = \frac{K \cdot Q}{r}$$

$$V = \frac{16}{0.3} = 53.3 \text{ V}$$

Sol. of Skill Builder on Pg. 88

(*a*) Charge on first sphere,

$$Q_1 = 4\sigma\pi(2R)^2 = 16\,\sigma\pi R^2$$

Charge on second sphere,

$$Q_2 = 4\sigma\pi(4R)^2 = 64\sigma\pi R^2$$

When they are brought in cantact with each other, the total charge will be

$$Q_t = Q_1 + Q_2 = 80\sigma\pi R^2$$

when two bodies are connected,

$$V_1 = V_2$$

$$\frac{Q_1'}{4\pi\varepsilon_0(2R)} = \frac{Q_2'}{4\pi\varepsilon_0(4R)}$$

$$\Rightarrow \quad \frac{Q_1'}{Q_2'} = \frac{1}{2} \Rightarrow Q_1' = \frac{1}{3} Q_t \text{ and } Q_2' = \frac{2}{3} Q_t$$

After separation, new surface charge density will be

$$\sigma_1 = \frac{Q_1'}{4\pi(2R)^2} = \frac{1}{3} \cdot \frac{Q_t}{(4\pi)(2R)^2} = \frac{80\sigma\pi R^2}{24\pi R^2} = \frac{10}{3}\sigma$$

$$\sigma_2 = \frac{Q_2'}{4\pi(4R)^2} = \frac{2}{3} \cdot \frac{Q_t}{4\pi(4R)^2} = \frac{2}{3} \cdot \frac{80\sigma\pi R^2}{4\pi 16R^2} = \frac{5}{6}\sigma$$

For deeper insight
Scan the QR Code

Chapter 3

Capacitance

Learning Objectives

Module-I

- Electrostatics of Conductors
- Dielectrics and Polarisation
- Capacitors and Capacitance
- Parallel Plate Capacitor
- Effect of Dielectric on Various Parameters of Capacitor

Module-II

- Capacitors in Series
- Capacitors in Parallel

Module-III

- Energy Stored in Charged Capacitor
- Common Potential (Redistribution of Charge)
- Loss of Energy During Redistribution of Charge

Chapter Overview with NEET Connection

- This chapter is one step ahead of previous chapter towards the electrostatic conductance. Without having good hold on this chapter, it will be difficult to understand whole electrostatic section. It is also helpful for the understanding of other chapter like current electricity, electromagnetic induction.

Special format questions can be easily framed on the following topics of this chapter

- Capacitance of a capacitor and effect of variation in different parameters on capacitance.
- Dielectric inside capacitor.
- Equivalent capacitance in different combinations of capacitors.
- Potential at different points in combinations of capacitors.
- Energy stored, energy dissipated in contact cases of capacitors.

For better understanding of this chapter

- Knowledge of potential and potential difference should be revisited.
- Voltage and current distribution behaviour in series and parallel circuits should be studied (class 10th).
- Charge and energy conservation laws should be revisited.

Introduction

Some electric components has ability to collect and store energy in the form of electric charge. These components are known as **capacitor** and this property is known as **capacitance**.

In this chapter, we will study about conceptualisation of capacitors, their combinations and energy prospectus of capacitor.

Module 1

Electrostatics of Conductors and Capacitors

- Electrostatics of Conductors • Dielectrics and Polarisation • Capacitors and Capacitance
- Parallel Plate Capacitor • Effect of Dielectric on Various Parameters of Capacitor

Electrostatics of Conductors

The substances such as metals which allow the charge to flow freely through them are called conductors. Conductors contain large number of free electrons which can move freely inside it.

Conductor Placed in Electric Field

Whenever a conductor is placed in an external electric field, the free electrons in it experience a force due to it and start moving opposite to the field. This movement makes one side of conductor positively charged and the other as negatively charged. This creates an electric field in the conductor in a direction opposite to external electric field (called induced field). The movement of electrons continues till the net electric field (resultant of external electric field and induced field) becomes zero. This is a state of electrostatic equilibrium.

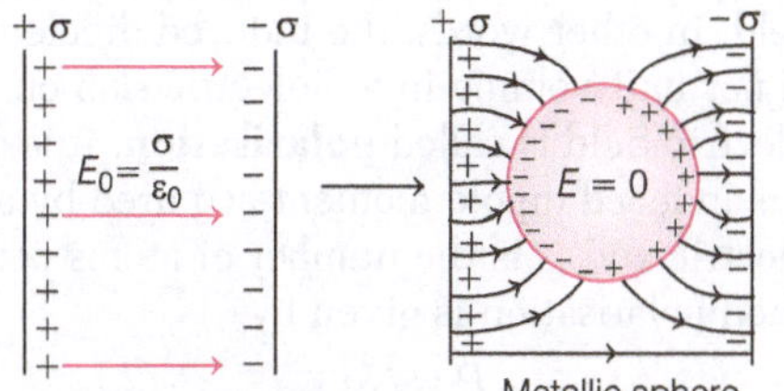

Electric field between two charged plates

Metallic sphere in electric field

1. When a conductor is charged by induction, induced charge (which is free to move) is equal and opposite to the inducing charge, *i.e.* $q' = -q$.
2. In electrostatic, conductors are equipotential surfaces, *i.e.* potential on the surface or inside the conductor is same.
3. Charge given to conductor resides on its outer surface. However, distribution of charge on the surface is such that surface density of charge varies inversely as the radius of curvature of that part of the conductor, *i.e.*, $\sigma \propto 1/R$.

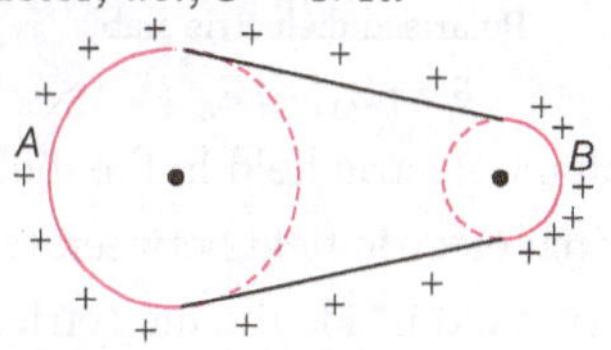

$\sigma_B > \sigma_A$

4. The dielectric constant of conductors in electrostatics is infinite, *i.e.*, $\varepsilon_r = \infty$.
5. Electric field intensity inside a conductor is zero, so electrostatic field lines never exist within the conducting object.
6. Electric field and hence, lines of force are normal to the surface of a conductor.
7. Electric field intensity near a conducting surface is given as $\mathbf{E} = \frac{\sigma}{\varepsilon_0}\,\hat{\mathbf{n}}$.
8. **Electrostatic Shielding** A cavity surrounded by conducting walls is a field free region as long as there are no charges inside the cavity. Whatever be the charge and field configuration, the field inside the cavity is always zero. This is known as **electrostatic shielding**.

Concept ladder A cavity inside a metallic conductor is shielded from outside electrical disturbances. However, the electrostatic shielding does not work on the other way i.e. if we place charges inside the cavity, the exterior of the conductor cannot be shielded from the electric fields of the inside charges.

Dielectrics and Polarisation

Dielectrics are insulating (non-conducting) materials that can produce electric effect without conduction. Movement of free charges is not possible in a dielectric. So, they behave differently. When a dielectric material is kept in an electric field, then the external field induces dipole moment. Due to which, net charge on the surface of the dielectric appears and as a result electric field is produced that opposes the external field. Induced field is less in magnitude than the external field, so field inside the dielectric gets reduced.

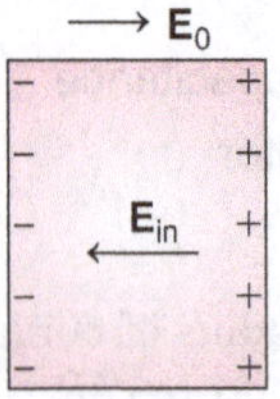

Polarised dielectric slab

$$\mathbf{E} = |\mathbf{E}_0| - |\mathbf{E}_{in}|$$

where, $\mathbf{E}$ = resultant electric field in the dielectric,

$\mathbf{E}_0$ = external electric field between two plates

and $\mathbf{E}_{in}$ = electric field inside the dielectric.

Types of Dielectrics

There are two types of dielectrics.

(i) Polar Dielectrics

A polar molecule is one in which the centres of positive and negative charges are separated (even when there is no external field). Such molecules have permanent dipole moment, *e.g.* HCl, H_2O. So, a polar dielectric is one which is having a net dipole moment zero in the absence of electric field due to the random orientation of polar molecules as shown in figure.

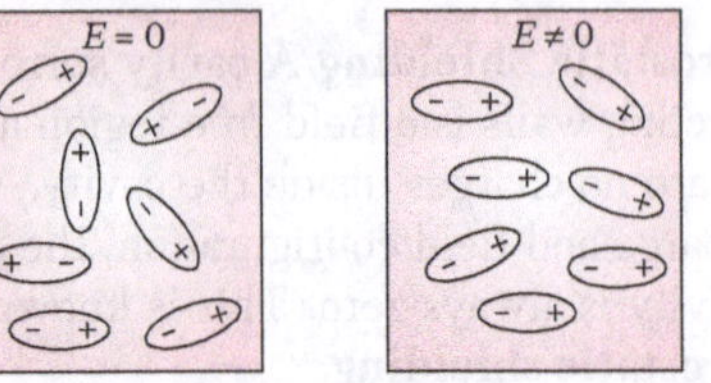

Behaviour of a polar dielectric in external field

In the presence of electric field, polar molecules tend to line up in the direction of electric field and now they have finite dipole moment.

(ii) Non-Polar Dielectrics

In a non-polar molecule, the centres of positive and negative charges coincide. The molecule thus has no permanent (or intrinsic) dipole moment, *e.g.*, oxygen (O_2) and hydrogen (H_2) molecules. In an external electric field, the positive and negative charges of a non-polar molecules are displaced in opposite direction. This occurs till the point where external force is balanced by the restoring force (due to internal field in the molecule). Thus, dipole moment is induced in non-polar molecules and dielectric is said to be **polarised.** The induced dipole moments of different molecules add up giving a net dipole moment of the dielectric in the presence of the external field.

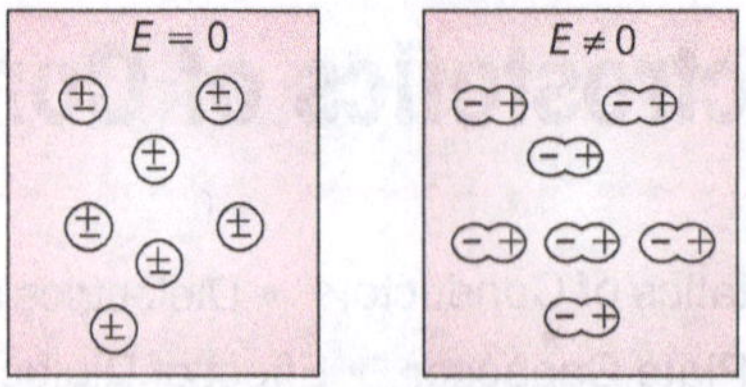

Behaviour of a non-polar dielectric in external field

Dielectric constant (*K*)

The ratio of the strength of the applied electric field to the strength of the reduced value of the electric field on placing the dielectric between the two charged plates called the dielectric constant of the dielectric medium.

It is also known as relative permittivity or specific inductive capacity and it is denoted by K (or ε_r).

$$K = \frac{E_0}{E}$$

Mentor's TIP

Dielectric constant is always greater than one for all materials and for air, it is 1.

Polarisation (*P*)

It is a process of inducing equal and opposite charges on the two faces of the dielectrics on the application of electric field. In other words, the induced dipole moment developed per unit volume in a dielectric slab on placing it, in an electric field is called **polarisation.** It is denoted by P. If p is induced dipole moment acquired by an atom of the dielectric and N is the number of atoms per unit volume, then polarisation is given by

$$P = Np$$

The induced dipole moment acquired by the atom is found to be directly proportional to the reduced value of electric field and is given by

$$P = \alpha\varepsilon_0 E_0$$

where, α is constant of proportionality and is called **atomic polarisability.**

Polarisation, $P = \sigma_i$ = induced surface charge density

Its unit is C/m^2 and dimension is $[L^{-2}T^1A^1]$.

Electric Susceptibility (χ)

The polarisation density of dielectric slab is directly proportional to the reduced value of the electric field and may be expressed as

$$P = \chi\varepsilon_0 E_0$$

where, χ is a constant of proportionality and is called electric susceptibility of the dielectric slab. It is a dimensionless constant.

Dielectric Strength

The maximum electric field that a dielectric can withstand without breakdown is called its dielectric strength.

Its SI unit is Vm^{-1} and its practical unit is kV $(mm)^{-1}$.

For air, it is about $3 \times 10^6\, Vm^{-1}$.

Capacitors and Capacitance

A capacitor is a device which is used to store electric charge or potential energy. It is made up of two isolated conductors carrying equal and opposite charges placed at small separation.

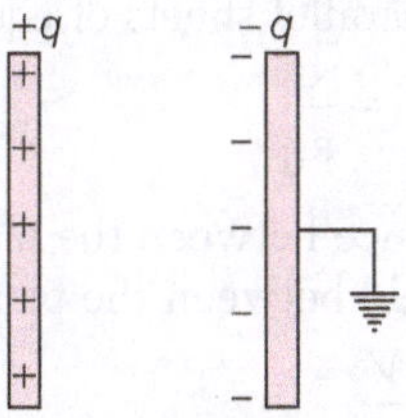

Capacitor

The space between the conductors may be vacuum or an insulating material. Capacitors is represented as

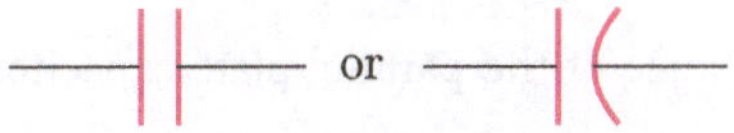

Symbol of capacitor

Capacitance of a Conductor

When a charge q is given to a conductor, it spreads over the outer surface of the conductor. The whole conductor comes to the same potential (say V). This potential V is directly proportional to the charge q, i.e.,

$$V \propto q$$

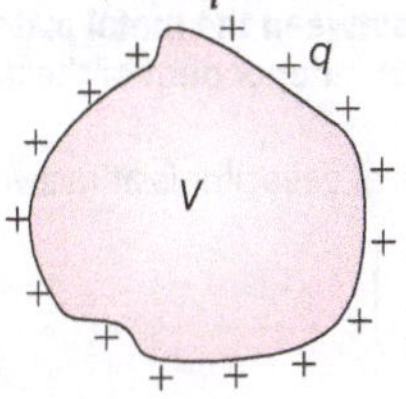

$$q = CV$$

or $$C = \frac{q}{V}$$

This C is constant of proportionality and is called the **capacitance** of the conductor.

The SI unit of capacitance is called **Farad** (F).

$\therefore$ 1 Farad (1 F) = 1 coulomb/volt (1 C/V)

Its dimensional formula is $[ML^{-2}T^4A^2]$.

Capacitance C depends on the shape, size and separation of the system of two conductors and is independent of the charge given to the body.

Example 1. *A capacitor of capacitance* $0.75\,\mu F$ *is charged to a voltage of* 16 V. *What is the magnitude of the charge on each plate of the capacitor?*

Sol. Using $q = CV$, we get

$$q = CV = (0.75 \times 10^{-6}\text{ F})(16\text{ V}) = 1.2 \times 10^{-5}\text{ C}$$

Capacitance of an Isolated Spherical Conductor

When a charge q is given to a spherical conductor of radius R, the potential on its surface is

$$V = \frac{1}{4\pi\varepsilon_0} \cdot \frac{q}{R}$$

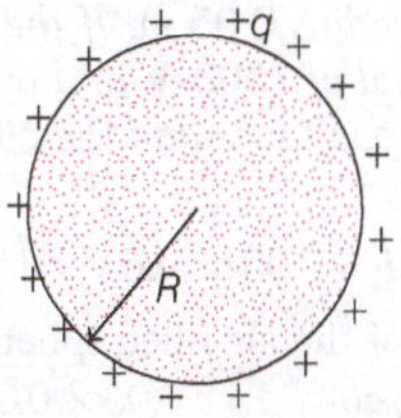

From this expression, we find that

$$\frac{q}{V} = 4\pi\varepsilon_0 R = C$$

Thus, capacitance of the spherical conductor is

$$C = 4\pi\varepsilon_0 R$$

From this expression, we can draw the following conclusions

(i) $C \propto R$ or C depends on R, which we have already stated that C depends on the dimensions of the conductor. Moreover, if two conductors have radii R_1 and R_2, then

$$\frac{C_1}{C_2} = \frac{R_1}{R_2}$$

(ii) Earth is also a spherical conductor of radius $R = 6.4 \times 10^6$ m. The capacity of earth is therefore,

$$C = \left(\frac{1}{9 \times 10^9}\right)(6.4 \times 10^6)$$

$$= 711 \times 10^{-6}\text{ F or } C = 711\,\mu\text{F}$$

From here, we can see that farad is a large unit. As capacity of such a huge conductor is only $711\,\mu$F.

Capacity of a Spherical Conductor Enclosed by an Earthed Concentric Spherical Shell

Let a system of two concentric conducting spheres of radii a and b, where a is less than b. Inner sphere is given charge q while outer sphere is earthed. Potential difference between the spheres is given by

$$V = \frac{q}{4\pi\varepsilon_0}\left(\frac{1}{a} - \frac{1}{b}\right) \quad \text{...(i)}$$

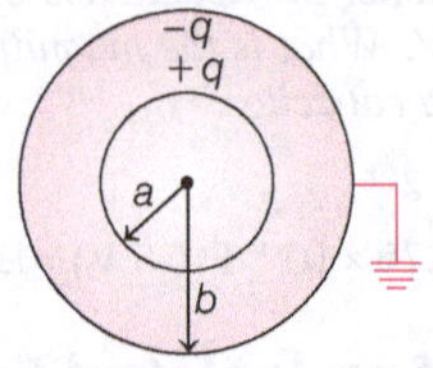

Hence, the capacitance of this system will be $C = \frac{q}{V}$

or $$C = 4\pi\varepsilon_0\left(\frac{ab}{b-a}\right) \quad \text{[from Eq. (i)]}$$

Example 2. *A sphere of radius 0.03 m is suspended within a hollow sphere of radius 0.05 m. If the inner sphere is charged to a potential of 1500 V and outer sphere is earthed, find the capacitance and the charge on the inner sphere.*

Sol. Here, $a = 0.03$ m, $b = 0.05$ m and $V = 1500$ V

The capacitance of the air-filled spherical capacitor,

$$C = \frac{4\pi\varepsilon_0 ab}{(b-a)} = \frac{0.03 \times 0.05}{9 \times 10^9 \times (0.05 - 0.03)}$$

$$= 8.33 \times 10^{-12} \text{ F} = 8.33 \text{ pF}$$

Charge, $q = CV = 8.33 \times 10^{-12} \times 1500 = 1.25 \times 10^{-8}$ C

Example 3. *The thickness of air layer between the two coatings of a spherical capacitor is 2 cm. The capacitor has the some capacitance as the sphere of 1.2 m diameter. Find the radii of its surface.*

Sol. Here, $\frac{4\pi\varepsilon_0 ab}{b-a} = 4\pi\varepsilon_0 R$

or $$\frac{ab}{b-a} = R$$

Now, $b - a = 2$ cm and $R = \frac{1.2}{2}$ m $= 60$ cm

$\therefore$ $$\frac{ab}{2} = 60$$

or $$ab = 120$$

$$(b+a)^2 = (b-a)^2 + 4ab$$

$$= 2^2 + 4 \times 120 = 484$$

or $$b + a = 22$$

or $$2 + a + a = 22 \quad (\because b - a = 2 \text{ cm})$$

$\therefore$ $$a = 10 \text{ cm and } b = 12 \text{ cm}$$

Parallel Plate Capacitor

A parallel plate air capacitor consists of two parallel metallic plates separated by a small distance.

Suppose, the area of each plate is A and the separation between the two plates is d. Also assume that the space between the plates contains vacuum. Suppose, the charge density on each of these surfaces has a magnitude

$$\sigma = q/A.$$

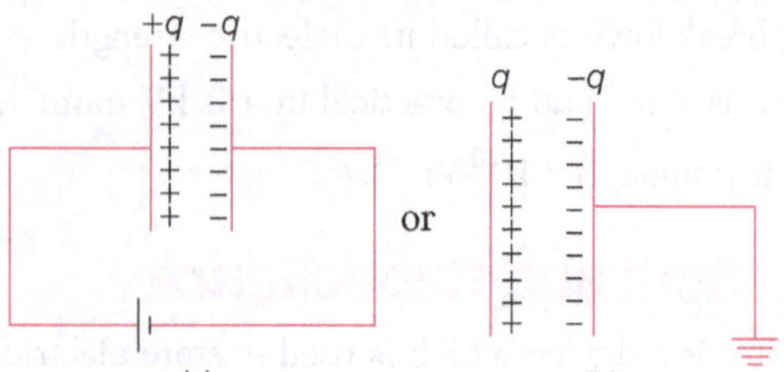

(a) (b)

We know that, the intensity of electric field at a point between two plane parallel sheets of equal and opposite charges is given by $E = \frac{\sigma}{\varepsilon_0}$.

The potential difference between the plates be V volt. Then, the electric field between the plates is given by

$$E = \frac{V}{d}$$

$\therefore$ $$V = Ed = \left(\frac{\sigma}{\varepsilon_0}\right)d = \frac{qd}{A\varepsilon_0}$$

$\therefore$ The capacitance of the parallel plate capacitor is given by

$$C = \frac{q}{V} = \frac{A\varepsilon_0}{d}$$

or $$C = \frac{\varepsilon_0 A}{d}$$

NEET Snapshot

The electrostatic force between the metal plates of an isolated parallel plate capacitor is independent of the distance between the plates. ***[NEET 2018]***

The force between plates of capacitor is attractive and can be expressed as

$$F = qE = q\left(\frac{\sigma}{2\varepsilon_0}\right)$$

or $$F = \frac{1}{2}\varepsilon_0 AE^2 \quad (\because q = \sigma A = \varepsilon_0 EA)$$

Scan for Video

If the space between the plates be filled with some dielectric medium of dielectric constant K, then the electric field between the plates is increased to K-times and given as,

$$C = \frac{K\varepsilon_0 A}{d} \text{ farad}$$

Example 4. *A parallel plate capacitor is constructed with plates of area 0.0280 m^2 and separation 0.550 mm. Find the magnitude of the charge on each plate of this capacitor when the potential difference between the plates is 20.1 V.*

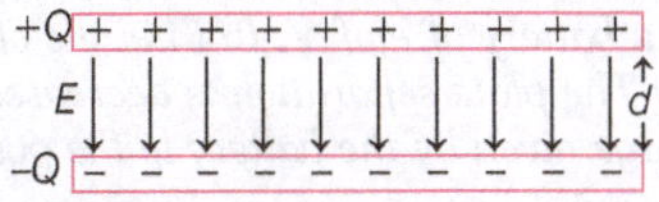

Sol. Using the formula,

$$C = \frac{\varepsilon_0 A}{d} = \frac{(8.85\times10^{-12})(0.0280)}{0.550\times10^{-3}}$$

$$= 4.51\times10^{-10}\,\text{F}$$

We obtain the capacitance of the parallel plate capacitor, $C = 4.51\times10^{-10}$ F

Capacitance of a Capacitor Partially Filled with Dielectric

Suppose, the space between parallel plates of capacitor is partially filled with a dielectric (dielectric constant = K) of thickness $t < d$, then the filling thickness between the plates is t in the dielectric and $(d - t)$ in vacuum (or air)

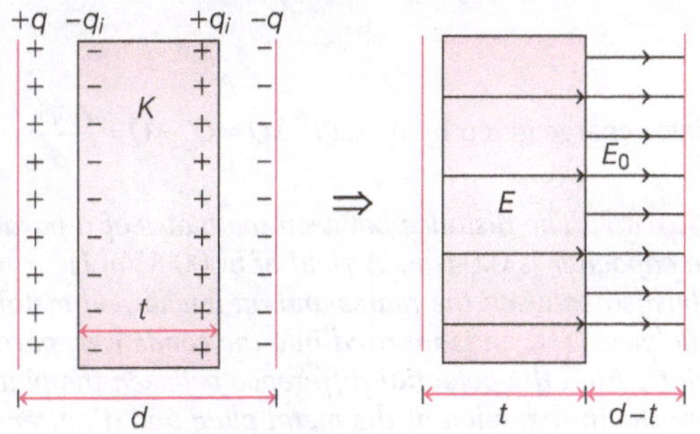

If $E_0 = \dfrac{q}{\varepsilon_0 A}$ is the electric field in the region, where dielectric is absent, then electric field inside the dielectric will be $E = E_0 / K$. The potential difference between the plates of the capacitor is

$$V = Et + E_0(d-t)$$

$$= \frac{E_0}{K}t + E_0(d-t)$$

$$= E_0\left(d - t + \frac{t}{K}\right)$$

$$= \frac{q}{A\varepsilon_0}\left(d - t + \frac{t}{K}\right)$$

Now, as per the definition of capacitance,

$$C = \frac{q}{V} = \frac{\varepsilon_0 A}{d - t + \dfrac{t}{K}}$$

or

$$\boxed{C = \frac{\varepsilon_0 A}{d - t + \dfrac{t}{K}}}$$

Special Cases

(i) If the slab completely fills the space between the plates, then $t = d$ and therefore

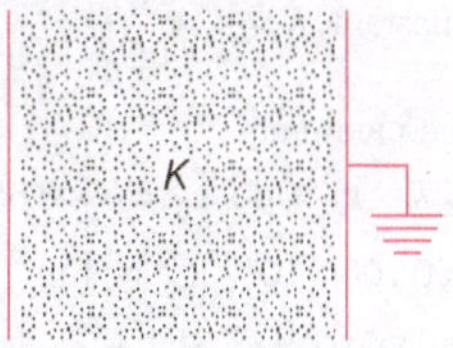

$$C = \frac{\varepsilon_0 A}{d/K} = \frac{K\varepsilon_0 A}{d} \text{ or } \frac{C}{C_0} = K$$

where, $C_0 = \dfrac{\varepsilon_0 A}{d}$ is capacitance without the dielectric.

(ii) If a conducting slab (*i.e.* $K = \infty$) is placed between the plates, then

$$C = \frac{\varepsilon_0 A}{d - t + t/\infty} = \frac{\varepsilon_0 A}{d - t}$$

This can also be understood from the following figure

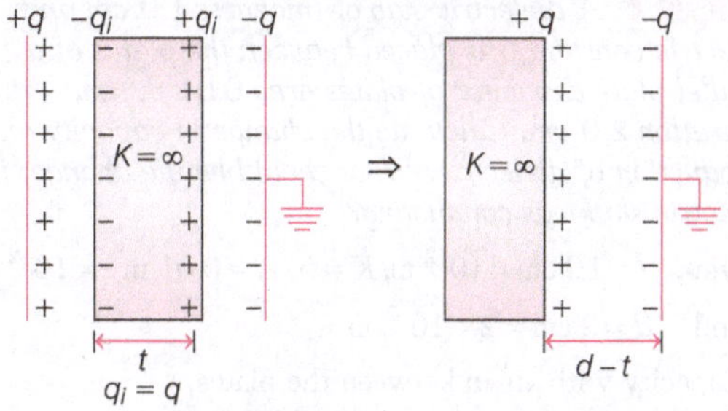

(iii) If the space between the plates is completely filled with a conductor, then $t = d$ and $K = \infty$.

$$C = \frac{\varepsilon_0 A}{d - d + \dfrac{d}{\infty}} = \infty$$

(iv) If more than one dielectric slabs are placed between the capacitor, then

$$C = \frac{\varepsilon_0 A}{d - t_1 - t_2 - \ldots - t_n + \dfrac{t_1}{K_1} + \dfrac{t_2}{K_2} + \ldots + \dfrac{t_n}{K_n}}$$

NEET Close-up

Example Similar to PYQ Asked in NEET 2020

The capacitance of a parallel plate capacitor with air as medium is 3 μF. With the introduction of a dielectric medium, the capacitance becomes 24 μF. The permittivity of the medium is

(a) 4.2×10^{-10} C² N⁻¹ m⁻² (b) 7.1×10^{-11} C²N⁻¹m⁻²

(c) 3.4×10^{-11} C² N⁻¹ m⁻² (d) 5.6×10^{-10} C² N⁻¹ m⁻²

Sol. (b) Given, $C_0 = 3\,\mu F$, $C_m = 24\,\mu F$

$\therefore$ As, dielectric constant, $K = \varepsilon_r = \dfrac{C_m}{C_0} = \dfrac{24}{3} = 8$

Permittivity of the medium,

$$\varepsilon_m = K \times \varepsilon_0 = 8 \times \varepsilon_0 = 8 \times 8.85 \times 10^{-12}$$
$$= 0.708 \times 10^{-10}\ C^2\ N^{-1}\ m^{-2}$$
$$= 7.1 \times 10^{-11}\ C^2\ N^{-1}\ m^{-2}$$

Skill Builder

The capacitance of a parallel plate capacitor with air as medium is 8 μF. When dielectric medium introduce, the capacitance becomes 48 μF. The permittivity of the medium is ($\varepsilon_0 = 8.85 \times 10^{-12}\ C^2N^{-1}m^{-2}$)

(a) $1.28 \times 10^{-12}\ C^2 N^{-1} m^{-2}$ (b) $0.53 \times 10^{-12}\ C^2N^{-1}m^{-2}$

(c) $0.53 \times 10^{-10}\ C^2N^{-1} m^{-2}$ (d) $0.44 \times 10^{-12}\ C^2 N^{-1} m^{-2}$

For more Practice Refer Q. No. 16 of step-up practice 1 and Q.No 14 of Gearing up for NEET.

Example 5. *A dielectric slab of thickness 1.0 cm and dielectric constant 5 is placed between the plates of a parallel plate capacitor of plates area 0.01 m² and separation 2.0 cm. Calculate the change in capacity on introduction of dielectric. What should be the change, if the dielectric slab was conducting?*

Sol. Given, $t = 1.0\ \text{cm} = 10^{-2}$ m, $K = 5$, $A = 0.01\ m^2 = 10^{-2}\ m^2$

and $d = 2\ \text{cm} = 2 \times 10^{-2}$ m

Capacity with air in between the plates,

$$C_0 = \frac{\varepsilon_0 A}{d} = \frac{8.85 \times 10^{-12} \times 10^{-2}}{2 \times 10^{-2}} = 4.425 \times 10^{-12} F$$

Capacity with dielectric slab in between the plates,

$$C = \frac{\varepsilon_0 A}{\left[d - \left(1 - \dfrac{1}{K}\right)t\right]} = \frac{8.85 \times 10^{-12} \times 10^{-2}}{2 \times 10^{-2} - 10^{-2}\left(1 - \dfrac{1}{5}\right)}$$
$$= 7.375 \times 10^{-12}\ F$$

Capacity with conducting slab in between the plates,

$$C' = \frac{\varepsilon_0 A}{d - t} = \frac{8.85 \times 10^{-12} \times 10^{-2}}{2 \times 10^{-2} - 1 \times 10^{-2}} = 8.85 \times 10^{-12}\ F$$

Increase in capacity on introduction of dielectric

$$= C - C_0 = 7.375 \times 10^{-12} - 4.425 \times 10^{-12}$$
$$= 2.95 \times 10^{-12}\ F$$

Increase in capacity on introduction of conducting slab

$$= C' - C_0 = 8.85 \times 10^{-12} - 4.425 \times 10^{-12} = 4.425 \times 10^{-12}\ F$$

Example 6. *A parallel plate capacitor has plate area A and separation d between the plates. The capacitor is connected to a battery of emf V. (i) Find the charge on the capacitor, (ii) The plate separation is decreased to d/2. Find the extra charge given by the battery to the positive plate.*

Sol. (i) Capacitance, $C = \dfrac{A\varepsilon_0}{d}$

$\therefore$ Charge, $Q = CV = \dfrac{A\varepsilon_0 V}{d}$

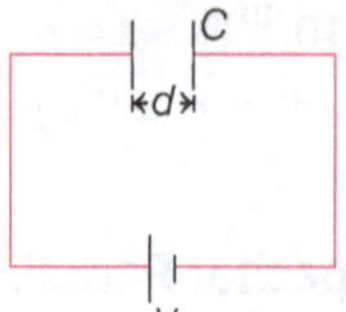

(ii) $C' = \dfrac{A\varepsilon_0}{d/2} = \dfrac{2A\varepsilon_0}{d} \Rightarrow Q' = C'V = \dfrac{2A\varepsilon_0 V}{d}$

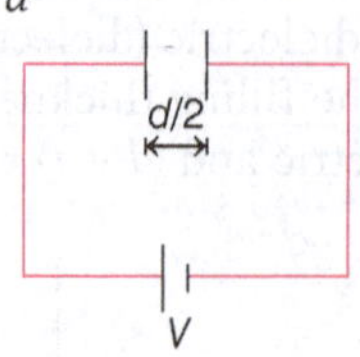

Extra charge given by battery, $\Delta Q = Q' - Q = \dfrac{A\varepsilon_0 V}{d}$

Example 7. *The distance between the plates of a parallel plate capacitor is 0.04 m. A field of 5000 V/m is established between the plates and an uncharged metal plate of thickness 0.01 m is inserted into the condenser, parallel to its plate. Find the potential difference between the plates (i) before the introduction of the metal plate and (ii) after its introduction. What would be the potential difference, if a plate of dielectric constant K = 2 is introduced in place of metal plate?*

Sol. (i) Potential difference across capacitor,

$$V = Ed = 5000 \times 0.04 = 200\ V$$

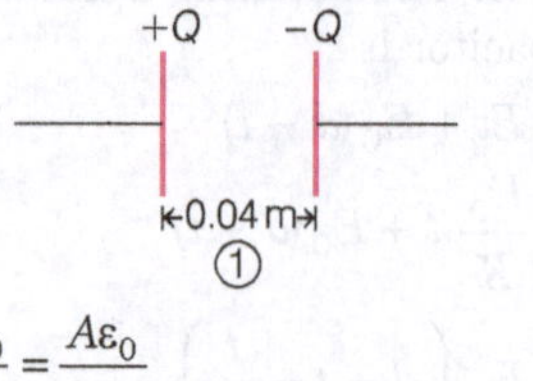

(ii) $C = \dfrac{A\varepsilon_0}{d} = \dfrac{A\varepsilon_0}{0.04}$

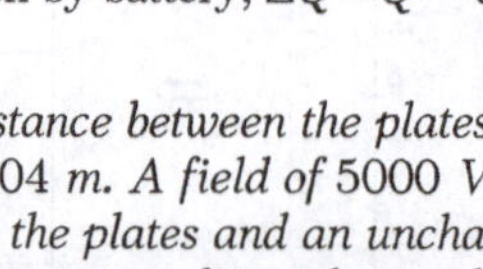

$$C' = \frac{A\varepsilon_0}{d - t + \dfrac{t}{K}} = \frac{A\varepsilon_0}{0.04 - 0.01 + \dfrac{0.01}{\infty}} = \frac{A\varepsilon_0}{0.03}$$

Since, charge remains same,

$$Q = CV = C'V' \Rightarrow \frac{A\varepsilon_0}{0.04} \times 200 = \frac{A\varepsilon_0}{0.03} V'$$

$\therefore$ Potential difference, $V' = 150$ V

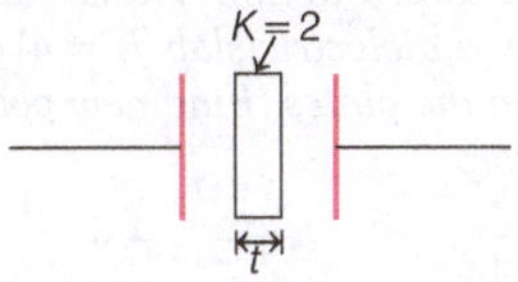

$$C'' = \frac{A\varepsilon_0}{d - t + \frac{t}{K}} = \frac{A\varepsilon_0}{0.04 - 0.01 + \frac{0.01}{2}} = \frac{A\varepsilon_0}{0.035}$$

$$Q = CV = C''V''$$

$$\frac{A\varepsilon_0}{0.04} \times 200 = \frac{A\varepsilon_0}{0.035} V''$$

$\therefore$ Potential, $V'' = 175$ V

NEET Close-up

Example Similar to PYQ Asked in NEET (Oct) 2020

A parallel plate capacitor having cross-sectional area $2a$ and separation d has air in between the plates. When an insulating slab of same area but thickness $\frac{d}{4}$ is inserted between the plates as shown in figure having dielectric constant K (= 2), then new capacitance of capacitor will be

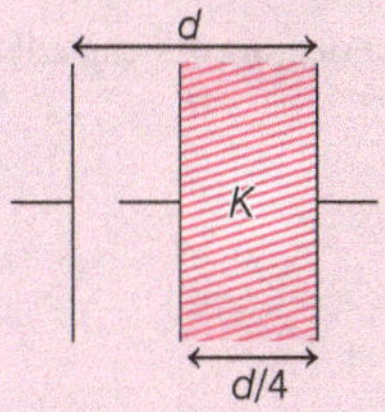

(a) $\frac{16\varepsilon_0 a}{7d}$ (b) $\frac{21\varepsilon_0 a}{8d}$ (c) $\frac{11\varepsilon_0 a}{7d}$ (d) $\frac{17\varepsilon_0 a}{9d}$

Sol. (a) Capacitor of parallel plate capacitor when medium is air

$$C_0 = \frac{\varepsilon_0 (2a)}{d}$$

According to second condition, $a' = 2a, t = \frac{d}{4}, K = 2$

$$\therefore \text{Capacitance, } C = \frac{\varepsilon_0 (2a)}{(d - t) + \frac{t}{K}} = \frac{\varepsilon_0 (2a)}{\left(d - \frac{d}{4}\right) + \frac{d/4}{2}} = \frac{2\varepsilon_0 a}{7d/8} = \frac{16\varepsilon_0 a}{7d}$$

Skill Builder

A parallel plate capacitor having cross-sectional area a and separation d has air in between the plates. Now, an insulating slab of same area but thickness $\frac{d}{3}$ is inserted between the plates having dielectric constant K (= 6). The new capacitance of parallel plate capacitor is

(a) $\frac{15}{7}\frac{\varepsilon_0 a}{d}$ (b) $\frac{18}{13}\frac{\varepsilon_0 a}{d}$ (c) $\frac{17}{12}\frac{\varepsilon_0 a}{d}$ (d) $\frac{13}{7}\frac{\varepsilon_0 a}{d}$

For more Practice Refer Q. No. 19 of step-up practice 1 and Q.No. 36, 37 of Gearing up for NEET.

Effect of Dielectric on Various Parameters

A parallel plate capacitor is charged by a battery which is then disconnected. A dielectric slab is then inserted to fill the space between the plates.

Let q_0, C_0, V_0 and E_0 be the charge, capacitance, potential difference and electric field respectively, before the dielectric slab is inserted.

Now, we will discuss two cases.

(i) Effect of Dielectric when the Battery is kept Disconnected from the Capacitor

As $q_0 = C_0 V_0$, $E_0 = \frac{V_0}{d}$ and $U_0 = \frac{1}{2} C_0 V_0^2$

- The charge on the plates of capacitor remains q_0.
- The electric field gets reduced, *i.e.*, $E = \frac{E_0}{K}$.
- The potential difference gets reduced, *i.e.*, $V = \frac{V_0}{K}$.
- The capacitance increases, *i.e.*, $C = KC_0$.
- The energy decreases, *i.e.*, $U = \frac{U_0}{K}$.

(ii) Effect of Dielectric when Battery Remains Connected across the Capacitor

- The charge now becomes Kq_0, *i.e.*, $q = Kq_0$.
- The electric field remains constant, *i.e.*, $E = E_0$.
- The potential difference remains constant at V_0, *i.e.*, $V = V_0$.
- The capacitance increases from C_0 to C, *i.e.*, $C = KC_0$.
- The energy increases, *i.e.*, $U = KU_0$.

Example 8. *An isolated 16 μF parallel plate air capacitor has a potential difference of 100 V. A dielectric slab having relative permittivity (i.e. dielectric constant) = 5 is introduced to fill the space between the two plates completely. Calculate*

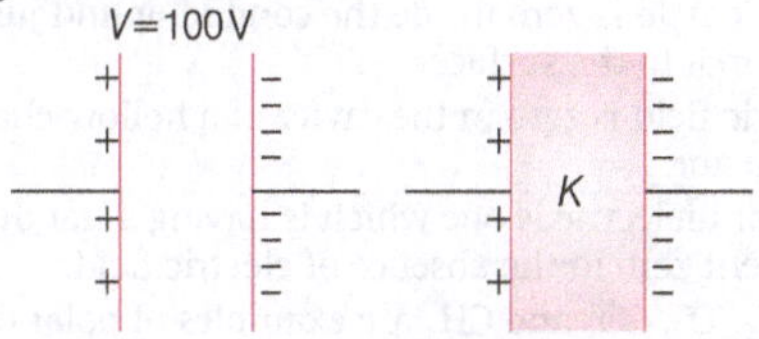

(i) the new capacitance of the capacitor.

(ii) the new potential difference between the two plates of capacitor.

Sol. (i) The new capacity of the capacitor, $C = KC_0$

$$= 5 \times 16 = 80\,\mu\text{F}$$

(ii) Since, the capacitor is isolated, therefore the charge on the capacitor remains the same, thus its capacity is increased on expense of its potential drop.

Therefore, the new potential difference,

$$V = \frac{V_0}{K} = \frac{100}{5} = 20\text{ V}$$

Example 9. *A capacitor ($C = 50\ \mu F$) is charged to a potential difference of 20 V. The charging battery is disconnected and the capacitor is connected to another cell of emf 10V with the positive plate of capacitor joined with the positive terminal of cell.*

(i) Find charge flown through 10V cell.

(ii) Is work done by the cell or is it done on the cell? Find its magnitude.

Sol. Circuit for 20 V battery,

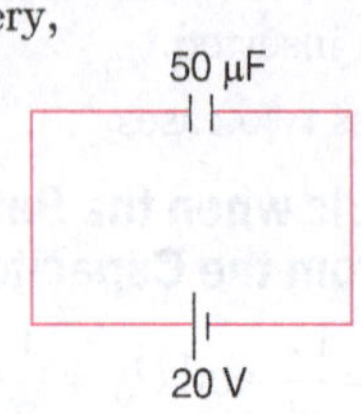

Charge on capacitor,

$$Q_1 = 50 \times 20 = 1000\ \mu C$$

Circuit for 10 V battery,

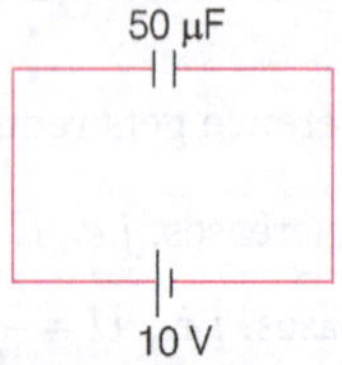

Charge on capacitor,

$$Q_2 = 50 \times 10 = 500\ \mu C,\ Q_2 < Q_1$$

(i) Charge flown through cell of emf 10 V,

$$\Delta Q = Q_1 - Q_2 = 500\ \mu C$$

(ii) Since, $Q_2 < Q_1$, work is done on the cell (W is negative)

$$W = \Delta Q V = 500 \times 10 \times 10^{-6}$$

$$= 5 \times 10^{-3}\ J$$

Example 10. *A parallel plate capacitor ($C = 50\ \mu F$, $d = 4$ mm) is charged to 200 V and then charging battery is removed. Now, a dielectric slab ($K = 4$) of thickness 2 mm is placed between the plates. Find new potential difference across capacitor.*

Sol.

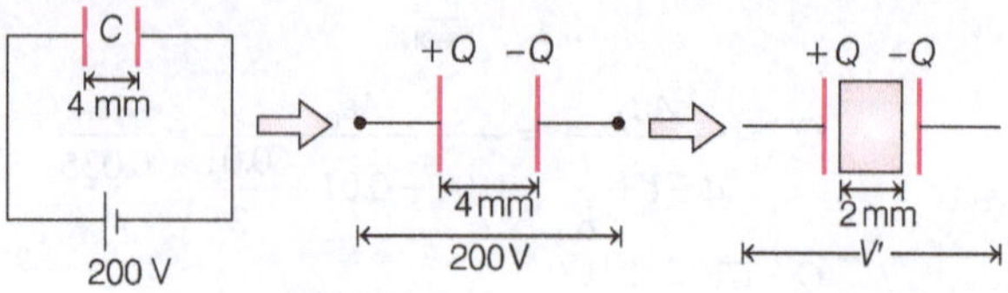

$$C = \frac{A\varepsilon_0}{d}$$

$$\Rightarrow \quad A\varepsilon_0 = Cd = 50 \times 10^{-6} \times 4 \times 10^{-3}$$

$$C' = \frac{A\varepsilon_0}{d - t + \frac{t}{K}} = \frac{Cd}{d - t + \frac{t}{K}}$$

$$= \frac{Cd}{(5/2) \times 10^{-3}}$$

$$= \frac{50 \times 10^{-6} \times 4 \times 10^{-3}}{(5/2) \times 10^{-3}} = 80 \times 10^{-6}\ F$$

Since, charge remains same

$$Q = CV = C'V' = 50 \times 200 = 80V'$$

$\Rightarrow$ Potential difference across capacitor,

$$V' = 125\ V$$

STEP UP Practice 1

1. Identify the false statement.
   (a) Electric field is zero inside the conductor and just outside, it is normal to the surface.
   (b) Electric field is zero in the cavity of a hollow charged conductor.
   (c) A polar dielectric is one which is having a net dipole moment zero in the absence of electric field.
   (d) H_2, N_2, O_2, CO_2 and CH_4 are examples of polar dielectric

2. When **P** is normal to the surface, the polarisation is numerically equal to the
   (a) surface density of the induced charge
   (b) dipole moemnt
   (c) Both (a) and (b)
   (d) Neither (a) nor (b)

3. The total dipole moment of dielectric with polar molecules in absence of an external electric field is
   (a) zero (b) negative
   (c) infinite (d) None of these

4. **Statement I** In the absence of an externally applied electric field, the displacement per unit volume of a polar dielectric material is constant.

   Statement II In polar dielectrics, each molecule has a permanent dipole moment and these are randomly oriented in the absence of an externally applied electric field.

   In the light of the above statements, choose the most appropriate answer from the options given below
   (a) Both Statement I and Statement II are incorrect.
   (b) Statement I is correct but Statement II is incorrect.
   (c) Statement I is incorrect but Statement II is correct.
   (d) Both Statement I and Statement II are correct.

5. Eight drops of mercury of equal radii possessing equal charges combine to form a big drop, then the capacitance of bigger drop compared to each individual small drop is
   (a) 8 times (b) 4 times
   (c) 2 times (d) 32 times

6. The earth has volume V and surface area A, then capacitance would be
(a) $4\pi\varepsilon_0 \frac{A}{V}$ (b) $2\pi\varepsilon_0 \frac{A}{V}$
(c) $12\pi\varepsilon_0 \frac{V}{A}$ (d) $12\pi\varepsilon_0 \frac{A}{V}$

7. If the circumference of a sphere is 2 m, then capacitance of sphere in water would be
(a) 2700 pF (b) 2760 pF
(c) 2780 pF (d) 2800 pF

8. Two charged spheres connected with a wire don't exchange their charges, if both spheres have
(a) equal potential (b) equal capacitance
(c) equal energy (d) unequal potential

9. Select wrong statement.
The capacitance of a capacitor depends upon
(a) shape of plates
(b) size of plates
(c) charge on plates
(d) separation between plates

10. **Statement I** A capacitor can be given only a limited quantity of charge.
Statement II A capacitor is an arrangement which can store sufficient quantity of charge.
In the light of the above statements, choose the most appropriate answer from the options given below.
(a) Both Statement I and Statement II are incorrect.
(b) Statement I is correct but Statement II is incorrect.
(c) Statement I is incorrect but Statement II is correct.
(d) Both Statement I and Statement II are correct.

11. As shown in the figure, a very thin sheet of aluminium is placed in between the plates of the condenser. Then, the capacity will

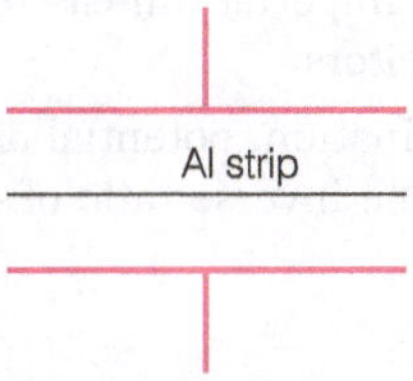

(a) increase
(b) decrease
(c) remains unchanged
(d) may increase or decrease

12. The capacity of parallel plate capacitor depends on
(a) the type of metal used
(b) the thickness of plates
(c) the potential applied across on the plates
(d) the separation between the plates

13. The capacitance of a parallel plate capacitor is 12 μF. If the distance between the plates is doubled and area is halved, then new capacitance will be
(a) 8 μF (b) 6 μF
(c) 4 μF (d) 3 μF

14. A parallel plate condenser has a capacitance 50 μF in air and 110 μF when immersed in an oil. The dielectric constant K of the oil is
(a) 0.45 (b) 0.55 (c) 1.10 (d) 2.20

15. **Statement I** Capacity of a parallel plate capacitor increases when distance between the plates is decreased.
Statement II Capacitance of capacitor is inversely proportional to distance between them.
In the light of the above statements, choose the most appropriate answer from the options given below
(a) Both Statement I and Statement II are incorrect.
(b) Statement I is correct but Statement II is incorrect.
(c) Statement I is the incorrect but Statement II is correct.
(d) Both Statement I and Statement II are correct.

16. There is an air filled 1 pF parallel plate capacitor. When the plate separation is doubled and the space is filled with wax, the capacitance increases to 2pF. The dielectric constant of wax is
(a) 2 (b) 4 (c) 6 (d) 8

17. **Statement I** If the distance between parallel plates of a capacitor is halved and dielectric constant is increase three times, then the capacitance becomes six times.
Statement II Capacitance of the capacitor does not depend upon the nature of the material of the plates.
In the light of the above statements, choose the most appropriate answer from the options given below.
(a) Both Statement I and Statement II are incorrect.
(b) Statement I is correct but Statement II is incorrect.
(c) Statement I is incorrect but Statement II is correct.
(d) Both Statement I and Statement II are correct.

18. A parallel plate capacitor with air between the plates has a capacitance of 9pF. The separation between its plates is d. The space between the plates is now filled with two dielectrics. One of the dielectrics has dielectric constant $K_1 = 3$ and thickness $d/3$ while the other one has dielectric constant $K_2 = 6$ and thickness $2d/3$. Capacitance of the capacitor is now
(a) 45 pF (b) 40.5 pF (c) 20.25 pF (d) 1.8 pF

19. Two parallel plate of area A are separated by two different dielectrics as shown in figure. The net capacitance is

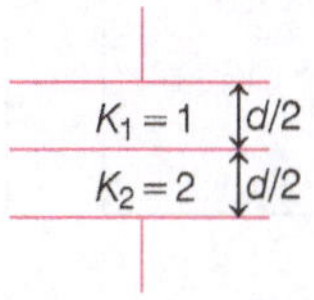

(a) $\frac{4\varepsilon_0 A}{3d}$ (b) $\frac{3\varepsilon_0 A}{R}$ (c) $\frac{2\varepsilon_0 A}{d}$ (d) $\frac{\varepsilon_0 A}{d}$

20. **Statement I** When air between the plates of a parallel plate condenser is replaced by an insulating medium of dielectric constant, its capacity decreases.
Statement II When dielectric material is inserted between the plates of parallel plate capacitor, then electric field intensity between the plates is reduced.

In the light of the above statements, choose the most appropriate answer from the options given below.
(a) Both Statement I and Statement II are incorrect.
(b) Statement I is correct but Statement II is incorrect.
(c) Statement I is incorrect but Statement II is correct.
(d) Both Statement I and Statement II are correct.

21. Select the incorrect pair.
(a) A parallel plate capacitor filled with metal — C become infinite
(b) A parallel circular plate capacitor — $C \propto R^2$
(c) A spherical capacitor — $C \propto R$
(d) A parallel plate capacitor filled with dielectric — C decreases

22. The potentials of the two plates of capacitor are +10 V and −10 V. The charge on one of the plates is 40 C. The capacitance of the capacitor is
(a) 2 F (b) 4 F (c) 0.5 F (d) 0.25 F

23. Two capacitors having equal charge and capacitances as C_1 and C_2 will have ratio of their potential as
(a) $C_1 : C_2$ (b) $C_2 : C_1$
(c) $C_1^2 : C_2^2$ (d) $C_2^2 : C_1^2$

24. A 500 μF capacitor is charged at a steady rate of 100 μC/s. The potential difference across the capacitor will be 10 V after an interval of
(a) 5 s (b) 25 s (c) 20 s (d) 50 s

Module 2

Combinations of Capacitors

• Capacitors in Series • Capacitors in Parallel

Capacitors in Series

In a series connection, charge on each capacitor remains same and equals to the main charge supplied by the battery but potential difference across each capacitor is different, such that $V = V_1 + V_2 + V_3$.

where, V_1, V_2, V_3 are the potential difference across capacitor C_1, C_2 and C_3, respectively.

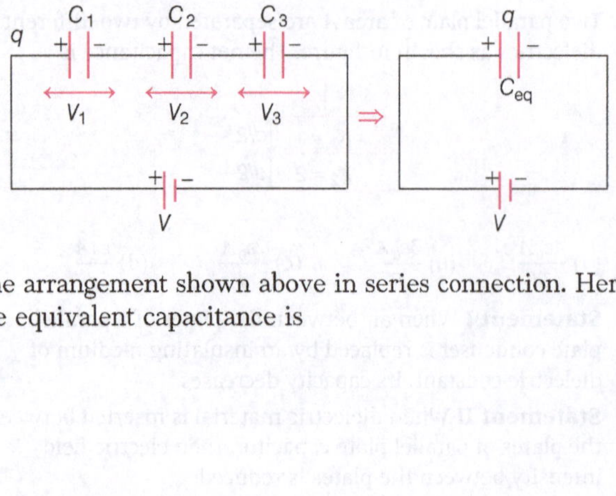

The arrangement shown above in series connection. Here, the equivalent capacitance is

$$\frac{1}{C_{eq}} = \frac{1}{C_1} + \frac{1}{C_2} + \frac{1}{C_3}$$

Following points are important in case of series combination of capacitors

(i) In series combination, potential difference distributes in the inverse ratio of capacitance, *i.e.*, $V \propto \frac{1}{C}$.

(ii) If two capacitors having capacitances C_1 and C_2 are connected in series, then $C = \frac{C_1 C_2}{C_1 + C_2}$

$$V_1 = \left(\frac{C_2}{C_1 + C_2}\right) V$$

and

$$V_2 = \left(\frac{C_1}{C_1 + C_2}\right) V$$

(iii) If n capacitors of equal capacity C are connected in series, with supply voltage V, then their equivalent capacitance is $\frac{C}{n}$ and potential difference across each capacitor is $V' = \frac{V}{n}$.

Mentor's TiP

If n identical plates are arranged as shown in figure, then they constitute $(n-1)$ capacitors in series. Each capacitor has capacitance $\frac{\varepsilon_0 A}{d}$

and $$C_{eq} = \frac{\varepsilon_0 A}{(n-1)\,d}$$

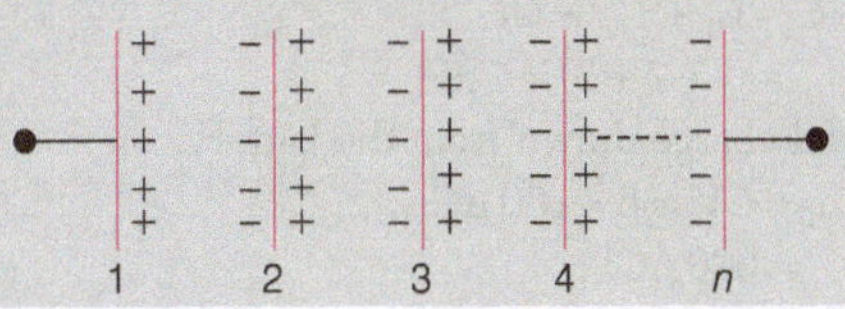

Example 11. *In the circuit shown in figure, find*

(i) the equivalent capacitance.

(ii) the charge stored in each capacitor and

(iii) the potential difference across each capacitor

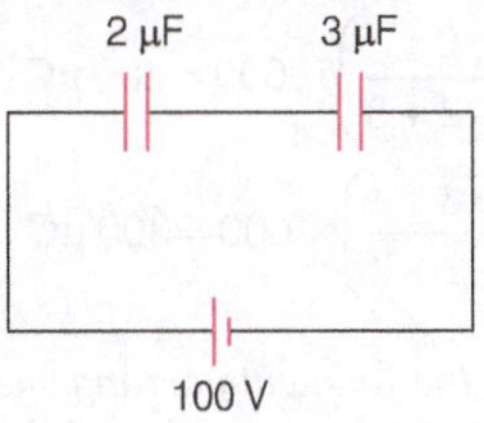

Sol. (i) The equivalent capacitance,

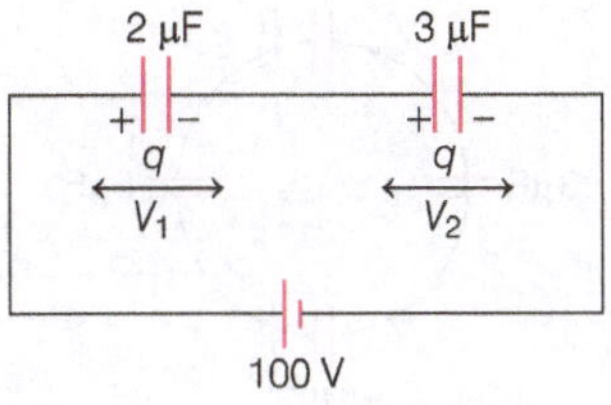

$$C = \frac{C_1 C_2}{C_1 + C_2}$$

or $$C = \frac{(2)(3)}{2+3} = 1.2\ \mu F$$

(ii) The charge, stored in each capacitor is

$$q = CV = (1.2 \times 10^{-6})(100)\ C = 120\ \mu C$$

(iii) In series combination, $V \propto \frac{1}{C}$

$$V_1 = \left(\frac{C_2}{C_1 + C_2}\right) V = \left(\frac{3}{2+3}\right)(100) = 60\ V$$

and $$V_2 = V - V_1 = 100 - 60 = 40\ V$$

Example 12. *Find the potential difference and charge on each capacitor.*

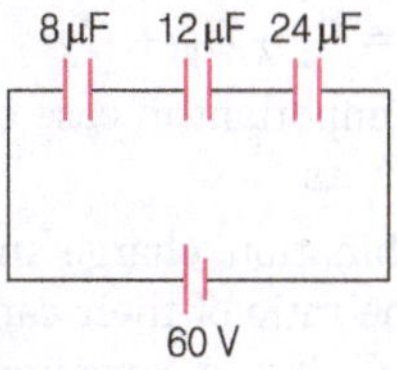

Sol.

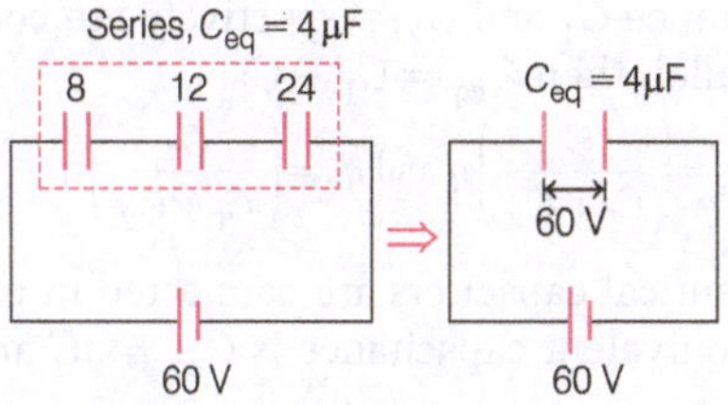

Charge on each capacitor,

$$C = C_{eq} V = 4 \times 60 = 240\ \mu C$$

Now, the individual potential can be shown as

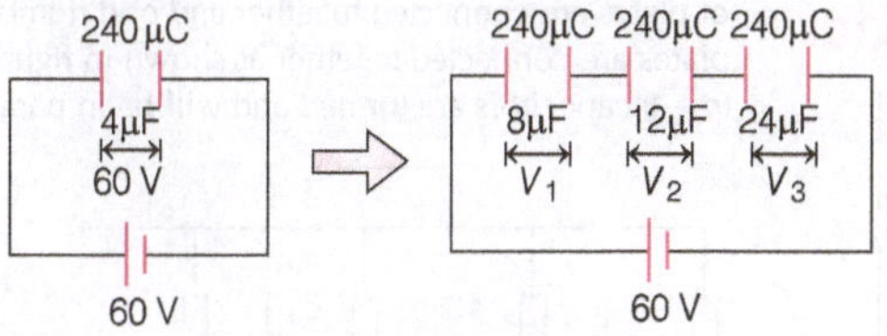

In series, charge on individual capacitors and equivalent capacitor is same and equal to 240 μC.

$$V_1 = \frac{240}{8} = 30\ V$$

$$V_2 = \frac{240}{12} = 20\ V$$

$$V_3 = \frac{240}{24} = 10\ V$$

Capacitors in Parallel

In a parallel connection, potential difference across each capacitor remains same and equal to be applied potential difference but charge gets distributed, *i.e.*, $q = q_1 + q_2 + q_3$ where, q_1, q_2 and q_3 are the charges across capacitor C_1, C_2 and C_3, respectively and q is the net charge flowing across the circuit.

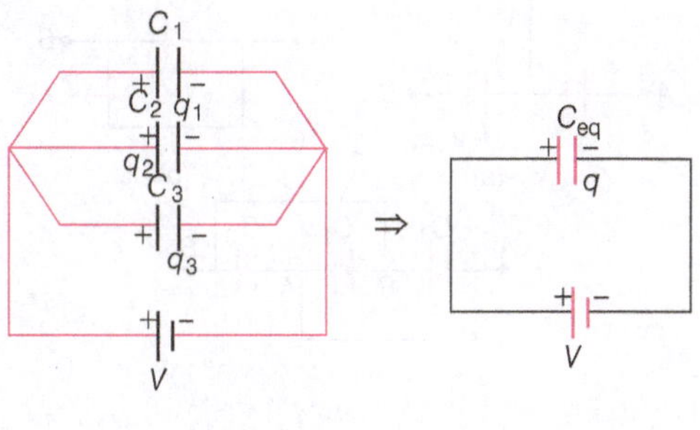

The arrangement shown in figure is called a parallel connection. Here, the equivalent capacitance is equal to

$$C_{eq} = C_1 + C_2 + C_3$$

Following points are important in case of parallel combination of capacitors

(i) In parallel combination, charge and energy distributes in the ratio of their capacitance, *i.e.*, $q \propto C$ and $U \propto C$. If two capacitors having capacitance C_1 and C_2, respectively are connected in parallel, then $C_{eq} = C_1 + C_2$

$$q_1 = \left(\frac{C_1}{C_1 + C_2}\right) q \text{ and } q_2 = \left(\frac{C_2}{C_1 + C_2}\right) q$$

(ii) If n identical capacitors are connected in parallel, then equivalent capacitance is $C_{eq} = nC$ and charge on each capacitor is $q' = \frac{q}{n}$.

Concept ladder

- If n identical plates are arranged such that even numbered of plates are connected together and odd number of plates are connected together as shown in figure, then $(n-1)$ capacitors are formed and will be in parallel.

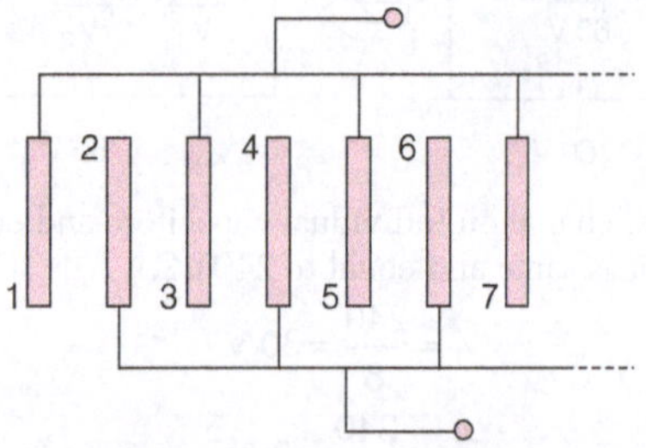

The capacitance of each capacitor in above combination is $\frac{\varepsilon_0 A}{d}$ and the equivalent capacitance, $C_{eq} = \frac{(n-1)\varepsilon_0 A}{d}$.

- If there are n identical capacitors, then $\frac{C_P}{C_S} = n^2$ where, C_P and C_S are the equivalent capacitances when n capacitors are connected in parallel and series, respectively.

Below are some of the examples of combination of capacitors arranged in parallel.

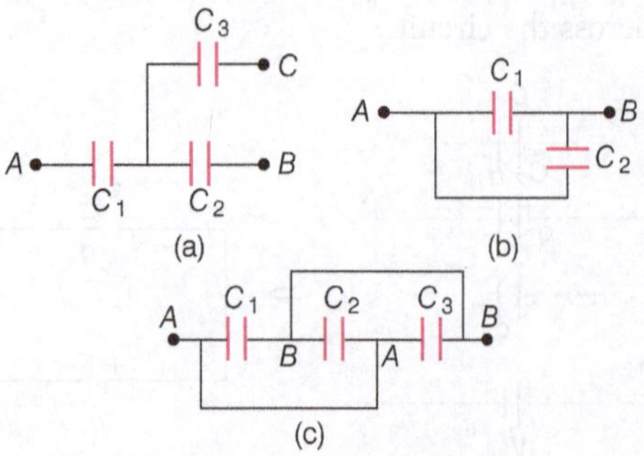

(a) (b) (c)

Example 13. *In the circuit shown in figure, find*
(i) the equivalent capacitance and
(ii) the charge stored in each capacitor.

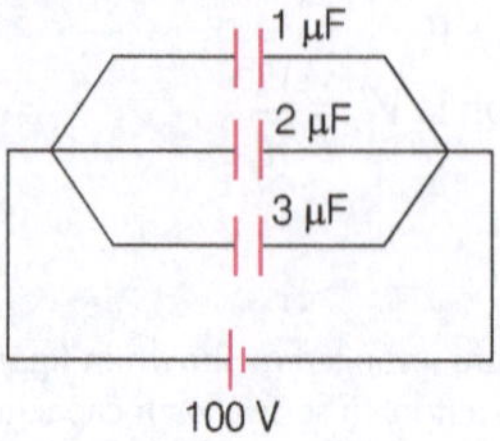

Sol. (i) The capacitors are in parallel, hence the equivalent capacitance,

$$C = C_1 + C_2 + C_3$$
$$= (1 + 2 + 3) = 6\ \mu F$$

(ii) Total charge drawn from the battery,

$$q = CV = 6 \times 100\ \mu C$$
$$= 600\ \mu C$$

This charge will be distributed in the ratio of their capacities, hence

$$q_1 : q_2 : q_3 = C_1 : C_2 : C_3 = 1 : 2 : 3$$

$$q_1 = \left(\frac{1}{1+2+3}\right) \times 600 = 100\ \mu C$$

$$q_2 = \left(\frac{2}{1+2+3}\right) \times 600 = 200\ \mu C$$

and $$q_3 = \left(\frac{3}{1+2+3}\right) \times 600 = 300\ \mu C$$

Example 14. *For the following arrangement, find the equivalent capacitance between A and B.*

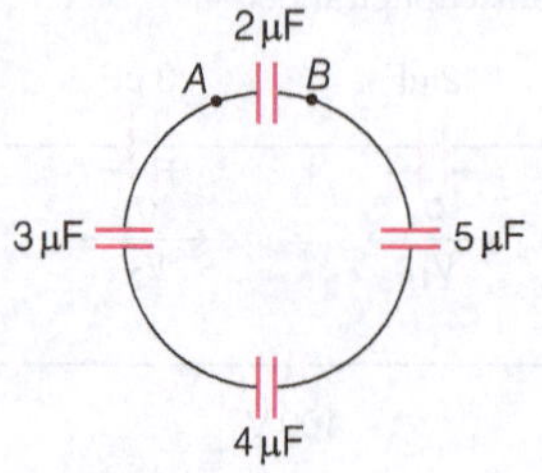

Sol. Here, the 3 μF, 4 μF and 5 μF capacitors are in series.

$$C_{eq} = \left(\frac{1}{3} + \frac{1}{4} + \frac{1}{5}\right) = \frac{60}{12 + 20 + 15} = \frac{60}{47}\ \mu F$$

Now, 2 μF and $\frac{60}{47}$ μF are in parallel, so we have

$$C_{eq} = C_1 + C_2 = \frac{154}{17}\ \mu F$$

Mentor's Tip

Series or parallel connectivity changes with change in points of measurement. Be careful in calculations.

Example 15. *Three capacitors connected in series and then parallel to each other gives equivalent capacitances of 0.5 μF and 5 μF respectively. If one of the capacitor is of 2 μF, find other two capacitances.*

Sol. Given, $\frac{1}{C_1}+\frac{1}{C_2}+\frac{1}{2}=2$

$$\Rightarrow \quad \frac{1}{C_1}+\frac{1}{C_2}=\frac{3}{2} \quad \text{...(i)}$$

and $\quad C_1+C_2+2=5$

$$\Rightarrow \quad C_1+C_2=3 \quad \text{...(ii)}$$

which gives $C_1=1\,\mu F$ and $C_2=2\,\mu F$

or $\quad C_1=2\,\mu F$ and $C_2=1\,\mu F$

NEET Close-up

Example Similar to PYQ Asked in NEET 2024, 23

Find equivalent capacitance of given circuit.

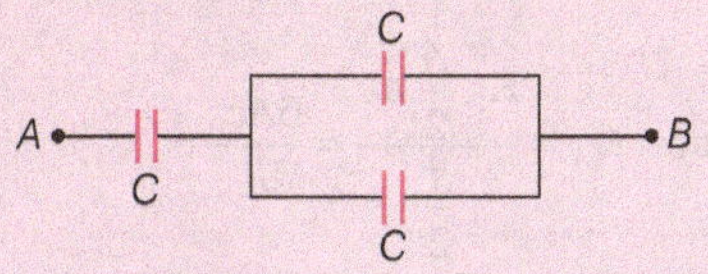

(a) $\frac{3}{2}C$ (b) $\frac{4}{3}C$ (c) $\frac{2}{3}C$ (d) $2C$

Sol. (c) Given, circuit is equivalent to

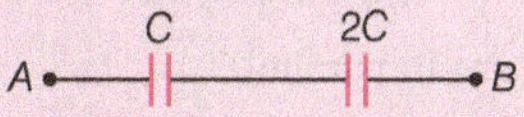

final equivalent capacitance,

$$C_{eq}=\frac{2C^2}{2C+C}=\frac{2}{3}C$$

Skill Builder

The equivalent capacitance of given circuit is

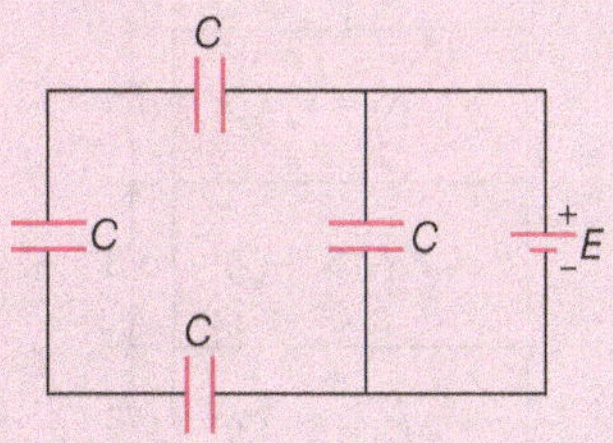

(a) C (b) $\frac{4C}{3}$ (c) $\frac{2C}{3}$ (d) $\frac{3C}{4}$

For more Practice Refer Q.No. 11, 12, 17 of step up practice 2 and Q.No. 17, 18 of Gearing up for NEET.

Example 16.

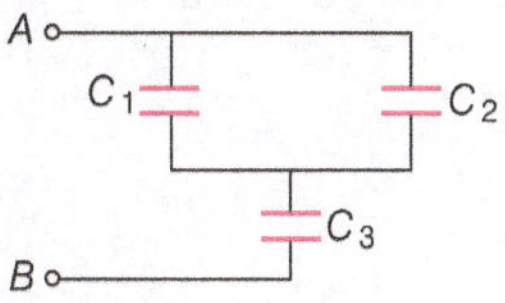

(a)

(i) Find the equivalent capacitance of the combination shown in the Fig. (a), when $C_1=2.0\,\mu F$, $C_2=4.0\,\mu F$ and $C_3=3.0\,\mu F$.

(ii) The input terminals A and B in Fig. (a) are connected to a battery of 12 V. Find the potential and the charge of each capacitor.

Sol. (i) C_1 and C_2 are in parallel, hence their equivalent capacitance is

Fig (b) shows the combination of C' and C_3 in series.

$$C'=C_1+C_2=2.0+4.0=6.0\,\mu F$$

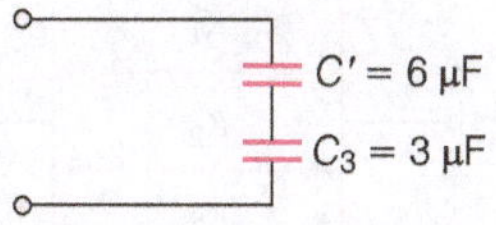

(b) C_1 and C_2 are replaced by C'

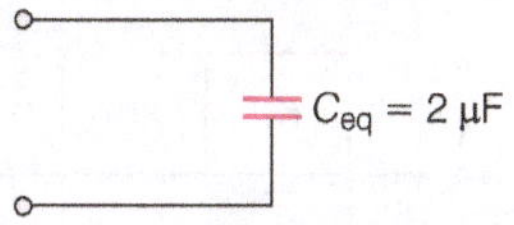

(c) C' and C_3 are replaced by C_{eq}

The final equivalent capacitance, shown in Fig. (c) is given by

$$\frac{1}{C_{eq}}=\frac{1}{C'}+\frac{1}{C_3}$$

$$=\frac{1}{6.0}+\frac{1}{3.0}=\frac{1}{2.0}$$

or $\quad C_{eq}=2.0\,\mu F$

(ii) To find the charge and potential difference, we retrace the path to the original in Fig. (a).

The charge supplied by the battery is $q=C_{eq}V$, when the inputs are joined to a V volt battery

$$=(2.0)(12.0)=24.0\,\mu C$$

The charge on each capacitor in series in Fig. (b),

$$q_3=q'=q=24.0\,\mu C$$

So, $\quad V_3=\frac{q_3}{C_3}=\frac{24.0\,\mu C}{3.0\,\mu F}=8\text{ V}$

Potential difference across C' in Fig. (b) is

$$V'=\frac{q'}{C'}=\frac{24.0\,\mu C}{6.0\,\mu C}=4V$$

The same potential difference V' appears across C_1 and C_2 in Fig. (a) and hence the charges on them are

$$q=C_1V_1$$
$$=(2.0\,\mu F)(4.0\text{ V})=8.0\,\mu C$$

and $\quad q_2=C_2V_2$
$$=(4.0\,\mu F)(4.0\text{ V})=16.0\,\mu C$$

Thus, we have $V_1=V_2=4.0\text{ V}, V_3=8\text{ V}$

and $\quad q_1=8.0\,\mu C, q_2=16.0\,\mu C, q_3=24.0\,\mu C$

Concept ladder

- Dielectrics filled inside the capacitor can be assumed as series/parallel combinations as follows

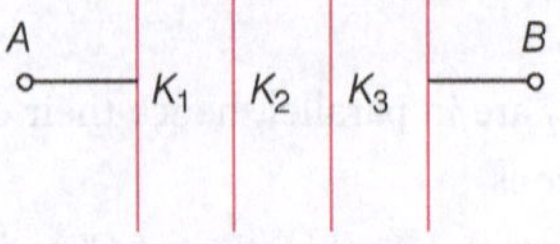

K_1, K_2 and K_3 are in series

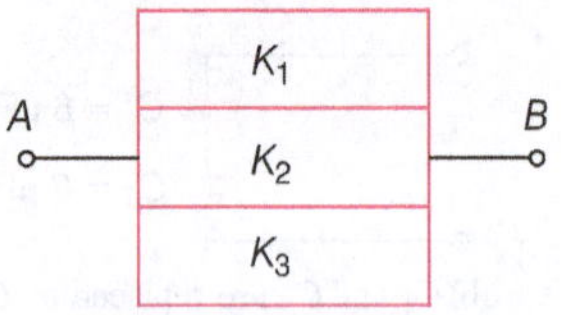

K_1, K_2 and K_3 are in parallel

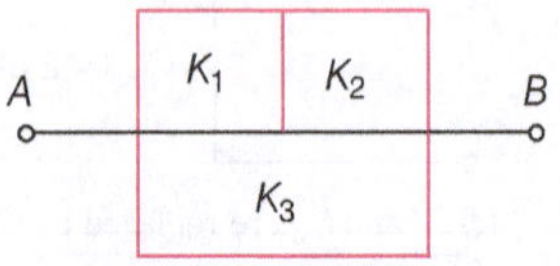

K_1, K_2 are in series and K_3 is parallel to K_1 and K_2

Example 17. *Find the equivalent capacitance between P and Q, there, A is area of each plate and d is separation between plates.*

(i)

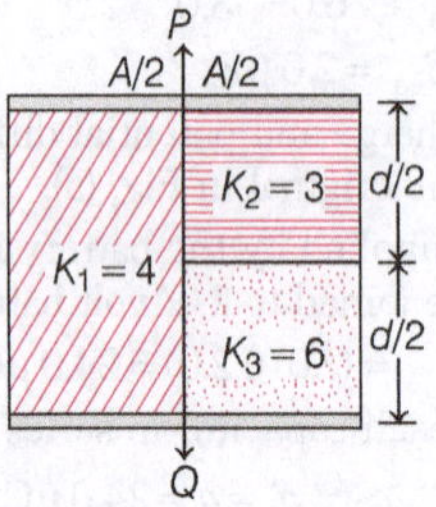

(ii)

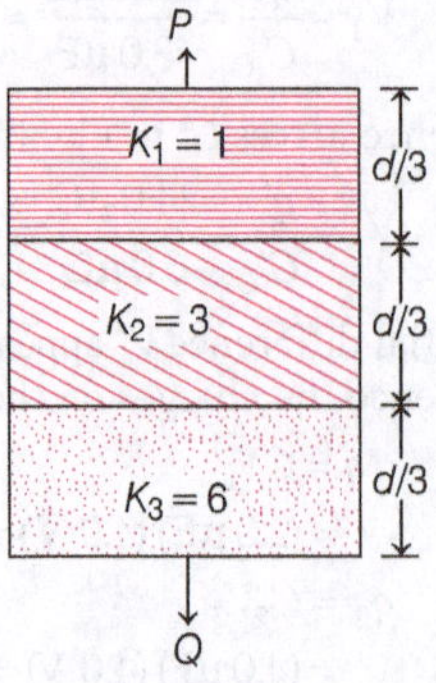

Sol. (i)

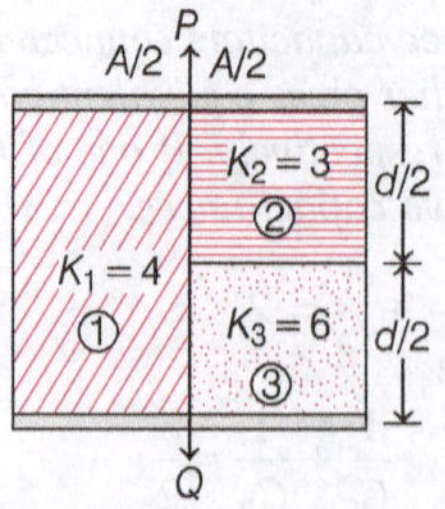

$$\text{Capacitance, } C_1 = \frac{K_1 \frac{A}{2} \varepsilon_0}{d} = \frac{4 \frac{A}{2} \varepsilon_0}{d} = \frac{2A\varepsilon_0}{d} \qquad \left(\because C = \frac{KA\varepsilon_0}{d}\right)$$

$$\text{Capacitance, } C_2 = \frac{K_2 \frac{A}{2} \varepsilon_0}{\frac{d}{2}} = \frac{3A\varepsilon_0}{d}$$

$$\text{Capacitance, } C_3 = \frac{K_3 \frac{A}{2} \varepsilon_0}{\frac{d}{2}} = \frac{6A\varepsilon_0}{d}$$

C_2 and C_3 are in series,

$$C' = \frac{C_2 C_3}{C_2 + C_3} = \frac{2A\varepsilon_0}{d}$$

and C' and C_1 are in parallel.

Hence, equivalent capacitance,

$$C_{eq} = C_1 + C' = \frac{2A\varepsilon_0}{d} + \frac{2A\varepsilon_0}{d} = \frac{4A\varepsilon_0}{d}$$

(ii) Capacitance, $C_1 = \dfrac{K_1 A\varepsilon_0}{d/3} = \dfrac{3A\varepsilon_0}{d}$

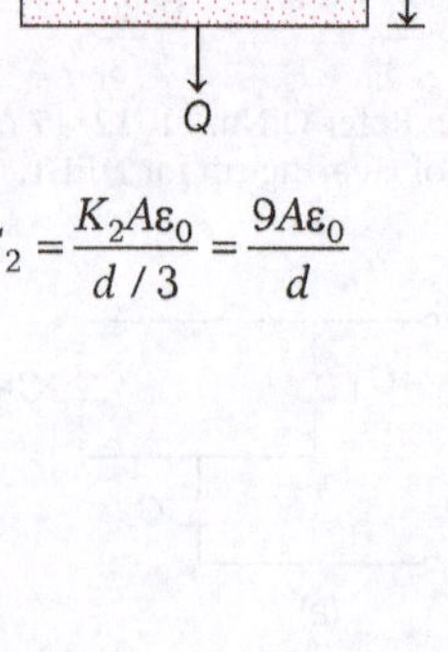

$$\text{Capacitance, } C_2 = \frac{K_2 A\varepsilon_0}{d/3} = \frac{9A\varepsilon_0}{d}$$

Capacitance, $C_3 = \dfrac{K_3 A\varepsilon_0}{d/3} = \dfrac{18A\varepsilon_0}{d}$

C_1, C_2 and C_3 are in series,

$$\frac{1}{C_{eq}} = \frac{1}{C_1} + \frac{1}{C_2} + \frac{1}{C_3}$$

Putting the values of C_1, C_2 and C_3, we get

Equivalent capacitance, $C_{eq} = \dfrac{2A\varepsilon_0}{d}$

Example 18. *Find the potential difference and charge on each capacitances. All capacitances are in μF.*

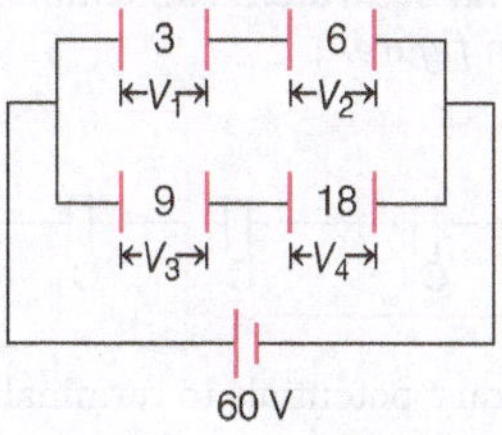

Sol. Here, two branches are in parallel. Potential difference across each branch is 60 V. There are two capacitors in series, use direct formulae as explained earlier.

$$V_1 = \left(\frac{6}{3+6}\right) \times 60 = 40\text{ V}$$

and $V_2 = 60 - V_1 = 20\text{ V}$

Similarly, $V_3 = \left(\dfrac{18}{9+18}\right) \times 60 = 40\text{ V}$

and $V_4 = 60 - V_3 = 20\text{ V}$

Charge on 3 μF capacitor, $q_1 = 3 \times 40 = 120\ \mu\text{C}$

Charge on 6 μF capacitor, $q_2 = 6 \times 20 = 120\ \mu\text{C}$

Charge on 9 μF capacitor, $q_3 = 9 \times 40 = 360\ \mu\text{C}$

and charge on 18 μF capacitor, $q_4 = 18 \times 20 = 360\ \mu\text{C}$

Example 19. *In the following figure, area of each plate is A and d is separation between adjacent plates. Find the capacitance of system between points A and B.*

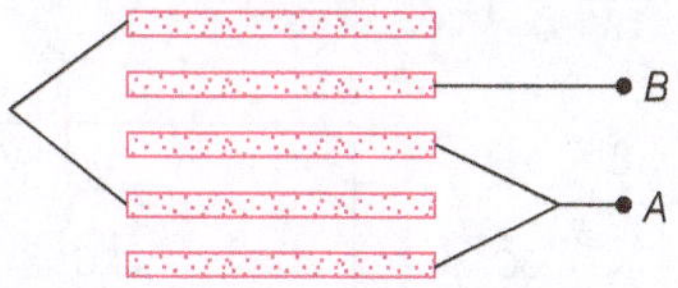

Sol. ∵ Area and distance are constant for each capacitor, so capacitance also remain constant. Let it is C.

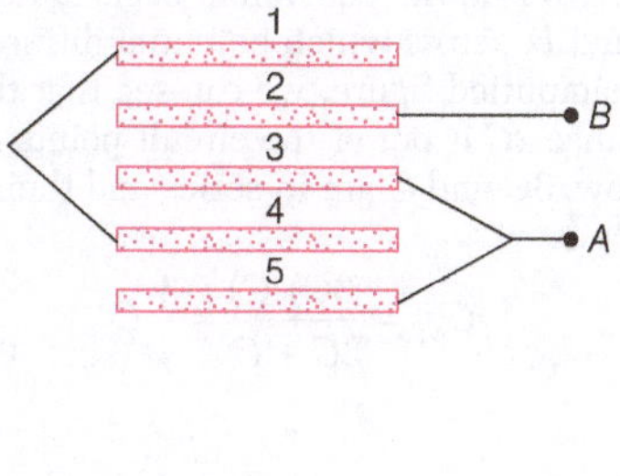

The equivalent circuit can be drawn as

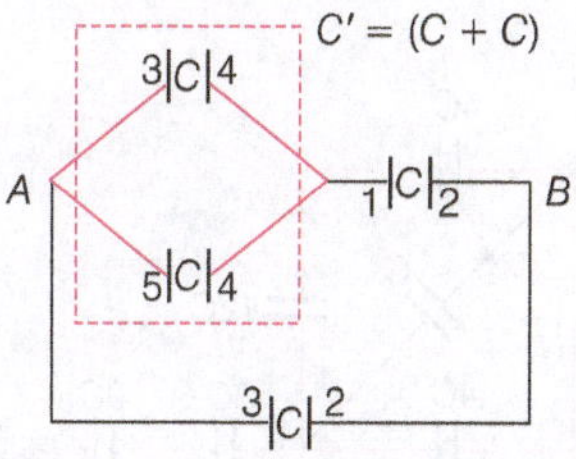

Hence, equivalent capacitance is

$$C_{AB} = \frac{(C+C)\times C}{(C+C)+C} + C = \frac{5C}{3}$$

Example 20. *Five identical capacitor plates each of area A are arranged, such that adjacent plates are at a distance d apart. The plates are connected to a source of emf V as shown below. What is the magnitude and nature of charge on plates 1 and 3, respectively?*

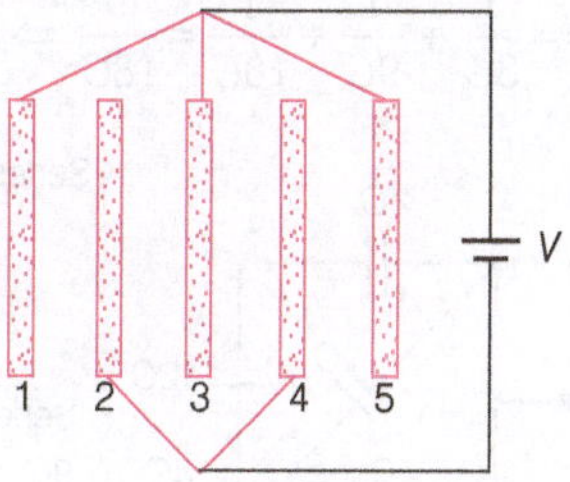

Sol.

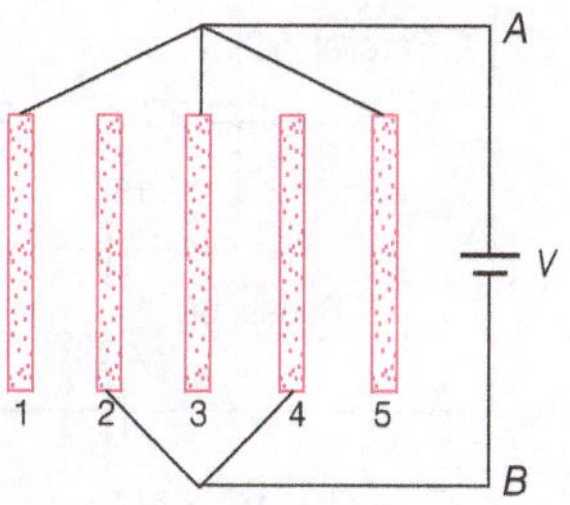

First, rearrange the plates,

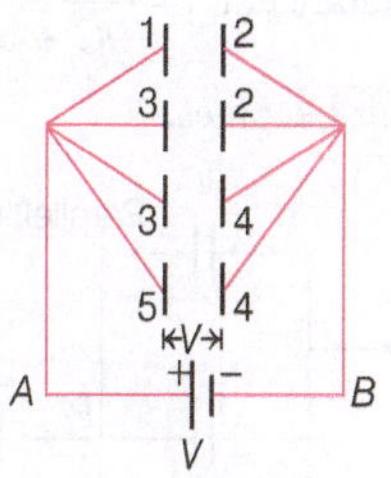

Charge on plate 1, $q = CV = \dfrac{A\varepsilon_0 V}{d}$

Charge on plate 3, $q' = CV + CV = 2CV$

$$= \frac{3A\varepsilon_0 V}{d}$$

Example 21. *Find the equivalent capacitance between A and B.*

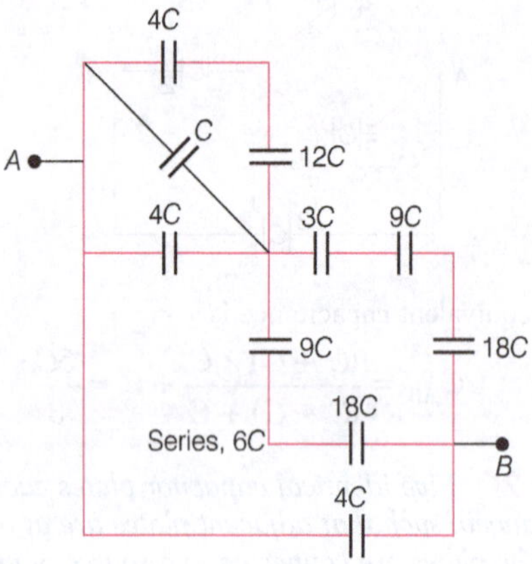

Sol. In series, capacitance, $C_1 = \dfrac{4C \times 12C}{4C + 12C} = 3C$

In series, $\dfrac{1}{C_2} = \dfrac{1}{3C} + \dfrac{1}{9C} + \dfrac{1}{18C} = \dfrac{9}{18C} \Rightarrow C_2 = 2C$

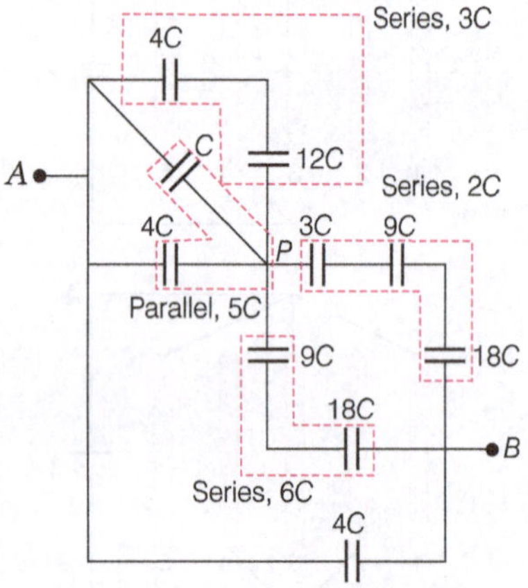

In parallel, $C_3 = C + 4C = 5C$

In series, capacitance, $C_4 = \dfrac{9C \times 18C}{9C + 18C} = 6C$

Now, the circuit becomes,

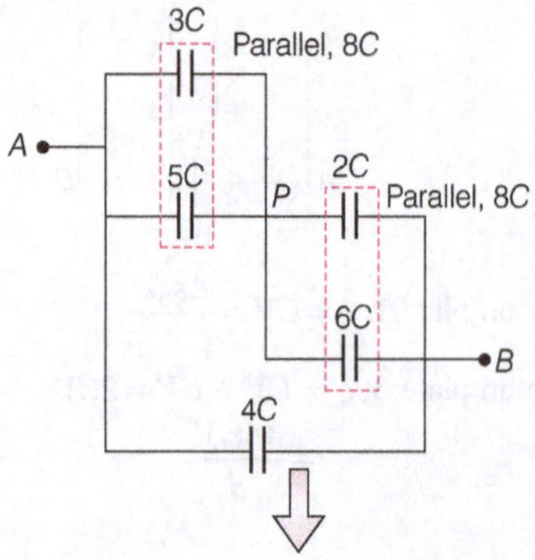

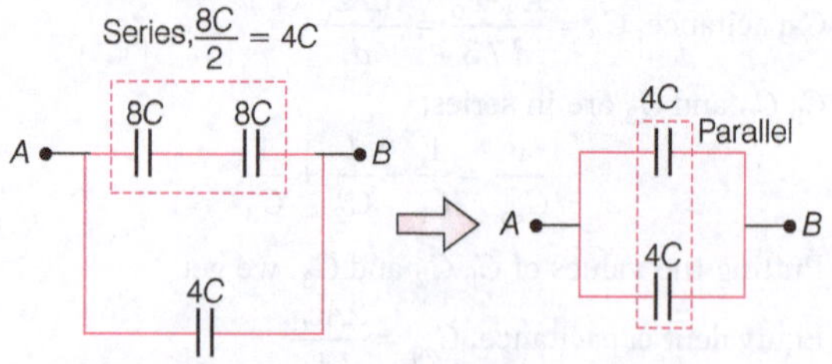

The equivalent capacitance between A and B,

$$C_{eq} = 4C + 4C = 8C$$

Example 22. *Find equivalent capacitance between points A and B shown in figure.*

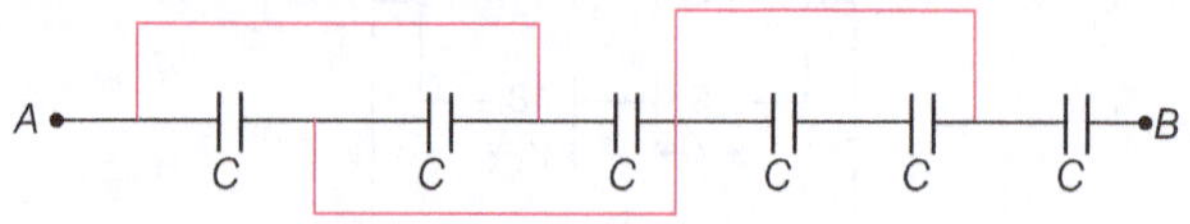

Sol. By giving arbitrary potentials to terminals, we get the following arrangement of potentials.

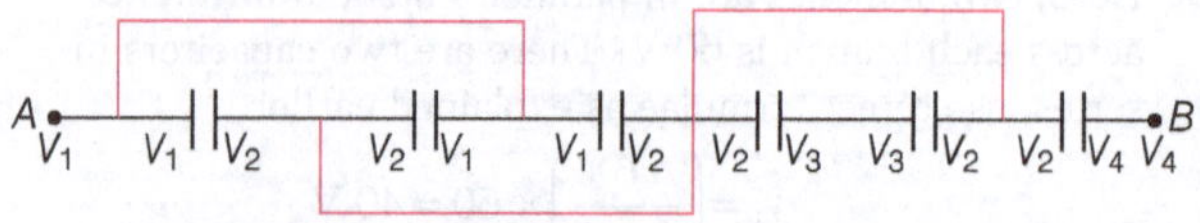

Three capacitors have potential difference $V_1 - V_2$, so they are in parallel. Their equivalent capacitance is $3C$. Two capacitors have potential difference $V_2 - V_3$, so their equivalent capacitance is $2C$ and lastly there is one capacitor across which potential difference is $V_2 - V_4$. So, let us make a table corresponding to this information.

Potential difference	Capacitance
$V_1 - V_2$	$3C$
$V_2 - V_3$	$2C$
$V_2 - V_4$	C

Now, corresponding to this table, we make a simple figure as shown in figure.

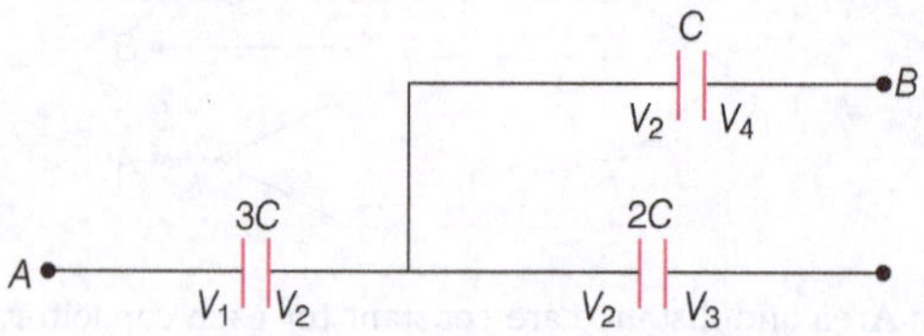

As we have to find the equivalent capacitance between points A and B, across which potential difference is $V_1 - V_4$. From the simplified figure, we can see that the capacitor of capacitance $2C$ is out of the circuit points A and B as shown. Now, $3C$ and C are in series and their equivalent capacitance is

$$C_{eq} = \frac{(3C)(C)}{3C + C} = \frac{3}{4}C$$

Mentor's Tip

The points connected with only conducting wires have same potentials.

Example 23. *Find equivalent capacitance between points A and B.*

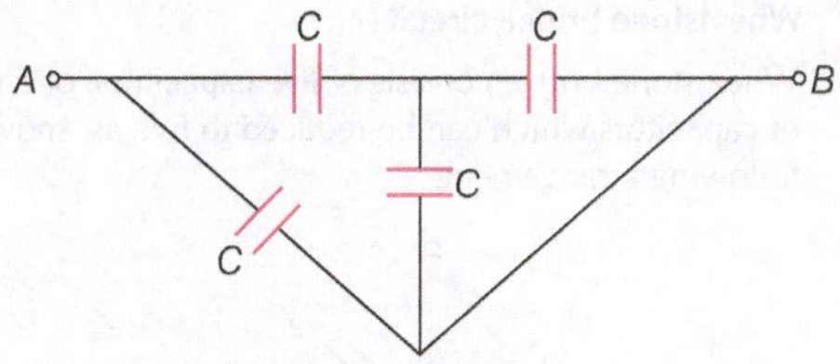

Sol. The circuit can be drawn as

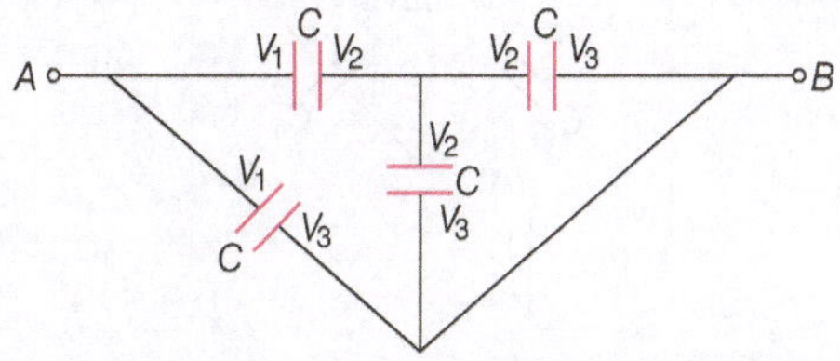

Two capacitors have potential difference $V_2 - V_3$, so their equivalent capacitance is $2C$. Let us make a corresponding table based on the potential each capacitor is having.

Potential difference	Capacitance
$V_1 - V_2$	C
$V_2 - V_3$	$2C$
$V_1 - V_3$	C

Now, corresponding to this table, we make a simple figure as shown below.

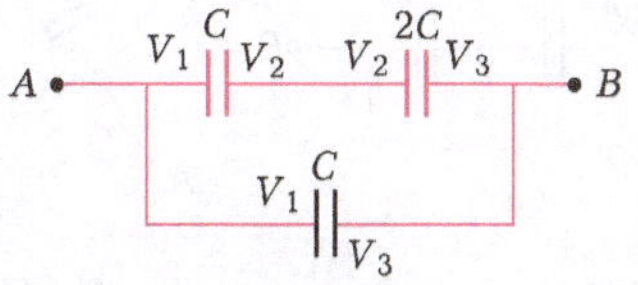

From the figure, we can see that, C and $2C$ are connected in series.

$$\therefore \quad C' = \frac{(C)(2C)}{C + 2C} = \frac{2}{3}C$$

This combination is connected in parallel with C, so net capacitance of the given circuit is

$$C_{\text{net}} = C + \frac{2}{3}C = \frac{5}{3}C$$

Example 24. *Find the equivalent capacitance between A and B.*

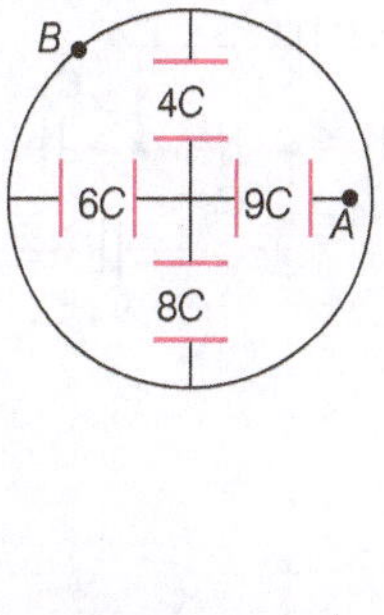

Sol. As, we have solved in above examples, we can solve here also using the same technique.

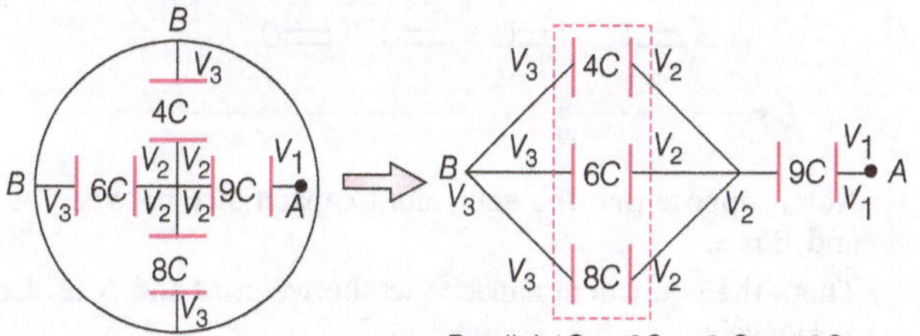

Parallel 4C + 6C + 8 C = 18C

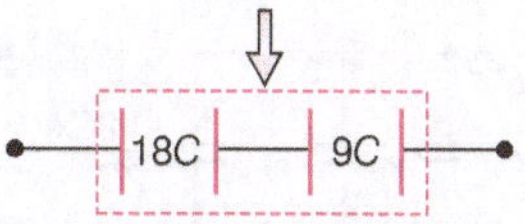

$$\text{Series capacitance} = \frac{9C \times 18C}{9C + 18C} = 6C \Rightarrow C_{eq} = 6C$$

Example 25. *Find equivalent capacitance of given circuit.*

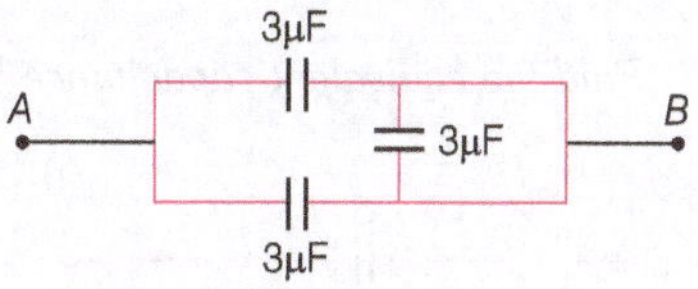

Sol.

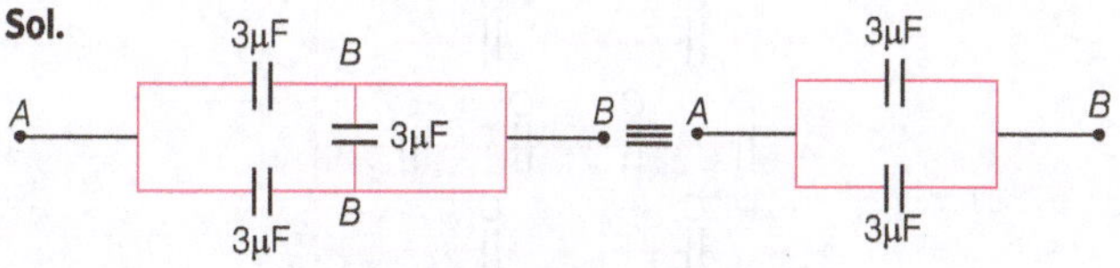

$$\because \quad C_{eq} = 3 + 3 = 6\,\mu F$$

Concept ladder

Infinite series problems

This consists of an infinite series of identical loops. To find C_{eq} of such a series network, first we consider by ourself a value (say x) C_{eq}.

Then, we break the chain in such a manner that only one loop is left with us and in place of the remaining portion we connect a capacitor x.

Then, we find the C_{eq} and put it equal to x. With this we get a quadratic equation in x. By solving this equation, we can find the desired value of x.

Example 26. *Find the equivalent capacitance of the infinite ladder shown in the figure btween the points A and B.*

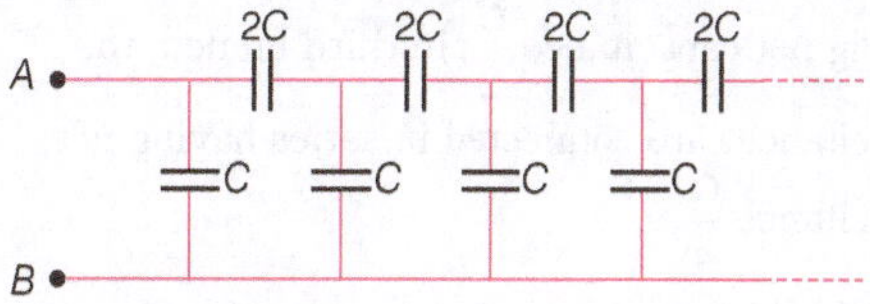

Sol. If we look at the infinite ladder between M and N, the arrangement obtained is exactly same as we have between A and B.

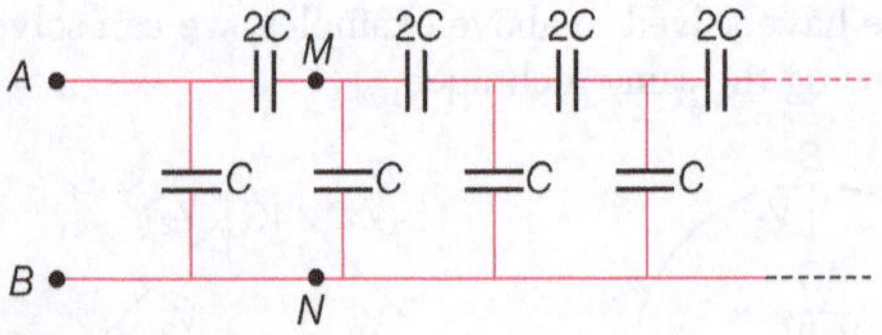

Now, suppose that the equivalent capacitance between A and B is x.

Then, the equivalent capacitance between M and N is also x. Hence,

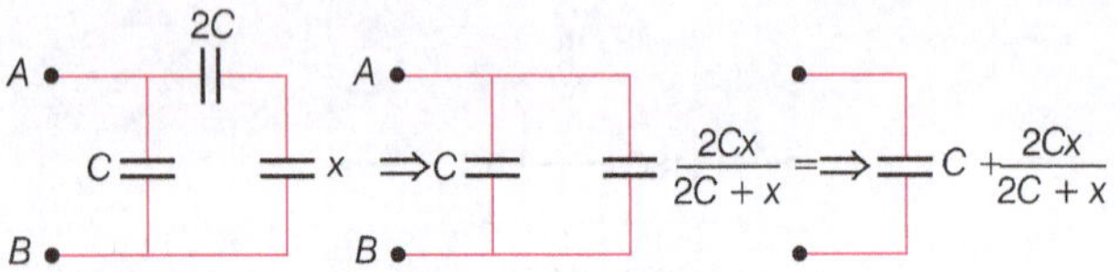

Thus, $x = C + \dfrac{2Cx}{2C + x} = \dfrac{2C^2 + 3Cx}{2C + x}$

or $x^2 - Cx - 2C^2 = 0$

Example 27. *Find the equivalent capacitance between A and B.*

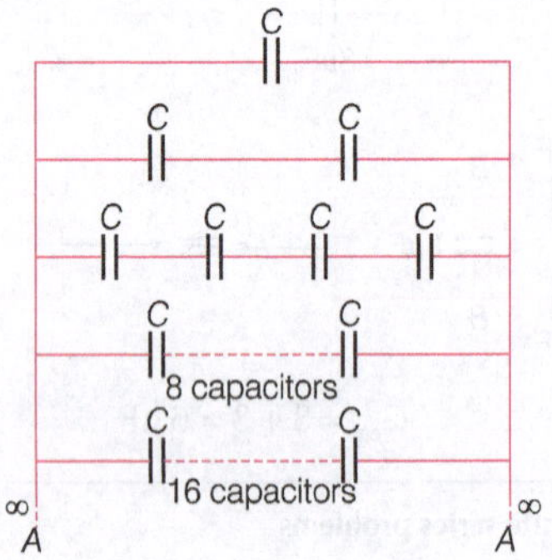

Sol.

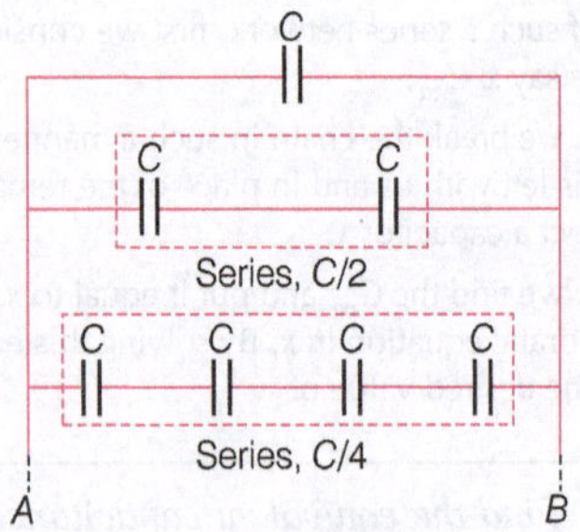

In second branch, the capacitances are connected in series having net capacitance $\dfrac{C}{2}$, in third branch, the capacitances are connected in series having net capacitance $\dfrac{C}{4}, \ldots$

$\therefore C, \dfrac{C}{2}, \dfrac{C}{4}, \ldots, \infty$ are in parallel, therefore

$$C_{eq} = C + \frac{C}{2} + \frac{C}{4} + \ldots \infty$$

$$= C\left(1 + \frac{1}{2} + \frac{1}{2^2} + \ldots \infty\right) = C\left(\frac{1}{1 - \frac{1}{2}}\right) = 2C$$

Concept ladder

Wheatstone bridge circuit

Wheatstone bridge consists of five capacitors, or a number of capacitors which can be reduced to five as, shown in the following arrangement,

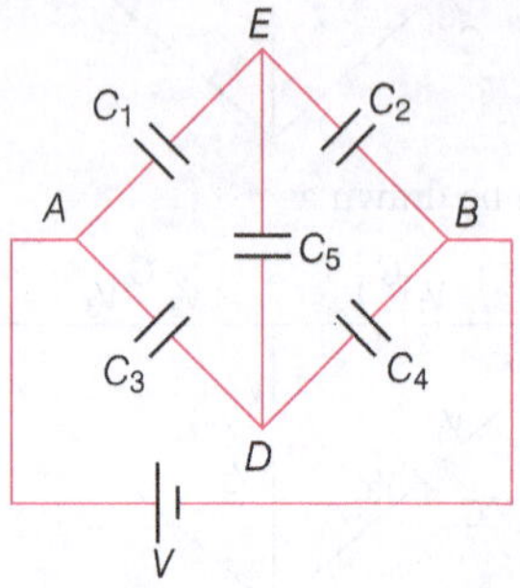

If $\dfrac{C_1}{C_2} = \dfrac{C_3}{C_4}$, bridge is said to be balanced and in that case

$$V_E = V_D \text{ or } V_E - V_D = 0 \text{ or } V_{ED} = 0$$

i.e. no change is stored in C_5. Hence, it can be removed from the circuit.

Some of the different forms of the Wheatstone bridge are given below.

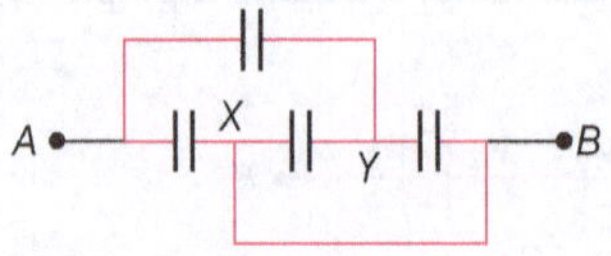

(a)

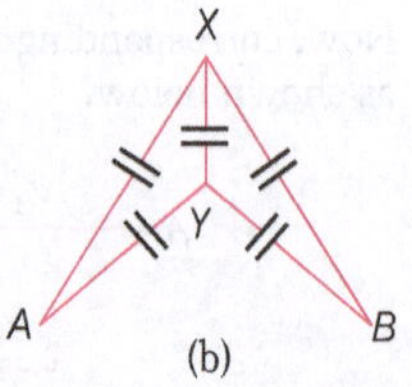

(b)

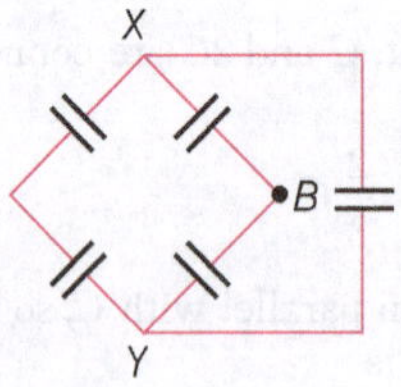

(c)

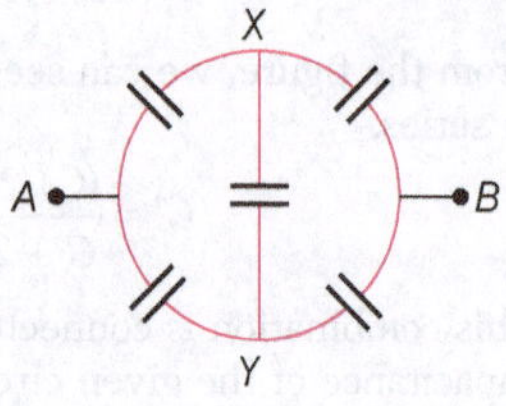

(d)

Example 28. *In the network of capacitors given below, find the effective capacitance between the points P and Q. (Take, $C_1 = C_2 = C_3 = C_4 = 4\,\mu F$)*

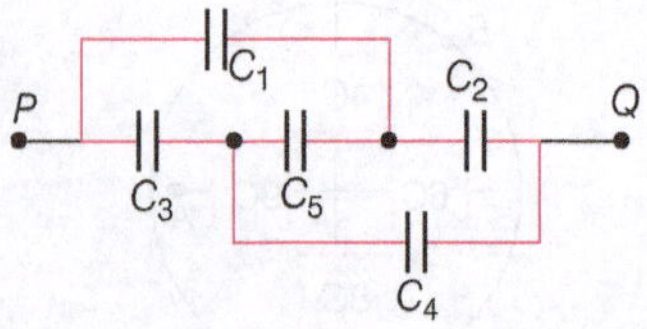

Sol. The given network consists of two closed capacitor circuits one containing C_1, C_3 and C_5, and the other containing C_2, C_4, C_5. Thus, C_5 is common in both. Hence, the network can be replaced as a Wheatstone bridge arrangement

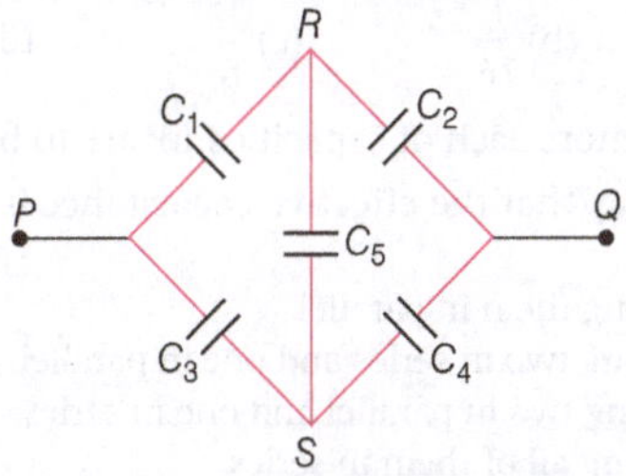

C_1 and C_2 are in series between the points P and Q. Similarly, C_3 and C_4 area also in series. Suppose the equivalent capacitance of C_1 and C_2 is C' and that of C_3 and C_4 is C''. Then, we have

$$C' = \frac{C_1C_2}{C_1 + C_2} = \frac{1 \times 4}{4+4} = 2\,\mu F$$

Similarly, $\quad C'' = 2\,\mu F$

Now, capacitors C' and C'' are in parallel between P and Q. Hence, the equivalent capacitance is given by

$$C = C' + C'' = 2 + 2 = 4\,\mu F$$

NEET Close-up

Example Similar to PYQ Asked in NEET 2021

A parallel-plate capacitor of area A, plate separation d and capacitance C is filled with three dielectric materials having dielectric constant K_1, K_2 and K_3 as shown in figure below. If a single dielectric material is to be used to have the same capacitance C in this capacitor, then its dielectric constant K will be

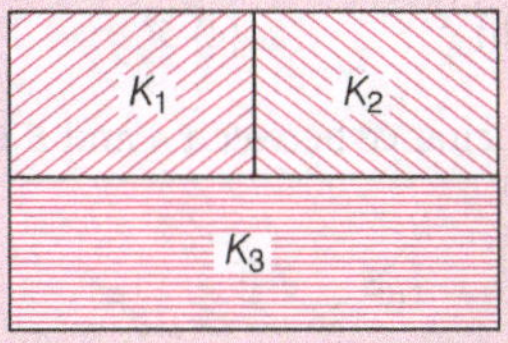

(a) $\dfrac{(K_1 + K_2)\, 2K_3}{K_1 + K_2 + 2K_3}$ (b) $\dfrac{(K_1 + K_2)K_3}{K_1 + K_2 + K_3}$

(c) $\dfrac{K_1K_3 + K_2K_3}{K_1K_2\, K_3}$ (d) $\dfrac{K_1K_2 + K_3}{(K_1 + K_2)\, K_3}$

Sol. (*a*) Here, $C_1 = \dfrac{\varepsilon_0 K_1 A}{d}$, $C_2 = \dfrac{\varepsilon_0 K_2 A}{d}$, $C_3 = \dfrac{2\varepsilon_0 K_3 A}{d}$

Given, system of C_1, C_2 and C_3 can be simplified as

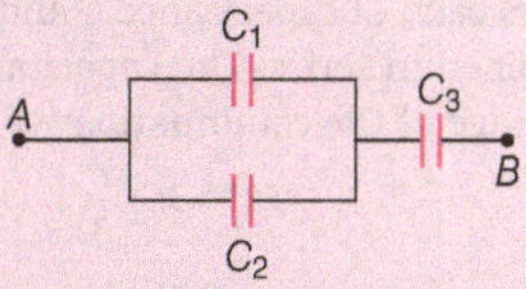

$$\therefore \quad \frac{1}{C_{AB}} = \frac{1}{C_1 + C_2} + \frac{1}{C_3}$$

Suppose, $\quad C_{AB} = \dfrac{K\varepsilon_0 A}{d}$

$$\frac{1}{K\left(\frac{\varepsilon_0 A}{d}\right)} = \frac{1}{\frac{\varepsilon_0 A}{d}(K_1 + K_2)} + \frac{1}{\frac{2\varepsilon_0 A}{d}K_3}$$

$$\Rightarrow \quad \frac{1}{K} = \frac{1}{K_1 + K_2} + \frac{1}{2K_3}$$

$$\therefore \quad K = \frac{(K_1 + K_2)\, 2K_3}{K_1 + K_2 + 2K_3}$$

Skill Builder

A parallel-plate capacitor of area A, plate separation d and capacitance C is filled with four dielectric materials having dielectric constant K_1, K_2, K_3 and K_4 as shown in figure below. If a single dielectric material is to be used to have the same capacitance C in this capacitor, then its dielectric constant K will be

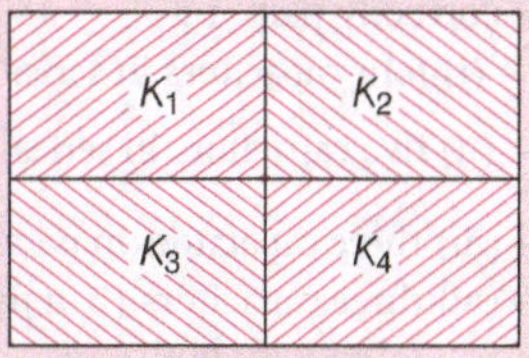

(a) $K = \dfrac{(K_1 + K_2)(K_3 + K_4)}{K_1 + K_2 + K_3 + K_4}$ (b) $K = \dfrac{K_1K_2K_3K_4}{K_1 + K_2 + K_3 + K_4}$

(c) $K = \dfrac{K_1/K_2 + K_3/K_4}{(K_1 + K_2)(K_3 + K_4)}$ (d) $K = \dfrac{K_1 + K_2 + K_3 + K_4}{(K_1K_2)(K_3K_4)}$

For more Practice Refer Q.No. 36, 37, 41 of Gearing up for NEET.

STEP UP Practice 2

1. Three capacitors each of capacitance C and of breakdown voltage V are joined in series. The capacitance and breakdown voltage of the combination will be
(a) $\frac{C}{3}, \frac{V}{3}$
(b) $3C, \frac{V}{3}$
(c) $\frac{C}{3}, 3V$
(d) $3C, 3V$

2. Three condensers each of capacitance 2 F are put in series. The resultant capacitance is
(a) 6 F
(b) $\frac{3}{2}$ F
(c) $\frac{2}{3}$ F
(d) 5 F

3. **Assertion** (A) Two condensers of same capacity are connected first in parallel and then in series. The ratio of resultant capacitance in the two cases will be 4 : 1.
Reason (R) In parallel capacitance increases and in series capacitance decreases.
In the light of the above statements, choose the correct answer from the options given below.
(a) Both A and R are true but R is not the correct explanation of A.
(b) A is true but R is false.
(c) A is false but R is true.
(d) Both A and R are true and R is the correct explanation of A.

4. By using n-different capacitors of 2 μF each. Which of the following is not correctly paired ?
(a) $C_{eq} = 10\,\mu F \rightarrow$ (i) four capacitors in series
(b) $C_{eq} = \frac{2}{5}\,\mu F \rightarrow$ (ii) five capacitors in series
(c) $C_{eq} = 6\,\mu F \rightarrow$ (iii) three capacitors in parallel
(d) $C_{eq} = 3\,\mu F \rightarrow$ (iv) three capacitors (2 in parallel and third in series with both)

5. Two capacitors of capacitance 2 μF and 3 μF are joined in series. Outer plate of first capacitor is at 1000 V and outer plate of second capacitor is earthed (grounded). Now, the potential on inner plate of each capacitor will be
(a) 700 V
(b) 200 V
(c) 600 V
(d) 400 V

6. A series combination of three capacitors of capacities 1 μF, 2 μF and 8 μF is connected to a battery of emf 13 V. The potential difference across the plates of 2 μF capacitor will be
(a) 1 V
(b) 8 V
(c) 4 V
(d) $\frac{13}{3}$ V

7. Four capacitors of equal capacitance have an equivalent capacitance C_1 when connected in series and an equivalent capacitance C_2 when connected in parallel. The ratio $\frac{C_1}{C_2}$ is
(a) $\frac{1}{4}$
(b) $\frac{1}{16}$
(c) $\frac{1}{8}$
(d) $\frac{1}{12}$

8. Three capacitors each of capacity 4 μF are to be connected in such a way that the effective capacitance is 6 μF. This can be done by
(a) connecting them in parallel
(b) connecting two in series and one in parallel
(c) connecting two in parallel and one in series
(d) connecting all of them in series

9. **Assertion** (A) In series combination, charges in two capacitors are always equal.
Reason (R) If charges are same, the total potential difference applied across two capacitors will be distributed in inverse ratio of capacities.
In the light of the above statements, choose the correct answer from the options given below.
(a) Both A and R are true but R is not the correct explanation of A.
(b) A is true but R is false.
(c) A is false but R is true.
(d) Both A and R are true and R is the correct explanation of A.

10. In the figure shown, the effective capacitance between the points A and B, if each has capacitance C, is

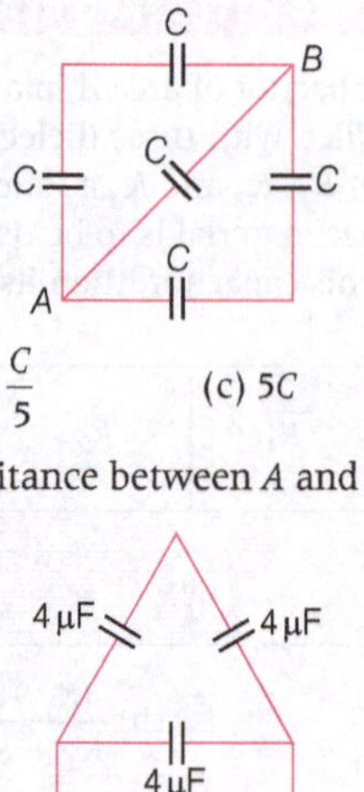

(a) $2C$
(b) $\frac{C}{5}$
(c) $5C$
(d) $\frac{C}{2}$

11. Equivalent capacitance between A and B is

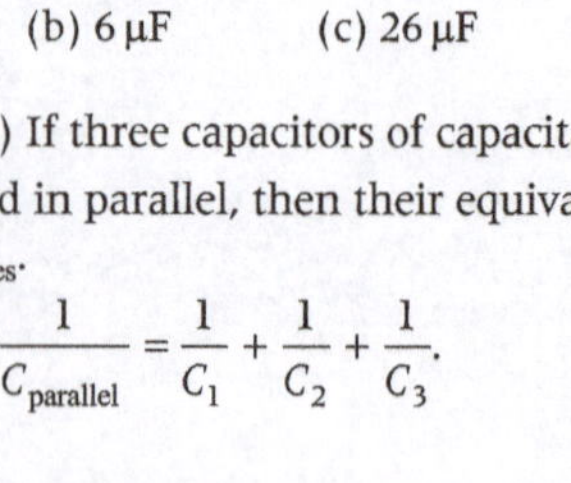

(a) 8 μF
(b) 6 μF
(c) 26 μF
(d) $\frac{10}{3}$ μF

12. **Assertion** (A) If three capacitors of capacitance $C_1 < C_2 < C_3$, are connected in parallel, then their equivalent capacitance $C_{parallel} > C_{series}$.
Reason (R) $\frac{1}{C_{parallel}} = \frac{1}{C_1} + \frac{1}{C_2} + \frac{1}{C_3}$.

In the light of the above statements, choose the correct answer from the options given below.

(a) Both A and R are true but R is not the correct explanation of A.

(b) A is true but R is false.

(c) A is false but R is true.

(d) Both A and R are true and R is the correct explanation of A.

13. If $C_2 = 10\,\mu F$ and rest all capacitors are of $3\,\mu F$, then the equivalent capacitance between X and Y

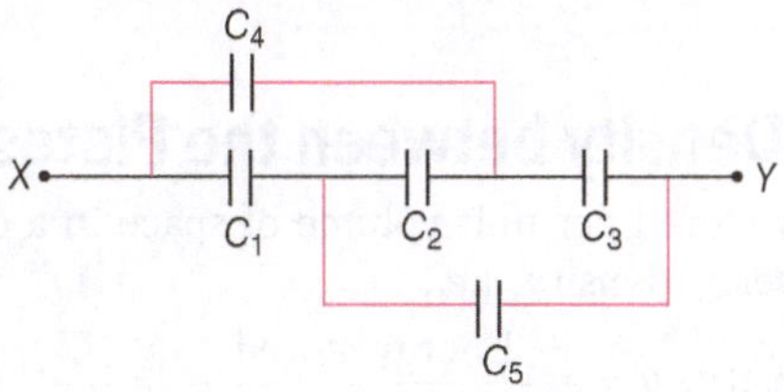

(a) $6\,\mu F$ (b) $2\,\mu F$
(c) $3\,\mu F$ (d) $10\,\mu F$

14. Assertion (A) In a parallel combination of capacitors, the total capacitance of the combination is the sum of capacitance of the individual capacitors.

Reason (R) In such a combination, voltage across each capacitor is same.

In the light of the above statements, choose the correct answer from the options given below.

(a) Both A and R are true but R is not the correct explanation of A.

(b) A is true but R is false.

(c) A is false but R is true.

(d) Both A and R are true and R is the correct explanation of A.

15. Find incorrect statement.

(a) Equivalent capacitance in parallel combination is larger than the largest capacitor of combination.

(b) Charge remains conserved in series combination of capacitors.

(c) Capacitance of a parallel plate capacitor decreases with increment in separation between the plates.

(d) Equivalent capacitance in series combination is larger than the capacitor of least value of capacitance.

16. In the circuit as shown in the figure, the effective capacitance between A and B is

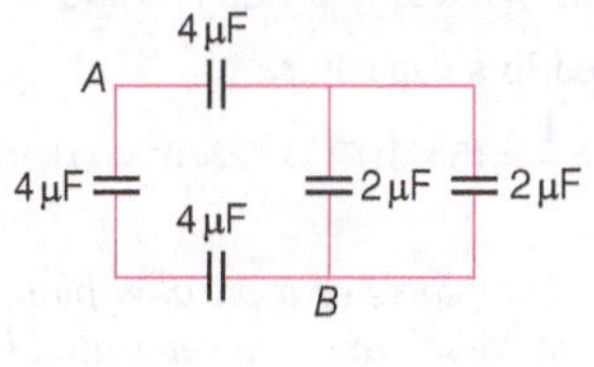

(a) $3\,\mu F$ (b) $2\,\mu F$
(c) $4\,\mu F$ (d) $8\,\mu F$

17. The charge on anyone of the $2\,\mu F$ capacitors and $1\,\mu F$ capacitor will be given respectively (in μC) as

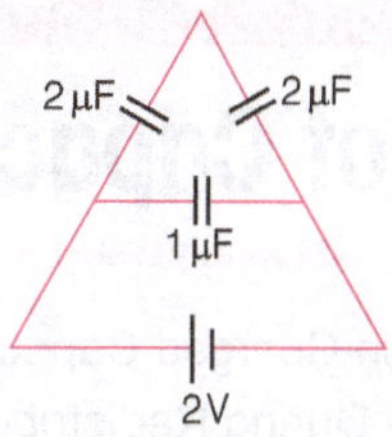

(a) 1, 2 (b) 2, 1 (c) 1, 1 (d) 2, 2

18. Equivalent capacitance between X and Y is

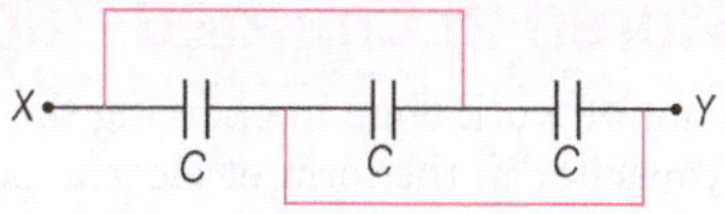

(a) $\frac{3}{2}C$ (b) $3C$

(c) $\frac{C}{3}$ (d) $\frac{2}{3}C$

19. Which of the following pair is not correctly paired ?

(a) 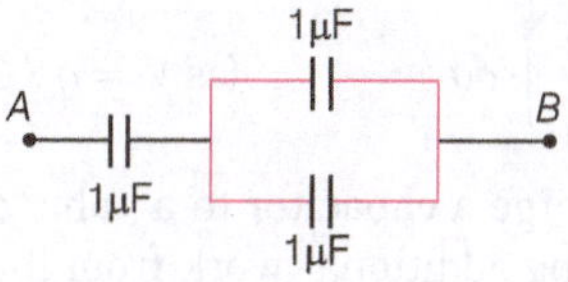

→ $C_{eq} = \frac{2}{3}\mu F$

(b) 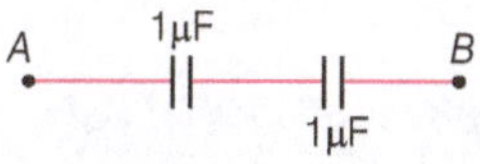

→ $C_{eq} = \frac{1}{2}\mu F$

(c) 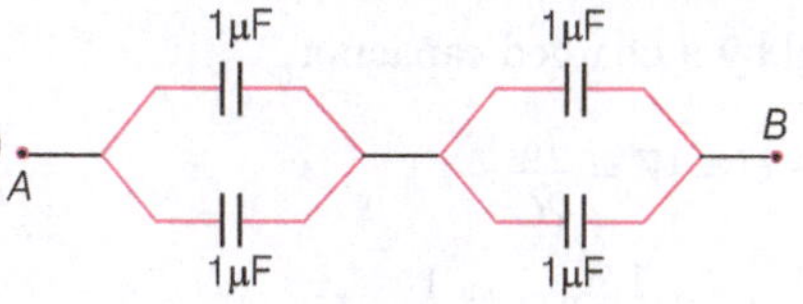

→ $C_{eq} = \mu F$

(d) 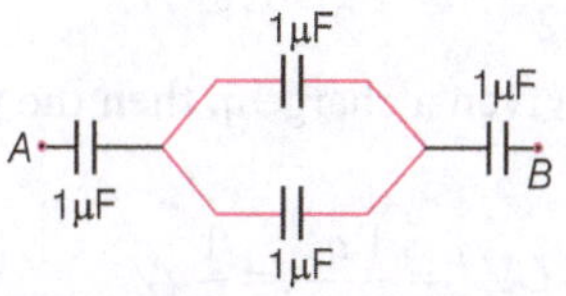

→ $C_{eq} = 3\mu F$

20. Assertion (A) Charge on all the condensers connected in series is the same.

Reason (R) Capacitance of capacitor is directly proportional to charge on it.

In the light of the above statements, choose the correct answer from the options given below.

(a) Both A and R are true but R is not the correct explanation of A.

(b) A is true but R is false.

(c) A is false but R is true.

(d) Both A and R are true and R is the correct explanation of A.

Module 3

Energy of Capacitors

- Energy Stored in Charged Capacitor • Common Potential (Redistribution of Charge)
- Loss of Energy During Redistribution of Charge

Energy Stored in Charged Capacitor

The total amount of work done in charging the capacitor is stored in the capacitor in the form of electric potential energy. Suppose, at time t, a charge q is present on the capacitor and V is the potential of the capacitor. If dq is the amount of charge that is brought against the forces of the field done to the charge already present on the capacitor, the additional work needed will be

$$dW = (dq)\,V = \left(\frac{q}{C}\right)\cdot dq \qquad (\text{as } V = q/C)$$

$\therefore$ Total work done to charge a capacitor to a value q_0, can be obtained by integrating additional work from limits 0 to q_0, we get

$$W = \frac{q_0^2}{2C}$$

$\therefore$ Energy stored by a charged capacitor,

$$U = W = \frac{q_0^2}{2C}$$

$$= \frac{1}{2}CV_0^2 = \frac{1}{2}q_0V_0$$

Thus, if a capacitor is given a charge q, then the potential energy stored in it is,

$$U = \frac{1}{2}CV^2 = \frac{1}{2}\frac{q^2}{C} = \frac{1}{2}qV$$

The above relation shows that the charged capacitor is the electrical analog of a stretched spring whose elastic potential energy is $\frac{1}{2}kx^2$. The charge q is analogous to the elongation x and the reciprocal of capacitance, *i.e.* $\frac{1}{C}$ to the force constant k.

Total energy stored in series combination or parallel combination of capacitors is equal to the sum of the energies stored in individual capacitors, *i.e.*,

$$U = U_1 + U_2 + U_3 + \ldots$$

Energy Density between the Plates

The energy stored per unit volume of space in a capacitor is called energy density, *i.e.*,

$$\text{Energy density, } u = \frac{\text{Energy stored}}{\text{Volume of capacitor}} = \frac{U}{Ad} \qquad \ldots\text{(i)}$$

Energy on either plate of capacitor is $Q = \sigma A = \varepsilon_0 EA$

Energy stored in the capacitor is

$$U = \frac{Q^2}{2C} = \frac{(\varepsilon_0 EA)^2}{2\varepsilon_0 A/d} = \frac{1}{2}\varepsilon_0 E^2\cdot Ad \qquad \ldots\text{(ii)}$$

By using Eqs. (i) and (ii), we get

$$u = \frac{1}{2}\varepsilon_0 E^2$$

Concept ladder

Change in energy on introducing a dielectric slab.

- When a dielectric slab is inserted between the plates of a charged capacitor, with battery connected to its plates. Then, the capacitance and energy stored in the capacitor becomes K (dielectric constant) times.
- When a dielectric slab is inserted between the plates of a charged capacitor and battery is disconnected. Then, the charge on this plates remains unchanged and energy stored in the capacitor becomes $\frac{U_0}{K}$, i.e., energy decreases.

Example 29. *Calculate energy stored in a capacitor of 5 μF when it is charged to a potential of 250 V?*

Sol. Given, $C = 5\,\mu\text{F} = 5\times10^{-6}$ F and $V = 250$ V

Energy stored in a capacitor,

$$U = \frac{1}{2}CV^2 = \frac{1}{2}\times(5\times10^{-6})\times(250)^2 = 0.156\text{ J}$$

Example 30. *The plates of a parallel plate capacitor have an area of 90 cm² each and are separated by 2.5 mm. The capacitor is charged to 400 V. How much electrostatic energy is stored in it? Find the value of electrostatic energy when it is filled with a dielectric medium $K = 3$ and, then charged If it is first charged as an air capacitor and, then filled with the dielectric.*

Sol. Capacitance of the parallel plate capacitor,

$$C_0 = \frac{\varepsilon_0 A}{d}$$

$$= \frac{8.85 \times 10^{-12} \times 90 \times 10^{-4}}{2.5 \times 10^{-3}}$$

$$= 3.19 \times 10^{-11}\ \text{F}$$

The energy stored in the air-capacitor,

$$U_0 = \frac{1}{2} C_0 V_0^2$$

$$= \frac{1}{2} \times (3.19 \times 10^{-11}) \times (400)^2$$

$$= 2.55 \times 10^{-6}\ \text{J}$$

The capacitance of the dielectric filled capacitor is

$$C = KC_0$$

$$\text{Energy, } U = \frac{1}{2} CV_0^2 = \frac{1}{2} KC_0 V_0^2$$

$$= KU_0 = 3 \times (2.55 \times 10^{-6})$$

$$= 7.65 \times 10^{-6}\ \text{J}$$

If the capacitor is first charged and, then filled with the dielectric, then the charge remains constant but the potential difference between the plates decreases. The potential difference is $V = \frac{V_0}{K}$.

The new energy of capacitor,

$$U = \frac{1}{2} CV^2 = \frac{1}{2} (KC_0)(V_0 / K)^2$$

$$= \frac{1}{K}\left(\frac{1}{2} C_0 V_0^2\right) = \frac{U_0}{K}$$

$$= \frac{2.55 \times 10^{-6}\ \text{J}}{3} = 8.5 \times 10^{-7}\ \text{J}$$

Example 31. *Two capacitors of capacitances $C_1 = 2\ \mu F$ and $C_2 = 8\ \mu F$ are connected in series and the resulting combination is connected across 300 V. Calculate the charge, potential difference and energy stored in the capacitors separately.*

Sol. If C is the equivalent capacitance, then

$$\frac{1}{C} = \frac{1}{C_1} + \frac{1}{C_2} = \frac{1}{2} + \frac{1}{8} = \frac{5}{8}$$

$$\therefore \quad C = \frac{8}{5} = 1.6\ \mu\text{F}$$

$$\text{Charge, } q = CV = 1.6 \times 10^{-6} \times 300$$

$$= 4.8 \times 10^{-4}\ \text{C}$$

Potential across capacitance,

$$C_1 = V_1 = \frac{q}{C_1} = 240\ \text{V}$$

Potential across capacitance,

$$C_2 = V_2 = \frac{q}{C_2} = 60\ \text{V}$$

Energy stored in capacitance C_1 is

$$U_1 = \frac{1}{2} C_1 V_1^2$$

$$= \frac{1}{2} \times 2 \times 10^{-6} \times (240)^2$$

$$= 5.76 \times 10^{-2}\ \text{J}$$

Energy stored in capacitance C_2 is

$$U_2 = \frac{1}{2} C_2 V_2^2$$

$$= \frac{1}{2} \times 8 \times 10^{-6} \times (60)^2$$

$$= 1.44 \times 10^{-2}\ \text{J}$$

Concept ladder

- When we store energy in a capacitor by connecting a battery with it, 50% of energy provided by battery gets wasted in form of heat.
- zattery's utilised energy = QV
- Capacitor's stored energy = $\frac{1}{2} QV$

Common Potential (Redistribution of Charge)

When two charged conductors or capacitors are joined together by a conducting wire and having different potentials, then charge flows from capacitor at higher potential to the capacitor at lower potential. This flow of charge continues till their potential becomes equal, this equal potential is called common potential.

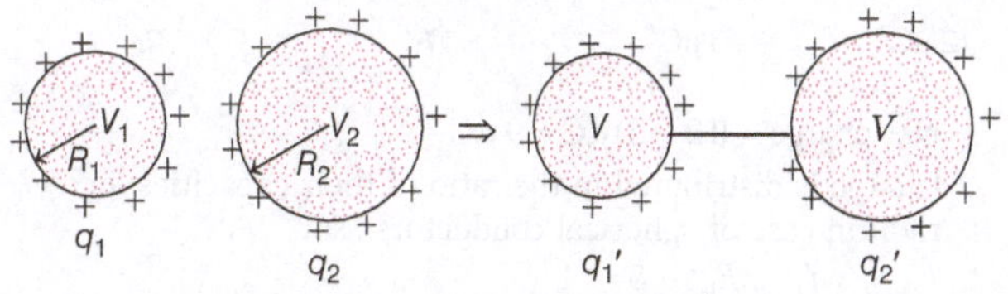

Suppose two conductors of capacities C_1 and C_2 have charges q_1 and q_2 respectively and raised to potential V_1 and V_2 respectively are joined together by a conducting wire, then charge redistributes in these conductors in the ratio of their capacities. Charge redistributes till potential of both the conductors becomes equal. Thus, let q'_1 and q'_2 be the final charges on them, then

$$q_1' = C_1 V \text{ and } q_2' = C_2 V$$

or

$$\frac{q_1'}{q_2'} = \frac{C_1}{C_2}$$

and if they are spherical conductors, then $\frac{C_1}{C_2} = \frac{R_1}{R_2}$

$$\therefore \quad \frac{q_1'}{q_2'} = \frac{C_1}{C_2} = \frac{R_1}{R_2}$$

where, R_1 and R_2 are radius of capacitors.
Since, the total charge is $(q_1 + q_2)$. Therefore,

$$q'_1 = \left(\frac{C_1}{C_1 + C_2}\right)(q_1 + q_2)$$

and $$q'_2 = \left(\frac{C_2}{C_1 + C_2}\right)(q_1 + q_2)$$

Common potential,

$$V = \frac{\text{Total charge}}{\text{Total capacity}}$$

$$V = \frac{q_1 + q_2}{C_1 + C_2} = \frac{C_1V_1 + C_2V_2}{C_1 + C_2}$$

Mentor's TIP

If the two capacitors are connected in such a way that negative plate of one capacitor is connected to positive plate of another capacitor, then their common potential is

$$V = \frac{C_1V_1 - C_2V_2}{C_1 + C_2}$$

Example 32. *Two isolated spherical conductors have radii 5 cm and 10 cm, respectively. They have charges of 12 μC and −3 μC. Find the charge after they are connected by a conducting wire. Also, find the common potential after redistribution.*

Sol.

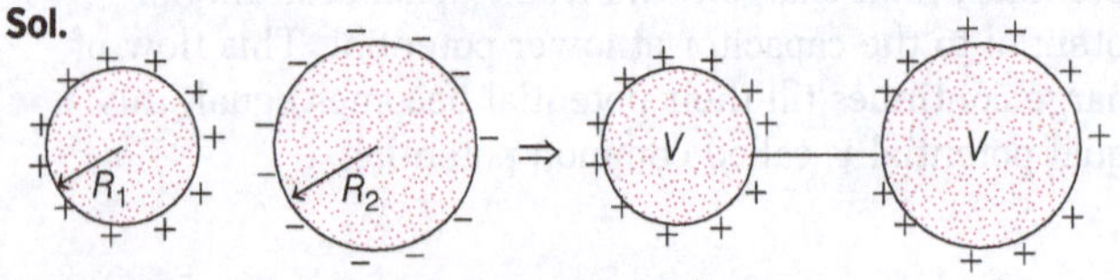

Net charge = (12 − 3) μC = 9 μC

Charge is distributed in the ratio of their capacities (or radii in case of spherical conductors), so

$$\frac{q'_1}{q'_2} = \frac{R_1}{R_2} = \frac{5}{10} = \frac{1}{2}$$

$$q'_1 = \left(\frac{1}{1+2}\right)(9) = 3\ \mu C$$

and $$q'_2 = \left(\frac{2}{1+2}\right)(9) = 6\ \mu C$$

Common potential,

$$V = \frac{q_1 + q_2}{C_1 + C_2} = \frac{(9 \times 10^{-6})}{4\pi\varepsilon_0(R_1 + R_2)}$$

$$= \frac{(9 \times 10^{-6})(9 \times 10^9)}{(15 \times 10^{-2})}$$

$$= 5.4 \times 10^5\ V$$

Example 33. *Two parallel plates capacitors A and B having capacitance of 1 μF and 5 μF are charged separately to the some potential of 100 V. Now, the positive plate of A is connected to the negative plate of B and the negative plate of A to the positive plate of B. Find the final charges on each capacitor.*

Sol. As, for a capacitor, $q = CV$, so, initially the charge on each capacitor,

$$q_1 = C_1V_1 = (1 \times 10^{-6}) \times 100 = 100\ \mu C$$

and $$q_2 = C_2V_2 = (5 \times 10^{-6}) \times 100 = 500\ \mu C$$

Now, when two capacitors are joined to each other such that positive plate of one is connected with the negative of the other, by conservation of charge

$$q = q_1 + q_2$$

$$\Rightarrow \quad |q| = |q_1 - q_2|$$

$$= (500 - 100)\ \mu C = 400\ \mu C$$

So, common potential,

$$V = \frac{(q_1 + q_2)}{(C_1 + C_2)}$$

$$= \frac{400 \times 10^{-6}}{(1+5) \times 10^{-6}} = \frac{200}{3}\ V$$

and, hence after sharing, charge on each capacitor

$$q'_1 = C_1V$$

$$= (1 \times 10^{-6}) \times \frac{200}{3} = \frac{200}{3}\ \mu C$$

$$q'_2 = C_2V$$

$$= (5 \times 10^{-6}) \times \frac{200}{3} = \frac{1000}{3}\ \mu C$$

Example 34. *A capacitor of capacitance 5 μF is charged to potential 20 V and, then isolated. Now, an uncharged capacitor is connected in parallel to it. If the charge distributes equally on these capacitors, find total energy stored in capacitors.*

Sol. Let C be unknown capacitance,

$$Q'_1 = Q'_2 \Rightarrow C_1V\ CV$$

$$5V = CV \Rightarrow C = 5\ \mu F$$

Common potential, $$V = \frac{C_1V_1 + C_2V_2}{C_1 + C_2}$$

$$= \frac{5 \times 20 + 5 \times 0}{5 + 5} = 10\ V$$

Total energy stored in capacitors,

$$U_f = \frac{1}{2}(C_1 + C_2)V^2$$

$$= \frac{1}{2}(5 + 5)(10)^2 \times 10^{-6}\ J$$

$$= 500 \times 10^{-6}$$

$$= 500\ \mu J$$

NEET Close-up

Example Similar to PYQ Asked in NEET 2016

A capacitor of 3 μF is charged as shown in the figure. When the switch S is turned to position b, the percentage of its stored energy dissipated is

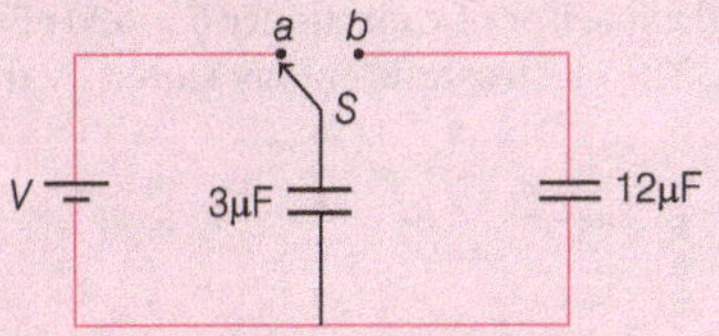

(a) 90% (b) 60%
(c) 80% (d) 50%

Sol. (c) From the given figure,

When the switch S is connected to point a, then initial energy stored in the capacitor can be given as

$$U = \frac{1}{2}(3\,\mu\text{F}) \times V^2$$

When the S is connected to point b, energy dissipated on connection across 8 μF will be

$$\Delta U = \frac{1}{2}\left(\frac{C_1 C_2}{C_1 + C_2}\right) \cdot V^2$$

$$= \frac{1}{2}\left(\frac{3 \times 12}{15}\right) V^2 = \frac{1}{2}\left(\frac{36}{15}\right) V^2 = \left(\frac{18}{15}\,\mu\text{F}\right) V^2$$

Therefore, loss of energy,

$$\frac{\Delta U}{U} \times 100\% = \frac{36}{45} \times 100 = 80\%$$

Skill Builder

A capacitor of $2C$ is charged as show in the figure. When the switch S is turned to position b, the percentage of its stored energy dissipated is

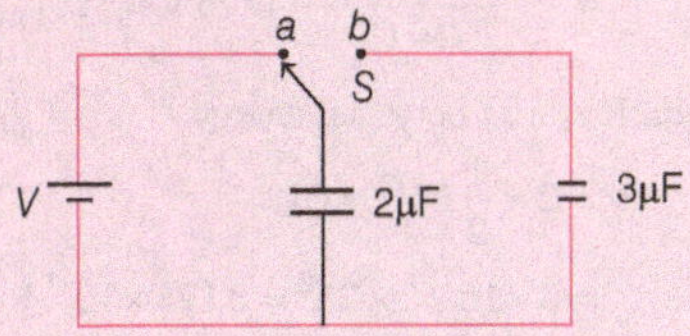

(a) 50% (b) 60%
(c) 80% (d) 75%

For more Practice Refer Q.No. 97 of Gearing up for NEET.

Example 35. *A capacitor C is charged with battery V. Then, it is disconnected from battery and connected with another capacitor of capacitance C and potential difference $2V$. Find electrostatic energy stored by the system.*

Sol. Common potential after connection

$$V_C = \frac{C_1 V_1 + C_2 V_2}{C_1 + C_2} = \frac{CV + 2CV}{2C}$$

$$\Rightarrow \quad V_C = \frac{3}{2} V$$

So, energy of system

$$U = \frac{1}{2} C_1 V^2 + \frac{1}{2} C_2 V^2 = \frac{1}{2}(C_1 + C_2) V^2$$

$$= \frac{1}{2} \times 2C \times \frac{9}{4} V^2 = \frac{9}{4} CV^2$$

Loss of Energy During Redistribution of Charge

The initial charge on the capacitor C_1 is q and after joining it becomes q'. The transferred charge from the capacitor C_1 to the capacitor C_2 is $q - q'$.

Now, $$q - q' = C_1 V_1 - C_1 V$$

$$= C_1\left(V_1 - \frac{C_1 V_1 + C_2 V_2}{C_1 + C_2}\right)$$

$$q - q' = \frac{C_1 C_2 (V_1 - V_2)}{C_1 + C_2}$$

This is the quantity of the transferred charge.

The loss of energy due to redistribution of charge is given by

$$\Delta U = \frac{C_1 C_2}{2(C_1 + C_2)}(V_1 - V_2)^2$$

Now, as C_1, C_2 and $(V_1 - V_2)^2$ are always positive. $U_i > U_f$, *i.e.*, there is a decrease in energy. Hence, energy is always lost in redistribution of charge. Further,

$$\Delta U = 0, \text{ if } V_1 = V_2$$

This is because no flow of charge takes place when both the conductors are at same potential.

Example 36. *A capacitor A of capacitance 4 μF is charged to 30 V and another capacitor B of capacitance 2 μF is charged to 15 V. Now, the positive plate of A is connected to the negative plate of B and negative plate of A to the positive plate of B. Find the final charge of each capacitor and loss of electrostatic energy in the process.*

Sol.

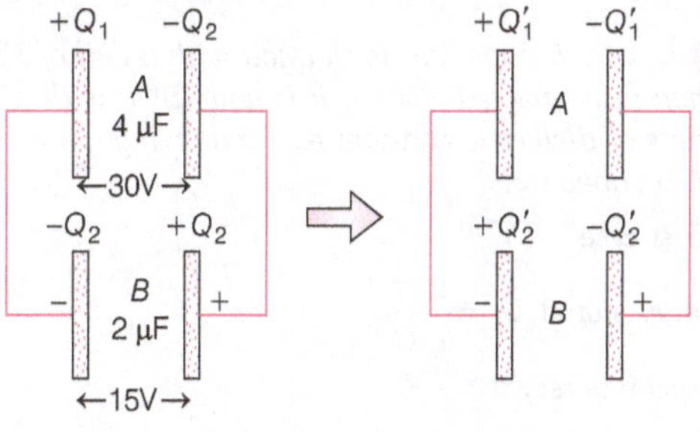

Here, charges on A,

$$Q_1 = C_1 V_1 = 4 \times 30 = 120\,\mu\text{C}$$

Charge on B,

$$Q_2 = C_2 V_2 = 2 \times 15 = 30\,\mu\text{C}$$

When positive plate is connected to negative plate, we find net charge as,

$$|Q_1 - Q_2| = 120 - 30 = 90\,\mu C$$

The charge 90 μC will be redistributed in such a manner that capacitors acquire same potential.

Common potential,

$$V = \frac{|C_1V_1 - C_2V_2|}{C_1 + C_2}$$

$$= \frac{4 \times 30 - 2 \times 15}{4 + 2} = 15\text{ V}$$

Hence, $Q'_1 = C_1V = 4 \times 15 = 60\,\mu C$

and $Q'_2 = C_2V = 2 \times 15 = 30\,\mu C$

Loss of energy,

$$\Delta U = \frac{1}{2}\frac{C_1C_2}{C_1 + C_2}(V_1 - V_2)^2$$

$$= \frac{1}{2}\cdot\frac{4 \times 2}{4 + 2}(30 - 15)^2 \times 10^{-6}\text{ J} = 150\,\mu J$$

Example 37. *A capacitor is charged by a battery. The battery is removed and another identical uncharged capacitor is connected in parallel. Energy of the system decreases by factor of x. Find x.*

Sol. Initially, energy of capacitor

$$U_i = \frac{1}{2}CV^2$$

Common potential

$$V_C = \frac{CV + 0}{2C} = \frac{V}{2}$$

Total energy of system

$$U_f = \frac{1}{2}(C + C) \times \left(\frac{V}{2}\right)^2$$

$$= \frac{1}{2}\left(\frac{1}{2}CV^2\right)$$

$$\Rightarrow \quad U_f = \frac{1}{2}U_i$$

Clearly, energy of system decreases by factor of 2.

Example 38. *A capacitor is charged with a cell of EMF V and then disconnected from it. It is now filled with dielectric materials of dielectric constant K. Find change in energy stored in capacitor.*

Sol. In first case,

Energy stored $U_1 = \frac{1}{2}\frac{q^2}{C}$

In second case,

Energy stored $U_2 = \frac{1}{2}\frac{q^2}{KC}$

Change in energy stored

$$\Delta U = U_2 - U_1 = \frac{1}{2}\frac{q^2}{C}\left[\frac{1}{K} - 1\right]$$

NEET Close-up

Example Similar to PYQ Asked in NEET 2021

A capacitor of capacitance $C = 500$ pF is charged fully by 50 V battery B as shown in figure (a). Then, it is disconnected from the battery and connected to another uncharged capacitor of capacitance $C = 500$ pF as shown in figure (b). The electrostatic energy stored by the system (b) is

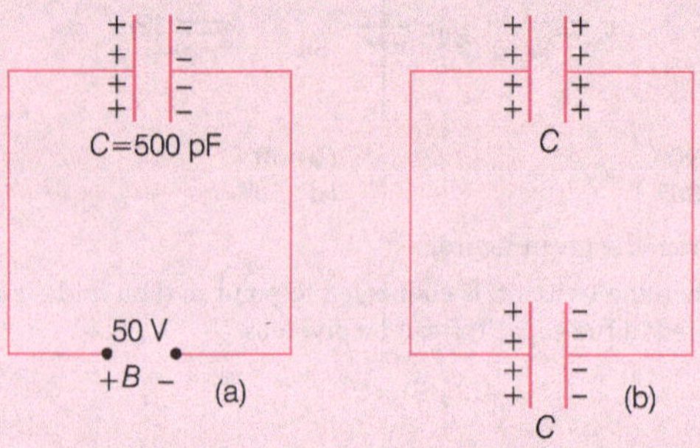

(a) 2.28×10^{-8} J (b) 3.125×10^{-7} J
(c) 1.782×10^{-8} J (d) 4.5×10^{-6} J

Sol. (*b*)

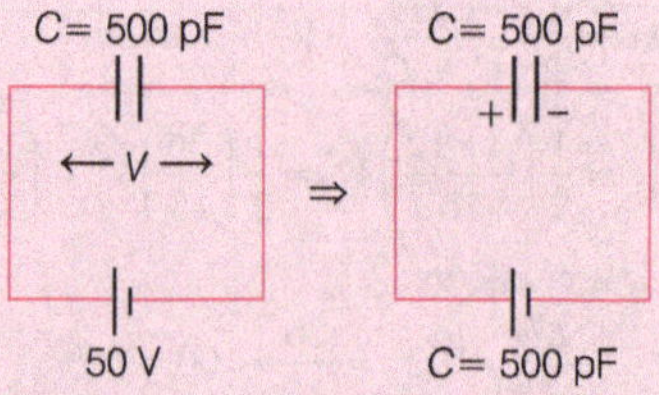

After combination,

Common potential,

$$V = \frac{C_1V_1 + C_2V_2}{C_1 + C_2}$$

$$= \frac{C \times 50 + C \times 0}{C + C} = 25\text{ V}$$

∴ Electrostatic stored potential energy

$$U = 2 \times \frac{1}{2}CV^2 = CV^2$$

$$= 5 \times 10^{-10} \times 25^2 = 3.125 \times 10^{-7}\text{ J}$$

Skill Builder

A capacitor of capacitance $C = 800$ pF is charged fully by a battery, which has capacity of 120 V. Then, it is disconnected from the battery and connected to another uncharged capacitor of capacitance $C = 800$ pF. The electrostatic energy stored by the system when battery is disconnected and capacitor is connected is

(a) 2×10^{-6} J (b) 3.8×10^{-8} J
(c) 2.8×10^{-6} J (d) 2.5×10^{-9} J

For more Practice Refer Q.No. 15 of Gearing up for NEET.

STEP UP Practice 3

1. The energy stored in a capacitor of capacitance 100 μF is 50 J. Its potential difference is
(a) 50 V (b) 500 V
(c) 1000 V (d) 1500 V

2. A series combination of n_1 capacitors, each of value C_1, is charged by a source of potential difference $4V$. When another parallel combination of n_2 capacitors, each of value C_2, is charged by a source of potential difference V, it has the same (total) energy stored in it, as the first combination has. The value of C_2, in terms of C_1 is, then
(a) $\frac{16C_1}{n_1 n_2}$ (b) $\frac{2C_1}{n_1 n_2}$
(c) $16 \frac{n_2}{n_1} C_1$ (d) $2 \frac{n_2}{n_1} C_1$

3. Putting a dielectric substance between plates of capacitor affect is capacitance and potential energy respectively
(a) both increases (b) increases, decreases
(c) decreases, increases (d) both decreases

4. If there are n capacitors in parallel connected to V volt source, then energy stored is equal to
(a) CV (b) CV^2
(c) $\frac{1}{2n} CV^2$ (d) $\frac{1}{2} nCV^2$

5. **Assertion** (A) When an uncharged capacitor is charged by a battery, only 50% of the energy supplied by a battery is stored in the capacitor.
Reason (R) Rest 50% is lost.
In the light of the above statements, choose the correct answer from the options given below.
(a) Both A and R are true but R is not the correct explanation of A.
(b) A is true but R is false.
(c) A is false but R is true.
(d) Both A and R are true and R is the correct explanation of A.

6. When dielectric medium of constant K is filled between the plates of a charged parallel plate condenser, then the energy stored becomes, as compared to its previous value
(a) K times (b) K^{-1} times
(c) K^{-2} times (d) K^2 times

7. If potential difference on a capacitor is kept constant and different mediums are filled between two plates, then stored energy is
(a) remains constant
(b) inversely proportional to dielectric constant of medium
(c) directly proportional to dielectric constant of medium
(d) None of the above

8. A capacitor of 20 μF and charged to 500 V is connected in parallel with another capacitor of 10 μF charged to 200 V. The common potential will be
(a) 400 V (b) 300 V
(c) 200 V (d) 100 V

9. **Assertion** (A) A capacitor is connected to a battery. If we move its plate further apart, work will be done against the electrostatic attraction between the plates and the energy of the capacitor gets increased.
Reason (R) The energy stored in a capacitor is dissipated in the form of heat energy.
In the light of the above statements, choose the correct answer from the options given below.
(a) Both A and R are true but R is not the correct explanation of A.
(b) A is true but R is false.
(c) A is false but R is true.
(d) Both A and R are true and R is the correct explanation of A.

10. Find correct statement.
(a) Capacitors are connected in series for maximum storage of energy.
(b) Charge remains common in redistribution process.
(c) Voltage becomes common in redistribution process.
(d) Capacitance becomes common in redistribution process.

11. Find incorrect statement.
(a) Half of the energy supplied by battery to a capacitor is lost in the process of charging of capacitor.
(b) Energy is always lost in redistribution of charges.
(c) Energy lost in redistribution is proportional to average of potentials of both capacitors.
(d) Redistribution of charges continue until potential of both capacitors become same.

12. Two conductor spheres of radii R_1 and R_2 having charges Q_1 and Q_2, respectively are connected to each other. There is
(a) no change in the energy of the system
(b) energy of the system
(c) energy of the system continuously
(d) a decrease in the energy of the system unless $Q_1 R_2 = Q_2 R_1$

13. If the charge on a capacitor is increased by 2 C, then the energy stored in it increases by 21%. The original charge on the capacitor is
(a) 10 C
(b) 20 C
(c) 30C
(d) 40 C

14. A capacitor of capacitance value 1 μF is charged to 30V and the battery is, then disconnected. If it is connected across a 2 μF capacitor, then the energy lost by the system is

(a) 300 μJ (b) 450 μJ
(c) 225 μJ (d) 150 μJ

15. Assertion (A) If a battery remains connected, potential of capacitor will not change.

Reason (R) When a capacitor is kept connected with a battery and a dielectric slab is inserted between the plates, both the charge on capacitor and the energy stored gets decreased.

In the light of the above statements, choose the correct answer from the options given below.

(a) Both A and R are true but R is not the correct explanation of A.
(b) A is true but R is false.
(c) A is false but R is true.
(d) Both A and R are true and R is the correct explanation of A.

16. The two parallel plates of condenser have been connected to a battery of 300 V and the charge collected at each plate is 1 μC. The energy supplied by the battery is

(a) 6×10^{-4} J (b) 3×10^{-4} J
(c) 1.5×10^{-4} J (d) 45×10^{-4} J

17. A parallel plate capacitor is charged and then, the battery is removed. A mica sheet is inserted between its plates. Consequently

	Charge	Potential difference	Energy
(a)	decreases	increases	decreases
(b)	remains constant	increases	decreases
(c)	remains constant	decreases	decreases
(d)	increases	decreases	increases

18. A parallel plate capacitor is charged to a potential difference of 50 V. It is then discharged through a resistance for 2 s and its potential drops by 10 V. Calculate the fraction of energy stored in the capacitance

(a) 0.14 (b) 0.25
(c) 0.50 (d) 0.64

19. Assertion (A) A charged capacitor is disconnected from a battery. Now, if its plate are separated further, the potential energy will fall.

Reason (R) Energy stored in a capacitor is not equal to the work done in charging it.

In the light of the above statements, choose the correct answer from the options given below.

(a) Both A and R are true but R is not the correct explanation of A.
(b) A is true but R is false.
(c) A is false but R is true.
(d) Both A and R are true and R is the correct explanation of A.

20. What fraction of energy drawn from the charging battery is stored in a capacitor

(a) 100% (b) 75%
(c) 50% (d) 25%

21. A capacitor C_1 of capacitance C is charged to a potential difference V_0. The terminals of the charged capacitor are, then connected to an unchared capacitor C_2 of capacitance $\frac{C}{2}$.

Which of the below pair is not correctly paired?

(a) Final energy of capacitor $C_1 \rightarrow \left(\frac{2}{9}\right) CV_0^2$

(b) Final energy of capacitor $C_2 \rightarrow \left(\frac{1}{8}\right) CV_0^2$

(c) Final energy of the system $\rightarrow \left(\frac{1}{3}\right) CV_0^2$

(d) Change in energy on joining the capacitors $\rightarrow -\left(\frac{1}{6}\right) CV_0^2$

NEET Exclusive EXTRA BYTES

- Farad is very large unit of capacitance. We normally use smaller unit of capacitance (μF, nF).
- Capacitance of earth is approximately 711 F which is normally taken as infinite for numerical problems.
- Capacitance is inherent property and do not depend upon applied potential.
- If one plate of capacitor is grounded, its capacitance increases.
- In series combination of capacitors $V \propto \frac{1}{C}$.
- In parallel combination of capacitors $Q \propto C$.
- Breakdown voltage in series combination of N identical capacitors is N times of breakdown voltage of each capacitor.
- Cylindrical capacitor consists of two co-axial cylinders of radii a and b ($a < b$), inner cylinder is given charge $+q$ while outer cylinder is earthed.

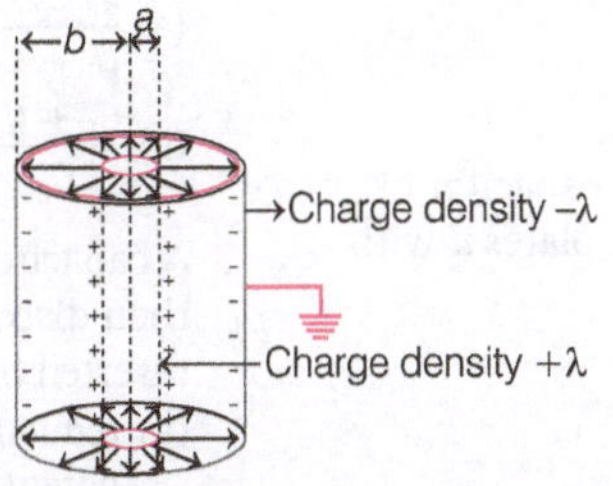

Common length of the cylinder is l, then capacity of a cylindrical capacitor is given by

$$C = \frac{2\pi\varepsilon_0 l}{\log_e(b/a)}$$

- Capacitors must be connected in parallel to each other to store maximum energy in the system.
- The relation $\frac{q^2}{2C}$ shows that the charged capacitor is the electrical analog of a stretched spring whose elastic potential energy is $\frac{1}{2}kx^2$. The charge q is analogous to the elongation x and reciprocal of capacitance to the force constant k.

GEARING UP FOR NEET

Single Option Correct

1 The potential energy of a charged parallel plate capacitor is U_0. If a slab of dielectric constant K is inserted between the plates, then the new potential energy will be

(a) $\frac{U_0}{K}$ (b) $U_0 K^2$

(c) $\frac{U_0}{K^2}$ (d) U_0^2

2 The force between the plates of a parallel plate capacitor of capacitance C and distance of separation of the plates d with a potential difference V between the plates, is

(a) $\frac{CV^2}{2d}$ (b) $\frac{C^2V^2}{2d^2}$

(c) $\frac{C^2V^2}{d^2}$ (d) $\frac{V^2d}{C}$

3 A capacitor of capacity C has charge Q and stored energy is W. If the charge is increased to $2Q$, then the stored energy will be

(a) $2W$ (b) $\frac{W}{2}$

(c) $4W$ (d) $\frac{W}{4}$

4 A 2 μF capacitor is charged to 100 V and then its plates are connected by a conducting wire. The heat produced is

(a) 1 J (b) 0.1 J

(c) 0.01 J (d) 0.001 J

5 If there are n capacitors in parallel connected to V volt source, then the energy stored is equal to

(a) nCV^2 (b) $\frac{1}{2}nCV^2$

(c) $\frac{CV^2}{n}$ (d) $\frac{1}{2n}CV^2$

6 A variable condenser is permanently connected to 100 V battery. If the capacity is changed from 2 μF to 10 μF, then change in energy is equal to

(a) 2×10^{-2} J (b) 2.5×10^{-2} J

(c) 3.5×10^{-2} J (d) 4×10^{-2} J

7 Two condensers of capacity 0.3 μF and 0.6 μF respectively are connected in series. The combination is connected across a potential of 6 V. The ratio of energies stored by the condensers will be

(a) $\frac{1}{2}$ (b) 2 (c) $\frac{1}{4}$ (d) 4

8 A capacitor of capacity C_1, is charged by connected it across a battery of emf V_0. The battery is then removed and the capacitor is connected in parallel with an uncharged capacitor of capacity C_2. The potential difference across this combination is

(a) $\frac{C_2}{C_1 + C_2}V_0$ (b) $\frac{C_1}{C_1 + C_2}V_0$

(c) $\frac{C_1 + C_2}{C_2}V_0$ (d) $\frac{C_1 + C_2}{C_1}V_0$

9 A capacitor is charged by using a battery which is then disconnected. A dielectric slab is then inserted between the plates which results in

(a) reduction of charges on the plates and increase of potential difference across the plates

(b) increase in the potential difference across the plates, reduction in stored energy,but no change in the charge on the plates

(c) decrease in the potential difference across the plates, reduction in stored energy, but no change in the charge on the plates

(d) None of the above

10 A parallel plate air capacitor is charged to a potential difference of V. After disconnecting the battery, distance between the plates of the capacitor is increased using an insulating handle. As a result, the potential difference between the plates

(a) decreases (b) increases

(c) becomes zero (d) does not change

11 Two spherical conductors each of capacity C are charged to potential V and $-V$. These are then connected by means of a fine wire. The loss of energy is

(a) zero (b) $\frac{1}{2}CV^2$

(c) CV^2 (d) $2CV^2$

12 Two spheres A and B of radius 4 cm and 6 cm are given charges of 80 μC and 40 μC, respectively. If they are connected by a fine wire, then the amount of charge flowing from one to the other is

(a) 20 μC from A to B

(b) 20 μC from B to A

(c) 32 μC from B to A

(d) 32 μC from A to B

13 A parallel plate capacitor has a uniform electric field E (V/m) in the space between the plates. If the distance between the plates is d (m) and area of each plates is A (m^2), then the energy (J) stored in the capacitor is

(a) $\frac{1}{2}\varepsilon_0 E^2$
(b) $\varepsilon_0 EAd$
(c) $\frac{1}{2}\varepsilon_0 E^2 Ad$
(d) $E^2 Ad / \varepsilon_0$

14 In a parallel plate capacitor the separation between the plates is 3 mm with air between them. Now a 1 mm thick layer of a material of dielectric constant 2 is introduced between the plates due to which the capacity increases. In order to bring its capacity to the original value the separation between the plates must be made

(a) 1.5 mm (b) 2.5 mm
(c) 3.5 mm (d) 4.5 mm

15 A capacitor of 2 μF charged to 50 V is connected parallel with another capacitor of 1 μF charged to 20V. The common potential and loss of energy will be

(a) 40 V, 300 μJ (b) 50V, 400 μJ
(c) 40 V, 600 μJ (d) 50 V, 700 μJ

16 A spherical condenser has inner and outer spheres of radii a and b, respectively. The space beween the two is filled with air. The difference between the capacities of two condensers formed when outer sphere is earthed and when inner sphere is earthed will be

(a) zero (b) $4\pi\varepsilon_0 a$
(c) $4\pi\varepsilon_0 b$ (d) $4\pi\varepsilon_0 a\left(\frac{b}{b-a}\right)$

17 Five capacitors of 10 μF capacity each are connected to a DC potential of 100 V as shown in the adjoining figure. The equivalent capacitance between the points A and B will be equal to

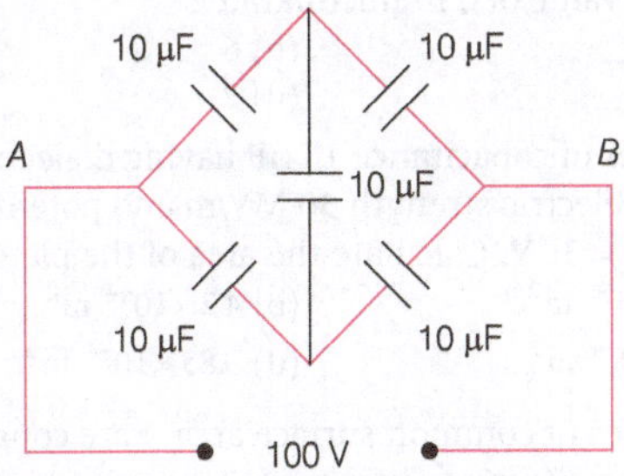

(a) 40 μF (b) 20 μF
(c) 30 μF (d) 10 μF

18 Three capacitors of capacitances 3 μF, 9 μF and 18 μF are connected once in series and another time in parallel. The ratio of equivalent capacitance in the two cases $\left(\frac{C_S}{C_P}\right)$ will be

(a) 1 : 15 (b) 15 : 1 (c) 1 : 1 (d) 1 : 3

19 In the circuit diagram shown in the adjoining figure, the resultant capacitance between points P and Q is

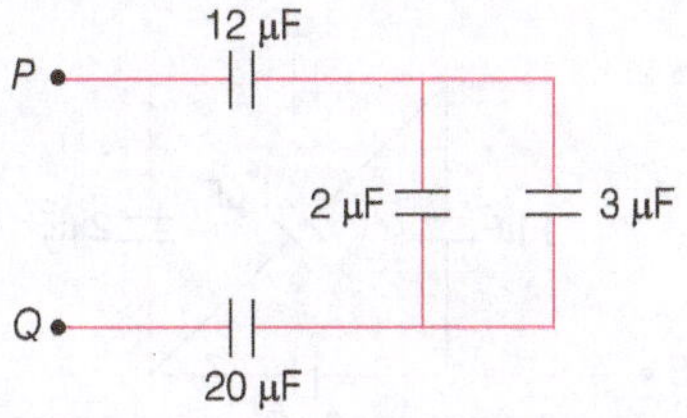

(a) 47 μF (b) 3 μF
(c) 60 μF (d) 10 μF

20 Four capacitors each of capacity 3 μF are connected as shown in the adjoining figure. The ratio of equivalent capacitance between A and B and between A and C will be

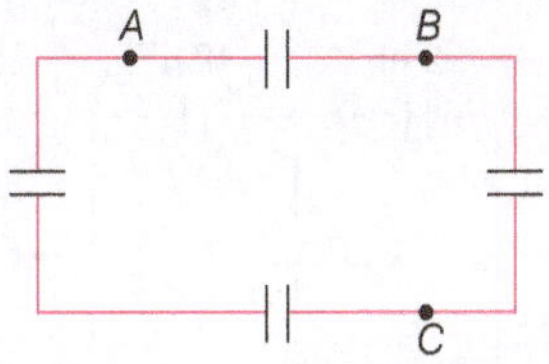

(a) 4 : 3 (b) 3 : 4
(c) 2 : 3 (d) 3 : 2

21 What is the equivalent capacitance between A and B in the given figure (all are in micro farad)?

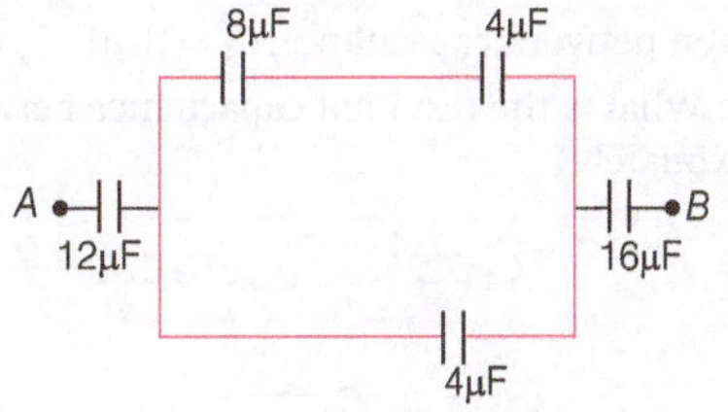

(a) $\frac{13}{18}$ F (b) $\frac{48}{13}$ F
(c) $\frac{1}{31}$ F (d) $\frac{240}{71}$ F

22 Four capacitors are connected as shown. The equivalent capacitance between the points P and Q is

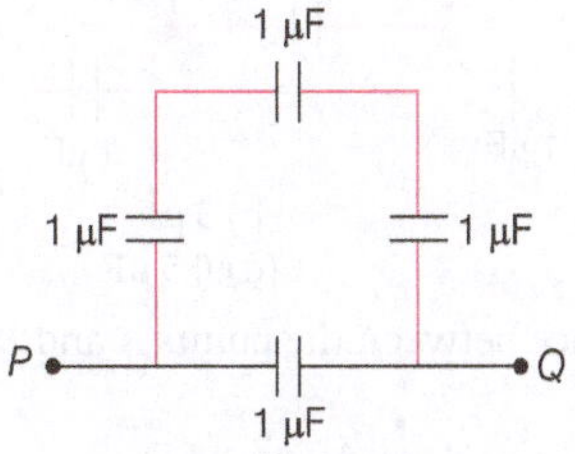

(a) 4 μF (b) $\frac{1}{4}$ μF
(c) $\frac{3}{4}$ μF (d) $\frac{4}{3}$ μF

23 The total capacity of the system of capacitors shown in the adjoining figure between the points A and B.

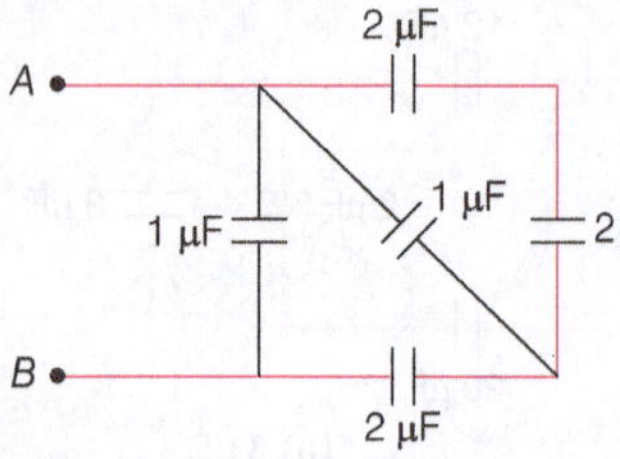

(a) 1 μF (b) 2 μF
(c) 3 μF (d) 4 μF

24 Four capacitors are connected in a circuit as shown in the figure. The effective capacitance between points A and B will be

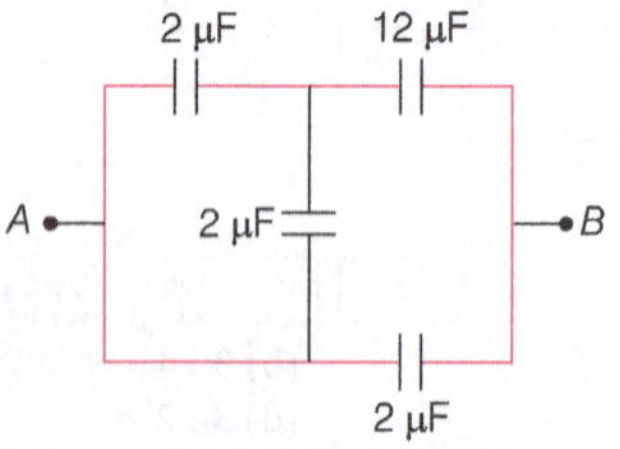

(a) $\frac{28}{9}$ μF (b) 4 μF
(c) 5 μF (d) 18 μF

25 In the given network capacitance, $C_1 = 10\,\mu F$, $C_2 = 5\,\mu F$ and $C_3 = 4\,\mu F$. What is the resultant capacitance between A and B (approximately)

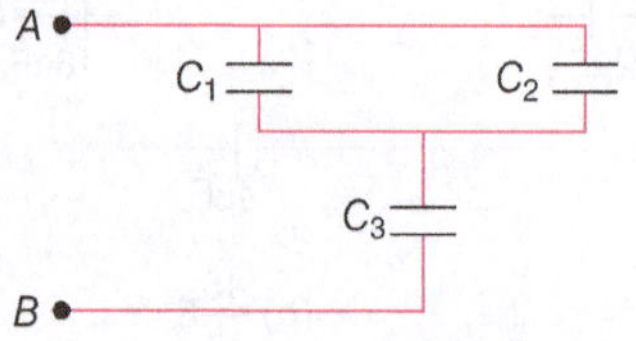

(a) 2.2 μF (b) 3.2 μF
(c) 1.2 μF (d) 4.7 μF

26 The equivalent capacitance between points A and B is

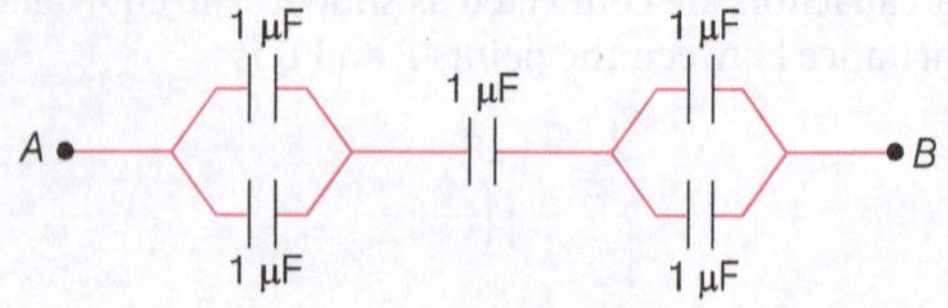

(a) 2 μF (b) 3 μF
(c) 5 μF (d) 0.5 μF

27 The capacitance between the points A and B in the given circuit will be

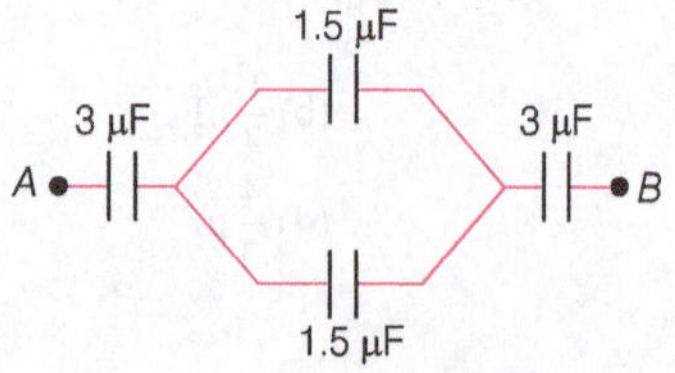

(a) 1 μF (b) 2 μF
(c) 3 μF (d) 4 μF

28 Four equal capacitors, each of capacity C, are arranged as shown. The effective capacitance between points A and B is

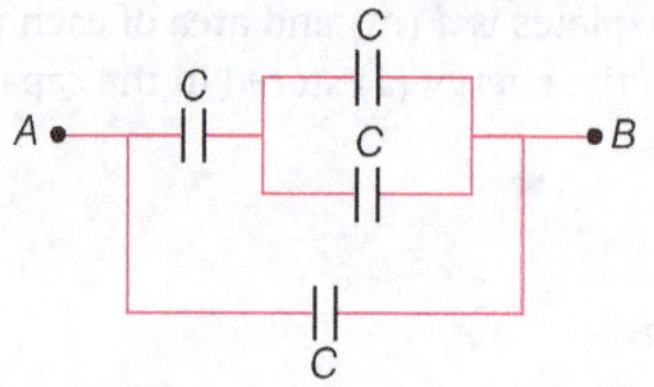

(a) $\frac{5}{8}C$ (b) $\frac{3}{5}C$ (c) $\frac{5}{3}C$ (d) C

29 There are seven identical capacitors. The equivalent capacitance when they are connected in series is C. The equivalent capacitance when they are connected in parallel is

(a) $\frac{C}{49}$ (b) $\frac{C}{7}$
(c) $7C$ (d) $49C$

30 The capacitance of a parallel plate capacitor is 16 μF. When a glass slab is placed between the plates, the potential difference reduces to1/8th of the original value. What is the dielectric constant of glass?

(a) 4 (b) 8
(c) 16 (d) 32

31 A parallel plate condenser with air between the plates possesses the capacity of 10^{-12} F. Now the plates are removed apart, so that the separation is twice the original value. The space between the plates is filled with a material of dielectric constant 4.0. Then, new value of the capacity is (in farad)

(a) 4×10^{-12} (b) 3×10^{-12}
(c) 2×10^{-12} (d) 0.5×10^{-12}

32 Three condensers each of capacity C μF are connected in series. An exactly similar set is connected in parallel to the first one. The effective capacity of the combination is 4 μF. Then, the value of C in microfarad is

(a) 8 (b) 6
(c) 4 (d) 2

33 A capacitor of capacitance 15 nF having dielectric slab of $\varepsilon_r = 2.5$, dielectric strength 30 MV/m and potential difference = 30 V. Calculate the area of the plate.

(a) $6.7 \times 10^{-4}\ m^2$ (b) $4.2 \times 10^{-4}\ m^2$
(c) $8.0 \times 10^{-4}\ m^2$ (d) $9.85 \times 10^{-4}\ m^2$

34 Three plates of common surface area A are connected as shown. The effective capacitance between points P and Q will be

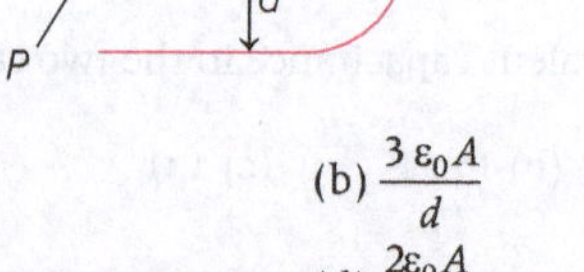

(a) $\frac{\varepsilon_0 A}{d}$ (b) $\frac{3\varepsilon_0 A}{d}$
(c) $\frac{3}{2}\frac{\varepsilon_0 A}{d}$ (d) $\frac{2\varepsilon_0 A}{d}$

35 Eight drops of mercury of equal radii combine to form a big drop. The capacitance of the bigger drop as compared to each smaller drop is

(a) 2 times (b) 8 times
(c) 4 times (d) 16 times

36 Consider a parallel plate capacitor of capacity 10 μF with air filled in the gap between the plates. Now, one-half of the space between the plates is filled with a dielectric of dielectric constant 4, as shown in the figure. The capacity of the capacitor changes to

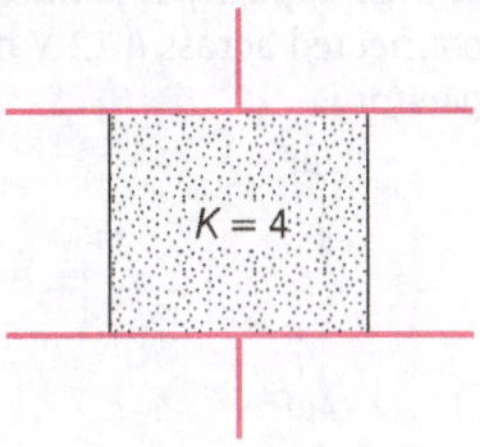

(a) 25 μF (b) 20 μF
(c) 40 μF (d) 5 μF

37 Find the capacitance as shown in the figure.

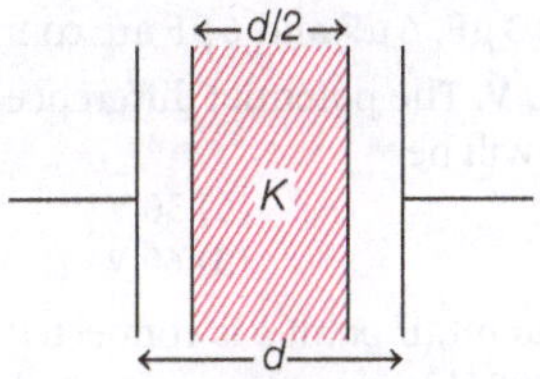

(a) $\dfrac{2KA\varepsilon_0}{(K+1)\,d}$ (b) $\dfrac{2KA\varepsilon_0}{d}$
(c) $\dfrac{(K+1)\,A\varepsilon_0}{2d}$ (d) $\dfrac{2KA\varepsilon_0}{(K^2+1)\,d}$

38 A capacitor of capacity C is connected with a battery of potential V. The distance between its plates is reduced to half, assuming that the battery remains the same. Then, the new energy given by the battery will be

(a) $\dfrac{CV^2}{4}$ (b) $\dfrac{CV^2}{2}$
(c) $\dfrac{3CV^2}{4}$ (d) CV^2

39 A parallel plate capacitor has plate separation d and capacitance 25 μF. If a metallic foil of thickness $\dfrac{2}{7}d$ is introduced between the plates, the capacitance would become

(a) 25 μF (b) 35 μF
(c) $\dfrac{125}{7}$ μF (d) $\dfrac{175}{2}$ μF

40 The capacity and the energy stored in a charged parallel plate condenser with air between its plates are respectively, C_0 and W_0. If the air is replaced by glass (dielectric constant = 5) between the paltes, the capacity of the plates and the energy stored in it will respectively be

(a) $5C_0, 5W_0$ (b) $5C_0, \dfrac{W_0}{5}$
(c) $\dfrac{C_0}{5}, 5W_0$ (d) $\dfrac{C_0}{5}, \dfrac{W_0}{5}$

41 A slab of copper of thickness b is inserted in between the plates of parallel plate capacitor as shown in figure. The separation of the plates is d. If $b = d/2$, then the ratio of capacities of the capacitor after and before inserting the slab will be

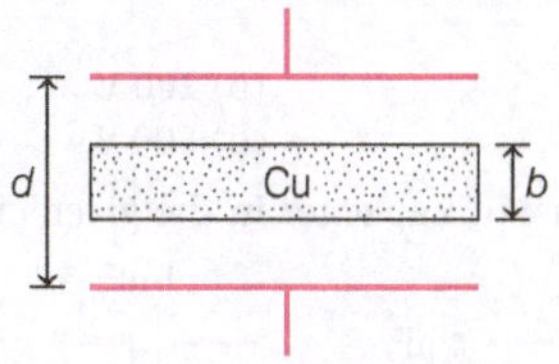

(a) $\sqrt{2}:1$ (b) 2 : 1
(c) 1 : 1 (d) $1:\sqrt{2}$

42 A charged capacitor when filled with a dielectric $K = 3$ has charge Q_0, voltage V_0 and field E_0. If the dielectric is replaced with another one having $K = 9$, the new values of charge, voltage and electric field will be respectively

(a) $3Q_0, 3V_0, 3E_0$ (b) $Q_0, 3V_0, 3E_0$
(c) $Q_0, \dfrac{V_0}{3}, 3E_0$ (d) $Q_0, \dfrac{V_0}{3}, \dfrac{E_0}{3}$

43 In the adjoining figure, four capacitors are shown with their respective capacities and the potential difference is applied. The charge and the potential difference across the 4 μF capacitor will be

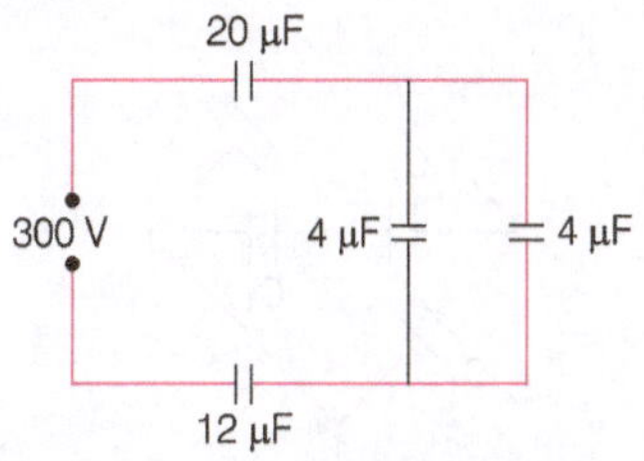

(a) 600 μC, 150 V (b) 300 μC, 75 V
(c) 800 μC, 200 V (d) 580 μC, 145 V

44 Two condensers C_1 and C_2 in a circuit are joined shown in figure. The potential of point A is V_1 and that of B is V_2. The potential of point D will be

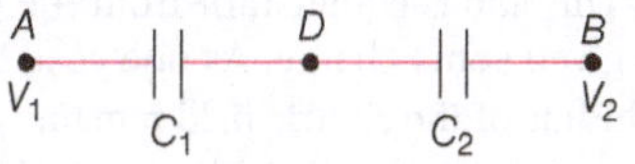

(a) $\dfrac{1}{2}(V_1 + V_2)$ (b) $\dfrac{C_2V_1 + C_1V_2}{C_1 + C_2}$
(c) $\dfrac{C_1V_1 + C_2V_2}{C_1 + C_2}$ (d) $\dfrac{C_2V_1 - C_1V_2}{C_1 + C_2}$

45 Three capacitors of 2 μF, 3 μF and 6 μF are joined series and the combination is charged by means of 24 V battery. The potential difference between the plates of the 6 μF capacitor is

(a) 4 V (b) 6 V
(c) 8 V (d) 10 V

46 In the figure a potential of +1200 V is given to point A and point B is earthed, what is the potential at the point P?

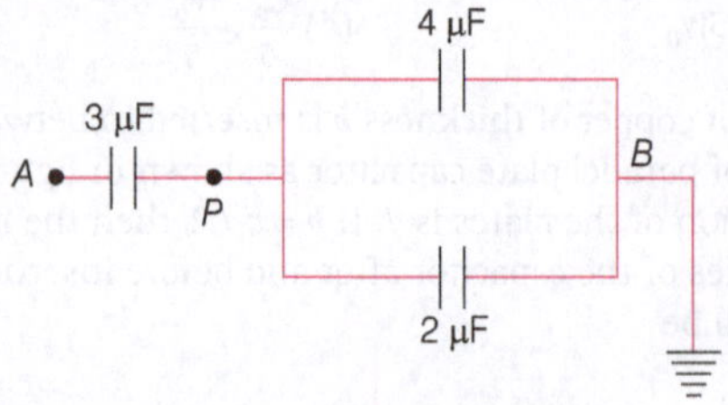

(a) 100 V (b) 200 V
(c) 400 V (d) 800 V

47 The charge on 4 μF capacitor in the given circuit is (in μF)

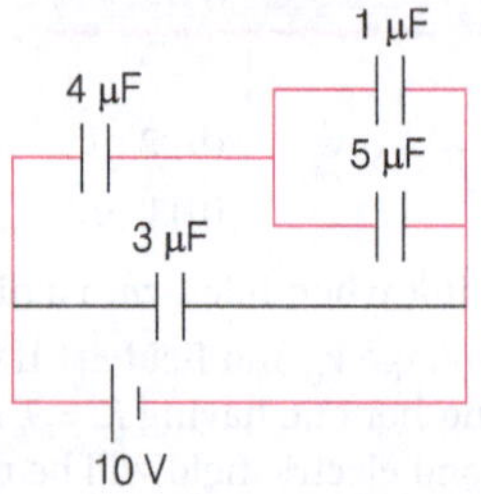

(a) 12 (b) 24
(c) 36 (d) 32

48 Four identical capacitors are connected as shown in diagram. When a battery of 6 V is connected between A and B, then the charge stored is found to be 1.5 μC. The value of C_1 is

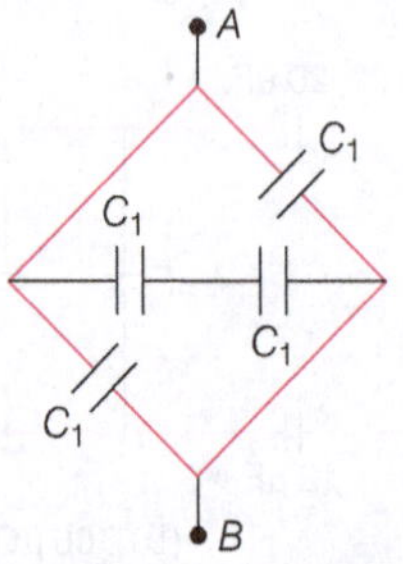

(a) 2.5 μF (b) 15 μF
(c) 1.5 μF (d) 0.1 μF

49 A dielectric slab of thickness d is inserted in a parallel plate capacitor whose negative plate is at $x = 0$ and positive plate is at $x = 3d$. The slab is equidistant from the plates. The capacitor is given some charge. As one goes from 0 to $3d$

(a) the magnitude of the electric field remains the same
(b) the direction of the electric field remains the same
(c) the electric potential decrease continuously
(d) the electric potential increases at first, then decreases and again increases

50 2 μF condenser is charged upto 200 V and then battery is removed. On combining this with another uncharged condenser in parallel, the potential differences between two plates are found to be 40 V. The capacity of second condenser is

(a) 2 μF (b) 4 μF
(c) 8 μF (d) 16 μF

51 Consider two conductors. One of them has a capacity of 2 units and the capacity of the other is unknown. They are charged until their potentials are 4 and 5 units, respectively. The two conductors are now connected by a wire when their common potential is found to be 4.6 units. Then, the unknown capacity has the value (in the same units as above)

(a) 6 (b) 5
(c) 4 (d) 3

52 Two capacitors 2 μF and 4 μF are connected in parallel. A third capacitor of 6 μF capacity is connected in series. The combination is connected across a 12 V battery. The voltage across a 2 μF capacitor is

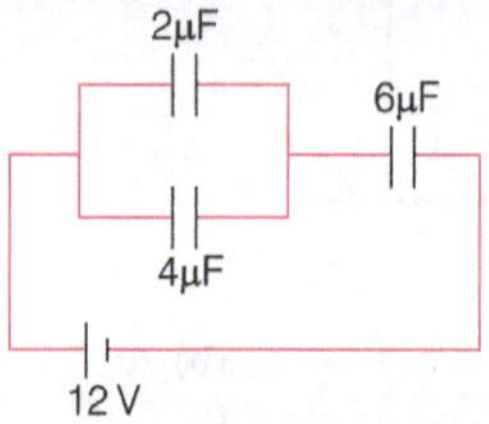

(a) 2 V (b) 6 V
(c) 8 V (d) 1 V

53 The capacitors 3 μF, 6 μF and 6 μF are connected in series to a source of 120 V. The potential difference in volt, across the 3 μF capacitor will be

(a) 24 V (b) 30 V
(c) 40 V (d) 60 V

54 In the given circuit, if point b is connected to earth and a potential of 1200 V is given to a point a, the charge on 4 μF capacitor is

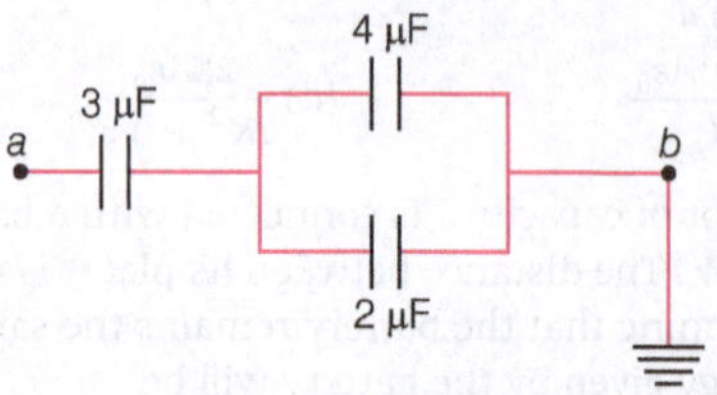

(a) 800 μC (b) 1600 μC
(c) 2400 μC (d) 3000 μC

55 A circuit is shown in the given figure. Find out the charge on the condenser having capacity 5 μF.

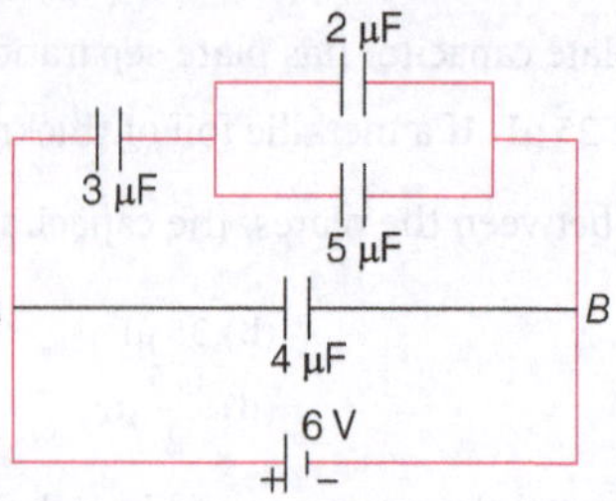

(a) 4.5 μC (b) 9 μC
(c) 7 μC (d) 30 μC

56 A potential of $V = 3000$ V is applied to a combination of four initially uncharged capacitors as shown in the figure. Capacitors A, B, C and D have capacitances $C_A = 6.0$ μF,

$C_B = 5.2\,\mu F$, $C_C = 1.5\,\mu F$ and $C_D = 3.8\,\mu F$, respectively. If the battery is disconnected, then potential difference across capacitor B is (approximately)

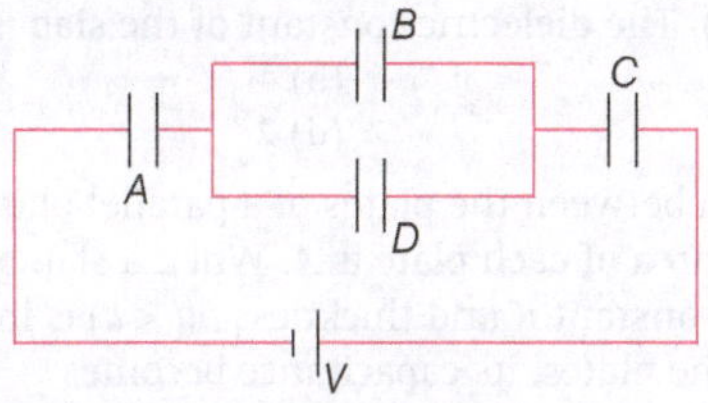

(a) 3000 V (b) zero
(c) 530 V (d) 350 V

57 Four capacitors are arranged as shown in below figure. All are initially uncharged. A 30 V battery is placed across terminal PQ to charge the capacitors and is then removed. The voltage across the terminals RS is then (in volt)

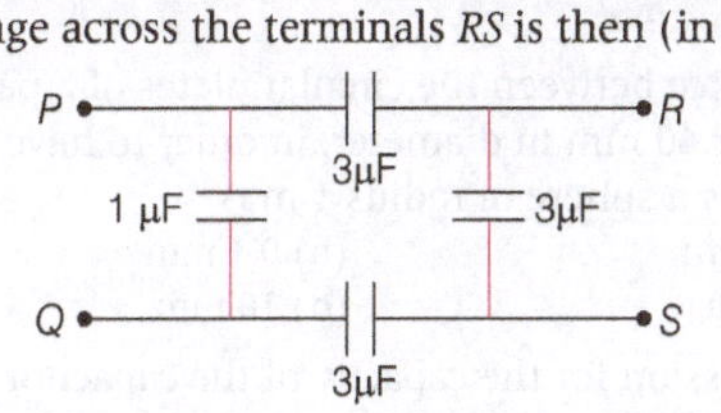

(a) 10 (b) 20
(c) 30 (d) 40

58 If the equivalent capacitance between points P and Q of the combination of the capacitors shown in figure below is $30\,\mu F$, the capacitor C is

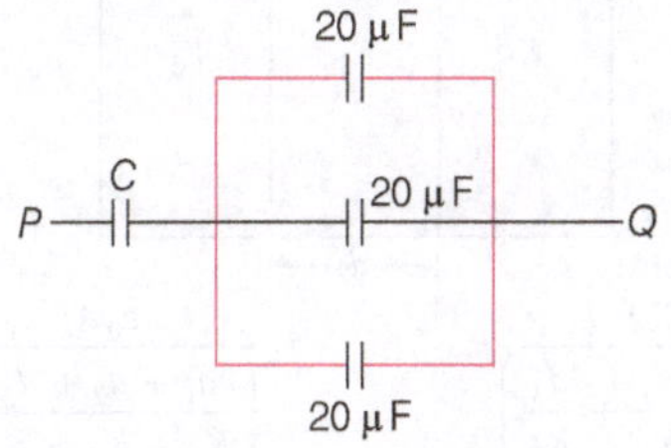

(a) $60\,\mu F$ (b) $30\,\mu F$
(c) $10\,\mu F$ (d) $5\,\mu F$

59 In the circuit shown in figure $C = 6\,\mu F$. The charge stored in the capacitor of capacity C is

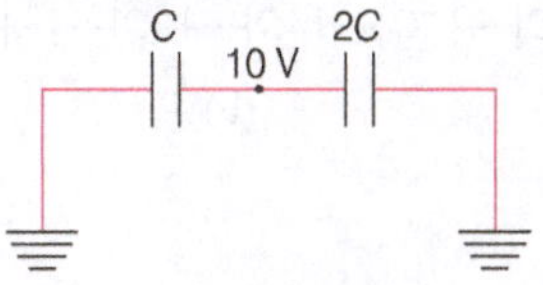

(a) zero (b) $90\,\mu C$
(c) $40\,\mu C$ (d) $60\,\mu C$

60 In the circuit shown in figure. Charge stored in $6\,\mu F$ capacitor will be

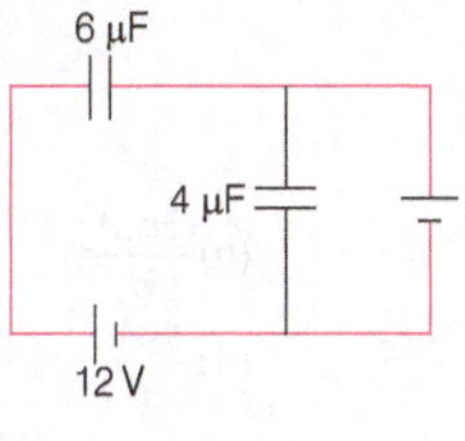

(a) $18\,\mu C$ (b) $54\,\mu C$
(c) $36\,\mu C$ (d) $72\,\mu C$

61 In the given circuit, if point C is connected to the earth of and a potential of $+2000$ V is given to the point A, the potential at B is

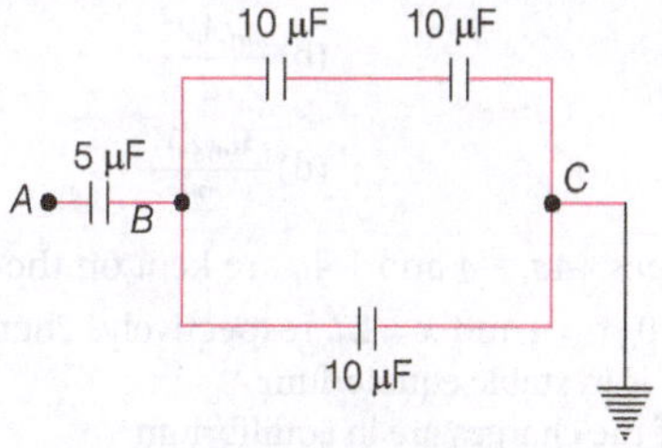

(a) 1500 V (b) 1000 V
(c) 500 V (d) 400 V

62 Two condensers, one of capacity C and the other capacity $\frac{C}{3}$, are connected to a V volt battery as shown. The work done in charging fully both the condensers is

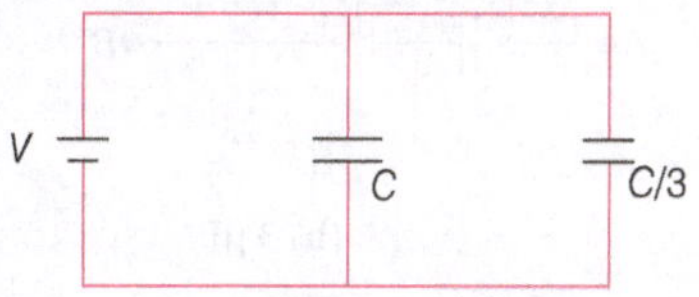

(a) $2CV^2$ (b) $\left(\frac{1}{4}\right) CV^2$
(c) $\left(\frac{2}{3}\right) CV^2$ (d) $\frac{1}{2} CV^2$

63 Two capacitors C and $C/2$ are connected to a battery of V volts, as shown below.

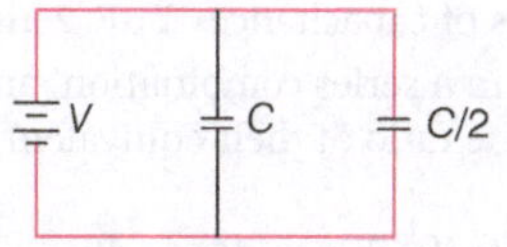

The work done in charging both the capacitor fully is

(a) $2CV^2$ (b) $\left(\frac{1}{2}\right) CV^2$
(c) $\left(\frac{3}{4}\right) CV^2$ (d) $\left(\frac{1}{4}\right) CV^2$

64 In the circuit shown here $C_1 = 6\,\mu F$, $C_2 = 3\,\mu F$ and battery $B = 20$ V. The switch S_1, is first closed. It is then opened and afterwards S_2 is closed. What is the charge finally on C_2?

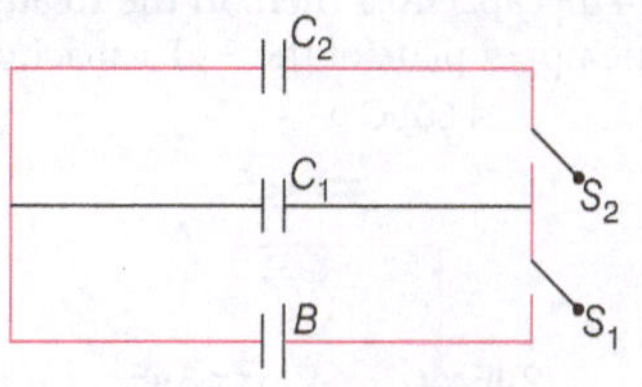

(a) $120\,\mu C$ (b) $80\,\mu C$
(c) $40\,\mu C$ (d) $20\,\mu C$

65 Consider the arrangement of three plates X, Y and each of area A and separation d. The energy stored when the plates are fully charged is

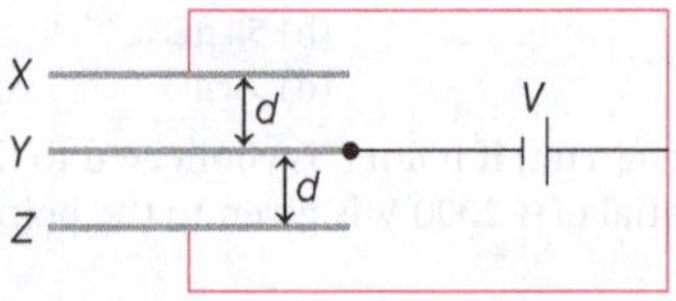

(a) $\frac{\varepsilon_0 AV^2}{2d}$ (b) $\frac{\varepsilon_0 AV^2}{d}$

(c) $\frac{2\varepsilon_0 AV^2}{d}$ (d) $\frac{3\varepsilon_0 AV^2}{2d}$

66 Point charges $+4q, -q$ and $+4q$ are kept on the X-axis at points $x = 0$, $x = a$ and $x = 2a$, respectively. Then,
(a) only $-q$ is in stable equilibrium
(b) none of the charges are in equilibrium
(c) all the charges are in unstable equilibrium
(d) all the charges are in stable equilibrium

67 In the figure below, the capacitance of each capacitor is 3 μF. The effective capacitance between points A and B is

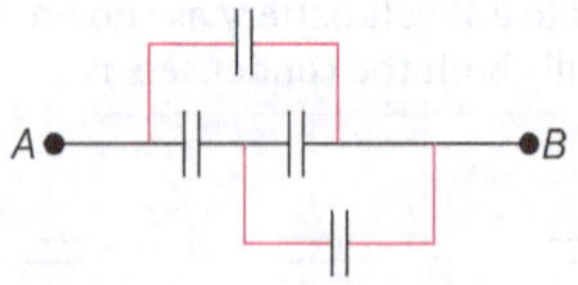

(a) $\frac{3}{4}$ μF (b) 3 μF
(c) 6 μF (d) 5 μF

68 A 500 μF capacitor is charged at the steady rate of 100 μC/s. How long will it take to raise the potential difference between the plates of the capacitor to 10 V ?
(a) 5 s (b) 10 s
(c) 50 s (d) 100 s

69 Three capacitors of capacitances 1 μF, 2 μF and 4 μF are connected first in a series combination, and then in parallel combination. The ratio of their equivalent capacitances will be
(a) 2 : 49 (b) 49 : 2 (c) 4 : 49 (d) 49 : 4

70 Three capacitor of capacitance C (μF) are connected in parallel to which a capacitor of capacitance C is connected in series. Effective capacitance is 3.75, then capacity of each capacitor is
(a) 4 μF (b) 5 μF
(c) 6 μF (d) 8 μF

71 In the given circuit, a charge of +80 μC is given to the upper plate of the 4 μF capacitor. Then, in the steady state, the charge on the upper plate of the 3 μF capacitor is

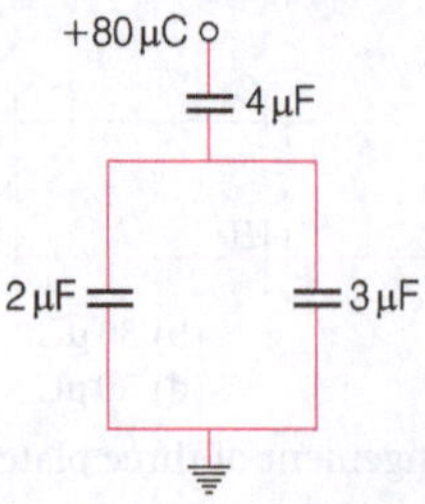

(a) +32 μC (b) +40 μC
(c) +48 μC (d) +80 μC

72 Capacitance of a parallel plate capacitor becomes 4/3 times its original value, if a dielectric slab of thickness $t = d/2$ is inserted between the plates (d is the separation between the plates). The dielectric constant of the slab is
(a) 8 (b) 4
(c) 6 (d) 2

73 Separation between the plates of a parallel plate capacitor is d and the area of each plate is A. When a slab of material of dielectric constant K and thickness t ($t < d$) is introduced between the plates, its capacitance becomes

(a) $\frac{\varepsilon_0 A}{d + t\left(1 - \frac{1}{K}\right)}$ (b) $\frac{\varepsilon_0 A}{d + t\left(1 + \frac{1}{K}\right)}$

(c) $\frac{\varepsilon_0 A}{d - t\left(1 - \frac{1}{K}\right)}$ (d) $\frac{\varepsilon_0 A}{d - t\left(1 + \frac{1}{K}\right)}$

74 The distance between the circular plates of a parallel plate condenser 40 mm in diameter, in order to have same capacity as a sphere of radius 1 m is
(a) 0.01 mm (b) 0.1 mm
(c) 1.0 mm (d) 10 mm

75 The expression for the capacity of the capacitor formed by compound dielectric placed between the plates of a parallel plate capacitor as shown in figure, will be (area of plate = A)

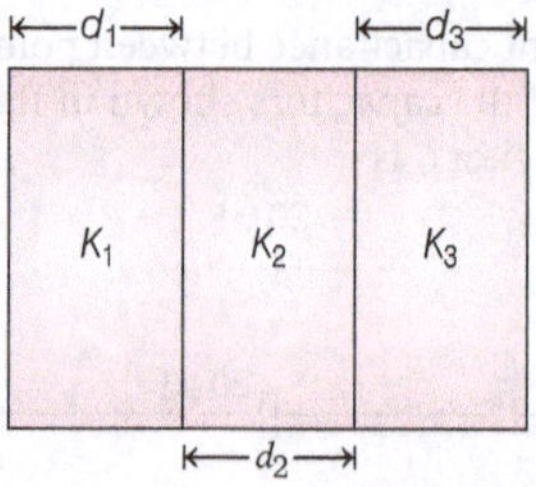

(a) $\frac{\varepsilon_0 A}{\left(\frac{d_1}{K_1} + \frac{d_2}{K_2} + \frac{d_3}{K_3}\right)}$ (b) $\frac{\varepsilon_0 A}{\left(\frac{d_1 + d_2 + d_3}{K_1 + K_2 + K_3}\right)}$

(c) $\frac{\varepsilon_0 A(K_1 K_2 K_3)}{d_1 d_2 d_3}$ (d) $\varepsilon_0 \left(\frac{AK_1}{d_1} + \frac{AK_2}{d_2} + \frac{AK_3}{d_3}\right)$

76 The equivalent capacitance between A and B will be

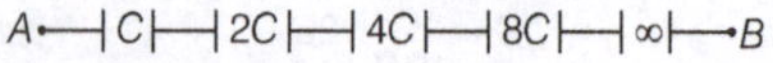

(a) $2C$ (b) $\frac{C}{2}$

(c) $3C$ (d) $\frac{2}{C}$

77 Four plates of equal area A are separated by equal distances d and are arranged as shown in the figure. The equivalent capacity is

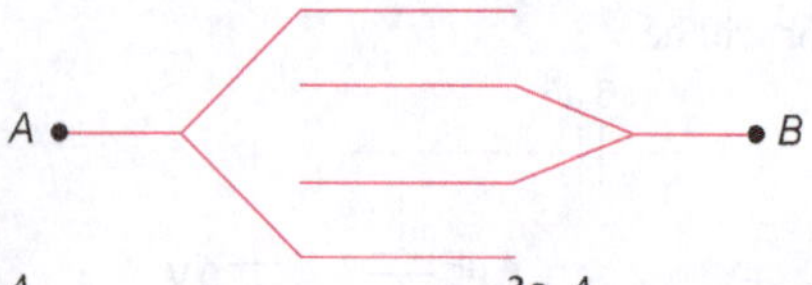

(a) $\frac{2\varepsilon_0 A}{d}$ (b) $\frac{3\varepsilon_0 A}{d}$

(c) $\frac{4\varepsilon_0 A}{d}$ (d) $\frac{\varepsilon_0 A}{d}$

78 Four plates of the same area of cross-section are joined as shown in the figure. The distance between each plate is d. The equivalent capacity across A and B will be

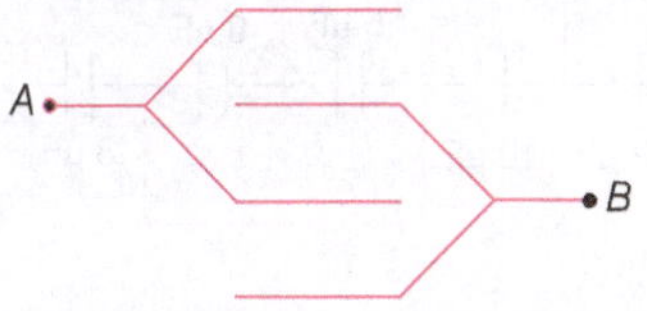

(a) $\frac{2\varepsilon_0 A}{d}$ (b) $\frac{3\varepsilon_0 A}{d}$ (c) $\frac{3\varepsilon_0 A}{2d}$ (d) $\frac{\varepsilon_0 A}{d}$

79 The equivalent capacity between points A and B in figure will be, while capcitance of each capacitor is $3\mu F$.

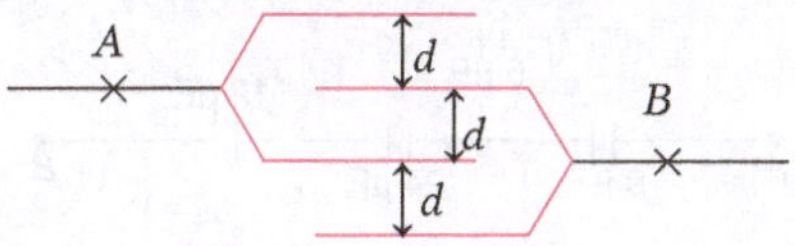

(a) $2\,\mu F$ (b) $4\,\mu F$
(c) $7\,\mu F$ (d) $9\mu F$

80 In the arrangement of capacitors shown in figure, each capacitor is of $9\,\mu F$, then the equivalent capacitance between the points A and B is

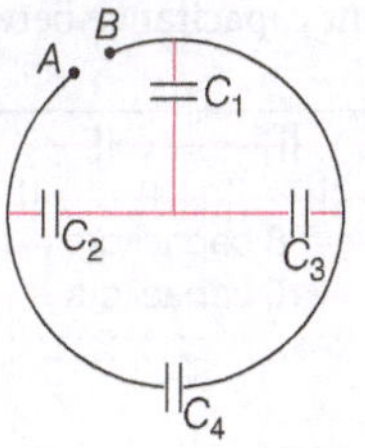

(a) $9\,\mu F$ (b) $18\,\mu F$
(c) $4.5\,\mu F$ (d) $15\,\mu F$

81 Three equal capacitors, each with capacitance C are connected as shown in figure. Then, the equivalent capacitance between point A and B is

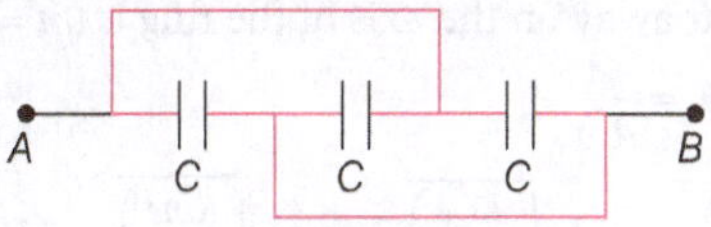

(a) C (b) $3C$
(c) $\frac{C}{3}$ (d) $\frac{3C}{2}$

82 Four capacitors each of capacity $8\,\mu F$ are connected with each other as shown in figure. The equivalent capacitance between points X and Y will be

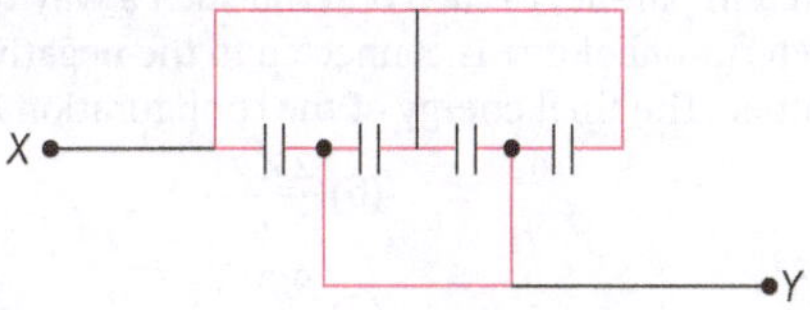

(a) $2\,\mu F$ (b) $8\,\mu F$
(c) $16\,\mu F$ (d) $32\,\mu F$

83 If a slab of insulating material 4×10^{-3}m thick is introduced between the plates of a parallel plate capacitor, the separation between plates has to be increased by 3.5×10^{-3} m to restore the capacity to original value. The dielectric constant of the material will be

(a) 6 (b) 8
(c) 10 (d) 12

84 In this figure, the equivalent capacitance between A and B will be

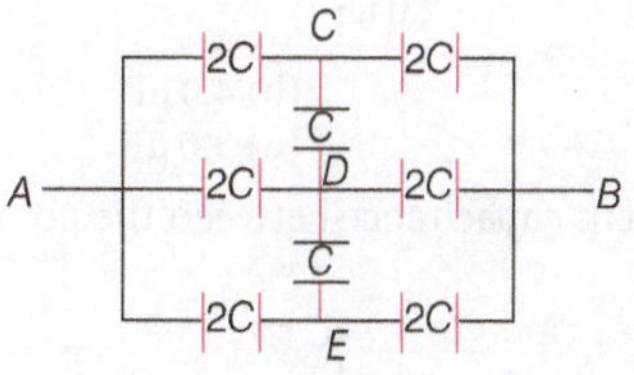

(a) $\frac{C}{2}$ (b) $\frac{C}{3}$
(c) $3C$ (d) $2C$

85 The resultant capacitance of given circuit between points P and Q is

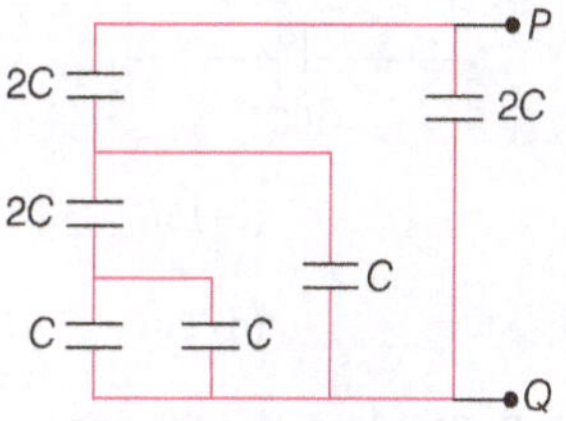

(a) $3C$ (b) $2C$
(c) C (d) $\frac{C}{3}$

86 In the figure, a capacitor is filled with dielectrics. The resultant capacitance is

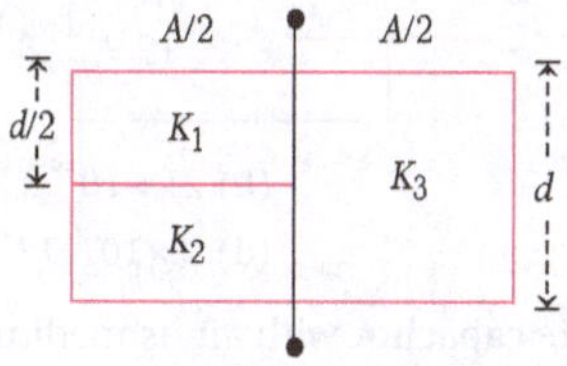

(a) $\frac{2\varepsilon_0 A}{d}\left[\frac{1}{K_1}+\frac{1}{K_2}+\frac{1}{K_3}\right]$ (b) $\frac{\varepsilon_0 A}{d}\left[\frac{1}{K_1}+\frac{1}{K_2}+\frac{1}{K_3}\right]$

(c) $\frac{2\varepsilon_0 A}{d}[K_1+K_2+K_3]$ (d) None of these

87 The equivalent capacitance between points A and B in the circuit will be

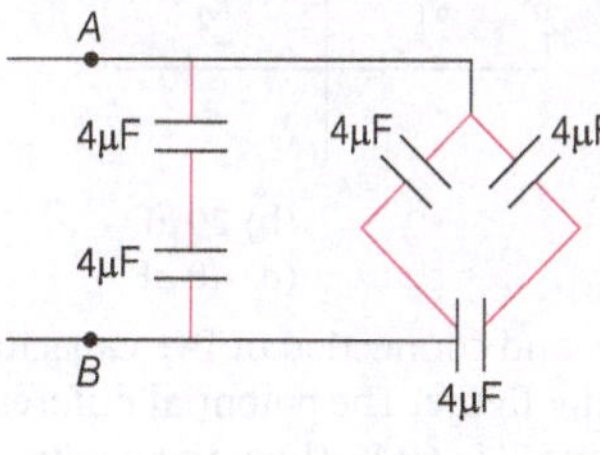

(a) $\frac{10}{3}\mu F$ (b) $4\,\mu F$

(c) $6\,\mu F$ (d) $8\,\mu F$

88 The equivalent capacitance between A and B for the combination of capacitors shown in figure, where all capacitances are in microfarad is

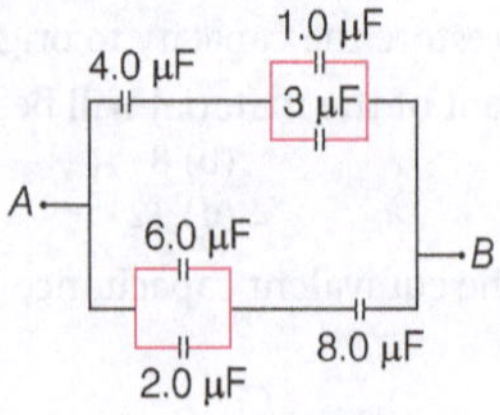

(a) 6.0 μF (b) 4.0 μF
(c) 2.0 μF (d) 3.0 μF

89 The equivalent capacitance between the points A and C is given by

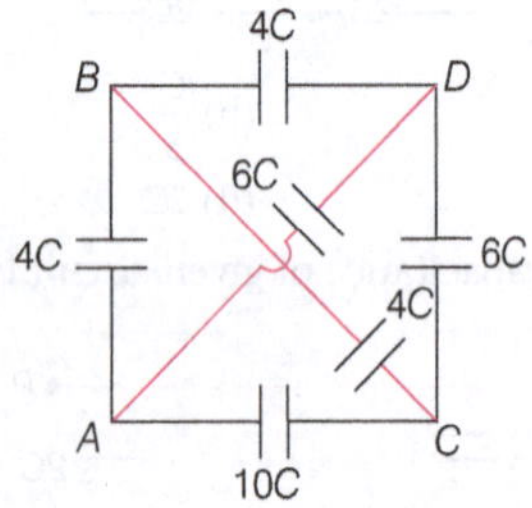

(a) $\frac{10}{3}C$ (b) $15C$
(c) $\frac{3}{10}C$ (d) $20C$

90 Three plates A, B, C each of area 50 cm^2 have separation 3 mm between A and B and 3 mm between B and C. The energy stored when the plates are fully charged is

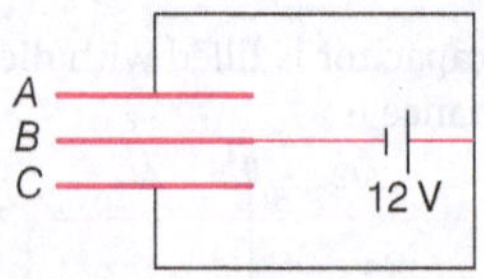

(a) 1.6×10^{-9} J (b) 2.1×10^{-9} J
(c) 5×10^{-9} J (d) 7×10^{-9} J

91 A parallel plate capacitor with air as medium between the plates has a capacitance of 10 μF. The area of capacitor is divided into two equal halves and filled with two media as shown in the figure having dielectric constant $K_1 = 2$ and $K_2 = 4$. The capacitance of the system will now be

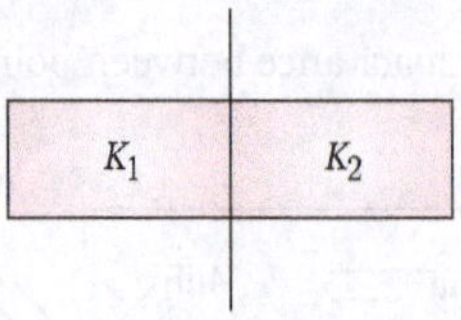

(a) 10 μF (b) 20 μF
(c) 30 μF (d) 40 μF

92 The capacities and connection of five capacitors are shown in the adjoining figure. The potential difference between the points A and B is 60 V. Then, the equivalent capacity between A and B and the charge on 5 μF capacitance will be respectively.

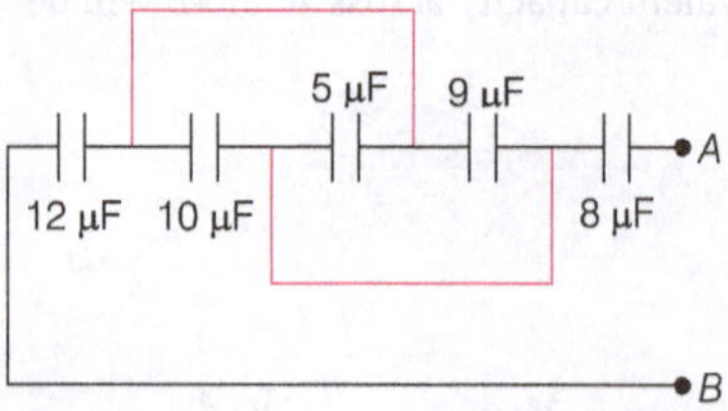

(a) 44 μF, 300 μC (b) 16 μF, 150 μC
(c) 15 μF, 200 μC (d) 4 μF, 50 μC

93 The equivalent capacitance between points A and B will be

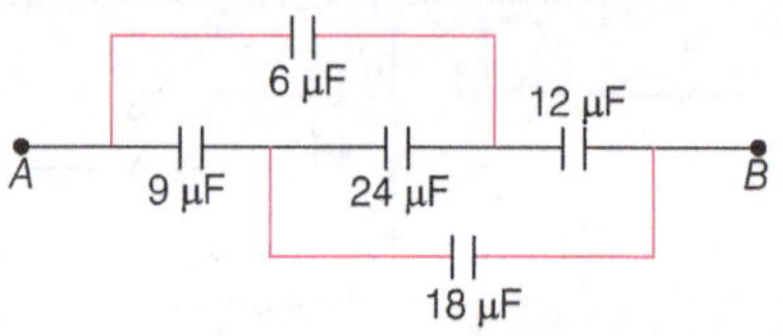

(a) 10 μF (b) 15 μF
(c) 10.8 μF (d) 69 μF

94 An infinite number of identical capacitor each of capacitance 1 μF are connected as shown in the figure. Then, the equivalent capacitance between A and B is

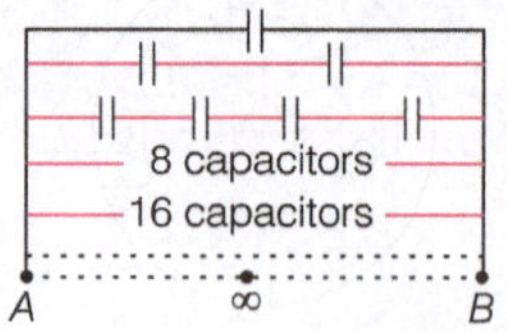

(a) 1 μF (b) $\frac{1}{2}$ μF
(c) 2 μF (d) ∞

95 A charge $+Q$ is uniformly distributed over a thin ring of the radius R. The velocity of an electron at the moment when it passes through the center O of the ring, if the electron was initially far away on the axis of the ring is (m = mass of electron, $K = \frac{1}{4\pi\varepsilon_0}$)

(a) $\sqrt{\left(\frac{2KQe}{mR}\right)}$ (b) $\sqrt{\left(\frac{KQe}{m}\right)}$ (c) $\sqrt{\left(\frac{Kme}{QR}\right)}$ (d) $\sqrt{\left(\frac{KQe}{mR}\right)}$

96 A parallel plate capacitor of capacitance C is connected to a battery and is charged to a potential difference V. Another capacitor of capacitance $2C$ is connected to another battery and is charged to potential difference $2V$. The charging batteries are now disconnected and the capacitors are connected in parallel to each other in such a way that the positive terminal of one is connected to the negative terminal of the other. The final energy of the configuration is

(a) zero (b) $\frac{25CV^2}{6}$
(c) $\frac{3CV^2}{2}$ (d) $\frac{9CV^2}{2}$

97 A battery charges a parallel plate capacitor separated by distance d so, that the energy V_0 is stored in the system. A slab of dielectric constant K and thickness d is then introduced between the plates of capacitor. The new energy of the system is given by

(a) KV_0 (b) K^2V_0 (c) $\frac{V_0}{K}$ (d) $\frac{V_0}{K^2}$

98 Condenser A has a capacity of 15 μF when it is filled with a medium of dielectric constant 15. Another condenser B has a capacity of 1 μF with air between the plates. Both are charged separately by a battery 100 V. After charging, both are connected in parallel without the battery and the dielectric medium being removed. The common potential now is

(a) 400 V (b) 800 V (c) 1200 V (d) 1600 V

99 In the given circuit if point C is connected to the earth and a potential of +2000 V is given to the point A, the potential at B is

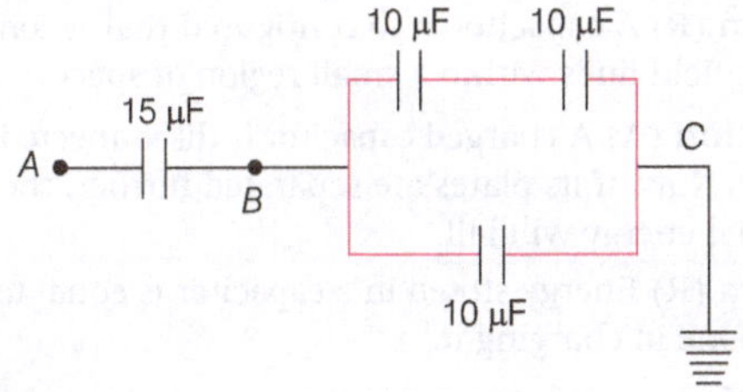

(a) 1500 V (b) 1000 V
(c) 500 V (d) 400 V

100 A network of four capacitors of capacity equal to $C_1 = C$, $C_2 = 2C$, $C_3 = 3C$ and $C_4 = 4C$ are connected to a battery as shown in the figure. The ratio of the charges on C_2 and C_4 is

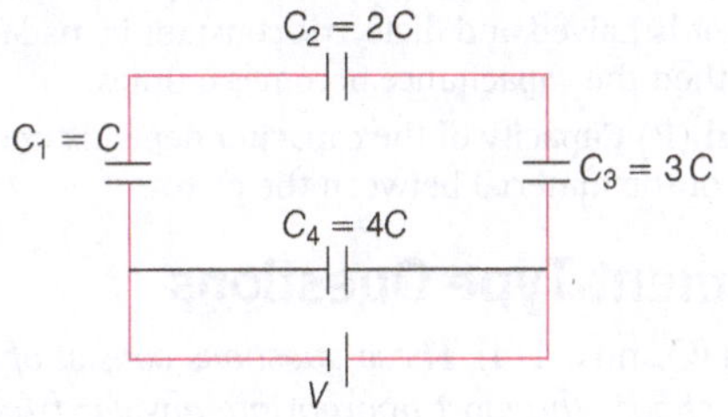

(a) $\frac{22}{3}$ (b) $\frac{3}{22}$
(c) $\frac{7}{4}$ (d) $\frac{4}{7}$

101 A parallel plate capacitor is made of two dielectric blocks in series. One of the blocks has thickness d_1 and dielectric constant K_1 and the other has thickness d_2 and dielectric constant K_2 as shown in figure. This arrangement can be thought as a dielectric slab of thickness d (= $d_1 + d_2$) and effective dielectric constant K. The K is ***[NCERT Exemplar]***

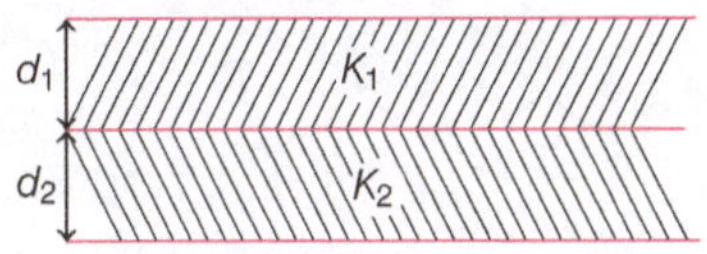

(a) $\frac{K_1d_1 + K_2d_2}{d_1 + d_2}$ (b) $\frac{K_1d_1 + K_2d_2}{K_1 + K_2}$

(c) $\frac{K_1K_2(d_1 + d_2)}{K_1d_2 + K_2d_1}$ (d) $\frac{2K_1K_2}{K_1 + K_2}$

102 A number of condensers, each of the capacitance 1 μF and each one of which gets punctured if a potential difference just exceeding 500 V is applied, are provided. An arrangement suitable for giving capacitance of 2 μF across which 3000 V may be applied requires at least

(a) 6 component capacitors
(b) 12 component capacitors
(c) 72 component capacitors
(d) 2 component capacitors

103 The resultant capacitance between A and B in the following figure is equal to

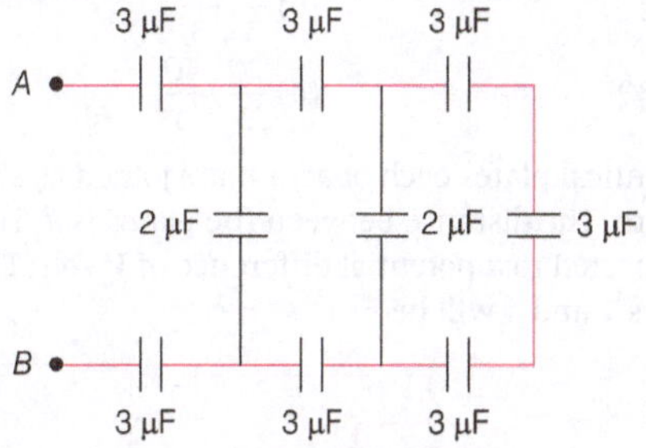

(a) 1 μF (b) 3 μF
(c) 2 μF (d) 1.5 μF

104 In the following circuit, the resultant capacitance between A and B is 1 μF. The value of C is

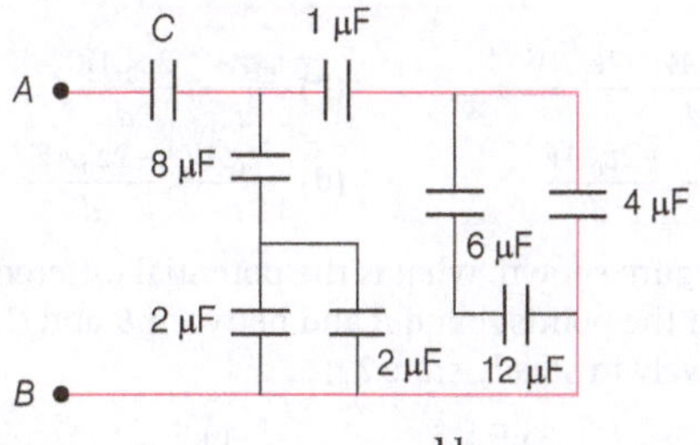

(a) $\frac{32}{11}$ μF (b) $\frac{11}{32}$ μF
(c) $\frac{23}{32}$ μF (d) $\frac{32}{23}$ μF

105 Seven capacitors each of capacity 2 μF are to be connected to have a total capacity 10/11 μF. Which will be the necessary figure as shown ?

(a) 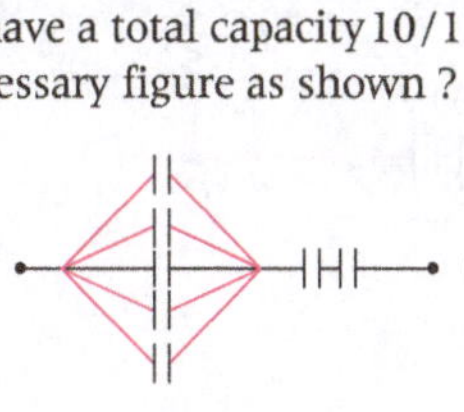 (b) 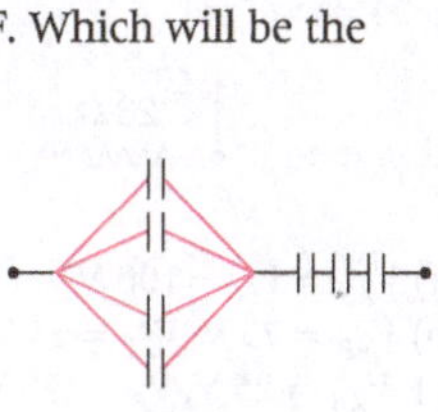

(c) 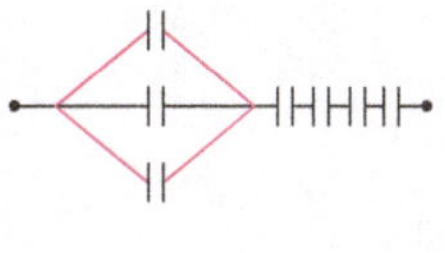 (d) 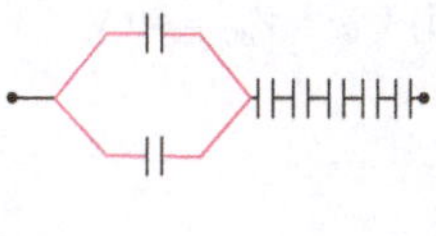

106 Two capacitors C_1 and $C_2 = 2C_1$ are connected in a circuit with a switch between them as shown in the figure. Initially the switch is open and C_1 holds charge Q. The switch is closed. At steady state, the charge on each capacitor will be

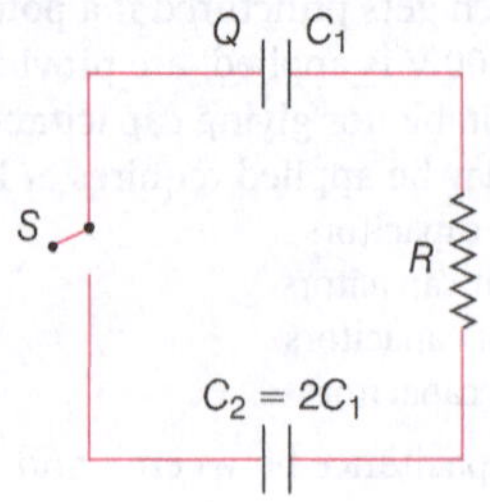

(a) $Q, 2Q$ (b) $\frac{Q}{3}, \frac{2Q}{3}$

(c) $\frac{3Q}{2}, 3Q$ (d) $\frac{2Q}{3}, \frac{4Q}{3}$

107 Five identical plates each of area A are joined as shown in the figure. The distance between the plates is d. The plates are connected to a potential difference of V volt. The charge on plates 1 and 4 will be

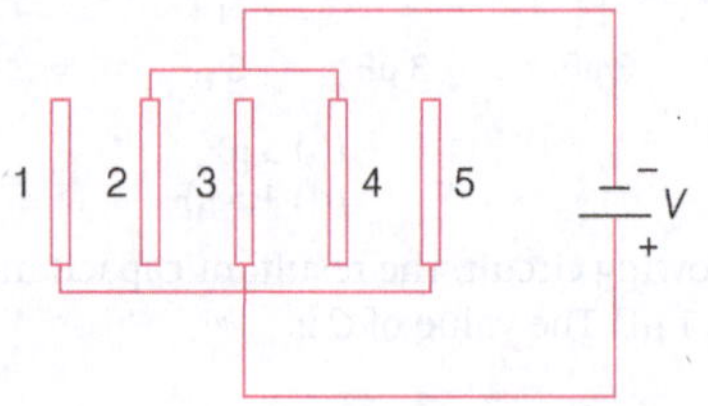

(a) $-\frac{\varepsilon_0 AV}{d}, \frac{2\varepsilon_0 AV}{d}$ (b) $\frac{\varepsilon_0 AV}{d}, \frac{2\varepsilon_0 AV}{d}$

(c) $\frac{\varepsilon_0 AV}{d}, \frac{-2\varepsilon_0 AV}{d}$ (d) $\frac{-\varepsilon_0 AV}{d}, \frac{-2\varepsilon_0 AV}{d}$

108 In the figure shown, what is the potential difference between the points A and B and between B and C respectively in steady state ?

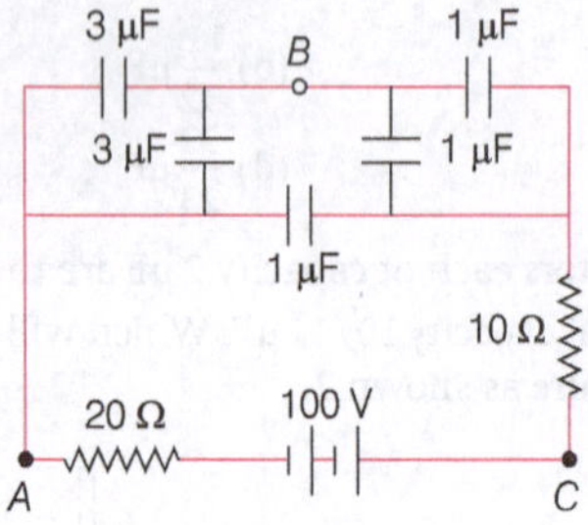

(a) $V_{AB} = V_{BC} = 100$ V
(b) $V_{AB} = 75$ V, $V_{BC} = 25$ V
(c) $V_{AB} = 25$ V, $V_{BC} = 75$ V
(d) $V_{AB} = V_{BC} = 50$ V

Assertion and Reason

Directions (Q. Nos. 1-5) *These questions consist of two statement each linked as Assertion (A) and Reason (R). While answering these questions you are required to choose any one of the following four responses.*

(a) Both A and R are true but R is not the correct explanation of A.
(b) A is true but R is false.
(c) A is false but R is true.
(d) Both A and R are true and R is the correct explanation of A.

1 **Assertion** (A) The capacity of a given conductor remains same even if charge is varied on it.
Reason (R) Capacitance depends upon nearly medium as well as size and shape of conductor.

2 **Assertion** (A) The potential difference between the two conductors of a capacitor is small.
Reason (R) A capacitor is so configured that it confines the electric field lines within a small region of space.

3 **Assertion** (A) A charged capacitor is disconnected from a battery. Now, if its plates are separated further, the potential energy will fall.
Reason (R) Energy stored in a capacitor is equal to the work done in charging it.

4 **Assertion** (A) When a capacitor is charged by a battery, half of the energy supplied by the battery is stored in the capacitor and rest half is lost.
Reason (R) If resistance in the circuit is zero, then there will be no loss of energy.

5 **Assertion** (A) If the distance between parallel plates of a capacitor is halved and dielectric constant is made three times, then the capacitance becomes 6 times.
Reason (R) Capacity of the capacitor depends upon the nature of the material between the plates.

Statement Type Questions

Directions (Q. nos. 1-4) *These questions consist of two statements, choose the most appropriate answer from the options given below.*

(a) Both Statement I and Statement II are incorrect.
(b) Statement I is correct but Statement II is incorrect.
(c) Statement I is incorrect but Statement II is correct.
(d) Both Statement I and Statement II are correct.

1 **Statement I** Charge never flows from a condenser of higher capacity to the condenser of lower capacity.
Statement II Flow of charge between two bodies connected by a thin wire is determined by the charges on them.

2 **Statement I** A capacitor of a certain capacity, whenever charged, will always store the same amount of charge.

Statement II A definite capacity implies always a same definite value of charge.

3 **Statement I** The force between the plates of a parallel plate capacitor is proportional to charge on it.

Statement II Electric force is equal to charge per unit area.

4 **Statement I** When a capacitor is connected to a battery it is charged instantly.

Statement II Current travels in a wire at a speed of light.

Match the Columns

1 Match the Column I (parameter of capacitor) with Column II (value) and select the correct answer from the codes given below. Consider a dielectric inserted between the plates fully occupying the intervening region. The surface charge densities on the charged plates are $\pm\sigma$.

Column I		Column II	
A.	Electric field E	I.	$Qd/A\varepsilon_0K$
B.	Potential difference across the plates V	II.	$(\sigma - \sigma_p)/\varepsilon_0$
C.	The capacitance C, with dielectric between the plates	III.	C/C_0
D.	Dielectric constant of the substance K	IV.	ε_0KA/d

Choose the correct answer from the option given below.

(a) A-(I), B-(II), C-(III), D-(IV)
(b) A-(III), B-(IV), C-(I), D-(II)
(c) A-(IV), B-(II), C-(III), D-(I)
(d) A-(II), B-(I), C-(IV), D-(III)

2 A dielectric slab of thickness 1.0 cm and dielectric constant 5 is placed between the plates of a parallel plate capacitor of plates area 0.01 m^2 and separation 2.0 cm.

Column I		Column II	
A.	Capacity with air in between the plates	I.	2.95×10^{-12}F
B.	Capacity with dielectric slab in between the plates	II.	8.85×10^{-12} F
C.	Capacity with conducting slab in between the plates	III.	7.375×10^{-12} F
D.	Increase in capacity on introduction of dielectric	IV.	4.425×10^{-12} F

Choose the correct answer from the options given below

(a) A-(I), B-(IV), C-(II), D-(III)
(b) A-(IV), B-(III), C-(II), D-(I)
(c) A-(III), B-(IV), C-(I), D-(II)
(d) A-(II), B-(I), C-(IV), D-(III)

3 The area of parallel plates of an air-filled capacitor is 0.20 m^2 and the distance between them is 0.01 m. The potential difference across the plates is 3000 V. When a 0.01 m thick dielectric sheet is introduced between the plates, then the potential difference decreases to 1000 V.

Column I		Column II	
A.	Capacitance of air-filled capacitor (in F)	I.	5.31×10^{-7}
B.	Charge on each plate (in C)	II.	5.31×10^{-10}
C.	Dielectric constant of the material	III.	3
D.	Capacitance after the dielectric sheet is introduced (in F)	IV.	1.77×10^{-10}

Choose the correct answer from the option given below.

(a) A-(I), B-(III), C-(IV), D-(II)
(b) A-(II), B-(IV), C-(I), D-(III)
(c) A-(IV), B-(I), C-(III), D-(II)
(d) A-(III), B-(II), C-(I), D- (IV)

4 Match the Column I (charge on capacitor) with Column II (value).

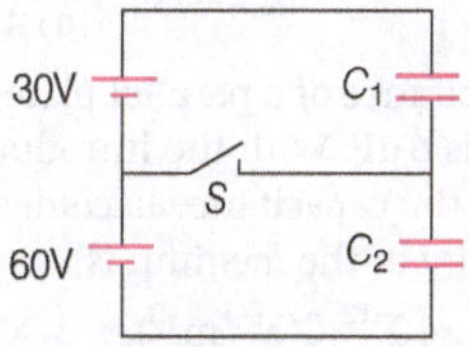

Column I		Column II	
A.	Charges on both the capacitors (S open)	I.	108 μC
B.	Charge on C_2 (S closed)	II.	240 μC
C.	Charge on C_1 (S closed)	III.	60 μC
D.	Charge on C_1 and C_2 (S closed)	IV.	180 μC

Choose the correct answer from the options given below.

(a) A-(II), B-(III), C-(I), D-(IV)
(b) A-(IV), B-(II), C-(I), D-(III)
(c) A-(I), B-(IV), C-(III), D-(II)
(d) A-(I), B-(II), C-(III), D-(IV)

Final Check Through PYQs

Module-I Electrostatics of Conductors and Capacitors

1 A parallel plate capacitor having cross-sectional area A and separation d has air in between the plates. Now, an insulating slab of same area but thickness $d/2$ is inserted between the plates as shown in figure having dielectric constant K (= 4). The ratio of new capacitance to its original capacitance will be

[NCERT (New) Pg. 68, NEET (Oct.) 2020]

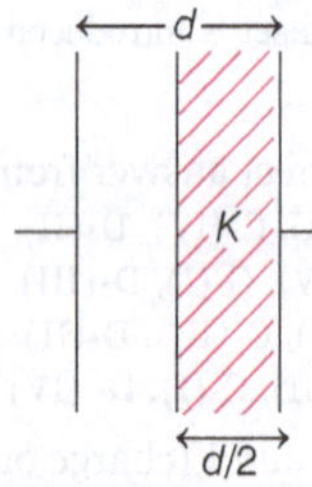

(a) 2 : 1
(b) 8 : 5
(c) 6 : 5
(d) 4 : 1

2 The capacitance of a parallel plate capacitor with air as medium is 6 μF. With the introduction of a dielectric medium, the capacitance becomes 30 μF. The permittivity of the medium is

($\varepsilon_0 = 8.85 \times 10^{-12}\ C^2N^{-1}m^{-2}$)

[NCERT (New) Pg. 68, NEET (Sep.) 2020]

(a) $1.77 \times 10^{-12}\ C^2N^{-1}m^{-2}$
(b) $0.44 \times 10^{-10}\ C^2N^{-1}m^{-2}$
(c) $5.00\ C^2N^{-1}m^{-2}$
(d) $0.44 \times 10^{-13}\ C^2N^{-1}m^{-2}$

3 The electrostatic force between the metal plates of an isolated parallel plate capacitor C having a charge Q and area A, is ***[NCERT (New) Pg. 68, NEET 2018]***

(a) proportional to the square root of the distance between the plates
(b) linearly proportional to the distance between the plates
(c) independent of the distance between the plates
(d) inversely proportional to the distance between the plates

4 A parallel plate air capacitor has capacity C, distance of separation between plates is d and potential difference V is applied between the plates. Force of attraction between the plates of the parallel plate air capacitor is

[NCERT (New) Pg. 68, AIPMT 2015]

(a) $\frac{C^2V^2}{2d}$
(b) $\frac{CV^2}{2d}$
(c) $\frac{CV^2}{d}$
(d) $\frac{C^2V^2}{2d^2}$

Module-II Combination of Capacitors

5 In the following circuit, the equivalent capacitance between terminal A and terminal B is

[NCERT (New) Pg. 72, NEET 2024]

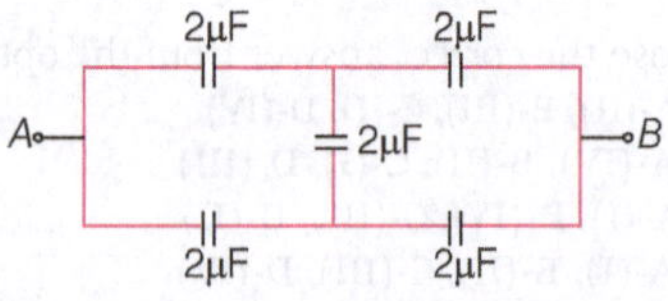

(a) 2 μF
(b) 1 μF
(c) 0.5 μF
(d) 4 μF

6 The equivalent capacitance of the system shown in the following circuit is ***[NCERT (New) Pg. 72, NEET 2023]***

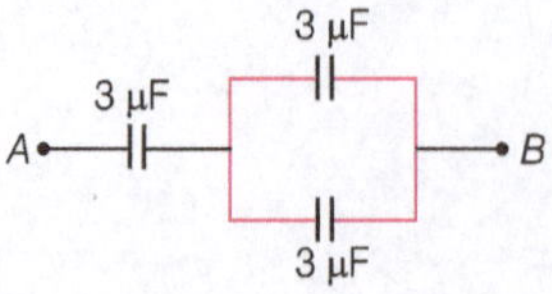

(a) 3 μF
(b) 6 μF
(c) 9 μF
(d) 2 μF

7 A parallel plate capacitor of area A, plate separation d and capacitance C is filled with four dielectric materials having dielectric constants K_1, K_2, K_3 and k_4 as shown in the figure below. If a single dielectric material is to be used to have the same capacitance C in this capacitor, then its dielectric constant k is given by

[NCERT (New) Pg. 70, NEET 2021]

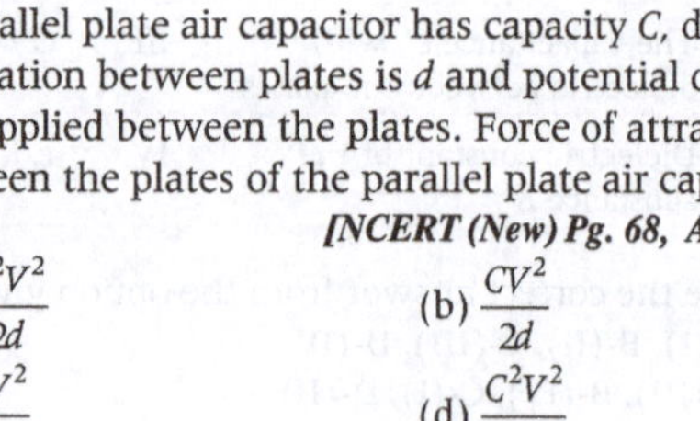

(a) $K = K_1 + K_2 + K_3 + 3K_4$
(b) $K = \frac{2}{3}(K_1 + K_2 + K_3) + 2K_4$

(c) $\frac{2}{K} = \frac{3}{K_1 + K_2 + K_3} + \frac{1}{K_4}$

(d) $\frac{1}{K} = \frac{1}{K_1} + \frac{1}{K_2} + \frac{1}{K_3} + \frac{3}{2K_4}$

8 The equivalent capacitance of the combination shown in the figure is *[NCERT (New) Pg. 72, NEET 2021]*

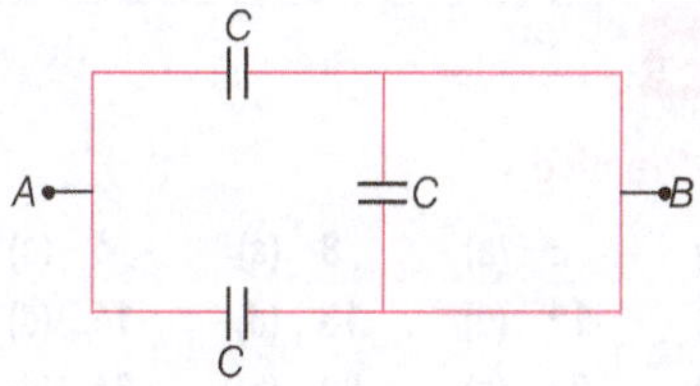

(a) $3C$ (b) $2C$ (c) $\frac{C}{2}$ (d) $\frac{3C}{2}$

Module-III Energy of Capacitors

9. If the plates of a parallel plate capacitor connected to a battery are moved close to each other, then *[NCERT (New) Pg. 74, NEET 2024]*

A. the charge stored in it, increases.
B. the energy stored in it, decreases.
C. its capacitance increases.
D. the ratio of charge to its potential remains the same.
E. the product of charge and voltage increases.

Choose the most appropriate answer from the options given below

(a) A, B and E only (b) A, C and E only
(c) B, D and E only (d) A, B and C only

10 A capacitor of capacitance $C = 900$ pF is charged fully by 100 V battery B as shown in figure (i). Then, it is disconnected from the battery and connected to another uncharged capacitor of capacitance $C = 900$ pF as shown in figure (ii). The electrostatic energy stored by the system (ii) is *[NCERT (New) Pg. 74, NEET 2021]*

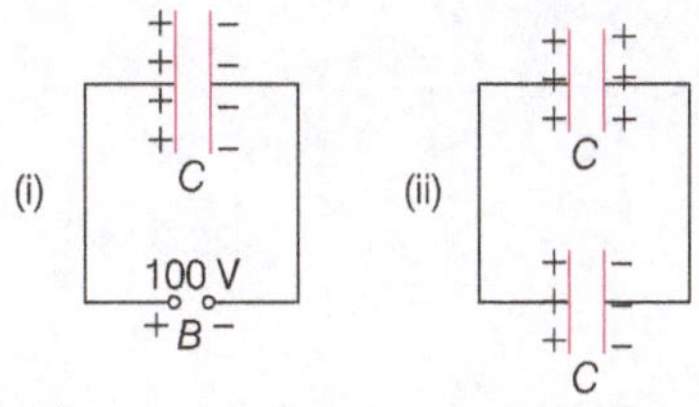

(a) 3.25×10^{-6} J (b) 2.25×10^{-6} J
(c) 1.5×10^{-6} J (d) 4.5×10^{-6} J

11 A parallel plate capacitor has a uniform electric field **E** in the space between the plates. If the distance between the plates is d and the area of each plate is A, the energy stored in the capacitor is
(ε_0 = permittivity of free space). *[NCERT (New) Pg. 74, NEET 2021]*

(a) $\frac{1}{2}\varepsilon_0 E^2$ (b) $\varepsilon_0 EAd$
(c) $\frac{1}{2}\varepsilon_0 E^2 Ad$ (d) $\frac{E^2 Ad}{\varepsilon_0}$

12 Two identical capacitors C_1 and C_2 of equal capacitance are connected as shown in the circuit. Terminals a and b of the key k are connected to charge capacitor C_1 using battery of emf V volt. Now, disconnecting a and b the terminals b and c are connected. Due to this, what will be the percentage loss of energy? *[NCERT (New) Pg. 74, NEET (Odisha) 2019]*

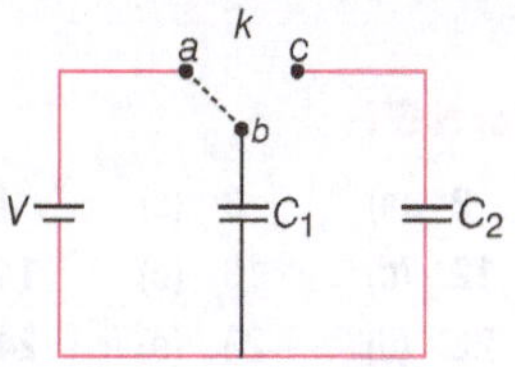

(a) 75% (b) 0%
(c) 50% (d) 25%

13 A capacitor is charged by a battery. The battery is removed and another identical uncharged capacitor is connected in parallel. The total electrostatic energy of resulting system *[NCERT (New) Pg. 74, NEET 2017]*

(a) increases by a factor of 4
(b) decreases by a factor of 2
(c) remains the same
(d) increases by a factor of 2

14 A capacitor of 2 μF is charged as shown in the figure. When the switch S is turned to position 2, the percentage of its stored energy dissipated is *[NCERT (New) Pg. 74, NEET 2016]*

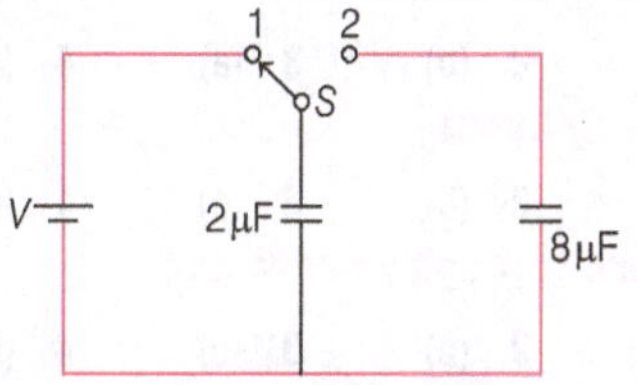

(a) 20% (b) 75%
(c) 80% (d) 0%

15 A parallel plate air capacitor of capacitance C is connected to a cell of emf V and then disconnected from it. A dielectric slab of dielectric constant K, which can just fill the air gap of the capacitor, is now inserted in it. Which of the following is incorrect ? *[NCERT (New) Pg. 74, AIPMT 2015]*

(a) The potential difference between the plates decreases K times.
(b) The energy stored in the capacitor decreases K times.
(c) The change in energy stored is $\frac{1}{2}CV^2\left(\frac{1}{K} - 1\right)$.
(d) The charge on the capacitor is not conserved.

Answers

Step up Practice 1

1 (d)	2 (a)	3 (a)	4 (c)	5 (c)	6 (c)	7 (d)	8 (a)	9 (c)	10 (d)
11 (c)	12 (d)	13 (d)	14 (d)	15 (d)	16 (b)	17 (b)	18 (b)	19 (a)	20 (c)
21 (d)	22 (a)	23 (b)	24 (d)						

Step up Practice 2

1 (c)	2 (c)	3 (a)	4 (a)	5 (d)	6 (c)	7 (b)	8 (b)	9 (d)	10 (a)
11 (a)	12 (b)	13 (c)	14 (d)	15 (d)	16 (c)	17 (d)	18 (b)	19 (d)	20 (b)

Step up Practice 3

1 (c)	2 (a)	3 (b)	4 (d)	5 (d)	6 (b)	7 (c)	8 (a)	9 (c)	10 (c)
11 (c)	12 (d)	13 (b)	14 (a)	15 (b)	16 (b)	17 (c)	18 (d)	19 (c)	20 (c)
21 (b)									

Gearing up for NEET

1 (a)	2 (a)	3 (c)	4 (c)	5 (b)	6 (d)	7 (b)	8 (b)	9 (c)	10 (b)
11 (c)	12 (d)	13 (c)	14 (c)	15 (a)	16 (c)	17 (d)	18 (a)	19 (b)	20 (a)
21 (d)	22 (d)	23 (b)	24 (c)	25 (b)	26 (d)	27 (a)	28 (c)	29 (d)	30 (b)
31 (c)	32 (b)	33 (a)	34 (d)	35 (a)	36 (a)	37 (a)	38 (d)	39 (b)	40 (b)
41 (b)	42 (d)	43 (d)	44 (c)	45 (a)	46 (c)	47 (b)	48 (d)	49 (b)	50 (c)
51 (d)	52 (b)	53 (d)	54 (b)	55 (b)	56 (d)	57 (a)	58 (a)	59 (d)	60 (a)
61 (c)	62 (c)	63 (c)	64 (c)	65 (b)	66 (c)	67 (d)	68 (c)	69 (c)	70 (b)
71 (c)	72 (d)	73 (c)	74 (b)	75 (a)	76 (b)	77 (a)	78 (b)	79 (d)	80 (d)
81 (b)	82 (d)	83 (b)	84 (c)	85 (a)	86 (d)	87 (d)	88 (a)	89 (b)	90 (b)
91 (c)	92 (d)	93 (a)	94 (c)	95 (a)	96 (c)	97 (a)	98 (b)	99 (b)	100 (b)
101 (c)	102 (c)	103 (a)	104 (d)	105 (a)	106 (b)	107 (c)	108 (c)		

Assertion and Reason

1 (d)	2 (d)	3 (c)	4 (b)	5 (a)

Statement Type Questions

1 (a)	2 (b)	3 (a)	4 (c)

Match the Columns

1 (d)	2 (b)	3 (c)	4 (c)

Final Check Through PYQs Module-I

1 (b)	2 (b)	3 (c)	4 (b)

Final Check Through PYQs Module-II

5 (a)	6 (d)	7 (c)	8 (b)

Final Check Through PYQs Module-III

9 (b)	10 (b)	11 (c)	12 (c)	13 (b)	14 (c)	15 (d)

Hints and Solutions

Step up Practice 1

1. (*d*) H_2, O_2, N_2 etc., are not polar dielectrics.

3. (*a*) In the absence of an external electric field, the dipole moment of dielectric with polar molecules is zero because the dipoles of polar dielectric is randomly positioned.

4. (*c*) Statement I is incorrect but Statement II is correct.

In the absence of an externally applied electric field, the displacement per unit volume of a polar dielectric material is always zero.

5. (*c*) Volume of 8 small drops = Volume of big drop

$$8 \times \frac{4}{3}\pi r^3 = \frac{4}{3}\pi R^3 \Rightarrow R = 2r$$

As, capacity is proportional to *r*, hence capacity become 2 times.

6. (*c*) For spherical conductor,

$$C = 4\pi\varepsilon_0 R$$

$$\because \quad V = \frac{4}{3}\pi R^3 \text{ and } A = 4\pi R^2$$

$$\therefore \quad R = \frac{3V}{A}$$

$$\therefore \text{Capacitance, } C = 12\pi\varepsilon_0 \frac{V}{A}$$

7. (*d*) Given, $2\pi R = 2 \Rightarrow R = \frac{1}{\pi}$

For sphere, $C = 4\pi\varepsilon_0 KR$

$$\Rightarrow \quad C = \frac{1}{9 \times 10^9} \times \frac{1}{\pi} \times 80 \qquad \text{(for water } K = 80\text{)}$$

Capacitance of sphere,

$$C = 2828.28 \text{ pF} \approx 2800 \text{ pF}$$

8. (*a*) Charge flows from high potential to low potential. Equal potential will not allow flow of charge in any direction.

10. (*d*) Both Statement I and Statement II are correct.

A capacitor can be given only a limited quantity of charge because every dielectric is limited by the dielectric strength of medium between the plates. The dielectric strength is a maximum value of electric field that it can handle without breakdown. Beyond this field the dielectric no more behave as dielectric but it conduct electric and become conductor.

11. (*c*) Since, aluminium is a metal and very thin, therefore field inside this will be zero. Hence, it would not affect the field in between the two plates, so capacity $= \frac{q}{V} = \frac{q}{Ed}$, remains unchanged.

12. (*d*) We have, $C = \frac{\varepsilon_0 A}{d} \Rightarrow C \propto \frac{1}{d}$

Therefore, the capacity of parallel plate condenser depends on the separation between the plates.

13. (*d*) $C = \frac{\varepsilon_0 A}{d}$. As $A \to \frac{1}{2}$ times and $d \to 2$ times

So, $C \to \frac{1}{4}$ times, *i.e.* $C' = \frac{1}{4}C = \frac{12}{4} = 3\,\mu\text{F}$

14. (*d*) Capacitance, $C_{\text{medium}} = KC_{\text{air}}$

$$\Rightarrow K = \frac{C_{\text{medium}}}{C_{\text{air}}} = \frac{110}{50} = 2.20$$

15. (*d*) Both Statement I and Statement II are correct.

Capacitance of parallel plate capacitor is $C = \frac{\varepsilon_0 A}{d}$.

Thus, distance decreases and capacitance of capacitor increases.

16. (*b*) $C = \frac{\varepsilon_0 A}{d} = 1 \text{ pF}$

and $\quad C = \frac{K\varepsilon_0 A}{2d} = 2 \text{ pF}$

$\therefore \quad K = 4$

17. (*b*) Statement I is correct but Statement II is incorrect.

The capacitance *C*, with dielectric between the plates is given as

$$C = \frac{\varepsilon_0 KA}{d}$$

As, $\quad d' = \frac{d}{2}, K' = 3K$

Then new capacitance is

$$C' = \frac{\varepsilon_0 3KA}{d/2} = 6C$$

The capacitance *C* depends only on the geometrical configuration of the system of two conductors.

18. (*b*)

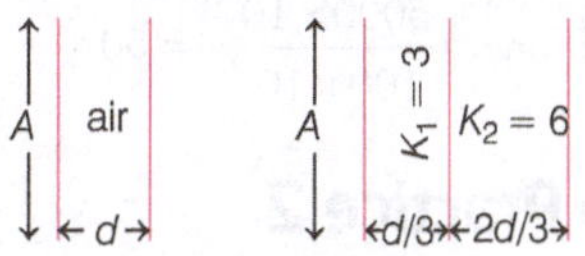

Capacitance in air, $C_{\text{air}} = \frac{\varepsilon_0 A}{d} = 9$

Capacitance in medium,

$$\frac{1}{C_{\text{medium}}} = \frac{1}{C_1} + \frac{1}{C_2}$$

$$= \frac{d_1}{K_1\varepsilon_0 A} + \frac{d_2}{K_2\varepsilon_0 A}$$

$$\Rightarrow \quad C_{\text{medium}} = \frac{K_1K_2\varepsilon_0A}{K_1d_2 + K_2d_1}$$

$$= \frac{3 \times 6 \times \varepsilon_0 A}{3 \times 2d/3 + 6 \times d/3}$$

$$= \frac{18}{4} \times 9 = 40.5 \text{ pF}$$

19. (*a*) Parallel plate capacitor,

$$C = K\varepsilon_0 A/d$$

As, given in figure, for series combination,

$$\frac{1}{C'} = \frac{1}{\dfrac{\varepsilon_0 A}{\frac{d}{2}}} + \frac{1}{\dfrac{2\varepsilon_0 A}{\frac{d}{2}}}$$

$$\Rightarrow \quad C = \frac{4}{3}\frac{\varepsilon_0 A}{d}$$

20. (*c*) Statement I is incorrect but Statement II is correct.
The capacity of a parallel plate condenser is,

$$C = \frac{q}{V}$$

Electric field intensity becomes $\frac{1}{K}$ times, therefore potential V also becomes $\frac{1}{K}$ times.
Hence, from above equation capacity becomes K times.
Thus electric field decreases and capacitance increases.

22. (*a*) The potential difference across the parallel plate capacitor

$$V = 10 - (-10) = 20 \text{ V}$$

$$\therefore \quad \text{Capacitance} = \frac{Q}{V} = \frac{40}{20} = 2 \text{ F}$$

23. (*b*) $Q = CV \Rightarrow C \propto \frac{1}{V}$ or $\frac{V_1}{V_2} = \frac{C_2}{C_1}$

24. (*d*) Charge on capacitor, when its potential becomes 10 V,

$$Q = CV = 500 \times 10^{-6} \times 10$$

$$= 5000 \times 10^{-6} \ \mu\text{C}$$

$$\therefore \text{Required time} = \frac{5000 \times 10^{-6}}{100 \times 10^{-6}} = 50 \text{ s}$$

Step up Practice 2

1. (*c*) Capacitor are in series,

$$\frac{1}{C'} = \frac{1}{C} + \frac{1}{C} + \frac{1}{C} = \frac{3}{C}$$

$$\therefore \text{ Capacitance, } C' = \frac{C}{3}$$

Total voltage of the series combination,

$$V' = V_1 + V_2 + V_3$$

$$= V + V + V = 3V$$

2. (*c*) In series, $\frac{1}{C} = \frac{1}{2} + \frac{1}{2} + \frac{1}{2}$

$$\Rightarrow \text{Capacitance, } C = \frac{2}{3} \text{ F}$$

3. (*a*) Both A and R are true but R is not correct explanation of A.
The equivalent capacitance in series combination,

$$\frac{1}{C_s} = \frac{1}{C} + \frac{1}{C} = \frac{2}{C}$$

$$\Rightarrow \quad C_s = \frac{C}{2}$$

Equivalent capacitance in parallel combination,

$$C_p = C + C = 2C$$

So, required ratio

$$\frac{C_p}{C_s} = \frac{2C}{C/2} = 4:1$$

4. (*a*) For four capacitors in series, the C_{eq} is $\frac{1}{2}$ μF not 10 μF.

5. (*d*) Equivalent capacitance $= \frac{2 \times 3}{2 + 3} = \frac{6}{5}$ μF

Total charge by $Q = CV = \frac{6}{5} \times 1000 = 1200$ μC

Potential V across 2 μF is,

$$V = \frac{Q}{C} = \frac{1200}{2} = 600 \text{ V}$$

$\therefore$ Potential on inner plates $= 1000 - 600 = 400$ V

6. (*c*) Capacitors are in series,

$$\frac{1}{C_{\text{eq}}} = \frac{1}{1} + \frac{1}{2} + \frac{1}{8} \Rightarrow C_{\text{eq}} = \frac{8}{13} \ \mu\text{F}$$

Total charge, $Q = C_{\text{eq}}V = \frac{8}{13} \times 13 = 8$ μC

Potential difference across 2 μF capacitor $= \frac{8}{2} = 4$ V

7. (*b*) Capacitance, $C_1 = \frac{C}{4}$ (series)

Capacitance, $C_2 = 4C$ (parallel)

The ratio of capacitance, $\frac{C_1}{C_2} = \frac{C/4}{4C} = \frac{1}{16}$

8. (*b*) The given circuit can be drawn as follows

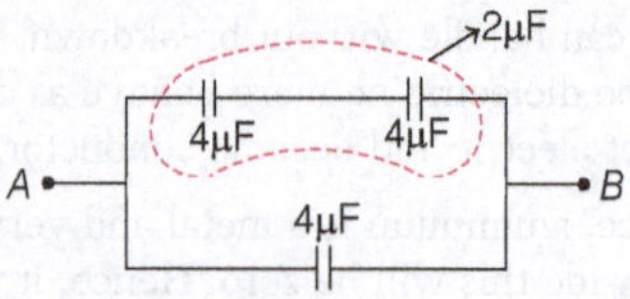

Effective capacitance, $C_{AB} = 2 + 4 = 6$ μF

9. (*d*) Both A and R are true but R is the correct explanation of A.

In series the capacitors will have same charge, if they are initially uncharged.

Also, $V = \dfrac{q}{C}$

If q same, then $V \propto \dfrac{1}{C}$.

10. (*a*) The given circuit can be simplified as follows

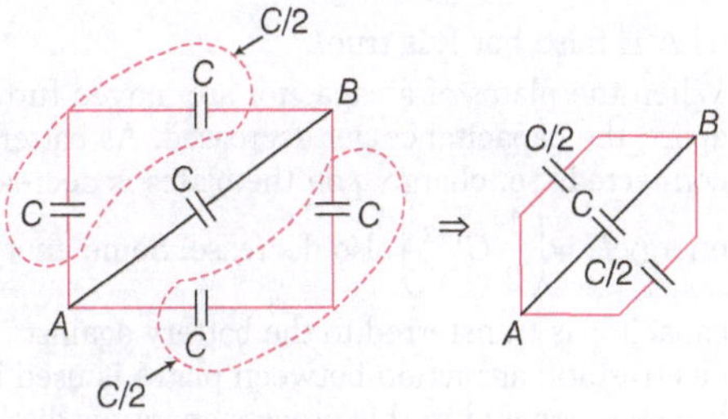

Equivalent capacitance between A and B is

$$C_{AB} = \frac{C}{2} + \frac{C}{2} + C = 2C$$

11. (*a*)

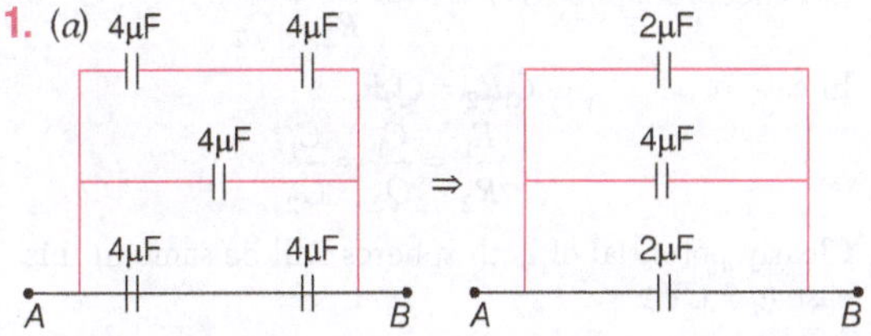

Therefore, capacitor 2 μF, 4 μF and 2 μF are in parallel.
So, equivalent capacitance between A and B

$$C_{AB} = 2 + 4 + 2 = 8\ \mu\text{F}$$

12. (*b*) In parallel, capacitance will increase because

$$C_{\text{parallel}} = C_1 + C_2 + C_3$$

$$\frac{1}{C_{\text{series}}} = \frac{1}{C_1} + \frac{1}{C_2} + \frac{1}{C_3}$$

So, $C_{\text{parallel}} > C_{\text{series}}$

Therefore, A is true and R is false.

13. (*c*) Given, circuit is special case of Wheatstone bridge. So, C_2 can be treated as open circuit.

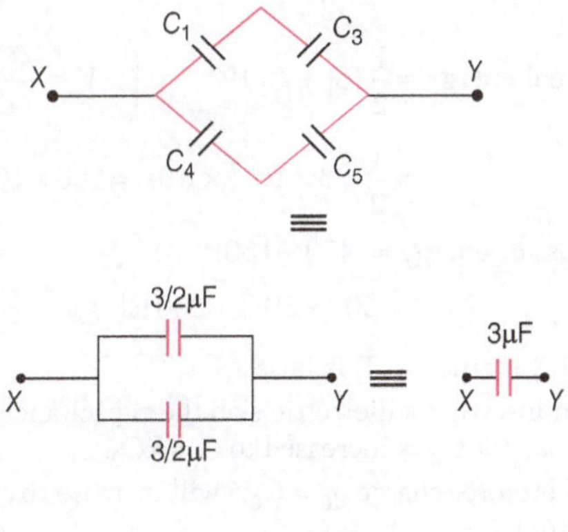

14. (*d*) Both A and R are true and R is the correct explanation of A.

16. (*c*) The given circuit can be simplified as follows

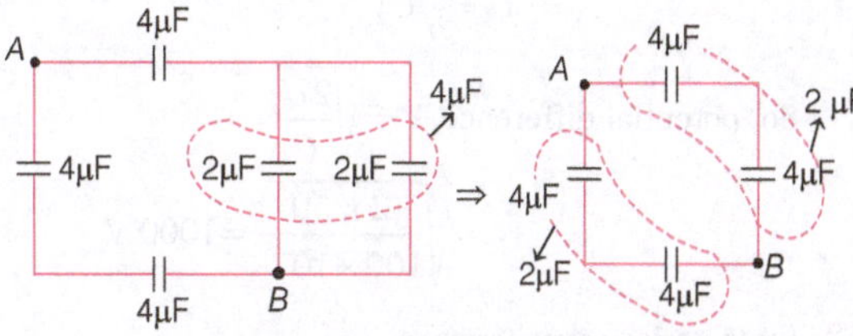

Equivalent capacitance between A and B is

$$C_{AB} = 2 + 2 = 4\ \mu\text{F}$$

17. (*d*) Potential difference across both the lines is same. Hence, charge flowing in line (2).

$$Q = \frac{2 \times 2}{2 + 2} = 2\ \mu\text{C}$$

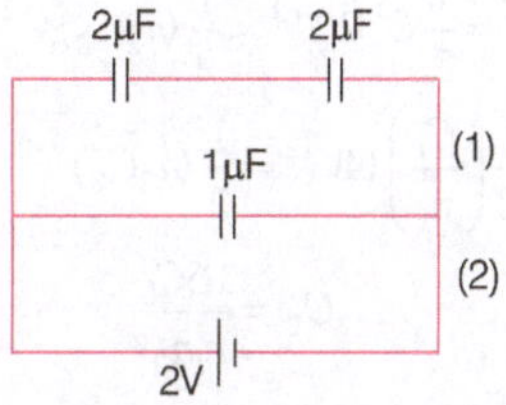

So, charge on each capacitor in line (2) is 2 μC and charge in line (1) is $Q = 2 \times 1 = 2\ \mu\text{C}$.

18. (*b*) Using same potential method

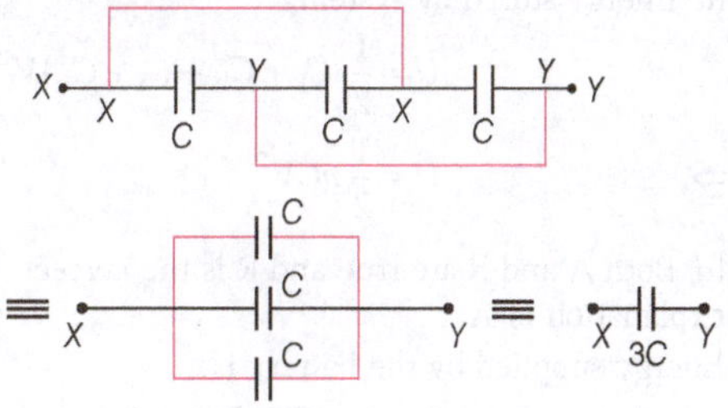

19. (*d*) For (d), C_{eq} is $\dfrac{2}{5}$ μF.

20. (*b*) A is true but R is false.

Let two capacitors are connected in series. If $+q$ charge is installed on left plate of the first capacitor, then $-q$ charge will be induced on right plate of this capacitor. This charge comes from electron drawn from the left plate of second capacitor. Thus, there will be equal charge $+q$ on the left plate of second capacitor and $-q$ charge induced on the right plate of second capacitor. Thus, each capacitor has same charge q when connected in series. Capacitance is depends on construction of capacitor and independent of charge on it.

Step up Practice 3

1. (c) The energy stored in a capacitor is

$$U = \frac{1}{2} CV^2$$

So, potential difference, $V = \sqrt{\frac{2U}{C}}$

$$= \sqrt{\frac{2 \times 50}{100 \times 10^{-6}}} = 1000 \text{ V}$$

2. (a) In series capacitance,

$$C' = \left(\frac{C_1}{n_1}\right) \text{ and } V' = 4V$$

Energy, $U' = \frac{1}{2} C'V'^2 = \frac{1}{2}\left(\frac{C_1}{n_1}\right)(4V)^2$

In parallel capacitance,

$$C'' = n_2 C_2 \text{ and } V'' = V$$

$$U'' = \frac{1}{2} C''V''^2 = \frac{1}{2}(n_2 C_2)V^2$$

Given, $\frac{1}{2}\left(\frac{C_1}{n_1}\right)(4V)^2 = \frac{1}{2}(n_2 C_2)V^2$

$$\Rightarrow \quad C_2 = \frac{16C_1}{n_1 n_2}$$

3. (b)

$$C' = KC$$

$$U' = \frac{U}{K} \quad (K > 1)$$

4. (d) Energy stored by system,

$$U = \frac{1}{2}(C_1 + C_2 + \dots + C_n)V^2$$

$$\Rightarrow \quad U = \frac{1}{2} nCV^2$$

5. (d) Both A and R are true and R is the correct explanation of A.

Energy supplied by the battery is

$$\Delta qV = (CV)(V) = CV^2$$

Energy stored in the capacitor is $\frac{1}{2} CV^2$.

6. (b) Energy, $E = \frac{1}{2}\frac{q^2}{C}$

Since, $C' = CK$

$$\Rightarrow \quad E' = \frac{1}{2}\frac{q^2}{CK} = \frac{1}{K}(E)$$

7. (c) Since, V is constant

$$U = \frac{1}{2} CV^2 \Rightarrow U \propto C$$

We know that, $C \propto K$

$$\therefore \quad U \propto K$$

8. (a) Common potential,

$$V_C = \frac{C_1V_1 + C_2V_2}{C_1 + C_2}$$

$$= \frac{(20 \times 500 + 10 \times 200)}{(20 + 10) \times 10^{-6}} \times 10^{-6}$$

$$V_C = \frac{10000 + 2000}{30} = \frac{12000}{30} = 400 \text{ V}$$

9. (c) A is false but R is true.

When the plates of a capacitor are moved further apart, the capacitance get decreased. As battery remain connected. So, charge q on the plates is decreased and energy $U = \left(\frac{1}{2} CV^2\right)$ also decrease. Some energy of capacitor is transferred to the battery against electrostatic attraction between plates is used in the transference and in this process energy is dissipated in the form of heat. Hence, work done decreased.

12. (d) Since, for spheres $C \propto R \Rightarrow \frac{R_1}{R_2} = \frac{C_1}{C_2}$

In case of

$$Q_1R_2 = Q_2R_1$$

$$\frac{R_1}{R_2} = \frac{Q_1}{Q_2} = \frac{C_1}{C_2}$$

Clearly potential of both spheres will be same in this case $(q = CV)$.

13. (b) Energy of capacitor, $U = \frac{1}{2}\frac{Q^2}{C}$

$$\therefore \quad 1.21U = \frac{1}{2}\frac{(Q+2)^2}{C}$$

$$\therefore \quad \frac{1.21}{1} = \frac{(Q+2)^2}{Q^2}$$

$$\Rightarrow \quad \sqrt{\frac{1.21}{1}} = \frac{Q+2}{Q}$$

$$\Rightarrow \quad 1.1Q = Q + 2$$

$\Rightarrow$ Charge on the capacitor, $Q = 20$ C

14. (a) Initial energy $= \frac{1}{2} \times 1 \times 10^{-6} \times (30)^2 = 450 \times 10^{-6}$ J

Final energy $= \frac{1}{2}(C_1 + C_2)V^2 \quad \left(\because V = \frac{V_1C_1 + V_2C_2}{C_1 + C_2}\right)$

$$= \frac{1}{2} \times 3 \times 10^{-6} \times (10)^2 = 150 \times 10^{-6} \text{ J}$$

Loss of energy $= (450 - 150) \times 10^{-6}$ J

$$= 300 \times 10^{-6} = 300 \ \mu\text{J}$$

15. (b) A is true but R is false.

On inserting a dielectric slab the capacitance of the capacitor C_0 is increased to $C = KC_0$.

Therefore, charge $q_0 = C_0V$ will increase to $q = Kq_0$.

Initial potential energy,

$$U_0 = \frac{1}{2} C_0 V^2$$

Final potential energy,

$$U = \frac{1}{2} CV^2$$
$$= \frac{1}{2} KC_0 V^2 = KU_0$$

16. (*b*) Energy supplied by battery

$$E = qV = 10^{-6} \times 300$$
$$\Rightarrow \quad E = 3 \times 10^{-4} \text{ J}$$

17. (*c*) Charge follows conservation law

$$C' = KC \text{ and } q = CV \Rightarrow V \propto \frac{1}{C}$$

Clearly potential, $V' = \frac{V}{K}$

Energy, $E = \frac{1}{2}\frac{q^2}{C} \Rightarrow E' = \frac{E}{K}$

18. (*d*) Initial energy stored in the capacitor,

$$U_i = \frac{1}{2} CV^2$$
$$= \frac{1}{2} C \times (50)^2 = \frac{1}{2} C(50)^2 \quad \text{...(i)}$$

After 2 s, when the potential drops by 10 V, the final potential is 40 V.
Final energy stored in the capacitor,

$$U_f = \frac{1}{2} C(40)^2 \quad \text{...(ii)}$$

Fraction of energy stored $= \frac{U_f}{U_i}$

$$= \frac{\frac{1}{2} C(40)^2}{\frac{1}{2} C(50)^2} = \left(\frac{40}{50}\right)^2 = 0.64$$

19. (*c*) A is false but R is true.
Battery is disconnected from the capacitor.
So, Q = constant

$$\text{Energy} = \frac{Q^2}{2C} = \frac{Q^2 d}{2\varepsilon_0 A}$$

$\Rightarrow$ Energy $\propto d$

20. (*c*) Energy supplied by battery, $E = qV$

Energy stored in capacitor, $U = \frac{1}{2} qV$

Clearly, $U = \frac{E}{2}$ or 50% of E

21. (*b*) (a) As, $\frac{Q_1}{C_1} = \frac{Q_2}{C_2}$,

$$Q_2 = \left(\frac{C_2}{C_1}\right) Q_1 = \frac{(C/2)}{C} Q_1 = \frac{Q_1}{2}$$

Further as, $Q = Q_1 + Q_2 = Q_1 + \frac{Q_1}{2} = \frac{3}{2} Q_1$

$$Q_1 = \frac{2}{3} Q \text{ and } Q_2 = \frac{1}{3} Q$$

Final energy of capacitor C_1,

$$U_1 = \frac{Q_1^2}{2C_1} = \frac{\left(\frac{2}{3}Q\right)^2}{2C}$$
$$= \frac{2}{9}\left(\frac{Q^2}{C}\right) = \frac{2}{9}\left(\frac{C^2 V_0^2}{C}\right)$$
$$= \frac{2}{9} CV_0^2 \quad (\text{as } Q = CV_0)$$

(b) Final energy of capacitor C_2,

$$U_2 = \frac{Q_2^2}{2C_2} = \frac{\left(\frac{1}{3}Q\right)^2}{2(C/2)}$$
$$= \frac{1}{9}\left(\frac{Q^2}{C}\right) = \frac{1}{9} CV_0^2$$

(c) Final energy of system,

$$U_{\text{final}} = U_1 + U_2 = \frac{1}{3} CV_0^2$$

(d) Initial energy of system,

$$U_{\text{initial}} = \frac{Q^2}{2C} = \frac{(CV_0)^2}{2C} = \frac{1}{2} CV_0^2$$

Change in energy,

$$\Delta U = U_{\text{final}} - U_{\text{initial}} = -\frac{1}{6} CV_0^2$$

Gearing up for NEET

1. (*a*) $U = \frac{Q^2}{2C}$

When a slab of dielectric constant K is inserted, then $C' = CK$

$$U' = \frac{Q^2}{2C'} = \frac{Q^2}{2CK}$$
$$\Rightarrow \quad U' = \frac{U_0}{K}$$

2. (*a*) Force between the plates of a parallel plate capacitor is given by

$$|F| = \frac{\sigma^2 A}{2\varepsilon_0} = \frac{Q^2}{2\varepsilon_0 A} = \frac{CV^2}{2d}$$

3. (*c*) Energy stored, $W = \frac{Q^2}{2C}$

$$\therefore \quad W \propto Q^2 \quad [\text{if } C \text{ is constant}]$$

or $$\frac{W}{W'} = \frac{Q^2}{(2Q)^2} = \frac{Q^2}{4Q^2}$$

$$\therefore \quad W' = 4W$$

4. (c) Heat produced in capacitor = Energy of charged capacitor

$$= \frac{1}{2} CV^2 = \frac{1}{2} \times (2 \times 10^{-6}) \times (100)^2 = 0.01 \text{ J}$$

5. (b) The energy stored, $U = \frac{1}{2}(nC)V^2$

6. (d) Change in energy of condenser,

$$\Delta U = U_2 - U_1 = \frac{1}{2} C_2V^2 - \frac{1}{2} C_1V^2$$

$$= \frac{V^2}{2}(C_2 - C_1)$$

$$= \frac{(100)^2}{2}(10 \times 10^{-6} - 2 \times 10^{-6})$$

$$= 4 \times 10^{-2} \text{ J}$$

7. (b) In series, charge remains same on both capacitors

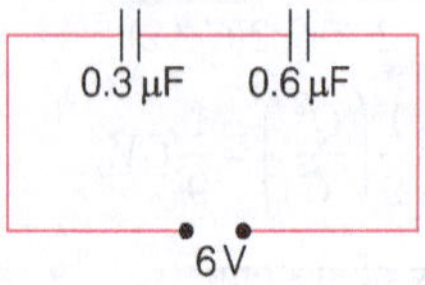

$$\therefore \quad U = \frac{Q^2}{2C} \text{ or } U \propto \frac{1}{C} \qquad (\because Q_1 = Q_2)$$

$$\therefore \quad \frac{U_1}{U_2} = \frac{C_2}{C_1} = \frac{0.6}{0.3}$$

$\therefore \quad U_1 : U_2 = 2 : 1$

8. (b) In parallel combination,

$$C_{\text{net}} = C_1 + C_2$$

$$V = \frac{q_{\text{net}}}{C_{\text{net}}} = \frac{C_1V_0}{C_1 + C_2}$$

9. (c) Let Q_0, C_0, V_0 and U_0 be the charge, capacitance, potential difference and stored energy, respectively before the dielectric slab of dielectric constant K is inserted.

After inserting dielectric slab, charge will remain same, i.e. $Q' = Q_0$.

Potential difference will decrease as $V' = \frac{V_0}{K}$

Stored energy will decrease as, $U = \frac{V_0}{K}$.

10. (b) Potential on parallel plate capacitor, $V = \frac{Q}{C}$.

Also, capacity of parallel plate capacitor is given by

$$C = \frac{\varepsilon_0 KA}{d}$$

$$\therefore \quad V = \frac{Qd}{\varepsilon_0 KA}$$

$$\Rightarrow \quad V \propto d$$

So, on increasing the distance between plates of capacitor, the potential difference between plates also increases.

11. (c) Both the conductors carry equal and opposite charges. So, after connecting by a wire, there will be no charge in any conductor. Hence, all the stored energy will be neutralised.

$$\text{Loss of energy} = 2\left(\frac{1}{2} CV^2\right) = CV^2$$

12. (d) Net charge distributes in direct ratio of capacity (or radius in case of spherical conductor)

$$\therefore \quad q'_A = q_{\text{net}}\left[\frac{4}{4+6}\right] = 120\left[\frac{4}{4+6}\right]$$

$$= 48 \, \mu\text{C}$$

So, $\quad \Delta q = 80 - 48 = 32 \, \mu\text{C}$ from A to B.

13. (c) The energy stored in the capacitor,

$$U = \frac{1}{2} CV^2$$

$$U = \frac{1}{2}\left(\frac{A\varepsilon_0}{d}\right)(Ed)^2$$

$$\left(\because C = \frac{A\varepsilon_0}{d} \text{ and } V = Ed\right)$$

$$U = \frac{1}{2} \varepsilon_0 E^2 Ad$$

14. (c) We have, $K = \frac{t}{t - d'}$

$$2 = \frac{1}{1 - d'} \Rightarrow d' = \frac{1}{2} \text{ mm}$$

So, now distance $= 3 + \frac{1}{2} = 3.5$ mm

15. (a) Given, $C_1 = 2 \, \mu\text{F}, V_1 = 50 \text{ V}$

$$C_2 = 1 \, \mu\text{F}, V_2 = 20 \text{ V}$$

Common potential,

$$V = \frac{C_1V_1 + C_2V_2}{C_1 + C_2}$$

$$= \frac{(2 \times 50 + 1 \times 20) \times 10^{-6}}{(2 + 1) \times 10^{-6}} = 40 \text{ V}$$

Loss of energy,

$$\Delta u = \frac{1}{2} \frac{C_1C_2}{C_1 + C_2}(V_1 - V_2)^2$$

$$= \frac{1}{2} \frac{2 \times 1}{(2 + 1)}(50 - 20)^2 \times 10^{-6}$$

$$= 300 \times 10^{-6}$$

$$= 300 \, \mu\text{J}$$

16. (*c*) Capacitance of spherical condenser, when outer sphere is earthed,

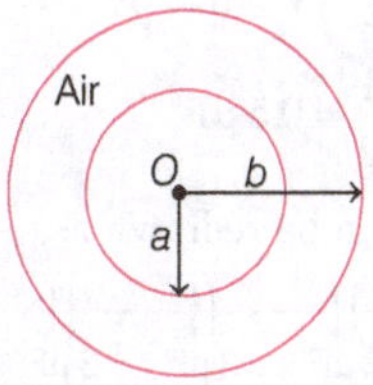

$$C_1 = 4\pi\varepsilon_0 \cdot \frac{ab}{b-a}$$

Capacitance of spherical condenser when inner sphere is earthed, $C_2 = 4\pi\varepsilon_0 b + \dfrac{4\pi\varepsilon_0 ab}{b-a}$

$\therefore$ Difference in their capacity

$$= C_2 - C_1 = 4\pi\varepsilon_0 b$$

17. (*d*) Given circuit is balanced Wheatstone bridge circuit.

For branch *ACB*, $C' = \dfrac{10 \times 10}{10+10} = 5\,\mu F$

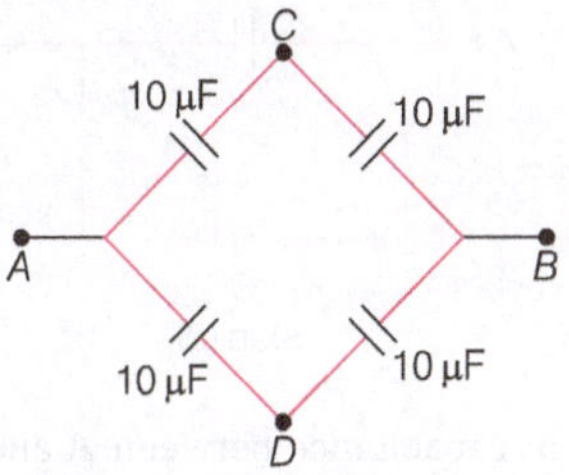

For branch *ADB*, $C'' = \dfrac{10 \times 10}{10+10} = 5\,\mu F$

Their is no flow of charge in branch *CD*.

So, equivalent capacitance between *AB*,

$C_{AB} = C' + C'' = 5 + 5 = 10\,\mu F$

18. (*a*) When capacitors are connected in series, then

$$\frac{1}{C_S} = \frac{1}{C_1} + \frac{1}{C_2} + \frac{1}{C_3} = \frac{1}{3} + \frac{1}{9} + \frac{1}{18}$$

$$\frac{1}{C_S} = \frac{1}{2} \Rightarrow C_S = 2\,\mu F$$

When capacitors are joined in parallel, then

$$C_P = 3 + 9 + 18 = 30\,\mu F$$

$$\therefore \quad \frac{C_S}{C_P} = \frac{2}{30} = \frac{1}{15}$$

19. (*b*) In circuit, capacitors of capacitance 2 μF and 3 μF are in parallel. Their resultant capacitance is 5 μF.

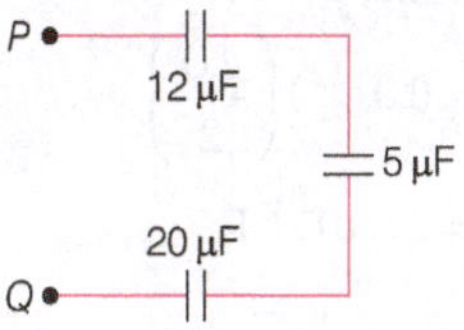

Now, capacitor 12 μF, 5 μF and 20 μF are in series. So, their resultant capacity,

$$\frac{1}{C} = \frac{1}{5} + \frac{1}{20} + \frac{1}{12} = \frac{1}{3}$$

$$\therefore \quad C = 3\,\mu F$$

20. (*a*) Capacitance between *A* and *B*,

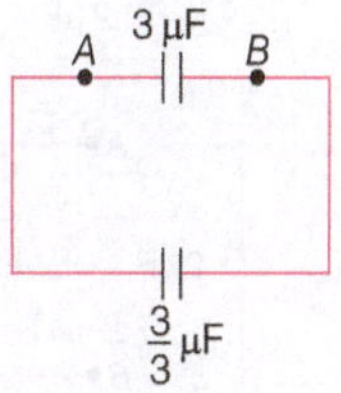

$$C_{AB} = 3 + 1 = 4\,\mu F$$

Capacitance between *A* and *C*,

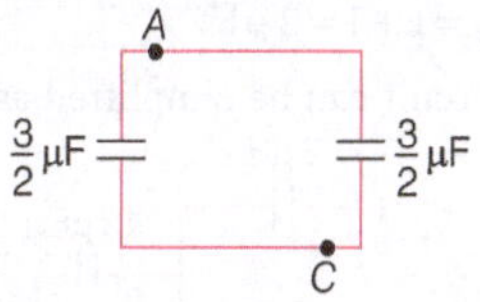

$$C_{AC} = \frac{3}{2} + \frac{3}{2} = 3\,\mu F$$

$$\therefore \quad \frac{C_{AB}}{C_{AC}} = \frac{4}{3}$$

21. (*d*) Given circuit can be reduced as following

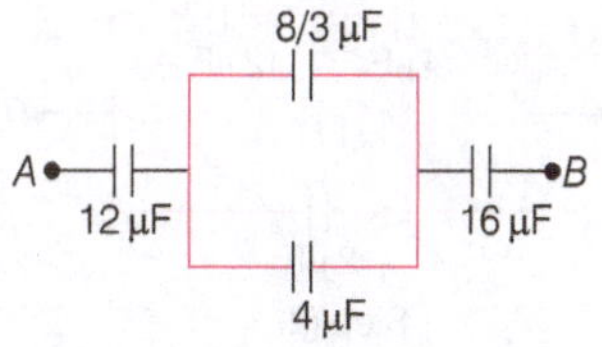

Step (1)

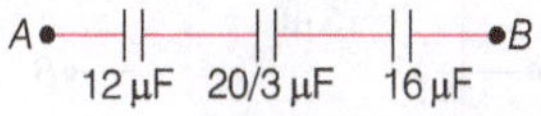

Step (2)

Hence, equivalent capacitance between *A* and *B*,

$$\frac{1}{C_{AB}} = \frac{1}{12} + \frac{1}{20/3} + \frac{1}{16}$$

$$\therefore \quad C_{AB} = \frac{240}{71}\,F$$

22. (*d*) Given circuit can be simplified as shown,

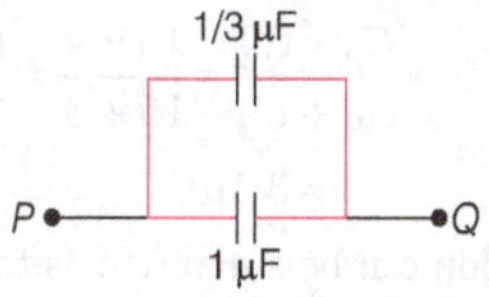

$$\therefore \quad C_{PQ} = \frac{1}{3} + 1 = \frac{4}{3}\,\mu F$$

23. (*b*) Given circuit can be simplified as follows

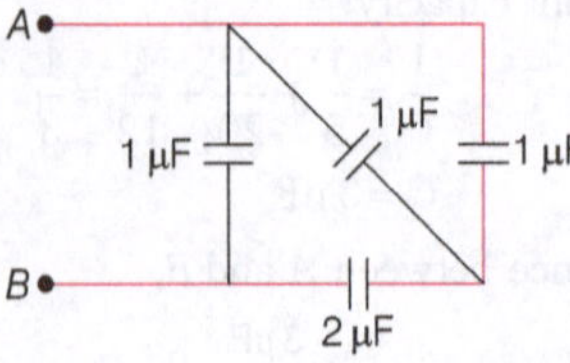

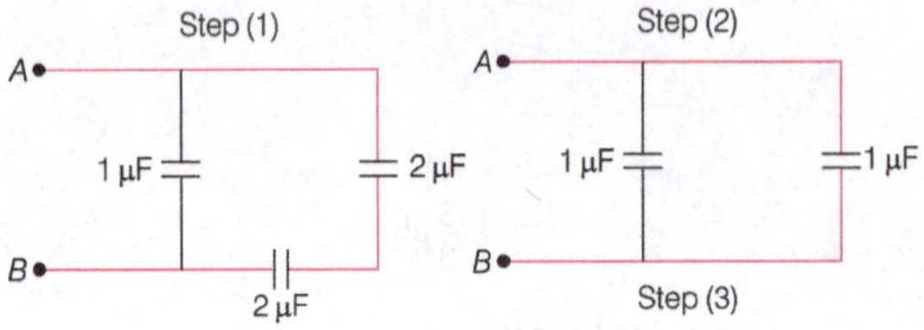

So, equivalent capacitance between A and B,

$$C_{AB} = 1 + 1 = 2\,\mu\text{F}$$

24. (*c*) Given circuit can be simplified as,

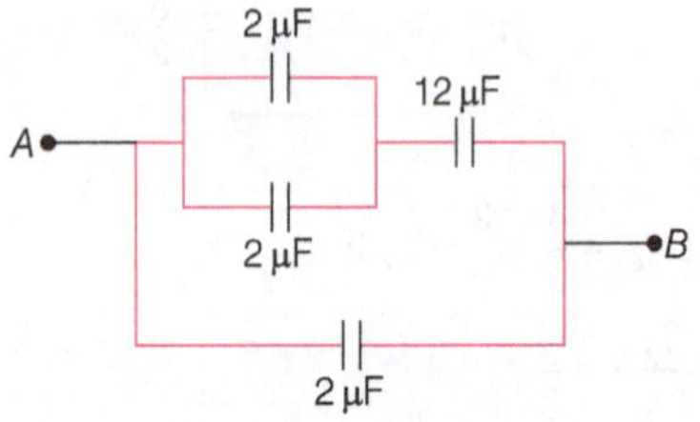

Step (1)

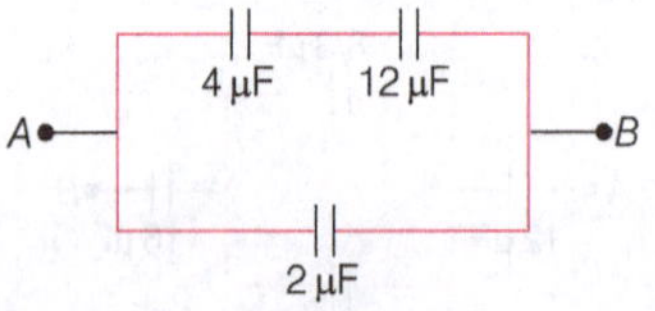

Step (2)

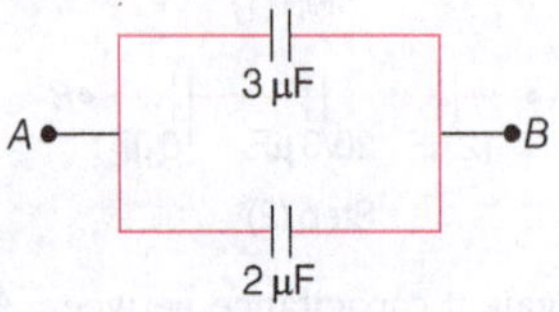

Step (3)

So, net capacitance between AB,

$$C_{AB} = 3 + 2 = 5\,\mu\text{F}$$

25. (*b*) Capacitors C_1 and C_2 and in parallel and they are in series with C_3, then equivalent capacity between A and B

$$C = \frac{C_P \times C_3}{C_P + C_3} = \frac{15 \times 4}{15 + 4} = \frac{60}{19}$$

$$= 3.2\,\mu\text{F}$$

26. (*d*) The situation can be simplified as follows,

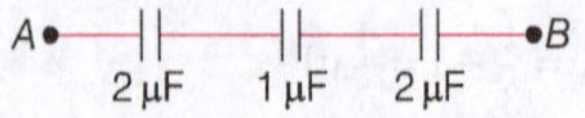

∴ Equivalent capacity between A and B,

$$\frac{1}{C_{AB}} = \frac{1}{2} + \frac{1}{1} + \frac{1}{2} = \frac{4}{2} = 2$$

$$\Rightarrow \quad C_{AB} = \frac{1}{2} = 0.5\,\mu\text{F}$$

27. (*a*) The circuit can be redrawn as,

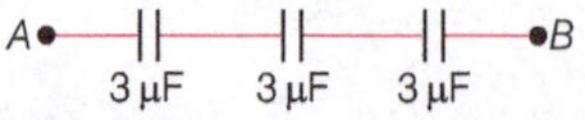

So, the capacitance between the piont A and B,

$$C_{AB} = \frac{1}{3} + \frac{1}{3} + \frac{1}{3} = \frac{3}{3} = 1\,\mu\text{F}$$

28. (*c*) Given circuit can be redrawn as follows,

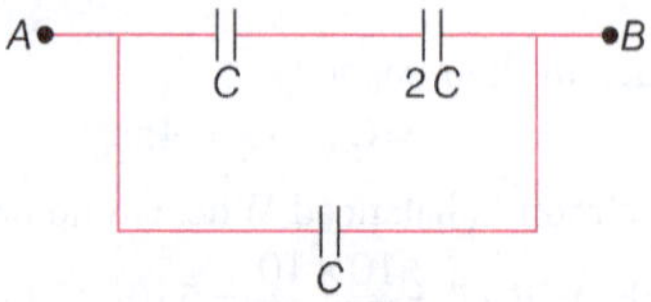

Step (1)

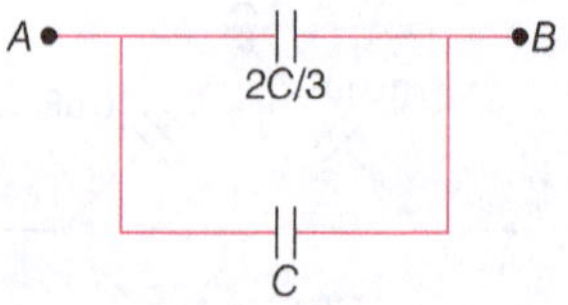

Step (2)

Equivalent capacitance between A and B,

$$C_{AB} = \frac{2C}{3} + C = \frac{5}{3}C$$

29. (*d*) Let, here, C_0 = capacity of one capacitor.

$$C_S = \frac{C_0}{7} \Rightarrow C_0 = 7C_S$$

and $\quad C_P = 7C_0$

∴ $\quad C_P = 49C_S = 49C$

30. (*b*) Potential, $V = \frac{q}{C}$ or $V \propto \frac{1}{C}$

V has reduced to $\frac{1}{8}$th its original value. Therefore, C has increased 8 times, *i.e.* $K = 8$.

31. (*c*) Capacitance, $C' = \frac{K\varepsilon_0 A}{d}$ or $C' \propto \frac{K}{d'}$

$$\therefore \quad \frac{C'}{C} = \frac{Kd}{d'}$$

Here, $K = 4.0$, $d' = 2d$

$$\therefore \quad C' = (10^{-12})\left(\frac{4.0}{2}\right)$$

$$= 2 \times 10^{-12}\ \text{F}$$

32. (b)

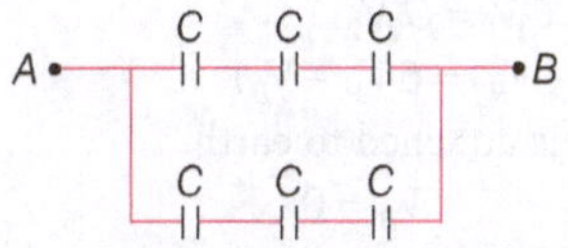

The effective capacity of the combination, $\frac{2C}{3} = 4\,\mu F$

$\therefore$ Capacitance, $C = 6\,\mu F$

33. (a) Given, capacitance of a capacitor,

$$C = 15\text{ nF} = 15 \times 10^{-9}\text{ F}, \varepsilon_r = 2.5$$

Electric field, $E = 30 \times 10^6$ V/m

Potential difference, $V = 30$ V

Area of plate = ?

If d be the distance between the plates, then

$$d = \frac{V}{E} = \frac{30}{30 \times 10^6} = 10^{-6}\text{ m}$$

Capacitance of capacitor, $C = \frac{\varepsilon_0 \varepsilon_r A}{d}$

$$15 \times 10^{-9} = \frac{8.85 \times 10^{-12} \times 2.5 \times A}{10^{-6}}$$

$$\Rightarrow \quad A = 6.7 \times 10^{-4}\text{ m}^2$$

34. (d) By the given arrangement, two capacitors are formed such a way that they are in parallel.

$$\therefore \quad C_{\text{net}} = 2C = 2\left(\frac{\varepsilon_0 A}{d}\right)$$

35. (a) According to the question, $8\left(\frac{4}{3}\pi r^3\right) = \frac{4}{3}\pi R^3$

$\therefore$ Radius, $R = 2r$

Capacitance, $C = 4\pi\varepsilon_0 r$

$$C' = 4\pi\varepsilon_0 2r \Rightarrow C' = 2C$$

Therefore, the capacitance of the bigger drop as compared to each smaller drop is 2 times.

36. (a) Given, $C = 10\,\mu F = 10^{-5}$ F

$$\Rightarrow \quad \frac{\varepsilon_0 A}{D} = 10^{-5}\text{ F} \quad \text{...(i)}$$

Now, both capacitors are in parallel.

$$\therefore \quad C' = C_1 + C_2$$

$$= \frac{\varepsilon_0 (A/2)}{d} + \frac{K\varepsilon_0 (A/2)}{D}$$

$$\Rightarrow \quad C' = \frac{\varepsilon_0 A}{d}\left(\frac{1}{2} + 2\right)$$

$$= \frac{5}{2}\frac{\varepsilon_0 A}{d} = \frac{5}{2} \times 10^{-5} \quad \text{[from Eq. (i)]}$$

$$= 25\,\mu F$$

37. (a) This combination is same as the two capacitors are connected in series and distance between plate of each capacitor is $d/2$. So,

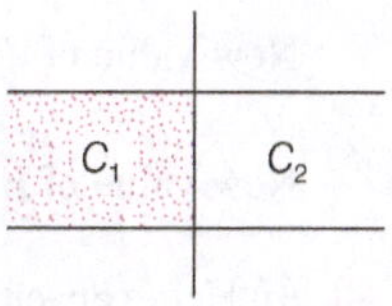

$$C_1 = \frac{K\varepsilon_0 A}{d/2} \text{ and } C_2 = \frac{\varepsilon_0 A}{d/2}$$

Hence, $C_{\text{net}} = \frac{C_1 C_2}{C_1 + C_2}$

$$= \frac{\left(\frac{2K\varepsilon_0 A}{d}\right)\left(\frac{2\varepsilon_0 A}{d}\right)}{\left(\frac{2K\varepsilon_0 A}{d} + \frac{2\varepsilon_0 A}{d}\right)}$$

$$C_{\text{net}} = \frac{2KA\varepsilon_0}{(K+1)d}$$

38. (d) Capacity of capacitor, $C = \frac{\varepsilon_0 A}{d}$

$$\Rightarrow \quad C \propto \frac{1}{d}$$

$\therefore$ Capacitance, $C' = 2C$

$\therefore$ Extra charge flow,

$$q = (2CV - CV) = CV$$

$\therefore$ Work done, $W = qV$

$$= (CV)V = CV^2$$

39. (b) $\frac{C'}{C} = \frac{\varepsilon_0 A/(d-t)}{\varepsilon_0 A/d} = \frac{d}{d-t}$

$$\Rightarrow \quad \frac{d}{(5/7)d} = \frac{7}{5}$$

$\therefore$ Capacitance, $C' = \frac{7}{5} \times 25\,\mu F = 35\,\mu F$

40. (b) On introducing dielectric K in a parallel plate capacitor, its capacity becomes,

$$C' = KC_0$$

$$\therefore \quad C' = 5C_0$$

Also, energy stored, $W_0 = \frac{q^2}{2C_0}$

$$\therefore \quad W' = \frac{q^2}{2C'} = \frac{q^2}{2 \times 5C_0}$$

$$\therefore \quad \frac{W_0}{W'} = \frac{5}{1}$$

$$\therefore \quad W' = \frac{W_0}{5}$$

41. (b) $\frac{C'}{C} = \frac{\varepsilon_0 A/d-t}{\varepsilon_0 A/d} = \frac{d}{d-t} = \frac{d}{d/2} = 2:1$

$$\left[\because \text{In question, thickness } (t) \text{ is } b = \frac{d}{2}\right]$$

42. (d) When charged capacitor is filled with a dielectric material of dielectric constant K, then charge remains constant, V becomes $\frac{1}{K}$ times and E becomes $\frac{1}{K}$ times.

So, new value of charge is Q_0.

New value of $V = \dfrac{V_0 \times 3}{9} = \dfrac{V_0}{3}$

New value of $E = \dfrac{E_0 \times 3}{9} = \dfrac{E_0}{3}$

43. (*d*) Here capacitors of capacity 4 μF each are in parallel, their equivalent capacity is 8 μF. Now, there is a combination of three capacitors in series of capacity 20 μF, 8 μF and 12 μF so, their resultant capacity,

$$\frac{1}{C} = \frac{1}{20} + \frac{1}{8} + \frac{1}{12}$$

$$\therefore \quad C = \frac{120}{31}\ \mu\text{F}$$

Total charge, $Q = CV$

$$= \frac{120}{31} \times 300 = 1161\ \mu\text{C}$$

$\therefore$ Charge through 4 μF capacitor $= \dfrac{1161}{2} = 580\ \mu\text{C}$

and potential difference across 4 μF condenser,

$$V = \frac{q}{C} = \frac{580}{4} = 145\ \text{V}$$

44. (*c*) As capacitors C_1 and C_2 are in series, then there should be equal charge on them, i.e.

Charge on C_1 = charge on C_2

$\therefore \quad C_1(V_A - V_D) = C_2(V_D - V_B)$

or $\quad C_1(V_1 - V_D) = C_2(V_D - V_2)$

or $\quad C_1V_1 - C_1V_D = C_2V_D - C_2V_2$

or $\quad V_D(C_1 + C_2) = C_1V_1 + C_2V_2$

$\therefore$ The potential difference of point D,

$$V_D = \frac{C_1V_1 + C_2V_2}{C_1 + C_2}$$

45. (*a*) Equivalent capacitance of circuit,

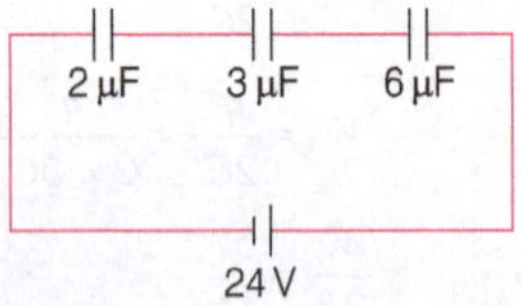

$$C_{eq} = \frac{6}{3+2+1} = 1\ \mu\text{F}$$

Total charge, $Q = 1 \times 24 = 24\ \mu\text{C}$

Now, potential difference across 6 μF capacitor

$$= \frac{24}{6} = 4\ \text{V}$$

46. (*c*) Given, circuit can be reduced as,

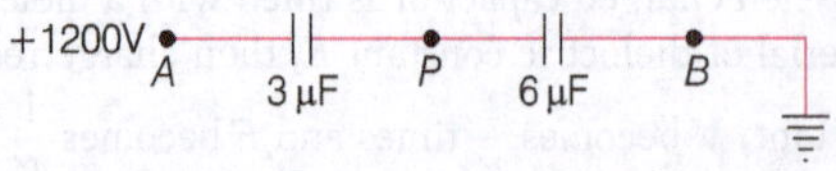

Let potential at P be V_P and potential at B be V_B.

As capacitors 3 μF and 6 μF are in series, they have same charge.

$\therefore$ Charge on 3 μF = Charge on 6 μF

$\therefore \quad C_1V_1 = C_2V_2$

or $\quad 3(1200 - V_P) = 6(V_P - V_B)$

As B point is attached to earth.

So, $\quad V_B = 0$

$\therefore \quad 1200 - V_P = 2V_P$

$\quad V_P = 400\ \text{V}$

47. (*b*) The circuit can be redrawn as,

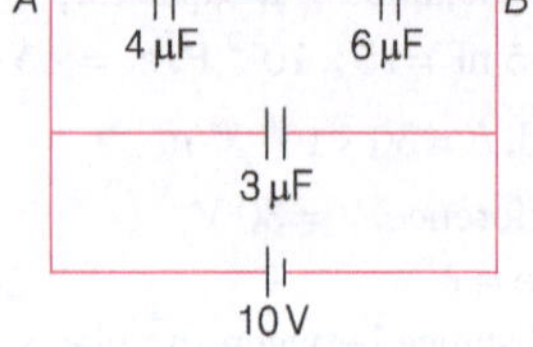

Here, 4 μF and 6 μF are in series. So, charge is same on both.

Now, equivalent capacity between A and B,

$$C_{AB} = \frac{6 \times 4}{6+4} = 2.4\ \mu\text{F}$$

So, charge on 4 μF capacitor,

$$Q = C_{AB} \times 10 = 2.4 \times 10 = 24\ \mu\text{C}$$

48. (*d*) Equivalent capacitance between A and B,

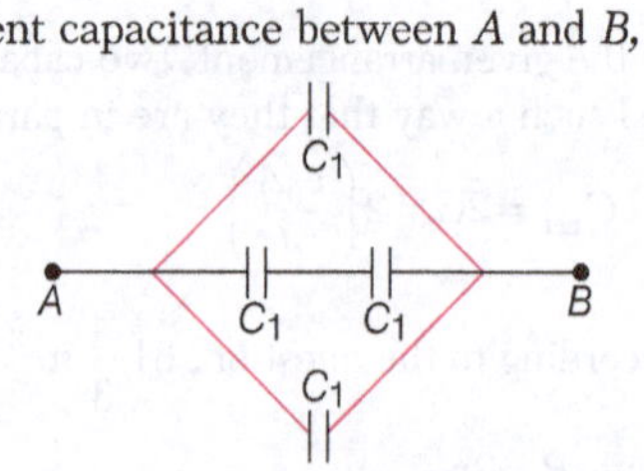

$$C_{AB} = C_1 + \frac{C_1}{2} + C_1 = \frac{5}{2}C_1$$

As charge, $\quad Q = CV$

So, $\quad 1.5 \times 10^{-6} = \dfrac{5}{2}C_1 \times 6$

$\Rightarrow \quad C_1 = \dfrac{1.5}{15} \times 10^{-6}$

$$= 0.1 \times 10^{-6}\ \text{F} = 0.1\ \mu\text{F}$$

49. (*b*) After the introduction of dielectric slab, direction of electric field remains perpendicular to plate and is directed from positive to negative plate.

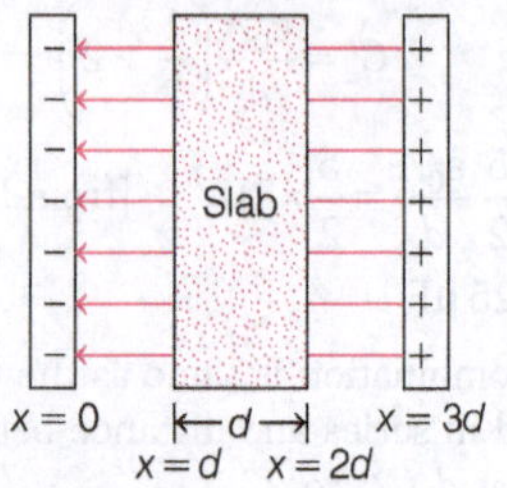

Electric field in air $= \dfrac{\sigma}{\varepsilon_0}$

and electric field in dielectric $= \dfrac{\sigma}{K\varepsilon_0}$

Positive plate is at higher potential and negative plate is at lower potential. So, electric potential increases continuously as we more from $x = 0$ to $x = 3d$.

50. (c) Potential, $V = \dfrac{q_{net}}{C_{net}}$

$$\Rightarrow \quad 40 = \frac{(2)(200)}{2 + C} \Rightarrow 80 + 40C = 400$$

$\therefore$ Capacity of second condenser, $C = 8\,\mu F$

51. (d) We have, $q_i = q_f$

$$C_1V_1 + C_2V_2 = (C_1 + C_2)V$$

$$\therefore \quad (2)(4) + (C)5 = (2 + C)\,4.6$$

$$0.4C = 1.2$$

$$C = 3 \text{ units}$$

52. (b) The simplified circuit will be as under.

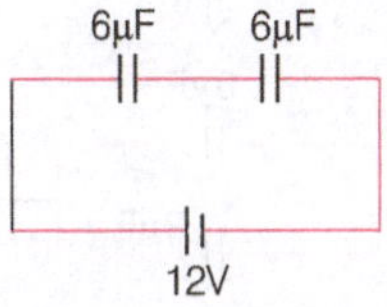

The potential drop 12 V will be equally distributed. Potential difference across capacitor of 6 μF is 6 V. So, the voltage across a 2 μF capacitor is 6 V.

53. (d) For the combination of three capacitors in series,

$$\frac{1}{C} = \frac{1}{C_1} + \frac{1}{C_2} + \frac{1}{C_3}$$

$$\Rightarrow \quad \frac{1}{C} = \frac{1}{3} + \frac{1}{6} + \frac{1}{6}$$

$$\Rightarrow \quad C = \frac{6}{4} = 1.5\,\mu F$$

The charge stored in this circuit,

$$q = CV = 1.5 \times 120 = 180\,\mu C$$

The potential difference across the 3 μF

$$q = CV, V = \frac{q}{C} = \frac{180}{3} = 60 \text{ V}$$

54. (b) Potential difference across 6 μF capacitor,

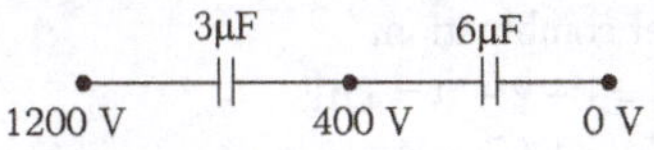

$$V_2 = \left(\frac{3}{3+6}\right) \times 1200$$

$$= \frac{3}{9} \times 1200 = 400 \text{ V}$$

$\therefore$ Charge, $q = 4 \times 400 = 1600\,\mu C$

55. (b) In parallel, potential difference is same and in series, it distributes in inverse ratio of capacity.

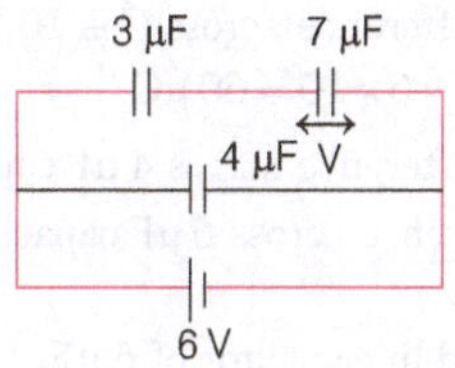

Potential difference,

$$V = 6\left(\frac{3}{3+7}\right) = 1.8 \text{ V}$$

$\therefore$ Charge stored in 5 μF capacitor will be

$$q = CV = (5)(1.8) = 9\,\mu C$$

56. (d) In series, potential difference distributes in inverse ratio of capacities. Hence,

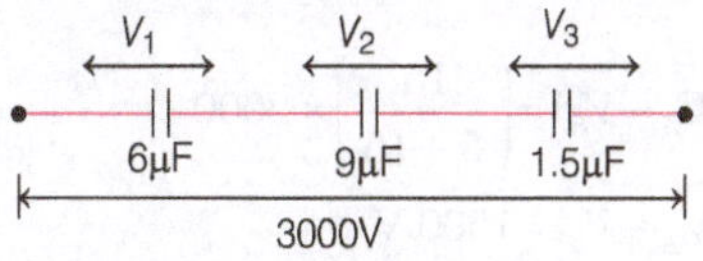

$$V_1 : V_2 : V_3 = \frac{1}{6} : \frac{1}{9} : \frac{1}{1.5} = 1.5 : 1 : 6$$

$$V_2 = (3000)\left(\frac{1}{1 + 1.5 + 6}\right) = 352.9 \text{ V}$$

$$\simeq 350 \text{ V}$$

57. (a) In the given figure capacitors 3 μF, 3 μF and 3 μF (between R and S) are in series. If Q is the charge on each of these capacitors, then

$$30 = \frac{Q}{3} + \frac{Q}{3} + \frac{Q}{3}$$

$$Q = 30\,\mu C$$

Potential difference between R and S

$$V = \frac{Q}{C} = \frac{30}{3}$$

$$\Rightarrow \quad V = 10 \text{ V}$$

58. (a)

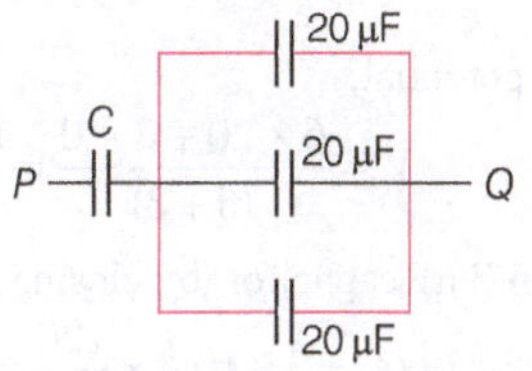

$$C' = C_1 + C_2 + C_3$$

$$= 20 + 20 + 20 = 60\,\mu F$$

$$\frac{1}{C''} = \frac{1}{C} + \frac{1}{C'}$$

$$\frac{1}{30} = \frac{1}{C} + \frac{1}{60}$$

$$\frac{1}{C} = \frac{1}{30} - \frac{1}{60} \Rightarrow \frac{1}{C} = \frac{2-1}{60}$$

$$\frac{1}{C} = \frac{1}{60} \Rightarrow C = 60\,\mu F$$

59. (*d*) Potential difference across C is 10 V.

$\therefore \quad q = CV = 6 \times 10 = 60\,\mu C$

60. (*a*) Potential difference across 4 μF capacitor is 9 V and potential difference across 6 μF capacitor will be $(12 - 9)\text{ V} = 3\text{ V}$

∴ Charge stored in capacitor of 6 μF,

$$q = CV = 6 \times 3 = 18\,\mu C$$

61. (*c*) The given circuit can be redrawn as follow

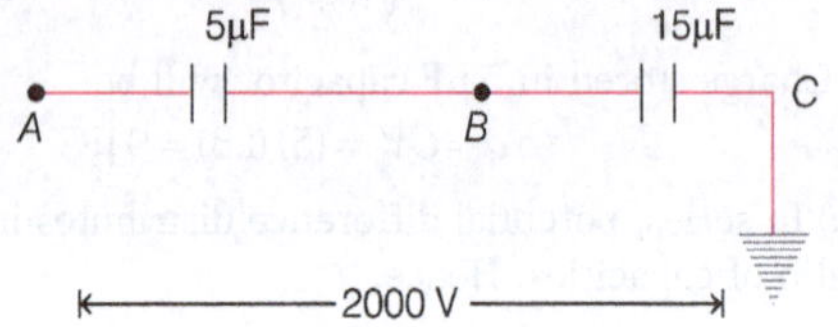

$$(V_A - V_B) = \left(\frac{15}{5+15}\right) \times 2000$$

$$(V_A - V_B) = 1500\text{ V}$$

$$2000 - V_B = 1500\text{ V}$$

$$V_B = 500\text{ V}$$

62. (*c*) Work done $= \frac{1}{2}\left(\frac{4C}{3}\right)V^2 = \frac{2CV^2}{3}$

63. (*c*) The two capacitors are connected in parallel. The equivalent capacitance,

$$C' = C + \frac{C}{2} = \frac{3C}{2}$$

Work done in charging the equivalent capacitor is stored in the form of potential energy,

$$W = U = \left(\frac{1}{2}\right)C'V^2$$

$$W = \frac{1}{2} \times \frac{3C}{2} \times V^2$$

$$W = \frac{3}{4}CV^2$$

64. (*c*) Common potential,

$$V = \frac{6 \times 20 + 3 \times 0}{(6+3)} = \frac{120}{9}\text{ V}$$

So, charge on 3 μF capacitor (by closing S_2)

$$Q_2 = 3 \times 10^{-6} \times \frac{120}{9} = 40\,\mu C$$

65. (*b*) The energy stored when the plates are fully charged,

$$U = \frac{1}{2}(2C)V^2 = CV^2 = \left(\frac{\varepsilon_0 A}{d}\right)(V^2)$$

66. (*c*) At the given positions all the charges are in equilibrium. But when they displaced slightly from their given position, they do not return back. So, they are in unstable equilibrium position.

67. (*d*)

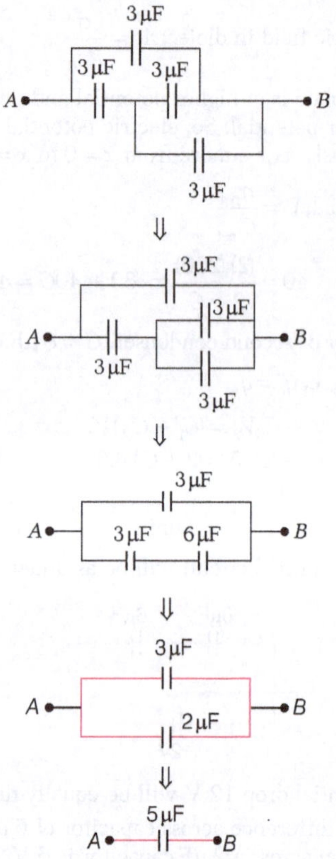

The effective capacitance between point A and B is 5 μF.

68. (*c*) Charge, $Q = CV = 500 \times 10^{-6} \times 10$

$$= 5 \times 10^{-3}\text{ C}$$

Now, $\quad Q = qt \text{ or } t = \frac{Q}{q}$

or $\quad t = \frac{5 \times 10^{-3}}{100 \times 10^{-6}} = \frac{1}{20} \times 1000 = 50\text{ s}$

69. (*c*) In series combination,

$$\frac{1}{C_1} = \frac{1}{1} + \frac{1}{2} + \frac{1}{4} = \frac{4+2+1}{4} = \frac{7}{4}$$

$$\Rightarrow \quad C_1 = \frac{4}{7}\,\mu F$$

In parallel combination,

$$C_2 = 1 + 2 + 4 = 7\,\mu F$$

$$\therefore \quad \frac{C_1}{C_2} = \frac{4/7}{7} = \frac{4}{49}$$

70. (*b*) When capacitors are connected in parallel, then

$$C_P = C + C + C = 3C$$

According to question,

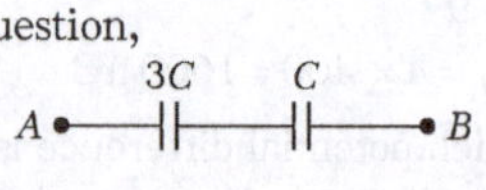

$\therefore$ In series, $C_s = \dfrac{3C \times C}{3C + C}$

$\Rightarrow \quad 3.75 = \dfrac{3C \times C}{4C} \Rightarrow C = 5\,\mu\text{F}$

71. (c) Charge 80 μC divided in both capacitors of capacitances 2 μF and 3 μF.

Charge on $3\mu F$

$$q_3 = \left(\frac{C_3}{C_2 + C_3}\right) \times Q$$

$$\Rightarrow \quad q_3 = \left(\frac{3}{3+2}\right) \times 80 = \frac{3}{5} \times 80 = 48\,\mu\text{C}$$

72. (d) $C_{\text{air}} = \dfrac{\varepsilon_0 A}{d}$, with dielectric slab $C' = \dfrac{\varepsilon_0 A}{\left(d - t + \dfrac{t}{K}\right)}$

Given, $\quad C' = \dfrac{4}{3} C$

$$\Rightarrow \quad \frac{\varepsilon_0 A}{\left(d - t + \dfrac{t}{K}\right)} = \frac{4}{3} \times \frac{\varepsilon_0 A}{d}$$

The dielectric constant of the slab,

$$K = \frac{4t}{4t - d} = \frac{4(d/2)}{4(d/2) - d} = 2$$

73. (c) Potential difference between plates A and B,

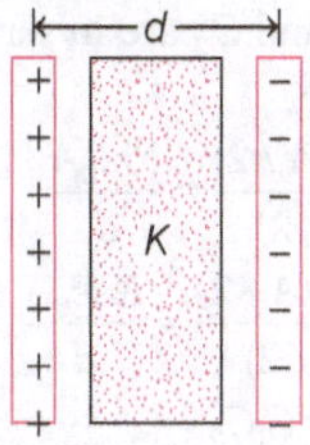

V = Potential difference in air + Potential difference in medium

$$V = \frac{q}{\varepsilon_0}(d - t) + \frac{\sigma}{K\varepsilon_0} t$$

$$\therefore \quad V = \frac{\sigma}{\varepsilon_0}\left[d - t + \frac{t}{K}\right]$$

$$= \frac{Q}{A\varepsilon_0}\left(d - t + \frac{t}{K}\right) \qquad \left(\because \sigma = \frac{Q}{A}\right)$$

$$\therefore \text{Capacitance, } C = \frac{Q}{V} = \frac{Q}{\dfrac{Q}{A\varepsilon_0}\left(d - t + \dfrac{t}{K}\right)}$$

$$= \frac{\varepsilon_0 A}{d - t + \dfrac{t}{K}} = \frac{\varepsilon_0 A}{d - t\left(1 - \dfrac{1}{K}\right)}$$

74. (b) According to question,

capacity of spherical condenser = capacity of parallel plate capacitor

$$\therefore \quad 4\pi\varepsilon_0 r = \frac{\varepsilon_0 A}{d}$$

$$\therefore \quad d = \frac{A}{4\pi r} = \frac{\pi R^2}{4\pi r}$$

$$= \frac{\pi (20 \times 10^{-3})^2}{4\pi \times 1} = 0.1\text{ mm}$$

75. (a) Three capacitors are in series therefore, their resultant capacity is given by

$$\frac{1}{C_S} = \frac{1}{\left(\dfrac{\varepsilon_0 K_1 A}{d_1}\right)} + \frac{1}{\left(\dfrac{\varepsilon_0 K_2 A}{d_2}\right)} + \frac{1}{\left(\dfrac{\varepsilon_0 K_3 A}{d_3}\right)}$$

or $\quad \dfrac{1}{C_S} = \dfrac{d_1}{\varepsilon_0 K_1 A} + \dfrac{d_2}{\varepsilon_0 K_2 A} + \dfrac{d_3}{\varepsilon_0 K_3 A}$

$$\frac{1}{C_S} = \frac{1}{\varepsilon_0 A}\left(\frac{d_1}{K_1} + \frac{d_2}{K_2} + \frac{d_3}{K_3}\right)$$

$$\therefore \quad C_S = \frac{\varepsilon_0 A}{\left(\dfrac{d_1}{K_1} + \dfrac{d_2}{K_2} + \dfrac{d_3}{K_3}\right)}$$

76. (b) $\dfrac{1}{C_{\text{eq}}} = \dfrac{1}{C} + \dfrac{1}{2C} + \dfrac{1}{4C} + \ldots \infty$

$$= \frac{1}{C}\left[1 + \frac{1}{2} + \frac{1}{2^2} + \ldots \infty\right]$$

$$= \frac{1}{C}\left[\frac{1}{1 - \dfrac{1}{2}}\right] = \frac{2}{C}$$

The equivalent capacitance between A and B,

$$C_{\text{eq}} = \frac{C}{2}$$

77. (a) The given figure is equivalent to two identical capacitors in parallel combination,

$$C = \frac{\varepsilon_0 A}{d} + \frac{\varepsilon_0 A}{d} = \frac{2\varepsilon_0 A}{d}$$

$\because$ Both the middle plates have same potential V_B.

78. (b) Given plates are equivalent to 3 identical capacitors in parallel combination. Hence, equivalent capacitance

$$C_P = C + C + C$$

$$= 3C = 3\frac{\varepsilon_0 A}{d}$$

79. (d) It will act like three capacitors which are connected in parallel, so equivalent capacitance,

$$C = C_1 + C_2 + C_3 = 3 + 3 + 3 = 9\,\mu\text{F}$$

80. (d) Here, $C_{13} = C_1 + C_3 = 9 + 9 = 18\,\mu\text{F}$

$$C_{2\text{-}13} = \frac{C_2 \cdot C_{13}}{C_2 + C_{13}} = \frac{9 \times 18}{9 + 18} = 6\,\mu\text{F}$$

Equivalent capacitance between the point A and B,

$C_{\text{eq}} = C_{2\text{-}13} + C_4 = 6 + 9 = 15\,\mu\text{F}$

81. (*b*) Here, three capacitors are connected in parallel. So, their equivalent capacity

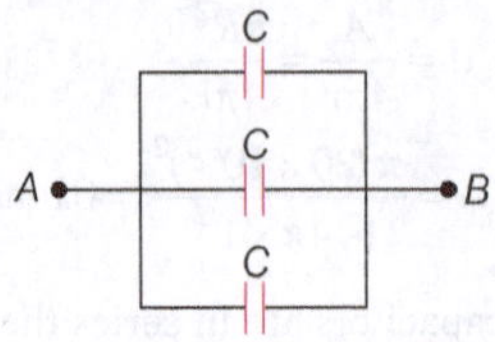

$$C_P = C + C + C = 3C$$

82. (*d*) The given circuit can be redrawn as

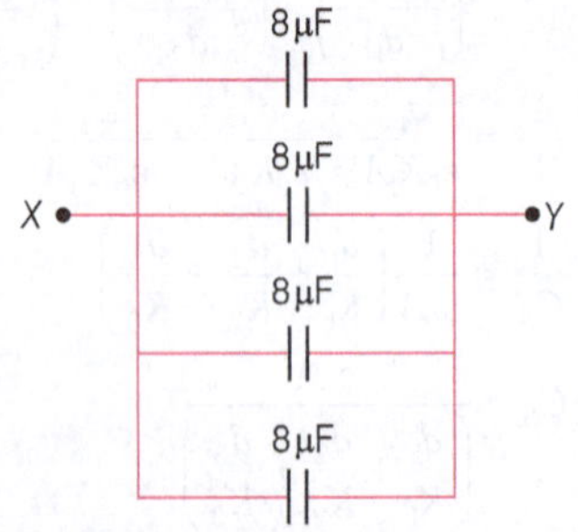

$$\therefore \quad C_{XY} = 4 \times 8 = 32\ \mu\text{F}$$

83. (*b*) We have, $\dfrac{\varepsilon_0 A}{d} = \dfrac{\varepsilon_0 A}{(d + \Delta d) - t + \dfrac{t}{K}}$ or $K = \dfrac{t}{t - \Delta d}$

Dielectric constant, $K = \dfrac{4 \times 10^{-3}}{4 \times 10^{-3} - 3.5 \times 10^{-3}}$

$$K = \frac{4 \times 10^{-3}}{0.5 \times 10^{-3}} = \frac{40}{5} = 8 \Rightarrow K = 8$$

84. (*c*) This diagram is symmetrical about line *AB*, hence point on perpendicular of *AB*, *i.e.* *C*, *D* and *E* are at same potential. So, remove capacitor between *C* and *D*, *D* and *E*.

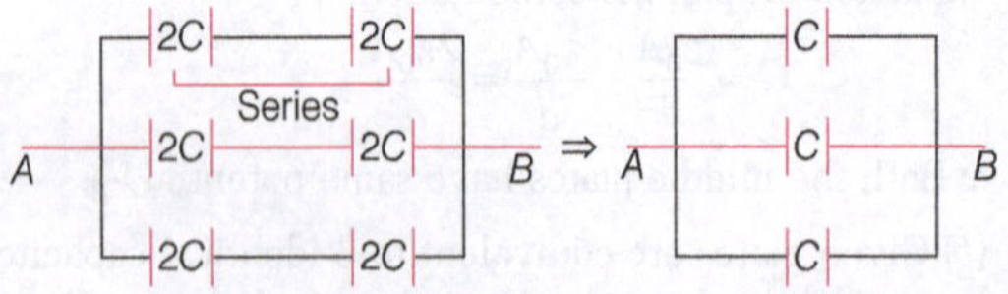

The equivalent capacitance, $C_{eq} = C + C + C = 3C$

85. (*a*) The given circuit can be simplified in following way.

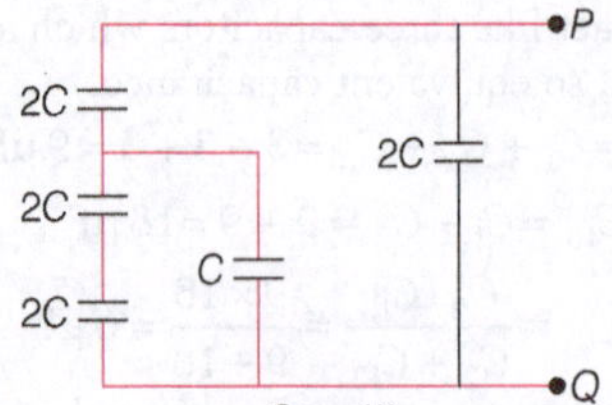

Step (1)

⇓

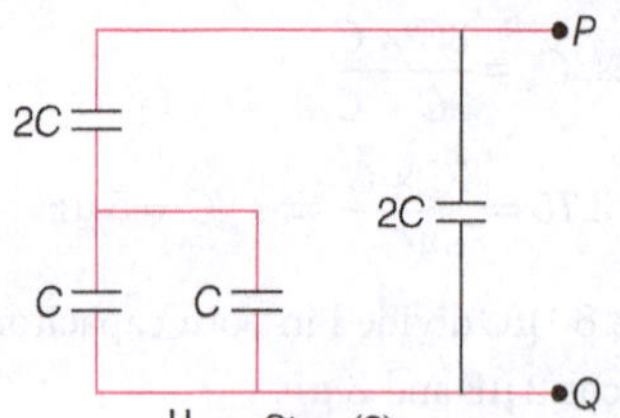

⇓ Step (2)

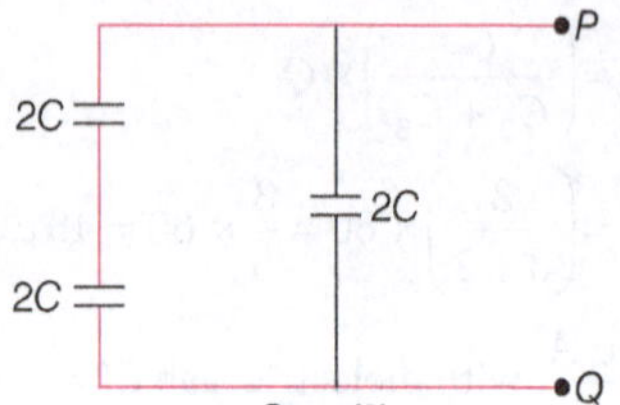

Step (3)

⇓

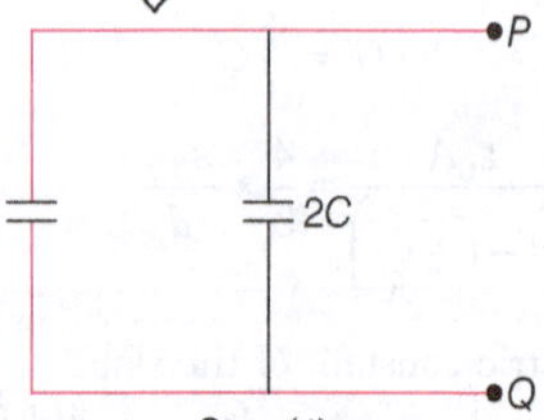

Step (4)

So, capacity between *P* and *Q*,

$$C_{PQ} = 2C + C = 3C$$

86. (*d*) Capacitors C_1 and C_2 are in series with C_3 in parallel with them.

Now, $C_1 = \dfrac{K_1 \varepsilon_0 (A/2)}{(d/2)} = \dfrac{K_1 \varepsilon_0 A}{d}$

$C_2 = \dfrac{K_2 \varepsilon_0 (A/2)}{(d/2)} = \dfrac{K_2 \varepsilon_0 A}{d}$ and $C_3 = \dfrac{K_3 \varepsilon_0 A}{2d}$

$$C_{\text{equivalent}} = C_3 + \frac{C_1 C_2}{C_1 + C_2}$$

$$= \frac{K_3 \varepsilon_0 A}{2d} + \frac{\left(\dfrac{K_1 \varepsilon_0 A}{d}\right)\left(\dfrac{K_2 \varepsilon_0 A}{d}\right)}{\dfrac{K_1 \varepsilon_0 A}{d} + \dfrac{K_2 \varepsilon_0 A}{d}}$$

$$= \frac{\varepsilon_0 A}{d}\left(\frac{K_3}{2} + \frac{K_1 K_2}{K_1 + K_2}\right)$$

So, option (d) is correct.

87. (*d*) The simple circuit is as shown below,

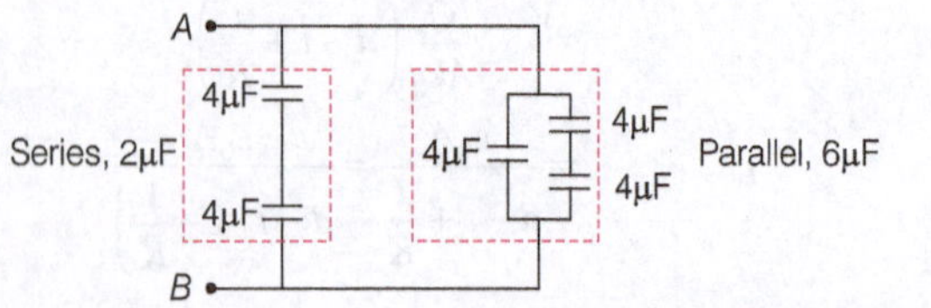

$$C_{AB} = (2 + 6)\ \mu\text{F} = 8\ \mu\text{F}$$

88. (a) In given figure, C_2 and C_3 are in parallel.

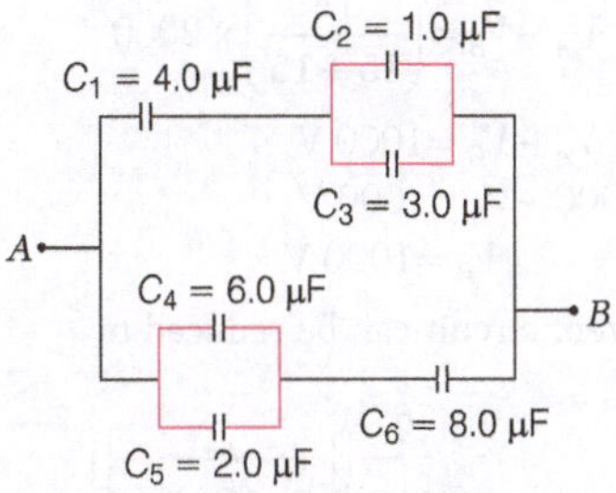

$$\therefore \quad C' = C_2 + C_3 = 4\,\mu F$$

As C' and C_1 are in series,

$$\frac{1}{C_{S_1}} = \frac{1}{C'} + \frac{1}{C_1} = \frac{1}{4} + \frac{1}{4}$$

$$\Rightarrow \quad C_{S_1} = 2\,\mu F$$

Similarly, C_4 and C_5 are in parallel,

$$C'' = 6 + 2 = 8\,\mu F$$

C'' and C_6 are in series,

$$\frac{1}{C_{S_2}} = \frac{1}{C''} + \frac{1}{C_6} = \frac{1}{8} + \frac{1}{8}$$

$$\Rightarrow \quad C_{S_2} = 4\,\mu F$$

Now, C_{S_1} and C_{S_2} are in parallel,

$$C = 4 + 2 = 6\,\mu F$$

89. (b) The given combination is a balanced Wheatstone bridge in parallel with 10 C.

Capacitance, $C_1 = \dfrac{6 \times 6}{6 + 6} = 3C$

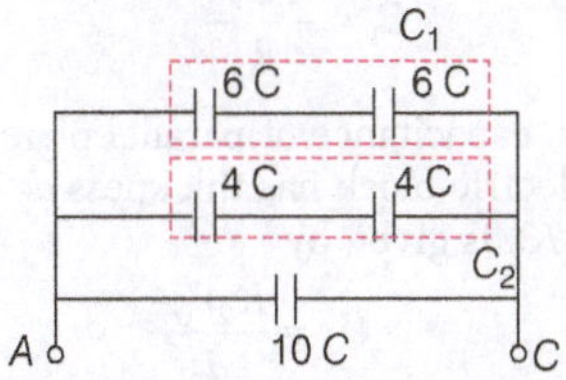

Capacitance, $C_2 = \dfrac{4 \times 4}{4 + 4} = 2C$

The equivalent capacitance between the points A and C.

$$C_{AC} = (3 + 2 + 10)\,C \Rightarrow C_{AC} = 15\,C$$

90. (b) Here, circuit is equivalent to two capacitors in parallel,

$$\therefore \quad C_{eq} = C_1 + C_2$$

$$= \frac{\varepsilon_0 A}{d} + \frac{\varepsilon_0 A}{d} = \frac{2\varepsilon_0 A}{d}$$

$$\therefore \text{Energy stored} = \frac{1}{2} C_{eq} V^2 = \frac{1}{2}\left(\frac{2\varepsilon_0 A}{d}\right) V^2$$

$$= \frac{8.85 \times 10^{-12} \times 50 \times 10^{-4} \times 12 \times 12}{3 \times 10^{-3}}$$

$$= 2.1 \times 10^{-9}\,J$$

91. (c) In figure, there is combination of two capacitors in parallel,

$$\therefore \quad C_P = C_1 + C_2 = \frac{K_1 \varepsilon_0 (A/2)}{d} + \frac{K_2 \varepsilon_0 (A/2)}{d}$$

$$= \frac{2\varepsilon_0 (A/2)}{d} + \frac{4\varepsilon_0 (A/2)}{d}$$

$$= 2 \times \frac{10}{2} + 4 \times \frac{10}{2} = 30\,\mu F$$

92. (d) Given circuit can be redrawn as follows

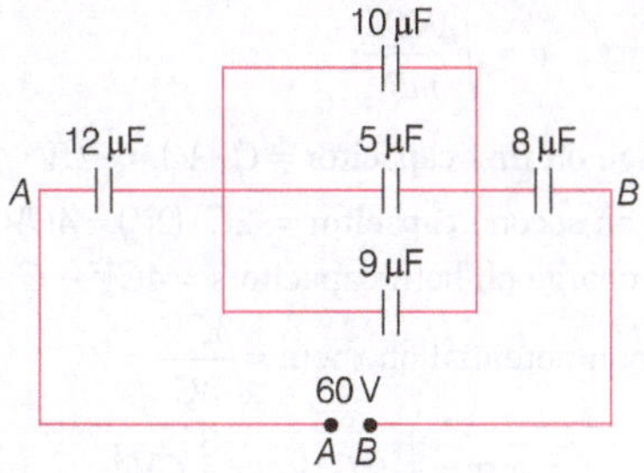

Equivalent capacitance of the circuit,

$$C_{AB} = \frac{24}{2 + 1 + 3} = 4\,\mu F$$

Total charge given by battery,

$$q = C_{AB} \cdot V = 4 \times 60 = 240\,\mu C$$

Charge on 5 μF capacitor,

$$q_2 = \left(\frac{5}{10 + 5 + 9}\right) \times 240 = 50\,\mu C$$

93. (a) The given circuit can be redrawn as,

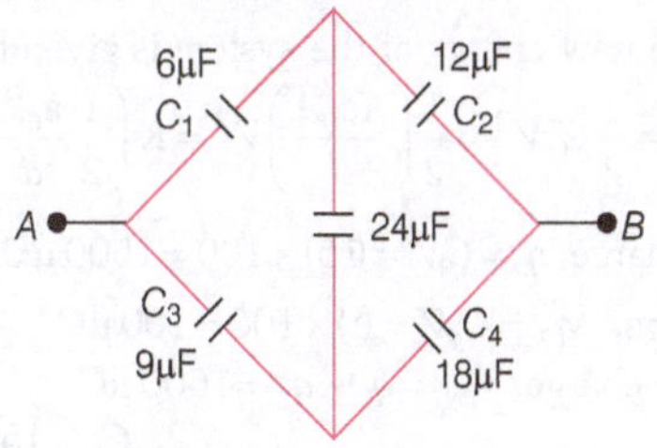

It is a balance Wheatstone bridge type network,

i.e., $\dfrac{C_1}{C_2} = \dfrac{C_3}{C_4} = \dfrac{1}{2}$

$\therefore$ 24 μF capacitor can be neglected.

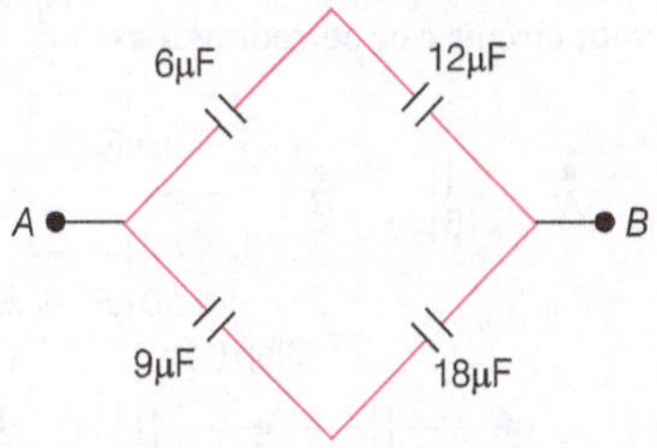

Hence, equivalent capacitance between A and B

$$= 4 + 6 = 10\,\mu F$$

94. (c) This combination forms a GP, $S = 1 + \frac{1}{2} + \frac{1}{4} + \frac{1}{8} + \ldots$

Sum of infinite GP, $S = \frac{a}{1-r} \Rightarrow S = \frac{1}{1-1/2} = \frac{1}{\frac{1}{2}} = 2$

Hence, capacitance of combination, $C_\infty = 2 \times 1\,\mu\text{F} = 2\,\mu\text{F}$

95. (a) we have, $K_i + U_i = K_f + U_f$

$$0 + 0 = \frac{1}{2}mv^2 + (-e)\frac{KQ}{R}$$

$\therefore$ Velocity, $v = \sqrt{\frac{2KQe}{mR}}$

96. (c) Charge on first capacitor $= C(-V) = -CV$

Charge on second capacitor $= (2C)(2V) = 4CV$

$\therefore$ Total charge on both capacitors $= 4CV - CV = 3CV$

$\therefore$ Common potential on them $= \frac{3CV}{3C} = V$

$\therefore$ $\quad$ Energy $= \frac{1}{2}(3C)V^2 = \frac{3}{2}CV^2$

97. (a) Energy stored in a parallel plate capacitor of capacitance C and separated by a distance d is

$$V_0 = \frac{1}{2}CV^2 = \frac{1}{2}\left(\frac{\varepsilon_0 A}{d}\right)V^2$$

If a slab of dielectric constant K and thickness d is introduced between plates of capacitor, then

$$C' = \frac{\varepsilon_0 A}{d - d\left(1 - \frac{1}{K}\right)} = \frac{K\varepsilon_0 A}{d}$$

$\therefore$ The new energy of the system is given by

$$U' = \frac{1}{2}C'V^2 = \frac{1}{2}\left(\frac{K\varepsilon_0 A}{d}\right)V^2 = K\left(\frac{1}{2}\frac{\varepsilon_0 A}{d}V^2\right) = KV_0$$

98. (b) Charge, $q_1 = C_1V = (15) \times 100 = 1500\,\mu\text{C}$

Charge, $q_2 = C_2V = (1) \times 100 = 100\,\mu\text{C}$

$\therefore$ Net charge, $q_{\text{net}} = q_1 + q_2 = 1600\,\mu\text{C}$

When dielectric is removed, $C'_1 = \frac{C_1}{K} = \frac{15}{15} = 1\,\mu\text{F}$

Now, common potential,

$$V = \frac{q_{\text{net}}}{C'_1 + C_2} = \frac{1600}{1+1} = 800\text{ V}$$

99. (b) Given, circuit can be redrawn as

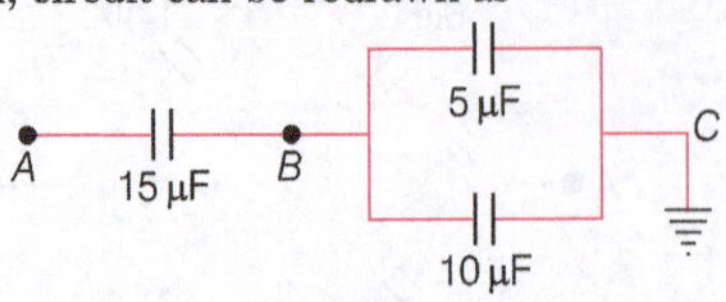

Step (1)

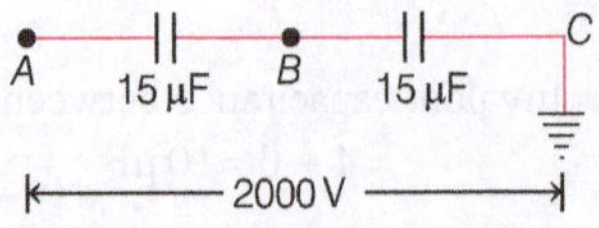

Step (2)

Potential difference between A and B,

$$V_A - V_B = \left(\frac{15}{15+15}\right) \times 2000$$

$\therefore$ $\quad V_A - V_B = 1000\text{ V}$

$\therefore$ $\quad 2000 - V_B = 1000\text{ V}$

$\therefore$ $\quad V_B = 1000\text{ V}$

100. (b) Given, circuit can be reduced to

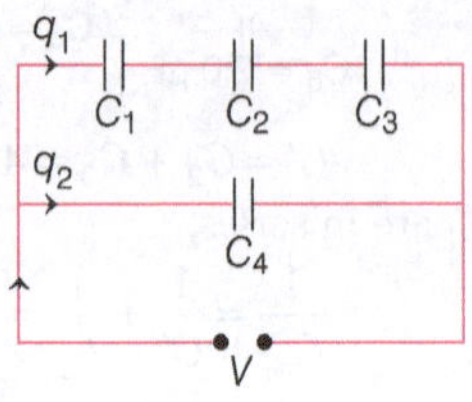

For series combination of C_1, C_2, C_3 resultant capacitance are

$$C_S = \frac{6C}{6C + 3C + 2C}$$

or $\quad C_S = \frac{6C}{11}$

Now, the ratio of the charges on C_2 and C_4,

$$\frac{q_1}{q_2} = \frac{C_S}{C_4} = \frac{6C/11}{4C} = \frac{3}{22}$$

101. (c) The capacitance of parallel plate capacitor filled with dielectric block has thickness d_1 and dielectric constant K_1 is given by

$$C_1 = \frac{K_1\varepsilon_0 A}{d_1}$$

Similarly, capacitance of parallel plate capacitor filled with dielectric block has thickness d_2 and dielectric constant K_2 is given by

$$C_2 = \frac{K_2\varepsilon_0 A}{d_2}$$

Since, the two capacitors are in series combination, the equivalent capacitance is given by

$$\frac{1}{C} = \frac{1}{C_1} + \frac{1}{C_2}$$

or $\quad C = \frac{C_1C_2}{C_1 + C_2} = \frac{\frac{K_1\varepsilon_0 A}{d_1}\,\frac{K_2\varepsilon_0 A}{d_2}}{\frac{K_1\varepsilon_0 A}{d_1} + \frac{K_2\varepsilon_0 A}{d_2}}$

$$= \frac{K_1K_2\varepsilon_0 A}{K_1d_2 + K_2d_1} \quad \ldots\text{(i)}$$

But, the equivalent capacitances is given by

$$C = \frac{K\varepsilon_0 A}{d_1 + d_2}$$

On comparing, we have

$$K = \frac{K_1K_2(d_1 + d_2)}{K_1d_2 + K_2d_1}$$

102. (c) Minimum number of condensers in each row

$$=\frac{3000}{500}=6$$

If C_S is capacity of 6 condensers in a row,

$$\frac{1}{C_S}=\frac{1}{1}+\frac{1}{1}+\frac{1}{1}+\frac{1}{1}+\frac{1}{1}+\frac{1}{1}=6$$

$$\Rightarrow \quad C_S=\frac{1}{6}\mu F$$

Let there be m such rows in parallel.

Total capacity $=m\times C_s$

$$2=m\times\frac{1}{6}$$

$$\therefore \quad m=12$$

Total number of capacitors $=6\times12=72$

103. (a) The given circuit can be reduced in following manner

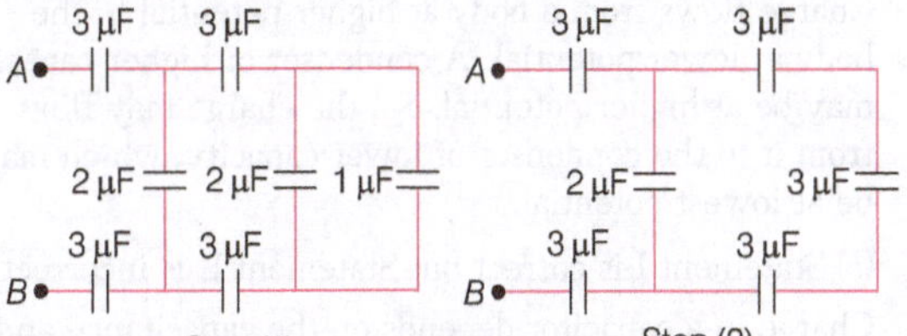

Step (1) Step (2)

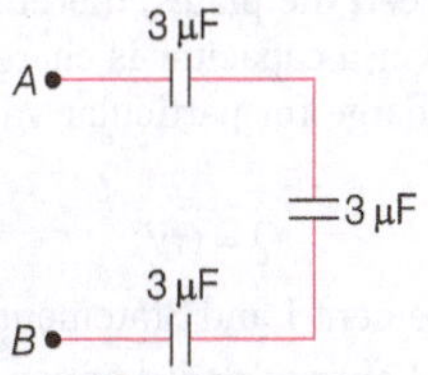

Step (3)

$\therefore$ Resultant capacity between A and B, $C_{AB}=1\,\mu F$

104. (d) Given, circuit can be reduced in following manner

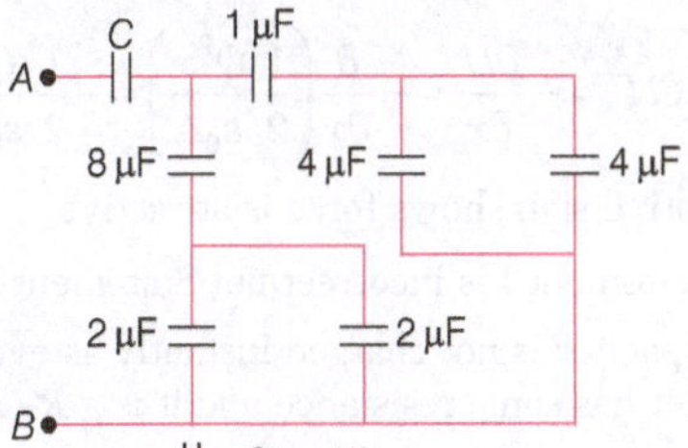

⇓ Step (1)

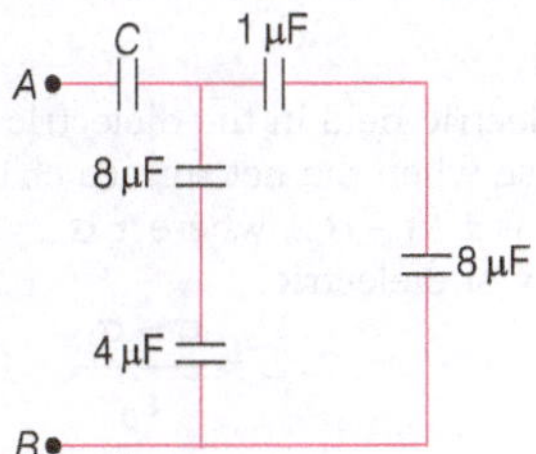

⇓ Step (2)

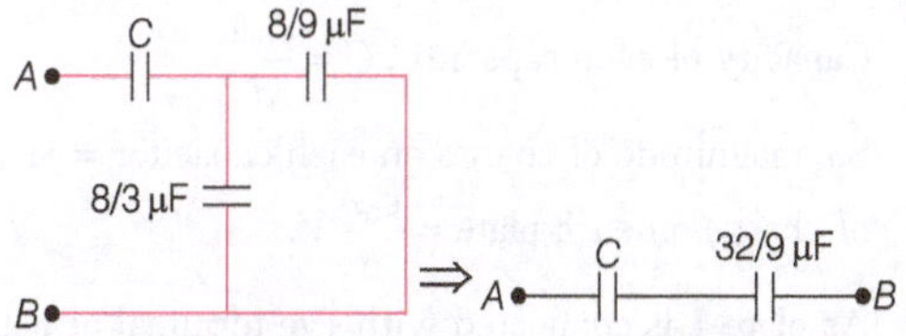

Step (3) Step (4)

So, equivalent capacitance between A and B,

$$C_{eq}=1=\frac{\frac{32}{9}\times C}{\frac{32}{9}+C}$$

$\therefore$ The value of $C=\frac{32}{23}\,\mu F$

105. (a) From concept of series and parallel combination, we can easily find that in option (a) the resultant capacity is $\frac{10}{11}\,\mu F$.

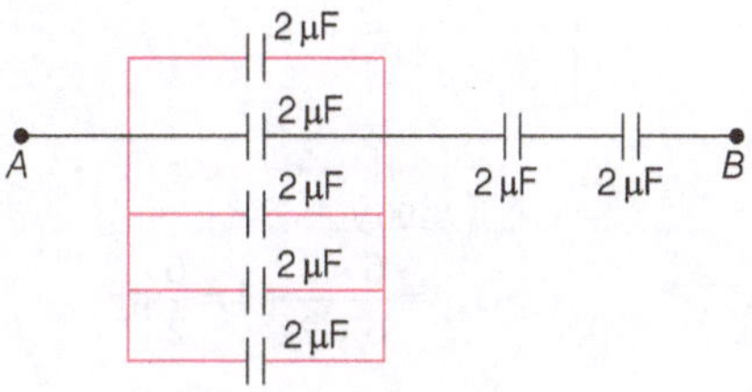

The circuit can be redrawn as

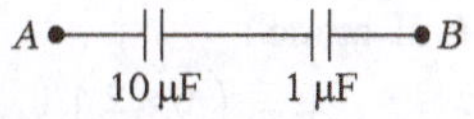

$\therefore$ Equivalent capacity,

$$C_{eq}=\frac{10\times1}{10+1}=\frac{10}{11}\,\mu F$$

106. (b) Applying charge distribution law on C_1 and C_2 at steady state. Charge on C_1,

$$Q_1=\left(\frac{C_1}{C_1+2C_1}\right)\times Q=\frac{Q}{3}$$

Charge on C_2,

$$Q_2=\left(\frac{2C_1}{C_1+2C_1}\right)\times Q=\frac{2}{3}Q$$

107. (c) Given circuit can be redrawn as shown

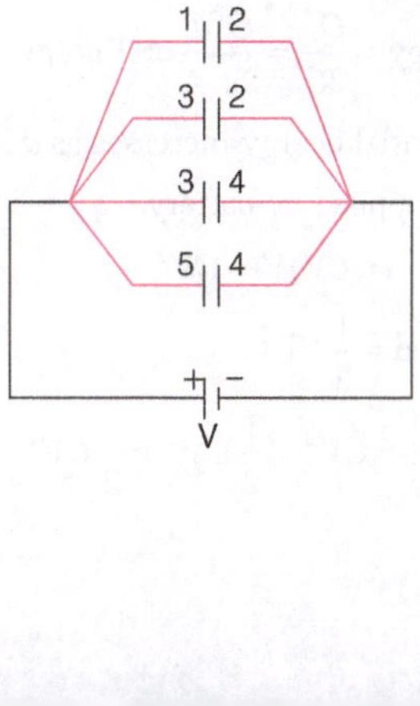

Capacity of each capacitor, $C = \frac{\varepsilon_0 A}{d}$

So, magnitude of charge on each capacitor = Magnitude of charge on each plate $= \frac{\varepsilon_0 A}{d} V$.

As plate 1 is connected with +ve terminal of battery, so charge on plate 1 $= + \frac{\varepsilon_0 A}{d} V$.

Plate 4 comes twice and it is connected with negative terminal of battery. So, charge on plate 4 $= -\frac{2\varepsilon_0 AV}{d}$.

108. (c) The given circuit can be reduced as follows. (Resistance does not matter in considering equivalent capacitance)

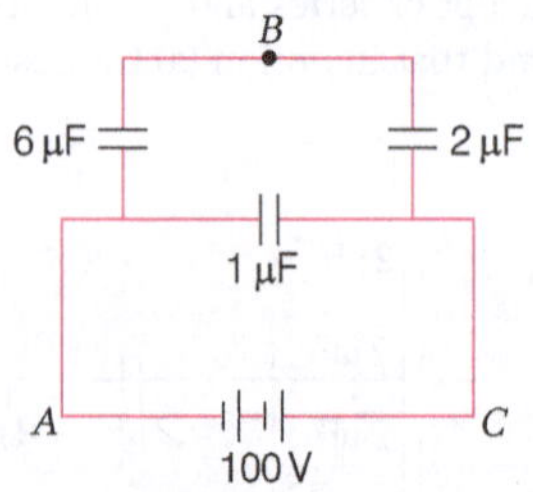

$$C_{eq} = \frac{6 \times 2}{6+2} + 1 = \frac{5}{2} \, \mu F$$

Total charge, $Q = CV = \frac{5}{2} \times 100 = 250 \, \mu C$

So, charge in 6 μF branch

$$= CV = \left(\frac{6 \times 2}{6+2}\right) \times 100 = 150 \, \mu C$$

$$\therefore \quad V_{AB} = \frac{150}{6} = 25 \text{ V}$$

and $\quad V_{BC} = 100 - V_{AB} = 100 - 25 = 75 \text{ V}$

Assertion and Reason

1. (d) Capacitance is basically a geometrical quantity.
2. (d) Even though field may have considerable strength, the potential difference between the two conductors of a capacitor is small because the field lines are confined within a small region of space.
3. (c) Battery is disconnected from the capacitor.

So, $\quad Q = \text{constant}$

$$\text{Energy} = \frac{Q^2}{2C} = \frac{Q^2 d}{2\varepsilon_0 A} \Rightarrow \text{Energy} \propto d$$

Hence, potential energy increases as d increased.

4. (b) Energy supplied by battery $= qV$

$$= (CV)V = CV^2$$

Energy stored $= \frac{1}{2} CV^2$

$\therefore$ Energy lost $= CV^2 - \frac{1}{2} CV^2 = \frac{1}{2} CV^2$

Therefore, half energy is lost.

As, we have seen in the above case, half of the energy is lost by changing a capacitor. Hence, we can say that, capacitor also consumes energy.

5. (a) $C = \frac{\varepsilon_0 KA}{d} \Rightarrow C \propto \frac{K}{d}$

$$\therefore \quad \frac{C_1}{C_2} = \frac{K_1}{d_1} \times \frac{d_2}{K_2} = \frac{K}{d} \times \frac{d/2}{3K} = \frac{1}{6}$$

$$C_2 = 6C_1$$

Again for capacity of a capacitor, $C = \frac{K \varepsilon_0 A}{d}$

Therefore, capacity of a capacitor depends upon the medium between two plates of capacitor.

Statements Type Questions

1. (a) Both Statement I and Statement II are incorrect.

Charge flows from a body at higher potential to the body at lower potential. A condenser of higher capacity may be at higher potential. So, the charge may flow from it to the condenser of lower capacity, which may be at lowest potential.

2. (b) Statement I is correct but Statement II is incorrect.

Charge in a capacitor depends on the capacitance and voltage between the plates, therefore Statement II is false whenever a capacitor is charged it will always have same charge for particular values of voltage and capacitance.

$$Q = CV$$

3. (a) Both Statement I and Statement II are incorrect.

The potential energy stored between the plates of capacitor,

$$U = \frac{1}{2}\frac{Q^2}{C} = \frac{1}{2}\frac{Q^2}{\varepsilon_0 A} x \qquad \left(\because C = \frac{\varepsilon_0 A}{x}\right)$$

$$\text{Force, } F = -\frac{\partial U}{\partial x} = -\frac{\partial}{\partial x}\left(\frac{1}{2}\frac{Q^2 x}{\varepsilon_0 A}\right) = -\frac{1}{2}\frac{Q^2}{\varepsilon_0 A}$$

Negative sign shows force is attractive.

4. (c) Statement I is incorrect but Statement II is correct.

A capacitor is not charged instantly as every practical circuit has some resistance and it is a R-C circuit.

Match the Columns

1. (d)

A. The electric field in the dielectric corresponds to the case when the net surface charge density on the plates is $\pm(\sigma - \sigma_p)$, where $\pm \sigma_p$ = surface charge density of dielectric.

i.e. $$E = \frac{\sigma - \sigma_p}{\varepsilon_0} \qquad \text{...(i)}$$

B. So the potential difference across the plates is

$$V = Ed = \frac{\sigma - \sigma_p}{\varepsilon_0} d \qquad \text{...(ii)}$$

For linear dielectric, we except σ_p to be proportional to E_0, *i.e.*, to σ. Thus, $(\sigma - \sigma_p)$ is proportional to σ and we can write

$$\sigma - \sigma_p = \frac{\sigma}{K} \quad ...(iii)$$

where, K is a constant characteristic of the dielectric. Clearly, $K > 1$, then we have

$$V = \frac{\sigma d}{\varepsilon_0 K} = \frac{Qd}{A\varepsilon_0 K} \quad ...(iv)$$

C. The capacitance C with dielectric between the plates is

$$C = \frac{Q}{V} = \frac{\varepsilon_0 KA}{d} \quad ...(v)$$

D. The product $\varepsilon_0 K$ is called the permittivity of the medium and is denoted by ε.

$$\varepsilon = \varepsilon_0 K \quad ...(vi)$$

For vacuum, $K = 1$ and $\varepsilon = \varepsilon_0$.

The dimensionless ratio, $K = \frac{\varepsilon}{\varepsilon_0}$ ...(vii)

is called the dielectric constant of the substance. As remarked before, from Eq. (iii), it is clear that K is greater than 1.

From equations, $\left(C_0 = \varepsilon_0 \frac{A}{d}\right)$

and $C = \frac{\varepsilon_0 KA}{d}$,

$$K = \frac{C}{C_0} \quad ...(viii)$$

Hence, A-(II), B-(I), C-(IV), D-(III)

2. (*b*) Given, $t = 1.0 \text{ cm} = 10^{-2}\text{m}, k = 5$

$A = 0.01\text{m}^2 = 10^{-2}\text{m}^2, d = 2 \text{ cm} = 2 \times 10^{-2}\text{m}$

A. Capacity with air in between the plates $C_o = \frac{\varepsilon_o A}{d}$

$$= \frac{8.85 \times 10^{-12} \times 10^{-2}}{2 \times 10^{-2}} = 4.425 \times 10^{-12} \text{ F}$$

B. Capacity with dielectric slab in between the plates

$$C = \frac{\varepsilon_o A}{d - t\left(1 - \frac{1}{k}\right)} = \frac{8.85 \times 10^{-12} \times 10^{-2}}{2 \times 10^{-2} - 10^{-2}\left(1 - \frac{1}{5}\right)}$$

$$= 7.375 \times 10^{-12} \text{ F}$$

C. Capacity with conducting slab in between the plates

$$C' = \frac{\varepsilon_o A}{d - t} = \frac{8.85 \times 10^{-12} \times 10^{-2}}{2 \times 10^{-2} - 1 \times 10^{-2}}$$

$$= 8.85 \times 10^{-12} \text{ F}$$

D. Increase in capacitance on introduction of dielectric

$$= C - C_o = 7.375 \times 10^{-12} - 4.425 \times 10^{-12}$$

$$= 2.95 \times 10^{-12} \text{ F}$$

Hence, A-IV, B-III, C-II, D-I

3. (*c*) (A) Capacitance, $C = \frac{\varepsilon_0 A}{d}$

$$= \frac{8.85 \times 10^{-12} \times 0.20}{0.01} = 1.77 \times 10^{-10} \text{ (SI unit)}$$

(B) Charge on each plate, $q = CV$

$$= 3000 \times 1.77 \times 10^{-10}$$

$$= 5.31 \times 10^{-7} \text{ (SI unit)}$$

(C) $\therefore C = \frac{\varepsilon_0 A}{d - t + \frac{t}{K}}$

$$\Rightarrow \quad 5.31 \times 10^{-10} = \frac{8.85 \times 10^{-12} \times 0.20}{0.01 - 0.01 + \frac{0.01}{K}}$$

$$\Rightarrow \quad K = \frac{5.31 \times 10^{-10} \times 0.01}{8.85 \times 10^{-12} \times 0.20} = 3$$

Dielectric constant, $K = 3$

(D) Capacitance, $C = \frac{q}{V}$

$$\Rightarrow \quad C = \frac{5.31 \times 10^{-7}}{1000}$$

$$\Rightarrow \quad C = 5.31 \times 10^{-10} \text{ (SI unit)}$$

Hence, A-IV, B-I, C-III, D-II.

4. (*c*) A. When S is open, then

$$C_{eq} = \frac{C_1 C_2}{C_1 + C_2} = \frac{(2\,\mu\text{F})(3\,\mu\text{F})}{(2\,\mu\text{F} + 3\,\mu\text{F})} = \frac{6}{5}\,\mu\text{F}$$

Charge q on both the capacitors will be the same (as these are in series), *i.e.*

$$q = C_{eq} V = \left(\frac{6}{5}\,\mu\text{F}\right)(30 + 60)\text{ V} = 108\,\mu\text{C}$$

B. Charge on C_2, *i.e.*, $q_2 = C_2 V_2$

$$= (3\,\mu\text{F})(60\text{ V}) = 180\,\mu\text{C}$$

C. When S is closed, charge on C_1, *i.e.*,

$$q_1 = C_1 V_1 = (2\,\mu\text{F})(30\text{ V}) = 60\,\mu\text{C}$$

D. Charge on C_1 and C_2

$$= 60\,\mu\text{C} + 180\,\mu\text{C} = 240\,\mu\text{C}$$

$\therefore$ A-(I), B-(IV), C-(III), D-(II)

Final Check Through PYQ

1. (*b*) Capacitance of parallel plate capacitor when medium is air

$$C_0 = \frac{\varepsilon_0 A}{d} \quad ...(i)$$

According to second condition,

$$A' = A, t = \frac{d}{2}, K = 4$$

$\therefore$ Capacitance, $C = \frac{\varepsilon_0 A}{(d - t) + \frac{t}{K}}$

$$= \frac{\varepsilon_0 A}{\left(d - \frac{d}{2}\right) + \frac{d/2}{4}} = \frac{8}{5} \cdot \frac{\varepsilon_0 A}{d}$$

$$\therefore \quad \frac{C}{C_0} = \frac{\frac{8}{5} \cdot \frac{\varepsilon_0 A}{d}}{\frac{\varepsilon_0 A}{d}} \Rightarrow C : C_0 = 8 : 5$$

2. (*b*) Given, $C_0 = 6\ \mu F$, $C_m = 30\ \mu F$

$\therefore$ As, dielectric constant

$$K = \varepsilon_r = \frac{C_m}{C_0} = \frac{30}{6} = 5$$

Permittivity of the medium,

$$\varepsilon_m = K \times \varepsilon_0 = 5 \times \varepsilon_0$$
$$= 5 \times 8.85 \times 10^{-12}$$
$$= 0.44 \times 10^{-10}\ C^2 N^{-1} m^{-2}$$

3. (*c*) As we know that, the total work done in transferring a charge to a parallel plate capacitor is given as

$$W = \frac{Q^2}{2C} \quad \text{...(i)}$$

Since, $\quad W = F \cdot d \quad$ ...(ii)

where, F is the electrostatic force between the plates of capacitor and d is the distance between the plates.

From Eqs. (i) and (ii), we get

$$W = \frac{Q^2}{2C} = Fd \Rightarrow F = \frac{Q^2}{2Cd} \quad \text{...(iii)}$$

As, the capacitance of a parallel plate is given as,

$$C = \frac{\varepsilon_0 A}{d}$$

Substituting the value of C in Eq. (iii), we get,

$$F = \frac{Q^2 d}{2\varepsilon_0 A d} = \frac{Q^2}{2\varepsilon_0 A}$$

This means, electrostatic force is independent of the distance between the plates.

4. (*b*) Force between plates of parallel capacitor,

$$F = qE = q\left[\frac{\sigma}{2\varepsilon_0}\right]$$

$\because$ Surface charge density

$$\sigma = \frac{q}{A}$$

$$\therefore \quad F = q\left[\frac{q}{2A\varepsilon_0}\right]$$

$$\Rightarrow \quad F = \frac{q^2}{2A\varepsilon_0}$$

So, net charge across a capacitor,

$$q = CV$$

$$F = \frac{C^2 V^2}{2A\varepsilon_0} \quad \left[C = \frac{A\varepsilon_0}{d}\right]$$

$$\Rightarrow \quad F = \frac{\left(\frac{A\varepsilon_0}{d}\right) \times CV^2}{2A\varepsilon_0} = \frac{CV^2}{2d}$$

5. (*a*) Given combination of capacitors represent Wheatstone bridge, thus central capacitor can be removed.

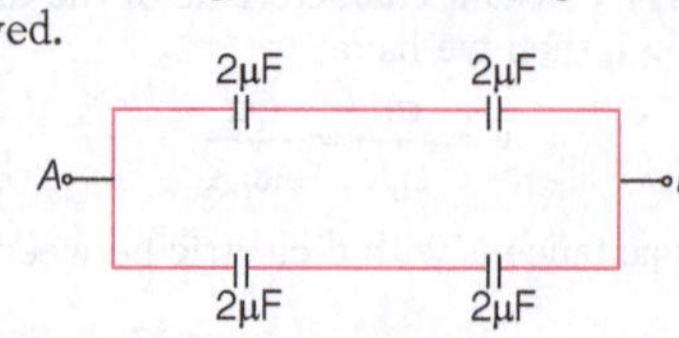

Capacitance of each branch,

$$C = \frac{2}{2} = 1\ \mu F$$

Capacitance between A and B, $C_{net} = 1 + 1 = 2\ \mu F$

6. (*d*) Equivalent capacitance of the system,

$$C_{AB} = \frac{3 \times (3+3)}{3 + (3+3)} = \frac{18}{9} = 2\ \mu F$$

7. (*c*) Here, $C_1 = \frac{2\varepsilon_0 K_1 A}{3d}, C_2 = \frac{2\varepsilon_0 K_2 A}{3d}$

$$C_3 = \frac{2\varepsilon_0 K_3 A}{3d}, C_4 = \frac{2\varepsilon_0 K_4 A}{d}$$

Given system of C_1, C_2, C_3 and C_4 can be simplified

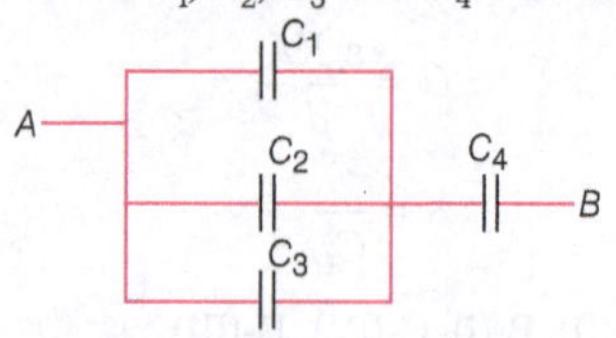

$$\therefore \quad \frac{1}{C_{AB}} = \frac{1}{C_1 + C_2 + C_3} + \frac{1}{C_4}$$

Suppose, $C_{AB} = \frac{K\varepsilon_0 A}{d}$

$$\frac{1}{K\left(\frac{\varepsilon_0 A}{d}\right)} = \frac{1}{\frac{2}{3}\frac{\varepsilon_0 A}{d}(K_1 + K_2 + K_3)} + \frac{1}{\frac{2\varepsilon_0 A}{d} K_4}$$

$$\Rightarrow \quad \frac{1}{K} = \frac{3}{2(K_1 + K_2 + K_3)} + \frac{1}{2K_4}$$

$$\Rightarrow \quad \frac{2}{K} = \frac{3}{K_1 + K_2 + K_2} + \frac{1}{K_4}$$

8. (*b*) Consider the nodes be A, B, E and F as shown in the figure

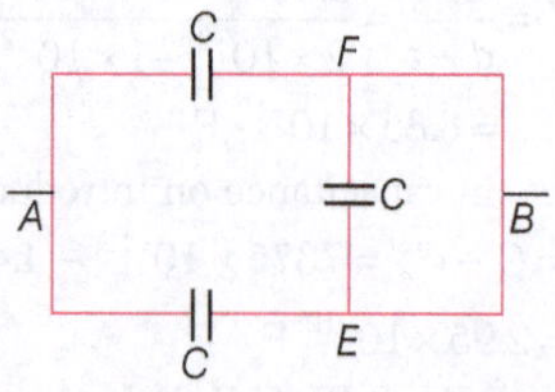

The potential at F is equal to the potential at node E. So, EF behave as open circuit.

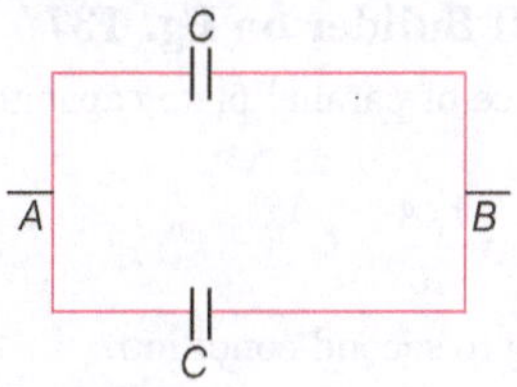

Now, the two capacitors are arranged in parallel. The net equivalent capacitors,

$$C_{eq} = C_1 + C_2$$

$$\Rightarrow \quad C_{eq} = C + C$$

$$\Rightarrow \quad C_{eq} = 2C$$

9. (b) We know that,

$$C = \frac{\varepsilon_0 A}{d}$$

$$E = \frac{1}{2} CV^2$$

and $\quad Q = C \cdot V$

As the distance between the plates decreases capacitance increases, therefore energy increases and also charge stored is increased.

Hence, A, C, and E are correct.

10. (b) The given situation is shown below.

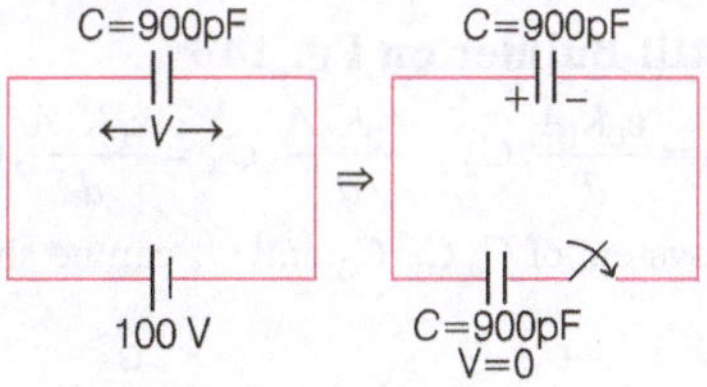

After combination,

Common potential,

$$V = \frac{C_1V_1 + C_2V_2}{C_1 + C_2} = \frac{C \times 100 + C \times 0}{C + C}$$

$$= 50 \text{ V}$$

∴Electrostatic stored potential energy,

$$U = 2 \times \frac{1}{2} CV^2 = CV^2$$

$$= 9 \times 10^{-10} \times 50^2 = 2.25 \times 10^{-6} \text{ J}$$

11. (c) The energy stored in the capacitor,

$$U = \frac{1}{2} CV^2$$

$$U = \frac{1}{2}\left(\frac{\varepsilon_0 A}{d}\right)(Ed)^2 \qquad \left[\because C = \frac{\varepsilon_0 A}{d} \text{ and } V = Ed\right]$$

$$U = \frac{1}{2}(\varepsilon_0 A)(E)^2 d$$

$$= \frac{1}{2}\varepsilon_0 E^2 Ad$$

12. (c) When C_1 is connected to voltage source, it is charged to a potential V and this will be stored as a potential energy in the capacitor given by

$$U = \frac{1}{2} CV^2$$

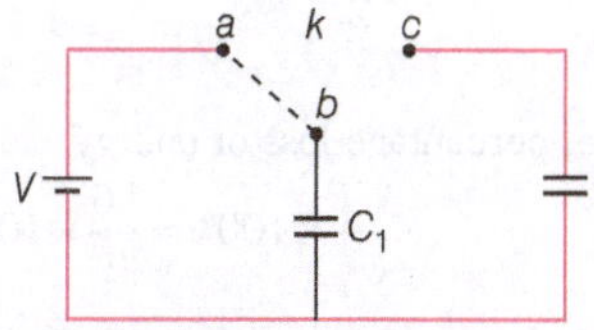

When key is disconnected from battery and b and c are connected, the charge will be transformed from the capacitor C_1 to capacitor C_2, then

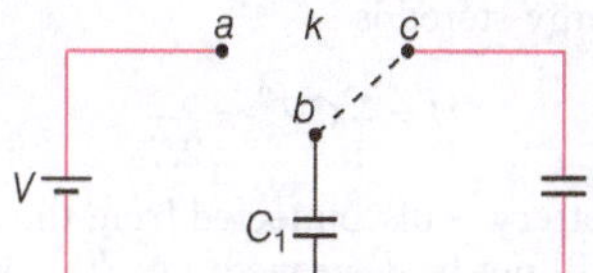

The loss of energy due to redistribution of charge is given by

$$\Delta U = \frac{C_1C_2}{2(C_1 + C_2)}(V_1 - V_2)^2$$

$$= \frac{C \times C}{2(C + C)}(V - 0)^2 = \frac{1}{4} CV^2 \qquad [\because C_1 = C_2]$$

$$\therefore \text{ Percentage loss} = \frac{\Delta U}{U} \times 100$$

$$= \frac{\frac{1}{4}CV^2}{\frac{1}{2}CV^2} \times 100 = 50\%$$

13. (b) $U_i = \frac{1}{2} CV^2$

$$V' = \frac{CV + 0}{2C} = V/2$$

$$U_f = \frac{1}{2}(2C)\left(\frac{V}{2}\right)^2$$

$$= \frac{1}{2} U_i$$

14. (c) Consider the given figure,

When the switch S is connected to point 1, then initial energy stored in the capacitor can be given as

$$U = \frac{1}{2}(2\ \mu\text{F}) \times V^2$$

When the switch S is connected to point 2, energy dissipated on connection across 8 μF will be

$$\Delta U = \frac{1}{2}\left(\frac{C_1C_2}{C_1 + C_2}\right).V^2$$

$$= \frac{1}{2} \times \frac{2\,\mu\text{F} \times 8\,\mu\text{F}}{10\,\mu\text{F}} \times V^2$$

$$= \frac{1}{2} \times (1.6\,\mu\text{F}) \times V^2$$

Therefore, percentage loss of energy

$$\frac{\Delta U}{U} \times 100\% = \frac{1.6}{2} \times 100 = 80\%$$

15. (*d*) When a parallel plate air capacitor connected to a cell of emf V, then charge stored will be

$$q = CV \Rightarrow V = \frac{q}{C}$$

Also, energy stored is

$$U = \frac{1}{2}CV^2 = \frac{q^2}{2C}$$

As the battery is disconnected from the capacitor the charge will not be destroyed, *i.e.* $q' = q$ with the introduction of dielectric in the gap of capacitor the new capacitance will be

$$C' = CK$$

$$\Rightarrow \quad V' = \frac{q}{C'} = \frac{q}{CK}$$

The new energy stored will be

$$U' = \frac{1}{2}C'(V')^2 = \frac{q^2}{2CK}$$

$$\Rightarrow \quad \Delta U = U' - U$$

$$= \frac{q^2}{2C}\left(\frac{1}{K} - 1\right)$$

$$= \frac{1}{2}CV^2\left(\frac{1}{K} - 1\right)$$

Skill Builder

■ Sol. of Skill Builder on Pg. 136

(*c*) Given $C_0 = 8 \times 10^{-6}$ F

$$C_m = 48 \times 10^{-6}\ \text{F}$$

$\therefore$ As, dielectric constant,

$$K = \varepsilon_r = \frac{C_m}{C_0} = \frac{48}{8} = 6$$

Permittivity of the medium,

$$\varepsilon_m = k \times \varepsilon_0 = \times \varepsilon_0$$

$$= 6 \times 8.85 \times 10^{-12}$$

$$= 0.53 \times 10^{-10}\,\text{C}^2\text{N}^{-1}\text{m}^{-2}$$

■ Sol. of Skill Builder on Pg. 137

(*b*) Capacitance of parallel plate capacitor when medium is air

$$C_0 = \frac{\varepsilon_0 A}{d}$$

According to second condition,

$$A' = A,\ t = \frac{d}{3},\ k = 6$$

$$\therefore \text{ Capacitance, } C = \frac{\varepsilon_0 a}{\left(d - \frac{d}{3}\right) + \frac{d/3}{6}} = \frac{\varepsilon_0 a}{\frac{13d}{18}} = \frac{18}{13}\frac{\varepsilon_0 a}{d}$$

■ Sol. of Skill Builder on Pg. 143

(*b*) Given circuit is equivalent to

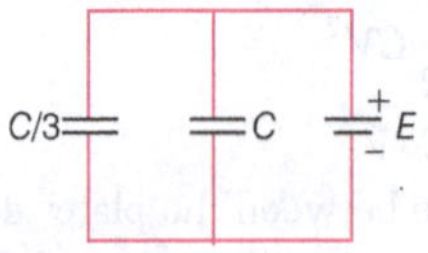

Final equivalent capacitance

$$C_{\text{eq}} = \frac{C}{3} + C = \frac{C + 3C}{3} = \frac{4C}{3}$$

■ Sol. of Skill Builder on Pg. 149

(*a*) Here $C_1 = \frac{\varepsilon_0 K_1 A}{d}, C_2 = \frac{\varepsilon_0 K_2 A}{d}, C_3 = \frac{\varepsilon_0 K_3 A}{d}, C_4 = \frac{\varepsilon_0 K_4 A}{d}$

Given, system of C_1, C_2, C_3 and C_4 can be simplified as

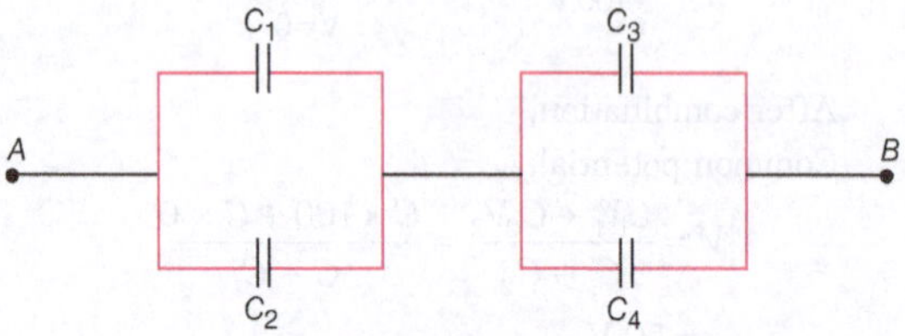

$$\frac{1}{C_{AB}} = \frac{1}{C_1 + C_2} + \frac{1}{C_3 + C_4}$$

Suppose, $C_{AB} = \frac{K\varepsilon_0 A}{d}$

$$\frac{1}{K\left(\frac{\varepsilon_0 A}{d}\right)} = \frac{1}{\frac{\varepsilon_0 A}{d}(K_1 + K_2)} + \frac{1}{\frac{\varepsilon_0 A}{d}(K_3 + K_4)}$$

$$\frac{1}{K} = \frac{1}{(K_1 + K_2)} + \frac{1}{(K_3 + K_4)}$$

$$K = \frac{(K_1 + K_2)(K_3 + K_4)}{K_1 + K_2 + K_3 + K_4}$$

■ Sol. of Skill Builder on Pg. 155

(*b*) From the given figure

When the switch *S* is connected to point *A*, then initial energy stored in the capacitor can be given as

$$U = \frac{1}{2}(2\mu F) \times V^2$$

When *S* is connected to point *B*, energy dissipated on connection across 3μF will be

$$\Delta U = \frac{1}{2}\left(\frac{C_1C_2}{C_1 + C_2}\right)V^2$$

$$= \frac{1}{2}\left(\frac{2 \times 3}{2 + 3}\right)V^2$$

$$= \frac{1}{2}\left(\frac{6}{5}\right)V^2 = \left(\frac{3}{5}\mu F\right)V^2$$

Therefore, loss of energy,

$$\frac{\Delta U}{U} \times 100 = \frac{\left(\frac{3}{5}\mu F\right)V^2}{(1\mu F)V^2} \times 100$$

$$= \frac{3}{5} \times 100 = 60\%$$

■ Sol. of Skill Builder on Pg. 156

(*c*)

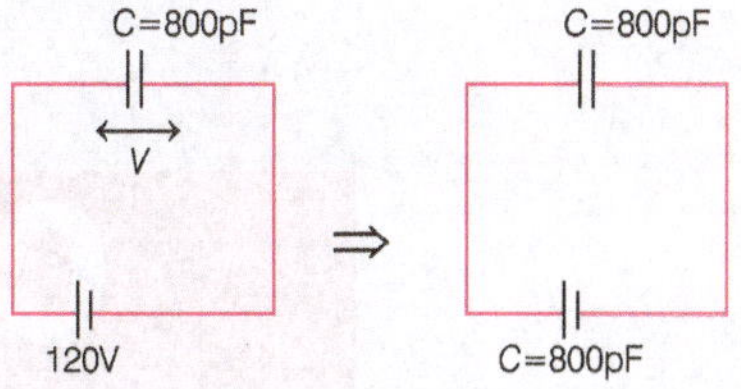

After combination, common potential,

$$V = \frac{C_1V_1 + C_2V_2}{C_1 + C_2}$$

$$= \frac{C \times 120 + C \times 0}{C + C}$$

$$= 60 \text{ V}$$

∴Electrostatic stored potential energy

$$u = 2 \times \frac{1}{2}CV^2 = CV^2$$

$$= 8 \times 10^{-10} \times (60)^2$$

$$= 28800 \times 10^{-10}$$

$$= 2.8 \times 10^{-6}\text{J}$$

For deeper insight
Scan the QR Code

Chapter 4

Current Electricity

Learning Objectives

Module-I

- Electric Current
- Electric Current in Conductors
- Ohm's Law

Module-II

- Series Combination
- Parallel Combination

Module-III

- Cell
- Grouping of Cells

Module-IV

- Kirchhoff's Laws
- Electrical Energy and Power
- Heating Effects of Current
- Wheatstone Bridge
- Meter Bridge

Chapter Overview with
NEET Connection

The concept of current electricity is one of the most important topic of NEET syllabus. Without gripping this chapter, it will be difficult to learn and understand the chapter like moving charge and magnetism, electromagnetic induction and alternating current etc.

Special format questions can be easily framed on the following topics of this chapter

- Relation among different parameters related to electric current.
- Combination of resistors and calculation of potential difference as well as current in different resistors.
- Solution of combination of batteries.
- Kirchhoff's laws.
- Wheatstone bridge and meter bridge.

For better understanding of this chapter

- Basic understanding of conductors is required.
- Basic idea of resistance, conductance, resistivity and conductivity will be helpful.
- Laboratory exposure of ammeter, voltmeter, batteries, rheostat, meter bridge will be more helpful.

Introduction

In previous chapters, we learnt that charge flows from high potential to low potential. This flow of charge inside a conductor constitutes an electric current in the conductors.

In this chapter, we will discuss about properties related to flow of electric current, role of resistance and batteries in flow of charge, their different combinations in the circuit and different methods of solving electric current related problems in circuits.

Module 1

Electric Current and Ohm's Law

- Electric Current • Electric Current in Conductors • Ohm's Law

Electric Current

Electric current is defined as the rate of flow of charge through any cross-sectional area of the conductor. It is denoted by I.

If electric current is steady, then it can be expressed as

$$I = \frac{\text{Total charge flowing } (q)}{\text{Total time taken } (t)} \Rightarrow \boxed{I = \frac{q}{t} = \frac{ne}{t}}$$

where, n = number of carriers (electrons) of electricity and e = electronic charge.

But current is not always steady, so it can be defined in two ways

(i) **Average current** If a charge Δq flows through a conductor in the time interval t to $(t + \Delta t)$, then average current is defined as $I_{av} = \frac{\Delta q}{\Delta t}$.

(ii) **Instantaneous current** Current at any instant of time passing through a conductor is called instantaneous current. If a small charge dq flows through a conductor in small time dt, i.e. limit of Δt tending to zero, then $I_{ins} = \lim_{\Delta t \to 0} \frac{\Delta q}{\Delta t} = \frac{dq}{dt}$.

Mentor's Tip

- Net electric field inside the conductor when electric current is flowing through it, $E = \frac{V}{l}$
- Net electric field outside the conductor = 0 $(\because q_{net} = 0)$

Important points about electric current

(i) Current is a scalar quantity.

(ii) Its SI unit is ampere (A) and CGS unit is emu and is also called biot (Bi) or ab ampere, i.e.

$$|A| = \left(\frac{1}{10}\right) \text{Bi (ab amp)}$$

(iii) One ampere is the current through a wire, if a charge of one coulomb flows through any cross-section of the wire in one second, i.e.

$$1 \text{ ampere (A)} = \frac{1 \text{ coulomb (C)}}{1 \text{ second (s)}}$$

$$= 1 \text{ coulomb per second} = 1 \text{ Cs}^{-1}$$

(iv) As a matter of convention, the direction of flow of positive charge gives the direction of current. This is called **conventional current**. The direction of flow of electrons gives the direction of **electronic current**. Therefore, the direction of electronic current is opposite to that of conventional current.

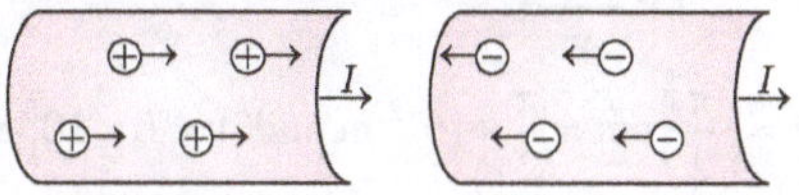

Flow of electronic current is equivalent to the flow of conventional current in opposite direction

(v) As charge is conserved and current is the rate of flow of charge, *i.e.* charge entering per second at one end of conductor is equal to the charge leaving per second to the other end.

Concept ladder

- In case, a charge q is revolving in a circle of radius r with uniform velocity v, current is given by
$$I = \frac{q}{t} = qf = q \cdot \frac{\omega}{2\pi} = \frac{qv}{2\pi r}$$
- Total charge in time interval t_1 to t_2 can be given as
$$Q = \int_{t_1}^{t_2} I \cdot dt$$
- Area under the graph I *versus* t in the interval t_1 to t_2 as shown in the figure gives amount of total charge (Q).

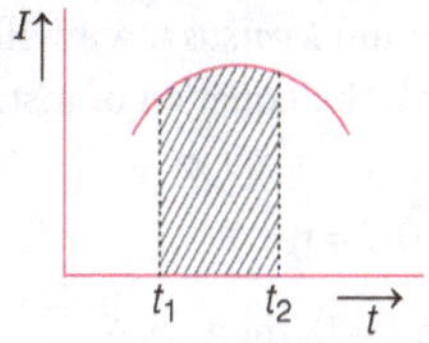

I versus t graph

So, average current in this interval,

$$I_{av} = \frac{Q}{t_2 - t_1} = \frac{\int_{t_1}^{t_2} I \cdot dt}{t_2 - t_1} = \frac{\text{Area under the } I \text{ versus } t \text{ graph}}{\text{Time interval}}$$

Example 1. *How many electrons pass through a bulb in 1 min, if the current is 400 mA? (Take, $e = 1.6 \times 10^{-19}$ C)*

Sol. Given, current, $I = 400 \text{ mA} = 400 \times 10^{-3}$ A

Time, $t = 1 \text{ min} = 60$ s

Charge, $e = 1.6 \times 10^{-19}$ C

Thus, charge passing through a bulb in 1 min is

$$q = I \times t = 400 \times 10^{-3} \times 60 = 24\text{ C}$$

Also, $q = ne$

$\therefore$ Number of electrons,

$$n = \frac{q}{e} = \frac{24}{1.6 \times 10^{-19}}$$

$$= 1.5 \times 10^{20} \text{ electrons}$$

Example 2. *If an electron revolves in a circle of radius $\pi/2$ cm with uniform speed 6×10^5 m/s. Find the electric current. (Take, $\pi^2 = 10$)*

Sol. Time period is given by

$$t = \frac{2\pi r}{v}$$

Here, $r = \left(\frac{\pi}{2}\right)\text{cm} = \frac{\pi}{2} \times 10^{-2}$ m and $v = 6 \times 10^5$ m/s

So, electric current, $i = \frac{ev}{2\pi r} = \frac{1.6 \times 10^{-19} \times 6 \times 10^5}{2\pi \times \frac{\pi}{2} \times 10^{-2}}$

$$= 9.6 \times 10^{-13}\text{ A}$$

Example 3. *If the amount of charge flowed in time t through a cross-section of wire is $q = \beta t - \gamma t^2$, where β and γ are constants.*

(i) Find the current in terms of t.

(ii) Sketch I versus t graph.

Sol. Given, $q = \beta t - \gamma t^2$

(i) As we know, current in a wire is given by

$$I = \frac{dq}{dt} = \frac{d}{dt}(\beta t - \gamma t^2) = \beta - 2\gamma t$$

(ii) To plot a graph I *versus* t, we will compare the given current with the equation of a straight line, i.e.

$$y = mx + c$$

So, at $t = 0$, $I = \beta$

and when $I = 0$, then $t = \frac{\beta}{2\gamma}$.

which means the graph for given current equation is a straight line with negative slope, *i.e.* -2γ and positive intercept, *i.e.* β.

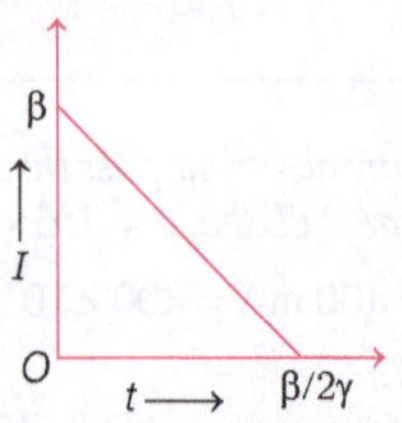

So, the plot will be as shown in the figure.

Example 4. *Charge passing through a conductor is given by $Q = \alpha t - \beta t^2$, where α and β are constants. Find*

(i) time for which current is passing through conductor.

(ii) total amount of charge flow through the conductor.

Sol. (i) $Q = \alpha t - \beta t^2 \Rightarrow I = \frac{dQ}{dt} = \alpha - 2\beta t = 0 \Rightarrow t = \frac{\alpha}{2\beta}$

(ii) Total charge flow through the conductor

$$I = \frac{dQ}{dt} = \alpha - 2\beta t \Rightarrow \int dQ = \int_0^{\alpha/2\beta} (\alpha - 2\beta t)\,dt \Rightarrow Q = \frac{\alpha^2}{4\beta}$$

Current Density

Current density at any point inside a conductor is defined as *"the amount of charge flowing per second through a unit area held normal to the direction of the flow of charge at that point".*

Current density is a vector quantity and its direction is along the motion of the positive charge as shown in fig. (a).

$$\text{Current density, } \mathbf{J} = \frac{q/t}{\mathbf{A}} = \frac{I}{\mathbf{A}}$$

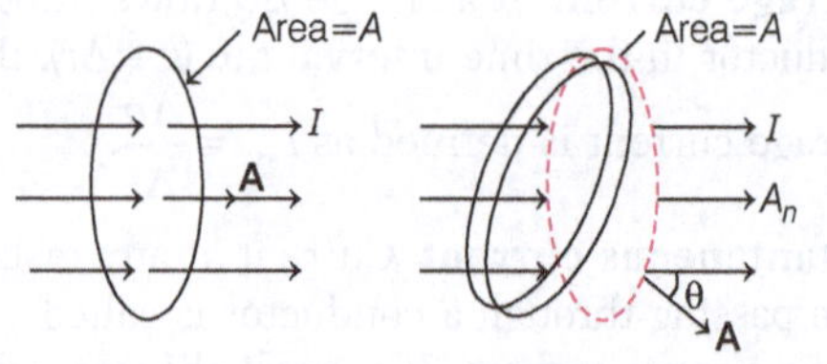

If the cross-sectional area A is not perpendicular to the current and normal to the area makes an angle θ with the direction of the current as shown in Fig. (b), then

$$A_n = A\cos\theta$$

$\therefore$ Current density, $\mathbf{J} = \frac{I}{A_n} = \frac{I}{A\cos\theta}$

or $I = \mathbf{J} \cdot \mathbf{A}$

If area is finite,

$$I = \int \mathbf{J} \cdot d\mathbf{A}$$

where, $d\mathbf{A}$ is a small element of the given surface.

The SI unit of current density is ampere per square metre, i.e. Am^{-2} and its dimensional formula is $[\text{AL}^{-2}]$.

Example 5. *An electron beam has an aperture of 2 mm². A total of 7×10^{16} electrons flow through any perpendicular cross-section per second. Calculate the current density in the electron beam.*

Sol. As we know, current density in the electron beam,

$$J = \frac{I}{A} = \frac{ne}{t} / A = \frac{ne}{tA}$$

Substituting the values, we get

$$J = \frac{7\times 10^{16} \times 1.6 \times 10^{-19}}{1 \times 2 \times 10^{-6}} = 5.6 \times 10^{3} \text{Am}^{-2}$$

Electric Current in Conductors

The electric current in a conductor can be explained by free electron theory. In an atom of a substance, the electrons in the orbits close to the nucleus are bound to it under the strong attraction of the nuclear positive charge, but the electrons far from the nucleus experience a very feeble force.

Hence, the outer electrons can be removed easily from the atom (by rubbing or by heating the substance). In fact, a few outer electrons, leave their atoms and move freely within the substance (in the vacant spaces between the atoms). These electrons, called **free electrons** or **conduction electrons**, carry the charge in the substance from one place to the other.

Mentor's TiP

- Since, the number of electrons travelling in any direction will be equal to number of electrons travelling in opposite direction. Thus, in the absence of external electric field, movements of free electrons cancel out each other and resulting zero net current inside the conductor.

Therefore, the electrical conductivity of a solid substance depends upon the number of free electrons in it. In metals, this number is quite large ($\approx 10^{29}\ /\text{m}^3$). Hence, metals are good conductors of electricity. **Silver is the best conductor of electricity** than copper, gold and aluminium, respectively.

There are some other materials in which the electrons will be bound and they will not be accelerated, even if the electric field is applied, *i.e.* **no current flow on applying electric field.** Such materials are called **insulators,** *e.g.* wood, plastic, rubber, etc.

Drift Velocity

It is defined as "the average velocity with which the free electrons in a conductor get drifted towards the positive end of the conductor under the influence of an electric field applied across the conductor".

It is given by $v_d = \frac{eE}{m}\tau$

where, e = charge on electron, E = electric field,

m = mass of the electron and τ = relaxation time.

The electric current relates with drift velocity as

$$I = neAv_d$$

$$\Rightarrow \quad v_d = \frac{I}{neA} = \frac{J}{ne}$$

Hence, current density is also given by

$$J = \frac{I}{A} = nev_d$$

The direction of drift velocity for electrons in a metal is opposite to that of applied electric field. The drift velocity of electron is very small of the order of $10^{-4}\ \text{ms}^{-1}$ as compared to thermal speed ($\approx 10^5$ m/s) of electron at room temperature.

Relaxation Time

Average time taken by free electron between two successive collisions is called time of relaxation.

($\tau \approx 10^{-14}$ s in metals)

With increase in temperature, relaxation time decreases.

Mobility of Free Electrons (μ)

Drift velocity of free electron per unit electric field represenst mobility.

i.e., $\quad \mu = \frac{v_d}{E}$

$$\Rightarrow \quad \mathbf{v}_d = \mu\mathbf{E} = \frac{eE\tau}{m} \Rightarrow \mu = \frac{e\tau}{m}$$

Its unit is m^2/V-s.

Example 6. *Find the current flow through a copper wire of length 0.2 m, area of cross-section 1 mm², when connected to a battery of 4 V. (Take, electron mobility is $4.5 \times 10^{-6} m^2V^{-1}s^{-1}$, charge on an electron is 1.6×10^{-19} C and density of electrons in copper is $8.5 \times 10^{28}\ m^{-3}$)*

Sol. Given, length of copper wire, $l = 0.2$ m

Cross-sectional area, $A = 1\ \text{mm}^2 = 10^{-6}\text{m}^2$

Potential difference, $V = 4$ V

Electron mobility, $\mu = 4.5 \times 10^{-6}\ \text{m}^2\ \text{V}^{-1}\text{s}^{-1}$

Charge on an electron, $e = 1.6 \times 10^{-19}$C

Density of electrons in copper, $n = 8.5 \times 10^{28}\text{m}^{-3}$

We know that, electric field set up across the conductor,

$$E = \frac{V}{l} = \frac{4}{0.2} = 20\ \text{Vm}^{-1}$$

Mobility of electrons, $\mu = \frac{v_d}{E}$

$$\Rightarrow \quad v_d = 4.5 \times 10^{-6} \times 20 = 9 \times 10^{-5}\ \text{m/s}$$

So, the current flow through the copper wire is

$$I = nev_d A = 8.5 \times 10^{28} \times 1.6 \times 10^{-19} \times 9 \times 10^{-5} \times 10^{-6}$$
$$= 1.224\ \text{A}$$

NEET Close-up

Example Similar to PYQ Asked in NEET 2020

A charged particle having drift velocity of 6.6×10^{-4} ms^{-1} in an electric field of 3×10^{-10} Vm^{-1}. Then, the mobility of the particle would be.

(a) 2.5×10^5 m^{2}V^{-1}s^{-1} (b) 2.2×10^6 m^{2}V^{-1}s^{-1}
(c) 3.2×10^5 m^{2}V^{-1}s^{-1} (d) 3.3×10^5 m^{2}V^{-1}s^{-1}

Sol. (*b*) Given, drift velocity,

$$v_d = 6.6 \times 10^{-4} \text{ ms}^{-1}$$

Electric field, $E = 3 \times 10^{-10}$ Vm^{-1}

As, mobility, $\mu = \frac{v_d}{E} = \frac{6.6 \times 10^{-4}}{3 \times 10^{-10}}$

$$= 2.2 \times 10^6 \text{ m}^2 \text{ V}^{-1} \text{ s}^{-1}$$

Skill Builder

A charged particle having drift velocity of 9.5×10^{-2} m/s in an electric field of 4×10^{-10} Vm^{-1}. Then, the mobility of the particle would be

(a) 3.5×10^6 m^2 V^{-1} s^{-1} (b) 2.375×10^8 m^2 V^{-1} s^{-1}
(c) 3.358×10^8 m^2 V^{-1} s^{-1} (d) 2.5×10^6 m^2 V^{-1} s^{-1}

For more Practice Refer Q. No. 8 of Gearing up for NEET.

Example 7. *An aluminium wire of diameter 0.24 cm is connected in series to a copper wire of diameter 0.16 cm. The wire carry an electric current of 10 A. Find (i) current density in the aluminium wire (ii) and drift velocity of electrons in the copper wire.*
(Take, number of electrons per cubic metre volume of copper, $n = 8.4 \times 10^{28}$.)

Sol. (i) Radius of Al wire, $r = \frac{0.24}{2} = 0.12 \text{ cm} = 0.12 \times 10^{-2}$ m

Area of cross-section of Al wire, $A = \pi r^2$

$$= 3.14 \times (0.12 \times 10^{-2})^2$$

$$= 4.5 \times 10^{-6} \text{ m}^2$$

$\therefore$ Current density, $J = \frac{I}{A} = \frac{10}{4.5 \times 10^{-6}} = 2.2 \times 10^6$ Am^{-2}

(ii) Radius of copper wire, $r = \frac{0.16}{2}$ cm $= 0.08 \times 10^{-2}$ m

Area of cross-section of copper wire,

$$A = \pi r^2 = 3.14 \times (0.08 \times 10^{-2})^2 = 2 \times 10^{-6} \text{ m}^2$$

Also, $n = 8.4 \times 10^{28}$ m^{-3}, $e = 1.6 \times 10^{-19}$ C, $I = 10$ A

$\therefore$ Drift velocity of electrons in the copper wire,

$$v_d = \frac{I}{enA} = \frac{10}{1.6 \times 10^{-19} \times 8.4 \times 10^{28} \times 2 \times 10^{-6}}$$

$$= 3.7 \times 10^{-4} \text{ ms}^{-1}$$

Ohm's Law

It states that, "the current *I* flowing through a conductor is always directly proportional to the potential difference *V* across the ends of the conductor", provided that the physical conditions (temperature, mechanical strain, etc) are kept constant.

Mathematically, $I \propto V$

or $V \propto I$

or $\boxed{V = IR}$

where, *R* is resistance of the conductor.

Graph between *V* and *I* for a metallic conductor is a straight line as shown. At different temperature, *V-I* curves are different.

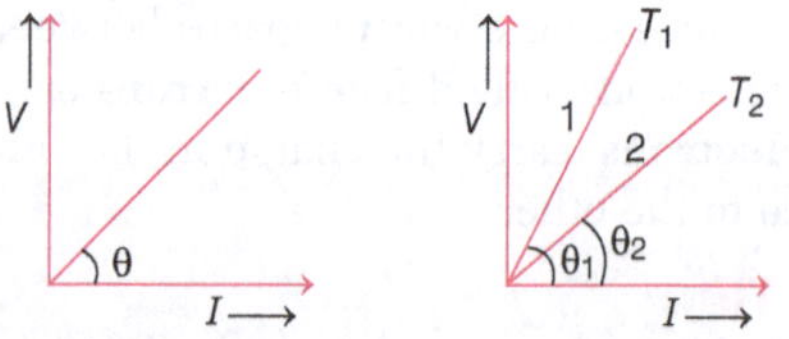

(a) Slope of the line $= \tan\theta = \frac{V}{I} = R$

(b) Here, $\tan\theta_1 > \tan\theta_2$
So, $R_1 > R_2$
i.e. $T_1 > T_2$

Concept ladder

- The substances which obey Ohm's law, e.g. copper, silver, aluminium are known as **ohmic substances.**
- The devices or substances which do not obey Ohm's law, e.g. gases, crystal rectifiers, thermionic valve, transistors, etc., are known as **non-ohmic** or **non-linear conductors.**

Resistance and Resistivity

The property of a substance by virtue of which it opposes the flow of current through it, is known as the **resistance.**

It is defined as 'the ratio of the potential difference applied across the ends of the conductor to the current flowing through".

Mathematically, $\boxed{R = \frac{V}{I}}$

The resistance of the conductor depends upon the following factors

(i) It is directly proportional to the length of the conductor,

i.e. $R \propto l$ ...(i)

(ii) It is inversely proportional to the area of the cross-section of the conductor,

i.e. $R \propto \frac{1}{A}$ ...(ii)

From Eqs. (i) and (ii), we get

$R \propto \frac{l}{A} \Rightarrow \boxed{R = \rho \frac{l}{A}}$ ...(iii) where, ρ is the constant of proportionality known as **resistivity** or **specific resistance** of the conductor.

Resistivity is the intrinsic property of the substance. It is independent of shape and size of the body and depends upon the nature of the material.

Example 8. *Resistance of a conductor of length l and area of cross-section A is R. If its length is doubled and area of cross-section is halved, then find its new resistance.*

Sol. Initial length $= l$, area $= A$

So, initial resistance, $R = \rho \frac{l}{A}$ ... (i)

Final length, $l' = 2l$, area, $A' = \frac{A}{2}$

New resistance, $R' = \rho \frac{l'}{A'} = \rho \frac{2l}{\left(\frac{A}{2}\right)} = 4\rho \frac{l}{A} = 4R$ [from Eq. (i)]

Mentor's TIP

If length of a conductor is increased to n times by drawing it, i.e. $l_2 = nl_1$, then its new resistance, $R_2 = n^2 R_1$

Similarly, if $r_2 = \frac{1}{n} r_1 \Rightarrow R_2 = n^4 R_1$

Unit and Dimensional Formula of Resistance

The SI unit of resistance is ohm and is denoted by symbol Ω.

$$1 \text{ ohm } (\Omega) = \frac{1 \text{ volt (V)}}{1 \text{ ampere (A)}} = 1 \text{ volt/ampere (or V/A)}$$

The resistance of a conductor is said to be one ohm, if one ampere of current flows when a potential difference of one volt is applied across the ends of the conductor.

Its dimensional formula is $[ML^2T^{-3}A^{-2}]$.

Conductance and Conductivity

Conductance

Reciprocal of resistance is known as conductance (G), *i.e.*

$$\boxed{G = \frac{1}{R}}$$

Its unit is $1/\Omega$ or Ω^{-1} or siemen.

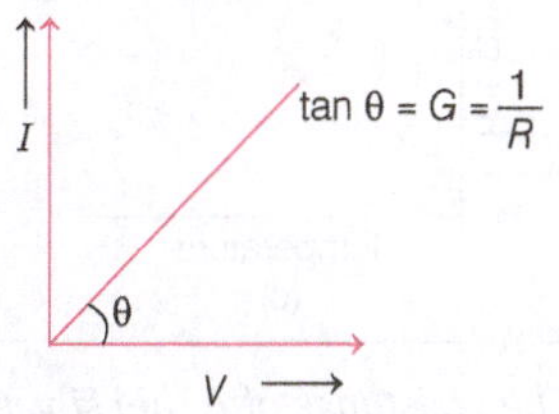

Conductivity

Reciprocal of resistivity is called conductivity (σ), i.e.

$$\boxed{\sigma = \frac{1}{\rho}}$$

Its unit is mho/m.

The dimensional formula of conductivity is $[M^{-1}L^{-3}T^3A^2]$.

Vector form of Ohm's Law

Electric field in a conductor of length l and having potential difference V at its ends is given by

$$V = El$$

Also, $$V = IR \Rightarrow El = \frac{I\rho l}{A}$$

$$\Rightarrow \quad E = \frac{I}{A}\rho$$

$$\therefore \quad \mathbf{E} = \rho \mathbf{J}$$

or $$\boxed{\mathbf{J} = \sigma \mathbf{E}} \quad ...(i)$$

The above equation is the vector form of Ohm's law.

Also, current density,

$$J = nev_d = ne\left(\frac{eE\tau}{m}\right) = \left(\frac{ne^2\tau}{m}\right)E$$

Comparing with Eq. (i), we get

$$\text{Conductivity, } \sigma = \frac{ne^2\tau}{m}$$

$$\text{and resistivity, } \rho = \frac{1}{\sigma} = \frac{m}{ne^2\tau}$$

Example 9. *Resistivity of a wire is 2×10^{-6} Ω-m. Find its conductivity.*

Sol. Given, $\rho = 2 \times 10^{-6}$ Ω-m

Conductivity, $\sigma = \frac{1}{\rho} = \frac{1}{2 \times 10^{-6}} = 5 \times 10^5$ mho/m

Example 10. *A conductor wire of length 1 m and radius 7×10^{-2} m has electric resistance of 10 Ω for electric field of 1 V/m, find current density of the wire.*

Sol. Since, $R = \rho \frac{l}{A} \Rightarrow \rho = \frac{RA}{l} \Rightarrow \sigma = \frac{l}{RA}$

Clearly, current density, $J = \sigma E = \frac{lE}{RA}$

$$= \frac{1 \times 1}{7 \times 10^{-2} \times \frac{22}{7} \times 7 \times 10^{-2} \times 10}$$

$$\Rightarrow \quad J = \frac{10^3}{22 \times 7} = 6.49 \text{ A/m}^2$$

Example 11. *Calculate the electric field in a copper wire of cross-sectional area 2.0 mm^2 carrying a current of 1 A. The conductivity of copper is 6.25×10^7 Sm^{-1}.*

Sol. Given, area, $A = 2 \text{ mm}^2 = 2 \times 10^{-6} \text{ m}^2$

Current, $I = 1$ A, Conductivity, $\sigma = 6.25 \times 10^7$ Sm^{-1}

As, current density, $J = \frac{I}{A} = \sigma E$

$\therefore$ Electric field, $E = \frac{I}{A\sigma} = \frac{1}{2\times10^{-6}\times6.25\times10^{7}}$

$= 8\times10^{-3}\ \text{Vm}^{-1}$

Example 12. *A copper wire has a resistance of 10 Ω and an area of cross-section 1 mm². A potential difference of 10 V exists across the wire. Calculate the drift velocity of electrons, if the number of electrons per cubic metre in copper is 8×10^{28} electrons.*

Sol. Given, $R = 10\,\Omega$, $A = 1\ \text{mm}^2 = 10^{-6}\ \text{m}^2$

$V = 10\ \text{V}$, $n = 8\times10^{28}$ electrons/m³

Now, electric current, $I = enAv_d$

Using Ohm's law,

$$\frac{V}{R} = enAv_d \quad \text{or} \quad v_d = \frac{V}{enAR}$$

$$= \frac{10}{1.6\times10^{-19}\times8\times10^{28}\times10^{-6}\times10}$$

$$= 0.078\times10^{-3}\ \text{ms}^{-1} = 0.078\ \text{mm/s}$$

Example 13. *A current of 1A is flowing through a copper wire of length 0.1 m and cross-section $1\times10^{-6}\,m^2$.*

(i) If the specific resistance of copper is 1.7×10^{-8} Ω-m, then calculate the potential difference across the ends of the wire.

(ii) Determine current density in the wire.

(Take, density of copper = 8.9×10^{3} kg m^{-3}, atomic weight = 63.5 and N = 6.02×10^{26} per kg-atom)

Sol. Given, $I = 1\ \text{A}$, $l = 0.1\ \text{m}$, $A = 1\times10^{-6}\ \text{m}^2$,

$\rho = 1.7\times10^{-8}\ \Omega\text{-m}$, $d = 8.9\times10^{3}\ \text{kg m}^{-3}$.

(i) Resistance of wire, $R = \frac{\rho l}{A} = \frac{1.7\times10^{-8}\times0.1}{1\times10^{-6}}$

$= 1.7\times10^{-3}\ \Omega$

$\therefore$ Potential difference, $V = IR = 1\times1.7\times10^{-3}$

$= 1.7\times10^{-3}\ \text{V}$

(ii) Current density, $J = \frac{I}{A} = \frac{1}{1\times10^{-6}}\ \text{Am}^{-2}$

Temperature Dependence of Resistivity

Resistivity of a material depends on relaxation time as follows.

$$\rho \propto \frac{1}{\tau}$$

When temperature increases in a conductor, average speed of free electrons increases, hence relaxation time decreases. Thus, resistivity increases.

Resistivity of a metal conductor is given by

$$\rho = \rho_0[1 + \alpha(T - T_0)]$$

where, ρ = resistivity at temperature T, ρ_0 = resistivity at temperature T_0 and α = temperature coefficient of resistivity.

i.e. $\alpha = \frac{\rho - \rho_0}{\rho_0(T - T_0)}$

In terms of resistance, $R \propto \rho$

$\therefore \quad R = R_0[1 + \alpha(T - T_0)]$

$\Rightarrow \quad \alpha = \frac{R - R_0}{R_0(T - T_0)}$

where, R_0 = resistance of conductor at 0°C

and R_t = resistance of conductor at t°C.

Concept ladder

- **For metals**, α is positive as their resistivity increases with rise in temperature. The graph of ρ plotted against T would be a straight line as shown in fig. (a).

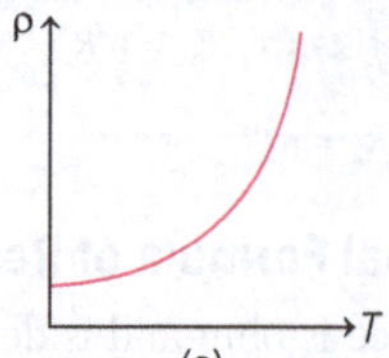

(a)

- **For semiconductors**, α is negative as their resistivity decreases with rise in temperature. Variation in resistivity with the temperature for semiconductor is shown in fig. (b).

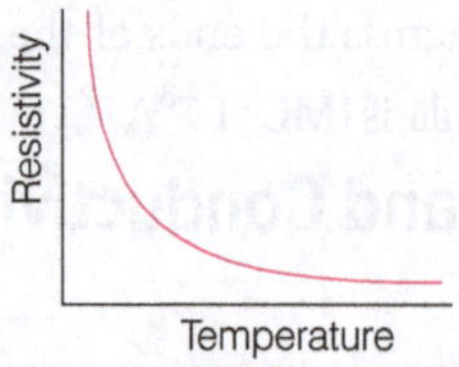

(b)

- The resistivity of **alloys** also increases with rise in temperature. The graph between resistivity and temperature is shown in fig. (c).

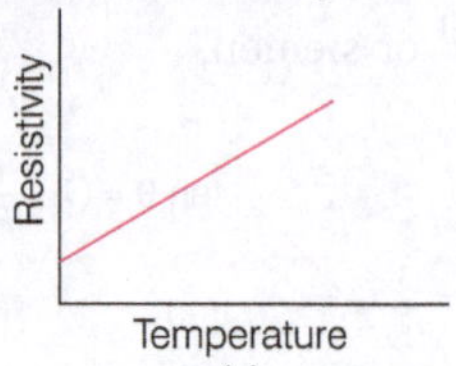

(c)

Example 14. *The resistance of a thin silver wire is 1.0 Ω at 20°C. The wire is placed in a liquid bath and its resistance rises to 1.2 Ω. What is the temperature of the bath? (Take, α for silver = 3.8×10^{-3} per °C)*

Sol. We know that, $R(T) = R_0[1 + \alpha(T - T_0)]$

Here, $R(T) = 1.2\Omega$, $R_0 = 1.0\Omega$,

$\alpha = 3.8 \times 10^{-3}$ per °C and $T_0 = 20°C$

Substituting the values, we get

$$1.2 = 1.0[1 + 3.8 \times 10^{-3}(T - 20)]$$

or $3.8 \times 10^{-3}(T - 20) = 0.2$

Solving this, we get $T = 72.6°C$

Example 15. *The temperature coefficient of resistance of a wire is 0.00145 $°C^{-1}$. At 100 °C, its resistance is 2 Ω. At what temperature, the resistance of the wire will be 3 Ω?*

Sol. Using the relation, $R = R_0[1 + \alpha T]$

$$R_1 = R_0[1 + \alpha t_1]$$

$\therefore$ $2 = R_0[1 + 0.00145 \times 100]$ ...(i)

and $R_2 = R_0[1 + \alpha t_2]$

$\therefore$ $3 = R_0[1 + 0.00145 \times t_2]$ ...(ii)

On dividing Eq. (ii) by Eq. (i), we get

$$\frac{3}{2} = \frac{1 + 0.00145 \times t_2}{1 + 0.00145 \times 100}$$

or $t_2 = 494.8°C = 767.8K$

Mentor's TiP

- If R_1 and R_2 are resistances at θ_1 and θ_2°C, then

$$\frac{R_1}{R_2} = \frac{1 + \alpha\theta_1}{1 + \alpha\theta_2}$$

NEET Close-up

Example Similar to PYQ Asked in NEET 2023

A resistance of platinum wire at 0°C is 5 Ω and 8.5 Ω at 70°C. The temperature coefficient of resistance of the wire.

(a) 0.1×10^{-2} °C^{-1}
(b) 0.01×10^{-2} °C^{-1}
(c) 1×10^{-2} °C^{-1}
(d) 1×10^{-3} °C^{-1}

Sol. (c) Given, $R_0 = 5\Omega$

At $t = 70°C$, $R_t = 8.5\Omega$

$$R_t = R_0(1 + \alpha t)$$

$\Rightarrow$ $R_t = R_0 + R_0\alpha t$

$\Rightarrow$ $\alpha = \dfrac{R_t - R_0}{R_0 t}$

$$= \frac{8.5 - 5}{5 \times 70} = \frac{3.5}{5 \times 70}$$

$$= 0.01 = 1 \times 10^{-2} °C^{-1}$$

Skill Builder

A resistance of copper wire at 0°C is 3 Ω and 5.2 Ω at 80°C. The temperature coefficient of resistance of the wire is

(a) 4.5×10^{-2}°C^{-1} (b) 4×10^{-2}°C^{-1}
(c) 5.5×10^{-3}°C^{-1} (d) 9.2×10^{-3}°C^{-1}

For more Practice Refer Q. No. 18, 19 of step-up practice 1 and Q. No. 23 of Gearing up for NEET.

STEP UP Practice 1

1. The current through wire depends on time as $I = 3t^2 + 2t + 5$. The charge flowing through the cross-section of the wire in time interval between $t = 0$ to $t = 2$ s is

(a) 22 C (b) 20 C (c) 18 C (d) 5 C

2. The charge on an electron is 1.6×10^{-19} C. How many electrons strike the screen of a cathode-ray tube each second, when the beam current is 16 mA?

(a) 10^{17} (b) 10^{19} (c) 10^{-19} (d) 10^{-17}

3. A conductor carries a current of 0.2 A. In 30 s, how many electrons will flow through the cross-section of the conductor? (Take, $q = 1.6 \times 10^{-19}$ C)

(a) 0.375×10^{19} (b) 375×10^{19}
(c) 3.75×10^{19} (d) 37.5×10^{19}

4. Assertion (A) The drift velocity of electrons in a metallic wire will decrease, if the temperature of the wire is increased.

Reason (R) On increasing temperature, conductivity of metallic wire decreases.

In the light of the above statements, choose the correct answer from the options given below

(a) Both A and R are true but R is not the correct explanation of A.
(b) A is true but R is false.
(c) A is false but R is true.
(d) Both A and R are true and R is the correct explanation of A.

5. In a closed circuit, the current I (in ampere) at an instant of time t (in second) is given by $I = 4 - 0.08t$. The number of electrons flowing in 50 s through the cross-section of the conductor is

(a) 1.25×10^{19} (b) 6.25×10^{20}
(c) 5.25×10^{19} (d) 2.25×10^{20}

6. Drift velocity v_d varies with the intensity of electric field as per the relation

(a) $v_d \propto E$ (b) $v_d \propto \dfrac{1}{E}$
(c) v_d = constant (d) $v_d \propto E^2$

7. When current flows through a conductor, then the order of drift velocity of electrons will be

(a) 10^{10} cms^{-1} (b) 10^{-2} cms^{-1} (c) 10^4 cms^{-1} (d) 10^{-1} cms^{-1}

8. Assertion (A) Insulators do not allow flow of current through them.

Reason (R) Insulators have no free charge carrier.

In the light of the above statements, choose the correct answer from the options given below.
(a) Both A and R are true but R is not the correct explanation of A.
(b) A is true but R is false.
(c) A is false but R is true.
(d) Both A and R are true and R is the correct explanation of A.

9. The number density of free electron in a copper conductor is $8.5 \times 10^{28}\ m^{-3}$. How long does an electron take to drift from one end of a wire, 3.0 m long to its other end? If the area of cross-section of the wire is $2.0 \times 10^{-6}\ m^2$ and it is carrying a current of 3.0 A.
(a) 2.73×10^4 s (b) 4.73×10^4 s
(c) 5×10^4 s (d) 6×10^8 s

10. The total momentum of electrons in a straight wire of length $l = 1000$ m carrying a current $I = 70$ A, will be (in N-s)
(a) 0.6 μ (b) 0.4 μ (c) 0.6 m (d) 0.4 m

11. The resistance between two rectangular faces of a block of dimensions 4 cm × 4 cm × 10 cm of manganin ($\rho = 48 \times 10^{-8}\ \Omega$-m), will be
(a) 1.2 μΩ (b) 2.4 μΩ (c) 3.6 μΩ (d) 4.8 μΩ

12. Which of the following pair is incorrect?
(a) Mobility — (i) m^2/V-s
(b) Resistivity — (ii) Ω/m
(c) Conductivity — (iii) mho/m
(d) Drift velocity — (iv) m/s

13. If resistance of a wire formed by 1 cc of copper be 2.46 Ω. The diameter of wire is 0.32 mm, then the specific resistance of wire will be
(a) 1.59×10^{-6} Ω-cm (b) 2.18×10^{-6} Ω-cm
(b) 1.59×10^{-5} Ω-cm (d) 1.59×10^{-7} Ω-cm

14. A given piece of wire length l, cross-sectional area A and resistance R is stretched uniformly to a wire of length $2l$. The new resistance will be
(a) R (b) $2R$ (c) $4R$ (d) $\frac{R}{2}$

15. A given piece of wire of length l, radius r and resistance R is stretched uniformly to a wire of radius $(r/2)$. The new resistances will be
(a) $4R$ (b) $16R$ (c) $\frac{R}{4}$ (d) $\frac{R}{16}$

16. **Assertion (A)** The temperature coefficient of resistance is always positive only for metals and alloys.
Reason (R) On increasing the temperature, the resistance of metal and alloys increases.
In the light of the above statements, choose the correct answer from the options given below.
(a) Both A and R are true but R is not the correct explanation of A.
(b) A is true but R is false.
(c) A is false but R is true.
(d) Both A and R are true and R is the correct explanation of A.

17. Curve between current and potential difference for a conductor at temperature T_1 and T_2 are as shown in figure. Compare T_1 and T_2.

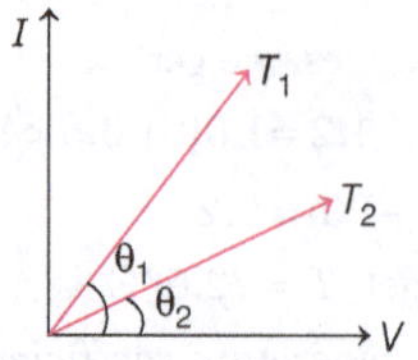

(a) $T_1 = T_2$ (b) $T_1 > T_2$
(c) $T_2 > T_1$ (d) $T_1 \geq T_2$

18. As temperature increases resistance of conductor also increases, so $T_2 > T_1$. Resistance of a conducting wire at 27°C is 1 Ω. If the temperature coefficient of resistance is $\alpha = 0.00125$/°C, then find the temperature at which resistance of wire is 2 Ω.
(a) 54°C (b) 254°C
(c) 554°C (d) 854°C

19. Resistance of a conducting wire at 20°C is 120 Ω. If α for the resistance is 0.01/°C then what will be the resistance of 50°C?
(a) 300 Ω (b) 150 Ω
(c) 240 Ω (d) 180 Ω

20. **Assertion** (A) Specific resistance is independent of cross-section of material used.
Reason (R) When the radius of a copper wire is doubled, its specific resistance gets increased.
In the light of the above statements, choose the correct answer from the options given below
(a) Both A and R are true but R is not the correct explanation of A.
(b) A is true but R is false.
(c) A is false but R is true.
(d) Both A and R are true and R is the correct explanation of A.

21. Calculate the amount of charge flowed in 2 min through a wire of resistance 10 Ω, when the potential difference of 20 V is applied across its ends.
(a) 120 C (b) 240 C
(c) 20 C (d) 4 C

22. If e, τ and m respectively, represent the electron density, relaxation time and mass of the electron, then the resistance R of a wire of length l and area of cross-section A will be
(a) $\frac{ml}{ne^2\tau A}$ (b) $\frac{m\tau^2 A}{ne^2 l}$
(c) $\frac{ne^2\tau A}{2ml}$ (d) $\frac{ne^2 A}{2m\tau l}$

23. Four wires are made of the same material and are at the same temperature. Which one of them has highest electrical resistance?
(a) Length = 50 cm, diameter = 0.5 mm
(b) Length = 10 cm, diameter = 1 mm
(c) Length = 200 cm, diameter = 2 mm
(d) Length = 300 cm, diameter = 3 mm

Module 2

Combination of Resistors

- Series Combination
- Parallel Combination

There are two types of combination of resistances, i.e. series combination and parallel combination.

Series Combination

In this combination, resistors are connected end-to-end, *i.e.* second end of first resistor is connected to first end of the second resistor and so on.

In series combination, same current flows through each resistance but potential difference distributes in the ratio of their resistance, *i.e.* $V \propto R$. So, the total potential difference is equal to the sum of potential difference applied across the combination of resistors.

Equivalent resistance in series combination is given by

$$R_{eq} = R_1 + R_2 + R_3$$

i.e. equivalent resistance is greater than the maximum value of resistance in the combination.

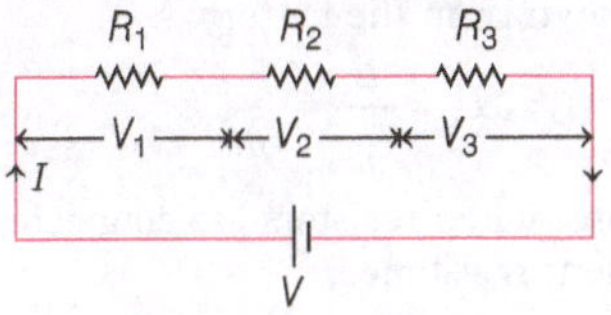

Resistances in Series

Parallel Combination

In this combination, first end of all resistors are connected to one point and second end of all resistors are connected to other point.

Same potential difference appears across each resistor but current distributes in the reverse ratio of their resistance. *i.e.* $I \propto \dfrac{V}{R}$. So, the total current is equal to the sum of currents through each resistance.

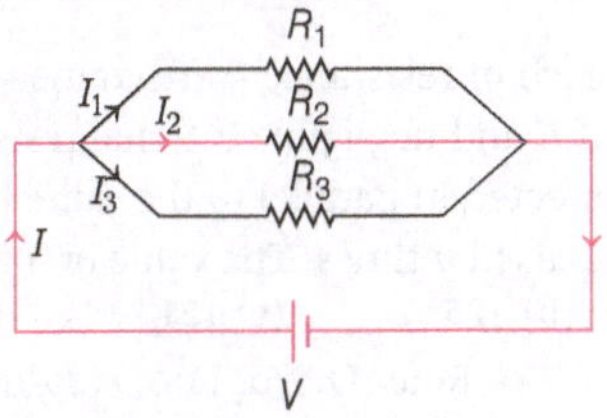

Resistances in parallel

Equivalent resistance in parallel combination is given by

$$\frac{1}{R_{eq}} = \frac{1}{R_1} + \frac{1}{R_2} + \frac{1}{R_3}$$

i.e. equivalent resistance is less than the minimum value of resistance in the combination.

Mentor's Tip

If n identical resistors of resistance R each, are connected in series, then equivalent resistance, $R_{eq} = nR$ and potential difference across each resistor is $V' = V/n$.

If n identical resistors of resistance R each, are connected in parallel, then equivalent resistance, $R_{eq} = \dfrac{R}{n}$ and current through each resistor is $I' = \dfrac{I}{n}$

Example 16. *A wire of resistance 6R is bent in the form of a circle. What is the effective resistance between the ends of the diameter ?*

Sol.

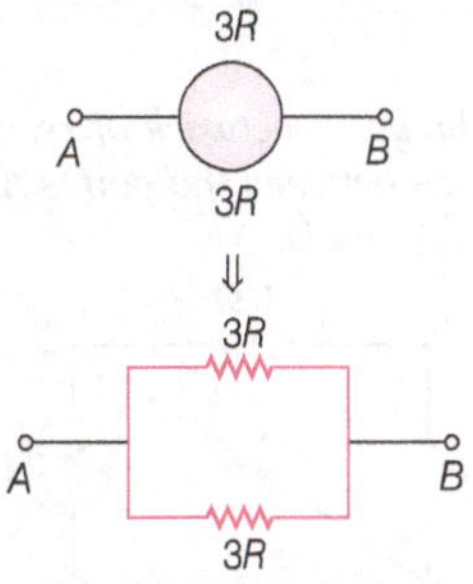

As shown in figure, the two resistances of value $3R$ each are in parallel with each other. So, the resistance between the ends A and B of a diameter is

$$R' = \frac{R_1 \times R_2}{R_1 + R_2} = \frac{3R \times 3R}{3R + 3R} = \frac{9R^2}{6R} = \frac{3}{2}R$$

Example 17. *Find the equivalent resistance between A and B in the following cases.*

(*i*)

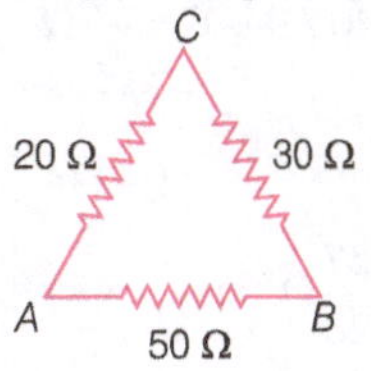

(*ii*)

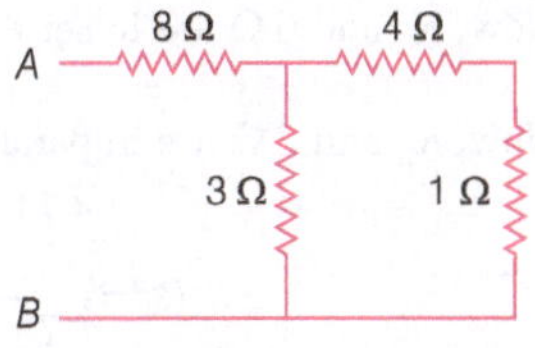

Sol. (i)

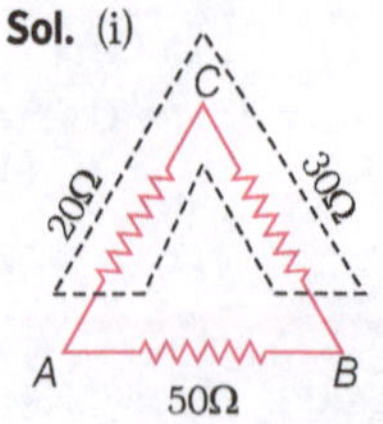

From the above dotted region, 20 Ω and 30 Ω are in series,
$\Rightarrow R = 20 + 30 = 50\ \Omega$

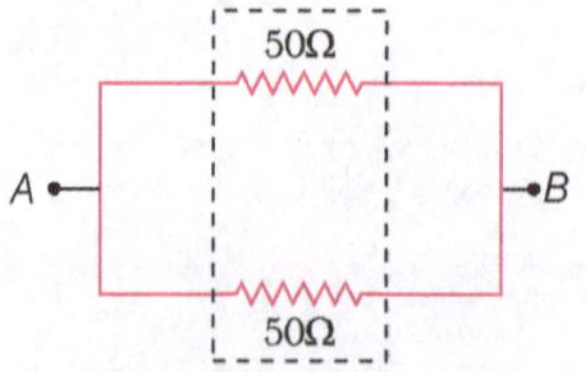

From the above dotted region, 50 Ω and 50 Ω are in parallel,
$\Rightarrow R_{eq} = \dfrac{50 \times 50}{50 + 50} = \dfrac{2500}{100} = 25\ \Omega$

(ii)

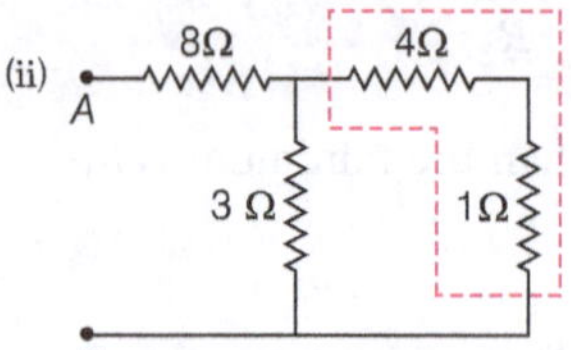

From the above dotted region, 4 Ω and 1Ω are in series,
$\Rightarrow R = 4 + 1 = 5\ \Omega$

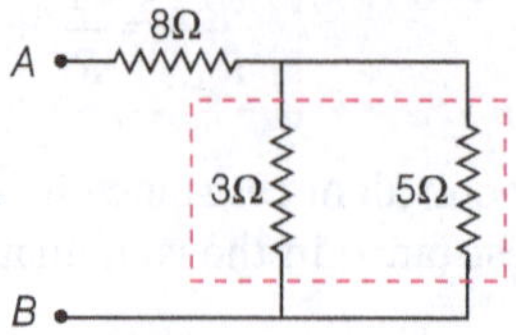

From the above dotted region, 3 Ω and 5Ω are in parallel,
$\Rightarrow \dfrac{1}{R} = \dfrac{1}{R_1} + \dfrac{1}{R_2} = \dfrac{1}{3} + \dfrac{1}{5} \Rightarrow R = \dfrac{15}{8}\Omega$

$\Downarrow$

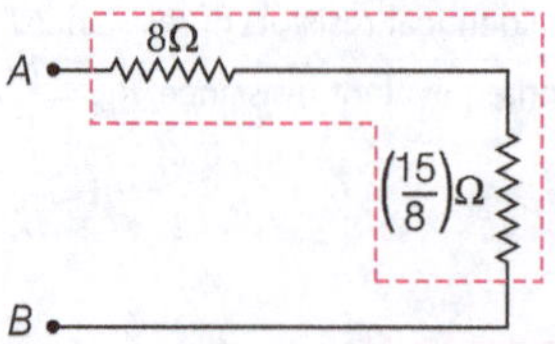

From the above dotted region, we have 8 Ω and (15/8)Ω are in series,
$\Rightarrow R_{eq} = 15/8 + 8 = 79/8\Omega$

Example 18. *In the given network of resistors, find the equivalent resistance between the points A and B and between the points A and D.*

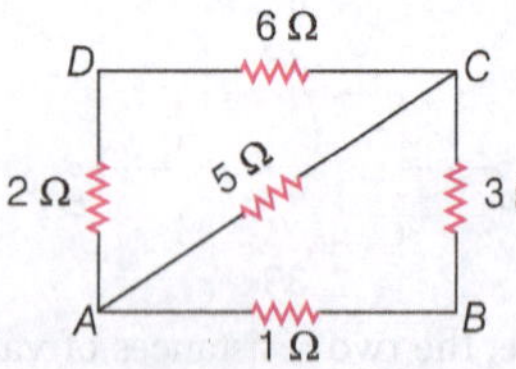

Sol. *Resistance between A and D,*

As we can see from the circuit, 1 Ω and 3Ω are in series,

$$R_1 = 1 + 3 = 4\Omega$$

Now, R_1 and 5 Ω are in parallel, $R_2 = \dfrac{4 \times 5}{4 + 5} = \dfrac{20}{9}\Omega$

Now, R_2 and 6 Ω are in series, $R_3 = 20/9 + 6 = \dfrac{74}{9}\Omega$

Now, R_3 and 2 Ω are in parallel,

$$R_4 = \frac{\frac{74}{9} \times 2}{\left(\frac{74}{9} + 2\right)} = \frac{37}{23}\Omega$$

Resistance between A and B,

The resistors $AD\ (= 2\,\Omega)$ and $DC (= 6\,\Omega)$ are in series to give a total resistance $R' = 8\,\Omega$. The resistance $R' (= 8\,\Omega)$ and the resistor $AC\ (= 5\,\Omega)$ are in parallel. Their equivalent resistance is, $R'' = \dfrac{5 \times 8}{5 + 8} = \dfrac{40}{13}\Omega$

Now, R'' and 3Ω are in series,

$$R''' = R'' + 3 = \frac{40}{13} + 3 = \frac{79}{13}\Omega$$

Now, R''' and 1 Ω are in parallel, so resistance between A and B,

$$(R'''') = \frac{1 \times 79/13}{1 + 79/13} = \frac{79}{92}\Omega$$

NEET Close-up

Example Similar to PYQ Asked in NEET 2023

5 resistors, each of resistance R are connected in series to a battery of emf E and negligible internal resistance. Then, those are connected in parallel to the same battery, the current is increased n times. The value of n is

(a) 25 (b) 30 (c) 22 (d) 20

Sol. (*a*) When 5 resistors, each of resistance R is connected in series, then equivalent resistance,

$$R_S = 5R$$

$\therefore$ Current drawn from the battery,

$$I_S = \frac{E}{R_S} = \frac{E}{5R}$$

In second case, when resistors are connected in parallel, then equivalent resistance,

$$\frac{1}{R_P} = \frac{1}{R} + \frac{1}{R} \ldots 5 \text{ times}$$

$$= \frac{5}{R} \Rightarrow R_P = \frac{R}{5}$$

$\therefore$ Current drawn from the battery,

$$I_P = \frac{E}{R_P} = \frac{E}{R/5} = 5 \times \frac{E}{R} = 25 \times \frac{E}{5R}$$

$\Rightarrow \quad I_P = 25 I_S$

$\therefore \quad n = 25$

Skill Builder

11 resistors, each of resistance R are connected in series to a battery of emf E and negligible internal resistance. Then those are connected in parallel to the same battery, the current is increased n times. The value of n is

(a) 120 (b) 125 (c) 121 (d) 122

For more Practice Refer Q. No. 11 of step-up practice 2 and Q. No. 20, 21, 25 of Gearing up for NEET.

Example 19. *Find the equivalent resistance between A and B.*

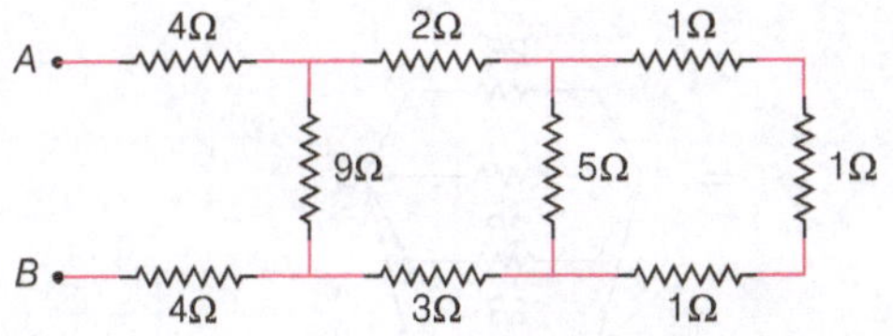

Sol.

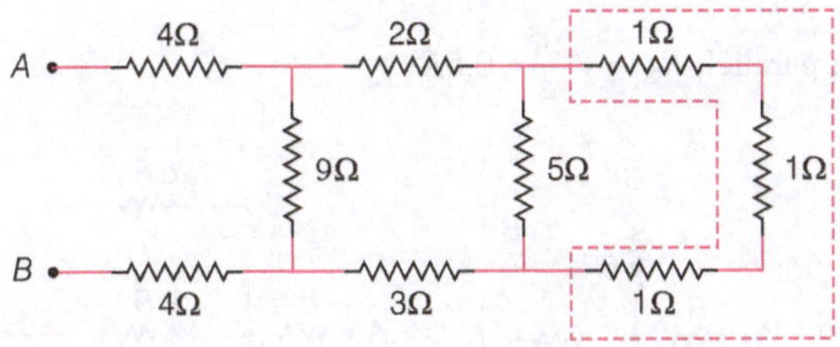

As per the dotted region, 1Ω, 1Ω and 1Ω are in series,

$$R = 1 + 1 + 1 = 3\,\Omega$$

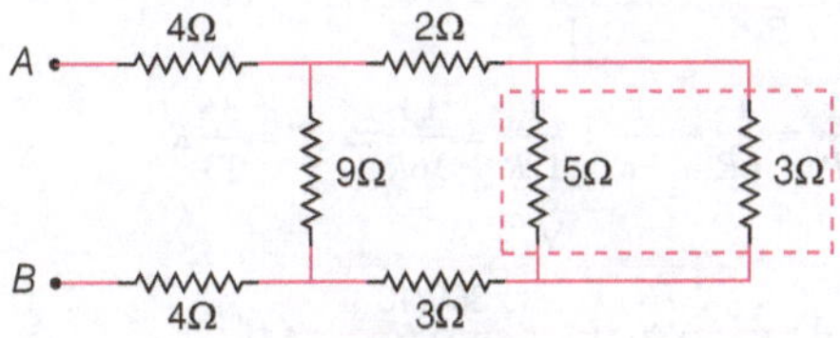

In dotted region, 3Ω and 5Ω are in parallel,

$$\Rightarrow R_1 = \frac{3\times5}{3+5} = \frac{15}{8}\Omega$$

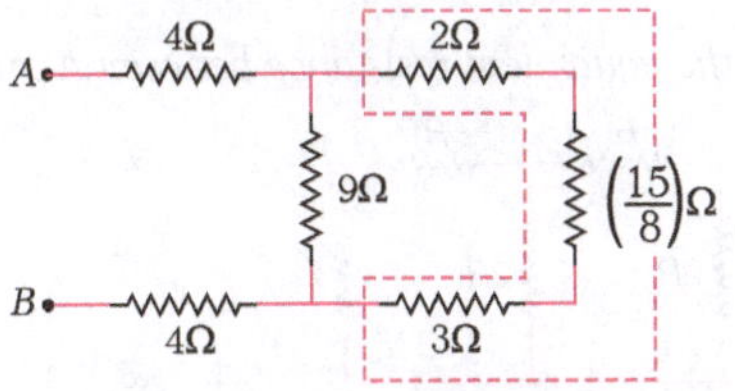

In dotted region, 2Ω, 3Ω and $(15/8)\Omega$ are in series,

$$\Rightarrow \quad R_2 = 2+3+\frac{15}{8} = \frac{55}{8}\,\Omega$$

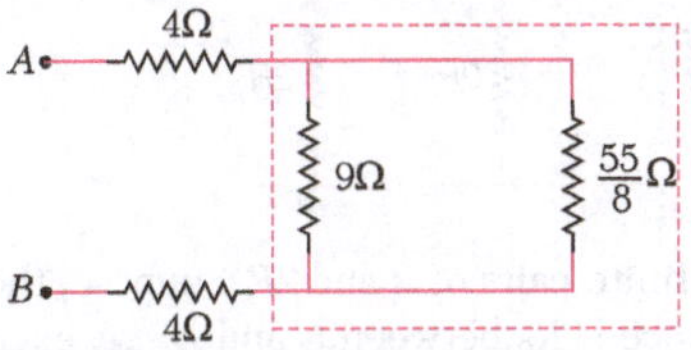

In dotted region, $(55/8)\,\Omega$ and $9\,\Omega$ are in parallel,

$$\Uparrow \quad R_3 = \frac{\frac{55}{8}\times9}{\frac{55}{8}+9} = \frac{495}{127}\,\Omega$$

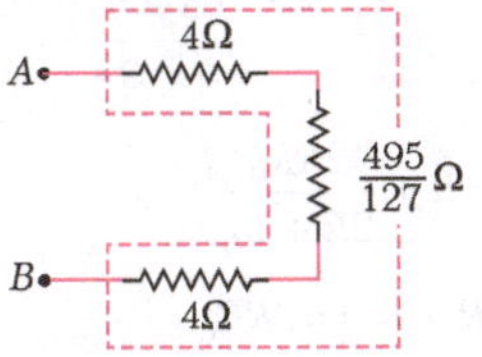

In dotted region, 4Ω, 4Ω and $(495/127)\Omega$ are in series,

$$\Rightarrow \quad R_{eq} = 4 + 4 + (495/127) \Rightarrow R_{eq} = \frac{1511}{127}\,\Omega$$

NEET Close-up

Example Similar to PYQ Asked in NEET 2021

4 resistors having resistances r_1, r_2, r_3 and r_4 are connected as shown in the given circuit. The ratio of I_4/I_1 of current in the circuit is

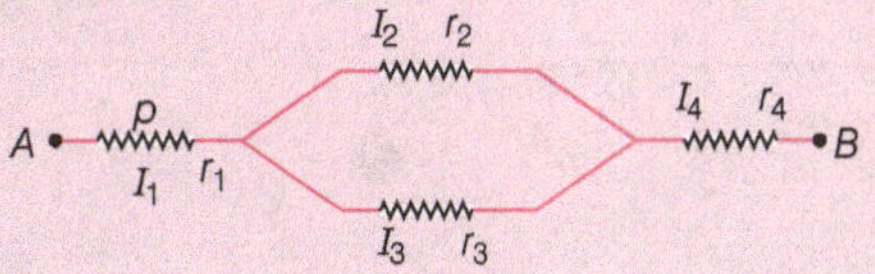

(a) 1 (b) 3 (c) 2 (d) 4

Sol. (*a*) According to the given circuit diagram in question,

$$I_1 = I_2 + I_3 = I_4 \quad \text{...(i)}$$

In parallel arrangement of the electrical circuit, the voltage remain same,

$$V = Ir$$

$$\Rightarrow \quad I_2 r_2 = I_3 r_3$$

$$\Rightarrow \quad I_2 = \frac{I_3 r_3}{r_2}$$

Substituting the value in the Eq. (i) we get

$$I_1 = \frac{I_3 r_3}{r_2} + I_3$$

$$\Rightarrow \quad \frac{I_1}{I_3} = \frac{r_3}{r_2} + 1$$

$$\Rightarrow \quad \frac{I_3}{I_1} = \frac{r_2}{r_3 + r_2}$$

Similarly, $\frac{I_3}{I_4} = \frac{r_2}{r_3 + r_2}$

$$\Rightarrow \quad \frac{I_4}{I_1} = 1$$

Skill Builder

3 resistors having resistances r_1, r_2 and r_3 are connected as shown in the given circuit. The ratio of $\frac{I_2}{I_1}$ of current in term of resistances used in the circuit is

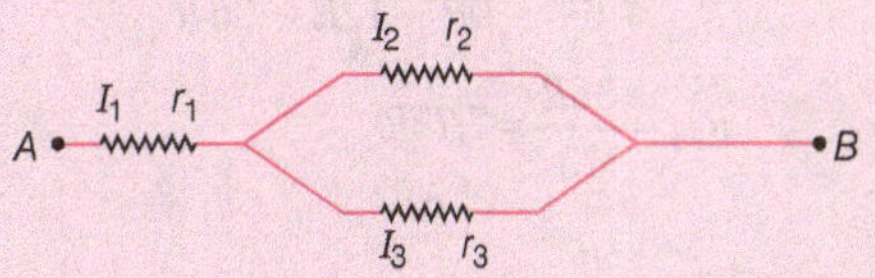

(a) $\frac{r_3}{r_3 + r_2}$ (b) $\frac{r_3}{r_1 + r_2}$ (c) $\frac{r_2}{r_2 + r_3}$ (d) $\frac{r_2}{r_3 + r_2}$

For more Practice Refer Q. No. 6 of step-up practice 2 and Q. No. 16 of Gearing up for NEET.

Example 20. *Find the equivalent resistance between A and B.*

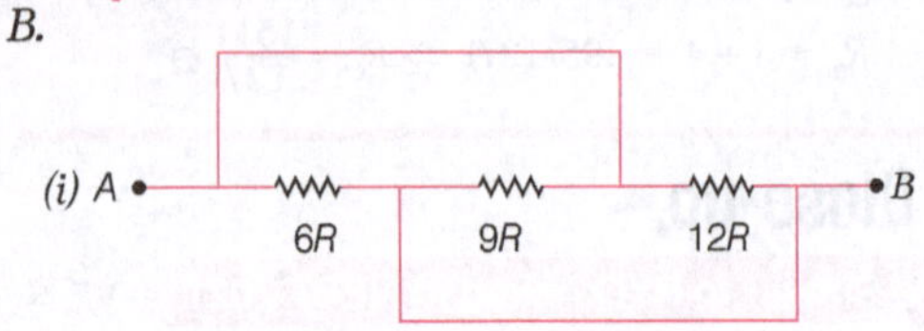

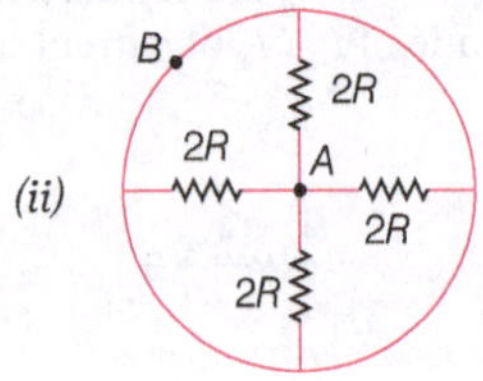

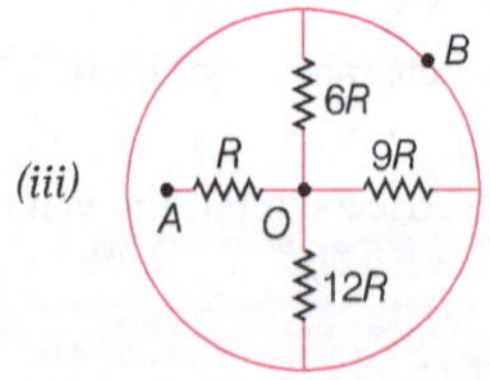

Sol. (i) The points connected by a conducting wire are at same potential. Then, redraw the diagram, by placing the points of same potential at one place and then solve for equivalent resistance.

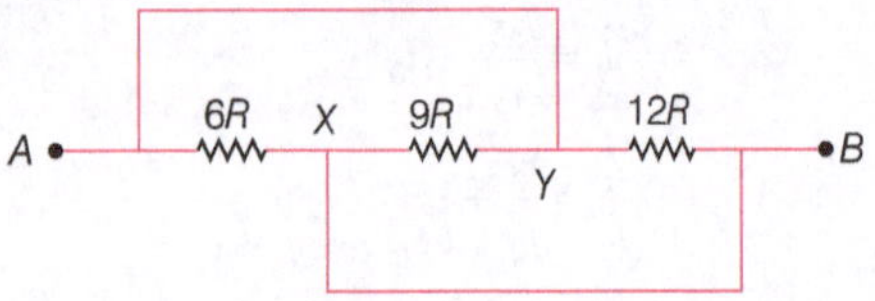

⇓

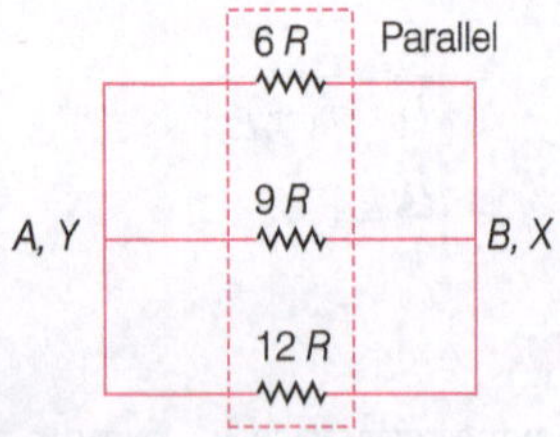

Hence, from the new figure, A and Y are at same potential; B and X are at same potential.

$$\Rightarrow \quad \frac{1}{R_{eq}} = \frac{1}{6R} + \frac{1}{9R} + \frac{1}{12R} = \frac{13}{36R}$$

$$\Rightarrow \quad R_{eq} = \frac{36R}{13} = 2.77R$$

(ii)

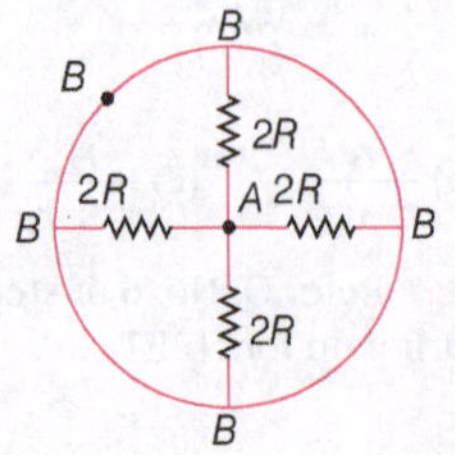

Similarly, placing the points of same potential at one place, then the equivalent resistance is

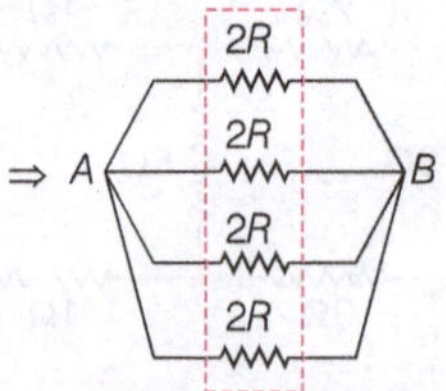

In parallel, $R_{eq} = \frac{2R}{4} = 0.5R$

(iii)

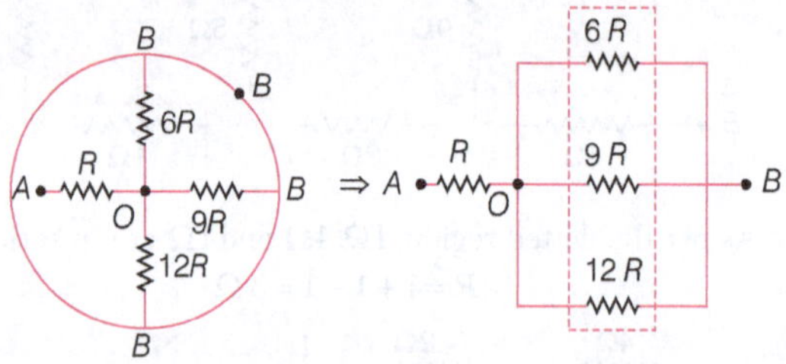

In parallel, $\frac{1}{R'} = \frac{1}{6R} + \frac{1}{9R} + \frac{1}{12R} = \frac{13}{36R} \Rightarrow R' = \frac{36}{13}R$

⇩

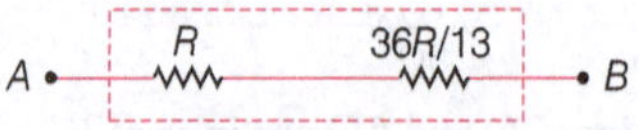

In series, $R_{eq} = R + \frac{36R}{13} = \frac{49}{13}R = 3.77R$

Example 21. *Find the equivalent resistance between A and B.*

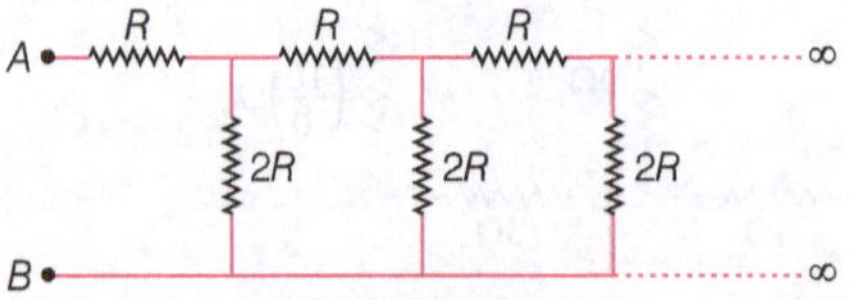

Sol.

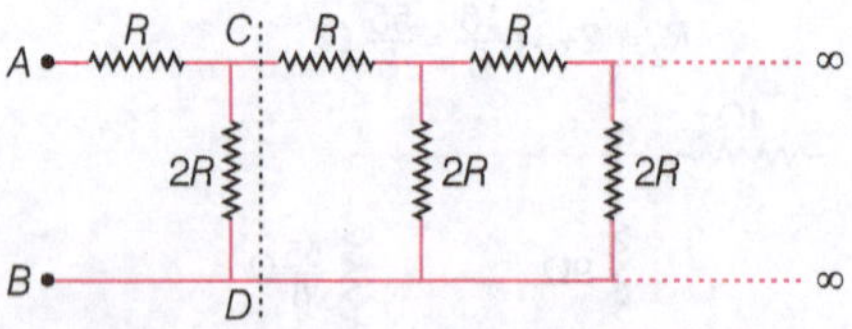

Here, we have infinite pairs of R and $2R$. Suppose, the equivalent resistance is R_0 between C and D, *i.e.* excluding one pair near AB (since, pairs are infinite, equivalent resistance will remain same, if we include pair near AB).

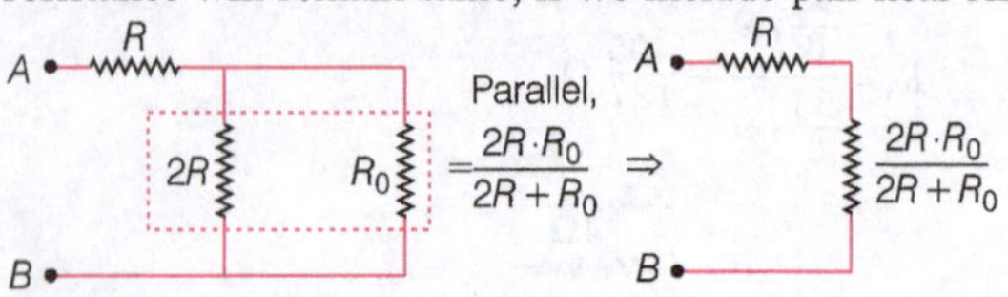

$$\Rightarrow \quad R_{eq} = R_0 = R + \frac{2RR_0}{2R + R_0}$$

$$(R_0 - R)(2R + R_0) = 2RR_0$$

$$2RR_0 - 2R^2 + R_0^2 - RR_0 = 2RR_0$$

$$R_0^2 - RR_0 - 2R^2 = 0$$

$$R_0 = \frac{R \pm \sqrt{R^2 + 8R^2}}{2} = \frac{R \pm 3R}{2} = 2R \text{ or } -R$$

Equivalent resistance between A and $B = 2R$ ($\because$ equivalent resistance cannot be negative).

Example 22. *N resistors of identical resistances are initially connected in series and then in parallel. If potential difference applied across them is same in both cases, find ratio of current of second case w.r.t. first case.*

Sol. Let each resistance $= R$

Let applied voltage $= V$

R_{eq} in first case,

$$R_{eq} = NR$$

So, current in circuit,

$$I_1 = \frac{V}{R_{eq}} = \frac{V}{NR} \quad \text{...(i)}$$

R_{eq} in second case,

$$R_{eq} = \frac{R}{N}$$

So, current in circuit,

$$I_2 = \frac{V}{R} \times N \quad \text{...(ii)}$$

Clearly,

$$\frac{I_2}{I_1} = \frac{V}{R} \times N \times \frac{RN}{V} = N^2$$

STEP UP Practice 2

1. The potential difference between points A and B of the following figure is

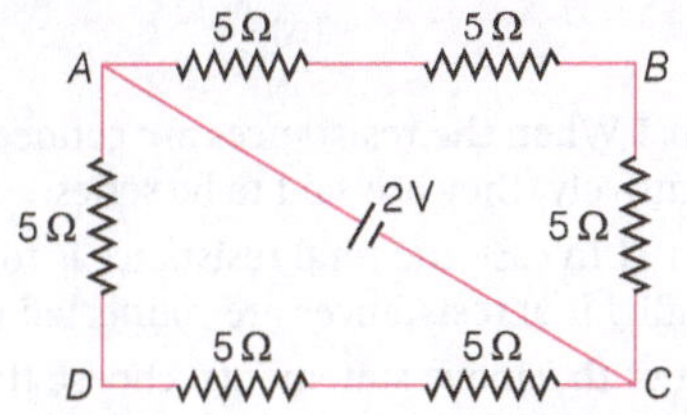

(a) $\frac{2}{3}$ V (b) $\frac{8}{9}$ V (c) $\frac{4}{3}$ V (d) 2 V

2. In the figure given below, the current passing through 6 Ω resistor is

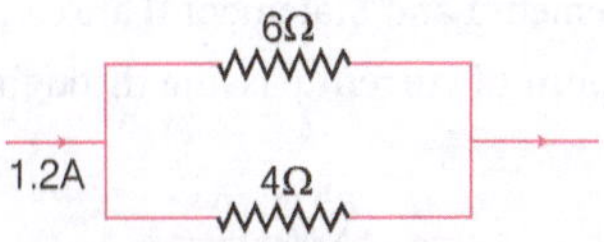

(a) 0.40 A (b) 0.48 A (c) 0.72 A (d) 0.80 A

3. In the figure given below, current passing through the 3 Ω resistor is 0.8 A, then potential drop through 4 Ω resistor is

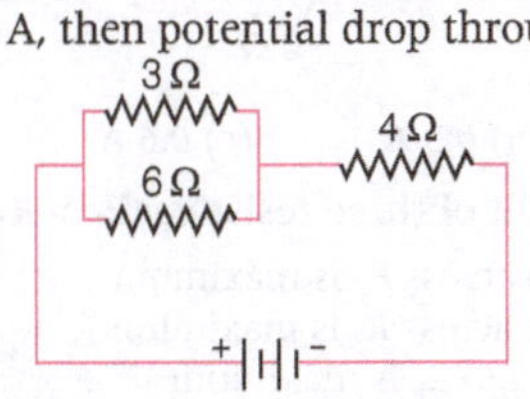

(a) 9.6 V (b) 2.6 V (c) 4.8 V (d) 1.2 V

4. Statement I In series combination of two resistors, the equivalent resistance is greater than the individual resistances.

Statement II In parallel combination of two resistors, the equivalent resistance is less than the individual resistances.

In the light of the above statements, choose the most appropriate answer from the options given below.

(a) Both Statement I and Statement II are incorrect.
(b) Statement I is correct but Statement II is incorrect.
(c) Statement I is incorrect but Statement II is correct.
(d) Both Statement I and Statement II are correct.

5. Current I as shown in the circuit will be

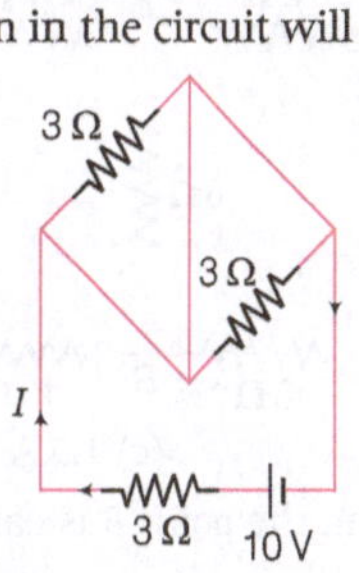

(a) 10 A (b) $\frac{10}{3}$ A (c) zero (d) infinite

6. In the figure given below, the current flowing through 10 Ω resistance is

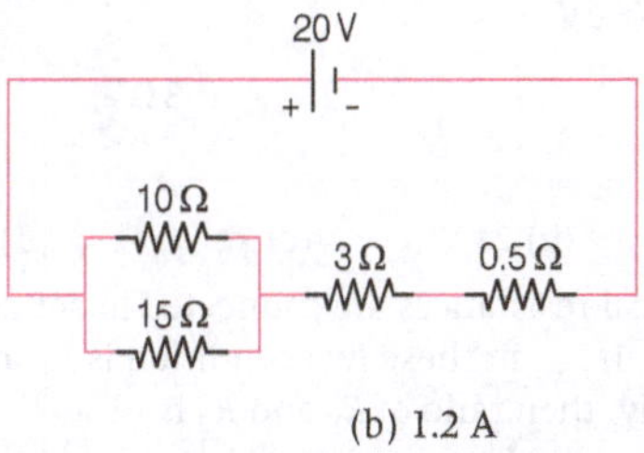

(a) 12 A (b) 1.2 A
(c) 0.8 A (d) 0.4 A

7. If all the resistors shown have the value 2 Ω each, the equivalent resistance over AB is

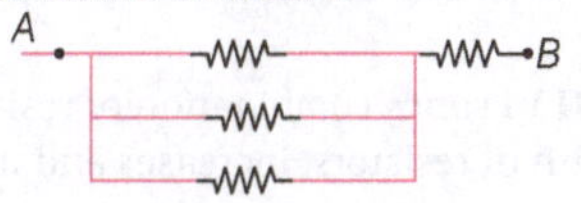

(a) 2 Ω (b) 4 Ω (c) $1\frac{2}{3}$ Ω (d) $2\frac{2}{3}$ Ω

8. In the following question, different arrangement of resistor and their equivalent resistance is given. Choose the incorrect pair from among them. (Each resistor of 1 Ω)

(a) 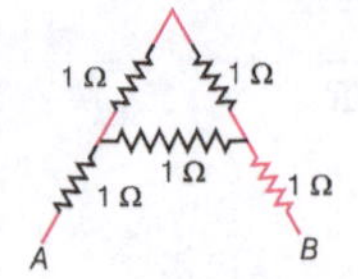

⟶ (i) $R_{eq.(AB)} = \frac{8}{3}\ \Omega$

(b) 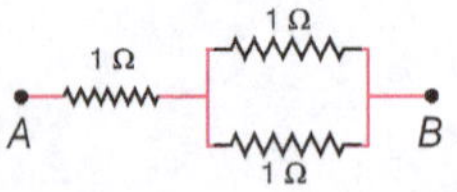

⟶ (ii) $R_{eq.(AB)} = \frac{3}{2}\ \Omega$

(c) 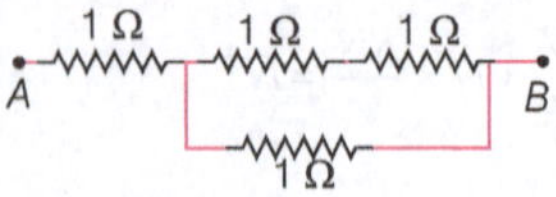

⟶ (iii) $R_{eq.(AB)} = \frac{7}{3}\ \Omega$

(d) 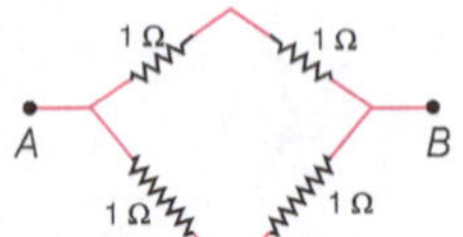

⟶ (iv) $R_{eq.(AB)} = 1\ \Omega$

9. The current drawn from the battery in circuit diagram shown is

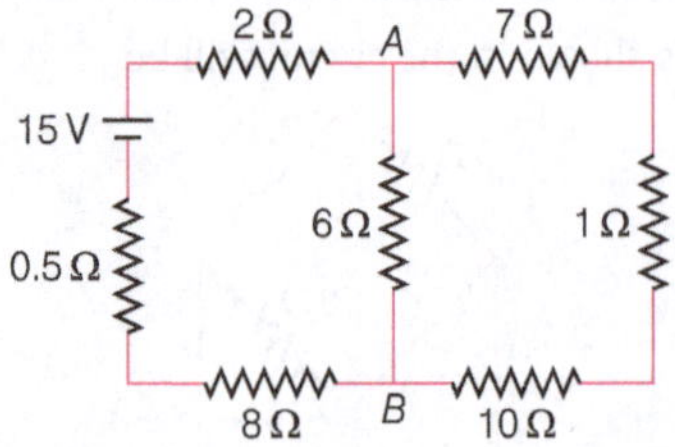

(a) 1 A (b) 2 A (c) 1.5 A (d) 3 A

10. In the circuit shown, the point B is earthed. The potential at the point A is

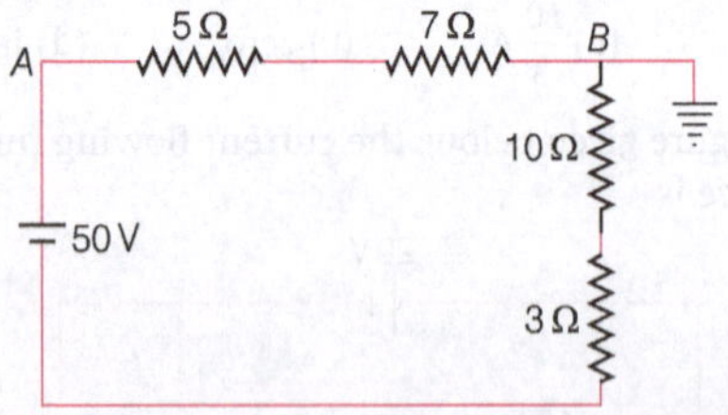

(a) 14 V (b) 24 V (c) 26 V (d) 50 V

11. If n identical resistances are connected in series first, then in parallel. If R_{eq} in these two condition is R_1 and R_2 respectively, then ratio of R_1 and R_2 is
(a) $n:1$ (b) $1:n$ (c) $1:n^2$ (d) $n^2:1$

12. **Statement I** The total resistance in series combination of resistors increases and in parallel combination of resistors decreases.

Statement II In series combination of resistors, the effective length of resistors, increases and in parallel combination of resistors, the area of cross-section of the resistors increases.

In the light of the above statements, choose the most appropriate answer from the options given below.
(a) Both Statement I and Statement II are incorrect.
(b) Statement I is correct but Statement II is incorrect.
(c) Statement I is incorrect but Statement II is correct.
(d) Both Statement I and Statement II are correct.

13. Infinite resistors of resistances $R, 2R, 4R, 8R, \ldots$, are connected in parallel combination, then calculate equivalent resistance.
(a) R (b) $\frac{R}{2}$
(c) $\frac{R}{4}$ (d) Zero

14. Calculate equivalent resistance between points P and Q.

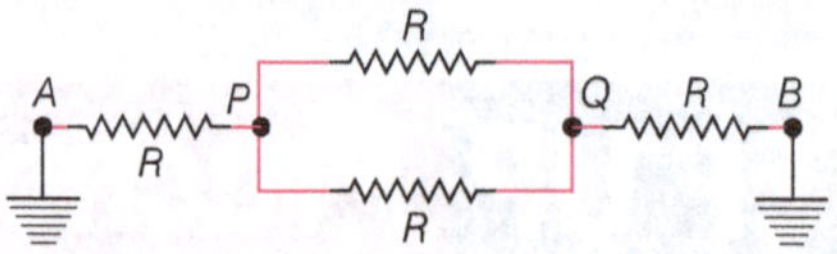

(a) $\frac{5}{2}R$ (b) $4R$
(c) $\frac{2R}{5}$ (d) $\frac{R}{2}$

15. **Statement I** When the resistances are connected end to end consecutively, they are said to be series.

Statement II In case the total resistance is to be increased, then the individual resistances are connected in series.

In the light of the above statements, choose the most appropriate answer from the options given below.
(a) Both Statement I and Statement II are incorrect.
(b) Statement I is correct but Statement II is incorrect.
(c) Statement I is incorrect but Statement II is correct.
(d) Both Statement I and Statement II are correct.

16. Find the amount of current passing through 60 Ω resistance.

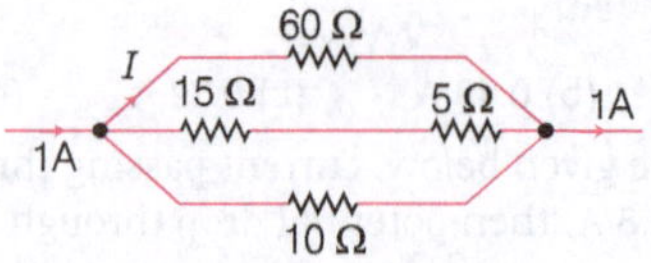

(a) 0.1 A (b) 0.3 A (c) 0.6 A (d) 1 A

17. In a series circuit of three resistors ($R_1 > R_2 > R_3$),
(a) voltage drop across R_1 is maximum
(b) voltage drop across R_3 is maximum
(c) current through R_1 is maximum
(d) current through R_3 is maximum

18. In a parallel circuit of three resistors ($R_1 > R_2 > R_3$),
(a) voltage across R_1 is maximum
(b) current across R_1 is maximum
(c) voltage across R_3 is maximum
(d) current across R_1 is minimum

Module 3

Cells and their Combinations

- Cell
- Grouping of Cells

Cell

An electric cell is a source of energy that maintains a continuous flow of charge in a circuit. Electric cell changes chemical energy into electrical energy.

It is a device which provide constant potential difference.

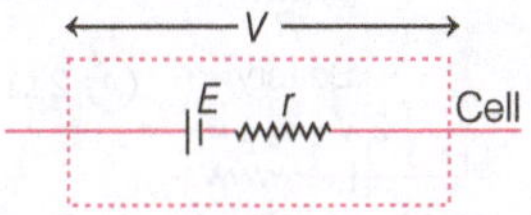

Electromotive Force [EMF (E)]

When cell is in open circuit or no current associates with cell, then potential difference across the terminals of cell represent emf of a cell.

$$V_A - E + 0 = V_B$$

$$\Rightarrow \quad V_A - V_B = E$$

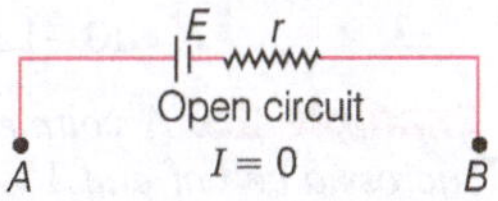

It depends upon nature of electrode and concentration of electrolyte.

Internal Resistance (r)

It is opposition provided by electrolytes of a cell to the flow of ions through it. Dependence of internal resistance (r) with various factors of a battery is shown below.

1. $r \propto$ distance between electrodes and concentration of electrolyte.
2. $r \propto \dfrac{1}{\text{temperature and area of electrode}}$
3. 'r' depends on the nature, concentration and temperature of the electrolyte. It increases with increment in concentration of electrolytes.

Terminal Potential Difference (V)

Terminal potential difference of a cell is defined as the potential difference between the two terminals of the cell in a closed circuit (*i.e.* when current is drawn from the cell). It is represented by V and its unit is volt.

Concept ladder

- Value of terminal potential difference may be less than, equal to or greater than EMF of cell. It can be understood by following cases :
- **Case-I** When current is drawn from cell (discharging of cell)

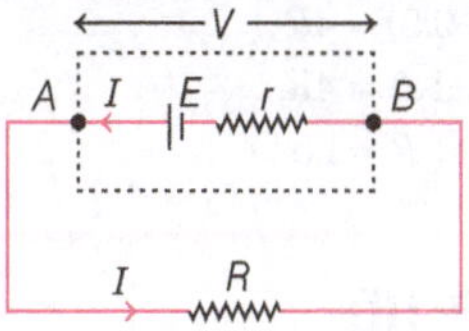

$$V_{AB} = V_A - V_B = E - Ir \Rightarrow V = E - Ir$$

$$\text{and } V_A - V_B = IR; I = \frac{E}{r + R}$$

$$V_{AB} < E$$

- **Case-II** When current is given to cell (charging of cell),

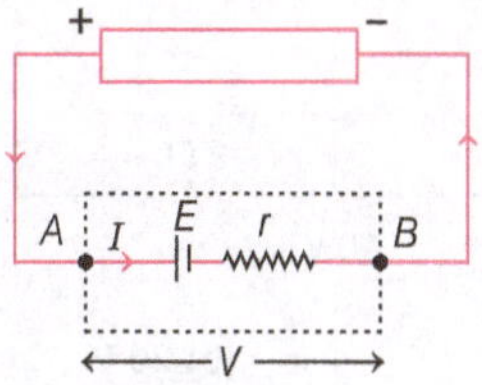

$$V_{AB} = V_A - V_B = E + Ir \Rightarrow V = E + Ir$$

$$V_{AB} > E$$

- **Case-III** When cell is in open circuit,

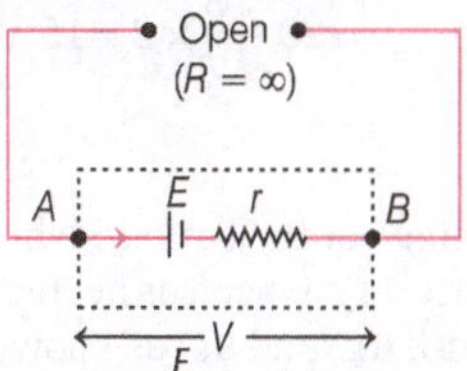

$$\Rightarrow R = \infty \qquad I = \frac{E}{R + r} = 0$$

$$V_A - V_B = E$$

$$V_{AB} = E$$

- **Case-IV** When cell is short-circuited ($R = 0$)

$$V_{AB} = V_A - V_B = E - Ir; \left[I = \frac{E}{r}\right]$$

$$V = E - \frac{E}{r} \times r = 0$$

$$V_{AB} = 0$$

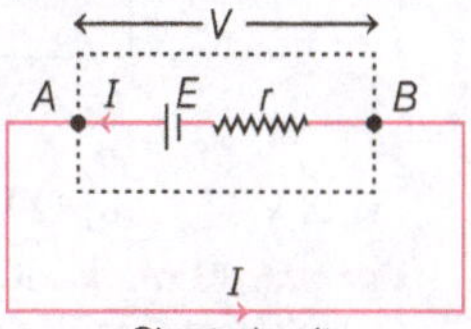

Short-circuit

Example 23. *A cell of emf 10 V and internal resistance 0.5 Ω gives terminal potential difference of 7.5 V when connected with an external resistance R. Find value of R.*

Sol. Here, $E = Ir + IR$

$$\Rightarrow \quad I = \frac{E}{R+r}$$

Again, $$V = IR$$

$$\Rightarrow \quad V = \left(\frac{E}{R+r}\right)R$$

$$\Rightarrow \quad 7.5 = \frac{10}{R+0.5} \times R$$

$$\Rightarrow \quad 3(R+0.5) = 4R$$

$$\Rightarrow \quad 3R + 1.5 = 4R$$

or $$R = 1.5\,\Omega$$

NEET Close-up

Example Similar to PYQ Asked in NEET 2024

The terminal voltage of the battery, whose emf is 20 V and internal resistance 2 Ω, when connected through an external resistance of 6 Ω as shown in the firgure is

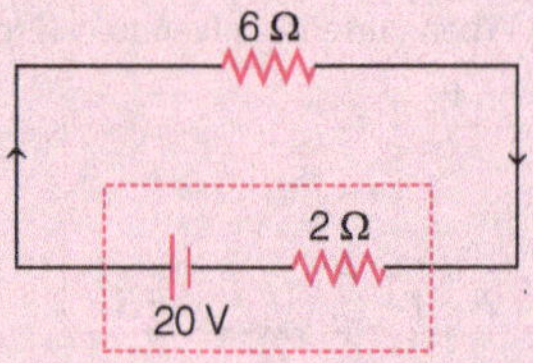

(a) 15 V
(b) 20 V
(c) 5 V
(d) 10 V

Sol. (*a*) Current in circuit $= \frac{20}{6+2} = \frac{5}{2}$ A

Terminal voltage $= E = iR$

$$= 20 - \frac{5}{2} \times 2 = 15 \text{ V}$$

Skill Builder

The terminal voltage of the battery, whose emf is 15 V and internal resistance 1 Ω, when connected through two external resistance 8 Ω and 8 Ω as shown in the figure is

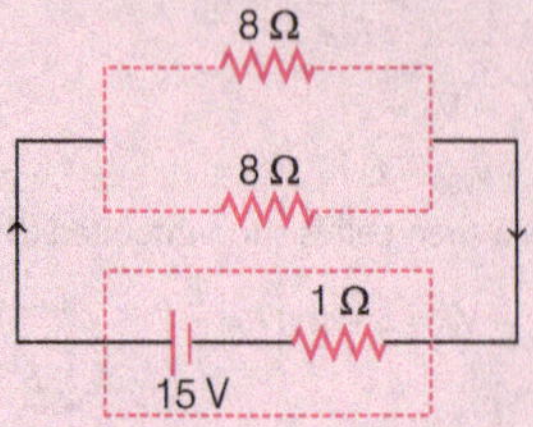

(a) 14 V (b) 12 V (c) 17 V (d) 18 V

For more Practice Refer Q. No. 6 of step-up practice 2 and Q. No. 16 of Gearing up for NEET.

Example 24. *The reading on a high resistance voltmeter when a cell is connected across it is 3 V. When the terminals of the cell are also connected to a resistance of 4 Ω, then the voltmeter reading drops to 1.2 V. Find the internal resistance of the cell.*

Sol. Given, $E = 3$ V, $R = 4\,\Omega$ and $V = 1.2$V

As, internal resistance,

$$r = R\left(\frac{E-V}{V}\right) = 4\left(\frac{3-1.2}{1.2}\right)\Omega = 6\,\Omega$$

Example 25. *A battery of emf 2V and internal resistance r is connected in series with a resistor of 10 Ω through an ammeter of resistance 2 Ω. The ammeter reads 50 mA. Draw the circuit diagram and calculate the value of r.*

Sol. Total resistance $= 10 + 2 + r = (12 + r)\,\Omega$

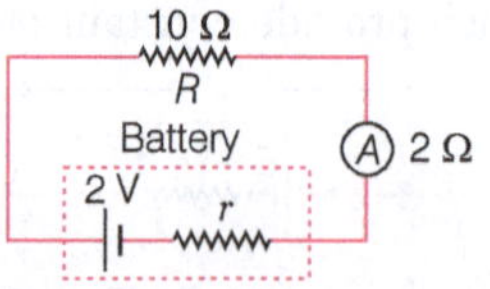

Now, current = 50 mA = 50×10^{-3}A and emf = 2 V.

So, $$\text{resistance} = \frac{\text{emf}}{\text{current}}$$

$$12 + r = \frac{2}{50 \times 10^{-3}} = 40$$

$$\Rightarrow \quad r = 40 - 12 = 28\,\Omega$$

Example 26. *A voltmeter of resistance 994 Ω is connected across a cell of emf 1 V and internal resistance 6 Ω. Find the potential difference across the voltmeter, that is across the terminals of the cell and percentage error in the reading of the voltmeter.*

Sol. Given, $E = 1$ V, $r = 6\,\Omega$

and resistance of voltmeter, $R = 994\,\Omega$

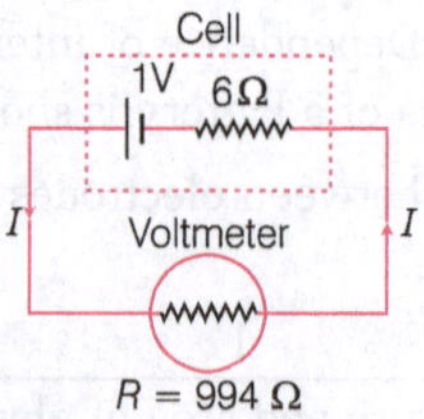

Current in the circuit is

$$I = \frac{E}{R+r} = \frac{1}{(994+6)} = 1 \times 10^{-3} \text{A}$$

The potential difference across the voltmeter is

$$V = IR = 1 \times 10^{-3} \times 994$$
$$= 9.94 \times 10^{-1} \text{V}$$

The same will be the potential difference across the terminals of the cell. The voltmeter used to measure the emf of the cell will read 0.994 V. Hence, the percentage error is

$$\frac{E-V}{E} \times 100 = \frac{1-0.994}{1} \times 100 = 0.6\%$$

Concept ladder

- Graph between V and I is a straight line as follows

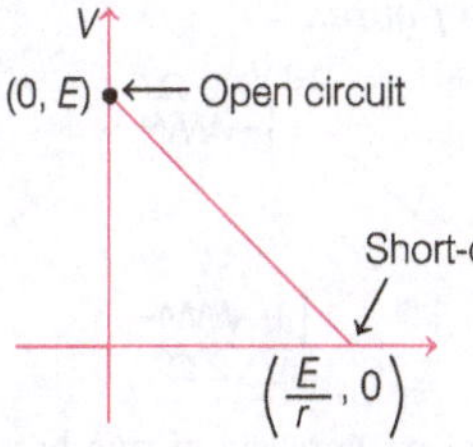

- Efficiency of cell is given by

$$\eta\% = \left(\frac{R}{R+r}\right) \times 100\% = \left(\frac{V}{E}\right) \times 100\%$$

Grouping of Cells

Series Grouping

In series grouping, anode of one cell is connected to cathode of other cell and so on as shown below.

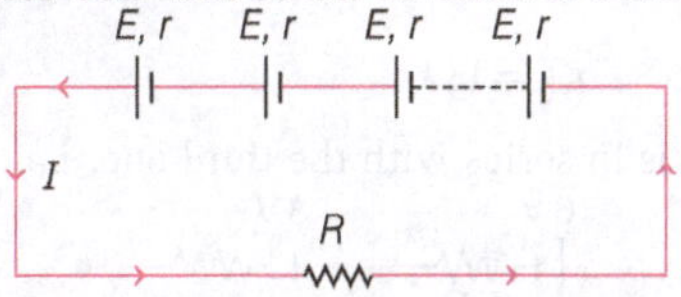

If n identical cells of emf E and internal resistance r each, are connected in series, then

(i) equivalent emf of the combination, $E_{eq} = nE$.

(ii) equivalent internal resistance of the combination, $r_{eq} = nr$.

(iii) main current = current from each cell = $I = \dfrac{nE}{R + nr}$.

(iv) potential difference across external resistance, $V = IR$.

(v) potential difference across each cell, $V' = \dfrac{V}{n}$.

Concept ladder

There are two special cases for point (iii) of the above discussion.

- If $nr >> R \Rightarrow I = E/r$, If $nr << R \Rightarrow I = nE/r$
- E_{eq} depends on polarity of cells while r_{eq} is independent of polarity.
- If external resistance is much higher than the total internal resistance, then cells should be connected in series to get the maximum current.
- If dissimilar plates of cells are connected together, then their emf's are added to each other while, if their similar plates are connected together their emf's are subtracted. While their internal resistances are always additive.

$E_{eq} = E_1 + E_2$
$r_{eq} = r_1 + r_2$

$E_{eq} = E_1 - E_2$ (when $E_2 < E_1$)
$r_{eq} = r_1 + r_2$

Parallel Grouping

In parallel grouping of cells, all anodes of cells are connected at one point and all cathodes of cells are connected together at other point as shown below.

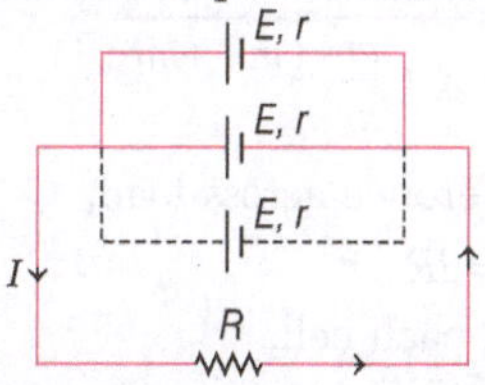

If n identical cells of emf E and internal resistance r each are connected in parallel, then

(i) equivalent emf of the combination, $E_{eq} = E$.

(ii) equivalent internal resistance, $R_{eq} = r/n$.

(iii) main current, $I = \dfrac{E}{R + r/n}$.

(iv) current from each cell, $I' = \dfrac{I}{n}$.

(v) potential difference across external resistance = potential difference across each cell = $V = IR$.

If external resistance is much smaller than the total internal resistance, then cells should be connected in parallel to get the maximum current.

Mentor's TIP

- If two non-identical cells are connected in parallel

$$E_{net} = \frac{E_1 r_2 + E_2 r_1}{r_1 + r_2}$$

- If two cells are connected with reverse polarity

$$E_{net} = \frac{(E_1 r_2 - E_2 r_1)}{r_1 + r_2}$$

Mixed Grouping

If n identical cells of emf E and internal resistance r each, are connected in a row and such m rows are connected in parallel as shown in Figure, then

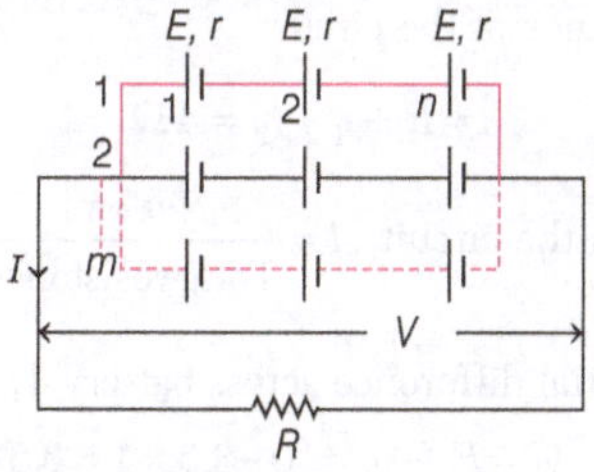

(i) Equivalent emf of the combination,

$$E_{eq} = nE$$

(ii) Equivalent internal resistance, $r_{eq} = \dfrac{nr}{m}$

(iii) Main current flowing through the load,

$$I = \frac{nE}{R + \frac{nr}{m}} = \frac{mnE}{mR + nr}$$

(iv) Potential difference across load,

$$V = IR$$

(v) Current from each cell,

$$I' = \frac{I}{n}$$

(vi) Potential difference across each cell,

$$V' = \frac{V}{n}$$

(vii) Total number of cells = mn

In mixed grouping of cells, the current through the external resistance would be maximum, if the external resistance is equal to the total internal resistance of the cells, *i.e.* $R = \dfrac{nr}{m}$.

Example 27. *In the circuit shown in figure,*

$E_1 = 10\,V, E_2 = 4\,V, r_1 = r_2 = 1\,\Omega$ *and* $R = 2\,\Omega$.

Find the potential difference across battery of emf E_1 and battery of emf E_2.

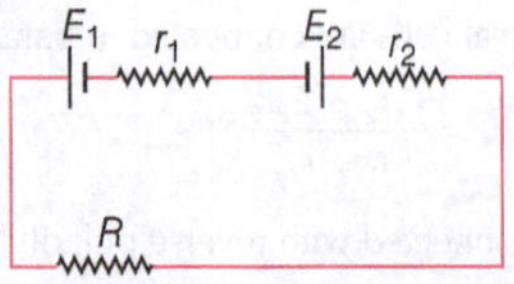

Sol. Net emf of the circuit $= E_1 - E_2 = 6\,V$

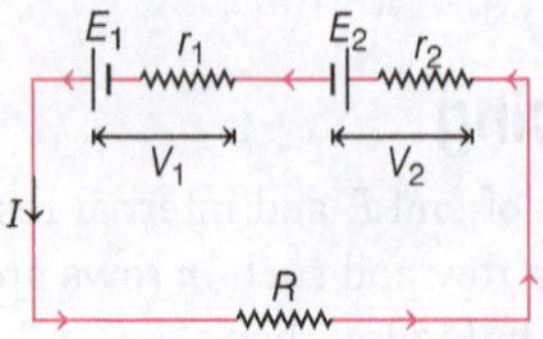

Total resistance of the circuit

$$= R + r_1 + r_2 = 4\,\Omega$$

$$\therefore \text{Current in the circuit, } I = \frac{\text{Net emf}}{\text{Total resistance}} = \frac{6}{4} = 1.5\text{ A}$$

Now, potential difference across battery 1,

$$V_1 = E_1 - Ir_1 = 10 - 1.5 \times 1 = 8.5\text{ V}$$

and potential difference across battery 2,

$$V_2 = E_2 + Ir_2 = 4 + 1.5 \times 1 = 5.5\text{ V}$$

Example 28. *Find the emf and internal resistance of a single battery which is equivalent to a combination of three batteries as shown in figure.*

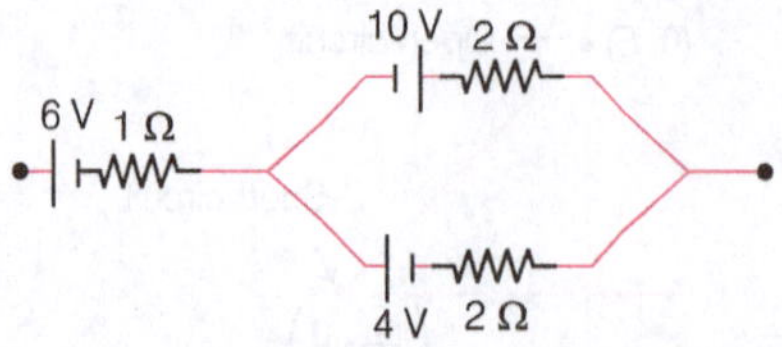

Sol. The given combination consists of two batteries in parallel and resultant of these two in series with the third one.

For parallel combination, we can apply,

$$E_{eq} = \frac{\frac{E_1}{r_1} - \frac{E_2}{r_2}}{\frac{1}{r_1} + \frac{1}{r_2}} = \frac{\frac{10}{2} - \frac{4}{2}}{\frac{1}{2} + \frac{1}{2}} = 3\text{ V}$$

Further, $\dfrac{1}{r_{eq}} = \dfrac{1}{r_1} + \dfrac{1}{r_2} = \dfrac{1}{2} + \dfrac{1}{2} = 1$

$\therefore \quad r_{eq} = 1\,\Omega$

Now, this is in series with the third one, *i.e.*

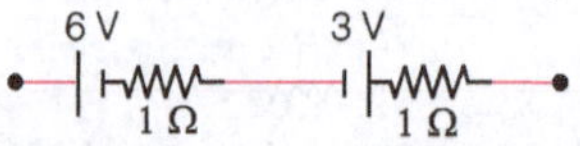

The equivalent emf of these two is (6 − 3) V or 3 V and the internal resistance will be (1 + 1)Ω or 2 Ω, *i.e.*

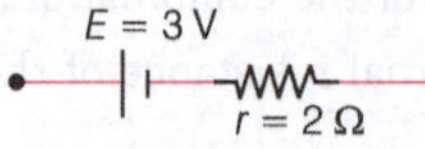

Example 29. *Find the minimum number of cells required to produce an electric current of 1.5 A through a resistance of 30 Ω. Given that the emf of each cell is 1.5 V and internal resistance is 1.0 Ω.*

Sol. As, $\dfrac{nr}{m} = R$

$$\therefore \quad \frac{n \times 1}{m} = 30 \text{ or } n = 30\,m \qquad \text{...(i)}$$

$$\text{Current,} \quad I = \frac{nE}{2R} \text{ or } 1.5 = \frac{n \times 1.5}{2 \times 30} \text{ or } n = 60 \qquad \text{...(ii)}$$

From Eqs. (i) and (ii), we get

$$m = 60/30 = 2 \quad \text{and} \quad mn = 120$$

Example 30. 36 *cells, each of internal resistance* 0.5 Ω *and emf of* 1.5 V, *are used to send maximum current through an external circuit of* 2 Ω *resistance. Find the best mode of grouping them and the maximum current through the external circuit.*

Sol. Given, $E = 1.5\,V$, $r = 0.5\,\Omega$ and $R = 2\,\Omega$

Total number of cells, $mn = 36$ ...(i)

For maximum current in the mixed grouping,

$$\frac{nr}{m} = R \text{ or } \frac{n \times 0.5}{m} = 2 \qquad \text{... (ii)}$$

Multiplying Eqs. (i) and (ii), we get

$$0.5n^2 = 72 \quad \text{or} \quad n^2 = 144$$

$$\therefore \quad n = 12 \quad \text{and} \quad m = \frac{36}{12} = 3$$

Thus, for maximum current, there should be three rows in parallel, each containing 12 cells in series.

$$\therefore \text{ Maximum current} = \frac{mnE}{mR + nr} = \frac{36 \times 1.5}{3 \times 2 + 12 \times 0.5} = 4.5 \text{ A}$$

Example 31. *12 cells, each of emf 1.5 V and internal resistance of 0.5 Ω, are arranged in m rows each containing n cells connected in series, as shown. Calculate the values of n and m for which this combination would send maximum current through an external resistance of 1.5 Ω.*

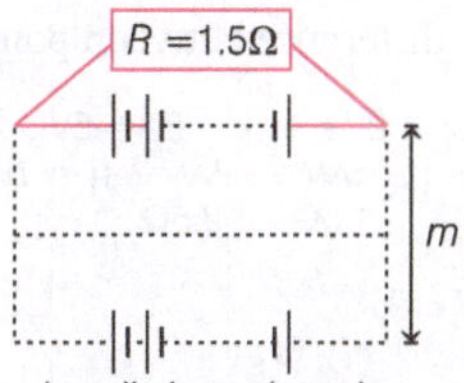

(n cells in each row)

Sol. For maximum current through the external resistance,

external resistance = total internal resistance of cells

$$\text{or} \quad R = \frac{nr}{m}$$

$$\therefore \quad 1.5 = \frac{n \times 0.5}{12/n} \quad (\because mn = 12)$$

$$\text{or} \quad 36 = n^2 \text{ or } n = 6 \text{ and } m = 2$$

STEP UP Practice 3

1. A current of 2 A passes through a cell of emf 1.5 V having internal resistance of 0.15 Ω. The potential difference measured in volt, across both the ends of the cell will be
   (a) 1.35 (b) 1.50 (c) 1.00 (d) 1.20

2. If V_{AB} is 4 V in the given figure, then resistance X will be

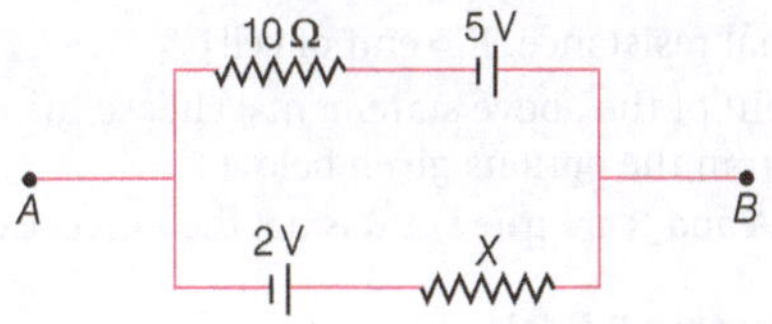

   (a) 5 Ω (b) 10 Ω (c) 15 Ω (d) 20 Ω

3. Two batteries of emf 4 V and 8 V with internal resistances 1 Ω and 2 Ω are connected in a circuit with a resistance of 9 Ω as shown in figure. The current and potential difference between the points P and Q are

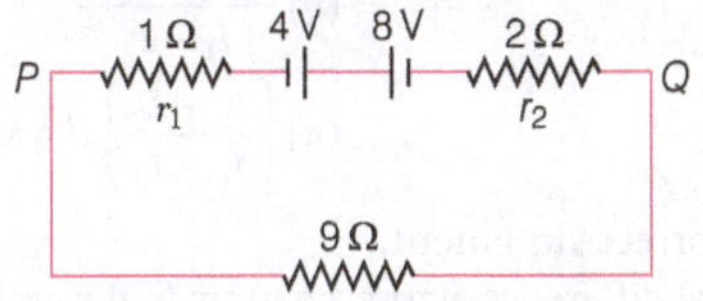

   (a) $\frac{1}{3}$ A and 3 V (b) $\frac{1}{6}$ A and 4 V
   (c) $\frac{1}{9}$ A and 9 V (d) $\frac{1}{2}$ A and 12 V

4. **Assertion** (A) Terminal voltage of a cell is greater than emf of the cell, during charging of the cell.
   Reason (R) The emf of a cell is always greater than its terminal voltage.

   In the light of the above statements, choose the correct answer from the options given below.
   (a) Both A and R are true but R is not the correct explanation of A.
   (b) A is true but R is false.
   (c) A is false but R is true.
   (d) Both A and R are true and R is the correct explanation of A.

5. The current flowing through 5 Ω resistance is

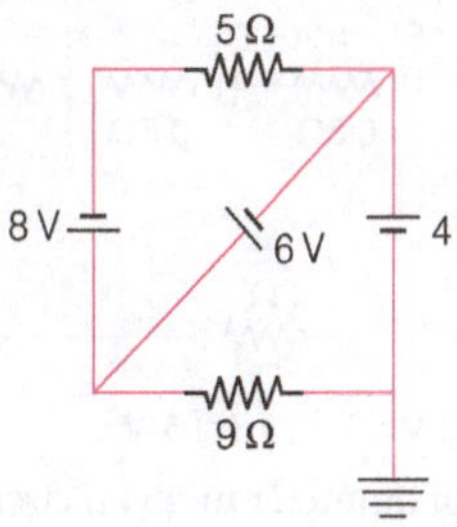

   (a) 10 A (b) 1 A
   (c) 2.5 A (d) 0.4 A

6. A battery of emf 10 V and internal resistance 3 Ω is connected to a resistor. If the current in the circuit is 0.5 A, then find resistance of resistor and terminal potential difference (TPD) of cell when circuit is closed.
   (a) 18Ω, 10 V (b) 17Ω, 8.5 V (c) 16Ω, 8.5 V (d) 12Ω, 10 V

7. The cell has an emf of 2V and the internal resistance of this cell is 0.1 Ω, it is connected to resistance of 3.9 Ω, the voltage across the cell will be
   (a) 1.95 V (b) 1.5 V
   (c) 2 V (d) 1.8 V

8. What is potential difference between points a and b in given circuit?

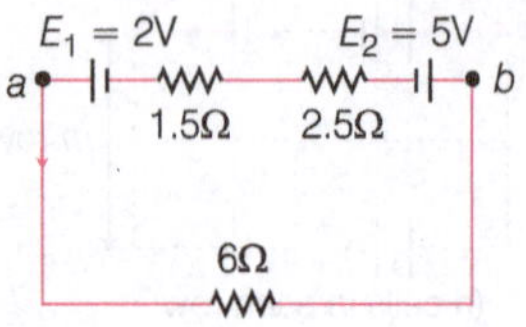

(a) 1.8 V (b) –1.8 V (c) 0.3 V (d) –0.3 V

9. Consider two identical cells each of emf E and internal resistance r connected to a load R. Which of the following pair is not correctly paired?

(a) Main current in series combinations of cells	(i) $\dfrac{nE}{R+nr}$
(b) Main current in parallel combinations of cells	(ii) $\dfrac{E}{R+r/n}$
(c) Equivalent internal resistance in series combination of cells	(iii) nr
(d) Equivalent internal resistance in parallel combination of cells	(iv) $\dfrac{rE}{n}$

10. If 10 identical cells are connected in series, then current passing through a load resistance is I. If polarity of some cells are reversed, then current through load resistance is $I/5$. Find the number of cells whose polarity has been changed.

(a) 2 (b) 3
(c) 4 (d) 5

11. Four identical cells, emf of each 4 V and internal resistance 0.5 Ω and connected as shown in figure. Find the TPD across cell E_4.

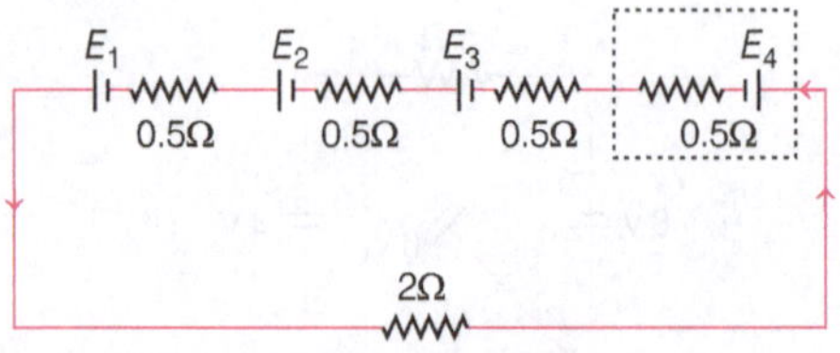

(a) 8 V (b) 2 V (c) 5 V (d) –2V

12. Find the reading of ammeter in given circuit.

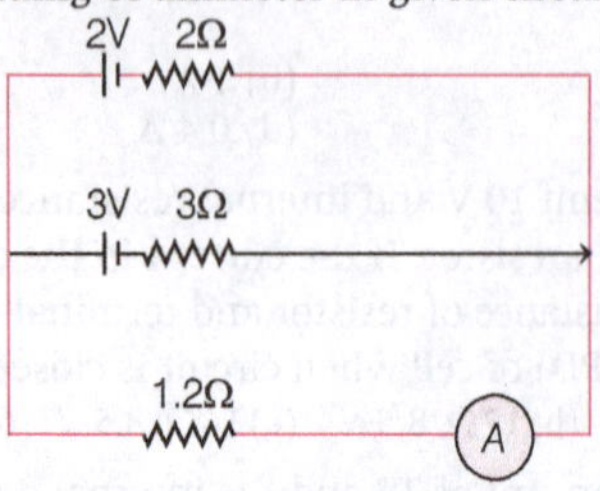

(a) 1 A (b) 1.2 A
(c) 2.4 A (d) 0.8 A

13. A cell of emf E and internal resistance r is connected in series with an external resistance nr. Then, the ratio of the terminal potential difference to emf is

(a) $\dfrac{n+1}{n}$ (b) $n+1$ (c) $\dfrac{n}{n+1}$ (d) n

14. **Assertion** (A) When n cells, each of internal resistance r are arbitrary connected in series, the total external resistance of cells may be zero.

Reason (R) The internal resistance does not depends in polarity of cell connected in circuit.

In the light of the above statements, choose the correct answer from the options given below.

(a) Both A and R are true but R is not the correct explanation of A.
(b) A is true but R is false.
(c) A is false but R is true.
(d) Both A and R are true and R is the correct explanation of A.

15. If E is the emf of a cell of internal resistance r and external resistance R, then potential difference across R is given as

(a) $V = E/(R+r)$ (b) $V = E$
(c) $V = E/(1 + r/R)$ (d) $V = E/(1 + R/r)$

16. There are n cells, each of emf E and internal resistance r, connected in series with an external resistance R. One of the cells is wrongly connected, so that it sends current in the opposite direction. The current flowing in the circuit is

(a) $\dfrac{(n-1)E}{(n+1)r+2}$ (b) $\dfrac{(n-1)E}{nr+R}$
(c) $\dfrac{(n-2)E}{nr+R}$ (d) $\dfrac{(n-2)E}{(n-2)r+R}$

17. **Assertion** (A) Parallel connection of cells is preferred to draw less current at low potential difference.

Reason (R) In parallel connection, current $I = \dfrac{nE}{r}$. [where, r = internal resistance, E = emf of cell]

In the light of the above statements, choose the correct answer from the options given below.

(a) Both A and R are true but R is not the correct explanation of A.
(b) A is true but R is false.
(c) A is false but R is true.
(d) Both A and R are true and R is the correct explanation of A.

18. A cell supplies a current I_1 through a resistance R_1 and a current I_2 through a resistance R_2. The internal resistance of this cell is

(a) $R_2 - R_1$ (b) $\dfrac{I_1R_2 - I_2R_1}{I_1 - I_2}$
(c) $\dfrac{I_2R_2 - I_1R_1}{I_1 - I_2}$ (d) $\left(\dfrac{I_1 + I_2}{I_1 - I_2}\right)\sqrt{R_1R_2}$

19. Find the correct statement.

(a) Potential difference across a battery is always less than or equal to EMF of the battery.
(b) Potential difference across a battery is always greater than or equal to EMF of the battery.
(c) Potential difference across a battery can never be zero.
(d) None of the above statement is correct.

20. Find the incorrect statement.

(a) In series combination of cells, $r_{eq} = r_1 + r_2 + \dots,$
(b) In series combination of cells, $E_{eq} = E_1 \pm E_2 \pm E_3 \pm \dots,$
(c) In parallel combination of cells, $\dfrac{1}{r_{eq}} = \dfrac{1}{r_1} + \dfrac{1}{r_2} + \dots$
(d) Parallel combination of n cells has less current than series combination of n cells.

Module 4

Kirchhoff's Laws and its Applications

- Kirchhoff's Laws
- Electrical Energy and Power
- Heating Effects of Current
- Wheatstone Bridge
- Meter Bridge

Kirchhoff's Laws

Many electric circuits cannot be reduced to simple series-parallel combinations. Kirchhoff's laws (or rules) are used to solve these complicated electric circuits. These rules are basically the expressions of conservation of electric charge and of energy. e.g. two circuits that cannot be broken down are shown in figure.

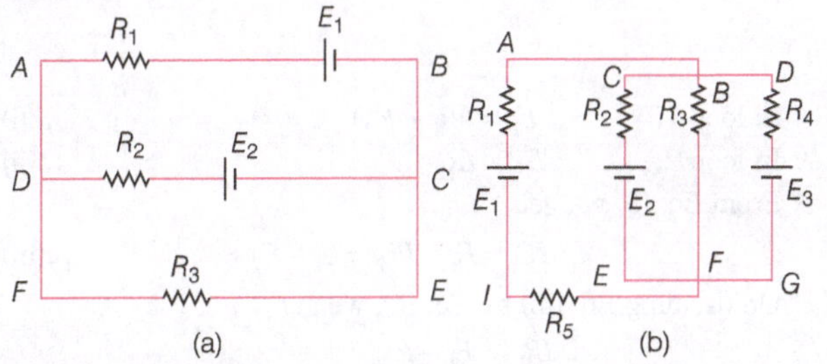

(a) (b)

However, it is always possible to analyse such circuits by applying two rules, derived by Kirchhoff in 1845 and 1846. The two terms related to Kirchhoff's laws are given below

Junction

A junction in a circuit is a point, where three or more conductors meet. Junctions are also called **nodes** or **branch points**. For example, in Fig. (a), points *D* and *C* are junctions. Similarly, in Fig. (b), points *B* and *F* are junctions.

Loop

A loop is any closed conducting path. For example, in Fig. (a), *ABCDA*, *DCEFD* and *ABEFA* are loops. Similarly, in Fig. (b), *CBFEC*, *BDGFB* are loops.

Kirchhoff's Junction Rule

The algebraic sum of the currents meeting at a point or at a junction in an electric circuit is always zero.

i.e. $$\sum_{\text{junction}} I = 0$$

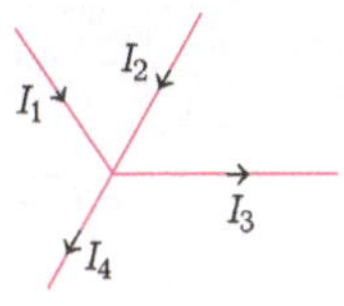

According to junction rule,
$I_1 + I_2 = I_3 + I_4$

This law can also be written as, "the sum of all the currents directed towards a point (node) in a circuit is equal to the sum of all the currents directed away from that point (node)".

This law is also known as **Kirchhoff's Current Law (KCL)**.

The junction rule is based on **conservation of electric charge**.

Kirchhoff's Loop Rule

This law states that, the algebraic sum of change in potential around any closed loop involving resistors and cells in the loop, is zero. It means that, in any closed part of an electrical circuit, the algebraic sum of the emfs is equal to the algebraic sum of the products of the resistances and currents flowing through them. It is also known as **loop rule**. i.e. $\sum_{\text{closed loop}} \Delta V = 0$

This law is also known as **Kirchhoff's Voltage Law (KVL)**.

The loop rule is based on **conservation of energy**.

Sign Conventions for the Application of Kirchhoff's Laws

For the application of Kirchhoff's laws, the following sign conventions are to be considered.

(i) The change in potential in traversing a resistance in the direction of current is $-IR$, while in the opposite direction is $+IR$.

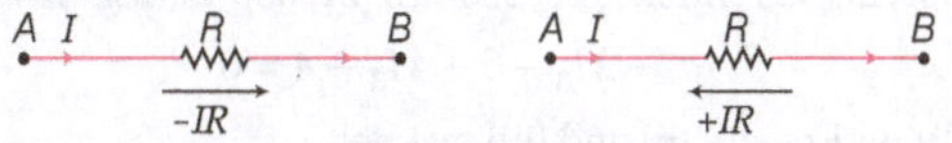

(ii) The change in potential in traversing an emf source from negative to positive terminal is $+E$, while in the opposite direction is $-E$, irrespective of the direction of current in the circuit.

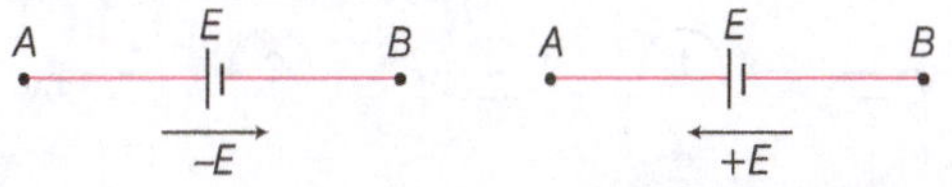

To calculate potential difference between two points by using Kirchhoff's law

While using Kirchhoff's laws to calculate the potential difference, the following points should be considered

(i) Start from a point on the loop and go along the loop, either anti-clockwise or clockwise, to reach the same point again, but balance currents at junction as per KCL.

(ii) If moving along the direction of the current, there will be potential drop across a resistance and if moving in the opposite direction, there will be potential gain.

(iii) The net sum of all these potential differences should be zero, using the KVL rule.

Now, let us consider a circuit as shown in Figure.

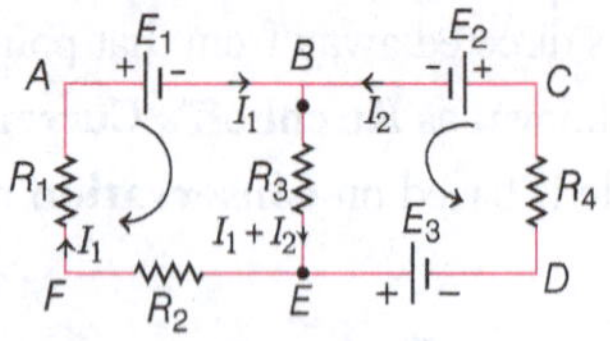

In closed loop $ABEFA$,

$$-E_1 - (I_1 + I_2)R_3 - I_1R_2 - I_1R_1 = 0$$

In closed loop $BCDEB$,

$$E_2 + I_2R_4 + E_3 - (I_1 + I_2)R_3 = 0$$

Example 32. *Find currents in different branches of the electric circuit shown in figure.*

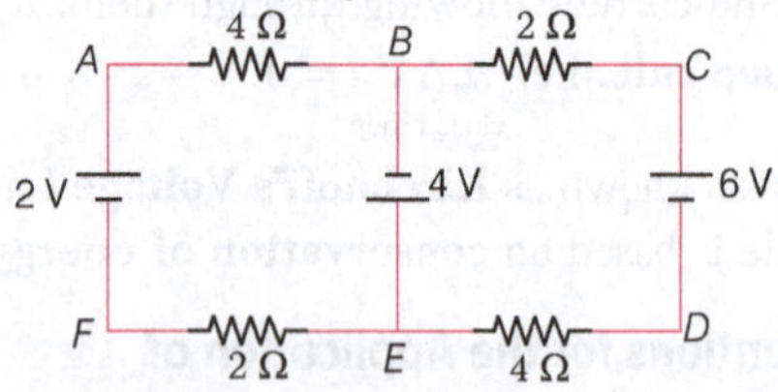

Sol. Applying Kirchhoff's first law (junction law) at junction B,

$$I_1 = I_2 + I_3 \quad \text{...(i)}$$

Applying Kirchhoff's second law in loop 1 ($ABEFA$),

$$-4I_1 + 4 - 2I_1 + 2 = 0 \quad \text{...(ii)}$$

Applying Kirchhoff's second law in loop 2 ($BCDEB$),

$$-2I_3 - 6 - 4I_3 - 4 = 0 \quad \text{...(iii)}$$

Solving Eqs. (i), (ii) and (iii), we get

$$I_1 = 1 \text{ A}$$

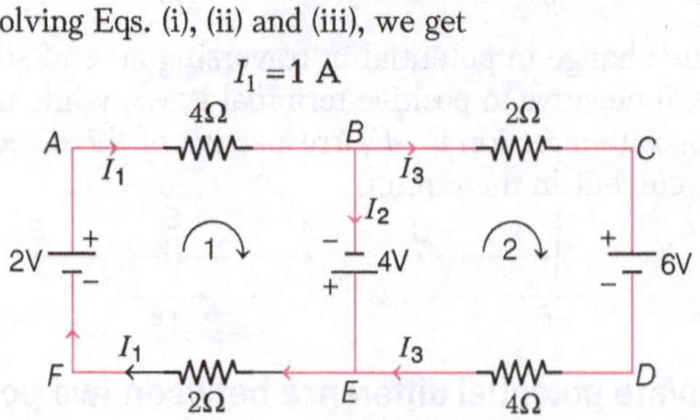

$$I_3 = -\frac{5}{3} \text{ A} \Rightarrow I_2 = \frac{8}{3} \text{ A}$$

Here, negative sign of I_3 implies that current I_3 is in opposite direction of what we have assumed.

NEET Close-up

Example Similar to PYQ Asked in NEET 2023

If reading in galvanometer is zero. Then, ratio of R_1 and R_2 is

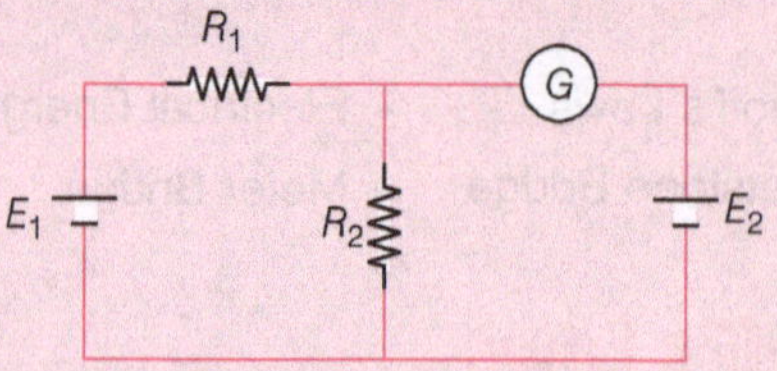

(a) $\frac{E_1 - E_2}{E_2}$ (b) $\frac{E_2 - E_1}{E_2}$ (c) $\frac{E_1 - E_2}{E_1}$ (d) $\frac{E_2 - E_1}{E_1}$

Sol. (*a*) There is no potential difference across galvanometer.

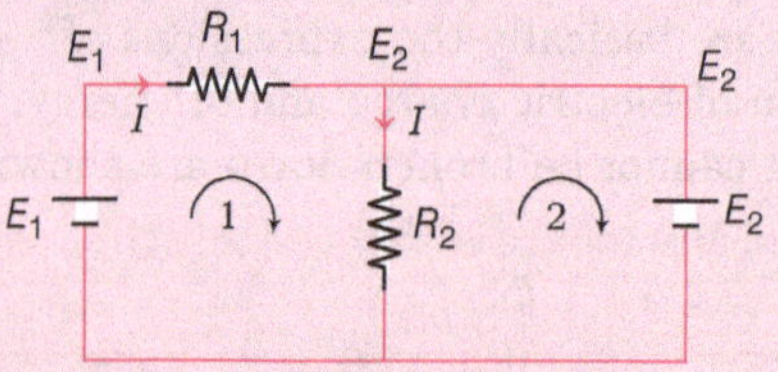

In loop 1, $E_1 = I(R_1 + R_2)$ ...(i)

In loop 2, $E_2 = IR_2$ ...(ii)

From Eq. (i), we get

$$IR_1 = E_1 - IR_2 = E_1 - E_2 \quad \text{...(iii)}$$

On dividing Eq. (iii) by Eq. (ii), we get

$$\frac{IR_1}{IR_2} = \frac{E_1 - E_2}{E_2}$$

$$\Rightarrow \quad \frac{R_1}{R_2} = \frac{E_1 - E_2}{E_2}$$

Skill Builder

Current through 10 Ω resistor in the given circuit is

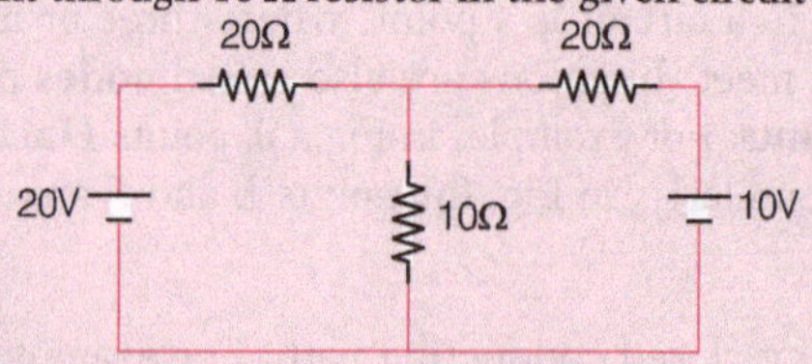

(a) 0.5 A (b) 0.75 A (c) 1.00 A (d) 1.25 A

For more Practice Refer Q. No. 60, 90, 123 of Gearing up for NEET.

Example 33. *Find the potential difference between points F and C of an electric circuit shown in below figure.*

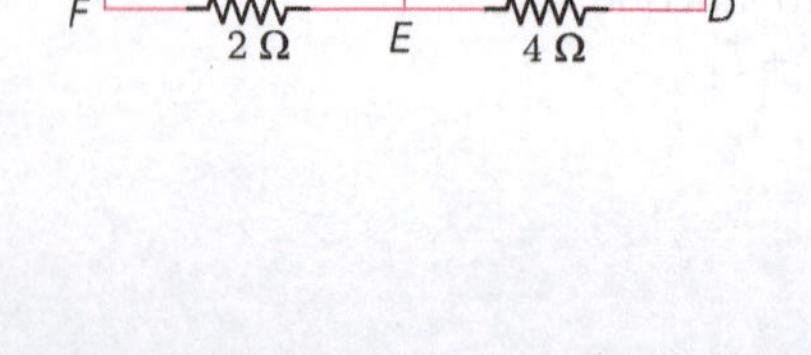

Sol. Let us reach from F to C *via* A and B,

$$V_F + 2 - 4I_1 - 2I_3 = V_C$$

$\therefore$ $$V_F - V_C = 4I_1 + 2I_3 - 2$$

Substituting, $I_1 = 1$ A

and $I_3 = -(5/3)$ A, we get

$$V_F - V_C = -(4/3)\text{ V}$$

Here, negative sign implies that $V_F < V_C$.

Example 34. *Find the potential difference between the points A and B.*

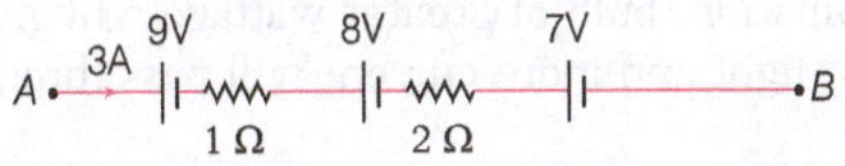

Sol. According to given figure, when we move from A to B, using KVL,

$$V_A - 9 - 3\times 1 - 8 - 3\times 2 - 7 = V_B$$

$$\Rightarrow \quad V_A - V_B = 33\text{ V}$$

Example 35. *(a) Find the potential difference between the points A and B.*

(b) Find current through 20 V cell, if points A and B are connected.

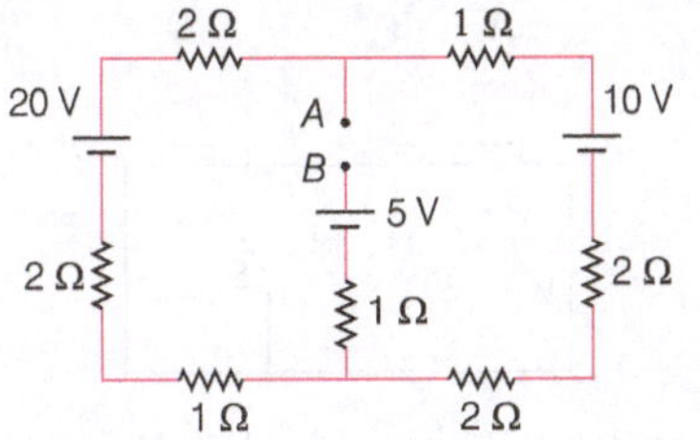

Sol. (a)

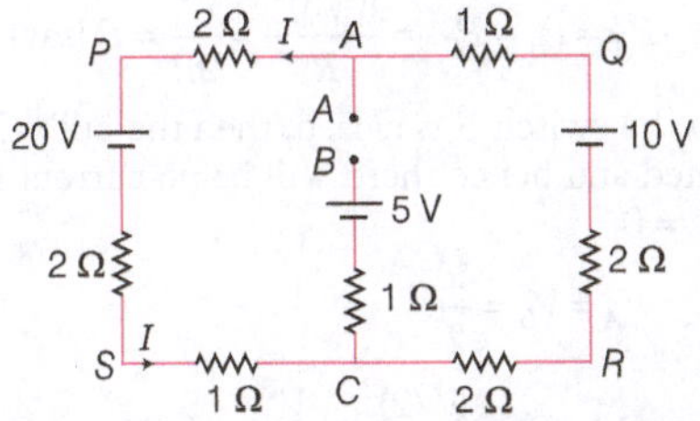

No current flows in the branch CB as AB is not connected.

Let current in the circuit $APSCRQA$ be I.

Using KVL,

$$V_A - I\times 2 - 20 - I\times 2 - I\times 1 - I\times 2 - I\times 2 + 10 - I\times 1 = V_A$$

$$\Rightarrow 10I = -10 \Rightarrow \quad I = -1\text{ A}$$

i.e., direction of I is opposite.

Now, A to B path will be $APSCB$,

$$V_A - I\times 2 - 20 - I\times 2 - I\times 1 + 5 = V_B$$

$$V_A - V_B = 15 + 5I = 15 + 5\times(-1) = 10\text{ V}$$

(b) Now, if the points A and B are connected.

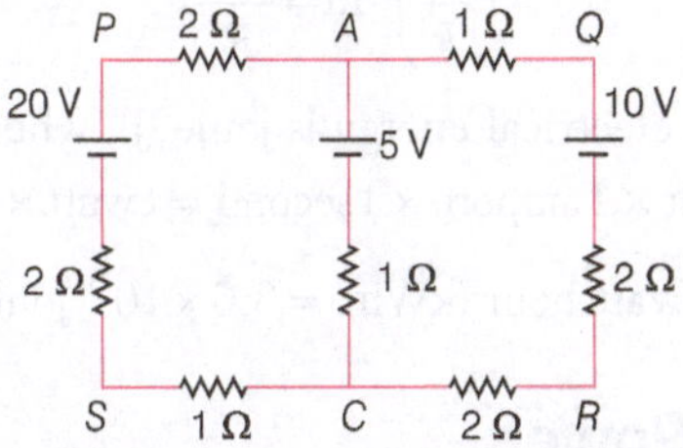

Resistances 2 Ω, 2 Ω and 1 Ω are in series along $APSC$ and resistances 1 Ω, 2Ω and 2Ω are also in series along $AQRC$.

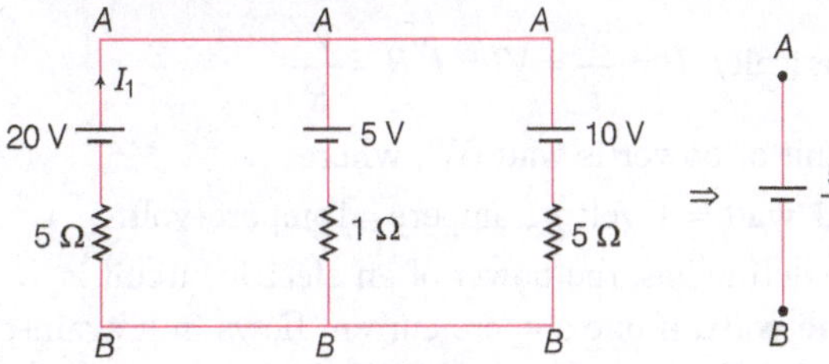

So, the equivalent voltage will be

$$E = \frac{\frac{20}{5} + \frac{5}{1} + \frac{10}{5}}{\frac{1}{5} + \frac{1}{1} + \frac{1}{5}} = \frac{4+5+2}{\frac{1+5+1}{5}} = \frac{11\times 5}{7} = \frac{55}{7}\text{ V}$$

$\therefore$ Potential difference between points A and B,

$$V_A - V_B = \frac{55}{7}\text{ V}$$

For cell of emf 20 V,

$$V_A - V_B = 20 - 5I_1$$

$$\Rightarrow \quad \frac{55}{7} = 20 - 5I_1 \Rightarrow 5I_1 = 20 - \frac{55}{7} \simeq 12\text{ A}$$

$\therefore$ Current through cell of 20 V, $I_1 = 2.4$ A

Electrical Energy and Power

Electrical energy and power in electrical circuits or components are described below

Electrical Energy

It is defined as the total work done W by the source of emf V in maintaining the electric current I in the circuit for a specified time t.

According to Ohm's law, we have $V = IR$

Total charge that crosses the resistor is given by $q = It$

Energy gained is given by $E = W = Vq = VIt$

$$= (IR)\,It = I^2Rt \qquad [\because V = IR]$$

$$= \left(\frac{V}{R}\right)^2 Rt = \frac{V^2 t}{R} \qquad \left[\because I = \frac{V}{R}\right]$$

The SI unit of electrical energy is joule (J), where

$$1 \text{ joule} = 1 \text{ volt} \times 1 \text{ ampere} \times 1 \text{ second} = 1 \text{ watt} \times 1 \text{ second}.$$

$$1 \text{ kilowatt hour (kWh)} = 3.6 \times 10^6 \text{ joule}$$

Electrical Power

It is defined as the rate of electrical energy supplied per unit time to maintain the flow of electric current through a conductor.

Mathematically, $P = \frac{W}{t} = VI = I^2 R = \frac{V^2}{R}$

The SI unit of power is watt (W), where

$$1 \text{ watt} = 1 \text{ volt} \times 1 \text{ ampere} = 1 \text{ ampere-volt}.$$

It can be defined as, the power of an electric circuit is called **one watt**, if one ampere current flows in it against a potential difference of one volt. The bigger units of electrical power are kilowatt (kW) and megawatt (MW) where, $1 \text{kW} = 1000$ W and $1 \text{ MW} = 10^6 \text{W}$.

Commercial unit of electrical power is horse power (HP), where, $1\text{HP} = 746$ W.

Power consumption in a combination of bulbs

Series Combination of Bulbs

(i) Total power consumed is given by

$$\frac{1}{P_{eq}} = \frac{1}{P_1} + \frac{1}{P_2} + \ldots$$

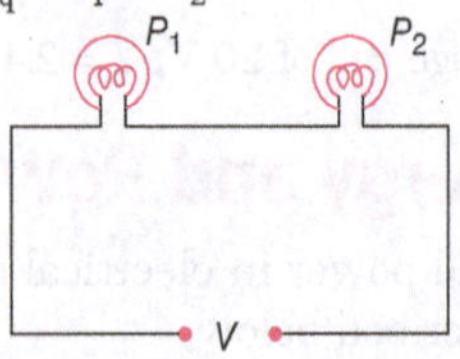

Series combination of two bulbs

(ii) P_{consumed} (brightness) $\propto V \propto R \propto \frac{1}{P_{\text{rated}}}$, *i.e.* in series combination bulb of lesser wattage will give more bright light and potential difference appearing across it will be more.

Parallel Combination of Bulbs

(i) Total power consumed is given by

$$P_{\text{total}} = P_1 + P_2 + \ldots$$

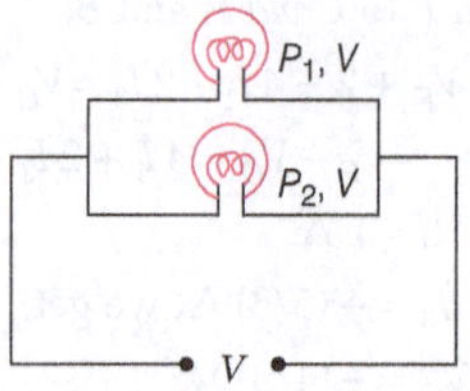

Parallel combination of two bulbs

(ii) P_{consumed} (brightness) $\propto P_{\text{rated}} \propto I \propto \frac{1}{R}$, *i.e.* in parallel combination, bulb of greater wattage will give more bright light and more current will pass through it.

Mentor's Tip

To solve questions related to power consumption in a combination of other electric appliances. Such as a heater, we can use the same rules as for bulb combinations.

Example 36. *Figure shows three identical bulbs A, B and C, which are connected to a battery of supply voltage V. When the switch S is closed, then discuss the change in*

(i) the illumination of the three bulbs.

(ii) the power dissipated in the circuit.

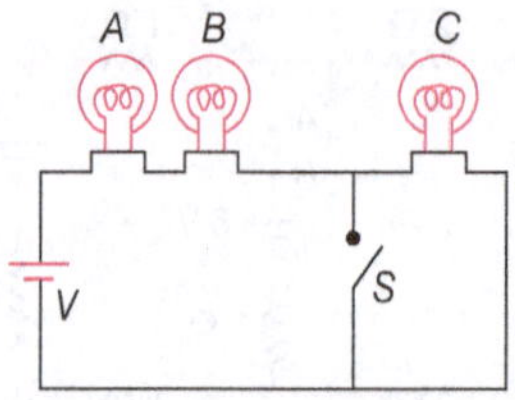

Sol. When the switch S is open, $V_A = V_B = V_C = V/3$

and $\quad P_A = P_B = P_C = \frac{(V/3)^2}{R} = \frac{V^2}{9R} = P$ (say)

(i) When the switch S is closed, then the bulb C is short circuited and hence there will be no current through C.

So, $P_C = 0$

$$V_A = V_B = \frac{V}{2}$$

So, $\quad P_A = P_B = \frac{(V/2)^2}{R} = \frac{V^2}{4R} = \frac{9}{4}P$

Therefore, the intensity of illumination of each of the bulb A and B become 9/4 times of the initial value but the intensity of the bulb C becomes zero.

(ii) The power dissipated in the circuit before closing the switch is

$$P_i = P_A + P_B + P_C = 3P$$

The power dissipated after closing the switch is

$$P_f = P_A + P_B + P_C$$
$$= \frac{9}{4}P + \frac{9}{4}P + 0$$
$$= \frac{9}{2}P$$

NEET Close-up

Example Similar to PYQ Asked in NEET 2024

Two heaters A and B have power rating of 6 kW and 2 kW, respectively. Those two are first connected in series and then in parallel to a fixed source. The ratio of power output of these two cases is

(a) $\frac{7}{16}$ (b) $\frac{3}{16}$
(c) $\frac{5}{16}$ (d) $\frac{5}{18}$

Sol. (b) Given, $P_1 = 6$ kW

$$P_2 = 2\text{ kW}$$

$$P_{\text{series}} = \frac{P_1P_2}{P_1 + P_2} \text{ and } P_{\text{Parallel}} = P_1 + P_2$$

According to question, $\frac{P_{\text{series}}}{P_{\text{parallel}}} = \frac{\frac{6\times 2}{6+2}}{6+2} = \frac{12}{8\times 8} = \frac{3}{16}$

Skill Builder

Two electric water boiler B_1 and B_2 have power rating of 4 kW and 6 kW, respectively. First both boiler are connected in series and then in parallel to a fixed power source. The ratio of power outputs for these two cases is

(a) $\frac{6}{25}$ (b) $\frac{8}{18}$ (c) $\frac{5}{22}$ (d) $\frac{3}{20}$

For more Practice Refer Q.No. 13 of step up exercise 4 and Q.No. 88 of Gearing up for NEET.

Heating Effects of Current

An electric current through a resistor increases its thermal energy. Also, there are other situations in which an electric current can produce or absorb thermal energy. This effect is called heating effect of electric current.

When some potential difference V is applied across a resistance R, charge q flows through the circuit in time t, then the heat absorbed or produced is given by

$$W = qV = VIt = I^2Rt = \frac{V^2t}{R}\text{ joule}$$

or $$W = \frac{VIt}{J} = \frac{I^2Rt}{J} = \frac{V^2t}{JR}\text{ cal}$$

where, J is the joule's mechanical equivalent of heat (4.18 J/cal).

These relations are also called **Joule's law of heating.**

Example 37. *In the given network of resistors, find the heat developed across each resistance in 2s.*

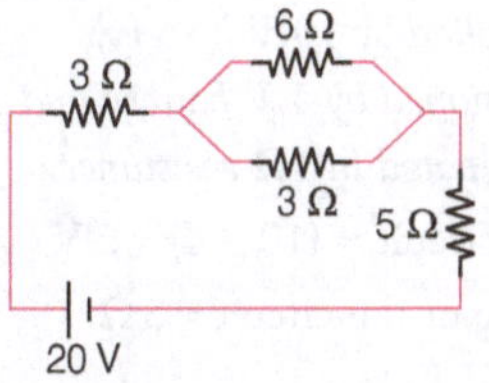

Sol. The 6 Ω and 3 Ω resistances are in parallel. So, their combined resistance is $\frac{1}{R} = \frac{1}{6} + \frac{1}{3} = \frac{1}{2}$ or $R = 2\,\Omega$

The equivalent simple circuit can be drawn as shown.

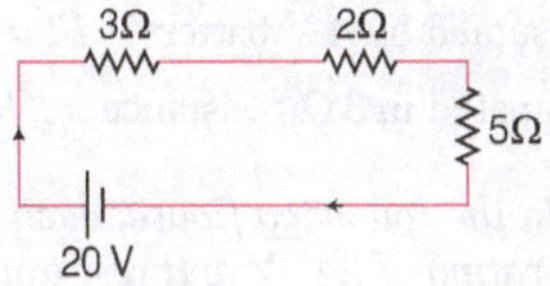

Current in the circuit,

$$I = \frac{\text{Net emf}}{\text{Total resistance}} = \frac{20}{3+2+5} = 2\text{ A}$$

$$\therefore \quad V = IR = (2)(2) = 4\text{ V}$$

i.e. potential difference across 6 Ω and 3 Ω resistances same as 4 V. Now,

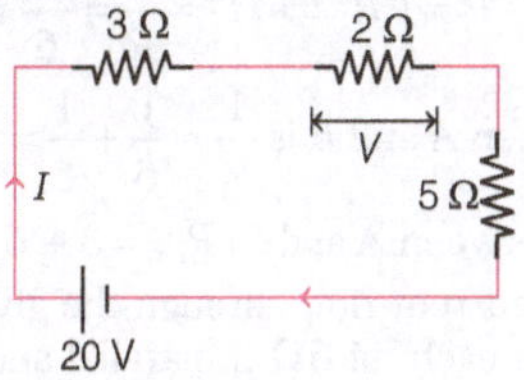

$$H_{3\Omega} = I^2Rt = (2)^2(3)(2) = 24\text{ J}$$

$$H_{6\Omega} = \frac{V^2}{R}t = \frac{(4)^2}{6}(2) = \frac{16}{3}\text{ J}$$

$$H_{3\Omega} = \frac{V^2}{R}t = \frac{(4)^2(2)}{3} = \frac{32}{3}\text{ J}$$

and $$H_{5\Omega} = I^2Rt = (2)^2(5)(2) = 40\text{ J}$$

Mentor's TiP

Bulbs in series follows brightness $\propto V \propto R$

Bulbs in parallel flows brightness $\propto I \propto \frac{1}{R}$

Example 38. *In the following figure, find*

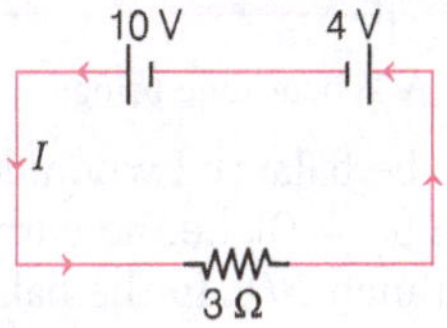

(i) the power supplied by 10 V battery,

(ii) the power consumed by 4 V battery and

(iii) the power dissipated in 3 Ω resistance.

Sol. Net emf of the circuit = (10 − 4) = 6 V

Total resistance of the circuit = 3 Ω

$\therefore$ Current in the circuit, $I = \frac{\text{Net emf}}{\text{Total resistance}} = \frac{6}{3} = 2\text{ A}$

(i) Power supplied by 10 V battery $= EI = (10)(2) = 20\text{ W}$

(ii) Power consumed by 4 V battery $= EI = (4)(2) = 8\text{ W}$

(iii) Power dissipated in 3 Ω resistance $= I^2R = (2)^2(3) = 12\text{ W}$

Example 39. *In the following figure, each of the three resistances, has rating of 24 W and resistance of 6 Ω. Find the maximum power rating of the circuit.*

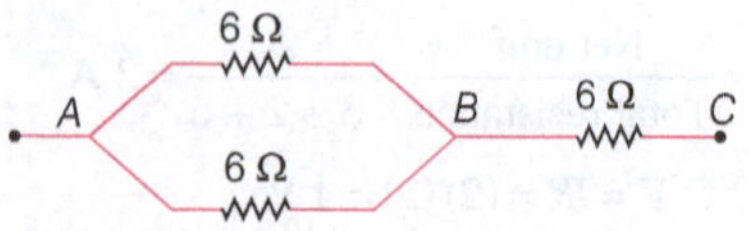

Sol. To find maximum current I,

we use, $P = I^2R \Rightarrow I^2 = \frac{P}{R} = \frac{24}{6} = 4 \Rightarrow I = 2\text{ A}$

Resistance between A and B is $\frac{1}{R_1} = \frac{1}{6} + \frac{1}{6} = \frac{1}{3} \Rightarrow R = 3\,\Omega$

and resistance between A and C, $R_{eq} = 3 + 6 = 9\,\Omega$

If we make 2 A current flow through the given circuit, 1 A will flow through each of 6Ω in parallel and 2 A through 6Ω in series. This is the maximum current the circuit can hold.

So, power of circuit $= I^2R = 2 \times 2 \times 9 = 36\text{ W}$

Wheatstone Bridge

It is an arrangement of four resistances used to measure one of them, in terms of the other three as shown in Figure.

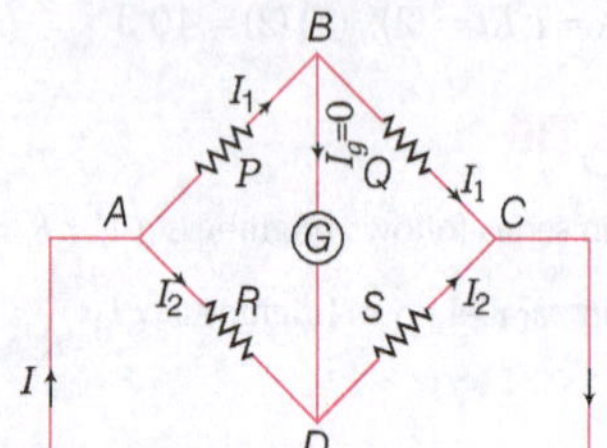

A Wheatstone bridge

The bridge is said to be balanced when deflection in galvanometer is zero ($I_g = 0$), i.e. no current flows through the galvanometer (branch BD). In the balanced condition,

$$\frac{P}{Q} = \frac{R}{S}$$

On mutually changing the position of cell and galvanometer, this condition will not change.

Note Different forms of Wheatstone bridge are shown below,

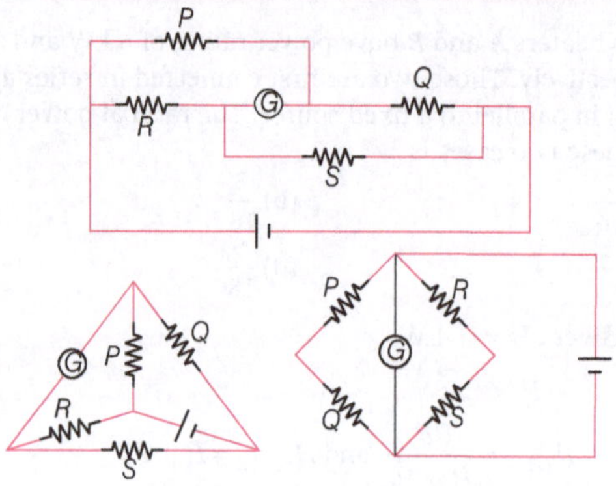

Example 40. *Find out the magnitude of resistance X in the circuit shown in figure, when no current flows through the 5 Ω resistor.*

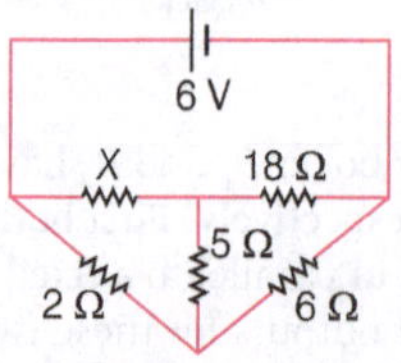

Sol. As no current flows through the middle 5 Ω resistor, the circuit represents a balanced Wheatstone bridge.

$$\therefore \quad \frac{X}{18} = \frac{2}{6} \quad \text{or} \quad X = \frac{2}{6} \times 18 = 6\,\Omega$$

Mentor's Tip

- A resistance through which no current flows can be removed from the circuit to simplify the circuit.

Example 41. *Calculate the current drawn from the battery by the network of resistors shown in figure.*

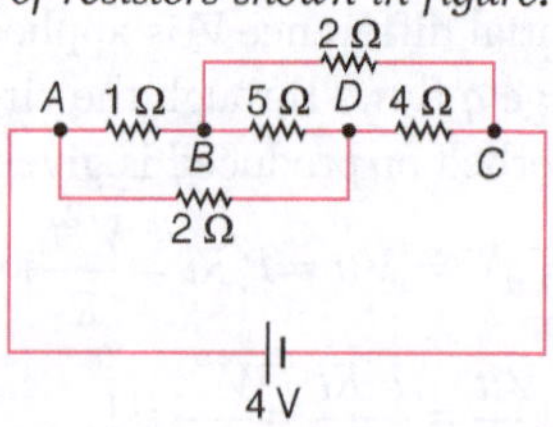

Sol. The given network is equivalent to the circuit shown in figure below

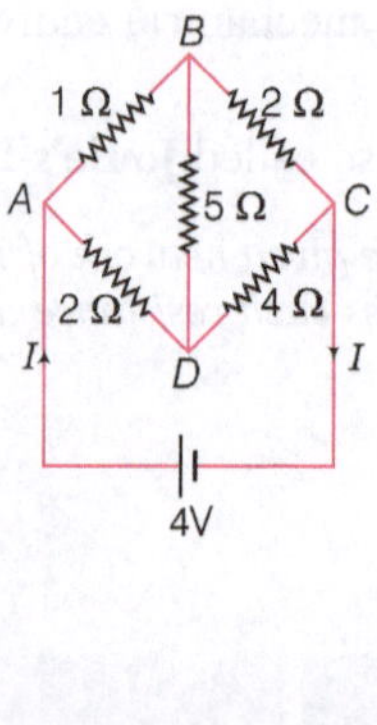

Now, the circuit represents a balanced Wheatstone bridge.

$$\therefore \quad \frac{1}{2} = \frac{2}{4}$$

The resistance of 5 Ω in arm BD is ineffective. The equivalent circuit reduces to the circuit shown in figure.

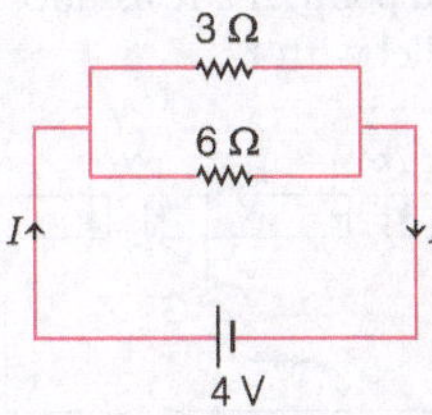

Equivalent resistance, $R_{eq} = \dfrac{6 \times 3}{6+3} = 2\,\Omega$

$\therefore$ Current drawn from the battery, $I = \dfrac{V}{R_{eq}} = \dfrac{4}{2} = 2\,\text{A}$

NEET Snapshot

For the most precise measurement of unknown resistance by Wheatstone bridge, the ratio of resistance in arms should be equal.
[NEET 2022]

The equal ratio of resistance in arms could decrease error in experiment. So, that wheatstone bridge gives precise measurement of unknown resistance.

Scan for Video

Meter Bridge

A meter bridge is **slide wire bridge** or **Carey Foster bridge**. It is an instrument that works on the principle of Wheatstone bridge.

It consists of a straight and uniform wire along a meter scale (AC) and by varying the taping point B as shown in Figure, the bridge is balanced.

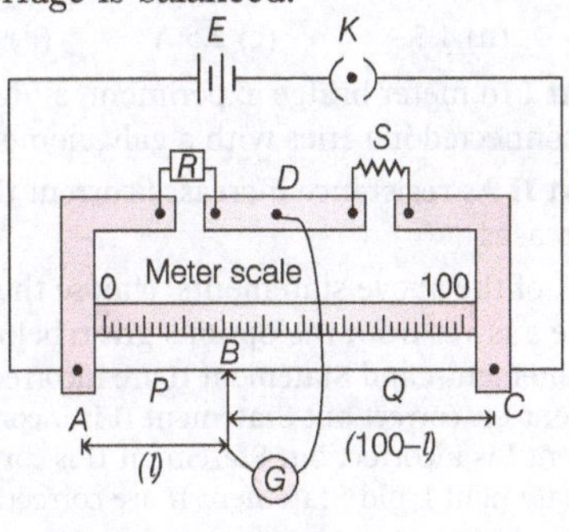

Measuring unknown resistance using meter bridge

$\therefore$ At balancing situation of bridge,

$$\frac{P}{Q} = \frac{R}{S} \quad \Rightarrow \quad \frac{l}{100-l} = \frac{R}{S}$$

$$\Rightarrow \quad S = \frac{100-l}{l} \times R$$

Applications of meter bridge

(i) It is used to measure an unknown resistance by using, $S = \dfrac{R(100-l)}{l}$

(ii) To compare the two unknown resistances by using, $\dfrac{R}{S} = \dfrac{l}{100-l}$

Example 42. *In the following circuit, a meter bridge is shown in its balanced state. The meter bridge wire has a resistance of 1 Ω-cm. Calculate the value of the unknown resistance X and the current drawn from the battery of negligible internal resistance.*

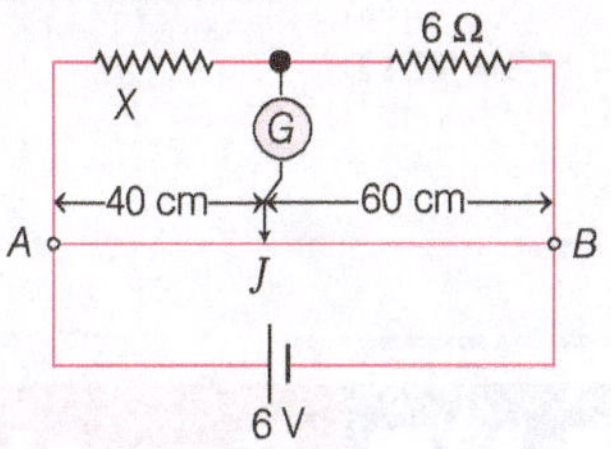

Sol. In balanced condition, no current flows through the galvanometer.

Here, P = resistance of wire $AJ = 40\Omega$

Q = resistance of wire $BJ = 60\Omega$, $R = X$, $S = 6\Omega$

In the balanced condition, $\dfrac{P}{Q} = \dfrac{R}{S}$

or $\quad \dfrac{40}{60} = \dfrac{X}{6}$ or $X = 4\,\Omega$

Total resistance of wire $AB = 100\Omega$

Total resistance of resistances X and 6 Ω connected in series $= 4 + 6 = 10\Omega$

This series combination is in parallel with wire AB.

$\therefore$Equivalent resistance $= \dfrac{10 \times 100}{10+100} = \dfrac{100}{11}\Omega$

emf of the battery = 6 V

$\therefore$ Current drawn from the battery,

$$I = \frac{\text{emf}}{\text{resistance}} = \frac{6}{100/11} = 0.66\text{ A}$$

NEET Close-up

Example Similar to PYQ Asked in NEET 2020

A meter bridge has left gap filled with 10 Ω resistor. Length of resistor in right gap of meter bridge is 2 m. Balance point is at 40 cm from left. Find resistance of 1 m length of unknown resistor.

(a) 7.5 Ω (b) 6.5 Ω
(c) 5 Ω (d) 9.2 Ω

Sol. (*a*) Unknown resistance

$$Q = \left(\frac{100 - l}{l}\right) R$$

$$\Rightarrow \quad Q = \left(\frac{100 - 40}{40}\right) \times 10 = 15\,\Omega$$

So, wire of 2 m length of unknown wire = 15 Ω

We know that, $R \propto l$

$$\Rightarrow \quad \frac{R_2}{R_1} = \frac{l_2}{l_1}$$

$$\Rightarrow \quad R_2 = \frac{1}{2} \times 15 = 7.5\,\Omega$$

Skill Builder

The given figure shows the experimental set up of a meter bridge. The null point is found to be 60 cm away from the end *A* with *X* and *Y* in position as shown. When a resistance of 15 Ω is connected in series with *Y*, then the null point is found to shift by 10 cm towards the end *A* of the wire. Find the position of null point, if a resistance of 30 Ω were connected in parallel with *Y*.

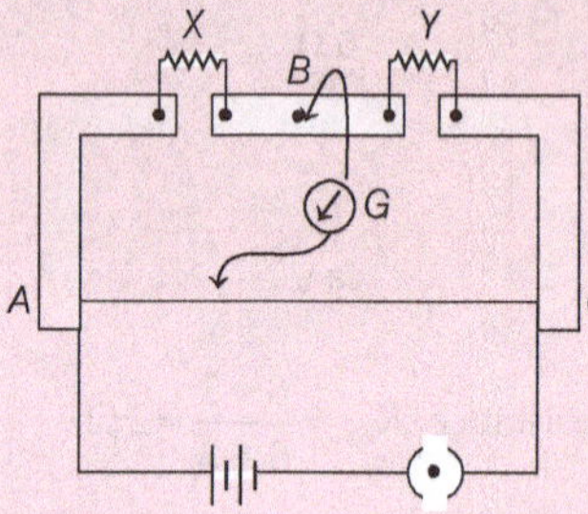

(a) 50 cm (b) 75 cm
(c) 40 cm (d) 60 cm

For more Practice Refer Q. No. 68 of Gearing up for NEET.

STEP UP Practice 4

1. The figure shows a network of currents. The current *I* will be

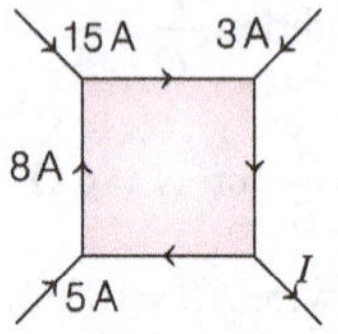

(a) 3 A (b) 13 A
(c) 23 A (d) −3A

2. In the circuit element given here, if the potential difference at point *B*, $V_B = 0$, then the potential difference between *A* and *D* are

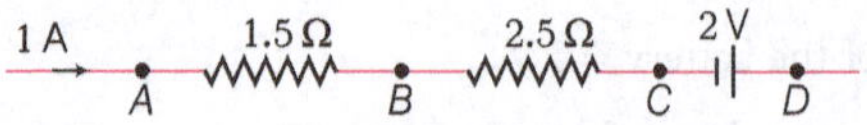

(a) $V_A = -1.5\text{ V}, V_D = +2\text{ V}$
(b) $V_A = -1.5\text{ V}, V_D = +0.5\text{ V}$
(c) $V_A = +1.5\text{ V}, V_D = +0.5\text{ V}$
(d) $V_A = +1.5\text{ V}, V_D = -0.5\text{ V}$

3. Three resistances are connected to form a *T*-shape as shown in the figure. Then, the current *I* in the 2 Ω resistor is

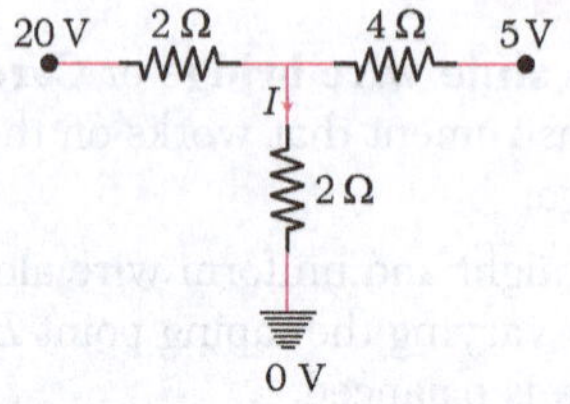

(a) 0.93 A (b) 4.5 A (c) 2.5 A (d) 1.57 A

4. **Statement I** In meter bridge experiment, a high resistance is always connected in series with a galvanometer.

Statement II As resistance increases current through the circuit increases.

In the light of the above statements, choose the most appropriate answer from the options given below

(a) Both Statement I and Statement II are incorrect.
(b) Statement I is correct but Statement II is incorrect.
(c) Statement I is incorrect but Statement II is correct.
(d) Both Statement I and Statement II are correct.

5. Two resistors *R* and 2*R* are connected in series in an electric circuit. The thermal energy developed in *R* and 2*R* are in the ratio

(a) 1 : 2 (b) 2 : 1 (c) 1 : 4 (d) 4 : 1

6. The resistor of resistance R is connected to 25 V supply and heat produced it is 25 Js^{-1}. The value of R is
(a) 225 Ω (b) 1 Ω
(c) 25 Ω (d) 50 Ω

7. Just as electricity is supplied at 220 V for domestic use in India, it is supplied at 110 V in USA. If the resistance of 60 W bulb for use in India is R, then that of 60 W bulb for use in USA will be
(a) $\frac{R}{4}$ (b) $\frac{R}{2}$
(c) R (d) $2R$

8. The electric bulb have tungsten filament of same length. If one of them gives 60 W and other 100 W, then
(a) 100 W bulb has thicker filament
(b) 60 W bulb has thicker filament
(c) Both filaments are of same thickness
(d) it is not possible to get different wattage unless the lengths are different

9. How many calories of heat will be produced approximately in 210 W electric bulb in 5 min?
(a) 800000 cal (b) 63000 cal
(c) 1050 cal (d) 15000 cal

10. **Statement I** The algebraic sum of currents meeting at junction in a closed circuit is zero.
Statement II The Kirchhoff's first law does not obey law of conservation of charge.
In the light of the above statements, choose the most appropriate answer from the options given below.
(a) Both Statement I and Statement II are incorrect.
(b) Statement I is correct but Statement II is incorrect.
(c) Statement I is incorrect but Statement II is correct.
(d) Both Statement I and Statement II are correct.

11. If in the circuit, power dissipation is 150 W, then R is

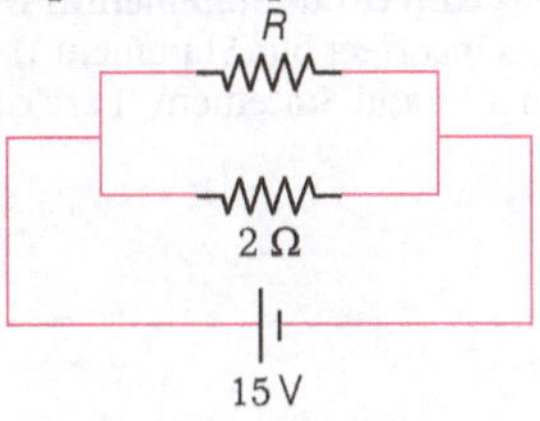

(a) 2 Ω (b) 6 Ω
(c) 5 Ω (d) 4 Ω

12. A wire when connected to 220 V mains supply has power dissipation P_1. Now, the wire is cut into two equal pieces, which are connected in parallel to the same supply. Power dissipation in this case is P_2. Then, $P_2 : P_1$ is
(a) 1 (b) 4
(c) 2 (d) 3

13. Three identical bulbs are connected in series and these together dissipate a power P. Now, if the bulbs are connected in a parallel, then the power dissipated will be
(a) $\frac{P}{3}$ (b) $3P$ (c) $9P$ (d) $\frac{P}{9}$

14. A and B are two bulbs connected in parallel. If A is glowing brighter than B, then the relation between R_A and R_B is
(a) $R_A = R_B$
(b) $R_B > R_A$
(c) $R_A > R_B$
(d) None of the above

15. Some electric bulbs are connected in series across a 220 V supply in a room. If one bulb is fused, then remaining bulbs are connected again in series (after removing the fused bulb) across the same supply. The illumination in the room will
(a) increase
(b) decrease
(c) remain the same
(d) not continuous

16. Consider the given Wheatstone bridge, let current in branch AD is I_2.

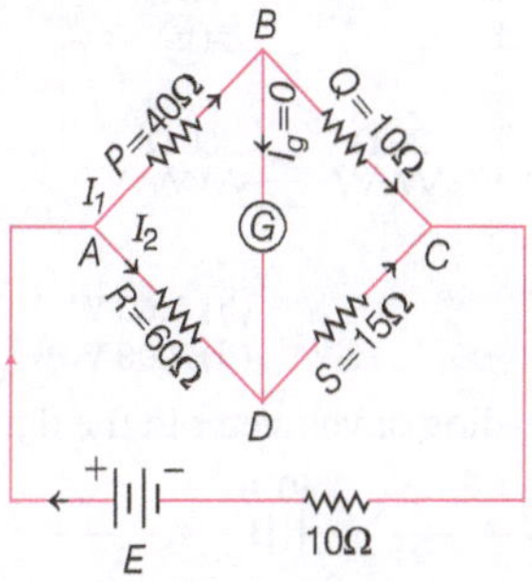

Which of the following pair is incorrect?
(a) Heat produced in t sec in branch $AB \rightarrow$ (i) $90I_2^2t$.
(b) Heat produced in t sec in branch $BC \rightarrow$ (ii) $30I_2^2t$.
(c) Heat produced in t sec in branch $AD \rightarrow$ (iii) $60I_2^2t$.
(d) Heat produced in t sec in branch $DC \rightarrow$ (iv) $15I_2^2t$.

17. Electric bulbs of 50 W-100 V glowing at full power are to be used in parallel with battery 120 V, 10 Ω. Maximum number of bulbs that can be connected, so that they glow in full power is
(a) 2 (b) 8
(c) 4 (d) 6

18. In the circuit shown, A and V are ideal ammeter and voltmeter, respectively. Reading of the voltmeter will be

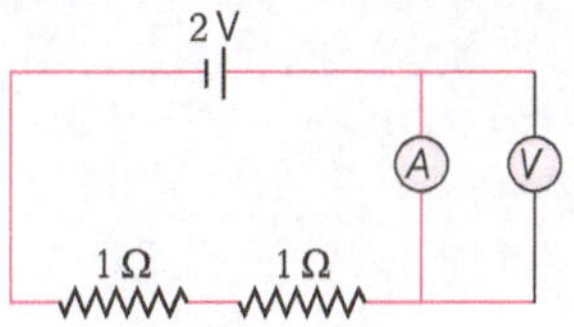

(a) 2 V (b) 1 V
(c) 0.5 V (d) zero

19. An ammeter A, a voltmeter V and a resistance R are connected as shown in the figure. If the voltmeter reading is 1.6 V and the ammeter reading is 0.4 A, then R is

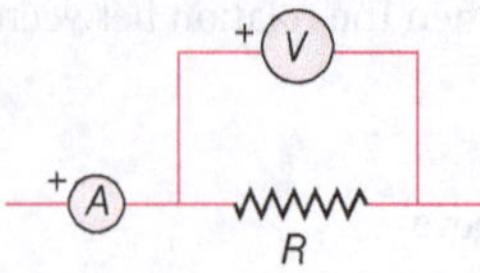

(a) equal to 4 Ω
(b) greater than 4 Ω
(c) less than 4 Ω
(d) between 3 Ω and 4 Ω

20. In the following circuit, the emf of the cell is 2 V and the internal resistance is negligible. The resistance of the voltmeter is 80 Ω. the reading of the voltmeter will be

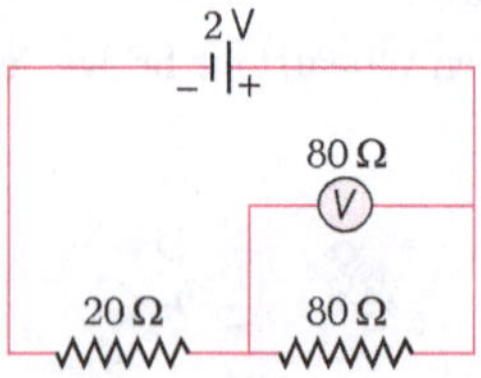

(a) 0.80 V (b) 1.60 V
(c) 1.33 V (d) 2.00 V

21. What is the reading of voltmeter in the figure?

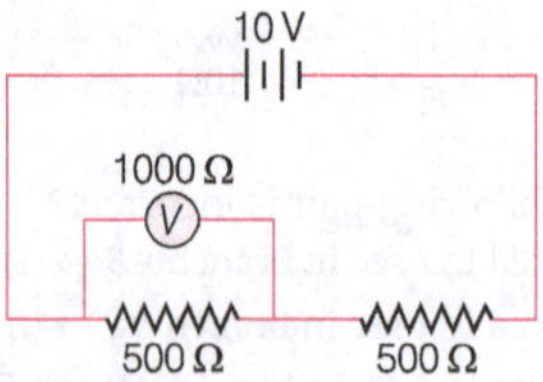

(a) 3 V (b) 2 V
(c) 5 V (d) 4 V

22. In the given circuit, it is observed that the current I is independent of the value of the resistance R_6. Then, the resistance values must satisfy

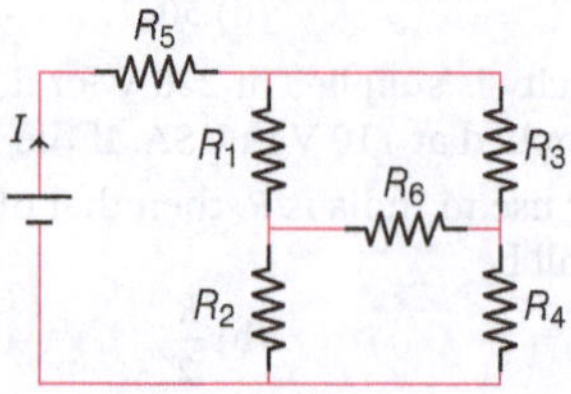

(a) $R_1R_2R_3 = R_3R_4R_5$
(b) $\dfrac{1}{R_5} + \dfrac{1}{R_6} = \dfrac{1}{R_1 + R_2} + \dfrac{1}{R_3 + R_4}$
(c) $R_1R_4 = R_2R_3$
(d) $R_1R_3 = R_2R_4 = R_5R_6$

23. **Statement I** In the balanced condition of a Wheatstone bridge, there is no current flow through the galvanometer.

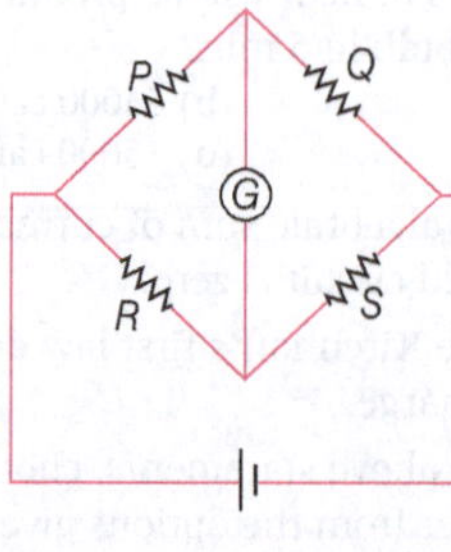

Statement II The potential of points B and D are the same.
In the light of the above statements, choose the most appropriate answer from the options given below.
(a) Both Statement I and Statement II are incorrect.
(b) Statement I is correct but Statement II is incorrect.
(c) Statement I is incorrect but Statement II is correct.
(d) Both Statement I and Statement II are correct.

NEET Exclusive EXTRA BYTES

- There are n cells each of emf E are connected in series as shown in figure. If polarity of m cells (where, $n > 2m$) is reversed, then net emf in the circuit is $(n-2m)E$ and resistance of the circuit is R.

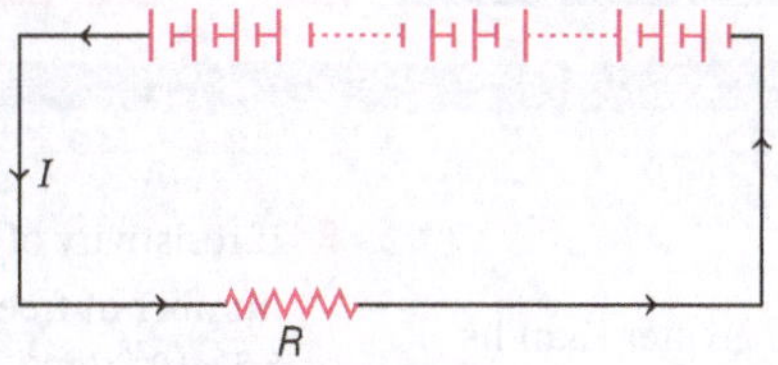

$$i = \frac{(n-2m)E}{R}$$

- Two points in an electric circuit directly connected by a conducting wire are called short-circulted. Under such condition, both points are at some potential.
  For example, resistance R_1 in the above circuit is short-circuited, *i.e.*, potential difference across it is zero. Hence, no current will flow through R_1 and the current through R_2 is therefore, E/R_2.

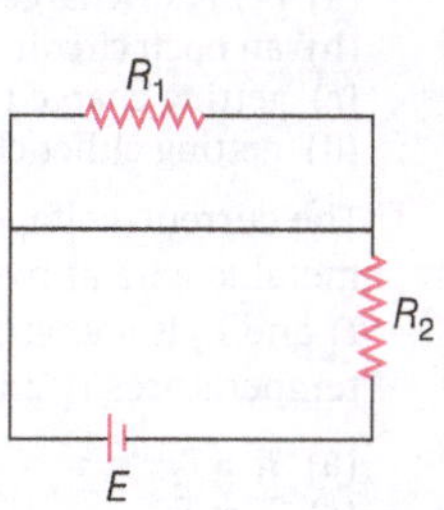

- **Earthing** If some point of a circuit is earthed, then its potential is taken to be zero.
  For example, in the adjoining figure,

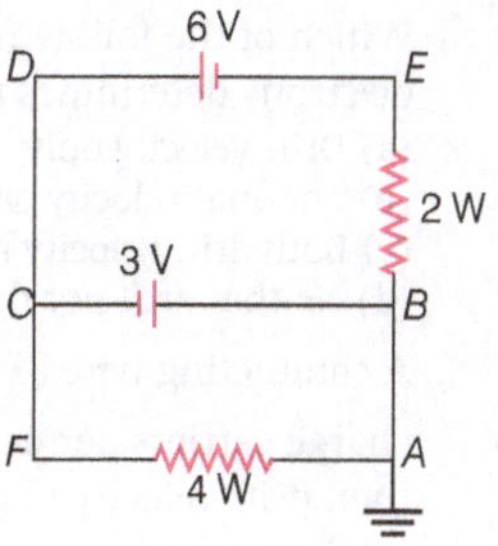

$$V_A = V_B = 0$$
$$V_F = V_C = V_D = -3\text{ V}$$
$$V_E = -9\text{ V}$$
$$\therefore \quad V_B - V_E = 9\text{ V}$$

or current through $2\,\Omega$ resistance is $\dfrac{V_B - V_E}{2}$ or $\dfrac{9}{2}$ A (from B to E)

Similarly, $V_A - V_F = 3\text{ V}$

the current through $4\,\Omega$ resistance is $\dfrac{V_A - V_F}{4}$ or $\dfrac{3}{4}$ A (from A to F)

- Relaxation of time decrease with rise in temperature.
- Bending or re-orienting the wire does not change the validity of Kirchhoff's Junction rule.
- Using n conductors of equal resistance, the maximum number of combination one can have, using all at a time is 2^{n-1}.
- Balanced position of meter bridge is not affected on interchanging the position of the battery and the galvanometer.

GEARING UP FOR NEET

Single Option Correct

1. The terminal potential difference of a cell is greater than its emf when it is
(a) being discharged
(b) an open circuit
(c) getting charged
(d) getting either charged or discharged

2. The current-voltage graph for a given metallic wire at two different temperatures T_1 and T_2 is shown in the figure. The temperatures T_1 and T_2 are related as

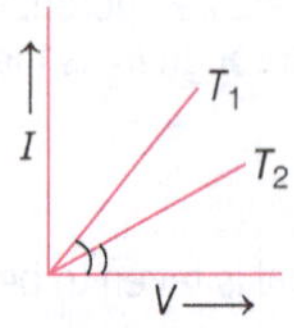

(a) $T_1 > T_2$ (b) $T_1 < T_2$
(c) $T_1 = T_2$ (d) $T_1 > 2T_2$

3 Which of the following characteristics of electrons determines the current in a conductor?
(a) Drift velocity only
(b) Thermal velocity only
(c) Both drift velocity and thermal velocity
(d) Neither drift nor thermal velocity

4. A conducting wire of cross-sectional area 1 cm^2 has 3×10^{23} charge carriers per metre^3. If wire carries a current 24 mA, then drift velocity of carriers is
(a) $5 \times 10^{-2}\ ms^{-1}$ (b) $0.5\ ms^{-1}$
(c) $5 \times 10^{-3} ms^{-1}$ (d) $5 \times 10^{-6} ms^{-1}$

5. Two wires of the same material but of different diameters carry the same current I. If the ratio of their diameters is 2 : 1, then the corresponding ratio of their mean drift velocities will be
(a) 4 : 1 (b) 1 : 1 (c) 1 : 2 (d) 1 : 4

6. For a wire $\frac{R}{l} = \frac{1}{2}$ and length of wire is $l = 5$ cm.

If potential difference of 1 V is applied across it, then current through wire will be
(a) 40 A (b) 4 A (c) 25 A (d) 2.5 A

7. A current of 10 A is passing through a metallic wire of cross-sectional area $4 \times 10^{-6}\ m^2$. If the density of the aluminium conductor is 2.7 g/cc, considering aluminium gives 1 electron per atom for conduction, then find the drift velocity of the electrons, if molecular weight of aluminium is 27 g.
(a) 1.6×10^{-4} m/s (b) 3.6×10^{-4} m/s
(c) 2.6×10^{-4} m/s (d) 1.5×10^{-4} m/s

8. If resistivity of copper is $1.72 \times 10^{-8}\ \Omega$-m and number of free electrons in copper is $8.5 \times 10^{28}\ /\ m^3$. Find the mobility.
(a) $4.25 \times 10^{-3} m^2 / C\Omega$ (b) $6.8 \times 10^{-3} m^2 / C\Omega$
(c) $8.5 \times 10^{-3} m^2 / C\Omega$ (d) $3.4 \times 10^{-3} m^2 / C\Omega$

9. A current I is flowing through the wire of diameter d having drift velocity of electrons v_d in it. What will be new drift velocity when diameter of wire is made $d/4$?
(a) $4v_d$ (b) $\frac{v_d}{4}$ (c) $16v_d$ (d) $\frac{v_d}{16}$

10. The temperature coefficient of the resistance of a wire is 0.00125 per °C. At 300 K, its resistance is 1 Ω. The resistance of wire will be 2 Ω at
(a) 1154 K (b) 1100 K
(c) 1400 K (d) 1127 K

11. Copper and carbon wires are connected in series and the combined resistor is kept at 0°C. Assuming the combined resistance does not vary with temperature, the ratio of the resistances of carbon and copper wires at 0°C is (temperature coefficients of resistivity of copper and carbon respectively are 4×10^{-3}/°C and -0.5×10^{-3} / °C)
(a) 4 (b) 8 (c) 6 (d) 2

12. When current i is flowing through a conductor, the drift velocity is v. If the value of current through the conductor and its area of cross-section is doubled, then new drift velocity will be
(a) $4v$ (b) $\frac{v}{2}$ (c) $\frac{v}{4}$ (d) v

13. At room temperature, copper has free electron density of $8.4 \times 10^{28}\ m^{-3}$. The electrons's drift velocity in a copper conductor of cross-sectional area of $10^{-6}\ m^2$ and carrying a current of 5.4 A, will be
(a) $4\ ms^{-1}$ (b) $0.4\ ms^{-1}$
(c) $4\ cms^{-1}$ (d) $0.4\ mms^{-1}$

14. A student has 10 resistors of resistance r each. The minimum resistance made by him from given resistors is
(a) $10r$ (b) $\frac{r}{10}$ (c) $\frac{r}{100}$ (d) $\frac{r}{5}$

15. The resistance of a wire is 10 Ω. Its length is increased by 10% by stretching. The new resistance will be

(a) 12 Ω (b) 1.2 Ω (c) 13 Ω (d) 11 Ω

16. Four resistances are connected in a circuit as shown in the given figure. The electric current flowing through 4 Ω and 6 Ω resistance is respectively

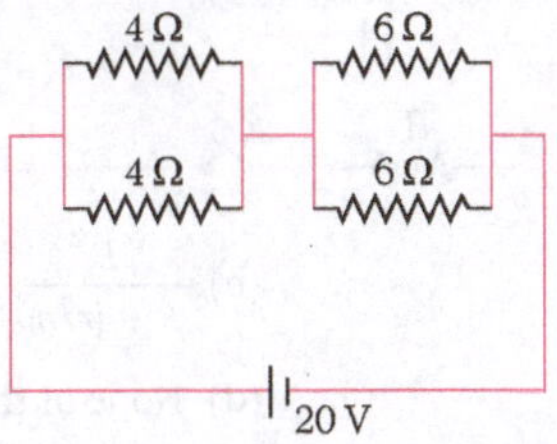

(a) 2 A and 4 A (b) 1 A and 2 A
(c) 1 A and 1 A (d) 2 A and 2 A

17. A piece of wire of resistance 4 Ω is bent through 180° at its mid-point and the two halves are twisted together, then the resistance is

(a) 8 Ω (b) 1 Ω (c) 2 Ω (d) 5 Ω

18. Three resistors each of 2 Ω are connected together in a triangular shape. The resistance between any two vertices will be

(a) 4/3 Ω (b) 3/4 Ω (c) 3 Ω (d) 6 Ω

19. The effective resistance between the points *A* and *B* in the figure is

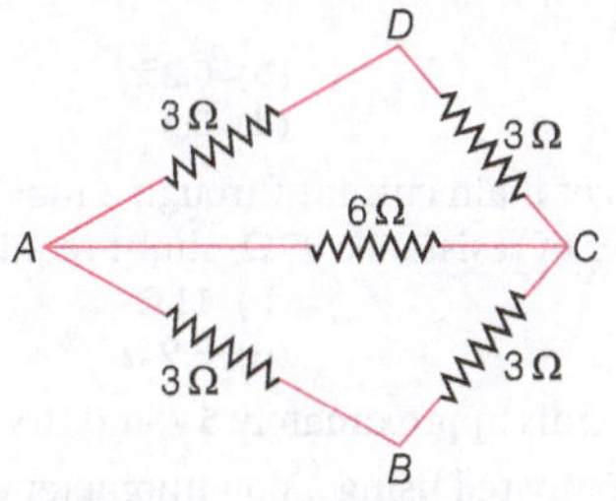

(a) 5 Ω (b) 2 Ω (c) 3 Ω (d) 4 Ω

20. Two resistances are joined in parallel whose resultant is $\frac{6}{8}$ Ω. One of the resistance wire is broken and the effective resistance becomes 2 Ω. Then, the resistance (in ohm) of the wire that got broken was

(a) 3/5 (b) 2 (c) 6/5 (d) 3

21. A wire of resistance 9Ω is broken in two parts. The length ratio being 1 : 2. The two pieces are connected in parallel. The net resistance will be

(a) 2 Ω (b) 3 Ω (c) 4 Ω (d) 6 Ω

22. In the network shown, the equivalent resistance between *A* and *B* is

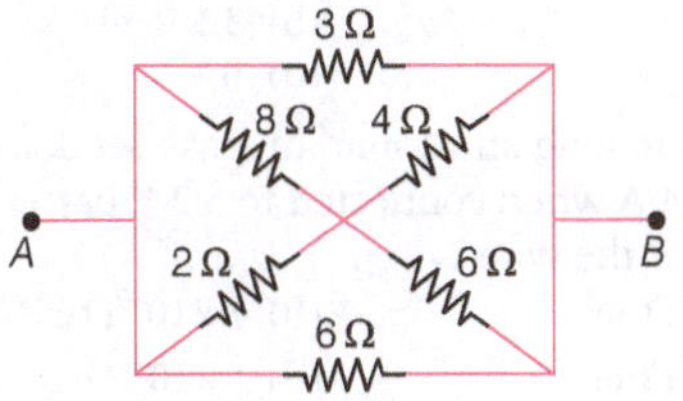

(a) $\frac{4}{3}$ Ω (b) $\frac{3}{4}$ Ω (c) $\frac{24}{17}$ Ω (d) $\frac{17}{24}$ Ω

23. The resistance of a wire at 20°C is 20Ω and at 500°C is 60Ω. At which temperature its resistance will be 25Ω?

(a) 50°C (b) 60°C (c) 70°C (d) 80°C

24. A metal rod of length 10 cm and a rectangular cross-section of 1cm × (1/2) cm is connected to a battery across opposite faces. The resistance will be

(a) maximum when the battery is connected across 1 cm × (1/2) cm faces
(b) maximum when the battery is connected across 10 cm × (1) cm faces
(c) maximum when the battery is connected across 10 cm × (1/2) cm faces
(d) same irrespective of the three faces

25. Out of five resistances of *R* Ω each, 3 are connected in parallel and are joined to the rest 2 in series. Find the resultant resistance.

(a) (3/7)*R*Ω (b) (7/3)*R*Ω
(c) (7/8)*R*Ω (d) (8/7)*R*Ω

26. Two wires of same metal have the same length but their cross-sections are in the ratio 3 : 1. They are joined in series. The resistance of the thicker wire is 10 Ω. The total resistance of the combination will be

(a) 40 Ω (b) $\frac{40}{3}$ Ω (c) $\frac{5}{2}$ Ω (d) 100 Ω

27. Two uniform wires *A* and *B* are of same metal and have equal masses. The radius of wire *A* is twice that of wire *B*. The total resistance of *A* and *B* when connected in parallel is

(a) 4 Ω when the resistance of wire *A* is 4.25 Ω
(b) 5 Ω when the resistance of wire *A* is 4 Ω
(c) 4 Ω when the resistance of wire *B* is 4.25 Ω
(d) 5 Ω when the resistance of wire *B* is 4 Ω

28. The potential drop across the 3 Ω resistor is

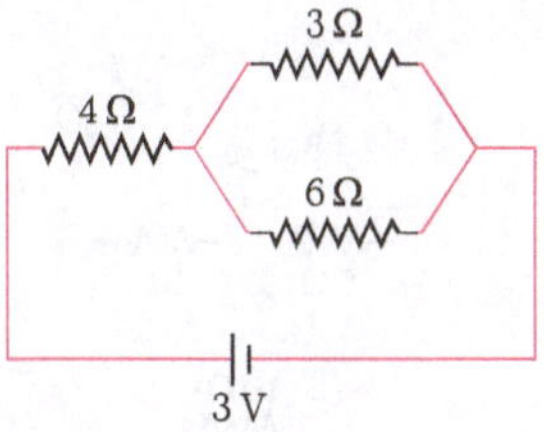

(a) 1 V (b) 1.5 V (c) 2 V (d) 3 V

29. Equivalent resistance between *A* and *B* will be

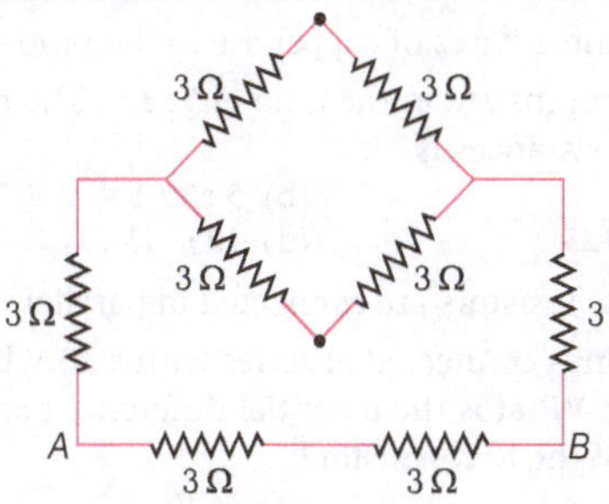

(a) 2 Ω (b) 18 Ω (c) 6 Ω (d) 3.6 Ω

30. In the network of resistors shown in the figure, the equivalent resistance between A and B is

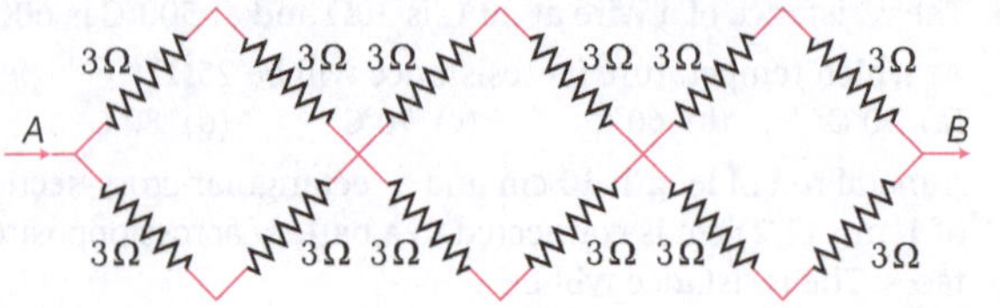

(a) 54Ω (b) 18Ω
(c) 36Ω (d) 9Ω

31. In the figure shown, the total resistance between A and B is

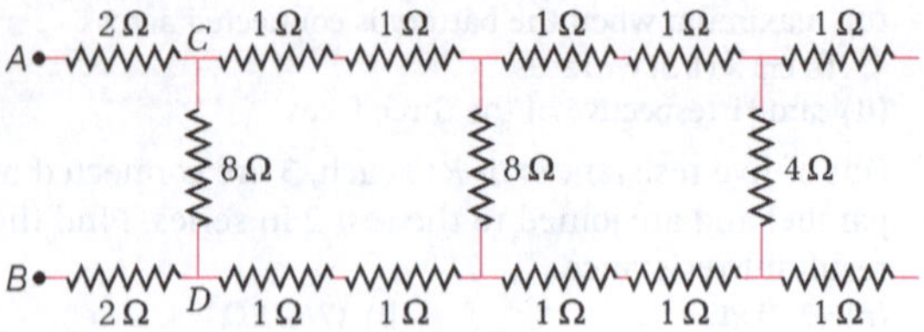

(a) 12Ω (b) 4Ω
(c) 6Ω (d) 8Ω

32. Find the equivalent resistance across AB.

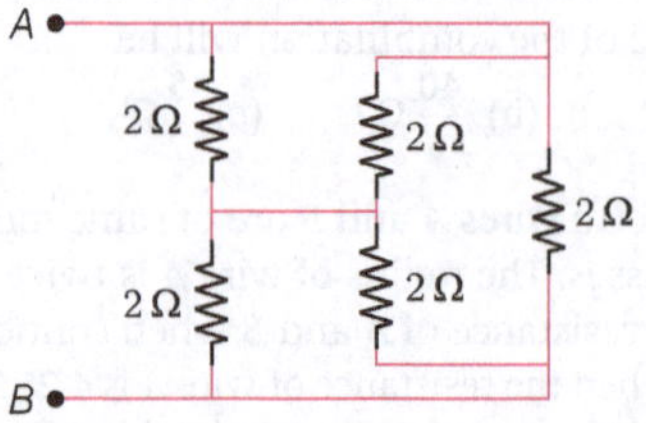

(a) 1Ω (b) 2Ω
(c) 3Ω (d) 4Ω

33. The equivalent resistance between P and Q in the figure is approximately

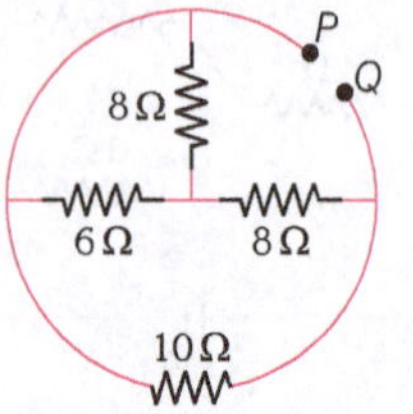

(a) 6Ω (b) 5Ω
(c) 7.5Ω (d) 20Ω

34. Masses of three wires of copper are in the ratio of 1 : 3 : 5 and their lengths are in the ratio of 5 : 3 : 1. The ratio of their electrical resistances is

(a) 1 : 3 : 5 (b) 5 : 3 : 1
(c) 1 : 15 : 125 (d) 125 : 15 : 1

35. 6Ω and 12Ω resistors are connected in parallel. This combination is connected in series with a 10 V battery and 6Ω resistor. What is the potential difference between the terminals of the 12Ω resistor?

(a) 4 V (b) 16 V
(c) 2 (d) 8 V

36. When n cells are joined in parallel combination as shown, the strength of the current I is given by

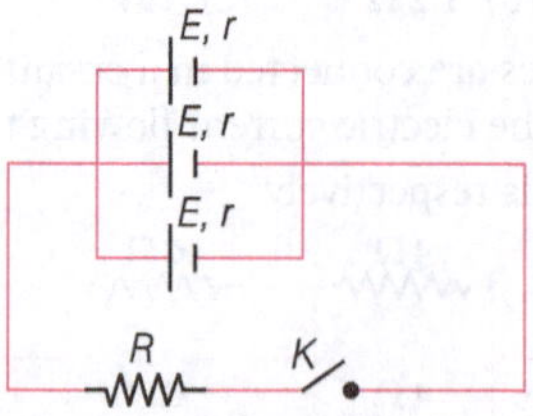

(a) $\frac{nE}{R+nr}$ (b) $\frac{E}{R+(r/n)}$
(c) $\frac{E}{r+Rn}$ (d) None of these

37. An ammeter and a voltmeter of resistance R are connected in series to an electric cell of negligible internal resistance. Their readings are A and V, respectively. If another resistance R is connected in parallel with the voltmeter, then potential across

(a) Both A and V will increase
(b) Both A and V will decrease
(c) A will decrease and V will increase
(d) A will increase and V will decrease

38. A cell which has an emf of 1.5 V is connected in series with an external resistance of 10Ω. If the potential difference across the cell is 1.25 V, then the internal resistance of the cell (in Ω) is

(a) 2 (b) 0.25
(c) 1.5 (d) 0.3

39. To send 10% of main current through a moving coil galvanometer of resistance 99Ω, shunt required is

(a) 9Ω (b) 11Ω
(c) 10Ω (d) 9.9Ω

40. Two cells of emfs approximately 5V and 10V are to be accurately compared using a potentiometer of length 400 cm.

(a) The battery that runs the potentiometer should have voltage of 8V
(b) The battery of potentiometer can have a voltage of 15 V and R adjusted, so that the potential drop across the wire slightly exceeds 10 V
(c) The first portion of 50 cm of wire itself should have a potential drop of 10 V
(d) Potentiometer is usually used for comparing resistances and not voltages

41. A voltmeter of resistance 998 Ω is connected across a cell of emf 2 V and internal resistance 2 Ω. The potential difference across the voltmeter is

(a) 1.99 V (b) 3.5 V
(c) 5 V (d) 6 V

42. A wire 50 cm long and 1 mm^2 in cross-section carries a current of 4 A when connected to a 2 V battery. The resistivity of the wire is

(a) 2×10^{-7}Ω-m (b) 5×10^{-7}Ω-m
(c) 4×10^{-6}Ω-m (d) 1×10^{-6}Ω-m

43. The electron with charge $q = (1.6 \times 10^{-19}$ C) moves in an orbit of radius 5×10^{-11} m with a speed of 2.2×10^6 ms^{-1}, around an atom. The equivalent current is
(a) 1.12×10^{-6} A (b) 1.12×10^{-3} A
(c) 1.12×10^{-9} A (d) 1.12 A

44. The n rows each containing m cells in series are joined in parallel. Maximum current is taken from this combination across an external resistance of 3 Ω. If the total number of cells used are 24 and internal resistance of each cell is 0.5 Ω, then
(a) $m = 8, n = 3$ (b) $m = 6, n = 4$
(c) $m = 12, n = 2$ (d) $m = 2, n = 12$

45. A 100 V voltmeter of internal resistance 20 kΩ in series with a high resistance R is connected to a 110 V line. The voltmeter reads 5 V, the value of R is
(a) 210 kΩ (b) 315 kΩ (c) 420 kΩ (d) 440 kΩ

46. Two batteries A and B each of emf 2V are connected in series to an external resistance $R = 1$ Ω. If the internal resistance of battery A is 1.9 Ω and that of B is 0.9 Ω. What is the potential difference between the terminals of battery A?

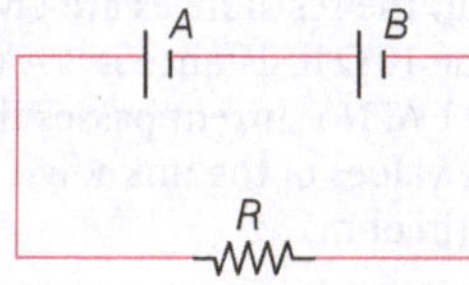

(a) 2 V (b) 3.8 V (c) Zero (d) 4.8 V

47. Two resistors 400Ω and 800Ω are connected in series with a 6 V battery. The potential difference measured by voltmeter of 10kΩ across 400Ω resistor is
(a) 2 V (b) 1.95 V (c) 3.8 V (d) 4 V

48. A battery of emf E has an internal resistance r. A variable resistance R is connected to the terminals of the battery. A current I is drawn from the battery. V is the terminal potential difference. If R alone is gradually reduced to zero, which of the following best describes I and V?
(a) I approaches zero, V approaches E
(b) I approaches $\frac{E}{r}$, V approaches zero
(c) I approaches $\frac{E}{r}$, V approaches E
(d) I approaches infinity, V approaches E

49. A battery of four cells in series, each having an emf of 1.4 V and an internal resistance of 2 Ω is to be used to charge a small 2 V accumulator of negligible internal resistance. What is the charging current?
(a) 0.1 A (b) 0.2 A (c) 0.3 A (d) 0.45 A

50. Consider a current carrying wire (current I) in the shape of a circle. Note that as the current progresses along the wire, the direction of J (current density) changes in an exact manner, while the current I remains unaffected. The agent that is essentially responsible for
(a) source of emf
(b) electric field produced by charges accumulated on the surface of wire
(c) the charges just behind a given segment of wire which push them just the right way by repulsion
(d) the charges ahead

51. Two batteries of emf ε_1 and $\varepsilon_2 (\varepsilon_2 > \varepsilon_1)$ and internal resistances r_1 and r_2 respectively are connected in parallel as shown in figure.

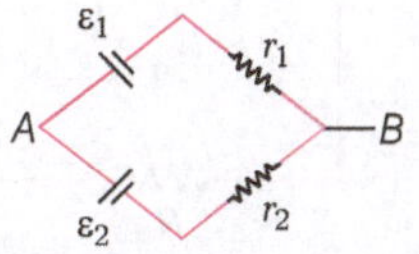

(a) The equivalent emf ε_{eq} of the two cells is between ε_1 and ε_2, *i.e.* $\varepsilon_1 < \varepsilon_{eq} < \varepsilon_2$
(b) The equivalent emf ε_{eq} is smaller than ε_1
(c) The ε_{eq} is given by $\varepsilon_{eq} = \varepsilon_1 + \varepsilon_2$ always
(d) ε_{eq} is independent of internal resistances r_1 and r_2

52. The potential difference (in volt) across the resistance R_3 in the circuit shown in figure, is ($R_1 = 15\Omega, R_2 = 15\Omega, R_3 = 30\Omega, R_4 = 35\Omega$)

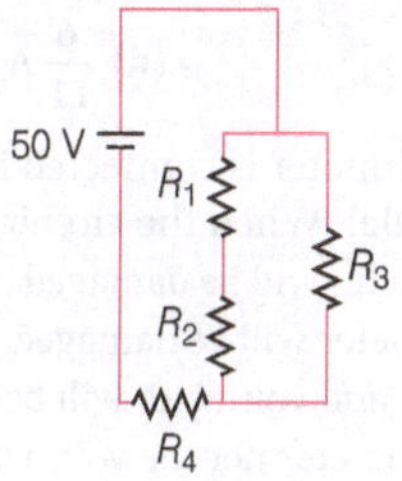

(a) 5 (b) 7.5 (c) 15 (d) 12.5

53. In the given circuit, the voltmeter records 5 V. The resistance of the voltmeter (in Ω) is

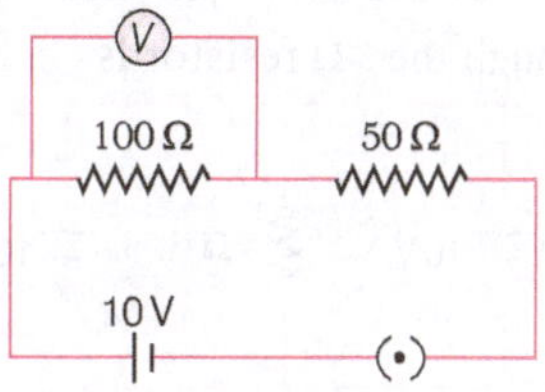

(a) 200 (b) 100 (c) 10 (d) 50

54. A source of emf $E = 15$ V and having negligible internal resistance is connected to a variable resistance, so that the current in the circuit increases with time as $I = 1.2t + 3$. Then, the total charge that will flow in first five second will be
(a) 10 C (b) 20 C
(c) 30 C (d) 40 C

55. The charge flowing in a conductor varies with time as $Q = at - bt^2$, then the current
(a) reaches a maximum and then decreases
(b) falls to zero after $t = \frac{a}{2b}$
(c) changes at a rate of $(-2b)$
(d) Both (b) and (c)

56. Under what conditions, current passing through the resistance R can be increased by short circuiting the battery of emf E_2? The internal resistances of the two batteries are r_1 and r_2, respectively.

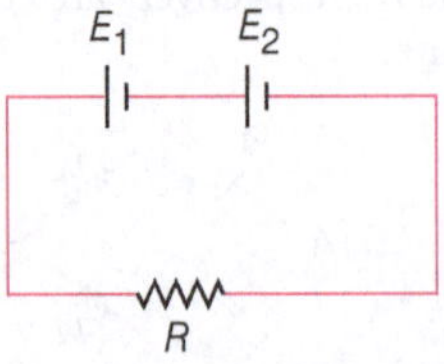

(a) $E_2 r_1 > E_1(R + r_2)$ (b) $E_1 r_2 < E_2(R + r_1)$
(c) $E_2 r_2 < E_1(R + r_2)$ (d) $E_1 r_2 > E_2(R + r_1)$

57. Three conductors draw currents of 1 A, 2 A snd 3 A respectively, when connected in turn across a battery. If they are connected in series and the combination is connected across the same battery, then the current drawn will be
(a) $\frac{2}{7}$ A (b) $\frac{3}{7}$ A
(c) $\frac{4}{7}$ A (d) $\frac{6}{11}$ A

58. By mistake, a voltmeter is connected in series and an ammeter in parallel. When the circuit is switched ON
(a) Only the ammeter will be damaged
(b) Only the voltmeter will be damaged
(c) Both ammeter and voltmeter will be damaged
(d) Neither the ammeter nor the voltmeter will be damaged

59. A wire has resistance 12 Ω. It is bent in the form of a circle. The effective resistance between the two points on any diameter is equal to
(a) 12 Ω (b) 6 Ω (c) 3 Ω (d) 24 Ω

60. Current through the 5 Ω resistor is

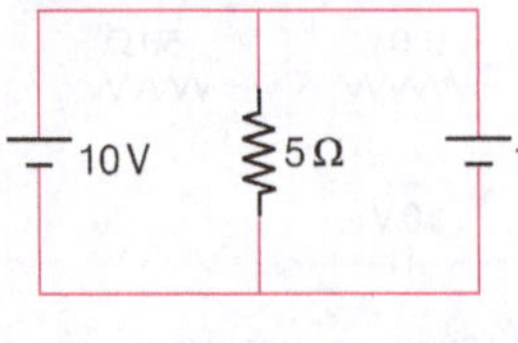

(a) 2A (b) 4A (c) zero (d) 1A

61. Three resistances P, Q, R each of 2Ω and an unknown resistance S form the four arms of a Wheatstone's bridge circuit. When a resistance of 6Ω is connected in parallel to S, the bridge gets balanced. What is the value of S?
(a) 2Ω (b) 3Ω
(c) 6Ω (d) 1Ω

62. Equivalent resistance between the points A and B is (in Ω)

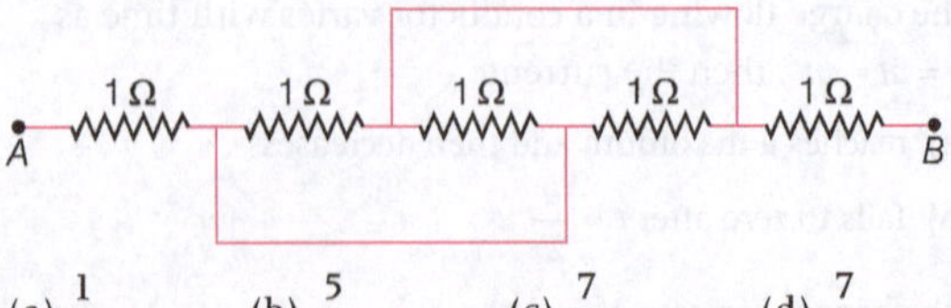

(a) $\frac{1}{5}$ (b) $\frac{5}{4}$ (c) $\frac{7}{3}$ (d) $\frac{7}{2}$

63. In the circuit shown here, what is the value of the unknown resistance R, so that the total resistance of the circuit between points P and Q is also equal to R?

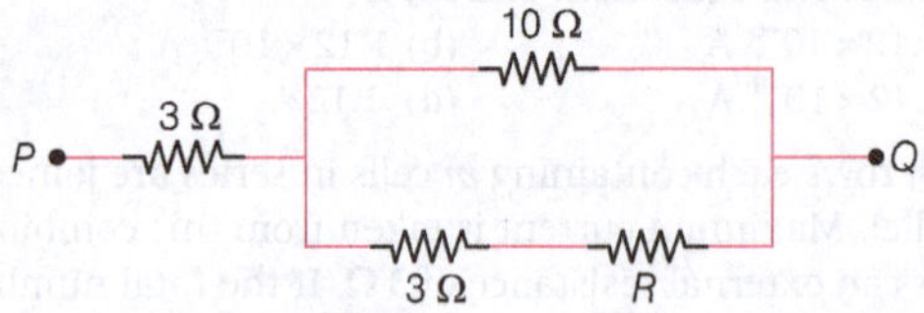

(a) 3Ω (b) $\sqrt{39}$Ω (c) $\sqrt{69}$Ω (d) 10Ω

64. The reading of the ammeter in the following figure will be

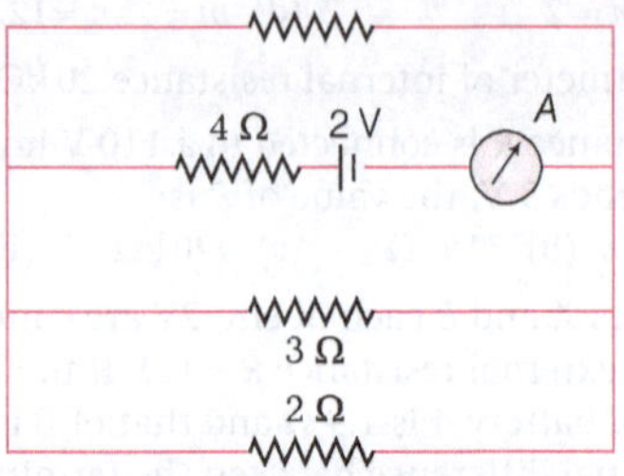

(a) 0.8 A (b) 0.6 A (c) 0.4 A (d) 0.2 A

65. In the given circuit, the resistances are given in ohm. The current through the 10 Ω resistance is 3 A while that through the resistance X is 1 A. No current passes through the galvanometer. The values of the unknown resistances X and Y are respectively (in ohm)

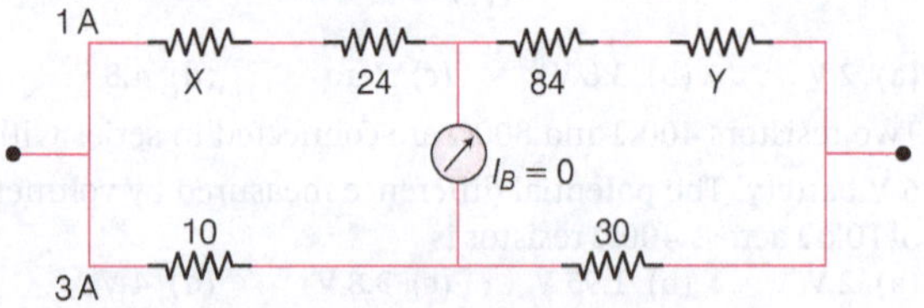

(a) 14 and 54 (b) 12 and 6 (c) 6 and 12 (d) 6 and 6

66. The current I drawn from the 5 V source will be

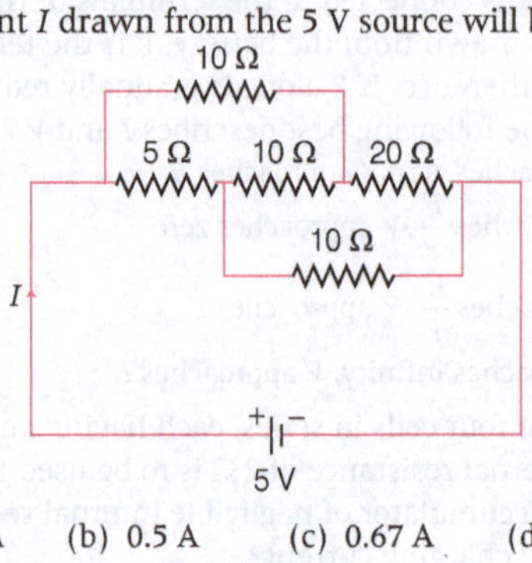

(a) 0.33 A (b) 0.5 A (c) 0.67 A (d) 0.17 A

67. The current in the given circuit is

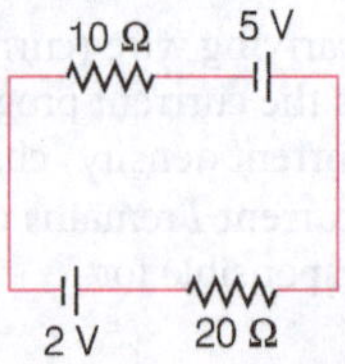

(a) 0.3 A (b) 0.4 A (c) 0.1 A (d) 0.2 A

68. Two resistances are connected in two gaps of a meter bridge. The balance point is 20 cm from the zero end. A resistance of 15 Ω is connected in series with the smaller of the two. The null point shifts to 40 cm. The value of the smaller resistance (in ohm) is
(a) 3 (b) 6 (c) 9 (d) 12

69. Two bulbs consume same power when operated at 200 V and 300 V, respectively. When these bulbs are connected in series across a DC source of 500 V, then
(a) ratio of potential differences across them is 3/2
(b) ratio of potential differences across them is 9/4
(c) ratio of powers consumed across them is 4/9
(d) ratio of powers consumed across them is 2/3

70. A factory is served by a 220 V supply line. In a circuit protected by a fuse marked 10 A, the maximum number of 100 W lamps in parallel that can be turned on, is
(a) 11 (b) 22 (c) 33 (d) 66

71. A tap supplies water at 22°C, a man takes 1 L of water per min at 37°C from the geyser. The power of geyser is
(a) 525 W (b) 1050 W (c) 1775 W (d) 2100 W

72. The mean free path of electrons in a metal is 4×10^{-8} m. The electric field which can give an average 2 eV energy to an electron in the metal will be in unit of Vm^{-1}?
(a) 8×10^{7} (b) 5×10^{-11} (c) 8×10^{-11} (d) 5×10^{7}

73. You are given two resistances R_1 and R_2. By using them singly, in series and in parallel, you can obtain four resistances of 1.5Ω, 2Ω, 6Ω and 8Ω. The values of R_1 and R_2 are
(a) 1Ω, 7Ω (b) 1.5Ω, 6.5Ω
(c) 3Ω, 5Ω (d) 2Ω, 6Ω

74. The tungsten filaments of two electric bulbs are of the same length. If one of them gives 25 W power and the other 60 W power, then
(a) Both the filaments are of same thickness
(b) 25 W bulb has thicker filament
(c) 60 W bulb has thicker filament
(d) Both the filaments have same cross-sectional area

75. Three unequal resistors in parallel are equivalent to a resistance 1 Ω. If two of them are in the ratio 1 : 2 and if no resistance value is fractional, then the largest of the three resistances (in ohm) is
(a) 4 (b) 6 (c) 8 (d) 12

76. In the circuit given here, the points A, B and C are at 70 V, zero, 10 V, respectively. Then,

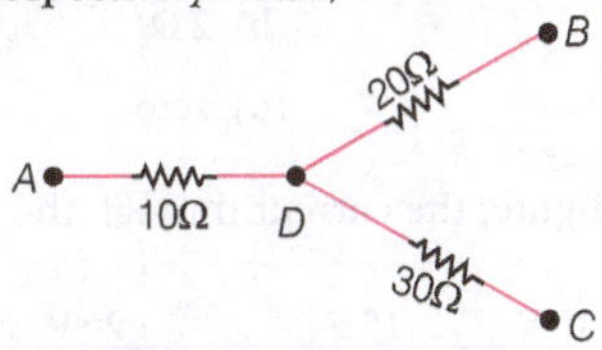

(a) the point D will be at a potential of 60 V
(b) the point D will be at a potential of 20 V
(c) currents in the paths AD, DB and DC are in the ratio of 1 : 2 : 3
(d) currents in the paths AD, DB and DC are in the ratio of 3 : 2 : 1

77. The current in the resistance R will be zero, if

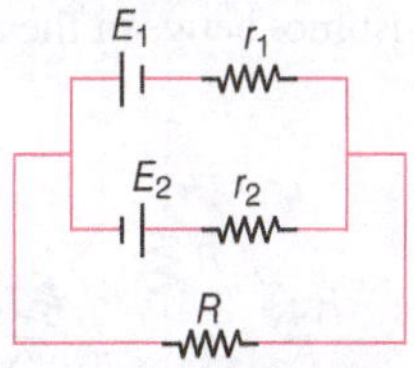

(a) $E_1 r_1 = E_2 r_2$ (b) $\frac{E_1}{r_1} = \frac{E_2}{r_2}$
(c) $(E_1 + E_2) r_1 = E_1 r_2$ (d) $(E_1 - E_2) r_1 = E_2 r_1$

78. The magnitude and direction of the current in the circuit shown will be

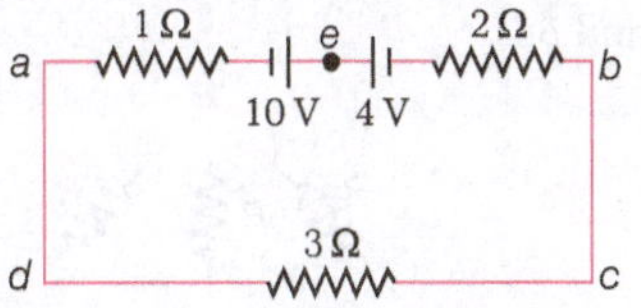

(a) $\frac{7}{3}$ A from a to e (b) $\frac{7}{3}$ A from b to e
(c) 1A from b to e (d) 1A from a to e

79. A resistance R is to be measured using a meter bridge, student chooses the standard resistance S to be 100 Ω. He finds the null point at $l_1 = 2.9$ cm. He is told to attempt to improve the accuracy.
Which of the following is a useful way?
(a) He should measure l_1 more accurately
(b) He should change S to 1000 Ω and repeat the experiment
(c) He should change S to 3 Ω and repeat the experiment
(d) He should given up hope of a more accurate measurement with a meter bridge

80. The current drawn from the battery shown in the figure is

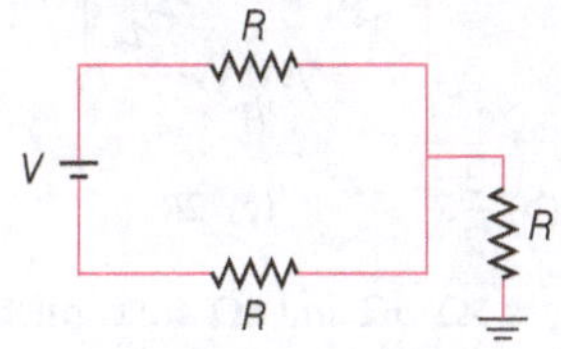

(a) $\frac{V}{R}$ (b) $\frac{V}{2R}$
(c) $\frac{2V}{R}$ (d) $\frac{3V}{2R}$

81. In the circuit shown below, the readings of the ammeter and voltmeter are

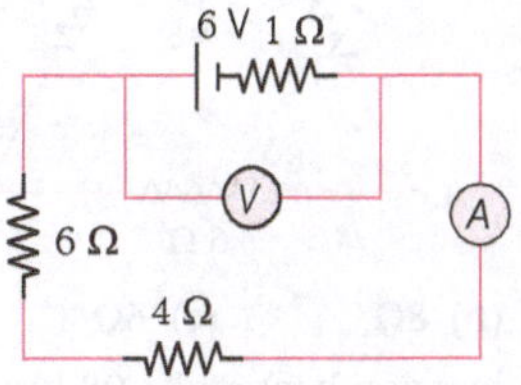

(a) 6 A, 60 V
(b) 0.6 A, 6 V
(c) 6 A, 6 V
(d) (6/11) A, $\frac{60}{11}$ V

82. Each of the resistance in the network shown in the figure is equal to R. The resistance between the terminals A and B is

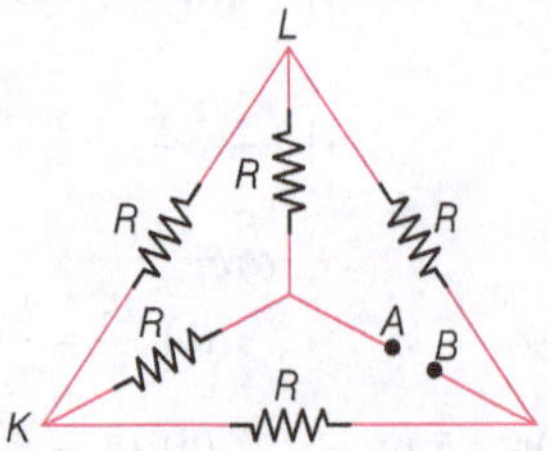

(a) R (b) $5R$ (c) $3R$ (d) $6R$

83. In the given network of resistances, the effective resistance between A and B is

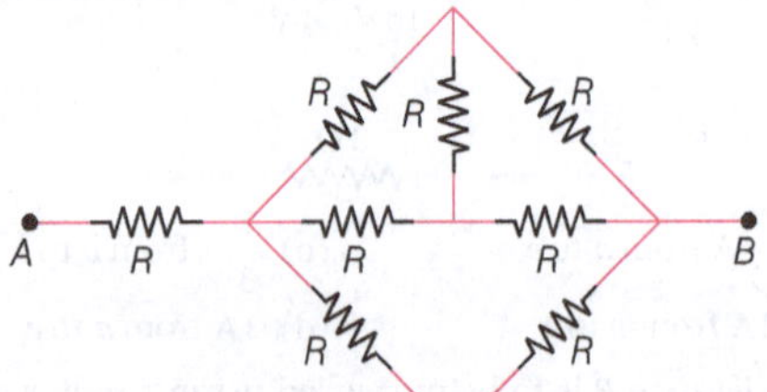

(a) $\frac{5}{3}R$ (b) $\frac{8}{3}R$ (c) $5R$ (d) $8R$

84. The effective resistance between points A and C for the network shown in figure is

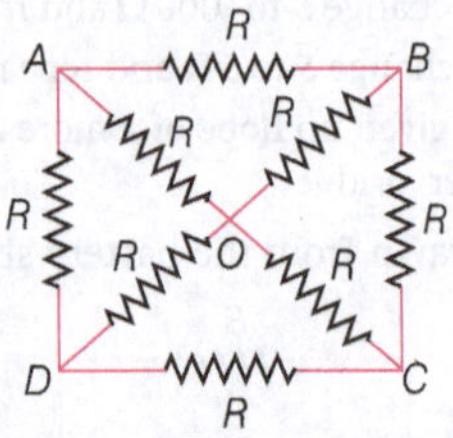

(a) $\frac{2}{3}R$ (b) $\frac{3}{2}R$ (c) $2R$ (d) $\frac{1}{2R}$

85. Three resistances 5Ω, 5Ω and 6Ω are connected as shown in figure. If the point S divides the resistance 6Ω into two equal halves, the resistance between points P and S is

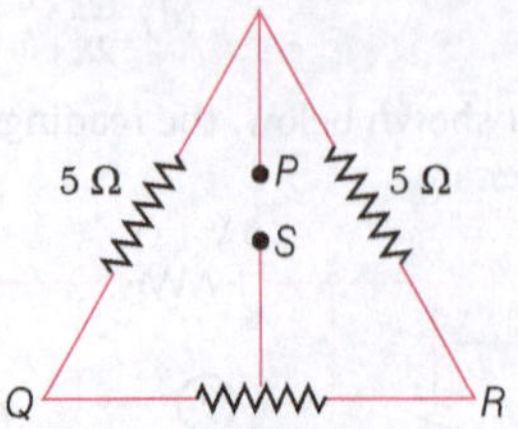

(a) 11Ω (b) 8Ω (c) 6Ω (d) 4Ω

86. An electric immersion heater of 1.08 kW is immersed in water. After the water has reached a temperature of 100°C, how much time will be required to produce 100 g of steam?

(a) 50 s (b) 420 s
(c) 105 s (d) 210 s

87. B_1, B_2 and B_3 are the three identical bulbs connected to a battery of steady emf with key K closed. What happens to the brightness of the bulbs B_1 and B_2 when the key is opened?

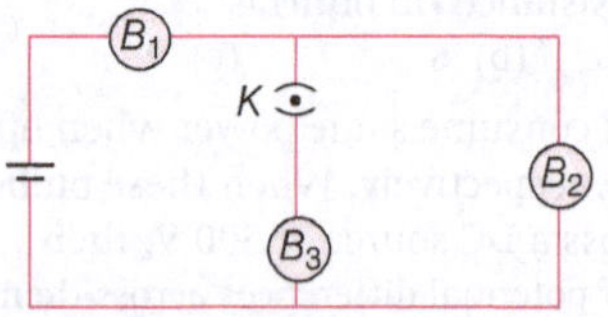

(a) Brightness of the bulb B_1 increases and that of B_2 decreases
(b) Brightness of the bulbs B_1 and B_2 increases
(c) Brightness of the bulb B_1 decreases and B_2 increases
(d) Brightness of the bulbs B_1 and B_2 decreases

88. Three electric bulbs of 200 W, 200 W and 400 W are connected as shown in figure. The resultant power of the combination is

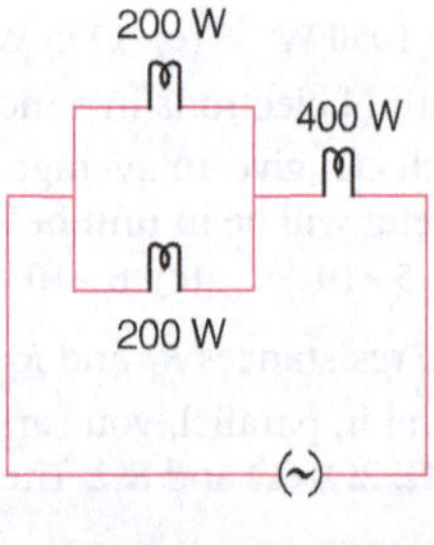

(a) 800 W (b) 400 W (c) 200 W (d) 600 W

89. Two electric bulbs rated 50 W and 100 V are glowing at full power, when used in parallel with a battery of emf 120 V and internal resistance 10Ω. The maximum number of bulbs that can be connected in the circuit when glowing at full power, is

(a) 6 (b) 4 (c) 2 (d) 8

90. The equivalent resistance between points A and B of an infinite network of resistances, each of 1 Ω, connected as shown, is

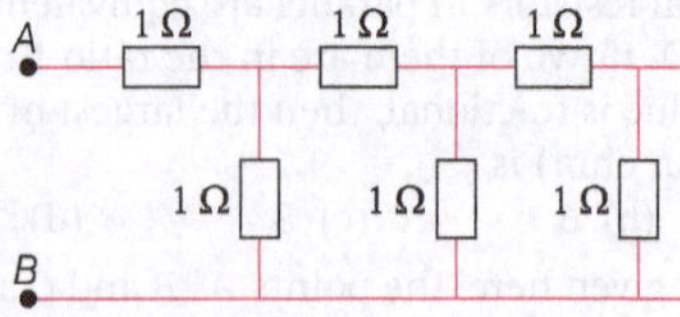

(a) infinite (b) 2Ω
(c) $\frac{1+\sqrt{5}}{2}$ Ω (d) zero

91. In the given figure, the current through the 20 V battery is

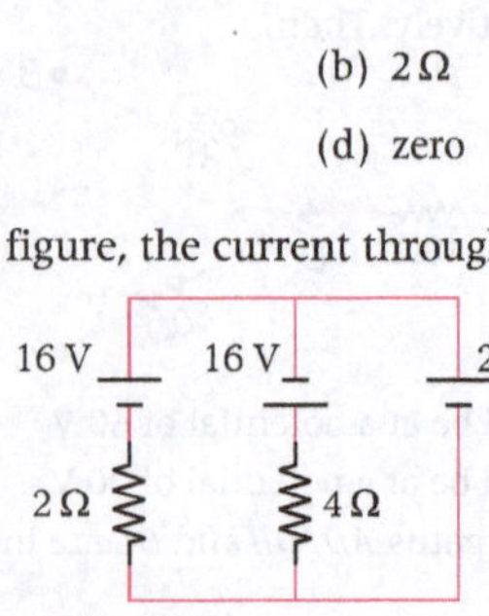

(a) 11 A (b) 12 A (c) 7 A (d) 14 A

92. The current in resistance R_3 in the given circuit is

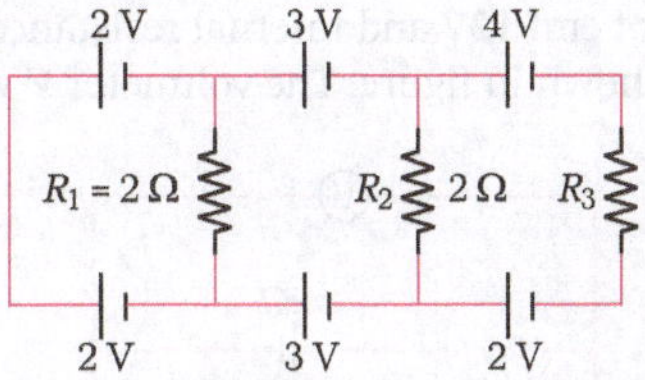

(a) 1 A (b) 2/3 A (c) 0.25 A (d) 0.50 A

93. In the circuit shown in figure, the resistance R has a value that depends on the current. Specifically R is 20Ω when I is zero and the amount of increase in resistance is numerically equal to one-half of the current.

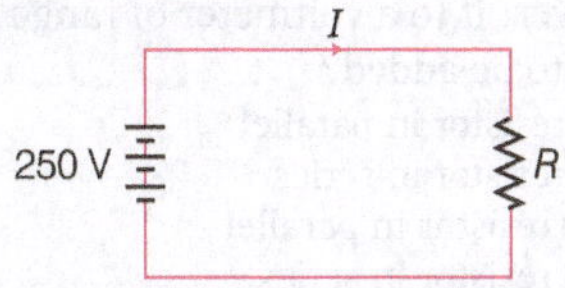

What is the value of current I in circuit?

(a) 15 A (b) 10 A (c) 20 A (d) 5 A

94. In the circuit shown in figure, ammeter and voltmeter are ideal. If $E = 4$ V, $R = 9\,\Omega$ and $r = 1\,\Omega$, then readings of ammeter and voltmeter are

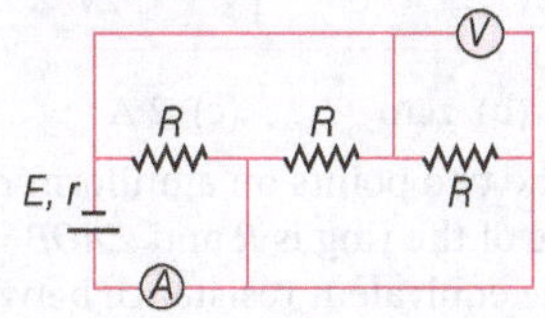

(a) 1 A, 3 V (b) 2 A, 3 V (c) 3 A, 4 V (d) 4 A, 4 V

95. In the circuit shown, the current in 3 Ω resistance is

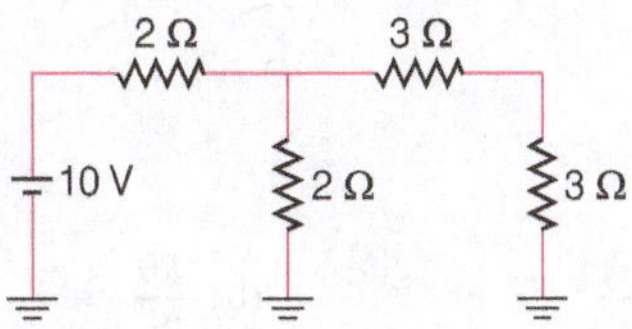

(a) 1 A (b) $\frac{1}{7}$ A (c) $\frac{5}{7}$ A (d) $\frac{15}{7}$ A

96. In the arrangement shown, the magnitude of each resistance is 1 Ω. The equivalent resistance between O and A is given by

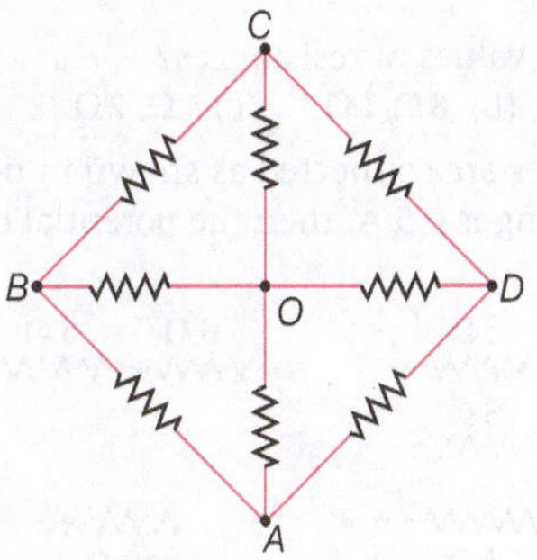

(a) $\frac{14}{13}\,\Omega$ (b) $\frac{3}{4}\,\Omega$ (c) $\frac{2}{3}\,\Omega$ (d) $\frac{5}{6}\,\Omega$

97. Find the reading of the ideal ammeter connected in the given circuit. Assume that the cells have negligible internal resistance.

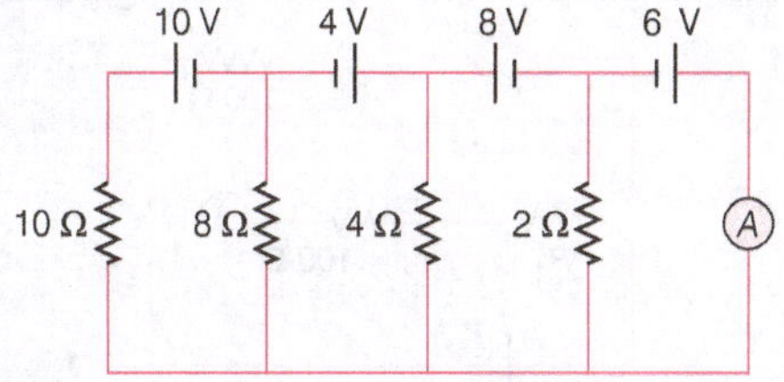

(a) 0.8 A (b) 0.25 A
(c) 1.95 A (d) 1.0 A

98. It takes 16 min to boil some water in an electric kettle. Due to some defect, it becomes necessary to remove 10% turns of heating coil of the kettle. After repairs, how much time will it take to boil the same mass of water?

(a) 17.7 min (b) 14.4 min
(c) 20.9 min (d) 13.9 min

99. Equivalent resistance between points A and B is

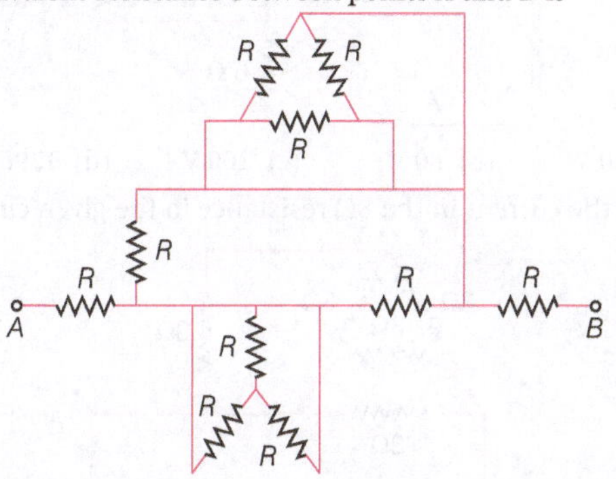

(a) $3R$ (b) $4R$ (c) $\frac{5R}{2}$ (d) $\frac{7R}{2}$

100. All resistances shown in circuit are 2 Ω each. The current in the resistance between D and E is

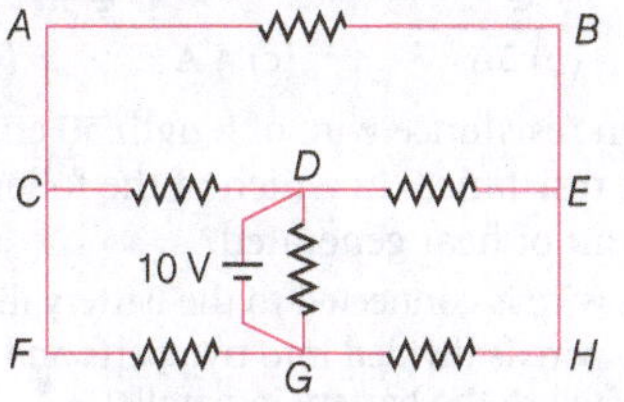

(a) 5 A (b) 2.5 A (c) 1 A (d) 7.5 A

101. A battery of emf 10 V is connected to a group of resistances as shown in figure. The potential difference $V_A - V_B$ between the points A and B is

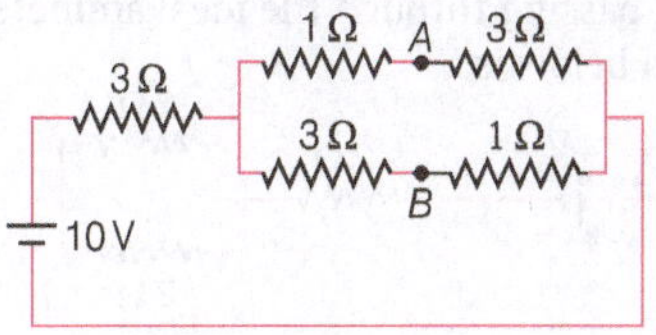

(a) −2 V (b) 2 V (c) 5 V (d) $\frac{20}{11}$ V

102. In the circuit shown, when key K_1 is closed, then the ammeter reads I_0 whether K_2 is open or closed. But when K_1 is open the ammeter reads $I_0/2$, when K_2 is closed.

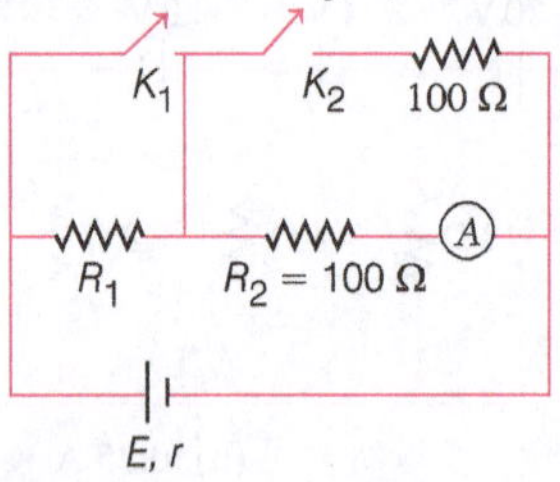

Assuming that, ammeter resistance is much less than R_2, the values of r and R_1 (in ohms) are

(a) 100, 50 (b) 50, 100 (c) 0, 100 (d) 0, 50

103. In the circuit shown in figure, V must be

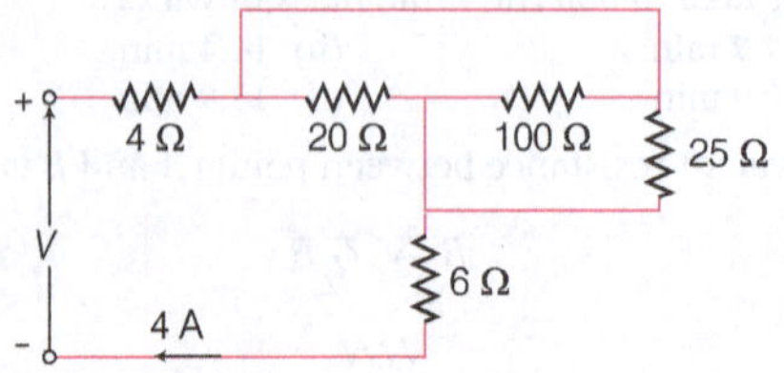

(a) 50 V (b) 80 V (c) 100 V (d) 1290 V

104. Find the current in the 8Ω resistance in the given circuit.

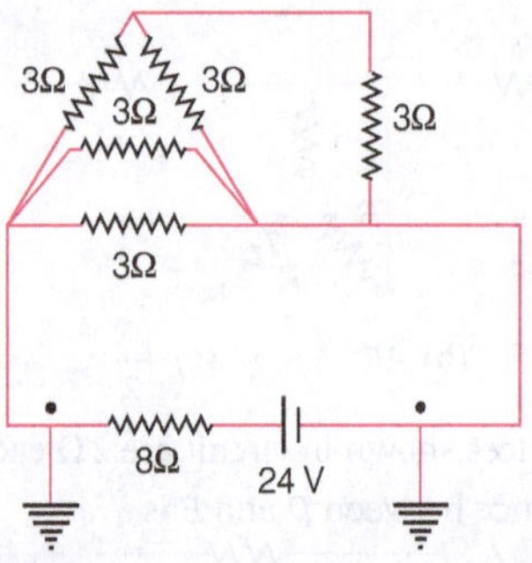

(a) 2 A (b) 3A (c) 4 A (d) 5 A

105. You are given resistance wire of length 50 cm and a battery of negligible resistance. In which of the following cases is largest amount of heat generated?

(a) When the wire is connected to the battery directly.
(b) When the wire is divided into two parts and both the parts are connected to the battery in parallel.
(c) When the wire is divided into four parts and all the four parts are connected to the battery in parallel.
(d) When only half of the wire is connected to the battery.

106. The current passing through the ideal ammeter in the circuit given below is

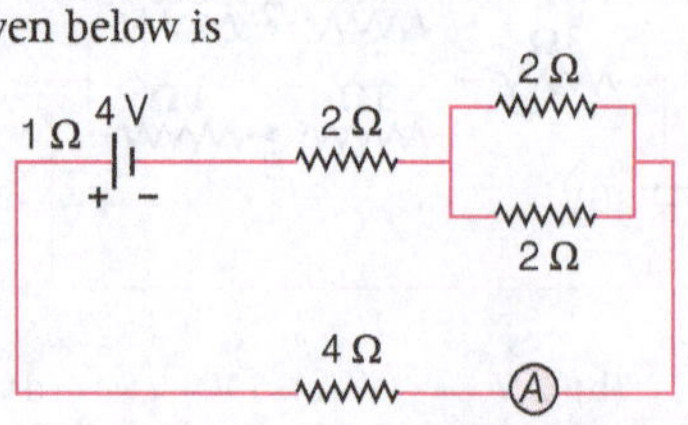

(a) 1.25A (b) 1A (c) 0.75A (d) 0.5 A

107. Two batteries, one of emf 18V and internal resistance 2Ω and the other of emf 12V and internal resistance 1Ω are connected as shown in figure. The voltmeter V will record a reading of

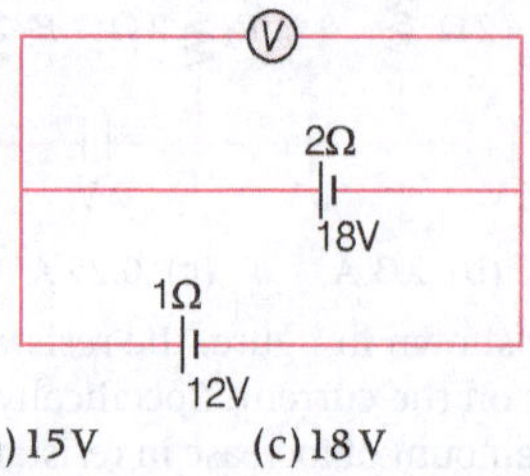

(a) 14 V (b) 15 V (c) 18 V (d) 30 V

108. The range of voltmeter is 10 V and its internal resistance is 50 Ω. To convert it to a voltmeter of range 15 V, how much resistance is to be added?

(a) Add 25Ω resistor in parallel
(b) Add 25Ω resistor in series
(c) Add 125Ω resistor in parallel
(d) Add 125Ω resistor in series

109. The current I shown in the circuit is

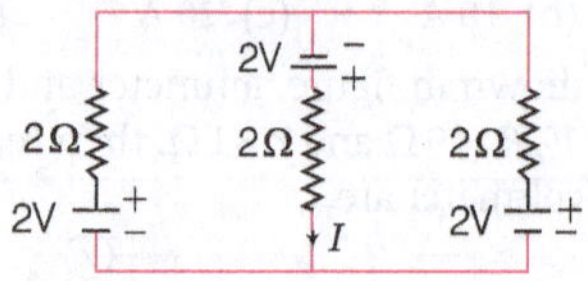

(a) 1.33 A (b) zero (c) 2 A (d) 1 A

110. A and B are the two points on a uniform ring of radius r. The resistance of the ring is R and $\angle AOB = \theta$ as shown in the figure. The equivalent resistance between points A and B is

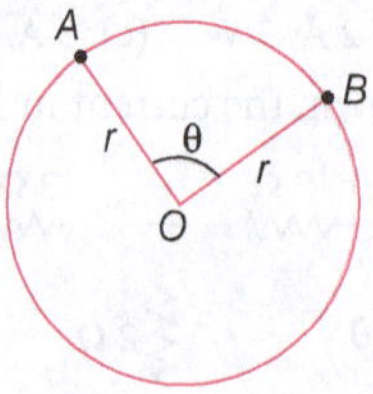

(a) $\frac{R(2\pi - \theta)}{4\pi}$ (b) $\frac{R\theta}{2\pi}$

(c) $R\left(1 - \frac{\theta}{2\pi}\right)$ (d) $\frac{R}{4\pi^2}(2\pi - \theta)\theta$

111. The equivalent resistance of two resistors connected in series is 6 Ω and their parallel equivalent resistance is $\frac{4}{3}$ Ω.

What are the values of resistances?

(a) 4 Ω, 6 Ω (b) 8 Ω, 1 Ω (c) 4 Ω, 2 Ω (d) 6 Ω, 2 Ω

112. Six resistances are connected as shown in figure. If total current flowing is 0.5 A, then the potential difference $V_A - V_B$ is

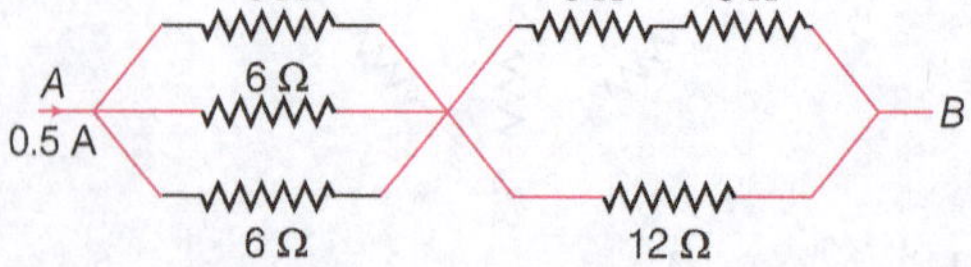

(a) 8 V (b) 6 V (c) 2 V (d) 4 V

113. A circuit consists of three batteries of emf $E_1 = 1$ V, $E_2 = 2$ V and $E_3 = 3$ V and internal resistance $1\,\Omega$, $2\,\Omega$ and $1\,\Omega$ respectively which are connected in parallel as shown in figure. The potential difference between points P and Q is

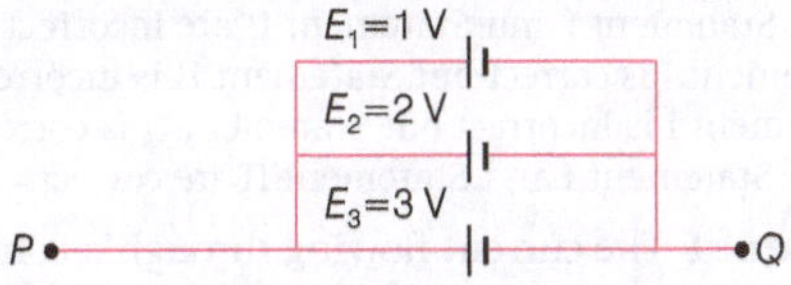

(a) 1.0 V (b) 2.0 V
(c) 2.2 V (d) 3.0 V

114. In Wheatstone bridge, three resistors P, Q and R are connected in three arms in order and 4th arm of resistance S, is formed by two resistors S_1 and S_2 connected in parallel. The condition for bridge to be balanced is, $\frac{P}{Q}$

(a) $\frac{R(S_1 + S_2)}{S_1 S_2}$ (b) $\frac{S_1 S_2}{R(S_1 + S_2)}$
(c) $\frac{R S_1 S_2}{(S_1 + S_2)}$ (d) $\frac{(S_1 + S_2)}{R S_1 S_2}$

115. A galvanometer has a coil of resistance $100\,\Omega$ and gives full scale deflection for 30 mA current. If it is to work as a voltmeter of 30 V, the resistance required to be added is
(a) $500\,\Omega$ (b) $900\,\Omega$
(c) $1000\,\Omega$ (d) $1800\,\Omega$

116. The emf of a cell E is 15 V as shown in the figure with an internal resistance of $0.5\,\Omega$. Then, the value of the current drawn from the cell is

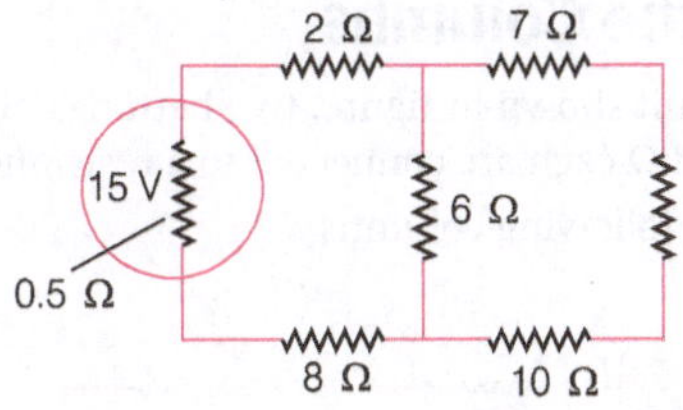

(a) 3 A (b) 2 A
(c) 5 A (d) 1 A

117. The variation between V-I has shown by graph for heating filament

(a) 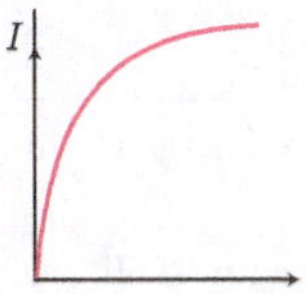

(b) 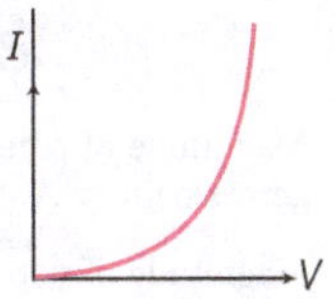

(c) 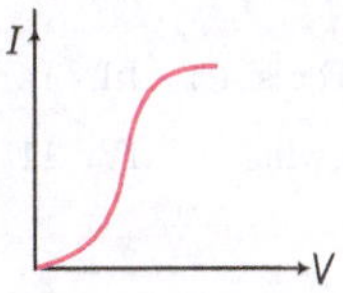

(d) 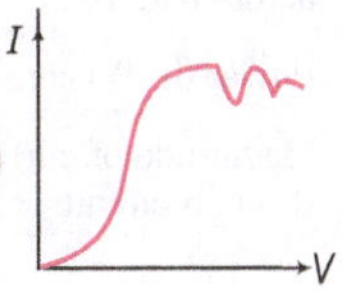

118. In the Wheatstone network given, $P = 10\,\Omega$, $Q = 20\,\Omega$, $R = 15\,\Omega$, $S = 30\,\Omega$, the current passing through the battery (of negligible internal resistance) is

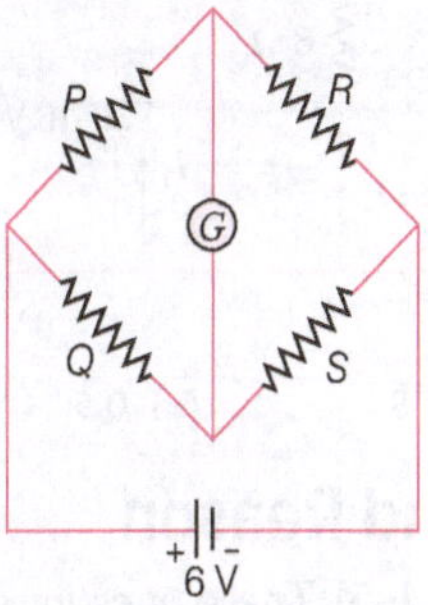

(a) 0.36 A (b) zero (c) 0.18 A (d) 0.72 A

119. Each resistance shown in figure is $2\,\Omega$. The equivalent resistance between A and B is

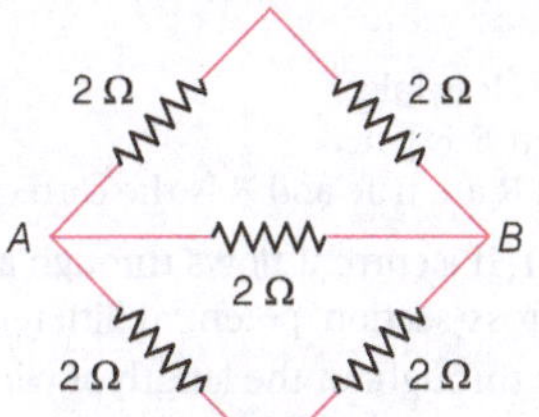

(a) $2\,\Omega$ (b) $1\,\Omega$ (c) $4\,\Omega$ (d) $5\,\Omega$

120. If a current of 2 A flows through resistances connected as shown in figure, the potential difference $V_A - V_B$ is

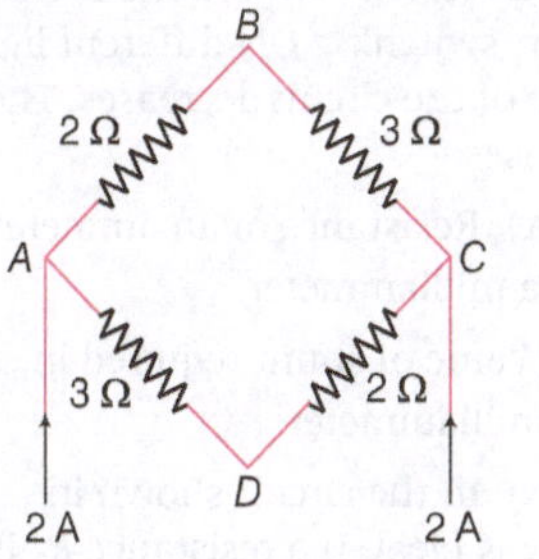

(a) –1 V (b) +1 V
(c) –2V (d) + 2V

121. Current through wire XY of circuit shown is

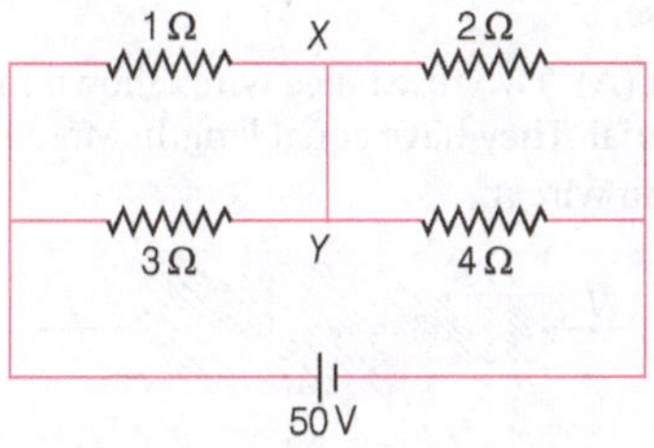

(a) 1 A (b) 4 A (c) 2 A (d) 3 A

122. In the circuit shown in figure, the ratio of currents I_1/I_2 is

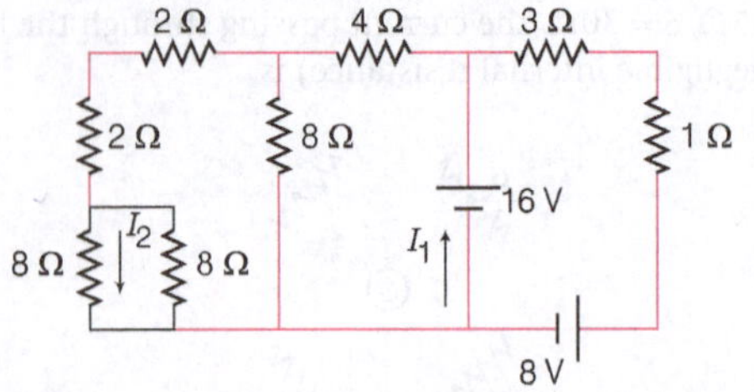

(a) 2 (b) 8 (c) 0.5 (d) 4

Assertion and Reason

Directions (Q. Nos. 1-5) *These questions consist of two statements each linked as Assertion and Reason. While answering these questions you are required to choose any one of the following four responses.*

(a) Both A and R are true but R is not the correct explanation of A.
(b) A is true but R is false.
(c) A is false but R is true.
(d) Both A and R are true and R is the correct explanation of A.

1. Assertion (A) If a current flows through a wire of non-uniform cross-section, potential difference per unit length of wire is same throughout the length of wire.

Reason (R) Current through the wire is same at all cross-sections.

2. Assertion (A) In our houses, when we start switching ON different light buttons, main current goes on increasing.

Reason (R) Different connections in houses are in parallel. When we start switching ON different light buttons, then net resistance of the circuit decreases. Therefore, main current increases.

3. Assertion (A) Resistance of an ammeter is less than the resistance of a milliammeter.

Reason (R) Value of shunt required in case of ammeter is more than a milliammeter.

4. Assertion (A) In the circuit shown in figure, battery is ideal. If a resistance R_0 is connected in parallel with R, then power across R will increase.

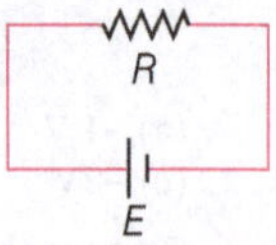

Reason (R) Current drawn from the battery will increase.

5. Assertion (A) Two resistance wires shown in figure are of same material. They have equal length. More heat is generated in wire A.

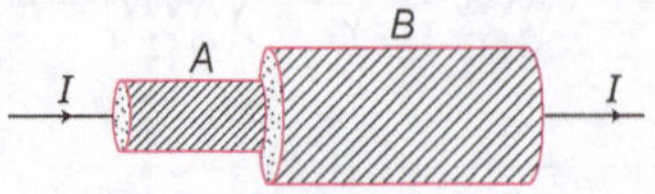

Reason (R) In series, $H \propto R$ and resistance of wire A is more.

Statement Type Questions

Directions (Q. Nos. 1-5) *These questions consist of two statements, choose the most appropriate answer from the options given below*

(a) Both Statement I and Statement II are incorrect.
(b) Statement I is correct but Statement II is incorrect.
(c) Statement I is incorrect but Statement II is correct.
(d) Both Statement I and Statement II are correct.

1. Statement I The current flowing through a conductor is directly proportional to the drift velocity.

Statement II As the drift velocity increases the current flowing through the conductor decreases.

2. Statement I It is advantageous to transmit electric power at high voltage.

Statement II High voltage implies high current.

3. Statement I Internal resistance of a cell decreases with increase the temperature of electrolyte.

Statement II Direction of the current is opposite to flow of electrons.

4. Statement I Bulb generally get fused when they switched ON or OFF.

Statement II When we switch On or OFF a circuit, current changes in it rapidly.

5. Statement I In a simple battery circuit, the point of the lowest potential is positive terminal of the battery.

Statement II The current flow towards the point of the higher potential, as it does in such a circuit from the negative to the positive terminal.

Match the Columns

1. In the circuit shown in figure, two batteries of internal resistance 1 Ω each are connected to a resistance of 3 Ω. Match the following columns.

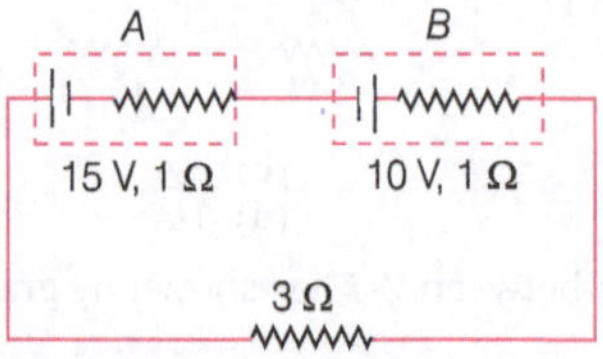

Column I	Column II
A. Magnitude of potential difference (in V) across battery A	I. 3
B. Magnitude of potential difference (in V) across battery B	II. 1
C. Power (in W) consumed by 3 Ω resistor	III. 14
D. Magnitude of current (in A) flowing through circuit	IV. 11

Choose the correct answer from the options given below.
(a) A-III, B-IV, C-I, D-II
(b) A-I, B-II, C-III, D-IV
(c) A-II, B-I, C-IV, D-III
(d) A-IV, B-I, C-II, D-III

2. In the circuit diagram shown in figure, potential difference across 3 Ω resistance is 20 V. Then, match the following two columns and choose the correct option from codes given below.

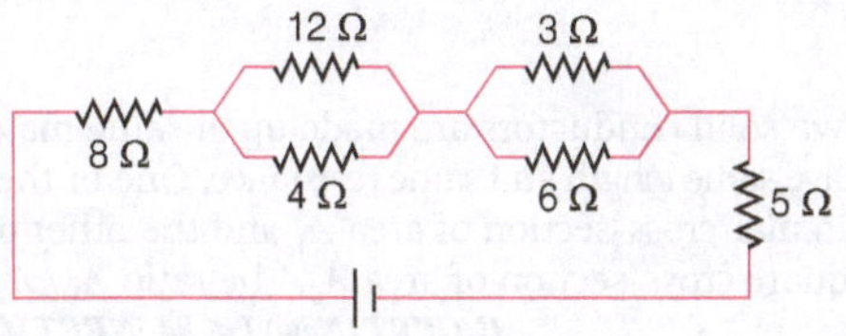

	Column I		Column II
A.	Potential difference across 6 Ω resistance	I.	30 V
B.	Potential difference across 4 Ω resistance	II.	50 V
C.	Potential difference across 5 Ω resistance	III.	20 V
D.	Potential difference across 8 Ω resistance	IV.	80 V

Choose the correct answer from the options given below.
(a) A-IV, B-III, C-II, D-I
(b) A-III, B-I, C-II, D-IV
(c) A-I, B-IV, C-III, D-II
(d) A-II, B-III, C-IV, D-I

3. Four bulbs of powers 25 W, 40 W, 60 W and 100 W are connected in series. Match Column I of watts of bulbs with potential difference across them in Column II.

	Column I		Column II
A.	25 W	I.	Highest potential difference
B.	40 W	II.	Lowest potential difference
C.	60 W	III.	Third highest potential difference
D.	100 W	IV.	Second highest potential difference

Choose the correct answer from the options given below.
(a) A-IV, B-II, C-I, D-III
(b) A-II, B-III, C-IV, D-I
(c) A-I, B-III, C-IV, D-II
(d) A-III, B-IV, C-I, D-II

4. Rated power of a bulb at V voltage is P. Now, same voltage V is applied in all conditions mentioned in Column I. Match this Column I with Column II in which actual total power consumed is given.

	Column I		Column II
A.	Two bulbs are connected in parallel.	I.	P
B.	Two bulbs are connected in series.	II.	$2P$
C.	Two bulbs are connected in parallel and one bulb in series with this combination.	III.	$\frac{P}{2}$
D.	A group of two-two bulbs in parallel are mutually connected in series.	IV.	$\frac{2}{3}P$

Choose the correct answer from the options given below.
(a) A-II, B-IV, C-III, D-I
(b) A-II, B-III, C-IV, D-I
(c) A-I, B-IV, C-II, D-III
(d) A-III, B-II, C-I, D-IV

Final Check Through PYQs

Module-I Electric Current and Ohm's Law

1. The resistance of platinum wire at 0°C is 2 Ω and 6.8 Ω at 80°C. The temperature coefficient of resistance of the wire is ***[NCERT (New) Pg. 90, NEET 2023]***
(a) $3\times10^{-3}\ °C^{-1}$ (b) $3\times10^{-2}\ °C^{-1}$
(c) $3\times10^{-1}\ °C^{-1}$ (d) $3\times10^{-4}\ °C^{-1}$

2. A copper wire of length 10m and radius $(10^{-2}/\sqrt{\pi})$ m has electrical resistance of 10Ω. The current density in the wire for an electric field strength of 10(V/m) is ***[NCERT (New) Pg. 86, NEET 2022]***
(a) 10^4 A/m^2 (b) 10^6 A/m^2
(c) 10^{-5} A/m^2 (d) 10^5 A/m^2

3. As the temperature increases, the electrical resistance ***[NCERT (New) Pg. 90, NEET 2022]***
(a) decreases for both conductors and semiconductors.
(b) increases for conductors but decreases for semiconductors.
(c) decreases for conductors but increases for semiconductors.
(d) increases for both conductors and semiconductors.

4. **Column I** Gives certain physical terms associated with flow of current through a metallic conductor.
Column II Gives some mathematical relations involving electrical quantities. Match Column I and Column II with appropriate relations. ***[NCERT (New) Pg. 86, NEET 2021]***

Column I		Column II
A. Drift velocity	I.	$\dfrac{m}{ne^2\rho}$
B. Electrical resistivity	II.	nev_d
C. Relaxation period	III.	$\dfrac{eE}{m}\tau$
D. Current density	IV.	E/J

Codes

	A	B	C	D
(a)	III	IV	I	II
(b)	III	IV	II	I
(c)	III	I	IV	II
(d)	III	II	IV	I

5. Two solid conductors are made up of same material, have same length and same resistance. One of them has a circular cross-section of area A_1 and the other one has a square cross-section of area A_2. The ratio A_1/A_2 is ***[NCERT (New) Pg. 84, NEET (Oct.) 2020]***
(a) 1.5 (b) 1 (c) 0.8 (d) 2

6. Which of the following graph represents the variation of resistivity (ρ) with temperature (T) for copper? ***[NCERT (New) Pg. 90, NEET (Sep.) 2020]***

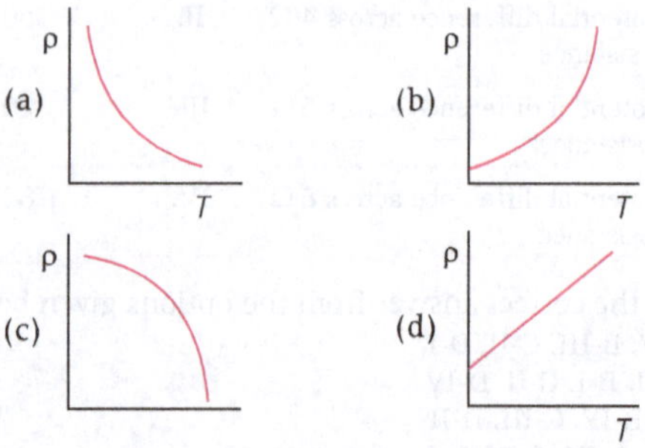

7. A charged particle having drift velocity of $7.5\times10^{-4}\ ms^{-1}$ in an electric field of $3\times10^{-10}\ Vm^{-1}$, has a mobility (in $m^2V^{-1}s^{-1}$) of ***[NCERT (New) Pg. 86, NEET (Sep.) 2020]***
(a) 2.5×10^{6} (b) 2.5×10^{-6}
(c) 2.25×10^{-15} (d) 2.25×10^{15}

8. Which of the following acts as a circuit protection device? ***[NCERT (New) Pg. 90, NEET (National) 2019]***
(a) Inductor (b) Switch
(c) Fuse (d) Conductor

9. In the circuits shown below, the readings of voltmeters and the ammeters will be ***[NCERT (New) Pg. 84, NEET (National) 2019]***

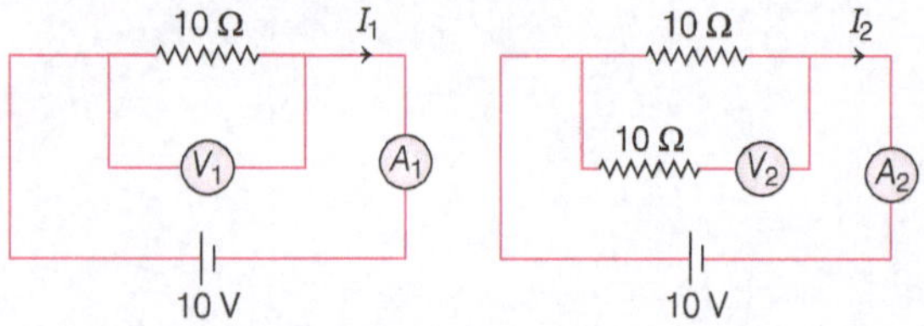

(a) $V_1 = V_2$ and $I_1 > I_2$ (b) $V_1 = V_2$ and $I_1 = I_2$
(c) $V_2 > V_1$ and $I_1 > I_2$ (d) $V_2 > V_1$ and $I_1 = I_2$

10. The resistance of a wire is R ohm. If it is melted and stretched to n times its original length, its new resistance will be *[NCERT (New) Pg. 84, NEET 2017]*

(a) nR (b) $\frac{R}{n}$
(c) n^2R (d) $\frac{R}{n^2}$

11. A, B and C are voltmeters of resistance R, $1.5R$ and $3R$ respectively as shown in the figure. When some potential difference is applied between X and Y, the voltmeter readings are V_A, V_B and V_C respectively. Then, *[NCERT (New) Pg. 98, AIPMT 2015]*

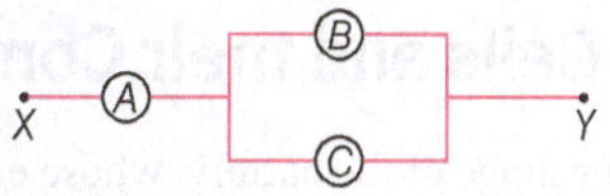

(a) $V_A = V_B = V_C$
(b) $V_A \neq V_B = V_C$
(c) $V_A = V_B \neq V_C$
(d) $V_A \neq V_B \neq V_C$

12. Across a metallic conductor of non-uniform cross-section, a constant potential difference is applied. The quantity which remain constant along the conductor is *[NCERT (New) Pg. 86, AIPMT 2015]*

(a) current density (b) current
(c) drift velocity (d) electric field

Module-II Combination of Resistors

13. A wire of length l and resistance $100\,\Omega$ is divided into 10 equal parts. The first 5 parts are connected in series while the next 5 parts are connected in parallel. The two combinations are again connected in series. The resistance of this final combination is *[NCERT (Old) Pg. 108, NEET 2024]*

(a) $26\,\Omega$ (b) $52\,\Omega$
(c) $55\,\Omega$ (d) $60\,\Omega$

14. 10 resistors, each of resistance R are connected in series to a battery of emf E and negligible internal resistance. Then, those are connected in parallel to the same battery, the current is increased n times. The value of n is *[NCERT (Old) Pg. 108, NEET 2023]*

(a) 100 (b) 1
(c) 1000 (d) 10

15. The effective resistance of a parallel connection that consists of four wires of equal length, equal area of cross-section and same material is $0.25\,\Omega$. What will be the effective resistance, if they are connected in series? *[NCERT (Old) Pg. 108, NEET 2021]*

(a) $0.25\,\Omega$ (b) $0.5\,\Omega$
(c) $1\,\Omega$ (d) $4\,\Omega$

16. Three resistors having resistances r_1, r_2 and r_3 are connected as shown in the given circuit. The ratio i_3/i_1 of currents in terms of resistances used in the circuit is *[NCERT (Old) Pg. 109, NEET 2021]*

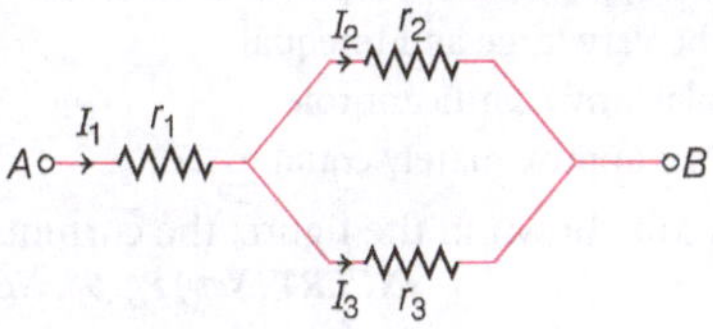

(a) $\frac{r_1}{r_2 + r_3}$ (b) $\frac{r_2}{r_2 + r_3}$
(c) $\frac{r_1}{r_1 + r_2}$ (d) $\frac{r_2}{r_1 + r_3}$

17. The equivalent resistance between A and B for the mesh shown in the figure is *[NCERT (Old) Pg. 109, NEET (Oct.) 2020]*

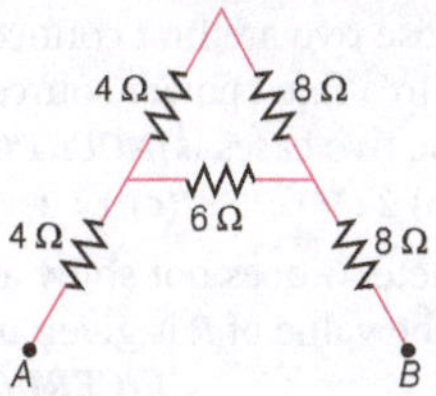

(a) 7.2Ω (b) 16Ω
(c) 30Ω (d) 4.8Ω

18. Two metal wires of identical dimensions are connected in series. If σ_1 and σ_2 are the conductivities of the metal wires respectively, the effective conductivity of the combination is *[NCERT (Old) Pg. 108, AIPMT 2015]*

(a) $\frac{2\sigma_1\sigma_2}{\sigma_1 + \sigma_2}$ (b) $\frac{\sigma_1 + \sigma_2}{2\sigma_1\sigma_2}$
(c) $\frac{\sigma_1 + \sigma_2}{\sigma_1\sigma_2}$ (d) $\frac{\sigma_1\sigma_2}{\sigma_1 + \sigma_2}$

19. A circuit contains an ammeter, a battery of 30 V and a resistance $40.8\,\Omega$ all connected in series. If the ammeter has a coil of resistance $480\,\Omega$ and a shunt of $20\,\Omega$, then reading in the ammeter will be *[NCERT (Old) Pg. 108, AIPMT 2015]*

(a) 0.5 A (b) 0.25 A
(c) 2 A (d) 1 A

Module-III Cells and their Combinations

20. The terminal voltage of the battery, whose emf is 10 V and internal resistance 1 Ω, when connected through an external resistance of 4 Ω as shown in the figure is *[NCERT (New) Pg. 94, NEET 2024]*

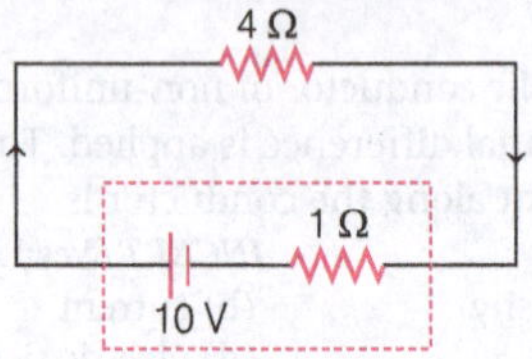

(a) 4 V (b) 6 V (c) 8 V (d) 10 V

21. A set of n equal resistors, of value R each are connected in series to a battery of emf E and internal resistance R. The current drawn is I. Now, the n resistors are connected in parallel to the same battery. Then, the current drawn from battery becomes $10I$. The value of n is *[NCERT (New) Pg. 95, NEET 2018]*

(a) 20 (b) 11 (c) 10 (d) 9

22. A battery consists of a variable number n of identical cells (having internal resistance r each) which are connected in series. The terminals of the battery are short-circuited and the current I is measured. Which of the graphs shows the correct relationship between I and n? *[NCERT (New) Pg. 95, NEET 2018]*

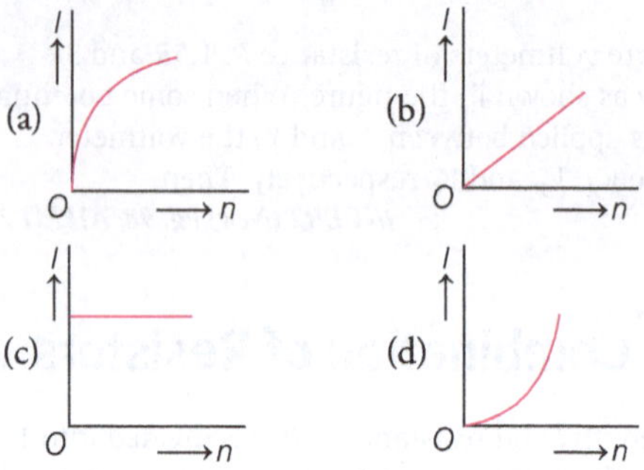

Module-IV Kirchhoff's Laws and its Applications

23. Two heaters A and B have power rating of 1 kW and 2kW respectively. Those two are first connected in series and then in parallel to a fixed power source. The ratio of power outputs for these two cases is *[NCERT (New) Pg. 92, NEET 2024]*

(a) 1 : 1 (b) 2 : 9 (c) 1 : 2 (d) 2 : 3

24. If the galvanometer G does not show any deflection in the circuit shown, the value of R is given by *[NCERT (New) Pg. 98, NEET 2023]*

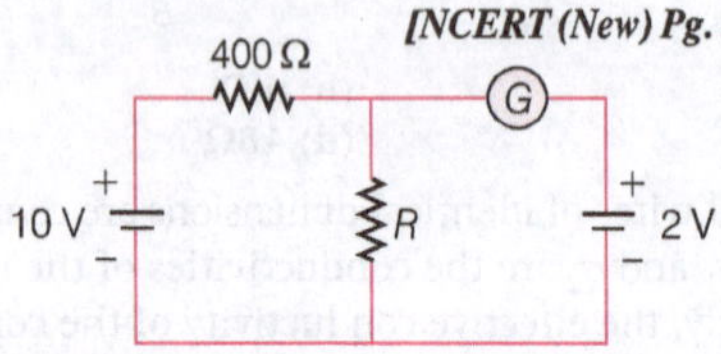

(a) 50 Ω (b) 100 Ω (c) 400 Ω (d) 200 Ω

25. The magnitude and direction of the current in the following circuit is *[NCERT (New) Pg. 98, NEET 2023]*

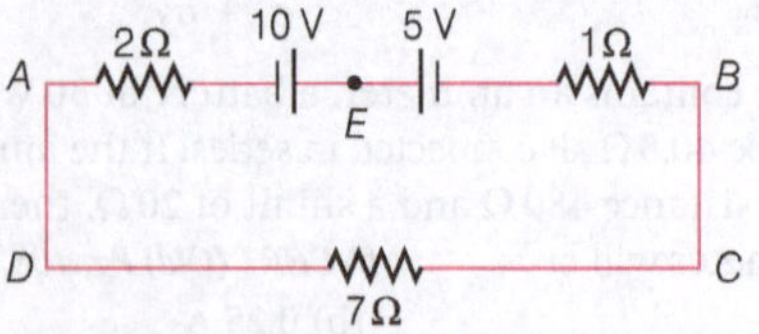

(a) 0.5 A from A to B through E
(b) 5/9 A from A to B through E
(c) 1.5 A from B to A through E
(d) 0.2 A from B to A through E

26. Two resistors of resistance, 100 Ω and 200 Ω are connected in parallel in an electrical circuit, The ratio of the thermal energy developed in 100 Ω to that in 200 Ω in a given time is *[NCERT (New) Pg. 92, NEET 2022]*

(a) 2 : 1 (b) 1 : 4
(c) 4 : 1 (d) 1 : 2

27. The energy that will be ideally radiated by a 100 kW transmitter in 1 hour is *[NCERT (New) Pg. 92, NEET 2022]*

(a) 36×10^4 J (b) 36×10^5 J (c) 1×10^5 J (d) 36×10^7 J

28. A Wheatstone bridge is used to determine the value of unknown resistance X by adjusting the variable resistance Y as shown in the figure. For the most precise measurement of X, the resistances P and Q *[NCERT (New) Pg. 101, NEET 2022]*

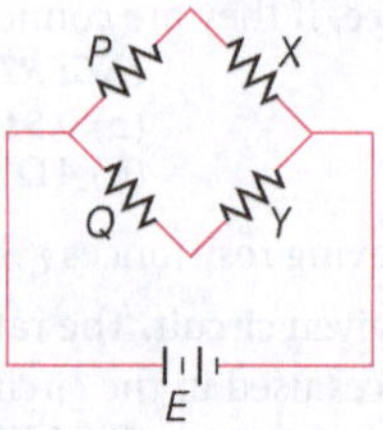

(a) should be approximately equal and are small
(b) should be very large and unequal
(c) do not play any significant role
(d) should be approximately equal to $2X$

29. For the circuit shown in the figure, the current I will be *[NCERT (New) Pg. 98, NEET (Oct.) 2020]*

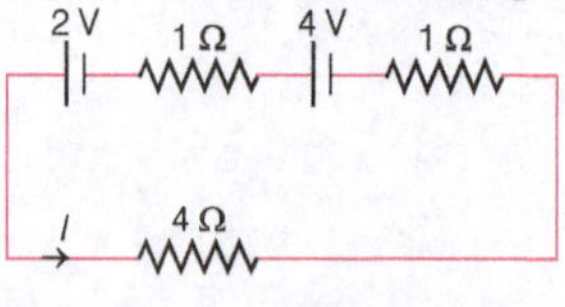

(a) 0.75 A (b) 1 A
(c) 1.5 A (d) 0.5 A

30. A resistance wire connected in the left gap of a meter bridge balances a 10 Ω resistance in the right gap at a point which divides the bridge wire in the ratio 3 : 2. If the length of the resistance wire is 1.5 m, then the length of 1 Ω of the resistance wire is *[NCERT (Old) Pg. 121, NEET (Sep.) 2020]*

(a) 1.0×10^{-1} m (b) 1.5×10^{-1} m
(c) 1.5×10^{-2} m (d) 1.0×10^{-2} m

31. For the circuit given below, the Kirchhoff's loop rule for the loop *BCDEB* is given by the equation *[NCERT (New) Pg. 98, NEET (Oct.) 2020]*

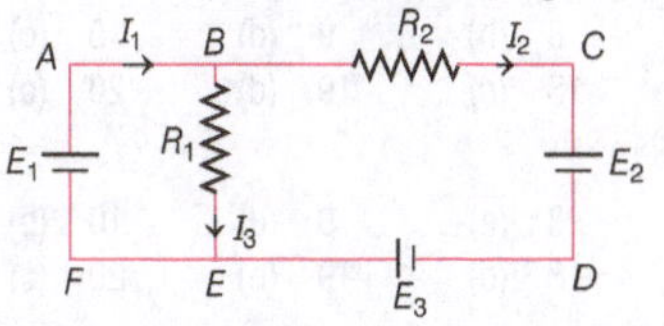

(a) $-I_2R_2 + E_2 - E_3 + I_3R_1 = 0$
(b) $I_2R_2 + E_2 - E_3 - I_3R_1 = 0$
(c) $I_2R_2 + E_2 + E_3 + I_3R_1 = 0$
(d) $-I_2R_2 + E_2 + E_3 + I_3R_1 = 0$

32. Six similar bulbs are connected as shown in the figure with a DC source of emf *E* and zero internal resistance. The ratio of power consumption by the bulbs when (i) all are glowing and (ii) in the situation when two from section *A* and one from section *B* are glowing, will be *[NCERT (New) Pg. 93, NEET (National) 2019]*

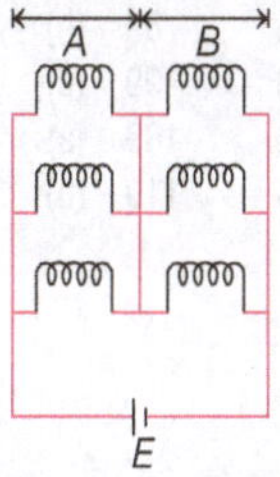

(a) 9 : 4 (b) 1 : 2 (c) 2 : 1 (d) 4 : 9

33. The meter bridge shown in the balance position with $\frac{P}{Q} = \frac{l_1}{l_2}$. If we now interchange the positions of galvanometer and cell, will the bridge work? If yes, what will be balanced condition? *[NCERT (Old) Pg. 121, NEET (Odisha) 2019]*

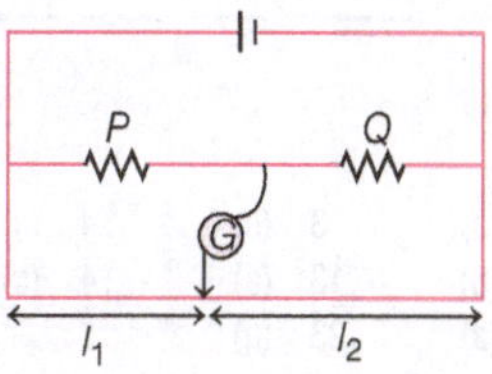

(a) Yes, $\frac{P}{Q} = \frac{l_2 - l_1}{l_2 + l_1}$ (b) No, no null point
(c) Yes, $\frac{P}{Q} = \frac{l_2}{l_1}$ (d) Yes, $\frac{P}{Q} = \frac{l_1}{l_2}$

34. The reading of an ideal voltmeter in the circuit shown is *[NCERT (New) Pg. 98, NEET (Odisha) 2019]*

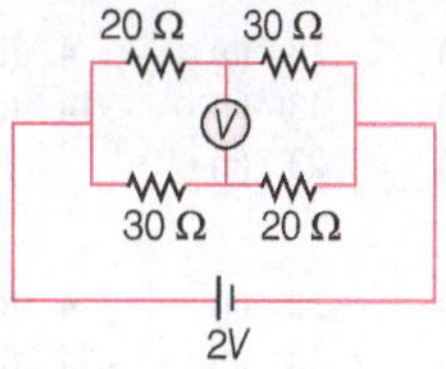

(a) 0.6 V (b) 0 V (c) 0.5 V (d) 0.4 V

35. The potential difference $(V_A - V_B)$ between the points *A* and *B* in the given figure is *[NCERT (New) Pg. 98, NEET 2016]*

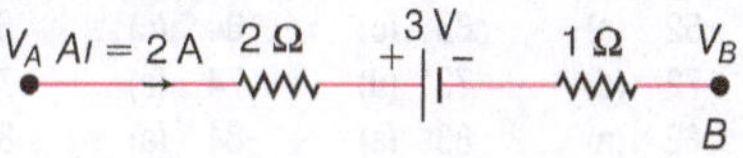

(a) −3 V (b) +3 V
(c) +6 V (d) +9 V

36. A filament bulb (500 W, 100 V) is to be used in a 230 V main supply. When a resistance *R* is connected in series, it works perfectly and the bulb consumes 500 W. The value of *R* is *[NCERT (New) Pg. 93, NEET 2016]*

(a) 230 Ω (b) 46 Ω
(c) 26 Ω (d) 13 Ω

37. The charge following through a resistance *R* varies with time *t* as $Q = at - bt^2$, where *a* and *b* are positive constants. The total heat produced in *R* is *[NCERT (New) Pg. 92, NEET 2016]*

(a) $\frac{a^3R}{3b}$ (b) $\frac{a^3R}{2b}$
(c) $\frac{a^3R}{b}$ (d) $\frac{a^3R}{6b}$

Answers

Step up Practice 1

1 (a)	2 (a)	3 (c)	4 (a)	5 (b)	6 (a)	7 (b)	8 (d)	9 (a)	10 (b)
11 (d)	12 (b)	13 (a)	14 (c)	15 (b)	16 (a)	17 (c)	18 (d)	19 (b)	20 (b)
21 (b)	22 (a)	23 (a)							

Step up Practice 2

1 (c)	2 (b)	3 (c)	4 (d)	5 (b)	6 (b)	7 (d)	8 (c)	9 (a)	10 (b)
11 (d)	12 (d)	13 (b)	14 (c)	15 (d)	16 (a)	17 (a)	18 (d)		

Step up Practice 3

1 (d)	2 (d)	3 (a)	4 (b)	5 (d)	6 (b)	7 (a)	8 (b)	9 (d)	10 (c)
11 (c)	12 (a)	13 (c)	14 (c)	15 (c)	16 (c)	17 (c)	18 (c)	19 (d)	20 (d)

Step up Practice 4

1 (c)	2 (d)	3 (b)	4 (b)	5 (a)	6 (c)	7 (a)	8 (a)	9 (d)	10 (b)
11 (b)	12 (b)	13 (c)	14 (b)	15 (a)	16 (b)	17 (c)	18 (d)	19 (b)	20 (c)
21 (d)	22 (c)	23 (d)							

Gearing up for NEET

1 (c)	2 (b)	3 (a)	4 (c)	5 (d)	6 (a)	7 (c)	8 (a)	9 (c)	10 (d)
11 (b)	12 (d)	13 (d)	14 (b)	15 (a)	16 (d)	17 (b)	18 (a)	19 (b)	20 (c)
21 (a)	22 (a)	23 (d)	24 (a)	25 (b)	26 (a)	27 (a)	28 (a)	29 (d)	30 (d)
31 (d)	32 (a)	33 (b)	34 (d)	35 (a)	36 (b)	37 (d)	38 (a)	39 (b)	40 (b)
41 (a)	42 (d)	43 (b)	44 (c)	45 (c)	46 (c)	47 (b)	48 (b)	49 (d)	50 (b)
51 (a)	52 (c)	53 (b)	54 (c)	55 (d)	56 (d)	57 (d)	58 (a)	59 (c)	60 (a)
61 (b)	62 (c)	63 (c)	64 (c)	65 (d)	66 (b)	67 (c)	68 (c)	69 (c)	70 (b)
71 (b)	72 (d)	73 (d)	74 (c)	75 (b)	76 (d)	77 (b)	78 (d)	79 (c)	80 (b)
81 (d)	82 (a)	83 (a)	84 (a)	85 (d)	86 (d)	87 (c)	88 (c)	89 (b)	90 (c)
91 (a)	92 (b)	93 (b)	94 (a)	95 (c)	96 (c)	97 (c)	98 (b)	99 (c)	100 (b)
101 (b)	102 (d)	103 (b)	104 (b)	105 (c)	106 (d)	107 (a)	108 (b)	109 (a)	110 (d)
111 (c)	112 (d)	113 (b)	114 (a)	115 (b)	116 (d)	117 (a)	118 (a)	119 (b)	120 (d)
121 (c)	122 (b)								

Assertion and Reason

1 (c)	2 (d)	3 (a)	4 (c)	5 (d)

Statement Type Questions

1 (b)	2 (b)	3 (d)	4 (d)	5 (a)

Match the Columns

1 (a)	2 (b)	3 (b)	4 (b)

Final Check through PYQs : Module-I

1 (b)	2 (d)	3 (b)	4 (a)	5 (b)	6 (b)	7 (a)	8 (c)	9 (b)	10 (c)
11 (a)	12 (b)								

Final Check through PYQs : Module-II

13 (b)	14 (a)	15 (d)	16 (b)	17 (b)	18 (a)	19 (a)

Final Check through PYQs : Module-III

20 (c)	21 (c)	22 (c)

Final Check through PYQs : Module-IV

23 (b)	24 (b)	25 (a)	26 (a)	27 (d)	28 (a)	29 (b)	30 (a)	31 (b)	32 (a)
33 (d)	34 (d)	35 (d)	36 (c)	37 (d)					

Hints and Solutions

Step up Practice 1

1. (a) Current, $I = \frac{dq}{dt} = 3t^2 + 2t + 5$

$$q = \int_{t=0}^{t=2} (3t^2 + 2t + 5)\, dt$$

Charge, $q = [t^3 + t^2 + 5t]_0^2$

$= [8 + 4 + 10] = 22$ C

2. (a) Current, $I = \frac{q}{t}$ or $I = \frac{ne}{t}$

$\Rightarrow 16 \times 10^{-3} = \frac{n \times 1.6 \times 10^{-19}}{1}$

$\therefore$ Number of electrons, $n = 10^{17}$

3. (c) We have, current, $I = \frac{ne}{t}$

$\therefore$ Number of electrons, $n = \frac{It}{e}$

$$= \frac{0.2 \times 30}{1.6 \times 10^{-19}} = 3.75 \times 10^{19}$$

4. (a) Both A and R are true but R is not the correct explanation of A.

On increasing temperature of wire, the kinetic energy of free electrons increase and so they collide more rapidly with each other and hence, their drift velocity decreases. Also, when temperature increases, resistance increase and resistance is inversely proportional to conductivity of material.

5. (b) Given, $I = 4 - 0.08t$

$\Rightarrow \frac{dq}{dt} = 4 - 0.08t$

$\Rightarrow q = \int_0^{50} (4 - 0.08t)\, dt$

$\Rightarrow ne = \left[4t - \frac{0.08t^2}{2}\right]_0^{50} = 100$

$\Rightarrow n = \frac{100}{e} = \frac{100}{1.6 \times 10^{-19}}$

$= 6.25 \times 10^{20}$ electrons

6. (a) Drift velocity, $v_d = \frac{eE\tau}{m}$

$\therefore \quad v_d \propto E$

7. (b) The order of drift velocity of electrons is

10^{-4} ms^{-1} $= 10^{-2}$ cms^{-1}

8. (d) Both A and R are true and R is the correct explanation of A.

Since, current arises due to continuous flow of charged particles. There is no free charge in insulator, hence no flow of charges are possible. Therefore, current do not flow through insulators.

9. (a) Drift velocity, $v_d = \frac{I}{neA}$

$$= \frac{3}{8.5 \times 10^{28} \times 1.6 \times 10^{-19} \times 2 \times 10^{-6}}$$

$= 0.11 \times 10^{-3}$ ms^{-1}

$\therefore$ Time, $t = \frac{\text{Length of the wire}}{v_d}$

$$= \frac{3}{0.11 \times 10^{-3}} = 2.73 \times 10^4 \text{ s}$$

10. (b) We know that, $I = neAv_d$

$\therefore$ Total number of electron, $N = nAl$

Total momentum (p) of electron $= Nmv_d$

or $\quad p = (nALm)\frac{I}{neA} = \frac{ILm}{e}$

$$= \frac{70 \times 1000 \times 9.1 \times 10^{-31}}{1.6 \times 10^{-19}} = 0.4\,\mu \text{ N-s}$$

11. (d) Given, $l = 4$ cm,

$A = 10 \text{ cm} \times 4 \text{ cm} = 40 \text{ cm}^2$,

$\rho = 48 \times 10^{-8}\ \Omega$-m

$\therefore R = \rho \times \frac{l}{A}$

$$= 48 \times 10^{-8} \times \frac{4 \times 10^{-2}}{40 \times 10^{-4}} = 4.8\ \mu\Omega$$

12. (b) Resistivity $\rightarrow \Omega$-m

13. (a) Given, $R = 2.46\ \Omega$,

$d = 0.32 \text{ mm} \Rightarrow r = 0.16$ mm

Volume, $V = 1$ cm^3

Clearly, length of wire, $l = \frac{\text{Volume}}{\pi r^2}$

$$= \frac{10^{-6}}{\pi \times 0.16 \times 0.16 \times 10^{-6}}$$

$\Rightarrow \quad l = \frac{625}{16\pi}$

So, specific resistance, $\rho = R \times \frac{A}{l}$

$$= 2.46 \times \frac{\pi \times 0.16 \times 0.16 \times 10^{-6}}{625} \times 16\pi$$
$$= 0.0159 \times 10^{-6}\ \Omega\text{-m}$$
$$= 1.59 \times 10^{-6}\ \Omega\text{-cm}$$

14. (*c*) Since, $l_2 = 2l$

$$R_2 = 4R \qquad \text{(If } l_2 = nl_1\text{, then } R_2 = n^2 R_1\text{)}$$

15. (*b*) Since, $r_2 = \frac{r}{2}$

$$\Rightarrow \quad R_2 = (2)^4 R \quad [\text{If } r_2 = r_1/n, \text{ then } R_2 = n^4 R_1]$$
$$= 16R$$

16. (*a*) Both A and R are true but R is not the correct explanation of A.

The value of temperature coefficient of resistance is positive only for metals and alloys and is negative for semiconductors and insulators.

17. (*c*) Slope of *I*-*V* curve, $\tan\theta = \frac{1}{R}$

$$\frac{R_1}{R_2} = \frac{\tan\theta_2}{\tan\theta_1} \Rightarrow R_2 > R_1$$

So, $\quad T_2 > T_1$

18. (*d*) $R_\theta = R_0(1 + \alpha\theta)$

$$1 = R_0(1 + 27\alpha) \qquad \text{...(i)}$$
$$2 = R_0(1 + \theta\alpha) \qquad \text{...(ii)}$$

Eqs. (i) and (ii) gives,

$$2 + 54\alpha = 1 + \alpha\theta$$
$$\Rightarrow \quad \alpha\theta = 1 + 54\alpha$$
$$\therefore \quad \theta = \frac{1}{\alpha} + 54 = \frac{1}{0.00125} + 54 = 854°\text{C}$$

19. (*b*) $R_\theta = R_0(1 + \alpha\theta)$

$$120 = R_0(1 + 20\alpha) \qquad \text{...(i)}$$
$$R_{50} = R_0(1 + 50\alpha) \qquad \text{...(ii)}$$

From Eqs. (i) and (ii), we get

$$\frac{R_{50}}{120} = \frac{1 + 50\alpha}{1 + 20\alpha}$$
$$\Rightarrow \quad \frac{R_{50}}{120} = \frac{1.5}{1.2} \Rightarrow R_{50} = 150\,\Omega$$

20. (*b*) A is true but R is false.

Specific resistance is independent of the dimensions of wire. Specific resistance of wire is given by $\rho = \frac{m}{ne^2\tau}$, where τ is relaxation time. From this, we find that the resistivity of a conductor depend upon the nature of material and temperature.

21. (*b*) We have, $\quad I = \frac{V}{R} = \frac{q}{t}$

$$\therefore \text{ Charge,} \quad q = \frac{Vt}{R}$$
$$= \frac{20 \times 2 \times 60}{10} = 240\text{ C}$$

22. (*a*) Resistance, $R = \rho\frac{l}{A}$ and resistivity, $\rho = \frac{m}{ne^2\tau}$

$$\therefore \quad R = \frac{ml}{ne^2\tau A}$$

23. (*a*) $R = \rho\frac{l}{A}$

Since, wires are made of same material, so resistivity ρ of all wires will be same.

Therefore, $\quad R \propto \frac{l}{A}$

$$\Rightarrow \quad R \propto \frac{l}{\pi r^2}$$
$$\Rightarrow \quad R \propto \frac{l}{\left(\frac{d}{2}\right)^2}$$

For length = 50 cm and diameter = 0.5 mm

Resistance will be maximum.

Step up Practice 2

1. (*c*) Given circuit can be redrawn as follows

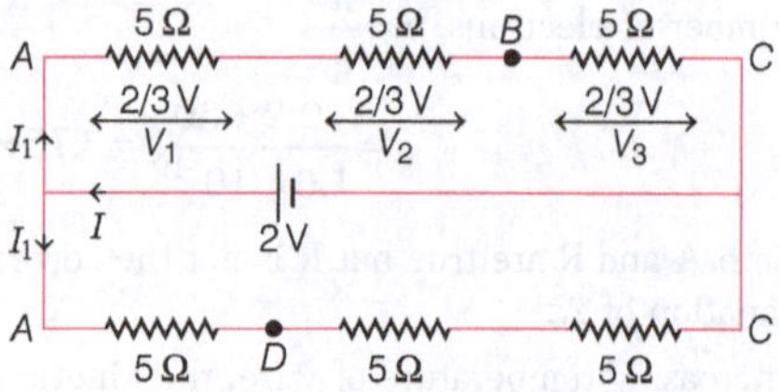

Here, $\quad I_1 = \frac{I}{2} = \frac{V}{2R_{eq}} = \frac{2}{2 \times \left(\frac{15}{2}\right)} = \frac{2}{15}\text{ A}$

So, potential across each resistance,

$$V' = I_1 R = \frac{2}{15} \times 5 = \frac{2}{3}\text{ V}$$

$\therefore$ Potential difference across

$$AB = \frac{2}{3} + \frac{2}{3} = \frac{4}{3}\text{ V}$$

2. (*b*) Potential difference across the circuit

$$= I\left(\frac{R_1 R_2}{R_1 + R_2}\right)$$
$$= 1.2 \times \left(\frac{6 \times 4}{6 + 4}\right) = 2.88\text{ V}$$

So, current through 6 Ω resistance $= \frac{2.88}{6} = 0.48$ A

3. (*c*) Current divides according to resistance, so current in 6 Ω resistance is $\frac{0.8}{2} = 0.4$ A

So, total current in circuit is $0.8 + 0.4 = 1.2$ A

$\therefore$ Potential drop across 4 Ω $= 1.2 \times 4 = 4.8$ V

4. (d) Both Statement I and Statement II are correct.
In series combination of two resistors,
$$R_{eq} = R_1 + R_2$$
So, the equivalent resistance is greater than the individual resistances.
In parallel combination,
$$R_{eq} = \frac{R_1R_2}{R_1 + R_2}$$
Which is less than the individual resistances.

5. (b) Two resistances are short-circuited.
So, only third resistance will be considered and hence,
$$I = \frac{V}{R} = \frac{10}{3} \text{ A}$$

6. (b) Net resistance, $R_{net} = \frac{10 \times 15}{10 + 15} + 3 + 0.5 = 9.5\,\Omega$
$$\therefore \quad I = \frac{V}{R_{net}} = \frac{20}{9.5} = 2.1 \text{ A}$$
According to current division rule, current through $10\,\Omega$ resistance is
$$I_1 = \left(\frac{15}{10 + 15}\right) \times 2.1 = 1.2 \text{ A}$$

7. (d) Resistance, $R_{AB} = \frac{R}{3} + R = \frac{2}{3} + 2$
$$\Rightarrow \quad R_{AB} = \frac{8}{3} = 2\frac{2}{3}\,\Omega$$

8. (c) $R_{eq(AB)} = \frac{5}{3}\,\Omega$

9. (a) The circuit can be reduced as follows

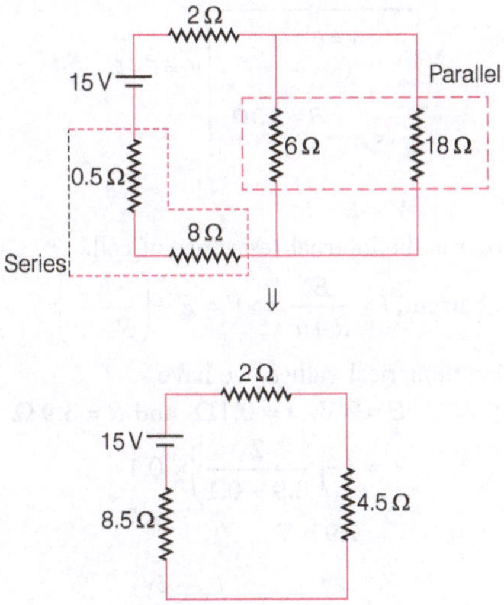

So, equivalent resistance across battery,
$$R_{eq} = 8.5 + 2 + 4.5 = 15\,\Omega$$
Hence, current from the battery,
$$I = \frac{15}{15} = 1 \text{ A}$$

10. (b) As B is connected to the earth, so potential at B is $V_B = 0$.
Now, current in the given circuit,
$$I = \frac{V}{R_{net}} = \frac{50}{5 + 7 + 10 + 3} = 2 \text{ A}$$
Potential difference between A and B is
$$V_A - V_B = 2 \times 12$$
or $\quad V_A \; 0 = 24$
or $\quad V_A = 24$ V

11. (d) In series combination, $R_1 = nR$
In parallel combination, $R_2 = \frac{R}{n}$
$$\therefore \quad \frac{R_1}{R_2} = \frac{nR}{R / n} = n^2 : 1$$

12. (d) Both Statement I and Statement II are correct.
when resistor are connected in parallel combination,
$$\frac{1}{R_{eq}} = \frac{1}{R_1} + \frac{1}{R_2} \ldots \frac{1}{R_n}$$
then net resistance will decrease.
When resistor are connected in series.
$$R_S = R_1 + R_2 \ldots\ldots R_n$$
then net resistance will increases,
As we know, $R = \frac{\rho l}{A}$
When resistor are connected in series, the length will increase, but the cross-section area will be same, so that net resistance will increase.
When resistor are connected in parallel, the cross-section area will increase, but length will be same, so that total resistance will decrease.

13. (b) $\frac{1}{R_{eq}} = \frac{1}{R_1} + \frac{1}{R_2} + \frac{1}{R_3} \ldots \frac{1}{R_n} = \frac{1}{R} + \frac{1}{2R} + \frac{1}{4R} + \ldots \frac{1}{R_\infty}$
$$\Rightarrow \quad \frac{1}{R_{eq}} = \frac{1}{R}\left[1 + \frac{1}{2} + \frac{1}{4} + \frac{1}{8} \ldots\right]$$
[Infinite GP, $S_\infty = \frac{a}{1 - r}$]; $\frac{1}{R_{eq}} = \frac{1}{R}\left[\frac{1}{1 - 1/2}\right] = \frac{2}{R}$
$$\Rightarrow \quad R_{eq} = \frac{R}{2}$$

14. (c) As points A and B are at same potential.
So, $\quad V_{AB} = 0 \Rightarrow R_{AB} = 0$

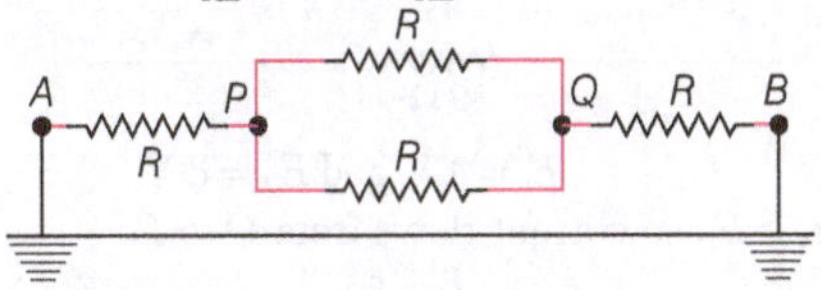

Net resistance between points P and Q,
$$R_{PQ} = \frac{(R / 2) \times 2R}{2R + (R / 2)} = \frac{2R}{5}$$

15. (*d*) Both Statement I and Statement II are correct.

We know that, the resistances can be combined in two different ways : In series and parallel. When two or more resistances are linked end to end in a row, they seem to be connected in series. When two or more resistances are linked between the same two points, they seem to connected in parallel. So, in a series combination, the effective resistance is the sum of all individual resistance that are connected in series.

16. (*a*) The equivalent circuit will be as following

Currents in 60 Ω, 20 Ω and 10 Ω resistors will be divided in inverse proportion.

i.e. $$I : I_1 : I_2 = \frac{1}{60} : \frac{1}{20} : \frac{1}{10} = 1:3:6$$

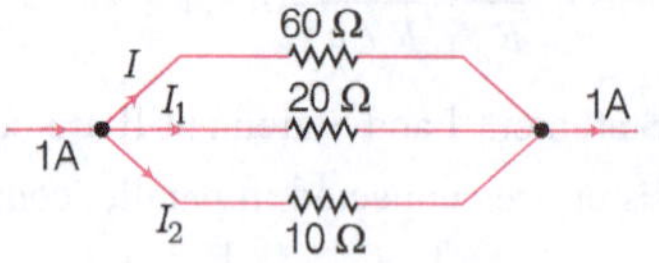

∴ $$I = \frac{1}{1+3+6} \times 1 = 0.1\text{ A}$$

17. (*a*) In series combination of resistors, the current through all resistors is equal and voltage, $V \propto R$.

∴ Voltage drop across R_1 is maximum.

18. (*d*) In the parallel combinations of resistors, the voltage through all resistors is equal and current, $I \propto \frac{1}{R}$.

∴ Current across R_1 is minimum.

Step up Practice 3

1. (*d*) We have, $V = E - Ir$

$$= 1.5 - 2 \times 0.15$$

⇒ $$V = 1.20\text{ V}$$

2. (*d*) Potential difference between *A* and *B* is given by

$$V_A - V_B = \frac{E_1 r_2 + E_2 r_1}{r_1 + r_2}$$

∴ $$4 = \frac{5X + 2 \times 10}{X + 10}$$

⇒ $$X = 20\,\Omega$$

3. (*a*)

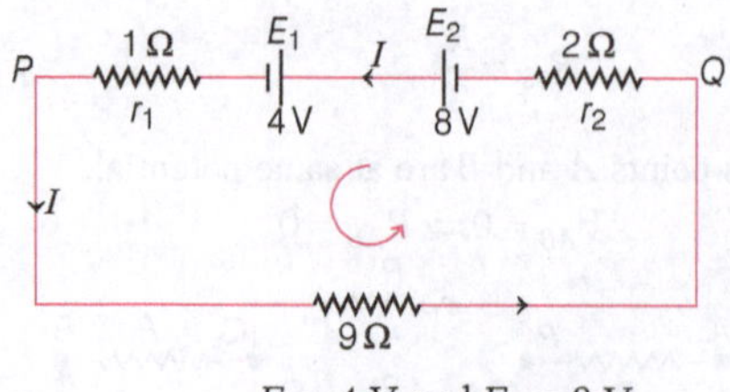

$$E_1 = 4\text{ V and } E_2 = 8\text{ V}$$

As $E_2 > E_1$, so current flows from *Q* to *P*.

∴ $$I = \frac{8-4}{12} = \frac{1}{3}\text{ A}$$

∴ Potential difference across $PQ = \frac{1}{3} \times 9 = 3\text{ V}$

4. (*b*) A is true but R is false.

During charging of the cell, current flows inside the cell from positive to negative, supporting the electrostatic field inside.

Therefore, $V > E$

Emf is greater than the terminal voltage only when the cell delivers the current to the external circuit.

5. (*d*) The potentials of different points are shown in below figure

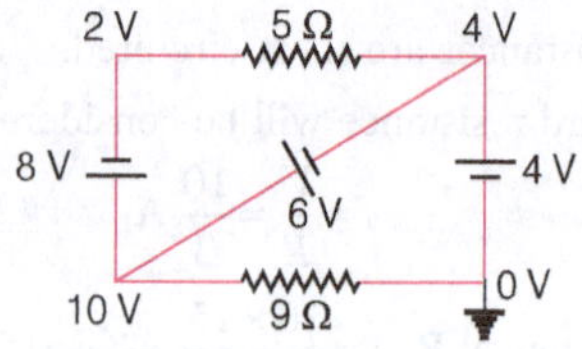

Current through 5 Ω resistance

$$= \frac{\text{Potential difference}}{\text{Resistance}}$$

$$= \frac{(4-2)}{5} = 0.4\text{ A}$$

6. (*b*) If current through cell is *I*, then

$$I = \frac{E}{R+r} \text{ or } R = \frac{E - Ir}{I}$$

$$= \frac{10 - 1.5}{0.5} = 17\,\Omega$$

TPD across cell, $V = E - Ir$

$$= 10 - 0.5 \times 3 = 8.5\text{ V}$$

7. (*a*) The situation can be drawn as

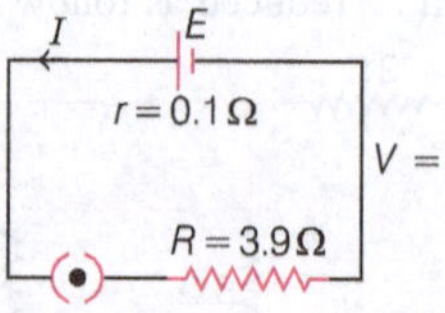

∴ $$V = E - Ir$$

where, *r* is the internal resistance of cell.

Also, current, $I = \frac{E}{R+r} \Rightarrow V = E - \left(\frac{E}{R+r}\right) r$

Putting numerical values, we have

$$E = 2\text{ V}, \; r = 0.1\,\Omega \text{ and } R = 3.9\,\Omega$$

⇒ $$V = 2 - \left(\frac{2}{3.9 + 0.1}\right) \times 0.1$$

⇒ $$V = 1.95\text{ V}$$

8. (*b*)

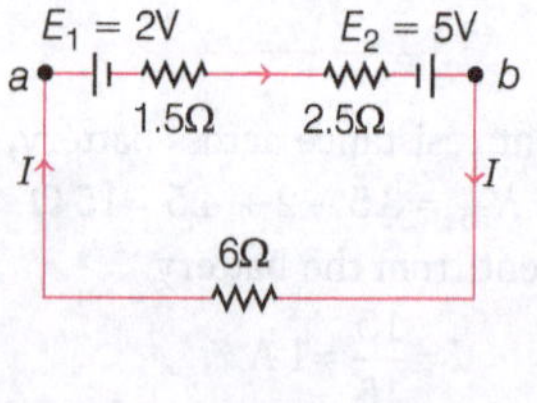

$$I = \frac{E_2 - E_1}{r_1 + r_2 + R}$$

$$I = \frac{5-2}{6+4} = \frac{3}{10} = 0.3 \text{ A}$$

$$V_a - V_b = -0.3 \times 6 = -1.8 \text{ V}$$

9. (*d*) Equivalent internal resistance in parallel combination of cells is $\frac{r}{n}$.

10. (*c*) If emf and internal resistance of each cells is E and r, respectively. Then,

$$10E = (R + 10r) I_1 \quad \text{[Here, } R \text{ is external resistance]}$$

If polarity of P cells have been changed, then

$$(10 - 2P) E = (R + 10r) I_2$$

$$\frac{I_1}{I_2} = \frac{10E}{(10-2P)E} \Rightarrow 5 = \frac{10}{10-2P}$$

$$\Rightarrow \quad 50 - 10P = 10 \Rightarrow P = 4 \text{ cells}$$

11. (*c*) $E_{net} = (4-2)\,4 = 8$ V

$$\Rightarrow r_{net} = 4 \times 0.5 = 2\,\Omega, R_{ext} = 2\,\Omega$$

$$I = \frac{8}{2+2} = 2 \text{ A}$$

So, $(\text{TPD})_4 = E + Ir = 4 + 2 \times 0.5 = 5$ V

12. (*a*) $E_{net} = \frac{E_1 r_2 + E_2 r_1}{r_1 + r_2} = \frac{2 \times 3 + 3 \times 2}{2+3} = 2.4$ V

$$\Rightarrow \quad r_{net} = \frac{r_1 r_2}{r_1 + r_2} = \frac{2 \times 3}{2+3} = \frac{6}{5}\,\Omega = 1.2\,\Omega$$

$$R_{eq} = 1.2 + 1.2 = 2.4\,\Omega$$

So, $$I = \frac{E}{r+R} = \frac{2.4}{2.4} = 1 \text{ A}$$

13. (*c*) $E = I(r + nr) \Rightarrow E = Ir(1+n)$

$$V = I(nr)$$

Clearly, $\frac{V}{E} = \frac{Inr}{Ir(n+1)} = \frac{n}{n+1}$

14. (*c*) A is false but R is true.

The total internal resistance is nr, there is no effect of connection of cells in circuit on total internal resistance.

Internal resistance depends only on nature and dimension of cell. It has same property as that of resistance.

$$r = r_1 + r_2 \quad \text{(connected in series)}$$

$$\Rightarrow \quad \frac{1}{r} = \frac{1}{r_1} + \frac{1}{r_2} \quad \text{(connected in parallel)}$$

15. (*c*) $V = E - Ir = E - \left(\frac{E}{R+r}\right) r = E\left(\frac{R}{R+r}\right) = \frac{E}{1 + r/R}$

16. (*c*) Out of n cells, two cells will cancel out each other's emf.

So, net emf $= (n-2)E$.

Total resistance $= R + nr$

Current, $I = \frac{(n-2)E}{nr + R}$

17. (*c*) A is false but R is true.

In parallel connection of cell, we get maximum current at low potential difference.

18. (*c*) We have, $I_1 = \frac{E}{r + R_1}$ and $I_2 = \frac{E}{r + R_2}$

From these two equations, we get

$$r = \frac{I_2 R_2 - I_1 R_1}{I_1 - I_2}$$

19. (*d*) Potential difference (V) in different cases;

(i) When cell is in open circuit, then

$$V = E$$

(ii) Discharging of cell when cell is supplying current, then

$$V < E$$

(iii) Charging of cell when cell is taking current, then

$$V > E$$

(iv) When the cell is short-circuited, then

$$V = 0$$

Here, E is emf of the cell in all cases.

20. (*d*) Parallel combination of cells has greater current because I and R are inversely proportional and series combination of cells has greater equivalent resistance.

Step up Practice 4

1. (*c*)

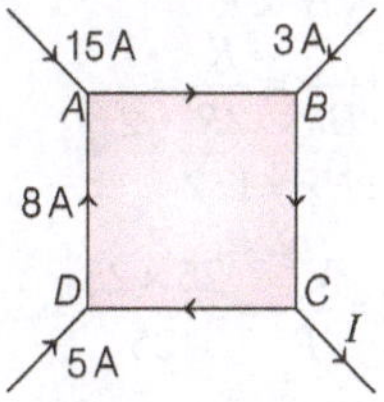

Applying Kirchhoff's first law at junction A, B, C, D.

At A, $\quad I_{AB} = 15 + 8 = 23$ A

At B, $\quad I_{BC} = 23 + 3 = 26$ A

At D, $\quad I_{CD} = 8 - 5 = 3$ A

At C, $\quad I_{CD} + I = I_{BC}$

or $\quad 3 + I = 26$

$\therefore \quad I = 23$ A

2. (*d*)

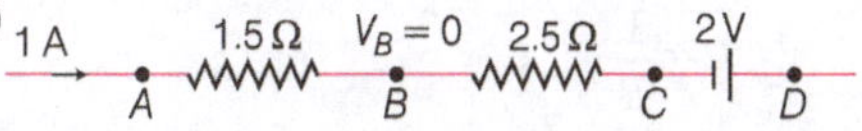

Potential difference between A and B,

$$V_A - V_B = 1 \times 1.5$$

or $\quad V_A - 0 = 1.5 \quad (\because V_B = 0, \text{ given})$

$\therefore \quad V_A = 1.5$ V

Now, potential difference between B and C,

$$V_B - V_C = 1 \times 2.5 = 2.5 \text{ V}$$

$\therefore \quad 0 - V_C = 2.5$ V

$\Rightarrow \quad V_C = -2.5$ V

Hence, potential difference between C and D,

$$V_C - V_D = -2 \text{ V or } -2.5 - V_D = -2$$

or $$V_D = -0.5 \text{ V}$$

3. (b) Let at junction C, potential is V.

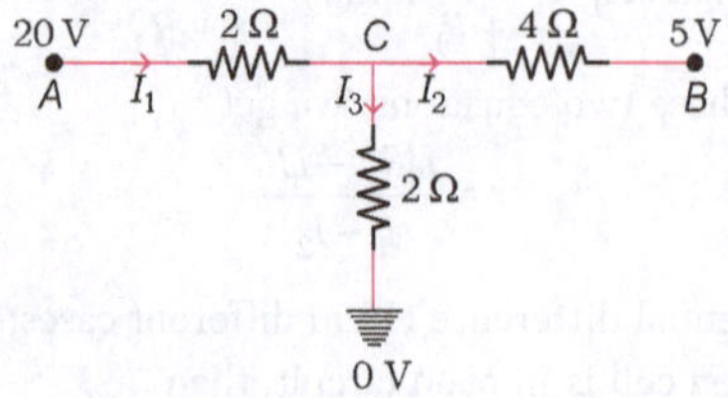

$$\therefore \quad \frac{V_A - V_C}{2} + \frac{V_B - V_C}{4} = \frac{V_C - 0}{2}$$

$$\Rightarrow \quad \frac{20 - V}{2} + \frac{5 - V}{4} = \frac{V - 0}{2}$$

$$\Rightarrow \quad V = 9 \text{ V}$$

Current, $I_3 = I = \frac{9}{2} = 4.5 \text{ A}$

4. (b) Statement I is correct but Statement II is incorrect.

The resistance of the galvanometer is fixed. In meter bridge experiments, to protect the galvanometer from a high current, high resistance is connected to the galvanometer in order to protect it from damage.

5. (a) In series, I is same, so $H = I^2Rt$. Therefore,

$$H \propto R$$

$$\therefore \quad \frac{H_1}{H_2} = \frac{R}{2R} = \frac{1}{2}$$

$$\Rightarrow \quad H_1 : H_2 = 1 : 2$$

6. (c) Resistance, $R = \frac{V^2}{P} = \frac{25 \times 25}{25} = 25 \, \Omega$

7. (a) Resistance, $R = \frac{V^2}{P}$ or $R \propto V^2$

$$\Rightarrow \quad \frac{R_1}{R_2} = \frac{V_1^2}{V_2^2} \Rightarrow \frac{R}{R_2} = \left(\frac{220}{110}\right)^2 = 4$$

$$\Rightarrow \quad R_2 = \frac{R}{4}$$

8. (a) Power, $P = \frac{V^2}{R}$

$$\therefore \quad P \propto \frac{1}{R}$$

Also, resistance of wire $\propto \frac{1}{(\text{radius of filament})^2}$

$\therefore P \propto (\text{radius of filament})^2$

So, 100 W bulb has thicker filament.

9. (d) $H = \frac{V^2 t}{R \times J} = \frac{Pt}{J} = \frac{210 \times 5 \times 60}{4.2} = 15000 \text{ cal}$

10. (b) Statement I is correct but Statement II is incorrect.

Current is rate of flow charges and source generate charges like cells, generator, etc. So, point in a circuit (or junction of the circuit) cannot act as source or sink of charge.

Therefore, the number of charges entering at the junction is equal to number of charges coming out of the junction. Thus, Kirchhoff's first law follows the law of conservation of charge.

11. (b) $P = \frac{V^2}{R} \Rightarrow 150 = \frac{(15)^2}{\left(\frac{2R}{2+R}\right)}$

$$\therefore \quad \frac{2+R}{2R} = \frac{2}{3}$$

$\therefore$ Resistance, $R = 6 \, \Omega$

12. (b) $R' = \frac{R}{4}$ and $P = \frac{V^2}{R}$

$$\therefore \quad P_2 = 4P_1 \Rightarrow \frac{P_2}{P_1} = 4$$

13. (c) When bulbs are in series,

$$P = \frac{V^2}{3R} \quad \text{...(i)}$$

When bulbs are connected in parallel,

$$P' = \frac{V^2}{(R/3)} = \frac{3V^2}{R} = 3 \times 3P \quad \text{[from Eq.(i)]}$$

$$= 9P$$

14. (b) It is known that in parallel combination,

$$P_{\text{consumed}} \propto \text{Brightness} \propto \frac{1}{R}$$

According to question, $P_A > P_B$ (given), therefore

$$R_B > R_A$$

15. (a) $P = \frac{V^2}{R}$. As, R_{net} will decrease, so P will increase.

16. (b) Wheatstone bridge is balanced.

As, $$\frac{P}{Q} = \frac{R}{S}$$

$$\Rightarrow \quad \frac{40}{10} = \frac{60}{15} = \frac{4}{1}$$

$$\Rightarrow \quad V_{AB} = V_{AD}$$

So, $$40I_1 = 60I_2$$

$$\Rightarrow \quad I_1 = 1.5I_2$$

Heat produced in $AB = I_1^2 Rt$

$$= (1.5I_2)^2 \times 40 \times t = 90I_2^2 t$$

Heat produced in $BC = I_1^2 Rt$

$$= (1.5I_2)^2 \times 10 \times t = 22.5I_2^2 t$$

Heat produced in $AD = I_2^2 Rt$

$$= I_2^2 \times 60 \times t = 60I_2^2 t$$

Heat produced in $DC = I_2^2 Rt$

$$= I_2^2 \times 15 \times t = 15I_2^2 t$$

17. (c) When each bulb is glowing at full power.

Current from each bulb,

$$I = \frac{50}{100} = \frac{1}{2}\text{ A}$$

So, main current, $I = \frac{n}{2}$ A (for parallel circuit)

Also, $E = V + Ir$

$\Rightarrow \quad 120 = 100 + \left(\frac{n}{2}\right) \times 100$

$\Rightarrow \quad n = 4$

18. (d) Ammeter is parallel with voltmeter, therefore its reading will be zero.

19. (b) If voltmeter is ideal, then R should be $\frac{1.6}{0.4} = 4\,\Omega$. If it is non-ideal, R should be greater than $4\,\Omega$.

20. (c) Total resistance of given circuit

$$= \frac{80}{1+1} + 20 = 40 + 20 = 60\,\Omega$$

$\therefore$ Main current, $I = \frac{2}{60} = \frac{1}{30}$ A

Now, in parallel, there are two resistances of $80\,\Omega$ each (one of voltmeter and other $80\,\Omega$ resistance). So, current is equally distributed in $80\,\Omega$ resistance and voltmeter, i.e. $\frac{1}{60}$ A of current flows through each.

$\therefore$ Potential difference across $80\,\Omega$ resistance or

voltmeter reading $= \frac{1}{60} \times 80 = 1.33$ V

21. (d) Equivalent resistance of circuit,

$$R_{eq} = 500 + \frac{1000}{3} = \frac{2500}{3}\,\Omega$$

$\therefore$ Current drawn from the cell,

$$I = \frac{10}{2500/3} = \frac{3}{250}\text{ A}$$

Reading of voltmeter $= \frac{3}{250} \times \frac{1000}{3} = 4$ V

22. (c) $\frac{R_3}{R_4} = \frac{R_1}{R_2}$ (balanced Wheatstone bridge)

or $\quad R_1 R_4 = R_2 R_3$

23. (d) Both Statement I and Statement II are correct. In the balanced condition of a Wheatstone bridge, there is no current flow through the galvanometer. This is also called null condition. So, the Statement I is correct. When the potential of points B and D are same, then only there is no current flow through the galvanometer.

Gearing up for NEET

1. (c) During the charging of battery, terminal potential difference is always greater than emf of circuit.

$$V = E + Ir$$

where, V is terminal potential difference and E is emf of cell.

2. (b) Slope of the V-I curve at any point is equal to reciprocal of resistance at that point.

From the curve, slope for $T_1 >$ slope for T_2.

$\Rightarrow \quad R_{T_1} < R_{T_2}$

Also, at higher temperature, resistance will be higher. So,

$$T_2 > T_1$$

3. (a) The relationship between current and drift speed is given by $\quad I = neAv_d$

Here, I is the current and v_d is the drift velocity.

So, $\quad I \propto v_d$

Thus, only drift velocity determines the current in a conductor.

4. (c) The current I crossing area of cross-section A, can be expressed in terms of drift velocity v_d and the moving charges as

$$I = nev_dA$$

where, n is number of charge carriers per unit volume and e the charge on the carrier.

$\therefore \quad v_d = \frac{I}{neA} = \frac{24 \times 10^{-3}}{(3\times 10^{23})(1.6\times 10^{-19})(10^{-4})}$

$= 5\times 10^{-3}\text{ms}^{-1}$

5. (d) Drift velocity, $v_d = \frac{I}{nAe} = \frac{I\times 4}{n\pi D^2 e}$

i.e. $\quad v_d \propto \frac{1}{D^2}$

$\therefore \quad \frac{v_{d_1}}{v_{d_2}} = \frac{D_2^2}{D_1^2} = \left(\frac{1}{2}\right)^2 = \frac{1}{4}$

6. (a) Given, for a wire, $\frac{R}{l} = \frac{1}{2}$

Length of wire, $l = 5\text{ cm} = 5 \times 10^{-2}$ m

$\therefore \quad R = \frac{l}{2} = 2.5 \times 10^{-2}\,\Omega$

Potential difference, $V = 1$ V or $IR = 1$

$\Rightarrow \quad I = \frac{1}{R} = \frac{1}{2.5\times 10^{-2}} = \frac{100}{2.5} = 40$ A

7. (c) Given, current, $I = 10$ A

Area of cross-section, $A = 4 \times 10^{-6}\text{ m}^2$

Density of conductors, $\rho = 2.7\text{ g/cc} = 2.7\times 10^3\text{ kg/m}^3$

Molecular weight of aluminium,

$$M_w = 27\text{g} = 27 \times 10^{-3}\text{ kg}$$

If n be the total number of electrons in the conductor per unit volume, then

$$n = \frac{\text{Total number of electrons}}{\text{Volume of conductor } (V)}$$

$$= \frac{\text{Number of atoms per mole} \times \text{Number of moles}}{V}$$

$$= \frac{\text{Avogadro number}}{V} \times \left(\frac{M}{M_w}\right)$$

$$= 6 \times 10^{23} \times \frac{\rho}{M_w}$$

$$= 6 \times 10^{23} \times \frac{2.7 \times 10^3}{27 \times 10^{-3}}$$

$$\therefore \quad n = 6 \times 10^{28}$$

We know that, drift velocity,

$$v_d = \frac{I}{neA} = \frac{10}{6 \times 10^{28} \times 1.6 \times 10^{-19} \times 4 \times 10^{-6}}$$

$$= 2.6 \times 10^{-4} \text{ m/s}$$

8. (*a*) Given, resistivity of copper, $\rho = 1.72 \times 10^{-8} \Omega$-m

Electrons density, $n = 8.5 \times 10^{28} / \text{m}^3$

$$\therefore \text{ Mobility } (\mu) = \frac{1}{\rho\, ne}$$

$$= \frac{1}{1.72 \times 10^{-8} \times 8.5 \times 10^{28} \times 1.6 \times 10^{-19}}$$

$$\simeq 4.25 \times 10^{-3} \text{ m}^2/\text{C}\,\Omega$$

9. (*c*) $\because$ Current, $I = nAev_d$

or $\quad v_d \propto \frac{1}{A}$

If diameter of wire is $d/4$, then area will be $A/16$, so new drift velocity $= 16\, v_d$.

10. (*d*) $\quad R_1 = R_0 (1 + \alpha t)$

$$1 = R_0 (1 + 0.00125 \times 27) \quad \text{...(i)}$$

$$2 = R_0 (1 + 0.00125 \times t) \quad \text{...(ii)}$$

From Eqs. (i) and (ii), we get

$$t = 854°\text{C} = 1127 \text{ K}$$

11. (*b*) Given, temperature coefficient of carbon,

$$\alpha_1 = 4 \times 10^{-3} /°\text{C}$$

Temperature coefficient of copper,

$$\alpha_2 = -0.5 \times 10^{-3} /°\text{C}$$

Hence, $R_1\alpha_1 = -R_2\alpha_2$

$$\frac{R_2}{R_1} = \frac{4 \times 10^{-3}}{0.5 \times 10^{-3}}$$

$$\Rightarrow \quad \frac{R_2}{R_1} = \frac{8}{1}$$

12. (*d*) The drift velocity, $v_d = \frac{J}{ne}$

(where, J is current density $= \frac{I}{A}$)

So, $\quad v_d \propto J$

$$\therefore \quad J_1 = \frac{I}{A} \text{ and } J_2 = \frac{2I}{2A} = \frac{I}{A} = J_1$$

So, $\quad (v_d)_1 = (v_d)_2 = v$

13. (*d*) Drift velocity in a copper conductor,

$$v_d = \frac{I}{neA} = \frac{5.4}{8.4 \times 10^{28} \times 1.6 \times 10^{-19} \times 10^{-6}}$$

$$= 0.4 \times 10^{-3} \text{ms}^{-1} = 0.4 \text{ mms}^{-1}$$

14. (*b*) The minimum resistance can be achieved when we connect all resistances in parallel.

So, equivalent resistance of combination $= \frac{r}{10}$.

15. (*a*) Resistance of wire, $R = \rho\, l/A$

On stretching the wire, the volume of the wire remains same.

$$\Rightarrow \quad \frac{A'}{A} = \frac{l}{l'}$$

So, new resistance, $R' = \rho l'/A'$

$$\Rightarrow \quad \frac{R'}{R} = \left(\frac{l'}{l}\right)\left(\frac{A}{A'}\right) = \frac{l'}{l} \cdot \frac{l'}{l} = \left(\frac{l'}{l}\right)^2 = \left(\frac{1.1\, l}{l}\right)^2 = 1.21$$

$$\therefore \quad R' = 1.21 R = 1.21 \times 10 = 12.1 \Omega \simeq 12 \Omega$$

16. (*d*) Circuit can be reduced as follows

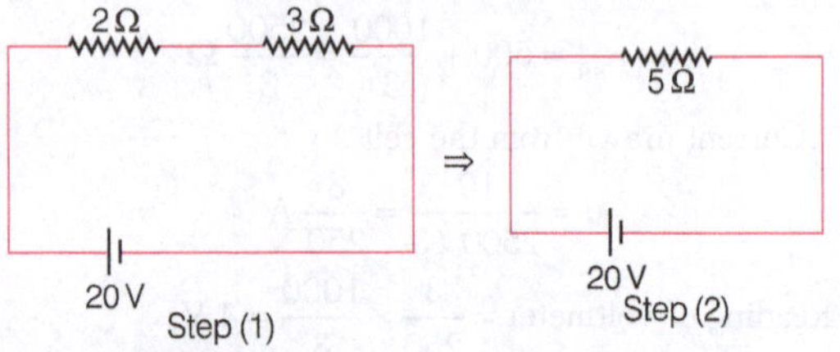

So, equivalent resistance of circuit, $R_{eq} = 5 \Omega$

$\therefore$ Current in the circuit $= \frac{20}{5} = 4$ A

As in parallel, current is divided according to resistance, so current flowing through each resistance $= 2$ A.

17. (*b*) For twisted wire, there are two halves each of resistance 2 Ω in parallel.

So, $\quad R_{eq} = \frac{2 \times 2}{2 + 2} = 1 \Omega$

18. (*a*) Equivalent resistance between B and C,

$$R_{BC} = \frac{(2+2) \times 2}{2+2+2} = \frac{8}{6} = \frac{4}{3} \Omega$$

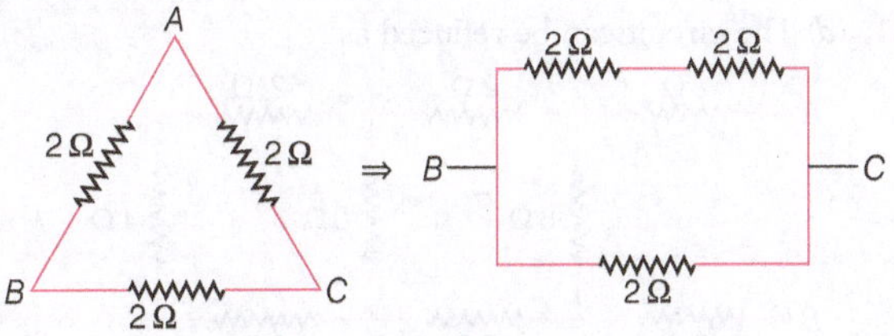

19. (*b*) Given circuit can be reduced to

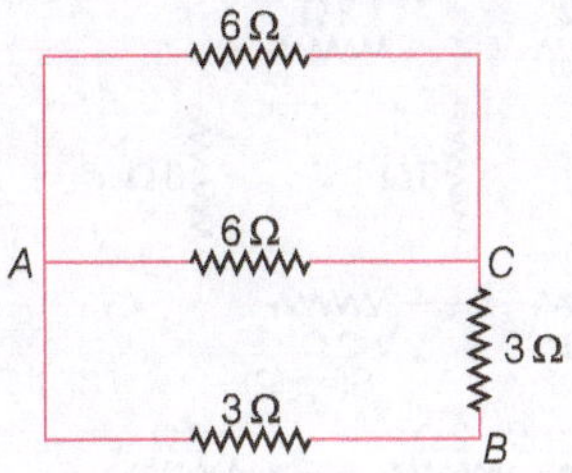

So, equivalent resistance between points *A* and *B* is equal to

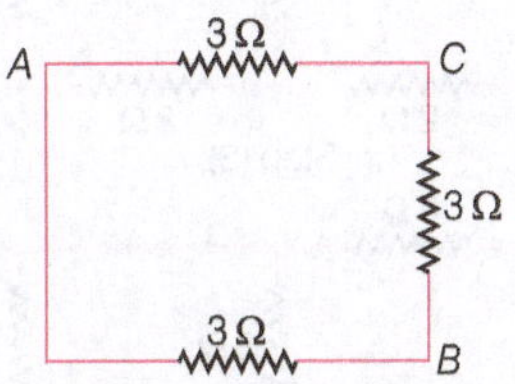

$$R_{eq} = \frac{6 \times 3}{6+3} = 2\Omega$$

20. (*c*) Given, $\dfrac{R_1 R_2}{R_1 + R_2} = \dfrac{6}{8}$ ...(i)

When one resistance say R_2 is broken, then

$$R_1 = 2\Omega \quad ...(ii)$$

From Eqs. (i) and (ii), we get

$$R_2 = \frac{6}{5}\Omega$$

21. (*a*) We have, $R = \rho \dfrac{l}{A}$

$$R \propto l$$

$$\frac{R_1}{R_2} = \frac{l_1}{l_2} = \frac{1}{2}$$

$\Rightarrow$ $R_2 = 2R_1$ ...(i)

$\because$ $R_1 + R_2 = 9$ ...(ii)

From Eqs. (i) and (ii), we get

$$R_1 + 2R_1 = 9$$

$\Rightarrow$ $R_1 = 3\Omega$

$\therefore$ $R_2 = 2R_1 = 2 \times 3 = 6\Omega$

Net resistance, $R_{net} = \dfrac{R_1 R_2}{R_1 + R_2} = \dfrac{3 \times 6}{3+6} = 2\Omega$

22. (*a*) The simplified circuit is as shown below

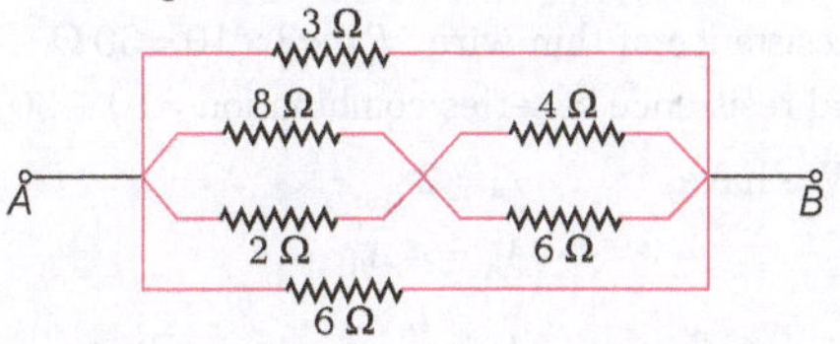

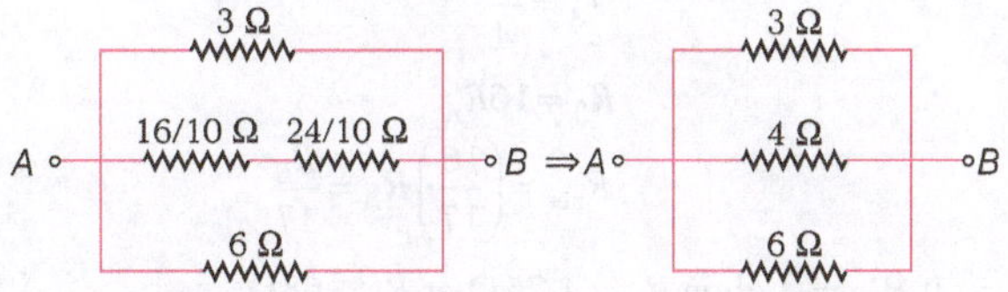

$$\Rightarrow \quad \frac{1}{R_{eq}} = \frac{1}{3} + \frac{1}{4} + \frac{1}{6} = \frac{4+3+2}{12} = \frac{9}{12}$$

$$R_{eq} = \frac{4}{3}\Omega$$

23. (*d*) Resistance, $R_t = R_0(1 + \alpha t)$

$$20 = R_0(1 + 20\,\alpha)$$

and $\quad 60 = R_0(1 + 500\,\alpha)$

From these equations, we can find

$$R_0 = 18.33\,\Omega,$$

$$\alpha = 4.54 \times 10^{-3}\ {}^\circ\text{C}^{-1},$$

$$R_t = 25\,\Omega$$

Again, $\quad R_t = R_0(1 + \alpha t)$

$$25 = 18.33(1 + 4.54 \times 10^{-3} t)$$

We find, $\quad t = 80^\circ\text{C}$

24. (*a*) The resistance of wire is given by, $R = \rho \dfrac{l}{A}$

For greater value of *R*, *l* must be higher and *A* should be lower and it is possible only when the battery is connected across $1\text{ cm} \times \left(\dfrac{1}{2}\right)$ cm (area of cross-section *A*).

25. (*b*) $\dfrac{1}{R_P} = \dfrac{1}{R} + \dfrac{1}{R} + \dfrac{1}{R} = \dfrac{3}{R}$

$\Rightarrow$ $R_P = \dfrac{R}{3}\Omega$

and $R_S = R + R = 2R\,\Omega$

$$R_{net} = R_P + R_S$$

$$R_{net} = 2R + \frac{R}{3} = \frac{7R}{3}\Omega$$

26. (*a*) Resistance, $R = \rho \cdot \dfrac{l}{A}$

For same material and same length, $\dfrac{R_2}{R_1} = \dfrac{A_1}{A_2} = \dfrac{3}{1}$

$\therefore$ $R_2 = 3R_1$

Resistance of thick wire, $R_1 = 10\Omega$ (given)

$\therefore$ Resistance of thin wire, $R_2 = 3 \times 10 = 30\Omega$

Total resistance of series combination $= 10 + 30 = 40\Omega$

27. (*a*) We have, $r_A = 2r_B$

$\therefore$ $A_A = 4A_B$

or $l_A = \dfrac{l_B}{4}$

$\therefore$ $R_B = 16R_A$

$$R_{\text{net}} = \left(\frac{16}{17}\right)R_A = \frac{R_B}{17}$$

If $R_{\text{net}} = 4$, then $R_A = 4.25\Omega$ or $R_B = 68\Omega$.

28. (*a*) Equivalent resistance of circuit,

$$R = 4 + \frac{3 \times 6}{3 + 6} = 6\Omega$$

and current through battery,

$$I = \frac{3}{6} = 0.5\text{ A}$$

Potential difference over

$$4\Omega = 0.5 \times 4 = 2\text{V}$$

Potential difference across the resistor of 3Ω over $6\Omega = 3 - 2 = 1\text{V}$

29. (*d*) The given circuit can be reduced to

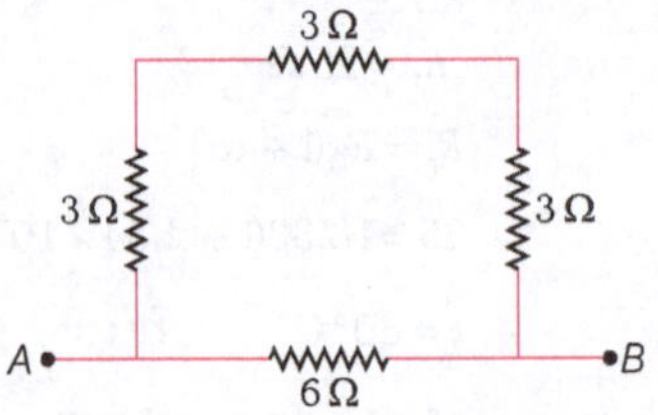

So, equivalent resistance between A and B,

$$R_{AB} = (3 + 3 + 3) \,||\, 6 = 9 \,||\, 6$$

$$= \frac{9 \times 6}{9 + 6} = \frac{9 \times 6}{15} = \frac{18}{5}\Omega$$

$\Rightarrow$ $R_{AB} = 3.6\Omega$

30. (*d*) The network can be redrawn as follows

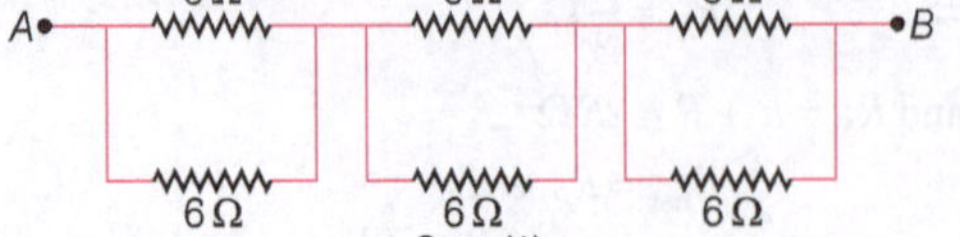

Step (1)

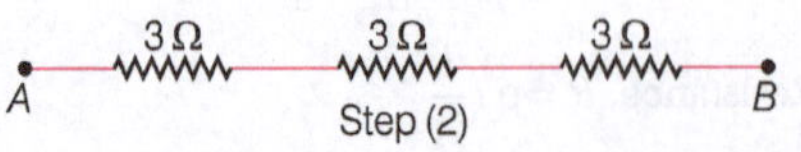

Step (2)

Now, there are three resistances in series.

So, equivalent resistance,

$$R_{\text{eq}} = 3 + 3 + 3 = 9\Omega$$

31. (*d*) The circuit can be reduced as,

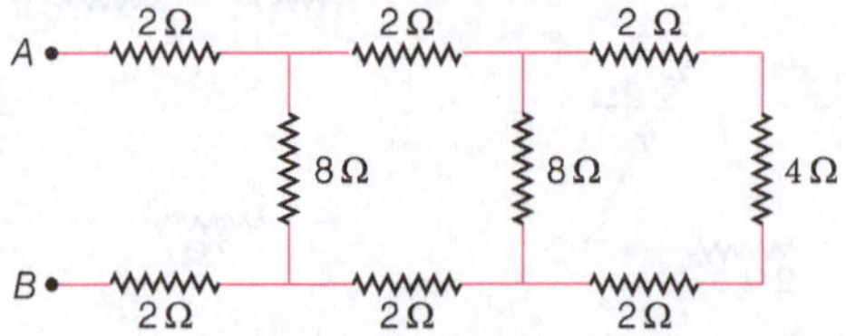

Step (1)

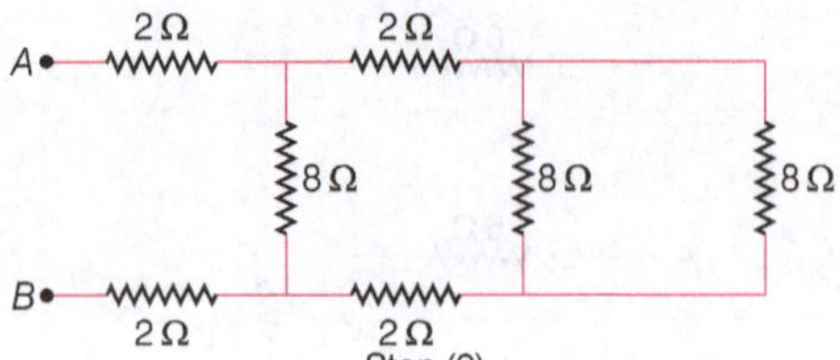

Step (2)

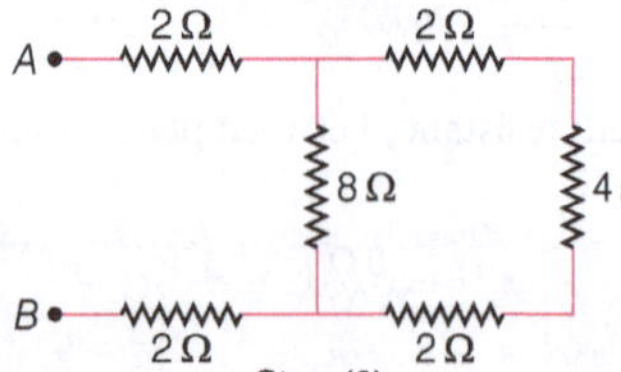

Step (3)

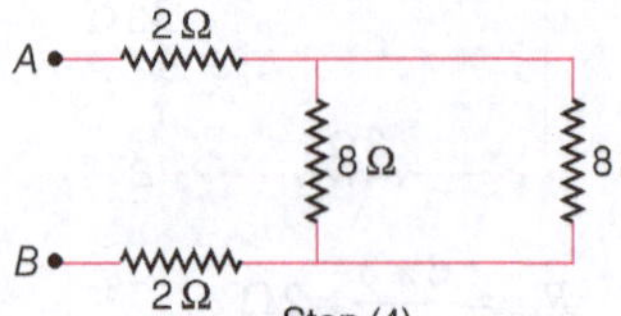

Step (4)

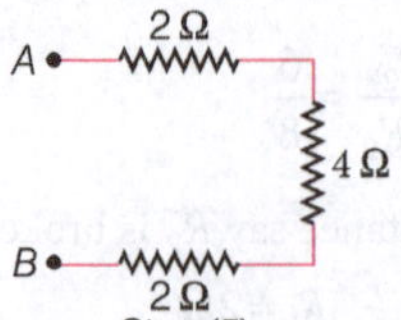

Step (5)

Now, equivalent resistance between A and B is

$$R_{\text{eq}} = 2 + 4 + 2 = 8\Omega$$

32. (*a*) The simple circuit is as shown below,

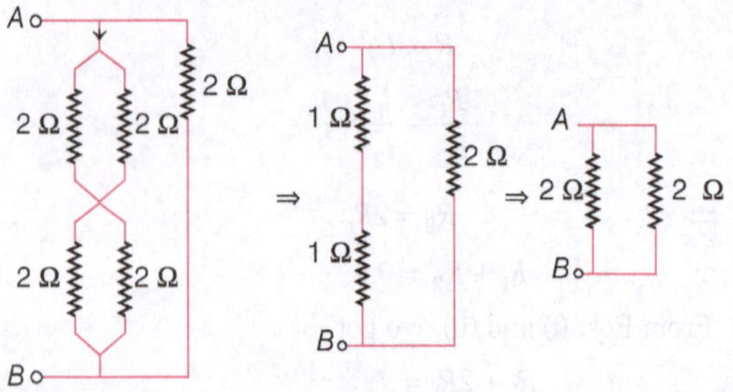

$\therefore$ The equivalent resistance across AB,

$$R_{\text{eq}} = \frac{2 \times 2}{2 + 2} = 1\Omega$$

33. (*b*) The simple circuit is as shown below

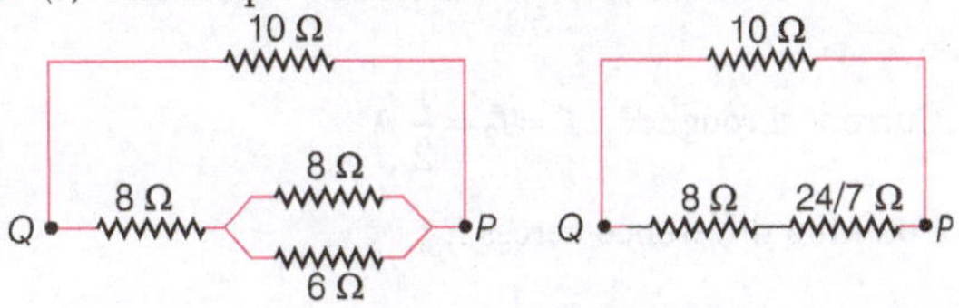

$$R_{\text{net}} = \frac{10 \times (8 + 24/7)}{10 + (8 + 24/7)}$$

$$= 5.3\Omega \simeq 5\Omega$$

34. (*d*) $R \propto l^2 / m \Rightarrow R_1 : R_2 : R_3 = \frac{l_1^2}{m_1} : \frac{l_2^2}{m_2} : \frac{l_3^2}{m_3}$

$$= \frac{25}{1} : \frac{9}{3} : \frac{1}{5} = 125 : 15 : 1$$

35. (*a*)

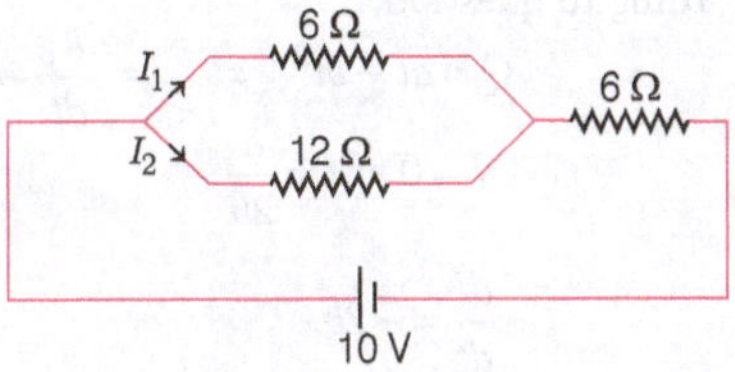

Resistance, $R = \frac{6 \times 12}{6 + 12} = \frac{6 \times 12}{18} = 4\,\Omega$

Total resistance, $R_{\text{eq}} = 6 + 4 = 10\,\Omega$

Current, $I = \frac{V}{R} = \frac{10}{10} = 1\,\text{A}$

The current in 12 Ω resistor is

$$I_2 = I\left(\frac{R_1}{R_1 + R_2}\right) = 1 \times \left(\frac{6}{6 + 12}\right) \Rightarrow I_2 = \frac{1}{3}\,\text{A}$$

The potential difference in 12 Ω resistor,

$$V = I \times 12 = \frac{1}{3} \times 12 = 4\,\text{V}$$

36. (*b*) $E_{\text{net}} = \dfrac{\frac{E_1}{r_1} + \frac{E_2}{r_2} + \frac{E_3}{r_3} + \ldots}{\frac{1}{r_1} + \frac{1}{r_2} + \frac{1}{r_3} + \ldots}$

$$\Rightarrow E_{\text{net}} = \frac{\frac{E}{r} + \frac{E}{r} + \frac{E}{r} + \ldots}{\frac{1}{r} + \frac{1}{r} + \frac{1}{r} + \ldots}$$

$$\Rightarrow E_{\text{net}} = \frac{\frac{nE}{r}}{n\left(\frac{1}{r}\right)} = E \Rightarrow \frac{1}{r_{\text{eq}}} = \frac{1}{r} + \frac{1}{r} + \frac{1}{r} + \ldots \frac{n}{r}$$

$$\Rightarrow \frac{1}{r_{\text{eq}}} = \frac{n}{r}$$

$$\therefore \quad I = \frac{E_{\text{net}}}{R_{\text{net}}} = \frac{E}{(R + r/n)} \Rightarrow r_{\text{eq}} = \frac{r}{n}$$

37. (*d*) Current in the circuit will increase because another resistance is connected in parallel to the circuit and hence, potential drop across the ammeter will increase. So, the potential difference over voltmeter will decrease because effective resistance decreases.

38. (*a*) Internal resistance, $r = R\left(\frac{E}{V} - 1\right)$

$$= (10)\left(\frac{1.5}{1.25} - 1\right) = 2\,\Omega$$

39. (*b*) Let resistance, $R = 100\,\Omega$

$$\therefore \quad R' = 100 + 100 \times \frac{10}{100} = 110\,\Omega$$

$\therefore$ Required shunt, $\Delta R = R' - R = 110 - 99 = 11\,\Omega$

40. (*b*) In potentiometer experiment, the emf of a cell can be measured, if the potential drop along the potentiometer wire is more than the emf of the cell to be determined. Here, value of emfs of two cells are given as 5V and 10V, therefore the potential drop along the potentiometer wire must be more than 10 V.

41. (*a*) From Ohm's law,

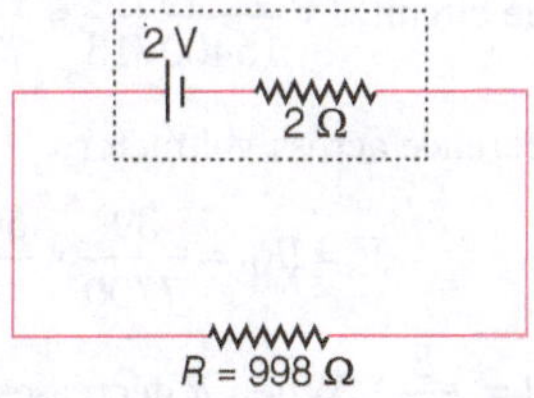

$$I = \frac{E}{R + r} = \frac{2}{998 + 2} = 2 \times 10^{-3}\,\text{A}$$

Potential difference across the voltmeter is

$$V = IR = (2 \times 10^{-3}) \times 998$$

$$= 1.996\,\text{V} \simeq 1.99\,\text{V}$$

42. (*d*) Resistance, $R = \frac{V}{I} = \frac{2}{4} = 0.5\,\Omega$

Resistance, $R = \frac{\rho l}{A} \Rightarrow 0.5 = \frac{\rho \times 0.5}{1 \times 10^{-6}}$

Resistivity of wire,

$$\rho = \frac{0.5 \times 10^{-6}}{0.5} = 1 \times 10^{-6}\,\Omega\text{-m}$$

43. (*b*) Current, $I = qf = q\left(\frac{v}{2\pi r}\right) = \frac{1.6 \times 10^{-19}\,(2.2 \times 10^{6})}{(2\pi)\,(5 \times 10^{-11})}$

$$= 1.12 \times 10^{-3}\,\text{A}$$

44. (*c*) Total cells $= m \times n = 24 \Rightarrow mn = 24$ ...(i)

For maximum current in the circuit,

$$R = \frac{mr}{n} \Rightarrow 3 = \frac{m}{n} \times (0.5)$$

$$\Rightarrow \quad m = 6n \qquad \text{...(ii)}$$

On solving Eqs. (i) and (ii), we get $m = 12$ and $n = 2$

45. (c) Current, $I_V = \frac{V_V}{R_V} = \frac{5}{20 \times 10^3} = 0.25 \times 10^{-3}$ A

$\therefore \quad V = I_V(R + r)$

$110 = 0.25 \times 10^{-3}(R + 20 \times 10^3)$

$R = 420\,\text{k}\Omega$

46. (c) $I = \frac{2+2}{1+1.9+0.9} = \frac{4}{3.8}$ A

For cell A, $E = V + Ir$

$\Rightarrow \quad V = E - Ir = 2 - \frac{4}{3.8} \times 1.9 \Rightarrow V = 0$

47. (b) Here, the resistances of 400 Ω and 10000 Ω are in parallel, so their effective resistance R_P will be

$$R_P = \frac{400 \times 10000}{400 + 10000} = \frac{5000}{13}\,\Omega$$

Total resistance of the circuit,

$$R = \frac{5000}{13} + 800 = \frac{15400}{13}\,\Omega$$

Current in the circuit, $I = \frac{6}{15400/13} = \frac{39}{7700}$ A

Potential difference across voltmeter,

$$V = IR_P = \frac{39}{7700} \times \frac{5000}{13} = 1.95\text{ V}$$

48. (b) Current, $I = \frac{E}{R+r}$. When R decreases to 0, $I = \frac{E}{r}$ and $V = IR = 0$.

49. (d) Effective voltage on charging, V

$= 4 \times 1.4 - 2 = 3.6$ V

Total resistance, $R = 8\Omega$

$\Rightarrow \quad I = V/R = 3.6/8 = 0.45$ A

50. (b) Electric field produced by charges accumulated on the surface of wire, provides force to the electrons to change the direction of current density.

51. (a) We know that in the given circuit,

$$\varepsilon_{eq} = \frac{\varepsilon_1 r_2 + \varepsilon_2 r_1}{r_1 + r_2}$$

Here, ε_{eq} is weighted average of ε_1 and ε_2.

Naturally, its value will lie between the value of ε_1 and ε_2,

i.e. ε_{eq} will be less than ε_2 and more than ε_1.

52. (c) Total resistance of the circuit,

$$R = R_4 + \frac{(R_1 + R_2) \times R_3}{(R_1 + R_2) + R_3} = 35 + \frac{(15+15) \times 30}{(15+15) + 30}$$

$$= 35 + \frac{30 \times 30}{30 + 30} = 50\,\Omega$$

Current in circuit, $I = \frac{50}{50} = 1$ A

Current through R_3, $I' = I_2 = \frac{1}{2}$ A

Potential difference across R_3,

$$V_3 = I' \times R_3 = \frac{1}{2} \times 30 = 15\text{ V}$$

53. (b) Potential difference across 100 Ω resistance is 5V. As voltmeter and 100 Ω resistance are in parallel. It means equivalent resistance of voltmeter and 100 Ω should be 50 Ω.

So, resistance of voltmeter must be 100 Ω.

54. (c) $q = \int_0^5 I\,dt = \int_0^5 (1.2t + 3)\,dt = 30$ C

55. (d) According to question,

$$Q = at - bt^2 \Rightarrow I = \frac{dQ}{dt} = a - 2bt$$

$$I = 0 \text{ at } t = \frac{a}{2b}$$

$$\frac{dI}{dt} = -2b$$

56. (d) Current, $I_1 = \frac{E_1 + E_2}{r_1 + r_2 + R}$ and $I_2 = \frac{E_1}{R + r_1}$

$\because \quad I_2 > I_1$

$\therefore \quad \frac{E_1}{R + r_1} > \frac{E_1 + E_2}{r_1 + r_2 + R}$ or $E_1 r_2 > E_2(R + r_1)$

57. (d) Let the three conductors having resistances R_1, R_2 and R_3 respectively, and the current drawn by them are 1 A, 2 A and 3 A respectively, when connected in turn across a battery.

$\therefore \quad V = R_1, \; V = 2R_2$ and $V = 3R_3$

So, $\quad R_1 = V, R_2 = \frac{V}{2}$ and $R_3 = \frac{V}{3}$

When the conductors are connected in series, across the same battery, then $V = I[R_1 + R_2 + R_3]$

$$\Rightarrow \quad V = I\left[V + \frac{V}{2} + \frac{V}{3}\right]$$

$$\Rightarrow \quad 1 = I\left[\frac{6+3+2}{6}\right] \text{ or } I = \frac{6}{11}\text{ A}$$

58. (a) Voltmeter has high resistance. So, most of the main current will flow through ammeter which is in parallel. So, it will burn out. No damage will occur to voltmeter.

59. (c) When wire is bent in the form of a circle, then between two points in any diameter,

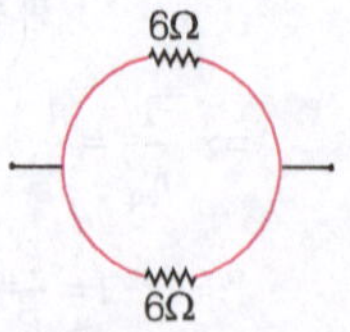

$$R_{eq} = \frac{6 \times 6}{6 + 6} = 3\Omega$$

60. (*a*) Potential difference = 10 V

So, $I = \frac{10}{5} = 2\text{ A}$

61. (*b*) In order to balance the bridge, the effective value of S must be equal to $2\,\Omega$.

So, $2 = \frac{S \times 6}{S + 6}$

$\Rightarrow \quad 2S + 12 = 6S \Rightarrow 4S = 12 \Rightarrow S = 3\,\Omega$

62. (*c*)

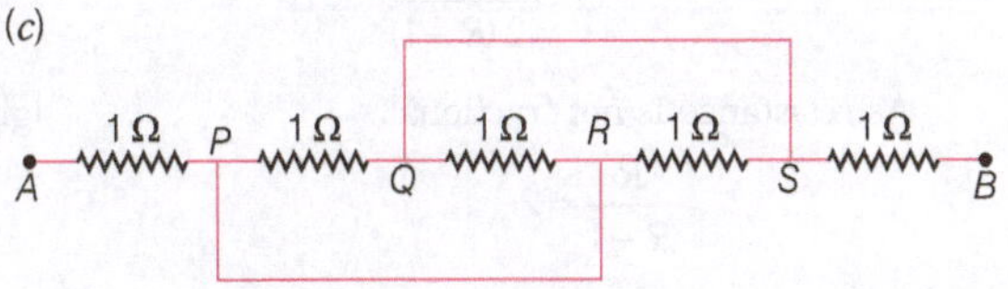

In circuit, resistance between PQ, QR and RS are in parallel. Now, circuit reduces to

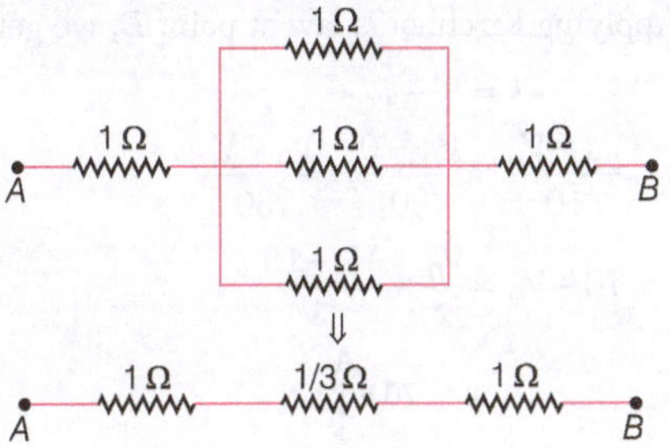

$\therefore \quad R_{AB} = 1 + 1 + \frac{1}{3} = \frac{7}{3}\,\Omega$

63. (*c*) Resistance, $R = 3 + 10 \| (3 + R) = 3 + \frac{10\,(3 + R)}{13 + R}$

Solving this equation, we get

$R = \sqrt{69}\,\Omega$

64. (*c*) The equivalent circuit can be drawn as

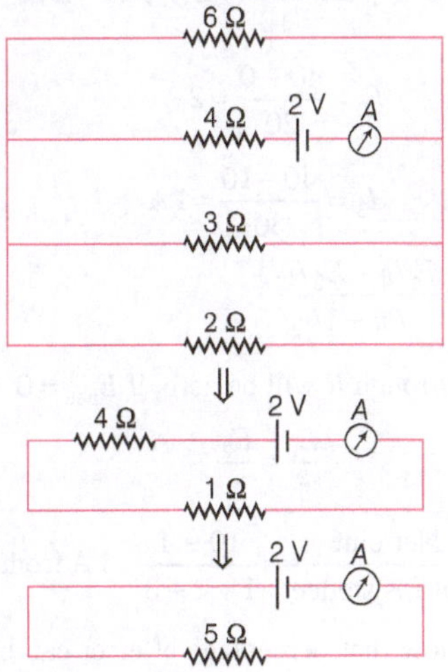

Current $= \frac{2}{5} = 0.4\text{ A}$

65. (*d*) Balanced condition for Wheatstone's bridge,

$$\frac{R_1}{R_2} = \frac{R_3}{R_4}$$

We have, $\frac{24 + X}{84 + Y} = \frac{10}{30} = \frac{1}{3}$ ...(i)

and $\frac{3}{1} = \frac{24 + 84 + X + Y}{10 + 30}$ $[\because V = IR]$

$= \frac{108 + X + Y}{40}$ ...(ii)

Solving Eqs. (i) and (ii), we get

$X = Y = 6\,\Omega$

66. (*b*) The given circuit can be redrawn as

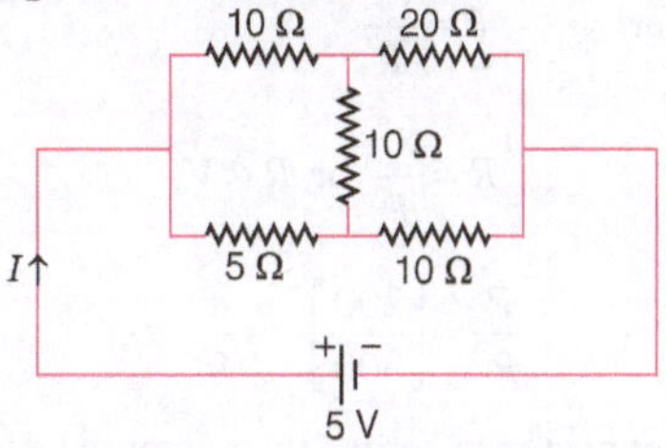

It is a balanced Wheatstone bridge and hence, no current flows in the middle resistor, so equivalent circuit would be as shown in figure.

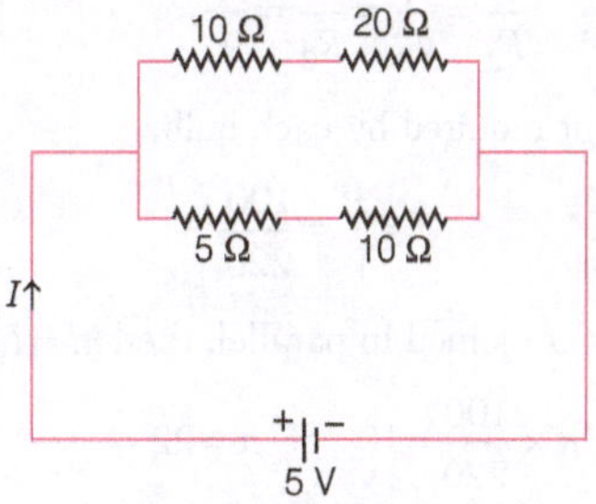

$10\,\Omega$ and $20\,\Omega$ resistances are in series,

$R' = 10\,\Omega + 20\,\Omega = 30\,\Omega$

Similarly, $5\,\Omega$ and $10\,\Omega$ are in series, $R'' = 15\,\Omega$

Now, R' and R'' are in parallel, $R = \frac{15 \times 30}{15 + 30} = 10\,\Omega$

So, $I = \frac{V}{R} = \frac{5}{10} = 0.5\text{ A}$

67. (*c*) We know that, when current flow is same, then resistors are connected in series, hence resultant resistance is

$R' = R_1 + R_2 = 10\,\Omega + 20\,\Omega = 30\,\Omega$

Also since, cells are connected in opposite polarities, the resultant emf is

$E = E_1 - E_2 = 5\text{ V} - 2\text{ V} = 3\text{ V}$

From Ohm's law, $E = IR \Rightarrow I = \frac{E}{R} = \frac{3}{30} = 0.1\text{ A}$

68. (c) Initially, $\frac{P}{Q}=\frac{l}{100-l}=\frac{20}{100-20}=\frac{20}{80}=\frac{1}{4}$

When a resistance of 15Ω is connected in series with the smaller of the two, i.e. with P, then

$$\frac{P+15}{Q}=\frac{40}{60} \Rightarrow \frac{P}{Q}+\frac{15}{Q}=\frac{2}{3}$$

$$\Rightarrow \quad \frac{1}{4}+\frac{15}{Q}=\frac{2}{3} \Rightarrow \frac{15}{Q}=\frac{5}{12}$$

$$\Rightarrow \quad Q=36\Omega$$

Resistance, $P=\frac{1}{4}\times 36=9\Omega$

69. (c) Power, $\quad P=\frac{V^2}{R}$

$$\Rightarrow \quad R=\frac{V^2}{P} \text{ or } R\propto V^2$$

i.e. $\quad \frac{R_1}{R_2}=\left[\frac{200}{300}\right]^2=\frac{4}{9}$

When connected in series, then potential drop and power consumed are in the ratio of their resistances. So,

$$\frac{P_1}{P_2}=\frac{V_1}{V_2}=\frac{R_1}{R_2}=\frac{4}{9}$$

70. (b) Current required by each bulb,

$$I=\frac{P}{V}=\frac{100}{220}\text{ A}$$

If n bulbs are joined in parallel, then $nI=I_{fuse}$

or $\quad n\times\frac{100}{220}=10$ or $n=22$

71. (b) Rise in temperature $=15°C$

Amount of water = 1L = 1000 cc = 1000 g

Heat supplied in cal $=1000\times 15\times 1$

$=1000\times 15\times 4.2$ (in form of joule)

$\therefore$ Power $=\frac{1000\times 15\times 4.2}{60}=1050$ W or (J/s)

72. (d) Average energy = 2 eV

$$\Rightarrow \quad eV_0=2eV_0$$

$$\Rightarrow \quad V_0=2\text{ V}$$

$\therefore$ Electric field, $E=\frac{V_0}{\text{Mean free path}}$

$$=\frac{2}{4\times 10^{-8}}=5\times 10^7\text{ V/m}$$

73. (d) By joining 2Ω and 6Ω in parallel, we get 1.5Ω and joining them in series, we get 8Ω.

So, values of R_1 and R_2 will be 2Ω and 6Ω.

74. (c) Higher the power, lower is the resistance and lower the resistance, thicker will be the element.

75. (b) Given, $\frac{R_1}{R_2}=\frac{1}{2}$

Let, third resistance is R.

So, $\quad \frac{1}{a}+\frac{1}{2a}+\frac{1}{R}=1$

$$\therefore \quad a=\frac{3R}{2(R-1)}$$

As resistance is not fractional. (given)

$$\therefore \quad \frac{R}{R-1}=2$$

So, $\quad R=2\Omega$

$\therefore \quad R_1=a=3\Omega$ and $R_2=2a=6\Omega$

76. (d) Applying Kirchhoff's law at point D, we get

$$I_1=I_2+I_3$$

$$\frac{V_A-V_D}{10}=\frac{V_D-0}{20}+\frac{V_D-V_C}{30}$$

or $\quad 70-V_D=\frac{V_D}{2}+\frac{V_D-10}{3}$

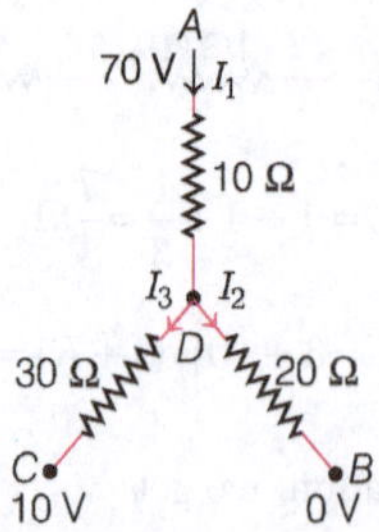

$$\Rightarrow \quad V_D=40\text{ V}$$

$$\Rightarrow \quad I_1=\frac{70-40}{10}=3\text{ A}$$

$$I_2=\frac{40-0}{20}=2\text{ A}$$

and $\quad I_3=\frac{40-10}{30}=1\text{ A}$

77. (b) $E_{net}=\frac{E_1/r_1-E_2/r_2}{1/r_1+1/r_2}$

Current through R will be zero, if $E_{net}=0$

$$\therefore \quad \frac{E_1}{r_1}=\frac{E_2}{r_2}$$

78. (d) $I=\frac{\text{Net emf}}{\text{Net resistance}}=\frac{10-4}{1+2+3}=1$ A from a to e.

79. (c) We know that percentage of error can be minimised by adjusting the balance point near the middle of the meter scale, i.e. around 50 cm. This can be achieved by adjusting the value of S. For balance point to be at 2.9 cm, we have the equation,

$$\frac{R}{S} = \frac{2.9}{97.1}$$

$$\Rightarrow \quad R = \frac{2.9}{97.1} \times 100 = 3\,\Omega$$

For balance point to be in the middle, the equation becomes

$$\frac{R}{S} = \frac{1}{1}$$

$$\Rightarrow \quad R = S$$

Here, $R = 3\Omega$

$$\Rightarrow \quad S = 3\Omega$$

So, the value of S should be changed from 100 Ω to 3 Ω to obtain reading in the mean position.

80 (*b*) No current will flow through the grounded wire.

$$\therefore \quad I = \frac{V}{2R}$$

81. (*d*) Net resistance of circuit, $R = 1 + 6 + 4 = 11\Omega$

$$I = \frac{6}{11}\text{A}$$

$$\therefore \quad V = 6 - 1 \times \frac{6}{11} = \frac{60}{11}\text{V}$$

82. (*a*) The given circuit forms a balanced Wheatstone bridge between points A and B.

i.e.

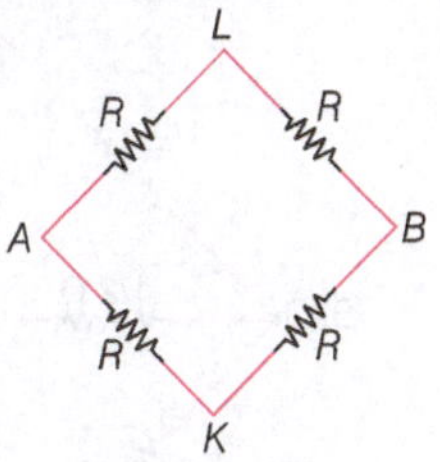

$$R_{AB} = (R + R) \,||\, (R + R)$$

$$= 2R \,||\, 2R$$

$$= \frac{2R \times 2R}{2R + 2R} = R$$

83. (*a*) The given circuit consists of a balanced Wheatstone bridge.

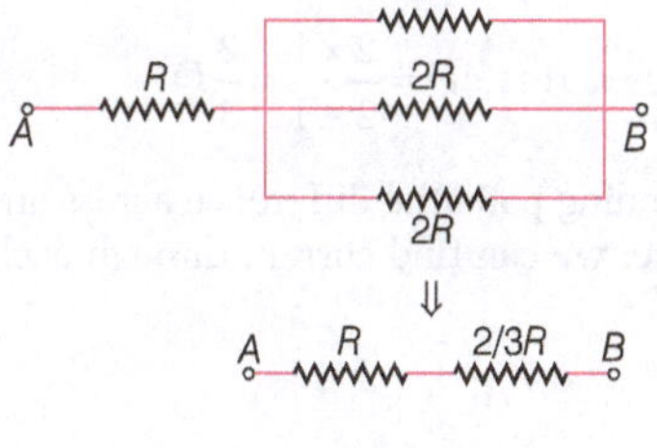

$$\therefore \quad R_{\text{net}} = R + \frac{2}{3}R = \frac{5}{3}R$$

84. (*a*) As $R_{AB} = R_{AO}$ and $R_{BC} = R_{OC}$, so points O and B will be at same potential and hence, resistance R_{OB} becomes ineffective. Similarly, as $R_{AO} = R_{AD}$ and $R_{OC} = R_{DC}$, resistance R_{OD} becomes ineffective.

So, excluding R_{BO} and R_{OD}, equivalent resistance R_{eq} of the given network between points A and C will be given by

$$\frac{1}{R_{\text{eq}}} = \frac{1}{2R} + \frac{1}{2R} + \frac{1}{2R}$$

$$\Rightarrow \quad R_{\text{eq}} = \frac{2}{3}R$$

85. (*d*) The circuit can be drawn as,

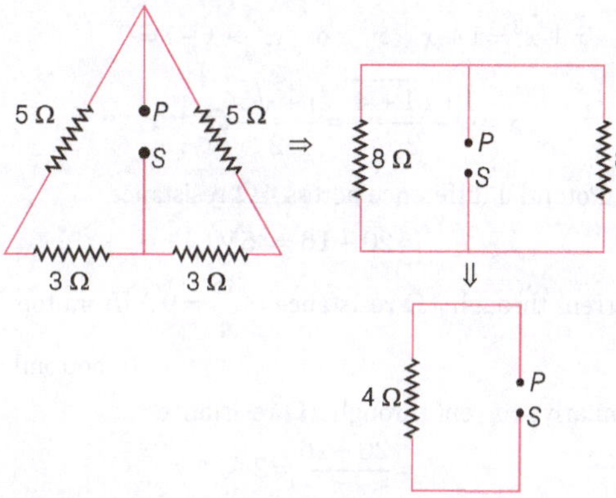

Resistance between points P and $S = 4\,\Omega$

86. (*d*) Power = 1.08 kW = 1080 W

$$P \times t = E \Rightarrow 1080 \times t = m \times L$$

$$1080 \times t = 100 \times 540 \times 4.2 \Rightarrow t = 210\text{ s}$$

87. (*c*) When key K is opened, bulb B_3 will not draw any current from the source. So the terminal voltage of source increases. Hence, power consumed by bulb increases. So, light of the bulb B_2 becomes more. The brightness of bulb B_1 decreases.

88. (*c*) $P' = P_1 + P_2 = 200 + 200 = 400\text{W}$

$$\frac{1}{P_{\text{eq}}} = \frac{1}{400} + \frac{1}{400}$$

$$P_{\text{eq}} = 200\text{ W}$$

89. (*b*) Maximum current possible in bulb

$$= \frac{50}{100} = 0.5\text{ A}$$

Resistance of each bulb

$$= \frac{V^2}{P} = \frac{100 \times 100}{50} = 200\,\Omega$$

If n be the number of bulbs possible, then total resistance of circuit $= \frac{200}{n} + 10$

Maximum current in the circuit $= 0.5 \times n$

So, $\frac{120}{\frac{200}{n} + 10} = 0.5n \Rightarrow n = 4$

90. (c) Let $R_{AB} = x$. Then,

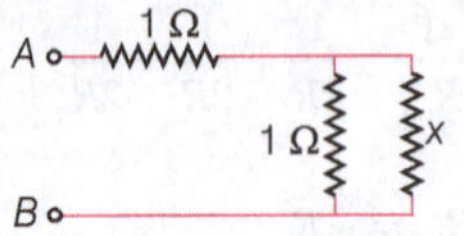

$$R_{AB} = 1 + \frac{x}{1+x} \quad \text{or} \quad x = 1 + \frac{x}{1+x}$$

$$\therefore \quad x + x^2 = 1 + x + x \quad \text{or} \quad x^2 - x - 1 = 0$$

$$\Rightarrow \quad x = \frac{1 + \sqrt{1+4}}{2} = \frac{1+\sqrt{5}}{2}\,\Omega$$

91. (a) Potential difference across 4Ω resistance

$$= 20 + 16 = 36\,\text{V}$$

Current through 4Ω resistance $= \frac{36}{4} = 9$ A [from top to bottom]

Similarly, current through 2Ω resistance

$$= \frac{20-16}{2} = 2\,\text{A}$$

Therefore, total current through 20 V battery will be 11 A.

92. (b) Current through R_1 and R_2 comes out to be zero (potential difference = 0).

$\therefore$ Current through $R_3 = \frac{\text{Net emf}}{\text{Total resistance}}$

$$= \frac{(4+3+2)-(2+3+2)}{3} = \frac{2}{3}\,\text{A}$$

93. (b) According to the question,

$$R = \left(20 + \frac{I}{2}\right)\Omega$$

Now, current, $I = \frac{250}{R} = \frac{250}{20 + (I/2)}$

$$\Rightarrow \quad I^2 + 40I - 500 = 0$$

Solving, we get $I = 10$ A

94. (a) The given three resistors are in parallel,

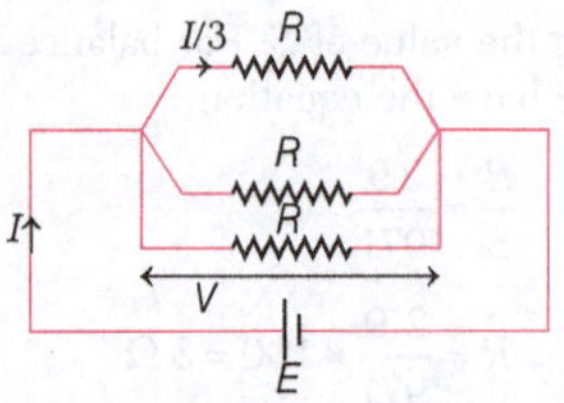

$$\therefore \quad \text{Current, } I = \frac{E}{r + R/3} = \frac{4}{1+3} = 1\,\text{A}$$

$$V = \frac{I}{3}R = E - Ir = 4 - 1(1) = 3\,\text{V}$$

95. (c) Resistance, $R_{\text{net}} = 2 + \frac{6 \times 2}{6+2} = \frac{7}{2}\,\Omega$

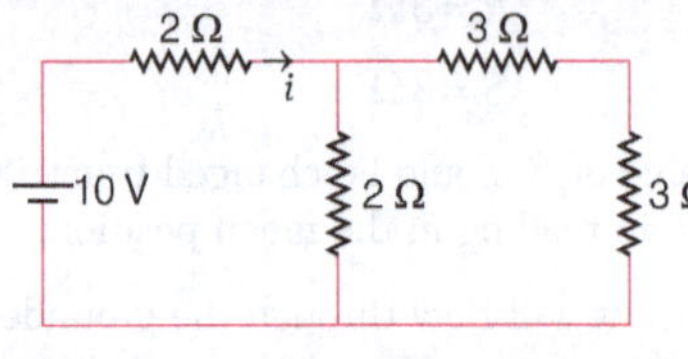

$$\therefore \quad I = \frac{10}{(7/2)} = \frac{20}{7}\,\text{A}$$

According to current division rule,

$$I_{3\,\Omega} = \left(\frac{2}{2+6}\right)I = \frac{1}{4}\cdot I = \frac{5}{7}\,\text{A}$$

96. (c) Both B and D are symmetrically located with respect to points O. Hence, the figure can be folded as shown in figure.

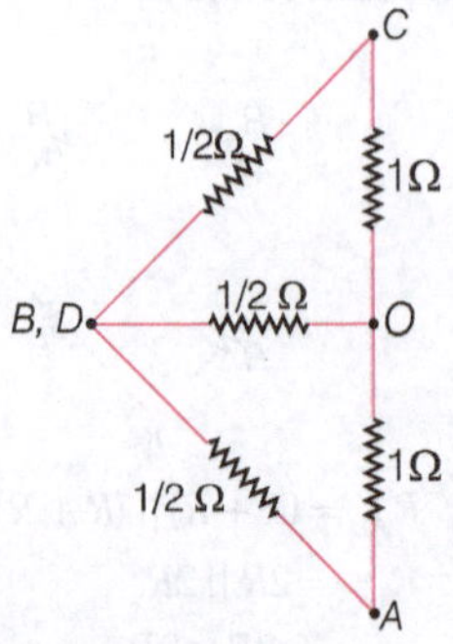

The given circuit forms Wheatstone bridge with DO or BO ineffective.

$$\therefore \quad R_S = 1 + \frac{1}{2} + \frac{1}{2} = 2\Omega$$

Resistance across $AO = \frac{2 \times 1}{2+1} = \frac{2}{3}\,\Omega$

97. (c) By finding potential difference across any resistance, we can find current through each resistance directly.

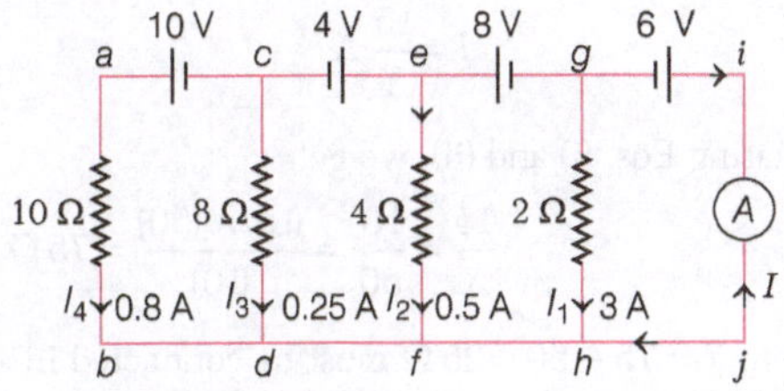

In loop *ghjig*, $-2I_1 - 6 = 0 \Rightarrow I_1 = -3$ A

In loop *efhge*, $-4I_2 + 2I_1 + 8 = 0 \Rightarrow I_2 = +\frac{1}{2}$ A

In loop *cdfec*, $-8I_3 + 4I_2 - 4 = 0 \Rightarrow I_3 = -\frac{1}{4}$ A

In loop *abdca*, $-10I_4 + 8I_3 + 10 = 0 \Rightarrow I_4 = \frac{4}{5}$ A

$\therefore \quad I = -3 - 0.25 + 0.5 + 0.8 = -1.95$ A

98. (*b*) We have, $\frac{V^2}{R} \times 16 = H \qquad (\because H = P \times t)$

$$\Rightarrow \quad \frac{V^2}{0.9R} \times t = H \Rightarrow \frac{V^2}{R} \times 16 = \frac{V^2}{0.9R} \times t$$

$\therefore$ Time, $t = 16 \times 0.9 = 14.4$ min

99. (*c*) Topmost and bottommost figures are short-circuited. Simplified circuit is shown below

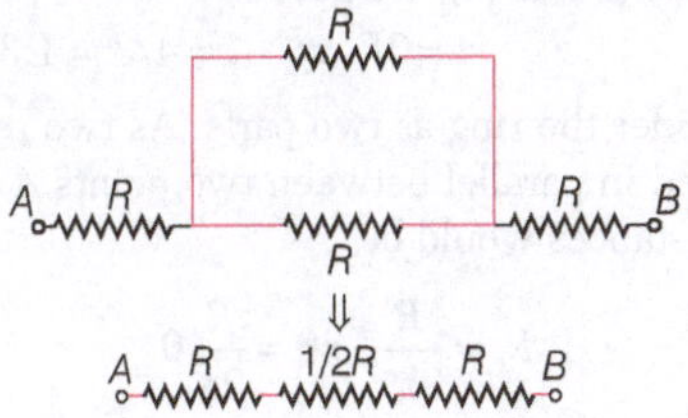

$$R_{eq} = R + R + \frac{R}{2} = \frac{5R}{2}$$

100. (*b*) Due to balanced Wheatstone bridge, resistance between *A* and *B* can be removed.

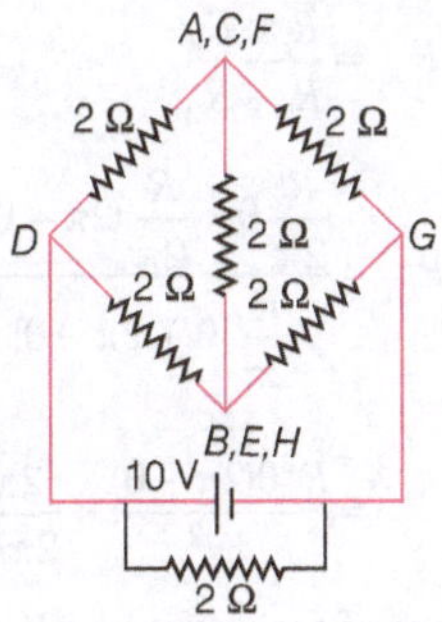

The current between *D* and *E*,

$$I_{DE} = \frac{10}{R_{DE} + R_{HG}} = \frac{10}{2+2} = 2.5 \text{ A}$$

101. (*b*) Resistance between upper branch and lower branch in parallel part is same, so equal amount of current flows through them.

Let main current is *I*.

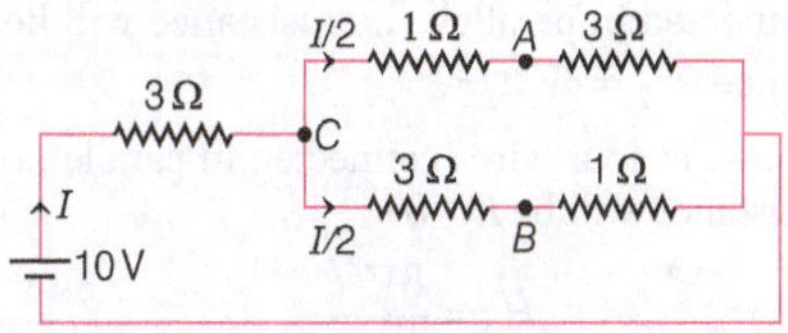

$$\therefore \qquad I = \frac{V}{R_{eq}}$$

Equivalent resistance of circuit,

$$R_{eq} = 3 + 2 = 5\,\Omega \Rightarrow I = \frac{10}{5} = 2 \text{ A}$$

So, current in each branch = 1 A

Now, $\quad V_C - V_A = 1 \times 1 = 1$ V ...(i)

and $\quad V_C - V_B = 1 \times 3 = 3$ V ...(ii)

Solving Eqs. (i) and (ii), we have

$$V_A - V_B = 3 - 1 = 2 \text{ V}$$

102. (*d*) When K_1 is closed, R_1 is short-circuited.

When K_2 is open, $I_0 = \frac{E}{r + R_2} = \frac{E}{r + 100}$ ...(i)

When K_2 is closed, $I_0 = \frac{1}{2}\left[\frac{E}{r + 50}\right]$ ...(ii)

From these two equations, we get $r = 0$

When K_1 is open and K_2 is closed,

$$\frac{I_0}{2} = \frac{E}{2(R_1 + 50)} \qquad \text{...(iii)}$$

From Eqs. (i) and (iii), we have

$$R_1 = 50\,\Omega$$

103. (*b*) In the circuit, we can see that 20 Ω, 100 Ω and 25 Ω are in parallel.

Net resistance of circuit $= 4 + 6 + \frac{1}{\frac{1}{20} + \frac{1}{100} + \frac{1}{25}}$

$$= 20\,\Omega$$

$$\therefore \qquad V = IR = 4 \times 20 = 80 \text{ V}$$

104. (*b*) As the other end of 8Ω resistor is grounded, which is at zero potential, the potential difference across 8 Ω resistor = 24 − 0 = 24 V

So, current in 8Ω resistor,

$$I = \frac{V}{R} = \frac{24 - 0}{8} = 3\text{A}$$

105. (c) Let R be the resistance of the wire, then

(i) The heat generated is $H_1 = \dfrac{V^2t}{R}$.

(ii) Resistance of each part will be $R/2$. When they are connected in parallel, the resistance will be $R/4$. Hence, $H_2 = 4V^2t/R$.

(iii) In case of four wires connected in parallel, the resistance will be $R/8$.

$$\therefore \quad H_3 = \frac{8V^2t}{R}$$

(iv) $H_4 = \dfrac{V^2t}{R/2} = \dfrac{2V^2 \cdot t}{R}$

Hence, largest amount of heat will be generated in case of four parts connected in parallel.

106. (d) Here, $2\,\Omega$ and $2\,\Omega$ are in parallel.

$$\therefore \quad \frac{1}{R} = \frac{1}{2} + \frac{1}{2}$$

$$\Rightarrow \quad R = \frac{2 \times 2}{2+2} = 1\,\Omega$$

Now, resistance $1\,\Omega$, $2\,\Omega$, $4\,\Omega$ and $1\,\Omega$ are in series.

$$\therefore \quad R_{net} = 1 + 2 + 4 + 1 = 8\,\Omega$$

Hence, current, $I = \dfrac{V}{R} = \dfrac{4}{8} = 0.5$ A

107. (a) It is clear that the two cells oppose each other, hence the effective emf in closed circuit is $18 - 12 = 6$V and net resistance is $1 + 2 = 3\Omega$ (because in the closed circuit, the internal resistance of two cells are in series).

The current in circuit will be in direction of arrow shown in figure

$$I = \frac{\text{effective emf}}{\text{total resistance}} = 6/3 = 2\text{A}$$

The potential difference across V will be same as the terminal voltage of either cell.

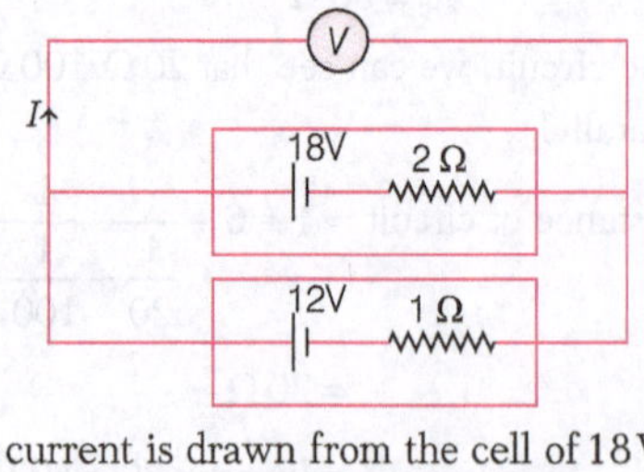

Since, current is drawn from the cell of 18 V, hence

$$V_1 = E_1 - Ir_1 = 18 - (2 \times 2)$$
$$= 18 - 4 = 14\text{V}$$

108. (b) The current in case of voltmeter of range 10 V and resistance $50\,\Omega$ is

$$I = \frac{10}{50}\text{ A} \quad \text{...(i)}$$

Let X be the resistance connected in order to make a voltmeter with range 15 V having current,

$$I = \frac{15}{X}\text{ A} \quad \text{...(ii)}$$

Equating Eqs. (i) and (ii), we get

$$\frac{15}{X} = \frac{10}{50} = \frac{(15) \times (50)}{(10)} = 75\,\Omega$$

Then, $R = 75 - 50 = 25\,\Omega$ must be connected in series, because $V \propto R$ when current is constant.

109. (a) The circuit diagram can be redrawn as the potential between A and B is

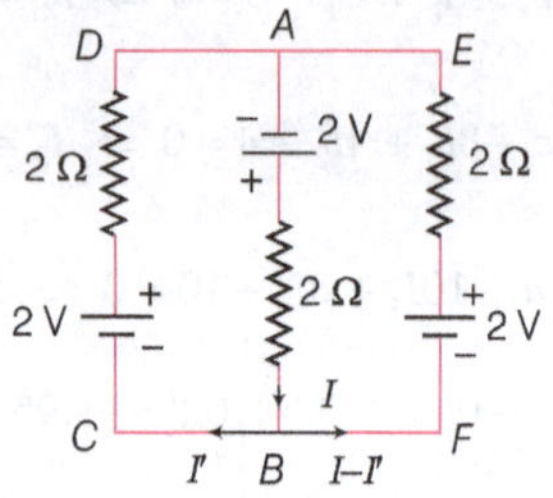

For the loop $ABCDA$, $+2 - 2I' + 2 - 2I = 0$

$$\Rightarrow \quad 2 = I + I' \quad \text{...(i)}$$

For the loop $ABFEA$,

$$2 - 2I + 2 - 2(I - I') = 0$$
$$\Rightarrow \quad 4 - 4I + 2I' = 0$$
$$\Rightarrow \quad 2 = 2I - I' \quad \text{...(ii)}$$

From Eqs. (i) and (ii), we get

$$4 = 3I \Rightarrow I = 4/3 = 1.33\text{ A}$$

110. (d) Consider the ring as two parts. As two resistances are joined in parallel between two points A and B, then two resistances would be

$$R_1 = \frac{R}{2\pi r} \cdot r\theta = \frac{R}{2\pi}\theta$$

and
$$R_2 = \frac{R}{2\pi r} r(2\pi - \theta) = \frac{R}{2\pi}(2\pi - \theta)$$

Now, equivalent or effective resistance between A and B,

$$R_{eq} = \frac{R_1 \times R_2}{R_1 + R_2}$$

$$\Rightarrow \quad R_{eq} = \frac{\frac{R}{2\pi}\theta \times \frac{R}{2\pi}(2\pi - \theta)}{\frac{R}{2\pi}[\theta + 2\pi - \theta]} = \left[\frac{\frac{R^2\theta(2\pi - \theta)}{4\pi^2}}{\frac{2\pi R}{2\pi}}\right]$$

$$= \frac{R^2\theta(2\pi - \theta)}{4\pi^2} \times \frac{2\pi}{2\pi R} = \frac{R\theta(2\pi - \theta)}{4\pi^2}$$

111. (c) Let the values of resistances be R_1 and R_2, respectively.

When R_1 and R_2 resistances are in series, then

$$R_1 + R_2 = 6 \text{ (according to question)} \quad \text{...(i)}$$

When R_1 and R_2 resistances in are parallel, then

$$\frac{R_1 R_2}{R_1 + R_2} = \frac{4}{3} \quad \text{...(ii)}$$

$$\frac{R_1 R_2}{6} = \frac{4}{3} \quad \text{[From Eq. (i), we get]}$$

$$\Rightarrow \quad R_1 R_2 = 4 \times 2$$

$$\Rightarrow \quad R_1 R_2 = 8 \quad \text{...(iii)}$$

We know that,

$$R_1 - R_2 = \sqrt{(R_1 + R_2)^2 - 4R_1R_2} = \sqrt{36 - 4 \times 8}$$

$$\Rightarrow \quad R_1 - R_2 = \sqrt{4}$$

$$\Rightarrow \quad R_1 - R_2 = 2 \quad \text{...(iv)}$$

From Eqs. (i) and (iv), we get

$$R_1 = 4\,\Omega, R_2 = 2\,\Omega$$

112. (*d*) Given, 6Ω, 6Ω and 6Ω are in parallel.

So, $$\frac{1}{R} = \frac{1}{6} + \frac{1}{6} + \frac{1}{6} = \frac{3}{6}$$

$$\therefore \quad R = \frac{6}{3} = 2\,\Omega$$

Now, 6Ω and 6Ω are in series.

So, $$R' = 6 + 6 = 12\,\Omega$$

$$\therefore \quad \frac{1}{R''} = \frac{1}{R'} + \frac{1}{12} = \frac{1}{12} + \frac{1}{12} = \frac{2}{12} \Rightarrow R'' = 6\,\Omega$$

The required resistance of the circuit $= 2 + 6 = 8\,\Omega$.

So, the potential difference,

$$V_A - V_B = IR = 0.5 \times 8 = 4\text{ V}$$

113. (*b*) As, resistances 1Ω, 2Ω and 1Ω are in parallel.

So, the required internal resistance,

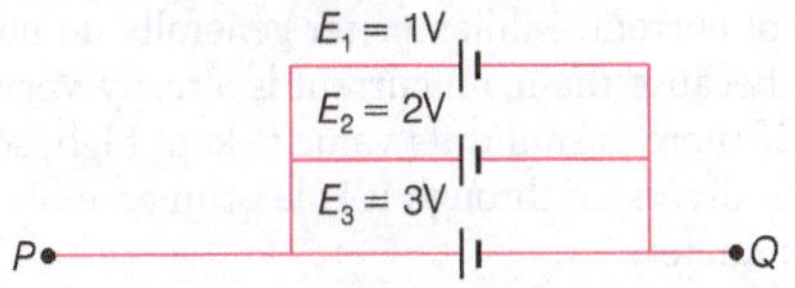

$$\frac{1}{r} = \frac{1}{r_1} + \frac{1}{r_2} + \frac{1}{r_3} = \frac{1}{1} + \frac{1}{2} + \frac{1}{1} = \frac{2+1+2}{2} \Rightarrow r = \frac{2}{5}\,\Omega$$

The potential difference between points P and Q,

$$E = \frac{\frac{E_1}{r_1} + \frac{E_2}{r_2} + \frac{E_3}{r_3}}{1/r} = \frac{\frac{1}{1} + \frac{2}{2} + \frac{3}{1}}{5/2}$$

$$= \frac{\frac{2+2+6}{2}}{5/2} = \frac{10/2}{5/2} = \frac{10}{5} \times \frac{2}{2} = 2\text{ V}$$

114. (*a*) Balanced condition for Wheatstone bridge,

$$\frac{P}{Q} = \frac{R}{S} \quad \text{...(i)}$$

where, $$\frac{1}{S} = \frac{1}{S_1} + \frac{1}{S_2} \Rightarrow S = \frac{S_1S_2}{S_1 + S_2} \quad \text{...(ii)}$$

From Eqs. (i) and (ii), we get

$$\frac{P}{Q} = \frac{R(S_1 + S_2)}{S_1S_2}$$

115. (*b*) Let, R_x resistance be connected in series to convert galvanometer to voltmeter.

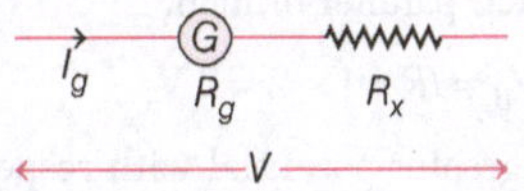

According to the question, $R_g = 100\,\Omega$, $I_g = 30\text{ mA}$

(Current corresponding to full scale deflection)

Now, we can write, $V = I_g \times R_g + I_gR_x = I_g(R_g + R_x)$...(i)

Given, $\quad V = 30\text{ V}$

From Eq. (i), we get

$$30 = (30 \times 10^{-3})\,(100 + R_x)$$

$$\Rightarrow \quad \frac{30}{30 \times 10^{-3}} = 100 + R_x \Rightarrow 10^3 = 100 + R_x$$

$$\Rightarrow \quad R_x = 1000 - 100 = 900\,\Omega$$

116. (*d*) We know that,

$$I = \frac{E}{r + R_{\text{eff}}} = \frac{15}{0.5 + 14.5} = \frac{15}{15} = 1\text{ A}$$

117. (*a*) As the current in heating filament increases, it gets more heated. Hence, its temperature increases and resistance also increases, due to which the current decreases.

118. (*a*) The balanced condition for Wheatstone bridge is $\frac{P}{Q} = \frac{R}{S}$.

As is obvious from the given values, no current flows through galvanometer.

Now, P and R are in series, so

Resistance, $R_1 = P + R = 10 + 15 = 25\,\Omega$

Similarly, Q and S are in series, so

Resistance, $R_2 = Q + S = 20 + 30 = 50\,\Omega$

Net resistance of the network, as R_1 and R_2 are in parallel, $\quad R_{\text{net}} = \frac{25 \times 50}{75} = \frac{50}{3}\,\Omega$

$$I = \frac{V}{R_{\text{net}}} = \frac{6 \times 3}{50} = 0.36\text{ A}$$

119. (*b*)

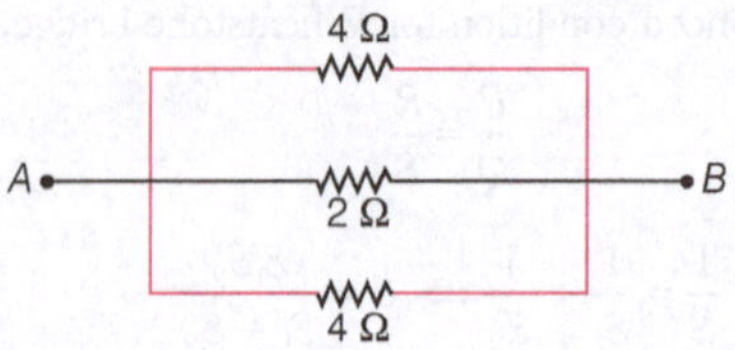

$$\frac{1}{R_{AB}} = \frac{1}{4} + \frac{1}{2} + \frac{1}{4}$$

$$R_{AB} = 1\Omega$$

120. (*d*) The resistances of branches *ABC* and *ADC* are in parallel. The current entering at node *A* will equally divided in each parallel branch.

$\therefore \quad V_A - V_B = IR = 1 \times 2 = 2\text{ V}$

Point *A* is at greater potential with respect to point *B*

So,

$$V_A - V_B = +2\text{ V}$$

121. (*c*) Let current through *XY* is I_3. Applying Kirchhoff's law to loops (1) and (2),

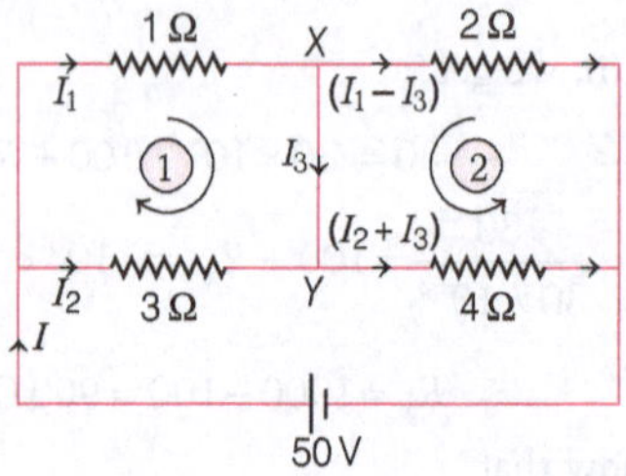

$$I_1 + 0 \times I_3 - 3I_2 = 0$$

$\therefore \quad I_1 = 3I_2 \quad$ ...(i)

and $\; -2(I_1 - I_3) + 4(I_2 + I_3) = 0$

So, $\quad 2I_1 - 4I_2 = 6I_3 \quad$ ...(ii)

Also, $\quad 50 = I_1 + 2(I_1 - I_3)$

$\therefore \quad 3I_1 - 2I_3 = 50 \quad$ ...(iii)

From Eqs. (i), (ii) and (iii), we get

$$I_3 = 2\text{ A}$$

122. (*b*) The simplified circuit can be drawn as,

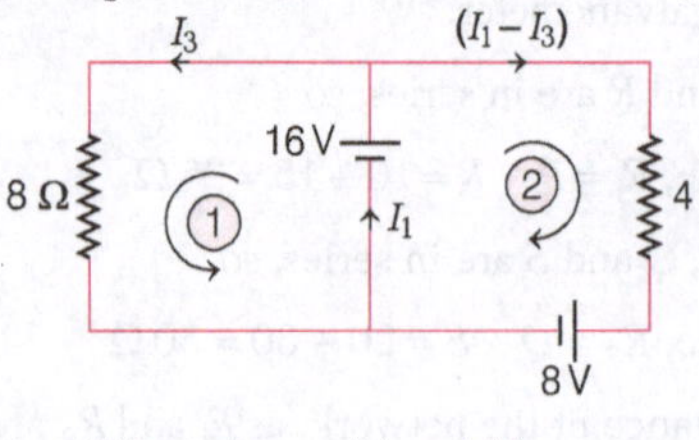

Applying KVL in loops (1) and (2), we get

$8I_3 = 16 \Rightarrow I_3 = 2\text{A} \quad$ ...(i)

and $4(I_1 - I_3) = 16 - 8 = 8$

$\Rightarrow \quad I_1 = 2 + I_3 = 4\text{ A} \quad$ [using Eq. (i)]

The current in a circuit is distributed depending on the value of resistance as shown below.

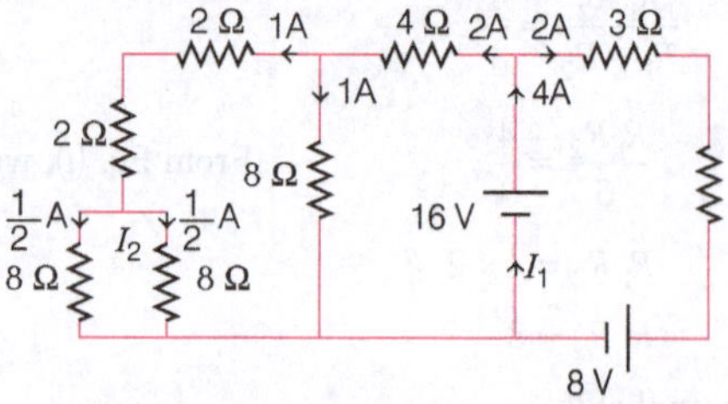

$$\therefore \quad I_2 = \frac{1}{2}\text{ A} \Rightarrow \frac{I_1}{I_2} = \frac{4}{(1/2)} = 8$$

Assertion and Reason

1. (*c*) R_1 and R_2 are resistances per unit length.

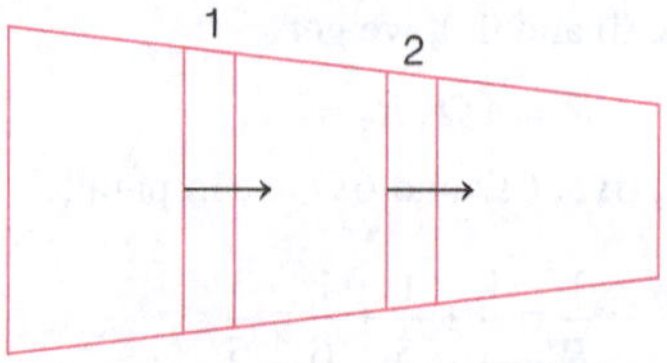

$$V_1 = I_1R_1$$

and $\quad V_2 = I_2R_2$

$$R_2 > R_1 \quad \left(\text{as } R \propto \frac{1}{A}\right)$$

As, $\quad I_1 = I_2$

Hence, $\quad V_2 > V_1$

2. (*d*) When we start switching ON different light buttons, then net resistance of the circuit decreases because all the connections are in parallel. Therefore, main current increases.

3. (*a*) The resistance of milliammeter becomes high because of increased number of turns of coil, so the torque produced in the coil is not decreased due to low value of current. Milliammeter generally do not have shunt because the main current is already very low. Even if there is shunt, its value is kept high, so that current diversion through it is least in case of milliammeter.

4 (*c*) In both cases potential difference across *R* is *E*.

$$\therefore \quad P = \frac{E^2}{R}$$

i.e., power remains same.

In second case, net resistance will decrease. Therefore, main current will increase.

5 (*d*) $\quad R = \rho\frac{l}{A}$ or $R \propto \frac{1}{A}$

Area of cross-section of wire *A* is less. Hence, its resistance is more.

Also, $H \propto R$, so more heat is generated in wire *A*.

Statement Type Questions

1. (b) Statement I is correct but Statement II is incorrect.

Consider a conductor of length l and area of cross-section A. Time taken by the free electrons to cross the conductor, $t = \frac{l}{v_d}$

Hence, current, $I = \frac{q}{t} = \frac{Al \times ne}{l \times v_d}$

$\Rightarrow \quad I = Anev_d$

$\Rightarrow \quad I \propto v_d$

Thus, current is directly proportional to drift velocity.

2. (b) Statement I is correct but Statement II is incorrect.

As $P = VI$, hence for the transmission of same power, high voltage implies less current.

Therefore heat energy loses ($H = I^2Rt/4.2$) are minimised if power is transmitted at high voltage.

3. (d) Both Statement I and Statement II are correct.

As we increase the temperature, more electrolyte dissociates and resistance decreases.

4. (d) Both Statement I and Statement II are correct.

Switching results in high decay/growth rate of current which result in a high current when bulb is turned ON or OFF (due to back emf). So, a bulb is most likely to get fused when it is just turned ON or OFF.

5. (a) Both Statement I and Statement II are incorrect.

In a battery circuit, the point of lowest potential is the negative terminal of the battery. And the current flows from higher potential to lower potential.

Match the Columns

1. (a) Suppose current i flows through the circuit.

$$10 - i - 3i - 15 - i = 0$$
$$-5 - 5i = 0$$

Current flowing, $i = -1$ A

Potential difference across battery A,

$$V_A = 15 - i \times 1 = 15 - 1 = 14 \text{V}$$

Potential difference across battery B,

$$V_B = -i - 10 = -1 - 10 = -11 \text{ V}$$

Power consumed by 3 Ω resistor

$$= I^2 R = (1)^2 \times 3 = 3 \text{ W}$$

2. (b) The simple circuit is shown in below figure

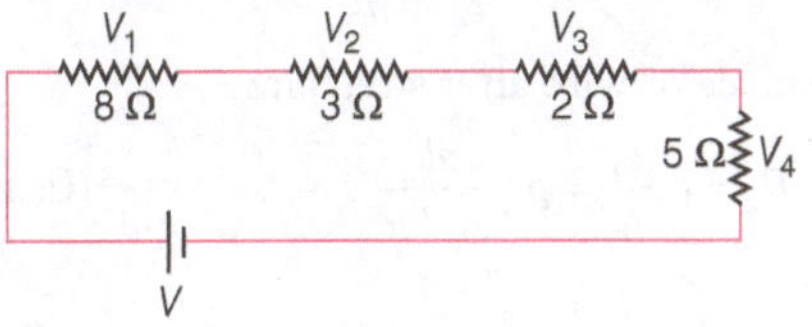

As, 3Ω and 6Ω are in parallel connection.

Hence, potential difference across 6Ω is also 20 V.

And, for 8Ω, $\frac{V_1}{8} = \frac{20}{3} + \frac{20}{6} = \frac{60}{6} = 10$

$\Rightarrow \quad V_1 = 80$ V

Similarly, for 12Ω and 4Ω,

$\Rightarrow \quad \frac{V_1}{8} = \frac{V_2}{3}$

$\Rightarrow \quad \frac{80}{8} = \frac{V_2}{3}$

$\Rightarrow \quad V_2 = 30$ V

$\Rightarrow \quad \frac{V_2}{3} = \frac{V_4}{5} \Rightarrow \frac{30 \times 5}{3} = V_4$

$\quad V_4 = 50$ V

Hence, A-(III), B-(I), C-(II) and D-(IV).

3. (b) In series, current is same and power of bulb $= I^2R = P$

and potential drop across and bulb is

$$V = IR$$

$\Rightarrow \quad V = I \cdot \frac{P}{I^2} = PI$

Clearly, when bulbs are in series, $V \propto P$

So, bulb of lowest power has lowest potential drop.

Hence, A-(II), B-(III), C-(IV) and D-(I).

4. (b) In parallel, $P = P_1 + P_2$

and in series $\frac{1}{P} = \frac{1}{P_1} + \frac{1}{P_2}$

Final Check Through PYQs

1. (b) Given, $R_0 = 2\,\Omega$

At $t = 80°$C, $R_t = 6.8\,\Omega$

We know that,

$$R_t = R_0 (1 + \alpha t)$$

$\Rightarrow \quad R_t = R_0 + R_0 \alpha t$

$\therefore \quad \alpha = \frac{R_t - R_0}{R_0 t} = \frac{6.8 - 2}{2 \times 80} = \frac{4.8}{2 \times 80}$

$$= 0.03 = 3 \times 10^{-2} \text{ °C}^{-1}$$

2. (d) Given, length, $l = 10$ m

Radius, $\quad r = \frac{10^{-2}}{\sqrt{\pi}}$ m

The current density,

$$J = \sigma E = \frac{E}{\rho} \qquad \text{...(i)}$$

So, $\quad \rho = \frac{RA}{l} = \frac{10 \times \pi \times \frac{10^{-4}}{\pi}}{10}$

$$= 10^{-4}\ \Omega\text{-m}$$

From Eq. (i), we get

$$J = \frac{10}{10^{-4}} = 10^5 \text{ A/m}^2$$

3. (*b*) Coefficient of thermal resistance α is positive for conductor and negative for semiconductor. Thus, on increasing temperature, resistance of conductor increases and resistance of semiconductor decreases.

4. (*a*) As we know that, the expression of the drift velocity,

$$v_d = \frac{eE}{m}\tau$$

Here, e is the electric charge,
E is the electric field,
m is the mass of an electron,
τ is the relaxation time.
Consider the conductor having length l, area of the cross-section A and the charge density n.

Electrical resistivity, $\rho = \dfrac{m}{ne^2\tau}$

Relaxation period, $\tau = \dfrac{m}{ne^2\rho}$

Current density, $J = \dfrac{I}{A} = \dfrac{neAv_d}{A} = nev_d$

Again, $\dfrac{E}{J} = \dfrac{E}{\sigma E} = \dfrac{1}{\sigma} = \rho$

$\therefore$ Electrical resistivity, $\rho = \dfrac{E}{J}$

The correct match is A-III, B-IV, C-I, D-II.

5. (*b*) Given, $R_1 = R_2, l_1 = l_2$

Since, resistance, $R = \rho \cdot \dfrac{l}{A}$

$$\Rightarrow \frac{R_1}{R_2} = \frac{l_1}{l_2} \cdot \frac{A_2}{A_1} \Rightarrow \frac{R_1}{R_1} = \frac{l_1}{l_1} \cdot \frac{A_2}{A_1}$$

$$\Rightarrow 1 = \frac{A_2}{A_1} \quad \left[\because R_1 = R_2 \text{ and } l_1 = l_2\right]$$

$$\Rightarrow \frac{A_1}{A_2} = 1$$

6. (*b*) Resistivity of copper (a metal) as a function of temperature increases with the increase in temperature as shown below

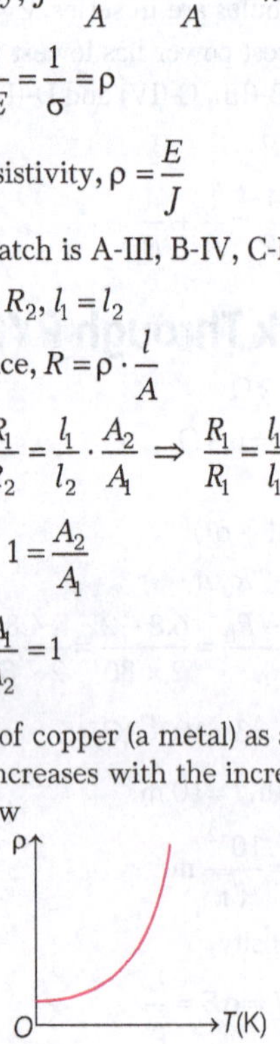

7. (*a*) Given, drift velocity,

$$v_d = 7.5 \times 10^{-4} \text{ m/s}$$

Electric field, $E = 3 \times 10^{-10}$ Vm^{-1}

As, mobility, $\mu = \dfrac{v_d}{E} = \dfrac{7.5 \times 10^{-4}}{3 \times 10^{-10}}$
$= 2.5 \times 10^6 \text{ m}^2\text{V}^{-1}\text{s}^{-1}$

8. (*c*) Among given devices, fuse is used in electric circuit as a protective device.
It helps in preventing excessive amount of current to flow in the circuit or from short-circuiting.
It has low melting point and low resistivity, so when excess amount of current flows in the circuit, it melts and breaks the circuit.

9. (*b*) For an ideal voltmeter, the resistance is infinite and for an ideal ammeter, the resistance is zero.
So, the current in circuit 1 is

$$R \times I = V$$

or $\quad 10 I_1 = 10$

$\Rightarrow \quad I_1 = \dfrac{10}{10} = 1 \text{ A}$

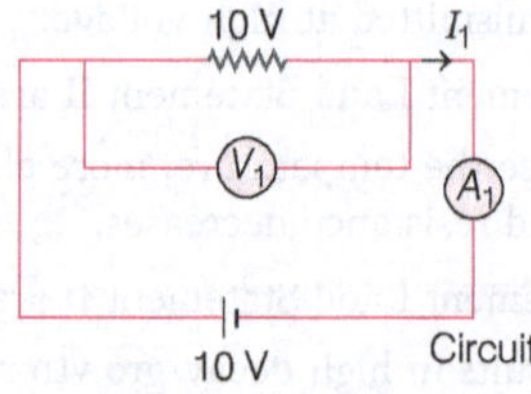

Circuit 1

$\therefore \quad V_1 = I_1 \times R$
$= 1 \times 10 = 10 \text{ V}$

Similarly, for circuit 2, the addition of 10Ω to voltmeter does not affect the current and hence,

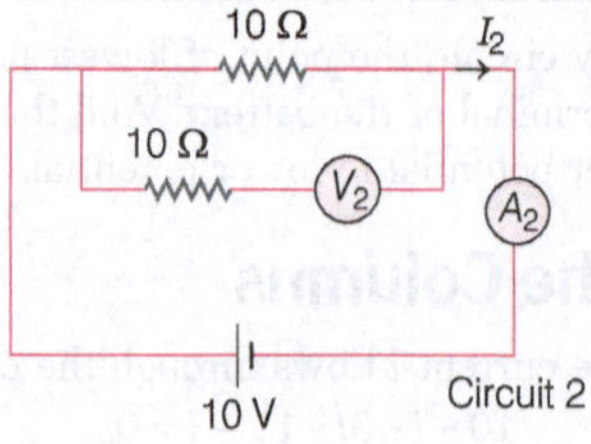

Circuit 2

$10 I_2 = 10$

$\Rightarrow \quad I_2 = \dfrac{10}{10} = 1 \text{ A}$

$V_2 = I_2 R = 1 \times 10 = 10 \text{ V}$

$\therefore \quad V_1 = V_2$

and $\quad I_1 = I_2$

10. (*c*) As volume remains same,

$$A_1 l_1 = A_2 l_2$$

Now, given $\quad l_2 = n l_1$

$\therefore$ New area, $\quad A_2 = \dfrac{A_1 l_1}{l_2} = \dfrac{A_1}{n} \quad$ ...(i)

Resistance of wire after stretching,

$$R_2 = \rho \frac{l_2}{A_2} = \rho \cdot \frac{n l_1}{A_1 / n} \quad \text{[Using Eq. (i)]}$$

$$= \left(\rho \frac{l_1}{A_1}\right) \cdot n^2 = n^2 \cdot R \quad \left[\because R = \left(\rho \frac{l_1}{A_1}\right)\right]$$

11. (*a*) The equivalent resistance between Q and S is given by

$$\frac{1}{R'} = \frac{1}{1.5R} + \frac{1}{3R} = \frac{2+1}{3R}$$

$\Rightarrow \quad R' = R$

Now, $\quad V_{PQ} = V_A = IR$

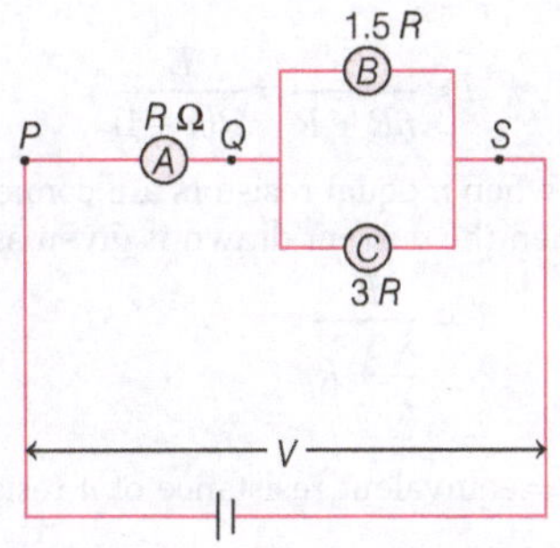

Also, $\quad V_{QS} = V_B = V_C = IR$

Hence, $V_A = V_B = V_C$

12. (*b*) As the cross-sectional area of the conductor is non-uniform, so current density will be different.

As, $\quad I = JA \quad$ ...(i)

It is clear from Eq. (i), when area increases, the current density decreases, so the number of flow of electrons will be same and thus, the current will be constant.

13. (*b*) Given, wire of length l is divided into 10 parts each having $\frac{100}{100}\Omega = 10\Omega$

According to question, 5 parts are connected in series,

i.e, $\quad R_1 = 5 \times 10 = 50\,\Omega$

5 parts are connected in parallel,

i.e, $\quad R_2 = \frac{R}{5} = \frac{10}{5} = 2\,\Omega$

When both R_1 and R_2 are connected in series

thus $\quad R_{\text{net}} = R_1 + R_2$

$\quad = 50 + 12 = 52\,\Omega$

14. (*a*) When 10 resistors, each of resistance R is connected in series, then equivalent resistance,

$R_s = R + R + R + \ldots$ 10 times

$\Rightarrow \quad R_s = 10R$

$\therefore$ Current drawn from the battery,

$$I_s = \frac{E}{R_S} = \frac{E}{10R}$$

$$\Rightarrow \quad I_s = \frac{E}{10R} \quad \text{...(i)}$$

In second case, when resistors are connected in parallel, then equivalent resistance,

$$\frac{1}{R_p} = \frac{1}{R} + \frac{1}{R} + \frac{1}{R} + \ldots 10 \text{ times}$$

$$= \frac{10}{R} \Rightarrow R_p = \frac{R}{10}$$

$\therefore$ Current drawn from the battery,

$$I_p = \frac{E}{R_p} = \frac{E}{R/10} = 10 \times \frac{E}{R} = 100 \times \frac{E}{10R}$$

$\Rightarrow \quad I_p = 100I$

$\therefore \quad n = 100$

15. (*d*) The four resistances have equal length, equal cross-sectional area and same material.

So, $\quad R_1 = R_2 = R_3 = R_4 = R$ (say)

Given, the effective resistance,

$R_{\text{eq}} = 0.25\,\Omega$

For parallel arrangement,

$$\frac{1}{R_{\text{eq}}} = \frac{1}{R_1} + \frac{1}{R_2} + \frac{1}{R_3} + \frac{1}{R_4}$$

$$\Rightarrow \quad \frac{1}{R_{\text{eq}}} = \frac{1}{R} + \frac{1}{R} + \frac{1}{R} + \frac{1}{R}$$

$$\Rightarrow \quad \frac{1}{0.25\,\Omega} = \frac{4}{R} \Rightarrow R = 1\,\Omega$$

For series combination,

$R_{\text{eq}} = R_1 + R_2 + R_3 + R_4$

$\Rightarrow \quad R_{\text{eq}} = R + R + R + R$

$\Rightarrow \quad R_{\text{eq}} = 4R$

$\Rightarrow \quad R_{\text{eq}} = 4(1) = 4\,\Omega$

16. (*b*) According to the given circuit diagram in question,

$I_1 = I_2 + I_3 \quad$ ...(i)

In parallel arrangement of the electrical circuit, the voltage remains same.

$\therefore \quad V = Ir \quad$ (using Ohm's law)

$\Rightarrow \quad I_2 r_2 = I_3 r_3$

$\Rightarrow \quad I_2 = \frac{I_3 r_3}{r_2}$

Substituting the values in the Eq. (i), we get

$$I_1 = \frac{I_3 r_3}{r_2} + I_3 \Rightarrow \frac{I_1}{I_3} = \frac{r_3}{r_2} + 1$$

$$\Rightarrow \quad \frac{I_3}{I_1} = \frac{r_2}{r_3 + r_2}$$

17. (*b*) Equivalent resistance between points A and B is given as

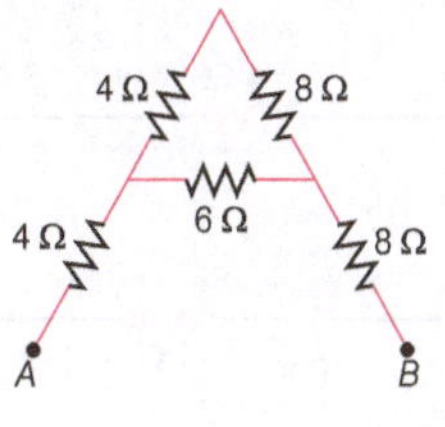

$$R_{AB} = [(4+8) \,||\, 6] + 4 + 8$$

$$= [12 \,||\, 6] + 12 = \left[\frac{12 \times 6}{12 + 6}\right] + 12$$

$$= [4] + 12 = 16\Omega$$

18. (a) Net resistance of a metal wire having resistivity ρ, we have

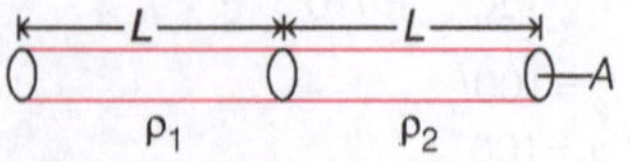

$$R_1 = \rho_1 \frac{L}{A}$$

Similarly, $R_2 = \rho_2 \frac{L}{A}$

Then, net effective resistance of two metal wires,

$$R_{eq} = R_1 + R_2$$

$$\Rightarrow \quad \rho \frac{2L}{A} = \rho_1 \frac{L}{A} + \rho_2 \frac{L}{A}$$

$$\Rightarrow \quad 2\rho = \rho_1 + \rho_2$$

As, conductivity, $\sigma = \frac{1}{\rho}$, we have

$$\frac{2}{\sigma} = \frac{1}{\sigma_1} + \frac{1}{\sigma_2} \Rightarrow \frac{2}{\sigma} = \frac{\sigma_1 + \sigma_2}{\sigma_1 \sigma_2}$$

$\Rightarrow$ Net effective conductivity of combined wires,

$$\sigma = \frac{2\sigma_1\sigma_2}{\sigma_1 + \sigma_2}$$

19. (a) Effective resistance of a circuit,

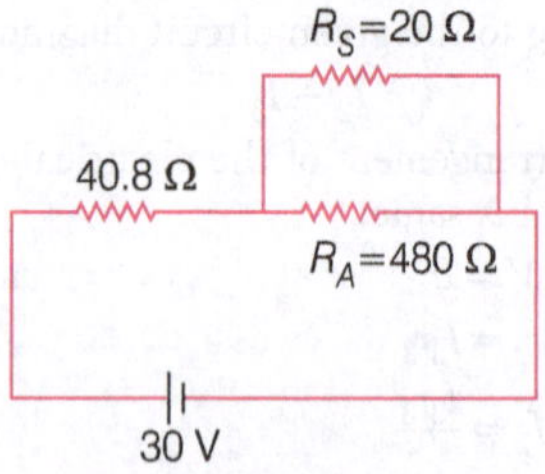

$$R_{eff} = 40.8 + \frac{480 \times 20}{480 + 20}$$

$$= 40.8 + 19.2 = 60\,\Omega$$

So, current flowing across ammeter,

$$I = \frac{V}{R} = \frac{30}{60} = \frac{1}{2} = 0.5\text{ A}$$

Hence, reading of ammeter = 0.5 A

20. (c) Given,

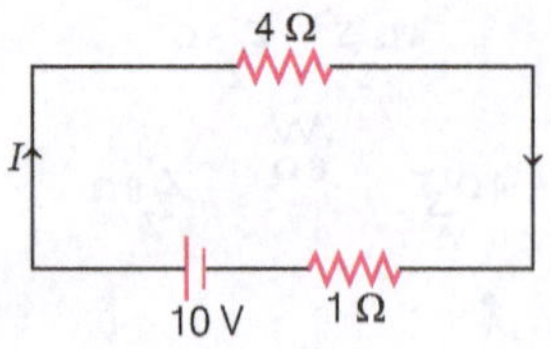

Current in circuit, $I = \frac{10}{4+1} = 2\text{ A}$

Terminal voltage $= E - Ir$

$$= 10 - 2 \times 1 = 8\text{ V}$$

21. (c) When n equal resistors of resistance R are connected in series, then the current drawn is given as

$$I = \frac{E}{nR + r}$$

where, nR = equivalent resistance of n resistors in series and r = internal resistance of battery.

Given, $\quad r = R$

$$\Rightarrow \quad I = \frac{E}{nR + R} = \frac{E}{R(n+1)} \quad \text{...(i)}$$

Similarly, when n equal resistors are connected in parallel, then the current drawn is given as

$$I' = \frac{E}{\frac{R}{n} + R}$$

where, $\frac{R}{n}$ = equivalent resistance of n resistors in parallel.

Given, $\quad I' = 10I$

$$\Rightarrow \quad 10I = \frac{E}{\frac{R}{n} + R} = \frac{nE}{(n+1)R} \quad \text{...(ii)}$$

Substituting the value of I from Eq. (i) in Eq. (ii), we get

$$10\left(\frac{E}{R(n+1)}\right) = \frac{nE}{R(n+1)}$$

$$\Rightarrow \quad n = 10$$

22. (c) If n identical cells are connected in series, then Equivalent emf of the combination,

$$E_{eq} = nE$$

Equivalent internal resistance,

$$r_{eq} = nr$$

$$\therefore \text{ Current, } I = \frac{E_{eq}}{r_{eq}} = \frac{nE}{nr}$$

or $\quad I = \frac{E}{r}$ = constant

Thus, current (I) is independent of the number of cells (n) present in the circuit.

Therefore, option (c) is correct.

23. (b) Given, $\quad P_1 = 1\text{ kW}$

$$P_2 = 2\text{ kW}$$

$$P_{series} = \frac{P_1P_2}{P_1 + P_2}$$

and $\quad P_{parallel} = P_1 + P_2$

According to question,

$$\frac{P_{series}}{P_{parallel}} = \frac{\frac{1 \times 2}{1+2}}{1+2} = \frac{2}{3 \times 3} = \frac{2}{9}$$

24. (*b*) The given situation is shown below,

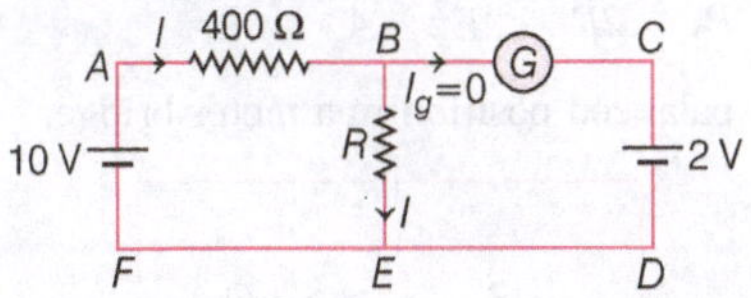

Applying Kirchhoff's voltage law in the loop *ABCDEFA*, we get

$$400I + 2 - 10 = 0$$

$$\Rightarrow \quad I = \frac{8}{400} = \frac{1}{50}\text{ A}$$

Applying Kirchhoff's voltage law in loop *ABEFA*, we get

$$400I + RI - 10 = 0$$

$$\Rightarrow \quad (400 + R)I = 10$$

$$\Rightarrow \quad (400 + R) \times \frac{1}{50} = 100$$

$$\Rightarrow \quad 400 + R = 500$$

$$\Rightarrow \quad R = 100\,\Omega$$

25. (*a*) The circuit diagram is shown as

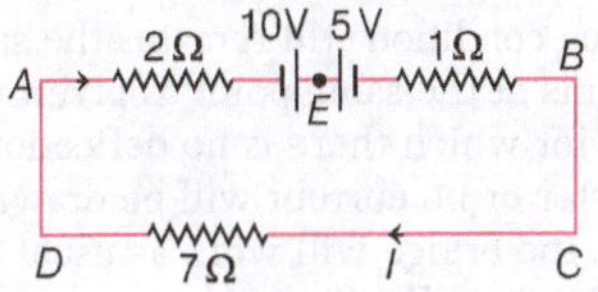

Applying KVL in the closed loop *AEBCDA*,

$$2I - 10 + 5 + I \cdot 1 + 7I = 0$$

$$\Rightarrow \quad 10I = 5$$

$$\Rightarrow \quad I = 0.5\text{ A}$$

Since, current is positive, hence direction of current is from *A* to *B* through *E*.

26. (*a*) The given situation is shown in the following circuit diagram.

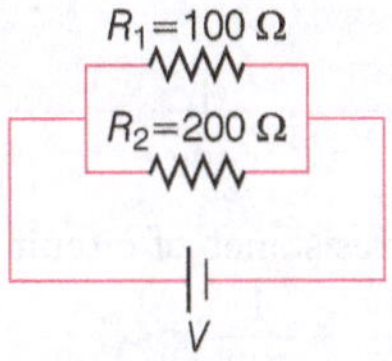

Let, these two resistors are connected with a battery of voltage *V* volts.

Hence, potential difference across R_1 and *R* are given as

$$V_1 = V_2 = V\text{ volts}$$

If H_1 and H_2 are thermal energy produced through resistances R_1 and R_2 in time *t*, then

$$H_1 = \frac{V_1^2}{R_1}t = \frac{V^2 t}{100}$$

and $$H_2 = \frac{V_2^2 t}{R_2} = \frac{V^2 t}{200}$$

Hence, $$\frac{H_1}{H_2} = \frac{V^2 t/100}{V^2 t/200} = \frac{200}{100} = \frac{2}{1}$$

$$\Rightarrow H_1 : H_2 = 2 : 1$$

27. (*d*) Given, power radiated by transmitter,

$$P = 100\text{ kW} = 10^5\text{ W}$$

$\therefore$ Time, $t = 1\text{ h} = 60 \times 60\text{ s} = 3.6 \times 10^3\text{ s}$

$\therefore$Energy radiated by the transmitter,

$$E = P \times t$$

$$= 10^5 \times 3.6 \times 10^3$$

$$= 3.6 \times 10^8\text{ J} = 36 \times 10^7\text{ J}$$

28. (*a*) For the most precise measurement of unknown resistance *X*, the resistances *P* and *Q* should be approximately equal and should be small, so that it could decrease error in experiment.

29. (*b*) The circuit diagram is shown below.

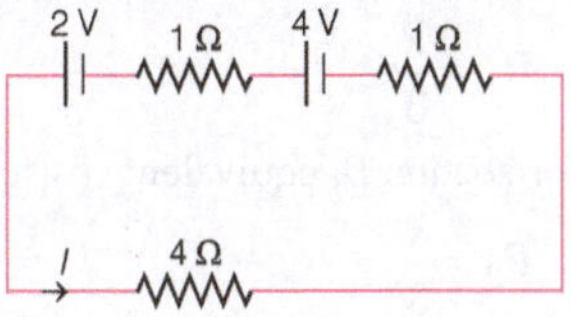

Applying KVL in the loop, we get

$$4I + I \cdot 1 - 4 + I \cdot 1 - 2 = 0$$

$$\Rightarrow \quad 6I = 6 \Rightarrow I = 1\text{ A}$$

30. (*a*) According to the question, the meter bridge is shown below

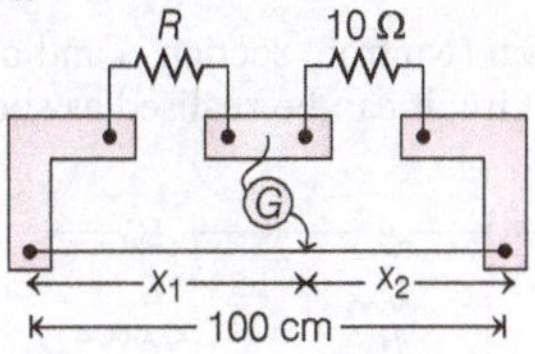

Given, $\frac{x_1}{x_2} = \frac{3}{2}$

At balance condition in meter bridge,

$$\frac{R}{10} = \frac{x_1}{x_2} \Rightarrow R = \frac{x_1}{x_2} \times 10 = \frac{3}{2} \times 10 = 15\,\Omega$$

Now, length of given wire whose resistance 15 Ω is 1.5 m.

Therefore, length of 1 Ω resistance wire is

$$= \frac{1.5}{15} = \frac{1}{10} = 0.1 = 1 \times 10^{-1}\text{ m}$$

31. (*b*) The circuit diagram is given below.

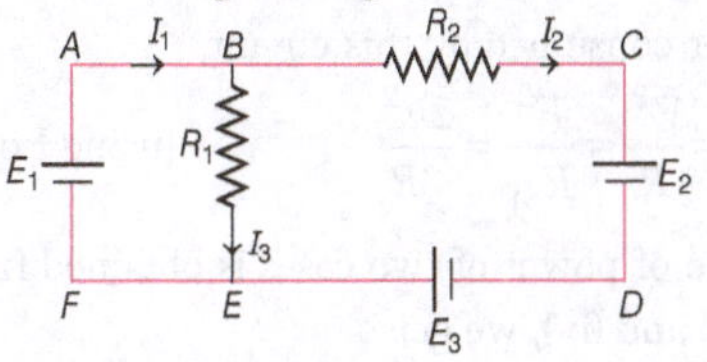

Applying KVL rule in loop *BCDEB*,

$$R_2I_2 + E_2 - E_3 - I_3 R_1 = 0$$

32. (*a*) **Case I** When all bulbs are glowing, then the circuit can be realised as shown in the figure.

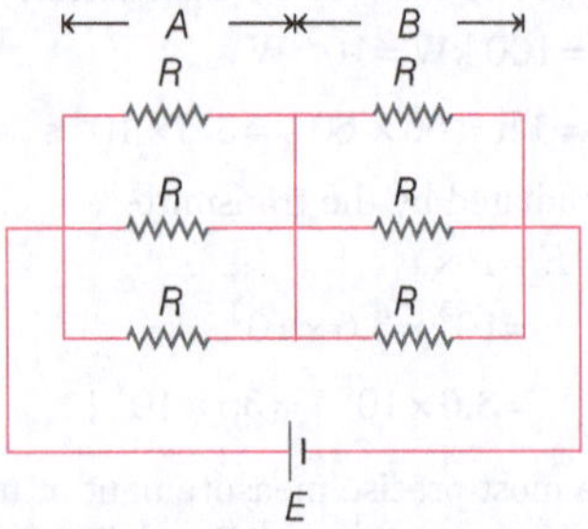

∴ The equivalent resistance of this circuit is

$$R_{eq} = R_A + R_B$$

As, section *A* has three parallel resistance, so equivalent resistance,

$$R_A = \frac{R}{3}$$

Similarly, for section *B*, equivalent resistance,

$$R_B = \frac{R}{3}$$

$$\therefore \quad R_{eq} = \frac{R}{3} + \frac{R}{3} = \frac{2R}{3} \quad \text{... (i)}$$

Thus, power consumed in this circuit,

$$P_1 = \frac{V^2}{R} = \frac{E^2}{R_{eq}} = \frac{3E^2}{2R} \quad \text{[using Eq. (i)] ...(ii)}$$

Case II When two from section *A* and one from section *B* glow, the circuit can be realised as shown in the figure below.

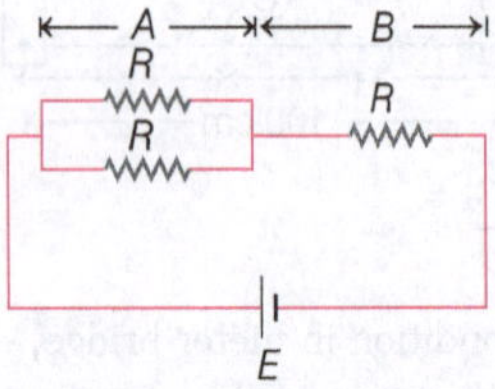

∴ Equivalent resistance of section *A*,

$$R_A = \frac{R}{2}$$

and of section *B*, $R_B = R$

Thus, equivalent resistance of the entire circuit becomes

$$R_{eq} = R_A + R_B = \frac{R}{2} + R = \frac{3R}{2} \quad \text{...(iii)}$$

∴ Power consumed by this circuit,

$$P_2 = \frac{V^2}{R} = \frac{E^2}{R_{eq}} = \frac{2E^2}{3R} \quad \text{[using Eq. (iii)] ...(iv)}$$

So, ratio of power of two cases is obtained from Eqs. (ii) and (iv), we get

$$\frac{P_1}{P_2} = \frac{3E^2}{2R} \times \frac{3R}{2E^2} = \frac{9}{4} \text{ or } 9:4$$

33. (*d*) For balanced position in a meter bridge,

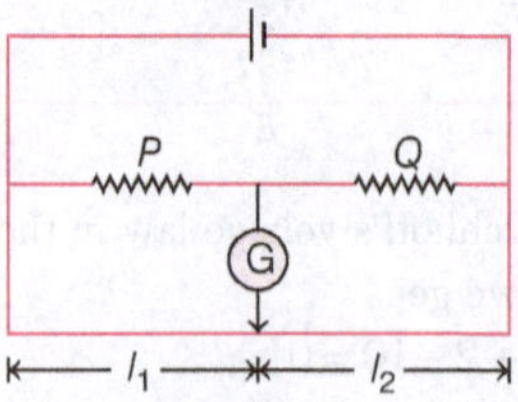

$$\frac{P}{Q} = \frac{l_1}{l_2}$$

Now, if position of *G* and cell is interchanged,

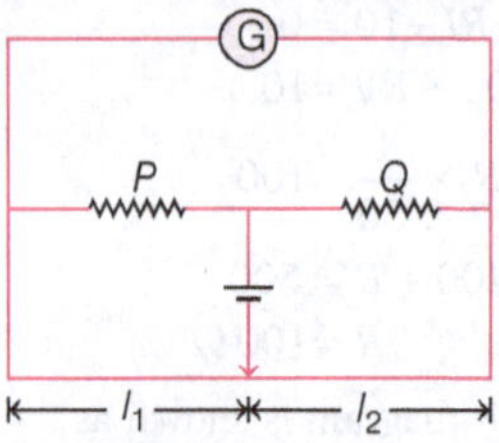

The balance condition still remains the same, if the jockey points at the same point as given in the initial condition, for which there is no deflection in the galvanometer or no current will be drawn from the cell. Thus, the bridge will work as usual and balance condition is same, $P / Q = l_1 / l_2$

34. (*d*) The given circuit diagram can be drawn as shown below

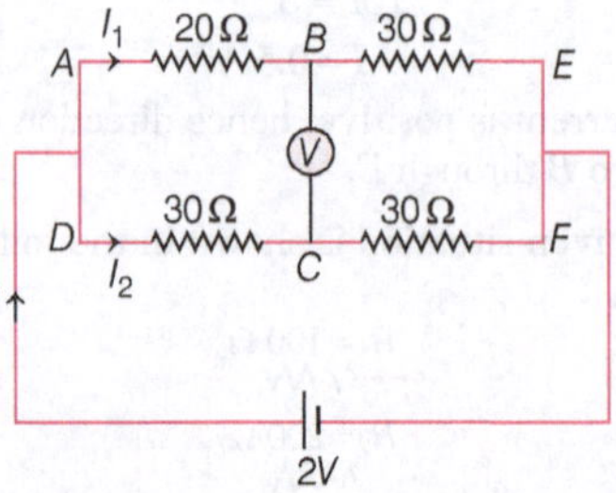

The equivalent resistance of circuit is given by

$$\frac{1}{R_{eq}} = \frac{1}{R_{AE}} + \frac{1}{R_{DF}}$$

$$= \frac{1}{(20+30)} + \frac{1}{(30+20)}$$

$$= \frac{1}{50} + \frac{1}{50} = \frac{2}{50}$$

$$\Rightarrow \quad R_{eq} = 25\,\Omega$$

The current in circuit, $I = \frac{V}{R} = \frac{2}{25}$ A

As the resistance of two branches is same, i.e. 50Ω. So, the current,

$$I_1 = I_2$$

$\Rightarrow \quad I = I_1 + I_2$

$\frac{2}{25} = 2I_1$

$\Rightarrow \quad I_2 = I_1 = \frac{1}{25} \text{ A}$

$\therefore$ The voltage across AB

$$V_1 = I_1 R_1 = \frac{1}{25} \times 20$$

and voltage across CD,

$$V_2 = I_2 R_2 = \frac{1}{25} \times 30$$

$\therefore$ Voltmeter reading $= V_2 - V_1$

$$= \frac{30}{25} - \frac{20}{25} = \frac{10}{25} = 0.4 \text{ V}$$

35. (*d*)

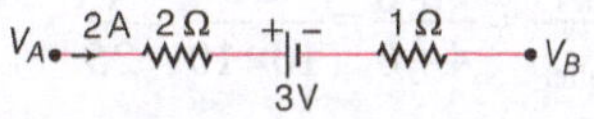

Applying KVL,

$$V_A - 3 = V_B + 2 \times 2 + 2 \times 1$$

$$V_A - V_B - 3 = 4 + 2$$

$$V_A - V_B = 9 \text{ V}$$

36. (*c*) $P_{\text{rated}} = \frac{V_{\text{rated}}^2}{R}$

$\therefore$ Current in the bulb, $I = \frac{P}{V}$ $\quad (\because P = VI)$

$$I = \frac{500}{100} = 5 \text{ A}$$

$\therefore$ Resistance of bulb,

$$R_b = \frac{100 \times 100}{500} = 20 \, \Omega$$

$\because$ Resistance R is connected in series.

$\therefore$ Current, $I = \frac{E}{R_{\text{net}}} = \frac{230}{R + R_b}$

$\Rightarrow \quad R + 20 = \frac{230}{5} = 46$

$\therefore \quad R = 26 \, \Omega$

37. (*d*) Given, charge $Q = at - bt^2$ $\quad$ ...(i)

$\because$ We know that current, $I = \frac{dQ}{dt}$

So, eq. (i) can be written as

$$I = \frac{d}{dt}(at - bt^2)$$

$\Rightarrow \quad I = a - 2bt$ $\quad$ ...(ii)

For maximum value of t, till the current exist is given by

$$I = 0$$

$\Rightarrow \quad a - 2bt = 0$

$\therefore \quad t = \frac{a}{2b}$ $\quad$ ...(iii)

$\because$ The total heat produced (H) can be given as

$$H = \int_0^t I^2 R \, dt$$

$$= \int_0^{a/2b} (a - 2bt)^2 R \, . \, dt \quad \left\{\because t = \frac{a}{2b}\right\}$$

$$= \int_0^{a/2b} (a^2 + 4b^2t^2 - 4abt) R dt$$

$$H = \left[a^2 t + 4b^2 \frac{t^3}{3} - \frac{4abt^2}{2}\right]_0^{a/2b} R$$

Solving above equation, we get

$\Rightarrow \quad H = \frac{a^3 R}{6b}$

Skill Builder

Sol. of Skill Builder on Pg. 202

(*b*) Given, drift velocity

$$v_d = 9.5 \times 10^{-2} \text{ m/s}$$

Electric field, $E = 4 \times 10^{-10} \text{ Vm}^{-1}$

As, mobility, $\mu = \frac{v_d}{E} = \frac{9.5 \times 10^{-2}}{4 \times 10^{-10}}$

$$= 2.375 \times 10^8 \text{ m}^2\text{V}^{-1}\text{s}^{-1}$$

Sol. of Skill Builder on Pg. 205

(*d*) Given, $R_0 = 3 \Omega$

At, $t = 80°\text{C}$, $R_t = 5.2 \, \Omega$

$$R_f = R_0(1 + \alpha t)$$

$$\Rightarrow R_t = R_0 + R_0 \, \alpha \, t$$

$$\alpha = \frac{R_t - R_0}{R_0 t} = \frac{5.2 - 3}{3 \times 80} = \frac{2.2}{240}$$

$$= 0.0092 = 9.2 \times 10^{-3} °\text{C}^{-1}$$

Sol. of Skill Builder on Pg. 208

(*c*) When, 11 resistances connected in series then,

$$R_S = 11R$$

$\therefore$ Current drawn from the battery,

$$I_S = \frac{E}{R_S} = \frac{E}{11R}$$

In second case, when resistances are connected in parallel, then equivalent resistance

$$\frac{1}{R_P} = \frac{1}{R} + \frac{1}{R} + \frac{1}{R} \text{........11 times}$$

$$R_P = \frac{R}{11}$$

Current drawn from the battery, $I_P = \frac{E}{R_P} = \frac{E}{R/11}$

$$= 11 \times \frac{E}{R} = 121 \times \frac{E}{11R}$$

$\Rightarrow \quad I_P = 121 I_S$

$\therefore \quad n = 121$

■ Sol. of Skill Builder on Pg. 209

(*a*) According to the given circuit diagram in question,

$$I_1 = I_2 + I_3$$

In parallel arrangement of the electrical circuit, the voltage remain same,

$$V = Ir$$

$$\Rightarrow \quad I_2 r_2 = I_3 r_3$$

$$\Rightarrow \quad I_3 = \frac{I_2 r_2}{r_3}$$

Substituting the value of I_3 in the Eq. (i) we get

$$I_1 = I_2 + \frac{I_2 r_2}{r_3}$$

$$\Rightarrow \quad \frac{I_1}{I_2} = 1 + \frac{r_2}{r_3}$$

$$\frac{I_2}{I_1} = \frac{r_3}{r_3 + r_2}$$

■ Sol. of Skill Builder on Pg. 214

(*b*) Current in circuit, $I = \dfrac{15}{\left(\dfrac{8 \times 8}{8+8}\right) + 1} = \dfrac{15}{5} = 3\text{ A}$

$\therefore$ Terminal voltage, $= E - IR$

$$= 15 - 3 \times 1 = 12\text{ V}$$

■ Sol. of Skill Builder on Pg. 220

(*b*)

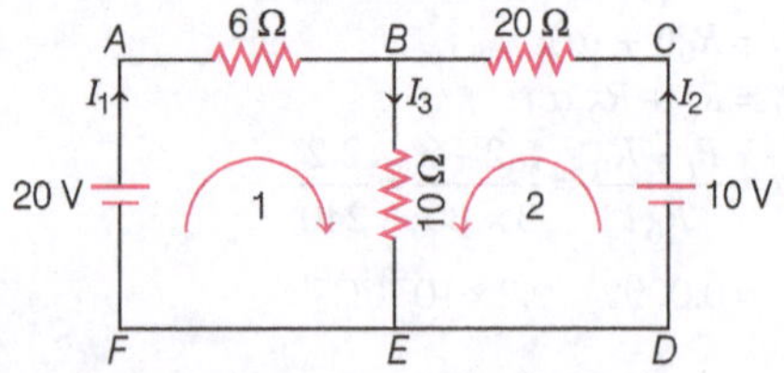

Applying Kirchhoff's first law at junction *B*,

$$I_3 = I_1 + I_2 \quad \text{... (i)}$$

Applying Kirchhoff's second law in loop 1 (*ABEFA*),

$$-20I_1 - 10(I_1 + I_2) + 20 = 0$$

$$30I_1 + 10I_2 = 20 \quad \text{... (ii)}$$

Applying Kirchhoff's second law in loop 2 (*BCDEB*),

$$10 - 20I_2 - 10(I_1 + I_2) = 0$$

$$10I_1 + 30I_2 = 10 \quad \text{... (iii)}$$

Solving Eqs. (ii) and (iii), we get

$$I_1 = \frac{5}{8}$$

$$I_2 \approx \frac{1}{8}$$

Put the value of I_1 and I_2 ion eq. (i), we get

$$I_3 = 0.75\text{ A}$$

■ Sol. of Skill Builder on Pg. 223

(*a*) Given,

$$P_1 = 4\text{ kW}$$

$$P_2 = 6\text{ kW}$$

$$P_{\text{series}} = \frac{P_1 P_2}{P_1 + P_2} \text{ and } P_{\text{parallel}} = P_1 + P_2$$

According to question,

$$\frac{P_{\text{series}}}{P_{\text{parallel}}} = \frac{\frac{4 \times 6}{4+6}}{4+6} = \frac{24}{10 \times 10} = \frac{6}{25}$$

■ Sol. of Skill Builder on Pg. 226

(*b*) In first case,

$$\frac{X}{Y} = \frac{60}{40} \text{ or } \frac{X}{Y} = \frac{3}{2} \quad \text{...(i)}$$

In second case,

$$\frac{X}{Y+15} = \frac{50}{50} = 1 \quad \text{...(ii)}$$

Dividing Eq. (i) by Eq. (ii), we get

$$\frac{X}{Y} \times \frac{Y+15}{X} = \frac{3}{2} \times 1$$

or $$1 + \frac{15}{Y} = \frac{3}{2} \text{ or } Y = 30\Omega$$

$$X = \frac{3}{2}Y = \frac{3}{2} \times 30 = 45\Omega$$

When a resistance of 30 Ω is connected in parallel with *Y*, then the resistance in the right gap becomes

$$Y' = \frac{30Y}{30+Y} = \frac{30 \times 30}{30+30} = 15\Omega$$

Suppose the null point occurs at *l* cm from end *A*. Then,

$$\frac{X}{15} = \frac{l}{100 - l}$$

or $$\frac{45}{15} = \frac{l}{100 - l}$$

or $300 - 3l = l$ or $4l = 300$ or $l = 75$ cm

For deeper insight
Scan the QR Code

Chapter 5

Moving Charges and Magnetism

Learning Objectives

Module-I

- Magnetic Field
- Biot-Savart's Law Magnetic Field Due to a Current Carrying Loop
- Rules of Find the Direction of Magnetic Field
- Applications of Biot-Savart's Law

Module-II

- Understanding the Ampere's Circuital Law
- Applications of Ampere's Circuital Law
- The Solenoid

Module-III

- Force on a Moving Charge in a Uniform Magnetic Field
- Motion of a Charged Particle in a Uniform Magnetic Field
- Motion of a Charged Particle in a Combined Electric and Magnetic Fields : Lorentz Force
- Force on a Current Carrying Conductor in a Magnetic Field
- Force between Two Parallel Current Carrying Conductors

Module-IV

- Magnetic Dipole Moment
- Torque on Current Carrying Loop in a Magnetic Field
- The Moving Coil Galvanometer

Chapter Overview with NEET Connection

For the perspective of NEET exam, this chapter helps NEET Aspirants to face the conceptual questions based on magnetism. This chapter is also useful for understanding other chapter like Magnetism and Matter, Electromagnetic Induction, Alternating Current and Electromagnetic Waves.

Special format questions can be easily framed on the following topics of this chapter

- Biot-Savart's law
- Ampere's law
- Forces between two current carrying wires
- Torque on rectangular loop in uniform magnetic field
- Conversion of galvanometer into voltmeter and ammeter

For better understanding of this chapter

- Conceptual study of chapter 4 is a must
- Revision of cross product of vectors is very important
- Determination of direction of vectors should be revisited (specially right hand rule and thumb rule)
- Basic idea and exposure to voltmeter and ammeter will be helpful.

Introduction

In continuation to static and moving charges as we have studied in previous chapters, we will study about magnetic effects of electric current and moving charges in this chapter. We will also study about magnetic fields due to charge flow through conductors, their related laws, magnetic forces, torque on current loop in magnetic field and tangent galvanometer in this chapter.

Module 1

Biot-Savart's Law

- Magnetic Field • Biot-Savart's Law Magnetic Field Due to a Current Carrying Conductor
- Rules to Find the Direction of Magnetic Field • Applications of Biot-Savart's Law

Magnetic Field

The space in the surroundings of a magnet, in which magnetic influence of moving charges or a current carrying conductor can be experienced is called **magnetic field**. Magnetic field is a vector quantity and is denoted by **B**. The SI unit of magnetic field is Wb/m^2 or tesla (T) and its CGS unit is gauss or $maxwell/cm^2$.

$$1\ T = 10^4\ G$$

Current Element

Length element (small part of length) of a thin current carrying wire is known as current element. It is a vector quantity which has direction in the direction of flow of current in the wire.

Its unit is Ampere-metre and dimensions are $[M^0L^1T^0A^1]$.

Biot-Savart's Law (Magnetic Field Due to a Current Carrying Conductor)

Biot-Savart's law is an experimental law predicted by Biot and Savart. This law deals with the magnetic field produced at a point due to a small current element (a part of any conductor carrying current).

Consider a wire *XY* carrying current *I*. Let *dl* be the infinitesimal element of the conductor, *dB* be the magnetic field at point *P* at a distance *r* from the element.

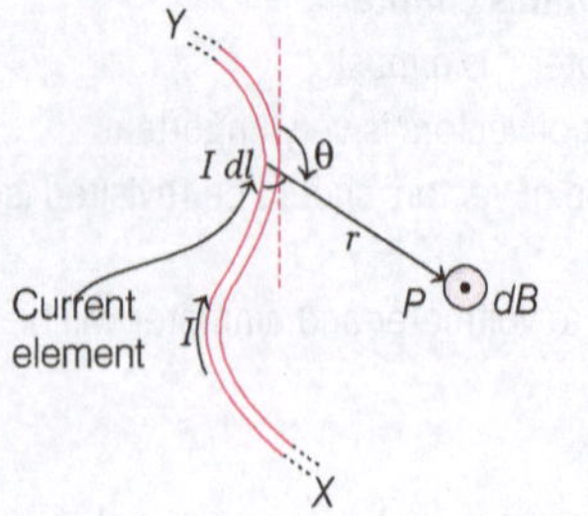

Magnetic field of a long current carrying conductor

Biot-Savart's law states that, the magnitude of the magnetic field induction *d***B** at the point *P* due to the current element is

- directly proportional to the current flowing through the conductor, *i.e.* $dB \propto I$ ...(i)
- directly proportional to the length of the element, *i.e.* $dB \propto dl$ ...(ii)
- directly proportional to the sine of angle between the length of element and line joining the element to the point, *i.e.* $dB \propto \sin\theta$ ...(iii)
- inversely proportional to the square of distance between the element and the point, *i.e.* $dB \propto 1/r^2$ ...(iv)

Combining all the above four relations, we get

$$dB \propto \frac{Idl\sin\theta}{r^2}$$

This relation is called **Biot-Savart's law.**

If conductor is placed in air or vacuum, then magnitude of magnetic field is given by

$$|d\mathbf{B}| = \frac{\mu_0}{4\pi}\frac{Idl\sin\theta}{r^2}$$

where, $\frac{\mu_0}{4\pi}$ is the **proportionality constant.**

μ_0 is called the **permeability of free space (or vacuum).**

In SI unit, $\mu_0 = 4\pi\times10^{-7}$ Tm/A or Wb/A-m and its dimensions are $[MLT^{-2}A^{-2}]$. The value of $\frac{\mu_0}{4\pi}$ in CGS system is unity.

In vector form, Biot-Savart's law can be written as

$$d\mathbf{B} \propto \frac{Id\mathbf{l}\times\mathbf{r}}{|\mathbf{r}|^3} = \frac{\mu_0}{4\pi}\cdot\frac{Id\mathbf{l}\times\mathbf{r}}{r^3}$$

The direction of *d***B** is represented by the right hand screw rule or right hand thumb rule.

Similarly, magnetic field induction at point *P* due to current through entire wire is

$$\mathbf{B} = \int\frac{\mu_0}{4\pi}\cdot\frac{Id\mathbf{l}\times\mathbf{r}}{r^3}$$

or

$$\mathbf{B} = \int\frac{\mu_0}{4\pi}\cdot\frac{Idl\sin\theta}{r^2}$$

Biot-Savart's Law in a Medium

If the conductor is placed in a medium, then vector form of Biot-Savart's law is given as

$$dB = \frac{\mu}{4\pi} \frac{Id\mathbf{l} \times \mathbf{r}}{|\mathbf{r}|^3} = \frac{\mu_0 \mu_r}{4\pi} \frac{I\, d\mathbf{l} \times \mathbf{r}}{r^3}$$

where, μ_r = relative permeability $= \frac{\mu}{\mu_0} = 1$

(for air or vacuum)

and μ = absolute permeability of the medium.

Biot-Savart's Law in Terms of Current Density J

$$d\mathbf{B} = \frac{\mu_0}{4\pi} \cdot \frac{(\mathbf{J} \times \mathbf{r})}{r^3} dV \quad \left(\because \mathbf{J} = \frac{I}{A} = \frac{Id\mathbf{l}}{Ad\mathbf{l}} = \frac{Id\mathbf{l}}{dV} \right)$$

Biot-Savart's Law in Terms of Charge (*q*) and its Velocity (*v*)

A moving charge constitutes current and the magnetic field associated with the charge is given as

$$d\mathbf{B} = \frac{\mu_0}{4\pi} \cdot \frac{q(\mathbf{v} \times \mathbf{r})}{r^3} \quad \left(\because Id\mathbf{L} = \frac{q}{dt} d\mathbf{L} = q\frac{d\mathbf{L}}{dt} = q\mathbf{v} \right)$$

Special Conditions of Biot-Savart's law

Special conditions of Biot-Savart's law are given below.

(i) The magnetic field due to the current element can also be written as $d\mathbf{B} = \frac{1}{4\pi\varepsilon_0 c^2} \frac{Id\mathbf{l} \times \mathbf{r}}{r^3}$

where, $c = \frac{1}{\sqrt{\mu_0 \varepsilon_0}}$ = speed of light in vacuum.

(ii) When $\theta = 0°$ or $180°$, then magnetic field produced due to the current will be zero.

(iii) When $\theta = 90°$, *i.e.* r is perpendicular to dl, then magnetic field will be $dB = \frac{\mu_0 idl}{4\pi r^2}$, which is maximum.

Rules to Find the Direction of Magnetic Field

(i) **Right Hand Palm Rule** If we spread our right hand in such a way that thumb is towards the direction of current and fingers are towards that point where we have to find the direction of magnetic field, then direction of magnetic field will be perpendicular to the palm.

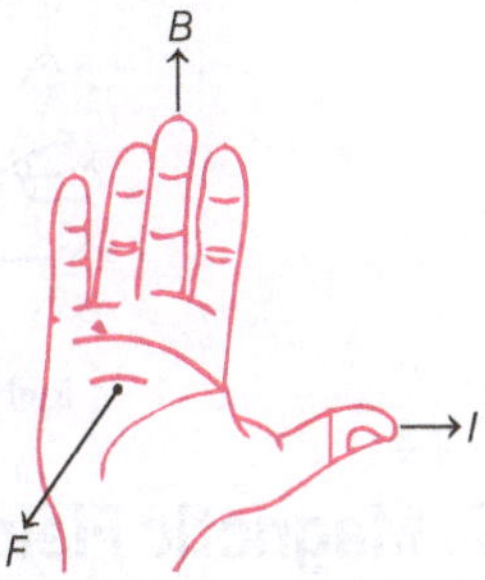

Right hand palm rule

(ii) **Maxwell's Right Handed Screw Rule** If a right handed cork screw is rotated such that its tip moves in the direction of flow of current through the conductor, then the rotation of head of the screw gives the direction of magnetic field.

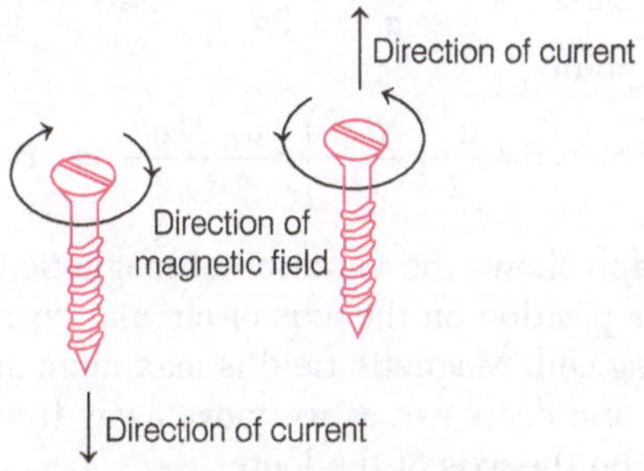

Right handed screw rule

(iii) **Right Hand Thumb Rule** If a straight current carrying conductor is held in the right hand such that the thumb represents the direction of flow of current, then the direction of the folding fingers will represent the direction of magnetic field around the conductor.

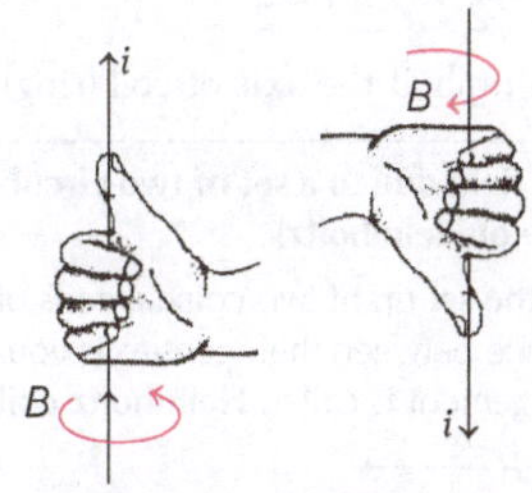

Right hand thumb rule

Mentor's Tip

Shape of magnetic field lines due to an infinite long straight current carrying conductor will be concentric circles considering wire as their principal axis.

Applications of Biot-Savart's Law

1. Magnetic Field on the Axis of a Circular Current Carrying Coil

If a coil of radius a is carrying current i, then magnetic field on its axis at a distance r from its centre is given by

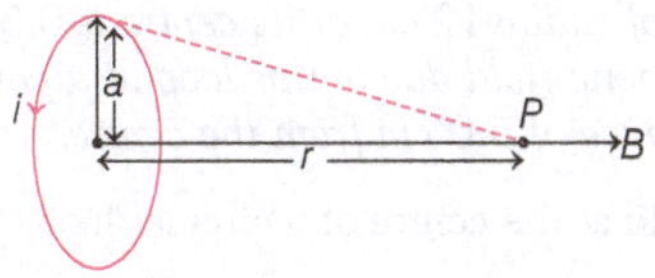

Magnetic field on the axis of a circular current carrying coil

$$B_{\text{axis}} = \frac{\mu_0}{2} \frac{Nia^2}{(a^2 + r^2)^{3/2}}$$

where, N = number of turns in coil.

(i) At centre, $r = 0$

$$\Rightarrow \quad B_{centre} = \frac{\mu_0}{2} \cdot \frac{Ni}{a} = \frac{\mu_0 Ni}{2a} = B_{max}$$

(ii) At far points,

$$r >> a, B \approx \frac{\mu_0}{2}\left(\frac{Nia^2}{r^3}\right) = \frac{\mu_0}{2}\frac{Nia^2}{r^3} \Rightarrow B \propto \frac{1}{r^3}$$

(iii) B-r graph shows the variation of magnetic field at various position on the axis of circular current carrying coil. Magnetic field is maximum at the centre and decreases as we move away from the centre on the axis of the loop.

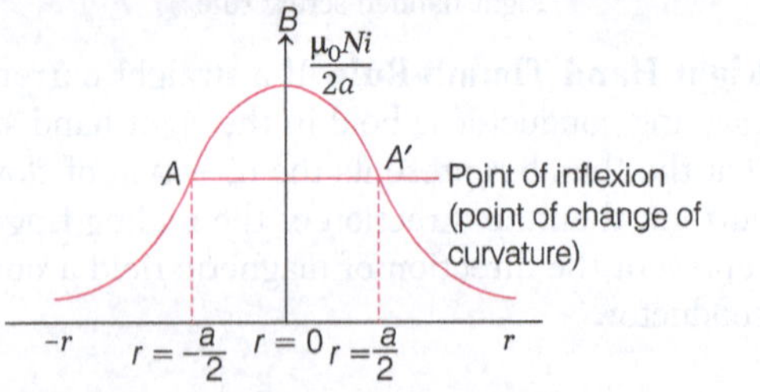

B-r graph at the axis of coil (ring)

Concept ladder

Magnetic field due to a set of two circular current carrying coils (case of Helmholtz)

Consider the set up of two coaxial coils of same radius such that distance between their centres is equal to their radius. This arrangement is called **Helmholtz coil.**

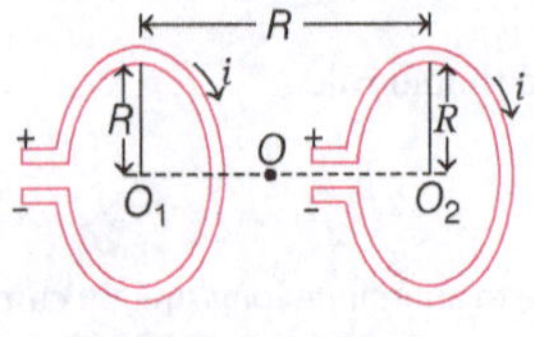

(a) Magnetic field due to two coaxial coils

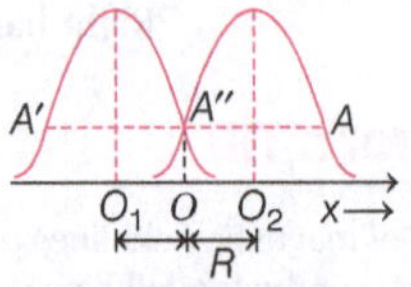

(b) B-x graph of two coaxial coils

At axial mid-point O, the magnetic field is given by

$$B = \frac{8\mu_0 Ni}{5\sqrt{5}R} = 0.716\frac{\mu_0 Ni}{R} = 1.432 B_{max}$$

where, $B_{max} = \frac{\mu_0 Ni}{2R}$

Example 1. *The magnetic field B due to a current carrying circular loop of radius 12 cm at its centre is 0.5×10^{-4} T. Find the magnetic field due to this loop at a point on the axis at a distance of 5.0 cm from the centre.*

Sol. Magnetic field at the centre of a circular loop, $B_1 = \frac{\mu_0 i}{2R}$

and that at an axial point, $B_2 = \frac{\mu_0 iR^2}{2(R^2 + x^2)^{3/2}}$

Thus, $\frac{B_2}{B_1} = \frac{R^3}{(R^2 + x^2)^{3/2}}$ or $B_2 = B_1\left[\frac{R^3}{(R^2 + x^2)^{3/2}}\right]$

Substituting the given values in above equation, we get

$$B_2 = (0.5 \times 10^{-4})\left[\frac{(12)^3}{(144 + 25)^{3/2}}\right]$$

$$= 3.9 \times 10^{-5} \text{ T}$$

NEET Close-up

Example Similar to PYQ Asked in NEET 2024

A coil of radius 20 cm has wounded 80 turns and carries a current of 5 A. Then, the magnitude of the magnetic field at the centre of the coil is

(a) 14.2×10^{-4} T (b) 12.6×10^{-3} T
(c) 12.6×10^{-4} T (d) 14.2×10^{-3} T

Sol. (c) The magnitude of magnetic field due to circular coil of N turns is given by

$$B_C = \frac{\mu_0 iN}{2R} = \frac{4\pi \times 10^{-7} \times 5 \times 80}{2 \times 0.2}$$

$$= 12.6 \times 10^{-4} \text{ T}$$

Skill Builder

A coil of radius 5 cm has wounded 40 turns and carries a current of 2 A. Then, the magnitude of the magnetic field at the centre of coil is

(a) 1 mT (b) 3 mT (c) 9 mT (d) 5 mT

For more Practice Refer Q. No. 7 of step up practice-1 and Q. No. 5 of Gearing up for NEET.

Direction of Magnetic field on the Axis of the Circular Coil

Direction of magnetic field on the axis of a circular loop can be obtained using the right hand thumb rule. This rule states that, if the fingers of right hand are curled along the current, then the stretched thumb will point towards the direction of magnetic field as shown in figures given below.

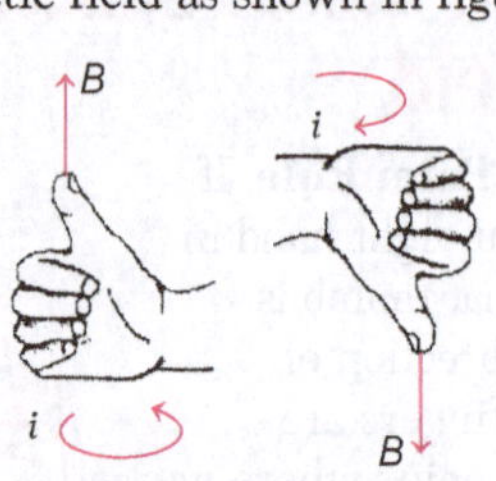

Right hand thumb rule

2. Magnetic Field at the Centre of a Circular Current Carrying Coil

Consider a circular current carrying coil of radius a and carrying current i. Magnetic field at the centre O due to the current element dl is

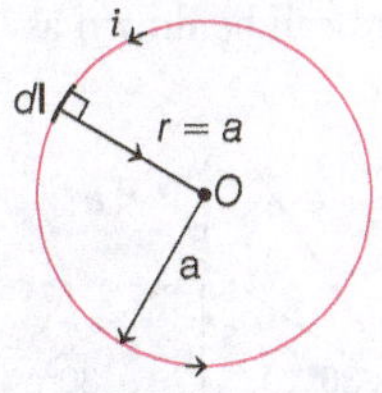

Current carrying circular coil

$$d\mathbf{B} = \frac{\mu_0 I}{4\pi} \cdot \frac{d\mathbf{l} \times \mathbf{r}}{r^3}$$

Here, $d\mathbf{l} \perp \mathbf{r}$, so $\theta = 90°$

$$dB = \frac{\mu_0}{4\pi} \frac{i\, dl \sin 90°}{a^2}$$

Therefore, magnetic field at the centre due to the whole circular loop, $B = \int dB = \frac{\mu_0 i}{4\pi a^2} \int dl = \frac{\mu_0 i}{4\pi a^2}(2\pi a)$

$$\boxed{B = \frac{\mu_0 i}{2a}}$$

Direction of this field is outward perpendicular to the plane of the paper.

If the loop has N turns, then magnetic field,

$$\boxed{B = \frac{\mu_0 NI}{2a}}$$

> **Concept ladder**
>
> **Magnetic Field due to an Arc**
>
> Magnetic field due to an arc of a circular current carrying coil at the centre is given by
>
> 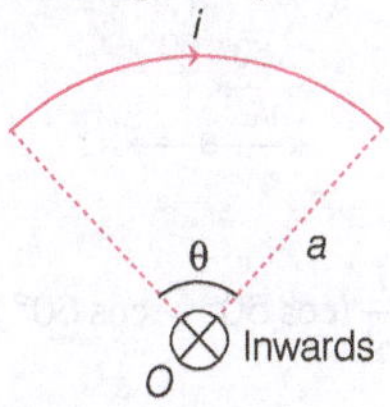
>
>
> Magnetic field due to an arc,
>
> $$B = \left(\frac{\theta}{2\pi}\right)\frac{\mu_0 i}{2a} = \frac{\mu_0}{4\pi}\left(\frac{i}{a}\right)\theta$$
>
> Here, θ is to be substituted in radians.

3. Magnetic Field Surrounding a thin, Straight Current Carrying Conductor

Magnetic field due to a current carrying wire at a point P which lies at a perpendicular distance d from the wire (as shown in figure) is given as

$$\boxed{B = \frac{\mu_0}{4\pi}\frac{i}{d}(\sin\alpha + \sin\beta)}$$

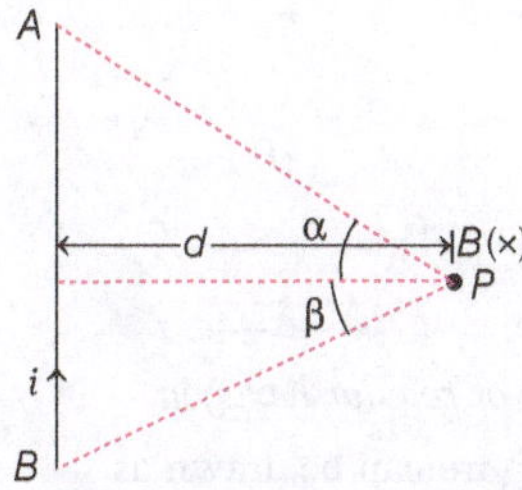

Magnetic field of a finite wire

Note down the following points regarding the above equation.

(i) For an infinitely long straight wire, $\alpha = \beta = 90°$

$$\therefore\ B = \frac{\mu_0 i}{4\pi d}(\sin 90° + \sin 90°) = \frac{\mu_0 i}{4\pi d}(1+1) = \frac{\mu_0}{2\pi}\frac{i}{d}$$

(ii) When wire is semi-infinite (at the foot of long wire),

$$\alpha = \frac{\pi}{2} \text{ and } \beta = 0°$$

$$\therefore\quad B = \frac{\mu_0 i}{4\pi d}\left(\sin 0° + \sin\frac{\pi}{2}\right) \Rightarrow B = \frac{\mu_0 i}{4\pi d}$$

(iii) For axial position of wire, *i.e.* when point P lies on axial position of current carrying conductor, then magnetic field at P,

$$B = 0 \qquad [\text{since, } \theta = 0°]$$

Example 2. *Evaluate magnitude and direction of magnetic field at point P in the following cases.*

(i)

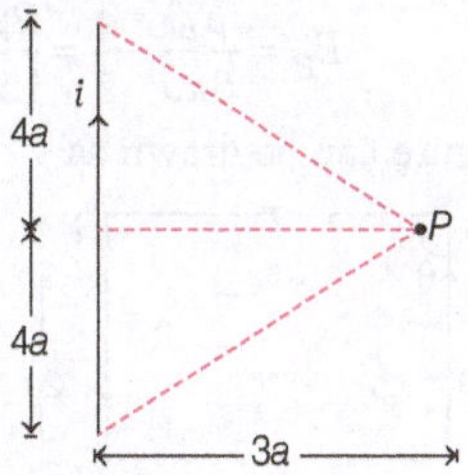

(ii)

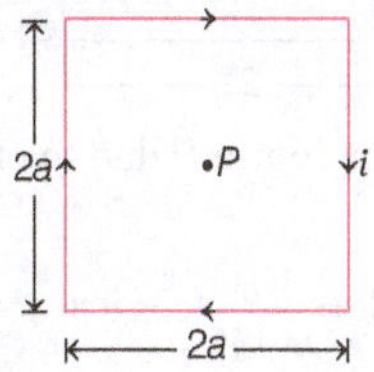

P is the centre of square.

(iii)

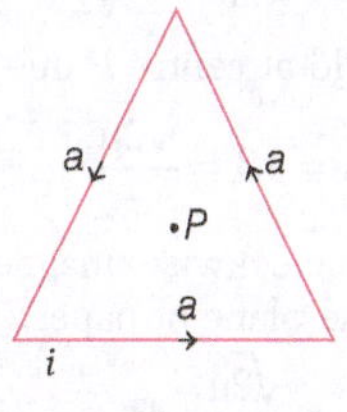

P is the centre of equilateral triangle.

(iv)

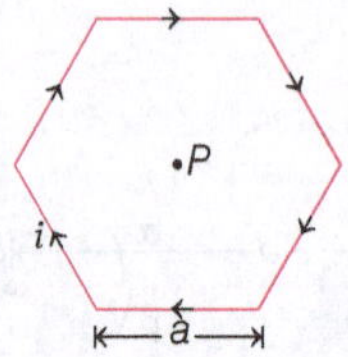

P is the centre of regular hexagon.

Sol. (i) The given figure can be drawn as

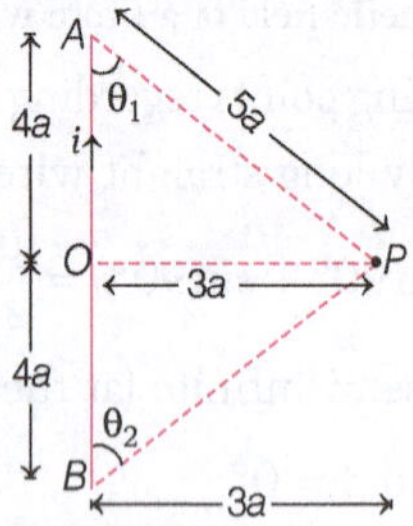

Magnetic field at centre P,

$$B_P = \frac{\mu_0 i}{4\pi(OP)}[\cos\theta_1 + \cos\theta_2]$$

$$= \frac{\mu_0 i}{4\pi(3a)}[\cos\theta + \cos\theta] = \frac{\mu_0 i}{6\pi a}\cos\theta$$

Use Pythagoras theorem, we find the value

$$PA = \sqrt{(3a)^2 + (4a)^2} = \sqrt{25a^2} = 5a$$

From the figure, $\cos\theta = \frac{PA}{OA} = \frac{4}{5}$

$$\therefore \quad B_P = \frac{\mu_0 i}{6\pi a}\cdot\frac{4}{5} = \frac{2\mu_0 i}{15\pi a} \otimes$$

(ii) The given figure can be drawn as

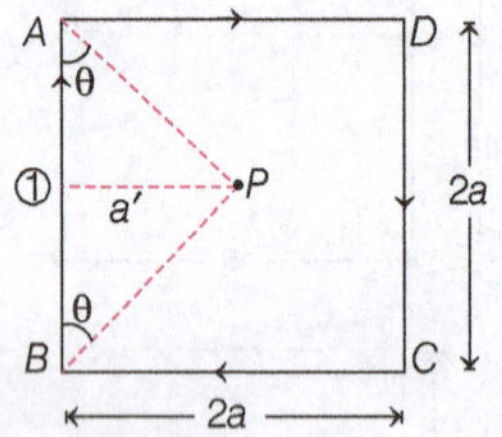

Magnetic field at centre P due to one side of square, say AB,

$$B_1 = \frac{\mu_0 i}{4\pi a'}(\cos\theta + \cos\theta) \quad (\because a' = a, \theta = 45°)$$

$$B_1 = \frac{\mu_0 i}{4\pi a}\cdot 2\cdot\frac{1}{\sqrt{2}} = \frac{\mu_0 i}{2\sqrt{2}\pi a}$$

So, magnetic field at centre P due to square loop,

$$B_P = 4B_1 = \frac{\sqrt{2}\mu_0 i}{\pi a}$$

Since, current is clockwise, magnetic field at centre P will be inside the plane of paper.

$$B_P = \frac{\sqrt{2}\mu_0 i}{\pi a} \otimes$$

(iii) The given figure can be drawn as

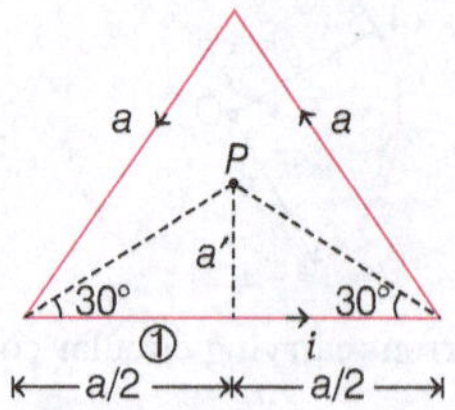

From the figure,

$$\tan 30° = \frac{a'}{a/2} \Rightarrow a' = \frac{a}{2\sqrt{3}}$$

and $\theta_1 = \theta_2 = 30°$

Magnetic field, $B_1 = \frac{\mu_0 i}{4\pi a'}[\cos 30° + \cos 30°]$

$$= \frac{\mu_0 i}{4\pi\cdot\frac{a}{2\sqrt{3}}}\cdot 2\cdot\frac{\sqrt{3}}{2} = \frac{3\mu_0 i}{2\pi a}$$

So, magnetic field at centre P due to triangular loop,

$$B_P = 3B_1 = \frac{9\mu_0 i}{2\pi a}$$

Since, current is anti-clockwise, magnetic field at centre P will be outside the plane of paper.

$$B_P = \frac{9\mu_0 i}{2\pi a} \odot$$

(iv)

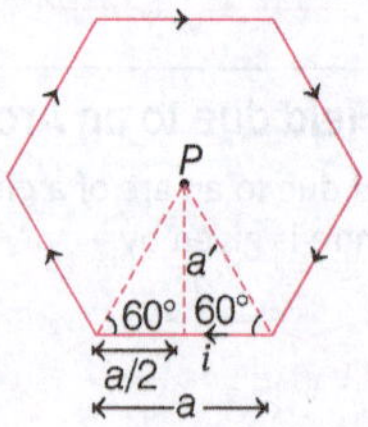

Magnetic field,

$$B_1 = \frac{\mu_0 i}{4\pi a'}(\cos 60° + \cos 60°)$$

$$= \frac{\mu_0 i}{4\pi\cdot\frac{a}{2}\cdot\tan 60°}\cdot 2\cos 60°$$

$$= \frac{\mu_0 i}{4\pi\cdot\frac{a}{2}\cdot\sqrt{3}}\cdot 2\times\frac{1}{2}$$

$$= \frac{\mu_0 i}{2\pi a\sqrt{3}}$$

Magnetic field at P = 6 times the magnetic field due to one side

$$\therefore \quad B_P = 6B_1 = \frac{\sqrt{3}\mu_0 i}{\pi a} \otimes$$

Example 3. *A wire shaped to a regular hexagon of side 2 cm carries a current of 2 A. Find the magnetic field at the centre of the hexagon.*

Sol.

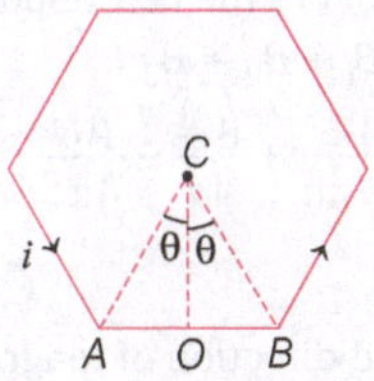

From geometry of the figure, we have

$$\Rightarrow \quad \frac{BC}{OC} = \tan\theta \qquad [\because BC = 1 \text{ cm (given)}]$$

$$\therefore \quad \frac{1}{r} = \tan 30° = \frac{1}{\sqrt{3}}$$

$$\Rightarrow \quad r = \sqrt{3} \text{ cm}$$

Net magnetic field at O = 6 times the magnetic field due to one side

$$\therefore \quad B_O = 6\left[\frac{\mu_0}{2\pi}\frac{i}{r}(\sin\theta + \sin\theta)\right]$$

$$= \frac{6\,(2\times10^{-7})(2)}{\sqrt{3}\times10^{-2}}\left(\frac{1}{2}+\frac{1}{2}\right) \qquad [\because \theta = 30°]$$

$$= 1.38\times 10^{-4} \text{ T}$$

Concept ladder

Magnetic field for different configurations of the circular coil

Magnitude and direction of magnetic fields associated with different configurations of the circular coil are given below.

(i)

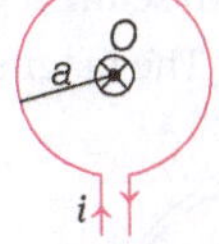

$B_O = \frac{\mu_0 i}{2a} \otimes$

(ii)

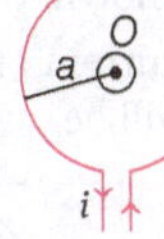

$B_O = \frac{\mu_0 i}{2a} \odot$

(iii)

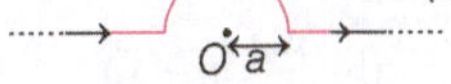

$B_O = \frac{\mu_0 i}{4a} \otimes$

(iv)

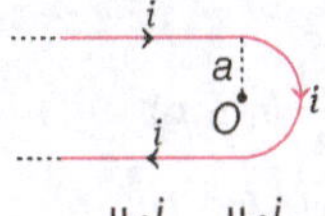

$B_O = \frac{\mu_0 i}{2\pi a} + \frac{\mu_0 i}{4a} \otimes$

(v)

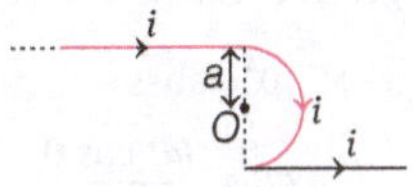

$B_O = \frac{\mu_0 i}{4a} \otimes$

(vi)

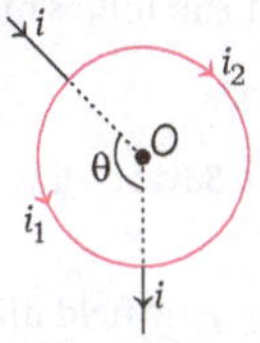

$B_O = 0$ (for any value of θ)

Example 4. *A current path shaped as shown in figure produces a magnetic field at P, the centre of the arc. If the arc subtends an angle of 30° and the radius of the arc is 0.6 m. What is the magnitude of the field at P, if the current is 3.0 A?*

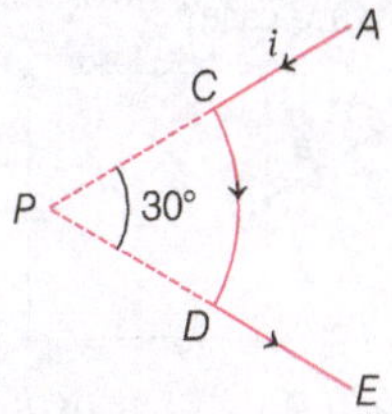

Sol. Here, point P is along the length of straight wires CA and DE, hence

$$B_{CA} = B_{DE} = 0$$

Magnetic field due to an arc of a circle at the centre,

$$B = \left(\frac{\theta}{2\pi}\right)\frac{\mu_0 i}{2R} = \left(\frac{\mu_0}{4\pi}\right)\left(\frac{i}{R}\right)\theta$$

Here, $\theta = 30° = \frac{\pi}{6}$ rad, $i = 3$ A and $R = 0.6$ m

$$B = \left(\frac{\mu_0}{4\pi}\right)\left(\frac{3}{0.6}\right)\left(\frac{\pi}{6}\right) = \frac{10^{-7}\times3\times\pi}{0.6\times6}$$

$$= 2.6\times10^{-7} \text{ T}$$

Example 5. *Figure shows a current loop having two circular arcs joined by two radial lines. Find the magnetic field B at the centre O.*

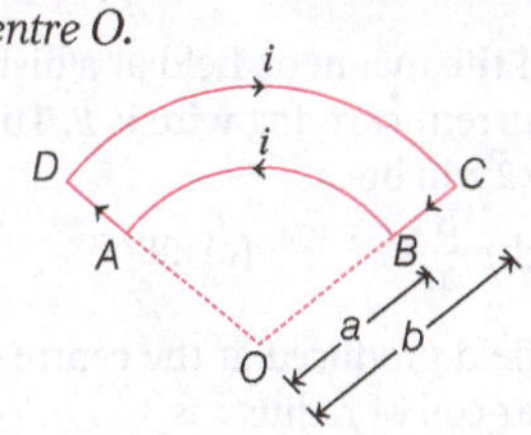

Sol. Magnetic field at O due to wires CB and AD will be zero.

Magnetic field due to arc BA,

$$B_1 = \left(\frac{\theta}{2\pi}\right)\left(\frac{\mu_0 i}{2a}\right)$$

Direction of field B_1 is out of the plane of the figure.

Similarly, magnetic field at O due to arc DC,

$$B_2 = \left(\frac{\theta}{2\pi}\right)\left(\frac{\mu_0 i}{2b}\right)$$

Direction of B_2 is into the plane of the figure.

The resultant field at O,

$$B = B_1 - B_2 = \frac{\mu_0\, i\,\theta\,(b-a)}{4\pi ab}, \text{ out of the plane of figure.}$$

NEET Close-up

Example Similar to PYQ Asked in NEET 2023

What is the magnitude and direction of magnetic field at point O in the following case?

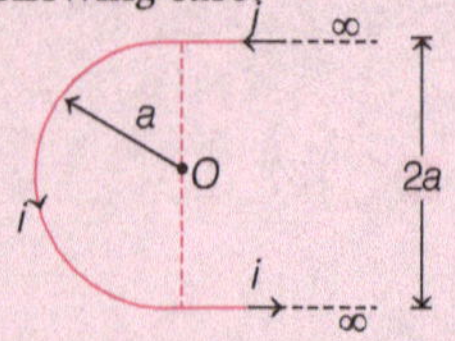

(a) $\frac{\mu_0 i}{2\pi a}\odot$ (b) $\frac{\mu_0 i}{4a}\left(\frac{2}{\pi}+1\right)\odot$ (c) $\frac{\mu_0 i}{4a}\odot$ (d) $\frac{\mu_0 i}{2a}\left(\frac{2}{\pi}+1\right)\odot$

Sol. (*b*) The given figure can be drawn as

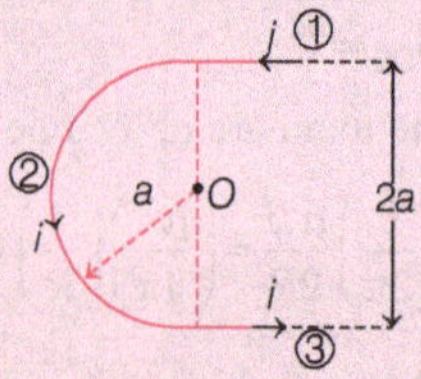

Since, point O is the foot of long wires 1 and 3,

$$\therefore \quad B_1 = B_3 = \frac{\mu_0 i}{4\pi a}\odot$$

Due to semicircle 2,

$$B_2 = \frac{\mu_0 i}{4a}\odot$$

Net magnetic field at the centre point O,

$$B_O = B_1 + B_2 + B_3$$

$$= \frac{\mu_0 i}{4\pi a} + \frac{\mu_0 i}{4a} + \frac{\mu_0 i}{4\pi a} = \frac{\mu_0 i}{4a}\left(\frac{2}{\pi}+1\right)\odot$$

Skill Builder

Find magnitude and direction of magnetic field at point O in the given case .

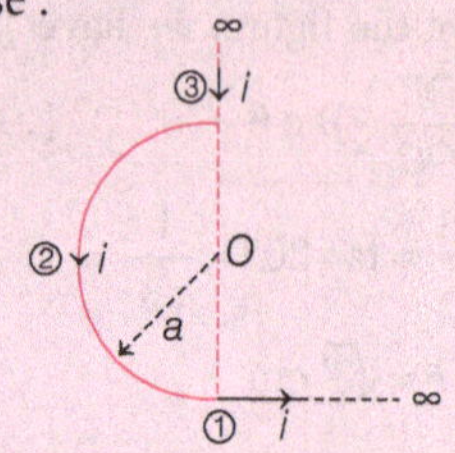

(a) $\frac{\mu_0 i}{4a}\left(\frac{1}{\pi}+1\right)\otimes$ (b) $\frac{\mu_0 i}{4a}\left(\frac{1}{\pi}-1\right)\otimes$

(c) $\frac{\mu_0 i}{4a}\left(\frac{1}{\pi}+1\right)\odot$ (d) $\frac{\mu_0 i}{4a}\left(\frac{1}{\pi}-1\right)\odot$

For more Practice Refer Q. No. 5 19, 20 of step up practice-1 and Q. No. 6, 7, 27, 28 of gearing up for NEET.

STEP UP Practice 1

1. The strength of the magnetic field at a distance r near a long straight current carrying wire is B. The magnetic field at a distance $r/2$ will be

(a) $\frac{B}{2}$ (b) $\frac{B}{4}$ (c) $2B$ (d) $4B$

2. The magnetic field produced at the centre of a current carrying circular coil of radius r is

(a) directly proportional to r (b) inversely proportional to r
(c) directly proportional to r^2 (d) inversely proportional to r^2

3. A particle carrying a charge equal to 100 times the charge on an electron, is rotating one rotation per second in a circular path of radius 0.8 m. The value of the magnetic field produced at the centre will be (μ_0 = permeability for vacuum)

(a) $\frac{10^{-7}}{\mu_0}$ T (b) $10^{-17}\mu_0$ T (c) $10^{-6}\mu_0$ T (d) $10^{-7}\mu_0$ T

4. **Assertion** (A) For a point on the axis of a circular coil carrying current, magnetic field is maximum at the centre of the coil.

Reason (R) Magnetic field is inversely proportional to the distance of point from the circular coil.

In the light of the above statements, choose the correct answer from the options given below.

(a) Both A and R are true but R is not the correct explanation of A.
(b) A is true but R is false.
(c) A is false but R is true.
(d) Both A and R are true and R is the correct explanation of A.

5. In the figure shown, there are two semicircles of radii r_1 and r_2 in which a current i is flowing. The magnetic induction at the centre O will be

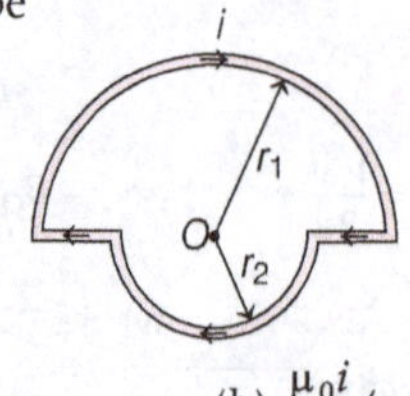

(a) $\frac{\mu_0 i}{4}(r_1 + r_2)$ (b) $\frac{\mu_0 i}{4}(r_1 - r_2)$

(c) $\frac{\mu_0 i}{4}\left[\frac{r_1 + r_2}{r_1 r_2}\right]$ (d) $\frac{\mu_0 i}{4}\left[\frac{r_2 - r_1}{r_1 r_2}\right]$

6. Which of the following pair given below is correct?

(a) 1 tesla → 10^4 gauss

(b) Biot-Savart's law → $dB \propto \frac{Idl\cos\theta}{r^2}$

(c) Magnetic field due to an arc → $B = \left(\frac{\mu_0}{\pi}\right)\left(\frac{i}{a}\right)\theta$

(d) SI unit of magnetic field → Maxwell/cm^2

7. A current of 0.1 A circulates around a coil of 100 turns and having a radius equal to 5 cm. The magnetic field set up at the centre of the coil is ($\mu_0 = 4\pi \times 10^{-7}$ Wb/A-m)
(a) $5\pi \times 10^{-5}$ T (b) $8\pi \times 10^{-5}$ T
(c) $4\pi \times 10^{-5}$T (d) $2\pi \times 10^{-5}$ T

8. A given length of a wire carries a steady current. It is bent first to form a circular plane coil of one turn. If a loop of same length is now bent more sharply to give a double loop of smaller radius, then the magnetic field at the centre caused by the same current is
(a) a quarter of its first value
(b) unaltered
(c) four times of its first value
(d) two times of its first value

9. **Assertion** (A) When the observation point lies along the length of the current element, magnetic field is zero.
Reason (R) Magnetic field close to current element is zero.
In the light of the above statements, choose the correct answer from the options given below.
(a) Both A and R are true but R is not the correct explanation of A.
(b) A is true but R is false.
(c) A is false but R is true.
(d) Both A and R are true and R is the correct explanation of A.

10. An arc of a circle of radius R subtends an angle $\pi/2$ at the centre. It carries a current i. The magnetic field at the centre will be
(a) $\frac{\mu_0 i}{2R}$ (b) $\frac{\mu_0 i}{8R}$
(c) $\frac{\mu_0 i}{4R}$ (d) $\frac{2\mu_0 i}{5R}$

11. The current is flowing in south direction along a power line. The direction of magnetic field above the power line (neglecting earth's field) is
(a) south (b) east
(c) north (d) west

12. Two infinitely long, thin, insulated, straight wires lie in the XY-plane along the X and Y-axes, respectively. Each wire carries a current i respectively in the positive x-direction and positive y-direction. The magnetic field will be zero at all points on the straight line with equation
(a) $y = x$ (b) $y = -x$
(c) $y = x - 1$ (d) $y = -x + 1$

13. **Assertion** (A) A circular loop carrying current lies in XY- plane with its centre at origin having a magnetic flux is negative Z-axis.
Reason (R) Magnetic flux direction is independent of the direction of current in conductor.
In the light of the above statements, choose the correct answer from the options given below.
(a) Both A and R are true but R is not the correct explanation of A.
(b) A is true but R is false.
(c) A is false but R is true.
(d) Both A and R are true and R is the correct explanation of A.

14. Magnetic field due to a ring having n turns at a distance x on its axis is proportional to (if r = radius of ring)
(a) $\frac{r}{(x^2 + r^2)}$ (b) $\frac{r}{(x^2 + r^2)^{3/2}}$
(c) $\frac{nr^2}{(x^2 + r^2)^{3/2}}$ (d) $\frac{n^2r^2}{(x^2 + r^2)^{3/2}}$

15. **Assertion** (A) The magnetic field intensity at the centre of circular coil carrying current changes, if the current through the coil is doubled.
Reason (R) The magnetic field intensity is dependent on current in conductor.
In the light of the above statements, choose the correct answer from the options given below.
(a) Both A and R are true but R is not the correct explanation of A.
(b) A is true but R is false.
(c) A is false but R is true.
(d) Both A and R are true and R is the correct explanation of A.

16. The ratio of the magnetic field at centre of a current carrying coil of the radius a and at a distance a from centre of the coil to the axis of coil is
(a) $\frac{1}{\sqrt{2}}$ (b) $\sqrt{2}$
(c) $\frac{1}{2\sqrt{2}}$ (d) $2\sqrt{2}$

17. A circular current carrying coil has a radius R. The distance from the centre of the coil on the axis of the coil, where the magnetic induction is (1/8)th of its value at the centre of coil is
(a) $\sqrt{3}R$ (b) $R/\sqrt{3}$
(c) $(2/\sqrt{3})R$ (d) $R/(2\sqrt{3})$

18. **Assertion** (A) Magnetic field is not associated with a stationary charge.
Reason (R) A magnetic field is detected by means of its effect on a current carrying conductor.
In the light of the above statements, choose the correct answer from the options given below.
(a) Both A and R are true but R is not the correct explanation of A.
(b) A is true but R is false.
(c) A is false but R is true.
(d) Both A and R are true and R is the correct explanation of A.

19. A current I flows through a closed loop as shown in figure. The magnetic field at the centre O is

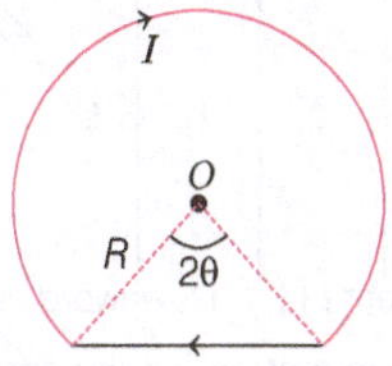

(a) $\frac{\mu_0 I}{2\pi R}(\pi - \theta + \tan\theta)$ (b) $\frac{\mu_0 I}{2\pi R}(\pi - \theta + \sin\theta)$
(c) $\frac{\mu_0 I}{2\pi R}(\theta + \sin\theta)$ (d) None of these

20. A current i A flows in a circular arc of radius R, which subtends an angle $3\pi/2$ rad at its centre. The magnetic induction B at the centre is

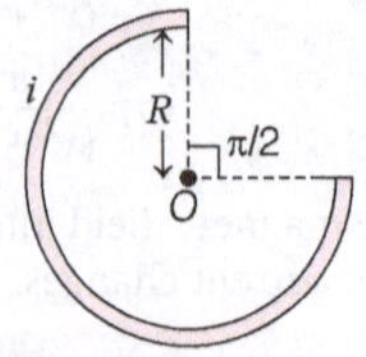

(a) $\frac{\mu_0 i}{R}$ (b) $\frac{\mu_0 i}{2R}$ (c) $\frac{2\mu_0 i}{R}$ (d) $\frac{3\mu_0 i}{8R}$

21. Two concentric coils each of 10 turns are situated in the same plane. Their radii are 2 cm and 4 cm and they carry 0.2 A and 0.3 A currents respectively in opposite directions. The magnetic field (in Wb/m^2) at the centre is

(a) $(35/4)\,\mu_0$ (b) $(\mu_0/80)$
(c) $(7/80)\,\mu_0$ (d) $(25/2)\,\mu_0$

Module 2

Ampere's Circuital Law

- Understanding the Ampere's Circuital Law
- Applications of Ampere's Circuital Law
- The Solenoid

Understanding the Ampere's Circuital Law

It states that, the line integral of magnetic field **B** around any closed path (Amperian loop) or circuit is equal to μ_0 times the total current crossing the area bounded by the closed path, provided that the magnetic field inside the loop remains constant. Thus,

$$\oint \mathbf{B} \cdot d\mathbf{l} = \mu_0 (i_{\text{net}})$$

In the above relation, we will use a sign convention given by right hand thumb rule. According to this rule, fingers of the right hand are curled in the sense that the boundary is traversed in the loop integral $\oint \mathbf{B} \cdot d\mathbf{l}$, then the direction of the thumb gives the sense in which the current i is treated as positive.

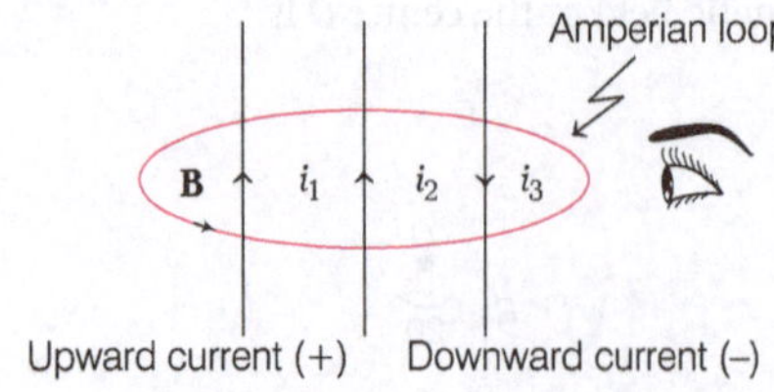

Sign convention for the current

In this way, currents i_1, i_2 and i_3 shown in the diagram are respectively taken as positive and negative.

$$\therefore \quad i_{\text{net}} = i_1 + i_2 - i_3$$

$$\Rightarrow \quad \oint \mathbf{B} \cdot d\mathbf{l} = \mu_0 (i_1 + i_2 - i_3)$$

Its simplified form is $Bl = \mu_0 i_{\text{net}}$.

This simplified equation can be used under the following conditions.

(i) At every point of the closed path, $\mathbf{B} \parallel d\mathbf{l}$.

(ii) Magnetic field has the same magnitude B at all places on the closed path.

(iii) Ampere's circuital law holds for steady currents which do not change with time.

Example 6. *Write equation for Ampere's circuital law for the Amperian loop as shown below.*
(Traverse in the direction shown by arrow mark put on it.)

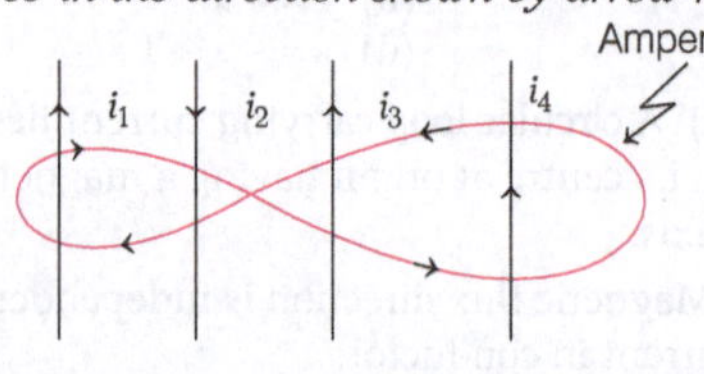

Sol. If observed from the top, then left side portion of the loop is traversed clockwise while the other portion is traversed anti-clockwise. Therefore, by sign convention

$$i_1 \longrightarrow (-),\ i_2 \longrightarrow (+)$$

$$i_3 \longrightarrow (+),\ i_4 \longrightarrow (+)$$

Thus, $\oint \mathbf{B} \cdot d\mathbf{l} = \mu_0 (i_2 + i_3 + i_4 - i_1)$

Applications of Ampere's Circuital Law

Ampere's circuital law can be applied to calculate magnetic field associated with symmetric distributed current carrying configurations which are discussed below.

Magnetic Field due to a Cylindrical Wire

(i) **Outside the cylinder** ($r > R$) To find magnetic field outside at point P, we will assume Amperian loops as shown below.

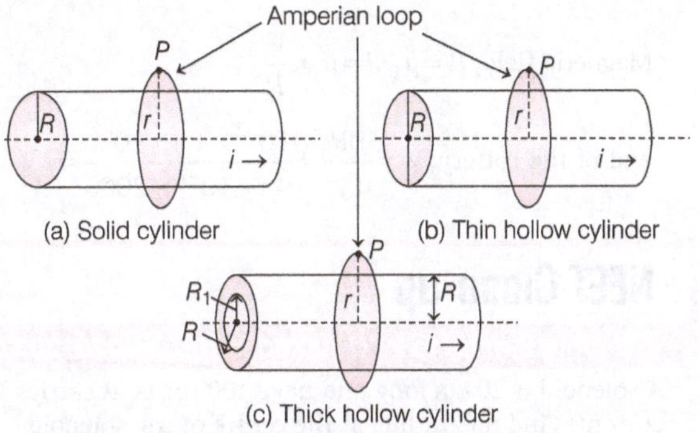

Applications of Ampere's circuital law for a point P outside the cylinder

In all the above cases, magnetic field outside the wire at P,

$$\oint \mathbf{B} \cdot d\mathbf{l} = B(2\pi r)$$

$$\Rightarrow \quad \boxed{B_{out} = \frac{\mu_0 i}{2\pi r}}$$

In all the above cases, $\boxed{B_{surface} = \frac{\mu_0 i}{2\pi R}}$

(ii) **Inside the hollow cylinder** ($r < R$) Magnetic field inside the hollow cylinder is zero because no current is enclosed by Amperian loops as shown below.

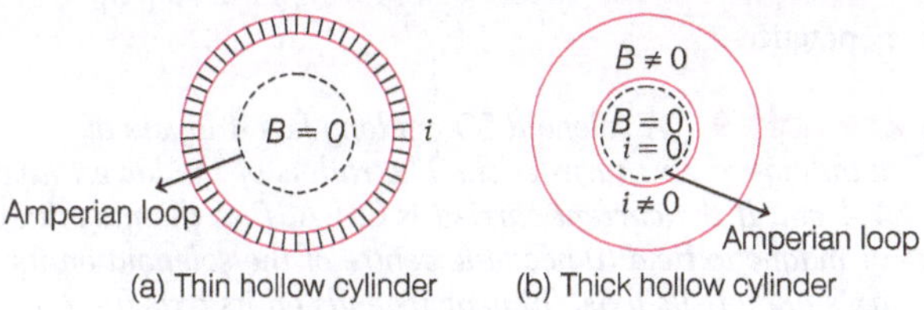

Magnetic field inside the hollow cylinder

(iii) **Inside the solid cylinder** ($r < R$) Current i' enclosed by Amperian loop is less than the total current i.

Current density is uniform, *i.e.* $J = J'$

$$\Rightarrow \quad i' = i \times \frac{A'}{A} = i\left(\frac{r^2}{R^2}\right)$$

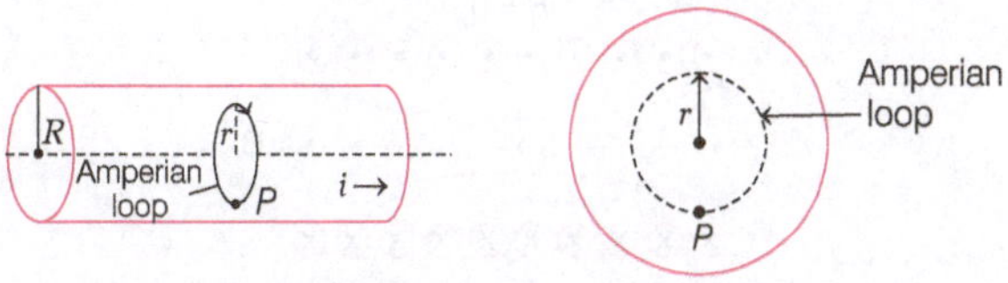

Amperian loop inside a solid cylinder

Hence, at inside point, $\oint \mathbf{B}_{in} \cdot d\mathbf{l} = \mu_0 i'$

$$\Rightarrow \quad \boxed{B_{in} = \frac{\mu_0}{2\pi} \cdot \frac{ir}{R^2}}$$

NEET Snapshot

The variation in magnetic field due to infinite long solid cylindrical conductor along its radius is as shown in figure *[NEET 2022, 21, 19]*

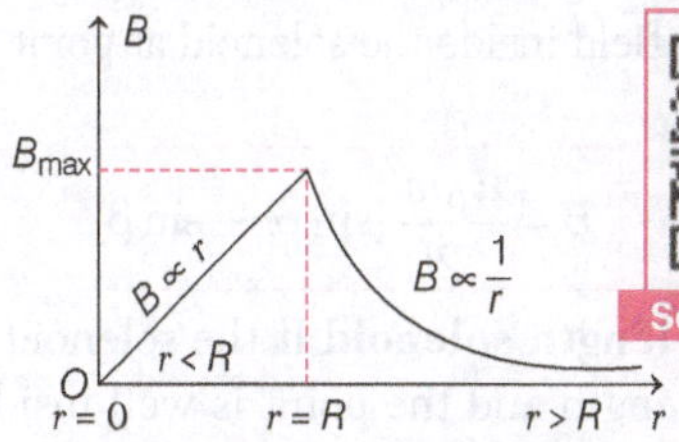

B-r graph for solid cylinder

Scan for Video

Magnetic field inside the cylinder is directly proportional to r and outside $B \propto \frac{1}{r}$, hence the graph is a straight line from centre to $r = R$ and after that it goes to zero.

Magnetic field inside the wire, $B = 0$ as $r = 0$.

Also, the magnetic field is continuous at the surface of the wire.

The Solenoid

A cylindrical coil of many wounded turns of insulated wire with diameter of the coil smaller than its length is called a **solenoid.**

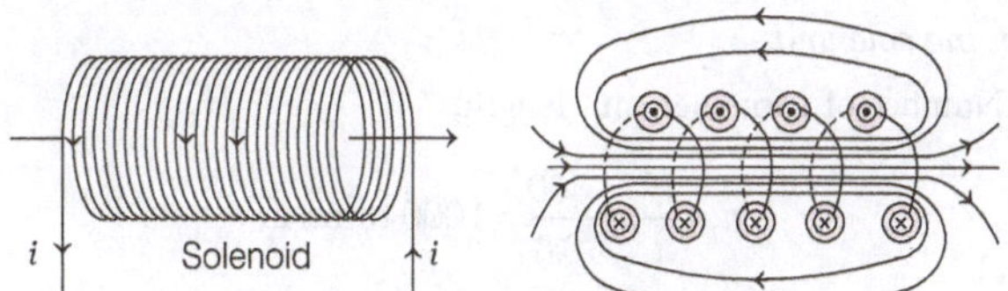

Solenoid and its magnetic field

A magnetic field is produced around and within the solenoid as shown in above figure. The magnetic field within the tightly wound solenoid (ideal solenoid) is uniform and parallel to the axis of solenoid.

Outside the ideal solenoid, magnetic field is zero as shown in the figure below

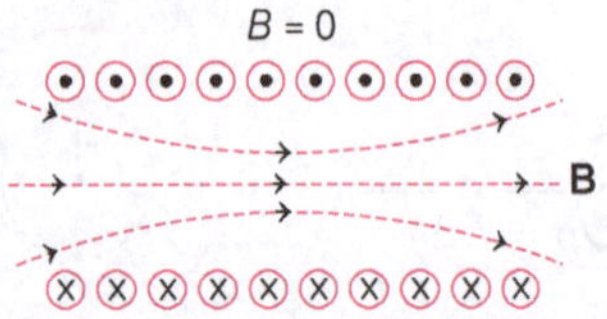

Magnetic field (outside) due to ideal solenoid

(i) **Finite length solenoid** If N = total number of turns, l = length of the solenoid and n = number of turns per unit length = N/l.

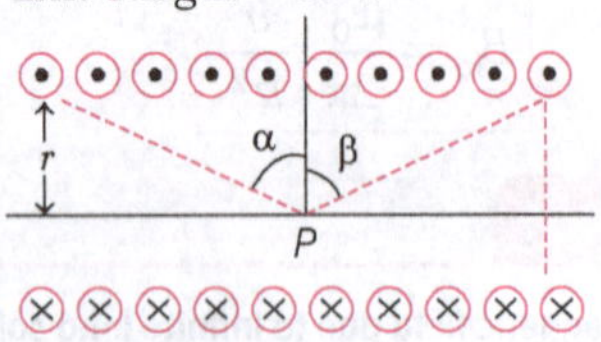

Magnetic field due to finite length solenoid

Magnetic field inside the solenoid at point P is given by

$$B = \frac{\mu_0 ni}{2} [\sin \alpha + \sin \beta]$$

(ii) **Infinite length solenoid** If the solenoid is of infinite length and the point is well inside it,

i.e. $\alpha = \beta = (\pi/2)$

Then, $B_{in} = \mu_0 ni$

If the solenoid is of infinite length and the point is near one end, *i.e.* $\alpha = 0$ and $\beta = (\pi/2)$, then

$$B_{end} = \frac{\mu_0 ni}{2}$$

Mentor's TIP

- Direction of magnetic field inside a solenoid is given by right hand thumb rule. This field is uniform.

Example 7. *A 0.8 m long solenoid has 800 turns and has a field density of 2.52×10^{-3} T at its centre. Find the current in the solenoid.*

Sol. Number of turns per unit length,

$$n = \frac{N}{l} = \frac{800}{0.8} = 1000 \text{ turns/m}$$

We know that, $B = \mu_0 ni$

$\therefore$ Current in the solenoid,

$$i = \frac{B}{\mu_0 n} = \frac{2.52 \times 10^{-3}}{4\pi \times 10^{-7} \times 1000} = 2.0 \text{ A}$$

Example 8. *A copper wire having a resistance of 0.01 Ω/m is used to wind a 400 turns solenoid of radius 1.0 cm and length 20 cm. Find the emf of a battery which when connected across the solenoid would produce a magnetic field of 10^{-2} T near the centre of the solenoid.*

Sol. Length of wire used $= 2\pi r \times$ Number of turns

$$= (2\pi \times 1.0 \times 10^{-2} \times 400) \text{m}$$

Resistance per unit length = 0.01 Ω/m

$\therefore$ Total resistance of wire,

$$R = 2\pi \times 1.0 \times 10^{-2} \times 400 \times 0.01$$
$$= 8\pi \times 10^{-2} \Omega$$

Number of turns per unit length,

$$n = N/l = \frac{400}{20 \times 10^{-2}} = 2000 \text{ turns/m}$$

Magnetic field, $B = \mu_0 ni = \mu_0 n \frac{V}{R}$

emf of the battery, $V = \frac{BR}{\mu_0 n} = \frac{10^{-2} \times 8\pi \times 10^{-2}}{4\pi \times 10^{-7} \times 2000} = 1 \text{ V}$

NEET Close-up

Example Similar to PYQ Asked in NEET 2020, 2022

A solenoid is 20 cm long and have 100 turns. It carries 1A current. Find magnitude at the centre of the solenoid.

(a) 6.28×10^{-4} T (b) 3.14×10^{-4} T
(c) 1.25×10^{-3} T (d) 1.5×10^{-4} T

Sol. (*a*) Here, $n = \frac{N}{L} = \frac{100}{20} \times 100 = 500 \frac{\text{turns}}{\text{m}}$

$$I = 1 \text{ A}$$

$\Rightarrow$ $B = \mu_0 nI$
$= 4\pi \times 500 \times 1 \times 10^{-7}$
$= 2 \times \pi \times 10^{-4}$
$= 2\pi \times 10^{-4} = 6.28 \times 10^{-4}$ T

Skill Builder

If number of turns, current through wire and radius of solenoid is doubled. Its magnetic field at the centre will be

(a) no change (b) doubled (c) four times (d) halved

For More Practice Refer Q. No. 15, 16, 17 of step up practice-2

Example 9. *A solenoid 50 cm long has 4 layers of windings of 350 turns each. The radius of the lowest layer is 1.4 cm. If the current carried is 6.0 A, find the magnitude of magnetic field (i) near the centre of the solenoid on its axis and off its axis, (ii) near its ends on its axis (iii) and outside the solenoid near its centre.*

Sol. (i) The magnitude of the magnetic field at (or near) the centre of the solenoid is given by

$$B = \mu_0 nI$$

where, n is the number of turns per unit length.

This expression for B can also be used, if the solenoid has more than one layer of windings because the radius of wire does not affect this equation. Therefore,

$$n = \frac{\text{Number of turns per layer} \times \text{Number of layers}}{\text{Length of the solenoid}}$$

$$= \frac{350 \times 4}{0.5} = 2800 \text{ turns/m}$$

Now, $I = 6.0\text{ A}, \mu_0 = 4\pi \times 10^{-7} \text{ TmA}^{-1}$

and $n = 2800$ turns/m

$\therefore \quad B = 4\pi \times 10^{-7} \times 2800 \times 6 = 2.1 \times 10^{-2}\text{T}$

Since, for an infinitely long solenoid, the internal field near the centre is uniform over the entire cross-section, therefore this value of B is for both on and off its axis.

(ii) Magnetic field at the ends of the solenoid,

$$B_{\text{end}} = \frac{\mu_0 nI}{2} = \frac{2.1 \times 10^{-2}}{2} = 1.05 \times 10^{-2}\text{T}$$

(iii) The outside field near the centre of a long solenoid is negligible as compared to the internal field.

STEP UP Practice 2

1. A current of i A flows along an infinitely long straight thin walled tube, then the magnetic induction at any point inside the tube is
(a) infinite
(b) zero
(c) $\frac{\mu_0 2i}{4\pi r}$ T
(d) $\frac{\mu_0 i}{2r}$ T

2. If a long hollow copper pipe carries a direct current, the magnetic field associated with the current will be
(a) only inside the pipe
(b) only outside the pipe
(c) both inside and outside the pipe
(d) neither inside nor outside the pipe

3. A current of $1/2\pi$ A is flowing in a long straight conductor. The line integral of magnetic induction around a closed path enclosing the current carrying conductor is
(a) 2×10^{-7} Wb/m
(b) $4\pi \times 10^{-7}$ Wb/m
(c) $16\pi^2 \times 10^{-7}$ Wb/m
(d) zero

4. **Statement I** If we consider two wires carrying currents I_1 and I_2, then for the Amperian loop shown

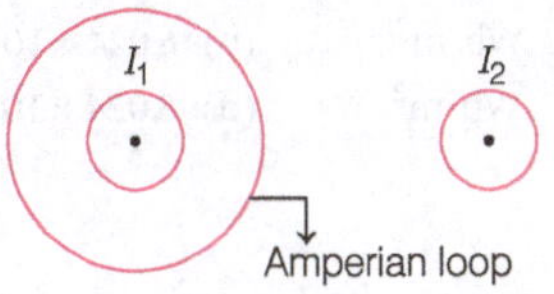

Then, $\int \mathbf{B} \cdot d\mathbf{l} = \mu_0 I_1$, even when the second wire is present or not.

Statement II At some points magnetic fields of both wires oppose each other and add up at some points and so, in sum over complete path these effects balance each other.

In the light of the above statements, choose the most appropriate answer from the options given below.
(a) Both Statement I and Statement II are incorrect.
(b) Statement I is correct but Statement II is incorrect.
(c) Statement I is incorrect but Statement II is correct.
(d) Both Statement I and Statement II are correct.

5. Rank the value of $\oint \mathbf{B} \cdot d\mathbf{l}$ for the closed paths shown in figure from the smallest to largest.

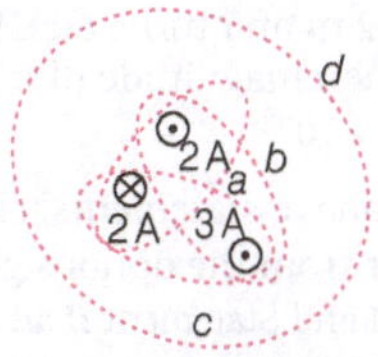

(a) a, b, c, d
(b) a, c, d, b
(c) a, d, c, b
(d) a, c, b, d

6. A current I flows along the length of an infinitely long, straight and thin-walled pipe. Then,
(a) the magnetic field at all points inside the pipe is the same but not zero.
(b) the magnetic field at any points inside the pipe is zero.
(c) the magnetic field is zero only on the axis of the pipe.
(d) the magnetic field is different at different points inside the pipe.

7. In the diagram shown, a wire carries current I. The loop has 25 turns and part of helical loop on which arrows are drawn is outside the plane of paper. What is the value of the $\oint \mathbf{B} \cdot d\mathbf{l}$ (as in Ampere's law) on the helical loop shown in the figure?

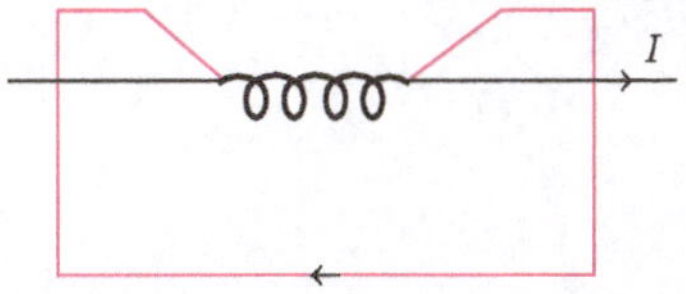

(a) $-\mu_0 NI$
(b) $\mu_0 I$
(c) $\mu_0 25I$
(d) Zero

8. **Statement I** A direct current flows through a metallic rod, produced magnetic field only outside the rod.

Statement II There is no flow of charge carriers inside the rod.

In the light of the above statements, choose the most appropriate answer from the options given below.
(a) Both Statement I and Statement II are incorrect.
(b) Statement I is correct but Statement II is incorrect.
(c) Statement I is incorrect but Statement II is correct.
(d) Both Statement I and Statement II are correct.

9. A direct current I flows along the length of an infinitely long straight thin walled pipe, then the magnetic field is
(a) uniform throughout the pipe but not zero
(b) zero only along the axis of the pipe
(c) zero at any point inside the pipe
(d) maximum at the centre and minimum at the edge

10. A large metal sheet carries an electric current along it surface. Current per unit length is λ.

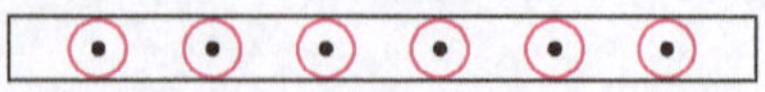

Magnetic field induction near the metal sheet is

(a) $\lambda\mu_0$ (b) $\frac{\lambda\mu_0}{2}$ (c) $\frac{\lambda\mu_0}{2\pi}$ (d) $\frac{\mu_0}{2\pi\lambda}$

11. **Statement I** Ampere's circuital law holds for steady current.
Statement II If a current of 5 A is flowing through a solenoid of length 2 m and turns 600. If the radius of solenoid is 2 cm, then magnitude of magnetic field inside the solenoid is 1.88×10^{-3} T.

In the light of the above statements, choose the most appropriate answer from the options given below :
(a) Both Statement I and Statement II are incorrect.
(b) Statement I is correct but Statement II is incorrect.
(c) Statement I is incorrect but Statement II is correct.
(d) Both Statement I and Statement II are correct.

12. Which of the following pair given below is incorrect?

(a) For finite length solenoid $\rightarrow B = \frac{\mu_0 ni}{2}(\sin\alpha + \sin\beta)$

(b) For infinite length solenoid $\rightarrow B = \mu_0 ni$

(c) Inside the solid cylinder $(r < R)$ $\rightarrow B_{in} = \frac{\mu_0}{2\pi} \cdot \frac{ir^2}{R}$

(d) Outside the solid cylinder $(r > R)$ $\rightarrow B_{out} = \frac{\mu_0 i}{2\pi r}$

13. Which of the following figures shows the magnetic flux density B at a distance r from a long straight rod carrying a steady current i?

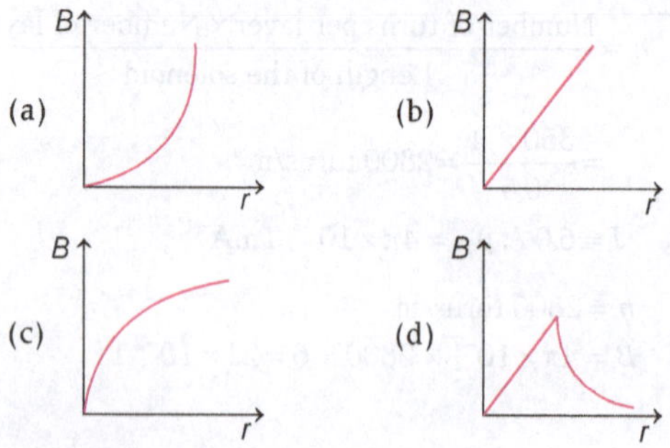

14. **Statement I** The magnetic field produced by a current carrying solenoid is independent of its length and cross-sectional area.
Statement II The magnetic field inside the solenoid is uniform.
In the light of the above statements, choose the most appropriate answer from the options given below.
(a) Both Statement I and Statement II are incorrect.
(b) Statement I is correct but Statement II is incorrect.
(c) Statement I is incorrect but Statement II is correct.
(d) Both Statement I and Statement II are correct.

15. A solenoid of length 0.5 m has a radius of 1 cm and is made up of 500 turns. It carries a current of 5A. What is the magnetic field inside the solenoid?
(a) 6.28×10^{-3} T (b) 6.28×10^{3} T
(c) 6.28×10^{-5} T (d) 6.28×10^{5} T

16. A long solenoid has 20 turns cm^{-1}. The current necessary to produce a magnetic field of 20 mT inside the solenoid is approximately
(a) 1A (b) 2A
(c) 4A (d) 8A

17. The magnetic field at a point on the axis of a long solenoid having 5 turns per cm length when a current of 0.8 A flows through it is
(a) 5.024×10^{-4} Wb/m^2 (b) 6.024×10^{-4} Wb/m^2
(c) 7.024×10^{-4} Wb/m^2 (d) 8.024×10^{-4} Wb/m^2

Module 3

Magnetic Forces

- Force on a Moving Charge in a Uniform Magnetic Field • Motion of a Charged Particle in a Uniform Magnetic Field • Motion of a Charged Particle in a Combined Electric and Magnetic Fields : Lorentz Force
- Force on a Current Carrying Conductor in a Magnetic Field • Force between Two Parallel Current Carrying Conductors

Force on a Moving Charge in a Uniform Magnetic Field

If a particle carrying a positive charge q and moving with velocity v enters in a magnetic field B, then it experiences a magnetic force F_m which is given by the expression

$$\mathbf{F}_m = q\,(\mathbf{v} \times \mathbf{B})$$

(i) The magnitude of $\mathbf{F}_m$ is

$$F_m = Bqv \sin\theta$$

where, θ is the angle between $\mathbf{v}$ and $\mathbf{B}$.

(ii) $\mathbf{F}_m$ is zero, when

(a) $B = 0$, *i.e.* no magnetic field is present.

(b) $q = 0$, *i.e.* particle is neutral.

(c) $v = 0$, *i.e.* charged particle is at rest.

(d) $\theta = 0°$ or $180°$, *i.e.* particle is moving parallel or anti-parallel to the direction of magnetic field.

(iii) $\mathbf{F}_m$ is maximum at $\theta = 90°$ and this maximum value is Bqv.

Concept ladder If $F_m \perp v \Rightarrow F \perp \frac{ds}{dt}$. Therefore, $F_m \perp ds$ or the work done by the magnetic force in a static magnetic field is zero.
i.e. $W_{F_m} = 0$

Example 10. *A charged particle of specific charge (i.e. charge per unit mass) 0.2 C/kg has velocity $(2\hat{\mathbf{i}} - 3\hat{\mathbf{j}})$ ms^{-1} at some instant in a uniform magnetic field $(5\hat{\mathbf{i}} + 2\hat{\mathbf{j}})$ T. Find the acceleration of the particle at this instant.*

Sol. The acceleration of the particle, $\mathbf{a} = \frac{\mathbf{F}}{m} = \frac{q}{m}(\mathbf{v} \times \mathbf{B})$

Given, $\frac{q}{m} = 0.2$ C/kg

$\mathbf{v} = (2\hat{\mathbf{i}} - 3\hat{\mathbf{j}})\,\text{ms}^{-1}$ and $\mathbf{B} = (5\hat{\mathbf{i}} + 2\hat{\mathbf{j}})$ T

Therefore, $\mathbf{a} = 0.2(2\hat{\mathbf{i}} - 3\hat{\mathbf{j}}) \times (5\hat{\mathbf{i}} + 2\hat{\mathbf{j}})$

$= 0.2\,[4\hat{\mathbf{k}} + 15\hat{\mathbf{k}}] = 3.8\,\hat{\mathbf{k}}\ \text{ms}^{-2}$

Mentor's Tip

- Use concept of cross product to find direction of force. It will be helpful in problem solving approach.

Example 11. *When a proton has a velocity $\mathbf{v} = (2\hat{\mathbf{i}} + 3\hat{\mathbf{j}}) \times 10^6\ ms^{-1}$, it experiences a force $\mathbf{F} = -(1.28 \times 10^{-13}\ \hat{\mathbf{k}})$ N. When its velocity is along the Z-axis, then it experiences a force along the X-axis. What is the magnetic field?*

Sol. Magnetic force, $\mathbf{F}_m = q\,(\mathbf{v} \times \mathbf{B})$

For $\mathbf{F}_m$ to be along $(-\hat{\mathbf{k}})$, magnetic field must be along $(-\hat{\mathbf{j}})$.

Now, substituting all the values in above equation, we get

$$-(1.28 \times 10^{-13}\ \hat{\mathbf{k}}) = (1.6 \times 10^{-19})\,[(2\hat{\mathbf{i}} + 3\hat{\mathbf{j}}) \times (-B\hat{\mathbf{j}})] \times 10^6$$

$$\therefore \quad 1.28 = 1.6 \times 2 \times B \quad \text{or} \quad B = \frac{1.28}{3.2} = 0.4$$

Therefore, the magnetic field, $\mathbf{B} = -B\,\hat{\mathbf{j}} = (-0.4\,\hat{\mathbf{j}})$ T

Example 12. *A charged particle is projected in a magnetic field*

$$\mathbf{B} = (3\hat{\mathbf{i}} + 4\hat{\mathbf{j}}) \times 10^{-2}\ T$$

and the acceleration of the particle is found to be

$$\mathbf{a} = (x\hat{\mathbf{i}} + 2\hat{\mathbf{j}})\ ms^{-2}.$$

Find the value of x.

Sol. As, $\mathbf{F}_m \perp \mathbf{B}$

i.e. the acceleration $\mathbf{a} \perp \mathbf{B} \Rightarrow \mathbf{a} \cdot \mathbf{B} = 0$

or $(x\hat{\mathbf{i}} + 2\hat{\mathbf{j}}) \cdot (3\hat{\mathbf{i}} + 4\hat{\mathbf{j}}) \times 10^{-2} = 0$

or $(3x + 8) \times 10^{-2} = 0$

$\therefore$ Value of $x = -\frac{8}{3}$

Motion of a Charged Particle in a Uniform Magnetic Field

As we know that, the magnetic force on a charged particle is perpendicular to its velocity. Thus, this force does not do any work on the particle. Hence, the kinetic energy or the speed of the particle does not change due to the magnetic force.

Let a charged particle q be thrown in magnetic field $\mathbf{B}$ with a velocity $\mathbf{v}$ as shown in the figure. The magnetic force acting on the particle is given by $F = Bqv \sin\theta$, where θ is the angle between the velocity and the magnetic field.

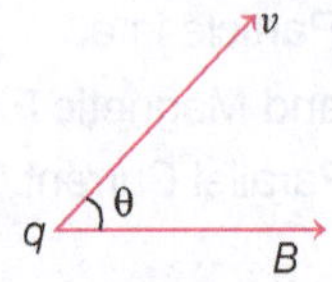

Charged particle thrown at angle θ with the magnetic field

Depending on the initial conditions, the charged particle can follow different trajectories in a region of uniform magnetic field. Let us take them one-by-one.

Case I When θ is 0° or 180°

When $\theta = 0°$ or $180°$, the magnetic force $F_m = 0$. Hence, path of the charged particle is a straight line (undeviated) when it enters parallel or anti-parallel to magnetic field as shown below.

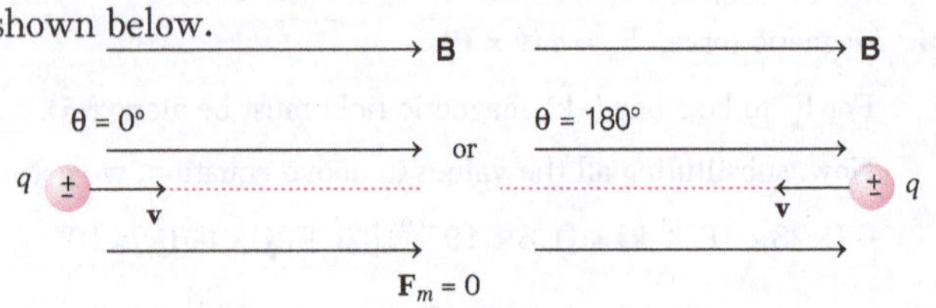

A charged particle moving parallel or anti-parallel to magnetic field

Case II When θ is 90°

When $\theta = 90°$, the magnetic force,

$$F_m = Bqv \sin 90° = Bqv$$

This magnetic force is perpendicular to the velocity at every instant. Hence, path of the charged particle is a circle. The necessary centripetal force is provided by the magnetic force.

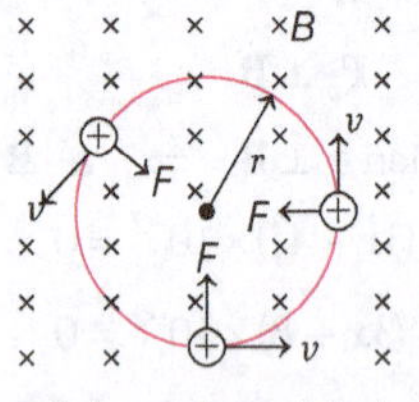

Circular motion of charged particle in magnetic field

Hence, if r be the radius of the circle, then

$$\frac{mv^2}{r} = Bqv \Rightarrow r = \frac{mv}{Bq}$$

This expression of r can be written in following different ways

$$r = \frac{mv}{Bq} = \frac{p}{Bq} = \frac{\sqrt{2Km}}{Bq}$$

Time Period and Frequency

- Further, time period of the circular path,

$$T = \frac{2\pi r}{v} = \frac{2\pi\left(\frac{mv}{Bq}\right)}{v} \Rightarrow \boxed{T = \frac{2\pi m}{Bq}}$$

- Angular speed of the particle, $\omega = \frac{2\pi}{T} = \frac{Bq}{m}$

$$\therefore \quad \boxed{\omega = \frac{Bq}{m}}$$

- Frequency of rotation, $f = \frac{1}{T}$

$$\Rightarrow \quad \boxed{f = \frac{Bq}{2\pi m}}$$

Concept ladder

- When a charged particle is projected perpendicular to a magnetic field, then
  (i) its path is circular in a plane perpendicular to the plane of magnetic field.
  (ii) the speed and kinetic energy of the particle remain constant.
  (iii) the velocity and momentum of the particle change only in direction.
  (iv) the time period of revolution, angular velocity and frequency of revolution are independent of velocity of the particle and radius of circular path.

Example 13. *What is the smallest value of B that can be set up at the equator to permit a proton having speed of 10^7 ms^{-1} to circulate around the earth? ($R = 6.4 \times 10^6$ m, $m_p = 1.67 \times 10^{-27}$ kg)*

Sol. From the relation, $R = \frac{mv}{Bq}$

$$\Rightarrow \quad B = \frac{mv}{qR}$$

Substituting the given values in above equation, we get

$$B = \frac{(1.67 \times 10^{-27})(10^7)}{(1.6 \times 10^{-19})(6.4 \times 10^6)}$$

$$= 1.6 \times 10^{-8} \text{ T}$$

Example 14. *A proton and an α-particle, accelerated through same potential difference, enter in a region of uniform magnetic field with their velocities perpendicular to the field. Compare the radii of circular paths followed by them.*

Sol. Let mass of proton be m and charge on proton be e.

Then, mass of α-particle = $4m$ and charge on α-particle = $2e$

When a charge q is accelerated by potential difference V, it acquires a kinetic energy, $E_k = qV$

$\therefore$ Momentum is given by $mv = \sqrt{2mE_k} = \sqrt{2mqV}$

Radius, $r = \frac{mv}{qB} = \frac{\sqrt{2mqV}}{qB} = \sqrt{\frac{2mV}{qB^2}}$

Thus, $\frac{r_p}{r_\alpha} = \sqrt{\frac{2mV}{eB^2}} \times \sqrt{\frac{2eB^2}{2(4m)V}} = \frac{1}{\sqrt{2}}$

Concept ladder

If charged particle enters in magnetic field at θ (0° < θ < 90° or 90° < θ < 180°), then path of charge will be helical.

In this case

(1) radius of path, $r = \frac{mv_1}{qB} = \frac{mv\sin\theta}{qB}$

(2) Time period, $T = \frac{2\pi m}{qB}$

Motion of a Charged Particle in a Combined Electric and Magnetic Fields : Lorentz Force

Consider a point charge q moving with velocity $\mathbf{v}$ and is located at position vector $\mathbf{r}$ at a given time t. If electric field $\mathbf{E}$ and magnetic field $\mathbf{B}$ are existing at that point, then force on the electric charge q is given by

$$\mathbf{F} = q[\mathbf{E} + \mathbf{v} \times \mathbf{B}] = \mathbf{F}_{\text{electric}} + \mathbf{F}_{\text{magnetic}}$$

This force was first given by H A Lorentz, hence it is called **Lorentz force.**

Here, magnetic force, $\mathbf{F}_m = q(\mathbf{v} \times \mathbf{B}) = Bqv\sin\theta$ and electric force, $\mathbf{F}_e = q\mathbf{E}$.

The direction of magnetic force is same as that of $\mathbf{v} \times \mathbf{B}$, if charge is positive and opposite to that of $\mathbf{v} \times \mathbf{B}$, if charge q is negative.

Case I When v , E and B are all Collinear

In this situation, the magnetic force on it will be zero and only electric force will act. So,

acceleration, $\mathbf{a} = \frac{\mathbf{F}_e}{m} = \frac{q\mathbf{E}}{m}$.

The particle will pass through the field following a straight line path (parallel field) with change in its speed. So, in this situation, speed, velocity, momentum and kinetic energy all will change without change in direction of motion as shown below.

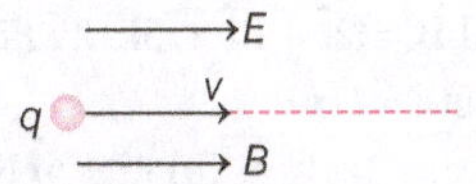

Motion of a charged particle with $\mathbf{v} \parallel \mathbf{E} \parallel \mathbf{B}$

Case II When v, E and B are Mutually Perpendicular

In this situation, if $\mathbf{E}$ and $\mathbf{B}$ are such that $\mathbf{F} = \mathbf{F}_e + \mathbf{F}_m = 0$, *i.e.* $\mathbf{a} = (\mathbf{F}/m) = 0$.

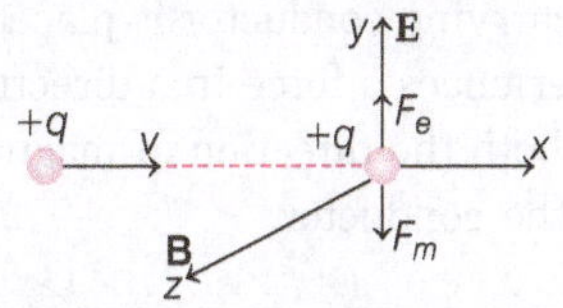

Motion of a charged particle with $\mathbf{v} \perp \mathbf{E} \perp \mathbf{B}$

The particle will pass through the field with same velocity without any deviation in its path as shown in figure.

In this situation, as $F_e = F_m$, *i.e.* $qE = qvB$

$$v = E/B$$

This principle is used in velocity-selector to get a charged beam having a specific velocity.

Mentor's TiP

If only magnetic field is present, we have to put

$\mathbf{E} = 0 \Rightarrow \mathbf{F} = q(\mathbf{v} \times \mathbf{B})$.

Similarly, if $\mathbf{B} = 0 \Rightarrow \mathbf{F} = q\mathbf{E}$

Example 15. *A charge particle having charge 2 C is thrown with velocity $(2\hat{\mathbf{i}} + 3\hat{\mathbf{j}})$ m/s inside a region having $\mathbf{E} = 2\hat{\mathbf{j}}$ V/m and magnetic field $5\hat{\mathbf{k}}$ T. Find the initial Lorentz force acting on the particle.*

Sol. Lorentz force is given by

$$\mathbf{F} = q(\mathbf{E} + \mathbf{v} \times \mathbf{B}) = 2[2\hat{\mathbf{j}} + (2\hat{\mathbf{i}} + 3\hat{\mathbf{j}}) \times 5\hat{\mathbf{k}}]$$
$$= 2[2\hat{\mathbf{j}} + 10(-\hat{\mathbf{j}}) + 15\hat{\mathbf{i}}]$$
$$= (30\hat{\mathbf{i}} - 16\hat{\mathbf{j}})\text{ N}$$

Example 16. *A proton beam passes without deviation through a region of space, where there are uniform transverse mutually perpendicular electric and magnetic fields with E = 220 kV/m and B = 50 mT. Then, the beam strikes a grounded target. Find the force imparted by the beam on the target if the beam current is equal to i = 0.80 mA.*

Sol. Since, proton is moving in a straight line, hence net force is zero.

$$\therefore \quad qE = Bqv \Rightarrow v = \frac{E}{B}$$

Also, current associated with the beam,

$$i = ne \Rightarrow n = i/e$$

where, n is number of protons/time.

Momentum of a proton $= mv$

Force, $F = nmv$

$$\Rightarrow \quad F = \frac{imE}{eB} = \frac{0.80 \times 10^{-3} \times 1.67 \times 10^{-27} \times 220 \times 10^3}{1.6 \times 10^{-19} \times 50 \times 10^{-3}}$$
$$= 3.67 \times 10^{-5}\text{ N}$$

Force on a Current Carrying Conductor in a Magnetic Field

When a current carrying conductor is placed in a magnetic field, then it experiences a force in a direction perpendicular to both the direction of magnetic field and that of length of the conductor.

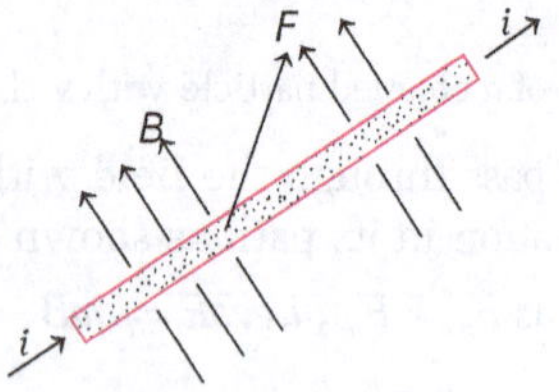

Current carrying conductor in a uniform magnetic field

The magnetic force, $F = ilB \sin\theta$

In vector form, $\boxed{\mathbf{F} = i\,(\mathbf{l} \times \mathbf{B})}$ ...(i)

where, B = intensity of magnetic field,
i = current in the conductor,
l = length of the conductor

and θ = angle between the length of conductor and direction of magnetic field.

Cases

I. When $\theta = 90^\circ$ or $\sin\theta = 1$, then $F = ilB \times 1 = ilB$ (maximum).

Therefore, force will be maximum when the current carrying conductor is perpendicular to magnetic field.

II. When $\theta = 0^\circ$ or $\sin\theta = 0$, then $F = ilB \times 0 = 0$.

Thus, the force will be zero when the current carrying conductor is parallel to the magnetic field.

Concept ladder

- Cross product of vectors can be explained using Fleming's left hand rule. Using this rule in the case of $\mathbf{F} = I(\mathbf{l} \times \mathbf{B})$, we get

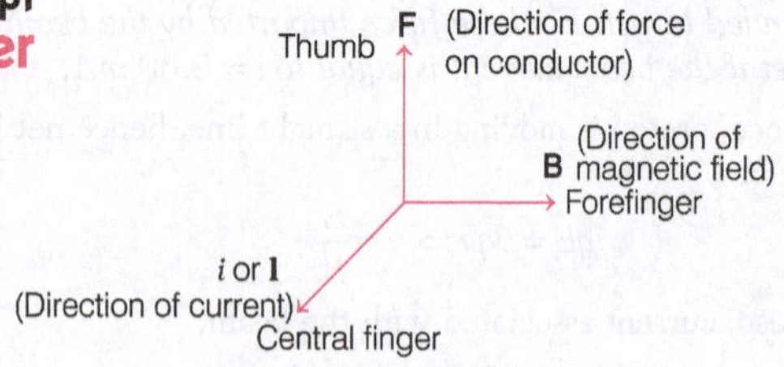

Fleming's left hand rule

- **Magnetic force on a closed current carrying loop**

When a closed current carrying loop is placed in uniform magnetic field, then the magnetic force on it is always zero. As the vector sum of $d\mathbf{l}$ is always zero, *i.e.* $\oint d\mathbf{l} = 0$.

$\therefore \quad \mathbf{F} = i\oint d\mathbf{l} \times \mathbf{B} = 0$

Magnetic Force on different Configurations of the Curve

Now, consider magnetic forces on current carrying conductors of different configurations as shown below. Here, magnetic force only depends upon effective length of the wires.

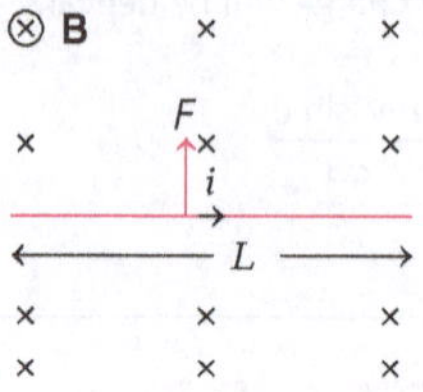

$F = BiL$

(a) Straight wire

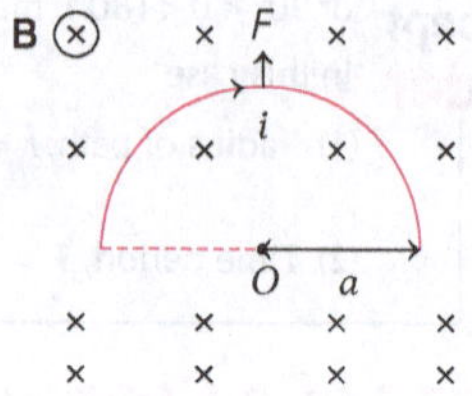

$F = i(2a)B$

(b) Semicircular wire

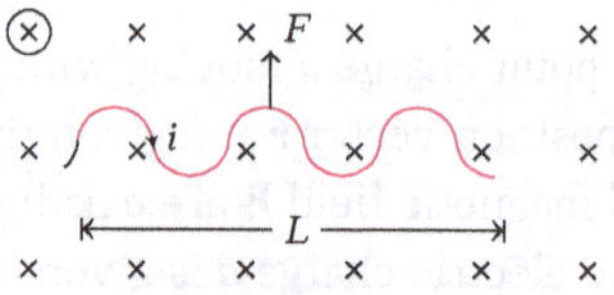

$F = BiL$

(c) Sinusoidal wire

NEET Close-up

Example Similar to PYQ Asked in NEET 2023

A wire of length a carries a current i along the Y-axis. A magnetic field exists which is given by

$$\mathbf{B} = B_0(3\,\hat{\mathbf{i}} + 2\hat{\mathbf{j}} + \hat{\mathbf{k}})\ \text{T}$$

The magnitude of magnetic force is

(a) $2\sqrt{2}B_0 ia$ (b) $3B_0 ia$ (c) $\sqrt{10}B_0 ia$ (d) $\sqrt{14}B_0 ia$

Sol. (c) Length of the wire, $\mathbf{l} = a\hat{\mathbf{j}}$

Magnetic force on the wire,

$$\mathbf{F} = i(\mathbf{l} \times \mathbf{B}) = i[a\,\hat{\mathbf{j}} \times B_0(3\hat{\mathbf{i}} + 2\hat{\mathbf{j}} + \hat{\mathbf{k}})]$$
$$= ia\,B_0[-3\hat{\mathbf{k}} + 0 + \hat{\mathbf{i}}]$$
$$= B_0 ia\,(\hat{\mathbf{i}} - 3\hat{\mathbf{k}})$$
$$\therefore \quad |\mathbf{F}| = F = B_0 ia\sqrt{(1)^2 + (-3)^2}$$
$$= \sqrt{10}\,B_0 ia$$

Skill Builder

A wire carries a current of 2A along z-direction is kept in a magnetic field $\mathbf{B} = (2\hat{\mathbf{i}} + 3\hat{\mathbf{j}} + 5\hat{\mathbf{k}})$ T. Find force on the wire (Take, length = 1 m)

(a) $4\hat{\mathbf{j}} + 6\hat{\mathbf{i}}$ N (b) $4\hat{\mathbf{j}} - 6\hat{\mathbf{i}}$ N
(c) $6\hat{\mathbf{j}} - 4\hat{\mathbf{i}}$ N (d) $6\hat{\mathbf{j}} - 4\hat{\mathbf{i}}$ N

For more Practice Refer Q. No.17 of Gearing up for NEET.

Example 17. *A square of side 2.0 m is placed in a uniform magnetic field of 2.0 T in a direction perpendicular to the plane of the square inwards. Equal current, i = 3.0 A is flowing in the directions shown in figure.*
Find the magnitude of magnetic force on the loop.

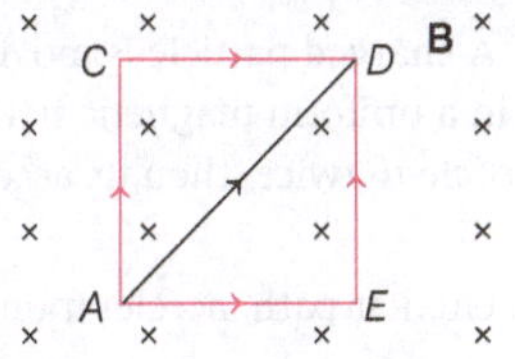

Sol. Force on wire ACD = Force on AD = Force on AED

All these forces are acting along EC.

$\therefore$ Net force on the loop $= 3\,(\mathbf{F}_{AD})$

or $\quad F_{\text{net}} = 3(i)(AD)(B)$

$= (3)(3.0)(2\sqrt{2})(2.0)\,\text{N} = 36\sqrt{2}\,\text{N}$

Force between Two Parallel Current Carrying Conductors

Consider two long wires 1 and 2 kept parallel to each other at a distance r and carrying currents i_1 and i_2 respectively in the same direction.

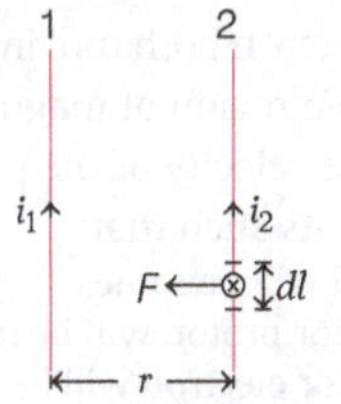

Two long parallel wires carrying currents in the same direction

Magnetic field on wire 2 due to current in wire 1,

$$B = \frac{\mu_0}{2\pi} \cdot \frac{i_1}{r} \quad \text{(in } \otimes \text{ direction)}$$

Magnetic force on a small element dl of wire 2 due to this magnetic field,

$$d\mathbf{F} = i_2 (d\mathbf{l} \times \mathbf{B})$$

Magnitude of this force,

$$dF = i_2\,[(dl)\,(B)\sin 90°] = i_2 (dl)\left(\frac{\mu_0}{2\pi}\,\frac{i_1}{r}\right) = \frac{\mu_0}{2\pi} \cdot \frac{i_1 i_2}{r} \cdot dl$$

Direction of this force is along $d\mathbf{l} \times \mathbf{B}$ or towards the wire 1.

The force per unit length of wire 2 due to wire 1,

$$\boxed{\frac{dF}{dl} = \frac{\mu_0}{2\pi}\,\frac{i_1 i_2}{r}}$$

The same force acts on wire 1 due to wire 2. The wires attract each other if currents in the wires are flowing in the same direction and they repel each other if the currents are flowing in opposite directions.

Example 18. *Currents of 10 A and 2 A are passed through two parallel wires A and B respectively in opposite directions. If the wire A is infinitely long and length of the wire B is 2 m, then find the force acting on the conductor B which is situated at 10 cm distance from A.*

Sol. Force on a conductor of length l carrying current i_2 and placed at a distance r parallel to another infinitely long conductor carrying current i_1,

$$F = \frac{\mu_0}{4\pi} \cdot \frac{2 i_1 i_2}{r}\, l \qquad \text{...(i)}$$

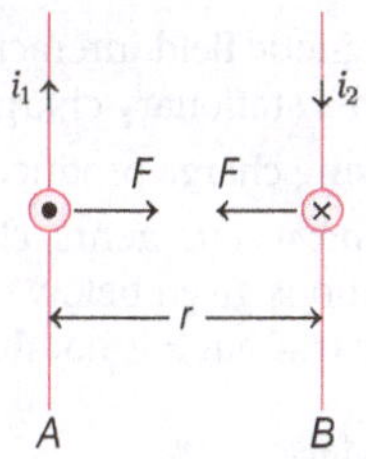

Here, $\quad i_1 = 10\,\text{A},\ i_2 = 2\,\text{A},\ l = 2\,\text{m},\ r = 10\,\text{cm} = 0.1\,\text{m}$

Substituting all these values in Eq. (i), we get

$$F = 10^{-7} \times \frac{2 \times 10 \times 2 \times 2}{0.1} = 8 \times 10^{-5}\,\text{N}$$

NEET Close-up

Example Similar to PYQ Asked in NEET 2017

Two long, straight and parallel wires are carrying current in same direction with magnitude of 2A and 5A. Find force acting per unit length between the two wires if distance between wires is 10 cm.

(a) 2×10^{-5} N/m

(b) 5.0×10^{-4} N/m

(c) 3×10^{-5} N/m

(d) 1.0×10^{-5} N/m

Sol. (a) $\dfrac{F}{l} = \dfrac{\mu_0 i_1 i_2}{2\pi d}$

$$= \frac{4\pi \times 10^{-7} \times 2 \times 5}{2\pi \times 10 \times 10^{-2}}$$

$$\Rightarrow \quad \frac{F}{l} = 2 \times 10^{-5}\,\text{N/m}$$

Skill Builder

If distance between two current carrying conductors is doubled, force per unit length acting between the two wires will gets

(a) not changed

(b) halved

(c) one-fourth times

(d) Doubled

For More Practice Refer Q. No. 23, 24 of step up practice-3 and Q. No. 56 of Gearing up for NEET.

STEP UP Practice 3

1. A strong magnetic field is applied on a stationary electron, then the electron
(a) moves in the direction of the field
(b) moves in an opposite direction of the field
(c) remains stationary
(d) starts spinning

2. **Assertion** (A) Magnetic field interacts with a moving charge and not with a stationary charge.
Reason (R) A moving charge produces a magnetic field.
In the light of the above statements, choose the correct answer from the options given below.
(a) Both A and R are true but R is not the correct explanation of A.
(b) A is true but R is false.
(c) A is false but R is true.
(d) Both A and R are true and R is the correct explanation of A.

3. A particle of mass m and charge Q moving with a velocity $\mathbf{v}$ enters a region of uniform magnetic field of induction $\mathbf{B}$. Then, its path in the region is
(a) always circular (b) circular, if $\mathbf{v} \times \mathbf{B} = 0$
(c) circular, if $\mathbf{v} \cdot \mathbf{B} = 0$ (d) None of these

4. An electron is moving in a circular path of radius r with speed v in a transverse magnetic field B. The value of e/m for it will be
(a) $\frac{v}{Br}$ (b) $\frac{B}{rv}$ (c) Bvr (d) $\frac{vr}{B}$

5. An electron and a proton with equal momentum enter perpendicularly into a uniform magnetic field, then
(a) the path of proton shall be more curved than that of electron
(b) the path of proton shall be less curved than that of electron
(c) Both are equally curved
(d) path of both will be straight line

6. A charged particle travels along a straight line with a speed v in a region, where both electric field $\mathbf{E}$ and magnetic field $\mathbf{B}$ are present. It follows that
(a) $|\mathbf{E}| = |\mathbf{B}|$ and the two fields are perpendicular.
(b) $|\mathbf{E}| = v|\mathbf{B}|$ and the two fields are perpendicular.
(c) $|\mathbf{B}| = v|\mathbf{E}|$ and the two fields are parallel.
(d) $|\mathbf{B}| = v|\mathbf{E}|$ and the two fields are perpendicular.

7. A proton, a deuteron and an α-particle having the same kinetic energy, are moving in circular trajectories in a uniform magnetic field. If r_p, r_d and r_α denote the radii of the trajectories of these particles respectively, then
(a) $r_\alpha = r_p < r_d$ (b) $r_\alpha > r_d > r_p$
(c) $r_\alpha = r_d > r_p$ (d) $r_p = r_d = r_\alpha$

8. When a charged particle enters a uniform magnetic field, then its kinetic energy
(a) remains constant (b) increases
(c) decreases (d) becomes zero

9. **Assertion** (A) A charged particle is moving in a circle with constant speed in a uniform magnetic field. If we increase the speed of particle to twice, then its acceleration becomes four times.
Reason (R) In circular path, acceleration of particle is given by $\frac{v^2}{r}$.
In the light of the above statements, choose the correct answer from the options given below.
(a) Both A and R are true but R is not the correct explanation of A.
(b) A is true but R is false.
(c) A is false but R is true.
(d) Both A and R are true and R is the correct explanation of A.

10. A proton of energy 8 eV is moving in a circular path in uniform magnetic field. The energy of an α-particle moving in the same magnetic field and along the same path will be
(a) 4 eV (b) 2 eV
(c) 8 eV (d) 6 eV

11. A proton and an electron both moving with the same velocity v enter into a region of magnetic field directed perpendicular to the velocity of the particles. They, will now move in circular orbits such that
(a) their time period will be same
(b) the time period for proton will be higher
(c) the time period for electron will be higher
(d) their orbital radii will be same

12. Which of the following pair given below is incorrect ?
(a) Magnetic force on a closed current carrying loop → $F = i\oint dl \times B = 0$
(b) Magnetic force on a straight wire → BiL
(c) Magnetic force on a sinusoidal wire → $2BiL$
(d) Magnetic force on a semicircular wire of radius → $i(2a)B$

13. If a charged particle is describing a circle of radius r in a magnetic field with a time period T. Then,
(a) $T^2 \propto r^3$ (b) $T^2 \propto r$
(c) $T \propto r^2$ (d) $T \propto r^0$

14. A particle is projected in a plane perpendicular to a uniform magnetic field. The area bounded by the path described by the particle is proportional to
(a) the velocity
(b) the momentum
(c) the kinetic energy
(d) None of the above

15. If electron velocity is $(2\hat{i} + 3\hat{j})$ and it is subjected to a magnetic field $4\hat{k}$, then
(a) speed of electron will change
(b) path of electron will change
(c) Both (a) and (b)
(d) None of the above

16. A beam of protons with a velocity of 4×10^5 ms^{-1} enters a uniform magnetic field of 0.3 T at an angle of 60° to the magnetic field. The radius of helical path taken by proton beam is
(a) 0.036 m (b) 0.012 m
(c) 0.024 m (d) 0.048 m

17. A proton and a deuteron, both having the same kinetic energy, enter perpendicularly into a uniform magnetic field B. For motion of proton and deuteron in circular path of radius R_p and R_d, respectively. The correct relation is
(a) $R_d = \sqrt{2}R_p$ (b) $R_d = R_p/\sqrt{2}$
(c) $R_d = R_p$ (d) $R_d = 2R_p$

18. Two ions having masses in the ratio 1 : 1 and charges in the ratio 1 : 2 are projected perpendicular to the field of a cyclotron with speeds in the ratio 2 : 3. The ratio of the radii of circular paths along which the two particles move is
(a) 4 : 3 (b) 2 : 3
(c) 3 : 1 (d) 1 : 4

19. Assertion (A) In a conductor, free electrons keep on moving but no magnetic force acts on a conductor in a magnetic field.
Reason (R) Force on free electron due to magnetic field always acts perpendicular to its direction of motion.
In the light of the above statements, choose the correct answer from the options given below.
(a) Both A and R are true but R is not the correct explanation of A.
(b) A is true but R is false.
(c) A is false but R is true.
(d) Both A and R are true and R is the correct explanation of A.

20. A conducting loop carrying a current I is placed in a uniform magnetic field pointing into the plane of the paper as shown. The loop will have a tendency to

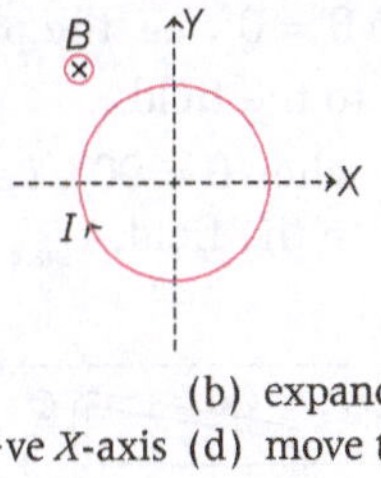

(a) contract (b) expand
(c) move towards +ve X-axis (d) move towards –ve X-axis

21. Two parallel wires carrying currents in the same direction attract each other because of
(a) potential difference between them
(b) mutual inductance between them
(c) electric force between them
(d) magnetic force between them

22. Two parallel conductor A and B of equal length carry currents I and $10I$, respectively, in the same direction, then
(a) A and B will repel each other with same force.
(b) A and B will attract each other with same force.
(c) A will attract B but B will repel A.
(d) A and B will attract each other with different forces.

23. Two thin long parallel wires, separated by a distance d carry a current i ampere in the same direction. They will
(a) attract each other with a force of $\mu_0 i / 2\pi d^2$
(b) repel each other with a force of $\mu_0 i^2 / 2\pi d^2$
(c) attract each other with a force of $\mu_0 i^2 / 2\pi d$
(d) repel each other with a force of $\mu_0 i / 2\pi d$

24. Two long conductors, separated by a distance d carry currents I_1 and I_2 in the same direction. They exert a force F on each other. Now the current in one of them is increased to two times and its direction is reversed. The distance is also increased to $3d$. The new value of the force between them is
(a) $-\frac{F}{3}$ (b) $\frac{F}{3}$
(c) $\frac{2F}{3}$ (d) $\frac{-2F}{3}$

25. Assertion (A) The work done by magnetic field on a moving charge is zero.
Reason (R) In magnetic field force is perpendicular to the velocity.
In the light of the above statements, choose the correct answer from the options given below.
(a) Both A and R are true but R is not the correct explanation of A.
(b) A is true but R is false.
(c) A is false but R is true.
(d) Both A and R are true and R is the correct explanation of A.

26. The force per unit length between two long parallel wires A and B carrying current is 0.004 Nm^{-1}. The conductors are 0.01 m apart. If the current in conductor A is twice that of conductor B, then the current in the conductor B would be
(a) 5 A (b) 50 A
(c) 10 A (d) 100 A

Module 4

Torque and Moving Coil Galvanometer

- Magnetic Dipole Moment
- Torque on Current Carrying Loop in a Magnetic Field
- The Moving Coil Galvanometer

Magnetic Dipole Moment

Magnetic dipole moment associated with a current carrying loop is given as $\mathbf{M} = Ni\mathbf{A} \Rightarrow |\mathbf{M}| = NiA$

where, N = number of turns in the loop,
i = current in the loop
and A = area of cross-section of the loop.

It is a vector quantity directed along area vector $\mathbf{A}$ of the loop with anti-clockwise sense as positive. Its SI unit is A-m^2.

Example 19. *Find the magnetic moment of a thin round loop with current i, if the radius of the loop is equal to $R = 100$ mm and the magnetic induction at its centre is equal to $B = 8.0\mu T$.*

Sol. Magnetic field at centre O,

$$B = \frac{\mu_0 i}{2R} \Rightarrow i = \frac{2RB}{\mu_0}$$

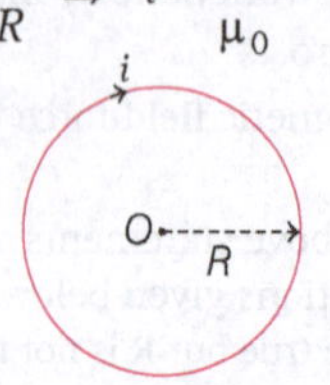

Magnetic moment of loop,

$$M = iA = i \cdot \pi R^2 = \frac{2RB}{\mu_0} \pi R^2$$

$$= \frac{2BR^3}{\mu_0/\pi} = \frac{2 \times 8 \times 10^{-6} \times (0.1)^3}{4 \times 10^{-7}}$$

$$= 4 \times 10^{-2}\ \text{Am}^{-2}$$

Example 20. *In the Bohr model of the hydrogen atom, the electron circulates around the nucleus in a path of radius 5.1×10^{-11} m at a frequency of 6.8×10^{15} Hz.*

(i) What value of magnetic field is set-up at the centre of the orbit?

(ii) What is the equivalent magnetic moment?

Sol. (i) An electron moving around the nucleus is equivalent to a current, $i = qf$

Magnetic field at the centre, $B = \dfrac{\mu_0 i}{2R} = \dfrac{\mu_0 q f}{2R}$

Substituting the given values in above equation, we get

$$B = \frac{(4\pi \times 10^{-7})(1.6 \times 10^{-19})(6.8 \times 10^{15})}{2 \times 5.1 \times 10^{-11}} = 13.4\ \text{T}$$

(ii) The current carrying circular loop is equivalent to a magnetic dipole, with magnetic moment,

$$M = NiA = Nqf\,\pi R^2$$

Substituting all the values in above equation, we get

$$M = (1)(1.6 \times 10^{-19})(6.8 \times 10^{15})(3.14)(5.1 \times 10^{-11})^2$$
$$= 8.9 \times 10^{-24}\ \text{A-m}^2$$

Torque on Current Carrying Loop in a Magnetic Field

When a current carrying coil is placed in a magnetic field, the coil experiences a torque.

Consider a rectangular current carrying coil $PQRS$ having N turns and area A. When this coil is placed in a uniform field $\mathbf{B}$ in such a way that the normal $\hat{\mathbf{n}}$ to the coil makes an angle θ with the direction of $\mathbf{B}$. The coil experiences a torque which is given by $\tau = NBiA \sin\theta$

In vector form, $\tau = \mathbf{M} \times \mathbf{B}$

Special cases

(i) τ is zero when $\theta = 0°$, *i.e.* the plane of the coil is perpendicular to the field.

(ii) τ is maximum when $\theta = 90°$, *i.e.* the plane of the coil is parallel to the field, $\tau_{max} = NBiA$

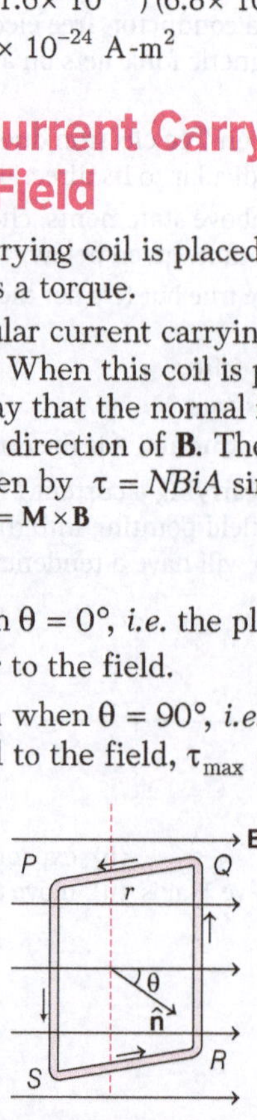

Torque on a Current Carrying Loop

Mentor's Tip

- Expression of torque is applicable for all shapes.
- Axis of rotation is parallel to τ, for loops rotating freely in magnetic field.

Example 21. *A uniform magnetic field of 3000 G is established along the positive z-direction. A rectangular loop of sides 10 cm and 5 cm carries a current of 12 A. What is the torque on the loop in the different cases shown in figure. What is the force in each case ? Which case corresponds to stable equilibrium?*

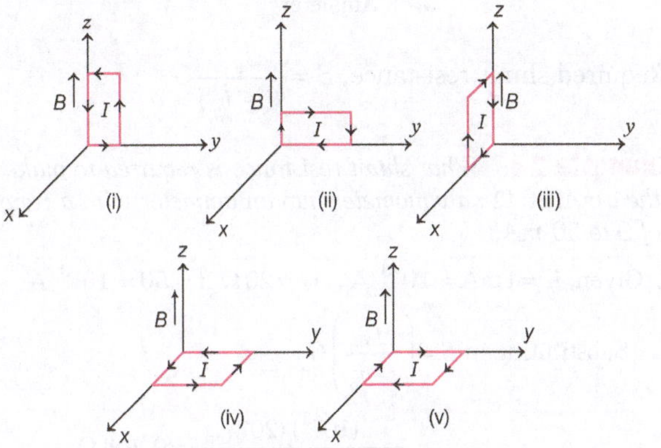

Sol. Here, B = uniform magnetic field = 3000 G along Z-axis

$$= 3000 \times 10^{-4}\ \text{T} = 0.3\ \text{T}$$

$\therefore$ Area of rectangular loop,

$$A = l \times b = 10 \times 5 = 50\ \text{cm}^2 = 50 \times 10^{-4}\ \text{m}^2$$

Torque on the loop, $\tau = IAB \sin\theta$

where, θ is the angle between the normal to the plane of the loop and the direction of magnetic field.

(i) Here, $\theta = 90°$

$$\therefore \quad \tau = 12 \times 50 \times 10^{-4} \times 0.3 \times \sin 90° = 1.8 \times 10^{-2}\ \text{N-m}$$

and acts along negative y-direction.

(ii) Here, $\theta = 90°$

$$\therefore \quad \tau = 12 \times 50 \times 10^{-4} \times 0.3 \times \sin 90° = 1.8 \times 10^{-2}\ \text{N-m}$$

and acts along y-direction.

(iii) Here, $\theta = 90°$

$$\therefore \quad \tau = 12 \times 50 \times 10^{-4} \times 0.3 \times \sin 90° = 1.8 \times 10^{-2}\ \text{N-m}$$

and acts along negative x-direction.

(iv) Here, $\theta = 0°$

$$\therefore \quad \tau = BIA \sin 0° = 0$$

(v) Here, $\theta = 180°$

$\therefore \tau = 0$

Net force on a planar loop in a uniform magnetic field is always zero, so force is zero in each case.

Case (iv) corresponds to stable equilibrium as M is aligned with B.

The Moving Coil Galvanometer (MCG)

It is a device which is based on the principle that when a current carrying coil is placed in a uniform magnetic field, then it experiences a torque.

The MCG consists of a multi-turn coil free to rotate about a vertical axis, in a uniform radial magnetic field. There is a cylindrical soft iron core to increase the sensitivity of the MCG.

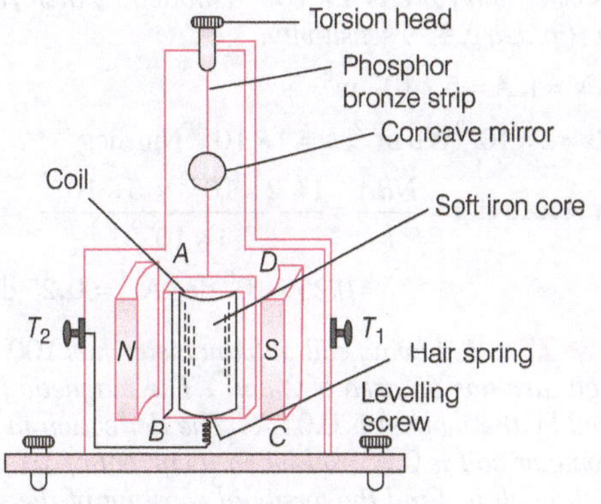

Moving coil galvanometer

The plane of the coil always remains parallel to the direction of magnetic field, therefore $\theta = 90°$. The deflecting torque has maximum value,

$$\tau = NIAB \quad \text{...(i)}$$

where, the symbols have their usual meaning. Since, the magnetic field is radial by design, we have taken $\sin\theta \approx 1$ in the above expression for the torque.

As the coil deflects, a restoring torque is set-up in the suspension fibre. If α is the angle of twist, the restoring torque,

$$\tau_{rest} = k\alpha \quad \text{...(ii)}$$

where, k is the torsional constant of the fibre. When the coil is in equilibrium, $NBIA = k\alpha$

$$\Rightarrow \quad I = G\alpha \Rightarrow \boxed{\alpha \propto I}$$

where, $G = \dfrac{k}{NBA}$ is the galvanometer constant.

This linear relationship between I and α makes the moving coil galvanometer useful for current measurement and detection.

Current sensitivity is the deflection per unit current flowing through it. It is given by $I_s = \dfrac{\alpha}{I} = \left(\dfrac{NAB}{k}\right)$

Its SI unit is rad/A or div/A.

Voltage sensitivity is the deflection per unit voltage.

It is given by $V_s = \dfrac{\alpha}{V} = \left(\dfrac{NAB}{k}\right)\dfrac{I}{V}$

$$\Rightarrow \qquad V_s = \frac{NAB}{k} \times \frac{I}{IR} = \frac{NAB}{kR} \qquad (\because V = IR)$$

$$\text{Voltage sensitivity} = \frac{\text{Current sensitivity}}{R}$$

Its SI unit is rad/V or div/V.

Example 22. *The coil of a moving coil galvanometer has an effective area of $5 \times 10^{-2}\,m^2$. It is suspended in a magnetic field of 2×10^{-2} Wb m^{-2}. If the torsional constant of the suspension fibre is 4×10^{-9} Nm deg^{-1}, then find its current (in deg μA^{-1}) sensitivity.*

Sol. Here, $N = 1, A = 5 \times 10^{-2} \text{m}^2$,

$$B = 2 \times 10^{-2} \text{Wb m}^{-2}, k = 4 \times 10^{-9} \text{ Nm deg}^{-1}$$

$$\text{Current sensitivity} = \frac{NBA}{k} = \frac{1 \times 2 \times 10^{-2} \times 5 \times 10^{-2}}{4 \times 10^{-9}}$$

$$= 0.25 \times 10^6 \text{ deg A}^{-1} = 0.25 \text{ deg } \mu \text{ A}^{-1}$$

Example 23. *A moving coil galvanometer has 100 turns and each turn has an area of 2 cm^2. The magnetic field produced by the magnet is 0.01 T. The deflection in the galvanometer coil is 0.05 rad when a current of 10 mA is passed through it. Find the torsional constant of the spiral spring.*

Sol. Current, $i = \frac{k}{NAB}\theta \Rightarrow k = \frac{NABi}{\theta}$

or $$k = \frac{100 \times 2 \times 10^{-4} \times 0.01 \times 10 \times 10^{-3}}{0.05}$$

$\therefore$ $$k = 4.0 \times 10^{-5} \text{ Nm rad}^{-1}$$

Concept ladder

Galvanometer

It is an instrument used to detect small current passing through it by showing deflection. It can be converted into voltmeter (for measuring voltage) and ammeter (for measuring current).

Ammeter

It is an instrument used to measure current and is always connected in series with the circuit element through which current is to be measured. Smaller the resistance of an ammeter, more accurate will be its reading, as it will not change the circuit current. An ammeter is said to be ideal, if its resistance r is zero.

Voltmeter

It is an instrument used to measure potential difference and is always connected in parallel with the circuit element across which potential difference is to be measured. Greater the resistance of voltmeter, more accurate will be its reading, as only small amount of current pass through it, by not changing the circuit current. A voltmeter is said to be ideal, if its resistance is infinite.

Conversion of Galvanometer into Ammeter

A galvanometer can be converted into an ammeter by **connecting a low resistance (called shunt S) in parallel to the galvanometer of resistance G.**

Hence, only a small amount of current pass through galvanometer and remaining will pass through the shunt. G and S are parallel and hence have equal potential difference, *i.e.* $i_g G = (i - i_g)S$.

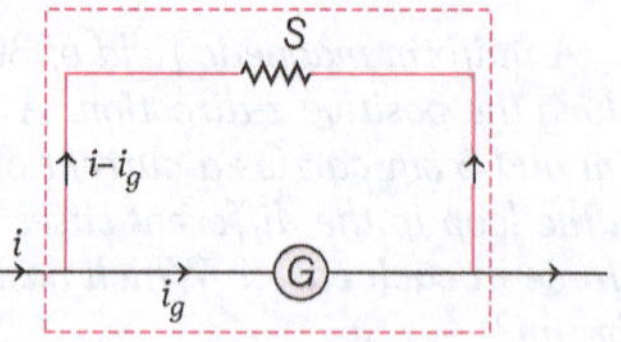

Ammeter

$$\therefore \text{ Required shunt resistance, } S = \frac{i_g}{(i - i_g)} G$$

Example 24. *What shunt resistance is required to make the 1 mA, 20 Ω galvanometer into an ammeter with a range of 0 to 50 mA?*

Sol. Given, $i_g = 1\text{mA} = 10^{-3}$ A, $G = 20\,\Omega, i = 50 \times 10^{-3}$ A

$$\text{Substituting in } S = \left(\frac{i_g}{i - i_g}\right) G$$

$$= \frac{(10^{-3})(20)}{(50 \times 10^{-3}) - (10^{-3})} = 0.408\,\Omega$$

Conversion of Galvanometer into Voltmeter

A galvanometer can be converted into voltmeter by **connecting a large resistance R in series with the galvanometer.**

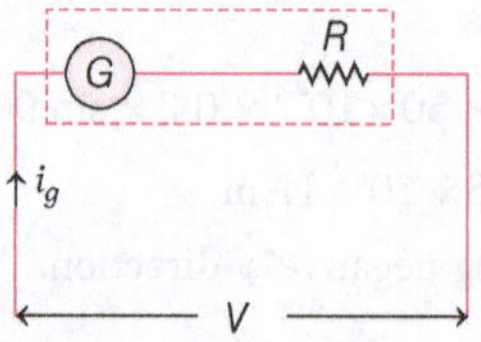

Voltmeter

According to Ohm's law, $V = i_g(G + R)$

$$\text{or required resistance, } \quad R = \frac{V}{i_g} - G$$

Example 25. *How can we make a galvanometer with $G = 20\,\Omega$ and $i_g = 1$ mA into a voltmeter with a maximum range of 10 V?*

Sol. Using, $R = \frac{V}{i_g} - G$

$$\text{We have, } R = \frac{10}{10^{-3}} - 20 = 9980\,\Omega$$

Thus, a resistance of 9980 Ω is to be connected in series with the galvanometer to convert it into the voltmeter of desired range.

STEP UP Practice 4

1. Current i is carried in a wire of length L. If the wire is turned into a circular coil, the maximum magnitude of torque in a given magnetic field B will be

(a) $\frac{L^2B^2}{2}$ (b) $\frac{L^2B}{2}$
(c) $\frac{L^2iB}{4\pi}$ (d) $\frac{L^2B}{4\pi}$

2. A circular coil of 20 turns and radius 10 cm is placed in uniform magnetic field of 0.10 T normal to the plane of the coil. If the current in coil is 5 A, then the torque acting on the coil will be

(a) 31.4 N-m (b) 3.14 N-m
(c) 0.314 N-m (d) zero

3. Two wires of same length are shaped into a square and a circle. If they carry same current, then the ratio of the magnetic moment is

(a) $2 : \pi$ (b) $\pi : 2$
(c) $\pi : 4$ (d) $4 : \pi$

4. Statement I Two long insulated wires carrying equal currents cross at right angles to each other. Then, the net magnetic force on either wire is zero, but net torque is non-zero.

Statement II Force between two long conductors is

$$F = \frac{\mu_0 I_1 I_2}{2\pi d} l$$

and torque = $\mathbf{M} \times \mathbf{B}$

In the light of the above statements, choose the most appropriate answer from the options given below.

(a) Both Statement I and Statement II are incorrect.
(b) Statement I is correct but Statement II is incorrect.
(c) Statement I is incorrect but Statement II is correct.
(d) Both Statement I and Statement II are correct.

5. A wire of length 2 m carrying a current of 1 A is bend to form a circle. The magnetic moment (in A-m^2) of the coil is

(a) 2π (b) $\pi/2$
(c) $\pi/4$ (d) $1/\pi$

6. The ratio of magnitude of magnetic field at the centre of a circular current carrying wire to its magnetic moment is N. If the current and radius both were doubled, the ratio will become

(a) $N/8$ (b) $N/4$
(c) $2N$ (d) $4N$

7. A moving coil galvanometer of resistance 40 Ω gives full scale deflection with a current of 2 mA. To convert ammeter of range 0-10A, amount of shunt resistance is

(a) 18 mΩ (b) 4 mΩ
(c) 12 mΩ (d) 8 mΩ

8. A 100 turns coil shown in figure carries a current of 2 A in a magnetic field $B = 0.2$ Wb/m^2. The torque acting on the coil is

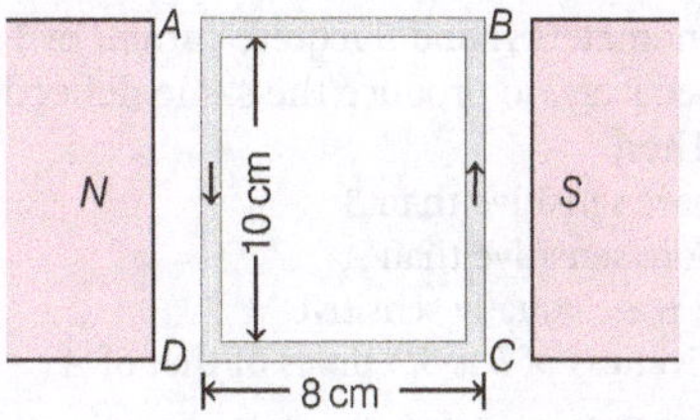

(a) 0.32 N-m tending to rotate the side AD out of the page.
(b) 0.32 N-m tending to rotate the side AD into the page.
(c) 0.0032 N-m tending to rotate the side AD out of the page.
(d) 0.0032 N-m tending to rotate the side AD into the page.

9. Statement I When a magnetic dipole is placed in a non-uniform magnetic field, only a torque acts on the dipole.

Statement II Force would act on dipole if magnetic field is uniform.

In the light of the above statements, choose the most appropriate answer from the options given below.

(a) Both Statement I and Statement II are incorrect.
(b) Statement I is correct but Statement II is incorrect.
(c) Statement I is incorrect but Statement II is correct.
(d) Both Statement I and Statement II are correct.

10. If a shunt of $\frac{1}{10}$th of the coil resistance is applied to a moving coil galvanometer, then its sensitivity becomes

(a) 10 fold (b) 11 fold (c) $\frac{1}{10}$ fold (d) $\frac{1}{11}$ fold

11. Which of the following pair given below is correct?

(a)	Torque on a current carrying loop in magnetic field	→	$\tau = NBIA \cos\theta$
(b)	At $\theta = 0°$	→	τ is maximum
(c)	At $\theta = 90°$	→	τ is minimum
(d)	At the axis of current carrying wire	→	$B = 0$

12. A voltmeter has a resistance of G Ω and range V volt. The value of resistance used in series to convert it into voltmeter of range nV volt is

(a) nG (b) $(n-1)G$
(c) G/n (d). $G/n - 1$

13. Statement I Voltmeter is connected in parallel with the circuit.

Statement II Resistance of a voltmeter is very large

In the light of the above statements, choose the most appropriate answer from the options given below.

(a) Both Statement I and Statement II are incorrect.
(b) Statement I is correct but Statement II is incorrect.
(c) Statement I is incorrect but Statement II is correct.
(d) Both Statement I and Statement II are correct.

14. An ammeter reads up to 1 A. Its internal resistance is $0.81\,\Omega$. To increase the range to 10 A, the value of the required shunt is
(a) $0.03\,\Omega$ (b) $0.3\,\Omega$
(c) $0.9\,\Omega$ (d) $0.09\,\Omega$

15. Two galvanometers *A* and *B* require current of 3 mA and 5 mA respectively, to produce the same deflection of I_0 division. Then,
(a) *A* is more sensitive than *B*
(b) *B* is more sensitive than *A*
(c) *A* and *B* are equally sensitive
(d) sensitiveness of *B* is 5/3 times of that of *A*

16. **Statement I** A moving coil galvanometer is based on heating effect of current.
Statement II On heating the coil starts to rotate in moving coil galvanometer.
In the light of the above statements, choose the most appropriate answer from the options given below.
(a) Both Statement I and Statement II are incorrect.
(b) Statement I is correct but Statement II is incorrect.
(c) Statement I is incorrect but Statement II is correct.
(d) Both Statement I and Statement II are correct.

17. In order to increase the sensitivity of a moving coil galvanometer one should decrease
(a) the strength of its magnet
(b) the torsional constant of its suspension
(c) the number of turns in its coil
(d) the area of its coil

18. In a moving coil galvanometer, the deflection of the coil θ is related to the electrical current *i* by the relation
(a) $i \propto \tan\theta$ (b) $i \propto \theta$
(c) $i \propto \theta^2$ (d) $i \propto \sqrt{\theta}$

19. **Statement I** A galvanometer can be used in electric circuit to detect the electric current.
Statement II A galvanometer can be used as an ammeter only.
In the light of the above statements, choose the most appropriate answer from the options given below.
(a) Both Statement I and Statement II are incorrect.
(b) Statement I is correct but Statement II is incorrect.
(c) Statement I is incorrect but Statement II is correct.
(d) Both Statement I and Statement II are correct.

20. The pole pieces of the magnet used in a pivoted coil galvanometer are
(a) plane surfaces of a bar magnet
(b) plane surfaces of a horse-shoe magnet
(c) cylindrical surfaces of a bar magnet
(d) cylindrical surfaces of a horse-shoe magnet.

21. In an ammeter, 0.5% of main current passes through a galvanometer. If the resistance of galvanometer is *G*, then the resistance of ammeter will be
(a) $G/200$ (b) $G/199$
(c) $199\,G$ (d) $200\,G$

NEET Exclusive EXTRA BYTES

- If magnetic field is directed perpendicular and into the plane of the paper, it is represented by ⊗ (cross) whereas if magnetic field is directed perpendicular and out of the plane of the paper, it is represented by ⊙ (dot).

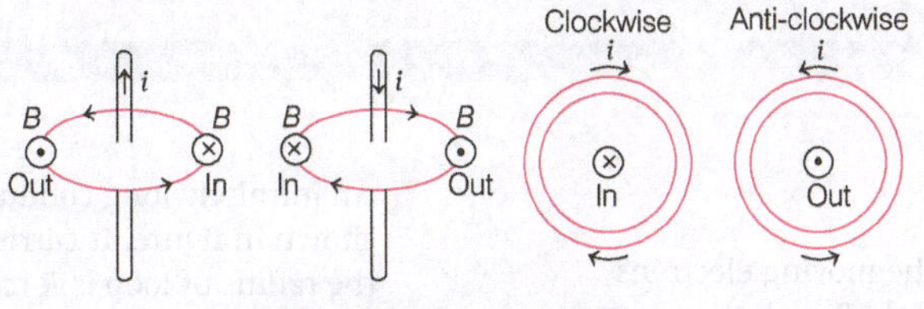

Direction of magnetic field

In Magnetic field is away from the observer or perpendicular inwards.

Out Magnetic field is towards the observer or perpendicular outwards.

- Direction of magnetic field vector in Biot-Savart law is perpendicular to current element (**Idl**) and **r**.
- Magnetic field at the axis of current carrying wire is always zero.
- If current is in straight line, magnetic field will be circular and vice-verse.
- For any symmetric circuital loop (made by same wire) has zero magnetic field at the centre. Examples :-

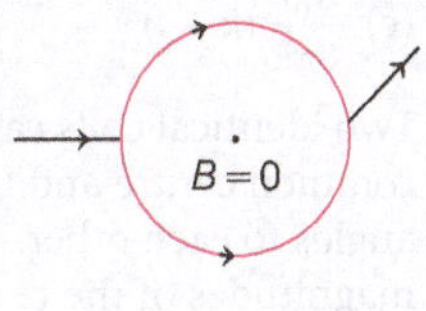

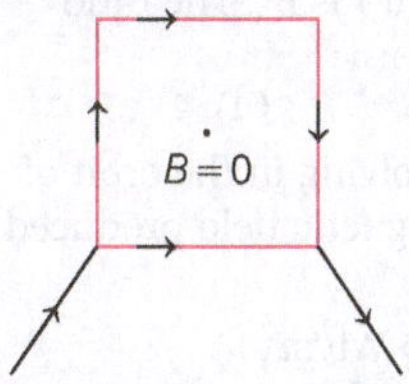

- Any coil (symmetric/assymetric) or loop kept in uniform magnetic field experiences zero net magnetic force, while torque may or may not be zero.
- Magnetic field inside the hollow cylinder is zero due to absence of current.
- Magnetic field inside the thick portion of hollow cylinder.

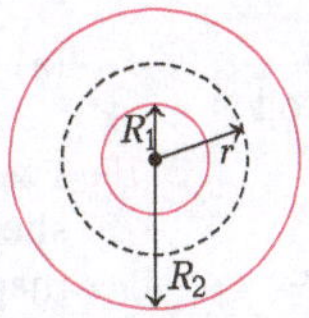

$$R_1 < r < R_2$$

$$B = \frac{\mu_0 i}{2\pi r} \cdot \frac{(r^2 - R_1^2)}{(R_2^2 - R_1^2)}$$

- Magnetic field outside the cylindrical conductor does not depend upon nature (thick/thin or solid/hollow) of the conductor as well as its radius of cross-section.

GEARING UP FOR NEET

Single Option Correct

1. Biot-Savart's law indicates that the moving electrons (velocity, **v**) produce a magnetic field **B** such that *[NCERT Exemplar]*
   (a) **B** is perpendicular to **v**
   (b) **B** is parallel to **v**
   (c) it obeys inverse cube law
   (d) it is along the line joining the electron and point of observation

2. The magnetic field at the centre of a circular coil of radius r carrying current I is B_1. The field at the centre of another coil of radius $2r$ carrying same current I is B_2. The ratio B_1/B_2 is
   (a) 1/2 (b) 1 (c) 2 (d) 4

3. In hydrogen atom, an electron is revolving in the orbit of radius 0.53 Å with 6.6×10^{15} rot/s. Magnetic field produced at the centre of the orbit is
   (a) 0.125 Wb/m^2 (b) 1.25 Wb/m^2
   (c) 12.5 Wb/m^2 (d) 125 Wb/m^2

4. A current carrying conductor of length l is bent into two loops one by one. First loop has one turn of wire and the second loop has two turns of wire.
   Compare the magnetic fields at the centre of the loops.
   (a) $B' = 4B$ (b) $4B' = B$ (c) $2B' = B$ (d) $B' = 2B$

5. When a certain length of wire is turned into one circular loop, then the magnetic field produced at the centre of coil due to some current flowing, is B_1. If the same wire is turned into three loops to make a circular coil, then the magnetic induction at the centre of this coil for the same current will be
   (a) B_1 (b) $9B_1$ (c) $3B_1$ (d) $27B_1$

6. An equilateral triangle of side length l is formed from a piece of wire of uniform resistance. The current I is fed as shown in the figure. Then, the magnitude of the magnetic field at its centre O is

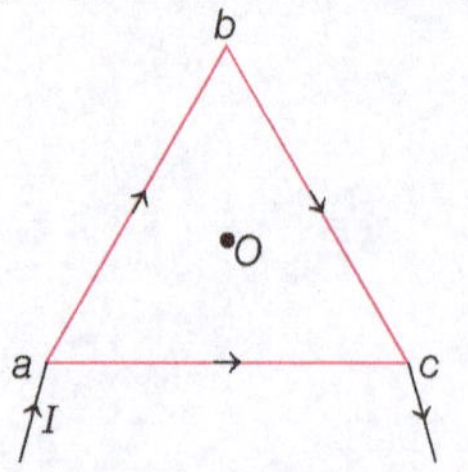

   (a) $\frac{\sqrt{3}\mu_0 I}{2\pi l}$ (b) $\frac{3\sqrt{3}\mu_0 I}{2\pi l}$ (c) $\frac{\mu_0 I}{2\pi l}$ (d) zero

7. An infinitely long conductor is bent into a circle as shown in figure. It carries a current I ampere and the radius of loop is R metre. The magnetic induction at the centre of loop is

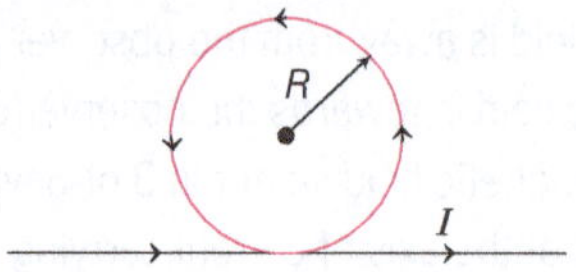

   (a) $\frac{\mu_0 2I}{4\pi R}(\pi + 1)$ (b) $\frac{\mu_0 2I}{4\pi R}(\pi - 1)$
   (c) $\frac{\mu_0 I}{8\pi R}(\pi + 1)$ (d) zero

8. Two identical coils carrying equal currents have a common centre and their planes are at right angles to each other. Find the ratio of the magnitudes of the resultant magnetic field at the centre and the field due to one coil alone.
   (a) 2 : 1 (b) 1 : 1
   (c) $1 : \sqrt{2}$ (d) $\sqrt{2} : 1$

9. An electron moves in a circular orbit with a uniform speed v. It produces a magnetic field B at the centre of the circle. The radius of the circle is proportional to
   (a) $\frac{B}{v}$ (b) $\frac{v}{B}$ (c) $\sqrt{\frac{v}{B}}$ (d) $\sqrt{\frac{B}{v}}$

10. Two long thin wires ABC and DEF are arranged as shown in the figure. The magnitude of the magnetic field at O is

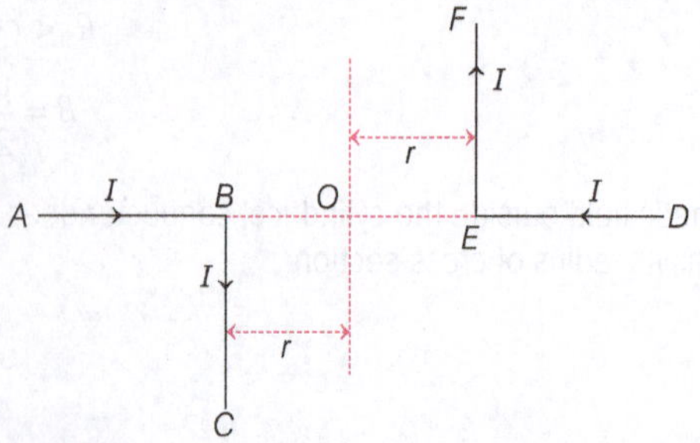

   (a) $\frac{\mu_0 I}{4\pi r}$ (b) $\frac{\mu_0 I}{2\pi r}$ (c) $\frac{\mu_0 I}{2\sqrt{2}\pi r}$ (d) zero

11. A circular conductor of uniform resistance per unit length, is connected to a battery of 4 V. The total resistance of the conductor is 4 Ω. The net magnetic field at the centre of the conductor is

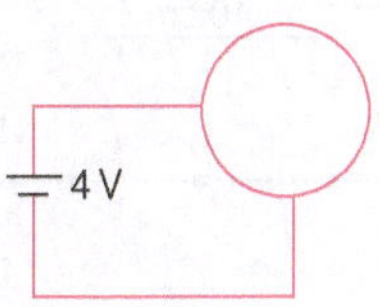

(a) $\frac{\mu_0}{2}$ (b) $\frac{8\mu_0}{3}$ (c) $2\mu_0$ (d) zero

12. An ionised gas contains both positive and negative ions initially at rest. If it is subjected simultaneously to an electric field along the $+x$-direction and a magnetic field along the $+z$-direction, then

(a) positive ions deflect towards $+y$-direction and negative ions $-y$-direction
(b) all ions deflect towards $+y$-direction
(c) all ions deflect towards $-y$-direction
(d) positive ions deflect towards $-y$-direction and negative ions towards $+y$-direction

13. Two infinitely long conductors carrying equal currents are shaped as shown in figure. All the short sections are of equal lengths. The point P is located symmetrically with respect to the two conductors. The magnetic field at P due to any one conductor is B. The total field at P is

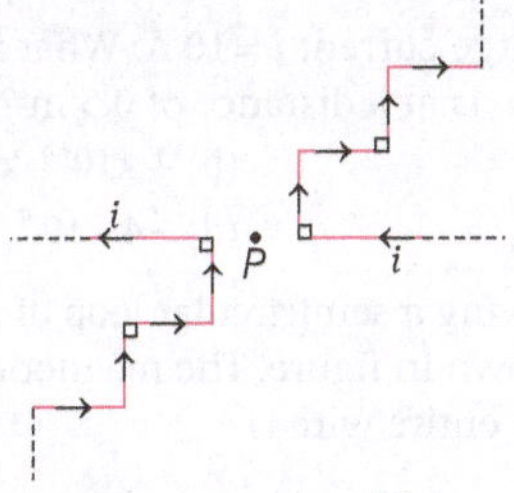

(a) zero (b) B (c) $\sqrt{2}\,B$ (d) $2B$

14. A disc of radius R rotates with constant angular velocity ω about its own axis. Surface charge density of this disc varies as $\sigma = \alpha r^2$, where r is the distance from the centre of disc. Determine the magnetic field intensity at the centre of disc.

(a) $\mu_0 \alpha \omega R^3$ (b) $\frac{\mu_0 \alpha \omega R^3}{6}$ (c) $\frac{\mu_0 \alpha \omega R^3}{8}$ (d) $\frac{\mu_0 \alpha \omega R^3}{3}$

15. Two circular coils 1 and 2 are made from the same wire but the radius of the 1st coil is twice that of the 2nd coil. What is the ratio of potential difference applied across them, so that the magnetic field at their centres is the same?

(a) 3 : 1 (b) 4 : 1 (c) 6 : 1 (d) 2 : 1

16. A square frame of side 1 m carries a current I, produces a magnetic field B at its centre. The same current is passed through a circular coil having the same perimeter as the square. The magnetic field at the centre of the circular coil is B'. The ratio B/B' is

(a) $\frac{8}{\pi^2}$ (b) $\frac{8\sqrt{2}}{\pi^2}$ (c) $\frac{16}{\pi^2}$ (d) $\frac{16}{\sqrt{2}\pi^2}$

17. A conducting stick of length $2L$ and mass m is moving down a smooth inclined plane of inclination 60° with constant speed 5 m/s. A current 2A is flowing in the conductor perpendicular to the paper inwards. A vertically upward magnetic field B exists in space there. The magnitude of magnetic field **B** is

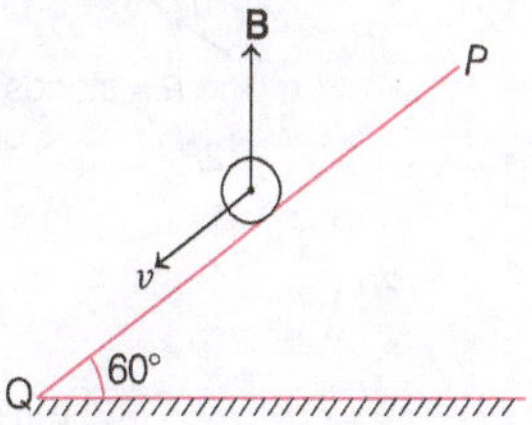

(a) $\frac{mg}{4L}$ (b) $\frac{mg}{L}$ (c) $\frac{\sqrt{3}mg}{4L}$ (d) $\frac{\sqrt{3}mg}{2L}$

18. Two straight infinitely long current carrying wires are kept along Z-axis at the coordinates $(0, a, 0)$ and $(0, -a, 0)$ respectively, as shown in the figure. The current in each of the wire is equal and along negative Z-axis (into the plane of the paper).

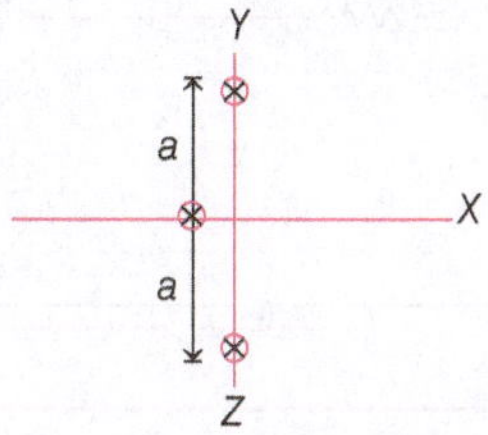

The variation of magnetic field on the X-axis will be approximately

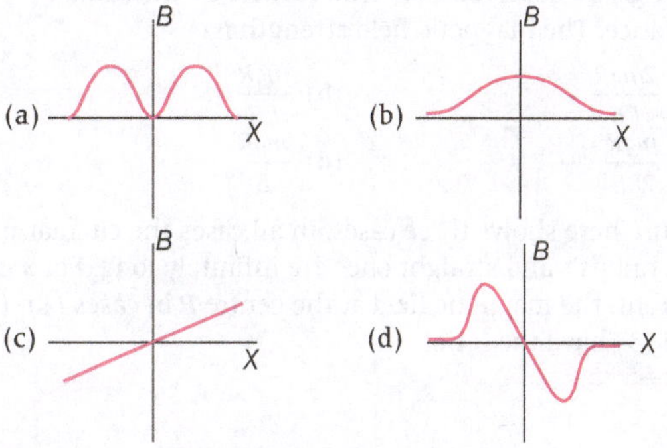

19. A wire is bent in the form of a regular polygon of n sides, is inscribed in a circle of radius a. If i ampere is the current flowing in the wire, then the magnetic field at the centre of the circle is

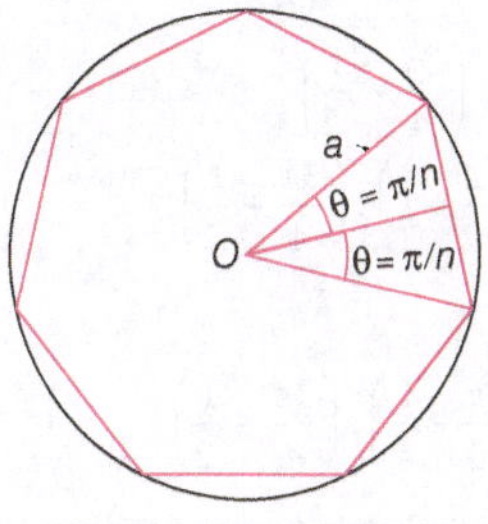

(a) $\frac{\mu_0 i}{2\pi a} \tan \frac{\pi}{n}$ (b) $\frac{\mu_0 n i}{2\pi a} \tan \frac{\pi}{n}$
(c) $\frac{2}{\pi} \frac{ni}{a} \mu_0 \tan \frac{\pi}{n}$ (d) $\frac{ni}{2a} \mu_0 \tan \frac{\pi}{n}$

20. The magnetic field at the centre of square of side a is

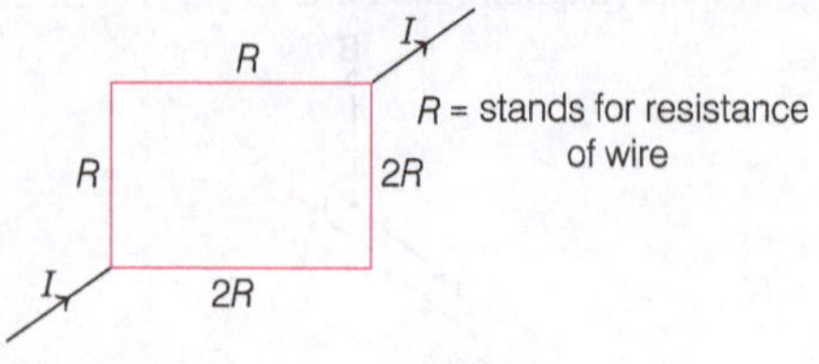

(a) $\frac{\sqrt{2}\mu_0}{\pi a}$ (b) $\frac{\sqrt{2}\mu_0 I}{3\pi a}$

(c) $\frac{2}{3}\frac{\mu_0 I}{a}$ (d) zero

21. A straight rod of mass m and length L is suspended from the identical springs as shown in figure. The spring is stretched a distance x_0 due to the weight of the wire.

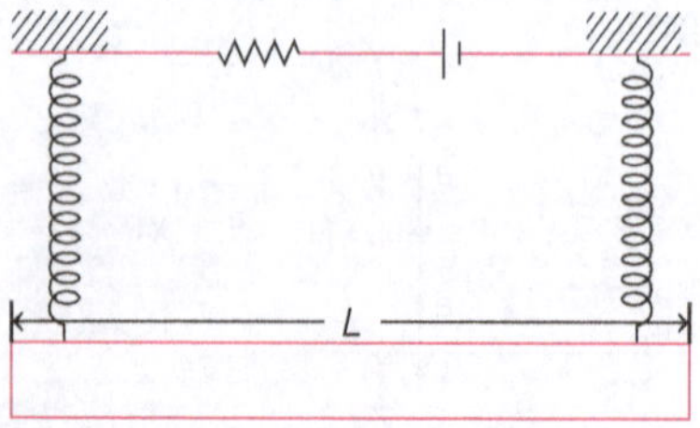

The circuit has total resistance R. When the magnetic field perpendicular to the plane of paper is switched on, then springs are observed to extend further by the same distance. The magnetic field strength is

(a) $\frac{2mgR}{LE}$ (b) $\frac{mgR}{LE}$

(c) $\frac{mgR}{2LE}$ (d) $\frac{mgR}{E}$

22. Figure here shows three cases, in all cases the circular path has radius r and straight ones are infinitely long. For same current, the magnetic field at the centre P in cases (1), (2) and (3) have the ratio

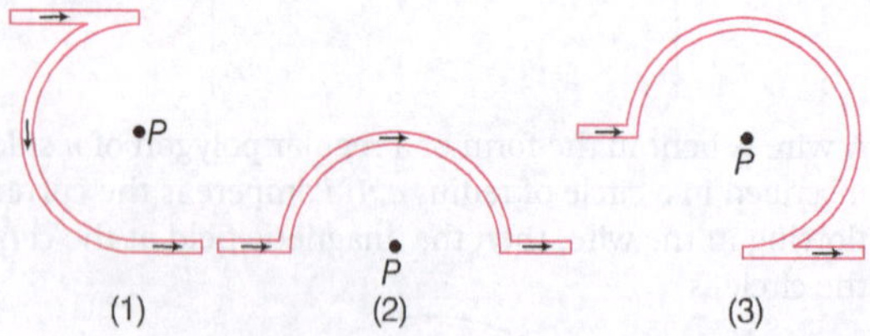

(a) $\left(-\frac{\pi}{2}\right):\left(\frac{\pi}{2}\right):\left(\frac{3\pi}{4}-\frac{1}{2}\right)$

(b) $\left(-\frac{\pi}{2}+1\right):\left(\frac{\pi}{2}+1\right):\left(\frac{3\pi}{4}+\frac{1}{2}\right)$

(c) $-\frac{\pi}{2}:\frac{\pi}{2}:3\frac{\pi}{4}$

(d) $\left(-\frac{\pi}{2}-1\right):\left(\frac{\pi}{2}-\frac{1}{4}\right):\left(\frac{3\pi}{4}+\frac{1}{2}\right)$

23. Two circular loops having same radius ($R = 10$ cm) and same current $\frac{7}{2}$ A are placed along same axis as shown in the figure. If distance between their centres is 10 cm, find the value of net magnetic field at point P.

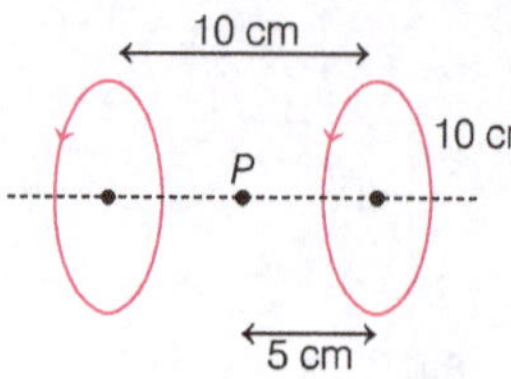

(a) $\frac{50\mu_0}{\sqrt{5}}$ T (b) $\frac{28\mu_0}{\sqrt{5}}$ T

(c) $\frac{56\mu_0}{\sqrt{5}}$ T (d) $\frac{56\mu_0}{\sqrt{3}}$ T

24. A long straight wire carrying current I is bent at its mid-point to form an angle of 45°. Induction of magnetic field (in tesla) at point P, distant R from point of bending, is equal to

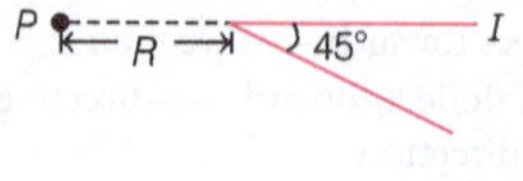

(a) $\frac{(\sqrt{2}-1)\mu_0 I}{4\pi R}$ (b) $\frac{(\sqrt{2}+1)\mu_0 I}{4\pi R}$

(c) $\frac{(\sqrt{2}-1)\mu_0 I}{4\sqrt{2}\pi R}$ (d) $\frac{(\sqrt{2}+1)\mu_0 I}{4\sqrt{2}\pi R}$

25. An element $dl = dx\hat{\mathbf{i}}$ (where $dx = 1$ cm) is placed at the origin and carries a large current $i = 10$ A. What is the magnetic field on the Y-axis at a distance of 0.5 m?

(a) $2\times10^{-8}\ \hat{\mathbf{k}}$T (b) $4\times10^{-8}\ \hat{\mathbf{k}}$T

(c) $-2\times10^{-8}\ \hat{\mathbf{k}}$T (d) $-4\times10^{-8}\ \hat{\mathbf{k}}$T

26. A long wire having a semicircular loop of radius r carries a current i as shown in figure. The magnetic induction at the centre O due to entire wire is

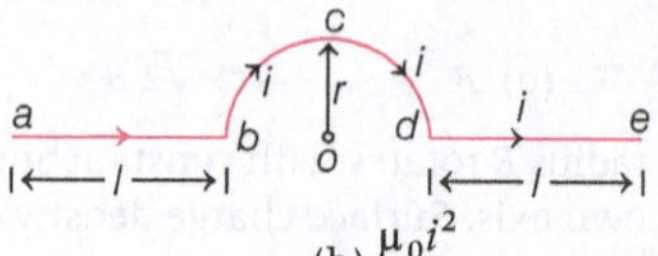

(a) $\frac{\mu_0 i}{4r}$ (b) $\frac{\mu_0 i^2}{4r}$

(c) $\frac{\mu_0 i}{4r^2}$ (d) None of these

27. In the given figure, what is the magnetic field induction at point O?

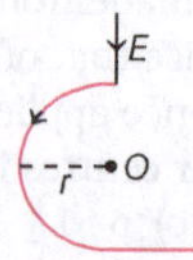

(a) $\frac{\mu_0 I}{4\pi r}$ (b) $\frac{\mu_0 I}{4r}+\frac{\mu_0 I}{2\pi r}$ (c) $\frac{\mu_0 I}{4r}+\frac{\mu_0 I}{4\pi r}$ (d) $\frac{\mu_0 I}{4r}-\frac{\mu_0 I}{4\pi r}$

28. Consider the circular loop having current i and with central point O. The magnetic field at the central point O is

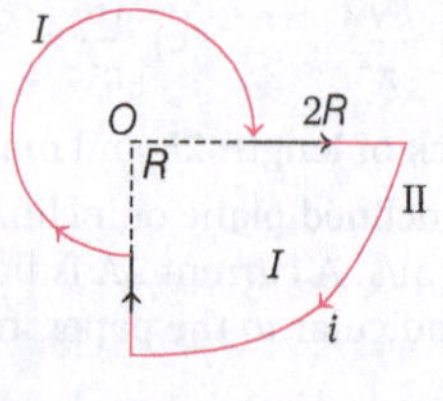

(a) $\frac{2\mu_0 i}{3\pi R}$ acting downward

(b) $\frac{5\mu_0 i}{12 R}$ acting downward

(c) $\frac{6\mu_0 i}{11 R}$ acting downward

(d) $\frac{3\mu_0 i}{7 R}$ acting upward

29. The magnetic field at the centre of a circular coil carrying current I ampere is B. If the coil is bent into smaller circular coil of $2n$ turns, then its magnetic field at the centre is B'. The ratio between B' and B is

(a) 1 : 1 (b) n:1 (c) $(2n)^2$:1 (d) $2n$:1

30. There is a ring of radius r having linear charge density λ and rotating with a uniform angular velocity ω. The magnetic field produced by this ring at its own centre would be

(a) $\frac{\lambda\omega^2}{2-\mu_0}$ (b) $\frac{\mu_0 \lambda^2 \omega}{\sqrt{2}}$ (c) $\frac{\mu_0 \lambda \omega}{2}$ (d) $\frac{\mu_0 \lambda}{2\omega^2}$

31. Two concentric coils each of radius equal to 2π cm are placed at right angles to each other. If 3A and 4A are the currents flowing through the two coils, respectively. The magnetic induction (in Wb/m^2) at the centre of the coils will be

(a) 5×10^{-5} (b) 12×10^{-5} (c) 7×10^{-5} (d) 10^{-5}

32. Two identical long conducting wires AOB and COD are placed at right angle to each other with one above other such that O is the common point for the two. The wires carry I_1 and I_2 currents, respectively. Point P is lying at distance d from O along a direction perpendicular to the plane containing the wires. The magnetic field at the point P will be

(a) $\frac{\mu_0}{2\pi d}\left(\frac{I_1}{I_2}\right)$ (b) $\frac{\mu_0}{2\pi d}(I_1 + I_2)$

(c) $\frac{\mu_0}{2\pi d}(I_1^2 - I_2^2)$ (d) $\frac{\mu_0}{2\pi d}(I_1^2 + I_2^2)^{1/2}$

33. The magnetic field due to a current carrying circular loop of radius 3 cm at a point on the axis at a distance of 4 cm from the centre is 54 μT. What will be its value at the centre of the loop?

(a) 200 μT (b) 250 μT (c) 125 μT (d) 75 μT

34. If the velocity of charged particle has both perpendicular and parallel components while moving through a magnetic field, then what is the path followed by a charged particle?

(a) Circular (b) Elliptical
(c) Linear (d) Helical

35. A long conducting wire carrying a current I is bent at 120° (see figure). The magnetic field B at a point P on the right bisector of bending angle at a distance d from the bend is (μ_0 is the permeability of free space)

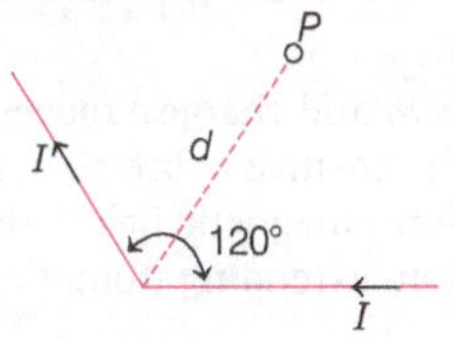

(a) $\frac{2\mu_0 I}{2\pi d}$ (b) $\frac{\mu_0 I}{2\pi d}$

(c) $\frac{\mu_0 I}{\sqrt{3}\pi d}$ (d) $\frac{\sqrt{3}\mu_0 I}{2\pi d}$

36. A current of 2 A is made to flow through a coil which has only one turn. The magnetic field produced at the centre is $4\pi\times10^{-6}$ Wb/m^2. The radius of the coil is

(a) 0.0001m (b) 0.01m
(c) 0.1m (d) 0.001 m

37. In the diagram, I_1, I_2 are the strength of the currents in the loop and straight conductors respectively, $OA = AB = R$. The net magnetic field at the centre O is zero, then the ratio of the currents in the loop and the straight conductor is

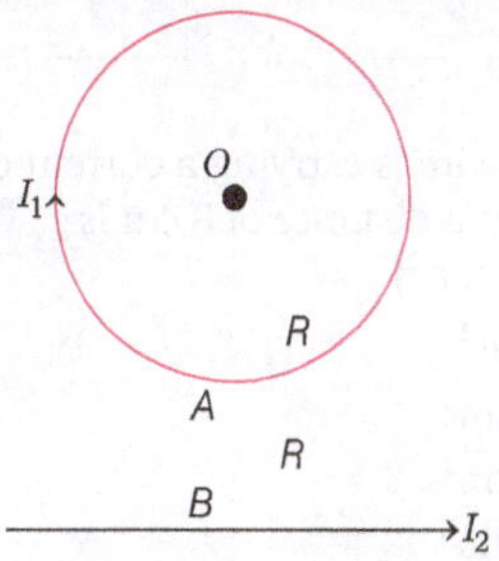

(a) π (b) 2π
(c) $\frac{1}{\pi}$ (d) $\frac{1}{2\pi}$

38. Two similar coils of radius R are lying concentrically with their planes at right angles to each other. The current flowing in them are I and $2I$, respectively. The resultant magnetic field induction at the centre will be

(a) $\frac{\sqrt{5}\mu_0 I}{2R}$ (b) $\frac{3\mu_0 I}{2R}$

(c) $\frac{\mu_0 I}{2R}$ (d) $\frac{\mu_0 I}{R}$

39. A wire of one metre length carries a constant current. The wire is bent to form a circular loop. The magnetic field at the centre of this loop is B. The same is now bent to form a circular loop of smaller radius having four turns. The magnetic field at the centre of this new loop will be

(a) $\frac{B}{2}$ (b) $4B$ (c) $\frac{B}{4}$ (d) $16B$

40. Two parallel long wires carry currents i_1 and i_2 with $i_1 > i_2$. When the currents are in the same direction, then the magnetic field midway between the wires is 10 μT. When the direction of i_2 is reversed, then it becomes 40 μT. Then, ratio of i_1/i_2 is

(a) 3 : 4 (b) 5 : 3
(c) 7:11 (d) 11 : 7

41. If a steel wire of length l and magnetic moment M is bent into a semicircular arc, the new magnetic moment is

(a) $M\times l$ (b) $\frac{M}{l}$

(c) $\frac{2M}{\pi}$ (d) M

42. A long thin hollow metallic cylinder of radius R has a current i ampere. The magnetic induction B away from the axis at a distance r from the axis varies as shown in

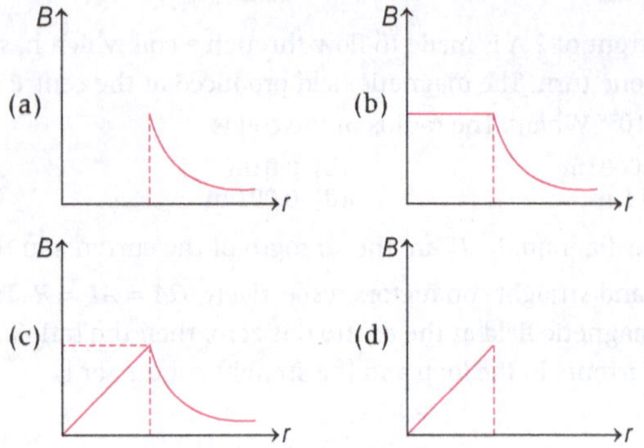

43. A long straight wire is carrying a current of 12 A. The magnetic field at a distance of 8 cm is
($\mu_0 = 4\pi \times 10^{-7}$ N A^2)
(a) 2×10^{-4} Wb/m^2
(b) 3×10^{-5} Wb/m^2
(c) 4×10^{-4} Wb/m^2
(d) 4×10^{-5} Wb/m^2

44. The adjacent figure shows the cross-section of a long rod with its length perpendicular to the plane of the paper. It carries constant current flowing along its length. B_1, B_2, B_3 and B_4 respectively, represent the magnetic fields due to the current in the rod at points 1, 2, 3 and 4 lying at different separations from the centre O, as shown in the figure. Which of the following shall hold true?

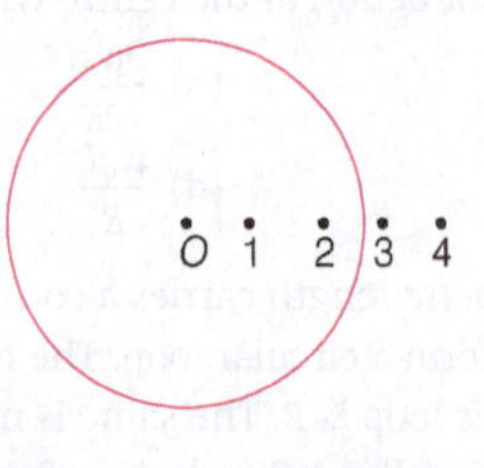

(a) $B_1 > B_2 \neq 0$ (b) $B_2 > B_3 \neq 0$
(c) $B_1 = B_2 = B_3 \neq 0$ (d) $B_3 > B_4 \neq 0$

45. A current i ampere flows along the inner conductor of a coaxial cable and returns along the outer conductor of the cable, then the magnetic induction at any point outside the conductor at a distance r metre from the axis is
(a) ∞ (b) zero
(c) $\frac{\mu_0}{4\pi}\frac{2i}{r}$ (d) $\frac{\mu_0}{4\pi}\frac{2\pi i}{r}$

46. A proton is moving along the negative direction of X-axis in a magnetic field directed along the positive direction of Y-axis. The proton will be deflected along the negative direction of
(a) X-axis
(b) Y-axis
(c) Z-axis
(d) None of the above

47. Three long straight wires A, B and C are carrying currents as shown in figure. Then, the resultant force on B is directed

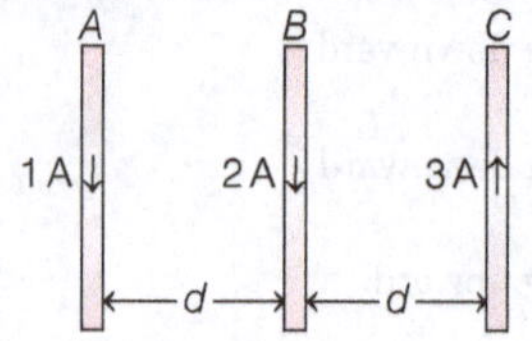

(a) towards A
(b) towards C
(c) perpendicular to the plane of paper and outward
(d) perpendicular to the plane of paper and inward

48. A circular flexible loop of wire of radius r carrying a current I is placed in a uniform magnetic field B perpendicular to the plane of the circle, so that wire comes under tension. If B is doubled, then tension in the loop
(a) remains unchanged
(b) is doubled
(c) is halved
(d) becomes 4 times

49. Two charged particles traverse identical helical paths in a completely opposite sense in a uniform magnetic field $\mathbf{B} = B_0\hat{\mathbf{k}}$. Then, *[NCERT Exemplar]*
(a) they have equal z-components of moment
(b) they must have equal charges
(c) they necessarily represent a particle, anti-particle pair
(d) the charge to mass ratio satisfy
$$\left(\frac{e}{m}\right)_1 + \left(\frac{e}{m}\right)_2 = 0$$

50. A long solenoid carrying a current I is placed with its axis vertical as shown in the figure. A particle of mass m and charge q is released from the top of the solenoid. Its acceleration is (g being acceleration due to gravity)

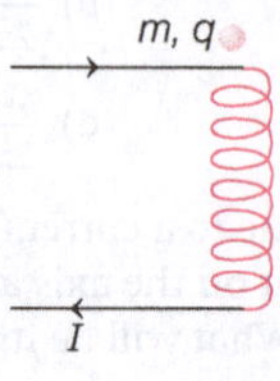

(a) greater than g (b) less than g
(c) equal to g (d) None of these

51. An electric current i enters and leaves a uniform circular wire of radius a through diametrically opposite points. A charged particle q moving along the axis of the circular wire passes through its centre at speed v. The magnetic force acting on the particle when it passes through the centre has a magnitude
(a) $qv\frac{\mu_0 i}{2a}$ (b) $qv\frac{\mu_0 i}{2\pi a}$
(c) $qv\frac{\mu_0 i}{a}$ (d) zero

52. A particle of mass m and charge q moves with a constant velocity v along the positive x-direction. It enters a region containing a uniform magnetic field B directed along the negative z-direction, extending from $x = a$ to $x = b$. The minimum value of v required, so that the particle can just enter the region $x > b$ is

(a) qbB/m (b) $q(b-a)\,B/m$
(c) qaB/m (d) $q(b+a)\,B/2m$

53. A proton of mass 1.67×10^{-27} kg and charge 1.6×10^{-19} C is projected in XY-plane with a speed of 2×10^{6} m/s at an angle of 60° to the X-axis. If a uniform magnetic field of 0.14 T is applied along the Y-axis, then the path of the proton is

(a) a circle of radius 0.2 m and time period $\pi \times 10^{-7}$ s
(b) a circle of radius 0.1 m and time period $2\pi \times 10^{-7}$ s
(c) a helix of radius 0.075 m and time period 0.5×10^{-6} s
(d) a helix of radius 0.14 m and time period 1.0×10^{-7} s

54. Figure shows, three long straight wires parallel and equally spaced with identical currents as shown below. Then, the force acting on each wire F_a, F_b and F_c due to the other are related as

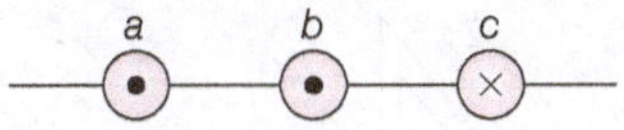

(a) $F_a > F_b > F_c$ (b) $F_b > F_c > F_a$
(c) $F_c > F_a > F_b$ (d) $F_b > F_a > F_c$

55. A, B and C are parallel conductors of equal length carrying currents I, I and $2I$, respectively. Distance between A and B is x. Distance between B and C is also x. F_1 is the force exerted by B on A and F_2 is the force exerted by C on A. Choose the correct answer.

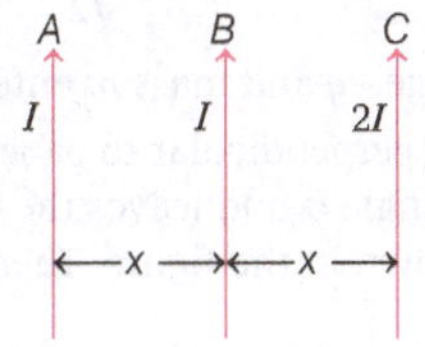

(a) $F_1 = 2F_2$ (b) $F_2 = 2F_1$
(c) $F_1 = F_2$ (d) $F_1 = -F_2$

56. Three long, straight and parallel wires carrying currents are arranged as shown in figure. The force experienced by 10 cm length of wire Q is

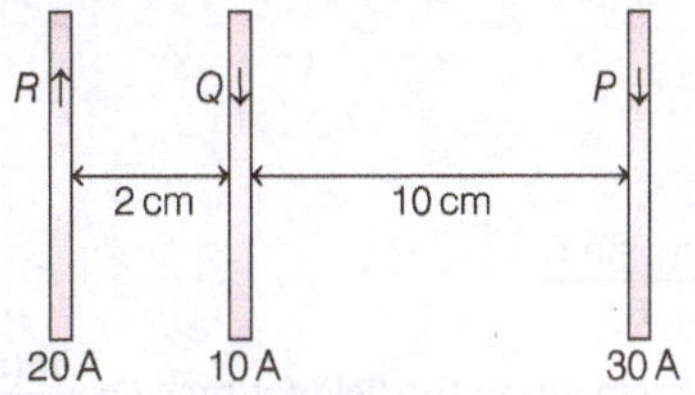

(a) 1.4×10^{-4} N towards the right
(b) 1.4×10^{-4} N towards the left
(c) 2.6×10^{-4} N towards the right
(d) 2.6×10^{-4} N towards the left

57. A current of 10 A is flowing in a wire of length 1.5 m. A force of 15 N acts on it when it is placed in a uniform magnetic field of 2 T. The angle between the magnetic field and the direction of the current is

(a) 30° (b) 45° (c) 60° (d) 90°

58. A charged particle P leaves the origin with speed $v = v_0$, at some inclination with the X-axis. There is a uniform magnetic field B along the X-axis. P strikes a fixed target T on the X-axis for a minimum value of $B = B_0$. P will also strike T, if

(a) $B = 2B_0,\ v = 2v_0$ (b) $B = 2B_0,\ v = v_0$
(c) Both are correct (d) Both are wrong

59. A particle of mass m and having a positive charge q is projected from origin with speed v_0 along the positive X-axis in a magnetic field $\mathbf{B} = -B_0\hat{\mathbf{k}}$, where B_0 is a positive constant. If the particle passes through $(0, y, 0)$, then y is equal to

(a) $-\dfrac{2mv_0}{qB_0}$ (b) $\dfrac{mv_0}{qB}$
(c) $-\dfrac{mv_0}{qB}$ (d) $\dfrac{2mv_0}{qB_0}$

60. A circular loop which is in the form of a major arc of a circle is kept in the horizontal plane and a constant magnetic field B is applied in the vertical direction such that the magnetic lines of forces go into the plane. If R is the radius of circle and it carries a current I in the clockwise direction, then the force on the loop will be

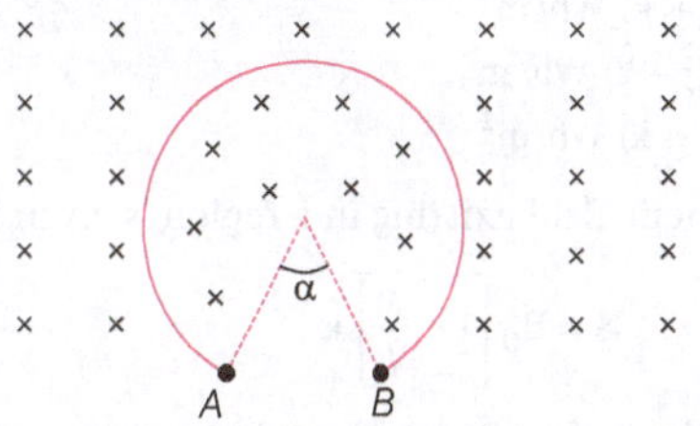

(a) $BIR \tan \alpha$ (b) $2\,BIR \cos(\alpha/2)$
(c) $2\,BIR \sin(\alpha/2)$ (d) None of these

61. Two protons are projected simultaneously from a fixed point with the same velocity v into a region, where there exists a uniform magnetic field. The magnetic field strength is B and it is perpendicular to the initial direction of v. One proton starts at time $t = 0$ and another proton at $t = \dfrac{\pi m}{2qB}$.

The separation between them at time $t = \dfrac{\pi m}{qB}$ (where, m and q are the mass and charge of proton), will be approximately

(a) $2\dfrac{mv}{qB}$ (b) $\dfrac{\sqrt{2}\,mv}{qB}$
(c) $\dfrac{mv}{qB}$ (d) $\dfrac{mv}{2qB}$

62. A charged particle with specific charge (charge per unit mass $= \dfrac{q}{m} = S$) moves undeflected through a region of space containing mutually perpendicular uniform electric and magnetic fields E and B. When the E field is switched off, then the particle will move in a circular path of radius

(a) $\dfrac{E}{BS}$ (b) $\dfrac{ES}{B}$
(c) $\dfrac{ES}{B^2}$ (d) $\dfrac{E}{B^2S}$

63. A current $i = 2$ A is flowing in a wire frame as shown in figure. The frame is a combination of two equilateral triangles *ACD* and *CDE* of side 1 m. It is placed in uniform magnetic field $B = 4$ T acting perpendicular to the plane of frame. The magnitude of magnetic force acting on the frame is

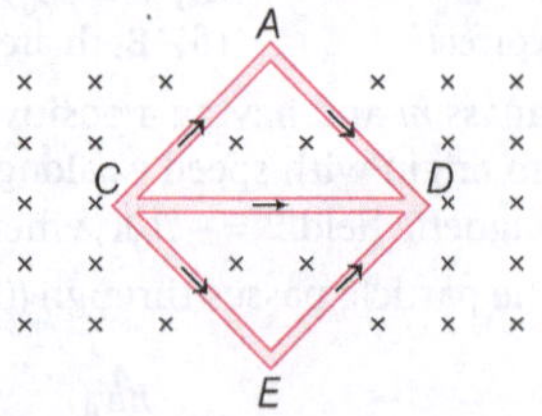

(a) 24 N (b) zero
(c) 16 N (d) 8 N

64. A charge q is moving with a velocity $\mathbf{v}_1 = \hat{\mathbf{i}}$ m/s at a point in a magnetic field and experiences a force $\mathbf{F} = q[-\hat{\mathbf{j}} + \hat{\mathbf{k}}]$ N. If the charge is moving with a velocity $\mathbf{v}_2 = \hat{\mathbf{j}}$ m/s at the same point, then it experiences a force $\mathbf{F}_2 = q(\hat{\mathbf{i}} - \hat{\mathbf{k}})$ N. The magnetic induction **B** at that point is
(a) $(\hat{\mathbf{i}} + \hat{\mathbf{j}} + \hat{\mathbf{k}})$ Wb/m²
(b) $(\hat{\mathbf{i}} - \hat{\mathbf{j}} + \hat{\mathbf{k}})$ Wb/m²
(c) $(-\hat{\mathbf{i}} + \hat{\mathbf{j}} - \hat{\mathbf{k}})$ Wb/m²
(d) $(\hat{\mathbf{i}} + \hat{\mathbf{j}} - \hat{\mathbf{k}})$ Wb/m²

65. The magnetic field existing in a region is given by

$$\mathbf{B} = \mathbf{B}_0\left[1 + \frac{x}{l}\right]\hat{\mathbf{k}}$$

A square loop of edge l and carrying current I is placed with its edges parallel to the X and Y-axes. The magnitude of the net magnetic force experienced by the loop is
(a) $2B_0Il$ (b) zero
(c) B_0Il (d) $4B_0Il$

66. A wire *PQRS* carrying a current I runs along three edges of a cube of side l as shown in figure. There exists a uniform magnetic field of magnitude B along one of the sides of the cube. The magnitude of the force acting on the wire is

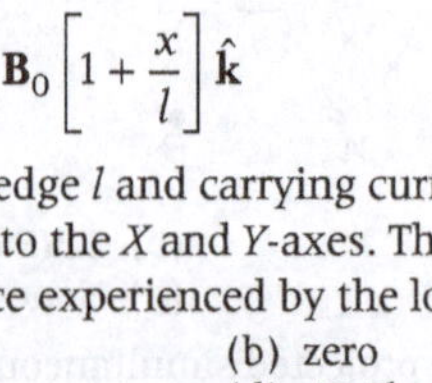

(a) zero (b) $\sqrt{3}\, IB$
(c) $\sqrt{2}IlB$ (d) $2IlB$

67. A particle of specific charge $q/m = \pi$ C/kg is projected from the origin towards positive X-axis with a velocity of 10 m/s in a uniform magnetic field $\mathbf{B} = -2\hat{\mathbf{k}}$T. The velocity **v** of the particle after time $t = \frac{1}{6}$ s will be
(a) $(5\hat{\mathbf{i}} + 5\sqrt{3}\,\hat{\mathbf{j}})$ m/s (b) $10\hat{\mathbf{j}}$ m/s
(c) $(5\sqrt{3}\,\hat{\mathbf{i}} + 5\hat{\mathbf{j}})$ m/s (d) $-10\hat{\mathbf{j}}$ m/s

68. A charged particle enters into a uniform magnetic field with velocity v_0 perpendicular to it, the length of magnetic field is $x = (\sqrt{3}/2)\,R$, where R is the radius of the circular path of the particle in the field. The magnitude of change in velocity of the particle when it comes out of the field is
(a) $2v_0$ (b) $\frac{v_0}{2}$ (c) $\frac{\sqrt{3}v_0}{2}$ (d) v_0

69. A proton moving with a constant velocity passes through a region of space without any change in its velocity. If **E** and **B** represent the electric and magnetic fields respectively, then this region of space may not have
(a) $E = 0, B = 0$ (b) $E = 0, B \neq 0$
(c) $E \neq 0, B = 0$ (d) $E \neq 0, B \neq 0$

70. A non-planar loop of conducting wire carrying a current I is placed as shown in the figure. Each of the straight sections of the loop is of length $2a$. The magnetic field due to this loop at the point P $(a, 0, a)$ is in the direction

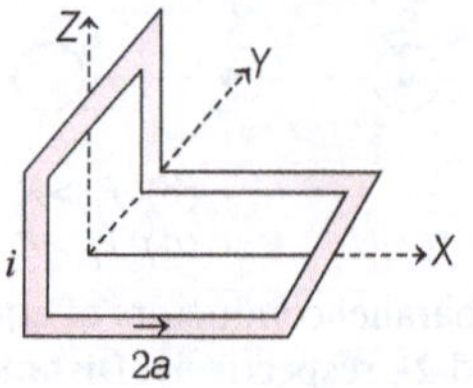

(a) $\frac{1}{\sqrt{2}}(-\hat{\mathbf{j}} + \hat{\mathbf{k}})$ (b) $\frac{1}{\sqrt{3}}(-\hat{\mathbf{j}} + \hat{\mathbf{k}} + \hat{\mathbf{i}})$
(c) $\frac{1}{\sqrt{3}}(\hat{\mathbf{i}} + \hat{\mathbf{j}} + \hat{\mathbf{k}})$ (d) $\frac{1}{\sqrt{2}}(\hat{\mathbf{i}} + \hat{\mathbf{k}})$

71. A particle of charge $-q$ and mass m enters a uniform magnetic field **B** (perpendicular to paper inwards) at P with a speed v_0 at an angle α and leaves the field at Q with speed v at angle β as shown in the figure. Then,

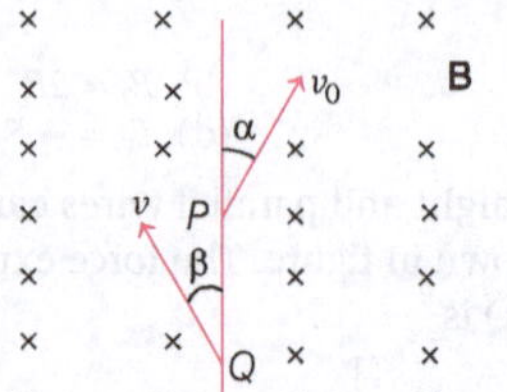

(a) $\alpha \neq \beta$
(b) $v \neq v_0$
(c) $PQ = \frac{mv_0 \sin\alpha}{Bq}$
(d) particle remains in the field for time $t = \frac{2m(\pi - \alpha)}{Bq}$

72. A long straight wire along the Z-axis carries a current I in the negative z-direction. The magnetic field vector **B** at a point having coordinates (x, y) in the $z = 0$ plane is
(a) $\frac{\mu_0 I(y\hat{\mathbf{i}} - x\hat{\mathbf{j}})}{2\pi(x^2 + y^2)}$ (b) $\frac{\mu_0 I(x\hat{\mathbf{i}} + y\hat{\mathbf{j}})}{2\pi(x^2 + y^2)}$
(c) $\frac{\mu_0 I(x\hat{\mathbf{j}} - y\hat{\mathbf{i}})}{2\pi(x^2 + y^2)}$ (d) $\frac{\mu_0 I(x\hat{\mathbf{i}} - y\hat{\mathbf{j}})}{2\pi(x^2 + y^2)}$

73. A proton moves at a speed $v = 2\times10^6$ m/s in a region of constant magnetic field of magnitude $B = 0.05$ T. The direction of the proton when it enters this field is $\theta = 30°$ to the field. When you look along the direction of the magnetic field, then the path is a circle, projected on a plane perpendicular to the magnetic field. How far will the proton move along the direction of B when two projected circles have been completed?
(a) 4.35 m (b) 0.209 m
(c) 2.82 m (d) 2.41 m

74. Two particles A and B having equal charges, after being accelerated through the same potential difference enter into a region of uniform magnetic field and the particles describe circular paths of radii R_1 and R_2, respectively. The ratio of the masses of A and B is
(a) $\sqrt{R_1/R_2}$ (b) R_1/R_2
(c) $(R_1/R_2)^2$ (d) $(R_2/R_1)^2$

75. A proton of mass m and charge q is moving in a plane with kinetic energy E. If there exists a uniform magnetic field B perpendicular to the plane motion, the proton will move in a circular path of radius
(a) $\frac{2Em}{qB}$ (b) $\frac{\sqrt{2Em}}{qB}$
(c) $\frac{\sqrt{Em}}{2qB}$ (d) $\frac{\sqrt{2Eq}}{qB}$

76. A charged particle of mass m and charge q moves along a circular path of radius r that is perpendicular to a magnetic field B. The time taken by the particle to complete one revolution is
(a) $\frac{2\mu mq}{B}$ (b) $\frac{2\pi q^2 B}{m}$
(c) $\frac{2\pi qB}{m}$ (d) $\frac{2\pi m}{qB}$

77. When a magnetic field is applied on a stationary electron, then it
(a) remains stationary
(b) spins about its own axis
(c) moves in the direction of the field
(d) moves perpendicular to the direction of the field

78. Two charged particles have charges and masses in the ratio 2 : 3 and 1 : 4, respectively. If they enter a uniform magnetic field and move with the same velocity, then the ratio of their respective time periods of revolution is
(a) 3 : 8 (b) 1 : 4
(c) 3 : 5 (d) 1 : 6

79. Two straight wires each 10 cm long are parallel to one another and separated by 2 cm. When the current flowing in them is 30 A and 40 A respectively, then the force experienced by either of the wires is
(a) 1.2×10^{-3} N (b) 12×10^{-3} N
(c) 11.2×10^{-3} N (d) 10.2×10^{-3} N

80. A charged particle with a velocity 2×10^3 ms^{-1} passes undeflected through electric field and magnetic fields in mutually perpendicular directions. The magnetic field is 15 T. The magnitude of electric field will be
(a) 1.5×10^3 NC^{-1} (b) 2×10^3 NC^{-1}
(c) 3×10^3 NC^{-1} (d) 1.33×10^3 NC^{-1}

81. A proton is moving in a uniform magnetic field B in a circular path of radius a in a direction perpendicular to Z-axis along which field B exists. Calculate the angular momentum, if the radius is a and charge on proton is e.
(a) $\frac{Be}{a^2}$ (b) eB^2a
(c) a^2eB (d) aeB

82. A proton travelling at 23° w.r.t. the direction of a magnetic field of strength 2.6 mT experiences a magnetic force of 6.5×10^{-17} N. What is the speed of the proton?
(a) 2×10^5 ms^{-1}
(b) 4×10^5 ms^{-1}
(c) 6×10^5 ms^{-1}
(d) 6×10^{-5} ms^{-1}

83. What uniform magnetic field applied perpendicular to a beam of electrons moving at 1.3×10^6 ms^{-1}, is required to make the electrons travel in a circular arc of radius 0.35 m?
(a) 2.1×10^{-5} G (b) 6×10^{-5} T
(c) 2.1×10^{-5} T (d) 6×10^{-5} G

84. Two very long straight parallel wires carry currents i and $2i$ in opposite directions. The distance between the wires is r. At a certain instant of time, a point charge q is at a point equidistant from the two wires in the plane of the wires. Its instantaneous velocity v is perpendicular to this plane. The magnitude of the force due to the magnetic field acting on the charge at this instant is
(a) zero (b) $\frac{3\mu_0}{2\pi}\frac{iqv}{r}$
(c) $\frac{\mu_0}{\pi}\frac{iqv}{r}$ (d) $\frac{\mu_0}{2\pi}\frac{iqv}{r}$

85. A current carrying circular loop of radius R is placed in the XY-plane with centre at the origin. Half of the loop with $x > 0$ is now bent, so that it now lies in the YZ-plane. Then, ***[NCERT Exemplar]***
(a) the magnitude of magnetic moment now diminishes.
(b) the magnetic moment does not change.
(c) the magnitude of **B** at $(0,0,z)$, $z > R$ increases.
(d) the magnitude of **B** at $(0,0,z)$, $z >> R$ is unchanged.

86. The rectangular coil of area A is in a field B. Find the torque about the Z-axis when the coil lies in the position shown and carries a current I.

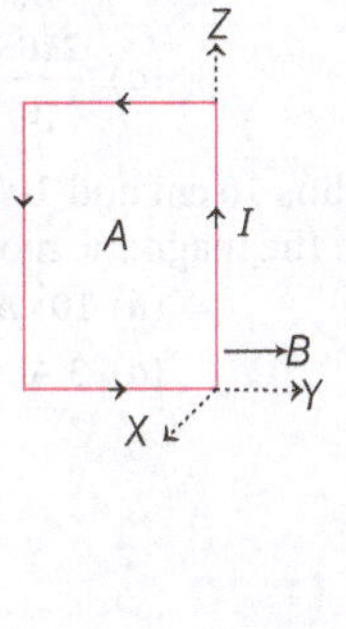

(a) IAB in negative Z-axis
(b) IAB in positive Z-axis
(c) $2IAB$ in positive Z-axis
(d) $2IAB$ in negative Z-axis

87. A rectangular loop consists of N closed wrapped turns and has dimensions $a \times b$. The loop is hinged along the Y-axis. What is the magnitude of the torque exerted on the loop by a uniform magnetic field $B = B_0$ directed along the X-axis when current $i = i_0$ in the direction shown. The torque acting on the loop is

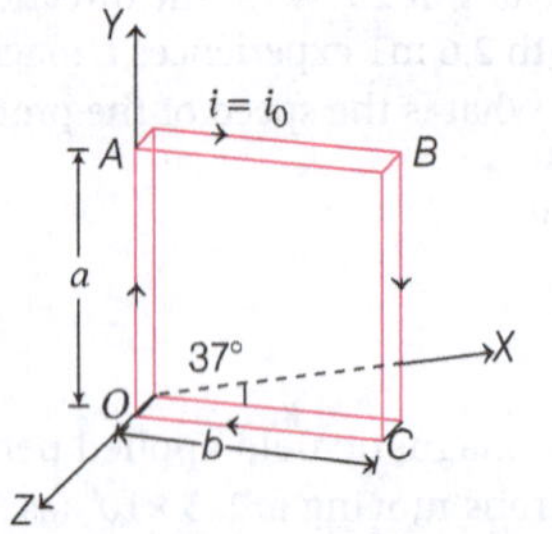

(a) $-\dfrac{4Ni_0abB_0\,\hat{\mathbf{j}}}{5}$ (b) $\dfrac{4Ni_0abB_0\,\hat{\mathbf{i}}}{5}$
(c) $-\dfrac{4Ni_0abB_0J}{3}\hat{\mathbf{j}}$ (d) $\dfrac{-2Ni_0abB_0\hat{\mathbf{j}}}{5}$

88. A square coil of edge L having n turns carries a current i. It is kept on a smooth horizontal plate. A uniform magnetic field B exists in a direction parallel to an edge. The total mass of the coil is M. What should be the minimum value of B for which the coil will start tipping over?
(a) $\dfrac{Mg}{niL}$ (b) $\dfrac{Mg}{2niL}$
(c) $\dfrac{Mg}{4niL}$ (d) $\dfrac{2Mg}{niL}$

89. A current carrying loop is placed in a uniform magnetic field. The torque acting on it does not depend upon
(a) shape of loop
(b) area of loop
(c) value of current
(d) magnetic field

90. Magnetic induction produced at the centre of a circular loop carrying current is B. The magnetic moment of the loop of radius R is
(where, μ_0 = permeability of free space)
(a) $\dfrac{BR^2}{2\pi\mu_0}$ (b) $\dfrac{2\pi BR^3}{\mu_0}$
(c) $\dfrac{BR^2}{2\pi\mu_0}$ (d) $\dfrac{2\pi BR^2}{\mu_0}$

91. A circular coil of radius 10 cm and 100 turns carries a current 1 A. What is the magnetic moment of the coil?
(a) 3.142×10^4 A-m^2 (b) 10^4 A-m^2
(c) 3.142 A-m^2 (d) 3 A-m^2

92. A wire of length L metre carrying a current I ampere is bent in the form of a circle. The magnitude of the magnetic moment is
(a) $\dfrac{L^2I^2}{4\pi}$ (b) $\dfrac{LI}{4\pi}$
(c) $\dfrac{L^2I}{4\pi}$ (d) $\dfrac{LI}{4\pi}$

93. A current loop in a magnetic field
(a) experiences a torque whether the field is uniform or non-uniform in all orientations.
(b) can be in equilibrium in one orientation.
(c) can be equilibrium in two orientations, both the. equilibrium states are unstable.
(d) can be in equilibrium in two orientations, one stable while the other is unstable

94. The torque required to hold a small circular coil of 10 turns, area 1 mm^2 and carrying a current of (21 / 44) A in the middle of a long solenoid of 10^3 turns/m carrying a current of 2.5 A with its axis perpendicular to the axis of the solenoid is

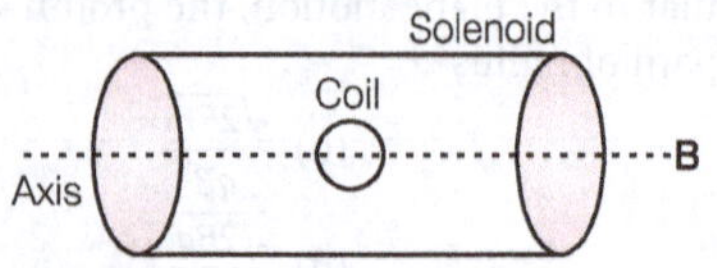

(a) 1.5×10^{-6} N-m
(b) 1.5×10^{-8} N-m
(c) $1.5 \times 10^{+6}$ N-m
(d) $1.5 \times 10^{+8}$ N-m

Assertion and Reason

Directions (Q. Nos. 1-6) *These questions consist of two statements each linked as Assertion and Reason. While answering these questions you are required to choose any one of the following four responses.*
(a) Both A and R are true but R is not the correct explanation of A.
(b) A is true but R is false.
(c) A is false but R is true.
(d) Both A and R are true and R is the correct explanation of A.

1. Assertion (A) Two infinitely long wires A and B carry unequal currents both in inward direction.

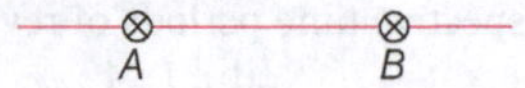

Then, there is only one point (excluding the points at infinity), where net magnetic field is zero.
Reason (R) That point lies between points A and B.

2. Assertion (A) When a charged particle moves perpendicular to a uniform magnetic field, then its momentum remains constant.
Reason (R) Magnetic force acts perpendicular to the velocity of the particle.

3. **Assertion** (A) An α-particle and a deuteron having same kinetic energy enter in a uniform magnetic field perpendicular to the field. Then, radius of circular path of α-particle will be more.

Reason (R) $\frac{q}{m}$ ratio of an α-particle is equal to the $\frac{q}{m}$ ratio of a deuteron.

4. **Assertion** (A) In a uniform magnetic field $\mathbf{B} = B_0\hat{\mathbf{k}}$, if velocity of a charged particle is $v_0\hat{\mathbf{i}}$ at $t = 0$, then it can have the velocity $v_0\hat{\mathbf{j}}$ at some other instant.

Reason (R) In uniform magnetic field, acceleration of a charged particle is always zero.

5. **Assertion** (A) If velocity of charged particle in a uniform magnetic field at same instant is $(a_1\hat{\mathbf{i}} - a_2\hat{\mathbf{j}})$ and at some other instant is $(b_1\hat{\mathbf{i}} + b_2\hat{\mathbf{j}})$, then

$$a_1^2 + a_2^2 = b_1^2 + b_2^2$$

Reason (R) Magnetic force cannot change velocity of a charged particle.

6. **Assertion** (A) Upper wire shown in figure is fixed. At a certain distance x, lower wire can remain in equilibrium.

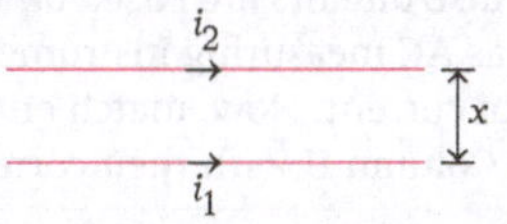

Reason (R) The above equilibrium of lower wire is stable equilibrium.

Statement Type Questions

Directions (Q. Nos. 1-5) *These questions consists of two statements, choose the most appropriate answer from the options given below.*

(a) Both Statement I and Statement II are incorrect.
(b) Statement I is correct but Statement II is incorrect.
(c) Statement I is incorrect but Statement II is correct.
(d) Both Statement I and Statement II are correct.

1. **Statement I** Inside a thick conductor, magnetic field increases linearly with the distance from the axis of conductor.

Statement II Current enclosed increases linearly with the distance from the axis of conductor.

2. **Statement I** Force experienced by moving charge will be maximum if direction of velocity of charge is parallel to applied magnetic field.

Statement II Force on moving charge is independent of direction of applied magnetic field.

3. **Statement I** A magnetic field produces a force on a moving charge but not on a static charge.

Statement II A moving charge produces a magnetic field.

4. **Statement I** When radius of circular wire carrying current becomes half its magnetic moment becomes four times.

Statement II Magnetic moment does not depend on areas of the loop.

5. **Statement I** Higher the range, greater is the resistance of ammeter.

Statement II To increase the range of ammeter, larger value of shunt needs to be use across it.

Match the Columns

1. Four particles; α-particle, deuteron, electron and a Cl^- ion enter in a transverse magnetic field perpendicular to it with same kinetic energy. Their paths are as shown in figure. Now, match the Column I with Column II and mark the correct option from the codes given below.

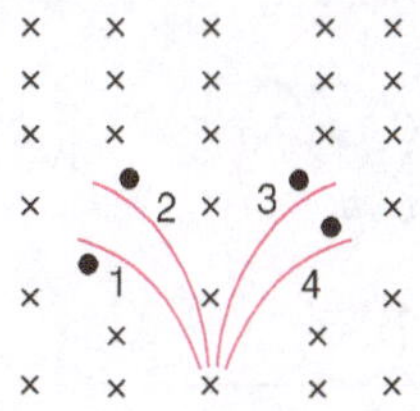

	Column I		Column II
A.	Deuteron	I.	Path-1
B.	α-particle	II.	Path-2
C.	Electron	III.	Path-3
D.	Cl^-	IV.	Path-4

Choose the correct answer from the options given below.
(a) A-II, B-I, C-IV, D-III
(b) A-III, B-II, C-I, D-IV
(c) A-IV, B-III, C-II, D-I
(d) A-I, B-II, C-III, D-IV

2. Match the figure in Column I with their magnitude of magnetic field at point O in Column II.

Column I		Column II
A.	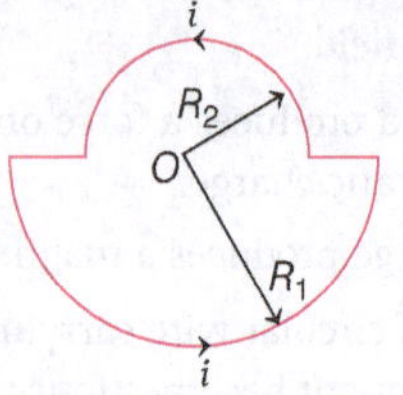	I. $\frac{\mu_0 i}{2\pi a}\left(\tan\frac{\theta}{2}+\pi-\frac{\theta}{2}\right)$
B.	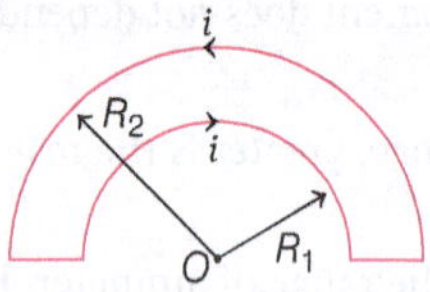	II. $\frac{\mu_0 i}{4R}\left(\frac{1}{\pi}+\frac{3}{2}\right)$
C.	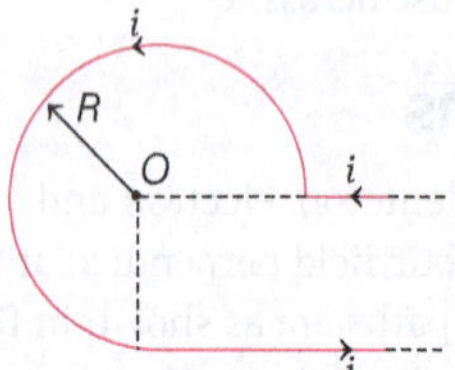	III. $\frac{\mu_0 i}{4}\left(\frac{1}{R_1}+\frac{1}{R_2}\right)$
D.	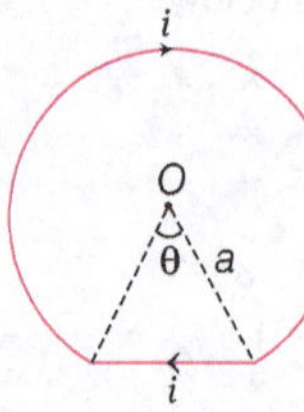	IV. $\frac{\mu_0 i}{4}\left(\frac{1}{R_1}-\frac{1}{R_2}\right)$

Choose the correct answer from the options given below.
(a) A-III, B-IV, C-II, D-I
(b) A-III, B-IV, C-I, D-II
(c) A-I, B-II, C-III, D-IV
(d) A-II, B-I, C-III, D-IV

3. A square current carrying loop *abcd* is placed near an infinitely long another current carrying wire *ef*. Now, match the Column I with Column II and mark the correct option from the codes given below.

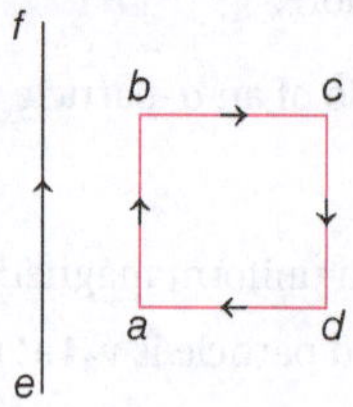

Column I	Column II
A. Net force on *bc* and *da*	I. zero
B. Net force on *ab* and *cd*	II. non-zero and unequal
C. Net force on complete loop *abcd*	III. rightwards
D. Net force on *ef*	IV. leftwards

Choose the correct answer from the options given below.
(a) A-I, B-II, C-III, D-IV
(b) A-IV, B-III, C-II, D-I
(c) A-III, B-IV, C-I, D-II
(d) A-I, B-II, C-IV, D-III

4. DC measuring instruments are based on magnetic effect of current, whereas AC measuring instruments are based on heating effect of current. Now, match entries of Column I with entries of Column II with their correct proportionality.

Column I	Column II
A. Deflection of AC ammeter	I. V
B. Deflection of DC ammeter	II. V^2
C. Deflection of AC voltmeter	III. I
D. Deflection of DC voltmeter	IV. I^2

Choose the correct answer from the options given below.
(a) A-IV, B-III, C-II, D-I
(b) A-III, B-II, C-I, D-IV
(c) A-IV, B-II, C-III, D-I
(d) A-I, B-II, C-IV, D-III

Final Check Through PYQs

Module-I Biot-Savart's Law

1. A tightly wound 100 turns coil of radius 10 cm carries a current of 7 A. The magnitude of the magnetic field at the centre of the coil is (Take, permeability of free space as $4\pi \times 10^{-7}$ SI units)
[NCERT (New) Pg. 116, NEET 2024]
(a) 44 mT (b) 4.4 T (c) 4.4 mT (d) 44 T

2. A very long conducting wire is bent in a semi-circular shape from A to B as shown in figure. The magnetic field at point P for steady current configuration is given by *[NCERT (New) Pg. 115, NEET 2023]*

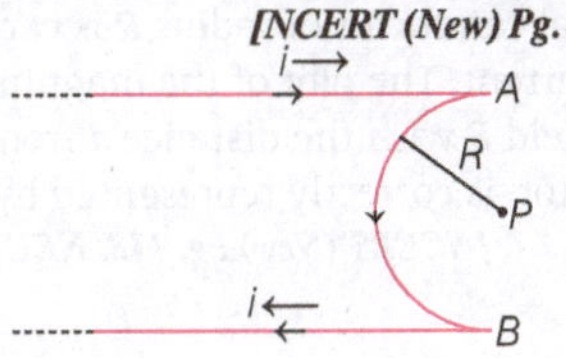

(a) $\frac{\mu_0 i}{4R}$ pointed away from the page
(b) $\frac{\mu_0 i}{4R}\left[1-\frac{2}{\pi}\right]$ pointed away from page
(c) $\frac{\mu_0 i}{4R}\left[1-\frac{2}{\pi}\right]$ pointed into the page
(d) $\frac{\mu_0 i}{4R}$ pointed into the page

3. Given below are two statements
Statement I Biot-Savart's law gives us the expression for the magnetic field strength of an infinitesimal current element (Idl) of a current carrying conductor only.
Statement II Biot-Savart's law is analogous to Coulomb's inverse square law of charge q, with the former being related to the field produced by a scalar source, Idl while the latter being produced by a vector source, q.
In light of above statements choose the most appropriate answer from the options given below.
[NCERT (New) Pg. 113, NEET 2022]
(a) Both Statement I and Statement II are incorrect.
(b) Statement I is correct and Statement II is incorrect.
(c) Statement I is incorrect and Statement II is correct.
(d) Both Statement I and Statement II are correct.

4. A straight conductor carrying current i splits into two parts as shown in the figure. The radius of the circular loop is R. The total magnetic field at the centre P at the loop is *[NCERT (New) Pg. 115, NEET (Odisha) 2019]*

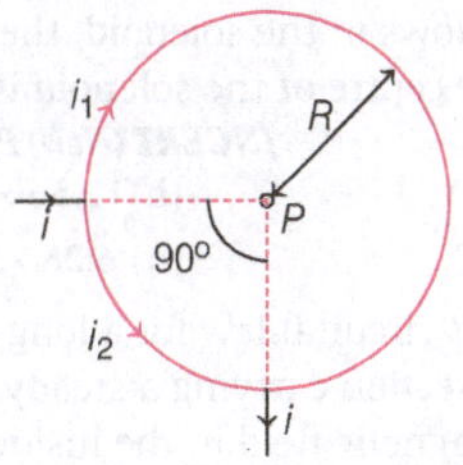

(a) zero (b) $3\mu_0 i/32R$, outward
(c) $3\mu_0 i/32R$, inward (d) $\frac{\mu_0 i}{2R}$, inward

5. A long wire carrying a steady current is bent into a circular loop of one turn. The magnetic field at the centre of the loop is B. It is then bent into a circular coil of n turns. The magnetic field at the centre of this coil of n turns will be *[NCERT (New) Pg. 115, NEET 2016]*
(a) nB (b) n^2B
(c) $2nB$ (d) $2n^2B$

6. A wire carrying current I has the shape as shown in adjoining figure. Linear parts of the wire are very long and parallel to X-axis while semicircular portion of radius R is lying in Y-Z plane. Magnetic field at point O is *[NCERT (New) Pg. 116, AIPMT 2015]*

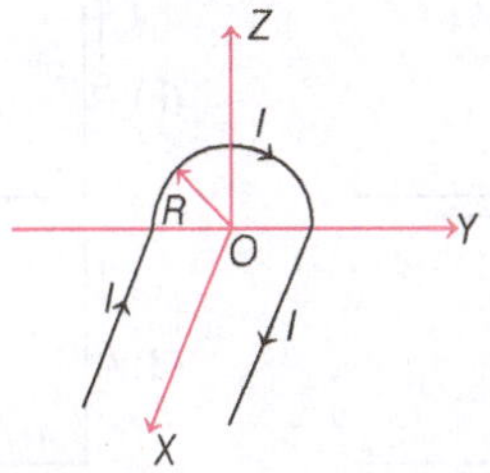

(a) $B = \frac{\mu_0}{4\pi}\frac{I}{R}(\pi\hat{i} + 2\hat{k})$ (b) $B = -\frac{\mu_0}{4\pi}\frac{I}{R}(\pi\hat{i} - 2\hat{k})$
(c) $B = -\frac{\mu_0}{4\pi}\frac{I}{R}(\pi\hat{i} + 2\hat{k})$ (d) $B = \frac{\mu_0}{4\pi}\frac{I}{R}(\pi\hat{i} - 2\hat{k})$

7. An electron moving in a circular orbit of radius r makes n rotations per second. The magnetic field produced at the centre has magnitude
[NCERT (New) Pg. 113, AIPMT 2015]
(a) $\frac{\mu_0 ne}{2\pi r}$ (b) zero
(c) $\frac{\mu_0 n^2 e}{r}$ (d) $\frac{\mu_0 ne}{2r}$

8. Two identical long conducting wires *AOB* and *COD* are placed at right angle to each other, such that one is above the other and *O* is their common point. The wires carry I_1 and I_2 currents, respectively. Point *P* is lying at distance *d* from *O* along a direction perpendicular to the plane containing the wires. The magnetic field at the point *P* will be *[NCERT (New) Pg. 113, AIPMT 2014]*

(a) $\frac{\mu_0}{2\pi d}\left(\frac{I_1}{I_2}\right)$ (b) $\frac{\mu_0}{2\pi d}(I_1 + I_2)$

(c) $\frac{\mu_0}{2\pi d}(I_1^2 - I_2^2)$ (d) $\frac{\mu_0}{2\pi d}(I_1^2 + I_2^2)^{1/2}$

Module-II Ampere's Circuital Law

9. A long solenoid of radius 1 mm has 100 turns per mm. If 1A current flows in the solenoid, the magnetic field strength at the centre of the solenoid is *[NCERT (New) Pg. 122, NEET 2022]*

(a) 12.56×10^{-2}T (b) 12.56×10^{-4}T

(c) 6.28×10^{-4}T (d) 6.28×10^{-2}T

10. From Ampere's circuital law for a long straight wire of circular cross-section carrying a steady current, the variation of magnetic field in the inside and outside region of the wire is *[NCERT (New) Pg. 118, NEET 2022]*

(a) a linearly increasing function of distance upto the boundary of the wire and then linearly decreasing for the outside region.

(b) a linearly increasing function of distance *r* upto the boundary of the wire and then decreasing one with $1/r$ dependence for the outside region.

(c) a linearly decreasing function of distance upto the boundary of the wire and then a linearly increasing one for the outside region.

(d) uniform and remains constant for both the regions.

11. A thick current carrying cable of radius *R* carries current *I* uniformly distributed across its cross-section. The variation of magnetic field *B* due to the cable with the distance *r* from the axis of the cable is represented by *[NCERT (New) Pg. 118, NEET 2021]*

(a)
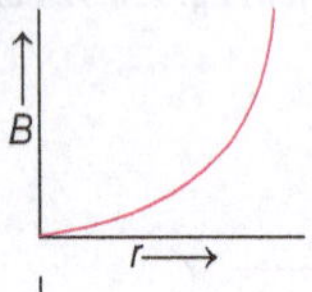

(b)
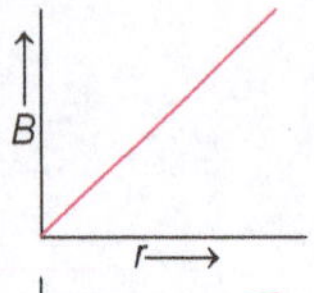

(c)
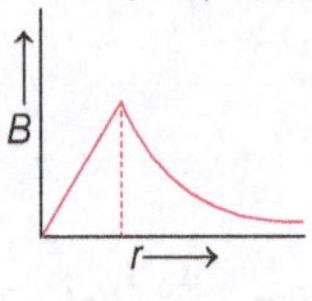

(d)
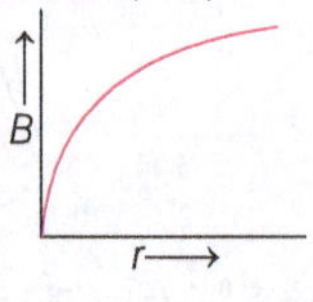

12. A long solenoid of 50 cm length having 100 turns carries a current of 2.5 A. The magnetic field at the centre of solenoid is (Take, $\mu_0 = 4\pi \times 10^{-7}$ T m A^{-1}) *[NCERT (New) Pg. 122, NEET (Sep.) 2020]*

(a) 3.14×10^{-4} T

(b) 6.28×10^{-5} T

(c) 3.14×10^{-5} T

(d) 6.28×10^{-4} T

13. A cylindrical conductor of radius *R* is carrying a constant current. The plot of the magnitude of the magnetic field *B* with the distance *d* from the centre of the conductor, is correctly represented by the figure *[NCERT (New) Pg. 118, NEET (National) 2019]*

(a)
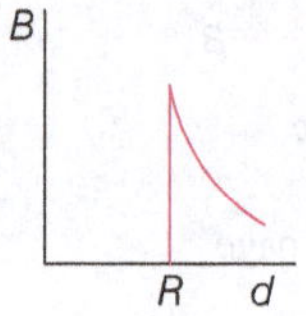

(b)
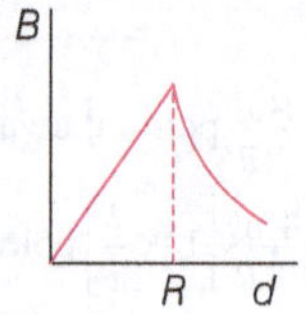

(c)
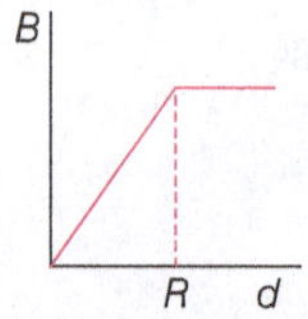

(d)
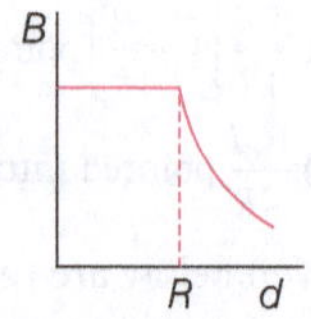

14. A long straight wire of radius *a* carries a steady current *I*. The current is uniformly distributed over its cross-section. The ratio of the magnetic fields *B* and *B'* at radial distances $a/2$ and $2a$ respectively, from the axis of the wire is *[NCERT (New) Pg. 116, NEET 2016]*

(a) $\frac{1}{2}$ (b) 1

(c) 4 (d) $\frac{1}{4}$

Module-III Magnetic Forces

15. A wire carrying a current *I* along the positive *X*-axis has length *L*. It is kept in a magnetic field $\mathbf{B} = (2\hat{i} + 3\hat{j} - 4\hat{k})$ T. The magnitude of the magnetic force acting on the wire is. *[NCERT (New) Pg. 110, NEET 2023]*

(a) $\sqrt{5}\,IL$ (b) $5\,IL$

(c) $\sqrt{3}\,IL$ (d) $3\,IL$

16. In the product $\mathbf{F} = q(\mathbf{v} \times \mathbf{B}) = q\mathbf{v} \times (B\hat{i} + B\hat{j} + B_0\hat{k})$

For $q = 1$ and $\mathbf{v} = 2\hat{i} + 4\hat{j} + 6\hat{k}$ and $\mathbf{F} = 4\hat{i} - 20\hat{j} + 12\hat{k}$

What will be the complete expression for **B**? *[NCERT (New) Pg. 109, NEET 2021]*

(a) $-8\hat{i} - 8\hat{j} - 6\hat{k}$ (b) $-6\hat{i} - 6\hat{j} - 8\hat{k}$

(c) $8\hat{i} + 8\hat{j} - 6\hat{k}$ (d) $6\hat{i} + 6\hat{j} - 8\hat{k}$

Final Check

17. An infinitely long straight conductor carries a current of 5 A as shown. An electron is moving with a speed of 10^5 m/s parallel to the conductor. The perpendicular distance between the electron and the conductor is 20 cm at an instant. Calculate the magnitude of the force experienced by the electron at that instant **[NCERT (New) Pg. 109, NEET 2021]**

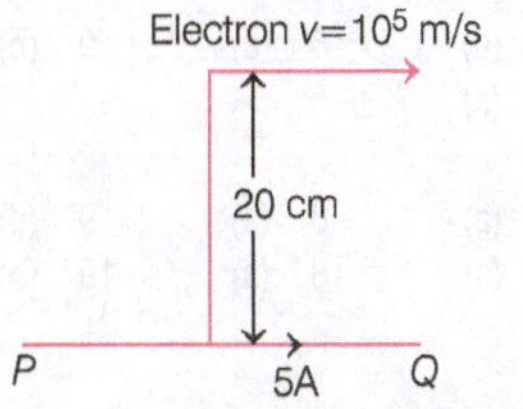

(a) 8×10^{-20} N (b) 4×10^{-20} N
(c) $8\pi\times10^{-20}$ N (d) $4\pi\times10^{-20}$ N

18. Ionised hydrogen atoms and α -particles with same momenta enters perpendicular to a constant magnetic field, B. The ratio of their radii of their paths $r_H : r_\alpha$ will be **[NCERT (New) Pg. 109, NEET (National) 2019]**

(a) 1 : 2 (b) 4 : 1 (c) 1 : 4 (d) 2 : 1

19. A metallic rod of mass per unit length 0.5 kg m^{-1} is lying horizontally on a smooth inclined plane which makes an angle of 30° with the horizontal. The rod is not allowed to slide down by flowing a current through it when a magnetic field of induction 0.25 T is acting on it in the vertical direction. The current flowing in the rod to keep it stationary is **[NCERT (New) Pg. 109, NEET 2018]**

(a) 14.76 A (b) 5.98 A
(c) 7.14 A (d) 11.32 A

20. An arrangement of three parallel straight wires placed perpendicular to plane of paper carrying same current I along the same direction is shown in figure. Magnitude of force per unit length on the middle wire B is given by **[NCERT (New) Pg. 123, NEET 2017]**

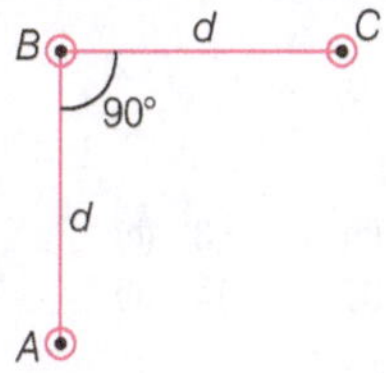

(a) $\frac{\mu_0 I^2}{2\pi d}$ (b) $\frac{2\mu_0 I^2}{\pi d}$
(c) $\frac{\sqrt{2}\mu_0 I^2}{\pi d}$ (d) $\frac{\mu_0 I^2}{\sqrt{2}\,\pi d}$

21. A square loop *ABCD* carrying a current *i*, is placed near and coplanar with a long straight conductor *XY* carrying a current *I*, the net force on the loop will be **[NCERT (New) Pg. 123, NEET 2016]**

(a) $\frac{\mu_0 Ii}{2\pi}$ (b) $\frac{2\mu_0 IiL}{3\pi}$
(c) $\frac{\mu_0 IiL}{2\pi}$ (d) $\frac{2\mu_0 Ii}{3\pi}$

22. An electron is moving in a circular path under the influence of a transverse magnetic field of 3.57×10^{-2} T. If the value of *e*/*m* is 1.76×10^{11} C/kg, the frequency of revolution of the electron is **[NCERT (New) Pg. 109, NEET 2016]**

(a) 1 GHz (b) 100 MHz
(c) 62.8 MHz (d) 6.28 MHz

23. A proton and an alpha particle both enter a region of uniform magnetic field *B*, moving at right angles to field *B*. If the radius of circular orbits for both the particles is equal and the kinetic energy acquired by proton is 1 MeV the energy acquired by the alpha particle will be **[NCERT (New) Pg. 109, AIPMT 2015]**

(a) 0.5 MeV (b) 1.5 MeV
(c) 1 MeV (d) 4 MeVs

Module-IV Torque and Moving Coil Galvanometer

24. Current sensitivity of a moving coil galvanometer is 5 div/mA and its voltage sensitivity (angular deflection per unit voltage applied) is 20 div/V. The resistance of the galvanometer is **[NCERT (New) Pg. 130, NEET 2018]**

(a) 250 Ω
(b) 25 Ω
(c) 40 Ω
(d) 500 Ω

25. A rectangular coil of length 0.12 m and width 0.1 m having 50 turns of wire is suspended vertically in a uniform magnetic field of strength 0.2 Wb/m². The coil carries a current of 2 A. If the plane of the coil is inclined at an angle of 30° with the direction of the field, the torque required to keep the coil in stable equilibrium will be **[NCERT (New) Pg. 125, AIPMT 2015]**

(a) 0.15 N-m (b) 0.20 N-m
(c) 0.24 N-m (d) 0.12 N-m

Answers

Step up Practice 1

1 (c)	2 (b)	3 (b)	4 (d)	5 (c)	6 (a)	7 (c)	8 (c)	9 (b)	10 (b)
11 (b)	12 (a)	13 (b)	14 (c)	15 (d)	16 (d)	17 (a)	18 (a)	19 (a)	20 (d)
21 (d)									

Step up Practice 2

1 (b)	2 (b)	3 (a)	4 (d)	5 (b)	6 (b)	7 (c)	8 (a)	9 (c)	10 (b)
11 (d)	12 (c)	13 (d)	14 (d)	15 (a)	16 (d)	17 (a)			

Step up Practice 3

1 (c)	2 (d)	3 (c)	4 (a)	5 (c)	6 (b)	7 (a)	8 (a)	9 (d)	10 (c)
11 (b)	12 (c)	13 (d)	14 (c)	15 (b)	16 (b)	17 (a)	18 (a)	19 (b)	20 (b)
21 (d)	22 (b)	23 (c)	24 (d)	25 (d)	26 (c)				

Step up Practice 4

1 (c)	2 (d)	3 (c)	4 (d)	5 (d)	6 (a)	7 (d)	8 (a)	9 (a)	10 (d)
11 (d)	12 (b)	13 (d)	14 (d)	15 (a)	16 (a)	17 (b)	18 (b)	19 (b)	20 (d)
21 (a)									

Gearing up for NEET

1 (a)	2 (c)	3 (c)	4 (a)	5 (b)	6 (d)	7 (a)	8 (d)	9 (c)	10 (b)
11 (d)	12 (d)	13 (a)	14 (b)	15 (b)	16 (b)	17 (c)	18 (d)	19 (b)	20 (b)
21 (b)	22 (a)	23 (c)	24 (a)	25 (b)	26 (a)	27 (c)	28 (b)	29 (c)	30 (c)
31 (a)	32 (d)	33 (b)	34 (d)	35 (d)	36 (c)	37 (d)	38 (a)	39 (d)	40 (b)
41 (c)	42 (a)	43 (b)	44 (d)	45 (b)	46 (c)	47 (a)	48 (b)	49 (d)	50 (c)
51 (d)	52 (b)	53 (c)	54 (b)	55 (c)	56 (c)	57 (a)	58 (c)	59 (d)	60 (c)
61 (b)	62 (d)	63 (a)	64 (a)	65 (c)	66 (c)	67 (a)	68 (d)	69 (c)	70 (d)
71 (d)	72 (a)	73 (a)	74 (c)	75 (b)	76 (d)	77 (a)	78 (a)	79 (a)	80 (c)
81 (c)	82 (b)	83 (c)	84 (a)	85 (a)	86 (b)	87 (a)	88 (b)	89 (a)	90 (b)
91 (c)	92 (c)	93 (d)	94 (b)						

Assertion and Reason

1 (a)	2 (c)	3 (c)	4 (b)	5 (b)	6 (b)

Statement Type Questions

1 (b)	2 (a)	3 (d)	4 (a)	5 (a)

Match the Columns

1 (a)	2 (a)	3 (d)	4 (a)

Final Check through PYQs : Module-I

1 (c)	2 (b)	3 (b)	4 (a)	5 (b)	6 (c)	7 (d)	8 (d)

Final Check through PYQs : Module-II

9 (a)	10 (b)	11 (c)	12 (d)	13 (b)	14 (b)

Final Check through PYQs : Module-III

15 (b)	16 (b)	17 (a)	18 (d)	19 (d)	20 (d)	21 (d)	22 (a)	23 (c)

Final Check through PYQs : Module-IV

24 (a)	25 (b)

Hints and Solutions

Step up Practice 1

1. (c) Magnetic field at a distance r near a long straight current carrying wire is given by

$$B = \frac{\mu_0}{4\pi} \cdot \frac{2i}{r} \Rightarrow B \propto \frac{1}{r}$$

$$\therefore \quad \frac{B_1}{B_2} = \frac{r_2}{r_1} \text{ or } \frac{B}{B_2} = \frac{r/2}{r}$$

$$\Rightarrow \quad B_2 = 2B$$

2. (b) Magnetic field at the centre of a current carrying circular coil of N turns is given by

$$B = \frac{\mu_0 Ni}{2r} \Rightarrow B \propto \frac{1}{r}$$

3. (b) Current produced in wire, $i = \frac{q}{t} = \frac{100 \times e}{1}$

$$\therefore \quad i = 100\, e$$

Magnetic field at the centre of circular path,

$$= \frac{\mu_0}{4\,\pi} \cdot \frac{2\pi i}{r} = \frac{\mu_0}{4\,\pi} \cdot \frac{2\pi \times 100\, e}{r} = \frac{\mu_0 \times 200e}{4r}$$

$$= \frac{\mu_0 \times 200 \times 1.6 \times 10^{-19}}{4 \times 0.8} = 10^{-17} \mu_0 \text{ T}$$

4. (d) Both A and R are true and R is the correct explanation of A.

The magnitude of the magnetic field produced due to flow of current through a circular loop at a point on its axis is given by

$$\Rightarrow \quad B = \frac{\mu_0}{4\pi} \frac{2\pi I a^2}{(a^2 + x^2)^{3/2}}$$

This is maximum at centre of loop, where $x = 0$

$$\Rightarrow \quad B = \frac{\mu_0}{4\pi} \frac{2\pi I}{a} = \frac{\mu_0 I}{2a}$$

5. (c) The direction of magnetic field produced due to both semicircular parts will be perpendicular to the paper and inwards.

Magnetic induction at the centre O,

$$B = B_1 + B_2 = \frac{\mu_0 i}{4 r_1} + \frac{\mu_0 i}{4 r_2}$$

$$= \frac{\mu_0 i}{4} \left(\frac{r_1 + r_2}{r_1 r_2} \right)$$

6. (a) 1 tesla $= 10^4$ gauss. Hence, option (a) is correct.

Biot savart's law $\rightarrow dB \propto \frac{Idl \sin \theta}{r^2}$

Magnetic field due to an arc $\rightarrow B = \left(\frac{\mu_0}{4\pi} \right) \left(\frac{i}{a} \right) \theta$

SI unit of magnetic field $\rightarrow$ Weber/m^2

7. (c) Magnetic field at the centre of circular coil of N turns is given by

$$B = \frac{4\pi \times 10^{-7} \times 100 \times 0.1}{2 \times 5 \times 10^{-2}} = 4\pi \times 10^{-5} \text{ T}$$

8. (c) The magnetic field, $B = \frac{\mu_0 Ni}{2R}$ or $B \propto \frac{N}{R}$

$$\frac{B_2}{B_1} = \frac{N_2}{N_1} \times \frac{R_1}{R_2} = \frac{2N_1}{N_1} \times \frac{R_1}{R_1/2} = 4$$

$$\Rightarrow \quad B_2 = 4B_1 = 4B$$

$$B' = 4B$$

9. (b) A is true but R is false.

Since $dB \propto \sin \theta$, where θ is angle between the direction of the flow of current and the line joining the elementary portion to the observation point which is zero in this case, so the magnetic field is also zero (because $\sin \theta$ is equal to zero).

10. (b) Magnetic field at the centre of arc,

$$B = \frac{\mu_0}{4\pi} \frac{\theta i}{r}$$

$$= \frac{\mu_0}{4\pi} \times \frac{\pi}{2} \times \frac{i}{R} = \frac{\mu_0 i}{8R}$$

11. (b) Using Fleming's right hand rule, the direction of magnetic field is towards east.

12. (a) According to right hand screw rule,

Along the line $x = y$, magnetic field due to two wires will be equal and opposite.

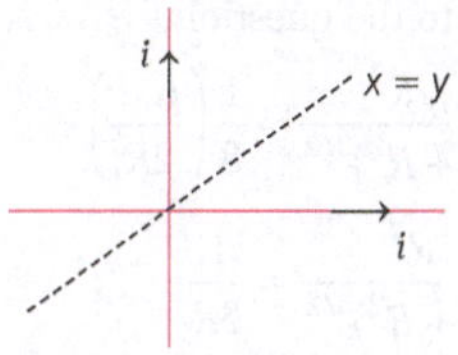

13. (b) A is true but R is false.

The direction of magnetic field due to a current carrying conductor can be found by applying right hand thumb rule. When electric current is passed through a circular conductor, the magnetic field lines near the centre of the conductor are almost straight lines. Magnetic flux direction is determined only by the direction of current.

14. (c) Magnetic field due to a ring having n turns at a distance x on its axis is given by

$$B = \frac{\mu_0}{2} \cdot \frac{nir^2}{(x^2 + r^2)^{3/2}}$$

$$\therefore \quad B \propto \frac{nr^2}{(x^2 + r^2)^{3/2}}$$

15. (d) Both A and R are true and R is the correct explanation of A.

The magnetic field at the centre of circular coil is given by $B = \frac{\mu_0}{4\pi} \cdot \frac{2\pi nI}{a}$.

So, if current through coil is doubled. The magnetic field is directly proportional to the current in conductor.

16. (d) Magnetic field at the centre of a current carrying coil having current I and radius a is given as

$$B_1 = \frac{\mu_0 I}{2a} \quad \text{...(i)}$$

Magnetic field on the axis of circular current carrying coil of radius a and current I at a distance x from the centre is given as

$$B_2 = \frac{\mu_0 I a^2}{2(x^2 + a^2)^{3/2}}$$

Here, $x = a$

$$\therefore \quad B_2 = \frac{\mu_0 I a^2}{2(a^2 + a^2)^{3/2}}$$

$$= \frac{\mu_0 I a^2}{2^{5/2} \cdot a^3}$$

$$= \frac{\mu_0 I}{2^{5/2} \cdot a} \quad \text{...(ii)}$$

From Eqs. (i) and (ii), we get

$$\therefore \quad \frac{B_1}{B_2} = \frac{\mu_0 I / 2a}{\mu_0 I / 2^{5/2} a} = \frac{2^{5/2}}{2}$$

$$= 2^{3/2} = 2 \cdot 2^{1/2} = 2\sqrt{2}$$

17. (a) According to the question,

$$\frac{\mu_0 I R^2}{2(x^2 + R^2)^{3/2}} = \frac{1}{8}\left(\frac{\mu_0 I}{2R}\right)$$

$$\therefore \quad \frac{R^2}{(x^2 + R^2)^{3/2}} = \frac{1}{8R}$$

or $\quad (x^2 + R^2)^{3/2} = 8R^3$

or $\quad x^2 + R^2 = 4R^2$

$$\therefore \quad x = \sqrt{3}R$$

18. (a) Both A and R are true but R is not the correct explanation of A.

A moving charge always produce a magnetic field whether it is accelerated or not accelerated. But once the charge becomes stationary, it does not produce any magnetic field.

19. (a) The magnetic field at the centre O,

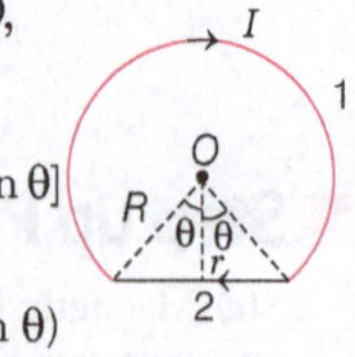

$$B_O = B_1 + B_2$$

$$= \frac{\mu_0 I}{2R}\left[\frac{2\pi - 2\theta}{2\pi}\right] + \frac{\mu_0 I}{4\pi r}[\sin\theta + \sin\theta]$$

$$= \frac{\mu_0 I}{2R}\left[\frac{\pi - \theta}{\pi}\right] + \frac{\mu_0 I}{4\pi (R\cos\theta)}(2\sin\theta)$$

$$= \frac{\mu_0 I}{2\pi R}[\pi - \theta + \tan\theta]$$

20. (d) Magnetic field induction at centre O is given by

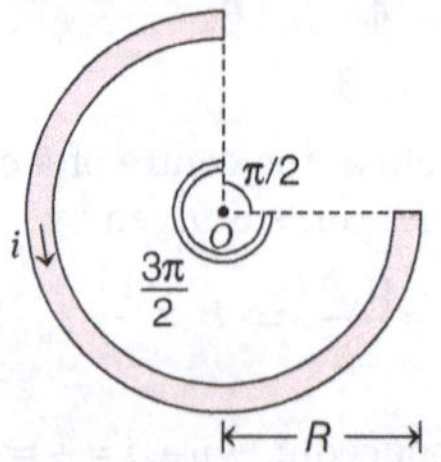

$$B = \frac{3}{4} \text{ (Magnetic field due to whole circle)}$$

$$= \frac{3}{4}\left(\frac{\mu_0 i}{2R}\right) = \frac{3\mu_0 i}{8R}$$

21. (d) The given situation is shown below

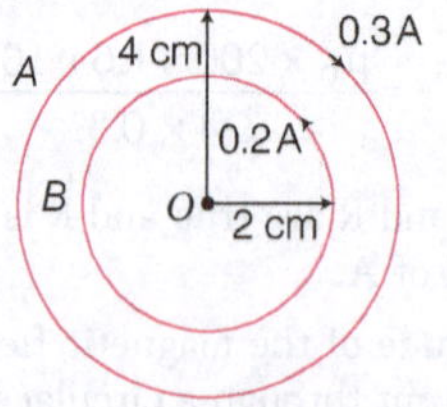

At centre O, magnetic field due to inner circular coil,

$$B_1 = \frac{\mu_0 N i_1}{2r_1} = \frac{\mu_0 (10) \times (0.2)}{2 \times (2 \times 10^{-2})} = 50\mu_0 \odot$$

Similarly, at centre O, magnetic field due to outer circular coil,

$$B_2 = \frac{\mu_0 N i_2}{2r_2} = \frac{\mu_0 (10) \times (0.3)}{2(4 \times 10^{-2})} = \frac{75\mu_0}{2} \otimes$$

Net magnetic field, $B_O = B_1 - B_2 = 50\mu_0 - \frac{75\mu_0}{2}$

$$= \frac{100\mu_0 - 75\mu_0}{2} = \frac{25}{2}\mu_0 \text{ Wb/m}^2 \odot$$

Step up Practice 2

1. (b) For a point inside the tube, using Ampere's law, $\int B \cdot dl = \mu_0 i$. Here, we have $i = 0$ for inside the tube.

$$\therefore \quad B = 0$$

2. (b) As we know, according to Ampere's law

$$\oint \mathbf{B} \cdot d\mathbf{l} = \mu_0 I$$

Only for outside point, path of line integration will enclose the current. Hence, magnetic field inside the pipe is zero.

3. (a) $\oint \mathbf{B}\cdot d\mathbf{l} = \mu_0 I$

$$= 4\pi \times 10^{-7} \times \frac{1}{2\pi}$$

$$= 2\times 10^{-7}\ \text{Wb/m}$$

4. (d) Both Statement I and Statement II are correct.

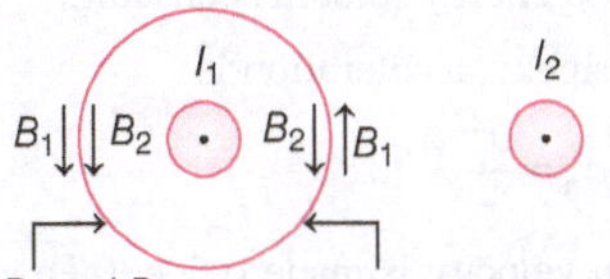

In $\mathbf{B}\cdot d\mathbf{l} = \mu_0 I_{net}$, **B** the magnetic field exists due to both wires whereas I_{net} is current enclosed.

At some points of path enclosed, $B_{net} = B_1 + B_2$ and at some points $B_{net} = B_1 - B_2$ and when we sum $\mathbf{B}\cdot d\mathbf{l}$, these effects balance each other and sum does not have effect of B_2. So, $\mathbf{B}\cdot d\mathbf{l} = \mu_0 I_1$ with or without the other wire.

5. (b) We shall use $\oint \mathbf{B}\cdot d\mathbf{l} = \mu_0 I$, where I is the current enclosed by loop.

Net current enclosed by these path,

For, path a is zero.

For, path c is 1A.

For, path d is 3A.

For, path b is 5A.

6. (b) By applying Ampere's law, $\oint \mathbf{B}\cdot d\mathbf{l} = \mu_0 I$ to any closed path. Inside the pipe we do not find any enclosed current. Hence, $B = 0$.

7. (c) Here **B** (due to I) and **dl** will be in same direction.

So, $$\oint \mathbf{B}\cdot d\mathbf{l} = \oint \mathbf{B}\cdot d\mathbf{l}\cos 0°$$

$$= \oint \mathbf{B}\cdot d\mathbf{l} = B\oint d\mathbf{l} = BN\,2\pi r$$

$$= 25(B2\pi r) = 25\mu_0 I$$

8. (a) Both Statement I and Statement II are incorrect.

In the case of metallic rod, the charge carriers flow through whole of the cross-section.

Therefore, the magnetic field exists both inside as well as outside. However, magnetic field inside the rod will go on decreasing as we go towards the axis.

9. (c) Required arrangement is shown in the following figure. According to Ampere's circuital law,

$$B_{outside} = \frac{\mu_0}{4\pi}\frac{2I}{r}$$

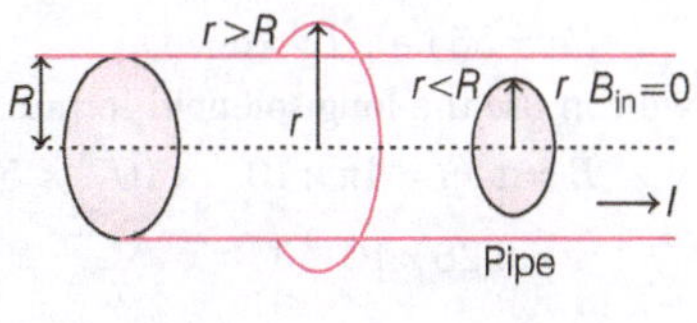

For an internal point, $r < R$

$$B_{internal} = \frac{\mu_0(0)}{2\pi r} = 0$$

For a point on pipe, $r = R$

$$B = \frac{\mu_0 I}{2\pi r}$$

For an external point, $r < R$

$$B_{external} = \frac{\mu_0 I}{2\pi r}$$

Hence, magnetic field is zero only inside the pipe at any point.

10. (b) Applying Ampere's circuital law in the closed loop as shown in the figure below.

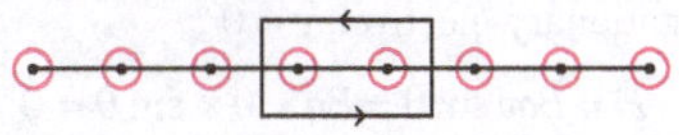

$$2Bl = \mu_0(\lambda \cdot l)$$

$$\therefore \quad B = \frac{\mu_0 \lambda}{2}$$

11. (d) Ampere's circuital law holds good for steady current which do not change with time.

Magnetic field inside solenoid,

$$B = \mu_0 nI = 4\pi \times 10^{-7} \times \frac{600}{2} \times 5$$

$$= 1.88 \times 10^{-3}\ \text{T}$$

12. (c) Magnet field inside the solid cylinder $(r < R)$

$$B_{in} = \frac{\mu_0}{2\pi}\cdot\frac{ir}{R^2}$$

13. (d) Inside the rod, $B \propto r$ and outside it, $B \propto \frac{1}{r}$.

Thus, graph (d) is correct option.

14. (d) Both Statement I and Statement II are correct.

The magnetic field produced by solenoid is given by,

$$B = \frac{1}{2}\mu_0 nI[\cos\theta_1 - \cos\theta_2]$$

Which is independent of its length and cross-sectional area.

15. (a) The number of turns per unit length is

$$n = \frac{500}{0.5} = 1000\ \text{turns/m}$$

The length $l = 0.5$ m and radius, $r = 0.01$ m.

Thus, $l/a = 50$ i.e., $l >> a$.
Hence, we can use the long solenoid formula, namely.

$$B = \mu_0 nI = 4\pi \times 10^{-7} \times 10^{-3} \times 5$$
$$= 6.28 \times 10^{-3}\ \text{T}$$

16. (*d*) By the formula,

$$B = \mu_0 nI$$

or $20 \times 10^{-3} = 4\pi \times 10^{-7} \times 2000 \times I$

or $$I = \frac{20 \times 10^{-3}}{4\pi \times 10^{-7} \times 2000}$$

$\Rightarrow I \simeq 8$ A

17. (*a*) Given, $\mu_0 = 4\pi \times 10^{-7}$ N/A^2,

$n = 500$ turns/m, $I = 0.8$ A

We know that, $B = \mu_0 nI$

$$B = 5.024 \times 10^{-4}\ \text{Wb/m}^2$$

Step up Practice 3

1. (*c*) For stationary electron, $v = 0$

$\therefore$ $F = Bqv \sin\theta = Bq \times 0 \times \sin\theta = 0$

Hence, on a static charge, there is no effect of magnetic field, so electron remains stationary.

2. (*d*) Both A and R are true and R is the correct explanation of A.

An electric current is equivalent to the charges (or electrons) in motion. Such charges produce magnetic interaction. The magnetic field produced by the conductor current thus interacts with magnetic needle and deflects it.

3. (*c*) Path is circular when $\mathbf{v} \perp \mathbf{B}$ or $\mathbf{v} \cdot \mathbf{B} = 0$.

4. (*a*) Radius of circular path, $r = \dfrac{mv}{qB}$

For electron, $r = \dfrac{mv}{eB}$

$\therefore$ $\dfrac{e}{m} = \dfrac{v}{Br}$

5. (*c*) Radius of circular path of charged particle,

$$r = \frac{mv}{qB} = \frac{p}{qB}$$

Since, electron and proton both have same momentum, therefore, the circular path of both will have the same radius.

6. (*b*) As, $\mathbf{F}_e = \mathbf{F}_m$, $q\mathbf{E} = q(\mathbf{v} \times \mathbf{B})$

$\therefore$ $\mathbf{E} = \mathbf{v} \times \mathbf{B} \Rightarrow |\mathbf{E}| = v|\mathbf{B}|$

Therefore, the two fields (**E** and **B**) are perpendicular.

7. (*a*) Radius, $r = \dfrac{\sqrt{2Km}}{Bq}$ or $r \propto \dfrac{\sqrt{m}}{q}$

$$\left(\frac{\sqrt{m}}{q}\right)_\alpha : \left(\frac{\sqrt{m}}{q}\right)_p : \left(\frac{\sqrt{m}}{q}\right)_d = \frac{\sqrt{4}}{2} : \frac{\sqrt{1}}{1} : \frac{\sqrt{2}}{1} = 1:1:\sqrt{2}$$

Hence, $r_\alpha = r_p < r_d$.

8. (*a*) Work done by magnetic force is zero, hence according to work-energy theorem,

Change in kinetic energy = Work done
$= 0$

So, kinetic energy remains constant.

9. (*d*) Centripetal acceleration is

$$a_c = \frac{v^2}{r}$$

So, when velocity is made twice, then acceleration is four times.

10. (*c*) Radius of circular path of proton,

$$r = \frac{\sqrt{2Km}}{Bq} \text{ or } K \propto \frac{q^2}{m} \quad \text{(for same radius)}$$

$$\Rightarrow \quad K_\alpha = K\left(\frac{q'}{q}\right)^2\left(\frac{m}{m'}\right) = 8(2)^2\left(\frac{1}{4}\right) = 8\ \text{eV}$$

11. (*b*) When charged particle moving in circular path enters into a region of magnetic field, then the time period of charged particle is given by

$$T = \frac{2\pi m}{qB}$$

$\therefore$ $T \propto m$ (q and B are same)

$\because$ $m_p > m_e$

$\therefore$ Time period of proton > Time period of electron.

12. (*c*) As we know that,

Magnetic field on a straight wire is equal to that on a sinusoidal wire

$\therefore$ $F = BiL$, Hence option (c) is incorrect.

13. (*d*) Time period of charged particle,

$$T = \frac{2\pi m}{Bq}$$

Hence, T is independent of r.

14. (*c*) Radius of particle, $r = \dfrac{\sqrt{2Km}}{Bq}$

$\therefore$ Area bounded by the path,

$$A = \pi r^2 = \frac{2\pi Km}{B^2 q^2}$$

or $A \propto K$

15. (*b*) Velocity is in XY-plane and magnetic field along Z-axis. Therefore, path of the electron in magnetic field will be a circle. Magnetic force cannot change the speed of a particle but direction of its motion continuously changes. Hence, path of electron will change.

16. (b) Radius of helical path taken by proton beam,

$$r = \frac{mv\sin 60^\circ}{Bq} = \frac{(1.67\times10^{-27})\times(4\times10^{5})\sin 60^\circ}{0.3\times1.6\times10^{-19}}$$

$$=0.012\text{ m}$$

17. (a) For charged particle on circular path,

$$\frac{mv^2}{r} = qvB$$

$$\therefore \quad r = \frac{mv}{qB} = \frac{\sqrt{2mE}}{qB}$$

For proton, $R_p = \dfrac{\sqrt{2m_pE}}{qB}$ ...(i)

For deuteron, $R_d = \dfrac{\sqrt{2m_dE}}{qB}$ ...(ii)

Dividing Eq. (ii) by Eq. (i), we get

$$\frac{R_d}{R_p} = \sqrt{\frac{m_d}{m_p}} = \sqrt{2} \qquad [\because m_d = 2m_p]$$

$$\therefore \quad R_d = \sqrt{2}R_p$$

18. (a) Radius of the circular path,

$$r = \frac{mv}{qB}$$

$$\Rightarrow \quad \frac{r_1}{r_2} = \frac{m_1v_1}{m_2v_2}\times\frac{q_2}{q_1}$$

$$= \frac{1\times2}{1\times3}\times\frac{2}{1} = \frac{4}{3}$$

19. (b) A is true but R is false.

In a conductor, the average velocity of electrons is zero. Hence, no current flows through the conductor. Hence, no force acts on this conductor.

20. (b) Applying Fleming's left hand rule, if magnetic field is perpendicular to paper inwards and current in the loop is clockwise, the magnetic force F on each element of loop is radially outwards and loop has a tendency to expand outwards.

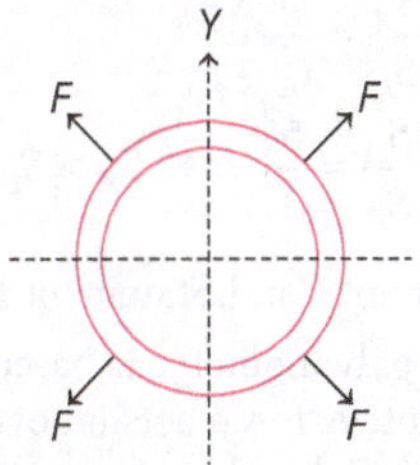

Also, when a current carrying loop is placed in uniform magnetic field, then net force on it is zero and loop cannot have translation motion.

21. (d) The parallel wires carrying currents in the same direction attract each other because magnetic forces on the two wires act towards each other.

22. (b) Two parallel conductor A and B of equal length carry currents I and $10I$, respectively in the same direction, then A and B attract each other with same force.

23. (c) Force per unit length,

$$\frac{F}{l} = \frac{\mu_0}{4\pi}\cdot\frac{2i_1i_2}{d}$$

$$\frac{F}{l} = \frac{\mu_0}{4\pi}\cdot\frac{2i^2}{d} \qquad (\because i = i_1 = i_2)$$

$$\frac{F}{l} = \frac{\mu_0}{2\pi}\cdot\frac{i^2}{d} \qquad \text{(attractive)}$$

24. (d) Force between two conductors, $F \propto \dfrac{I_1I_2}{d}$

When I_1 is changed to $2I_1$ and d is changed to $3d$.

$$\therefore \quad F' \propto \frac{(2I_1)(I_2)}{3d} \propto \frac{2}{3}F$$

As, direction of current is reversed, so $F' = -2F/3$.

25. (d) Both A and R are true and R is the correct explanation of A.

We know that, work done, $W = \mathbf{F}\cdot\mathbf{s} = Fs\cos\theta$, since force is acting perpendicular to the velocity (i.e., displacement). Therefore, $\theta = 90^\circ$ and $\cos 90^\circ = 0$

$\therefore\ W = 0$

Therefore, work done by magnetic field on a moving charge is zero.

26. (c) Force per unit length, $\dfrac{F}{l} = \dfrac{\mu_0}{2\pi}\dfrac{i_Ai_B}{r}$

Given, $i_A = 2i_B$

$$\therefore \quad (0.004) = \frac{2\times10^{-7}}{0.01}(2i_B^2)$$

$$\therefore \quad i_B = 10\text{ A}$$

Step up Practice 4

1. (c) Torque, $\tau_{max} = NiAB = 1\times i\times\pi r^2\times B$

$$\left(\because 2\pi r = L \Rightarrow r = \frac{L}{2\pi}\right)$$

$$\therefore \quad \tau_{max} = \pi i\left(\frac{L}{2\pi}\right)^2 B = \frac{L^2iB}{4\pi}$$

2. (d) Torque acting on the coil is given by

$$\tau = NiBA\sin\theta$$

As, magnetic field is normal to the plane of coil.

So, $\theta = 0^\circ$

$\therefore\ \tau = 0$

3. (c) Let length of each wire be L.

For square, length of each side is $L/4$

Area of square $= \left(\dfrac{L}{4}\right)^2 = \dfrac{L^2}{16}$

For circle,

$$L = 2\pi r$$

$\therefore \quad r = \dfrac{L}{2\pi}$

Area of circle $= \pi r^2 = \pi\left(\dfrac{L}{2\pi}\right)^2 = \dfrac{L^2}{4\pi}$

As, magnetic moment, $M = iA$

$$\therefore \quad \frac{M_{\text{square}}}{M_{\text{circle}}} = \frac{A_{\text{square}}}{A_{\text{circle}}} = \frac{L^2/16}{L^2/4\pi} = \frac{\pi}{4}$$

4. (*d*) Both Statement I and Statement II are correct.

Magnetic forces exerted by a wire on each other tend to align the wires. The net force on each wire is zero but net torque is not zero.

5. (*d*) $2\pi R = 2.0$ m

$$\therefore \quad R = \frac{1.0}{\pi} \text{ m}$$

$$M = iA = (i)(\pi R^2) = (1)(\pi)\left(\frac{1.0}{\pi}\right)^2 = \frac{1}{\pi} \text{ A-m}^2$$

6. (*a*) $N = \dfrac{\left(\dfrac{\mu_0 i}{2R}\right)}{i(\pi R^2)} = \left(\dfrac{\mu_0}{2\pi}\right)\left(\dfrac{1}{R^3}\right)$

or $\quad N \propto \dfrac{1}{R^3}$ and independent of current.

Therefore, if current and radius both were doubled, then the ratio will become $N/8$.

7. (*d*) $R_g = 40\Omega$, $I_g = 2\text{mA} = 2\times10^{-3}$A, $I = 10$A

$$R_S = \frac{I_g}{I - I_g}\times R_g = \frac{2\times10^{-3}\times40}{10-2\times10^{-3}} = 8\times10^{-3}\Omega = 8\text{ mA}$$

8. (*a*) Torque acting on the coil, $\tau = NiBA$

$$= 100\times0.2\times2\times(0.08\times0.1) = 0.32 \text{ N-m}$$

Direction of torque τ is given by the vector $\mathbf{M}\times\mathbf{B}$.

9. (*a*) Both Statement I and Statement II are incorrect.

In a non-uniform magnetic field, a torque and a net force both act on the dipole. If magnetic field is uniform, net force on dipole would be zero.

10. (*d*) Given, if a shunt of $\dfrac{1}{10}$th of the coil resistance is applied to a moving coil galvanometer, then

$$\frac{I_g}{I} = \frac{S}{S+G}$$

$$\frac{I_g}{I} = \frac{(G/10)}{(G/10+G)} = \frac{1}{11}$$

Initially, sensitivity of a galvanometer,

$$\alpha_I = \theta/I_g \quad \text{...(i)}$$

Finally after shunt, it becomes

$$\alpha_f = \theta/I \quad \text{...(ii)}$$

On dividing Eq. (ii) by Eq. (i), we get

$$\therefore \quad \frac{\alpha_f}{\alpha_I} = \frac{\theta/I}{\theta/I_g} = \frac{1}{11}$$

11. (*d*) As we know that

$$\tau = NBiA \sin\theta$$

At $\quad \theta = 0°$, τ is minimum

At $\quad \theta = 90°$, τ is maximum

Magnetic field inside a current carrying wire is given by

$$B = \frac{\mu_0}{2\pi}\frac{ir}{R^2}$$

At the axis, $r = 0 \Rightarrow B = 0$

12. (*b*) We know that resistance across voltmeter

$$R = \frac{V'}{I_g} - G$$

The voltmeter gives full scale deflection for potential difference of V volt. Its resistance is G.

Hence, $I_g = V/G$, given that $V' = nV$

$$R = \frac{nV}{(V/G)} - G = (n-1)G$$

13. (*d*) Both Statement I and Statement II are correct.

A voltmeter is always connected in parallel. This has a large resistance.

14. (*d*) Given, $I_g = 1$ A, $G = 0.81\Omega$, $I = 10$ A

So, value of the required shunt,

$$S = \frac{I_g G}{I - I_g} = \frac{1\times0.81}{10-1} = 0.09\Omega$$

15. (*a*) Sensitivity, $S = \dfrac{\theta}{i}$

$$\frac{S_A}{S_B} = \frac{i_B}{i_A}$$

$$\Rightarrow \quad \frac{S_A}{S_B} = \frac{5}{3} \Rightarrow S_A > S_B$$

16. (*a*) Both Statement I and Statement II are incorrect.

A moving coil galvanometer is based on magnetic effect of current. A force acts on evey side of the coil due to magnetic field when current is passed through the coil. Due to these force, a couple is exerted on the coil.

17. (*b*) We have sensitivity of a moving coil galvanometer

$$S = \frac{NAB}{k}$$

Hints and Solutions

where, k is the torsional constant of its suspension.

In order to increase the sensitivity of a moving coil galvanometer, one should decrease the torsional constant of its suspension.

18. (*b*) The electrical current in moving coil galvanometer

$$i = \frac{k\theta}{NAB}$$

$$\Rightarrow \quad i \propto \theta$$

19. (*b*) Statement I is correct but Statement II is incorrect.

A galvanometer can be used both as ammeter and voltmeter. It can be used as a ammeter by joining a low resistance in parallel with it and as a voltmeter by joining a high resistance in series with it.

20. (*d*) The pole pieces of the magnet used in a pivoted coil galvanometer are cylindrical surfaces of a horse-shoe magnet.

21. (*a*) Here, current across ammeter,

$$I_g = 0.5\% \text{ of } I = 0.005\, I$$

and current across shunt resistance,

$$I_s = I - I_g = I - 0.005 I = 0.995 I$$

∴ Resistance across shunt,

$$S = \frac{I_g G}{I_s} = \frac{0.005 I \times G}{0.995\, I} = \frac{G}{199}$$

Thus, resistance of ammeter will be

$$= \frac{GS}{G+S} = \frac{\frac{G}{199} \times G}{G + \frac{G}{199}} = \frac{G}{200}$$

Gearing up for NEET

1. (*a*) In Biot-Savart's law, magnetic field $\mathbf{B} \parallel i d\mathbf{l} \times \mathbf{r}$ and $id\mathbf{l}$ due to flow of electron is in opposite direction of $\mathbf{v}$, so by direction of cross product of two vectors, $\mathbf{B} \perp \mathbf{v}$

2. (*c*) We have, $B_1 = \frac{\mu_0 I}{2r}$, $B_2 = \frac{\mu_0 I}{4r}$

$$\therefore \quad \frac{B_1}{B_2} = 2$$

3. (*c*) Magnetic field produced at the centre of the orbit,

$$B = \frac{\mu_0}{4\pi} \frac{2\pi i}{r}$$

Now, $i = \frac{q}{t} = qf$

$$\therefore \quad B = \frac{\mu_0}{4\pi} \frac{2\pi (q f)}{r}$$

$$= \frac{4\pi \times 10^{-7} \times 2 \times 3.14 \times 1.6 \times 10^{-19} \times 6.6 \times 10^{15}}{4\pi \times 0.53 \times 10^{-10}}$$

$$= 12.5 \text{ Wbm}^{-2}$$

4. (*a*) **In Ist case**

$$l = 2\pi r_1 \quad \text{... (i)}$$

At centre, $B = \frac{\mu_0 i}{2r_1}$

In IInd case

$$l = 2 \times 2\pi r_2 \quad \text{...(ii)}$$

From Eqs. (i) and (ii), we get

$$2 \times 2\pi r_2 = 2\pi r_1$$

$$\Rightarrow \quad r_2 = \frac{r_1}{2}$$

$$\therefore \quad B' = \frac{2 \times \mu_0 i}{2r_2} \quad (\because \text{there are 2 turns})$$

$$\Rightarrow \quad \frac{B'}{B} = \frac{2r_1}{r_2} = 4 \Rightarrow B' = 4B$$

5. (*b*) When wire is turned into n circular loops, then magnetic field produced is $B' = n^2 B = (3)^2 B_1 = 9\, B_1$.

6. (*d*) Distribution of current will be as shown below.

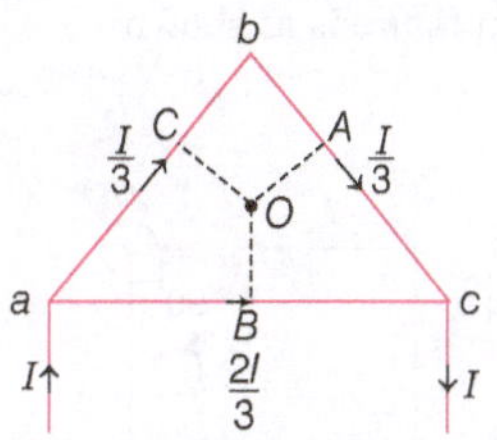

Net magnitude of magnetic field at the centre O is given by

$$B_{net} = B_{ab} + B_{bc} - B_{ac}$$

$$= \frac{\mu_0}{2\pi} \cdot \frac{I/3}{CO} + \frac{\mu_0}{2\pi} \cdot \frac{I/3}{AO} - \frac{\mu_0}{2\pi} \cdot \frac{2I/3}{BO}$$

$$= \frac{\mu_0}{2\pi} \cdot \frac{I/3}{r} + \frac{\mu_0}{2\pi} \cdot \frac{I/3}{r} - \frac{\mu_0}{2\pi} \cdot \frac{2I/3}{r}$$

$$[\because AO = BO = CO = r]$$

$$= 0$$

7. (*a*) $B =$ (due to circular wire) + (due to straight wire)

$$= \frac{\mu_0 I}{2R} + \frac{\mu_0}{2\pi} \frac{I}{R}$$

$$= \frac{\mu_0 I}{2R}\left(1 + \frac{1}{\pi}\right) = \frac{2\mu_0 I}{4R\pi}(1 + \pi)$$

8. (*d*) The magnitude of the resultant magentic field at the common centre of coil is given as $B_{net} = \sqrt{2}B$

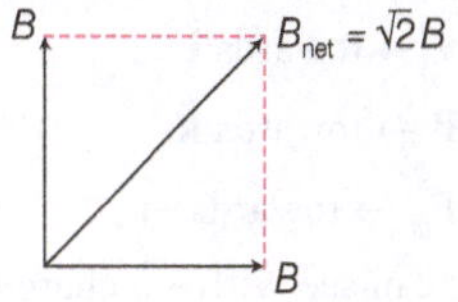

The ratio of the magnitude of the resultant magnetic field at the common centre and the magnetic field due to one coil alone at common centre.

$$\Rightarrow \quad \frac{B_{\text{net}}}{B_{\text{at centre}}} = \frac{\sqrt{2}B}{B} = \frac{\sqrt{2}}{1}$$

9. (c) Magnetic field, $B = \frac{\mu_0 i}{2R} = \frac{\mu_0 (ef)}{2R} = \frac{(\mu_0)(e)\left(\frac{v}{2\pi R}\right)}{2R}$

$$\Rightarrow \quad R^2 = \frac{\mu e v}{4\pi B}$$

$$\Rightarrow \quad R^2 \propto \frac{v}{B} \quad \Rightarrow \quad R \propto \sqrt{\frac{v}{B}}$$

10. (b) At O, due to wire AB and DE, magnetic field will be zero. The combined effect of BC and EF is equivalent to that of an infinitely long wire, *i.e.* both fields are in same direction.

$$\Rightarrow \quad B_O = \frac{2\mu_0 I}{4\pi r} = \frac{\mu_0 I}{2\pi r}$$

11. (d) The given figure is as shown

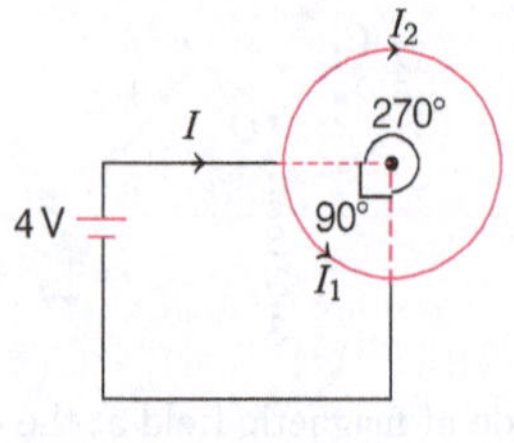

$$\frac{R_1}{R_2} = \frac{1}{3} \quad [\because \text{Resistance, } R \propto l]$$

$$\Rightarrow \quad \frac{I_1}{I_2} = \frac{R_2}{R_1} = 3 \quad [\because V = 4\text{V}]$$

$$\therefore \quad B_1 = \frac{\mu_0 I_1}{2r} \times \frac{90°}{360°} \otimes$$

and $$B_2 = \frac{\mu_0 I_2}{2r} \times \frac{270°}{360°}$$

$$\therefore \quad \frac{B_1}{B_2} = \frac{I_1}{I_2} \times \frac{90°}{270°}$$

$$= 3 \times \frac{1}{3} = 1 \text{ or } B_1 \otimes = B_2 \odot$$

$\therefore$ Net magnetic field at centre of conductor is zero.

12. (d) If charge q is positive, then due to electric field their velocity will be towards positive X-axis.

Now, $\mathbf{F}_m = q(\mathbf{v} \times \mathbf{B})$

where, $\mathbf{v} \rightarrow$ towards $\hat{\mathbf{i}}$

and $\mathbf{B} \rightarrow$ towards $\hat{\mathbf{k}}$

$\therefore$ $\mathbf{F}_m \rightarrow$ towards $-\hat{\mathbf{j}}$ (*i.e.* $-$ y-direction)

Similarly, we can see with $-q$ charge.

13. (a) All magnetic fields are cancelling each other.

14. (b) As, $dA = (2\pi r)\, dr$

$$\therefore \quad dq = \sigma \cdot dA = (2\pi\alpha r^3) \cdot dr$$

Current, $i = (dq) f = (dq) \frac{\omega}{2\pi} = (\alpha\omega r^3)\, dr$

Now, $dB = \frac{\mu_0 i}{2r} = \frac{\alpha\mu_0\omega r^2 dr}{2}$

$$\therefore \quad B = \int_0^R dB = \frac{\mu_0 \alpha\omega R^3}{6}$$

15. (b) At, the centre of coil 1,

$$B_1 = \frac{\mu_0}{4\pi} \times \frac{2\pi i_1}{r_1} \quad \text{...(i)}$$

At the centre of coil 2,

$$B_2 = \frac{\mu_0}{4\pi} \times \frac{2\pi i_2}{r_2} \quad \text{...(ii)}$$

But $B_1 = B_2$

$$\therefore \quad \frac{\mu_0}{4\pi} \frac{2\pi i_1}{r_1} = \frac{\mu_0}{4\pi} \frac{2\pi i_2}{r_2} \text{ or } \frac{i_1}{r_1} = \frac{i_2}{r_2}$$

As, $r_1 = 2r_2$

$$\therefore \quad \frac{i_1}{2r_2} = \frac{i_2}{r_2} \text{ or } i_1 = 2i_2$$

Now, ratio of potential differences,

$$\frac{V_2}{V_1} = \frac{i_2 \times R_2}{i_1 \times R_1} = \frac{i_2 \times R_2}{2i_2 \times 2R_2} = \frac{1}{4}$$

[$\because$ Resistance, $R \propto r$ (radius)]

$$\Rightarrow \quad \frac{V_1}{V_2} = \frac{4}{1}$$

16. (b) According to question,

$$l = 2\pi R \Rightarrow R = \frac{l}{2\pi}$$

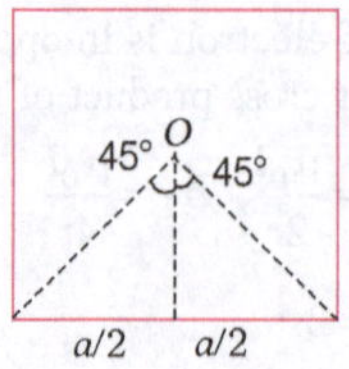

and $l = 4a \Rightarrow a = \frac{l}{4}$

$$B' = \frac{\mu_0 i}{2R} = \frac{\mu_0 i}{2 \cdot \frac{l}{2\pi}} = \frac{\mu_0 \pi i}{l}$$

$$B = 4\left[\frac{\mu_0}{4\pi} \cdot \frac{i}{a/2} (\sin 45° + \sin 45°)\right]$$

$$= \frac{2\sqrt{2}\,\mu_0 i}{\pi a} = \frac{8\sqrt{2}\,\mu_0 i}{\pi l} \quad \left[\because a = \frac{l}{4}\right]$$

$$\therefore \quad \frac{B}{B'} = \frac{8\sqrt{2}}{\pi^2}$$

17. (c) According to the question,

$$mg \sin \theta = IlB \cos \theta$$

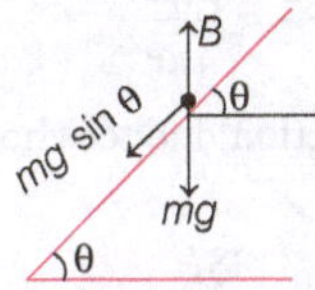

∴ Magnitude of magnetic field,

$$B = \frac{mg}{Il} \tan \theta = \frac{mg \tan 60°}{2 \times (2L)} = \frac{\sqrt{3}mg}{4L}$$

18. (d) At centre, $B = 0$.

As, $x \to a, B \to 0$ between centre and $x = a$, there will be a maximum value.

Along X-axis for $x > 0$, B_{net} is downwards.

Along X-axis for $x < 0$, B_{net} is upwards.

19. (b) Radius, $r = a \cos \frac{\pi}{n}$

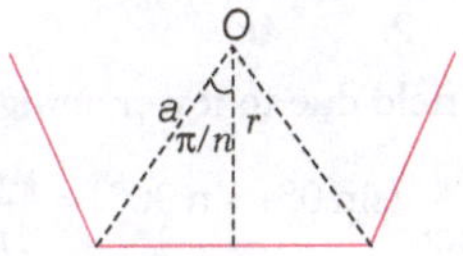

∴ Magnetic field,

$$B = n\left[\frac{\mu_0}{4\pi} \cdot \frac{i}{a \cos \pi/n}\left(\sin \frac{\pi}{n} + \sin \frac{\pi}{n}\right)\right]$$

$$= \frac{\mu_0 ni}{2\pi a} \tan\left(\frac{\pi}{n}\right)$$

20. (b) Magnetic field at O,

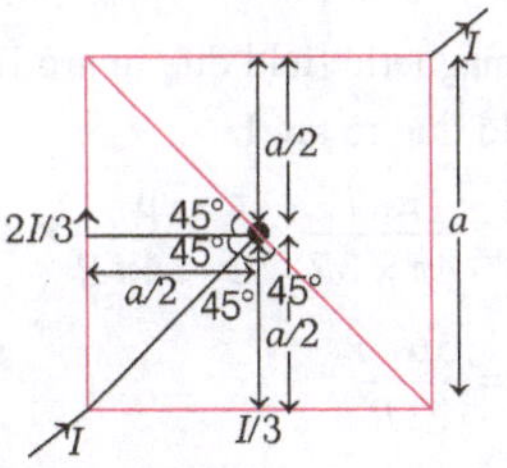

$$B = 2\left[\frac{\mu_0}{4\pi}\frac{2I/3}{a/2}(\sin 45° + \sin 45°) - \frac{\mu_0}{4\pi} \cdot \frac{I/3}{a/2}(\sin 45° + \sin 45°)\right]$$

$$= \frac{\sqrt{2}\mu_0 I}{3\pi a}$$

21. (b) As, $kx_0 = mg = ILB = \left(\frac{E}{R}\right) \cdot LB$

∴ The magnetic field, $B = \frac{mgR}{EL}$

22. (a) For first figure,

Magnetic field at P due to straight part (a), $B_a = \frac{\mu_0}{4\pi} \cdot \frac{i}{r}$

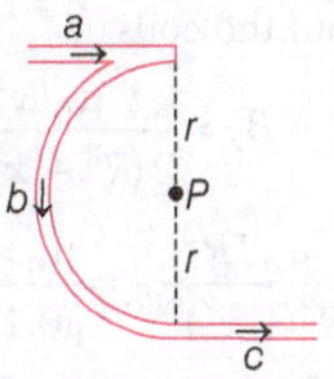

Magnetic field at P due to circular part (b), $B_b = \frac{\mu_0}{4\pi} \frac{\pi i}{r}$

Magnetic field at P due to straight part (c),

$$B_c = \frac{\mu_0}{4\pi} \frac{i}{r}$$

So, net magnetic field at the centre of first figure,

$$B_1 = B_b + B_c - B_a = \frac{\mu_0}{4\pi} \frac{\pi i}{r} \quad \text{....(i)}$$

For second figure, magnetic field at P due to two straight and one circular part,

$$B_2 = \frac{\mu_0}{4\pi} \frac{\pi i}{r} \quad \text{....(ii)}$$

For third figure, magnetic field at P due to straight part (a),

$$B_a = 0$$

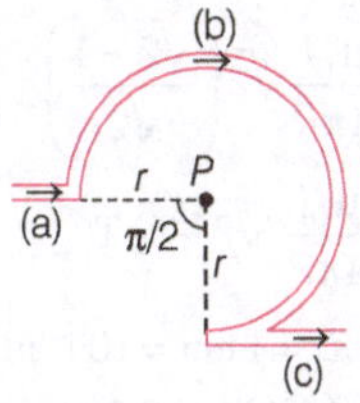

Magnetic field at P due to circular part (b),

$$B_b = \frac{\mu_0}{4\pi} \frac{(2\pi - \pi/2)i}{r} = \frac{\mu_0}{4\pi} \cdot \frac{3\pi}{2r} \cdot i$$

Magnetic field at C due to straight part (c), $B_c = \frac{\mu_0}{4\pi} \frac{i}{r}$

So, net magnetic field at centre of third figure,

$$B_3 = \frac{\mu_0}{4\pi} \cdot \frac{i}{r}\left(\frac{3\pi}{2} - 1\right) \quad \text{...(iii)}$$

From Eqs. (i), (ii) and (iii), we get

$$B_1 : B_2 : B_3 = \pi : \pi : \left(\frac{3\pi}{2} - 1\right)$$

$$= \frac{\pi}{2} : \frac{\pi}{2} : \left(\frac{3\pi}{4} - \frac{1}{2}\right)$$

23. (c) Given, radius of identical circular loops,

$$R = 10 \text{ cm} = 10^{-1} \text{ m}$$

Current, $I = \frac{7}{2}$ A

Distance from both circular loops at point P,

$$x_1 = x_2 = x = 5 \text{ cm} = 5 \times 10^{-2} \text{ m}$$

From figure, according to Maxwell's right hand thumb rule, it is clear that magnetic field will be in same direction by both the coils,

i.e. $$B = B_1 + B_2 = \frac{\mu_0 IR^2}{2(R^2 + x^2)^{3/2}} + \frac{\mu_0 IR^2}{2(R^2 + x^2)^{3/2}}$$

$$= \frac{\mu_0 IR^2}{(R^2 + x^2)^{3/2}} = \frac{\mu_0 \times 7/2 \times (10^{-1})^2}{[(0.1)^2 + (0.05)^2]^{3/2}}$$

$$= \frac{56}{\sqrt{5}} \mu_0 \text{T}$$

24. *(a)* $\because B \text{ (at } P) = \frac{\mu_0 I}{4\pi d}(\cos\theta_1 - \cos\theta_2)$

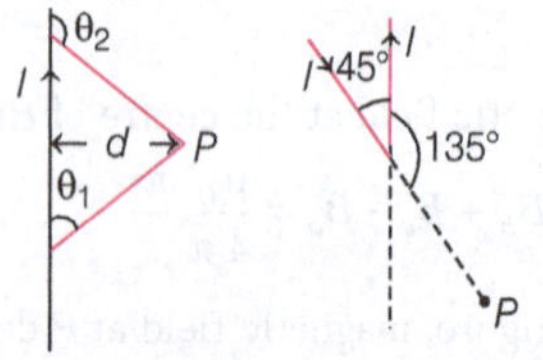

In given case, $d = R \sin 45° = R/\sqrt{2}$

$$\theta_1 = 135°, \theta_2 = 180°$$

$$\therefore B \text{ (at } P) = \frac{\mu_0 I}{4\pi(R/\sqrt{2})}[\cos 135° - \cos 180°]$$

$$= \frac{\mu_0 I}{4\pi R}\sqrt{2}\left[\frac{-1}{\sqrt{2}} - (-1)\right]$$

$$= \frac{\mu_0 I}{4\pi R}\sqrt{2}\left(\frac{\sqrt{2} - 1}{\sqrt{2}}\right)$$

$$\Rightarrow B \text{ (at } P) = \frac{\mu_0 I}{4\pi R}(\sqrt{2} - 1) \text{ T}$$

25. *(b)* Here, $dl = dx = 1 \text{ cm} = 10^{-2}$ m,

$$i = 10 \text{ A}, r = 0.5 \text{ m}$$

$$\therefore \quad dB = \frac{\mu_0}{4\pi} \cdot \frac{i(dl \times r)}{r^3} = \frac{\mu_0}{4\pi} \cdot \frac{idl}{r^2}(\hat{\mathbf{i}} \times \hat{\mathbf{j}})$$

$$= \frac{\mu_0}{4\pi} \cdot \frac{idl}{r^2}\hat{\mathbf{k}}$$

$$= \frac{10^{-7} \times 10 \times 10^{-2}}{(0.5)^2}\hat{\mathbf{k}} = 4 \times 10^{-8}\hat{\mathbf{k}}\text{T}$$

26. *(a)* According to Biot-Savart's law, the magnetic induction at a point to a current carrying element $i\delta l$ is given

by $$B = \frac{\mu_0}{4\pi} \cdot \frac{i\delta l \sin\theta}{r^2}$$

Directed normal to plane containing $\delta \mathbf{l}$ and $\mathbf{r}$, θ being angle between $\delta \mathbf{l}$ and $\mathbf{r}$.

Field due to semicircular arc

Now, angle between a current element $\delta \mathbf{l}$ of semicircular arc and the radius vector of the element to point c is $\pi/2$.

Therefore, the magnitude of magnetic induction B at O due to this element,

$$\delta B = \frac{\mu_0}{4\pi} \cdot \frac{i\delta l \sin \pi/2}{r^2} = \frac{\mu_0 i\delta l}{4\pi r^2}$$

Hence, magnetic induction due to whole semicircular loop is

$$B = \Sigma\delta B = \Sigma\frac{\mu_0}{4\pi} \cdot \frac{i\delta l}{r^2}$$

$$= \frac{\mu_0}{4\pi}\frac{i}{r^2}\Sigma\delta l = \frac{\mu_0 i}{4\pi r^2}(\pi r) = \frac{\mu_0 i}{4r}$$

The magnetic field due to ab and de is zero, because $\theta = 0°$ or $180°$, so net magnetic field is

$$B = \frac{\mu_0 i}{4r}$$

27. *(c)* Magnetic field due to straight wire above O is zero, i.e. $B_1 = 0$ (since, $\theta = 0°$)

The magnetic field due to semicircular part,

$$B_2 = \frac{1}{2} \times \frac{\mu_0 I}{2r} = \frac{\mu_0 I}{4r}$$

The magnetic field due to lower straight portion,

$$B_3 = \frac{\mu_0 I}{4\pi r}(\sin 0° + \sin 90°) = \frac{\mu_0 I}{4\pi r} \quad \text{(upward)}$$

Net magnetic field,

$$B = B_1 + B_2 + B_3 = 0 + \frac{\mu_0 I}{4r} + \frac{\mu_0 I}{4\pi r}$$

$$= \frac{\mu_0 I}{4r} + \frac{\mu_0 I}{4\pi r} \quad \text{(upwards)}$$

28. *(b)* The angle subtended by circular part of the conductor is $3\pi/2$ or $270°$.

Net magnetic field at point O, $B_{\text{net}} = B_1 + B_2$

where, B_1 = magnetic field due to arc II and B_2 = magnetic field due to arc I.

$$B_{\text{net}} = \frac{\mu_0 i}{4\pi \times 3R} \times \frac{\pi}{2} + \frac{\mu_0 i}{4\pi R} \times 3\frac{\pi}{2}$$

$$= \frac{5\mu_0 i}{12R} \quad \text{(downward)}$$

29. *(c)* Magnetic field at the centre of circular coil,

$$B = \frac{\mu_0 I}{2r} \quad \text{...(i)}$$

Now, magnetic field at the centre of smaller circular

coil, $$B' = \frac{\mu_0 (2n)I}{\left(\frac{2r}{2n}\right)} \Rightarrow B' = \frac{\mu_0 (2n)^2 I}{2r}$$

From Eq. (i), we get

$$B' = (2n)^2 B \Rightarrow \frac{B'}{B} = \frac{(2n)^2}{1}$$

30. (*c*) The magnetic field produced by the ring at its centre,

$$B = \frac{\mu_0 I}{2r} \quad \text{...(i)}$$

where, I = current through the ring

$$= \frac{Q}{T} = Q/(2\pi/\omega) = \frac{Q\omega}{2\pi} \quad \text{...(ii)}$$

Here, Q = total change on the ring

and T = time period of the ring.

According to the question, $\lambda = \frac{Q}{2\pi r}$

$$\Rightarrow \quad Q = \lambda \times 2\pi r \quad \text{...(iii)}$$

From Eqs. (i), (ii) and (iii), we get

$$B = \frac{\mu_0 \lambda \omega}{2}$$

31. (*a*) Given, $I_1 = 3\,A$, $I_2 = 4\,A$, $R = 2\pi\,\text{cm} = 2\pi \times 10^{-2}\,\text{m}$

Magnetic field at the centre of a coil, $B = \frac{\mu_0 I}{2R}$

$$\text{Now, } B_1 = \frac{\mu_0 I_1}{2R} = \frac{\mu_0}{2} \times \frac{3}{2\pi \times 10^{-2}} = \frac{\mu_0}{4\pi} \times \frac{3}{10^{-2}}$$

$$= 10^{-7} \times \frac{3}{10^{-2}} = 3 \times 10^{-5}\,\text{T}$$

$$\text{Similarly, } B_2 = \frac{\mu_0 I_2}{2R} = \frac{\mu_0}{2} \times \frac{4}{2\pi \times 10^{-2}}$$

$$= \frac{\mu_0}{4\pi} \times \frac{4}{10^{-2}}$$

$$= 10^{-7} \times \frac{4}{10^{2}} = 4 \times 10^{-5}\,\text{T}$$

Now, net magnetic field at centre of the coils,

$$B = \sqrt{B_1^2 + B_2^2}$$

$$\Rightarrow \quad B = \sqrt{(3 \times 10^{-5})^2 + (4 \times 10^{-5})^2}$$

$$\Rightarrow \quad B = \sqrt{10^{-10}\,(9 + 16)}$$

$$\Rightarrow \quad B = 5 \times 10^{-5}\,\text{T} = 5 \times 10^{-5}\,\text{Wb/m}^2$$

32. (*d*) The point P is lying at a distance d along the Z-axis.

$$|\mathbf{B}_1| = \frac{\mu_0}{2\pi}\frac{I_1}{d} \text{ and } |\mathbf{B}_2| = \frac{\mu_0}{2\pi}\frac{I_2}{d}$$

$$B_{\text{net}} = \sqrt{B_1^2 + B_2^2}$$

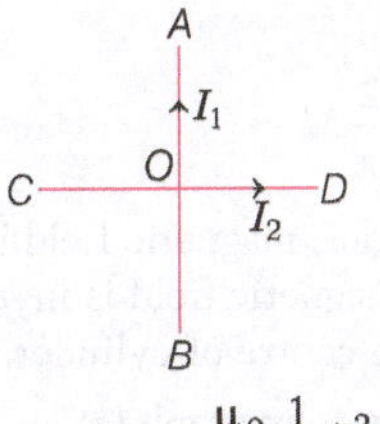

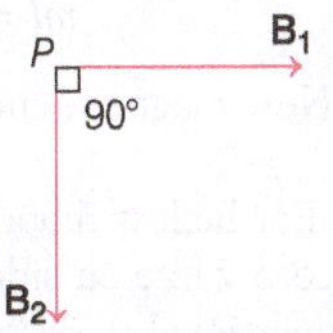

$$B_{\text{net}} = \frac{\mu_0}{2\pi}\frac{1}{d}(I_1^2 + I_2^2)^{1/2}$$

33. (*b*) The magnetic field at axis of current carrying loop is given by

$$B = \frac{\mu_0 i r^2}{2(r^2 + d^2)^{3/2}} \quad \text{...(i)}$$

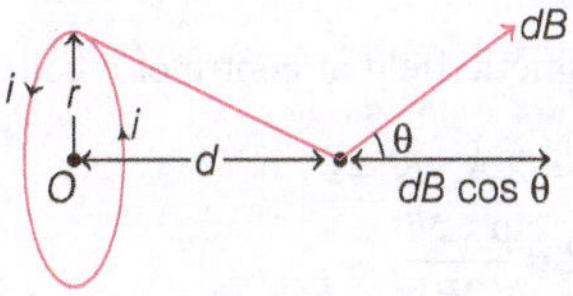

where, i = current in loop, r = radius of loop

d = distance on axis

and B = magnetic field of current carrying loop.

Let B_1 be the magnetic field at centre ($d = 0$).

$$\text{Now, } B_1 = \frac{\mu_0 i r^2}{2(r^2 + 0^2)^{3/2}} = \frac{\mu_0 i r^2}{2r^3} = \frac{\mu_0 i}{2r} \quad \text{...(ii)}$$

On dividing Eqs. (i) and (ii), we get

$$\frac{B}{B_1} = \frac{\mu_0 i r^2 \times 2r}{2\,(r^2 + d^2)^{3/2} \times \mu_0 i}$$

$$\Rightarrow \quad \frac{B}{B_1} = \frac{r^3}{(r^2 + d^2)^{3/2}} = \frac{3^3}{(3^2 + 4^2)^{3/2}}$$

$$\Rightarrow \quad \frac{B}{B_1} = \frac{27}{(25)^{3/2}} \Rightarrow \frac{54\,\mu\text{T}}{B_1} = \frac{27}{5^3}$$

$$B_1 = \frac{54 \times 125}{27}$$

$$\Rightarrow \quad B_1 = 250\,\mu\text{T}$$

34. (*d*) Let the velocity v of the particle entering the field **B**, instead of being perpendicular to **B** makes an angle with it.

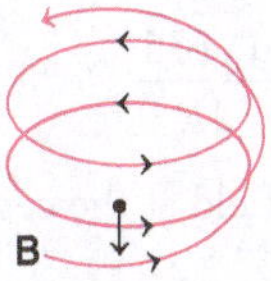

Then, v may be resolved into two components. $v_{\parallel} = v\cos\theta$ parallel to **B** and $v_{\perp} = v\sin\theta$ perpendicular to **B**. The component $v_{\parallel}$ gives a linear path and the component $v_{\perp}$ gives a circular path to the particle. The resultant of these two is a helical path whose axis is parallel to the magnetic field.

35. (*d*) The given figure can be drawn as follows.

The magnetic field at point P,

$$B_{\text{net}} = 2\left[\frac{\mu_0 I}{4\pi r}(\sin\theta_1 + \sin\theta_2)\right]$$

$$= 2\left[\frac{\mu_0}{4\pi} \times \frac{I}{\frac{d\sqrt{3}}{2}} \times (\sin 90° + \sin 30°)\right]$$

$$= 2\left[\frac{\mu_0}{4\pi} \times \frac{2I}{d\sqrt{3}} \times \left(1 + \frac{1}{2}\right)\right]$$

$$= 2\left[\frac{\mu_0}{4\pi} \times \frac{2I}{d\sqrt{3}} \times \frac{3}{2}\right] = \frac{\sqrt{3}\mu_0 I}{2\pi d}$$

36. (*c*) The magnetic field at centre of a coil, $B = \frac{\mu_0 Ni}{2R}$

Given, $i = 2$ A, $N = 1$

So, $R = \frac{\mu_0 Ni}{2B}$

$$R = \frac{4\pi \times 10^{-7} \times 1 \times 2}{2 \times 4\pi \times 10^{-6}}$$

$$\Rightarrow R = \frac{1}{10} = 0.1 \text{ m}$$

37. (*d*) Given that, the net magnetic field at the centre O is zero. Therefore, magnetic field at O due to circular coil and straight conductor must be equal and opposite in direction.

$$\therefore \frac{\mu_0 I_1}{2R} = \frac{\mu_0 I_2}{2\pi(2R)} \Rightarrow \frac{I_1}{I_2} = \frac{1}{2\pi}$$

38. (*a*) The magnetic field B at the centre of circular current carrying coil of radius R and current I,

$$B = \frac{\mu_0 I}{2R}$$

Similarly, if current $= 2I$, then

Magnetic field $= \frac{\mu_0 2I}{2R} = 2B$

So, resultant magnetic field

$$= \sqrt{B^2 + (2B)^2}$$

$$= \sqrt{5B^2} = \sqrt{5}B$$

$$= \frac{\mu_0 I\sqrt{5}}{2R}$$

39. (*d*) The magnetic field at the centre of new loop

$$B' = n^2 B$$

where, n is the number of turns in the loop.

$$\therefore B' = (4)^2 B \text{ or } B' = 16B$$

40. (*b*) When the currents in the wires are in same direction. Magnetic field at mid-point O due to I and II wires are respectively

$$B_{\text{I}} = \frac{\mu_0}{4\pi}\frac{2i_1}{x} \otimes \text{ and } B_{\text{II}} = \frac{\mu_0}{4\pi}\cdot\frac{2i_2}{x} \odot$$

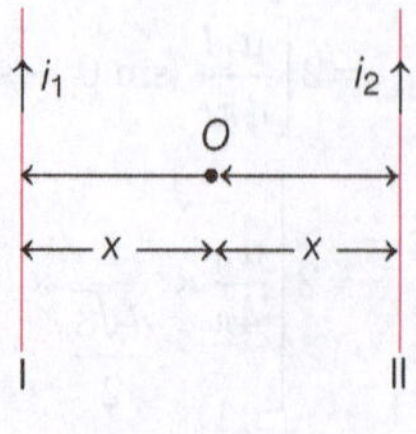

So, the net magnetic field at O,

$$B_{\text{net}} = \frac{\mu_0}{4\pi}\cdot\frac{2}{x}(i_1 - i_2)$$

$$\Rightarrow 10 \times 10^{-6} = \frac{\mu_0}{4\pi}\cdot\frac{2}{x}(i_1 - i_2) \quad \text{...(i)}$$

When the direction of i_2 is reversed,

$$B_{\text{I}} = \frac{\mu_0}{4\pi}\cdot\frac{2i_1}{x} \otimes$$

and

$$B_{\text{II}} = \frac{\mu_0}{4\pi}\cdot\frac{2i_2}{x} \otimes$$

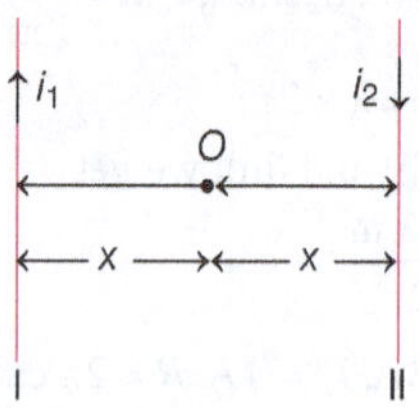

So, net magnetic field at O,

$$B_{\text{net}} = \frac{\mu_0}{4\pi}\cdot\frac{2}{x}(i_1 + i_2)$$

$$\Rightarrow 40 \times 10^{-6} = \frac{\mu_0}{4\pi}\cdot\frac{2}{x}(i_1 + i_2) \quad \text{...(ii)}$$

On dividing Eq. (ii) by Eq. (i), we get

$$\frac{i_1 + i_2}{i_1 - i_2} = \frac{4}{1} \Rightarrow \frac{i_1}{i_2} = \frac{5}{3}$$

41. (*c*) When wire is bent in the form of semicircular arc, then $l = \pi r$

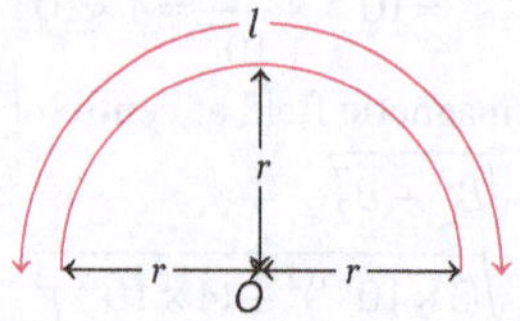

$\therefore$ The radius of semicircular arc, $r = l/\pi$

Distance between two end points of semicircular wire

$$= 2r = \frac{2l}{\pi}$$

$\therefore$ Magnetic moment of semicircular wire

$$= m \times 2r = m \times \frac{2l}{\pi} = \frac{2}{\pi}ml$$

But ml is the magnetic moment of straight wire,

i.e. $ml = M$

$\therefore$ New magnetic moment $= \frac{2}{\pi}M$

42. (*a*) For hollow metallic cylinder, magnetic field inside is zero while outside it the magnetic field is inversely proportional to distance from centre of cylinder.

So, variation is correctly shown by graph (a).

43. (b) Magnetic field, $B=\dfrac{\mu_0 I}{2\pi r}$

Given, $\mu_0 = 4\pi\times10^{-7}$ N/A^2, $r = 8$ cm $= 8\times10^{-2}$m, $I = 12$ A

$$B=\frac{4\pi\times10^{-7}}{2\pi}\times\frac{12}{8\times10^{-2}}$$

$$\Rightarrow \quad B = 3\times10^{-5}\ \text{Wb/m}^2$$

44. (d) The given figure is shown below

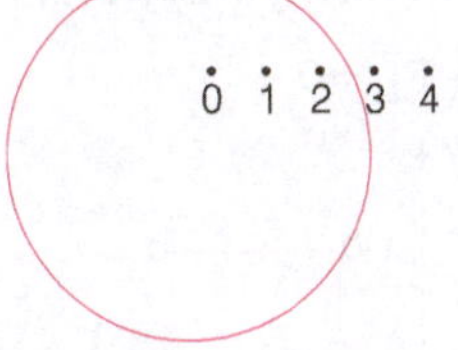

Magnetic field outside the long rod,

$$B=\frac{\mu_0 i}{2\pi r} \quad [\text{for rod 3 and rod 4, } r_3 < r_4]$$

$$\therefore \quad B_3 > B_4 \neq 0$$

45. (b) The described condition can be shown as

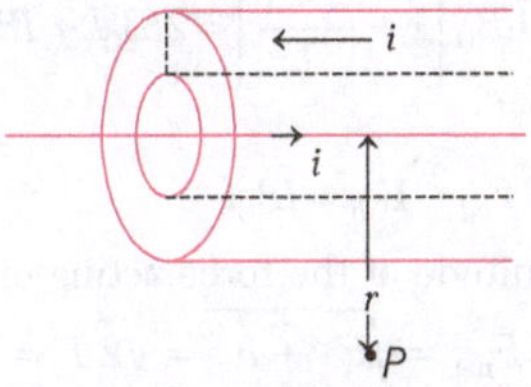

The magnetic field at P due to inner and outer conductors are equal and opposite. Hence, the net magnetic field at P will be zero.

46. (c) $\because$ Force, $\mathbf{F}_m = q(\mathbf{v}\times\mathbf{B})$

$\because$ A proton is moving along the negative direction of X-axis in a magnetic field directed along the positive direction of Y-axis. Therefore, according to Fleming's left hand rule, force on proton in magnetic field, will act along negative direction of Z-axis.

So, the proton will be deflected along the negative direction of Z-axis

47. (a) Magnetic force on wire B from both the wires is towards A.

48. (b) Force or tension in the loop, $F = Bil$

$$\Rightarrow \quad F \propto B$$

If B is doubled, then tension in the loop is double.

49. (d) For a given pitch x corresponding to charge particle,

we have $\dfrac{q}{m}=\dfrac{2\pi v\cos\theta}{Bx}=$ constant

Since, charged particles traverse identical helical paths in a completely opposite sense in a uniform magnetic field **B**, so LHS of above equation for two particles should be same and of opposite sign. Therefore,

$$\left(\frac{e}{m}\right)_1+\left(\frac{e}{m}\right)_2=0$$

50. (c) As magnetic field and velocity of charge is in same direction, so magnetic force on it is zero. Hence, it falls with acceleration equal to g.

51. (d) Velocity vector is parallel to magnetic field vector.

$$\therefore \quad \theta = 0^\circ$$

Hence, force, $F = Bqv\sin 0 = 0$

52. (b) We have, $\quad (b-a) = r = \dfrac{mv}{Bq}$

$$\therefore \quad v_{\min}=\frac{(b-a)Bq}{m}$$

53. (c) Radius of circular path,

$$r=\frac{mv\sin\theta}{Bq}$$

$$=\frac{(1.67\times10^{-27})(2\times10^6)\sin 30^\circ}{0.14\times1.6\times10^{-19}}=0.075\ \text{m}$$

$$[\because \theta = 90^\circ - 60^\circ = 30^\circ]$$

and $\quad T=\dfrac{2\pi m}{Bq}=\dfrac{(2\pi)(1.67\times10^{-27})}{0.14\times1.6\times10^{-19}}=0.5\times10^{-6}$ s

54. (b) $F_a = F_{ab} - F_{ac} = \dfrac{\mu_0 I^2 l}{2\pi d}-\dfrac{\mu_0 I^2 l}{2\pi(2d)}=\dfrac{\mu_0 I^2 l}{4\pi d}$

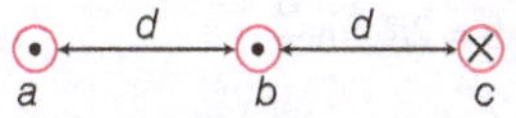

$$F_b = F_{ba}+F_{bc}=\frac{\mu_0 I^2 l}{2\pi d}+\frac{\mu_0 I^2 l}{2\pi d}=\frac{\mu_0 I^2 l}{\pi d}$$

$$F_c = F_{ca}+F_{cb}=\frac{\mu_0 I^2 l}{2\pi(2d)}+\frac{\mu_0 I^2 l}{2\pi d}=\frac{3\mu_0 I^2 l}{4\pi d}$$

On comparing values as F_a, F_b and F_c, we get

$$F_b > F_c > F_a$$

55. (c) $F_1=\dfrac{\mu_0}{4\pi}\dfrac{I^2\times l}{x}$, towards A and $F_2=\dfrac{\mu_0}{4\pi}\dfrac{2I^2\times l}{2x}$, towards A

$$\therefore \quad F_1 = F_2$$

56. (c) Force on wire Q due to wire R,

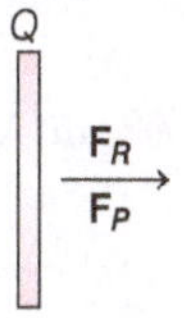

$$F_R=\frac{4\pi\times10^{-7}}{4\pi}\times\frac{2\times20\times10}{0.02}\times0.1$$

$$=20\times10^{-5}\ \text{N} \quad \text{(towards right)}$$

Force on wire Q due to wire P,

$$F_P=\frac{4\pi\times10^{-7}}{4\pi}\times\frac{2\times30\times10}{0.1}\times0.1$$

$$=6\times10^{-5}\ \text{N} \quad \text{(towards right)}$$

Net force on Q,

$$F = F_R + F_P = 20 \times 10^{-5} + 6 \times 10^{-5}$$

$$= 26 \times 10^{-5} \text{ N}$$

$$= 2.6 \times 10^{-4} \text{ N} \quad \text{(towards right)}$$

57. (*a*) Force on the wire, $F = ilB \sin\theta$

$$\sin\theta = \frac{F}{ilB} = \frac{15}{10 \times 1.5 \times 2} = \frac{1}{2} \Rightarrow \theta = 30°$$

$\therefore$ The angle between the magnetic field and direction of the current, $\theta = 30°$.

58. (*c*) For minimum value of B, it is colliding after one pitch. It will collide the target again, if pitch is halved or remains same.

$$p = (v\cos\theta)\left(\frac{2\pi m}{Bq}\right) \quad \text{or} \quad p \propto \frac{v}{B}$$

For $p/p_0 = 1$ and $\frac{1}{2}$, both options (a) and (b) are correct.

59. (*d*) Here, diameter of circular path, $y = 2r = 2\frac{mv_0}{qB_0}$

60. (*c*) From the figure,

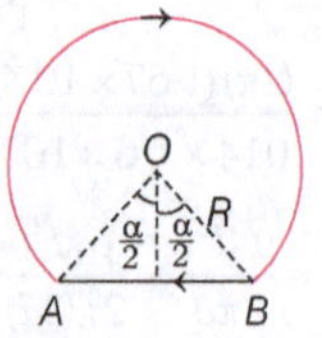

$$AB = 2R\sin\frac{\alpha}{2}$$

$$\therefore \text{ Force} = IB\left(2R\sin\frac{\alpha}{2}\right) = 2BIR\sin\frac{\alpha}{2}$$

61. (*b*) Given, time, $t = \frac{\pi m}{Bq} = \frac{T}{2}$ of proton

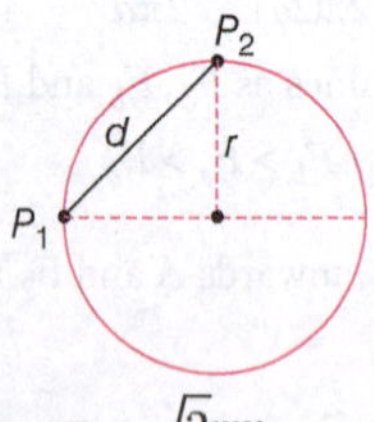

Sepearation, $d = \sqrt{2}r = \frac{\sqrt{2}mv}{Bq}$

62. (*d*) Velocity, $v = \frac{E}{B}$ and radius of path,

$$r = \frac{mv}{Bq} = \frac{v}{B \cdot q/m} = \frac{E/B}{B \cdot S} = \frac{E}{B^2 S}$$

63. (*a*) We have, $\mathbf{F}_{CAD} = \mathbf{F}_{CD} = \mathbf{F}_{CED}$

$\therefore$ Net force on frame $= 3\,\mathbf{F}_{CD}$

$$= 3\,(Bil) = 3 \times 4 \times 2 \times 1 = 24 \text{ N}$$

64. (*a*) Let the magnetic field,

$$\mathbf{B} = B_1\hat{\mathbf{i}} + B_2\hat{\mathbf{j}} + B_3\hat{\mathbf{k}}$$

Applying $\mathbf{F}_m = q(\mathbf{v} \times \mathbf{B})$ two times, we have

$$q[-\hat{\mathbf{j}} + \hat{\mathbf{k}}] = q[(\hat{\mathbf{i}}) \times (B_1\hat{\mathbf{i}} + B_2\hat{\mathbf{j}} + B_3\hat{\mathbf{k}})] = q[B_2\hat{\mathbf{k}} - B_3\hat{\mathbf{j}}]$$

On comparing two sides, we get

$$B_2 = 1 \text{ and } B_3 = 1$$

Further, $q[\hat{\mathbf{i}} - \hat{\mathbf{k}}] = q[(\hat{\mathbf{j}}) \times (B_1\hat{\mathbf{i}} + B_2\hat{\mathbf{j}} + B_3\hat{\mathbf{k}})]$

$$= q[-B_1\hat{\mathbf{k}} + B_3\hat{\mathbf{i}}]$$

Again comparing, we get

$$B_1 = 1 \text{ and } B_3 = 1$$

$$\therefore \quad \mathbf{B} = (\hat{\mathbf{i}} + \hat{\mathbf{j}} + \hat{\mathbf{k}}) \text{ Wb/m}^2$$

65. (*c*) Here, $\mathbf{F}_{bc} + \mathbf{F}_{da} = 0$

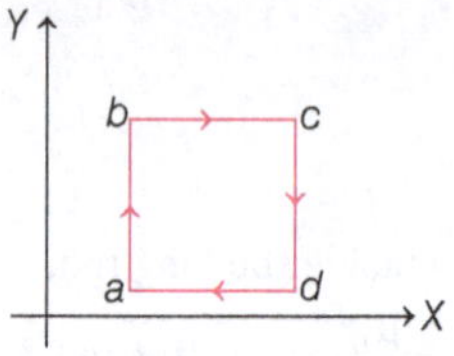

Force, $\mathbf{F}_{ab} = IlB_0\left(1 + \frac{x}{l}\right) = IB_0 l + IB_0 x$ (towards right)

Force, $\mathbf{F}_{cd} = IlB_0\left[1 + \frac{x+l}{l}\right] = 2IB_0 l + IB_0 x$

(towards left)

$\therefore \quad \mathbf{F}_{\text{net}} = \mathbf{F}_{cd} - \mathbf{F}_{ab} = IB_0 l$ (towards left)

66. (*c*) The magnitude of the force acting on the wire,

$$F_{\text{net}} = \sqrt{F^2 + F^2} = \sqrt{2}\,F = \sqrt{2}\,IlB$$

67. (*a*) Motion of charged particle in magnetic field ($\mathbf{B} = -2\hat{\mathbf{k}}$T) is shown below

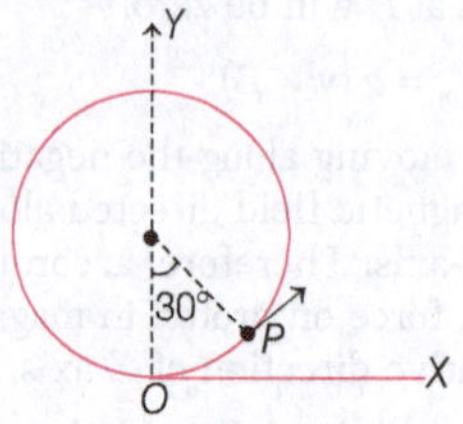

Time period, $T = \frac{2\pi m}{Bq} = \frac{2\pi}{B \cdot \frac{q}{m}} = \frac{2\pi}{2 \cdot \pi} = 1 \text{ s}$

Since, the particle will be at point P after time,

$$t = \frac{1}{6}\text{ s} = \frac{T}{6}\text{ s}$$

Hence, if it is deviated by angle θ, then $\theta = \frac{2\pi}{6} = 60°$.

Therefore, velocity of the particle after $t = \frac{1}{6}$ s, is given by

$$\mathbf{v} = 10\,(\cos 60°\,\hat{\mathbf{i}} + \sin 60°\,\hat{\mathbf{j}})$$

$$= 10\left(\frac{\hat{\mathbf{i}}}{2} + \frac{\hat{\mathbf{j}}\sqrt{3}}{2}\right)$$

$$= (5\hat{\mathbf{i}} + 5\sqrt{3}\,\hat{\mathbf{j}})\text{m/s}$$

68. (*d*) Deviation, $\theta = \sin^{-1}\left(\frac{x}{R}\right) = \sin^{-1}\left(\frac{\sqrt{3}}{2}\right) = 60°$

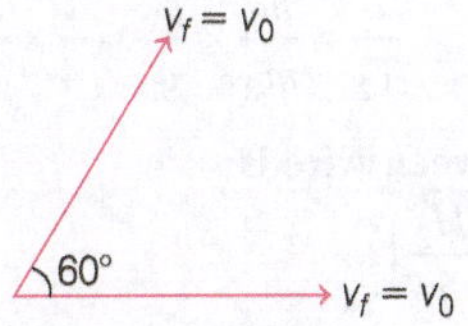

Velocity of the particle when it comes out of the field,

$$|\Delta \mathbf{v}| = 2v_0 \sin\frac{\theta}{2}$$

$$= 2v_0 \sin 30° = v_0$$

69. (*c*) As proton is moving with constant velocity, so acceleration is zero.

When $E \neq 0$, $B = 0$, then proton will move with a acceleration. Hence, this region of space for the motion proton in given condition does not satisfy.

So, $E = 0$ and $B = 0$

When $E = 0$ and $B \neq 0$ but proton is moving in parallel to the direction of magnetic field, then there will be no net force acting on proton.

When, $E \neq 0$ and $B \neq 0$ but electric force and magnetic force cancel each other, then also velocity will remain unchanged.

70. (*d*) We can consider the non-planar loop as made by two loops *ABCDA* and *AQRBA* as shown in figure.

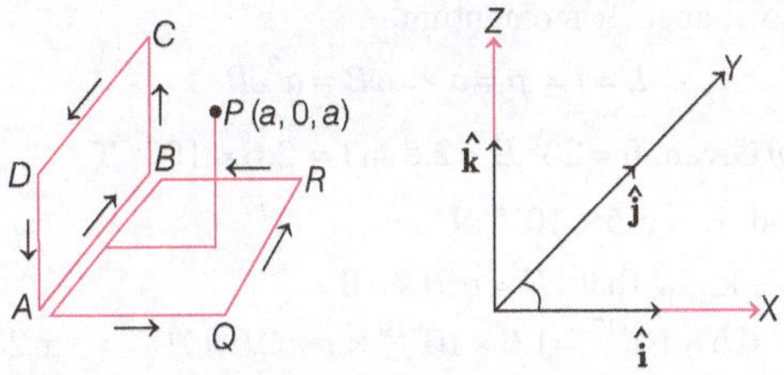

Magnetic field due to loop *ABCDA* will be along *X*-axis and due to loop *AQRBA* along *Z*-axis. Magnitude of magnetic field due to both loops will be equal.

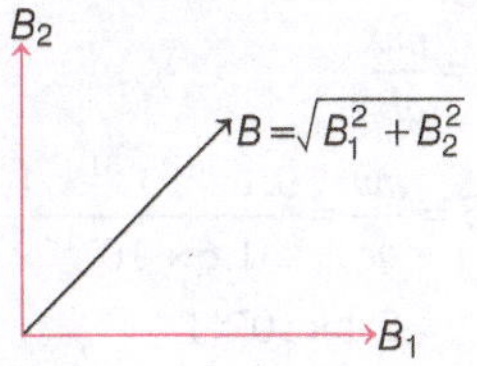

Therefore, direction of resultant magnetic field at *P* will be along $\frac{1}{\sqrt{2}}(\hat{\mathbf{i}} + \hat{\mathbf{k}})$.

71. (*d*) From the question, $PQ = 2r\sin\alpha = \frac{2mv_0}{Bq}\sin\alpha$

$\because \quad \theta = (2\pi - 2\alpha)$

Here, $\alpha = \beta$ and $v = v_0$

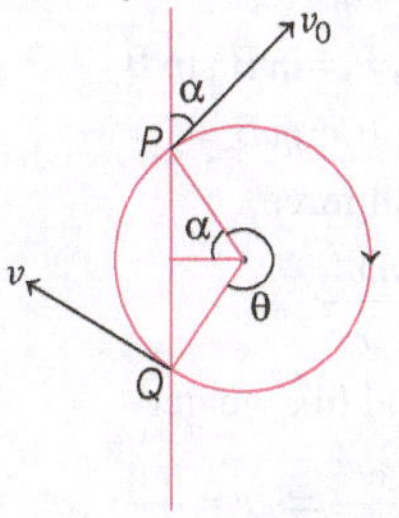

$$\therefore \quad t = \frac{\theta}{\omega} = \frac{2(\pi - \alpha)}{(Bq/m)} = \frac{2m(\pi - \alpha)}{Bq}$$

72. (*a*) In the $z = 0$ plane, the situation is as follows

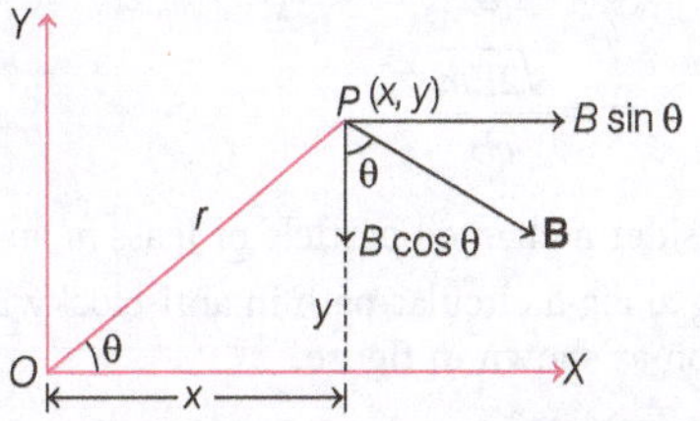

Here, $P(x, y)$ is the point and $r = \sqrt{x^2 + y^2}$

Magnetic field at *P* is perpendicular to *OP*, as it is shown in figure.

So, $\quad \mathbf{B} = B\sin\theta\,\hat{\mathbf{i}} - B\cos\theta\,\hat{\mathbf{j}}$

Here, $\quad B = \frac{\mu_0 I}{2\pi r}$

$$\sin\theta = \frac{y}{r},\ \cos\theta = \frac{x}{r}$$

$$\therefore \quad \mathbf{B} = \frac{\mu_0 I}{2\pi r}\left(\frac{y}{r}\hat{\mathbf{i}} - \frac{x}{r}\hat{\mathbf{j}}\right) = \frac{\mu_0}{2\pi}\frac{I(y\hat{\mathbf{i}} - x\hat{\mathbf{j}})}{(x^2 + y^2)}$$

73. (*a*) Distance $= 2$ (pitch) $= 2\left(\frac{2\pi m}{Bq}\right)v\cos\theta$

$$= \frac{4 \times \pi \times 1.6 \times 10^{-27} \times 2 \times 10^6 \times \cos 30°}{0.05 \times 1.6 \times 10^{-19}}$$

$$= 4.35\text{ m}$$

74. (*c*) Let the masses of two particles are m_1 and m_2.

As the charges are of the same magnitude and being accelerated through same potential difference,

$$R = \frac{1}{B}\sqrt{\frac{2mV}{q}}$$

$$\left(\frac{R_1}{R_2}\right)^2 = \frac{m_1}{m_2}$$

$$\Rightarrow \quad \frac{m_1}{m_2} = \left|\frac{R_1}{R_2}\right|^2$$

75. (*b*) Given, kinetic energy $= E$

Mass $= m$

Magnetic field $= B$

and charge $= q$

Magnetic force, $F = qvB \sin\theta$

If $\theta = 90°$, then $F = qvB$ ...(i)

Now, centripetal force,

$$F = \frac{mv^2}{r} \quad ...(ii)$$

From Eqs. (i) and (ii), we get

$$qvB = \frac{mv^2}{r} \Rightarrow r = \frac{mv}{qB}$$

$$\therefore \quad r = \frac{m\sqrt{\frac{2E}{m}}}{qB} \qquad \left(\because E = \frac{1}{2}mv^2, v = \sqrt{\frac{2E}{m}}\right)$$

$$\Rightarrow \quad r = \frac{\sqrt{2Em}}{qB}$$

76. (*d*) Consider a charged particle of mass m and charge q moving along a circular path in anti-clockwise direction as shown in figure.

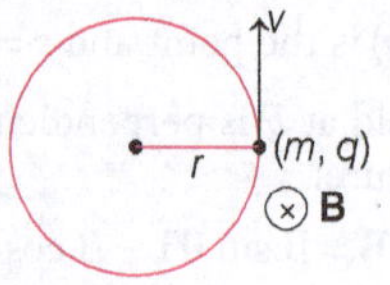

The magnetic field B is assumed to be into plane of paper and of constant magnitude.

Clearly, centripetal force required for the circular motion of the charge will be provided by magnetic Lorentz force $q(v \times B)$.

Hence, $\frac{mv^2}{r} = qvB \sin 90°$

$$\Rightarrow \quad \frac{mv^2}{r} = qvB$$

$$\Rightarrow \quad \text{Speed, } v = \frac{qBr}{m}$$

$$\Rightarrow \quad r = \frac{mv}{qB} \quad ...(i)$$

Let T be the time period of the periodic motion, *i.e.* time taken to complete one revolution.

$$\Rightarrow \quad T = \frac{2\pi}{\omega} = \frac{2\pi}{v/r} = \frac{2\pi r}{v} = \frac{2\pi}{v}\left(\frac{mv}{qB}\right) \quad \text{[from Eq. (i)]}$$

$$= \frac{2\pi m}{qB}$$

77. (*a*) When a magnetic field is applied on a stationary electron, then it remains stationary.

Because, $\mathbf{F} = q(\mathbf{v} \times \mathbf{B})$

If $v = 0 \Rightarrow F = 0$

78. (*a*) Time period, $T = \frac{2\pi m}{Bq} \Rightarrow T = \frac{m}{q}$

or $\frac{T_1}{T_2} = \frac{m_1}{m_2} \times \frac{q_2}{q_1} = \frac{1}{4} \times \frac{3}{2} = \frac{3}{8}$ or 3 : 8

79. (*a*) Force between wire is

$$F = \frac{\mu_0}{2\pi}\frac{I_1 I_2}{r} l$$

$$= \frac{2 \times 10^{-7} \times 30 \times 40 \times (0.1)}{0.02} = 1.2 \times 10^{-3}\text{ N}$$

80. (*c*) The charged particle goes undeflected through both the fields, therefore force experience by charged particle due magnetic field must be equal to the force experienced by the charge particle due to electric field, *i.e.* $F_m = F_e$

or $evB \sin\theta = eE$

Given, $v = 2 \times 10^3\text{ ms}^{-1}$

$B = 1.5$ T and $\theta = 90°$

Hence, $E = vB \sin\theta = 2 \times 10^3 \times 1.5 \times \sin 90°$

$= 3 \times 10^3$ V/m or N/C

81. (*c*) Under uniform magnetic field, force evB acts on proton and provides the necessary centripetal force $\frac{mv^2}{a}$.

$$\therefore \quad \frac{mv^2}{a} = evB \Rightarrow v = \frac{aeB}{m}$$

Now, angular momentum,

$$L = r \times p = a \times aeB = a^2eB$$

82. (*b*) Given, $\theta = 23°, B = 2.6\text{ mT} = 2.6 \times 10^{-3}$ T

and $F = 6.5 \times 10^{-17}$N

We know that, $F = qvB \sin\theta$

$$6.5 \times 10^{-17} = 1.6 \times 10^{-19} \times v \times 2.6 \times 10^{-3} \times \sin 23°$$

$$v = \frac{6.5 \times 10^{-17}}{2.6 \times 10^{-3} \times 1.6 \times 10^{-19} \times 0.39}$$

$$= 4 \times 10^5\text{ ms}^{-1}$$

83. (*c*) Radius, $r = \frac{mv}{qB}$

or $B = \frac{mv}{qr} = \frac{9.1 \times 10^{-31} \times 1.3 \times 10^6}{1.6 \times 10^{-19} \times 0.35}$

$= 2.1 \times 10^{-5}$T

84. (a) The magnetic field induction at P due to currents through both the wires,

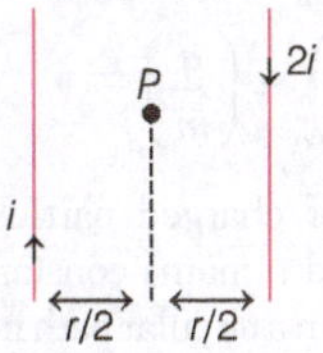

$$B = \frac{\mu_0}{4\pi}\frac{2i}{r/2} + \frac{\mu_0}{4\pi}\frac{2(2i)}{r/2} = \frac{\mu_0}{4\pi}\cdot\frac{12i}{r}$$

It is acting perpendicular to plane of wire inwards. Now, B and v are acting in the same direction, *i.e.* $\theta = 0°$.

$\therefore$ Force on charged particle is

$$F = qvB \sin\theta = qvB \times 0 = 0.$$

85. (a) The direction of magnetic moment of circular loop of radius R is placed in the XY-plane is along z-direction and its magnitude is given by $M = I(\pi R^2)$.

When half of the loop with $x > 0$ is bent, such that it now lies in the YZ-plane, the magnitudes of magnetic moment of each semi-circular loop of radius R lie in the XY-plane and the YZ-plane having magnitude $M' = I(\pi R^2)/4$ each and the direction of magnetic moments are along z-direction and x-direction, respectively.

Their resultant, $M_{net} = \sqrt{M'^2 + M'^2}$

$$= \sqrt{2}\, M'$$

$$= \sqrt{2}\, I(\pi R^2)/4$$

So, $M_{net} < M$ or M diminishes.

86. (b) $\tau = \mathbf{M} \times \mathbf{B} = IAB$

Magnetic moment is in positive x-direction and the magnetic field in positive y-direction. So, the torque (IAB) must be in positive z-direction.

87. (a) Area vector, $\mathbf{A} = \mathbf{CO} \times \mathbf{OA}$

$$= (-b\cos 37°\hat{\mathbf{i}} - b\sin 37°\hat{\mathbf{k}}) \times (a\hat{\mathbf{j}})$$

$$= -\frac{ab}{5}[4(\hat{\mathbf{i}} \times \hat{\mathbf{j}}) + 3(\hat{\mathbf{k}} \times \hat{\mathbf{j}})]$$

$$\left[\because \cos 37° = \frac{4}{5} \text{ and } \sin 37° = \frac{3}{5}\right]$$

$$= -\frac{ab}{5}[4\hat{\mathbf{k}} - 3\hat{\mathbf{i}}]$$

$$= \frac{ab}{5}[3\hat{\mathbf{i}} - 4\hat{\mathbf{k}}]$$

Magnetic moment, $\mathbf{M} = Ni_0\mathbf{A}$

$$= \frac{Ni_0ab}{5}(3\hat{\mathbf{i}} - 4\hat{\mathbf{k}})$$

$$\mathbf{B} = B_0\hat{\mathbf{i}}$$

$\therefore$ Torque, $\tau = \mathbf{M} \times \mathbf{B} = \frac{Ni_0ab}{5}(3\hat{\mathbf{i}} - 4\hat{\mathbf{k}}) \times B_0\hat{\mathbf{i}}$

$$= \frac{Ni_0abB_0}{5}[3(\hat{\mathbf{i}} \times \hat{\mathbf{i}}) - 4(\hat{\mathbf{k}} \times \hat{\mathbf{i}})]$$

$$= -\frac{4Ni_0abB_0}{5}\hat{\mathbf{j}}$$

88. (b)

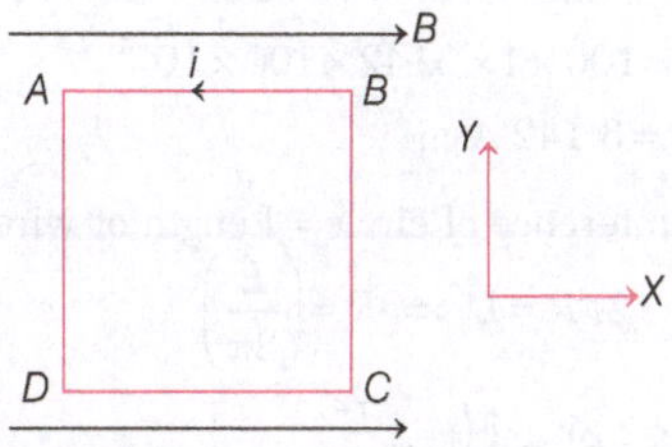

Deflecting torque due to current,

$$\tau_1 = (niA)B \sin 90° = niL^2B$$

Restoring torque,

$$\tau_2 = \text{force} \times \text{perpendicular distance}$$

$$= Mg \times \frac{L}{2}$$

$$\Rightarrow \quad \tau_1 \geq \tau_2$$

$$niL^2B \geq Mg\frac{L}{2}$$

$$\Rightarrow \quad B \geq \frac{Mg}{2niL}$$

$$\therefore \quad B_{min} = \frac{Mg}{2niL}$$

Note **M** is along + Z-axis and **B** is along + X-axis. The magnetic moment vector **M** tries to align along **B** through smaller angle to have minimum potential energy, so coil rotates clockwise about line BC.

89. (a) The torque acting on a current carrying loop is given by

$$\tau = MB\cos\theta$$

$$= NiAB\cos\theta \quad [\because M = NiA]$$

where, N = number of turns,

i = current of loop,

A = area of loop

and B = magnetic field.

Thus, torque does not depend on shape of loop.

90. (b) Magnetic moment,

M = Current × Area of enclosed by loop

$$= I \times A \quad \text{...(i)}$$

Magnetic induction at the centre of circular loop,

$$B = \frac{\mu_0 I}{2R} \Rightarrow I = \frac{2BR}{\mu_0} \quad \text{...(ii)}$$

Here, $A = \pi R^2$ ...(iii)

Substituting Eqs. (ii) and (iii) in Eq. (i), we get

$$M = \frac{2BR}{\mu_0} \times \pi R^2 = \frac{2\pi BR^3}{\mu_0}$$

91. (c) Given, radius of coil, $r = 10\text{ cm} = 10 \times 10^{-2}\text{ m}$
Number of turns, $N = 100$ turns, current in coil, $i = 1\text{ A}$
Magnetic moment, $M = ?$
Now, $M = NiA$, where $A = \pi r^2$

$$M = Ni\pi r^2 = 100 \times 1 \times 3.142 \times (10 \times 10^{-2})^2$$
$$= 100 \times 1 \times 3.142 \times 100 \times 10^{-4}$$
$$= 3.142\text{ A-m}^2$$

92. (c) Circumference of circle = Length of wire

$$\therefore \quad 2\pi R = L \Rightarrow R = \left(\frac{L}{2\pi}\right)$$

Area, $A = \pi R^2 = \frac{\pi L^2}{4\pi^2} = \frac{L^2}{4\pi}$

Magnetic moment, $M = IA = \frac{IL^2}{4\pi}$

93. (d) If the direction of dipole moment of the loop is parallel to the direction of magnetic field, then loop is in stable equilibrium and if the direction of dipole moment of the loop is anti-parallel to the direction of magnetic field, then it is in unstable equilibrium.

94. (b) We have, $M = N_1 I_1 A$, $B = \mu_0 n_2 I_2$

Torque, $\tau = MB$

Here, $\tau = (n_1 I_1 A)(\mu_0 n_2 I_2)$

$$= \left(10 \times \frac{21}{44} \times 10^{-6}\right)\left(4 \times \frac{22}{7} \times 10^{-7} \times 10^3 \times 2.5\right)$$
$$= 1.5 \times 10^{-8}\text{ N-m}$$

Assertion and Reason

1. (a) To the right of B, both fields are downwards and to the left of A, both fields are upwards. At mid-point between wires A and B, magnetic field due to current carrying wire A is equal and opposite to the magnetic field due to current carrying wire B. Hence, they cancel to each other.

2. (c) Velocity will change but speed will remain constant. Hence, momentum will change.

3 (c) As, $r = \frac{\sqrt{2Km}}{Bq}$

or $$r \propto \frac{\sqrt{m}}{q}$$

$$\left(\frac{\sqrt{m}}{q}\right)_\alpha = \frac{\sqrt{4}}{2} = 1$$

and $$\left(\frac{\sqrt{m}}{q}\right)_d = \frac{\sqrt{2}}{1} = \sqrt{2}$$

$$\therefore \quad r_d > r_\alpha$$

Further, $$\left(\frac{q}{m}\right)_\alpha = \frac{2}{4} = \frac{1}{2}$$

and $$\left(\frac{q}{m}\right)_d = \frac{1}{2}$$

$$\therefore \quad \left(\frac{q}{m}\right)_\alpha = \left(\frac{q}{m}\right)_d$$

4. (b) Acceleration of charged particle in uniform field is non-zero but speed remains constant. In given condition, particle will rotate in a circular path in XY-plane. Therefore, if velocity is $v_0\hat{\mathbf{i}}$ at some instant, then it can have the value $v_0\hat{\mathbf{j}}$ at other instant also.

5. (b) Magnetic force can change the velocity but not the speed. Speeds at two instants must be same.

6. (b) Magnetic force of attraction on lower wire is upwards while its weight is downwards. At a certain distance x, these two forces are equal. If the lower wire is displaced upwards from this position, then magnetic force will increase but weight will remain same. Therefore, net force is upwards or equilibrium is unstable.

Statement Type Questions

1. (b) Statement I is correct but Statement II is incorrect.
Inside a conductor, B proportional to r is correct but current enclosed (by an Amperian loop) is given by

$$I_{\text{enclosed}} = JA_{\text{enclosed}}$$
$$\Rightarrow \quad I_{\text{enclosed}} = J\pi r^2$$
or $$I \propto r^2$$

So, Statement I is correct, whereas Statement II is incorrect.

2. (a) Both Statement I and Statement II are incorrect.
From equation $F = qvB \sin\theta$. Force on moving charge will be maximum if direction of velocity of charge is perpendicular to direction of magnetic field (when $\theta = 90°$).

3. (d) Both Statement I and Statement II are correct.
A magnetic field interacts with a moving charge as a moving charge produces a magnetic field.

4. (a) Both Statement I and Statement II are incorrect.
Magnetic dipole moment of the current loop
= Total Current × area of the loop

So, $$M = NI\pi r^2$$

$$M_1 = NI\left(\frac{r}{2}\right)^2 = \frac{M}{4}$$

So, magnetic moment becomes one-fourth when radius becomes half.

5. (a) Both Statement I and Statement II are incorrect.
To increase the range of ammeter smaller value of shunt is used. So, the resistance of ammeter will be smaller.

Match the Columns

1. (*a*) As, $r = \dfrac{\sqrt{2Km}}{Bq} \Rightarrow r \propto \dfrac{\sqrt{m}}{q}$

$\Rightarrow r_d > r_\alpha$ (towards left) and $r_e < r_{Cl^-}$ (towards right)

Hence, A-II, B-I, C-IV, D-III.

2. (*a*) (A)

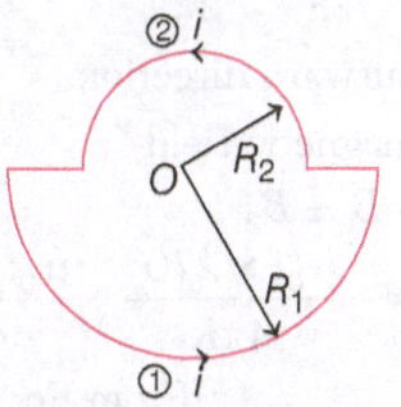

Magnetic field at O due to straight wires is zero

$$B_1 = \frac{\mu_0 i}{4R_1} \Rightarrow B_2 = \frac{\mu_0 i}{4R_2},$$

B_1 and B_2 both directed outward

Magnetic field at the centre point O,

$$B_O = B_1 + B_2 = \frac{\mu_0 i}{4}\left(\frac{1}{R_1} + \frac{1}{R_2}\right), \text{(outward)}$$

(B)

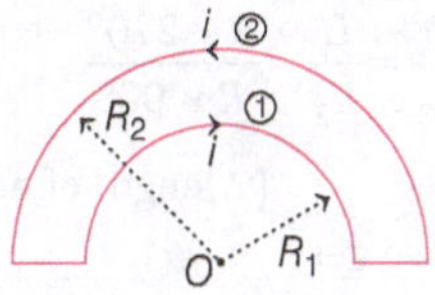

Magnetic field at O due to straight wire,

$$B_1 = \frac{\mu_0 i}{4R_1} \text{ and } B_2 = \frac{\mu_0 i}{4R_2},$$

B_1 is directed inward and B_2 is directed outward.

$$B_1 > B_2$$

Magnetic field at the centre O,

$$B_O = B_1 - B_2$$
$$= \frac{\mu_0 i}{4}\left(\frac{1}{R_1} - \frac{1}{R_2}\right), \text{(inward)}$$

(C)

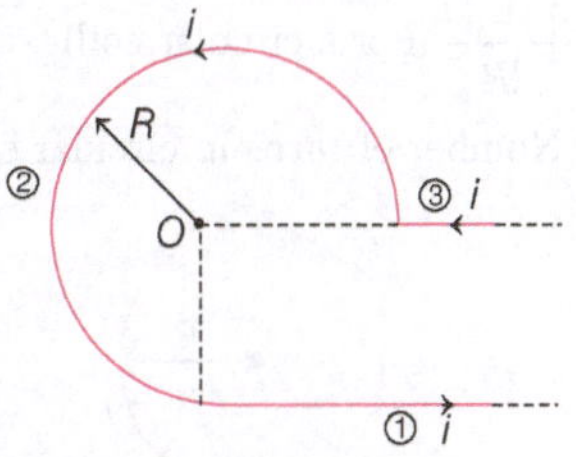

Magnetic field, $B_1 = \dfrac{\mu_0 i}{4\pi R}$, (outward)

Magnetic field, $B_2 = \dfrac{\mu_0 i}{2R} \cdot \dfrac{3}{4}$, (outward)

Magnetic field, $B_3 = 0$

Magnetic field at the centre, $B_O = B_1 + B_2$

$$= \frac{\mu_0 i}{4R}\left(\frac{1}{\pi} + \frac{3}{2}\right), \text{(outward)}$$

(D)

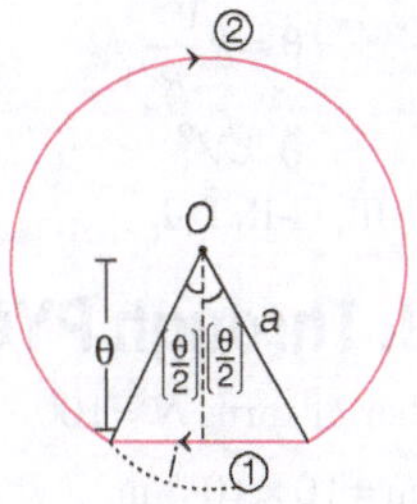

From the figure, $d = a \cos \dfrac{\theta}{2}$

$$B_1 = \frac{\mu_0 i}{4\pi d}\left(\sin\frac{\theta}{2} + \sin\frac{\theta}{2}\right)$$
$$= \frac{\mu_0 i}{4\pi a \cos\frac{\theta}{2}} \cdot 2 \sin\frac{\theta}{2}$$
$$= \frac{\mu_0 i}{2\pi a} \tan\left(\frac{\theta}{2}\right), \text{(inward)}$$
$$B_2 = \frac{\mu_0 i}{2a} \frac{(2\pi - \theta)}{2\pi}, \text{(inward)}$$

Magnetic field at the centre O,

$$B_O = B_1 + B_2$$
$$= \frac{\mu_0 i}{2\pi a}\left(\tan\frac{\theta}{2} + \pi - \frac{\theta}{2}\right), \text{(inward)}$$

Hence, A-III, B-IV, C-II, D-I.

3. (*d*) Magnetic field over the loop due to straight wire is perpendicular to paper inwards.

Force, $\mathbf{F} = i(d\mathbf{l} \times \mathbf{B})$

(A) Force on *bc* is equal to force and on *da* hence, net force is zero.

(B) Distance of *ab* from *ef* is not same as distance of *cd* from *ef* hence, net force is non-zero and unequal.

(C) According to the above explanation, net force on *abcd* is leftward because force on *ba* is greater than *cd*.

(D) According to Newton's third law, force on *ef* will be rightward.

Hence, A-I, B-II, C-IV, D-III.

4. (*a*) For a DC ammeter or voltmeter, a moving coil galvanometer is used. So, deflection of coil $\theta = \dfrac{BNA}{k} I$

or $\theta \propto I$

Also, $\theta = \dfrac{BNA}{kR} IR$

$$= \frac{BNA}{kR} V$$

or $\theta \propto V$

For an AC ammeter or voltmeter, a hot wire deflection instrument is used.

$\therefore \qquad \theta = kI^2R$

$\Rightarrow \qquad \theta \propto I^2$

and $\qquad \theta = k\dfrac{V^2}{R}$

$\Rightarrow \qquad \theta \propto V^2$

Hence, A-IV, B-III, C-II, D-I.

Final Check Through PYQs

1. (c) Given, number of turns $N = 100$

radius, $r = 10 \text{ cm} = 10 \times 10^{-2}$ m

current, $I = 7$ A

Magnetic field at the centre of a solenoid,

$$B = \frac{\mu_0 NI}{2r} = \frac{4\pi \times 10^{-7} \times 100 \times 7}{2 \times 10 \times 10^{-2}}$$

$$= 44 \times 10^{-4}$$

$$= 4.4 \times 10^{-3} \text{ T}$$

$$= 4.4 \text{ mT}$$

2. (b)

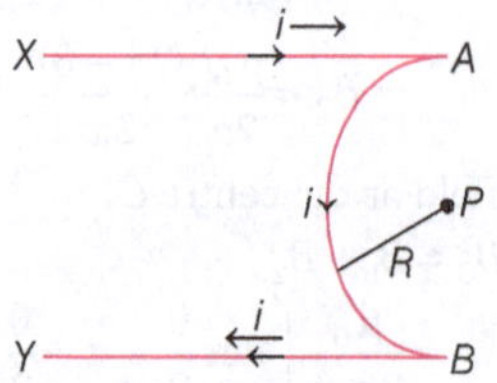

Net magnetic field at point P,

$$B = B_{\text{semicircle}} - B_{XA} - B_{YB}$$

$$= \frac{\mu_0 i}{4R} - \frac{\mu_0 i}{4\pi R} - \frac{\mu_0 i}{4\pi R} = \frac{\mu_0 i}{4R}\left[1 - \frac{2}{\pi}\right]$$

pointed away from the page.

3. (b) According to Biot-Savart's law, magnetic field due to small current element Idl, at a distance r from it is given as

$$dB = \frac{\mu_0 (Idl \times r)}{4\pi r^3}$$

Thus, current element Idl is a vector quantity. Hence, Statement I is correct and Statement II is incorrect.

4. (a) The magnetic field at the centre of an arc subtended at an angle θ is given by

$$B = \frac{\mu_0 i}{2R} \times \frac{\theta}{2\pi}$$

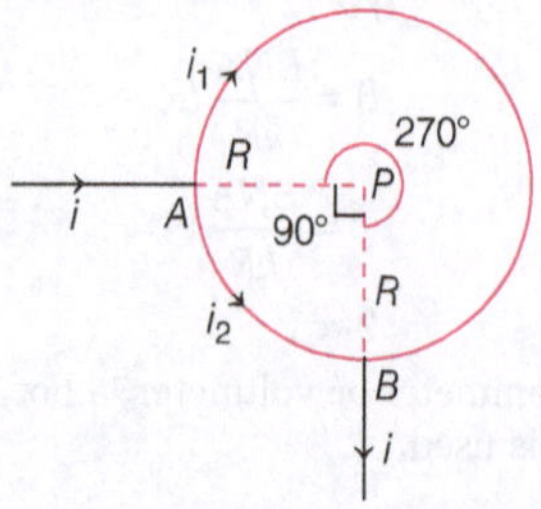

Then, the magnetic field due to larger arc AB is

$$B_1 = \frac{\mu_0 i_1}{2R} \times \frac{270°}{2\pi} \qquad \text{...(i)}$$

which acts in inward direction according to right hand thumb rule and magnetic field due to smaller arc AB is

$$B_2 = \frac{\mu_0 i_2}{2R} \times \frac{90°}{2\pi} \qquad \text{...(ii)}$$

which acts in outward direction.

The resultant magnetic field

$$B_R = B_1 + B_2$$

$$= -\frac{\mu_0 i_1 \times 270°}{4\pi R} + \frac{\mu_0 i_2 \times 90°}{4\pi R}$$

[From Eq. (i) and (ii)] ...(iii)

which acts in inward direction as $B_1 > B_2$.

Two arcs can also be seen as the two resistances in parallel combination.

So, the potential across them will be same i.e.

$$V_1 = V_2$$

$$i_1 R_1 = i_2 R_2 \qquad \text{...(iv)}$$

where, R_1 and R_2 = Resistance of respective segments

The wire is uniform so

$$\frac{R_1}{R_2} = \frac{L_1}{L_2} = \frac{R \times 270°}{R \times 90°}$$

[$\because$ length of arc = radius × angle]

From Eq. (iv), we get

$$\Rightarrow \qquad \frac{i_1}{i_2} = \frac{R_2}{R_1} = \frac{90°}{270°} = \frac{1}{3}$$

or $\qquad 3i_1 = i_2 \qquad$ ...(v)

From Eq. (iii) and (v), we get

$$B_R = \frac{\mu_0}{4\pi R}(-270° i_1 + 90° i_2)$$

$$= \frac{\mu_0}{4\pi R}[-270° i_1 + 90° (3i_1)]$$

$$= \frac{\mu_0}{4\pi R}[-270° i_1 + 270° i_1] = 0$$

5. (b) $B_{\text{centre}} = \dfrac{n \cdot \mu_0 i}{2R}$ (For a circular coil)

where, n = Number of turns in circular coil

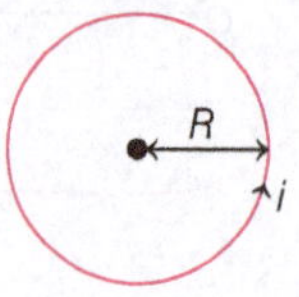

$$B = \frac{\mu_0 i}{2R} = \frac{\mu_0 i(2\pi)}{2(l)} = \frac{\mu_0 \pi i}{l}$$

$$= \frac{\mu_0 n i}{2\left(\dfrac{l}{2n\pi}\right)} = \frac{n^2 \mu_0 \pi i}{l} = n^2 B$$

6. (*c*) The magnetic field in the different regions is given by

$$\mathbf{B}_1 = \frac{\mu_0}{4\pi} \times \frac{I}{R}(-\hat{\mathbf{k}})$$

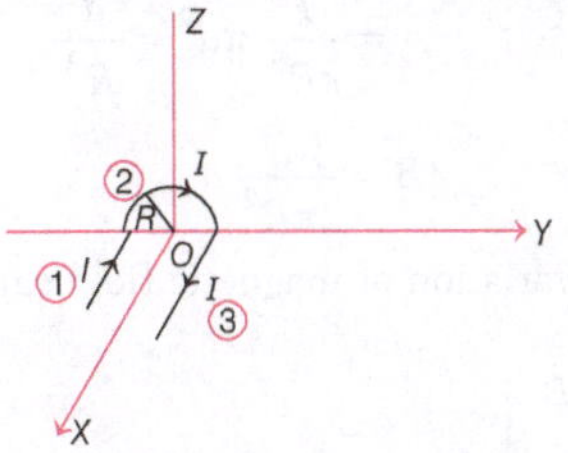

$$\mathbf{B}_3 = \frac{\mu_0 I}{4\pi R}(-\hat{\mathbf{k}})$$

$$\mathbf{B}_2 = \frac{\mu_0 I}{4R}(-\hat{\mathbf{i}})$$

The net magnetic field at the centre O is

$$\mathbf{B} = \mathbf{B}_1 + \mathbf{B}_2 + \mathbf{B}_3$$

$$= \frac{\mu_0 I}{4\pi R}(-2\hat{\mathbf{k}}) + \frac{\mu_0 I}{4R}(-\hat{\mathbf{i}})$$

$$= -\frac{\mu_0 I}{4\pi R}(2\hat{\mathbf{k}} + \pi\hat{\mathbf{i}})$$

7. (*d*) As $I = \frac{q}{t}$. So, for an electron revolving in a circular orbit of radius r

$q = e$ and $t = T$

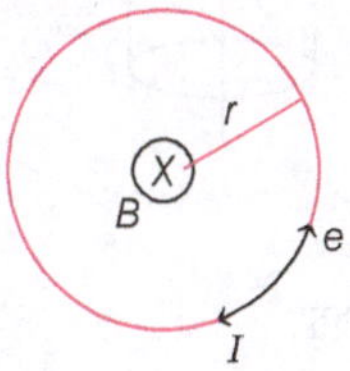

$$\Rightarrow \quad I = \frac{e}{T} = \frac{e}{2\pi/\omega} = \frac{\omega e}{2\pi} = \frac{2\pi ne}{2\pi} = ne$$

The magnetic field produced at the centre is

$$B = \frac{\mu_0 I}{2R} = \frac{\mu_0 ne}{2r}$$

8. (*d*) As from question,

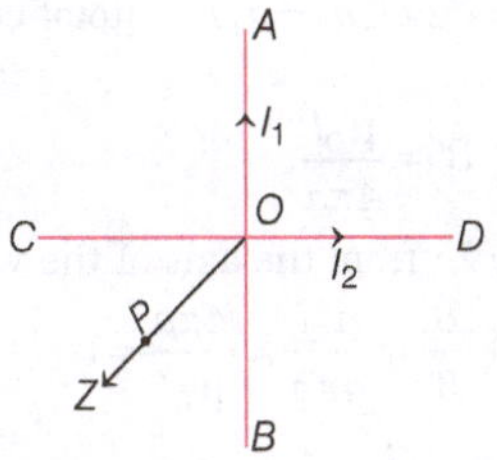

The point P is lying at a distance d along the Z-axis.

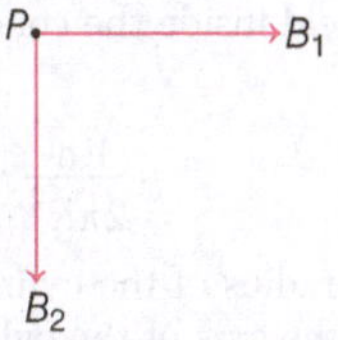

As magnetic field B_1 is given by

$$= \frac{\mu_0}{2\pi}\frac{I_1}{d}$$

and magnetic field B_2 is given by

$$= \frac{\mu_0}{2\pi}\frac{I_2}{d}$$

B_1 and B_2 are perpendicular to each other

So, B_{net} is given by

$$B_{net} = \sqrt{B_1^2 + B_2^2},$$

$$B_{net} = \frac{\mu_0}{2\pi}\frac{1}{d}(I_1^2 + I_2^2)^{1/2}$$

9. (*a*) Given, radius of solenoid,

$r = 1$ mm

$$\text{Number of turns per mm} = \frac{100}{1\text{ mm}}$$

$$\therefore \text{ Number of turns per metre} = \frac{100}{1 \times 10^{-3}\text{ m}}$$

i.e., $n = 10^5$ turns/m

Current flowing through the solenoid,

$I = 1$ A

$\therefore$Magnetic field strength at the centre of the solenoid

$$B = \mu_0 nI$$

$$= 4\pi \times 10^{-7} \times 10^5 \times 1$$

$$= 4\pi \times 10^{-2}\text{ T} = 12.56 \times 10^{-2}\text{ T}$$

10. (*b*) According to Ampere's circuital law, magnetic field inside the current carrying long straight wire of circular cross-section is a linearly increasing function of distance $r (r < R)$ upto the boundary of the wire and magnetic field outside the wire at distance $r (r > R)$ from its axis is decreasing one with $\frac{1}{r}$ dependence as shown in figure.

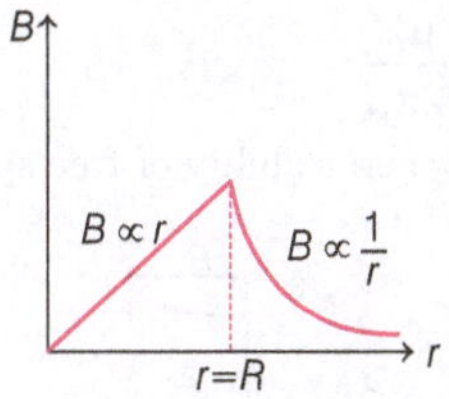

where, R is radius of circular cross-section of wire.

11. (c) Magnetic field inside the conducting cylindrical cable,

$$B = \frac{\mu_0 I}{2\pi R^2} r$$

Here, R is the radius of the cylindrical cable, r is the distance from the axis of the cylinder,

I is the current carrying in the cylindrical cable.

$\Rightarrow \quad B \propto r$

$\therefore$ The graph of magnetic field B with r is a straight line passing through origin.

For a point outside the cylinder,

$$B = \frac{\mu_0 I}{2\pi r} \Rightarrow B \propto \frac{1}{r}$$

The graph of magnetic field B with r is a rectangular hyperbola passing through the outer surface of the cylinder.

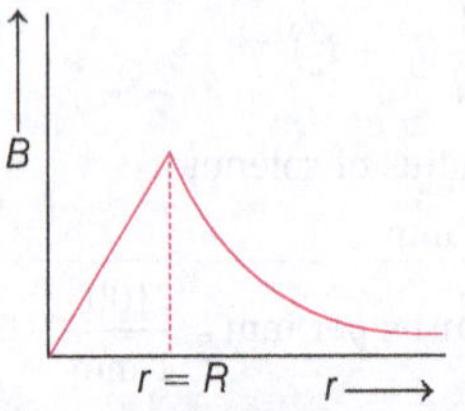

$\therefore$ The variation of the magnetic field B due to the cable with the distance r from the axis of the cylindrical cable is as shown in the figure.

12. (d) Given,

$l = 50$ cm $= 0.5$ m,

$N = 100$ turns and $I = 2.5$ A

$\therefore$ Magnetic field at the centre of solenoid is

$$= \mu_0 nI = \mu_0 \left(\frac{N}{l}\right) \cdot I$$

$$= 4\pi \times 10^{-7} \times \frac{100}{0.5} \times 2.5 = 6.28 \times 10^{-4} \text{ T}$$

Hence, correct option is (d).

13. (b) The cylinder can be considered to be made from concentric circles of radius R.

(i) The magnetic field at point outside cylinder, i.e. $d > R$

$$\Rightarrow \quad B = \frac{\mu_0 I}{2\pi d}$$

where, μ_0 = permeability of free space.

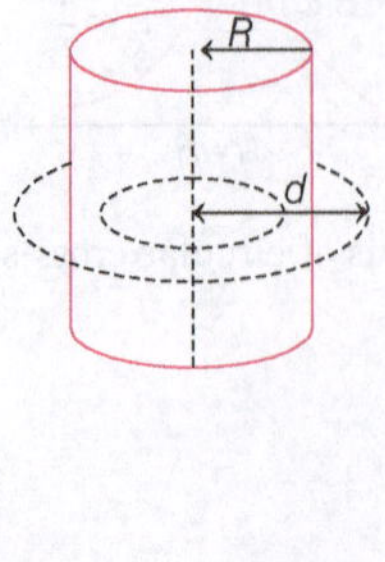

(ii) The magnitude field at surface, i.e. $d = R$

$$B = \frac{\mu_0 I}{2\pi R}$$

(iii) The magnetic field at inside point.

$$= \frac{I}{\pi R^2} \pi d^2 = \frac{Id^2}{R^2}$$

$$\therefore \quad B = \frac{\mu_0 I}{2\pi R^2} d$$

So, the variation of magnetic field can be plotted as

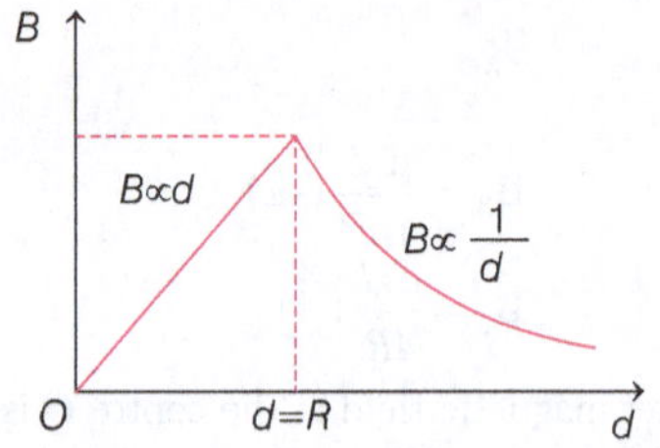

14. (b) Consider two Amperian loops of radius $\frac{a}{2}$ and $2a$ as shown in the diagram.

Applying Ampere's circuital law for these loops we get,

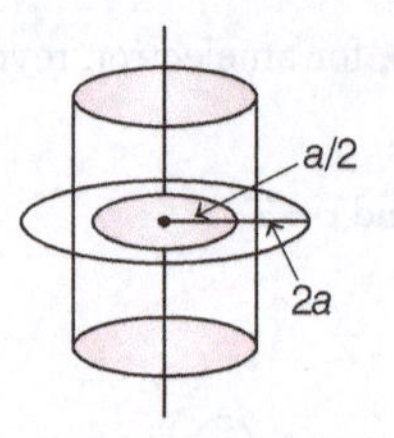

$$\oint \mathbf{B} \cdot d\mathbf{l} = \mu_0 I_{\text{enclosed}}$$

For the smaller loop

$$\Rightarrow B \times 2\pi \frac{a}{2} = \mu_0 \times \frac{I}{\pi a^2} \times \pi \left(\frac{a}{2}\right)^2$$

$$= \mu_0 I \times \frac{1}{4} = \frac{\mu_0 I}{4}$$

$\Rightarrow \quad B = \frac{\mu_0 I}{4\pi a}$, at distance $\frac{a}{2}$ from the axis of the wire.

Similarly, for bigger Amperian loop.

$B' \times 2\pi (2a) = \mu_0 I$ [total current enclosed by Amperian loop is 2]

$$\Rightarrow \quad B' = \frac{\mu_0 I}{4\pi a},$$

at distance $2a$ from the axis of the wire.

So, ratio of $\frac{B}{B'} = \frac{\mu_0 I}{4\pi a} \times \frac{4\pi a}{\mu_0 I} = 1$

15. (b) Given, $\mathbf{L} = L\hat{\mathbf{i}}$

$$\mathbf{B} = 2\hat{\mathbf{i}} + 3\hat{\mathbf{j}} - 4\hat{\mathbf{k}}$$

$$\therefore \quad \mathbf{F} = \mathbf{I}\,(\mathbf{L} \times \mathbf{B})$$

$$= I[L\hat{i} \times (2\hat{i} + 3\hat{j} - 4\hat{k})]$$
$$= I[2L(\hat{i} \times \hat{i}) + 3L(\hat{i} \times \hat{j}) - 4L(\hat{i} \times \hat{k})]$$
$$= I[0 + 3L\hat{k} + 4L\hat{j}]$$
$$= I[4L\hat{j} + 3L\hat{k}]$$
$$\therefore F = |\mathbf{F}| = \sqrt{(4LI)^2 + (3LI)^2} = 5LI$$

16. (*b*) Given, velocity,
$$\mathbf{v} = 2\hat{i} + 4\hat{j} + 6\hat{k}$$
Force, $\mathbf{F} = 4\hat{i} - 20\hat{j} + 12\hat{k}$

As we know, $\mathbf{F} = q(\mathbf{v} \times \mathbf{B})$

Here, $q = 1$ (given)

Substituting the values in the above equation, we get
$$4\hat{i} - 20\hat{j} + 12\hat{k} = (1)[(2\hat{i} + 4\hat{j} + 6\hat{k}) \times (B\hat{i} + B\hat{j} + B_0\hat{k})]$$
$$4\hat{i} - 20\hat{j} + 12\hat{k} = \begin{pmatrix} \hat{i} & \hat{j} & \hat{k} \\ 2 & 4 & 6 \\ B & B & B_0 \end{pmatrix}$$
$$\Rightarrow 4\hat{i} - 20\hat{j} + 12\hat{k} = \hat{i}(4B_0 - 6B) - \hat{j}(2B_0 - 6B) + \hat{k}(2B - 4B)$$
Comparing the LHS and RHS of the above equation, we get

$\hat{i}$ terms $\quad 4B_0 - 6B = 4$ ...(i)

$\hat{j}$ terms
$$2B_0 - 6B = 20 \quad \text{...(ii)}$$
$\hat{k}$ terms
$$2B - 4B = 12$$
$$\Rightarrow B = -6$$
Substituting the value of B in the Eq. (ii), we get
$$2B_0 - 6(-6) = 20$$
$$\Rightarrow B_0 = -8$$
Thus, the magnetic field vector,
$$B = -6\hat{i} - 6\hat{j} - 8\hat{k}$$

17. (*a*) Magnetic field due to a current carrying wire at a distance r from the wire.
$$\text{or, } B = \frac{\mu_0 2i}{4\pi r} = \frac{10^{-7} \times 2 \times 5}{20 \times 10^{-2}}$$
$$= \frac{1}{2} \times 10^{-5} \text{ T}$$
Upward to the plane of paper

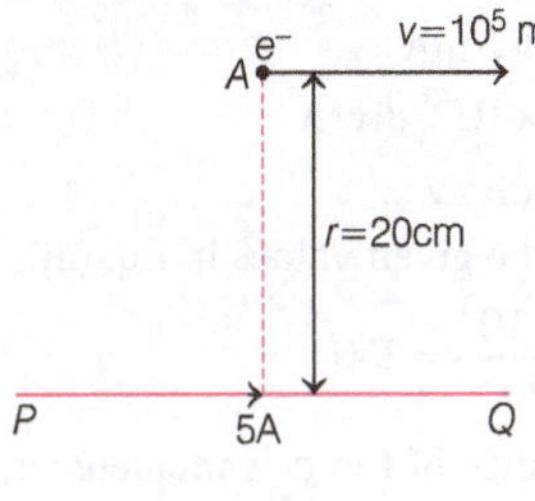

Therefore, force acting on electron
$$\mathbf{F} = q(\mathbf{v} \times \mathbf{B})$$
$$|\mathbf{F}| = 1.6 \times 10^{-19} \times 10^5 \times \frac{1}{2} \times 10^{-5}$$
$$= 8 \times 10^{-20} \text{ N}$$

18. (*d*) The centripetal force required for circular motion is provided by magnetic force
$$\Rightarrow \frac{mv_p^2}{r} = Bqv_p$$
$$\Rightarrow r = \frac{mv_p}{qB} \quad \text{...(i)}$$
where, v_p = perpendicular velocity of particle and q = charge on particle.

As, momentum, $p = mv_p$
$$\therefore r = \frac{p}{qB} \quad \text{[from Eq. (i)]}$$
According to the question, moment of both particle is same.
$$\Rightarrow r \propto \frac{1}{q}$$
For ionised hydrogen atom, $q_H = e$

and for α-particle, $q_\alpha = 2e$
$$\Rightarrow \frac{r_H}{r_\alpha} = \frac{q_\alpha}{q_H} = \frac{2e}{e} = \frac{2}{1} \text{ or } 2:1$$

19. (*d*) As, the system is in equilibrium,
$$\Sigma F_x = 0$$
$$\text{or} \quad mg \sin\theta = F\cos\theta \quad \text{...(i)}$$
where, F is the magnitude of force experienced by the rod when placed in a magnetic field and current I is flowing through it.

But the force experienced by the given rod in a uniform magnetic field is
$$F = ILB$$
$\therefore$ Eq. (i) becomes,
$$mg \sin\theta = ILB\cos\theta$$
$$\Rightarrow I = \frac{mg\sin\theta}{LB\cos\theta} = \frac{mg}{LB}\tan\theta$$
$$I = \left(\frac{m}{L}\right)\frac{g\tan\theta}{B} \quad \text{...(ii)}$$
According to the question,

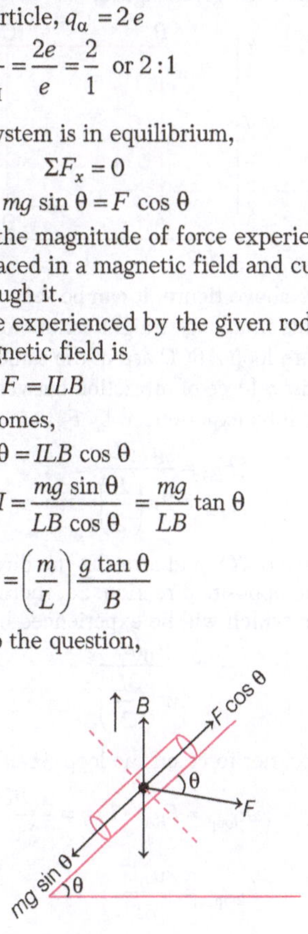

Here, $\frac{m}{L} = 0.5 \text{ kg m}^{-1}$, $g = 9.8 \text{ ms}^{-2}$,

$\theta = 30°, \ B = 0.25$ T

Substituting the given values in Eq. (ii), we get

$$I = \frac{0.5 \times 9.8}{0.25} \tan 30°$$

$$= \frac{0.5 \times 9.8}{0.25} \times \frac{1}{\sqrt{3}} = 11.32 \text{ A}$$

20. (*d*) As force on wire *B* due to *A* and *C* are attractive, so we have following condition

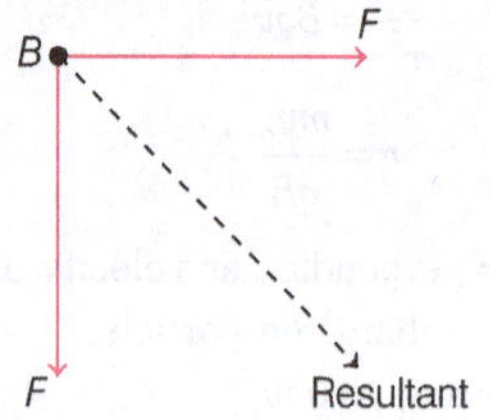

$$F = \frac{\mu_0 I^2}{2\pi d}$$

Resultant force on *B*

$$= \sqrt{F_1^2 + F_2^2} = \sqrt{2}\,F = \sqrt{2} \times \frac{\mu_0 I^2}{2\pi d} = \frac{\mu_0 I^2}{\sqrt{2}\pi d}$$

21. (*d*) Consider the given figure,

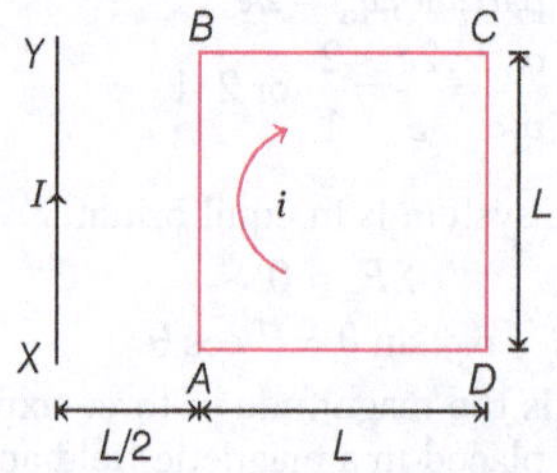

From the above figure, it can be seen that the direction of currents in a long straight conductor *XY* and arm *AB* of a square loop *ABCD* are in the same direction. So, there exist a force of attraction between the two, which will be experienced by F_{BA} as

$$F_{BA} = \frac{\mu_0 IiL}{2\pi\left(\frac{L}{2}\right)}$$

In the case of *XY* and arm *CD*, the direction of currents are in the opposite direction. So, there exist a force of repulsion which will be experienced by *CD* as

$$F_{CD} = \frac{\mu_0 IiL}{2\pi\left(\frac{3L}{2}\right)}$$

Therefore, net force on the loop *ABCD* will be

$$F_{\text{loop}} = F_{BA} - F_{CD} = \frac{\mu_0 IiL}{2\pi}\left[\frac{1}{(L/2)} - \frac{1}{(3L/2)}\right]$$

$$F_{\text{loop}} = \frac{2\mu_0 iI}{3\pi}$$

22. (*a*) As we know that, radius of a charged particle in a magnetic field *B* is given by

$$r = \frac{mv}{qB} \quad \text{...(i)}$$

∴ The time taken to complete the circle,

$$T = \frac{2\pi r}{v}$$

$$\Rightarrow \quad \frac{T}{2\pi} = \frac{m}{qB} \quad \text{[from Eq. (i)]}$$

$$\therefore \quad \omega = \frac{2\pi}{T} = \frac{qB}{m}$$

$$\because \quad q = e \text{ and } \frac{e}{m} = 1.76 \times 10^{11} \text{ C/kg}$$

$$B = 3.57 \times 10^{-2} \text{ T}$$

$$\Rightarrow \quad \frac{2\pi}{T} = \frac{eB}{m} \Rightarrow f = \frac{1}{2\pi}\frac{e}{m}B \quad \left(\because \frac{1}{T} = f\right)$$

$$= \frac{1}{2\pi} \times 1.76 \times 10^{11} \times 3.57 \times 10^{-2}$$

$$= 1.0 \times 10^9 \text{Hz} = 1 \text{ GHz}$$

23. (*c*) $F = qvB = \frac{mv^2}{r}$

$$\therefore \quad r = \frac{mv}{qB} = \frac{\sqrt{2m(\text{KE})}}{qB}$$

Since *r* is same so, $\text{KE} \propto \frac{q^2}{m}$

Therefore KE of α-particle $= \frac{q^2}{m} = \frac{(2)^2}{4} = 1$ MeV

24. (*a*) Current sensitivity of a moving coil galvanometer is the deflection θ per unit current *I* flowing through it, i.e.

$$I_S = \frac{\theta}{I} = \frac{NAB}{k} \quad \text{...(i)}$$

where, *N* = number of turns in the coil,
A = Area of each turn of coil, *B* = magnetic field
k = restoring torque per unit twist of the fibre strip.

Similarly, voltage sensitivity is the deflection per unit voltage, i.e.

$$V_S = \frac{\theta}{V} = \left(\frac{NAB}{k}\right)\frac{I}{V} = \frac{NAB}{kR_G} \quad \text{...(ii)}$$

where, R_G is the resistance of the galvanometer.

From Eqs. (i) and (ii), we get

$$R_G = \frac{I_S}{V_S} \quad \text{...(iii)}$$

Here, $I_S = 5$ div/mA
$= 5 \times 10^{+3}$ div/A

and $V_S = 20$ div/V

Substituting the given values in Eq. (iii), we get

$$R_G = \frac{5 \times 10^3}{20} = 250$$

∴ The resistance of the galvanometer is 250 Ω.

25. (*b*) Given, $N = 50$

$B = 0.2\ \text{Wb/m}^2, I = 2\text{A}$

$\theta = 60°, A = 0.12 \times 0.1 = 0.012\ \text{m}^2$

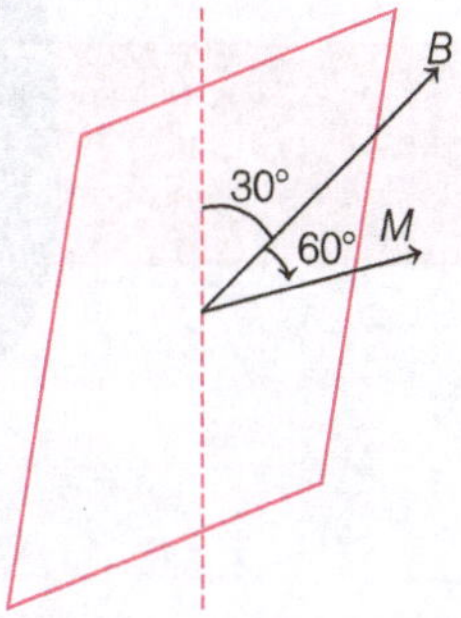

Thus, torque required to keep the coil in stable equilibrium, i.e.

$$\tau = NIAB \sin\theta$$
$$= 50 \times 2 \times 0.012 \times 0.2 \times \sin 60°$$
$$= 50 \times 2 \times 0.12 \times 0.2 \times \frac{\sqrt{3}}{2} = 0.20\ \text{N-m}$$

Skill Builder

■ Sol. of Skill Builder on Pg. 278

(*a*) The magnitude of magnetic field due to circular coil of N turns is given by $B_C = \frac{\mu_0 iN}{2R}$

$$= \frac{4\pi \times 10^{-7} \times 40 \times 2}{2 \times 0.05} = 1 \times 10^{-3}\ \text{T} = 1\ \text{mT}$$

■ Sol. of Skill Builder on Pg. 282

(*c*)

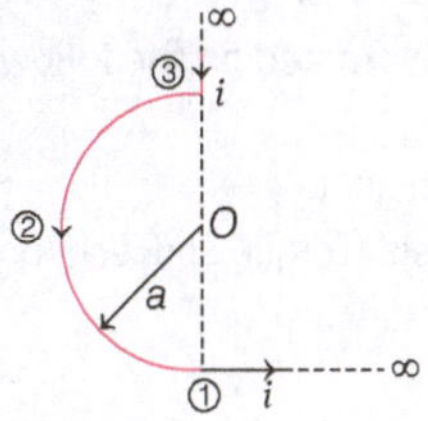

Magnetic field, $B_1 = \frac{\mu_0 i}{4\pi a}$, (outward)

Magnetic field, $B_2 = \frac{\mu_0 i}{4a}$, (outward)

Magnetic field, $B_3 = 0$

Magnetic field at the centre point O,

$$B_0 = B_1 + B_2 = \frac{\mu_0 i}{4\pi a} + \frac{\mu_0 i}{4a}$$
$$= \frac{\mu_0 i}{4a}\left(\frac{1}{\pi} + 1\right), \text{(outward)}$$

■ Sol. of Skill Builder on Pg. 286

(*c*) Magnetic field of solenoid, $B = \mu_0 nI$

If number of turns, current through wire and radius of solenoid is doubled then,

$$B = 4\mu_0 nI$$

Then, magnetic field becomes 4 times.

■ Sol. of Skill Builder on Pg. 292

(*b*) Given,

Length of the wire,

$$\mathbf{l} = 1\hat{\mathbf{k}}$$
$$\mathbf{B} = (2\hat{\mathbf{i}} + 3\hat{\mathbf{j}} + 5\hat{\mathbf{k}})$$
$$i = 2\ \text{A}$$

Magnetic force on wire,

$$\mathbf{F} = I(\mathbf{l} \times \mathbf{B})$$
$$= 2[1\hat{\mathbf{k}} \times (2\hat{\mathbf{i}} + 3\hat{\mathbf{j}} + 5\hat{\mathbf{k}})]$$
$$= 2[2\hat{\mathbf{j}} - 3\hat{\mathbf{i}}]$$
$$= [4\hat{\mathbf{j}} - 6\hat{\mathbf{i}}]\ \text{N}$$

■ Sol. of Skill Builder on Pg. 293

(*b*) We know that,

$$\frac{F}{l} = \frac{\mu_0 i_1 i_2}{2\pi d}$$

If d is doubled then,

$$\frac{F}{l} = \frac{\mu_0 i_1 i_2}{2\pi(2d)} = \frac{\mu_0 i_1 i_2}{2 \times 2\pi d}$$

i.e. force per unit length will be halved, if distance between two current carrying conductors is doubled.

For deeper insight
Scan the QR Code

Chapter 6

Magnetism and Matter

Learning Objectives

Module-I

- Bar Magnet
- Magnetic Field Lines
- Bar Magnet as an Equivalent Solenoid
- Magnetic Field Strength at a Point due to Magnetic Dipole or Bar Magnet
- Bar Magnet in a Uniform Magnetic Field
- Magnetism and Gauss' Law

Module-II

- Some Important Terms Used in Magnetism
- Classification of Substances on the Basis of Magnetic Behaviour
- Curie's Law

Chapter Overview with *NEET Connection*

Some natural materials have magnetic properties. These materials get attracted towards any magnet, while there are some other materials which are repelled by a magnet. All the magnetic properties and their temperature dependance are discussed in this chapter.

Without mastery over this chapter, it will be difficult to understand other chapters like Electromagnetic Induction and Electromagnetic Waves.

Special format questions can be easily framed on the following topics of this chapter

- Magnetic field strength due to bar magnet.
- Bar magnet in a uniform magnetic field (Torque and work done).
- Magnetic properties and their inter-relations.
- Magnetic materials.

For better understanding of this chapter

- Proper understanding of vector products is required.
- Quick revision of magnetic field and magnetic dipole moment of chapter 5 will be helpful.

Introduction

In previous chapter, we studied about magnetic effects of electric current with explanation how conductors behave like magnets.

In this chapter, we will study about magnets and magnetic materials in terms of magnetism and magnetisation of matter. It will be followed by knowledge of types of magnets, magnetic dipole and their magnetic fields.

Module 1

Magnet, Magnetic Dipole and Magnetic Field

- Bar Magnet • Magnetic Field Lines • Bar Magnet as an Equivalent Solenoid
- Magnetic Field Strength at a Point due to Magnetic Dipole or Bar Magnet
- Bar Magnet in a Uniform Magnetic Field • Magnetism and Gauss' Law

Bar Magnet

A bar magnet consists of two equal and non-separable magnetic poles. One pole is designated as north pole (*N*) and the other as south pole (*S*). These poles are separated at a small distance but they are not exactly at the ends. The distance between two poles of a bar magnet is known as **magnetic length of a magnet.** Its direction is from *S*-pole of the magnet to *N*-pole and is represented by $2l$. This length is sometimes also known as **effective length** (L_e) of the magnet and is less than its geometric length (L_g).

Mentor's TiP

For a bar magnet, $L_e = \left(\frac{5}{6}\right) L_g$

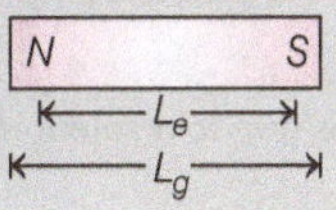

Pole Strength

Like electric charge, we have equivalent analogous in magnetism which is known as pole strength. Thus, **pole strength can be defined as the strength of a magnetic pole to attract magnetic materials towards itself.** It is a scalar quantity and its SI unit is ampere-metre (A-m). The strength of *N*-pole and *S*-pole of a magnet is conventionally represented by $+m$ and $-m$, respectively. It depends on the nature of material and area of cross-section of the magnet.

Strength of *N*-pole and *S*-pole of a magnet is always equal and opposite ($+m$ and $-m$).

General Properties of Magnet

Properties of a magnet are discussed below.

1. Directional Property

When a magnet is suspended freely, then it points in the earth's *N*-*S* direction (in magnetic meridian).

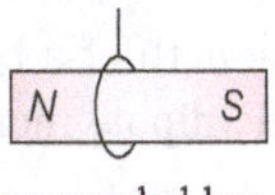

Freely suspended bar magnet

2. Monopole Non-existence Property

If a magnet is broken into number of pieces, then each piece behaves as an individual magnet rather than isolated poles. This means that monopoles do not exist.

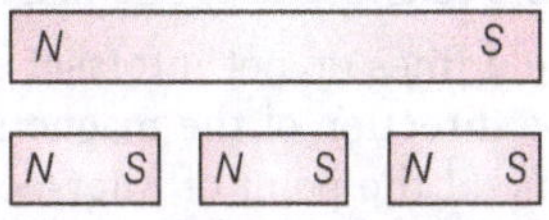

If a bar magnet is broken, each piece behaves as a small magnet

3. Attractive/Repulsive Property

Like magnetic poles repel each other and unlike magnetic poles attract each other.

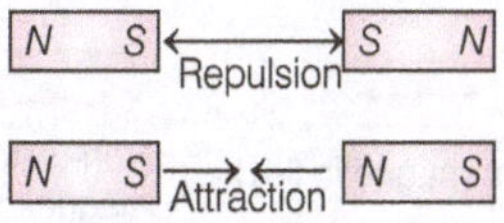

Like poles repel and unlike poles attract

Note Repulsion is a sure test of magnetism.

4. Earth behaves like a magnet with magnetic field from south to north (approx.)

5. Magnets can be made using iron and its alloys.

Magnetic Dipole Moment

It is the product of the strength of either of the pole strength and the magnetic length of the magnet. It is a vector quantity and it is represented by **M**.

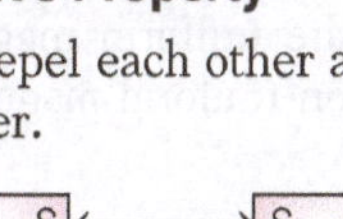

Magnetic moment of dipole

The direction of magnetic dipole moment is same as that of $2\mathbf{l}$. Therefore, $\mathbf{M} = m(2\mathbf{l})$

Its SI unit is ampere-metre^2 (A-m^2).

Magnetic Field Lines

The magnetic field lines of a magnetic field are the imaginary lines which continuously represent the direction of that magnetic field.

Properties of Magnetic Field Lines

(i) The magnetic field lines of a magnet form closed continuous loops. This property is unlike electric field lines, which begin from a positive charge and terminate at the negative charge or escape to infinity.

(ii) At any point, tangent to the magnetic field line represents the direction of net magnetic field (**B**) at that point.

(iii) Larger the number of field lines crossing per unit area, stronger is the magnitude of the magnetic field B.

(iv) Magnetic field lines do not intersect each other, if they did, the direction of the magnetic field would not be unique at the point of intersection.

(v) The direction of field lines is from N to S, if they are outside the magnet and from S to N, if they are inside the magnet.

(vi) Fig. (a) shows the uniform magnetic field lines and Fig. (b) shows non-uniform magnetic field lines.

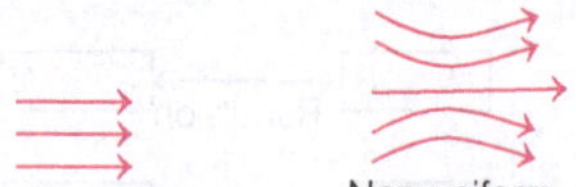

Uniform magnetic field (a) Non-uniform magnetic field (b)

(vii) Magnetic field lines can come out and go into a magnetic material at any angle.

Different Patterns of Magnetic Field Lines

Few patterns of magnetic field lines around a magnet or a pair of magnets are shown below

(a)

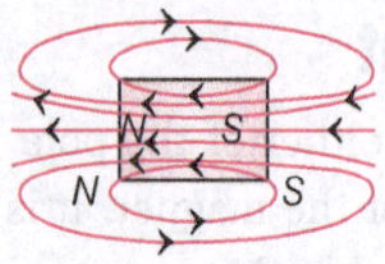

Magnetic field lines due to a bar magnet (form closed loops)

(b)

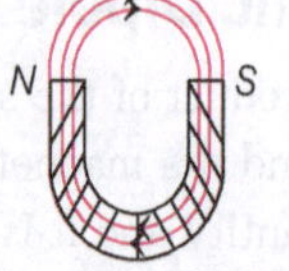

Magnetic field lines due to a horse shoe magnet (form closed loops)

(c)

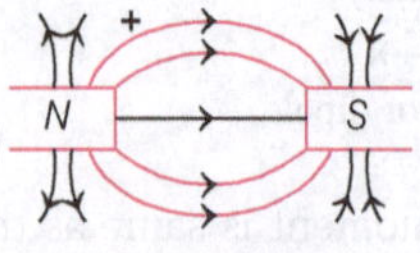

Magnetic field lines between two unlike poles (contract longitudinally)

(d)

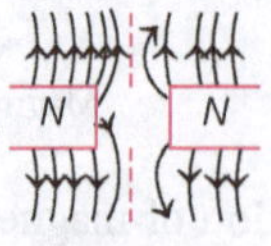

Magnetic field lines between two like poles (repel each other laterally)

Mentor's Tip

While comparing bar magnet with magnetic dipole, we can easily understand that bar magnet acts like magnetic dipole.

Bar Magnet as an Equivalent Solenoid

The magnetic field lines for a bar magnet and a current carrying solenoid resembles very closely. Therefore, a bar magnet can be thought as a large number of circulating currents in analogy with a solenoid. The expression for the magnetic field due to a solenoid,

$$B = \frac{\mu_0}{4\pi} \cdot \frac{2m}{r^3}$$

where, r is the distance between the centre of solenoid to the required point.

This expression is same as the expression for magnetic field of a bar magnet at its axial point. Thus, a bar magnet and a solenoid produce similar magnetic fields.

Therefore magnetic field lines associated with a solenoid are also similar to a bar magnet as shown in the figure.

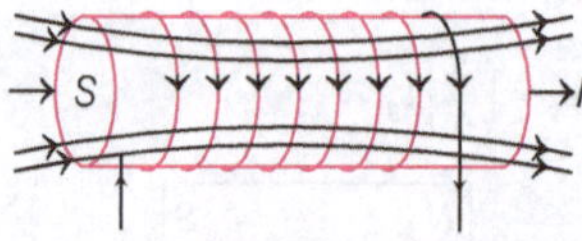

Magnetic field lines due to a solenoid carrying current

Magnetic Field Strength at a Point due to Magnetic Dipole or Bar Magnet

The strength of a magnetic field at any point is defined as the force experienced by a hypothetical unit strength north pole placed at that point.

i.e. $\mathbf{B} = \frac{\mathbf{F}}{m}$, where m is the pole strength of hypothetical north pole. Magnetic field strength is a vector quantity.

The direction of magnetic field **B** is the direction along which hypothetical north pole would tend to move, if free to do so. We have used the word hypothetical north pole in the above discussion because an isolated magnetic pole does not exist.

Let us now calculate the magnetic field strength at different points of magnetic dipole (or bar magnet).

1. When Point lies on Axial Line of a Bar Magnet

Let $2l$ be the magnetic length of a bar magnet with its centre at O. The magnetic dipole moment of the magnet is

M, where $M = m \times 2l$. The distance of the observation point P on the axial line from the centre of the magnet be $OP = r$.

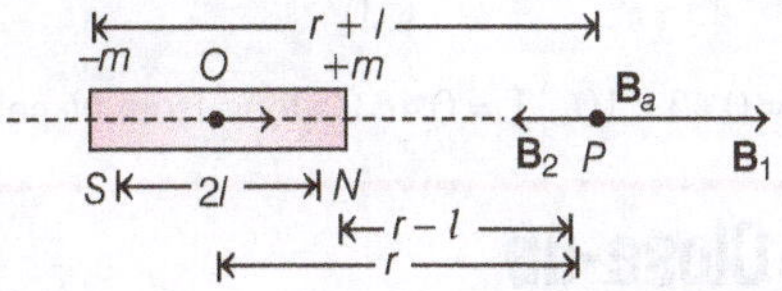

Magnetic field of bar magnet on axial line

If m is the strength of each pole, then magnetic field strength at P due to N-pole of magnet is given by

$$\mathbf{B}_1 = \frac{\mu_0}{4\pi} \times \frac{m}{(NP)^2} = \frac{\mu_0}{4\pi} \frac{m}{(r-l)^2}, \text{ along } OP$$

Magnetic field strength at P due to S-pole of magnet,

$$\mathbf{B}_2 = \frac{\mu_0}{4\pi} \times \frac{m}{(SP)^2} = \frac{\mu_0}{4\pi} \frac{m}{(r+l)^2}, \text{ along } PO$$

$\therefore$ Magnetic field strength at P due to the bar magnet,

$$\mathbf{B}_a = B_1 - B_2 = \frac{\mu_0}{4\pi} \frac{2Mr}{(r^2 - l^2)^2} \qquad (\because M = 2ml)$$

(Here, - ve sign is due to opposite direction)

When the magnet is short, $l^2 << r^2$, such that l^2 is neglected, then

$$\mathbf{B}_a = \frac{\mu_0}{4\pi} \frac{2\mathbf{M}r}{r^4} \Rightarrow \boxed{\mathbf{B}_a = \frac{\mu_0}{4\pi} \frac{2\mathbf{M}}{r^3}} \qquad \text{...(i)}$$

The direction of $\mathbf{B}_a$ is along OP.

2. When Point lies on Equatorial Line of a Bar Magnet

In figure given below, the point P is shown on equatorial line of the same bar magnet, where $OP = r$.

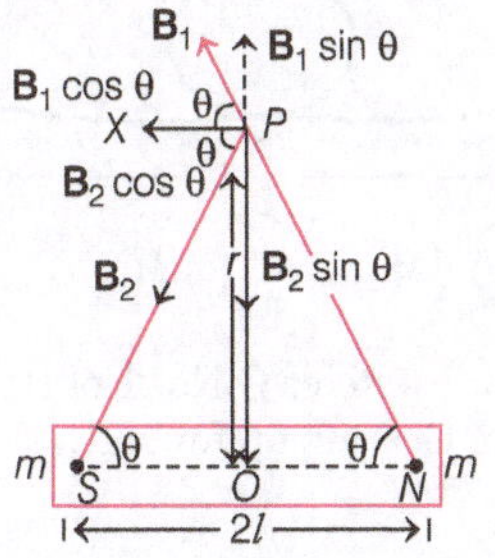

Magnetic field of bar magnet on equitorial line

Magnetic field strength at P due to N-pole of magnet,

$$\mathbf{B}_1 = \frac{\mu_0}{4\pi} \frac{m}{(NP)^2} = \frac{\mu_0}{4\pi} \frac{m}{(r^2 + l^2)}, \text{ from } N\text{- pole to point } P$$

Magnetic field strength at P due to S-pole of magnet,

$$\mathbf{B}_2 = \frac{\mu_0}{4\pi} \frac{m}{(SP)^2} = \frac{\mu_0}{4\pi} \frac{m}{(r^2 + l^2)}, \text{ from point } P \text{ to } S\text{-pole}$$

As, $B_1 = B_2$ in magnitude, their vertical components $B_1 \sin\theta$ along OP produced and $B_2 \sin\theta$ along PO will cancel out. However, horizontal components along PX will add. Therefore, magnetic field strength at P due to the bar magnet,

$$\mathbf{B}_e = \mathbf{B}_1 \cos\theta + \mathbf{B}_2 \cos\theta = 2\, B_2 \cos\theta, \text{ along } PX$$

$$\therefore \quad \mathbf{B}_e = \frac{\mu_0}{4\pi} \frac{\mathbf{m} \times 2\mathbf{l}}{(r^2 + l^2)^{3/2}}$$

$$\Rightarrow \quad \mathbf{B}_e = \frac{\mu_0}{4\pi} \frac{\mathbf{M}}{(r^2 + l^2)^{3/2}}$$

If the magnet is short, $l^2 << r^2$, such that l^2 is neglected.

$$\therefore \quad \mathbf{B}_e = \frac{\mu_0}{4\pi} \frac{\mathbf{M}}{(r^2)^{3/2}}$$

$$\Rightarrow \quad \boxed{\mathbf{B}_e = \frac{\mu_0}{4\pi} \frac{\mathbf{M}}{r^3}} \qquad \text{...(ii)}$$

The direction of $\mathbf{B}_e$ is along PX, a line parallel to line joining N-pole to S-pole.

On dividing Eq. (i) by Eq. (ii), we get

$$\frac{B_a}{B_e} = 2$$

$$\Rightarrow \quad B_a = 2B_e$$

Hence, magnitude of magnetic field due to a short bar magnet at any point on the axial line of magnet is twice the magnetic field at a point at the same distance on the equatorial line of the magnet.

> **Concept ladder** Magnetic field at an angle θ with the axis at distance r from the centre of magnet can calculated as
>
> $$\mathbf{B} = \frac{\mu_0}{4\pi} \frac{M}{r^3} \sqrt{(1 + 3\cos^2\theta)}$$

Example 1. *Consider a short magnetic dipole of magnetic length 10 cm. Find its geometric length.*

Sol. Geometric length of a magnet is $\frac{6}{5}$ times its magnetic length.

$$\therefore \text{ Geometric length} = \frac{6}{5} \times 10 = 12 \text{ cm}$$

Example 2. *A thin bar magnet of length 2L is bent at the mid-point, so that the angle between them is 60°. Find the new length of the magnet.*

Sol. On bending the magnet, the length of the magnet,

$AC = AO + OC$

$= L\sin\left(\frac{\theta}{2}\right) + L\sin\left(\frac{\theta}{2}\right)$

$= 2L\sin 30° = 2L \times \frac{1}{2} = L$

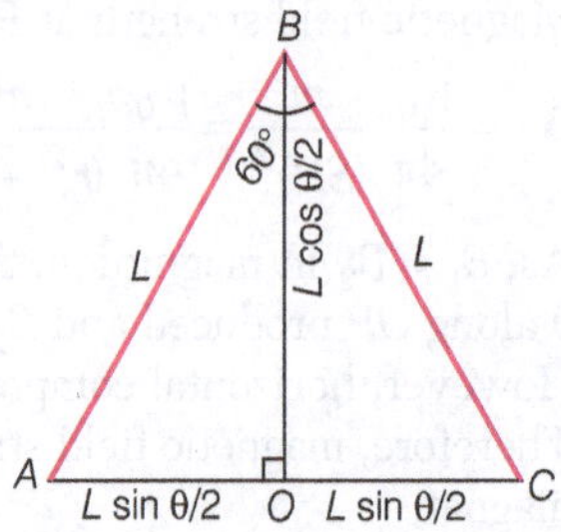

Example 3. *A bar magnet of length 0.1 m has pole strength of 50 A-m. Calculate the magnetic field at a distance of 0.2 m from its centre on (i) its axial line (ii) and its equatorial line.*

Sol. Here, $m = 50$ A-m, $r = 0.2$ m, $2l = 0.1$ m or $l = 0.05$ m

$\therefore$ Magnetic dipole moment,

$$M = m(2l) = 50 \times 0.1 = 5 \text{ A-m}^2$$

$$\text{(i) } B_{\text{axial}} = \frac{\mu_0}{4\pi}\frac{2Mr}{(r^2 - l^2)^2} = \frac{10^{-7} \times 2 \times 5 \times 0.2}{(0.2^2 - 0.05^2)^2}$$

$$= 1.42 \times 10^{-4}\text{T}$$

$$\text{(ii) } B_{\text{equi}} = \frac{\mu_0}{4\pi}\frac{M}{(r^2 + l^2)^{3/2}} = \frac{10^{-7} \times 5}{(0.2^2 + 0.05^2)^{3/2}}$$

$$= 5.71 \times 10^{-5}\text{T}$$

We can replace $r^2 - l^2 \approx r^2 \approx r^2 + l^2$ in case of $r >> l$. Here, we have not used it because l is not negligible w.r.t. r.

Example 4. *Calculate the magnetic induction at a point 1 Å away from a proton, measured along its axis of spin. The magnetic moment of the proton is 1.4×10^{-26} A-m^2.*

Sol. On the axis of a magnetic dipole, magnetic induction is given by

$$B = \frac{\mu_0}{4\pi} \cdot \frac{2M}{r^3}$$

Substituting the values, we get

$$B = \frac{(10^{-7})(2)(1.4 \times 10^{-26})}{(10^{-10})^3}$$

$$= 2.8 \times 10^{-3}\text{ T} = 2.8\text{ mT}$$

Example 5. *A short bar magnet has a magnetic moment of 0.48 JT^{-1}. Give the direction and magnitude of the magnetic field produced by the magnet at a distance of 10 cm from the centre of magnet on (i) the axial and (ii) the equatorial lines (normal bisector) of the magnet.*

Sol. (i) When the point lies on the axial line, then let B_1 be the magnetic field at P.

$$r = 10\text{ cm} = 0.1\text{ m}$$

$$\therefore \quad B_1 = \frac{\mu_0}{4\pi} \cdot \frac{2M}{r^3} = 10^{-7} \times \frac{2 \times 0.48}{(0.1)^3}$$

$$= 0.96 \times 10^{-4}\text{T from } S\text{-pole to } N\text{-pole}$$

(ii) Let B_2 be the magnetic field at point P on the equatorial line.

$$\therefore B_2 = \frac{\mu_0}{4\pi} \cdot \frac{M}{r^3} = 10^{-7} \times \frac{0.48}{(0.1)^3}$$

$$= 0.48 \times 10^{-4}\text{T} = 0.48\text{ G along from } N\text{-pole to } S\text{-pole}$$

NEET Close-up

Example Similar to PYQ Asked in NEET 2024

The length of a magnetised steel wire is $6l$ and its magnetic moment is M. It is bent into the middle of its length such that the two arms make an angle of 74° with each other. Then, the magnetic moment of this new magnet is

(a) $\frac{17}{5}M$ (b) $\frac{16}{3}M$ (c) $\frac{16}{9}M$ (d) $\frac{18}{5}M$

Sol. (*d*)

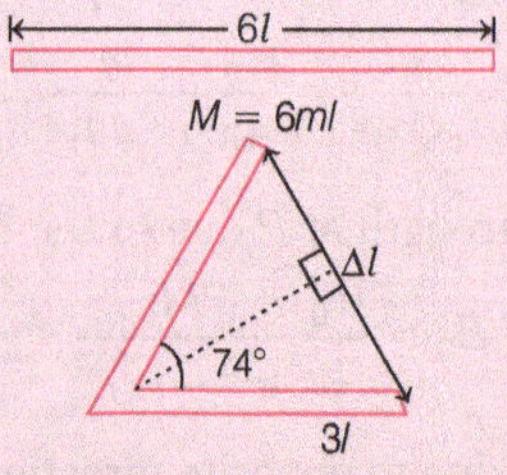

$$\Delta l = 2 \times 3l \times \sin 37°$$

$$\Delta l = 2 \times 3l \times \frac{3}{5} = \frac{18l}{5}$$

$$M' = m\left(\frac{18l}{5}\right)$$

$$M' = \frac{18}{5}M$$

Skill Builder

An iron bar of length $2L$ has magnetic moment M is bent in a weired shape as shown in the diagram. Its magnetic moment will be

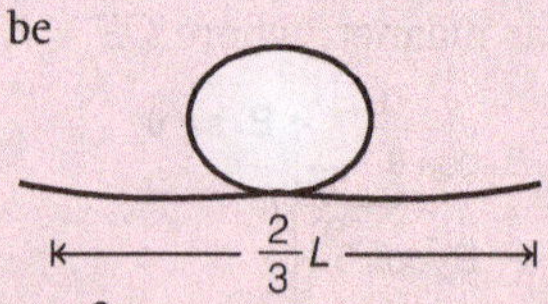

(a) $\frac{M}{3}$ (b) $\frac{2}{3}M$ (c) M (d) $\frac{M}{2}$

For More Practice Refer Q.No. 1 of step up practice 1 and Q.No. 15 of Gearing up for NEET.

Bar Magnet in a Uniform Magnetic Field

When a bar magnet is placed in a uniform magnetic field, torque acts on it. Also, magnetic potential energy is associated with the magnet due to its orientation, which is discussed in following sections.

Torque on Bar Magnet in a Uniform Magnetic Field

Let us consider a bar magnet of length $2l$ placed in a uniform magnetic field B. Let the magnetic axis of the bar magnet makes angle θ with the field $\mathbf{B}$, as shown in the figure.

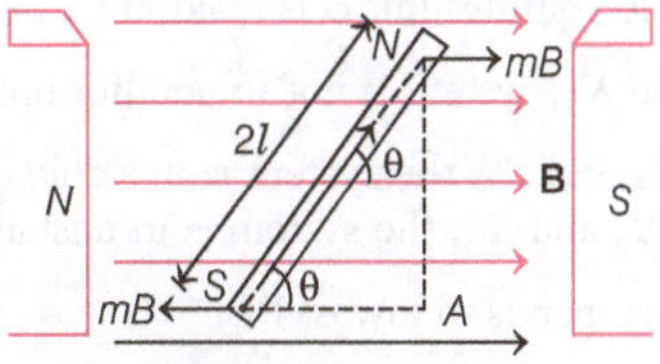

Torque on a bar magnet

Then, force on N-pole $= mB$, along $\mathbf{B}$

and force on S-pole $= mB$, opposite to $\mathbf{B}$

where, m = strength of each pole

and B = strength of magnetic field.

These forces being equal and opposite form a couple, which tends to rotate the magnet clockwise, so as to align it along $\mathbf{B}$. So, the moment of couple or torque is given by

$$\tau = \text{Force} \times \text{Perpendicular distance}$$

$$\Rightarrow \quad \tau = mB \times NA \quad \text{...(i)}$$

In ΔNAS, $\sin\theta = \dfrac{NA}{NS} = \dfrac{NA}{2l}$

$\therefore \quad NA = 2l \sin\theta$

Eq. (i) becomes, $\tau = mB \times 2l \sin\theta$

Also, $M = m \times 2l$

$$\Rightarrow \quad \boxed{\tau = MB\sin\theta} \quad \text{...(ii)}$$

In vector form, we can rewrite this equation as $\boxed{\boldsymbol{\tau} = \mathbf{M} \times \mathbf{B}}$

The direction of τ is perpendicular to the plane containing $\mathbf{M}$ and $\mathbf{B}$ and is given by right handed screw rule.

Work Done or Potential Energy of a Magnetic Dipole (Bar Magnet) in a Magnetic Field

The torque acting on the dipole tends to align it in the direction of the field. Work has to be done in rotating the dipole against the action of the magnetic torque. This work done is stored in the form of potential energy of the dipole. Now, a small amount of work done in rotating the dipole through a small angle $d\theta$ is given by

$$dW = \tau\, d\theta = MB\sin\theta \cdot d\theta \quad \text{[from Eq. (ii)]}$$

Total work done in rotating the dipole from $\theta = \theta_0$ to $\theta = \theta$ can be obtained by integrating the above expression.

$\therefore$ The potential energy of the dipole is given by

$$U = W = -MB(\cos\theta - \cos\theta_0)$$

Let us assume that, $\theta_0 = 90°$

So, $U = W = -MB(\cos\theta - \cos 90°)$

Therefore, $\boxed{U = -MB\cos\theta}$

In vector notation, we may rewrite this equation as

$$\boxed{U = -\mathbf{M} \cdot \mathbf{B}}$$

Special Cases

(i) When dipole is perpendicular to magnetic field its potential energy is zero, *i.e.* when $\theta = 90°$.

$$\Rightarrow \quad U = -MB\cos\theta = -MB\cos 90° = 0$$

(ii) When the magnetic dipole is aligned along the magnetic field, then it is in stable equilibrium having minimum potential energy, *i.e.* when $\theta = 0°$.

$$\Rightarrow \quad U = -MB\cos\theta = -MB\cos 0° = -MB$$

(iii) When $\theta = 180°$, (unstable equilibrium)

$$U = -MB\cos\theta = -MB\cos 180° = MB$$

In this condition, potential energy is maximum.

Example 6. *A magnet of magnetic moment $50\hat{\mathbf{i}}$ A-m^2 is placed along the X-axis in a magnet field $\mathbf{B} = (0.5\hat{\mathbf{i}} + 3\hat{\mathbf{j}})T$. Find the torque acting on the magnet.*

Sol. $\because$ Torque, $\boldsymbol{\tau} = \mathbf{M} \times \mathbf{B}$

where, $\mathbf{M}$ is magnetic moment and $\mathbf{B}$ is magnetic field.

Given, $\mathbf{M} = 50\hat{\mathbf{i}}$ A-m^2, $B = (0.5\hat{\mathbf{i}} + 3\hat{\mathbf{j}})$ T

$\therefore \quad \tau = 50\hat{\mathbf{i}} \times (0.5\hat{\mathbf{i}} + 3\hat{\mathbf{j}}) = 150(\hat{\mathbf{i}} \times \hat{\mathbf{j}})$

Using $\hat{\mathbf{i}} \times \hat{\mathbf{j}} = \hat{\mathbf{k}}$, we have $\tau = 150\,\hat{\mathbf{k}}$ N-m

Example 7. *A bar magnet when placed at an angle of 30° to the direction of magnetic field of 5×10^{-2} T, experiences a moment of couple 2.5×10^{-6} N-m. If the length of the magnet is 5 cm, then what will be its pole strength?*

Sol. Here, $\theta = 30°$, $B = 5 \times 10^{-2}$ T,

$\tau = 2.5 \times 10^{-6}$ N-m and $2l = 5\text{cm} = 0.05$ m

$\therefore$ Torque, $\tau = MB\sin\theta = m(2l)B\sin\theta$

$$\Rightarrow \quad m = \frac{\tau}{B(2l)\sin\theta} = \frac{2.5 \times 10^{-6}}{5 \times 10^{-2}(0.05)\sin 30°}$$

$\therefore \quad m = 2 \times 10^{-3}$ A-m

Example 8. *The work done in turning a magnet of magnetic moment M by an angle 90° from the meridian is n times the corresponding work done to turn it through an angle of 60°. What is the value of n?*

Sol. Here, $W_1 = MB(\cos 0° - \cos 90°) = MB(1-0) = MB$

Similarly, $W_2 = MB(\cos 0° - \cos 60°) = MB\left(1 - \dfrac{1}{2}\right) = \dfrac{MB}{2}$

$\therefore \quad W_1 = 2W_2 \Rightarrow n = 2$

Example 9. *A bar magnet of magnetic moment 2.0 A-m^2 is free to rotate about a vertical axis through its centre. The magnet is released from rest from the east-west position. Find the kinetic energy of the magnet as it takes the north-south position. The horizontal component of the earth's* magnetic field is $B = 25\ \mu T$. Earth's magnetic field is from south to north.

Sol. Gain in kinetic energy = Loss in potential energy

Thus, $\quad KE = U_i - U_f$

As, $\quad U = -MB\cos\theta$

Initially, $\theta_i = \frac{\pi}{2}$ (for east-west direction)

and finally, $\theta_f = 0°$ (for north-south direction)

$\therefore \quad KE = -MB\cos\left(\frac{\pi}{2}\right) - (-MB\cos 0°) = -0 + MB = MB$

Substituting the values, we have

$$KE = (2.0)(25 \times 10^{-6})\ J = 50\ \mu J$$

Example 10. *A short bar magnet of magnetic moment $m = 0.32\ JT^{-1}$ is placed in a uniform magnetic field 0.15T. If the bar magnet is free to rotate in the plane of the field, which orientation would correspond to its (i) stable and (ii) unstable equilibrium? What is the potential energy of the magnet in each case?*

Sol. (i) When **m** is parallel to **B**, then the magnet is in stable equilibrium, *i.e.* $\theta = 0°$

$\therefore$ PE in this case is given by

$$U = -\mathbf{m}\cdot\mathbf{B} = -mB\cos\theta = -0.32 \times 0.15 \times 1 = -0.048\ J$$

(ii) When **m** is anti-parallel to **B**, then the magnet will be in unstable equilibrium, *i.e.* $\theta = 180°$

Thus potential energy in this case is given by

$$U = -\mathbf{m}\cdot\mathbf{B} = -mB\cos 180°$$
$$= -0.32 \times 0.15 \times (-1) = +0.048\ J$$

Example 11. *Consider the situation shown in the diagram, where a small magnetised needle A is placed at a centre marked as O. The direction of its magnetic moment is indicated by arrow. The other arrows show different positions (and orientations of the magnetic moment) of another identical magnetised needle X.*

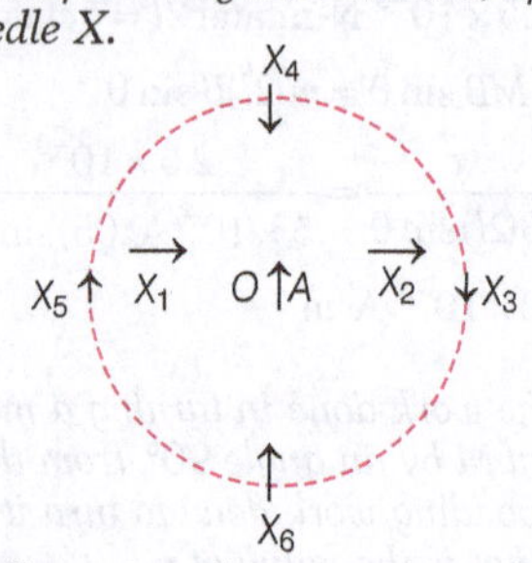

(i) In which configuration, the system is not in equilibrium?

(ii) In which configuration is the system in (a) stable and (b) unstable equilibrium?

(iii) Which configuration corresponds to the lowest potential energy among all the configurations shown?

Sol. Potential energy arises due to the position of dipole X in magnetic field of A.

Magnetic field due to A,

On end position, $\mathbf{B}_A = \frac{\mu_0}{4\pi}\cdot\frac{2M}{r^3}$, along **M**

On broadside position, $\mathbf{B}_P' = \frac{\mu_0}{4\pi}\cdot\frac{\mathbf{M}}{r^3}$, opposite to **M**

The PE, $U = -\mathbf{M}\cdot\mathbf{B} = -MB\cos\theta$

For stable equilibrium, U is minimum, *i.e.* $\theta = 0°$

For unstable equilibrium, U is maximum, *i.e.* $\theta = 180°$

(i) In X_1 and X_2, system is not in equilibrium.

(ii) (a) In X_5 and X_6, the system is in stable equilibrium and (b) in X_4 and X_3, the system is in unstable equilibrium.

(iii) X_6 corresponds to lowest PE,

$$U = -MB\cos\theta = -M\cdot\frac{\mu_0}{4\pi}\frac{2M}{r^3}\cos 0° = -\frac{\mu_0 \cdot 2M^2}{4\pi r^3} = U_{min}$$

Concept ladder A bar magnet freely suspended in a uniform magnetic field freely with period,

$$T = 2\pi\sqrt{\frac{I}{MB}}$$

Here, I = moment of inertia of bar magnet,
M = magnetic dipole moment
and B = uniform magnetic field.

Comparison between an Electric Dipole and a Magnetic Dipole

The behaviour of a magnetic dipole (may be a bar magnet also) is similar to the behaviour of an electric dipole. The only difference is that the electric dipole moment **p** is replaced by magnetic dipole moment **M** and the constant $\frac{1}{4\pi\varepsilon_0}$ is replaced by $\frac{\mu_0}{4\pi}$.

The table given below gives a comparison between an electric dipole and a magnetic dipole.

Physical quantity to be compared	Electric dipole	Magnetic dipole
Dipole moment	$p = q(2l)$	$M = m(2l)$
Direction of dipole moment	From negative charge to the positive charge	From south pole to north pole
Net force in uniform field	0	0
Net torque in uniform field	$\tau = \mathbf{p} \times \mathbf{E}$	$\tau = \mathbf{M} \times \mathbf{B}$
Field at far away point on the axis	$\frac{1}{4\pi\varepsilon_0}\cdot\frac{2p}{r^3}$ (along **p**)	$\frac{\mu_0}{4\pi}\cdot\frac{2M}{r^3}$ (along **M**)
Field at far away point on perpendicular bisector	$\frac{1}{4\pi\varepsilon_0}\cdot\frac{p}{r^3}$ (opposite to **p**)	$\frac{\mu_0}{4\pi}\cdot\frac{M}{r^3}$ (opposite to **M**)
Potential energy	$U_\theta = -\mathbf{p}\cdot\mathbf{E} = -pE\cos\theta$	$U_\theta = -\mathbf{M}\cdot\mathbf{B} = -MB\cos\theta$
Work done in rotating the dipole	$W_{\theta_1-\theta_2} = pE(\cos\theta_1 - \cos\theta_2)$	$W_{\theta_1-\theta_2} = MB(\cos\theta_1 - \cos\theta_2)$

In the table, θ is the angle between field (E or B) and dipole moment (p or M).

Magnetism and Gauss' Law

The Gauss's law of magnetism states that, "the surface integral of a magnetic field over a closed surface is zero, *i.e.* the net magnetic flux through any closed surface is always zero".

$$\oint \mathbf{B} \cdot d\mathbf{S} = 0$$

Consequences of Gauss' Law

(i) Consider a Gaussian surface (any closed surface) enclosing one of the poles (say south) of the magnet is shown in figure. Here, the number of field lines entering the Gaussian surface is same as the number of lines leaving it. *i.e.* Net magnetic flux for the whole Gaussian surface is zero.

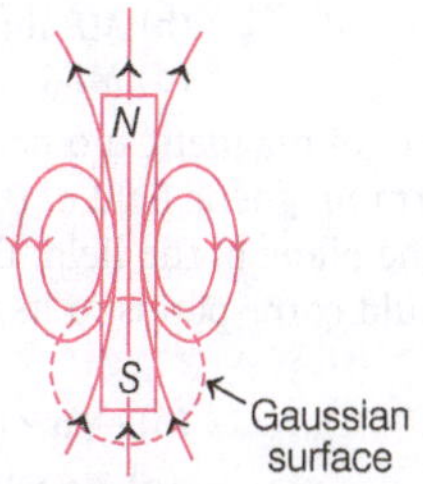

(ii) The Gauss's theorem in magnetism implies that isolated magnetic poles do not exist.

(iii) In case of open surface, $\int_S \mathbf{B} \cdot d\mathbf{S} = \phi_B$ (magnetic flux associated with the surface)

(iv) The magnetic poles always exist as unlike pairs of equal strengths.

STEP UP Practice 1

1. A magnet with moment m is given. If it is bent into a semi-circular form, its new magnetic moment will be

(a) $\frac{m}{\pi}$ (b) $\frac{m}{2}$ (c) m (d) $\frac{2m}{\pi}$

2. A bar magnet of magnetic moment M_1 is axially cut into two equal parts. If these two pieces are arranged perpendicular to each other, the resultant magnetic moment is M_2. The value of M_1 / M_2 is

(a) $\frac{1}{2\sqrt{2}}$ (b) 1 (c) $\frac{1}{\sqrt{2}}$ (d) $\sqrt{2}$

3. Two solenoids acting as short bar magnets P and Q are arranged such that centres are on the X-axis and are separated by a large distance. The magnetic axes of P and Q are along X and Y-axes, respectively. At a point R, mid-way between their centres, if B is the magnitude of induction due to Q, then the magnitude of total induction at R due to the both magnets is

(a) $3B$ (b) $\sqrt{5}B$ (c) $\frac{\sqrt{5}}{2}B$ (d) B

4. **Statement I** The poles of a bar magnet cannot be separated.

Statement II Magnetic monopoles do not exist.

In the light of the above statements, choose the most appropriate answer from the options given below.

(a) Both Statement I and Statement II are incorrect.
(b) Statement I is correct but Statement II is incorrect.
(c) Statement I is incorrect but Statement II is correct.
(d) Both Statement I and Statement II are correct.

5. If the bar magnet of magnetic moment 0.40 A-m^2 is replaced by a solenoid of cross-sectional area 2×10^{-4} m^2 and 1000 turns but of the same magnetic moment, the current flowing through the solenoid is

(a) −2 A (b) 2 A
(c) 20 A (d) 1 A

6. A bar magnet of magnetic moment **M**, is placed in a magnetic field of induction **B**. The torque exerted on it is

(a) $\mathbf{M} \times \mathbf{B}$ (b) $-\mathbf{B} \cdot \mathbf{M}$
(c) $\mathbf{M} \cdot \mathbf{B}$ (d) $\mathbf{M} + \mathbf{B}$

7. The couple acting on a magnet of length 10 cm and pole strength 15 A-m, kept in a field of $B = 2 \times 10^{-5}$ T, at an angle of 30° is

(a) 1.5×10^{-5} N-m (b) 1.5×10^{-3} N-m
(c) 1.5×10^{-2} N-m (d) 1.5×10^{-6} N-m

8. A bar magnet is held at right angle to a uniform magnetic field. The couple acting on the magnet is to be halved by rotating it from this position. The angle of rotation is

(a) 60° (b) 45° (c) 30° (d) 75°

9. Magnetic lines of force due to a bar magnet do not intersect because

(a) a point always has a single net magnetic field
(b) the lines have similar charges and so repel each other
(c) the lines always diverge from a single point
(d) None of the above

10. **Statement I** Magnetic field lines can be entirely confined within the core of a toroid but not within a straight solenoid.

Statement II The magnetic field inside the solenoid is non-uniform.

In the light of the above statements, choose the most appropriate answer from the options given below.

(a) Both Statement I and Statement II are incorrect.
(b) Statement I is correct but Statement II is incorrect.
(c) Statement I is incorrect but Statement II is correct.
(d) Both Statement I and Statement II are correct.

11. If a bar magnet of magnetic moment M is freely suspended in a uniform magnetic field of strength B, then the work done in rotating the magnet through an angle θ is

(a) $MB(1 - \sin\theta)$ (b) $MB \sin\theta$
(c) $MB \cos\theta$ (d) $MB(1 - \cos\theta)$

12. A short bar magnet of magnetic moment $m = 0.32\ JT^{-1}$ is placed in a uniform magnetic field of 0.15 T. If the bar is free to rotate in the plane of the field, then the potential energy which would corresponds to its unstable equilibrium is
(a) 4.8×10^{-2} J (b) -4.8×10^{-2} J
(c) 7.5×10^{-2} J (d) 3.6×10^{5} J

13. A thin bar magnet is placed in a uniform magnetic field and is aligned with the field. The needle is now rotated by an angle of 45° and the work done is W. The torque on the magnetic needle at this position is
(a) zero (b) $\frac{W}{\sqrt{2}-1}$
(c) $\frac{W}{\sqrt{2}}$ (d) $\sqrt{2}W$

14. A bar magnet having a magnetic moment of $2 \times 10^{4}\ JT^{-1}$ is free to rotate in a horizontal plane. A horizontal magnetic field $B = 6 \times 10^{-4}$ T exists in the space. The work done in taking the magnet slowly from a direction parallel to the field to a direction 60° from the field is
(a) 0.6 J (b) 12 J
(c) 6 J (d) 2 J

15. What is the magnitude of the equatorial and axial fields due to a bar magnet of length 5.0 cm at a distance of 50 cm from its mid-point? The magnet moment of the bar magnet is 0.40 A-m^2.
(a) 3.2×10^{-6} T, 6.4×10^{-7} T
(b) 4.2×10^{5} T, 6×10^{-7} T
(c) 5×10^{-6} T, 3.2×10^{-7} T
(d) 3.2×10^{-7} T, 6.4×10^{-7} T

16. With reference to magnetic dipole (M), choose the incorrect pair.

(a) Equatorial magnetic field for a short dipole	→	(i) $-\frac{\mu_0 M}{4\pi r^3}$
(b) Torque	→	(ii) $\mathbf{M} \times \mathbf{B}$
(c) Potential energy	→	(iii) $-\mathbf{M} \cdot \mathbf{B}$
(d) Axial magnetic field for a short dipole	→	(iv) $\frac{\mu_0 3M}{\pi r^3}$

17. Statement I When a magnetic dipole is placed in a non-uniform magnetic field, only a torque acts on the dipole.
Statement II Force would also acts on dipole, if magnetic field is uniform.
In the light of the above statements, choose the most appropriate answer from the options given below.
(a) Both Statement I and Statement II are incorrect.
(b) Statement I is correct but Statement II is incorrect.
(c) Statement I is incorrect but Statement II is correct.
(d) Both Statement I and Statement II are correct.

18. A dipole or current carrying loop is placed in a uniform magnetic field in four different orientations as shown in figure. The potential energy increases in order of

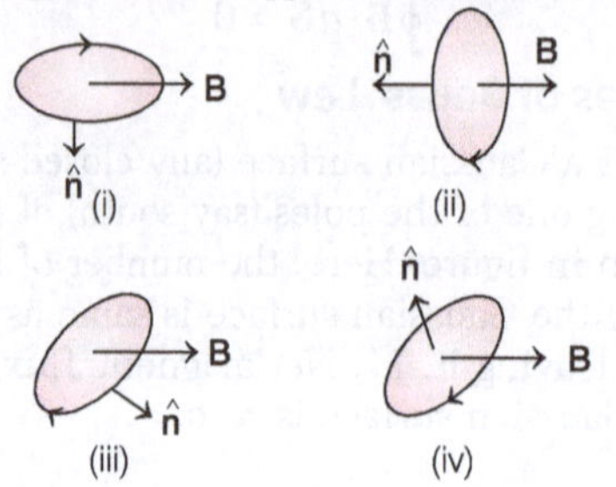

(a) (iii), (i), (iv) and (ii)
(b) (i), (ii), (iii) and (iv)
(c) (ii), (iii), (i) and (iv)
(d) (iv), (iii), (i) and (ii)

19. A bar magnet suspended freely in a uniform magnetic field is vibrating with a time period of 3 s. If the field strength is increased to 4 times of the earlier field strength, then the time period (in s) will be
(a) 12 (b) 6
(c) 1.5 (d) 0.75

20. The work done in turning a magnet of magnetic moment M by an angle of 90° from the meridian, is n times the corresponding work done to turn it through an angle of 60°. The value of n is given by
(a) 2 (b) 1
(c) 0.5 (d) 0.25

21. The net magnetic flux through any closed surface kept in a magnetic field is
(a) zero (b) $\frac{\mu_0}{4\pi}$
(c) $4\pi\mu_0$ (d) $\frac{4\mu_0}{\pi}$

22. Statement I Torque experienced by the bar magnet is maximum when field is applied perpendicular to magnetic moment.
Statement II Torque on a bar magnet depends on the angle between applied magnetic field and magnetic dipole moment.
In the light of the above statements, choose the most appropriate answer from the options given below.
(a) Both Statement I and Statement II are incorrect.
(b) Statement I is correct but Statement II is incorrect.
(c) Statement I is incorrect but Statement II is correct.
(d) Both Statement I and Statement II are correct.

Module 2

Properties of Magnetic Materials

- Some Important Terms Used in Magnetism • Classification of Substances on the Basis of Magnetic Behaviour
- Curie's Law

Some Important Terms Used in Magnetism

Magnetic materials have different properties, so some important terms which are used to define them, are given below

1. Magnetic Induction (*B*)

The number of magnetic lines of force inside a magnetic substance crossing per unit area normal to their direction is called the **magnetic induction** or **magnetic flux density** inside the substance. It is denoted by **B**.

The SI unit of **B** is tesla (T) or weber/metre^2 (Wb/m^2). The CGS unit is gauss (G).

$$1 \text{ Wb/m}^2 = 1 \text{ T} = 10^4 \text{ G}$$

2. Intensity of Magnetisation (*I*)

It is defined as the magnetic moment per unit volume of the magnetised substance. This basically represents the extent to which the substance is magnetised.

Thus, $$\mathbf{I} = \frac{\mathbf{M}}{V}$$

The SI unit of **I** is ampere/metre (A/m). Its dimensional formula is $[M^0L^{-1}T^0A]$.

Note For bar magnet, $I = m/A$.

Example 12. *The magnetic moment of a magnet* (15 *cm* × 2 *cm* × 1 *cm*) *is* 1.2 *A-m*^{2}. *Calculate its intensity of magnetisation.*

Sol. Given, magnetic moment, $M = 1.2$ A-m^2

Volume, $V = (15 \times 2 \times 1) \times 10^{-6} \text{m}^3 = 30 \times 10^{-6} \text{ m}^3$

∴ Intensity of magnetisation,

$$I = \frac{M}{V} = \frac{1.2}{30 \times 10^{-6}} = 4 \times 10^4 \text{Am}^{-1}$$

3. Magnetic Intensity or Magnetic Field Strength (*H*)

The capability of the magnetising field to magnetise the substance is expressed by means of a vector **H**, called the magnetic intensity of the field. It is defined through the vector relation, $\mathbf{H} = \frac{\mathbf{B}}{\mu_0} - \mathbf{I}$

The SI unit of **H** is same as that of **I**, *i.e.* ampere/metre (A/m). The CGS unit is oersted.

Mentor's Tip

- In vacuum, $I = 0$
  $\therefore H = \frac{B}{\mu_0}$.
- The magnetic field intensity of solenoid is $H = nI$. It is independent of the material of the core of a solenoid.
- When magnetic material is kept inside the solenoid, then
  $\mathbf{B} = \mathbf{B}_0 + \mathbf{B}_M$
  where, $\mathbf{B}_0$ = magnetic field due to magnetising field
  and $\mathbf{B}_m$ = magnetic field due to magnetisation of the material.

4. Magnetic Permeability (μ)

It is defined as the ratio of the magnetic induction **B** inside the magnetised substance to the magnetic intensity **H** of the magnetising field.

i.e. $$\mu = \frac{\mathbf{B}}{\mathbf{H}}$$

It is basically a measure of conduction of magnetic lines of force through a substance. The SI unit of magnetic permeability is weber/ampere-metre (Wb/A-m) or tesla metre-ampere^{-1} (TmA^{-1}).

5. Relative Magnetic Permeability (μ_r)

It is the ratio of the magnetic permeability μ of the substance to the permeability of free space.

Thus, $$\mu_r = \frac{\mu}{\mu_0}$$

μ_r is a pure ratio, hence dimensionless. For vacuum, its value is 1.

μ_r can also be defined as the ratio of the magnetic field B in the substance, when placed in magnetic field B_0. Thus,

$$\mu_r = \frac{B}{B_0}$$

6. Magnetic Susceptibility (χ_m)

It is the property of the substance which shows how easily a substance can be magnetised when kept in a magnetising field. It can also be defined as the ratio of intensity of magnetisation (I) in a substance to the magnetic intensity (H) applied to the substance, *i.e.* $\chi_m = \frac{I}{H}$.

It is a scalar quantity with no units and dimensions.

7. Relation between μ_r and χ_m

We have, $\mathbf{B} = \mu_0(\mathbf{I}+\mathbf{H})$

or $\quad B = \mu_0 H\left(\frac{I}{H}+1\right)$ or $B = B_0(\chi_m + 1)$

$$\Rightarrow \quad \frac{B}{B_0} = \chi_m + 1$$

But $\quad \frac{B}{B_0} = \frac{\mu}{\mu_0} = \mu_r$ = relative permeability

$$\therefore \quad \mu_r = \chi_m + 1$$

NEET Close-up

Example Similar to PYQ Asked in NEET 2020

A magnetic material of susceptibility 5499 is subjected to magnetising field of 1200 A/m. The permeability (in TmA^{-1}) of the material is

(a) $22\pi \times 10^{-4}$
(b) $26\pi \times 10^{-5}$
(c) $30\pi \times 10^{-2}$
(d) $48\pi \times 10^{-4}$

Sol. (a) $\mu_r = 1 + \chi_m$

$\Rightarrow \quad \mu_r = 1 + 5499 = 5500$

So, $\quad \mu = \mu_0 \mu_r$

$= 4\pi \times 10^{-7} \times 5500$

$\mu = 22\pi \times 10^{-4}\ TmA^{-1}$

Skill Builder

Relative permeability of iron is 5500, what will be its magnetic susceptibility?

(a) 5400
(b) 5499
(c) 5501
(d) 5599

For more Practice Refer Q. No. 8 of step-up practice 2 and Q. No. 70 of Gearing up for NEET.

Example 13. *The magnetising field of 20 CGS units produces a flux of 2400 CGS units in a bar of iron of cross-section 0.2 cm². Calculate the (i) permeability and (ii) susceptibility of the bar.*

Sol. Given, $H = 20$ oersted $= \frac{20 \times 10^3}{4\pi}$ A/m

$\phi = 2400$ Maxwell $= 2400 \times 10^{-8}$ Wb

and $\quad A = 0.2\ cm^2 = 0.2 \times 10^{-4}\ m^2$

$\therefore$ Magnetic field, $B = \frac{\phi}{A} = \frac{2400 \times 10^{-8}}{0.2 \times 10^{-4}} = 1.20\ Wb/m^2$

(i) The permeability of the bar material,

$$\mu = \frac{B}{H} = \frac{1.20}{(20/4\pi) \times 10^3} = 7.54 \times 10^{-4}\ H/m$$

(ii) The magnetic susceptibility and permeability of a material are related with each other as

$$\mu = \mu_0(1 + \chi_m) \quad \text{or} \quad \chi_m = \frac{\mu}{\mu_0} - 1$$

$$= \frac{7.54 \times 10^{-4}}{4\pi \times 10^{-7}} - 1 = 599$$

Example 14. *A solenoid having 2000 turns/m has a core of a material with relative permeability 220. The area of core is 4 cm² and carries a current of 5A. Calculate (i) magnetic intensity, (ii) magnetic field (iii) and magnetisation of the core. Also, calculate the pole strength developed.*

Sol. Given, $n = 2000$ turns/m, $i = 5A$,

$\mu_r = 220$, $A = 4\ cm^2 = 4 \times 10^{-4}$ m

(i) Magnetic intensity, $H = ni = 2000 \times 5 = 10000$ A/m

(ii) Magnetic field, $B = \mu H = \mu_0 \mu_r H$

$= 4\pi \times 10^{-7} \times 220 \times 10000 = 88\pi \times 10^{-2}$ T

(iii) As we know, $B = \mu_0(H + I)$

$88\pi \times 10^{-2} = 4\pi \times 10^{-7}(10000 + I)$

$\Rightarrow \quad 2.20 \times 10^6 = 10^4 + I$

$\therefore \quad I = (2.20 \times 10^6 - 10^4) = 2.19 \times 10^6$ A/m

Pole strength, $m = IA = (2.19 \times 10^6)(4 \times 10^{-4}) = 876$ A-m

Example 15. *The space within a current carrying solenoid is filled with magnesium having magnetic susceptibility, $\chi_{Mg} = 1.2 \times 10^{-5}$. What will be the percentage increase in magnetic field?*

Sol. Magnetic field without magnesium, $B_0 = \mu_0 H$

With magnesium, $B = \mu H = \mu_0(1 + \chi)H$

$\therefore$ % increase $= \left(\frac{B}{B_0} - 1\right) \times 100 = \chi_{Mg} \times 100$

$= 1.2 \times 10^{-5} \times 100 = 1.2 \times 10^{-3}$

Classification of Substances on the Basis of Magnetic Behaviour

All substances (whether solids, liquids or gases) may be classified into three categories in terms of their magnetic behaviour (i) paramagnetic, (ii) diamagnetic and (iii) ferromagnetic. In the following section, we will discuss them in details

1. Diamagnetic Substances

Diamagnetic substances are those which are repelled by a magnetic field. Examples of such substances are bismuth, antimony, gold, quartz, water, alcohol, etc.

They have following properties

(i) These substances when placed in a magnetic field, acquire feeble magnetisation in a direction opposite to that of the applied field. Thus, the magnetic lines of induction inside the substance is smaller than that outside of it.

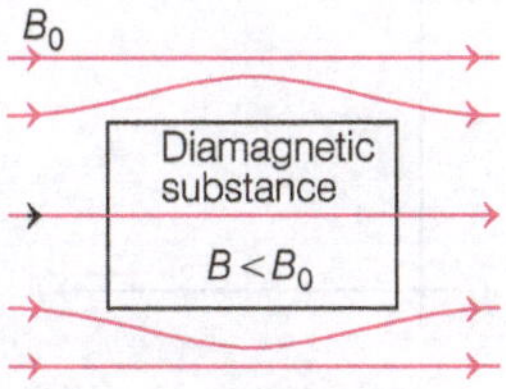

Magnetic field inside a diamagnetic substance

(ii) In a non-uniform magnetic field, these substances move from stronger to weaker parts of the external magnetic field. As, they acquire magnetisation in opposite direction, hence these are weakly repelled by the magnetic field.

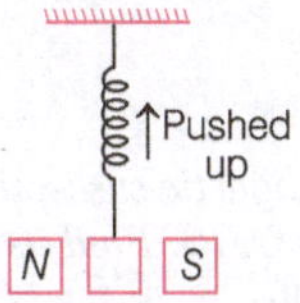

Diamagnetic substance in external field

(iii) If a diamagnetic liquid is filled in a narrow U-tube and one limb is placed in between the pole of an electromagnet, then the level of liquid depresses when the field is switched ON.

(iv) The relative permeability μ_r is slightly less than 1, *i.e.* $\mu_r < 1$.

(v) The susceptibility χ_m of such substances is always small and negative. It is constant and does not vary with field or the temperature as shown in figure.

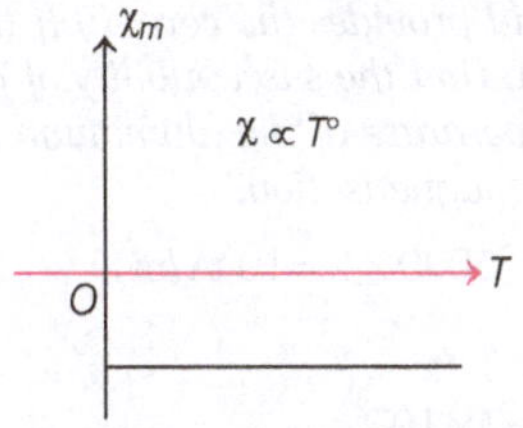

χ_m *versus* T graph for diamagnetic substance

(vi) Here, intensity of magnetisation varies inversely with magnetic field strength, *i.e.* $-I \propto H$ as shown in figure.

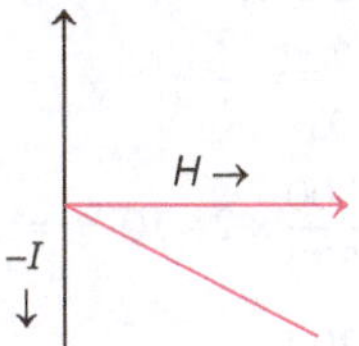

I versus H graph for diamagnetic substance

Mentor's Tip

- Diamagnetism is a universal property but in most of the substances, it is so weak that they behave like paramagnetic or ferromagnetic, etc.

2. Paramagnetic Substances

Paramagnetic substances are those which are attracted by a magnetic field. Examples of such substances are platinum, aluminium, chromium, manganese, $CuSO_4$ solution, etc.

They have following properties :

(i) These substances when placed in a magnetic field, acquire a feeble magnetisation in the same sense as the applied field.

Thus, the magnetic lines of induction inside the substance is slightly greater than outside of it.

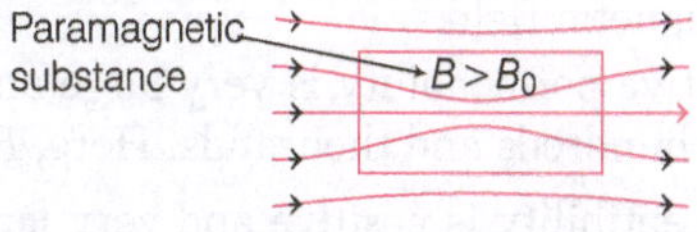

Magnetic field inside a paramagnetic substance

(ii) These substances are attracted towards regions of stronger magnetic field when placed in a non-uniform magnetic field.

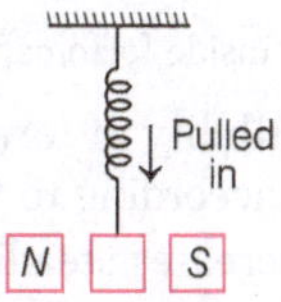

Paramagnetic substance in external field

Thus, they move from weaker to stronger parts of the field.

(iii) If a paramagnetic liquid is filled in a narrow U-tube and one limb is placed in between the pole pieces of an electromagnet such that the level of the liquid is in line with the field, then the liquid will rise in the limb as the field is switched ON.

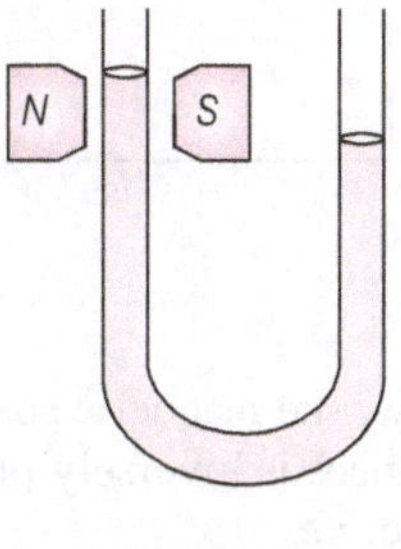

(iv) For paramagnetic substances, the relative permeability μ_r is slightly greater than one.

(v) Magnetic susceptibility is positive.

(vi) *I-H* curve is drawn below

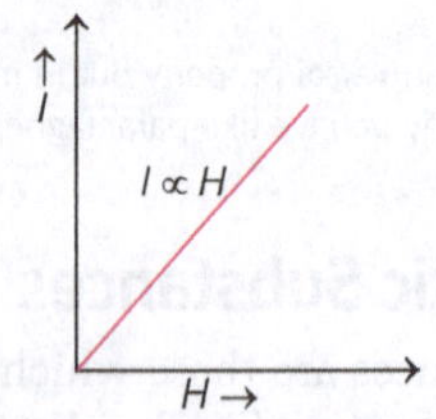

3. Ferromagnetic Substances

Ferromagnetic substances are those which are strongly attracted by a magnetic field. Examples of such substances are iron, nickel, steel, cobalt and their alloys. These substances resemble to a higher degree with paramagnetic substances as regard with their behaviour.

They have the following properties

(i) These substances are strongly magnetised by even a weak magnetic field.

(ii) The relative permeability is very large and is of the order of hundreds and thousands. Here, $B >> B_0$.

(iii) The susceptibility is positive and very large.

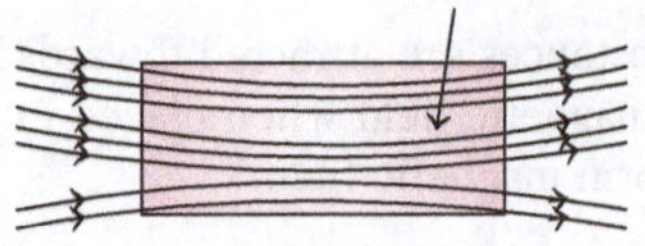

Magnetic field inside ferromagnetic substance

(iv) Magnetic susceptibility of ferromagnetic substance does not change according to Curie law.

(v) Susceptibility decreases steadily with the rise in temperature. Above a certain temperature known as **Curie temperature,** the ferromagnetic substances become paramagnetic. It is 1000°C for iron, 770°C for steel, 360°C for nickel and 1150°C for cobalt.

(vi) Its *I-H* curve can be drawn as

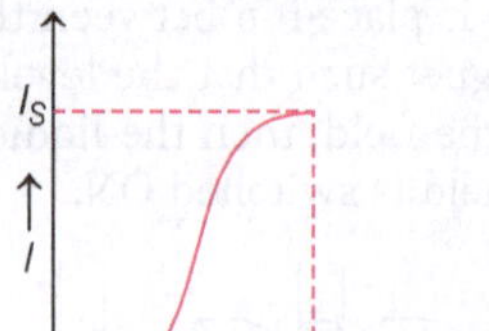

Curie's Law

According to this law, the magnetic susceptibility of paramagnetic substances is inversely proportional to its absolute temperature, *i.e.*

$$\chi_m \propto \frac{1}{T} \Rightarrow \chi_m = \frac{C}{T}$$

where, C is Curie constant and T = absolute temperature in kelvin. On increasing temperature, the magnetic susceptibility of paramagnetic material decreases and *vice-versa* as shown is figure. This variation can be shown as

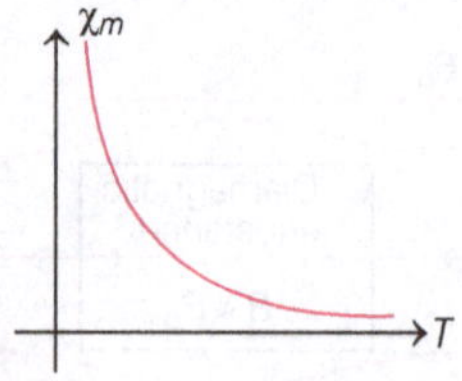

NEET Snapshot

Magnetic susceptibility is negative only for diamagnetic materials.
[NEET 2016]

The relation between magnetic permeability and susceptibility of a material is $\mu_r = 1 + \chi_m$
Since, μ_r is negative for diamagnetic material, hence χ_m is negative.

Scan for Video

Example 16. *The magnetic susceptibility of a paramagnetic material at −73°C is 0.0075. Find its value at −173°C.*

Sol. Magnetic susceptibility,

$$\chi_{m_1} = 0.0075, T_1 = -73°\text{C} = (-73 + 273)\text{ K} = 200\text{ K}$$

$$\chi_{m_2} = ?, T_2 = -173°\text{C} = (-173 + 273)\text{ K} = 100\text{ K}$$

According to Curie's law, $\chi_m \propto \frac{1}{T}$

$\therefore$ Ratio of magnetic susceptibilities, $\frac{\chi_{m_2}}{\chi_{m_1}} = \frac{T_1}{T_2} = \frac{200}{100} = 2$

$$\Rightarrow \quad \chi_{m_2} = 2\chi_{m_1} = 2 \times 0.0075 = 0.015$$

Example 17. *A solenoid having 5000 turns/m carries a current of 2A. An aluminium ring at temperature 300K inside the solenoid provides the core. (i) If the magnetisation I is 2×10^{-2} A/m, find the susceptibility of aluminium at 300K. (ii) If temperature of the aluminium ring is 320K, what will be the magnetisation?*

Sol. (i) Here, $H = ni = 5000 \times 2 = 10^4$ A/m

$$\because \quad I = \chi H$$

$$\therefore \quad \chi = \frac{I}{H} = \frac{2 \times 10^{-2}}{10^4} = 2 \times 10^{-6}$$

(where, I = intensity of magnetisation)

(ii) According to Curie's law,

$$\chi = \frac{C}{T} \Rightarrow \frac{\chi_2}{\chi_1} = \frac{T_1}{T_2}$$

$$\chi_2 = \frac{T_1}{T_2}\chi_1 = \frac{300}{320} \times 2 \times 10^{-6} = 1.875 \times 10^{-6}$$

Magnetisation at 320 K,

$$I = \chi_2 H = 1.875 \times 10^{-6} \times 10^4 = 1.875 \times 10^{-2}\text{ A/m}$$

Curie-Weiss Law

When temperature increases above the Curie temperature, a ferromagnetic substance becomes an ordinary paramagnetic substance whose magnetic susceptibility obeys the Curie-Weiss law as given below.

$$\chi_m = \frac{C'}{T - T_C}$$

where, T_C = Curie temperature and C' = constant.
Variation of χ_m *versus* T is shown below.

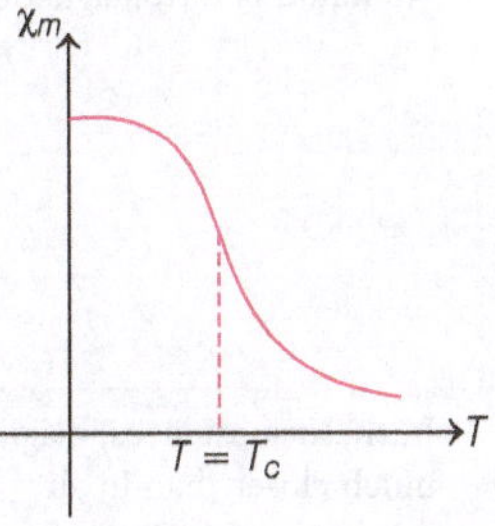

χ_m *versus* T graph for a magnetic substance

Concept ladder

Hysteresis Loop

- The word hysteresis means delayed. The phenomenon of the lagging of magnetic induction behind the magnetising field is called **hysteresis.**
- The plot of intensity of magnetisation (I) of ferromagnetic substances *versus* magnetic intensity (H) for a complete cycle of magnetisation and demagnetisation is called **hysteresis loop.**

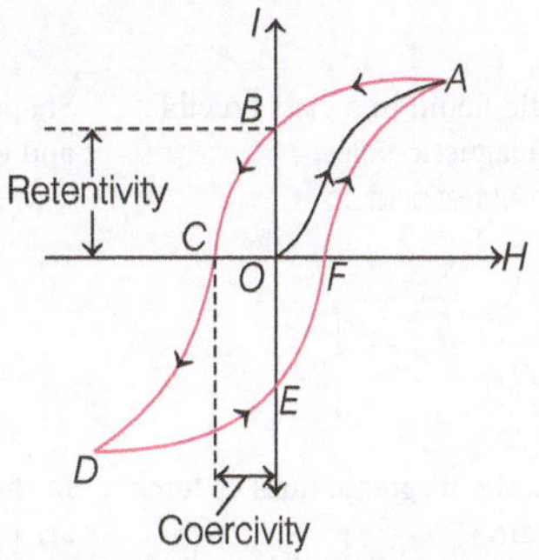

Comparative Study of Magnetic Materials

Diamagnetic substances	Paramagnetic substances	Ferromagnetic substances
These substances when placed in a magnetic field, acquire feeble magnetism opposite to the direction of the magnetic field.	These substances when placed in a magnetic field, acquire feeble magnetism in the direction of the magnetic field.	These substances when placed in a magnetic field are strongly magnetised in the direction of the field.
These substances are repelled by a magnet.	These substances are feebly attracted by a magnet.	These substances are strongly attracted by a magnet.
When a diamagnetic solution is poured into a U-tube and one arm is placed between the poles of strong magnet, then the level of solution in that arm is lowered. 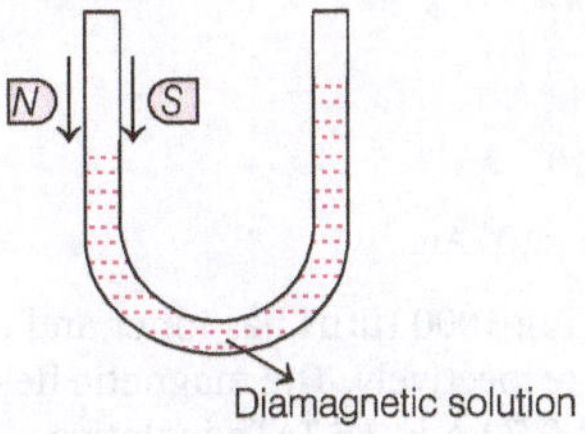	When one arm of a U-tube is placed between the poles of strong magnet, then the level of the paramagnetic solution in that arm rises. 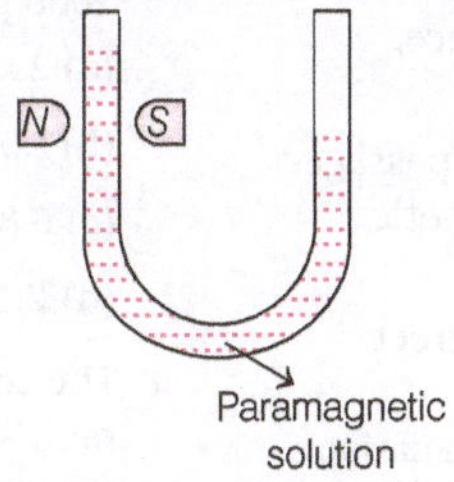	No liquid is ferromagnetic.
If a rod of diamagnetic material is suspended freely between two magnetic poles, then its axis becomes perpendicular to the magnetic field. 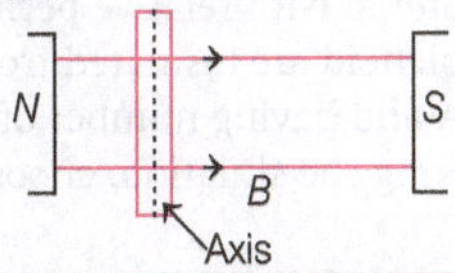	In case of paramagnetic rod, its axis becomes parallel to the magnetic field. 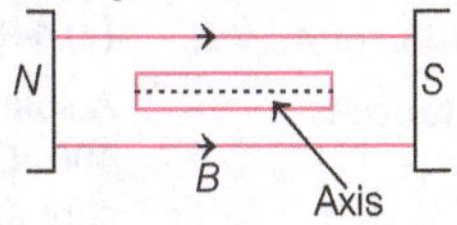	Also, in case of ferromagnetic rod, its axis becomes parallel to the magnetic field. 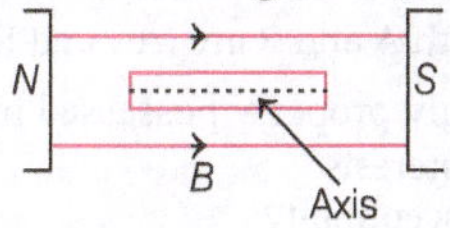
In non-uniform magnetic field, the diamagnetic substances are attracted towards the weaker fields, *i.e.* they move from stronger to weaker magnetic field.	In non-uniform magnetic field, they move from weaker to stronger part of the magnetic field slowly.	In non-uniform magnetic field, they move from weaker to stronger magnetic field rapidly.

Diamagnetic substances	Paramagnetic substances	Ferromagnetic substances
Their permeability is less than one ($\mu < 1$). $0 < \mu_r < 1, \mu < \mu_0$	Their permeability is slightly greater than one ($\mu > 1$). $1 < \mu_r < 1 + \varepsilon, \mu > \mu_0$	Their permeability is much greater than one ($\mu >> 1$). $\mu_r >> 1, \mu >> \mu_0$
Their susceptibility is small and negative $[-1 < \chi_m < 0]$. It is independent of temperature.	Their susceptibility is small and positive $(0 < \chi_m < \varepsilon)$. It is inversely proportional to absolute temperature which is Curie's law, *i.e.* $\chi \propto \frac{1}{T}$.	Their susceptibility is large and positive ($\chi_m >> 1$). They also follow Curie's law, *i.e.* $\chi \propto \frac{1}{T - T_C}$. At Curie temperature, ferromagnetic substances change into paramagnetic substances.
Shape of diamagnetic liquid in a glass crucible and kept over two magnetic poles. 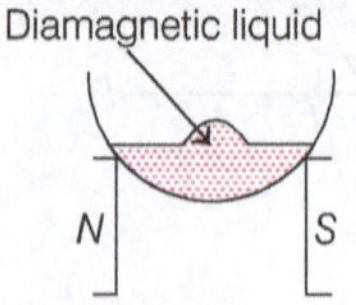	Shape of paramagnetic liquid in a glass crucible and kept over two magnetic poles. 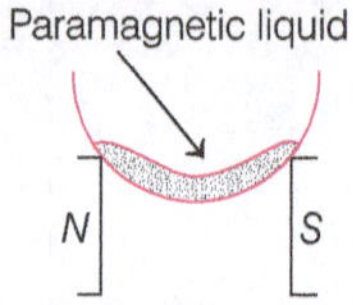	No liquid is ferromagnetic.
In these substances, the magnetic lines of force are farther than in air.	In these substances, the magnetic lines of force are closer than in air.	In these substances, magnetic lines of force are much closer than in air.
The resultant magnetic moment of these substances is zero.	These substances have a permanent magnetic moment.	These substances also have a permanent magnetic moment.

STEP UP Practice 2

1. The SI unit of magnetic permeability is
(a) Am^{-1} (b) Am (c) Hm^{-1}
(d) No unit, it is a dimensionless number

2. **Assertion** (A) For a perfectly diamagnetic substance, permeability is zero.
Reason (R) The ability of a material to permit the passage of magnetic lines of force through it, is called magnetic permeability.
In the light of the above statements, choose the correct answer from the options given below.
(a) Both A and R are true but R is not the correct explanation of A.
(b) A is true but R is false.
(c) A is false but R is true.
(d) Both A and R are true and R is the correct explanation of A.

3. The only property possessed by ferromagnetic substance is
(a) hysteresis
(b) susceptibility
(c) directional property
(d) attracting magnetic substances

4. A rod of ferromagnetic material has dimension 10 cm × 0.5 cm × 0.2 cm. It is placed in a magnetic field of strength 0.5×10^4 Am^{-1}. The magnetic moment produced in the rod is 5 A-m^2. The value of magnetic induction will be
(a) 0.54 T (b) 6.28 T (c) 0.358 T (d) 2.591 T

5. A solenoid has core of a material with relative permeability 400. The windings of the solenoid are insulated from the core and carry a current of 2 A. If the number of turns is 1000 per metre, calculate H and M.
(a) 2×10^3 Am^{-1}, 8×10^5 Am^{-1}
(b) 1.0 Am^{-1}, 1.5×10^5 Am^{-1}
(c) 6.8×10^{-5} Am^{-1}, 1.2×10^{-5} Am^{-1}
(d) 2.1×10^{-4} Am^{-1}, -2.6×10^5 Am^{-1}

6. The core of a toroid having 3000 turns has inner and outer radii 11 cm and 12 cm, respectively. The magnetic field in the core for a current of 0.70 A is 2.5 T. The relative permeability of the core is
(a) 685 (b) 880
(c) 448 (d) 790

7. A solenoid has a core of material with relative permeability 400. The windings of the solenoid are insulated from the core and carry a current 2 A and having number of turns 1000 per metre. By considering the situation, choose the incorrect pair.
(a) Magnetic intensity (H) → 2×10^3 Am^{-1}
(b) Magnetic field (B) → 1 T
(c) Magnetisation (I) → 4×10^5 Am^{-1}
(d) Magnetising current (I_m) → 794 A

8. An iron rod of 0.2 cm^2 cross-sectional area is subjected to a magnetising field of 1200 Am^{-1}. The susceptibility of iron is 1874. The permeability will be
(a) 7.9×10^5 TmA^{-1}
(b) 8.0×10^{22} TmA^{-1}
(c) 7.5×10^{-4} TmA^{-1}
(d) 1.8×10^{-5} TmA^{-1}

9. The *M*-*H* curve for a paramagnetic material is represented by figure

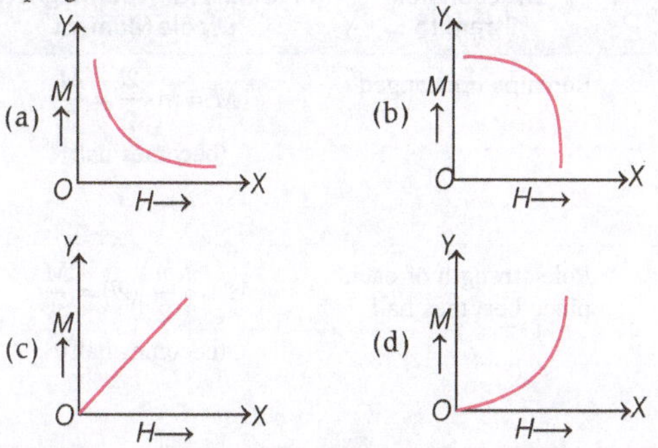

10. A domain in ferromagnetic iron is in the form of a cube of side length 1 μm. Estimate the number of iron atoms in the domain. The molecular mass of iron is 55 g/mol and its density is 7.9 g cm^{-3}.
(a) 8.65×10^{-10} atoms
(b) 8.0×10^{-13} atoms
(c) 8.0×10^5 atoms
(d) 8.65×10^{10} atoms

11. A sample of paramagnetic salt contains 2.0×10^{24} atomic dipoles, each of dipole moment 1.5×10^{-23} JT^{-1}. The sample is placed under a homogeneous magnetic field of 0.84 T and cooled to a temperature of 4.2 K. The degree of magnetic saturation achieved is equal to 15%. The total dipole moment of the sample for a magnetic field of 0.98 T and a temperature of 2.8 K is
(a) 3×10^3 JT^{-1}
(b) $4\pi \times 10^{-6}$ JT^{-1}
(c) 7.9 JT^{-1}
(d) 7×10^4 JT^{-1}

12. Property of a bulk material called intensity of magnetisation is
(a) magnetic moment per unit area
(b) magnetic moment per unit volume
(c) a vector quantity and having unit of Am^{-1}
(d) Both (b) and (c)

13. **Assertion** (A) Susceptibility is defined as the ratio of intensity of magnetisation *I* to magnetic intensity *H*.
Reason (R) Greater the value of susceptibility, smaller the value of intensity of magnetisation *I*.
In the light of the above statements, choose the correct answer from the options given below.
(a) Both A and R are true but R is not the correct explanation of A.
(b) A is true but R is false.
(c) A is false but R is true.
(d) Both A and R are true and R is the correct explanation of A.

14. A paramagnetic substance in the form of a cube with sides 1 cm has a magnetic dipole moment of 20×10^{-6} J/T when a magnetic intensity of 60×10^3 A/m is applied. Its magnetic susceptibility is
(a) 3.3×10^{-4} (b) 3.3×10^{-2} (c) 4.3×10^{-2} (d) 2.3×10^{-2}

15. The variation of magnetic susceptibility χ with absolute temperature *T* for a ferromagnetic material is given in figure by

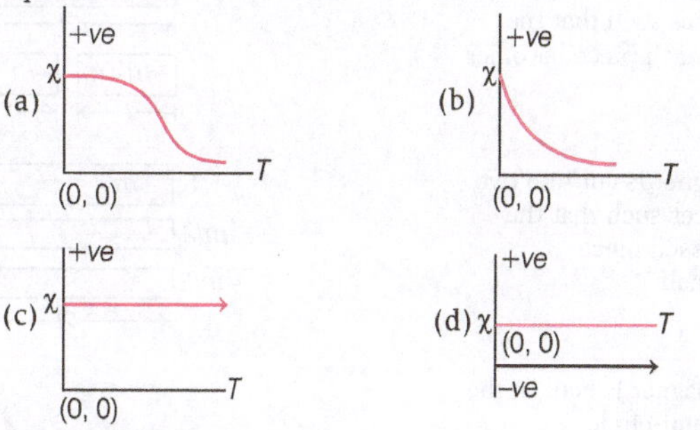

16. Choose the incorrect pair.
(a) Pole strength → LA
(b) Intensity of magnetisation → $L^{-1}A$
(c) Magnetic moment → L^2A
(d) Relative permeability → LA^2

17. **Assertion** (A) The properties of paramagnetic and ferromagnetic substance are not effected by heating.
Reason (R) As temperature rises, the alignment of molecular magnets gradually decreases.
In the light of the above statements, choose the correct answer from the options given below.
(a) Both A and R are true but R is not the correct explanation of A.
(b) A is true but R is false.
(c) A is false but R is true.
(d) Both A and R are true and R is the correct explanation of A.

18. **Assertion** (A) The ferromagnetic substance do not obey curie's law.
Reason (R) At curie point, a ferromagnetic substance starts behaving as a paramagnetic substance.
In the light of the above statements, choose the correct answer from the options given below.
(a) Both A and R are true but R is not the correct explanation of A.
(b) A is true but R is false.
(c) A is false but R is true.
(d) Both A and R are true and R is the correct explanation of A.

NEET Exclusive EXTRA BYTES

- Some special shapes of bar magnet and their magnetic dipole moment are shown below.

Special Cases	Figure	Effect on Pole Strength	Formula for New Magnetic Dipole Moment
If bar magnet is cut into two equal pieces such that the length of each piece becomes half	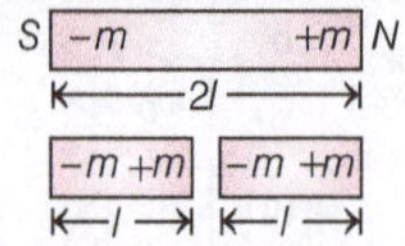	Remains unchanged	$M' = m \cdot \frac{2l}{2} = \frac{M}{2}$ (becomes half)
If bar magnet is cut into two equal pieces such that the width of each piece becomes half	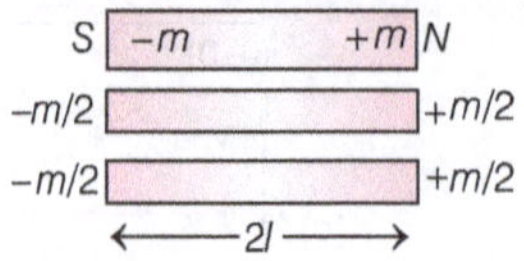	Pole strength of each piece becomes half	$M' = \left(\frac{m}{2}\right)(2l) = \frac{M}{2}$ (becomes half)
If a bar magnet is bent in the form of semi-circle	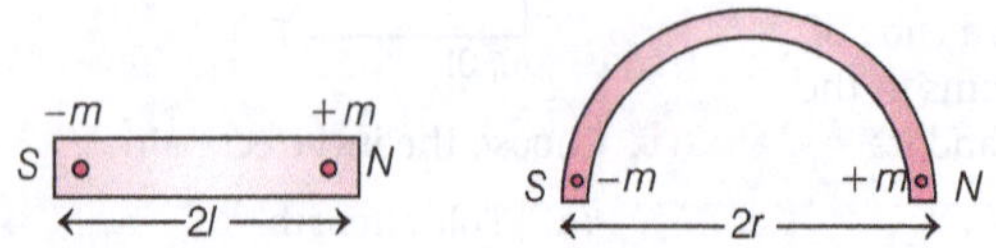	Remains unchanged	$M' = m(2r)[\because 2l = \pi r]$ $M' = m \times 2\left(\frac{2l}{\pi}\right) = \frac{2M}{\pi}$ $\left(\text{becomes } \frac{2}{\pi} \text{ times}\right)$
When two identical bar magnets are joined perpendicular to each other	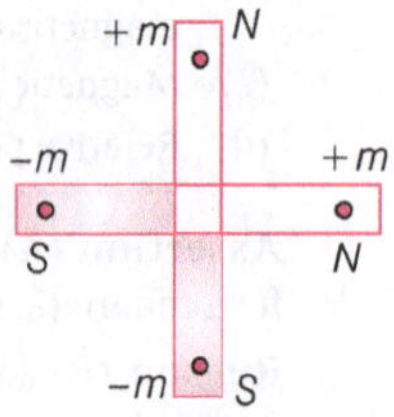	Remains unchanged	$M = \sqrt{M_1^2 + M_2^2} = \sqrt{2}M$
When two bar magnets are inclined at an angle θ	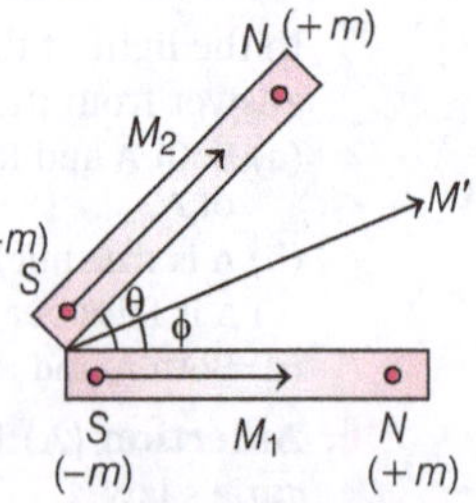	Remains unchanged	Resultant magnetic moment, $M' = \sqrt{M_1^2 + M_2^2 + 2M_1M_2\cos\theta}$ Angle made by resultant magnetic moment (M') with M_1 is given by $\tan\phi = \frac{M_2 \sin\theta}{M_1 + M_2\cos\theta}$

- Pole strength of bar magnet is proportional to cross-section area of magnet. *i.e.* $m \propto A$.
- Centre of bar magnet is neutral point.
- Force between two magnetic poles follows inverse square law.
- Diamagnetism is due to orbital velocity of electrons, paramagnetism is due to spin motion of electron and ferromagnetism is due to domain formation in magnetic materials.
- Torque on a magnetic dipole is an axial vector.

GEARING UP FOR NEET

Single Correct Options

1. Unit of magnetic flux density (or magnetic induction) is
   (a) tesla (b) weber/metre^2
   (c) newton/ampere-metre (d) All of these

2. Magnetic field intensity is defined as
   (a) magnetic moment per unit volume
   (b) magnetic induction force acting on a unit magnetic pole
   (c) number of lines of force crossing per unit area
   (d) number of lines of force crossing per unit volume

3. A magnetic needle kept in a non-uniform magnetic field experiences
   (a) a force and torque
   (b) a force but not a torque
   (c) a torque but not a force
   (d) Neither a torque nor a force

4. The mathematical equation for magnetic field lines of force is
   (a) $\nabla \cdot \mathbf{B} = 0$ (b) $\nabla \cdot \mathbf{B} \neq 0.1$
   (c) $\nabla \cdot \mathbf{B} > 0$ (d) $\nabla \cdot \mathbf{B} < 0$

5. Two lines of force due to a bar magnet
   (a) intersect at the neutral point
   (b) intersect near the poles of the magnet
   (c) intersect on the equatorial axis of the magnet
   (d) do not intersect at all

6. What happens to the force between magnetic poles when their pole strength and the distance between them both gets doubled?
   (a) Force increases to two times the previous value
   (b) No change
   (c) Force decreases to half the previous value
   (d) Force increases to four times the previous value

7. If a magnet of pole strength m is divided into four parts such that the length and width of each part is half that of initial one, then the pole strength of each part will be
   (a) $m/4$ (b) $m/2$
   (c) $m/8$ (d) $4m$

8. Two magnets have the same length and the same pole strength but one of the magnets has a small hole at its centre, then
   (a) both have equal magnetic moment
   (b) one with hole has smaller magnetic moment
   (c) one with hole has larger magnetic moment
   (d) one with hole loses magnetism through the hole

9. The magnetic field at a distance d from a short bar magnet in longitudinal and transverse positions are in the ratio
   (a) 1:1 (b) 2:3 (c) 2:1 (d) 3:2

10. The magnetic field lines due to a bar magnet are correctly shown in

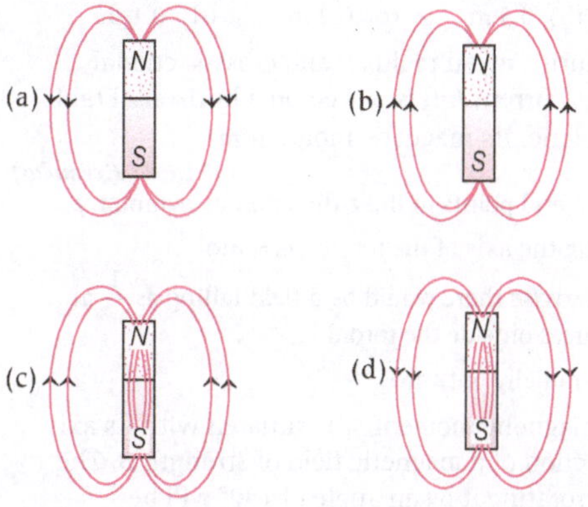

11. Torques τ_1 and τ_2 are required for a magnetic needle to remain perpendicular to the magnetic fields B_1 and B_2 at two different places. The ratio of B_1 / B_2 is
   (a) $\frac{\tau_2}{\tau_1}$ (b) $\frac{\tau_1}{\tau_2}$ (c) $\frac{\tau_1 + \tau_2}{\tau_1 - \tau_2}$ (d) $\frac{\tau_1 - \tau_2}{\tau_1 + \tau_2}$

12. The tangents deflection produced in tan A and tan B positions by a short magnet at equal distances are in the ratio
   (a) 1 : 1 (b) 2 : 1
   (c) 1 : 2 (d) None of these

13. The magnetic moment of a magnet of length 10 cm and pole strength 4.0 A-m will be
   (a) 0.4 A-m^2 (b) 1.6 A-m^2
   (c) 20 A-m^2 (d) 8.0 A-m^2

14. A magnet of magnetic moment M and pole strength m is cut in two equal parts along the axis of magnet, then magnetic moment of each part will be
   (a) M (b) $M/2$
   (c) $M/4$ (d) $2M$

15. Two identical thin bar magnets each of length l and pole strength m are placed at right angles to each other with north pole of one touching south pole of the other. Magnetic moment of the system is
   (a) ml (b) $2ml$ (c) $\sqrt{2}ml$ (d) $\frac{1}{2}ml$

16. A short bar magnet placed with its axis at 30° with a uniform external magnetic field of 0.16 T experiences a torque of magnitude 0.032 J. The magnetic moment of the bar magnet will be

(a) $0.23\ JT^{-1}$ (b) $0.40\ JT^{-1}$ (c) $0.80\ JT^{-1}$ (d) zero

17. A bar magnet when placed at an angle of 30° to the direction of magnetic field induction of 5×10^{-2} T, experiences a moment of couple 25×10^{-6} N-m. If the length of the magnet is 5 cm, its pole strength is

(a) 2×10^{-2} A-m (b) 5×10^{-2}A-m
(c) 2 A-m (d) 5 A-m

18. A bar magnet of magnetic moment 3 A-m^2 is placed in a uniform magnetic field induction of 2×10^{-5} T. If each pole of the magnet experiences a force of 6×10^{-4} N, the length of the magnet is

(a) 0.5 m (b) 0.3 m (c) 0.2 m (d) 0.1 m

19. A toroid of n turns, mean radius R and cross-sectional radius a carries current I. It is placed on a horizontal table taken as XY-plane. Its magnetic moment **m**

[NCERT Exemplar]

(a) is non-zero and points in the z-direction by symmetry
(b) points along the axis of the toroid ($\mathbf{m} = m\hat{\phi}$)
(c) is zero, otherwise there would be a field falling as $\frac{1}{r^3}$ at large distances outside the toroid
(d) is pointing radially outwards

20. A magnet of magnetic moment M is situated with its axis along the direction of a magnetic field of strength B. The work done in rotating it by an angle of 180° will be

(a) $-MB$ (b) $+MB$ (c) zero (d) $+2MB$

21. A magnet of magnetic moment 2 J/T is aligned in the direction of magnetic field of 0.1 T. What is the net work done to bring the magnet normal to the magnetic field?

(a) 0.1 J (b) 0.2 J (c) 1 J (d) 2 J

22. A planar coil having 15 turns carries 20 A current. The coil is oriented with respect to the uniform magnetic field $\mathbf{B} = 0.5\hat{\mathbf{i}}$T such that its directed area is $\mathbf{A} = -0.04\ \hat{\mathbf{i}}\text{m}^2$. The potential energy of the coil in the given orientation is

(a) 0 (b) + 0.72 J (c) 6 J (d) −1.44 J

23. The magnetic field on the axis of a short bar magnet at a distance of 10 cm is 0.2 oersted. What will be the field at a point, distant 5 cm on the line perpendicular to the axis and passing through the magnet?

(a) 0.025 oersted (b) 0.2 oersted
(c) 0.4 oersted (d) 0.8 oersted

24. A long magnetic needle of length $2L$, magnetic moment M and pole strength m units is broken into two at the middle. The magnetic moment and pole strength of each piece will be

(a) $M/2, m/2$ (b) $M, m/2$
(c) $M/2, m$ (d) M, m

25. Consider the two idealised systems (i) a parallel plate capacitor with large plates with small separation and (ii) a long solenoid of length $L >> R$, radius of cross-section. In (i) **E** is ideally treated as a constant between plates and zero outside. In (ii) magnetic field is constant inside the solenoid and zero outside. These idealised assumptions, however contradict fundamental laws as below

[NCERT Exemplar]

(a) Case (i) contradicts Gauss' law for electrostatic fields
(b) Case (ii) contradicts Gauss' law for magnetic fields
(c) Case (i) agrees with $\oint \mathbf{E} \cdot d\mathbf{l} = 0$
(d) Case (ii) contradicts $\oint \mathbf{H} \cdot d\mathbf{l} = I_{em}$

26. Due to a small magnet, intensity at a distance x in the end on position is 9 G. What will be the intensity at a distance $\frac{x}{2}$ on broadside on position?

(a) 9 G (b) 4 G (c) 36 G (d) 4.5 G

27. Two short magnets of equal dipole moments M are fastened perpendicularly at their centres (figure). The magnitude of the magnetic field at a distance d from the centre on the bisector of the right angle is

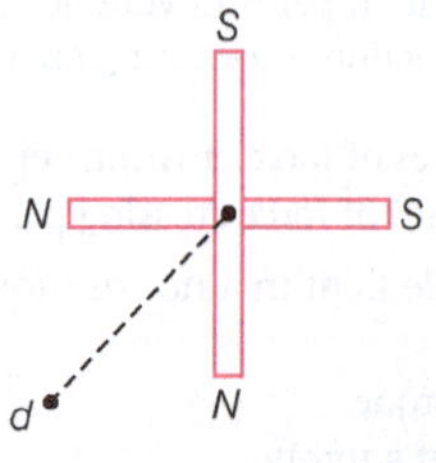

(a) $\frac{\mu_0}{4\pi} \frac{M}{d^3}$ (b) $\frac{\mu_0}{4\pi} \frac{\sqrt{2}\,M}{d^3}$
(c) $\frac{\mu_0}{4\pi} \frac{2\sqrt{2}\,M}{d^3}$ (d) $\frac{\mu_0}{4\pi} \frac{2M}{d^3}$

28. A thin rectangular magnet suspended freely has a period of oscillation 4 s. If it is broken into two halves each having half of their initial length. If they are suspended again, then the time period of oscillation of each part will be

(a) 4 s (b) 2 s (c) 1 s (d) $2\sqrt{2}$ s

29. Two magnets of same size and mass make respectively 10 and 15 oscillations per minute at certain place. The ratio of their magnetic moments is

(a) 4 : 9 (b) 9 : 4 (c) 2 : 3 (d) 3 : 2

30. Two like magnetic poles of strength 10 and 40 SI units are separated by a distance 30 cm. The intensity of magnetic field is zero on the line joining them

(a) at a point 10 cm from the stronger pole
(b) at a point 20 cm from the stronger pole
(c) at the mid-point
(d) at infinity

31. The figure shows the various positions (labelled by subscripts) of small magnetised needles P and Q. The arrows show the direction of their magnetic moment. Which configuration corresponds to the lowest potential energy of all the configurations shown?

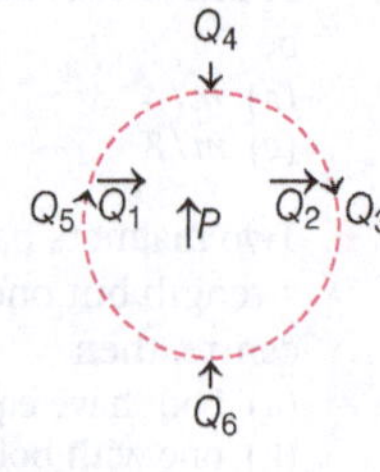

(a) PQ_3 (b) PQ_4 (c) PQ_5 (d) PQ_6

32. Two bar magnets having same geometry with magnetic moments M and $2M$ are placed in such a way that their similar poles are on the same side, then its time period of oscillation is T_1. Now, if the polarity of one of the magnets is reversed, then time period of oscillation is T_2, then

(a) $T_1 < T_2$ (b) $T_1 > T_2$
(c) $T_1 = T_2$ (d) $T_1 = \infty, T_1 = 0$

33. The length of a magnet is large compared to its width and breadth. The time period of its oscillation in a vibration magnetometer is 2 s. The magnet is cut along its length into three equal parts and three parts are then placed on each other with their like poles together. The time period of this combination will be

(a) 2s (b) $\frac{2}{3}$ s (c) $2\sqrt{3}$s (d) $\frac{2}{\sqrt{3}}$ s

34. A bar magnet has a coercivity of 4×10^3 Am^{-1}. It is placed inside a solenoid of length 12 cm having 60 turns in order to demagnetise it. The amount of current that should be passed through the solenoid is

(a) 16A (b) 8A (c) 4A (d) 2A

35. The effective length of magnet is 31.4 cm and its pole strength is 0.8 Am. The magnetic moment, if it is bent in the form of a semi-circle is ..... A-m^2.

(a) 1.2 (b) 1.6 (c) 0.16 (d) 0.12

36. Following figures show the arrangement of bar magnets in different configurations. Each magnet has magnetic dipole moment m. Which configuration has highest net magnetic dipole moment?

(a)
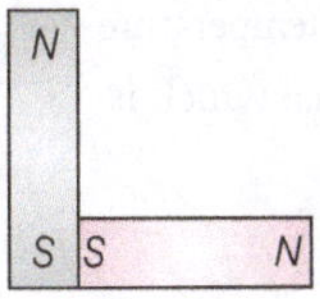

(b)
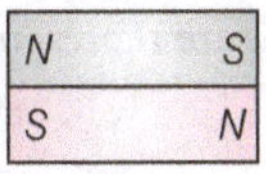

(c)
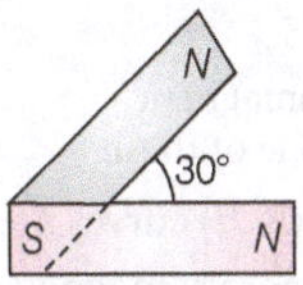

(d)
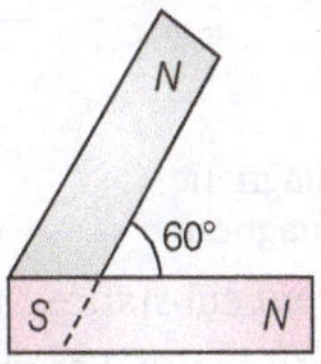

37. A bar magnet of moment M and pole strength m is cut into parts of equal lengths. The magnetic moment and pole strength of either part is

(a) $\frac{M}{2}, \frac{m}{2}$ (b) $M, \frac{m}{2}$ (c) $\frac{M}{2}, m$ (d) M, m

38. A bar magnet of length l and magnetic dipole moment M is bent in the form of an arc as shown in figure.

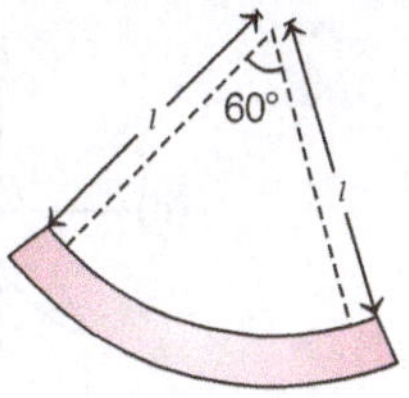

The new magnetic dipole moment will be

(a) M (b) $\frac{3}{\pi}M$
(c) $\frac{2}{\pi}M$ (d) $\frac{M}{2}$

39. A bar magnet of moment of inertia I is vibrated in a magnetic field of induction 0.4×10^{-4} T. The time period of vibration is 12 s. The magnetic moment of the magnet is 120 Am^2. The moment of inertia of the magnet is (in kg-m^2) approximately

(a) 172.8×10^{-4} (b) 2.1×10^{-2}
(c) 1.57×10^{-2} (d) 1728×10^{-2}

40. If a steel wire of length l and magnetic moment M is bent into a sem-circular arc, then the new magnetic moment is

(a) $M \times l$ (b) $\frac{M}{l}$
(c) $\frac{2M}{\pi}$ (d) M

41. An iron rod of volume 10^{-4}m^3 and relative permeability 1000 is placed inside a long solenoid having 5 turns/cm. If a current of 0.5 A is passed through the solenoid, then the magnetic moment of the rod is

(a) 20 A-m^2 (b) 25 A-m^2
(c) 30 A-m^2 (d) 35 A-m^2

42. A magnetic wire of dipole moment 4π A-m^2 is bent in the form of semi-circle. The new magnetic moment is

(a) 4π A-m^2 (b) 8 A-m^2
(c) 4 A-m^2 (d) None of these

43. Permeability is defined as the ratio between

(a) magnetic induction and susceptibility
(b) magnetic induction and magnetising field
(c) magnetising field and magnetic induction
(d) magnetising field and susceptibility

44. Hysteresis loss for steel is .... that for iron.

(a) lesser than (b) equal to
(c) greater than (d) Either (b) or (c)

45. Hysteresis is exhibited by a .... substance.

(a) paramagnetic (b) ferromagnetic
(c) diamagnetic (d) All of these

46. Which of the following materials has got the maximum retentivity?

(a) Copper (b) Zinc
(c) Soft iron (d) Hard iron

47. The area enclosed by a hysteresis loop is a measure of

(a) retentivity (b) susceptibility
(c) permeability (d) energy loss per cycle

48. The permeability of paramagnetic substance is

(a) slightly more than vacuum
(b) slightly less than vacuum
(c) much more than vacuum
(d) None of the above

49. The variation of magnetic susceptibility (χ) with temperature for a diamagnetic substance is best represented by

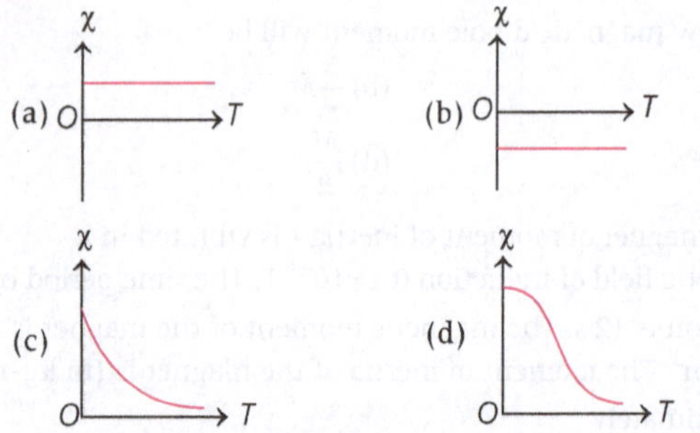

50. Which of the following statements are true about the magnetic susceptibility χ_m of paramagnetic substance?
(a) Value of χ_m is inversely proportional to the absolute temperature of the sample.
(b) χ_m is zero at all temperatures.
(c) χ_m is negative at all temperatures.
(d) χ_m does not depend on the temperature of the sample.

51. Resultant force acting on a diamagnetic material in a magnetic field is in direction
(a) from stronger to the weaker part of the magnetic field
(b) from weaker to the stronger part of the magnetic field
(c) perpendicular to the magnetic field
(d) in the direction making 60° to the magnetic field

52. When a diamagnetic substance is brought near north or south pole of a bar magnet, it is
(a) attracted by the poles
(b) repelled by the poles
(c) attracted by the north pole and repelled by the south pole
(d) repelled by the north pole and attracted by the south pole

53. Susceptibility is positive and large for a
(a) paramagnetic substance
(b) ferromagnetic substance
(c) non-magnetic substance
(d) diamagnetic substance

54. A curve between magnetic moment and temperature of magnet is

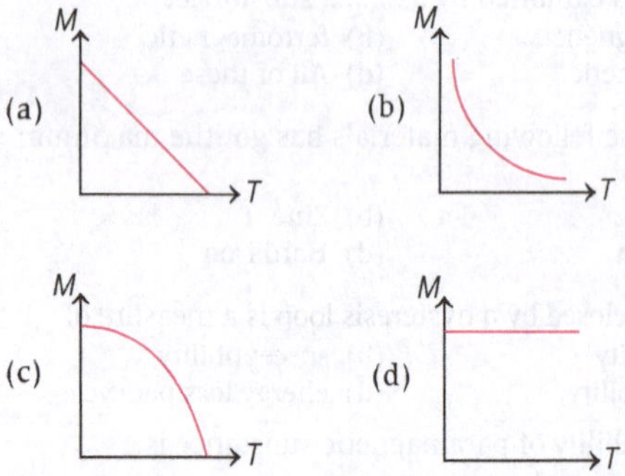

55. The relative permeability is represented by μ_r and the susceptibility is denoted by χ for a magnetic substance, then for a paramagnetic substance,
(a) $\mu_r < 1, \chi < 0$
(b) $\mu_r < 1, \chi > 0$
(c) $\mu_r > 1, \chi < 0$
(d) $\mu_r > 1, \chi > 0$

56. When a piece of a ferromagnetic substance is put in a uniform magnetic field,the flux density inside it is four times the flux density away from the piece. The magnetic permeability of the material is
(a) 1 (b) 2 (c) 3 (d) 4

57. If a diamagnetic solution is poured into a U-tube and one arm of this U-tube placed between the poles of a strong magnet with the meniscus in a line with the field, then the level of the solution will
(a) rise
(b) fall
(c) oscillate slowly
(d) remain as such

58. A paramagnetic liquid is filled in a U-tube, of which one limb is placed between the pole pieces of an electromagnet. When the field is switched ON, the liquid in the limb which is placed between the field will
(a) rise
(b) fall
(c) remain stationary
(d) first rise and then fall

59. A ferromagnetic material is heated above its curie temperature, which one is a correct statement?
(a) Ferromagnetic domains are perfectly arranged.
(b) Ferromagnetic domains become random.
(c) Ferromagnetic domains are not influenced.
(d) Ferromagnetic material changes into diamagnetic material.

60. Above the curie temperature, the susceptibility of a ferromagnetic substance varies
(a) directly as the absolute temperature
(b) inversely as the absolute temperature
(c) inversely as the square of absolute temperature
(d) directly as the square of absolute temperature

61. The given figure represents a material which is

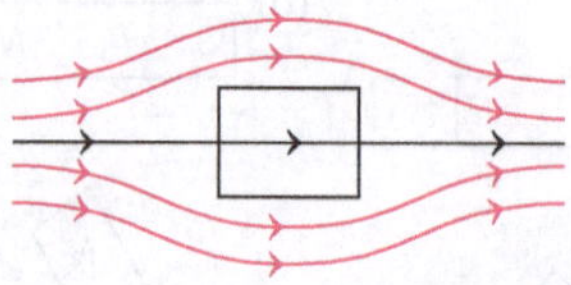

(a) paramagnetic
(b) diamagnetic
(c) ferromagnetic
(d) None of these

62. For different substances, hysteresis (B-H) curves are given as shown in figure. For making temporary magnet, which of the following is best?

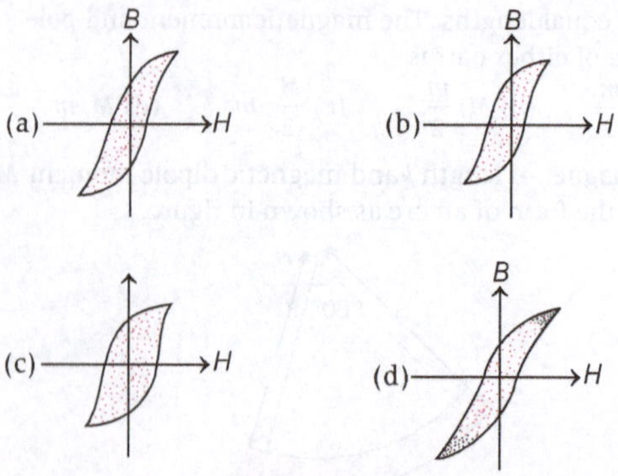

63. The magnetic moment produced in a substance of 1g is 6×10^{-7} Am^2. If its density is 5 g/cm^3, then the intensity of magnetisation in (A/m) will be
(a) 8.3×10^{6} (b) 3.0
(c) 1.2×10^{-7} (d) 3×10^{-6}

64. For ferromagnetic material, the relative permeability (μ_r) *versus* magnetic intensity (H) has the following shape

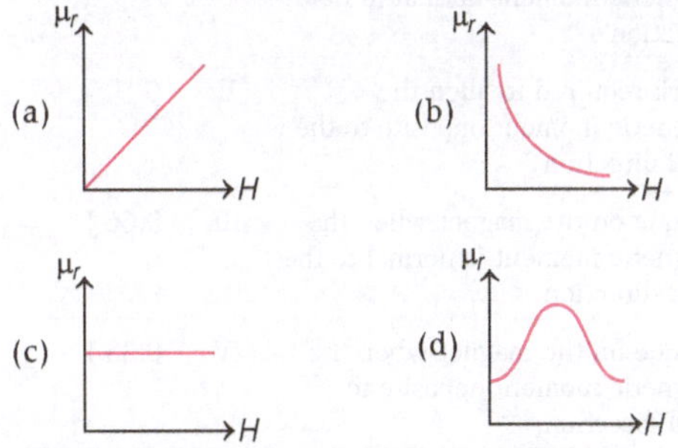

65. An iron rod of 0.2 cm^2 cross-sectional area is subjected to a magnetising field of 1200 Am^{-1}. The susceptibility of iron is 599. The magnetic flux produced is
(a) 0.904 Wb (b) 1.81×10^{-5} Wb
(c) 0.904×10^{-5} Wb (d) 5.43×10^{-5} Wb

66. A paramagnetic sample shows a net magnetisation of 8 A-m^{-1}, when placed in an external magnetic field of 0.6 T at a temperature of 4 K. When the same sample is placed in an external magnetic field of 0.2 T at a temperature of 16 K, the magnetisation will be *[NCERT Exemplar]*
(a) $\frac{32}{3}$ Am^{-1} (b) $\frac{2}{3}$ Am^{-1} (c) 6 Am^{-1} (d) 2.4 Am^{-1}

67. Two short magnets of magnetic moment 1000 A-m^2 are placed as shown at the corners of a square of side 10 cm. The net magnetic induction at P is

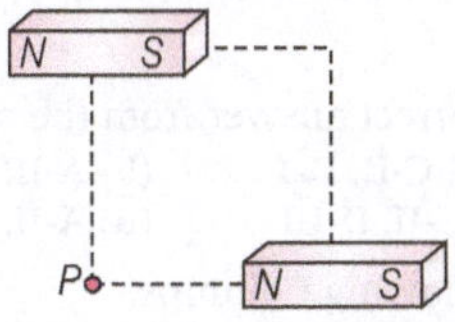

(a) 0.1 T (b) 0.2 T (c) 0.3 T (d) 0.4 T

68. Two identical short bar magnets, each having magnetic moment M, are placed a distance of $2d$ apart with axes perpendicular to each other in a horizontal plane. The magnetic induction at a point mid-way between them is
(a) $\frac{\mu_0}{4\pi}(\sqrt{2})\frac{M}{d^3}$ (b) $\frac{\mu_0}{4\pi}(\sqrt{3})\frac{M}{d^3}$
(c) $\left(\frac{2\mu_0}{\pi}\right)\frac{M}{d^3}$ (d) $\frac{\mu_0}{4\pi}(\sqrt{5})\frac{M}{d^3}$

69. A paramagnetic sample shows a net magnetisation of 0.8 Am^{-1}, when placed in an external magnetic field of strength 0.8 T at a temperature 5 K. When the same sample is placed in an external magnetic field of 0.4 T at a temperature of 20 K, the magnetisation is
(a) 0.8 Am^{-1} (b) 0.8 Am^2 (c) 0.1 Am^{-2} (d) 0.1 Am^{-1}

70. The magnetic susceptibility of a material of a rod is 299 and permeability of vacuum μ_0 is $4\pi\times10^{-7}$ Hm^{-1}. Absolute permeability of the material of the rod is
(a) 3771×10^{-7} Hm^{-1} (b) 3771×10^{-5} Hm^{-1}
(c) 3770×10^{-6} Hm^{-1} (d) 3771×10^{-8} Hm^{-1}

Assertion and Reason

Directions (Q. Nos. 1-5) *These questions consist of two statements each printed as Assertion (A) and Reason (R). While answering these questions, you are required to choose any one of the following four responses.*
(a) Both A and R are true but R is not the correct explanation of A.
(b) A is true but R is false.
(c) A is false but R is true.
(d) Both A and R are true and R is the correct explanation of A.

1. Assertion (A) The poles of a magnet cannot be separated by breaking it into two pieces.
Reason (R) The magnetic moment will be reduced to half when a magnet is broken into two equal pieces.

2. Assertion (A) The net magnetic flux coming out of a closed surface is always zero.
Reason (R) Unlike poles of equal strength exist together.

3. Assertion (A) Relative magnetic permeability has no units and no dimensions.
Reason (R) $\mu_r = \mu/\mu_0$, where the symbols have their standard meaning.

4. Assertion (A) χ_m-T graph for a diamagnetic material is a straight line parallel to T-axis.
Reason (R) This is because susceptibility of a diamagnetic material is not affected by temperature.

5. Assertion (A) A magnet suspended freely in a uniform magnetic field experiences no net force but a torque that tends to align the magnet along the field.
Reason (R) Net force, $mB - mB = 0$. But the forces on north and south poles being equal, unlike and parallel, make up a couple that tends to align the magnet, along the field.

Statement Type Questions

Directions (Q. Nos. 1-5) *These questions consist of two statements, choose the most appropriate answer from the options given below.*
(a) Both Statement I and Statement II are incorrect.
(b) Statement I is correct but Statement II is incorrect.
(c) Statement I is incorrect but Statement II is correct.
(d) Both Statement I and Statement II are correct.

1. Statement I In a non-uniform magnetic field, a magnetic needle experiences both torque and force.
Statement II The magnetic needle tries to move against the direction of the magnetic field.

2. Statement I Paramagnetic substances get poorly attracted in magnetic field.

Statement II Magnetic dipole are weakly aligned along external magnetic field.

3. **Statement I** Paramagnetic substances are those which get weakly magnetised when placed in an external magnetic field.

Statement II Paramagnetic substances have tendency to move from a region of weak magnetic field to strong magnetic field, *i.e.* they get weakly attracted to a magnet.

4. **Statement I** The permeability of a ferromagnetic material is independent of the magnetic field.

Statement II Permeability of a material is a constant quantity.

5. **Statement I** A paramagnetic sample displays greater magnetisation (for the same magnetising field) when cooled.

Statement II The magnetisation does not depends on temperature.

Match the Columns

1. Match Column I and Column II.

Column I		Column II	
A.	Magnetic moment	I.	A/m
B.	Magnetic induction	II.	H/m
C.	Magnetic permeability	III.	$NA^{-1} m^{-1}$
D.	Intensity of magnetisation	IV.	$\frac{N\text{-}m}{T}$

Choose the correct answer from the options given below.
(a) A-III, B-IV, C-I D-II
(b) A-IV, B-III, C-I D-II
(c) A-IV, B-III, C-II, D-I
(d) A-I B-III, C-IV, D-II

2. Match Column I with Column II, when lengths of magnets is considerably less than distance *x*.

Column I		Column II	
A.	Couple between two small magnets in the end on-position.	I.	$\frac{\mu_0}{4\pi} \cdot \frac{3MM'}{x^4}$
B.	Couple between two small magnets in the broadside-on-position.	II.	$\frac{\mu_0}{4\pi} \cdot \frac{6MM'}{x^4}$
C.	Force on a magnet when it is in end-on-position with respect to deflecting magnet.	III.	$\frac{\mu_0}{4\pi} \cdot \frac{MM'}{x^3}$
D.	Force on a magnet when it is in broadside-on-position with respect to deflecting magnet.	IV.	$\frac{\mu_0}{4\pi} \cdot \frac{2MM'}{x^3}$

Choose the correct answer from the options given below.
(a) A-I, B-II, C-III, D-IV
(b) A-II, B-I, C-IV D-III
(c) A-III, B-IV C-I, D-II
(d) A-IV B-III, C-II, D-I

3. A bar magnet of magnetic moment 1.5 JT^{-1} aligned with direction of uniform magnetic field of 0.22 T.

Match the scenarios (Column A) with corresponding values (Column B).

Column I		Column II	
A.	Work required to align the magnetic moment normal to field direction	I.	0.33 Nm
B.	Work required to align the magnetic moment opposite to the field direction	II.	0
C.	Torque on the magnet when the magnetic moment is normal to the field direction	III.	0.66 J
D.	Torque on the magnet when the magnetic moment opposite to field direction.	IV.	0.33 J

Choose the correct answer from the options given below.
(a) A-II, B-III, C-IV, D-I
(b) A-III, B-IV, C-II, D-I
(c) A-III, B-IV, C-I, D-II
(d) A-IV, B-III, C-I, D-II

4. Match the following Columns.

Column I		Column II	
A.	Intensity of Magnetisation (*I*)	I.	$\frac{I}{H}$
B.	Magnetic intensity (*H*)	II.	$\frac{B}{H}$
C.	Magnetic permeability (μ)	III.	$\frac{B}{\mu_0} - 1$
D.	Magnetic Susceptibility (χ_m)	IV.	$\frac{M}{V}$

Choose the correct answer from the options given below.
(a) A-IV, B-III, C-II, D-I
(b) A-III, B-IV, C-I, D-II
(c) A-I, B-IV, C-II, D-III
(d) A-II, B-III, C-IV, D-I

5. Match the following Columns.

Column I		Column II	
A.	Diamagnetic	I.	$\mu >> \mu_0 \mu_r >> 1$ and $\chi >> 1$
B.	Paramagnetic	II.	$-1 \le \chi < 0, 0 \le \mu_r < 1$ and $\mu < \mu_0$
C.	Ferromagnetic	III.	$0 < \chi < \varepsilon, 1 < \mu_r < 1 + \varepsilon$ and $\mu > \mu_0$
D.	Vacuum	IV.	$\mu_r = 1$

Choose the correct answer from the options given below.
(a) A-II, B-III, C-I, D-IV
(b) A-II, B-I, C-III, D-IV
(c) A-III, B-IV, C-I, D-II
(d) A-IV, B-III, C-II, D-I

Final Check Through PYQs

Module-I Magnet, Magnetic Dipole and Magnetic Field

1. An iron bar of length l has magnetic moment M. It is bent at the middle of its length such that the two arms make an angle 60° with each other. The magnetic moment of this new magnet is **[NCERT (Old) Pg. 178, NEET 2024]**

   (a) M (b) $\frac{M}{2}$ (c) $2M$ (d) $\frac{M}{\sqrt{3}}$

2. In a uniform magnetic field of 0.049 T, a magnetic needle performs 20 complete oscillations in 5 s as shown. The moment of inertia of the needle is 9.8×10^{-6} kg m^2. If the magnitude of magnetic moment of the needle is $x \times 10^{-5}$ Am^2, then the value of x is **[NCERT (Old) Pg. 178, NEET 2024]**

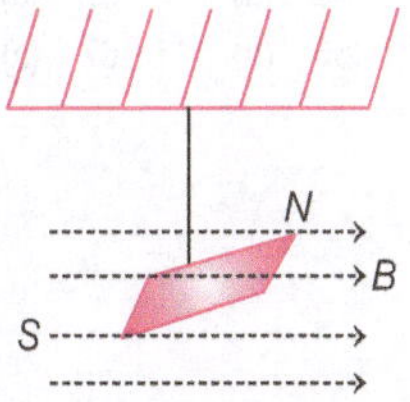

   (a) $5\pi^2$ (b) $128\pi^2$ (c) $50\pi^2$ (d) $1280\pi^2$

3. The net magnetic flux through any closed surface is **[NCERT (New) Pg. 138, NEET 2023]**

   (a) positive (b) infinity
   (c) negative (d) zero

4. A uniform conducting wire of length $12a$ and resistance R is wound up as a current (I) carrying coil in the shape of
   1. an equilateral triangle of side a.
   2. a square of side a.

   The magnetic dipole moments of the coil in each case respectively are **[NCERT (Old) Pg. 176, NEET 2021]**

   (a) $\sqrt{3}\,Ia^2$ and $3\,Ia^2$
   (b) $3\,Ia^2$ and Ia^2
   (c) $3\,Ia^2$ and $4\,Ia^2$
   (d) $4\,Ia^2$ and $3\,Ia^2$

5. A wire of length L metre carrying a current of I ampere is bent in the form of a circle. Its magnetic moment is **[NCERT (Old) Pg. 176, NEET (Oct.) 2020]**

   (a) $(IL^2/4)$ Am^2 (b) $(I\pi L^2/4)$ Am^2
   (c) $(2IL^2/\pi)$ Am^2 (d) $(IL^2/4\pi)$ Am^2

6. A 250 turn rectangular coil of length 2.1 cm and width 1.25 cm carries a current of 85 μA and subjected to a magnetic field of strength 0.85 T. Work done for rotating the coil by 180° against the torque is **[NCERT (Old) Pg. 178, NEET 2017]**

   (a) 9.1 μJ (b) 4.55 μJ
   (c) 2.3 μJ (d) 1.5 μJ

7. A bar magnet is hung by a thin cotton thread in a uniform horizontal magnetic field and is in equilibrium state. The energy required to rotate it by 60° is W. Now the torque required to keep the magnet in this new position is **[NCERT (New) Pg. 139, NEET 2016]**

   (a) $\frac{W}{\sqrt{3}}$ (b) $\sqrt{3}W$
   (c) $\frac{\sqrt{3}W}{2}$ (d) $\frac{2W}{\sqrt{3}}$

Module-II Properties of Magnetic Materials

8. The dimensions $[MLT^{-2}A^{-2}]$ belong to the **[NCERT (New) Pg. 146, NEET 2022]**

   (a) self-inductance (b) magnetic permeability
   (c) electric permittivity (d) magnetic flux

9. An iron rod of susceptibility 599 is subjected to a magnetising field of 1200 Am^{-1}. The permeability of the material of the rod is (Take, $\mu_0 = 4\pi \times 10^{-7}$ T m A^{-1}) **[NCERT (New) Pg. 146, NEET (Sep.) 2020]**

   (a) 8.0×10^{-5} T m A^{-1} (b) $24\pi \times 10^{-5}$ T m A^{-1}
   (c) $2.4\pi \times 10^{-7}$ T m A^{-1} (d) $2.4\pi \times 10^{-4}$ T m A^{-1}

10. A thin diamagnetic rod is placed vertically between the poles of an electromagnet. When the current in the electromagnet is switched ON, then the diamagnetic rod is pushed up, out of the horizontal magnetic field. Hence, the rod gains gravitational potential energy. The work required to do this comes from **[NCERT (New) Pg. 147, NEET 2018]**

    (a) the lattice structure of the material of the rod
    (b) the magnetic field
    (c) the current source
    (d) the induced electric field due to the changing magnetic field

11. The magnetic susceptibility is negative for **[NCERT (New) Pg. 147, NEET 2016]**

    (a) paramagnetic material only
    (b) ferromagnetic material only
    (c) paramagnetic and ferromagnetic materials
    (d) diamagnetic material only

Answers

Step up Practice 1

1 (d)	2 (d)	3 (b)	4 (d)	5 (b)	6 (a)	7 (a)	8 (a)	9 (a)	10 (b)
11 (d)	12 (a)	13 (b)	14 (c)	15 (d)	16 (d)	17 (a)	18 (a)	19 (c)	20 (a)
21 (a)	22 (d)								

Step up Practice 2

1 (c)	2 (a)	3 (a)	4 (b)	5 (a)	6 (a)	7 (c)	8 (c)	9 (c)	10 (d)
11 (c)	12 (d)	13 (b)	14 (a)	15 (a)	16 (d)	17 (c)	18 (a)		

Gearing up for NEET

1 (d)	2 (c)	3 (a)	4 (a)	5 (d)	6 (b)	7 (b)	8 (b)	9 (c)	10 (d)
11 (b)	12 (b)	13 (a)	14 (b)	15 (c)	16 (b)	17 (a)	18 (d)	19 (c)	20 (d)
21 (b)	22 (c)	23 (d)	24 (c)	25 (b)	26 (c)	27 (c)	28 (b)	29 (a)	30 (b)
31 (d)	32 (a)	33 (b)	34 (b)	35 (c)	36 (c)	37 (c)	38 (b)	39 (a)	40 (c)
41 (b)	42 (b)	43 (b)	44 (c)	45 (b)	46 (d)	47 (d)	48 (a)	49 (b)	50 (a)
51 (a)	52 (b)	53 (b)	54 (c)	55 (d)	56 (d)	57 (b)	58 (a)	59 (b)	60 (b)
61 (b)	62 (d)	63 (b)	64 (d)	65 (b)	66 (b)	67 (a)	68 (d)	69 (d)	70 (a)

Assertion and Reason

1 (a)	2 (a)	3 (d)	4 (d)	5 (d)

Statement Type Questions

1 (b)	2 (d)	3 (d)	4 (a)	5 (b)

Match the Columns

1 (c)	2 (d)	3 (d)	4 (a)	5 (a)

Final Check through PYQs : Module-I

1 (b)	2 (d)	3 (d)	4 (a)	5 (d)	6 (a)	7 (b)

Final Check through PYQs : Module-II

8 (b)	9 (d)	10 (c)	11 (d)

Hints and Solutions

Step up Practice 1

1. (*d*) As magnetic moment, $m = q_m \times 2l \Rightarrow q_m = \frac{m}{2l}$

Further, as length of semi-circular magnet, $\pi r = 2l$

or $$r = \frac{2l}{\pi}$$

Distance between the two poles,

$$2l' = 2r = \frac{4l}{\pi}$$

Magnetic moment, $m' = q_m \times 2l'$

$$= \left(\frac{m}{2l}\right)\left(\frac{4l}{\pi}\right) = \frac{2m}{\pi}$$

2. (*d*) Initial magnetic moment $= M_1$

When cut in two parts, magnetic moment of each part,

$$M' = \frac{M_1}{2}$$

When these pieces are placed perpendicular, effective magnetic moment,

$$M_2 = \sqrt{2}M' = \sqrt{2} \times \frac{M_1}{2}$$

$$\therefore \quad \frac{M_1}{M_2} = \frac{2}{\sqrt{2}} = \sqrt{2}$$

3. (*b*) Since, for magnet *P*, axis lies along *X*-axis and for magnet *Q*, axis is along *Y*-axis. The point *R* is along axial line w.r.t. magnet *P* and is along equatorial line w.r.t. magnet *Q*.

Hence, magnetic field due to magnet *Q*,

$$B_Q = \frac{\mu_0}{4\pi}\frac{M}{x^3} = B \quad [R \text{ at equatorial point}] \quad \text{...(i)}$$

Magnetic field due to magnet P,

$$B_P = \frac{\mu_0}{4\pi} \frac{2M}{x^3} = 2B \qquad [R \text{ at axial point}] \quad ...(ii)$$

As, at point R, magnetic field due to P and Q magnet are perpendicular to each other and B_R = net magnetic field at R due to magnet P and Q. *i.e.*

$$B_R = \sqrt{B_P^2 + B_Q^2}$$

$$= \sqrt{B^2 + (2B)^2} = \sqrt{5}B$$

4. (*d*) Both Statement I and Statement II are correct.

Magnetic poles cannot be separated as monopoles of a magnet do not exist.

5. (*b*) Given, magnetic moment of bar magnet,

$$m = 0.40 \text{ A - m}^2$$

Number of turns, $N = 1000$

and area, $A = 2 \times 10^{-4} \text{ m}^2$

Magnetic moment of solenoid, $m = NIA$

$$\Rightarrow \quad 0.40 = 1000 \times I \times 2 \times 10^{-4}$$

$$\Rightarrow \quad I = 0.40 \times 10^4 / (1000 \times 2) = 2 \text{ A}$$

Hence, the current flowing, $I = 2$ A.

6. (*a*) When a bar magnet of magnetic moment **M** is placed in a magnetic field of induction **B**, then net force on it is $F_R = mB + (-m)B = 0$

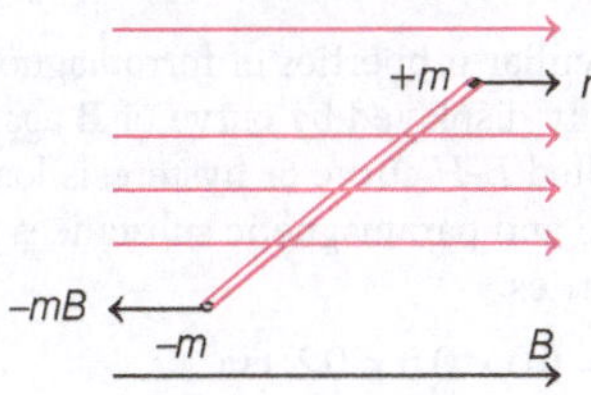

While torque, $\tau = mB \times 2l \sin\theta = MB \sin\theta$ (as, $M = 2ml$)

i.e. $\quad \tau = \mathbf{M} \times \mathbf{B}$

7. (*a*) As, $\tau = MB \sin\theta$

$$= (m \times 2l) \times 2 \times 10^{-5} \sin 30°$$

$$= 15 \times 10 \times 10^{-2} \times 2 \times 10^{-5} \times \frac{1}{2}$$

$$= 1.5 \times 10^{-5} \text{ N-m}$$

8. (*a*) As, $\tau = MB \sin\theta$

where, $\theta = 90° \Rightarrow \tau = MB$

Given, $\tau_2 = \frac{1}{2}\tau_1 \Rightarrow MB \sin\theta = \frac{1}{2} MB$

$$\Rightarrow \quad \sin\theta = \frac{1}{2} \Rightarrow \theta = 30°$$

$\therefore$ Angle of rotation $= 90° - 30° = 60°$

9. (*a*) Magnetic lines of force due to a bar magnet do not intersect because a point on magnetic lines always has a single net magnetic field. If they intersect, then it means, there are two directions of magnetic field intensity at that point, which is impossible.

10. (*b*) Statement I is correct but Statement II is incorrect.

Magnetic field lines can be totally confined to the core of toroid because toroid has no ends. It can confine the field within its core. A straight solenoid has two ends. If the entire flux were confined between these ends, the flux throughout the cross-section at each end would be non-zero.

The magnetic field inside the solenoid is uniform.

11. (*d*) Work done in rotating the magnet through an angle θ from initial position (*i.e.* $\theta_1 = 0°$) is given by

$$W = MB(\cos\theta_1 - \cos\theta)$$

$$= MB(\cos 0° - \cos\theta) = MB(1 - \cos\theta)$$

12. (*a*) For unstable equilibrium, **m** is to be anti-parallel to **B.** In this case, $\theta = 180°$, thus

$U = -mB \cos 180° = -mB(-1) = mB$

Given, $m = 0.32 \text{ JT}^{-1}$ and $B = 0.15$ T

Hence, $U = (0.32)(0.15) = 4.8 \times 10^{-2}$ J

13. (*b*) Given, work done $= W$ and $\theta = 45°$

We know that, $W = mB(\cos 0° - \cos\theta)$

$$= mB(1 - \cos 45°)$$

$$= mB\left(1 - \frac{1}{\sqrt{2}}\right) = \left(\frac{\sqrt{2}-1}{\sqrt{2}}\right) mB$$

$$\Rightarrow \qquad mB = \frac{\sqrt{2}W}{\sqrt{2}-1} \qquad ...(i)$$

Hence, torque, $\tau = mB \sin\theta$

$$\tau = mB \sin 45° = \frac{W \times \sqrt{2}}{\sqrt{2}-1} \times \frac{1}{\sqrt{2}} \qquad \text{[from Eq. (i)]}$$

$$= \frac{W}{\sqrt{2}-1}$$

14. (*c*) When magnetic dipole is rotated from initial position θ_1 to final position θ_2, then work done

$$= MB(\cos\theta_1 - \cos\theta_2)$$

Given, $\theta_1 = 0°$ and $\theta_2 = 60°$

Magnetic moment, $m = 2 \times 10^4 \text{ JT}^{-1}$

and magnetic field, $B = 6 \times 10^{-4}$ T

$$\therefore \qquad W = mB(\cos 0° - \cos 60°)$$

$$\Rightarrow \qquad W = mB\left(1 - \frac{1}{2}\right)$$

$$(\because \cos 0° = 1 \text{ and } \cos 60° = 1/2)$$

$$= \frac{2 \times 10^4 \times 6 \times 10^{-4}}{2} = 6 \text{ J}$$

$\therefore$ Work done to rotate bar magnet is 6 J.

15. (*d*) Given, $m = 0.40 \text{ A-m}^2$ and $r = 50 \text{ cm} = 0.5 \text{m}$

Magnetic field at equatorial line,

$$B_e = \frac{\mu_0 m}{4\pi r^3}$$

$$= \frac{10^{-7} \times 0.40}{(0.5)^3} = \frac{10^{-7} \times 0.40}{0.125} = 3.2 \times 10^{-7} \text{ T}$$

Magnetic field at axial line, $B_a = \frac{\mu_0 2m}{4\pi r^3} = 6.4 \times 10^{-7}$ T

16. (*d*) Axial magnetic field for a short dipole is $\frac{\mu_0 2M}{4\pi r^3}$.

17. (*a*) Both Statement I and Statement II are incorrect.

In a non-uniform magnetic field, both a torque and a net force acts on the dipole. If magnetic field is uniform, net force on dipole would be zero.

18. (*a*) The potential energy of a dipole or a current carrying coil in a magnetic field is.

$$U = -\mathbf{m} \cdot \mathbf{B} = -mB \cos \theta$$

where, θ is the angle between magnetic field **B** and magnetic moment **m** along normal vector $\hat{\mathbf{n}}$.

In given cases,

(i) $U = -mB \cos 90° = 0$ $[\because \cos 90° = 0]$

(ii) $U = -mB \cos 180° = mB$ $[\because \cos 180° = -1]$

(iii) $U = -mB \cos (360° - \theta) = -mB \cos \theta$ $[\because \cos (360° - \theta) = + \cos \theta]$

(iv) $U = -mB \cos (90° + \theta) = mB \sin \theta$ $[\because \cos (90° + \theta) = -\sin \theta]$

So, correct order of potential energy in increasing order is (iii) > (i) > (iv) > (ii).

19. (*c*) As, the time period, $T = 2\pi \sqrt{\frac{I}{MB}}$

or $T \propto \frac{1}{\sqrt{B}} \Rightarrow \frac{T_2}{T_1} = \sqrt{\frac{B_1}{B_2}}$

or $\frac{T_2}{3} = \sqrt{\frac{1}{4}} \Rightarrow T_2 = 1.5$ s

20. (*a*) Work done in rotating the dipole from θ_1 to θ_2,

$$W = -MB(\cos \theta_2 - \cos \theta_1)$$

Case I $W_1 = -MB(\cos 90° - \cos 0°) = MB$ ...(i)

Case II $W_2 = -MB(\cos 60° - \cos 0°)$

$$= -MB\left(\frac{1}{2} - 1\right) = \frac{1}{2} MB \quad \text{...(ii)}$$

From Eqs. (i) and (ii), we get

$$W_2 = \frac{1}{2} W_1 \quad \text{...(iii)}$$

Given, $W_1 = nW_2$ ...(iv)

By comparing Eqs. (iii) and (iv), we get

$\therefore$ $n = 2$

21. (*a*) According to Gauss' theorem in magnetism, surface integral of magnetic field intensity over a surface (closed or open) is always zero. *i.e.* $\int \mathbf{B} \cdot d\mathbf{A} = 0$.

22. (*d*) Both Statement I and Statement II are correct.

The torque on a bar magnetic,

$$\tau = MB \sin \theta$$

where,

M = magnetic dipole moment

and B = uniform magnetic field.

When $\theta = 90°$, then magnitude of the torque is maximum.

Step up Practice 2

1. (*c*) Magnetic permeability, $\mu = \frac{B}{H}$

Its SI unit is $\frac{\text{Wb/m}^2}{\text{A/m}} = \frac{\text{Wb}}{\text{A}} \cdot \frac{1}{\text{m}} = \text{Hm}^{-1}$

$$\left[\because \frac{\text{Wb}}{\text{A}} = \text{H (Henry)}\right]$$

2. (*a*) Both A and R are true and R is not the correct explanation of A.

For a perfectly diamagnetic substance,

$$B = \mu_0(H + I) = 0$$

$\therefore$ $I = -H$

Therefore, $\chi_m = \frac{I}{H} = -1$

Therefore, relative permeability

$$\mu_r = 1 + \chi_m = 1 - 1 = 0$$

$\therefore$ $\mu = \mu_0 \mu_r$ = zero

i.e. for a perfectly diamagnetic material, permeability is zero.

3. (*a*) Some peculiar properties of ferromagnetic materials are commonly displayed by curve of **B** against **H**, which is called *B-H* curve or hysteresis loop.

Diamagnetic and paramagnetic substances do not show these properties.

4. (*b*) Here, $V = (10 \times 0.5 \times 0.2)$ cm^3

$$= 1 \text{ cm}^3 = 10^{-6} \text{ m}^3$$

$H = 0.5 \times 10^4$ Am^{-1} and $m = 5$ Am^2

Intensity of magnetisation, $M = \frac{m}{V} = \frac{5}{10^{-6}}$

$$= 5 \times 10^6 \text{ Am}^{-1}$$

Magnetic induction, $B = \mu_0(M + H)$

$$B = 4\pi \times 10^{-7}(5 \times 10^6 + 0.5 \times 10^4) = 6.28 \text{ T}$$

Hence, the magnetic induction will be 6.28 T.

5. (*a*) Given, $\mu_r = 400$, $I = 2$ A and $n = 1000$

(i) The field H is depend on the material core and it is

$$H = nI = 1000 \times 2 = 2 \times 10^3 \text{ Am}^{-1}$$

(ii) Magnetisation, $M = (B - \mu_0 H)/\mu_0$

$\Rightarrow$ $M = (\mu_r \mu_0 H - \mu_0 H)/\mu_0$ $[\because B = \mu_r \mu_0 H]$

$$= (\mu_r - 1)H = (400 - 1)H = 399 \times H$$

$$= 399 \times 2 \times 10^3 \approx 8 \times 10^5 \text{ Am}^{-1}$$

Hence, the value of H and M are 2×10^3 Am^{-1} and 8×10^5 Am^{-1}, respectively.

6. (a) Given, $R_1 = 11$ cm, $R_2 = 12$ cm,

$I = 0.70$ A, $B = 2.5$ T and $N = 3000$

Mean radius of the toroid,

$$R = \frac{R_1 + R_2}{2} = \frac{(11 + 12)\text{ cm}}{2}$$

$$= 11.5 \times 10^{-2}\text{ m}$$

As we know, $B = \mu H$, $H = nI$ and $\mu_r = \mu / \mu_0$

So, $B = \mu_r \mu_0 nI$

$$\Rightarrow \quad \mu_r = \frac{B}{\mu_0 nI} = \frac{B}{\mu_0 (N / 2\pi R) I} \quad \left[\because n = \frac{N}{2\pi R}\right]$$

$$= \frac{2.5 \times 2\pi (11.5 \times 10^{-2})}{(4\pi \times 10^{-7})(3000) \times (0.70)} = 685$$

Hence, $\mu_r = 685$.

7. (c) (a) H = Number of turn × Current

$= 1000 \times 2.0 = 2 \times 10^3\text{ Am}^{-1}$

(b) $B = \mu_r \mu_0 H$

$= 400 \times 4\pi \times 10^{-7} \times 2 \times 10^3 = 1.0$ T

(c) $I = \frac{(B - \mu_0 H)}{\mu_0} = \frac{\mu_r \mu_0 H - \mu_0 H}{\mu_0}$

$= (\mu_r - 1) H$

$= 399 \times H$

$\simeq 8 \times 10^5$ A/m

(d) $B = \mu_r \times$ Number of turn (Current + Magnetic current)

Putting the values, $I = 2$ A and $B = 1$ T, we get magnetising current = 794 A

8. (c) Permeability of core,

$$\mu = \mu_0 \mu_r = \mu_0 (1 + \chi_m) \quad (\because \mu_r = 1 + \chi_m)$$

Given, $\chi_m = 1874$

$= (4\pi \times 10^{-7})(1 + 1874)$

$= 7.5 \times 10^{-4}\text{ TmA}^{-1}$

9. (c) In a paramagnetic material,

$$M = C\frac{B}{T} = C\frac{\mu H}{T} \quad [\because B = \mu H]$$

Hence, $M \propto H$. Therefore, the graph between H and M is a straight line represented by in figure

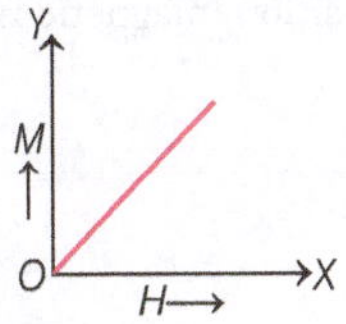

10. (d) The volume of cubic domain is

$$V = (10^{-6})^3\text{ m}^3 = 10^{-18}\text{ m}^3 = 10^{-12}\text{ cm}^3$$

[∵ side = 1 μm]

Mass = Density × Volume

$= 7.9\text{ gcm}^{-3} \times 10^{-12}\text{ cm}^3$ (∵ Density = 7.9 gcm^{-3})

$= 7.9 \times 10^{-12}$ g

It is given that Avogadro's number *i.e.* (6.023×10^{23}) of iron atoms have a mass of 55 g. Hence, the number of atoms in the domain,

$$N = \frac{\text{Mass}}{\text{Molecular mass}}$$

$$= \frac{7.9 \times 10^{-12} \times 6.023 \times 10^{23}}{55}$$

$= 8.65 \times 10^{10}$ atoms

11. (c) According to Curie's law, $\chi = \frac{C}{T}$ ...(i)

and magnetic susceptibility, $\chi = \frac{I}{H}$ ...(ii)

From Eqs. (i) and (ii), we get

$$\frac{C}{T} = \frac{I}{H} = \frac{m / V}{B / \mu} \quad \left[\because I = \frac{m}{V} \text{ and } H = \frac{B}{\mu}\right]$$

$$\Rightarrow \quad m = \frac{CV}{\mu}\left(\frac{B}{T}\right)$$

For a given sample, CV / μ = constant.

Thus, $m \propto B / T$

or $\frac{m_1}{m_2} = \frac{B_1 / T_1}{B_2 / T_2}$

Given, $B_1 = 0.84$ T, $B_2 = 0.98$ T

$T_1 = 4.2$ K and $T_2 = 2.8$ K

Thus, $\frac{m_1}{m_2} = \frac{0.84 / 4.2}{0.98 / 2.8} = 4 / 7$

or $m_2 = (7 / 4) m_1$

Initial total magnetic moment of the sample, *i.e.* $m_1 = 15\%$ of nm, where n is the number of atomic dipoles and m is the dipole moment of each dipole.

Given, $n = 2 \times 10^{24}$ and $m = 1.5 \times 10^{-23}\text{ JT}^{-1}$

∴ $m_1 = 15\%$ of $(2.0 \times 10^{24})(1.5 \times 10^{-23}) = 4.5\text{ JT}^{-1}$

Thus, $m_2 = (7 / 4)(4.5) = 7.9\text{ JT}^{-1}$

12. (d) Intensity of magnetisation of a bulk material is given by magnetic dipole moment developed per unit volume when it is placed in magnetic field, *i.e.*

$$I = \frac{m_{\text{net}}}{V}$$

where, m_{net} = magnetic moment and V = volume.

Unit of I = Am^{-1} and it is a vector quantity.

13. (b) A is true but R is false.

From the relation, susceptibility of the material,

$$\chi_m = \frac{I}{H} \Rightarrow \chi_m \propto I$$

Thus, it is obvious that, greater the value of susceptibility of a material, greater will be the value of intensity of magnetisation. *i.e.* More easily, it can be magnetised.

14. (*a*) Given, side of cube $= 1\text{ cm} = 10^{-2}\text{ m}$

$\therefore$ Volume, $V = 10^{-6}\text{ m}^3$

Dipole moment, $M = 20 \times 10^{-6}$ J/T

Applied magnetic intensity, $H = 60 \times 10^3$ A/m

Intensity of magnetisation,

$$I = \frac{M}{V} = \frac{20 \times 10^{-6}}{10^{-6}} = 20\text{ A/m}$$

Now, magnetic susceptibility χ,

$$\chi = \frac{\text{Intensity of magnetisation}}{\text{Applied magnetic intensity}} = \frac{I}{H}$$

$$= \frac{20}{60 \times 10^3}$$

$$\Rightarrow \quad \chi = \frac{1}{3} \times 10^{-3}$$

$$= 3.33 \times 10^{-4}$$

15. (*a*) As temperature of ferromagnetic material is raised its susceptibility χ remains constant upto curie temperature and then decreases as shown in figure.

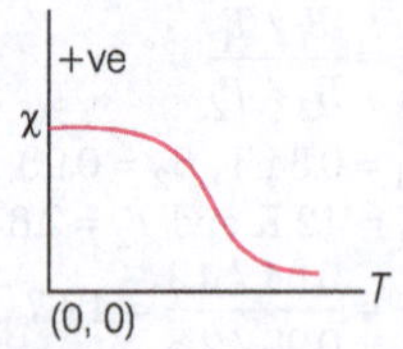

Hence, the correct variation is shown by figure in option (a).

16. (*d*) Dimension of relative permeability is L^0A^0.

17. (*c*) A is false but R is true.

The properties of substance is due to alignment of molecules in it. When these substances are heated, molecules acquire some kinetic energy. Due to this Kinetic energy, the alignment of molecular magnets gradually decreases. So, they loss their magnetic property or magnetism. Therefore, the properties of both ferromagnetic and paramagnetic are effected by heating.

18. (*a*) Both A and R are true and R is not the correct explanation of A.

The susceptibility of ferromagnetic substance decreases with the rise of temperature in a complicated manner. After curie point, the susceptibility of ferromagnetic substance varies inversely with its absolute temperature. Ferromagnetic substance obeys curie's law only above its curie point.

Gearing up for NEET

1. (*d*) SI unit of magnetic induction,

$$B = \frac{\text{Unit of } \phi}{\text{Unit of } \Delta A} = \frac{\text{Wb}}{\text{m}^2} = \text{tesla}$$

Also, SI unit of B is weber/metre^2 and newton/ampere-metre.

2. (*c*) Magnetic moment per unit volume is intensity of magnetisation and number of lines of force crossing per unit area is intensity of magnetic field.

3. (*a*) In non-uniform magnetic field, a magnetic needle experiences a force and a torque.

4. (*a*) From Gauss' law, $\oint \mathbf{B} \cdot d\mathbf{S} = 0$

or divergence of $B = \nabla \cdot \mathbf{B} = 0$

6. (*b*) Let pole strength be m_1 and m_2 and distance between them is r, then force between magnetic poles,

$$F \propto \frac{m_1 m_2}{r^2}$$

In second case, $F' \propto \dfrac{(2m_1)(2m_2)}{(2r)^2}$

$$\Rightarrow \quad F' \propto \frac{m_1 m_2}{r^2}$$

$$\therefore \quad F' = F$$

7. (*b*)

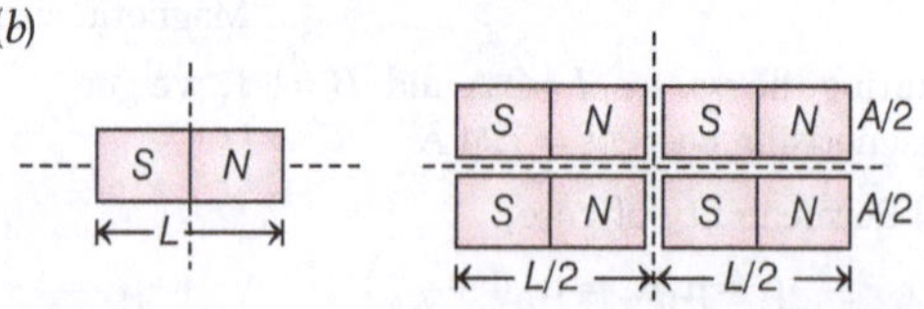

The situation is summarised in figure, we see that magnetic pole strength of each part becomes half, *i.e.* $m/2$.

8. (*b*) Due to hole, the effective length of magnet $(2l)$ is decreased, so magnetic moment of one with hole is smaller.

9. (*c*) For longitudinal position, magnetic field will be $B_1 \propto \dfrac{2M}{d^3}$.

For transverse position, magnetic field will be

$$B_2 \propto \frac{M}{d^3}$$

$$\therefore \quad \frac{B_1}{B_2} = 2:1$$

11. (*b*) Torque, $\tau = MB \sin\theta$

$\therefore \quad \tau_1 = MB_1 \sin 90° = MB_1$

and $\quad \tau_2 = MB_2 \sin 90° = MB_2$ or $\dfrac{MB_1}{MB_2} = \dfrac{\tau_1}{\tau_2}$

$$\therefore \quad \frac{B_1}{B_2} = \frac{\tau_1}{\tau_2}$$

12. (*b*) $$\frac{\tan A}{\tan B} = \frac{2d\,(d^2 + l^2)^{3/2}}{(d^2 - l^2)^2}$$

$$= \frac{2d \times d^3\,(1 + l^2/d^2)^{3/2}}{d^4\left(1 - \frac{l^2}{d^2}\right)^2}$$

$$\because \quad 1 >> \frac{l^2}{d^2} \Rightarrow \frac{\tan A}{\tan B} = 2:1$$

13. (*a*) As we know, $M = m(2l)$

$$\therefore \quad M = 4 \times 10 \times 10^{-2} = 0.4 \text{ A-m}^2$$

14. (*b*) If magnet is cut along the axis of magnet of length $2l$, then new pole strength becomes half, *i.e.* $m' = \frac{m}{2}$ and new length remains same,

i.e. $2l' = 2l$.

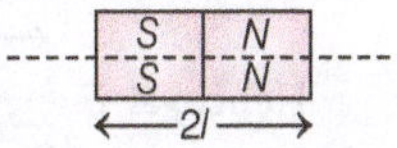

∴New magnetic moment,

$$M' = \frac{m}{2} \times 2l = \frac{m2l}{2} = \frac{M}{2}$$

15. (*c*) Net magnetic moment of the system is given by

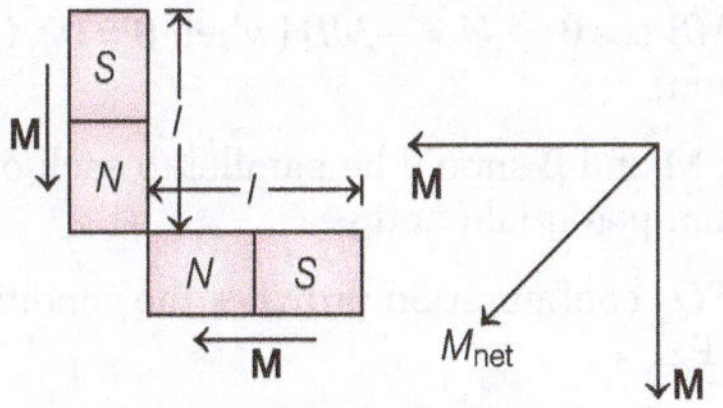

$$M = \sqrt{M^2 + M^2} = \sqrt{2}M = \sqrt{2}\, ml$$

16. (*b*) Magnetic moment of the bar magnet is given by

$$M = \frac{\tau}{B \sin \theta} \qquad (\because \tau = MB \sin \theta)$$

$$= \frac{0.032}{0.16 \times \sin 30^\circ} = \frac{0.032 \times 2}{0.16} = 0.4 \text{ J T}^{-1}$$

17. (*a*) As, $\tau = MB \sin \theta$

$$\tau = m(2l)\, B \sin \theta$$

$$\therefore \quad m = \frac{\tau}{(2l)\, B \sin \theta} = \frac{25 \times 10^{-6}}{(0.05)(5 \times 10^{-2}) \sin 30^\circ}$$

$$= 2 \times 10^{-2} \text{ A-m}$$

18. (*d*) Force experienced by each pole of bar magnet is given by

$$F = mB$$

where, m is pole strength of bar magnet.

But $\qquad M = mL$

$$\therefore \quad F = \frac{M}{L} \times B \Rightarrow 6 \times 10^{-4} = \frac{3}{L} \times 2 \times 10^{-5}$$

$$\therefore \quad L = 0.1 \text{ m}$$

19. (*c*) In case of toroid, the magnetic field is only confined inside the body of toroid in the form of concentric magnetic lines of force and there is no magnetic field outside the body of toroid. This is because, the loop encloses no current. Thus, the magnetic moment of toroid is zero.

In general, if we take r as a large distance outside the toroid, then $m \propto \frac{1}{r^3}$.

20. (*d*) Work done in rotating the magnet from angle θ_1 to angle θ_2 is given by

$$W = MB(\cos \theta_1 - \cos \theta_2)$$

Here, $\theta_1 = 0^\circ$ and $\theta_2 = 180^\circ$

$$W = MB\,(\cos 0^\circ - \cos 180^\circ) = 2MB$$

21. (*b*) Work done in rotating the magnet in uniform magnetic field is given by

$$W = MB(\cos \theta_1 - \cos \theta_2)$$

Here, $\theta_1 = 0^\circ, \theta_2 = 90^\circ$

$$\therefore \quad W = 2 \times 0.1\,(\cos 0^\circ - \cos 90^\circ)$$

$$= 2 \times 0.1\,(1 - 0) = 0.2 \text{ J}$$

22. (*c*) Here, $\mathbf{B} = 0.5\,\hat{\mathbf{i}}$T, $I = 20$ A, $N = 15$, $\mathbf{A} = -0.04\,\hat{\mathbf{i}}\text{m}^2$

Magnetic moment of the coil,

$$\mathbf{M} = NI\mathbf{A}$$

$$= (15)(20)(-0.04\,\hat{\mathbf{i}})$$

$$= -12\hat{\mathbf{i}} \text{ Am}^2$$

The potential energy of the coil in the given orientation,

$$U = -\mathbf{M} \cdot \mathbf{B} = -(-12\hat{\mathbf{i}}) \cdot (0.5\hat{\mathbf{i}}) = +6 \text{ J}$$

23. (*d*) $$\therefore \quad \frac{B}{0.2} = \frac{M/(5)^3}{2M/(10)^3} = \frac{(10/5)^3}{2} = 4 \text{ G}$$

$$\Rightarrow B = 4 \times 0.2 = 0.8 \text{ oersted}$$

25. (*b*) As, Gauss' law states that, $\oint_S \mathbf{E} \cdot d\mathbf{S} = \frac{q}{\varepsilon_0}$ for electrostatic field. It does not contradicts for electrostatic fields as the electric field lines do not form continuous closed path.

According to Gauss' law in magnetism, $\oint_S \mathbf{B} \cdot d\mathbf{S} = 0$.

which means that the number of magnetic field lines entering the Gaussian surface is equal to the number of field lines leaving it.

It contradicts for magnetic field because there is a magnetic field inside the solenoid and no field outside the solenoid carrying current but the magnetic field lines form the closed paths.

26. (*c*) In CGS, $B_{\text{axial}} = 9 = \frac{\mu_0}{4\pi} \frac{2M}{x^3}$ ...(i)

$$B_{\text{equatorial}} = \frac{\mu_0}{4\pi} \frac{M}{\left(\frac{x}{2}\right)^2} = \frac{\mu_0}{4\pi} \frac{8M}{x^3} \quad \text{...(ii)}$$

From Eqs. (i) and (ii), we get

$$B_{\text{equatorial}} = 4B_{\text{axial}} = 36 \text{ G}$$

27. (*c*) Resultant magnetic moment at point *O* is

$$M_{\text{net}} = \sqrt{M^2 + M^2} = \sqrt{2}M$$

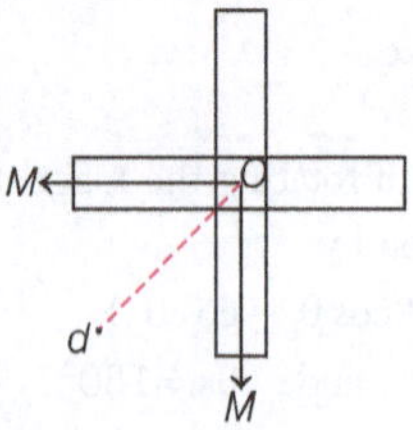

Suppose a dipole of magnetic moment $\sqrt{2}M$ is placed at point *O* along line *Od*. The point *d* is on the axial line of this dipole, hence magnetic field at point *d*,

$$B_{\text{net}} = \frac{\mu_0}{4\pi} \frac{2\sqrt{2}M}{d^3} \quad \left(\because B_{\text{axial}} = \frac{\mu_0}{4\pi} \frac{2M_{\text{net}}}{d^3}\right)$$

28. (*b*) Time period for oscillating magnet is

$$T = 2\pi\sqrt{\frac{I}{MB}} \quad \text{...(i)}$$

where *I* is the momentof inertia, *M* is the magnetic moment

$$M = 2m \times l$$

Where, m = pole strength

If the magnet is broken in two equal parts, the new magnetic dipole moment is

$$M' = \frac{2m \times l}{2} = \frac{M}{2}$$

$$I' = \frac{ML'^2}{12} = \frac{\frac{M}{2} \times \left(\frac{L}{2}\right)^2}{12} = \frac{ML^2}{12 \times 8} = \frac{I}{8}$$

New time period, $T' = 2\pi\sqrt{\frac{I'}{M'B}}$

$$\frac{T'}{T} = \sqrt{\frac{I'}{M'} \times \frac{M}{I}} = \sqrt{\frac{I \times 2}{8 \times M} \times \frac{M}{I}} = \frac{1}{2}$$

$$T' = \frac{T}{2} = \frac{4}{2} = 2 \text{ s}$$

29. (*a*) Time period of vibrating magnet is given by

$$T = 2\pi\sqrt{\left(\frac{I}{MB}\right)}$$

$$\therefore \quad \frac{T_1}{T_2} = \sqrt{\left(\frac{M_2}{M_1}\right)}$$

Frequency of oscillations of bar magnet,

$f_1 = 10$ oscillations/min

$f_2 = 15$ oscillations/min

$$\Rightarrow \quad T_1 = \frac{1}{f_2} = \frac{60}{10}$$

$$T_2 = \frac{1}{f_2} = \frac{60}{15}$$

$$\therefore \quad \frac{M_1}{M_2} = \frac{T_2^2}{T_1^2} = \frac{(60/15)^2}{(60/10)^2} = \frac{4}{9}$$

30. (*b*) Suppose magnetic field is zero at point *P* which lies at a distance *x* from 10 unit pole.

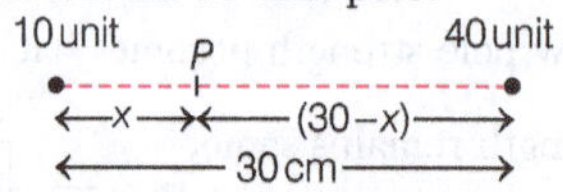

Hence, at *P*

$$\frac{\mu_0}{4\pi} \cdot \frac{10}{x^2} = \frac{\mu_0}{4\pi} \cdot \frac{40}{(30-x)^2} \Rightarrow x = 10 \text{ cm}$$

So, from stronger pole, distance is 20 cm.

31. (*d*) As potential energy is given as

$U = -MB\cos\theta \Rightarrow U = -MB$ [when $\theta = 0°$, U = minimum]

Hence, **M** and **B** should be parallel to each other for minimum potential energy.

Here, PQ_6 configuration provides the condition of lowest PE.

32. (*a*) Using the formula for time period for magnetic system,

$$T = 2\pi\sqrt{\left(\frac{I}{MB}\right)} \Rightarrow T \propto \frac{1}{\sqrt{M}} \quad \text{...(i)}$$

When similar poles placed at same side, then

$$M_1 = M + 2M = 3M$$

So, from Eq. (i), $T_1 \propto \frac{1}{\sqrt{3M}}$ ...(ii)

When the polarity of a magnet is reversed, then

$$M_2 = 2M - M = M$$

So, from Eq . (i),

$$T_2 \propto \frac{1}{\sqrt{M}} \quad \text{...(iii)}$$

Now, dividing Eq. (ii) by Eq. (iii), we get

$$\frac{T_1}{T_2} = \frac{\sqrt{M}}{\sqrt{3M}} = \frac{1}{\sqrt{3}} \Rightarrow T_2 = \sqrt{3}\,T_1$$

Hence, $T_1 < T_2$

33. (b) Initially, the time period of the magnet,

$$T = 2\pi\sqrt{\left(\frac{I}{MB}\right)}$$

For each part of magnet, its moment of inertia is $\frac{I}{27}$ and its magnetic moment $= M/3$.

When magnet is cut along its length into three equal parts and placed on each other, then new moment of inertia of system,

$$I' = \frac{I}{27} \times 3 = \frac{I}{9}$$

and magnetic moment of system, $M' = \frac{M}{3} \times 3 = M$

$\therefore$ Time period of system,

$$T' = 2\pi\sqrt{\frac{I'}{M'B}} = \frac{1}{3} \times 2\pi\sqrt{\frac{I}{MB}} = \frac{T}{3} = \frac{2}{3}\text{ s}$$

34. (b) The coercivity of bar magnet $= 4 \times 10^3\ \text{Am}^{-1}$

Length of solenoid $= 12\text{ cm} = 12 \times 10^{-2}\text{ m}$

and number of turns = 60

The coercivity of 12 cm length of solenoid

$$= 4 \times 10^3 \times 12 \times 10^{-2} = 480\ \text{Am}^{-1}$$

Now, current through each turn to demagnetise

$$= \frac{480}{60} = 8\text{ A}$$

35. (c) The effective length of magnet, $l = 31.4$ cm

$$= 31.4 \times 10^{-2}\text{ m}$$

Pole strength, $m = 0.8$ A-m

Length of semi-circle $= \pi\frac{D}{2} = l$

where, D = diameter of circle

$$\Rightarrow \quad D = \frac{2l}{\pi} = \frac{2 \times 31.4 \times 10^{-2}}{3.14}$$

$$\Rightarrow \quad D = 20 \times 10^{-2}\text{ m}$$

Now, the magnetic moment

$$= mD = 0.8 \times 20 \times 10^{-2}$$

$$= 16 \times 10^{-2} = 0.16\ \text{A-m}^2$$

36. (c) (a) $M_1 = m\sqrt{2}$

(b) $\overset{m}{\underset{m}{\leftrightarrows}} \Rightarrow M_2 = 0$

(c) $M_3 = m\sqrt{(1 + \cos 30°)^2}$

$$= m\sqrt{\left(1 + \frac{\sqrt{3}}{2}\right)^2} = m\sqrt{2 + \sqrt{3}}$$

(d) $M_4 = 2m\cos 30° = m\sqrt{3}$

Hence, option (c) has highest net magnetic dipole moment.

37. (c) The bar magnet is shown in the diagram.

For Figs. (a) and (b),

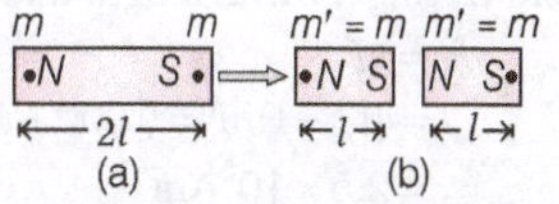

Magnetic moment for Fig. (a), $M = m\,(2l)$

Magnetic moment for Fig. (b), $M' = m'\,(l)$

Now, $\frac{M'}{M} = \frac{m'(l)}{m(2l)} = \frac{1}{2}\left(\frac{m'}{m}\right)$ ...(i)

When magnet is cut as shown in the diagram, pole strength will not be affected. Hence, $m' = m$

$\Rightarrow \frac{m'}{m} = 1 \Rightarrow M' = \frac{M}{2}$ [from Eq. (i)]

38. (b) Let magnetic pole strength be m, then $M = ml$.

$\therefore \quad M' = m\left[2r\sin\left(\frac{60°}{2}\right)\right]$, where $r\left(\frac{\pi}{3}\right) = l$.

$$\Rightarrow \quad M' = 2m\left(\frac{3l}{\pi}\right)\left(\frac{1}{2}\right) = \frac{3ml}{\pi} = \frac{3M}{\pi}$$

39. (a) Given, $M = 120\ \text{Am}^2$, $T = 12$ s and $B = 0.4 \times 10^{-4}$ T

We know that, $T = 2\pi\sqrt{\frac{I}{MB}}$ (squaring both sides)

So, $$I = \frac{T^2MB}{4\pi^2}$$

or $$I = \frac{(12)^2 \times (120) \times (0.4 \times 10^{-4})}{4 \times 3.14 \times 3.14}$$

$$I = 175.2 \times 10^{-4}\ \text{kg-m}^2$$

In this question, the option (a) is approximately equivalent to 175.2×10^{-4}, so the answer is $I = 172.8 \times 10^{-4}\ \text{kg-m}^2$

40. (c) When wire is bent in the form of semi-circular arc, then $l = \pi r$.

$\therefore$ The radius of sem-circular arc, $r = l/\pi$

Distance between two end points of semi-circular wire

$$= 2r = \frac{2l}{\pi}$$

$\therefore$ Magnetic moment of semicircular wire

$$= m \times 2r = m \times \frac{2l}{\pi} = \frac{2}{\pi}ml$$

But ml is the magnetic moment of wire, *i.e.* $ml = M$

$\therefore \quad$ New magnetic moment $= \frac{2}{\pi}M$

41. (*b*) We know that, $B = \mu_0 H + \mu_0 I$

$$\therefore \quad I = \frac{B - \mu_0 H}{\mu_0} = \frac{\mu H - \mu_0 H}{\mu_0} = \left(\frac{\mu}{\mu_0} - 1\right) H$$

$$I = (\mu_r - 1) H$$

For a solenoid having n turns/length and current I',

$$H = nI'$$

$$I = (\mu_r - 1) nI' = (1000 - 1) \times 500 \times 0.5 = 2.5 \times 10^5 \text{Am}^{-1}$$

$\therefore$ Magnetic moment, $M = IV$ (V = volume)

$$= 2.5 \times 10^5 \times 10^{-4} = 25 \text{ A-m}^2$$

42. (*b*) If length of wire is $2l$, then magnetic moment,

$$M = m \times 2l = 4\pi \text{ A-m}^2 \quad \text{(given)}$$

As wire is bent in the form of semi-circle, effective distance between the ends is $2r$.

So, new dipole moment, $M' = m \times 2r$

As, $\pi r = 2l$

$\Rightarrow$ $r = 2l/\pi$

So, $M' = m \times 2 \times \frac{2l}{\pi} = \frac{2}{\pi}(m \times 2l)$

$$= \frac{2}{\pi} M = \frac{2}{\pi} 4\pi = 8 \text{ A-m}^2$$

49. (*b*) For a diamagnetic substance, χ is small, negative and independent of temperature.

$\because$ Curve should be in negative direction with constant value *i.e.* graph (b).

54. (*c*) Magnetism of a magnet falls with rise of temperature and becomes practically zero above curie temperature as shown in Fig. (c).

56. (*d*) Given, $B = 4B_0$

$$\therefore \quad \frac{B}{B_0} = 4 \Rightarrow \mu_r = 4 \quad \left[\because \mu_r = \frac{B}{B_0}\right]$$

60. (*b*) Above the curie temperature, ferromagnetic substance become paramagnetic in nature. So, its susceptibility varies inversely as the absolute temperature.

62. (*d*) For a temporary magnet, the hysteresis loop should be long and narrow.

63. (*b*) Intensity of magnetisation, $I = \frac{M}{V} = -\frac{M}{\text{mass/density}}$

Given, mass $= 1 \text{ g} = 10^{-3}$ kg

and density $= 5 \text{g/cm}^3 = \frac{5 \times 10^{-3} \text{kg}}{(10^{-2})^3}$

$$= 5 \times 10^3 \text{kg/m}^3$$

Hence, $I = \frac{6 \times 10^{-7} \times 5 \times 10^3}{10^{-3}} = 3 \text{ A/m}$

65. (*b*) As, $\mu = \mu_0(1 + \chi)$ or $\mu = 4\pi \times 10^{-7}(1 + 599)$

or $\mu = 7.536 \times 10^{-4} \text{ TmA}^{-1}$

$$B = \mu H = (7.536 \times 10^{-4} \times 1200) \text{ T}$$

$\therefore$ Hence, $\phi = BA = (7.536 \times 10^{-4} \times 1200 \times 0.2 \times 10^{-4})$ Wb

$$= 1.81 \times 10^{-5} \text{ Wb}$$

66. (*b*) From curie's law, we can deduce a formula for the relation between magnetic field induction, temperature and magnetisation.

i.e. $I \text{ (magnetisation)} \propto \frac{B \text{ (magnetic field induction)}}{T \text{ (temperature in kelvin)}}$

$$\Rightarrow \quad \frac{I_2}{I_1} = \frac{B_2}{B_1} \times \frac{T_1}{T_2} \quad \text{...(i)}$$

Here, $I_1 = 8 \text{ Am}^{-1}$

$B_1 = 0.6\text{T}, T_1 = 4 \text{ K}$

$B_2 = 0.2 \text{ T}, T_2 = 16 \text{ K}, I_2 = ?$

Put values in Eq. (i)

$$\frac{0.2}{0.6} \times \frac{4}{16} = \frac{I_2}{8}$$

$$\Rightarrow \quad I_2 = 8 \times \frac{1}{12} = \frac{2}{3} \text{ Am}^{-1}$$

67. (*a*) Point P lies on equatorial line of magnet (1) and axial line of magnet (2) as shown

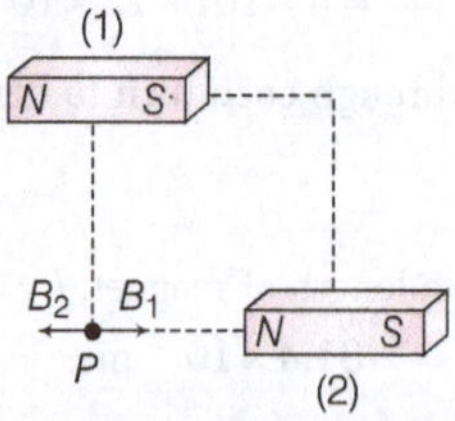

$$B_1 = \frac{\mu_0}{4\pi} \cdot \frac{M}{d^3}$$

$$= 10^{-7} \times \frac{1000}{(0.1)^3} = 0.1 \text{ T}$$

$$B_2 = \frac{\mu_0}{4\pi} \cdot \frac{2M}{d^3}$$

$$= 10^{-7} \times \frac{2 \times 1000}{(0.1)^3} = 0.2 \text{ T}$$

$$\therefore \quad B_{net} = B_2 - B_1 = 0.1 \text{ T}$$

68. (*d*) At point P, net magnetic field, $B_{net} = \sqrt{B_1^2 + B_2^2}$

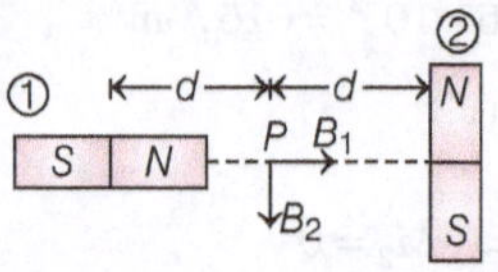

where, $B_1 = \frac{\mu_0}{4\pi} \cdot \frac{2M}{d^3}$ and $B_2 = \frac{\mu_0}{4\pi} \cdot \frac{M}{d^3}$

$$\Rightarrow \quad B_{net} = \frac{\mu_0}{4\pi} \cdot \frac{\sqrt{5}M}{d^3}$$

69. (*d*) For paramagnetic sample (curie's law), $I \propto B / T$

where, $I_1 = 0.8$ A/m, $B_1 = 0.8$ T,

$T_1 = 5$ K, $B_2 = 0.4$ T and $T_2 = 20$ K

$$\Rightarrow \frac{I_1}{I_2} = \frac{B_1 / T_1}{B_2 / T_2} \Rightarrow \frac{I_1}{I_2} = \frac{B_1 \times T_2}{B_2 \times T_1}$$

$$\Rightarrow \frac{0.8}{I_2} = \frac{0.8 \times 20}{0.4 \times 5} \Rightarrow I_2 = \frac{0.4 \times 5}{20} = 0.1 \text{ Am}^{-1}$$

70. (*a*) Given, $\chi_m = 299$

and $\mu_0 = 4\pi \times 10^{-7}$ Hm^{-1}

We know that, $\mu = \mu_0(1 + \chi_m)$

$$\therefore \quad \mu = 4\pi \times 10^{-7} (1 + 299)$$

$$\Rightarrow \quad = 4 \times \frac{22}{7} \times 10^{-7} \times 300$$

$$= \frac{26400}{7} \times 10^{-7} = 3771.4 \times 10^{-7} \text{ Hm}^{-1}$$

$$\Rightarrow \quad \mu \cong 3771 \times 10^{-7} \text{ Hm}^{-1}$$

Assertion and Reason

1 (*a*) When we break magnet into two pieces, its poles do not get separated as it again becomes a magnet. Also, when magnet is broken into two equal pieces, its magnetic moment gets reduced to half.

2. (*a*) According to Gauss' law in magnetism, $\oint \mathbf{B} \cdot d\mathbf{S} = 0$

It is because magnetic monopoles does not exist and unlike poles of equal strength exist together.

3 (*d*) Relative magnetic permeability is given by

$$\mu_r = \frac{\mu}{\mu_0}$$

It is a dimensionless quantity.

4. (*d*) The susceptibility of diamagnetic material is small and negative. It is independent of temperature, so the χ_m-T graph is a straight line parallel to T-axis.

5. (*d*) A magnet does not experience any force since net force, $mB - mB = 0$. The forces on north and south poles are equal, unlike and parallel, makes a couple to align the magnet along the field.

Statement Type Questions

1. (*b*) Statement I is correct but Statement II is incorrect. The magnetic needle tries to move in the direction of the magnetic field.

2. (*d*) Both Statement I and Statement II are correct.

If paramagnetic substances are kept in an external magnetic field, then it develops feeble magnetisation in the direction of externally applied magnetic field, *i.e.* magnetic dipoles are weakly aligned along external magnetic field.

3. (*d*) Both Statement I and Statement II are correct.

Paramagnetic substances are those which get weakly magnetised when placed in an external magnetic field because these substances have tendency to move from a region of weak magnetic field to strong magnetic field, *i.e.* they get weakly attracted to a magnet.

4. (*a*) Both Statement I and Statement II are incorrect.

The permeability of a ferromagnetic material is not independent of magnetic field, $\mathbf{B} = K_m \mathbf{B}_0$.

Where, B_0 is applied field. The total magnetic field **B** inside a ferromagnet may be 10^3 or 10^4 times the applied field B_0. The permeability K_m of a ferromagnetic material is not constant, neither the field **B** nor the magnetisation **M. M** increases linearly with **B** even at small value of B_0. From the hysteresis curves, magnetic permeability is greater for lower field.

5. (*b*) Statement I is correct but Statement II is incorrect.

The magnetisation of a paramagnetic material is inversely proportional to the absolute temperature T.

$M = C \dfrac{B_0}{T}$ (Curie's law]

where, C = Curie constant.

Thus, a paramagnetic sample displays greater magnetisation (for the same magnetic field) when cooled.

Match the Columns

1. (*c*) A. The unit of magnetic moment is $\dfrac{\text{N-M}}{\text{T}}$.

B. The unit of magnetic induction is NA^{-1}m^{-1}

C. The unit of magnetic permeability is H/m.

D. The unit of Intensity of magnetisation is A/m.

Hence, A-(IV), B-(III), C-(II), D-(I).

2. (*d*) Couple between two small magnets

A. The magnets being in the end-on-position.

$$\text{Couple} = \frac{\mu_0}{4\pi} \cdot \frac{2MM'}{x^3}$$

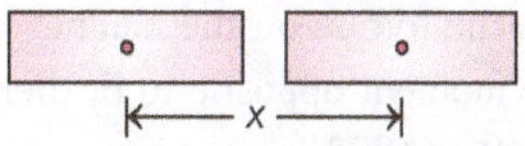

B. The magnets being in the broadside-on-position (two magnets are at right angle).

$$\text{Couple} = \frac{\mu_0}{4\pi} \cdot \frac{MM'}{x^3}$$

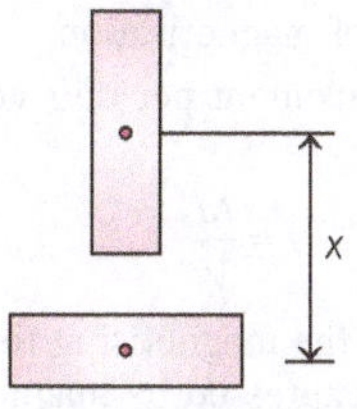

Force between two small magnets.

C. The magnet being in the end-on-position with respect to deflecting magnet.

$$F = \frac{\mu_0}{4\pi}\left[\frac{6MM'}{x^4}\right]$$

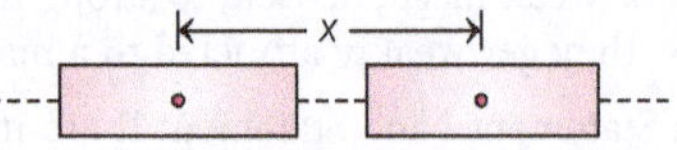

D. The magnet being in the broadside-on-position with respect to the deflecting magnet.

$$F = \frac{\mu_0}{4\pi}\left[\frac{3MM'}{x^4}\right]$$

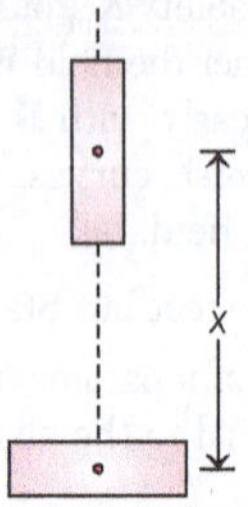

Hence, A-(IV), B-(III), C-(II), D-(I).

3. (*d*) $\theta_1 = 0°$ as the dipole is aligned with B.

A. When the bar magnet is displaced to perpendicular position, then $\theta_2 = 90°$.

$W = MB(\cos\theta_1 - \cos\theta_2)$, we get

$W = 1.5 \times 0.22\,(\cos 0° - \cos 90°) = 0.33\text{ J}$

B. When the magnet is displaced, so as to align M opposite to B, then

$\theta_2 = 180°$

$W = MB\,(\cos\theta_1 - \cos\theta_2)$

$= 1.5 \times 0.22\,(\cos 0° - \cos 180°) = 0.66\text{ J}$

C. Let τ_1 be the torque on the magnet when it is aligned perpendicular to B, then using the relation

$\tau = MB\sin\theta$, we get

$\tau_1 = MB\sin\theta_1$

$= 1.5 \times 0.22 \times \sin 90° = 0.33\text{ N-m}$

$(\because \theta_1 = 90°)$

D. Let τ_2 be the torque on the magnet when the magnetic moment opposite to B, then

$\theta_2 = 180°$

$\tau_2 = MB\sin\theta_2$

$= 1.5 \times 0.22 \times \sin 180° = 0$

Hence, A-(IV), B-(III), C-(I), D-(II).

4. (*a*) A. Intensity of magnetisation,

I = magnetic moment per unit volume of magnetised substance

$$I = \frac{M}{V}$$

B. Capability of the magnetising field to magnetise a substance is expressed by magnetic intensity vector H.

$$H = \frac{B}{\mu_0} - 1$$

C. Magnetic permeability,

$$\mu = \frac{B}{H}$$

D. Magnetic susceptibility,

$$\chi_m = \frac{I}{H}$$

Hence, A-(IV), B-(III), C-(II), D-(I).

5. (*a*)

Diamagnetic	Paramagnetic	Ferromagnetic
$-1 \le \chi < 0$	$0 < \chi < \varepsilon$	$\chi >> 1$
$0 \le \mu_r < 1$	$1 < \mu_r < 1 + \varepsilon$	$\mu_r >> 1$
$\mu < \mu_0$	$\mu > \mu_0$	$\mu >> \mu_0$
For vacuum $\mu_r = 1$		

Hence, A-(II), B-(III), C-(I), D-(IV).

Final Check Through PYQs

1. (*b*)

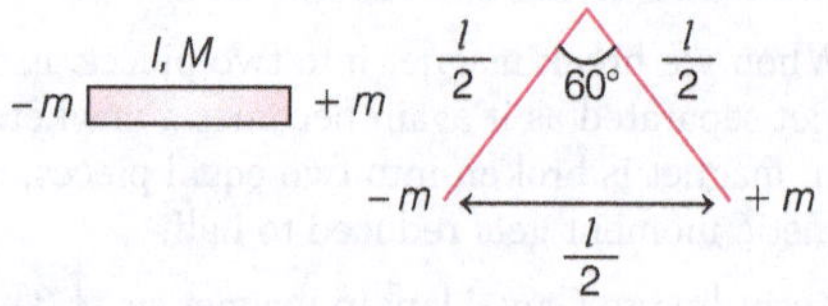

The magnetic moment is given by $M = m \cdot L$

New magnetic moment, $M' = m \cdot L'$

$$= m \cdot \frac{l}{2} = \frac{ml}{2}$$

Thus, $$M' = \frac{M}{2}$$

2. (*d*) Given, magnetic field $B = 0.049\text{ T}$

Time period, $T = \frac{5}{20} = \frac{1}{4}\text{ s}$

Moment of inertia, $I = 9.8 \times 10^{-6}\text{ kgm}^2$

The time period of oscillation of a magnetic needle in a magnetic field is given by $T = 2\pi\sqrt{\frac{I}{MB}}$

where, M is the magnetic moment of the needle.

Thus, $$T = 2\pi\sqrt{\frac{9.8 \times 10^{-6}}{M \times 0.049}}$$

$$\Rightarrow \left(\frac{1}{4}\right)^2 = (2\pi)^2\left(\frac{9.8 \times 10^{-6}}{M \times 4.9 \times 10^{-2}}\right)$$

$$\Rightarrow \frac{1}{16} = \frac{4\pi^2 \times 2 \times 10^{-4}}{M}$$

$$\Rightarrow M = 16 \times 8 \times \pi^2 \times 10^{-4}$$

$$= 128\pi^2 \times 10^{-4}\ \text{Am}^2$$
$$= 1280\pi^2 \times 10^{-5}\ \text{Am}^2$$

3. (*d*) Net magnetic flux through a closed surface is zero because the number of field lines leaving the surface are equal to the number of field lines entering the surface.

4. (*a*) We know that, magnetic dipole moment, $M = nIA$

For case (1)

An equilateral triangle of side a.

Total wire length

$$= n \times \text{Perimeter of the triangle}$$
$$12a = n \times 3a$$
$$\Rightarrow \quad n = 4$$

Area of the triangle,

$$A = \frac{\sqrt{3}}{4}a^2$$

Magnetic dipole moment,

$$M = nIA$$
$$\Rightarrow \quad M = 4I \times \frac{\sqrt{3}}{4}a^2$$
$$\Rightarrow \quad M = \sqrt{3}Ia^2$$

For case (2)

A square of side a.

Total wire length $= n \times$ Perimeter of the square

$$12a = n \times 4a$$
$$\Rightarrow \quad n = 3$$

Area of the square loop,

$$A = a^2$$

Magnetic dipole moment,

$$M = nIA$$
$$\Rightarrow \quad M = 3Ia^2$$

5. (*d*) When wire of length L is bent in the form of a circle of radius R, then

$$L = 2\pi R$$
$$\Rightarrow \quad R = \frac{L}{2\pi} \qquad \text{...(i)}$$

∴ Magnetic moment,

$$M = IA = I(\pi R^2)$$
$$= I \cdot \pi\left(\frac{L}{2\pi}\right)^2 \qquad \text{[from Eq. (i)]}$$
$$= \frac{I\pi L^2}{4\pi^2} = \frac{IL^2}{4\pi}\ \text{A-m}^2$$

6. (*a*) Work done for rotating the coil,

$$W = MB(\cos\theta_1 - \cos\theta_2)$$

where, M = magnetic moment

and B = magnetic field.

Given, $\theta_1 = 0°$, $\theta_2 = 180°$

$$\Rightarrow \quad W = MB(\cos 0° - \cos 180°)$$
$$= 2MB = 2 \times NIA \times B$$
$$= 2 \times 250 \times 85 \times 10^{-6} \times (2.1 \times 1.25 \times 10^{-4}) \times 0.85$$
$$= 9.48 \times 10^{-6}\ \text{J}$$
$$\approx 9.5 \times 10^{-6}\ \text{J}$$
$$= 9.5\ \mu\text{J}$$

The closest option is (a).

7. (*b*) ∵ Work done in rotating the magnet,

$$W = MB\ (\cos\theta_0 - \cos\theta)$$

where, M = magnetic moment of the magnet

and B = magnetic field.

$$W = MB\ (\cos 0° - \cos 60°)$$
$$= MB\left(1 - \frac{1}{2}\right) = \frac{MB}{2}$$
$$\therefore \quad MB = 2W \qquad \text{...(i)}$$

Torque on a magnet in this position is given by

$$\tau = \mathbf{M} \times \mathbf{B}$$
$$= MB \cdot \sin\theta = 2W \cdot \sin 60° \qquad \text{[from Eq. (i)]}$$
$$= 2W\frac{\sqrt{3}}{2} = W\sqrt{3}$$

8. (*b*) We know that, magnetic field due to current carrying solenoid,

$$B = \mu_0 nI$$
$$\Rightarrow \quad \mu_0 = \frac{B}{nI}$$
$$\Rightarrow \quad [\mu_0] = \frac{[B]}{[n][I]} = \frac{\left[\frac{F}{IL}\right]}{[n][I]} \qquad \left[\because F = IBL \Rightarrow B = \frac{F}{IL}\right]$$
$$= \frac{[F]}{[n][L][I^2]} = \frac{[\text{MLT}^{-2}]}{[\text{L}^{-1}]\,[\text{L}]\,[\text{A}^2]}$$
$$= [\text{MLT}^{-2}\text{A}^{-2}]$$

Dimensional formula of self-inductance,

$$[L] = [\text{M}^1\text{L}^2\text{T}^{-2}\text{A}^{-2}]$$

Dimensional formula of electric permittivity,

$$[\varepsilon_0] = [\text{M}^{-1}\text{L}^{-3}\text{T}^4\text{A}^2]$$

Dimensional formula of magnetic flux,

$$[\phi] = [\text{ML}^2\text{T}^{-2}\text{A}^{-1}]$$

Hence, option (b) is correct.

9. (*d*) Given, susceptibility, $\chi = 599$

Magnetic field, $B = 1200\ \text{Am}^{-1}$

Permeability of the material of the rod = ?

As, $\mu_m = \mu_0(1 + \chi)$

$$= 4\pi \times 10^{-7}(1 + 599)$$
$$= 2.4\pi \times 10^{-4}\ \text{TmA}^{-1}$$

10. (c) As the source of current is switched ON, a magnetic field sets up in between the poles of the electromagnet. As we know that, a diamagnetic substance when placed in a magnetic field acquires a feeble magnetism opposite to the direction of magnetic field.

Also, in the presence of the field (non-uniform), these substances are attracted towards the weaker field, *i.e.* they move from stronger to weaker magnetic field. Due to these reasons, the rod is repelled by the field produced to the current source. Hence, it is pushed up, out of horizontal field and gains gravitational potential energy. Hence, the current source is responsible for this work done.

11. (d) As we know, the relation between the magnetic permeability and susceptibility of material, *i.e.*

$$\mu_r = 1 + \chi_m \quad \text{...(i)}$$

∵ For diamagnetic substances, $\mu_r < 1$

So, according to Eq. (i), the magnetic susceptibility (χ_m) of diamagnetic substance will be negative.

While in the case of para and ferromagnetic substances, magnetic susceptibility is positive.

Skill Builder

Sol. of Skill Builder on Pg. 346

(a) On bending a rod its pole strength remains unchanged where as its magnetic moment changes.

Magnetic moment, $M = q_m (2L) \Rightarrow q_m = \dfrac{M}{2L}$

New magnetic moment,

$$M' = q_m \times \frac{2}{3}L$$

$$= \frac{M}{2L} \times \frac{2}{3}L = \frac{M}{3}$$

Sol. of Skill Builder on Pg. 352

(b) Relative permeability and magnetic susceptibility are related as follows

$$\mu_r = 1 + \chi_m$$

$$5500 = 1 + \chi_m$$

$$\Rightarrow \quad \chi_m = 5499$$

For deeper insight
Scan the QR Code

Chapter 7

Electromagnetic Induction (EMI)

Learning Objectives

Module-I

- Magnetic Flux
- Faraday's Laws of Electromagnetic Induction
- Lenz's Law and Conservation of Energy

Module-II

- Motional Electromotive Force
- Applications of EMI: Eddy Current

Module-III

- Inductance
- Self-Inductance
- Energy Stored in an Inductor
- Mutual Inductance

Chapter Overview with *NEET Connection*

In this chapter, we will study about the Lenz's law, motional emf and inductances. Without going through this chapter it will be difficult to understand other chapters like alternating current, electromagnetic waves and electronic devices.

Special format questions can be easily framed on the following topics of this chapter

- Calculation of magnetic flux
- Applications of Faraday's and Lenz's laws
- Induced emf and induced current
- Eddy current
- Self and mutual inductances

For better understanding of this chapter

- Study of electric flux will be helpful.
- Basic revision of electric potential and electric current will be helpful.

Introduction

The phenomenon of generating current/emf in a conducting circuit by changing the strength, position or orientation of an associated external magnetic field is called **electromagnetic induction (EMI).** The emf, so developed is called **induced emf.** It is the reverse process of magnetic field produced by electric current. This chapter includes various laws, like Faraday's law of electromagnetic induction, Lenz's law, Fleming's right hand thumb rule. All these laws explain how electric field can be produced by magnetic field. At the end, we will study about how inductor can store magnetic energy.

Module 1

Magnetic Flux and Laws of Electromagnetic Induction

- Magnetic Flux
- Faraday's Laws of Electromagnetic Induction
- Lenz's Law and Conservation of Energy

Magnetic Flux

The total number of magnetic field lines crossing through any surface, normally when it is placed in a magnetic field is known as the magnetic flux of that surface.

Consider an element of area $d\mathbf{S}$ on an arbitrary shaped surface as shown in figure. If the magnetic field at this element is **B**, then the magnetic flux through the element is

$$d\phi_B = \mathbf{B} \cdot d\mathbf{S} \Rightarrow d\phi_B = BdS\cos\theta$$

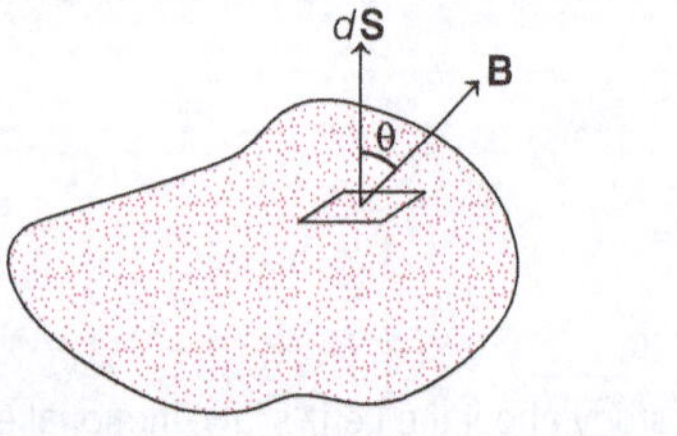

Here, $d\mathbf{S}$ is a vector that is perpendicular to the surface and has a magnitude equal to the area dS and θ is the angle between **B** and $d\mathbf{S}$ at that element. In general, $d\phi_B$ varies from element to element.

The total magnetic flux through the surface is the sum of the contributions from the individual area elements.

$$\therefore \quad \phi_B = \int BdS\cos\theta = \int \mathbf{B} \cdot d\mathbf{S}$$

A special case in which **B** is uniform over a plane surface with total area S, magnetic flux is given by

$$\phi_B = BS\cos\theta.$$

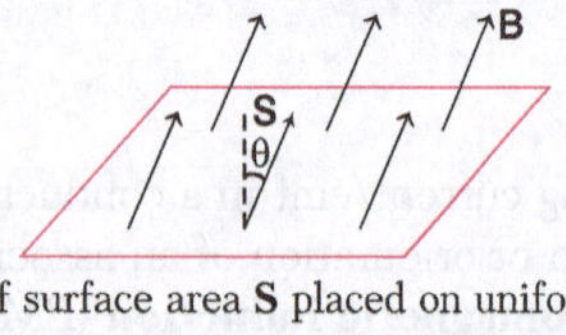

A plane of surface area **S** placed on uniform field **B**

Units and Dimensions of Magnetic Flux

(i) Magnetic flux is a scalar quantity.

(ii) The SI unit of magnetic flux is tesla-metre^2 (T-m^2). This unit is also called **weber (Wb).**

$$1 \text{ Wb} = 1 \text{ T-m}^2 = 1 \text{ N-m/A}$$

The CGS unit of magnetic flux is Maxwell (Mx).

$$1\text{Mx} = 1 \text{ G-cm}^2$$

$$1 \text{ Wb} = 1\text{T} \times 1\text{m}^2 = 10^4 \text{G} \times 10^4 \text{cm}^2$$

or $\quad 1 \text{ Wb} = 10^8 \text{ Mx}$

Thus, unit of magnetic field is also weber/metre^2 (1Wb/m^2)

or $\quad 1 \text{ T} = 1 \text{ Wb/m}^2$

(iii) The dimensional formula of magnetic flux is $[ML^2T^{-2}A^{-1}]$.

Example 1. *A uniform magnetic field exists in the space* $\mathbf{B} = B_1\hat{\mathbf{i}} + B_2\hat{\mathbf{j}} - B_3\hat{\mathbf{k}}$. *Find the magnetic flux through an area* **S**, *if the area* **S** *is in YZ-plane.*

Sol. Since, the magnetic field is uniform, we can use formula,

$$\phi_B = \mathbf{B} \cdot \mathbf{S}$$

Area **S** is in YZ-plane, it means $\mathbf{S} = S\hat{\mathbf{i}}$

Hence, $\phi_B = (B_1\hat{\mathbf{i}} + B_2\hat{\mathbf{j}} - B_3\hat{\mathbf{k}}) \cdot (S\hat{\mathbf{i}}) = B_1 S.$

NEET Close-up

Example Similar to PYQ Asked in NEET 2022

A square loop of side 1 m and resistance 1kΩ is placed such as its plane is perpendicular to the direction of magnetic field. Magnetic flux through the flux is 2 Wb. Find the value of magnetic field.

(a) 3T (b) 2T (c) 5T (d) 4T

Sol. (*b*) Magnetic flux, $\phi_B = \mathbf{B} \cdot \mathbf{S} = BS\cos 0°$

$$\Rightarrow \phi_B = BS \Rightarrow B = \phi_B / S \Rightarrow B = \frac{2}{(1)^2} = 2 \text{ T}.$$

Skill Builder

Plane of a square loop is at 60° angle with the direction of magnetic field. Side of square loop is 2m and magnetic field is 10 T. The magnetic flux through the loop is

(a) 10 Wb (b) 20 Wb
(c) 5 Wb (d) 40 Wb

For more Practice Refer Q.No. 17, 25 of Gearing up for NEET.

Example 2. *A long solenoid of radius 4 cm, length 400 cm carries a current of 3 A. The total number of turns is 100. Assuming ideal solenoid, find the flux passing through a circular surface having centre on axis of solenoid radius 3 cm and is perpendicular to the axis of solenoid inside.*

Sol.

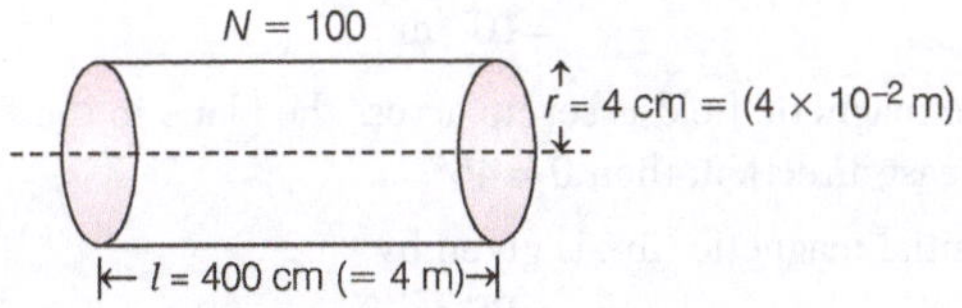

Number of turns per unit length is given by

$$n = \frac{N}{l} = \frac{100}{4} = 25 \text{ turns/m}$$

Magnetic field of a solenoid at a point inside is

$$B = \mu_0 nI, \; S = \pi r_1^2 \text{ and } \theta = 0°$$

Magnetic flux

$$\phi_B = BS \cos\theta = \mu_0 nI \, \pi r_1^2 \cos 0°$$

$$= 4\pi \times 10^{-7} \times 25 \times 3 \times \pi \times (3 \times 10^{-2})^2$$

$$= 0.27 \times 10^{-6} \text{ Wb} = 0.27 \mu \text{ Wb}$$

Faraday's Laws of Electromagnetic Induction

There are two laws of electromagnetic induction given by Faraday as below

Faraday's First Law

Whenever the amount of magnetic flux linked with a circuit changes, an emf is induced in the circuit.

The actual number of magnetic lines passing through the circuit does not matter to the value of the induced emf. Induced emf is determined by the rate at which the magnetic flux changes.

Faraday's Second Law

The magnitude of the induced emf in a circuit is equal to the rate of change of magnetic flux through the circuit. Mathematically, Faraday's second law can be expressed as,

Induced emf $\propto$ Rate of change of magnetic flux

$$e = \frac{-d\phi_B}{dt}$$

$$(\because \text{Rate of change of magnetic flux} = \frac{\phi_2 - \phi_1}{t_2 - t_1})$$

The negative sign in above relation indicates that the induced emf in the loop due to changing flux always opposes the change in the magnetic flux.

In the case of a closely wound coil of N turns, the change in flux associated with each turn, is same.

Therefore, the expression for the total induced emf is given by

$$e = -N\frac{d\phi_B}{dt}$$

The induced emf can be increased by increasing the number of turns N of a closed coil.

The magnetic flux can be changed in the following ways

(i) The magnitude of **B** can change with time, i.e. time-varying magnetic field, $B = B(t)$

(ii) The current producing the magnetic field can change with time, *i.e.* time varying current, $i = i(t)$.

(iii) The area enclosed by the loop can change with time. This can be done by pulling a loop inside (or outside) a magnetic field. By doing, so the area enclosed by loop (hatched area) can be changed.

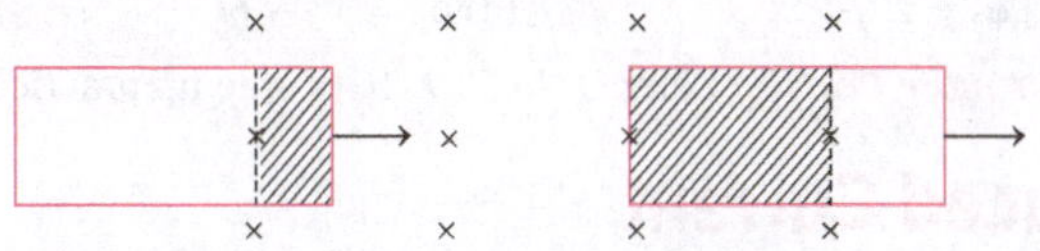

(iv) The angle θ between **B** and the normal to the loop can change with time. This can be done by rotating a loop in a magnetic field.

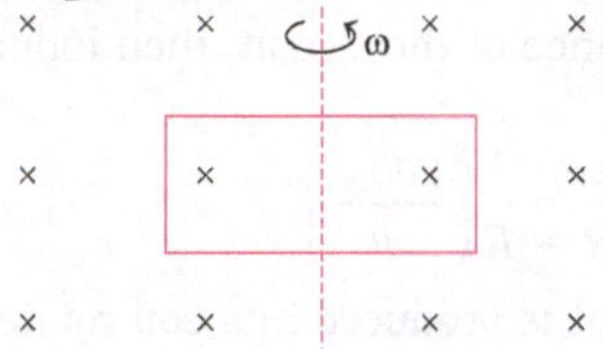

(v) Any combination of the above can occur.

Example 3. *A coil with an average diameter of 0.02 m is placed perpendicular to a magnetic field of 6000 T. If the induced emf is 11 V and the magnetic field is changed to 1000 T in 4 s, then what the number of turns in the coil?*

Sol. Given, radius of coil, $r = \frac{0.02}{2} = 0.01 \text{m}$

$$B_1 = 6000 \text{ T}, B_2 = 1000 \text{ T}, t = 4 \text{ s}, e = 11 \text{V}$$

Emf, $$e = N\frac{(\phi_2 - \phi_1)}{t} = NA\frac{(B_2 - B_1)}{t}$$

$$= N\pi r^2 \frac{B_2 - B_1}{t}$$

$$11 = N \cdot \frac{22}{7} \times (0.01)^2 \times \frac{(6000 - 1000)}{4}$$

$\therefore$ Number of turns, $$N = \frac{11 \times 7 \times 4}{22 \times (0.01)^2 \times 5000} = 28$$

NEET Close-up

Example Similar to PYQ Asked in NEET 2020

The magnetic flux linked to a coil is given by

$\phi = 3t^2 + 2t$

Find induced emf in the coil at $t = 2$s.

(a) −14 V (b) −16 V
(c) 15 V (d) −2V

Sol. (*a*) Emf, $e = \frac{-d\phi}{dt} = -6t - 2$

At $t = 2$ s, $e = -12 - 2 = -14$ V

Skill Builder

Magnitude of induced emf through a coil at $t = 5$ s is 200 V. Magnetic flux linked with the coil should be

(a) $\phi_B = 3t^2 + 6t$ (b) $\phi_B = 2t^3$
(c) $\phi_B = 2t^3 + 5t^2$ (d) $\phi_B = 3t^3 + 6t$

For more Practice Refer Q.No. 7, 9, 10 of step up practice 1.

Induced Current

When the magnetic flux passing through a loop is changed, an induced emf and hence an induced current is produced in the circuit.

If R is the resistance of the circuit, then induced current is given by

$$i = \frac{e}{R} = \frac{1}{R}\left(\frac{-d\phi_B}{dt}\right) \quad \text{...(i)}$$

If induced current is produced in a coil rotated in a uniform magnetic field, then $I = \frac{NBA\,\omega \sin\omega t}{R} = I_0 \sin\omega t$

where, $I_0 = \frac{NBA\,\omega}{R}$ = peak value of induced current,

N = number of turns in the coil,
B = magnetic field,
ω = angular velocity of rotation
and A = area of cross-section of the coil.

Concept ladder **Induced charge** When the current starts flowing in the circuit, flow of charges also takes place. Charge flown in a circuit in time dt will be given by

$$dq = i dt = \frac{1}{R}(-d\phi_B) \quad \text{[from Eq. (i)]}$$

Example 4. *A square loop of side 10 cm and resistance 0.5 Ω is placed vertically in the east-west plane. A uniform magnetic field of 0.10T is set up across the plane in the north-east direction. The magnetic field is decreased to zero in 0.70 s at a steady state. What is the magnitude of current in this time-interval?*

Sol. Given, magnetic field, $B = 0.10$ T

and area of square loop $= 10 \times 10 = 100\ \text{cm}^2$

$= 10^{-2}\text{m}^2$

As, the magnetic field is set up across the plane in the north-east direction, then $\theta = 45°$.

The initial magnetic flux is given by

$$\phi_B = BS\cos\theta$$

$$\therefore \quad \phi = \frac{0.1 \times 10^{-2}}{\sqrt{2}}\ \text{Wb}$$

Final flux, $\phi_{min} = 0$ (given)

The change in flux is brought about in 0.70 s, *i.e.* $\Delta t = 0.70$s.

The magnitude of the induced emf is

$$e = \frac{\Delta\phi_B}{\Delta t} = \frac{|\phi - 0|}{\Delta t} = \frac{10^{-3}}{\sqrt{2} \times 0.7} \cong 1\ \text{mV}$$

The magnitude of induced current is $I = \frac{e}{R} = \frac{10^{-3}}{0.5} = 2$ mA

Example 5. *A coil consists of 200 turns of wire having a total resistance of 2.0 Ω and each turn is a square of side 18 cm. A uniform magnetic field directed perpendicular to the plane of the coil is turned on. If the field changes linearly from 0 to 0.5 T in 0.80 s, then what is the magnitude of induced emf and current in the coil while the field is changing?*

Sol. Given, $N = 200$ turns, $R = 2.0\Omega$, change in magnetic field, $\Delta B = 0.5$ T, side of square, $l = 18$ cm $= 18 \times 10^{-2}$m and $\Delta t = 0.80$ s

From the Faraday's law,

Induced emf, $|e| = -\frac{Nd\phi_B}{dt} = (N \times S)\frac{\Delta B}{\Delta t}$

$[\because \phi_B = \mathbf{B} \cdot \mathbf{S}$ and area, $S = l^2 = (18 \times 10^{-2})^2]$

$$= \frac{(200)(18 \times 10^{-2})^2(0.5 - 0)}{0.8}$$

$$= 4.05\ \text{V}$$

$\therefore$ Further, induced current, $i = \frac{|e|}{R} = \frac{4.05}{2} \approx 2.0$ A

Example 6. *Suppose a coil of area 5 m^2, resistance 10 Ω and number of turns 200 held perpendicular to a uniform magnetic field of strength 0.4T. The coil is now turned through 180° in time 1s. What is*

(i) average induced emf,
(ii) average induced current
(iii) and total charge that flows through a given cross-section of the coil?

Sol. Given, area of coil, $S = 5\text{m}^2$, resistance, $R = 10\Omega$, number of turns, $N = 200$, magnetic field, $B = 0.4$T, $\Delta t = 1$s

When the plane of coil is perpendicular to the magnetic field, i.e. $\theta_i = 0°$ and after it is rotated through 180°, then $\theta_f = 180°$.

$\therefore$ Initial flux, $\phi_i = NBS\cos 0° = NBS$

$$= 200 \times 0.4 \times 5 = 400\ \text{Wb}$$

and final flux $= NBS \cos 180° = - NBS = -400\,\text{Wb}$

Change in flux, $|\Delta\phi_B|$

$= NBS - (-NBS) = 2NBS = 800\,\text{Wb}$

(i) Average induced emf $(e) = \dfrac{|\Delta\phi|}{\Delta t} = \dfrac{2NBS}{\Delta t} = 800\,\text{V}$

(ii) Average current $= \dfrac{e}{R} = \dfrac{2NBS}{R\Delta t} = 80\,\text{A}$

(iii) Total charge, $\Delta Q = \dfrac{2NBS}{R} = 80\,\text{C}$

Example 7. *A square loop ACDE of area 20 cm^2 and resistance 5 Ω is rotated in a magnetic field B = 2 T through 180°. Find the magnitude of e, i and Δq in both the cases.*

(i) in 0.01 s *(ii) in 0.02 s.*

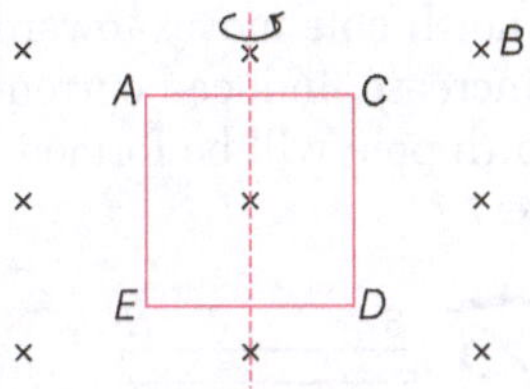

Sol. Let us take the area vector **S** perpendicular to plane of loop inwards.

Hence, initial flux passing through the loop,

$$\phi_i = BS \cos 0°$$
$$= (2)(20\times 10^{-4})(1)$$
$$= 4\times 10^{-3}\ \text{Wb}$$

Flux passing through the loop when it is rotated by 180°,

$$\phi_f = BS \cos 180° = (2)(20\times 10^{-4})(-1)$$
$$= -4\times 10^{-3}\ \text{Wb}$$

Therefore, change in flux,

$$\Delta\phi_B = \phi_f - \phi_i = -8\times 10^{-3}\ \text{Wb}$$

(i) Given at, $\Delta t = 0.01$ s, $R = 5\,\Omega$

Using the relation,

$$|e| = \left| -\frac{\Delta\phi_B}{\Delta t} \right| = \frac{8\times 10^{-3}}{0.01} = 0.8\ \text{V}$$

or induced current, $i = \dfrac{|e|}{R} = \dfrac{0.8}{5} = 0.16$ A

and charge, $\Delta q = i\Delta t = 0.16\times 0.01 = 1.6\times 10^{-3}$ C

(ii) Similarly, given at, $\Delta t = 0.02$ s, $R = 5\,\Omega$

$$\therefore \quad |e| = \left| -\frac{\Delta\phi_B}{\Delta t} \right| = \frac{8\times 10^{-3}}{0.02} = 0.4\ \text{V}$$

$$\therefore \quad i = \frac{|e|}{R} = \frac{0.4}{5} = 0.08\ \text{A}$$

and charge, $\Delta q = i\Delta t = (0.08)(0.02)$

$= 1.6\times 10^{-3}$ C

Lenz's Law and Conservation of Energy

The negative sign in Faraday's equation of electromagnetic induction describes the direction in which induced emf drives the current. This direction is easily determined with the help of Lenz's law, an associated principle with Faraday's law.

Lenz's law give the same result as the Faraday's law but it is often easier to use. Lenz's law states that, the direction of any magnetic induction effect is such as to oppose the cause of effect.

This law is based upon law of conservation of energy. As the induced emf opposes the change in flux, work has to be done against the opposition offered by induced emf/current in changing the flux. The work done appears as electrical energy in the circuit.

Direction of induced current can be determined by checking whether the flux through a conducting loop or circuit is increasing or decreasing.

If flux is decreasing, the magnetic field due to induced current will be along the existing magnetic field.

If flux is increasing, the magnetic field due to induced current will be opposite to existing magnetic field.

Mentor's TiP

- To apply Lenz's law, you can remember **RIN** or ⊗ **IN** (when the loop lies on the plane of paper).

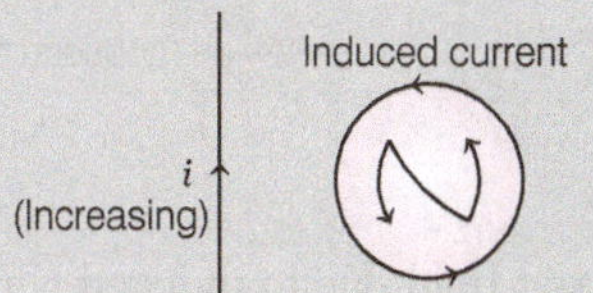

(i) In **RIN**, **R** stands for right, **I** stands for increasing and **N** for North pole (anti-clockwise). It means, if a loop is placed on the right side of a straight current carrying conductor and the current *i* in the conductor is increasing, then induced current in the loop is anti-clockwise (N).

(ii) In ⊗ **IN**, suppose the magnetic field in the loop is perpendicular to paper inwards (⊗) and this field is increasing, then induced current in the loop is anti-clockwise (N).

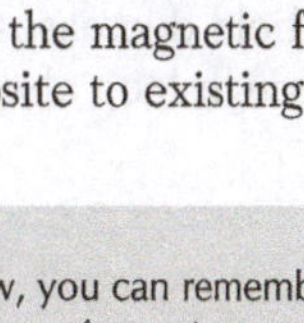

⊗ Increasing

Important Points Based on Lenz's Law

The following are some important points that will explain the direction of induced current according to Lenz's law

(i) Consider a conducting loop is being pulled inside a magnetic field, hence area of loop inside the magnetic field increases.

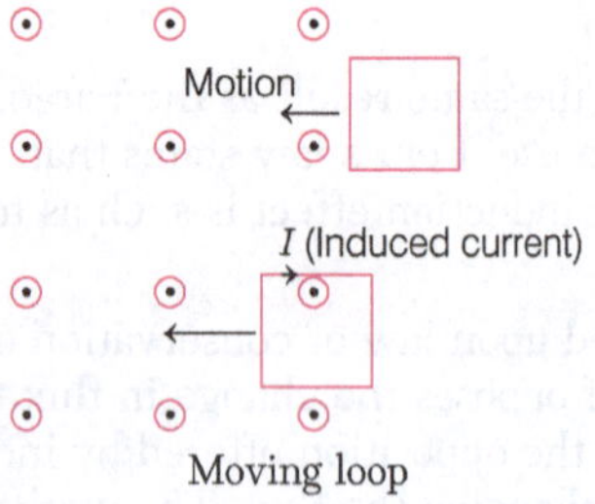

From the above figure, it is clear that the magnetic flux through loop is increasing and hence magnetic field due to induced current will be opposite to the existing magnetic field, *i.e.* inside the plane of paper, thus direction of induced current will be clockwise.

(ii) Consider a loop is being pulled out of magnetic field, area of loop inside field decreases and hence flux ($\phi = BS$) passing through loop also decreases.

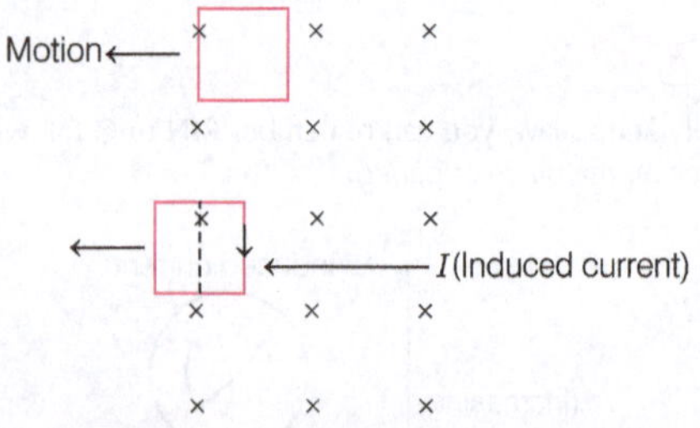

So, magnetic field due to induced current will be along the existing magnetic field, *i.e.* inside the plane of paper, thus direction of induced current will be clockwise.

(iii) Consider a loop is placed near a current carrying loop wire. The magnetic field due to long wire at distance x from it is given by

$$B = \frac{\mu_0 i}{2\pi x} \Rightarrow B \propto i \Rightarrow \phi \propto B \propto i$$

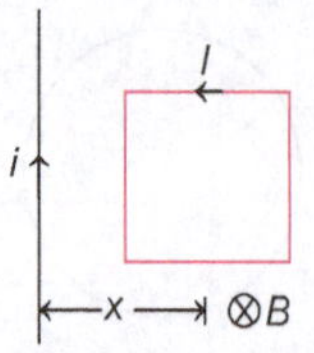

The direction of magnetic field due to long wire will be ⊗.

If the current in long wire increases, then ϕ increases and the magnetic field due to induced current will be opposite to existing magnetic field. Hence, direction of induced current is anti-clockwise.

(iv) If a conducting loop is brought away from a current carrying straight wire.

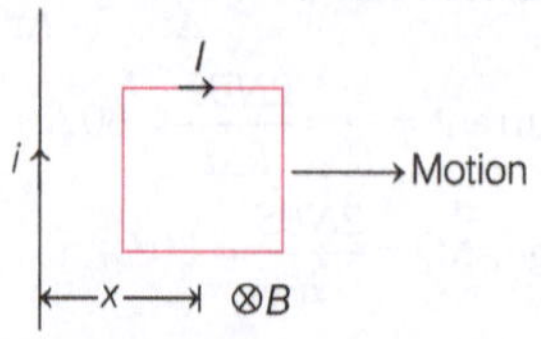

As the loop is moving away, so flux through the loop will decrease and the magnetic field due to induced current will be along the existing magnetic field, *i.e.* ⊗. Hence, direction of induced current is clockwise.

(v) (a) When north pole moves towards ring, then flux will increase, induced current will oppose this, so north pole will be formed in loop as seen by observer.

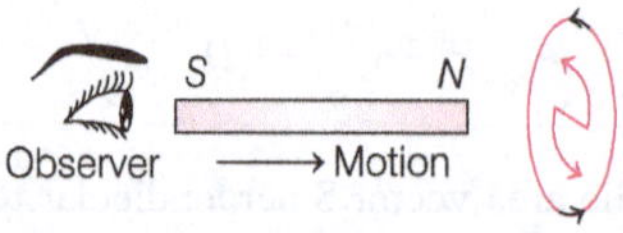

Induced current will be anti-clockwise.

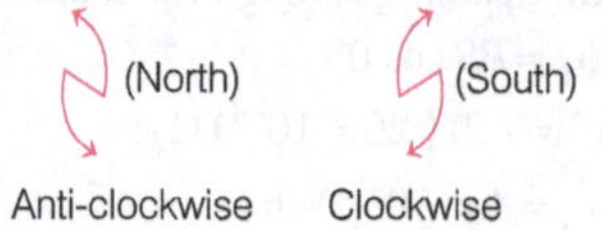

(b) When north pole moves away from ring, then flux will decrease, induced current will oppose this, so south pole will be formed in loop as seen by observer.

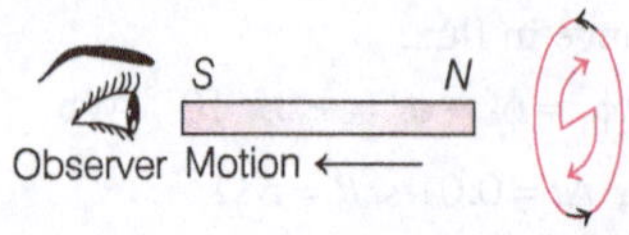

Induced current will be clockwise.

(c) Similar observations [as in case (a)] can be observed when south pole moves towards ring. So, induced current will be clockwise here.

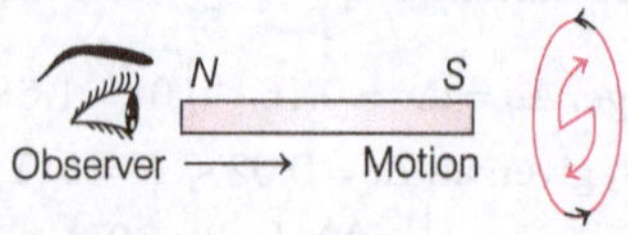

(d) Similar observations [as in case (b)] can be observed when south pole moves away from the ring. So, induced current in this case will be anti-clockwise.

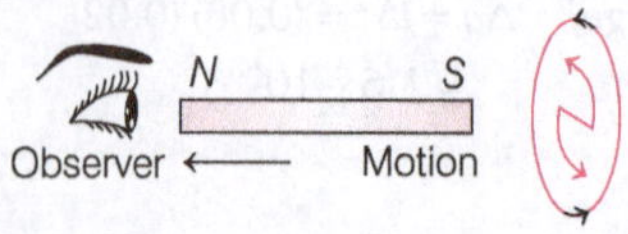

(vi) Two co-axial circular loops, identical to each other, carry equal amount of currents and circulating in the same direction.

(a) When loops approaches each other, then the flux linked with each coil will increase.

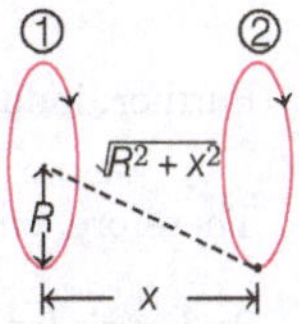

Magnetic field due to loop 1 at loop 2 will be given by

$$B = \frac{\mu_0 NiR^2}{2(R^2 + x^2)^{3/2}}$$

So, x decreases, B will increase ϕ also increases. The induced current in each coil will try to reduce flux and will be opposite to original current, so current in each coil will decrease.

(b) Now, loops move away from each other, then the flux linked with coil will decrease and so the induced current will try to increase the flux and hence current in each coil will increase.

Example 8. *A bar magnet is freely falling along the axis of a circular loop as shown in figure. State whether its acceleration a is equal to, greater than or less than the acceleration due to gravity g.*

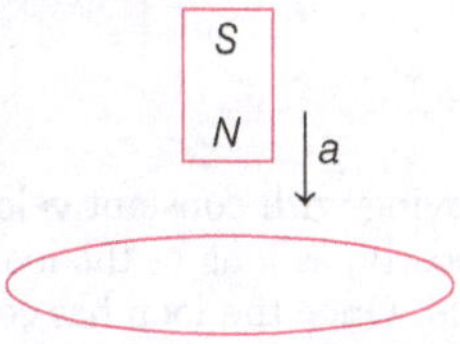

Sol. According to Lenz's law, whatever may be the direction of induced current, it will oppose the cause producting it. Here, the cause is the free fall of magnet and so the induced current will oppose it. So, the acceleration of magnet will be less than the acceleration due to gravity g.

Alternate method This can be understood in a different manner. When the magnet falls downwards with its north pole downwards, the magnetic field lines passing through the coil in the downward direction increase. Since, the induced current opposes this, the upper side of the coil will become north pole, so that field lines of coil's magnetic field are upwards. Now, like poles repel each other. Hence, $a < g$.

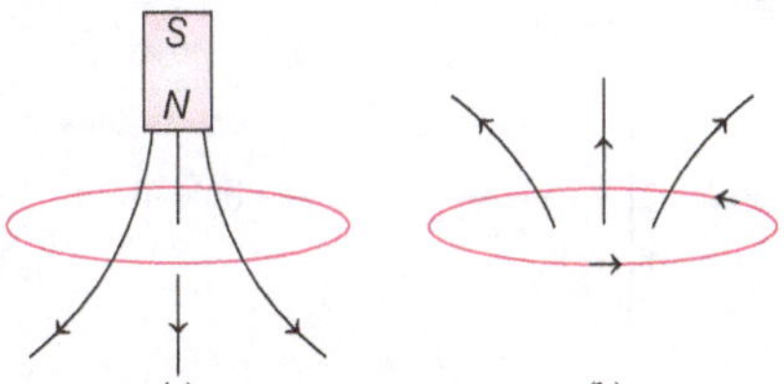

(a) (b)

Note If this circular loop had a slot, an emf in that case will be induced but no current will flow, *i.e.* $a = g$.

NEET Close-up

Example Similar to PYQ Asked in NEET 2024

In the figure, a bar magnet is moving towards solenoid-2 from solenoid-1. The direction of induced current in solenoid-1 and that in solenoid 2 respectively are through the directions

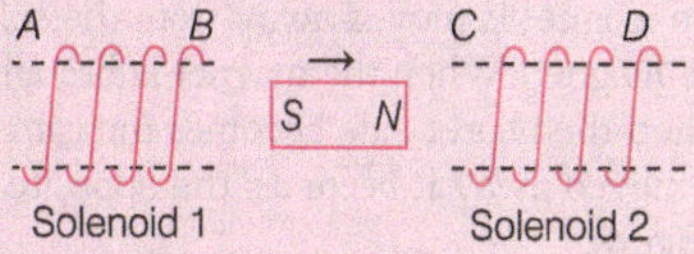

(a) BA and CD (b) BA and DC
(c) AB and CD (d) AB and DC

Sol. (*b*) When south pole of bar magnet leaving the coil, then induced current will be in anti-clockwise direction.

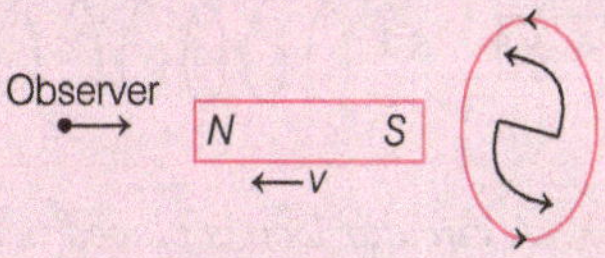

When north pole of bar magnet approaching the coil, then induced current will be in anti-clockwise direction.

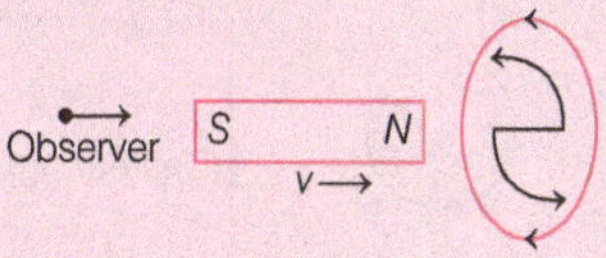

Skill Builder

In the figure, two solenoids are given. In both figures, a bar magnet going away from the solenoid. The direction of induced current in solenoid-1 and solenoid-2 respectively are through the directions

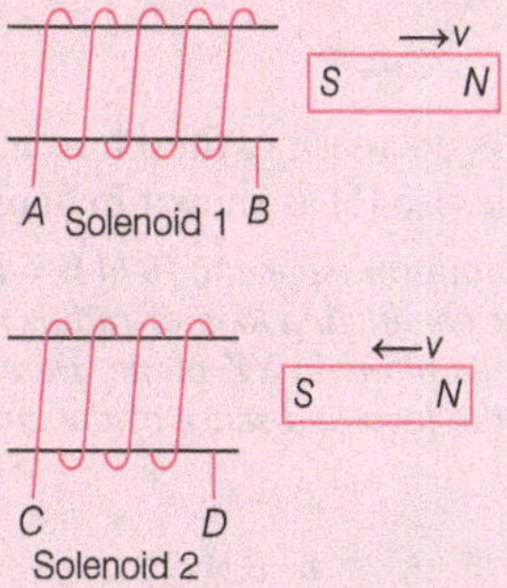

(a) AB and CD (b) AB and DC
(c) BA and CD (d) BA and DC

For more Practice Refer Q.No. 16, 17, 18, 19 of Step up practice 1 and Q.No. 11 of Gearing up for NEET.

Example 9. *A bar magnet is brought near a solenoid as shown in figure. Will the solenoid attract or repel the magnet?*

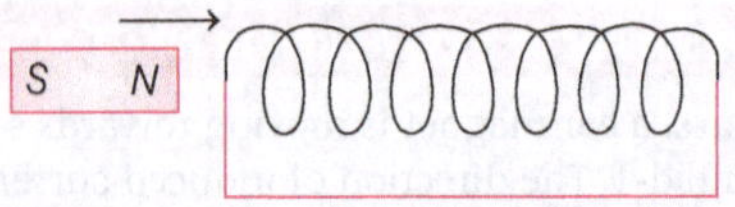

Sol. When the magnet is brought near the solenoid, then according to Lenz's law, both repel each other. On the other hand, if the magnet is moved away from the solenoid, then it attracts the magnet. When the magnet is brought near the solenoid, then the nearer side becomes the same pole and when it is moved away it becomes the opposite pole as shown in figure.

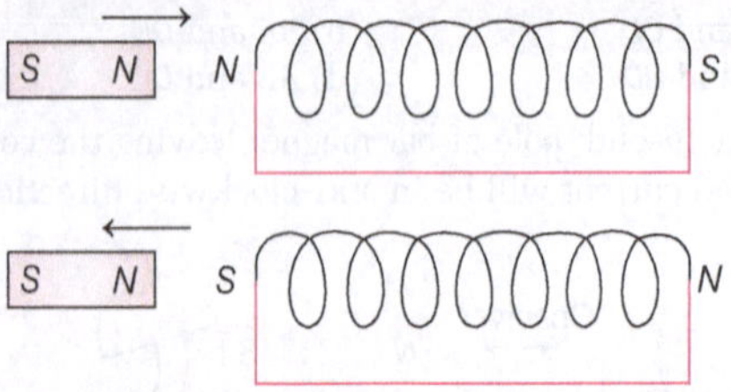

Example 10. *A circular loop is placed near a current carrying conductor as shown in figure. Find the direction of induced current, if the current, in the wire is decreasing.*

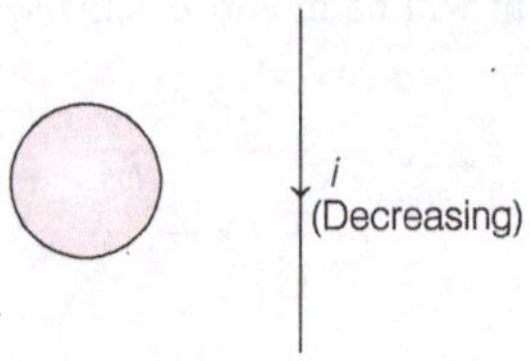

Sol. In this case, loop is placed to the right of current carrying wire (not to the left as it appears, because if you move in the direction of current, loop lies to the right).

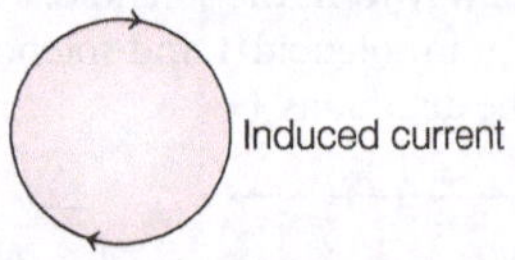

Now, the current is decreasing, therefore induced current in the loop is clockwise (S) as shown in above figure.

Example 11. *A uniform magnetic field $\mathbf{B} = B_0 t \hat{\mathbf{i}}$ in a region exists. A circular conducting loop of radius r and resistance R is placed with its plane in YZ-plane. Determine the current through the loop and sense of the current.*

Sol.

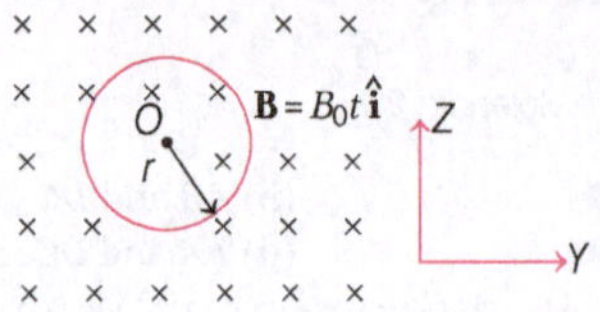

We know that, magnetic flux is given as

$$\phi_B = \mathbf{B} \cdot \mathbf{S} = (B_0 t)(\pi r^2)\cos 0°$$

$$\Rightarrow \quad \phi_B = B_0 \pi r^2 t \quad \text{and} \quad \frac{d\phi}{dt} = B_0 \pi r^2$$

Further, induced emf, $\varepsilon = \frac{-d\phi}{dt} = -B_0 \pi r^2$

Therefore, current, $i = \frac{|\varepsilon|}{R} = \frac{B_0 \pi r^2}{R}$

By Lenz's law, i should be anti-clockwise, so that it can oppose the increase in magnetic field.

Mentor's Tip

- Current (induced) should always oppose change in magnetic field associated with it. Here **B** was increasing according to the question, so current is anti-clockwise.

Example 12. *Through a uniform B field, a small rectangular loop is moving towards left with constant velocity as shown in the figure. Counting of time t begins at the moment, the loop starts entering the field.*
Plot the variation of flux through the loop with respect to time. Also, plot the variation of induced emf w.r.t. time t.

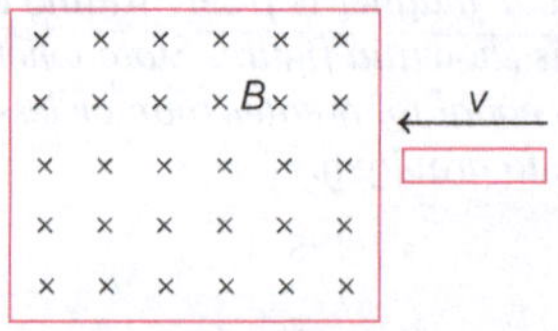

Sol. As the loop is moving with constant velocity, the flux will be increasing linearly, as long as the loop will be entering the magnetic field. Once the loop has completely entered the magnetic field the flux will become constant. Now, when the loop will start coming out the flux will linearly decrease to zero value.

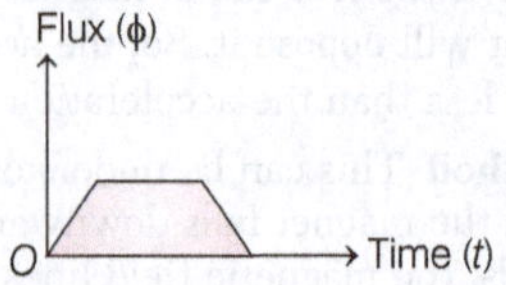

Since, emf induced, $\varepsilon = -\frac{d\phi}{dt}$, it means emf is negative of the slope of the ϕ-t graph. So, emf is negative in the beginning, then it becomes zero and then it becomes positive and again it becomes zero.

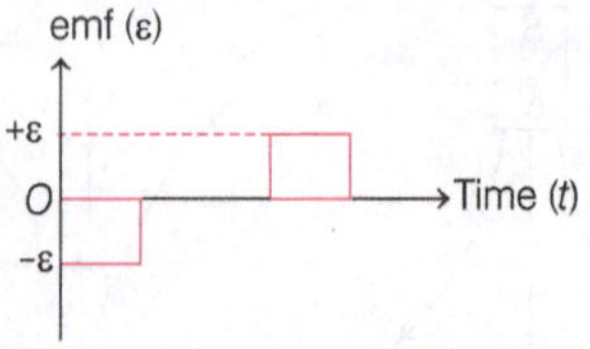

STEP UP Practice 1

1. The magnetic flux linked with a vector area **A** in a uniform magnetic field **B** is
(a) $\mathbf{B} \times \mathbf{A}$ (b) AB (c) $\mathbf{B} \cdot \mathbf{A}$ (d) $\frac{B}{A}$

2. The unit of magnetic flux is
(a) Wbm^{-2} (b) Wb (c) H (d) Am^{-1}

3. The dimensions of magnetic flux are
(a) $[MLT^{-2}A^{-2}]$ (b) $[ML^2T^{-2}A^{-2}]$
(c) $[ML^2T^{-1}A^{-2}]$ (d) $[ML^2T^{-2}A^{-1}]$

4. **Assertion** (A) An induced emf is generated when magnet is withdrawn from the solenoid.
Reason (R) The relative motion between magnet and solenoid induces emf in the solenoid.
In the light of the above statements, choose the correct answer from the options given below
(a) Both A and R are true but R is not the correct explanation of A.
(b) A is true but R is false.
(c) A is false but R is true.
(d) Both A and R are true and R is the correct explanation of A.

5. **Statement I** The induced emf in a conducting loop of wire will be non-zero when it rotates in a uniform magnetic field.
Statement II The emf is induced due to change in magnetic flux.
In the light of the above statements, choose the most appropriate answer from the options given below
(a) Both Statement I and Statement II are incorrect.
(b) Statement I is correct but Statement II is incorrect.
(c) Statement I is incorrect but Statement II is correct.
(d) Both Statement I and Statement II are correct.

6. **Assertion** (A) Changing magnetic flux can produce induced emf.
Reason (R) Faraday established induced emf experimentally.
In the light of the above statements, choose the correct answer from the options given below
(a) Both A and R are true but R is not the correct explanation of A.
(b) A is true but R is false.
(c) A is false but R is true.
(d) Both A and R are true and R is the correct explanation of A.

7. The magnetic flux linked with a coil (in weber) is given by the equation $\phi = 3t^2 + 4t + 9$, then, the magnitude of induced emf at $t = 2$ s will be
(a) 2 V (b) 4 V (c) 8 V (d) 16 V

8. A coil having an area A_0 is placed in a magnetic field which changes from B_0 to $4B_0$ in time interval t. The emf induced in the coil will be
(a) $3A_0B_0/t$ (b) $4A_0B_0/t$
(c) $3B_0/A_0t$ (d) $4B_0/A_0t$

9. The magnetic flux ϕ (in weber) in a closed circuit of resistance $10\,\Omega$ varies with time t (in second) according to equation $\phi = 6t^2 - 5t + 1$. The magnitude of induced current at $t = 0.25$ s is
(a) 1.2 A (b) 0.8 A
(c) 0.6 A (d) 0.2 A

10. The magnetic flux across a loop of resistance $10\,\Omega$ is given by $\phi = (5t^2 - 4t + 1)$ Wb. How much current is induced in the loop after 0.2 s?
(a) 0.4 A (b) 0.2 A
(c) 0.04 A (d) 0.02 A

11. **Assertion** (A) An induced current is developed when the number of magnetic lines of force associated with conductor is changed.
Reason (R) An induced current develop in a conductor moved in a direction parallel to the magnetic field.
In the light of the above statements, choose the correct answer from the options given below
(a) Both A and R are true but R is not the correct explanation of A.
(b) A is true but R is false.
(c) A is false but R is true.
(d) Both A and R are true and R is the correct explanation of A.

12. **Assertion** (A) Only a change in magnetic flux will induce current in the coil.
Reason (R) The presence of large magnetic flux through a coil maintains a current in the coil, if the current is continuous.
In the light of the above statements, choose the correct answer from the options given below
(a) Both A and R are true but R is not the correct explanation of A.
(b) A is true but R is false.
(c) A is false but R is true.
(d) Both A and R are true and R is the correct explanation of A.

13. In a circuit with a coil of resistance $2\,\Omega$, the magnetic flux changes from 2.0 Wb to 10.0 Wb in 0.2 s. The charge that flows in the coil during this time is
(a) 5.0 C (b) 4.0 C
(c) 1.0 C (d) 0.8 C

14. A circular ring of diameter 20 cm has a resistance $0.01\,\Omega$. How much charge will flow through the ring, if it is rotated from a position perpendicular to a uniform magnetic field of $B = 2$ T to a position parallel to field?
(a) 4 C (b) 6.28 C
(c) 3.14 C (d) 2.5 C

15. Which one of the following pair is incorrect?
(a) $\phi \rightarrow BA\cos\theta$
(b) $i_{\text{induced}} \rightarrow \frac{e}{R}$
(c) Charge flown $(\Delta q) \rightarrow \frac{\phi}{R}$
(d) $1\text{ Wb} \rightarrow 10^8$ maxwell

16. The direction of induced emf during electromagnetic induction is given by
(a) Faraday's law
(b) Lenz's law
(c) Maxwell's
(d) Ampere's law

17. Two different loops are concentric and lie in the same plane. The current in the outer loop is clockwise and increasing with time. The induced current in the inner loop is
(a) clockwise
(b) zero
(c) counter-clockwise
(d) in a direction that depends on the ratio of the loop radii

18. The north pole of a long horizontal bar magnet is being brought closer to a vertical conducting plane along the perpendicular direction. The direction of the induced current in the conducting plane will be
(a) horizontal
(b) vertical
(c) clockwise
(d) anti-clockwise

19. There is a uniform magnetic field directed perpendicular and into the plane of the paper. An irregular shaped conducting loop is slowly changing into a circular loop in the plane of the paper, then
(a) current is induced in the loop in the anti-clockwise direction
(b) current is induced in the loop in the clockwise direction
(c) AC is induced in the loop
(d) No current is induced in the loop

Module 2
Motional Electromotive Force and Eddy Current

- Motional Electromotive Force
- Applications of EMI : Eddy Current

Motional Electromotive Force

So far, we have considered the cases in which an emf is induced in a stationary circuit placed in a time-varying magnetic field. In this section, we will study about **motional emf**, *i.e.* the emf induced in a conductor when it is moving through a constant magnetic field. Now, let us consider, a straight conductor of length l as shown in figure, which is moving through a uniform magnetic field directed into the page. For simplicity, we assume that the conductor is moving in a direction perpendicular to the field with constant velocity under the influence of some external agent.

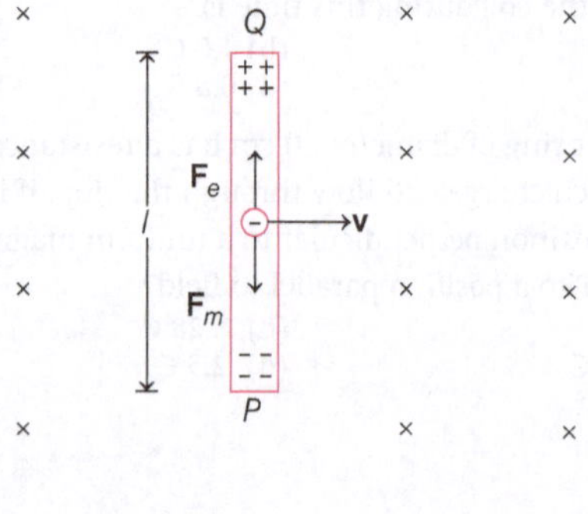

Due to motion of conductor in magnetic field, a potential difference is maintained between the ends of the conductor as long as the conductor continues to move through the uniform magnetic field.

This potential difference is called **motional electromagnetic force,** which is denoted by e and is given by

$$e = Bvl \quad \text{...(i)}$$

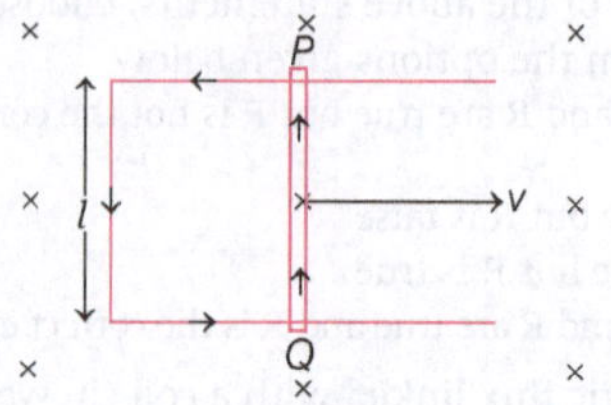

If R is the resistance of the circuit, then current will be written as

$$i = \frac{e}{R} = \frac{Bvl}{R} \quad \text{...(ii)}$$

General form of Motional EMF

To find motional emf for a conductor of any shape, moving in a uniform or non-uniform magnetic field, we will consider any small element $d\mathbf{l}$ of a conductor, then the contribution to the emf (de) is the magnitude of $d\mathbf{l}$ multiplied by the component of $(\mathbf{v}\times\mathbf{B})$ which is parallel to $d\mathbf{l}$.

i.e. $$de = (\mathbf{v}\times\mathbf{B})\cdot d\mathbf{l}$$

$$\Rightarrow \; e = \oint (\mathbf{v}\times\mathbf{B})\cdot d\mathbf{l} \text{ [motional emf, closed conducting loop]}$$

Important Points Related to Motional EMF

Some important points related to motional emf are given below

- For a semi-circular conducting loop of radius R with the centre at O and moving with velocity v, then the emf is given by

$$e = Bv(2R)$$

$$\Rightarrow \quad V_P - V_Q = 2BvR$$

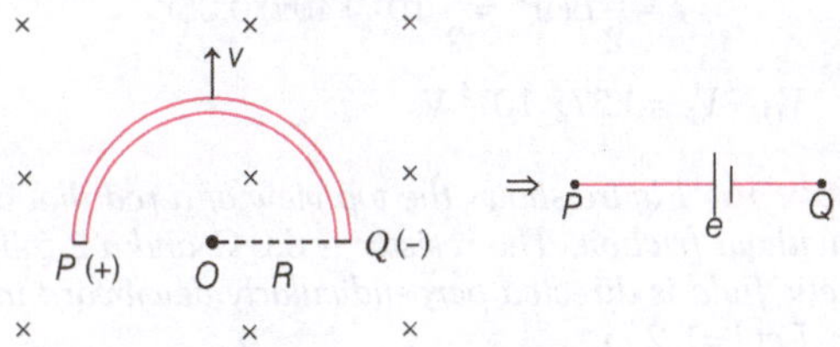

- If a conducting rod AB moves with a velocity v in XY-plane, then we can resolve the velocity vector in two components as shown in figure.

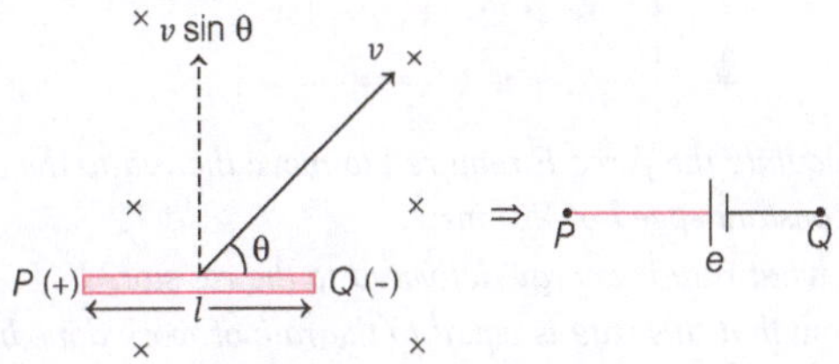

No emf will be induced, due to $v\cos\theta$. So, the net effect of emf will be due to $v\sin\theta$, which is given by $e = B(v\sin\theta)l$.

Concept ladder

For a circular loop of radius R moving with velocity v, we can replace its two ends lying on opposite sides of diameter with a battery of emf e. The emf is given by $e = Bv(2R) = 2BvR$

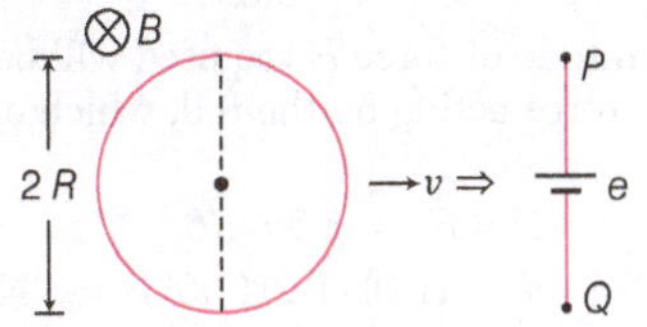

Motional EMF Induced in a Rotating Bar

(i) A conducting rod of length l rotates with a constant angular speed ω about a pivot at one end. A uniform magnetic field B is directed perpendicular to the plane of rotation as shown in figure.

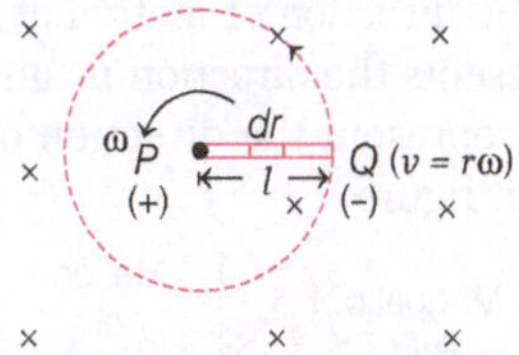

Let us suppose an element of length dr at a distance r from P. The induced emf in this segment is

$$de = Bvdr = B(r\omega)dr$$

Because every segment of the rod is moving perpendicular to B, an emf de of same form is generated across each.

So, summing the emfs induced across the ends of the rod is

$$e = \int_0^l de = \int_0^l Br\,\omega dr$$

$$\Rightarrow \quad e = \frac{1}{2}B\omega l^2$$

$$= Bl^2\pi\nu = \frac{Bl^2\pi}{T} \qquad (\because 2\pi\nu = \omega)$$

where, ν = frequency (revolution per second)

and T = time period.

(ii) A conducting disc of radius r rotates with constant angular velocity ω about its axis in a uniform magnetic field parallel to its axis of rotation as shown in figure.

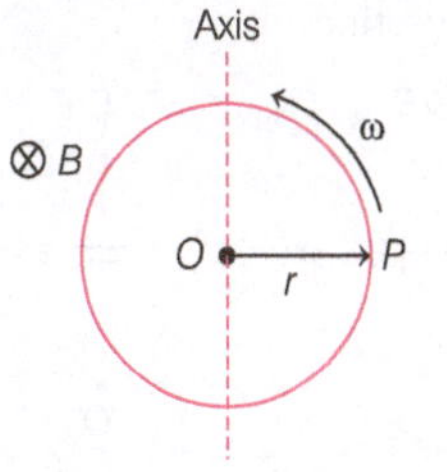

Take a rod between centre and point P.

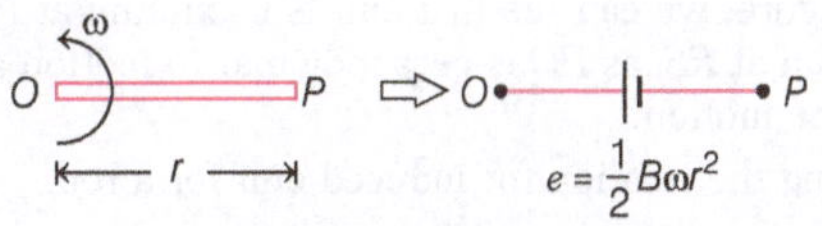

As, we have already deduced the emf for a rod rotating in a constant magnetic field.

So, the induced emf is given by $e = \frac{1}{2}B\omega r^2$.

That means, disc is equivalent to rod.

Fleming's Right Hand Thumb Rule

The direction of motional emf or current can be given by Fleming's right hand thumb rule. If we stretch the thumb, the forefinger and the central finger of right hand in such a way that all are mutually perpendicular to each other, so thumb represents the direction of motion of the conductor, the forefinger represents the direction magnetic field, then central finger will represent the direction of induced current as shown in figure.

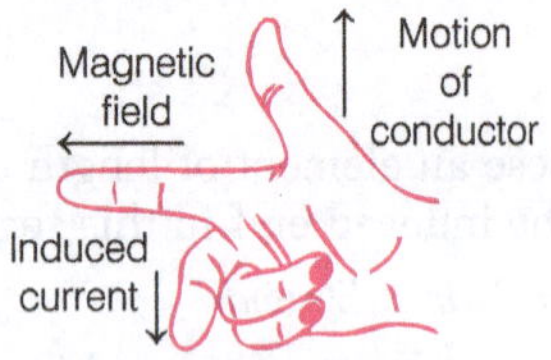

Example 13. *A conducting rod of length 1 m moves with a velocity of 5m/s in a direction perpendicular to its length and perpendicular to a uniform magnetic field of magnitude 0.4T. Find the emf induced between the ends of the stick.*

Sol. As we know that, induced emf for a moving rod is given by

$$\Rightarrow \quad e = Bvl = 0.4 \times 5 \times 1$$
$$= 2\text{ V}$$

Example 14. *A ring of radius 2m moves in its plane with a constant velocity 5m/s. A uniform magnetic field 0.1 T exists in the space in a direction perpendicular to the plane of the ring. Consider different pairs of diametrically opposite points on the ring.*

(i) Between which pair of points is the emf maximum and minimum?

(ii) What is the value of maximum and minimum emf?

Sol. Given, radius, $r = 2\text{m}$, velocity, $v = 5\text{ms}^{-1}$

Constant magnetic field, $B = 0.1\text{ T}$

(i) According to the question,

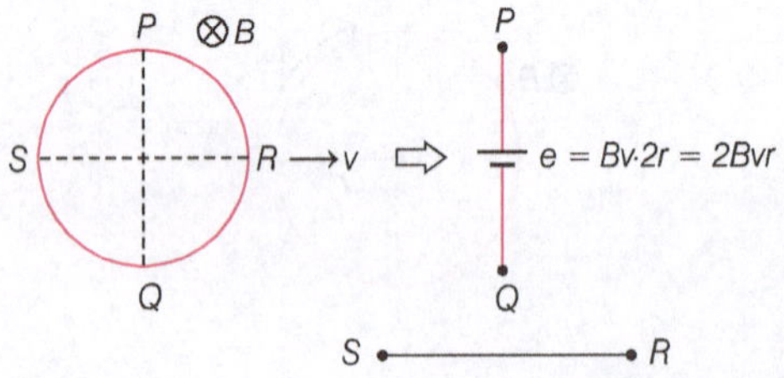

From figure, we can see that emf is maximum at PQ and minimum at RS, as PQ is perpendicular to motion and RS along the motion.

(ii) Using the relation for induced emf for a rod,

$$V_P - V_Q = 2Bvr$$
$$e_{\text{max}} = 2Bvr$$
$$= 2 \times 0.1 \times 5 \times 2 = 2\text{ V}$$
$$V_S - V_R = 0$$
$$\Rightarrow \quad e_{\text{min}} = 0$$

Example 15. *A vertical disc of diameter 10 cm makes 20 revolutions per second about a horizontal axis passing through its centre. A uniform magnetic field 10^{-1} T acts perpendicular to the plane of the disc. Calculate the potential difference between its centre and rim in volts.*

Sol. As, we know, disc is equivalent to a rod of length r. Divide disc into rods, each rod can be replaced by a battery and these batteries would be parallel in arrangement.

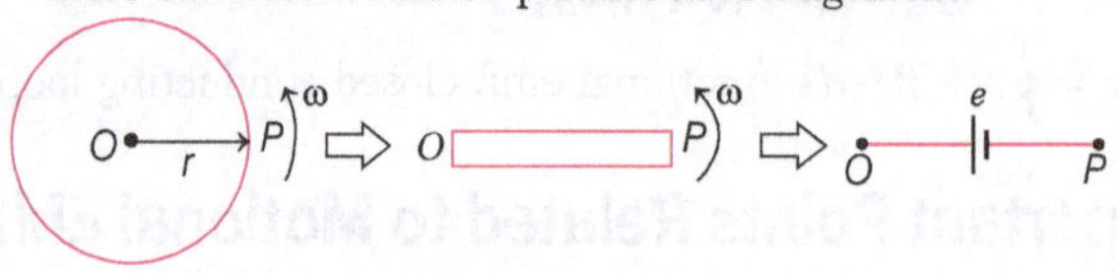

According to the question, radius of disc,

$$r = \frac{10}{2} = 5\text{ cm} = 0.05\text{m}$$

Angular velocity, $\omega = 20 \times 2\pi = 40\,\pi\text{ rad/s}$

Magnetic field, $B = 10^{-1}$ T

The emf of a disc is given as

$$e = \frac{1}{2}B\omega r^2 = \frac{1}{2}(10^{-1})(40\pi)(0.05)^2$$

$$\Rightarrow \quad V_O - V_P = 1.57 \times 10^{-2}\text{ V}$$

Example 16. *Figure shows the top view of a rod that can slide without friction. The resistor is 6.0 Ω and a 2.5 T magnetic field is directed perpendicularly downward into the paper. Let l = 1.2 m.*

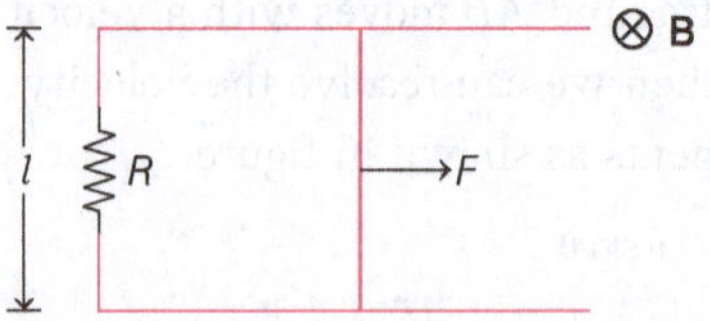

(i) Calculate the force F required to move the rod to the right at a constant speed of 2.0 ms^{-1}.

(ii) At what rate is energy delivered to the resistor?

(iii) Show that this rate is equal to the rate of work done by the applied force.

Sol. Given, resistance, $R = 6.0\,\Omega$

Magnetic field, $B = 2.5$ T

Length of the rod, $l = 1.20\text{m}$

The motional emf in the rod is given as, $e = Bvl$

or $\quad e = (2.5)\,(2.0)\,(1.2)\text{ V} = 6.0\text{ V}$

The current in the circuit, $i = \frac{e}{R} = \frac{6.0}{6.0} = 1.0\text{ A}$

(i) The magnitude of force F required will be equal to the magnetic force acting on the rod, which opposes the motion.

$$\therefore \quad F = F_m = qvB = ilB$$

or $\quad F = (1.0)\,(1.2)\,(2.5)\text{ N} = 3\text{ N}$

(ii) Rate by which energy is delivered to the resistor,

$$P_1 = i^2R = (1)^2\ (6.0) = 6\ \text{W}$$

(iii) The rate by which work is done by the applied force,

$$P_2 = Fv = (3)\ (2.0) = 6\ \text{W} \Rightarrow P_1 = P_2$$

Example 17. *A square loop of side l being moved towards right at a constant speed v as shown in figure. The front edge enters the magnetic field B at t = 0. The width of field is 4l. Sketch induced emf versus time graph.*

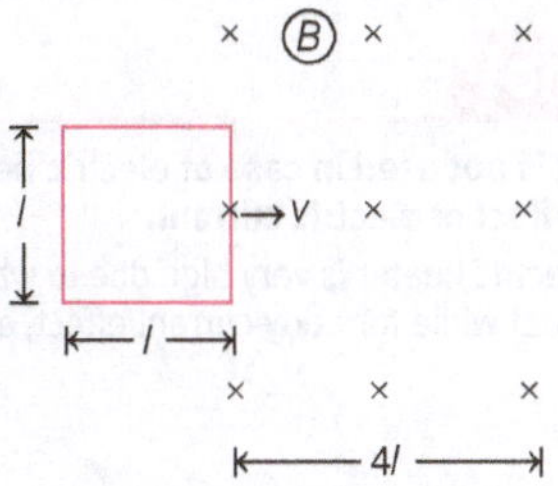

Sol.

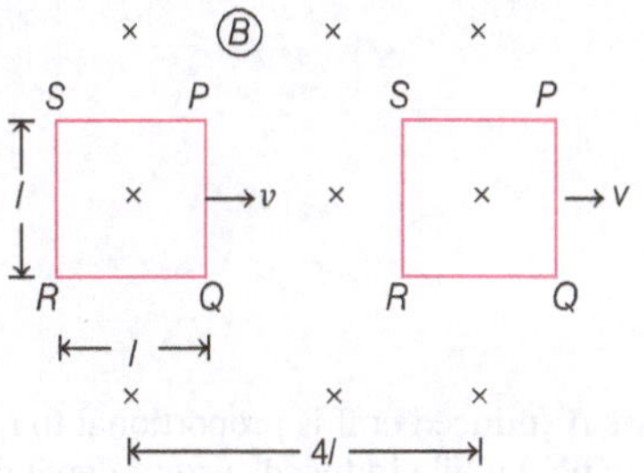

From $t = 0$ to $t = \frac{l}{v}$,

Induced emf, $e = Bvl$ and $I = \frac{e}{R} = \frac{Bvl}{R}$, which is anti-clockwise in direction.

Again from $t = \frac{l}{v}$ to $t = \frac{4l}{v}$, emf $e = 0$

$t = \frac{4l}{v}$ to $t = \frac{5l}{v}$, emf $e = Bvl$

So, induced current $I = \frac{e}{R} = \frac{Bvl}{R}$, which is clockwise in direction now.

So, the plot of induced emf *versus* time is given as

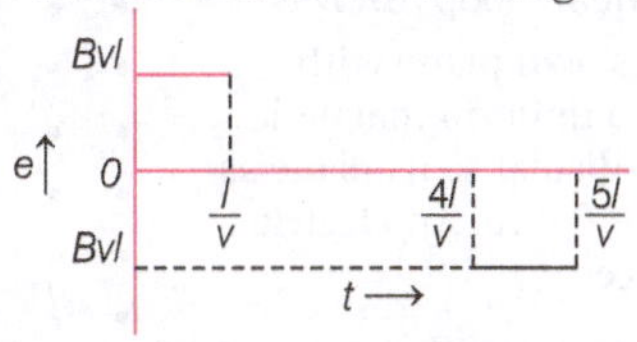

Applications of EMI : Eddy Current

When a changing magnetic flux is applied to a bulk piece of conducting material, then circulating currents induced in the body of the conductor, are called eddy currents. As the resistance of the bulk conductor is usually low, so the eddy currents often have large magnitudes and heat up the conductor.

Eddy currents are always produced in a plane perpendicular to the direction of magnetic field. This current shows both heating and magnetic effects.

The magnitude of eddy current is given by

$$i = \frac{\text{induced emf}}{\text{resistance}} = \frac{e}{R}$$

According to Faraday's law,

$$e = -\frac{d\phi}{dt}$$

$$i = -\frac{d\phi/dt}{R}$$

The direction of eddy currents can be given by Lenz's law or by Fleming's right hand rule.

However, their flow patterns resemble swirling eddies in water. That is why, they are called eddy currents. These were discovered by Foucault in the year 1895 and hence, they are also named as **Foucault current**. *e.g.* When we move a metal plate out of a magnetic field, then the relative motion of the field and the conductor again induces a current in the conductor. The conducting electrons building up the induced current whirl around within the plate as, if they were caught in an eddy of water.

Effects of Eddy Current

Eddy currents are produced inside the iron cores of the rotating armatures of electric motors and dynamos and also in the cores of transformers, which experience flux changes, when they are in use. The currents causes unnecessary heating and wastage of power and the heat produced may even damage the insulation of coils.

Methods to Reduce Eddy Current

Eddy currents are minimised by using laminations of metal to make a metal core. The laminations are separated by an insulating material. The plane of the laminations must be arranged parallel to the magnetic field, so that they cut across the eddy current paths. This arrrangement reduces the strength of eddy currents.

Applications of Eddy Current

Eddy currents are useful in many ways. Some of the important applications of eddy currents are given below

(i) Electromagnetic Damping

In order to bring the moving coil of a galvanometer immediately to rest, we make the use of electromagnetic damping which uses eddy currents to bring the coil to rest. When the coil oscillates, then the eddy currents generated in the core oppose the motion and bring the coil to rest.

(ii) Induction Furnace

In an induction furnace, high temperature can be produced by using eddy currents. We generally use induction furnace in preparation of alloys by melting the constituents of metal.

A coil is wound over the metal which needs to be melted and through the coil, we pass high frequency alternating current. The eddy current generated in the metal produces high temperature to melt the metal.

(iii) Electric Power Meter

Old electric power meters (analog type) had a metallic disc. The disc rotates due to generation of eddy currents which are produced due to sinusoidally varying current in the coil.

(iv) Magnetic Breaking in Electric Trains

Some electric powered trains make use of strong electromagnets which are situated above the rails. These electromagnets are used to produce eddy current in the rails which oppose the motion of the train and thus stop it. In this case, as there is no mechanical linkage, hence the breaking effect is smooth.

NEET Snapshot

Eddy current effect is not used in case of electric heater because it works on heating effect of electric current. ***[NEET 2019]***

The resistance of electric heater is very high due to which, electric current generates heat while for eddy current effect, a low resistance wire is used.

STEP UP Practice 2

1. A 10 m wire kept in east-west direction is falling with velocity 5 m/s perpendicular to the field 0.3×10^4 Wb/m^2. The induced emf across the terminal will be
(a) 0.15 V (b) 1.5 mV (c) 1.5 V (d) 15.0 V

2. The magnitude of the earth's magnetic field at a place is B_0 and the angle of dip is δ. A horizontal conductor of length l lying along the magnetic north-south moves eastwards with a velocity v. The emf induced across the conductor is
(a) zero (b) $B_0 lv \sin\delta$
(c) $B_0 lv$ (d) $B_0 lv \cos\delta$

3. A wire of length 50 cm moves with a velocity of 300 m/min, perpendicular to a magnetic field. If the emf induced in the wire is 2 V, then the magnitude of the field (in tesla) is
(a) 2 (b) 5 (c) 0.8 (d) 2.5

4. A boat is moving due east in a region, where the earth's magnetic field is 5.0×10^{-5} NA^{-1}m^{-1} due to north and horizontal. The boat carried a vertical aerial 2 m long. If the speed of the boat is 1.5 ms^{-1}, then the magnitude of the induced emf in the wire of aerial is
(a) 1 mV (b) 0.75 mV
(c) 0.50 mV (d) 0.15 mV

5. A 0.1 m long conductor carrying a current of 50 A is held perpendicular to a magnetic field of 1.25 mT. The mechanical power required to move the conductor with a speed of 1 ms^{-1} is
(a) 62.5 mW (b) 625 mW
(c) 6.25 mW (d) 12.5 mW

6. **Statement I** The induced emf and current will be same in two identical loops of copper and aluminium, when rotated with same speed in the same magnetic field.

Statement II Induced emf is proportional to rate of change of magnetic field while induced current depends on resistance of wire.

In the light of the above statements, choose the most appropriate answer from the options given below
(a) Both Statement I and Statement II are incorrect.
(b) Statement I is correct but Statement II is incorrect.
(c) Statement I is incorrect but Statement II is correct.
(d) Both Statement I and Statement II are correct.

7. A metal rod of length 2 m is rotating with an angular velocity of 100 rads^{-1} in a plane perpendicular to a uniform magnetic field of 0.3 T. The potential difference between the ends of the rod is
(a) 30 V (b) 40 V
(c) 60 V (d) 600 V

8. A metallic square loop $ABCD$ is moving in its own plane with velocity v in a uniform magnetic field perpen-dicular to its plane as shown in the figure. An electric field is induced

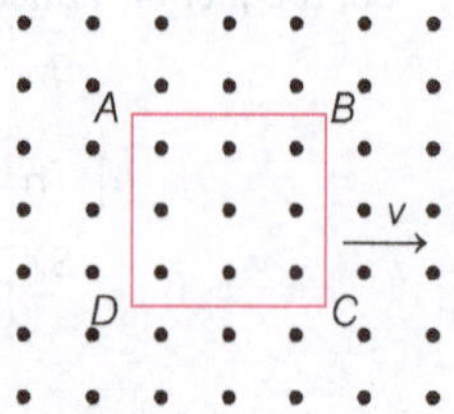

(a) in AD but not in BC
(b) in BC but not in AD
(c) neither in AD nor in BC
(d) in both AD and BC

9. A conducting rod of length l is moving perpendicular to magnetic field of strength B with velocity v. The resistance of the rod is R. The current in the rod is
(a) $\frac{Blv}{R}$ (b) Blv
(c) zero (d) $\frac{B^2v^2l^2}{R}$

10. **Statement I** A metallic surface is moved in and moved out in a magnetic field, then emf is induced in it.

Statement II Eddy current will be produced in a metallic surface moving in and out of magnetic field.

In the light of the above statements, choose the most appropriate answer from the options given below.

(a) Both Statement I and Statement II are incorrect.
(b) Statement I is correct but Statement II is incorrect.
(c) Statement I is incorrect but Statement II is correct.
(d) Both Statement I and Statement II are correct.

11. Eddy currents are produced when

(a) a metal is kept in varying magnetic field
(b) a metal is kept in a steady magnetic field
(c) a circular coil is placed in a magnetic field
(d) through a circular coil current is passed

12. Which of the following pair is incorrect?

(a) Eddy current → Soucault current
(b) Eddy current $(i) \rightarrow \frac{e}{R}$
(c) Eddy current → parallel to the direction of magnetic field
(d) According to Faraday's law $\rightarrow i = \frac{d\phi / dt}{R}$

13. **Statement I** The motion of a copper plate is damped, when it is allowed to oscillate between the pole pieces of a magnet.

Statement II A spark is produced in the switch of the fan when it is switched OFF.

In the light of the above statements, choose the most appropriate answer from the options given below

(a) Both Statement I and Statement II are incorrect.
(b) Statement I is correct but Statement II is incorrect.
(c) Statement I is incorrect but Statement II is correct.
(d) Both Statement I and Statement II are correct.

14. Which of the following is not an application of eddy currents?

(a) Induction furnace (b) Galvanometer damping
(c) Speedometer of automobiles (d) X-ray crystallography

Module 3

Inductance

Inductance • Self-Inductance • Energy Stored in an Inductor • Mutual Inductance

Inductance

Flow of charge (in form of induced current) in a coil due to change in flux connected with this coil is known as induction.

The flux associated to a coil is proportional to the current flowing in same coil or another coil.

$$\phi_B \propto I$$

Also, $\frac{d\phi_B}{dt} \propto \frac{dI}{dt}$ (in case of shape of coil do not change)

The constant of proportionality in the above equations is known as inductance.

It is a scalar quantity and its unit is henry.

Its dimensions are $[M^1L^2T^{-2}A^{-2}]$.

Inductance is of two types : Self-inductance and mutual inductance.

Self-Inductance

Self-induction is the property of a coil by virtue of which the coil opposes any change in the strength of current flowing through it by inducing an emf in itself.

This induced emf is also called **back emf.** When the current in a coil is switched ON, then the self-induction opposes the growth of the current and when it is switched OFF, then the self-induction opposes the decay of the current. Hence, self-induction is also known as **inertia of electricity.**

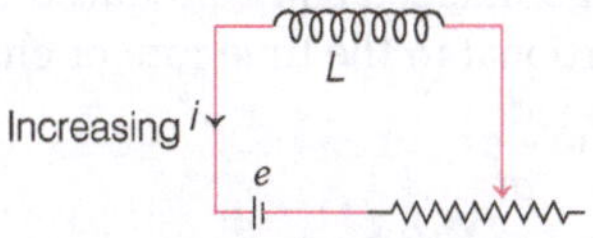

A circuit or part of a circuit, that is designed to have a particular induction is called an **inductor.** The usual symbol for an inductor is shown in figure.

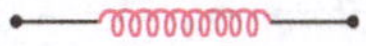

Thus, an inductor is a circuit element which opposes the change in current through it. It may be a circular coil, solenoid, etc.

When the proportionality sign is removed, the same constant L again comes here.

Hence, $e = -L\dfrac{di}{dt}$

The minus sign here is a reflection of Lenz's law. It says that the self-induced emf in a circuit opposes any change in the current in that circuit.

Average induced emf e is given by

$$e = -L\frac{di}{dt} = -\frac{L(i_2 - i_1)}{\Delta t}$$

From the above equation, we can write, $L = \left|\dfrac{-e}{di/dt}\right|$ ...(i)

If $\dfrac{di}{dt} = 1$, then $L = e$

So, when the coefficient of self-induction or self-inductance of a coil is equal to the emf induced in the coil, then time rate of change of current through the coil is unity.

Inductance is a scalar quantity.

Coefficient of Self-Induction

It can be defined in two ways as discussed below

1. Definition using Magnetic Flux

If i is the strength of current flowing through a coil at any time and ϕ is the amount of magnetic flux linked with all the turns of the coil at that time, then it is found that

$$\phi \propto i \text{ or } \phi = Li \Rightarrow L = \frac{\phi}{i}$$

where, L is a constant of proportionality and is called **coefficient of self-induction** or **self-inductance of the coil.** The value of L depends on number of turns N, area of cross-section A and nature of material of the core on which coil is wound.

For N number of turns in coil, $L = \dfrac{N\phi}{i}$.

2. Definition using Induced Emf

If a current i is passed in a circuit and it is changed with a rate di/dt, then the induced emf e produced in the circuit is directly proportional to the time rate of change of current. Thus, $e \propto \dfrac{di}{dt}$.

Example 18. *The inductor shown in figure has inductance 0.54 H and carries a current in the direction shown, which is decreasing at a uniform rate $\dfrac{di}{dt} = -0.03$ A/s.*

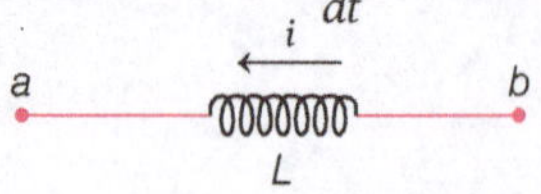

(i) Find the back emf.

(ii) Which end of the inductor a or b is at a higher potential?

Sol. (i) Given, inductance, $L = 0.54$ H

and rate, $\dfrac{di}{dt} = -0.03$ A/s

Self-induced emf (back emf) is given as

$$e = L\frac{di}{dt} = (0.54)(-0.03)\text{ V} = -1.62\times 10^{-2}\text{ V}$$

(ii) We know that, $V_{ba} = L\dfrac{di}{dt} = -1.62\times 10^{-2}$ V

Since, $V_{ba}\ (= V_b - V_a)$ is negative. It implies that $V_a > V_b$ or a is at higher potential.

Self-Inductance of a Coil

Consider a coil of radius r and current i is flowing through the coil. If number of turns in the coil is N, then magnetic field at the centre is given as

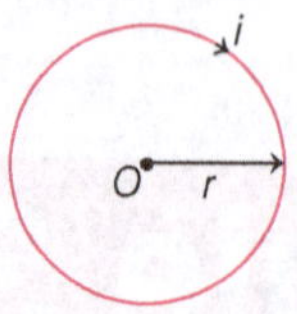

$$\Rightarrow \quad B_{\text{centre}} = \frac{\mu_0 Ni}{2r} \quad \text{and} \quad \phi_B = BS$$

where, S = area of cross-sectional of the coil = πr^2.

So, $$\phi_B = \frac{\mu_0 Ni}{2r}\times \pi r^2 \Rightarrow \phi_B = \frac{\mu_0 \pi Nir}{2}$$

Now, net flux for the coil of N number of turns,

$$\Rightarrow \quad \phi = N\phi_B = \frac{N\times \mu_0 \pi Nir}{2} = \frac{\mu_0 \pi N^2 ir}{2}$$

We know that, $L = \dfrac{\phi}{i} \Rightarrow \boxed{L = \dfrac{\mu_0 N^2 \pi r}{2}\text{ henry}}$

> **Concept ladder** **Combination of self-inductances**
>
> **In series** Equivalent inductance,
>
> $L = L_1 + L_2 + L_3$
>
> **In parallel** Equivalent inductance,
>
> $\dfrac{1}{L} = \dfrac{1}{L_1} + \dfrac{1}{L_2} + \dfrac{1}{L_3}$

Self-Inductance of a Solenoid

Let us find the inductance of a uniformly wound solenoid having N turns and length l. Assume that, l is much longer than the radius of the windings and that the core of the solenoid is air. We can assume that, the interior magnetic field due to a current i is uniform and given by equation,

$$B = \mu_0 ni = \mu_0 \left(\frac{N}{l}\right) i$$

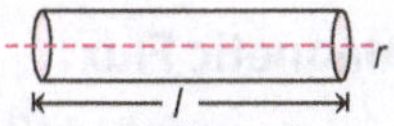

where, $n = \frac{N}{l}$ is the number of turns per unit length.

The magnetic flux through each turn, $\phi_B = BS = \mu_0 \frac{NS}{l} i$

Here, S is the cross-sectional area of the solenoid.

Now, as we know, $L = \frac{N\phi_B}{i} = \frac{N}{i}\left(\frac{\mu_0 NSi}{l}\right) = \frac{\mu_0 N^2 S}{l}$

$$\Rightarrow \quad \boxed{L = \frac{\mu_0 N^2 S}{l}}$$

This result shows that L depends on dimensions (S, l) and is proportional to the square of the number of turns.

$\therefore \quad L \propto N^2$

Because $N = nl$, we can also express the result in the form,

$$L = \mu_0 \frac{(nl)^2}{l} S = \mu_0 n^2 Sl = \mu_0 n^2 V \quad \text{or} \quad L = \mu_0 n^2 V$$

Here, $V = Sl$ is the volume of the solenoid.

Note If the space inside the solenoid is filled with a material of relative permeability μ_r, then $L = \mu_0 \mu_r n^2 Sl$.

Example 19.

(i) Calculate the inductance of an air core solenoid containing 300 turns, if the length of the solenoid is 25 cm and its cross-sectional area is 4 cm².

(ii) Calculate the self-induced emf in the solenoid, if the current through it is decreasing at the rate of 50 A/s.

Sol. (i) The inductance of a solenoid is given by $L = \frac{\mu_0 N^2 S}{l}$

where, S is the cross-sectional area of solenoid.

Substituting the values, we have

$$L = \frac{(4\pi \times 10^{-7})(300)^2 (4 \times 10^{-4})}{(25 \times 10^{-2})} \text{H} = 1.81 \times 10^{-4} \text{ H}$$

(ii) The self-induced emf is given by $e = -L\frac{di}{dt}$

Here, $\frac{di}{dt} = -50$ A/s

$\therefore \quad e = -(1.81 \times 10^{-4})(-50) = 9.05 \times 10^{-3}$ V

or $\quad e = 9.05$ mV

Energy Stored in an Inductor

The energy of a capacitor is stored in the electric field between its plates. Similarly, an inductor has the capability of storing energy in its magnetic field.

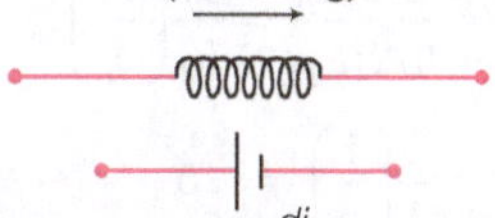

An increasing current in an inductor causes an emf between its terminals.

The work done per unit time is power, thus

$$P = \frac{dW}{dt} = -ei = -Li\frac{di}{dt}$$

From $dW = -dU$ or $\frac{dW}{dt} = -\frac{dU}{dt}$, we have

$$\frac{dU}{dt} = Li\frac{di}{dt} \quad \text{or} \quad dU = Li\, di$$

The total energy U supplied while the current increases from zero to a final value i, $U = L\int_0^i i\,di = \frac{1}{2}Li^2$

$$\therefore \quad \boxed{W = U = \frac{1}{2}Li^2}$$

Concept ladder Energy stored per unit volume in magnetic field is known as **energy density.**

$$\therefore \quad \text{Energy density} = \frac{U}{V} = \frac{1}{2}\frac{B^2}{\mu_0}$$

Example 20. *Two coils having self-inductances, $L_1 = 5$ mH and $L_2 = 1$ mH. The current in the coil is increasing at same constant rate at a certain instant and the power supplied to the coils is also same. Find the ratio of*

(i) induced voltage,

(ii) current

(iii) and energy stored in two coils at that instant.

Sol. Given, $L_1 = 5$ mH and $L_2 = 1$ mH

(i) As we know, induced voltage is given by $e = \frac{Ldi}{dt}$

$$\Rightarrow \quad \frac{e_1}{e_2} = \frac{L_1(di/dt)}{L_2(di/dt)} = \frac{L_1}{L_2} = \frac{5}{1} = 5:1 \quad \text{...(i)}$$

(ii) Power in the coil is given by $P = ei$

Here, $\quad P_1 = P_2 \Rightarrow e_1 i_1 = e_2 i_2 \Rightarrow \frac{i_1}{i_2} = \frac{e_2}{e_1}$

Using Eq. (i), we can write, $\frac{i_1}{i_2} = \frac{1}{5} = 1:5$

(iii) Energy stored in a coil is given by

$$U = \frac{1}{2}Li^2$$

$$\Rightarrow \quad \frac{U_1}{U_2} = \frac{(1/2)L_1 i_1^2}{(1/2)L_2 i_2^2} = \frac{L_1}{L_2}\left(\frac{e_2}{e_1}\right)^2$$

$$= \frac{5}{1}\left(\frac{1}{5}\right)^2 = 1:5$$

NEET Close-up

Example Similar to PYQ Asked in NEET 2023, 18

What inductance would be needed to store 1 kWh of energy in a coil carrying a 200 A current? (Take, 1 kWh = 3.6×10^6 J)

(a) 0 H (b) 90 H
(c) 180 H (d) 60 H

Sol. (c) We have, $i = 200$ A and $U = 1$ kWh $= 3.6 \times 10^6$ J

$\therefore$ Self-inductance, $L = \frac{2U}{i^2} = \frac{2(3.6 \times 10^6)}{(200)^2} = 180$ H $\quad \left(\because U = \frac{1}{2}Li^2\right)$

Skill Builder

The magnetic energy stored in an inductor of inductance 2H carrying current of 3A will be

(a) 3 J (b) 6 J (c) 9 J (d) 12 J

For more Practice Refer Q.No. 15, 16 of step up practice 3 and Q.No. 70 of Gearing up for NEET.

Mutual Inductance

Consider two neighbouring coils of wire as shown in figure. A current flowing in coil 1produces magnetic field and hence a magnetic flux through coil 2. If the current in coil 1 changes, then the flux through coil 2 changes as well. According to Faraday's law, this induces an emf in coil 2. In this way, a change in the current in one circuit can induce a current in a second circuit. This phenomenon is known as mutual induction.

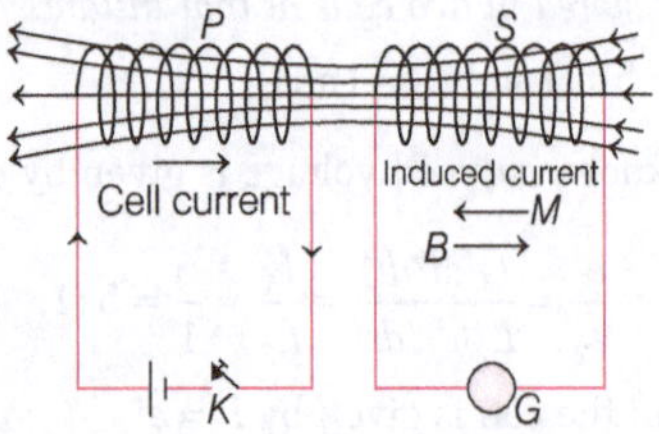

In other words, the phenomena of the production of an electromotive force in a circuit by a change in the current in an adjacent circuit which is linked to the first by the flux lines of a magnetic field is called mutual induction.

Like the self-inductance (L) of single circuit (coil), two circuits has mutual inductance (M).

Coefficient of Mutual Inductance

It can be defined in two ways as discussed below.

1. Definition Using Magnetic Flux

Suppose the circuit 1 has a current i_1 flowing in it, then total flux $N_2\phi_{B_2}$ linked with circuit 2 is proportional to the current in circuit 1.

Thus, $\quad N_2\phi_{B_2} \propto i_1$ or $N_2\phi_{B_2} = Mi_1$

Here, the proportionality constant M is known as **coefficient of mutual inductance** of the two circuits or coils.

Thus, $$M = \frac{N_2\phi_{B_2}}{i_1} \quad \text{...(i)}$$

From this expression, M can be defined as the total flux $N_2\phi_{B_2}$ linked with circuit 2 per unit current in circuit 1.

2. Definition Using Induced Emf

If we change the current in circuit 1 at a rate di_1/dt, an induced emf e_2 is developed in circuit 2, which is proportional to the rate di_1/dt.

Thus, $\quad e_2 \propto di_1/dt$

or $\quad e_2 = -M di_1/dt$ ...(ii)

Here, the proportionality constant is again M. Minus sign indicates that e_2 is in such a direction that it opposes any change in the current in circuit 1.

From the above equation, we can write $M = \left|\frac{-e_2}{di_1/dt}\right|$.

If $\frac{di}{dt} = 1$, then $M = e$. Thus, coefficient of mutual induction or mutual inductance of two coils is equal to the emf induced in one coil when time rate of change of current through the other coil is unity.

- **Reciprocity theorem** This theorem states that mutual inductance due to secondary coil on primary coil is equal to the mutual induction due to primary coil on secondary coil. *i.e.* $M_{21} = M_{12} = M$.
  Using Eq. (ii),
  $$e_2 = -M_{12}(di_1/dt)$$
  and $$e_1 = -M_{21}(di_2/dt)$$
  Using Eq. (i), $M_{12} = \frac{N_2\phi_{B_2}}{i_1}$ and $M_{21} = \frac{N_1\phi_{B_1}}{i_2}$
- Average induced emf, $\bar{e} = -M\frac{\Delta i}{\Delta t} = -\frac{M(i_2 - i_1)}{\Delta t}$.
- A good approach for calculating the mutual inductance of two circuits or coils consists of the following steps.

(a) Assume anyone of the circuits as primary (first) and the other as secondary (second).

(b) Suppose a current i_1 flows through the primary circuit.

(c) Determine the magnetic field **B** produced by the current i_1.

(d) Obtain the magnetic flux (ϕ_{B_2}) linked with secondary circuit.

(e) With the flux known, the mutual inductance can be found from

$$M = \frac{N_2 \phi_{B_2}}{i_1}$$

Mutual Inductances of Some Important Coil Configurations

1. Mutual Inductance for Two Concentric Coils

Let us consider a coil having N_1 turns and of radius r is surrounded by another coil having N_2 turns and of radius R as shown in the figure ($R >> r$).

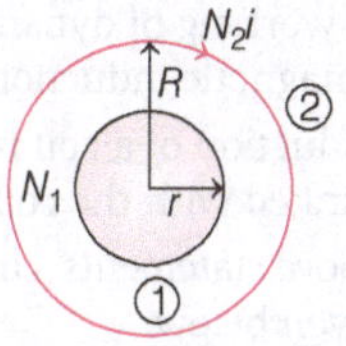

Magnetic field due to coil 2 at centre, $B_2 = \frac{\mu_0 N_2 i}{2R}$

Flux through coil 1, $\phi_{B_1} = N_1 B_2 S = \frac{N_1 \mu_0 N_2 i}{2R} \pi r^2 = Mi$

$$\Rightarrow \quad \boxed{M = \frac{\mu_0 N_1 N_2 \pi r^2}{2R}}$$

NEET Snapshot

If two conducting circular loops of radii R_1 and R_2 are placed in the same plane with their centre coinciding ($R_1 >> R_2$). Then, the mutual inductance M between them will be directly proportional to $\frac{R_2^2}{R_1}$.

[NEET 2021]

Magnetic flux, $\phi = Mi$ ... (i) [here, M is mutual inductance]

Also, the magnetic flux, $\phi = BA$ [here, B is magnetic field]

Magnetic field, $B = \frac{\mu_0 i}{2R_1}$

$\phi = \frac{\mu_0 i}{2R_1} \pi R_2^2$ ...(ii) [$\because \phi = BA, A = \pi R_2^2$]

Comparing Eqs. (i) and (ii), we get

$$M = \frac{\mu_0}{2R_1} \pi R_2^2$$

or $$M \propto \frac{R_2^2}{R_1}$$

Scan for Video

2. Mutual Inductance of Two Long Co-axial Solenoids

Figure shows two long co-axial solenoids, each of length l. Let n_1 be the number of turns per unit length of inner solenoid S_1 of radius r_1 and n_2 is number of turns per unit length of outer solenoid S_2 of radius r_2.

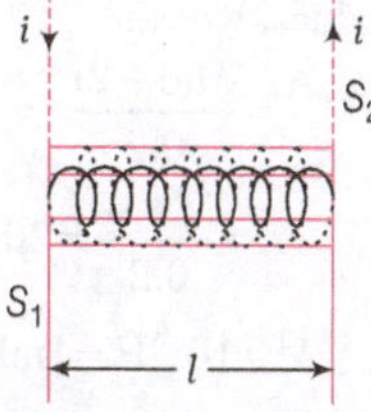

Magnetic field due to S_1, $B_1 = \mu_0 n_1 i$

Flux through S_2, $\phi_B = (n_2 l) B_1 \pi r_1^2$

$$= (n_2 l) \mu_0 n_1 i \pi r_1^2 = Mi$$

$$\Rightarrow \quad M = \mu_0 n_1 n_2 \pi r_1^2 l$$

$$\boxed{M = \frac{\mu_0 N_1 N_2 \times S}{l}}$$

where, S is the area of cross-section of inner solenoid.

Mentor's TiP

We do not take the area of cross-section of outer solenoid because there is no magnetic field between the two solenoids.

3. Mutual Inductance of a Solenoid Surrounded by a Coil

Let N_1 be the number of turns of solenoid of radius r_1 and N_2 be the number of turns of coil of radius r_2.

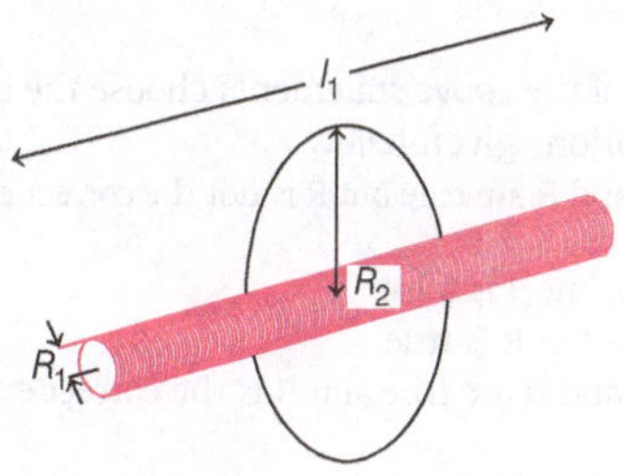

Magnetic field due to solenoid,

$$B = \mu_0 (N_1 / l) i$$

Then, flux through coil,

$$\phi_B = N_2 BS = N_2 \mu_0 \frac{N_1}{l} i \pi R_1^2 = Mi$$

$$\Rightarrow \quad \boxed{M = \frac{\mu_0 N_1 N_2 \pi R_1^2}{l}} \quad \left(\because M = \frac{N_2 \phi_B}{i}\right)$$

From the above relation, we see that, M is independent of radius R_2. This is because, solenoid's magnetic field is confined to the interior coil.

Example 21. *Calculate the mutual inductance between two coils when a current 2A changes to 6A in 0.2 s and induces an emf of 20mV in the secondary coil.*

Sol. We know that, emf is related to the mutual inductance by

$$e = M\frac{\Delta i}{\Delta t}$$

Substituting the given values, we get

$$20 \times 10^{-3} = \frac{M(6-2)}{0.2}$$

$$= \frac{M \times 4}{0.2} = 20M$$

$$\Rightarrow \quad M = 10^{-3}\text{H} = 1\text{mH}$$

Concept ladder

- If two coils of self-inductances L_1 and L_2 having mutual inductance M are **in series** and placed close to each other, then net inductance will be

$$L_S = L_1 + L_2 \pm 2M$$

- If two coils of self-inductances L_1 and L_2 having mutual inductance M, are connected **in parallel**, placed close to each other, then

$$L_P = \frac{L_1L_2 - M^2}{L_1 + L_2 \pm 2M}.$$

STEP UP Practice 3

1. Self-inductance of a coil is 50 mH. A current of 1 A passing through the coil reduces to zero at steady rate in 0.1 s, the self-induced emf is

(a) 5 V (b) 0.05 V (c) 50 V (d) 0.5 V

2. In a coil of self-inductance 0.5 H, the current varies at a constant rate from zero to 10 A in 2 s. The emf generated in the coil is

(a) 10 V (b) 5 V (c) 2.5 V (d) 1.25 V

3. **Assertion** (A) Inductor coils are made of copper.

Reason (R) Induced current is more in wire having less resistance.

In the light of the above statements choose the correct answer from the options given below

(a) Both A and R are true but R is not the correct explanation of A.
(b) A is true but R is false.
(c) A is false but R is true.
(d) Both A and R are true and R is the correct explanation of A.

4. The current passing through a choke coil of 5 H is decreasing at the rate of 2 A/s. The emf developing across the coil is

(a) 10 V (b) −10 V
(c) 2.5 V (d) −2.5 mV

5. During a current change from 2 A to 4 A in 0.5 s, 8 V of emf is developed in a coil. The coefficient of self-induction is

(a) 1 H (b) 2 H
(c) 4 H (d) 8 H

6. If a current of 10 A changes in one second through a coil, and the induced emf is 10 V,then the self-inductance of the coil is

(a) $\frac{2}{5}$ H (b) $\frac{4}{5}$ H
(c) $\frac{5}{4}$ H (d) 1 H

7. **Assertion** (A) The working of dynamo is based on the principle of electromagnetic induction.

Reason (R) Self-induction of a coil is numerically equal to the magnetic flux linked with the coil.

In the light of the above statements, choose the correct answer from the options given below

(a) Both A and R are true but R is not the correct explanation of A.
(b) A is true but R is false.
(c) A is false but R is true.
(d) Both A and R are true and R is the correct explanation of A.

8. A long solenoid has 500 turns. When a current of 2 A is passed through it, then the resulting magnetic flux linked with each turn of the solenoid is 4×10^{-3} Wb. The self-inductance of the solenoid is

(a) 1.0 H (b) 4.0 H (c) 2.5 H (d) 2.0 H

9. **Assertion** (A) The growth of current in *R-L* circuit is uniform.

Reason (R) Inductor (*L*) opposes the growth of current.

In the light of the above statements, choose the correct anser from the options given below

(a) Both A and R are true but R is not the correct explanation of A.
(b) A is true but R is false.
(c) A is false but R is true.
(d) Both A and R are true and R is the correct explanation of A.

10. The self-inductance of a long solenoid cannot be increased by

(a) increasing its area of cross-section
(b) decreasing the area of cross-section
(c) changing the medium with greater permeability
(d) increasing the current through it

11. The self-inductance of a coil is L. Keeping the length and area same, the number of turns in the coil is increased to four times. The self-inductance of the coil will now be
(a) $\frac{1}{4}L$ (b) L (c) $4L$ (d) $16L$

12. In circular coil, when number of turns is doubled and resistance becomes (1/4)th of initial, then inductance becomes
(a) 4 times (b) 2 times
(c) 8 times (d) No change

13. A solenoid has 2000 turns would over a length of 0.30 m. The area of its cross-section is $1.2\times10^{-3}\text{m}^2$. If an initial current of 2 A in the solenoid is reversed in 0.25 s, then the emf induced in the coil is
(a) 6×10^{-4} V (b) 4.8×10^{-3} V
(c) 6×10^{-2} V (d) 32.1×10^{-2} V

14. **Assertion** (A) When number of turns in a coil is doubled, coefficient of self-inductance of the coil become four times.
Reason (R) Coefficient of self-inductance is proportional to the square of number of turns.
In the light of the above statements, choose the correct answer from the options given below.
(a) Both A and R are true but R is not the correct explanation of A.
(b) A is true but R is false.
(c) A is false but R is true.
(d) Both A and R are true and R is the correct explanation of A.

15. A 50 mH coil carries a current of 2 A. The energy stored (in J) is
(a) 1 (b) 0.1 (c) 0.05 (d) 0.5

16. In an inductor of inductance $L = 100$ mH, a current of $i = 10$ A is flowing. The energy stored in the inductor is
(a) 5 J (b) 10 J
(c) 100 J (d) 1000 J

17. The SI unit of inductance, can be written as
(a) weber/(ampere)^2 (b) volt-second/ampere
(c) joule/(ampere)^2 (d) ohm-(second)^2

18. **Assertion** (A) The phenomenon of self-induction is helpful in working of a choke coil.
Reason (R) A choke coil is used for reducing energy loss in the circuit.
In the light of the above statements, choose the correct answer from the options given below
(a) Both A and R are true but R is not the correct explanation of A.
(b) A is true but R is false.
(c) A is false but R is true.
(d) Both A and R are true and R is the correct explanation of A.

19. Two pure inductors each of self-inductance L are connected in parallel but are well separated from each other. The total inductance is
(a) $2L$ (b) L (c) $\frac{L}{2}$ (d) $\frac{L}{4}$

20. Two coils X and Y are placed in a circuit such that when the current changes by 2 A in coil X. The magnetic flux changes by 0.4 Wb in Y. The value of mutual inductance of the coils is
(a) 0.2 H (b) 5 H
(c) 0.8 H (d) 4 H

21. Two coils have a mutual inductance of 0.005 H. The current changes in the first coil according to equation $i = i_0 \sin \omega t$, where $i_0 = 10$ A and $\omega = 100\pi$ rads^{-1}. The maximum value of emf in the second coil is (in volt)
(a) 2π (b) 5π
(c) π (d) 4π

22. The mutual inductance between a primary and secondary circuits is 0.5 H. The resistance of the primary and the secondary circuits are 20 Ω and 5 Ω, respectively. To generate a current of 0.4 A in the secondary, current in the primary must be changed at the rate of
(a) 4.0 As^{-1} (b) 1.6 As^{-1}
(c) 16.0 As^{-1} (d) 8.0 As^{-1}

23. Two circuits have coefficient of mutual induction of 0.09 H. Average emf induced in the secondary by a change of current from 0 to 20 A in 0.006 s in the primary will be
(a) 120 V (b) 80 V
(c) 200 V (d) 300 V

24. A current is varying at the rate of 3 A/s in a coil generates an emf of 8 mV in a nearby coil. The mutual inductance of the two coils is
(a) 2.66 mH (b) 2.66×10^{-3} mH
(c) 2.66 H (d) 0.266 H

25. A solenoid is placed inside another solenoid, the length of both being equal carrying same magnitude of current. The parameters like radius and number of turns are in the ratio 1: 2 for the two solenoids. The mutual inductance on each other would be
(a) $M_{12} = M_{21}$ (b) $M_{12} = 2M_{21}$
(c) $2M_{12} = M_{21}$ (d) $M_{12} = 4M_{21}$

26. Two coils of self-inductances L_1 and L_2 are placed closer to each other, so that total flux in one coil is completely linked with other. If M is mutual inductance between them, then
(a) $M = L_1L_2$ (b) $M = L_1/L_2$
(c) $M = \sqrt{L_1L_2}$ (d) $M = (L_1L_2)^2$

27. Two coils of self-inductances 2 mH and 8 mH are placed, so close together that the effective flux in one coil is completely linked with the other. The mutual inductance between these coils is
(a) 4 mH (b) 16 mH (c) 10 mH (d) 6 mH

28. Which of the following pair is correct?
(a) $U \rightarrow \frac{1}{2}Li$
(b) Energy density $= \frac{U}{V} = \frac{1}{2}\frac{B^2}{\mu_0}$
(c) Dimension of inductance $\rightarrow \text{M}^1\text{L}^1\text{T}^{-2}\text{A}^{-2}$
(d) L_S (mutual inductance) $\rightarrow L_1 + L_2$

NEET Exclusive EXTRA BYTES

- Induced emf is independent of the nature and resistance of coil.
- Induced emf is proportional to relative speed between coil and magnet.
- Induced current and induced charge depends on resistance of coil.
- Resistance opposes flow of the current while inductance opposes change in current, *i.e.* inductance has no importance in constant current cases.
- Mutual inductance in two concentric square loops, $M \propto \frac{b^2}{a}$

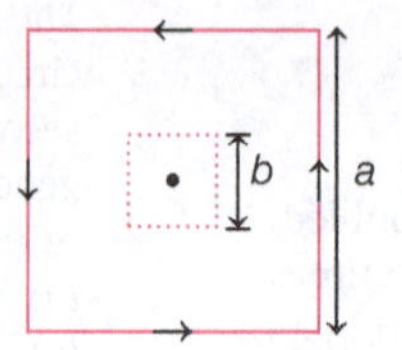

- Mutual inductance between a square and a circular concentric loops, $M \propto \frac{r^2}{a}$

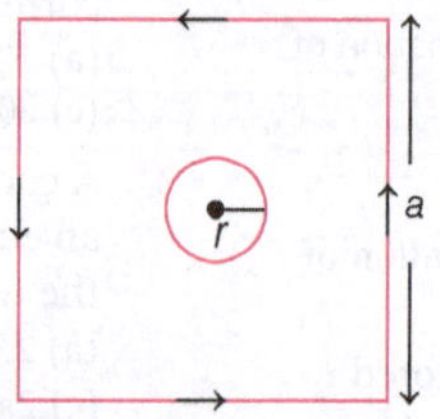

- Emf due to conducting rod rotating in a uniform magnetic field perpendicular to rod is given by
- **Kirchhoff's second law with an inductor**
  In Kirchhoff's second law (Loop rule), when we go through an inductor in the same direction as the assumed current, we encounter a voltage drop equal to $L\,di/dt$, where di/dt is to be substituted with sign.
  For example in the loop shown in the following figure, Kirchhoff's second law gives the equation.

$$E - iR - L\frac{di}{dt} = 0$$

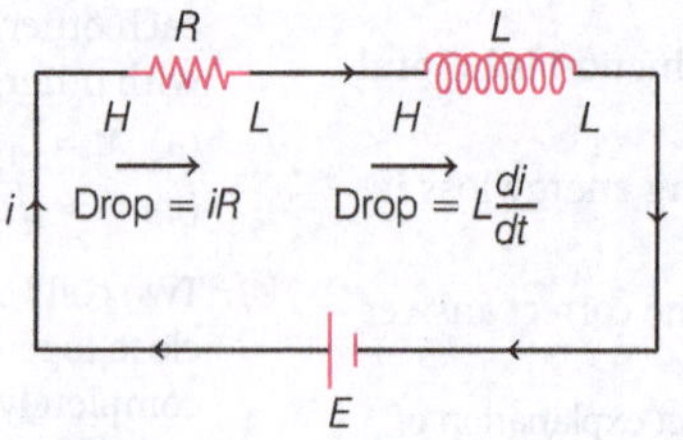

GEARING UP FOR NEET

Single Option Correct

1 In electromagnetic induction, the induced charge in a coil is independent of
(a) change in the flux
(b) time taken to change the flux
(c) resistance in the circuit
(d) None of the above

2 A magnet is brought towards a coil (i) speedly (ii) slowly, then the induced emf/induced charge will be respectively
(a) more in first case/more in first case
(b) more in first case/equal in both cases
(c) less in first case/more in second case
(d) less in first case/equal in both cases

3 A coil and a bulb are connected in series with a DC source, a soft iron core is then inserted in the coil, then
(a) intensity of the bulb remains the same
(b) intensity of the bulb decreases
(c) intensity of the bulb increases
(d) the bulb ceases to glow

4 The self-inductance L of a solenoid of length l and area of cross-section A, with a fixed number of turns N increases as
(a) Both l and A increase
(b) l decreases and A increases
(c) l increases and A decreases
(d) Both l and A decrease

5 In a coil of area 10 cm^2 and 10 turns, a magnetic field is directed perpendicular to the plane and is changing at the rate of 10^8 G/s. The resistance of the coil is 20 Ω. The current in the coil will be
(a) 5 A (b) 0.5 A (c) 0.05 A (d) 5×10^8 A

6 Two identical circular loops of metal wires are lying on a table without touching each other. Loop *A* carries a current which increases with time. In response, the loop *B*
(a) remains stationary
(b) is attracted by loop *A*
(c) is repelled by loop *A*
(d) rotates about its centre of mass with CM fixed

7 A coil having 500 square loops each of side 10 cm is placed normal to a magnetic flux which increases at the rate of 1.0 Ts^{-1}. The induced emf in volt is
(a) 0.1 (b) 0.5 (c) 1 (d) 5

8 A coil having an area 2 m^2 is placed in a magnetic field which changes from 1 Wbm^{-2} to 4 Wbm^{-2} in an interval of 2 s. The emf induced in the coil will be
(a) 4 V (b) 3 V
(c) 1.5 V (d) 2 V

9 The circular loops of equal radii are placed coaxially at some separation. The first is cut and a battery is inserted in between to drive a current in it. The current changes slightly because of the variation in resistance with temperature.
During this period, the two loops
(a) attract each other
(b) repel each other
(c) do not exert any force on each other
(d) attract or repel each other depending on the sense of the current

10 A small, conducting circular loop is placed inside a long solenoid carrying a current. The plane of the loop contains the axis of the solenoid.
If the current in the solenoid is varied, then the current induced in the loop is
(a) clockwise (b) anti-clockwise
(c) zero
(d) clockwise or anti-clockwise depending on whether the resistance is increased or decreased

11 The north pole of a magnet is brought near a metallic ring as shown in the figure. The direction of induced current in the ring will be

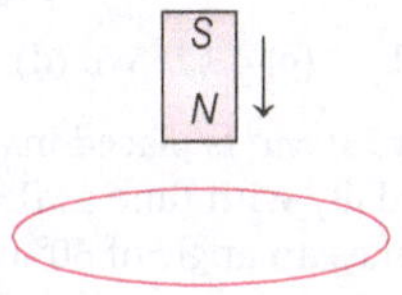

(a) anti-clockwise
(b) clockwise
(c) first anti-clockwise and then clockwise
(d) first clockwise and then anti-clockwise

12 Some magnetic flux is changed from a coil of resistance 10 Ω. As a result an induced current is developed in it, which varies with time as shown in figure. The magnitude of change in flux through the coil (in Wb) is
(a) 2
(b) 4
(c) 6
(d) None of the above

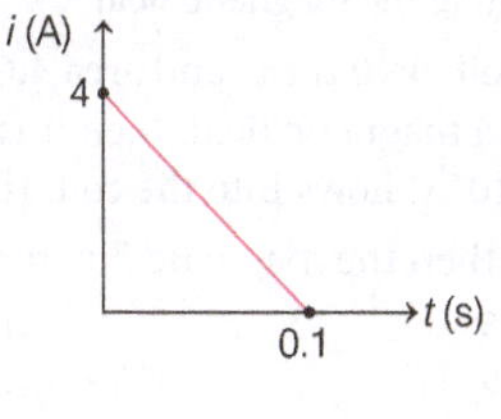

13 A coil of 40 Ω resistance, 100 turns and radius 6 mm is connected to ammeter of resistance 160 Ω. Coil is placed perpendicular to the magnetic field. When coil is taken out of the field, 32 μC charge flows through it. The intensity of magnetic field will be

(a) 6.55 T (b) 5.66 T (c) 2.55 T (d) 0.566 T

14 A coil has an area of 0.05 m^2 and it has 800 turns. It is placed perpendicularly in a magnetic field of strength 4×10^{-5} Wb m^{-2} and is rotated through 90° in 0.1 s. The average emf induced in the coil is

(a) 0.056 V (b) 0.046 V (c) 0.026 V (d) 0.016 V

15 In a magnetic field of 0.05 T, area of a coil changes from 101 cm^2 to 100 cm^2 without changing the resistance which is 2 Ω. The amount of charge that flows during this period is

(a) 2.5×10^{-6} C (b) 2×10^{-6} C
(c) 10^{-6} C (d) 8×10^{-6} C

16 An electron moves along the line *AB* which lies in the same plane as a circular loop of conducting wire as shown in figure. What will be the direction of the current induced (if any) in the loop?

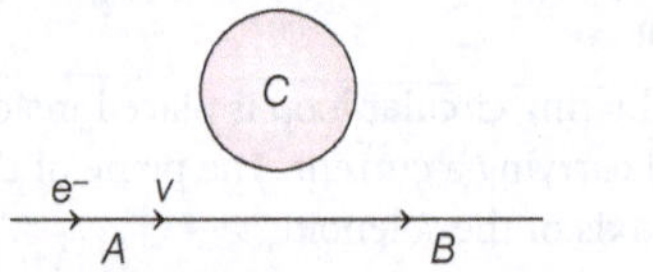

(a) No current will be induced
(b) The current will be clockwise
(c) The current will be anti-clockwise
(d) The current will change direction as the electron passes through

17 A square of side *L* metres lies in the *XY*-plane in a region, where the magnetic field is given by $\mathbf{B} = B_0(2\hat{\mathbf{i}} + 3\hat{\mathbf{j}} + 4\hat{\mathbf{k}})$ T, where B_0 is constant. The magnitude of flux passing through the square is ***[NCERT Exemplar]***

(a) $2B_0L^2$ Wb (b) $3B_0L^2$ Wb (c) $4B_0L^2$ Wb (d) $\sqrt{29}B_0L^2$ Wb

18 A conducting loop of area 5.0 cm^2 is placed in a magnetic field which varies sinusoidally with time as $B = 0.2\sin 300\,t$. The normal to the coil makes an angle of 60° with the field. The emf induced at $t = (\pi / 900)$ s

(a) 7.5×10^{-3} V (b) zero (c) 15×10^{-3} V (d) 20×10^{-3} V

19 An infinitely long cylinder is kept parallel to a uniform magnetic field **B** directed along positive *Z*-axis. The direction of induced current as seen from the *Z*-axis will be

(a) clockwise of the positive *Z*-axis
(b) anti positive *Z*-axis clockwise of the positive *Z*-axis
(c) zero
(d) along the magnetic field

20 If a coil of 40 turns and area 4.0 cm^2 is suddenly removed from a magnetic field, then it is observed that a charge of 2.0×10^{-4} C flows into the coil. If the resistance of the coil is 80 Ω, then the magnetic flux density (in Wb/m^2) is

(a) 0.5 (b) 1.0
(c) 1.5 (d) 2.0

21 A magnet *N-S* is suspended from a spring and while it oscillates, the magnet moves in and out of the coil *C*. The coil is connected to a galvanometer *G*.

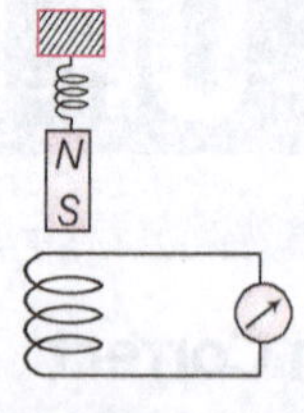

Then, as the magnet oscillates,

(a) *G* shows deflection to the left and right with constant amplitude
(b) *G* shows deflection on one side
(c) *G* shows no deflection
(d) *G* shows deflection to the left and right but the amplitude steadily decreases

22 The variation of induced emf (*E*) with time (*t*) in a coil, if a short bar magnet is moved along its axis with a constant velocity is best represented as

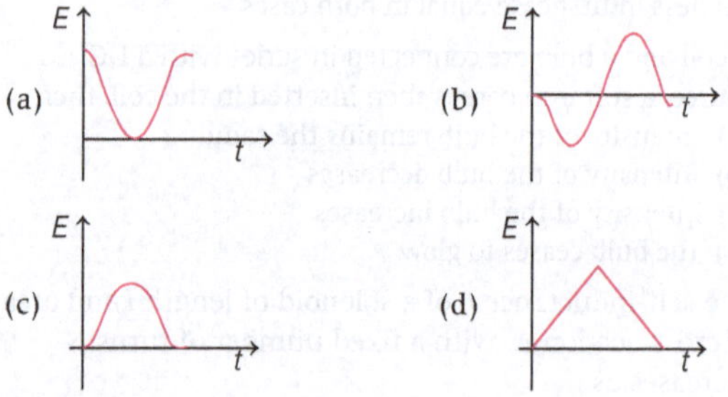

23 An infinitely long conductor *AB* lies along the axis of a circular loop of radius *R*. If the current in the conductor *AB* varies at the rate of *x* ampere/second, then the induced emf in the loop is

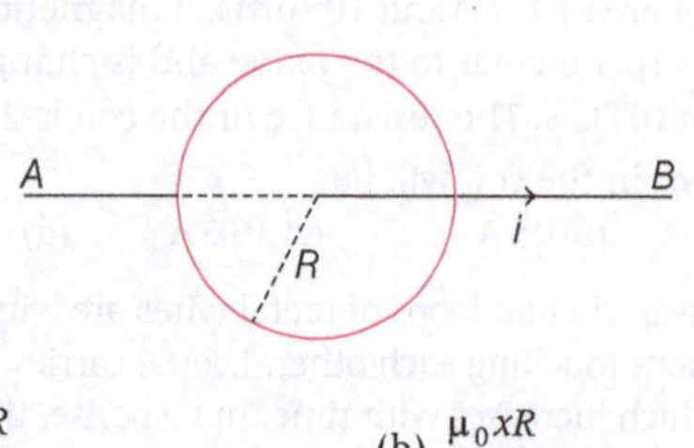

(a) $\frac{\mu_0 xR}{2}$ (b) $\frac{\mu_0 xR}{4}$
(c) $\frac{\mu_0 \pi xR}{2}$ (d) zero

24 A pair of coils of turns n_1 and n_2 are kept close together. Current passing through the first is reduced at the rate *r* and emf 3 mV is developed across the other coil. If the second coil carries current which is then reduced at the rate 2*r*, then the emf produced across the first coil will be

(a) $\frac{6n_1}{n_2}$ mV (b) $\frac{6n_2}{n_1}$ mV
(c) 6 mV (d) (3/2) mV

25 A loop made of straight edges has six corners at $A\,(0, 0, 0)$, $B\,(L, 0, 0)$, $C\,(L, L, 0)$, $D\,(0, L, 0)$, $E\,(0, L, L)$ and $F\,(0, 0, L)$. A magnetic field $\mathbf{B} = B_0(\hat{\mathbf{i}} + \hat{\mathbf{k}})$ T is present in the region. The flux passing through the loop $ABCDEFA$ (in that order) is *[NCERT Exemplar]*
(a) B_0L^2 Wb (b) $2B_0\,L^2$ Wb (c) $\sqrt{2}B_0L^2$ Wb (d) $4B_0L^2$ Wb

26 A magnetic field given by $B(t) = 0.2t - 0.05t^2$ tesla is directed perpendicular to the plane of a circular coil containing 25 turns of radius 1.8 cm and whose total resistance is 1.5 Ω. The power dissipation at 3 s is approximately
(a) 1.37 μW (b) 7 μW (c) zero (d) 4 μW

27 A small magnet M is allowed to fall through a fixed horizontal conducting ring R. Let g be the acceleration due to gravity. The acceleration of M, a will be

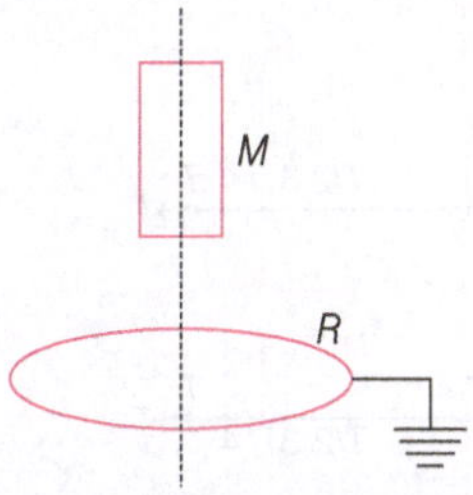

(a) $< g$ when it is above R and moving towards R
(b) $> g$ when it is above R and moving towards R
(c) $> g$ when it is below R and moving away from R
(d) None of the above

28 When the current in the portion of the circuit shown in the figure is 2 A and increasing at the rate of 1 As^{-1}, then the measured potential difference $V_{ab} = 8$ V. However, when the current is 2A and decreasing at the rate of 1As^{-1}, then the measured potential difference $V_{ab} = 4$ V.

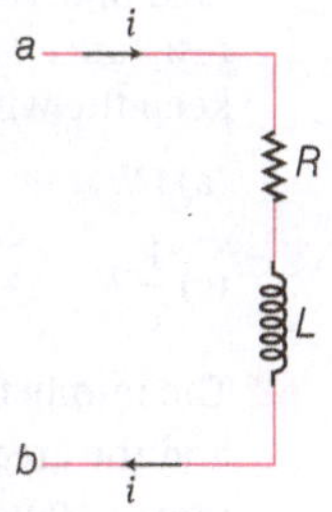

The values of R and L are
(a) 3 Ω and 2 H respectively
(b) 3 Ω and 3 H respectively
(c) 2 Ω and 1 H respectively
(d) 3 Ω and 1 H respectively

29 The coil A is made to rotate about a vertical axis (figure). No current flows in B, if A is at rest. The current in coil A, when the current in B (at $t = 0$) is counter-clockwise and the coil A is as shown at this instant, $t = 0$, is

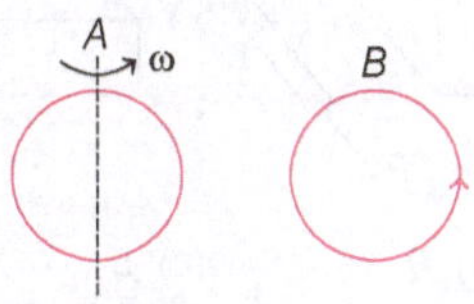

(a) constant current clockwise
(b) varying current clockwise
(c) varying current counter-clockwise
(d) constant current counter-clockwise

30 A rectangular loop of sides 10 cm and 5 cm with a cut is stationary between the pole pieces of an electromagnet. The magnetic field of the magnet is normal to the loop. The current feeding the electromagnet is reduced, so that the field decreased from its initial value of 0.2 T at the rate of 0.02 Ts^{-1}. If the cut is joined and the loop has a resistance of 2.0 Ω, then the power dissipated by the loop as heat is
(a) 5 nW (b) 4 nW (c) 3 nW (d) 2 nW

31 There are two coils A and B as shown in figure. A current starts flowing in B as shown, when A is moved towards B and stops when A stops moving. The current in A is counter-clockwise. B is kept stationary when A moves. We can infer that *[NCERT Exemplar]*

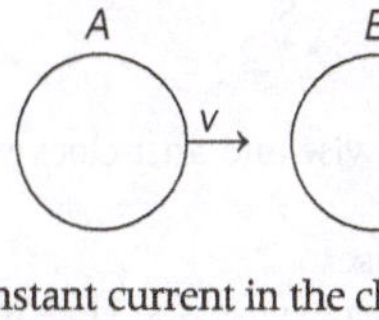

(a) there is a constant current in the clockwise direction in A
(b) there is a varying current in A
(c) there is no current in A
(d) there is a constant current in the counter-clockwise direction in A

32 An emf of 15 V is applied in a circuit coil containing 5 H inductance and 10 Ω resistance. The ratio of the currents at time $t = \infty$ and $t = 1$ s is
(a) $\dfrac{e^{1/2}}{e^{1/2} - 1}$ (b) $\dfrac{e^2}{e^2 - 1}$ (c) $1 - e^{-1}$ (d) e^{-1}

33 An aluminium ring B faces an electromagnet A. The current I through A can be altered

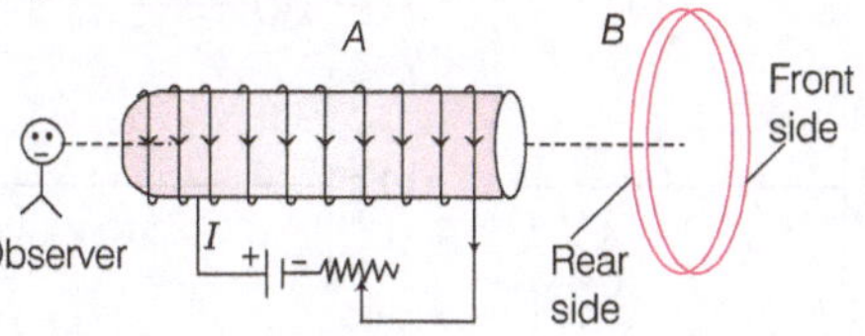

(a) whether I increases or decreases, B will not experience any force
(b) if I decreases, A will repel B
(c) if I increases, A will attract B
(d) if I increases, A will repel B

34 Which of the following figure correctly depicts the Lenz's law? The arrows show the movement of the labelled pole of a bar magnet into a closed circular loop and the arrows on the circle show the direction of the induced current.

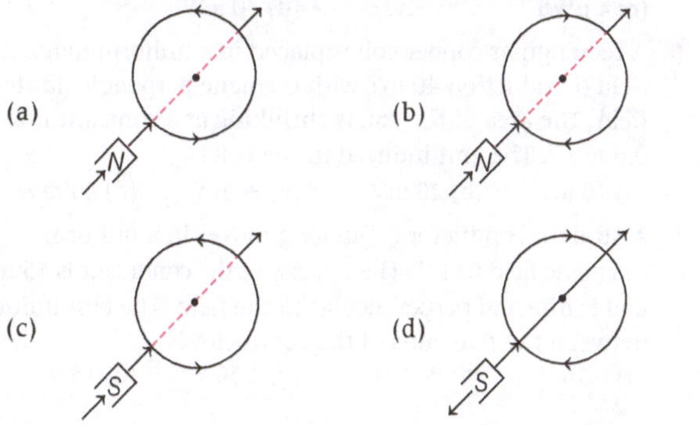

35 As shown in the figure, P and Q are two co-axial conducting loops separated by some distance. When the switch S is closed, a clockwise current I_P flows in P (as seen by E) and an induced current I_{Q_1} flows in Q. The switch remains closed for a long time. When S is opened, a current I_{Q_2} flows in Q. Then, the directions of I_{Q_1} and I_{Q_2} (as seen by E) are

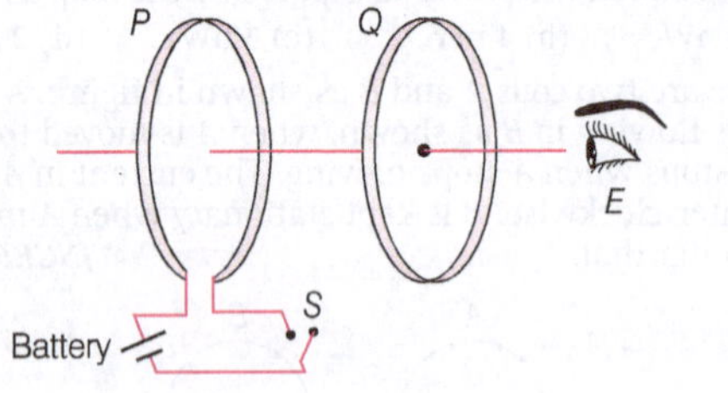

(a) respectively clockwise and anti-clockwise
(b) both clockwise
(c) both anti-clockwise
(d) respectively anti-clockwise and clockwise

36 A magnet is made to oscillate with a particular frequency, passing through a coil as shown in figure. The time variation of the magnitude of emf generated across the coil during one cycle.

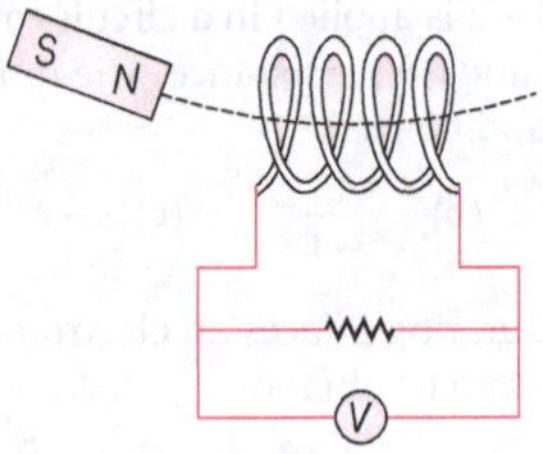

(a) 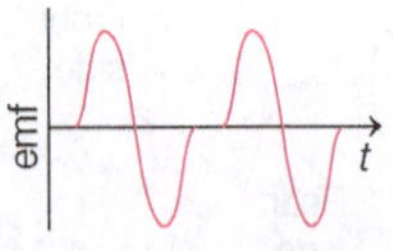

(b) 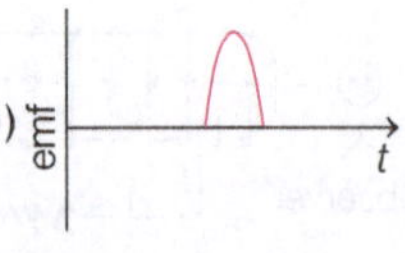

(c) 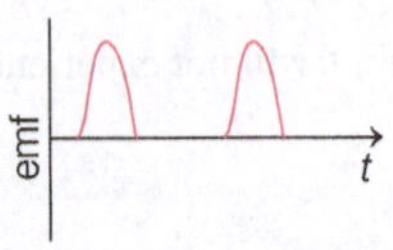

(d) 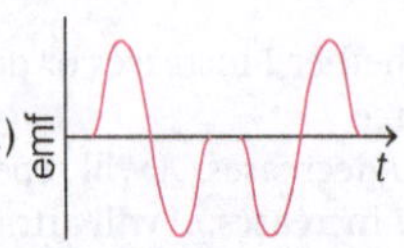

37 The self-inductance of a coil having 500 turns is 50 mH. The magnetic flux through the cross-sectional area of the coil while current through it is 8 mA is found to be
(a) 4×10^{-4} Wb (b) 0.04 Wb
(c) 4 μWb (d) 40 mWb

38 A rectangular copper coil is placed in a uniform magnetic field of induction 40 mT with its plane perpendicular to the field. The area of the coil is shrinking at a constant rate of 0.5 m^2s^{-1}. The emf induced in the coil is
(a) 10 mV (b) 20 mV (c) 80 mV (d) 40 mV

39 A straight conductor 0.1 m long moves in a uniform magnetic field 0. 1 T. The velocity of the conductor is 15 ms^{-1} and is directed perpendicular to the field. The emf induced between the two ends of the conductor is
(a) 0.10 V (b) 0.15 V (c) 1.50 V (d) 15 V

40 The current i in a coil varies with time as shown in the figure. The variation of induced emf with time would be

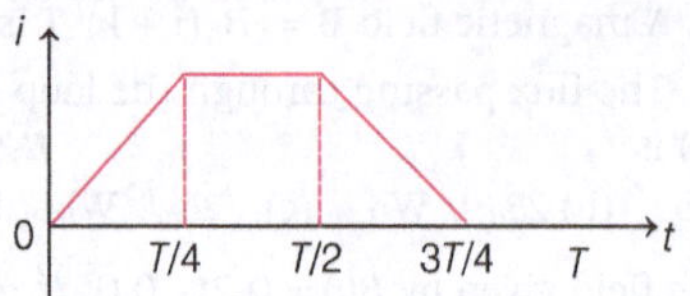

(a) 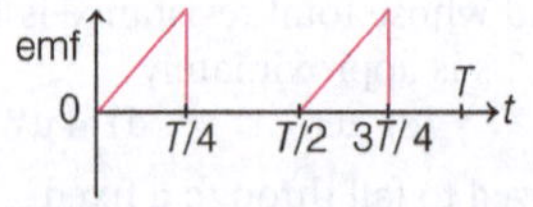

(b) 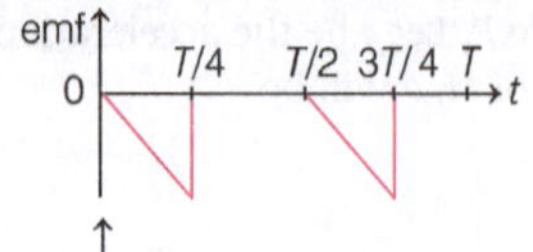

(c) 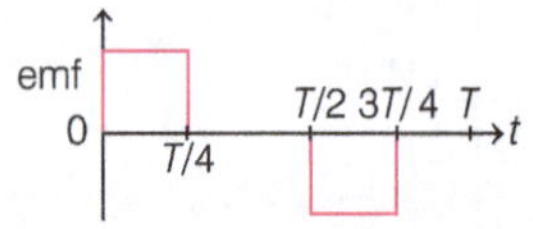

(d) 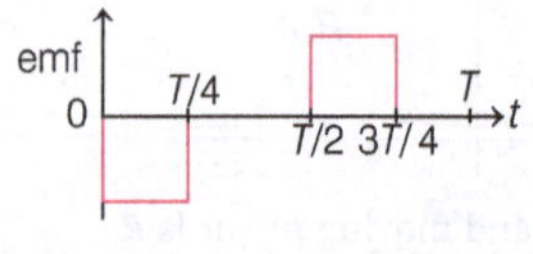

41 A wire of length 1m is moving at a speed of 2 ms^{-1} perpendicular to its length in a homogeneous magnetic field of 0.5T. If the ends of the wire are joined to a circuit of resistance 6 Ω, then the rate at which work is being done to keep the wire moving at constant speed is
(a) 1 W (b) $\frac{1}{3}$ W
(c) $\frac{1}{6}$ W (d) $\frac{1}{12}$ W

42 The number of turns in the coil of an AC generator is 5000 and the area of the coil is 0.25 m^2. The coil is rotated at the rate of 100 cycles/s in a magnetic field of 0.2 Wm^{-2}. The peak value of the emf generated is nearly
(a) 786 kV (b) 440 kV
(c) 220 kV (d) 157 kV

43 An electric potential difference will be induced between ends of the conductor as shown in the diagram, when the conductor moves in the direction

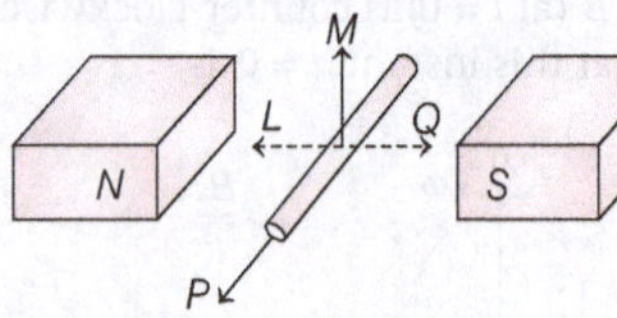

(a) P (b) Q (c) L (d) M

44 A long horizontal metallic rod with length along the east-west direction is falling under gravity. The potential difference between its two ends will
(a) be zero (b) be constant
(c) increase with time (d) decrease with time

45 A square loop of side l, resistance R is placed in a uniform magnetic field B acting normally to the plane of the loop. If we attempt to pull it out of the field with a constant velocity v, then the power needed is

(a) $BRlv$ (b) $\frac{B^2l^2v^2}{R}$ (c) $\frac{Bl^2v^2}{R}$ (d) $\frac{Bvl}{R}$

46 A rectangular coil is placed in a region having a uniform magnetic field B perpendicular to the plane of the coil. An emf will not be induced in the coil, if the

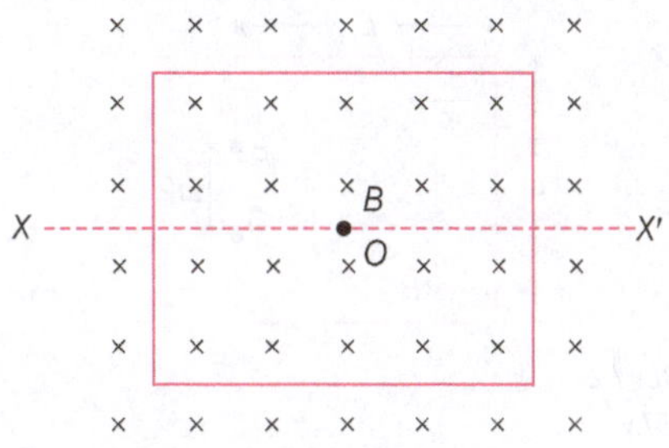

(a) magnetic field is increased uniformly
(b) magnetic field is switched OFF
(c) coil is rotated about an axis XX'
(d) coil is rotated about an axis perpendicular to the plane of the coil and passing through its centre O

47 The current carrying wire and the rod AB are in the same plane. The rod moves parallel to the wire with a velocity v. Which one of the following statements is true about induced emf in the rod?

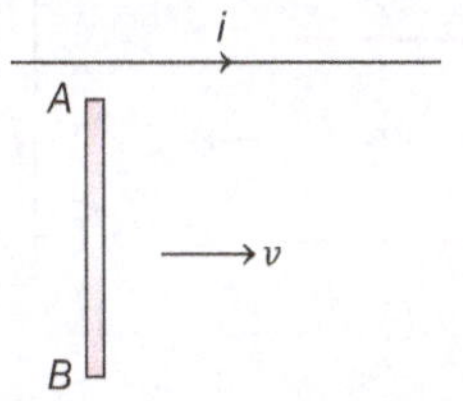

(a) End A will be at lower potential with respect to B.
(b) A and B will be at the same potential.
(c) There will be no induced emf in the rod.
(d) Potential at A will be higher than that at B.

48 A rectangular, a square, a circular and an elliptical loop, all in the XY-plane, are moving out of a uniform magnetic field with a constant velocity $\mathbf{v} = u\hat{\mathbf{i}}$. The magnetic field is directed along the negative Z-axis direction. The induced emf during the passage of these loops, out of the field region, will not remain constant for

(a) the rectangular, circular and elliptical loops
(b) the circular and the elliptical loops
(c) only the elliptical loop
(d) any of the four loops

49 A coil is suspended in a uniform magnetic field, with the plane of the coil parallel to the magnetic lines of force. When a current is passed through the coil it starts oscillating, then it is very difficult to stop. But, if an aluminium plate is placed near to the coil, then it stops. This is due to

(a) development of air current when the plate is placed
(b) induction of electrical charge on the plate
(c) shielding of magnetic lines of force as aluminium is a paramagnetic material
(d) electromagnetic induction in the aluminium plate give rise to electromagnetic damping

50 An aeroplane in which the distance between the tips of the wings is 50 m is flying horizontally from east to west with the speed of 360 kmh^{-1} over a place where the vertical component of the earth's magnetic field is 2.0×10^{-4} Wbm^{-2}. The potential difference between the tips of the wings would be

(a) 0.1 V (b) 0.01 V
(c) 0.2 V (d) 1.0 V

51 A conducting square loop of side l and resistance R is moving out of the plane with a uniform velocity v perpendicular to one of its sides. A uniform and constant magnetic field B exists along the perpendicular to the plane of the loop as shown in figure.

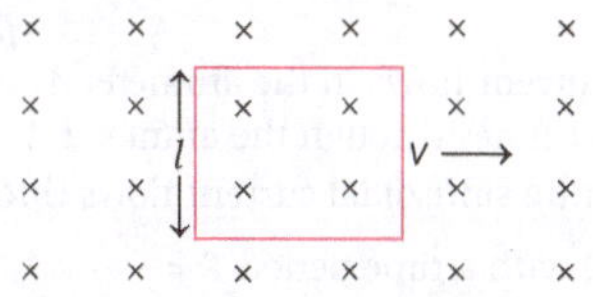

The current induced in the loop is

(a) $\frac{Blv}{R}$, clockwise (b) $\frac{Blv}{R}$, anti-clockwise
(c) $\frac{2Blv}{R}$, anti-clockwise (d) zero

52 Two rails of a railway track, insulated from each other and the ground, are connected to a millivoltmetre. What is the reading of the millivoltmetre when a train travels at a speed of 20 ms^{-1} along the track? Given that, the vertical component of earth's magnetic field is 0.2×10^{-4} Wb m^{-2} and the rails are separated by 1 m.

(a) 4 mV (b) 0.4 mV
(c) 80 mV (d) 10 mV

53 One conducting U-tube can slide inside another as shown in figure, maintaining electrical contacts between the tubes. The magnetic field B is perpendicular to the plane of the figure. If each tube moves towards the other at a constant speed v, then the emf induced in the circuit in terms of B, l and v, where l is the width of each tube, will be

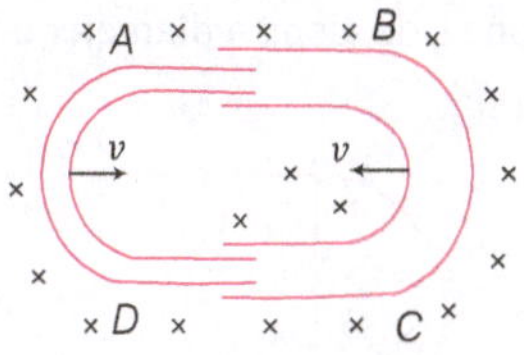

(a) zero (b) $2Blv$
(c) Blv (d) $-Blv$

54 A rectangular loop with a sliding connector of length 10 cm is situated in uniform magnetic field perpendicular to plane of loop. The magnetic induction is 0.1 T and resistance of connector (R) is 1Ω. The sides AB and CD have resistances 2Ω and $3\ \Omega$, respectively. Find the current in the connector during its motion with constant velocity $1\ ms^{-1}$.

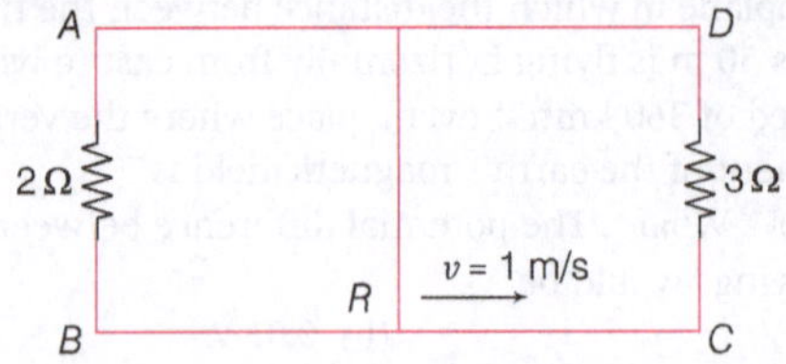

(a) $\frac{1}{242}$ A (b) $\frac{1}{220}$ A
(c) $\frac{1}{55}$ A (d) $\frac{1}{440}$ A

55 A cylindrical bar magnet is rotated about its axis. A wire is connected from the axis and is made to touch the cylindrical surface through a ammeter A, then **[NCERT Exemplar]**

(a) a direct current flows in the ammeter A
(b) no current flows through the ammeter A
(c) an alternating sinusoidal current flows through the ammeter A with a time period $T = \frac{2\pi}{\omega}$
(d) a time varying non-sinusoidal current flows through the ammeter A

56 The figure shows certain wire segments joined together to form a coplanar loop. The loop is placed in a perpendicular magnetic field in the direction going into the plane of the figure. The magnitude of the field increases with time, I_1 and I_2 are the currents in the segments ab and cd. Then,

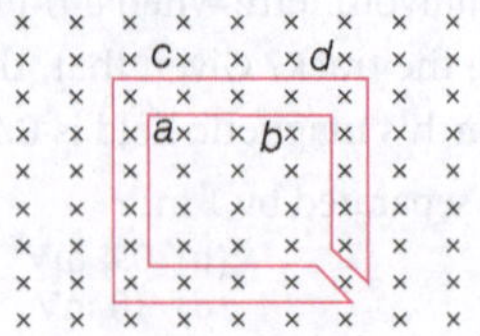

(a) $I_1 > I_2$
(b) $I_1 < I_2$
(c) I_1 is in the direction ba and I_2 is in the direction cd
(d) I_1 is in the direction ab and I_2 is in the direction dc

57 A uniform magnetic field B exists in a cylindrical region of radius 10 cm as shown in figure. A uniform wire of length 80 cm and resistance $4.0\,\Omega$ is bent into a square frame and is placed with one side along a diameter of the cylindrical region.

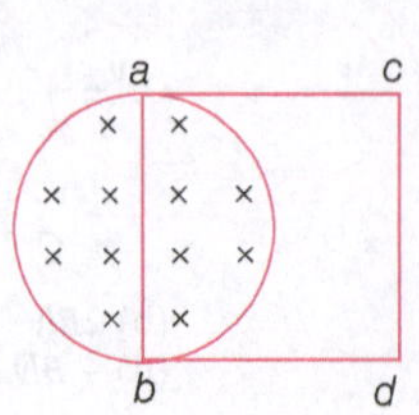

If the magnetic field increases at a constant rate of 0.01 T/s, then the current induced in the frame

(a) 3.9×10^{-5} A (b) 4.0×10^{5} A
(c) 4.1×10^{-5} A (d) 3.9×10^{-4} A

58 The loop shown moves with a velocity v in a uniform magnetic field of magnitude B, directed into the paper. The potential difference between P and Q is e.

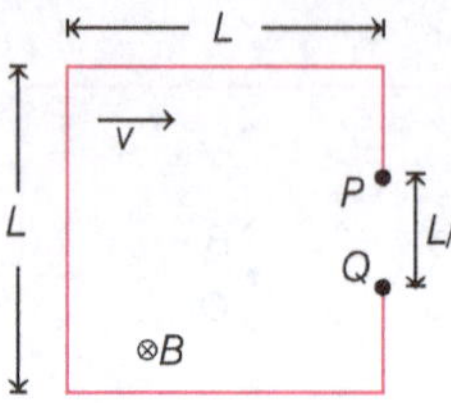

(i) $e = BLv/2$
(ii) $e = BLv$
(iii) P is positive with respect to Q
(iv) Q is positive with respect to P

(a) (ii), (iii) (b) (i), (iv)
(c) (i), (iii) (d) (ii), (iv)

59 A conducting loop being pulled out of magnetic field with a speed v. Which of the following plots may represent the power delivered by the pulling agent as a function of the speed v?

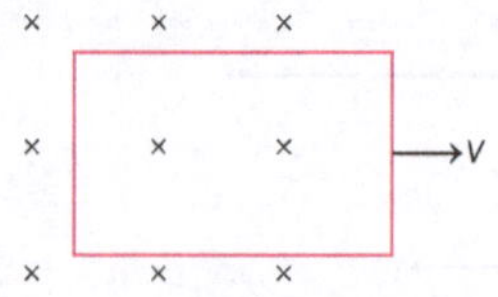

(i)

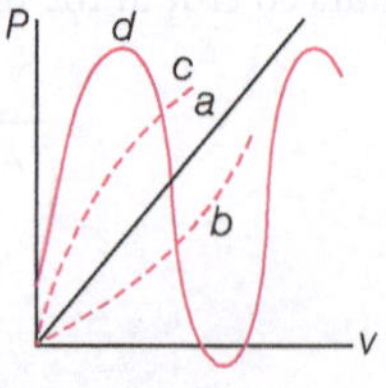

(ii)

(a) a (b) b (c) c (d) d

60 A rectangular loop has a sliding connector PQ of length l and resistance $R\,\Omega$ and it is moving with a speed v as shown. The set up is placed in a uniform magnetic field going into the plane of the paper. The three currents I_1, I_2 and I are

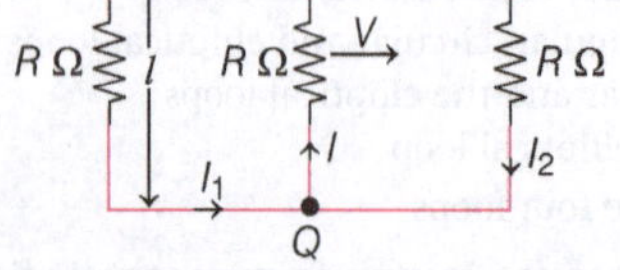

(a) $I_1 = I_2 = \frac{Blv}{6R}, I = \frac{Blv}{3R}$ (b) $I_1 = -I_2 = \frac{Blv}{R}, I = \frac{2Blv}{R}$
(c) $I_1 = I_2 = \frac{Blv}{3R}, I = \frac{2Blv}{3R}$ (d) $I_1 = I_2 = I = \frac{Blv}{R}$

61 The loop $ABCD$ is moving with velocity v towards right. The magnetic field is 4 T. The loop is connected to a resistance of 8 Ω. If steady current of 2 A flows in the loop, then value of v, if loop has resistance of 4 Ω, is (Given, $AB = 30$ cm, $AD = 30$ cm, $\sin 37° = \frac{3}{5}$)

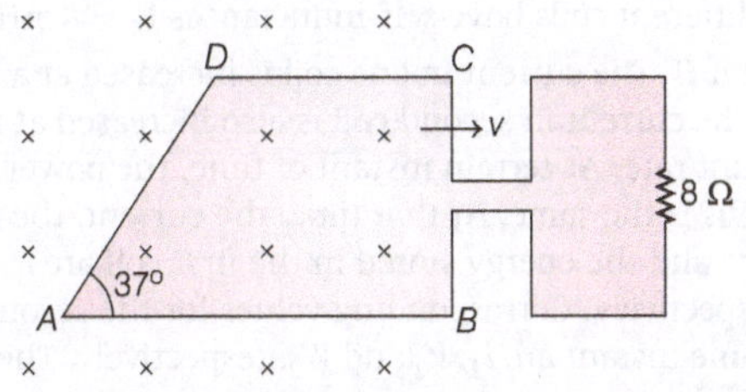

(a) $\frac{50}{3}$ ms^{-1} (b) 20 ms^{-1} (c) 10 ms^{-1} (d) $\frac{100}{3}$ ms^{-1}

62 A uniform but time varying magnetic field is present in a circular region of radius R. The magnetic field is perpendicular and into the plane of the loop and the magnitude of field is increasing at a constant rate α. There is a straight conducting rod of length $2R$ placed as shown in figure.

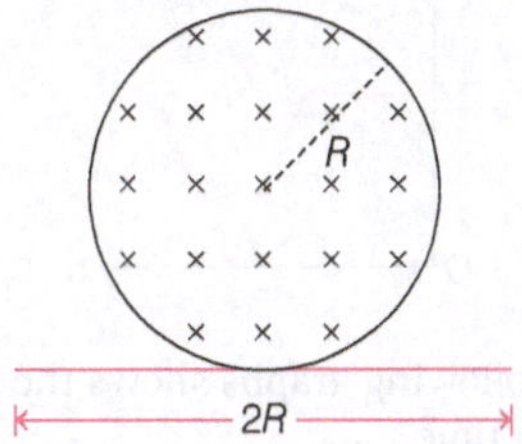

The magnitude of induced emf across the rod is

(a) $\pi R^2 \alpha$ (b) $\frac{\pi R^2 \alpha}{2}$

(c) $\frac{R^2 \alpha}{\sqrt{2}}$ (d) $\frac{\pi R^2 \alpha}{4}$

63 A conducting rod PQ of length, $L = 1.0$ m is moving with a uniform speed, $v = 2$ ms^{-1} in a uniform magnetic field, $B = 4.0$ T directed into the paper. A capacitor of capacity, $C = 10\,\mu$F is connected as shown in figure.

Then,

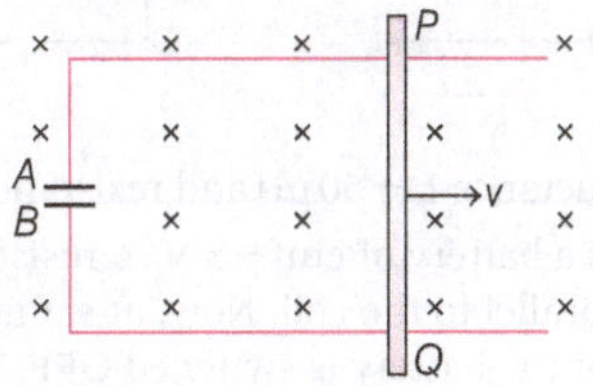

(a) $q_A = +80\,\mu$C and $q_B = -80\,\mu$C

(b) $q_A = -80\,\mu$C and $q_B = +80\,\mu$C

(c) $q_A = 0 = q_B$

(d) charge stored in the capacitor increases exponentially with time

64 A conducting rod AC of length $4l$ is rotated about a point O in a uniform magnetic field **B** directed into the paper. If $AO = l$ and $OC = 3l$, then

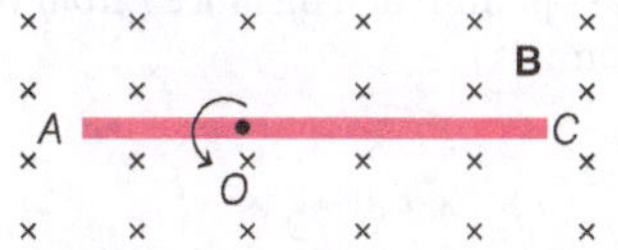

(a) $V_A - V_O = \frac{B\omega l^2}{2}$

(b) $V_O - V_C = \frac{7}{2} B\omega l^2$

(c) $V_A - V_C = 4B\omega l^2$

(d) $V_C - V_O = \frac{9}{2} B\omega l^2$

65 A rectangular coil $ABCD$ which is rotated at a constant angular velocity about an horizontal as shown in the figure. The axis of rotation of the coil as well as the magnetic field B are horizontal. Maximum current will flow in the circuit when the plane of the coil is

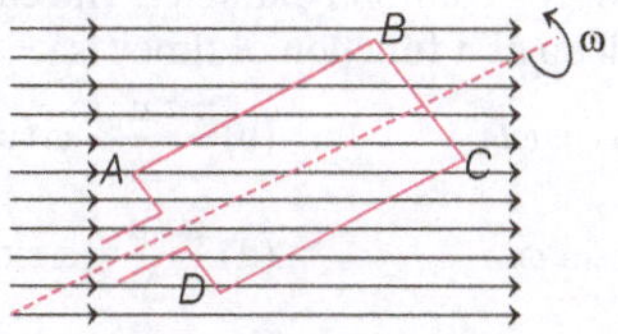

(a) inclined at 30° to the magnetic field

(b) perpendicular to the magnetic field

(c) inclined at 45° to the magnetic field

(d) parallel to the magnetic field

66 A metallic ring is dropped down, keeping its plane perpendicular to a constant and horizontal magnetic field. The ring enters the region of magnetic field at $t = 0$ and completely emerges out at $t = T$ second. The current in the ring varies as

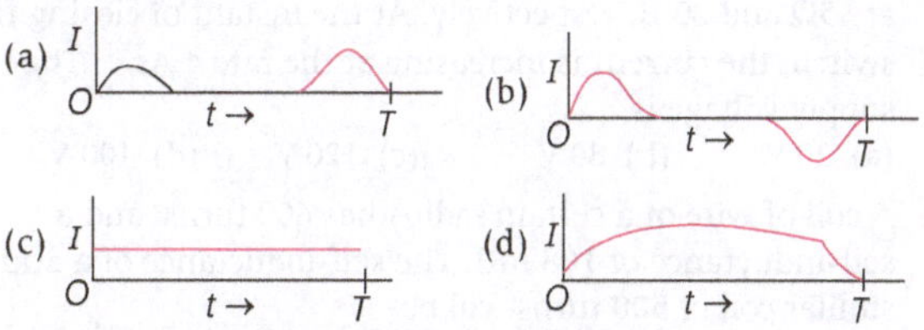

67 A circular coil of one turn of radius 5.0 cm is rotated about a diameter with a constant angular speed of 80 revolutions per minute. A uniform magnetic field $B = 0.01$ T exists in a direction perpendicular to the axis of rotation, the maximum emf induced, the average emf induced in the coil over a long period and the average of the squares of emf induced over a long period is

(a) 6.4×10^{-4} V, zero, 2.2×10^{-7} V^2

(b) 6.6×10^{-4} V, zero, 2.0×10^{-7} V^2

(c) 6.8×10^{-4} V, zero, 2.5×10^{-7} V^2

(d) 6.4×10^{-4} V, zero, 2.0×10^{-6} V^2

68 A uniform but time-varying magnetic field $B(t)$ exists in a cylindrical region of radius a and is directed into the plane of the paper as shown in figure. The magnitude of the induced electric field at point P at a distance r from the centre of the circular region

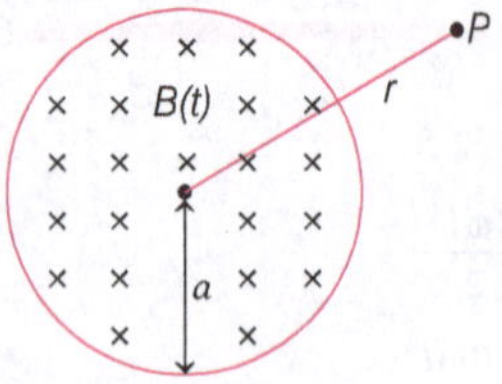

(a) is zero (b) decreases as $\frac{1}{r}$

(c) increases as r (d) decreases as $\frac{1}{r^2}$

69 A very small circular loop of radius a is initially (at $t = 0$) coplanar and concentric with a much larger fixed circular loop of radius b. A constant current I flows in the larger loop. The smaller loop is rotated with a constant angular speed ω about the common diameter. The emf induced in the smaller loop as a function of time t is

(a) $\frac{\pi a^2 \mu_0 I}{2b} \omega \cos \omega t$ (b) $\frac{\pi a^2 \mu_0 I}{2b} \omega \sin \omega^2 t^2$

(c) $\frac{\pi a^2 \mu_0 I}{2b} \omega \sin \omega t$ (d) $\frac{\pi a^2 \mu_0 I}{2b} \omega \sin^2 \omega t$

70 In the figure, magnetic energy stored in the coil is

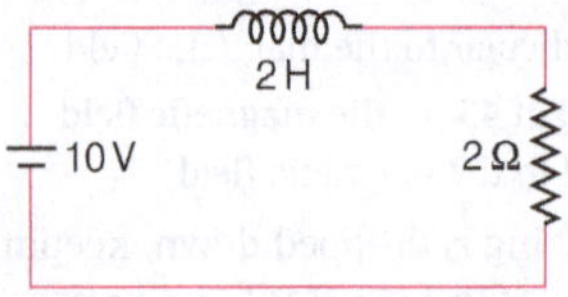

(a) zero (b) infinite
(c) 25 J (d) None of these

71 The resistance and inductance of series circuit are 5Ω and 20 H, respectively. At the instant of closing the switch, the current is increasing at the rate 4 As^{-1}. The supply voltage is

(a) 20 V (b) 80 V (c) 120 V (d) 100 V

72 A coil of wire of a certain radius has 600 turns and a self-inductance of 108 mH. The self-inductance of a 2nd similar coil of 500 turns will be

(a) 74 mH (b) 75 mH (c) 76 mH (d) 77 mH

73 Two circular coils can be arranged in any of the three situations shown in the figure. Their mutual inductance will be

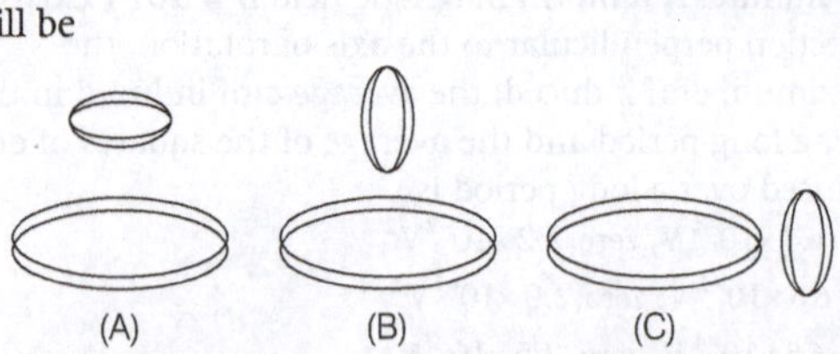

(a) maximum in situation (A) (b) maximum in situation (B)
(c) maximum in situation (C) (d) the same in all situations

74 Two conducting circular loops of radii R_1 and R_2 are placed in the same plane with their centres coinciding. If then $R_1 >> R_2$, then the mutual inductance M between them will be directly proportional to

(a) R_1 / R_2 (b) R_2 / R_1
(c) R_1^2 / R_2 (d) R_2^2 / R_1

75 Two different coils have self-inductances $L_1 = 8$ mH and $L_2 = 2$ mH. The current in one coil is increased at a constant rate. The current in second coil is also increased at the same constant rate. At certain instant of time, the power given to the coils is the same. At that time, the current, the induced voltage and the energy stored in the first coil are i_1, V_1 and W_1 respectively. Corresponding values for the second coil at the same instant are i_2, V_2 and W_2, respectively. Then, choose the wrong option.

(a) $\frac{i_1}{i_2} = \frac{1}{4}$ (b) $\frac{i_1}{i_2} = 4$

(c) $\frac{W_1}{W_2} = \frac{1}{4}$ (d) $\frac{V_2}{V_1} = \frac{1}{4}$

76 The current i in an induction coil varies with time t according to the graph shown in figure.

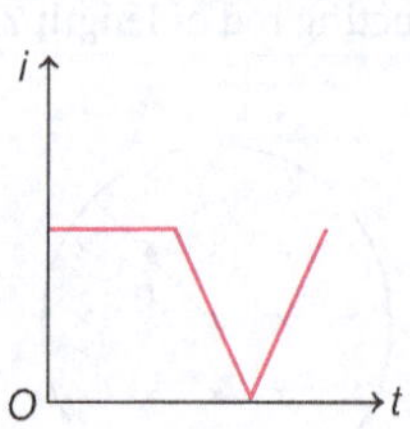

Which of the following graphs shows the induced emf (E) in the coil with time?

(a)
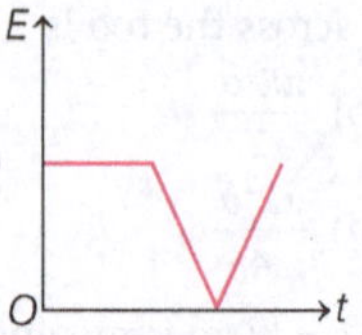

(b)
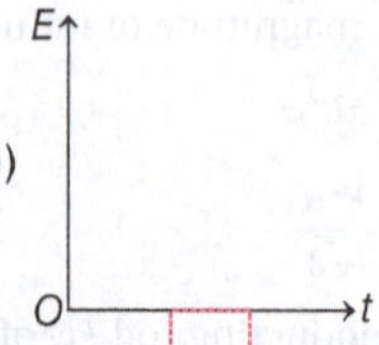

(c)
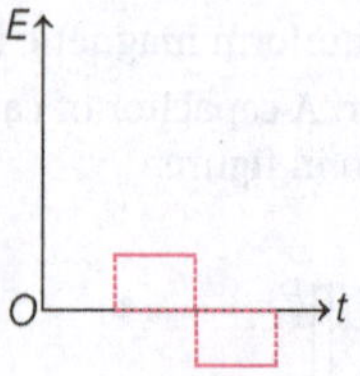

(d)
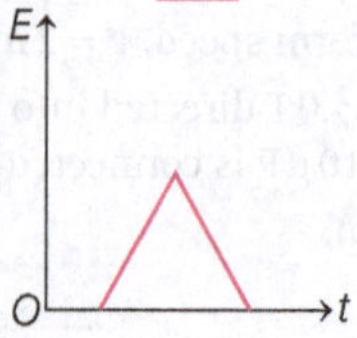

77 A coil of inductance $L = 50\,\mu$H and resistance $= 0.5\,\Omega$ is connected to a battery of emf = 5 V. A resistance of $10\,\Omega$ is connected parallel to the coil. Now, at same instant the connection of the battery is switched OFF. Then, the amount of heat generated in the coil after switching OFF the battery is

(a) 1.25 mJ
(b) 2.5 mJ
(c) 0.65 mJ
(d) 0.12 mJ

78 In the circuit shown, the coil has inductance and resistance. When X is joined to Y, the time constant is τ during growth of current. When the steady state is reached, then heat is produced in the coil at a rate P. If X is now joined to Z, then choose the correct statement.

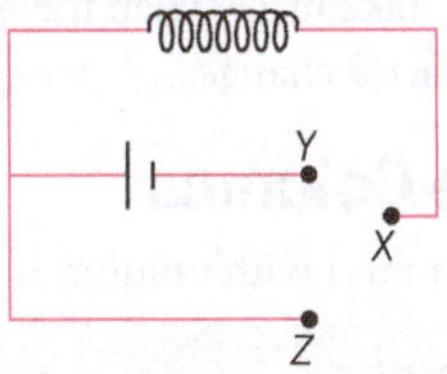

(a) The total heat produced in the coil is $P\tau$.

(b) The total heat produced in the coil is $\frac{1}{2}P\tau$.

(c) The total heat produced in the coil is $2P\tau$.

(d) The data given is not sufficient to reach a conclusion.

79 Three solenoid coils of same dimension, same number of turns and same number of layers of windings are taken. Coil 1 with inductance L_1 was wound using a wire of resistance $11\,\Omega/\text{m}$, coil 2 with inductance L_2 was wound using the similar wire but the direction of winding was reversed in each layer, coil 3 with inductance L_3 was wound using a superconducting wire. The self-inductance of the coils L_1, L_2 and L_3 are

(a) $L_1 = L_2 = L_3$

(b) $L_1 = L_2, L_3 = 0$

(c) $L_1 = L_3, L_2 = 0$

(d) $L_1 > L_2 > L_3$

80 A system S consists of two coils A and B. The coil A carries a steady current I while the coil B is suspended nearby as shown in figure. Now, if the system is heated, so as to raise the temperature of two coils steadily, then

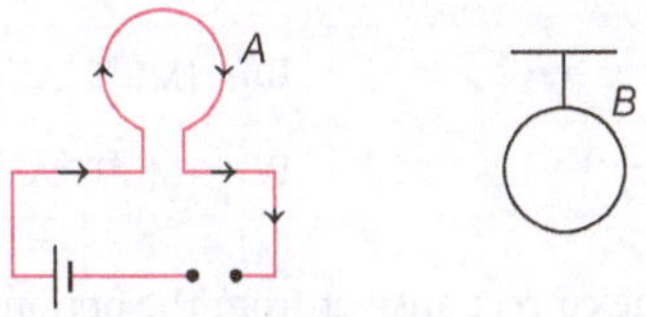

(a) the two coils shows attraction

(b) the two coils shows repulsion

(c) there is no change in the position of the two coils

(d) induced current are not possible in coil B

81 The current I in the inductance is varying with time according to the plot shown in figure.

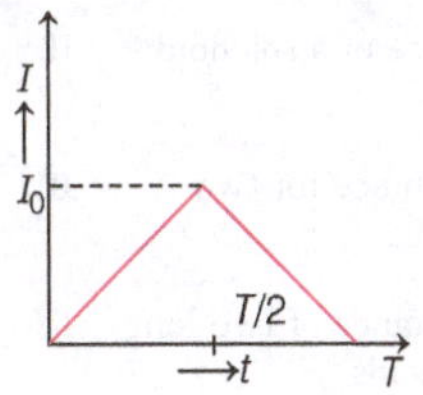

Which one of the following is the correct variation of voltage with time in the coil?

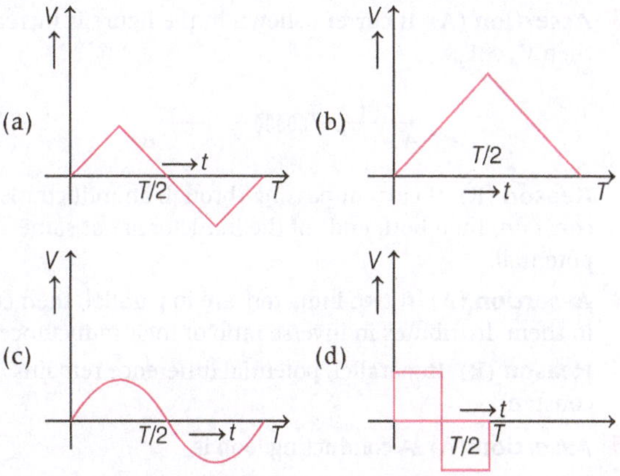

82 If emf induced in a coil is 2 V by changing the current in it from 8 A to 6 A in 2×10^{-3} s, then the coefficient of self-induction is

(a) 2×10^{-3} H (b) 10^{-3} H

(c) 0.5×10^{-3} H (d) 4×10^{-3} H

Assertion and Reason

Directions (Q. Nos. 1-5) *These questions consists of two statements each printed as Assertion and Reason. While answering these questions you are required to choose anyone of the following four responses.*

(a) Both A and R are true but R is not the correct explanation of A.

(b) A is true but R is false.

(c) A is false but R is true.

(d) Both A and R are true and R is the correct explanation of A.

1. Assertion (A) Coefficient of self-induction of an inductor depends upon the rate of change of current passing through it.

Reason (R) From, $e = -L\dfrac{di}{dt}$

We can see that, $L = \dfrac{-e}{(di/dt)}$

or $L \propto \dfrac{1}{(di/dt)}$

2. Assertion (A) In the figure, just after closing the switch, the potential drop across inductor is maximum.

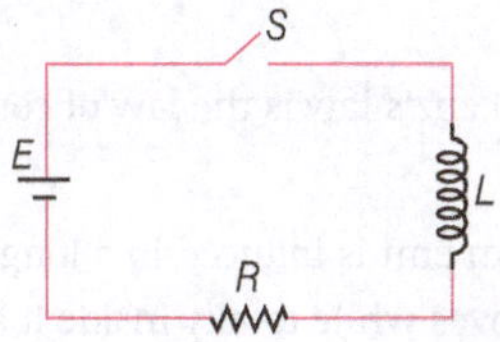

Reason (R) The rate of change of current just after closing the switch is maximum.

3. **Assertion** (A) If current shown in the figure is increasing, then $V_A > V_B$.

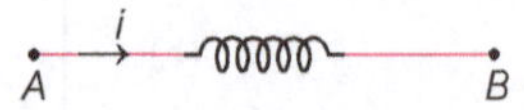

Reason (R) If current passing through an inductor is constant, then both ends of the inductor are at same potential.

4. **Assertion** (A) If two inductors are in parallel, then current in them distributes in inverse ratio of their inductance.

Reason (R) In parallel, potential difference remains constant.

5. **Assertion** (A) A conducting loop is rotated in a uniform magnetic field with constant angular velocity ω as shown in figure. At time $t = 0$, plane of the loop is perpendicular to the magnetic field. Induced emf produced in the loop is maximum when plane of loop is parallel to magnetic field.

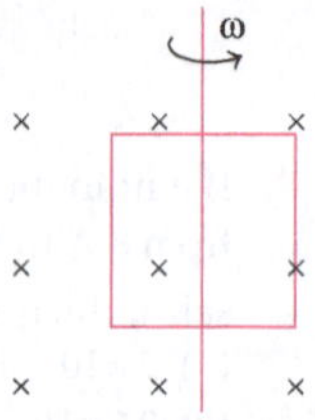

Reason (R) When plane of loop is parallel to magnetic field, then magnetic flux passing through the loop is zero.

Statement Type Questions

Directions (Q. Nos. 1-5) *These questions consist of two statements, choose the most appropriate answer from the options given below.*

(a) Both Statement I and Statement II are incorrect.
(b) Statement I is correct but Statement II is incorrect.
(c) Statement I is incorrect but Statement II is correct.
(d) Both Statement I and Statement II are correct.

1. **Statement I** An electrical motor converts mechanical energy into electrical energy.

Statement II An electrical motor works an the principle of mutual induction.

2. **Statement I** An emf is induced in a closed loop where magnetic flux is varied. The induced electric field in it, is not a conservative field.

Statement II The line integral around the closed loop is non-zero.

3. **Statement I** Lenz's law gives the direction of induced current in a coil in the phenomenon of electromagnetic induction.

Statement II Lenz's law is the law of conservation of energy.

4 **Statement I** An emf is induced in a long solenoid by a bar magnet that moves while totally inside it along the solenoid axis.

Statement II As the magnet moves inside the solenoid the flux through individual turns of the solenoid changes.

5 **Statement I** Emf is induced in a loop when it enters in a transverse magnetic field or comes out of the transverse magnetic field.

Statement II The phenomenon of electromagnetic induction only take place when the magnetic flux linked with the conductor changes.

Match the Columns

1. Match the Column I with Column II.

Column I	Column II
A. Faraday's law	I. Direction of force on current carrying conductor in magnetic field.
B. Lenz's law	II. Obeys principle of energy conservation.
C. Fleming's right hand rule	III. Direction of induced current.
D. Fleming's left hand rule	IV. EMI

Choose the correct answer from the options given below.

(a) A-IV, B-II, C-III, D-I
(b) A-I, B-II, C-III, D-IV
(c) A-IV, B-III, C-II, D-I
(d) A-II, B-III, C-I, D-IV

2. Match the Column I with Column II.

Column I	Column II
A. Tesla	I. $[ML^2T^{-2}A^{-2}]$
B. Weber	II. $[MT^{-2}A^{-1}]$
C. Volt	III. $[ML^2T^3A^{-1}]$
D. Henry	IV. $[ML^2T^{-2}A^{-1}]$

Choose the correct answer from the options given below.

(a) A-III, B-II, C-I, D-IV
(b) A-IV, B-III, C-II, D-I
(c) A-I, B-IV, C-II, D-III
(d) A-II, B-IV, C-III, D-I

3. Match the Column I with Column II.

Column I	Column II
A. Self inductance of a coil	I. $\frac{\mu_0 N_1 N_2 \times S}{l}$
B. Self-inductance of a solenoid	II. $\frac{\mu_0 N_1 N_2 \pi r^2}{2R}$
C. Mutual inductance for two concentric coils	III. $\frac{\mu_0 N^2 \pi r}{2}$
D. Mutual inductance of two long co-axial solenoids	IV. $\frac{\mu_0 N^2 S}{l}$

(a) A-III, B-IV, C-II, D-I
(b) A-III, B-I, C-IV, D-II
(c) A-II, B-III, C-IV, D-I
(d) A-IV, B-I, C-III, D-II

4. A square loop $ABCD$ whose area 20 cm^2 and resistance 5 Ω is rotated in a uniform field of $2T$ through 180° about an axis in plane of loop and passing through its centre.

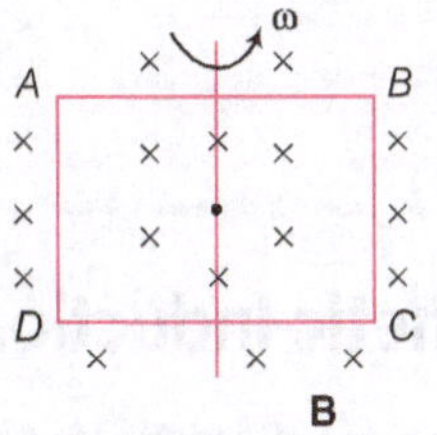

Match the Column I with Column II.

Column I	Column II
A. Current (in A) in loop at $t = 0.01$ s	I. 1.6
B. Current (in A) in loop at $t = 0.03$ s	II. 1.56
C. Magnitude of free charge (in mC) at= 0.01s	III. 0.052
D. Magnitude of free charge (in mC) at $t = 0.03$s	IV. 0.16

Choose the correct answer from the options given below.

(a) A-I, B-IV, C-III, D-II
(b) A-IV, B-III, C-I, D-II
(c) A-II, B-I, C-IV, D-III
(d) A-III, B-II, C-I, D-IV

5. Match the columns I and with Column II and mark the correct option from the codes given below.

Column I (Planar loops of different shapes)	Column II (Direction of Induced Current)
A. 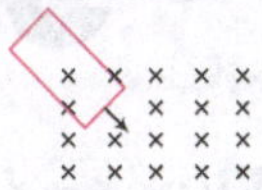	I. $bacb$
B. 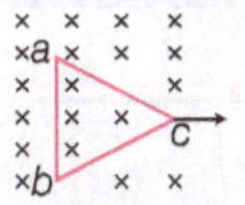	II. $cdabc$
C. 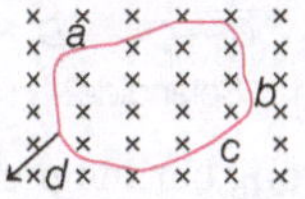	III. $bcdab$
D. 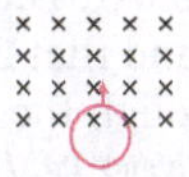	IV. Anti-clockwise

Choose the correct answer from the options given below.

(a) A-III, B-I, C-II, D-IV
(b) A-II, B-IIII, C-I, D-IV
(c) A-I, B-II, C-III, D-IV
(d) A-II, B-I, C-III, D-IV

Final Check Through PYQs

Module-I Magnetic Flux and Laws of Electromagnetic Induction

1. 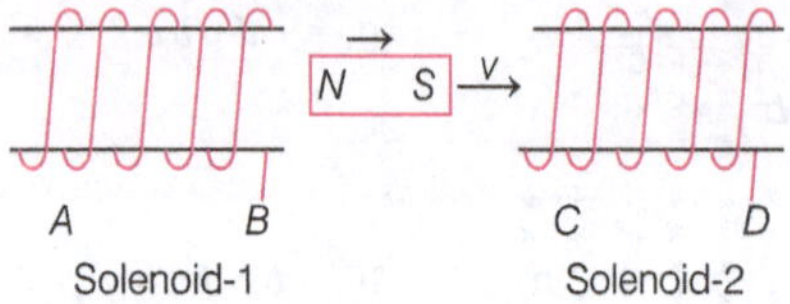

In the above figure, a strong bar magnet is moving towards solenoid-2 from solenoid-1. The direction of induced current in solenoid-1 and that in solenoid-2, respectively are through the directions

[NCERT (New) Pg. 160, NEET 2024]

(a) *AB* and *DC*
(b) *BA* and *CD*
(c) *AB* and *CD*
(d) *BA* and *DC*

2. A square loop of side 1 m and resistance 1 Ω placed in a magnetic field of 0.5 T. If the plane of loop is perpendicular to the direction of magnetic field, the magnetic flux through the loop is

[NCERT (New) Pg. 157, NEET 2022]

(a) 0.5 Wb
(b) 1 Wb
(c) zero Wb
(d) 2 Wb

3. A big circular coil of 1000 turns and average radius 10 m is rotating about its horizontal diameter at 2 rad s^{-1}. If the vertical component of earth's magnetic field at that place is 2×10^{-5} T and electrical resistance of the coil is 12.56 Ω, then the maximum induced current in the coil will be

[NCERT (New) Pg. 158, NEET 2022]

(a) 0.25 A
(b) 1.5 A
(c) 1 A
(d) 2 A

4. The magnetic flux linked with a coil (in Wb) is given by the equation $\phi = 5t^2 + 3t + 16$

The magnitude of induced emf in the coil at the fourth second will be **[NCERT (New) Pg. 158, NEET (Oct.) 2020]**

(a) 33 V (b) 43 V
(c) 108 V (d) 10 V

5. A coil of 800 turns effective area 0.05 m^2 is kept perpendicular to a magnetic field 5×10^{-5} T. When the plane of the coil is rotated by 90° around any of its co-planar axis in 0.1 s, the emf induced in the coil will be **[NCERT (New) Pg. 158, NEET (National) 2019]**

(a) 0.2 V (b) 2×10^{-3} V (c) 0.02 V (d) 2 V

6. A uniform magnetic field is restricted within a region of radius *r*. The magnetic field changes with time at a rate $\frac{d\mathbf{B}}{dt}$. Loop 1 of radius $R > r$ encloses the region *r* and loop 2 of radius *R* is outside the region of magnetic field as shown in the figure. Then, the emf generated is

[NCERT (New) Pg. 158, NEET 2016]

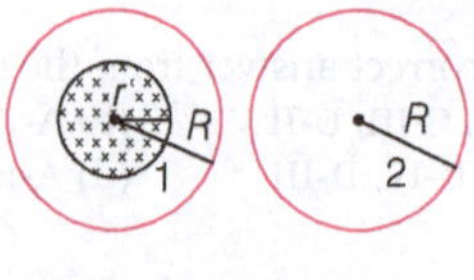

(a) zero in loop 1 and zero in loop 2
(b) $-\frac{d\mathbf{B}}{dt}\pi r^2$ in loop 1 and $-\frac{d\mathbf{B}}{dt}\pi r^2$ in loop 2
(c) $-\frac{d\mathbf{B}}{dt}\pi R^2$ in loop 1 and zero in loop 2
(d) $-\frac{d\mathbf{B}}{dt}\pi r^2$ in loop 1 and zero in loop 2

7. An electron moves on a straight line path *XY* as shown. The *abcd* is a coil adjacent in the path of electron. What will be the direction of current, if any induced in the coil? **[NCERT (New) Pg. 160, AIPMT 2015]**

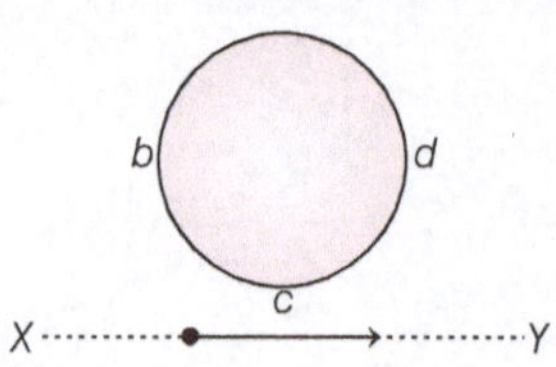

(a) *abcd* (b) *adcb*
(c) The current will reverse its direction as the electron goes past the coil
(d) No current induced

Module-II Motional Electromotive Force and Eddy Current

8. A sheet is placed in a horizontal surface in front of a strong magnetic pole. A force is needed to

A. hold the sheet there, if it is magnetic.

B. hold the sheet there, if it is non-magnetic.

C. move the sheet away from the pole with uniform velocity, if it is conducting.

D. move the sheet away from the pole with uniform velocity, if it is both non-conducting and non-polar.

Choose the correct statement(s) from the options given below. *[NCERT (New) Pg. 162, NEET 2024]*

(a) B and D only (b) A and C only
(c) A, C and D only (d) C only

9. A wheel with 20 metallic spokes each 1 m long is rotated with a speed of 120 rpm in a plane perpendicular to a magnetic field of 0.4 G. The induced emf between the axle and rim of the wheel will be ($1\ G = 10^{-4}\ T$) *[NCERT (New) Pg. 162, NEET (Oct.) 2020]*

(a) 2.51×10^{-4} V (b) 2.51×10^{-5} V
(c) 4.0×10^{-5} V (d) 2.51 V

10. A cycle wheel of radius 0.5 m is rotated with constant angular velocity of 10 rad/s in a region of magnetic field of 0.1 T which is perpendicular to the plane of the wheel. The emf generated between its centre and the rim is *[NCERT (New) Pg. 162, NEET (Odisha) 2019]*

(a) 0.25 V (b) 0.125 V (c) 0.5 V (d) zero

11. In which of the following devices, the eddy current effect is not used? *[NCERT (New) Pg. 160, NEET (National) 2019]*

(a) Magnetic braking in train
(b) Electromagnet
(c) Electric heater
(d) Induction furnace

Module-III Inductance

12. The magnetic energy stored in an inductor of inductance 4 μH carrying a current of 2 A is *[NCERT (New) Pg. 169, NEET 2023]*

(a) 4 mJ (b) 8 mJ (c) 8 μJ (d) 4 μJ

13. Two conducting circular loops of radii R_1 and R_2 are placed in the same plane with their centres coinciding. If $R_1 >> R_2$, the mutual inductance M between them will be directly proportional to *[NCERT (New) Pg. 167, NEET 2021]*

(a) $\frac{R_1}{R_2}$ (b) $\frac{R_2}{R_1}$ (c) $\frac{R_1^2}{R_2}$ (d) $\frac{R_2^2}{R_1}$

14. A light bulb and an inductor coil are connected to AC source through a key as shown in the figure below. The key is closed and after sometime an iron rod is inserted into the interior of the inductor. The glow of the light bulb *[NCERT (New) Pg. 167, NEET (Oct.) 2020]*

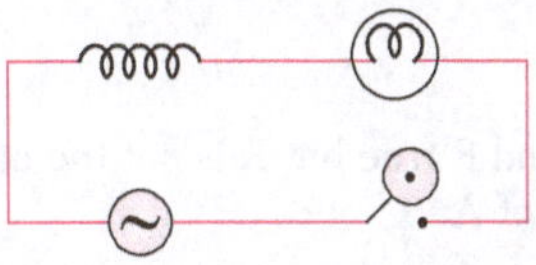

(a) decreases (b) remains unchanged
(c) will fluctuate (d) increases

15. The magnetic potential energy stored in a certain inductor is 25 mJ, when the current in the inductor is 60 mA. This inductor is of inductance *[NCERT (New) Pg. 169, NEET 2018]*

(a) 1.389 H (b) 138.88 H
(c) 0.138 H (d) 13.89 H

16. A long solenoid of diameter 0.1 m has 2×10^4 turns per metre. At the centre of the solenoid, a coil of 100 turns and radius 0.01 m is placed with its axis coinciding with the solenoid axis. The current in the solenoid reduces at a constant rate to 0 A from 4 A in 0.05 s. If the resistance of the coil is $10\pi^2\ \Omega$, the total charge flowing through the coil during this time is *[NCERT (New) Pg. 168, NEET 2017]*

(a) 32π μC (b) 16 μC
(c) 32 μC (d) 16π μC

17. A long solenoid has 1000 turns. When a current of 4A flows through it, the magnetic flux linked with each turn of the solenoid is 4×10^{-3} Wb. The self-inductance of the solenoid is *[NCERT (New) Pg. 168, NEET 2016]*

(a) 3 H (b) 2 H
(c) 1 H (d) 4 H

Answers

Step up Practice 1

1 (c)	2 (b)	3 (d)	4 (d)	5 (d)	6 (a)	7 (d)	8 (a)	9 (d)	10 (b)
11 (b)	12 (b)	13 (b)	14 (b)	15 (c)	16 (b)	17 (c)	18 (d)	19 (a)	

Step up Practice 2

1 (b)	2 (b)	3 (c)	4 (d)	5 (c)	6 (c)	7 (c)	8 (d)	9 (a)	10 (d)
11 (a)	12 (c)	13 (d)	14 (d)						

Step up Practice 3

1 (d)	2 (c)	3 (d)	4 (a)	5 (b)	6 (d)	7 (b)	8 (a)	9 (c)	10 (d)
11 (d)	12 (a)	13 (d)	14 (d)	15 (b)	16 (a)	17 (b)	18 (a)	19 (c)	20 (a)
21 (b)	22 (a)	23 (d)	24 (a)	25 (a)	26 (c)	27 (a)	28 (b)		

Gearing up for NEET

1 (b)	2 (b)	3 (b)	4 (b)	5 (a)	6 (c)	7 (d)	8 (b)	9 (a)	10 (c)
11 (a)	12 (a)	13 (d)	14 (d)	15 (a)	16 (d)	17 (c)	18 (a)	19 (c)	20 (b)
21 (d)	22 (b)	23 (d)	24 (c)	25 (b)	26 (d)	27 (a)	28 (a)	29 (a)	30 (a)
31 (d)	32 (b)	33 (d)	34 (a)	35 (d)	36 (a)	37 (a)	38 (b)	39 (b)	40 (d)
41 (c)	42 (d)	43 (d)	44 (c)	45 (b)	46 (d)	47 (d)	48 (b)	49 (d)	50 (d)
51 (a)	52 (b)	53 (b)	54 (b)	55 (b)	56 (d)	57 (a)	58 (c)	59 (b)	60 (c)
61 (d)	62 (d)	63 (a)	64 (c)	65 (d)	66 (b)	67 (b)	68 (b)	69 (c)	70 (c)
71 (b)	72 (b)	73 (a)	74 (d)	75 (b)	76 (c)	77 (d)	78 (b)	79 (a)	80 (a)
81 (d)	82 (a)								

Assertion and Reason

1 (d)	2 (d)	3 (a)	4 (d)	5 (a)

Statement Type Questions

1 (a)	2 (d)	3 (d)	4 (c)	5 (d)

Match the Columns

1 (a)	2 (d)	3 (a)	4 (b)	5 (a)

Final Check through PYQs : Module-I

1 (a)	2 (a)	3 (c)	4 (d)	5 (c)	6 (c)	7 (c)

Final Check through PYQs : Module-II

8 (b)	9 (a)	10 (b)	11 (c)

Final Check through PYQs : Module-III

12 (c)	13 (d)	14 (a)	15 (d)	16 (c)	17 (c)

Hints and Solutions

Step up Practice 1

1. (*c*) **B** · **A**

2. (*b*) Wb

3. (*d*) $[ML^2 T^{-2}A^{-1}]$

4. (*d*) Both A and R are true and R is the correct explanation of A.

   According to Faraday's law of electromagnetic induction, induced emf will be generated in the solenoid because of the relative motion between magnet and solenoid.

5. (*d*) Both Statement I and Statement II are correct.

   As the coil rotates, the magnetic flux linked with the coil (being **B** · **A**) will change and emf will be induced in the loop.

6. (*a*) Both A and R true but R is not the correct explanation of A.

   Emf induces, when there is change in magnetic flux. The magnitude of induced emf depends upon the rate at which the magnetic flux changes. When magnetic flux is steady or constant, no emf is induced. Faraday did experiment in which, there is relative motion between the coil and magnet, the flux linked with the coil changes and emf induces.

7. (*d*) Magnitude of induced emf,

$$e = -\frac{d\phi}{dt}$$

$$= -\frac{d}{dt}(3t^2 + 4t + 9) = -(6t + 4)$$

At $t = 2$ s, $e = -[6 \times (2) + 4] = -16$

$\therefore$ $|e| = 16$ V

8. (a) As, $|e| = \frac{\Delta\phi}{\Delta t} = \frac{4B_0A_0 - B_0A_0}{t} = \frac{3B_0A_0}{t}$

9. (d) Induced emf, $e = \left|\frac{d\phi}{dt}\right| = |12t - 5|$

At $t = 0.25$ s, $e = 2$ V

$\therefore$ Induced current, $i = \frac{e}{R} = 0.2$ A

10. (b) Magnetic flux, $\phi = (5t^2 - 4t + 1)$ Wb

$\therefore$ $\frac{d\phi}{dt} = (10t - 4)\,\text{Wbs}^{-1}$

Induced emf, $e = \frac{-d\phi}{dt} = -(10t - 4)$

At $t = 0.2$ s, $e = -(10 \times 0.2 - 4) = 2$ V

The induced current,

$$I = \frac{e}{R} = \frac{2\text{ V}}{10\,\Omega} = 0.2\text{ A}$$

11. (b) A is true but R is false.

12. (b) A is true but R is false.

Induced current (emf) in a coil is directly proportional to the rate of change in magnetic flux linked with the coil. If there is no change in the flux, there is no induced current also.

13. (b) As, charge,

$$\Delta Q = \frac{\Delta\phi}{R} = \frac{\phi_2 - \phi_1}{R} = \frac{(10-2)}{2} = 4\text{ C}$$

14. (b) As, charge,

$$|\Delta q| = \frac{\Delta\phi}{R} = \frac{BA}{R} = \frac{(2)\left(\frac{\pi}{4}\right)(0.2)^2}{0.01} = 6.28\text{ C}$$

15. (c) As we know that, charge flow, $\Delta q = \frac{\Delta\phi}{R}$

16. (b) Lenz's law

17. (c) According to Lenz's law, the induced current will be in such a direction, so that it opposes the change due to which it is produced. So, the induced current in the inner loop will be in counter-clockwise direction.

18. (d) According to Lenz's law, the direction of induced current is such as to attain north polarity. So, it will be anti-clockwise.

19. (a) Due to change in the shape of the loop, the magnetic flux linked with the loop increases. Hence, current is induced in the loop in such a direction that it opposes the increase in flux.

Therefore, induced current flows in the anti-clockwise direction.

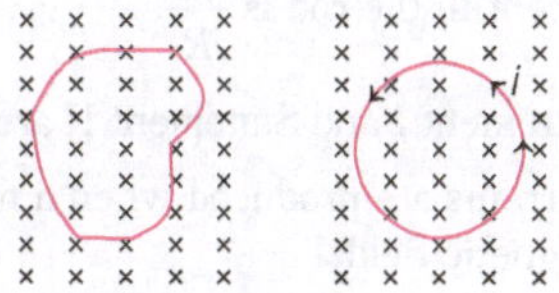

Step up Practice 2

1. (b) Induced emf $= Blv = 0.3 \times 10^{-4} \times 10 \times 5$

$= 1.5 \times 10^{-3}\text{V} = 1.5\text{ mV}$

2. (b) When a conductor lying along the magnetic north-south, then moves eastwards, it will cut vertical component of B_0.

So, induced emf, $e = vB_v\, l = lv(B_0 \sin\delta) = B_0 lv \sin\delta$.

3. (c) When a wire of length l moves with velocity v, perpendicular to a magnetic field B, then the emf is induced. The magnitude of induced emf is given by $|\varepsilon| = Blv$.

Given, $l = 50$ cm $= 0.5$ m, $v = 300$ m/min $= 5$ m/s

$$|\varepsilon| = 2\text{V or } B = \frac{|\varepsilon|}{lv} = \frac{2}{0.5 \times 5} = 0.8\text{ T}$$

4. (d) Induced emf $= B \times v \times l$

$= 5.0 \times 10^{-5} \times 1.5 \times 2$

$= 10.0 \times 10^{-5} \times 1.5$

$= 1.5 \times 10^{-4} = 0.15$ mV

5. (c) Here, $l = 0.1$m, $v = 1\text{ms}^{-1}$

$I = 50$ A and $B = 1.25$ mT $= 1.25 \times 10^{-3}$ T

We know that, induced emf, $\varepsilon = Blv$

The mechanical power,

$$P = \varepsilon I = BlvI = 1.25 \times 10^{-3} \times 0.1 \times 1 \times 50$$

$$= 6.25 \times 10^{-3}\text{W} = 6.25\text{mW}$$

6. (c) Statement I is incorrect but Statement II is correct. Since, both the loops are identical (same area and number of turns) and moving with a same speed in same magnetic field. Therefore, same emf is induced in both the coils but the induced current will be more in the copper loop as its resistance will be lesser as compared to that of the aluminium loop.

7. (c) Induced emf, when rod rotates in a vertical plane perpendicular to magnetic field is given as

$$e = \frac{1}{2}Bl^2\omega = \frac{1}{2} \times 0.3 \times 2^2 \times 100 = 60\text{ V}$$

8. (d) An electric field is induced in both AD and BC.

9. (a) The current in the rod is $\frac{Blv}{R}$.

10. (d) Both Statement I and Statement II are correct.

11. (a) Eddy currents are produced when a metal is kept in varying magnetic field.

12. (c) Eddy current always produced perpendicular to the direction of magnetic field.

13. (d) Both Statement I and Statement II are correct.

14. (d) X-ray crystallography is not an application of eddy current.

Step up Practice 3

1. (d) Here, $L = 50 \times 10^{-3}$ H

and $\frac{di}{dt} = \frac{(1-0)}{0.1} = 10$

emf, $|e| = \frac{L \cdot di}{dt} = 50 \times 10^{-3} \times 10 = 50 \times 10^{-2} = 0.5\,\text{V}$

2. (c) We have, $\frac{\Delta i}{\Delta t} = \frac{10}{2} = 5$ V

emf, $e = L\frac{\Delta i}{\Delta t} = 0.5 \times 5 = 2.5\,\text{V}$

3. (d) Both A and R are true and R is the correct explanation of A.

The inductor coils are made of copper will have very small ohmic resistance. Due to change in magnetic flux, a large induced current will be produced in such an inductance, which will effect appreciable opposition to the flow of current.

4. (a) Given, $\frac{di}{dt} = -2$ A/s and $L = 5$ H

$\therefore$ The emf developing across the coil,

$$e = -L\frac{di}{dt} = -5 \times (-2) = 10\,\text{V}$$

5. (b) Self-inductance, $L = \left|\frac{e}{di/dt}\right| = \frac{8}{(2/0.5)} = 2$ H

6. (d) Self-inductance of coil, $|e| = L\frac{di}{dt}$

$\therefore \quad 10 = L \times \frac{10}{1}$

$\therefore$ Self-inductance, $L = 1$ H

7. (b) A is true but R is false.

In a dynamo, a coil is rotated with a fixed frequency in a given magnetic field. As a result of this, magnetic flux linked with the coil changes continuously with respect to time at a constant rate and therefore induced is based on the principle of electromagnetic induction. The self induction of a coil is a proportionality constant and is not equal to the magnetic flux, it is given by I.

8. (a) We have, $N\phi_B = Li$

Self-inductance, $L = \frac{N\phi_B}{i} = \frac{500 \times 4 \times 10^{-3}}{2} = 1\,\text{H}$

9. (c) A is false but R is true.

The current in R-L circuit grows exponentially $I = I_0(1 - e^{-Rt/L})$.

10. (d) The self-inductance of a long solenoid is given by

$$L = \mu_r \mu_0 n^2 lA$$

It is clear that, the self-inductance of a long solenoid does not depend upon the current flowing through it.

11. (d) Self-inductance of coil is directly proportional to square of number of turns in the coil, i.e.

$$L \propto N^2$$

$\therefore \quad \frac{L_1}{L_2} = \frac{N_1^2}{N_2^2}$

$\therefore \quad \frac{L}{L_2} = \frac{N^2}{(4N)^2}$

$\therefore \quad L_2 = 16L$

12. (a) $L \propto N^2$

So, when number of turns is doubled, then L' will become 4 times of L, i.e. $L' = 4L$ or 4 times.

13. (d) Induced emf,

$e = L\frac{di}{dt} = \frac{\mu_0 N^2 S}{l}\frac{di}{dt}$

$= \frac{4\pi \times 10^{-7} \times (2000)^2 \times 1.2 \times 10^{-3}}{0.30} \times \left(\frac{2-(-2)}{0.25}\right)$

$= 32.1 \times 10^{-2}$ V

14. (d) Both A and R are true and R is the correct explanation of A.

The coefficient of self-inductance of the coil is given by $L = \frac{\mu_0 N^2 A}{l}$

where, N is number of turns, l is length of the coil and A is area of coil, so $L \propto N^2$.

15. (b) Energy stored in the coil,

$$E = \frac{1}{2}Li^2 = \frac{1}{2} \times 50 \times 10^{-3} \times 4 = 0.1\,\text{J}$$

16. (a) $E = \frac{1}{2}Li^2 = \frac{1}{2}(100 \times 10^{-3})(10)^2 = 5$ J

17. (b) $U = \frac{1}{2}Li^2$, $[L] = \left[\frac{U}{i^2}\right] = \frac{\text{joule}}{\text{ampere}^2}$

$[L] = \left[\frac{e}{di/dt}\right] = \text{ohm-second}$

$[L] = [\phi_B/i] = \text{weber/ampere}$

Hints and Solutions

$$[L] = [\phi/i] = [edt/di] = \frac{\text{volt-second}}{\text{ampere}}$$

Hence, SI unit of inductance is volt-second/ampere.

18. (*a*) Both A and R are true but R is not the correct explanation of A.
The phenomenon of self-induction is helpful in working of a choke coil because higher is the self-inductance of choke coil as compared to its resistance, less will be the dissipation of energy per cycle. The power in coil is $P_{av} = E_V I_V \cos\frac{\pi}{2}$ is zero because of which energy loss in coil is reduced.

19. (*c*) Equivalent inductance, $\frac{1}{L_{eq}} = \frac{1}{L} + \frac{1}{L}$

$\therefore$ The total inductance, $L_{eq} = \frac{L}{2}$

20. (*a*) We have, $M = \frac{\Delta\phi_2}{\Delta i_1} \Rightarrow M = \frac{0.4}{2}$

$\therefore$ Mutual inductance, $M = 0.2$ H

21. (*b*) Value of induced emf in coil,

$$e = M\frac{di}{dt} = 0.005 \times \frac{d}{dt}(i_0 \sin \omega t)$$

$$= 0.005 \times i_0\omega \cos \omega t \quad (\text{for } e_{max}, \cos\omega t = 1)$$

$\therefore e_{max} = 0.005 \times 10 \times 100\pi = 5\pi$

22. (*a*) emf, $e_2 = M\left(\frac{di}{dt}\right) = i_2 R_2$

$\therefore$ Current rate, $\frac{di_1}{dt} = \frac{i_2 R_2}{M} = \frac{(0.4)(5)}{0.5} = 4\text{As}^{-1}$

23. (*d*) Average emf, $e = M\frac{di}{dt} = 0.09 \times \frac{20}{0.006} = 300$ V

24. (*a*) As, $|e| = M\frac{di}{dt} \Rightarrow 8 \times 10^{-3} = M \times 3$

Mutual inductance, $M = 2.66$ mH

25. (*a*) We have, $M = \frac{\mu_0 N_1 N_2 S}{L}$

Here, S is area of inner solenoid. So, N_1, N_2 and S are same for both solenoids.

$\Rightarrow \quad M_{12} = M_{21}$

26. (*c*) Mutual inductance between two coils,

$$M = -\frac{e_2}{(di_1/dt)} = -\frac{e_1}{(di_2/dt)}$$

Also, $e_1 = -L_1\frac{di_1}{dt}$ and $e_2 = -L_2\frac{di_2}{dt}$

$$\therefore \quad M^2 = \frac{e_1 e_2}{\left(\frac{di_1}{dt}\right)\left(\frac{di_2}{dt}\right)} = L_1 L_2$$

$$\Rightarrow \quad M = \sqrt{L_1 L_2}$$

27. (*a*) Mutual inductance between coils is,

$$M = K\sqrt{L_1 L_2}$$

$$\Rightarrow \quad M = 1\sqrt{2 \times 10^{-3} \times 8 \times 10^{-3}} \quad (\because K = 1)$$

$$= 4 \times 10^{-3} = 4 \text{ mH}$$

28. (*b*) As, $U = \frac{1}{2}Li^2$

Energy density $= \frac{U}{V} = \frac{1}{2}\frac{B^2}{\mu_0}$

Dimension of inductance $= [\text{ML}^2\text{T}^{-2}\text{A}^{-2}]$

Mutual inductance $(L_S) = L_1 + L_2 \pm M^2$

[$\because M =$ Mutual Inductance.]

Gearing up for NEET

1. (*b*) Induced emf, $e = -\frac{d\phi}{dt}$

But $\quad e = iR$ and $i = \frac{dq}{dt}$

$\therefore \quad \frac{dq}{dt}R = -\frac{d\phi}{dt}$ or $dq = -\frac{d\phi}{R}$

So, induced charge in a coil is independent of time taken to change the flux.

2. (*b*) The magnitude of induced emf is directly proportional to the rate of change of magnetic flux.
Also, induced charge is $dq = -\frac{d\phi}{R}$, which is independent of time.
$\therefore$Induced emf and induced charge will be more in first case and equal in both cases, respectively.

3. (*b*) The value of self induction of coil increases when soft iron core is inserted in the coil, hence current decreases due to increase of its reactance. So, intensity of bulb decreases.

4. (*b*) The self-inductance of a long solenoid of cross-sectional area A and length l, having n turns per unit length, filled with a material of relative permeability (*e. g.* soft iron, which has a high value of relative permeability) inside the solenoid is given by

$$L = \mu_r \mu_0 n^2 Al = \frac{\mu_r \mu_0 N^2 A}{l}$$

5. (*a*) Induced current is given by

$$i = \frac{e}{R} = -\frac{N(d\phi/dt)}{R} = -\frac{N}{R}\left(\frac{d\phi}{dt}\right) = \frac{-N}{R}\cdot\frac{dB}{dt}\cdot A$$

$$= \frac{10 \times 10^8 \times 10^{-4} \times 10^{-4} \times 10}{20} = 5 \text{ A}$$

[$\because$ 1 Gauss $= 10^{-4}$T, 1 cm $= 10^{-2}$ m]

6. (*c*) Applying Lenz's law, the loop B is repelled by loop A.

7. (*d*) Induced emf, $e = -N\dfrac{d\phi}{dt}$

$$|e| = N\frac{d\phi}{dt} = N\frac{d}{dt}(BA\cos\theta)$$

$$= N\frac{dB}{dt}\cdot A\cos\theta$$

$$= 500 \times 1 \times (10\times10^{-2})^2 \cos 0° = 5\text{ V}$$

8. (*b*) Induced emf, $e = -\dfrac{d\phi}{dt}$

$$|e| = \frac{d}{dt}(BA) = A\frac{dB}{dt}$$

$$= 2\times\frac{(4-1)}{2} = 3\text{ V}$$

9. (*a*) During this period, the two loops attract each other.

10. (*c*) $\phi = \mathbf{B}\cdot\mathbf{A} = BA\cos 90° = 0$, therefore $d\phi = 0$ and $i = \dfrac{dq}{dt} = \dfrac{1}{R}\dfrac{d\phi}{dt} = 0$

11. (*a*) According to Lenz's law, the magnet gets repelled, therefore north pole is formed on the top side and hence current will flow in anti-clockwise direction.

12. (*a*) Charge induced in coil,

$$dq = \frac{d\phi_B}{R} = i\,dt = \text{Area under } i\text{-}t \text{ graph}$$

$$\therefore \quad d\phi_B = (\text{Area under } i\text{-}t \text{ graph})R$$

$$= \frac{1}{2}\times 4\times 0.1\times 10 = 2\text{ Wb}$$

13. (*d*) We have, $\Delta q = -\dfrac{N}{R}\Delta\phi$ and $\Delta\phi = \Delta B\cdot A\cos\theta$

$$\therefore \quad 32\times10^{-6} = -\frac{100}{(160+40)}(0-B)$$

$$\times \pi\times(6\times10^{-3})^2\times\cos 0°$$

$\therefore$ Intensity of magnetic field, $B = 0.566$ T

14. (*d*) Induced emf, $e = \left|\dfrac{-NBA(\cos\theta_2-\cos\theta_1)}{\Delta t}\right|$

$$= \left|\frac{800\times4\times10^{-5}\times0.05(\cos 90° - \cos 0°)}{0.1}\right|$$

$$= 0.016\text{ V}$$

15. (*a*) Magnetic flux, $\phi = B\cdot A$

$\therefore$ Change in flux, $d\phi = B\cdot dA$

$$= 0.05\,(101-100)\times10^{-4}$$

$$= 5\times10^{-6}\text{ Wb}$$

$$\therefore \quad \text{Charge, } dq = \frac{d\phi}{R} = \frac{5\times10^{-6}}{2} = 2.5\times10^{-6}\text{ C}$$

16. (*d*) If electron is moving from left to right, the flux linked with the loop (which is into the page) will first increase and then decrease as the electron passes through it. So, the induced current in the loop will be first anti-clockwise and will change direction as the electron passes through.

17. (*c*) The magnetic flux linked with a surface of area A in uniform magnetic field is given by

$$\phi = \mathbf{B}\cdot\mathbf{A}$$

Here, $A = L^2\hat{\mathbf{k}}$ and $B = B_0(2\hat{\mathbf{i}} + 3\hat{\mathbf{j}} + 4\hat{\mathbf{k}})$ T

$$\therefore \quad \phi = \mathbf{B}\cdot\mathbf{A} = B_0(2\hat{\mathbf{i}} + 3\hat{\mathbf{j}} + 4\hat{\mathbf{k}})\cdot L^2\hat{\mathbf{k}} = 4B_0L^2\text{ Wb}$$

18. (*a*) $\therefore$ Magnetic flux,

$$\phi = BA\cos\theta = 0.2\sin(300t)\times5\times10^{-4}\times\cos 60°$$

$$= 5\times10^{-5}\sin(300t)$$

$$\therefore \text{ emf, } e = \frac{d\phi}{dt} = 5\times10^{-5}\times300\cos(300t)$$

$$= 1.5\times10^{-2}\cos\left(300\times\frac{\pi}{900}\right) \quad \left(\because t = \frac{\pi}{900}\text{ s}\right)$$

$$= 1.5\times10^{-2}\cos(\pi/3) = 0.75\times10^{-2} = 7.5\times10^{-3}\text{ V}$$

19. (*c*) Since, the magnetic field is uniform, therefore there will be no change in flux, hence no current will be induced.

20. (*b*) Charge, $\Delta Q = \dfrac{\Delta\phi}{R} = \dfrac{N\times BA}{R}$

$\therefore$ Magnetic flux density,

$$B = \frac{\Delta Q\cdot R}{NA} = \frac{2\times10^{-4}\times80}{40\times4\times10^{-4}} = 1\text{ Wb/m}^2$$

21. (*d*) Since the magnet will perform SHM, its velocity both increase and decrease as it moves towards and away from the mean position and hence the galvanometer will show deflection on both sides. Since, the amplitude of the magnet will decrease due to eddy current losses, the amplitude of deflection will also decrease with time.

22. (*b*) As the magnet moves towards the coil, the magnetic flux increases (non-linearly). Also, there is a change in polarity of induced emf when the magnet passes on to the other side of the coil. So, correct variation is shown in (b).

23. (*d*) Magnetic lines on circular loop, due to current in wire AB are tangential to its plane.

$\therefore$ Magnetic flux, $\phi_B = 0$ or induced emf, $\varepsilon = \dfrac{d\phi_B}{dt} = 0$

24. (*c*) $\because M_{12} = M_{21}$, when rate of change of current is doubled, induced emf also becomes two times. Thus, emf produced across the first coil is 6 mV.

25. (*b*) Here, loop *ABCDA* lies in *XY*-plane whose area vector $\mathbf{A}_1 = L^2\hat{\mathbf{k}}$, whereas loop *ADEFA* lies in *YZ*-plane whose area vector $\mathbf{A}_2 = L^2\hat{\mathbf{i}}$.

Also, the magnetic flux linked with uniform surface of area *A* in uniform magnetic field is given by

$$\phi = \mathbf{B}\cdot\mathbf{A}$$

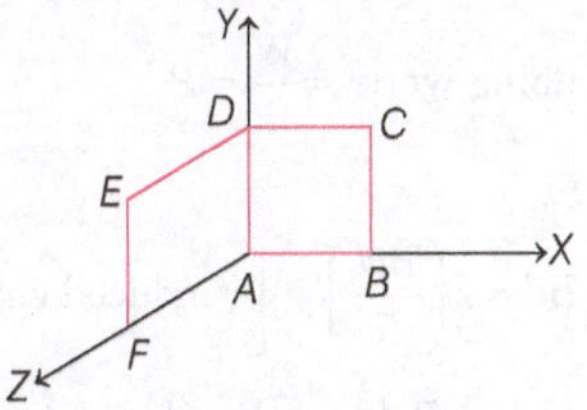

$$\mathbf{A} = \mathbf{A}_1 + \mathbf{A}_2 = (L^2\hat{\mathbf{k}} + L^2\hat{\mathbf{i}})$$

and $\mathbf{B} = B_0(\hat{\mathbf{i}} + \hat{\mathbf{k}})\,\text{T}$

Now, $\phi = \mathbf{B}\cdot\mathbf{A} = B_0(\hat{\mathbf{i}} + \hat{\mathbf{k}})\cdot(L^2\hat{\mathbf{k}} + L^2\hat{\mathbf{i}}) = 2B_0L^2$ Wb

26. (*d*) Magnetic flux,

$$\phi = NAB = (25)(\pi)(1.8\times10^{-2})^2[0.2t - 0.05t^2]$$
$$= 0.025\,(0.2t - 0.05t^2)$$

Induced emf, $e = \left|\frac{d\phi}{dt}\right| = |0.025\,(0.2 - 2\times0.05\,t)|$

At $t = 3$ s, $e = 0.0025$ V

$$i = \frac{e}{R} = 0.0016\ \text{A}$$

$\therefore$ Power dissipation, $P = ei = 4\times10^{-6}\ \text{W} = 4\ \mu\text{W}$

27. (*a*) In the case (a), the induced current in the ring will be in such a direction that it repels the magnet. *i.e.* $a < g$ and moving towards *R*.

In case (c), the induced current is such as to attract the magnet.

i.e. $a < g$ not $a > g$ and moving away from *R*. So, option (c) is incorrect.

28. (*a*) From the figure, $V_a - iR - L\frac{di}{dt} = V_b$

$$\therefore \quad V_a - V_b = iR + L\frac{di}{dt}$$

According to given conditions,

$$8 = 2R + L \quad \text{...(i)}$$
$$4 = 2R - L \quad \text{...(ii)}$$

Solving these two equations, we get

$$R = 3\,\Omega \text{ and } L = 2\,\text{H}$$

29. (*a*) When the current in *B* (at $t = 0$) is counter-clockwise and the coil *A* is considered above to it. The counter-clockwise flow of the current in *B* is equivalent to north pole of magnet and magnetic field lines are emanating upward to coil *A*. When coil *A* start rotating at $t = 0$, then the current in *A* is constant along clockwise direction by Lenz's rule.

30. (*a*) Here, area, $A = 10\times5 = 50\ \text{cm}^2 = 50\times10^{-4}\text{m}^2$

$$\frac{dB}{dt} = 0.02\ \text{Ts}^{-1} \text{ and } R = 2\,\Omega$$

$$\therefore \quad \text{emf, } e = \frac{d\phi}{dt} = A\cdot\frac{dB}{dt}$$
$$= 50\times10^{-4}\times0.02 = 10^{-4}\ \text{V}$$

Power dissipated in the form of heat

$$= \frac{e^2}{R} = \frac{10^{-4}\times10^{-4}}{2} = 0.5\times10^{-8}\text{W}$$
$$= 5\times10^{-9}\text{W} = 5\ \text{nW}$$

31. (*d*) When *A* stops moving, then current in *B* become zero, possible only if the current in *A* is constant in counter-clockwise direction. If the current in *A* would be variable, then there must be an induced emf (current) in *B* even, if *A* stops moving.

32. (*b*) Time constant,

$$\tau_L = \frac{L}{R} = \frac{5}{10} = \frac{1}{2}\ \text{s}$$

We have, $i = i_0\,(1 - e^{-t/\tau_L})$

$$\therefore \quad \frac{i_\infty}{i} = \frac{i_0}{i_0\,(1 - e^{-t/\tau_L})}$$

Substituting $t = 1$ s and $\tau_L = \frac{1}{2}$ s, we get

$$\frac{i_\infty}{i} = \frac{e^2}{e^2 - 1}$$

33. (*d*)

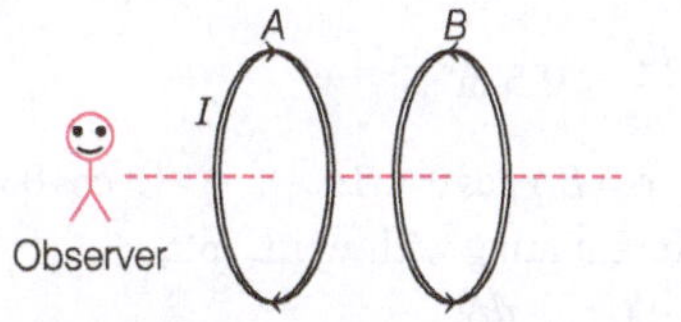

If current *I* through *A* increases, magnetic field linked with coil *B* increases. Hence, anti-clockwise current induces in coil *B*. As shown in figure, both the currents flowing in opposite directions produce repulsive effect.

34. (*a*) When the north pole of a bar magnet moves towards the coil, the induced current in the coil flows in a direction such that the coil presents its north pole to the bar magnet as shown in Fig. (a).

Therefore, the induced current flows in the coil in the anti-clockwise direction.

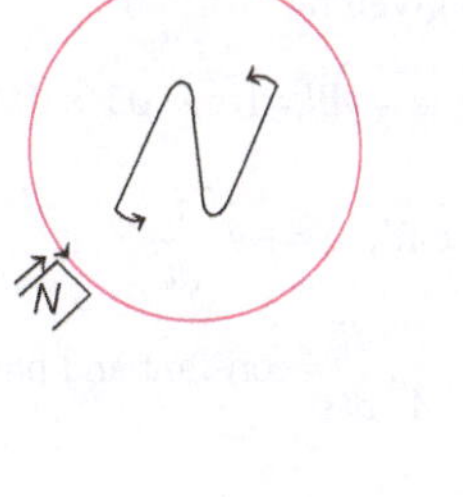

35. (d) When switch S is closed, then magnetic field lines passing through Q increases in the direction from right to left.

So, according to Lenz's law, induced current in Q, i.e. I_{Q_1} will flow in such a direction, so that the magnetic field lines due to I_{Q_1} passes from left to right through Q. This is possible when I_{Q_1} flows in anti-clockwise direction as seen by E. Opposite is the case when switch S is opened, i.e. I_{Q_2} will be clockwise as seen by E.

36. (a) As the north pole approaches, a north pole is developed at the face, i.e. the current flows anti-clockwise. Finally, when it completes the oscillation, no emf is present.

Now, south pole approaches the other side, i.e. RHS, the current flows clockwise to repel the south pole. This means the current is anti-clockwise at the LHS of the coil as before. The break occurs, when the pendulum is at the extreme and momentarily stationary position.

37. (a) Given, $n = 500$,

$$L = 50\text{ mH} = 50 \times 10^{-3}\text{ H}$$

and $$i = 8\text{ mA} = 8 \times 10^{-3}\text{ A}$$

The magnetic flux linked with the coil,

$$\phi = Li = 50 \times 10^{-3} \times 8 \times 10^{-3}$$
$$= 400 \times 10^{-6} = 4 \times 10^{-4}\text{ Wb}$$

38. (b) Given, $B = 40\text{ mT} = 40 \times 10^{-3}\text{T}$

Rate of shrinking of area $= 0.5\text{m}^2\text{s}^{-1}$

$$\Rightarrow \quad \frac{dA}{dt} = 0.5\text{ m}^2\text{s}^{-1}$$

As, $\phi = BA\cos\theta = BA$ $\quad (\because \cos\theta = \cos 0° = 1)$

On differentiating with w.r.t. to t,

$$\frac{d\phi}{dt} = B \cdot \frac{dA}{dt} = e$$

$$\Rightarrow \quad e = B \cdot \frac{dA}{dt} = 40 \times 10^{-3} \times 0.5$$
$$= 20 \times 10^{-3}\text{ V} = 20\text{ mV}$$

39. (b) Given, length of conductor, $l = 0.1$ m

Mangetic field, $B = 0.1$ T

Velocity of conductor, $v = 15\text{ms}^{-1}$

The angle between v and B is 90°.

When v and B are mutually perpendicular, then emf (induced) is given by

$$e = vBl = 15 \times 0.1 \times 0.1 = \frac{15}{100} = 0.15\text{ V}$$

40. (d) Induced emf, $e = -L\frac{di}{dt}$

During 0 to $\frac{T}{4}$, $\frac{di}{dt}$ = constant and positive,

so e = negative.

For $\frac{T}{4}$ to $\frac{T}{2}$, $\frac{di}{dt} = 0$, so $e = 0$.

For $T/2$ to $\frac{3T}{4}$, $\frac{di}{dt}$ = constant and negative, so e = positive.

This condition is satisfied only by graph in option (d).

41. (c) Rate of doing work $= \frac{W}{t} = P$

But $P = Fv$

Also, $F = Bil = B\left(\frac{Bvl}{R}\right)l \quad \left[\because \text{induced current, } i = \frac{Bvl}{R}\right]$

$$\therefore \text{ Power, } P = B\left(\frac{Bvl}{R}\right)lv = \frac{B^2v^2l^2}{R}$$
$$= \frac{(0.5)^2 \times (2)^2 \times (1)^2}{6} = \frac{1}{6}\text{ W}$$

42. (d) Peak value of emf generated in generator is given by

$$e_0 = \omega NBA = (2\pi v)NBA$$
$$= 2 \times 3.14 \times 100 \times 5000 \times 0.2 \times 0.25 = 157\text{ kV}$$

43. (d) **B**, **v** and **l** should be mutually perpendicular.

So, the conductor should more in the direction perpendicular to the plane of l and B, i.e. in the direction of M.

44. (c) Induced emf, $e = Bvl$

$$\therefore \quad e \propto v$$

Also, $$v = 0 + gt$$

$$\therefore \quad e \propto gt$$

So, potential difference between its two ends will increase with time.

45. (b) Power, $P = Fv = ilBv = \left(\frac{Bvl}{R}\right)lBv = \frac{B^2l^2v^2}{R}$

48. (b) Induced emf, $|e| = \frac{d\phi}{dt} = \frac{BdS}{dt}$

Now, as the square loop and rectangular loop move out of magnetic field, $\frac{BdS}{dt}$ is constant, therefore $|e|$ is constant. But in case of circular and elliptical loops, $\frac{dS}{dt}$ changes. Therefore, emf does not remain constant.

49. (d) Oscillating coil produces time varing magnetic field. Eddy current induced in aluminium plate create electromagnetic damping effect in coil.

50. (d) As, potential difference,

$$V = Bvl = (2.0 \times 10^{-4})\left(360 \times \frac{5}{18}\right)(50)$$
$$= 1.0\text{ V}$$

51. (a) If the loop remains inside the region of magnetic field, no current will be induced. But, if it moves out of the plane, then the induced current is given by $i = \dfrac{Blv}{R}$ and its direction will be clockwise (as per Lenz's law).

52. (b) $\because$ As, potential difference, $e = Bvl$

$$= (0.2 \times 10^{-4})(20)(1) \text{ V}$$
$$= 0.4 \text{ mV}$$

53. (b) Two emfs are induced in the closed circuit each of value Blv. These two emfs are additive, so $E_{net} = 2Blv$.

54. (b) Here, $e = Bvl = (0.1)(1)(0.1) = \dfrac{1}{100}$ V

Net resistance $= 1 + \dfrac{2 \times 3}{2 + 3} = \dfrac{11}{5}\ \Omega$

$\therefore$ Current, $i = \left(\dfrac{1/100}{11/5}\right) = \dfrac{1}{220}$ A

55. (b) When cylindrical bar magnet is rotated about its axis, no change in flux linked with the circuit takes place, consequently no emf induces and hence no current flows through the ammeter A.

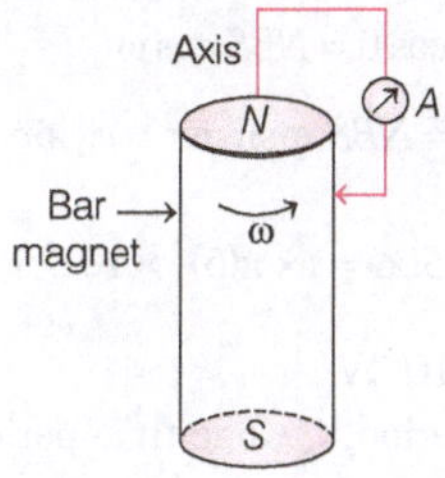

56. (d) The magnetic field ⊗ passing from the closed loop is increasing. Therefore, from Lenz's law, induced current will produce upward magnetic field. Hence, induced current is anti-clockwise, *i.e.* I_1 is in the direction ab and I_2 is in the direction dc.

57. (a) Since, here only half area of ring will be considered.

$\therefore\ \phi_B = B\,S = B \cdot \dfrac{\pi r^2}{2}$

$\therefore\ e = \dfrac{d\phi_B}{dt} = \dfrac{\pi r^2}{2} \cdot \dfrac{dB}{dt} = \dfrac{\pi (0.1)^2}{2} \times 0.01 = \dfrac{\pi}{2} \times 10^{-4}$ V

$\therefore\ i = \dfrac{e}{R} = \dfrac{\frac{\pi}{2} \times 10^{-4}}{4} = \dfrac{\pi}{8} \times 10^{-4} = 3.9 \times 10^{-5}$ A

58. (c) As, the potential due to a straight rod of length L in magnetic field B,

$$e = BLv$$

So, for $PQ = L/2$, $e = \dfrac{BLv}{2}$

Hence, current is from P to Q, *i.e.* P is at positive potential w.r.t. Q.

59. (b)

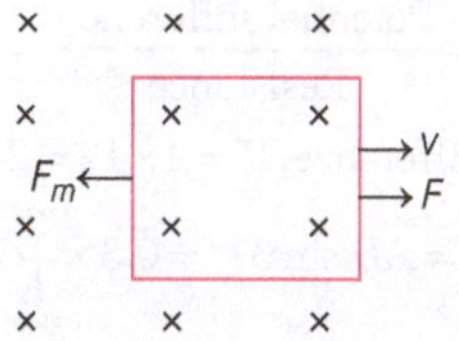

Induced emf $= Bvl$

Induced current, $i = \dfrac{Bvl}{R}$

Magnetic force on loop, $F_m = Bil = \dfrac{B^2vl^2}{R}$

Since, loop is moving with constant speed, $F = F_m$

Input power, $P = \mathbf{F} \cdot \mathbf{v} = Fv = \dfrac{B^2v^2l^2}{R}$

P *versus* v graph will be like,

$y \propto x^2$ (parabola, open upward)

60. (c) A moving conductor is equivalent to a battery of emf $= vBl$ [motion emf]

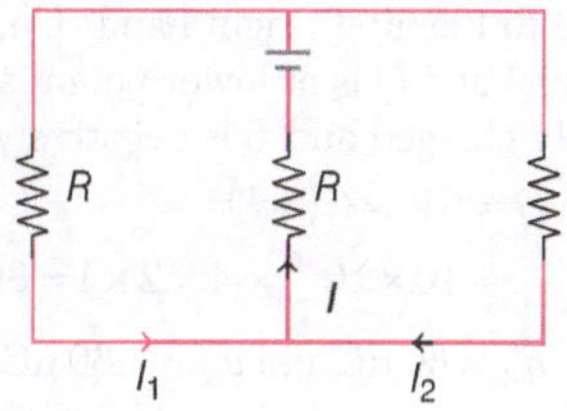

Equivalent circuit, $I = I_1 + I_2$ ...(i)

Applying Kirchhoff's law,

$I_1R + IR - vBl = 0$ ...(ii)

$I_2R + IR - vBl = 0$ ...(iii)

Adding Eqs. (ii) and (iii), we get

$I_1R + IR - vBl + I_2R + IR - vBl = 0$

$\Rightarrow\ 2IR + IR = 2vBl$ [From Eq. (i)]

$\Rightarrow\ I = \dfrac{2vBl}{3R}$

Subtracting Eq.(iii) from Eq.(ii), we get

$I_1R + IR - vBl = 0$

$\underline{{}_{-}I_2R +_{-} IR -_{+} vBl =_{-} 0}$

$I_1R - I_2R = 0$

$\Rightarrow\ R(I_1 - I_2) = 0$

$\Rightarrow\ I_1 - I_2 = 0$ $[\because R \neq 0]$

$\Rightarrow\ I_1 = I_2$ ...(iv)

From Eq. (i), we get

$I = 2I_1$ $[\because I_1 = I_2]$

$\Rightarrow\ 2I_1 = I$

$\Rightarrow\ I_1 = \dfrac{I}{2} = \dfrac{2vBl}{2 \times 3R} = \dfrac{vBl}{3R}$

$\therefore\ I_1 = I_2 = \dfrac{vBl}{3R}$

61. (*d*) Current, $I = \frac{\text{Potential difference}}{\text{Resistance}}$

$\therefore$ Potential difference, $V = 2 \times 12 = 24\text{ V} = Bvl$

Here, $l = AD \sin 37° = 0.3 \times \frac{3}{5} = 0.18\text{m}$

$\therefore$ Velocity, $v = \frac{V}{Bl} = \frac{24}{4 \times 0.18} = \frac{100}{3}\text{ ms}^{-1}$

62. (*d*) Induced emf, $V_{BA} = \frac{1}{4}\left(\frac{d\phi}{dt}\right)$

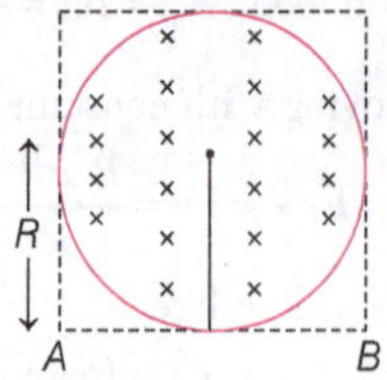

$$= \frac{1}{4}(\pi R^2) \cdot \frac{dB}{dt} = \frac{\pi R^2 \alpha}{4} \quad \left(\because \phi = B \cdot A \text{ and } \frac{dB}{dt} = \alpha\right)$$

63. (*a*) According to Fleming's right hand rule, *P* is at higher potential and *Q* is at lower potential. Therefore, *A* is positively charged and *B* is negatively charged. Also, charge, $Q = CV = C(Bvl)$

$$= 10 \times 10^{-6} \times 4 \times 2 \times 1 = 80\,\mu\text{C}$$

$\therefore$ $q_A = 80\,\mu\text{C}$ and $q_B = -80\,\mu\text{C}$

64. (*c*) For rotating rod, induced emf, $v = \frac{1}{2}Bl^2\omega$

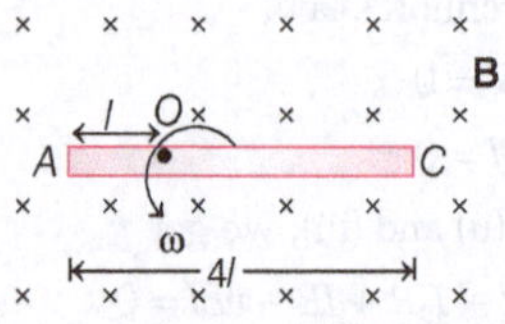

For part *AO*, $V_{OA} = V_O - V_A = \frac{1}{2}Bl^2\omega$

For part *OC*, $V_{OC} = V_O - V_C = \frac{1}{2}B(3l)^2\omega$

$\therefore V_A - V_C = V_{OC} - V_{OA} = (V_O - V_C) - (V_O - V_A) = 4Bl^2\omega$

65. (*d*) As, the coil is rotated, angle θ (angle which is normal to the coil makes with **B** at any instant *t*) changes, therefore magnetic flux φ linked with the coil changes and hence an emf is induced in the coil. At this instant *t*, if *e* is the emf induced in the coil, then

$$e = -\frac{d\phi}{dt} = -\frac{d}{dt}(NSB \cos \omega t)$$

where, *N* is number of turns in the coil.

or $e = -NSB\frac{d}{dt}(\cos \omega t) = -NSB(-\sin \omega t)\,\omega$

or $e = NSB\omega \sin \omega t$ ...(i)

The induced emf will be maximum, when $\sin \omega t$ is maximum.

$\therefore$ $e_{\max} = e_0 = NSB\omega \times 1$

or $e = e_0 \sin \omega t$

Therefore, *e* would be maximum, hence current is maximum (as $i_0 = e_0 / R$), when $\theta = 90°$, *i.e.* normal of plane of coil is perpendicular to the field or plane of coil is parallel to magnetic field.

66. (*b*) When ring enters and leaves, then the field polarity of induced emf is opposite. Also, during the stay of ring completely in the field, there is no induction. These variations are correctly shown in (b).

67. (*b*)

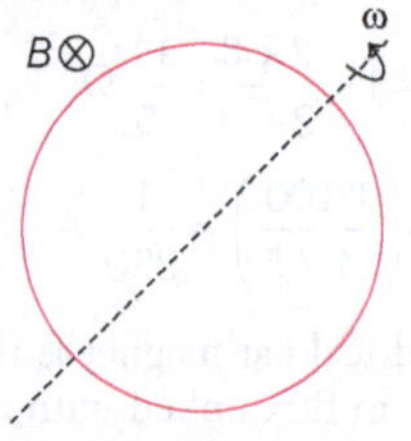

Let at any time, normal to loop makes an angle θ with magnetic field,

$$\phi_B = NBS \cos\theta = NBS \cos \omega t$$

$$e = -\frac{d\phi_B}{dt} = NBS\,\omega \sin \omega t = e_0 \sin \omega t$$

$$\therefore e_{\max} = e_0 = NSB\omega = 1 \times \pi(5)^2 \times 10^{-4} \times 0.01 \times \frac{80 \times 2\pi}{60}$$

$$= 6.6 \times 10^{-4}\text{V}$$

Over a long period, *i.e.* one time period, average of induced emf, $\bar{e} = \frac{\int_0^T e\,dt}{T} = 0$

and $\overline{e^2} = \frac{\int_0^T e^2 dt}{T} = \frac{e_0^2}{2} = 2.0 \times 10^{-7}\text{ V}^2$

68. (*b*)

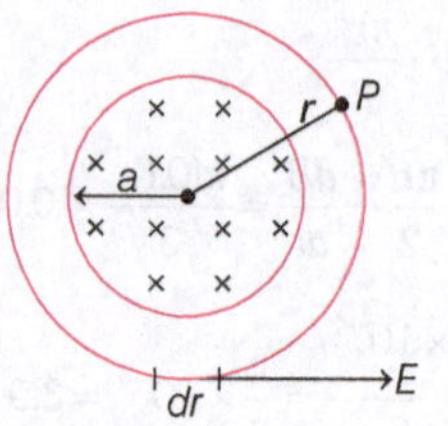

Draw a concentric circle of radius *r*. The induced electric field *E* at any point on the circle is equal to that at *P*.

For this circle, induced emf,

$$e = \oint \mathbf{E} \cdot d\mathbf{l} = \left|\frac{d\phi}{dt}\right| = S\left|\frac{dB}{dt}\right|$$

$\therefore \quad e = E\int dl = \pi a^2 \left|\frac{dB}{dt}\right| \quad$ (but $\oint dl = 2\pi r$)

$\therefore \quad E \times 2\pi r = \pi a^2 \left|\frac{dB}{dt}\right|$

$\therefore \quad E = \frac{a^2}{2r}\left|\frac{dB}{dt}\right|$

$\Rightarrow \quad E \propto \frac{1}{r}$

69. (c) We know that, $e = NBA\,\omega \sin \omega t$

where, N = number of loops = 1

$B = \frac{\mu_0 I}{2b}$ N/A-m

$\Rightarrow \quad A = \pi a^2\ \text{m}^2$

$\therefore \quad e = \frac{\mu_0 I}{2b}(\pi a^2)\,\omega \sin \omega t$

$\Rightarrow \quad = \frac{\pi a^2 \mu_0 I}{2b}\cdot \omega \sin \omega t$

70. (c) Current in the circuit, $i = V/R = 10/2 = 5\,\text{A}$

$\therefore$ Magnetic energy stored in the coil,

$U = \frac{1}{2}Li^2 = \frac{1}{2}\times 2 \times (5)^2 = 25\ \text{J}$

71. (b) For growth of current in L-R circuit, current is given by

$i = i_0(1 - e^{-Rt/L})$

$\therefore \quad \frac{di}{dt} = -i_0\left(-\frac{R}{L}\right)e^{-Rt/L}$

$= \frac{i_0 R}{L}e^{-Rt/L}$

At the instant of closing the switch, $\frac{di}{dt} = \frac{i_0 R}{L} = \frac{E}{L}$

$\Rightarrow \quad 4 = \frac{E}{20}$

$\therefore \quad E = 20 \times 4 = 80\ \text{V}$

72. (b) We have, $L \propto N^2$

$\frac{L_B}{L_A} = \left(\frac{N_B}{N_A}\right)^2$

Self-inductance, $L_B = \left(\frac{500}{600}\right)^2 \times 108 = 75\ \text{mH}$

73. (a) Mutual inductance between two coils depend on their degree of flux linkage, *i.e.* the fraction of flux linked with one coil when some current passes through the other coil. In Fig. (A), two coils with their planes are parallel. In this situation, maximum flux passes. So, mutual inductance will be maximum in this case.

74. (d) Mutual inductance between two coils in the same plane with their centres coinciding is given by

$M = \frac{\mu_0}{4\pi}\left(\frac{2\pi^2 R_2^2 N_1 N_2}{R_1}\right)$ henry $\Rightarrow M \propto \frac{R_2^2}{R_1}$

75. (b) $V = L\frac{di}{dt}$ or $V \propto L \quad \left(\because \frac{di}{dt} = \text{constant}\right)$

$\therefore \quad \frac{V_1}{V_2} = \frac{L_1}{L_2} = 4 \quad (\because P = Vi = \text{constant})$

$\therefore \quad i \propto \frac{1}{V}$ or $\frac{i_1}{i_2} = \frac{V_2}{V_1} = \frac{1}{4}$

$\therefore \quad \frac{W_1}{W_2} = \frac{L_1}{L_2}\left(\frac{i_1}{i_2}\right)^2 = (4)\left(\frac{1}{16}\right) = \frac{1}{4} \quad \left(\because W = \frac{1}{2}Li^2\right)$

$\because \quad \frac{i_1}{i_2} \neq 4$

Thus, wrong option is (b).

76. (c) Induced emf, $E = -L\frac{di}{dt}$

or induced emf $\propto$ − slope of i-t graph. So, initially emf is zero as slope of it curve is zero and then remaining two regions, slopes are constant but of opposite sign. So, graph (c) is correct.

77. (d) Energy, $U = \frac{1}{2}Li_0^2 = \frac{1}{2}L\left(\frac{V}{R}\right)^2$

$= \frac{1}{2}\times 50 \times 10^{-6}\left(\frac{5}{0.5}\right)^2\ \text{J} = 2.5\,\text{mJ}$

Now, after switching OFF the battery, this energy is dissipated in coil (resistance = 0.5 Ω) and resistance (10 Ω) in the ratio of their resistances ($H = i^2Rt$ or $H \propto R$). Therefore, heat generated in the coil.

$2.5 \times \left(\frac{0.5}{10 + 0.5}\right) = 0.12\,\text{mJ}$

78. (b) Power, $P = (i_0)^2 R$, *i.e.* $(i_0)^2 = \frac{P}{R}$ and $\tau = \frac{L}{R}$

Total heat produced, $U = \frac{1}{2}Li_0^2 = \frac{1}{2}(\tau R)\left(\frac{P}{R}\right) = \frac{1}{2}P\tau$

79. (a) The self-inductance of a solenoid, $L = \mu_0 n^2 Sl$,

where
μ_0 = permeability of air,
n = number of turns per unit length,
S = area of cross-section
and l = length of the solenoid.

This depends on the geometry of the inductor such as cross-sectional area, length and number of turns and not on the material, even if it is made of a superconducting material.

$\therefore \quad L_1 = L_2 = L_3$

80. (a) Coil A carries a steady current with increase in temperature, its resistance increases and so current is decreasing at a constant rate, this induces an emf in coil B which opposes this change, *i.e.* current in coil B is in same direction of A, therefore they attract to each other.

81. (*d*) For inductor, as we know induced voltage (for $t=0$ to $t=T/2$),

$$V=L\frac{dI}{dt}=L\frac{d}{dt}\left(\frac{2I_0t}{T}\right)=\text{constant}$$

(for $t=T/2$ to $t=T$),

$$V=\frac{LdI}{dt}\left(\frac{-2I_0t}{T}\right)=-\text{constant}$$

Therefore, correct variation will be represented by graph (d).

82. (*a*) Induced emf, $e=2$ V

$$i_1=8\text{ A},\ i_2=6\text{ A}$$

and $\Delta t=2\times10^{-3}$ s

Coefficient of self-induction,

$$L=\frac{-e}{\Delta i/\Delta t}=\frac{-2}{(6-8)/2\times10^{-3}}=\frac{-2\times2\times10^{-3}}{-2}=2\times10^{-3}\text{ H}$$

Assertion and Reason

1. (*d*) Self-inductance depends upon current flowing or change in current flowing through a circuit.

We have, $e=-L\dfrac{di}{dt}$

$$\Rightarrow\quad L=\frac{-e}{(di/dt)}\text{ or } L\propto\frac{1}{(di/dt)}$$

2. (*d*) If switch is closed in a circuit containing a pure inductor L and resistor R in series with a battery, then current through the circuit rises exponentially and reaches upto a certain maximum value. So, the corresponding potential drop across inductor is also maximum.

3. (*a*) If moving from left to right, current is increasing, then battery $\left(\text{induced emf}=L\cdot\dfrac{di}{dt}\right)$ will produce current from left to right current, *i.e.* its positive terminal is on left hand side or $V_A>V_B$.

Further $i=\text{constant}\Rightarrow\dfrac{di}{dt}=0$ or $V_A-V_B=V_L$.

$$\Rightarrow\quad V_A-V_B=0\Rightarrow V_A=V_B$$

4. (*d*) $V=L\dfrac{di}{dt}=\text{constant}$

$$\therefore\quad L\,(di)=\text{constant}\Rightarrow Li=\text{constant or } i\propto\frac{1}{L}$$

5. (*a*) We know that, $\phi=BA\cos\omega t$

At $t=0$, $\phi=\text{maximum}$

$$|e|=\left|\frac{d\phi}{dt}\right|=B\omega A\sin\omega t$$

For maximum value of $|e|$ is at, $\omega t=90°$, *i.e.* loop is rotated through 90° or it is parallel to magnetic field. At this instant, $\phi=0$.

Statement type Questions

1. (*a*) Both Statement I and Statement II are incorrect.

In an electric motor, current is passed through a coil mounted in magnetic field. Due to flow of current in the coil a torque acts on the coil which starts rotating it. Thus, electrical energy is converted into mechanical energy. It is based on a principle that current carrying coil experience a torque in magnetic field.

2. (*d*) Both Statement I and Statement II are correct.

3. (*d*) Both Statement I and Statement II are correct.

4. (*c*) Statement I is incorrect but Statement II is correct.

Even though flux through individual lines changes, it remains unchanged for the solenoid as a whole. Therefore, no emf is induced in the long solenoid.

5. (*d*) Both Statement I and Statement II are correct.

Match the Columns

1. (*a*) As, Faraday's laws are of EMI (Electromagnetic Induction) Lenz's law obeys the law of energy conservation. Fleming's right hand rule gives us the direction of induced current and Fleming's left hand rule gives us the direction of force on current carrying conductor in magnetic field.

Hence, A-(IV), B-(II), C-(III), D-(I).

2. (*d*) A. Tesla → II$[MT^{-2}A^{-1}]$

B. Weber → IV $[ML^2T^{-2}A^{-1}]$

C. Volt → III$[ML^2T^{-3}A^{-1}]$

D. Henry → I$[ML^2T^{-3}A^{-1}]$

Hence, A-(II), B-(IV), C-(III) and D-(I).

3. (*a*)

A.	Self-inductance of a coil	I.	$\dfrac{\mu_0N^2\pi r}{2}$
B.	Self inductance of a solenoid	IV.	$\dfrac{\mu_0N^2S}{l}$
C.	Mutual inductance for two concentric coils	II.	$\dfrac{\mu_0N_1N_2\pi r^2}{2R}$
D.	Mutual inductance of two long co-axial solenoids	I.	$\dfrac{\mu_0N_1N_2\times S}{l}$

Hence, A-(III), B-(IV), C-(II), D-(I).

4. (*b*) At $t = 0.01$s,

$$|e| = \frac{\Delta\phi_B}{\Delta t} = \frac{8\times10^{-3}}{0.01} = 0.8\text{ V}$$

$$i = \frac{|e|}{R} = \frac{0.8}{5} = 0.16\text{ A}$$

$$\Delta q = i\Delta t = 0.16\times 0.01 = 1.6\times10^{-3}\text{C} = 1.6\text{ mC}$$

At $t = 0.03$

$$|e| = \frac{8\times10^{-3}}{0.03} = 0.26\text{ V}$$

$$i = \frac{|e|}{R} = 0.052\text{ A}$$

$$\Delta q = i\Delta t = 0.052\times 0.03 = 1.56\times10^{-3}\text{C} = 1.56\text{ mC}$$

Hence, A-(IV), B-(III), C-(I), D-(II).

5. (*a*)

A. The magnetic flux through the rectangular loop *abcd* increases, due to the motion of the loop into the region of magnetic field. The induced current must flow along the path *bcdab*, so that it opposes the increasing flux.

B. Due to the outward motion, magnetic flux through the triangular loop *abc* decreases due to which the induced current flows along *bacb*, so as to oppose the change in flux.

C. As the magnetic flux decreases due to motion of the irregular shaped loop *abcd* out of the region of magnetic field, the induced current flows along *cdabc*, so as to oppose change in flux.

D. Circular loop is entering the magnetic field, so the flux linked with them increases. The direction of induced currents in this coils will be such as to oppose the increase in magnetic flux, hence the magnetic field due to current induced will be upward. *i.e.* Current induced will flow anti-clockwise.

Hence, A-(III), B-(I), C-(II), D-IV.

Final Check Through PYQs

1. (*a*) According to Lenz's law, the direction of induced current in a conductor by changing magnetic field is created by the induced current oppose the change in the initial magnetic field.

For solenoid-1, the magnet is moving away, hence at point *B*, *S*-pole will be generated. Thus, the direction of current is *AB*.

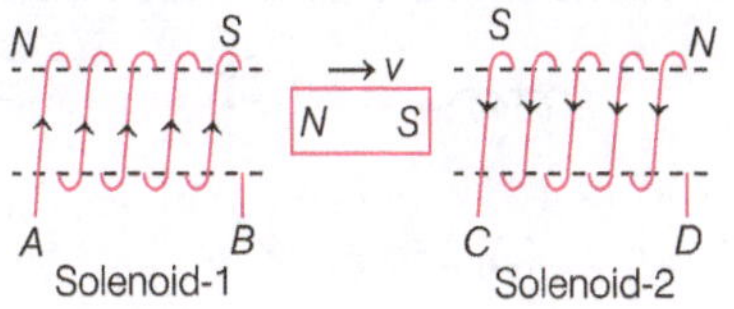

Similarly, in the solenoid-2, *S*-pole will be generated at point *C* and direction of current will be *DC*.

2. (*a*) Side of square loop, $a = 1$ m

$\therefore$ Area of square loop, $A = 1\text{ m}^2$

Resistance of square loop, $R = 1\,\Omega$

Magnetic field, $B = 0.5$ T

$\therefore$ Magnetic flux passing through the loop,

$$\phi = BA\cos\theta = 0.5\times1\times\cos0^\circ = 0.5\text{ Wb}$$

3. (*c*) Given, $N = 1000$, $r = 10$ m

$$\omega = 2\text{ rad s}^{-1}$$

$$B = 2\times10^{-5}\text{ T}$$

$$R = 12.56\,\Omega$$

Maximum induced emf $= N\omega AB$

Here area of the circular coil

$$A = \pi r^2$$

$$\varepsilon = N\omega\pi r^2 B$$

$$= 1000\times2\times3.14\times(10)^2\times2\times10^{-5}$$

$$\varepsilon = 12.56\text{ V}$$

The maximum induced current,

$$i_{max} = \frac{\varepsilon}{R} \Rightarrow i_{max} = \frac{12.56}{12.56} = 1\text{ A}$$

4. (*d*) Magnetic flux linked with coil,

$$\phi = (5t^2 + 3t + 16)\text{ Wb}$$

Magnitude of induced emf,

$$e = \left|-\frac{d\phi}{dt}\right| = \frac{d}{dt}(5t^2 + 3t + 16) = 10t + 3$$

For $t = 3$ s,

$$e_3 = 10\times3 + 3 = 33\text{ V}$$

For $t = 4$ s

$$e_4 = 10\times4 + 3 = 43\text{ V}$$

$\therefore$ Induced emf in coil at the fourth second is given as

$$e = e_4 - e_3 = 43 - 33 = 10\text{ V}$$

5. (*c*) Given, area of coil, $A = 0.05\text{ m}^2$

magnetic field, $B = 5\times10^{-5}$ T

and number of turns, $N = 800$.

The magnetic flux linked with the coil is

$$\phi = N(\mathbf{B}\cdot\mathbf{A}) = NBA\cos\theta \quad \text{...(i)}$$

where, θ is the angle between **B** and **A**.

The emf induced when coil is rotated from $\theta_1 = 0^\circ$ to $\theta_2 = 90^\circ$ is

$$e = -\frac{\Delta\phi}{\Delta t} = -\frac{\Delta}{\Delta t}(NBA\cos\theta) \quad \text{[using Eq. (i)]}$$

$$= -\frac{NBA}{\Delta t}(\cos\theta_2 - \cos\theta_1) \quad \text{...(ii)}$$

Here, $\Delta t = 0.1$ s

Thus, substituting the given values in Eq. (ii), we get

$$e = -\frac{800 \times 5 \times 10^{-5} \times 0.05 \times [\cos 90° - \cos 0°]}{0.1}$$

$$= 2000 \times 10^{-5} = 0.02 \text{ V}$$

6. (c) Induced emf in the region is given by $|e| = \frac{d\phi}{dt}$

where, $\phi = BA = \pi r^2 B \Rightarrow \frac{d\phi}{dt} = -\pi r^2 \frac{dB}{dt}$

Rate of change of magnetic flux associated with loop 1

$$e_1 = -\frac{d\phi_1}{dt} = -\pi r^2 \frac{dB}{dt}$$

Similarly e_2 = emf associated with loop 2

$$= -\frac{d\phi_2}{dt} = 0 \qquad (\because \phi_2 = 0)$$

7. (c) First current develops in direction of *abcd* but when electron moves away, then magnetic field inside loop decreases and current changes its direction.

8. (b)

A. Sheet will be attracted by the magnetic pole, hence a force is needed to hold the sheet.

B. The sheet will not experience any force, hence no external force is required to hold the sheet.

C. The sheet is conducting, hence eddy current will be produced in the sheet that will oppose the motion of the sheet. So, external for required to move the sheet with uniform velocity.

D. A non-conductcting and non-polar sheet do not interact with magnetic field hence, no force is required in this case.

9. (a) Given, magnetic field, $B = 0.4 \text{ G} = 0.4 \times 10^{-4}\text{T}$

$l = 1 \text{ m}$

Frequency, $f = 12 \text{ rpm} = \frac{120}{60} \text{ rps} = 2 \text{ Hz}$

Induced emf between the axle and rim of the wheel is given as

$$e = \frac{1}{2}B\omega l^2 = \frac{1}{2}B(2\pi f)l^2 = \pi B f l^2$$

$$= 3.14 \times 0.4 \times 10^{-4} \times 2 \times 1^2$$

$$= 2.51 \times 10^{-4}\text{V}$$

10. (b)

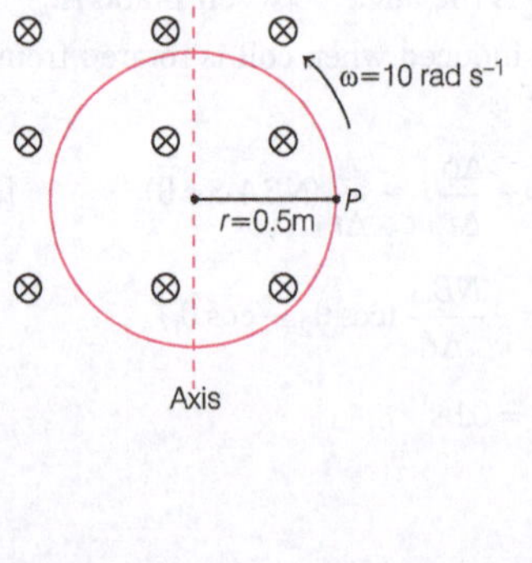

Induced emf is given by,

$$e = \frac{1}{2}B\omega r^2 \qquad \text{...(i)}$$

Here, $B = 0.1$ T, $\omega = 10$ rad/s,

$r = 0.5$ m

Substituting these values in Eq. (i), we get

$$\therefore e = \frac{1}{2} \times 0.1 \times 10 \times (0.5)^2 = \frac{1}{8} = 0.125 \text{ V}$$

11. (c) Electric heaters are not based on the eddy current effect. Rather their working is based on Joule's heating effect of current.

12. (c) Stored magnetic energy,

$$U = \frac{1}{2}LI^2$$

Here, $L = 4\mu\text{H} = 4 \times 10^{-6}$ H

$I = 2$ A

$$\therefore \quad U = \frac{1}{2} \times 4 \times 10^{-6} \times 2^2$$

$$= 8 \times 10^{-6} \text{ J} = 8 \mu\text{J}$$

13. (d) Since, both conducting circular loops are in same plane and their centres are coinciding.

Hence, magnetic flux, $\phi = Mi$ ...(i)

Here, M is the mutual inductance.

Also, the magnetic flux, $\phi = BA$

Here, B is the magnetic field and

$A (= \pi R_2^2)$ is the area of the inner circular loop. If the current passing through the outer loop is i, then the magnetic field,

$$B = \frac{\mu_0 i}{2R_1}$$

Magnetic flux, $\phi = BA$

$$\Rightarrow \quad \phi = \frac{\mu_0 i}{2R_1} \pi R_2^2 \qquad \text{...(ii)}$$

Comparing Eqs. (i) and (ii), we get

$$M = \frac{\mu_0}{2R_1} \pi R_2^2$$

Thus, the mutual inductance is directly proportional to the $\frac{R_2^2}{R_1}$.

14. (a) When an iron rod is inserted into the interior of the inductor, then inductance (L) of the coil increases.

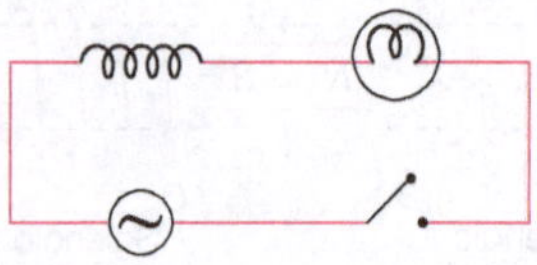

Hence, inductive reactance ($X_L = \omega L$) also increases.

$\therefore$ Current in the circuit is given as $I = \dfrac{e}{X_L}$

Hence, when X_L increases, then current I decreases. Therefore, glow of the light bulb will decrease.

15. (*d*) Given, magnetic potential energy stored in an inductor, $U = 25\text{ mJ} = 25 \times 10^{-3}$ J

Current in an inductor, $I_0 = 60\text{ mA} = 60 \times 10^{-3}$ A

As, the expression for energy stored in an inductor is given as $U = \dfrac{1}{2} L I_0^2$

where, L is the inductance of the inductor.

Substituting the given values in above equation., we get

$$(25 \times 10^{-3}) = \frac{1}{2} \times L \times (60 \times 10^{-3})^2$$

$$\Rightarrow \quad L = \frac{2 \times 25 \times 10^{-3}}{3600 \times 10^{-6}} = \frac{500}{36}$$

or $\quad L = 13.89\text{ H}$

16. (*c*) Given, resistance of the solenoid,

$$R = 10\pi^2\ \Omega$$

Radius of second and coil $r = 10^{-2}$

$$\Delta t = 0.05\text{ s}$$

$$\Delta i = 4 - 0 = 4\text{ A}$$

Charge flowing through the coil is given by

$$\Delta q = \left(\frac{\Delta \phi}{\Delta t}\right)\frac{1}{R}(\Delta t) = \mu_0 N_1 N_2 \pi r^2 \left(\frac{\Delta i}{\Delta t}\right)\frac{1}{R}\Delta t$$

$$= 4\pi \times 10^{-7} \times 2 \times 10^4 \times 100 \times \pi \times (10^{-2})^2 \times \left(\frac{4}{0.05}\right) \times \frac{1}{10\pi^2} \times 0.05$$

$$= 32 \times 10^{-6}\text{ C} = 32\ \mu\text{C}$$

17. (*c*) Given, number of turns of solenoid, $N = 1000$

Current, $I = 4$A

Magnetic flux,

$$\phi_B = 4 \times 10^{-3}\text{ Wb}$$

$\because$ Self-inductance of solenoid is given by

$$L = \frac{\phi_B \cdot N}{I} \quad \text{...(i)}$$

Substitute the given values in Eq. (i), we get

$$L = \frac{4 \times 10^{-3} \times 1000}{4} = 1\text{ H}$$

Skill Builder

Sol. of Skill Builder on Pg. 380

(b) Given, $\theta = 60°$

$$L = 2\text{ m}$$

$$B = 10\text{ T}$$

Magnetic flux,

$$\phi_B = \mathbf{B} \cdot \mathbf{S} = BS\cos\theta$$

$$\Rightarrow \quad \phi_B = 10 \times (2)^2 \cos 60°$$

$$\Rightarrow \quad \phi_B = 20\text{ Wb}$$

Sol. of Skill Builder on Pg. 382

(*c*) Given, $e = 200$ V

$$t = 5\text{ s}$$

emf, $\quad e = -\dfrac{d\phi}{dt}$

$$e = \frac{-d}{dt}(2t^3 + 5t^2)$$

$$e = -6t^2 - 10t$$

$$e\,(t = 5) = -6 \times (5)^2 - 10 \times 5$$

$$e\,(t = 5) = -200\text{ V}$$

Sol. of Skill Builder on Pg. 385

(*d*) When south pole of bar magnet leave the coil, then induced current will be in anti-clockwise direction.

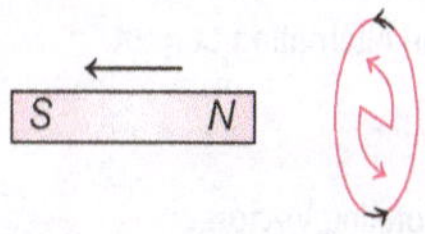

When south pole of bar magnet approaching the coil, then induced current will be in clockwise direction.

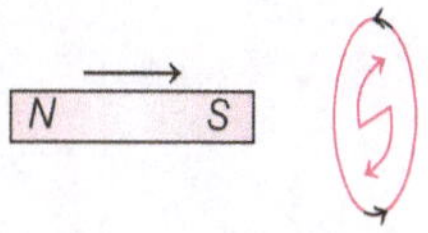

Sol. of Skill Builder on Pg. 396

(*c*) Given, $L = 2$ H

$$i = 3\text{ A}$$

Magnetic energy stored in an inductor,

$$U = \frac{1}{2} L i^2$$

$$U = \frac{1}{2} \times 2 \times (3)^2$$

$$U = 9\text{ J}$$

Chapter 8

Alternating Current

For deeper insight
Scan the QR Code

Learning Objectives

Module-I

- Types of Current
- Mean or Average Value of an Alternating Current
- Root Mean Square Value of an Alternating Current

Module-II

- Representation of *I* or *V* as Rotating Vectors-Phasors
- Different Types of AC Circuits
- AC Voltage Applied to a Series *L-C-R* Circuit

Module-III

- Power in AC Circuits
- Wattless Current

Module-IV

- Transformer
- Electric Generator or Dynamo

Chapter Overview with NEET Connection

This chapter is about generation and transmission of electric current and its properties. Concepts of this chapter are very important for NEET Exam.

Without gripping this chapter, it will be difficult to have strong hold on the concepts related to current and AC based devices. This chapter also helpful for the understanding of other chapter like electromagnetic induction, electronic devices etc.

Special format questions can be easily framed on the following topics of this chapter

- RMS values of current, voltage and power
- Calculation of Reactance, current in reactive circuits
- *L-C-R* circuits
- Resonance in *L-C-R* circuits
- Phasor diagram based solutions
- Power factor and wattless power
- AC generators

For better understanding of this chapter

- Knowledge of sin θ and cos θ functions from basic mathematics will be helpful.
- Knowledge of resultant of vectors will be helpful.
- Revision of resistors, capacitors and inductors is necessary.

Introduction

In previous chapters, we studied about storage of energy in electric and magnetic forms in capacitor and inductor respectively.

This chapter describes the process of transfer of this energy from one point to another point. In this chapter, we will study about representation of current and voltage in vector form, different types of circuit which can produce AC, wattless current and electric generators.

Module 1

Introduction to AC

- Types of Current
- Mean or Average Value of an Alternating Current
- Root Mean Square Value of an Alternating Current

Types of Current

There are two types of current which flows in any of the electrical appliances. These are as follows.

Direct Current (DC)

Current whose direction does not change with time through a load is known as direct current (DC) and this voltage is known as direct voltage (DC voltage). The graph given below shows that the direction of direct current (I) or voltage (V) does not change with time (t).

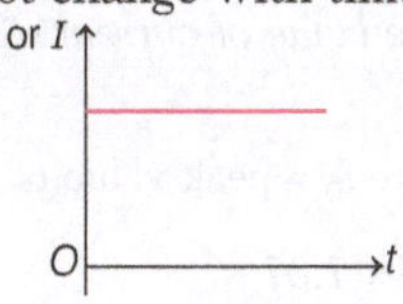

Voltage or current *versus* time graph for a DC

Alternating Current (AC)

Current whose direction changes periodically through a load is known as alternating current (AC) and the voltage is known as alternating voltage (AC voltage).

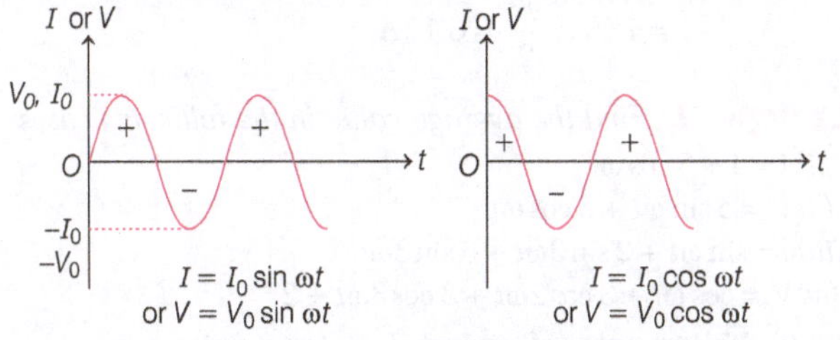

Voltage or current *versus* time graph of an AC

The instantaneous value of AC is given by

$$I = I_0 \sin\omega t$$

where, I = current at any instant t,

I_0 = maximum or peak value of AC

and ω = angular frequency.

Alternating emf or voltage

The instantaneous value of alternating emf or voltage is given by

$$V = V_0 \sin\omega t$$

where, V = voltage at any time t,

V_0 = maximum or peak value of alternating voltage

and ω = angular frequency.

Mentor's TIP

Alternating current, alternating voltage or emf, flux, etc., all are sinusoidal waves.

Some Definitions Related to Alternating Current or Voltage

(i) **Time period** The time taken to complete one cycle of variations is called time period or periodic time. It is given by the formula,

$$T = \frac{2\pi}{\omega}$$

where, 2π = angular displacement in a complete cycle

and ω = angular frequency.

(ii) **Frequency** The number of cycles completed per second by an alternating current is called its frequency and is denoted by f or ν.

$$f = \frac{1}{T} = \frac{\omega}{2\pi}$$

The frequency of AC in India is 50 Hz, *i.e.*

$$f = 50 \text{ Hz} = 50 \text{ cps}$$

or $\omega = 2\pi f \approx 314 \text{ rads}^{-1}$

(iii) **Peak value or amplitude** The maximum value of alternating current or alternating voltage is defined as peak value or amplitude. It is denoted by I_0 or V_0.

(iv) **Phase** Phase is a physical quantity representing both the instantaneous value and direction of alternating current at any instant. It is a dimensionless quantity and its unit is radian.
If $I = I_0 \sin(\omega t + \phi)$, then the argument of $\sin(\omega t + \phi)$ is called its phase.

(v) **Phase difference** The difference between the phases of current and voltage is called phase difference. If alternating voltage and current is given by the relation,

$$V = V_0 \sin(\omega t + \phi_1)$$

and $$I = I_0 \sin(\omega t + \phi_2)$$

Then, phase difference, $\phi = \phi_2 - \phi_1$ (relative to voltage)

and $\phi = \phi_1 - \phi_2$ (relative to current)

Some Important Points Related to Alternating Current

(i) An AC is produced by AC generator or AC dynamo and is represented by the symbol ⊝.

(ii) The AC is converted into DC with the help of rectifier while DC is converted into AC with the help of invertor.

(iii) It cannot produce electroplating or electrolysis.

(iv) It is measured with the help of 'hot wire ammeter'.

(v) An AC can be transmitted over long distances without much power loss.

(vi) In an AC (sinusoidal) current or voltage can have following four values.

(a) Instantaneous value

(b) Peak value (I_0 or V_0)

(c) rms value (I_{rms} or V_{rms})

(d) Average value

Mean or Average Value of an Alternating Current

Average or mean value of AC is defined as the value of direct current which sends the same amount of charge in a circuit in the same time as is sent by the given alternating current in its half-cycle (*i.e.*, $T/2$). It is denoted by I_{av} or I_m.

Let an alternating current be represented by $I = I_0 \sin \omega t$, where I_0 is the peak value. Clearly, the **mean value of the current over a complete cycle is zero.** It has no significance. Hence, the mean value of alternating current is defined as its average over half a cycle. For positive half cycle,

$$I_{mean} = \frac{1}{T/2} \int_0^{T/2} I \, dt$$

Putting $I = I_0 \sin \omega t$ and $T = (2\pi/\omega)$, we get

$$I_{mean} = \frac{2}{T} \int_0^{\pi/\omega} I_0 \sin \omega t \, dt = \frac{\omega}{\pi} \frac{I_0}{\omega} [-\cos \omega t]_0^{\pi/\omega}$$

$$= -\frac{I_0}{\pi} [\cos \pi - \cos 0] = -\frac{I_0}{\pi} [-1 - 1]$$

Thus, $$I_{mean} = \frac{2}{\pi} I_0 = 0.637 I_0 = 63.7\% \text{ of } I_0$$

[Mean current over positive half cycle]

In the same way, mean value of alternating emf,

$$E_{mean} = \frac{2E_0}{\pi} = 0.637 E_0 = 63.7\% \text{ of } E_0$$

Similarly, for negative half cycle the mean value of alternating current is $-2I_0/\pi$ and the average value of emf for negative half cycle is $-2E_0/\pi$.

Concept ladder Average values of some important expressions of current and voltage

- When $I = I_1 \sin \omega t + I_2 \cos \omega t$ and $V = V_1 \sin \omega t + V_2 \cos \omega t$ where I_1, I_2, V_1 and V_2 are constants, then $I_{av} = 0$ and $V_{av} = 0$
- Similarly, when $I = I_0 + I_1 \sin \omega t + I_2 \cos \omega t$ and $V = V_0 + V_1 \sin \omega t + V_2 \cos \omega t$ then $I_{av} = I_0$ and $V_{av} = V_0$

Example 1. *If the peak value of a current in 50Hz AC circuit is 7.07 A. What is the mean value of current over half a cycle and the value of current 1/300 s after it was zero?*

Sol. As, $I_m = \frac{2I_0}{\pi}$, where I_0 = peak value of current = 7.07A

$$\therefore \quad I_m = 0.637 \times 7.07 = 4.5\text{ A}$$

Also, at $t = \frac{1}{300}$ s

$$I = I_0 \sin \omega t = I_0 \sin 2\pi ft \qquad (\because \omega = 2\pi f)$$

$$\therefore \quad I = 7.07 \sin\left(2\pi \times 50 \times \frac{1}{300}\right) = 7.07 \sin \frac{\pi}{3}$$

$$= 7.07 \times \frac{\sqrt{3}}{2} = 6.12\text{ A}$$

Example 2. *Find the average value in the following cases*

(i) $i = 4 + 3\cos \omega t$

(ii) $V = 5 \sin \omega t + 3 \cos \omega t$

(iii) $i = \sin \omega t + 2 \sin 2\omega t + 3 \sin 3\omega t$

(iv) $V = \cos \omega t + 3 \cos 2\omega t + 3 \cos 3\omega t + 2$

Sol. (i) Average value of current, $I_{av} = I_0 = 4$ unit

(ii) Average value of voltage, $V_{av} = 0$

(iii) Average value of current, $I_{av} = 0$

(iv) Average value of voltage, $V_{av} = 2$ unit

Root Mean Square Value of an Alternating Current

It is defined as that value of a direct current which produces the same amount of heating effect in a given resistor as is produced by the given alternating current when passed for the same time during a complete cycle. It is denoted by I_{rms}, I_V or I_{eff}.

It is also called virtual value or effective value of AC.

Let instantaneous value of alternating current, $I = I_0 \sin \omega t$

If dH is small amount of heat produced in time dt in resistor R, then $dH = I^2R\,dt$. In complete cycle, the total heat produced is $\int dH = \int_0^T I^2R\,dt$

$$H = \int_0^T (I_0 \sin \omega t)^2 R\,dt$$

On solving, we get

$$H = \frac{I_0^2 RT}{2} \quad ...(i)$$

If I_{rms} is rms value of alternating current and H is the heat produced by rms current, then

$$H = I_{rms}^2 RT \quad ...(ii)$$

From Eqs. (i) and (ii), $I_{rms} = \frac{I_0}{\sqrt{2}}$

or $I_{rms} = 0.707 I_0$

or $I_{rms} = 70.7\%$ of I_0

In the same way, rms value of alternating emf

$$E_{rms} = \frac{E_0}{\sqrt{2}} = 0.707\,E_0 = 70.7\% \text{ of } E_0$$

AC ammeter and AC voltmeter always measure the virtual value of AC or alternating voltage. Also, the power supply which we are getting in our homes as 220 V AC is the rms voltage and its voltage amplitude is $V_0 = \sqrt{2} V_{rms} = 311$ V.

NEET Snapshot

Peak value of the AC source is $\sqrt{2}$ times of RMS value of the AC source. *[NEET 2022]*

The peak voltage only occurs twice in a cycle, once positive and once negative. The rest of the cycle, the voltage is less than the peak voltage.

Scan for Video

This is the reason why AC is more dangerous than DC as 311 V will cause more harm to the human body than 220 V DC. The different values I_0, I_{av} and I_{rms} are shown in figure below,

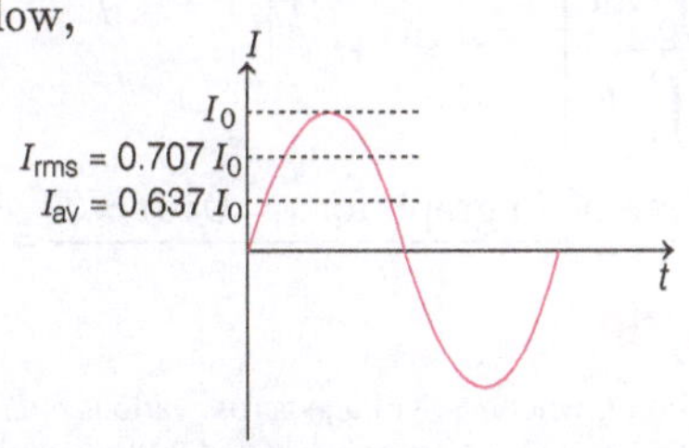

Peak, rms and average value on the same graph

Concept ladder

RMS values for some important expressions of current and voltage

- When $I = I_1 \sin \omega t + I_2 \cos \omega t$, where I_1 and I_2 are constant currents, then

$$I_{rms} = \sqrt{\frac{I_1^2}{2} + \frac{I_2^2}{2}}$$

Similarly, when $V = V_1 \sin \omega t + V_2 \cos \omega t$, where V_1 and V_2 are constant voltages, then

$$V_{rms} = \sqrt{\frac{V_1^2}{2} + \frac{V_2^2}{2}}$$

- When $I = I_0 + I_1 \sin \omega t + I_2 \cos \omega t$ and $V = V_0 + V_1 \sin \omega t + V_2 \cos \omega t$

$$I_{rms} = \sqrt{I_0^2 + \frac{I_1^2}{2} + \frac{I_2^2}{2}}$$

and $V_{rms} = \sqrt{V_0^2 + \frac{V_1^2}{2} + \frac{V_2^2}{2}}$

Example 3.

(i) The peak voltage of an AC supply is 300 V. What is the rms voltage?

(ii) The rms value of current in an AC circuit is 10 A. What is the peak current?

Sol. (i) Here, peak value of AC supply, $V_0 = 300$ V

$\therefore$ Using the relation, $V_{rms} = \frac{V_0}{\sqrt{2}}$

We get, $V_{rms} = \frac{300}{\sqrt{2}} = 212.1$ V

(ii) Let I_0 be the peak value of the current.

Here, I_{rms} = rms value of current = 10 A

Then, $I_{rms} = \frac{I_0}{\sqrt{2}}$

$\therefore$ $I_0 = \sqrt{2}\, I_{rms}$

$= 1.414 \times 10 = 14.14$ A

Example 4. *If $V = 220\sqrt{2} \sin(314t - \phi)$, calculate (i) peak and rms value of the voltage, (ii) average voltage for half time-period and (iii) frequency of AC.*

Sol. Given, $V = 220\sqrt{2} \sin(314t - \phi)$ ...(i)

Comparing with general equation, we get

(i) Peak voltage, $V_0 = 220\sqrt{2}$ V

rms voltage, $V_{rms} = \frac{V_0}{\sqrt{2}} = \frac{220\sqrt{2}}{\sqrt{2}} = 220$ V

(ii) Average voltage, $\bar{V} = \frac{2}{\pi} V_0 = \frac{2}{\pi} \times 220\sqrt{2} = \frac{440\sqrt{2}}{\pi}$ V

(iii) As, $\omega = 314$ rad s^{-1}

$\Rightarrow$ $\omega = 2\pi f = 314$

$\Rightarrow$ $f = 50$ Hz

Example 5. *If the current in an AC circuit is represented by the equation, $I = 5 \sin(300t - \pi/4)$*

Here, t is in second and I is in ampere. Calculate,

(i) peak and rms value of current,
(ii) frequency of AC,
(iii) and average current.

Sol. (i) Comparing the given equation with general equation, we have

$$I = I_0 \sin(\omega t \pm \phi)$$

$\therefore$ The peak value of current,

$$I_0 = 5\,\text{A}$$

and $$I_{rms} = \frac{I_0}{\sqrt{2}} = \frac{5}{\sqrt{2}} = 3.535\,\text{A}$$

(ii) Angular frequency,

$$\omega = 300\,\text{rads}^{-1}$$

$\therefore$ $$\nu = \frac{\omega}{2\pi} = \frac{300}{2\pi} \approx 47.75\,\text{Hz}$$

(iii) Average current, $I_{av} = \left(\frac{2}{\pi}\right) I_0 = \left(\frac{2}{\pi}\right)(5)$

$$= 3.18\,\text{A}$$

Example 6. *The voltage supplied to a circuit is given by $V = V_0 t^{3/2}$, where t is time in second. Find the rms value of voltage for the period, t = 0 to t = 1 s.*

Sol. The mean square voltage,

$$\overline{V^2} = \frac{1}{t}\int_0^t V^2 dt = \frac{1}{t}\int_0^1 V_0^2 t^3 dt$$

$$= \frac{V_0^2}{t}\left[\frac{t^4}{4}\right]_0^1 = \left[\frac{V_0^2 t^3}{4}\right]_0^1 = \frac{V_0^2}{4}$$

$\therefore$ $$V_{rms} = \sqrt{\overline{V^2}} = \frac{V_0}{2}$$

Calculation of Mean and RMS Value for Some Specific Cases of Alternating Current

Sinusoidal Waveform

(i) $I_{rms} = \frac{I_0}{\sqrt{2}}$

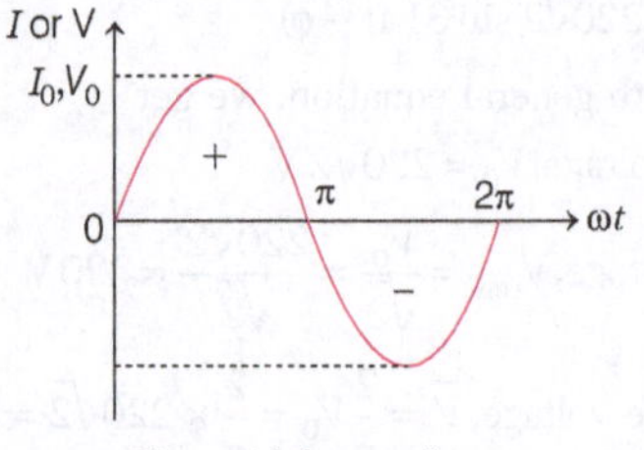

Sinusoidal waveform

(ii) $I_{av} = \frac{2I_0}{\pi}$, for half-cycle

$I_{av} = 0$, for one complete cycle

Square or Rectangular Waveform

(i) $I_{rms} = I_0$, for one complete cycle

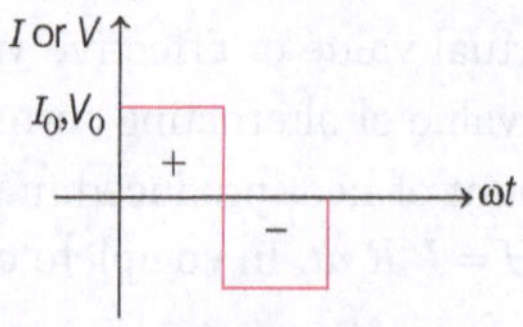

Square or rectangular waveform

(ii) $I_{av} = I_0$, for half-cycle

$I_{av} = 0$, for one complete cycle

Half-Wave Rectified

(i) $I_{rms} = \frac{I_0}{2}$, for one complete cycle

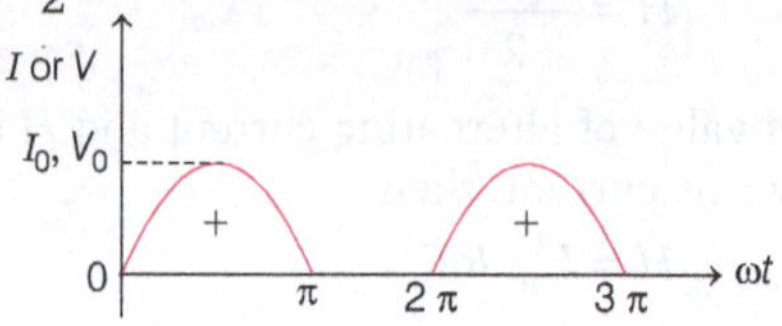

Half-wave rectified waveform

(ii) $I_{av} = \frac{I_0}{\pi}$, for one complete cycle

$I_{av} = \frac{2I_0}{\pi}$, for half-cycle

Full Wave Rectified

(i) $I_{rms} = \frac{I_0}{\sqrt{2}}$, for one complete cycle

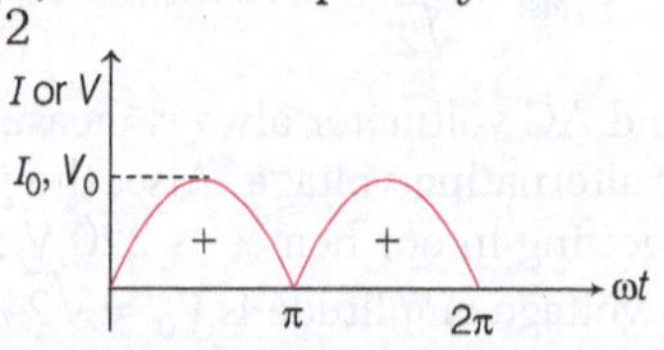

Full wave rectified waveform

(ii) $I_{av} = \frac{2I_0}{\pi}$

For a Current Varying Wave as Shown in the Graph

(i) $$I_{rms} = \left[\frac{\int_0^T I^2 dt}{\int_0^T dt}\right]^{1/2} = \frac{I_0}{\sqrt{3}}$$

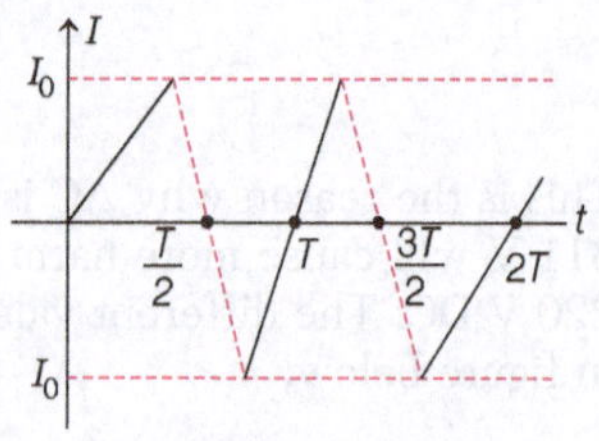

(ii) $$I_{av} = \left[\frac{\int_0^T I dt}{\int_0^T dt}\right]$$

$$= \frac{\text{Area of } I\text{-}t \text{ graph for } t = 0 \text{ to } t = T}{T} = \frac{I_0}{2}$$

Mentor's TIP

- In L-C-R circuit, whenever voltage across various elements is asked, always calculate rms values unless stated in the question for the peak or instantaneous value.

STEP UP Practice 1

1. Alternating current is transmitted to take place
   (a) at high voltage and low current
   (b) at high voltage and high current
   (c) at low voltage and low current
   (d) at low voltage and high current

2. An alternating current in a circuit is given by $I = 20 \sin(100\pi t + 0.05\pi)$ A. The rms value and the frequency of current respectively, are
   (a) 10 A and 100 Hz (b) 10 A and 50 Hz
   (c) $10\sqrt{2}$ A and 50 Hz (d) $10\sqrt{2}$ A and 100 Hz

3. If an alternating voltage is represented as $E = 141 \sin(628t)$V then the rms value of the voltage and the frequency are respectively
   (a) 141V, 628 Hz (b) 100 V, 50 Hz
   (c) 100 V, 100 Hz (d) 141 V, 100 Hz

4. **Assertion (A)** AC is more dangerous than DC.
   Reason (R) Frequency of AC is dangerous for human body.
   In the light of the above statements, choose the correct answer from the options given below.
   (a) Both A and R are true but R is not the correct explanation of A.
   (b) A is true but R is false.
   (c) A is false but R is true.
   (d) Both A and R are true and R is the correct explanation of A.

5. The peak value of an alternating current is 5 A and its frequency is 60 Hz. Find its rms value and time taken to reach the peak value of current starting from zero.
   (a) 3.536 A, 4.167 ms (b) 3.536 A, 15 ms
   (c) 6.07 A, 10 ms (d) 2.536 A, 4.167 ms

6. An alternating current of rms value 10 A is passed through a 12 Ω resistor. The maximum potential difference across the resistor is
   (a) 20 V (b) 90 V
   (c) 169.70 V (d) None of these

7. The instantaneous current in an AC circuit is $I = \sqrt{2} \sin(50t + \pi/4)$. The rms value of current is
   (a) $\sqrt{2}$ A (b) 50 A (c) 90 A (d) 1 A

8. 220 V, 50 Hz, AC is applied to a resistor. The instantaneous value of voltage is
   (a) $220\sqrt{2}\sin 100\pi t$ (b) $220\sin 100\pi t$
   (c) $220\sqrt{2}\sin 50\pi t$ (d) $220\sin 50\pi t$

9. **Assertion (A)** Average value of AC over a complete cycle is always zero.
   Reason (R) Average value of AC is always defined over half cycle.
   In the light of the above statements, choose the correct answer from the options given below.
   (a) Both A and R are true but R is not the correct explanation of A.
   (b) A is true but R is false.
   (c) A is false but R is true.
   (d) Both A and R are true and R is the correct explanation of A.

10. Which one of the following current given below is correct pair about alternating current?
    (a) $I_{mean} \rightarrow 70.7\%$ of I_0
    (b) $E_{mean} \rightarrow 63.7\%$ of E_0
    (c) $I_{rms} \rightarrow \sqrt{2}\, I_0$
    (d) $E_{rms} \rightarrow 63.7\%$ of E_0

11. A 220 V AC is more dangerous than 220 V DC because
    (a) peak voltage of DC is much larger than 220 V
    (b) the DC repels
    (c) the body offers less resistance to AC
    (d) peak voltage for AC is much larger than 220 V

12. **Assertion** (A) If the frequency of alternating current in an AC circuit consisting of an inductance coil is increased then current gets decreased.
    Reason (R) The current is inversely proportional to frequency of alternating current.
    In the light of the above statements, choose the correct answer from the options given below.
    (a) Both A and R are true but R is not the correct explanation of A.
    (b) A is true but R is false.
    (c) A is false but R is true.
    (d) Both A and R are true and R is the correct explanation of A.

13. Frequency of AC mains in India is
    (a) 30 Hz (b) 50 Hz (c) 60 Hz (d) 120 Hz

14. The frequency of a sinusoidal wave $E = 0.40 \cos[2000t + 0.80]$ would be
    (a) 1000 π Hz (b) 2000 Hz
    (c) 20 Hz (d) $1000/\pi$ Hz

15. **Assertion (A)** An alternating current does not show any magnetic effect.
    Reason (R) Alternating current varies with time.
    In the light of the above statements, choose the correct answer from the options given below.
    (a) Both A and R are true but R is not the correct explanation of A.
    (b) A is true but R is false.
    (c) A is false but R is true.
    (d) Both A and R are true and R is the correct explanation of A.

16. An alternating voltage given as, $V = 100\sqrt{2}\sin 100t$ V is applied to a capacitor of 1 μF. The current reading of the ammeter will be equal to .... mA.
    (a) 20 (b) 10 (c) 40 (d) 80

17. The electric current in AC circuit is given by the relation $i = 3\sin\omega t + 4\cos\omega t$. The rms value of the current in the circuit (in ampere) is
    (a) $\frac{5}{\sqrt{2}}$ (b) $5\sqrt{2}$
    (c) $\frac{\sqrt{2}}{5}$ (d) $\frac{1}{\sqrt{2}}$

Module 2

AC Circuits

- Representation of I or V as Rotating Vectors-Phasors
- Different Types of AC Circuits
- AC Voltage Applied to a Series L-C-R Circuit

Representation of I or V as Rotating Vectors-Phasors

To simplify the study of AC circuit, alternating quantities (*i.e.* I or V) are represented as rotating vectors, with the angle between the vectors equal to the phase difference between the current and emf or voltage. These rotating vectors representing current and alternating voltage are called **phasors**.

Some important points regarding phasors are as follows

- The length of the vector represents the maximum or peak value, *i.e.* I_0 and V_0.
- The projection of the vector on fixed axis gives the instantaneous value of alternating current and alternating emf.

  If $I = I_0 \sin\omega t$ and $V = V_0 \sin\omega t$, projection is taken on Y-axis. If $I = I_0 \cos\omega t$ and $V = V_0 \cos\omega t$, projection is taken on X-axis.
- A phasor is a geometric entity and not a real physical quantity that helps us to describe and analyse physical quantities that vary sinusoidally with time.
- A diagram representing alternating current and alternating emf (of same frequency) as rotating vectors (phasors) with the phase angle between them is called **phasor diagram.**

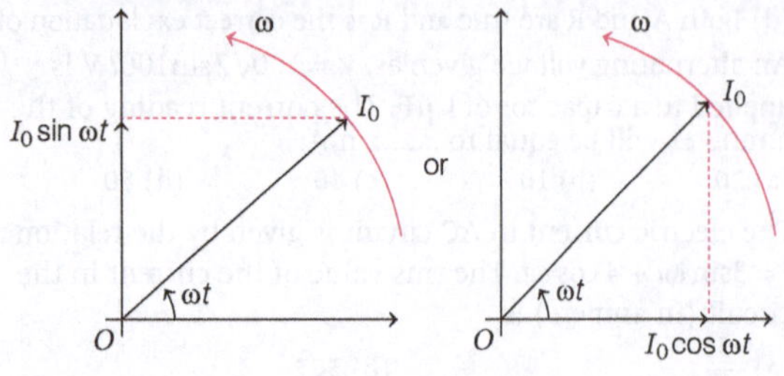

Phasor diagram

Different Types of AC Circuits

In this section, we will derive voltage-current relations for individual as well as combined circuit elements carrying a sinusoidal current. We will consider resistors, inductors and capacitors.

1. AC Voltage Applied to a Resistor (Resistive circuit or R-circuit)

Suppose a resistor of resistance R is connected to an AC source of emf with instantaneous value (E) is given by

$$E = E_0 \sin\omega t \quad \text{...(i)}$$

Variation of Resistance with Frequency of Source

Figure given below shows the graph of R as a function of angular frequency ω. The resistance R, does not depend upon angular frequency of the source.

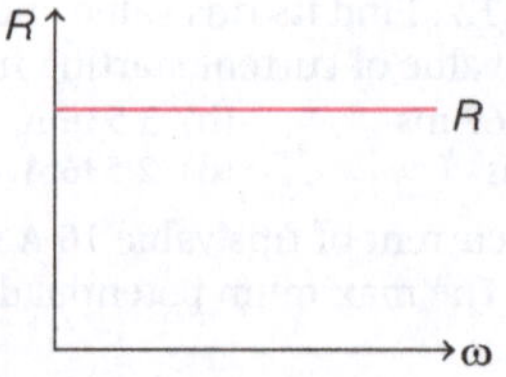

R remains constant with ω or f

Suppose E is the potential drop across resistance (R), then

$$E = IR \quad \text{...(ii)}$$

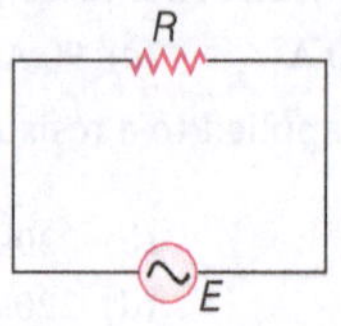

AC voltage applied to a resistor

Instantaneous emf = Instantaneous value of potential drop

∴ From Eqs. (i) and (ii), we have

$$IR = E = E_0 \sin\omega t$$

$$\text{or} \quad I = \frac{E}{R} = \frac{E_0 \sin\omega t}{R}$$

$$I = I_0 \sin\omega t \qquad \left(\because I_0 = \frac{E_0}{R}\right) \quad \text{...(iii)}$$

Comparing $I_0 = E_0 / R$ with Ohm's law, we find that resistors work equally well for both AC and DC voltages. From Eqs. (i) and (iii), we get that there is zero phase difference between instantaneous alternating current and instantaneous alternating emf (*i.e.* they are in same phase).

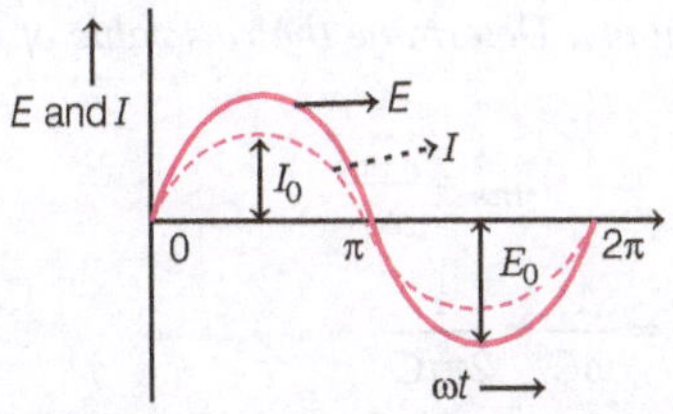

E and *I versus* ω*t* graph of a resistive circuit

Phasor Diagram

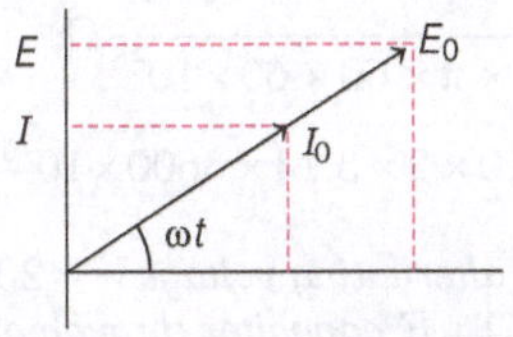

Phasor diagram for a purely resistive circuit

Here, peak values E_0 and I_0 are represented by vectors rotating with angular velocity ω with respect to horizontal reference. Their projections on vertical axis give their instantaneous values.

Example 7. *A 200 Ω resistor is connected to a 220 V, 50 Hz AC supply. Calculate rms value of current in the circuit. Also, find phase difference between voltage and the current.*

Sol. Given, $V_{rms} = 220$ V, $f = 50$ Hz, $R = 200\,\Omega$

Current in the purely resistive AC circuit, $I = \dfrac{V}{R}$

∴ rms value of current,

$$I_{rms} = \frac{V_{rms}}{R} = \frac{220}{200} = 1.1 \text{ A}$$

In purely resistive AC circuit, current and voltage are in phase. Therefore, phase difference is zero.

2. AC Voltage Applied to a Capacitor (Capacitive circuit or *C*-circuit)

Let us consider a capacitor with capacitance *C* be connected to an AC source with emf having instantaneous value.

$$E = E_0 \sin\omega t \quad \text{...(i)}$$

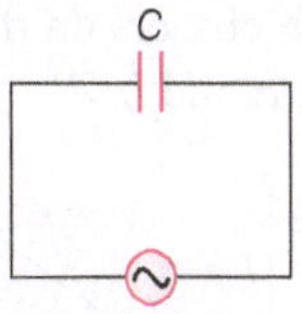

An AC source connected to a capacitor

Due to this emf, charge will be produced and it will charge the plates of capacitor with positive and negative charge. If potential difference across the plates of capacitor is *V*, then

$$V = \frac{q}{C} \text{ or } q = CV$$

The instantaneous value of current in the circuit,

$$I = \frac{dq}{dt} = \frac{d}{dt}(CE) \qquad (\because V = E)$$

$$= \frac{d}{dt}(CE_0 \sin\omega t) \qquad (\because E = E_0 \sin\omega t)$$

$$= CE_0 \cos\omega t \times \omega$$

$$= \frac{E_0}{1/\omega C}\cos\omega t$$

$$\Rightarrow \quad I = \frac{E_0}{1/\omega C}\sin(\omega t + \pi/2) \quad \text{...(ii)}$$

$[\because \cos\omega t = \sin(\pi/2 + \omega t)]$

I will be maximum when $\sin(\omega t + \pi/2) = 1$, so that $I = I_0$

where, peak value of current, $I_0 = \dfrac{E_0}{1/\omega C}$

$$\therefore \quad \boxed{I = I_0 \sin(\omega t + \pi/2)} \quad \text{...(iii)}$$

From Eqs. (i) and (iii), it is clear that in a perfect capacitor, the current leads the voltage by a phase angle of π/2 (90°) or the voltage lags behind the current by a phase angle of π/2 (90°).

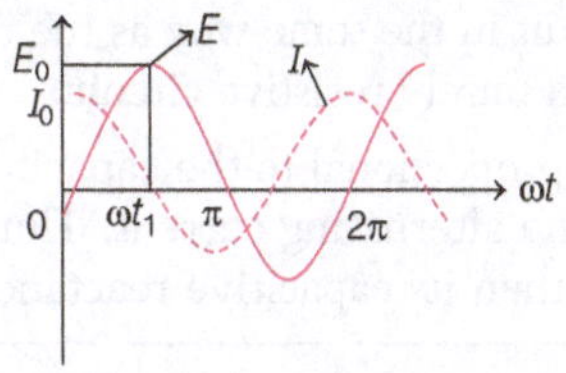

E and *I versus* ω*t* graph of a capacitive circuit

Phasor Diagram

The phase representing peak emf E_0 makes an angle ω*t* in anti-clockwise direction with respect to horizontal axis. As current leads the voltage by 90°, the phasor representing I_0 is turned 90° anti-clockwise with the phasor representing E_0.

The projections of these phasors on the vertical axis give instantaneous values of E and I.

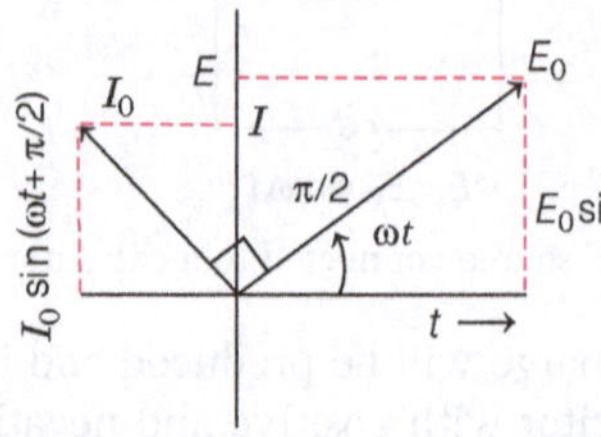

Phasor diagram for purely capacitive circuit

Mentor's TIP

In pure capacitive circuits, current leads voltage by $\frac{\pi}{2}$ phase.

Capacitive Reactance (X_C)

Instantaneous value of alternating current through a capacitor is given by

$$I = \frac{E_0}{1/\omega C} \sin (\omega t + \pi/2) = I_0 \sin\left(\omega t + \frac{\pi}{2}\right)$$

Comparing with Ohm's law, we get $I_0 = \dfrac{E_0}{1/\omega C}$

$$X_C = \frac{1}{\omega C}$$

where, X_C is called capacitive reactance.

The opposing nature of capacitor to the flow of alternating current is called **capacitive reactance.**

If f is the frequency of the alternating current, then

$$X_C = \frac{1}{2\pi f C}$$

The dimensions of capacitive reactance are same as that of resistance and its SI unit is ohm (Ω). The capacitive reactance limits the amplitude of the current in a purely capacitive circuit in the same way as the resistance limits the current in a purely resistive circuit.

It is inversely proportional to the capacitance and frequency of the alternating current. Thus, if frequency of AC increases, then its capacitive reactance decreases.

Concept ladder When capacitor is connected to DC source,

$$X_C = \frac{1}{\omega C} = \frac{1}{0} = \infty$$

($\because$ For DC, $\omega = 2\pi f = 0$, as $f = 0$)

Thus, capacitor blocks DC and acts as open circuit while passing AC of high frequency.

Variation of Capacitive Reactance with Frequency

The graph of X_C as function of angular frequency ω or frequency f can be drawn as

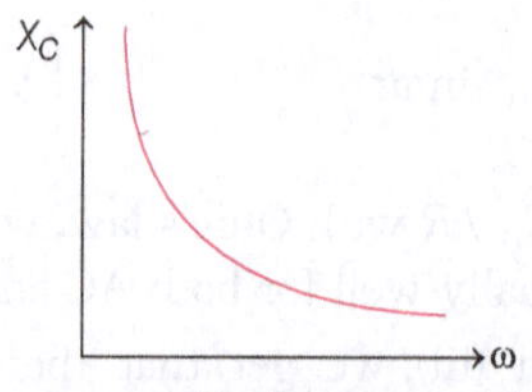

Capacitive reactance X_C decreases with frequency

Example 8. *A 60 μF capacitor is connected to a 110 V, 60 Hz AC supply. Determine the rms value of the current in the circuit.*

Sol. As, $I_{rms} = \dfrac{V_{rms}}{X_C}$

where, $X_C = \dfrac{1}{\omega C} = \dfrac{1}{2\pi f C}$

Here, $C = 60\,\mu F = 60 \times 10^{-6}\,F$,

$V_{rms} = 110\,V$, $f = 60\,Hz$

So, $X_C = \dfrac{1}{2 \times \pi \times 60 \times 60 \times 10^{-6}}\,\Omega$

$\therefore$ $I_{rms} = 110 \times 2 \times 3.14 \times 3600 \times 10^{-6} = 2.49\,A$

Example 9. *An alternating voltage $V = 200\sqrt{2} \sin (100t) V$ is connected to a 1 μF capacitor through an AC ammeter. What will be the reading of the ammeter?*

Sol. Consider the purely capacitive circuit as shown below.

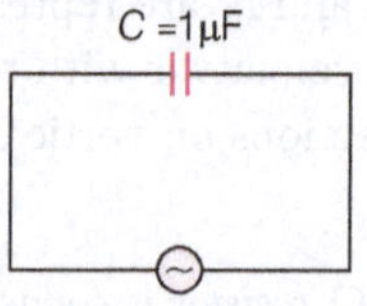

Given, $V = 200\sqrt{2} \sin (100\,t)\,V$

Comparing it with general equation, $V = V_0 \sin (\omega t)$

we get, $V_0 = 200\sqrt{2}\,V$, $\omega = 100\,rad\,s^{-1}$

$\therefore$ Reactance, $X_C = \dfrac{1}{\omega C} = \dfrac{1}{100 \times 10^{-6}} = 10^4\,\Omega$

Peak value of current, $I_0 = \dfrac{V_0}{X_C} = \dfrac{200\sqrt{2}}{10^4} = 2\sqrt{2} \times 10^{-2}\,A$

rms value of current, $I_{rms} = \dfrac{I_0}{\sqrt{2}} = \dfrac{2\sqrt{2} \times 10^{-2}}{\sqrt{2}}$

$= 20 \times 10^{-3}\,A = 20\,mA$

Reading of the ammeter will be same as, $I_{rms} = 20$ mA.

Mentor's TIP

- Treat Reactance as resistance while solving numericals.
- Please note that voltage and current do not reach to their peak values at the same time due to phase difference.

3. AC Voltage Applied to an Inductor (Inductive Circuit or L-Circuit)

Suppose an inductor with self-inductance (L) is connected to AC source with instantaneous emf (E) is given by

$$E = E_0 \sin\omega t \qquad \text{...(i)}$$

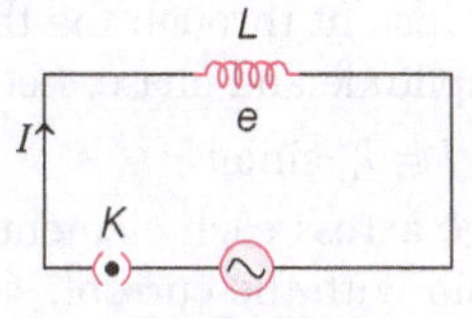

$E = E_0 \sin \omega t$

An AC source connected to an inductor

When key is closed, then current begins to grow because magnetic flux linked with it changes and an emf is induced which opposes the applied emf.

According to Lenz's law,

$$e = -L\frac{dI}{dt}$$

where, e is induced emf and $\frac{dI}{dt}$ is the rate of change of current.

To maintain the flow of current in the circuit, applied voltage must be equal and opposite to the induced emf.

$$E = -e$$

$$\therefore \qquad E = -\left(-\frac{LdI}{dt}\right) = \frac{LdI}{dt} \quad \text{or} \quad dI = \frac{E}{L}dt$$

Integrating the above equation on both sides, we get

$$\int dI = \int \frac{E}{L}dt$$

$$I = \int \frac{E_0 \sin\omega t}{L}dt \qquad [\because E = E_0 \sin\omega t]$$

$$\Rightarrow \qquad I = \frac{E_0}{L}\left[\frac{-\cos\omega t}{\omega}\right] = -\frac{E_0}{\omega L}\cos\omega t$$

$$\Rightarrow \qquad I = -\frac{E_0}{\omega L}\sin(\pi/2 - \omega t)$$

$$\left[\because \sin\left(\frac{\pi}{2} - \omega t\right) = \cos\omega t\right]$$

$$\Rightarrow \qquad I = \frac{E_0}{\omega L}\sin(\omega t - \pi/2) \qquad \text{...(ii)}$$

If $\quad \sin(\omega t - \pi/2) = \text{maximum} = 1$, then $I = I_0$

where, peak value of current, $I_0 = \dfrac{E_0}{\omega L}$

$$\Rightarrow \qquad \boxed{I = I_0 \sin(\omega t - \pi/2)} \qquad \text{...(iii)}$$

From Eqs. (i) and (iii), it is clear that in a pure inductor, the current lags behind the voltage by a phase angle of $\pi/2$ (90°) or the voltage leads the current by a phase angle of $\pi/2$ (90°).

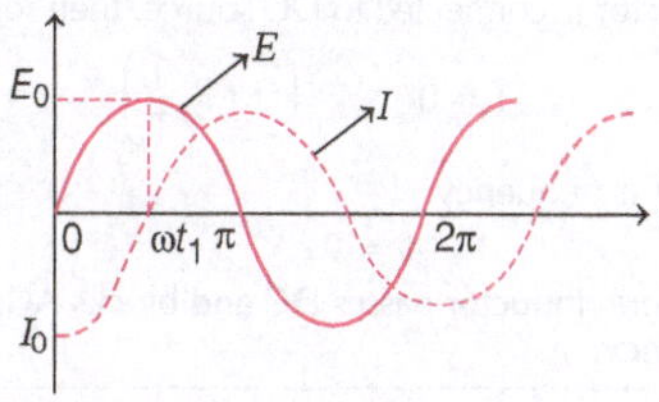

E and I *versus* ωt graph of an inductive circuit

Phasor Diagram

The phasor representing peak emf E_0 makes an angle ωt in anti-clockwise direction from horizontal axis. As current lags behind the voltage by 90°, so the phasor representing I_0 is turned 90° clockwise with the direction of E_0.

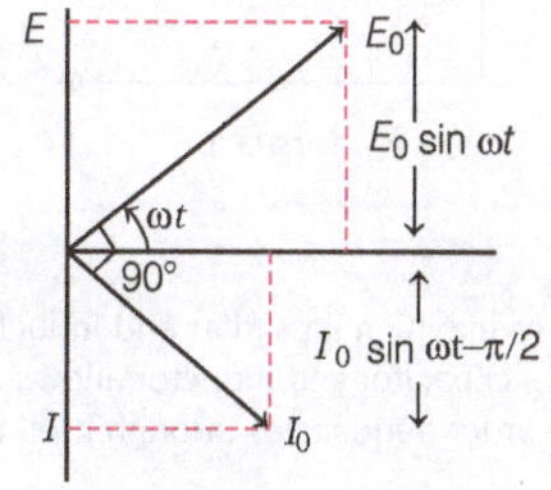

Phasor diagram for purely inductive circuit

Inductive Reactance (X_L)

The opposing nature of inductor to the flow of current is called **inductive reactance.**

As, $\qquad I = \dfrac{E_0}{\omega L}\sin(\omega t - \pi/2)$ or $I_0 = E_0/\omega L$

Comparing with Ohm's law, $I_0 = \dfrac{E_0}{R}$. The quantity ωL is analogous to the resistance and is denoted by X_L.

So, $\qquad X_L = \omega L$

X_L is called inductive reactance.

If f is the frequency of AC source, then

$$\boxed{X_L = \omega L = 2\pi f L} \qquad \left(\because \omega = \frac{2\pi}{T} = 2\pi f\right)$$

The dimensions of inductive reactance are same as that of resistance and its SI unit is ohm (Ω). The inductive reactance limits the current in a purely inductive circuit in the same way as the resistance limits the current in a purely resistive circuit.

Concept ladder The inductive reactance is directly proportional to the inductance and to the frequency of the AC current.

Thus, if the frequency of AC increases, its inductive reactance also increases.

If inductor is connected to DC source, then for DC,

$$f = 0 \qquad \left(\because f = \frac{1}{T}\right)$$

Here, f is frequency.

$$\therefore \qquad X_L = 0$$

Therefore, inductor passes DC and blocks AC of very high frequency.

Variation of Inductive Reactance with Frequency

The graph of X_L as function of angular frequency ω can be drawn as shown below. Clearly, X_L linearly increases with ω.

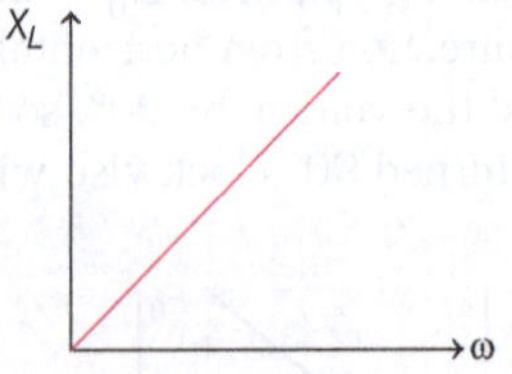

X_L *versus* ω

Mentor's TiP

- Capacitor behaves like high pass filter and inductor behaves like low pass filter i.e. capacitor and inductor allows to pass higher order and lower order frequencies through itself respectively.

Example 10. *An ideal inductor of inductance 50 μH is connected to an AC source of 220 V, 50 Hz. Find the inductive reactance.*

Sol. As inductive reactance, $X_L = \omega L = 2\pi f L$

where, L is inductance $= 50\,\mu\text{H} = 50 \times 10^{-6}$ H

and $\quad f =$ source frequency $= 50$ Hz

$$\therefore \; X_L = 2 \times \pi \times 50 \times 50 \times 10^{-6}$$
$$= 2\pi \times 25 \times 10^{-4}\,\Omega$$
$$= 5\pi \times 10^{-3}\,\Omega$$
$$= 5\pi\,\text{m}\Omega$$

Example 11. *A 44 mH inductor is connected to 220 V, 50 Hz AC supply. Determine the rms value of the current in the circuit.*

Sol. As, $I_{\text{rms}} = \dfrac{V_{\text{rms}}}{X_L}$

where, $X_L = \omega L = 2\pi f L$ is the reactance of the inductor.

Here, $f = 50$ Hz,

$$L = 44\text{mH} = 44 \times 10^{-3}\text{H},$$
$$V_{\text{rms}} = 220\text{V}$$
$$\therefore \quad X_L = 2\pi \times 50 \times 44 \times 10^{-3} = 13.82\ \Omega$$
$$\therefore \quad \text{RMS value of current, } I_{\text{rms}} = \frac{220}{13.82} = 15.9\text{A}$$

AC Voltage Applied to a Series *L-C-R* Circuit

Suppose that an inductor (L), capacitor (C) and resistor (R) are connected in series to an AC source. I is the current passed through this circuit. As R, L, C are in series, therefore at any instant through the three elements, AC has the same amplitude and phase. Let it be represented by

$$I = I_0 \sin\omega t$$

However, voltage across each element bears a different phase relationship with the current.

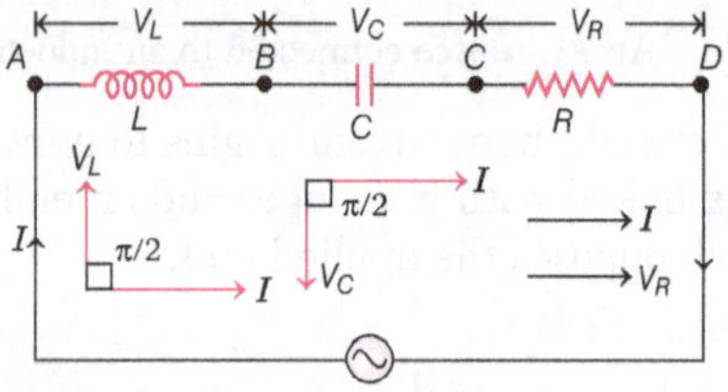

AC source, $E = E_0 \sin \omega t$

An AC source connected to series *L-C-R* circuit

$V_L = I_0 X_L$ (V_L is maximum voltage across L)

$V_C = I_0 X_C$ (V_C is maximum voltage across C)

$V_R = I_0 R$ (V_R is maximum voltage across R)

Inside phasor diagrams of each L, C and R are given. To form phasor diagram for series *L-C-R* circuit, combine all these phasor diagrams.

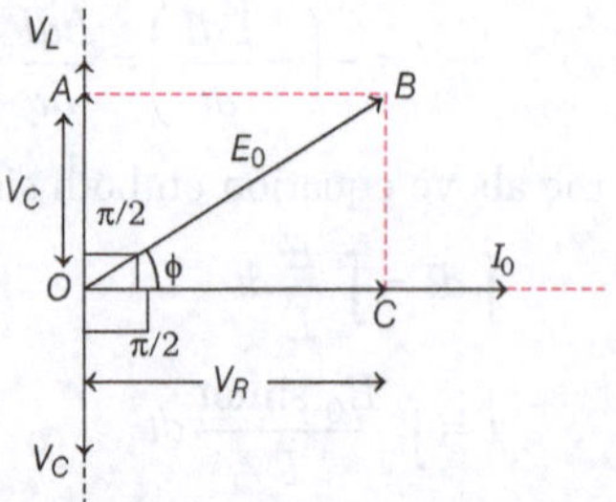

Phasor diagram of a series *L-C-R* circuit

Since, voltage (V_L) is in upward direction and voltage (V_C) in downward direction, so net voltage upto point A is ($V_L - V_C$) (assuming $V_L > V_C$) and net maximum voltage is E_0.

From phasor diagram,

$$OB = \sqrt{(OC)^2 + (CB)^2} = \sqrt{V_R^2 + (V_L - V_C)^2}$$

$$E_0 = \sqrt{(I_0 R)^2 + (I_0 X_L - I_0 X_C)^2} \qquad [\because OB = E_0]$$

$$E_0 = I_0\sqrt{R^2 + (X_L - X_C)^2}$$

$$\therefore \qquad Z = \frac{E_0}{I_0} = \sqrt{R^2 + (X_L - X_C)^2}$$

Here, Z is called **impedance**.

Impedance

It is the total resistance of a circuit, applied in the path of alternating current. It is given by

$$Z=\sqrt{R^2+(X_L-X_C)^2}$$

From phasor diagram, it is clear that voltage leads the current by angle ϕ.

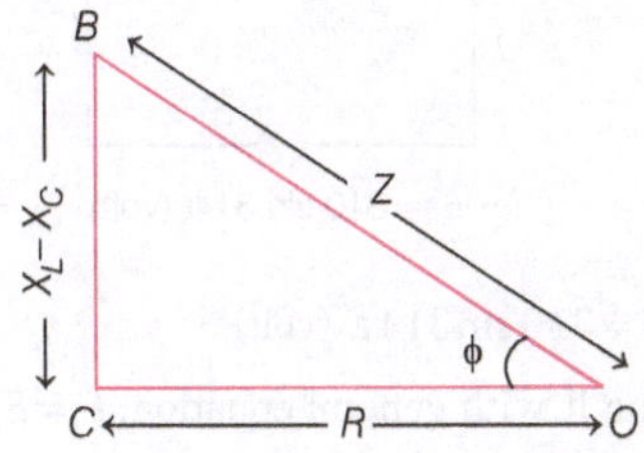

Impedance triangle of an *L-C-R* circuit

$\therefore$ From ΔOCB,

$$\tan\phi = \frac{CB}{OC} = \frac{V_L - V_C}{V_R}$$

$$= \frac{I_0X_L - I_0X_C}{I_0R}$$

$$\tan\phi = \frac{X_L - X_C}{R}$$

$\therefore$ The alternating emf in the series *L-C-R* circuit would be represented by $E = E_0 \sin(\omega t + \phi)$.

Special Cases

(i) When $X_L = X_C$,

$\therefore \quad Z = R$

and $\tan\phi = 0 \qquad (\because \phi = 0°)$

Hence, voltage and current are in the same phase. The AC circuit is non-inductive or resistive circuit.

(ii) When $X_L > X_C$, then $\tan\phi$ is positive.

Hence, voltage leads the current by a phase angle ϕ. The AC circuit is inductive circuit.

(iii) When $X_C > X_L$, then $\tan\phi$ is negative.

Hence, voltage lags behind the current by a phase angle ϕ. The AC circuit is capacitive circuit.

The variation of Z with frequency ω

At $\omega = \omega_0$, $X_L = X_C$, $Z = R$ = minimum.

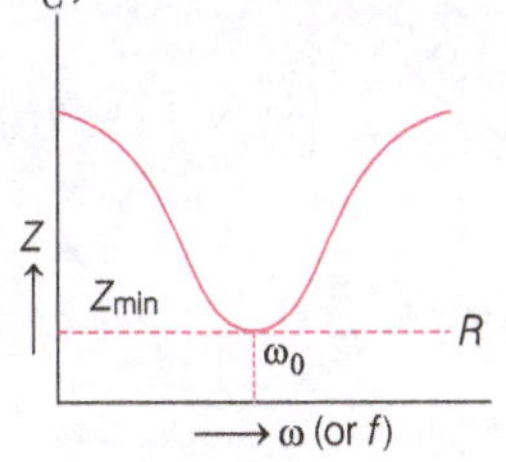

Z versus ω for a series *L-C-R* circuit

Concept ladder **Reduction of *L-C-R* circuit to *L-C*, *R-C*, *L-R* circuit**

The general formula of *L-C-R* series circuit can be reduced to apply it on *L-C*, *R-C*, *L-R*, circuit.

For *L-C-R* circuit, impedance $Z = \sqrt{R^2 + (X_L - X_C)^2}$

- ***L-C* circuit**

For *L-C* circuit, there is no *R*, so, we can ignore terms related to *R*.

$\therefore$ For *L-C* circuit, $Z = \sqrt{(X_L - X_C)^2}$ or $(X_L - X_C)$

(i) If $X_L > X_C$, then circuit will behave like pure inductive circuit and voltage will lead the current by $\pi/2$.

(ii) If $X_L < X_C$, then circuit will behave like pure capacitive circuit and voltage will lag behind the current by $\pi/2$.

(iii) If $X_L = X_C$, then $Z = R$ in this condition current in the circuit will be maximum.

- ***R-C* circuit**

For *R-C* circuit, there is no *L*, so we can ignore the term related to *L*.

$\therefore$ For *R-C* circuit, $Z = \sqrt{R^2 + X_C^2}$

The phase difference between current and emf,

$$\tan\phi = \frac{X_C}{R}$$

Here, the current leads the voltage by ϕ.

$\therefore \quad I = I_0 \sin(\omega t + \phi)$

- ***L-R* circuit**

In *L-R* circuit, there is no C, so we can ignore the term related to C.

$\therefore$ For *L-R* circuit, $Z = \sqrt{R^2 + X_L^2}$

The phase difference between current and emf,

$\tan\phi = X_L/R$

Here, the emf leads the current by ϕ.

$\therefore \quad I = I_0 \sin(\omega t - \phi)$

Example 12. *A 100 Ω resistance is connected in series with a 4 H inductor. The voltage across the resistor is $V_R = (2.0V)\sin(10^3 rads^{-1})t$.*

(i) Find the expression of circuit current.

(ii) Find the inductive reactance.

(iii) Derive an expression for the voltage across the inductor.

Sol. (i) Current in the circuit, $I = \frac{V_R}{R} = \frac{(2.0\text{ V})\sin(10^3 \text{ rad s}^{-1})t}{100}$

$$= (2.0\times 10^{-2}\text{ A})\sin(10^3\text{ rad s}^{-1})t$$

(ii) Inductive reactance, $X_L = \omega L = (10^3\text{ rad s}^{-1})(4\text{ H})$

$$= 4.0\times 10^3\,\Omega$$

(iii) The amplitude of voltage across inductor,

$$V_0 = I_0X_L = (2.0\times 10^{-2}\text{ A})(4.0\times 10^3\,\Omega) = 80\text{ V}$$

In an AC circuit, voltage across the inductor leads the current by 90° or $\frac{\pi}{2}$ rad. Hence,

$$V_L = V_0\sin\left(\omega t + \frac{\pi}{2}\right)$$

$$= (80\text{ V})\sin\left\{(10^3\text{ rad s}^{-1})t + \frac{\pi}{2}\text{ rad}\right\}$$

Mentor's TiP

- The amplitude of voltage across the resistor (= 2.0 V) is not same as the amplitude of the voltage across the inductor (= 80 V), even though the amplitude of the current through both elements is the same.

Example 13. *A long solenoid connected to a 12 V DC source passes a steady current of 2 A. When the solenoid is connected to an AC source of 12 V at 50 Hz, the current flowing is 1 A. Calculate inductance of the solenoid.*

Sol. Remember that the solenoid mentioned here is not just a solenoid but has the resistance also due to its wire material. Now, in DC, the solenoid doesn't offer any reactance after a few milliseconds, however in the beginning it offers infinite resistance. So, the current by a DC source into an inductor is, $I = \dfrac{V}{R}$

or $R = \dfrac{12}{2} = 6\,\Omega$

But when an AC source is connected to the same inductor, the reactance will also come into picture.

So, $I = \dfrac{V}{\sqrt{R^2 + \omega^2 L^2}}$

Here, $I = 1\text{ A}, V = 12\text{ V}, R = 6\,\Omega$

$\omega = 100\,\pi \text{ rads}^{-1}, L = ?$

or $1 = \dfrac{12}{\sqrt{6^2 + (100\,\pi L)^2}} \Rightarrow L = 33\text{ mH}$

Example 14. *A circuit containing of a capacitor and an active resistance $R = 110\,\Omega$ connected in series is fed an alternating voltage with amplitude $V_0 = 110$ V. In this case, the amplitude of current is equal to $I_0 = 0.50$ A. Find the phase difference between the current and the voltage fed.*

Sol. Consider an RC circuit as shown below.

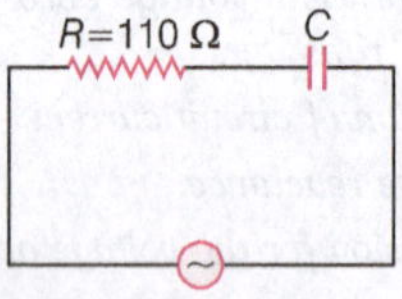

$V_0 = 110$V

Given, $I_0 = 0.50\text{ A}$

$\therefore \quad I_0 = \dfrac{V_0}{Z} \Rightarrow 0.5 = \dfrac{110}{Z} \Rightarrow Z = 220\,\Omega$

$\because \quad Z^2 = R^2 + X_C^2 \Rightarrow (220)^2 = (110)^2 + X_C^2$

$\Rightarrow \quad X_C^2 = (220)^2 - (110)^2 = 330 \times 110$

$\Rightarrow \quad X_C = 110\sqrt{3}\,\Omega$

Now we can write,

$$\tan\phi = \frac{X_C}{R} = \frac{110\sqrt{3}}{110} = \sqrt{3} \Rightarrow \phi = 60^\circ$$

Example 15. *A coil of inductance 0.01 H is connected in series with a capacitor of capacitance 25 μF with an AC source whose emf is given by $E = 310 \sin 314t$ V. What is the reactance of the circuit?*

Sol. Consider a series *L-C* circuit as shown below.

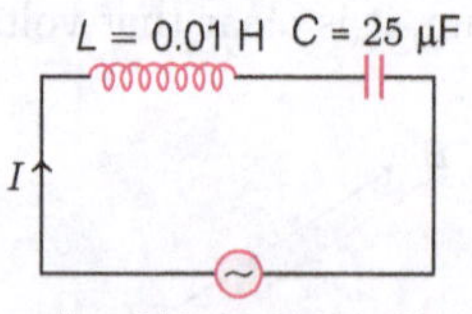

$E = 310 \sin 314t$ (volt)

Given, $E = 310 \sin 314t$ (volt)

Comparing it with general equation, $E = E_0 \sin \omega t$

We get,

$\omega = 2\pi f = 314$

or $f = \dfrac{314}{2\pi} = 50\text{ Hz}$

$\therefore$ Inductive reactance,

$X_L = \omega L = 2\pi f . L$

$= 314 \times 0.01 = 3.14\,\Omega$

Capacitive reactance,

$X_C = \dfrac{1}{\omega C} = \dfrac{1}{314 \times 25 \times 10^{-6}} = 127.3\,\Omega$

$\therefore$Net reactance, $X = X_C - X_L = (127.3 - 3.14)\,\Omega = 12416\,\Omega$

Example 16. *A series L-C-R circuit is connected across a source of emf $E = 20 \sin\left(100\pi t - \dfrac{\pi}{6}\right)$. The current from the supply is $I = 4 \sin\left(100\pi t + \dfrac{\pi}{12}\right)$. Draw the impedance triangle for the circuit.*

Sol. Given, $E_0 = 20$V and $I_0 = 4$A

$\therefore \quad Z = \dfrac{E_0}{I_0} = 5\,\Omega$

The current leads emf by $\phi = \dfrac{\pi}{12} - \left(-\dfrac{\pi}{6}\right) = \dfrac{\pi}{4}$

The impedance triangle can be drawn as

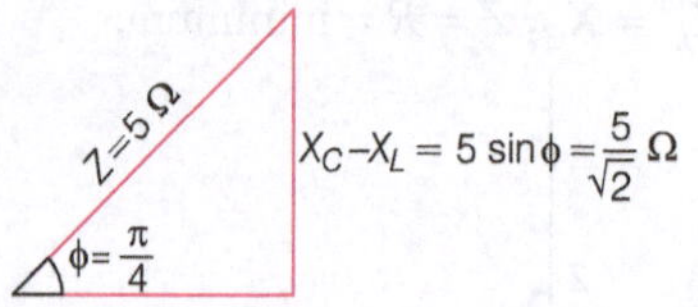

$R = 5 \cos\phi = \dfrac{5}{\sqrt{2}}\,\Omega$

NEET Close-up

Example Similar to PYQ Asked in NEET 2023

Impedance of the following circuit is

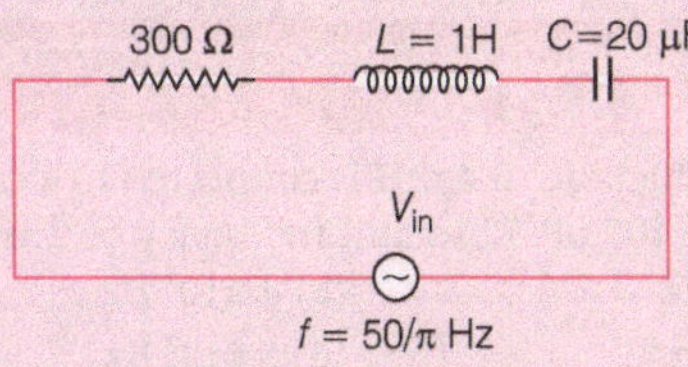

(a) 500 Ω (b) 400 Ω (c) 600 Ω (d) 300 Ω

Sol. (*a*) $Z = \sqrt{R^2 + (X_C - X_L)^2}$

$= \sqrt{(300)^2 + (500-100)^2}$

$\Rightarrow \quad Z = 500\Omega$

Skill Builder

In above question, if $L = 5$ H, then impedance of circuit will be

(a) 500 Ω (b) 300 Ω (c) 400 Ω (d) $300\sqrt{2}\Omega$

For more Practice Refer Q. No. 8 of step-up practice 2.

Example 17. *Find the voltage across the various elements, i.e. resistance, capacitance and inductance which are in series and having values* 1000 Ω, 1 μF *and* 2.0 H, *respectively.*
Given emf as, $V = 100\sqrt{2} \sin 1000\, t$ V

Sol. The rms value of voltage across the source, $V_{\text{rms}} = \dfrac{V_0}{\sqrt{2}}$

Comparing the given equation with general equation,

$V_0 = 100\sqrt{2}$ and $\omega = 1000 \text{ rad s}^{-1}$

Also, $R = 1000\Omega, C = 1\,\mu\text{F} = 1\times 10^{-6}\text{F}$

and $L = 2\text{H}$

$\therefore \quad V_{\text{rms}} = \dfrac{100\sqrt{2}}{\sqrt{2}} = 100 \text{ V}$

$$\therefore \quad I_{\text{rms}} = \frac{V_{\text{rms}}}{|Z|} = \frac{V_{\text{rms}}}{\sqrt{R^2 + (X_L - X_C)^2}}$$

$$= \frac{V_{\text{rms}}}{\sqrt{R^2 + \left(\omega L - \dfrac{1}{\omega C}\right)^2}}$$

$$= \frac{100}{\sqrt{(1000)^2 + \left(1000\times 2 - \dfrac{1}{1000\times 1\times 10^{-6}}\right)^2}}$$

$= 0.0707$ A

The current will be same everywhere in the circuit, therefore

PD across resistor,

$$V_R = I_{\text{rms}} R = 0.0707 \times 1000 = 70.7 \text{ V}$$

PD across inductor,

$$V_L = I_{\text{rms}} X_L = 0.0707 \times 1000 \times 2 = 141.4 \text{ V}$$

and PD across capacitor,

$$V_C = I_{\text{rms}} X_C = 0.0707 \times \frac{1}{1\times 1000 \times 10^{-6}} = 70.7 \text{ V}$$

Mentor's Tip

- The rms voltages do not add directly as, $V_R + V_L + V_C = 282.8$ V, which is not the source voltage 100 V. The reason is that these voltages are not in phase and can be added by vector or by phasor algebra.

Resonance

In series *L-C-R* circuit, when phase (φ) between current and voltage is zero, the circuit is said to be in resonance.

As, applied frequency increases, then

$X_L = \omega L$, X_L increases

and $X_C = \dfrac{1}{\omega C}$, X_C decreases.

At some frequency (ω_0), $X_L = X_C$

$\Rightarrow \quad X_L = \omega_0 L$

and $X_C = \dfrac{1}{\omega_0 C}$

The frequency at which X_C and X_L becomes equal is called **resonant frequency**.

$$\therefore \quad \omega_0 L = \frac{1}{\omega_0 C} \quad \text{or} \quad \omega_0^2 = \frac{1}{LC} \quad \text{or} \quad (2\pi f_0)^2 = \frac{1}{LC}$$

($\because \omega_0 = 2\pi f_0$, where f_0 is resonant frequency)

$$2\pi f_0 = \frac{1}{\sqrt{LC}}$$

or $$f_0 = \frac{1}{2\pi\sqrt{LC}}$$

Resonant frequency is independent of the resistance of the circuit. At resonating frequency,

$$Z = R = \text{Minimum}$$

Since, Z is minimum, therefore I will be maximum.

$$\therefore \quad I = \frac{V}{Z} = \text{Maximum}$$

These circuits are used for voltage amplification and as selector circuits in wireless telegraphy.

Mentor's Tip

- At resonance, we can say that

(i) $X_L = X_C$ or $\omega_0 = \dfrac{1}{\sqrt{LC}}$

(ii) $Z = Z_{\min} = R$

and (iii) I is maximum.

Example 18. *An inductor coil, a capacitor, a resistor and an AC source of rms voltage 24 V are connected in series. When the frequency of the sources is varied, a maximum rms current of 6 A is observed. Find the value of resistance. If this inductor coil of inductive reactance 4Ω is connected to a battery of emf 12 V and internal resistance 4.0 Ω. What will be the current?*

Sol. Consider an *L-C-R* series circuit as shown below

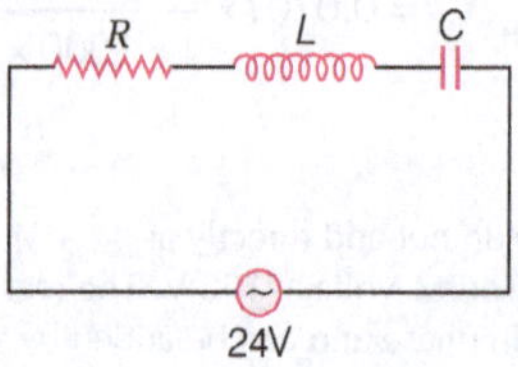

Maximum current will occur at series resonance.

At series resonance, $Z_{min} = R$ and $I_{max} = 6\text{A}$

$$\Rightarrow \quad I_{max} = \frac{V}{Z_{min}}$$

$$\Rightarrow \quad 6 = \frac{24}{R} \Rightarrow R = 4\Omega$$

Now, this inductor coil is connected with a battery of emf 12 V and internal resistance 4 Ω, so new circuit is

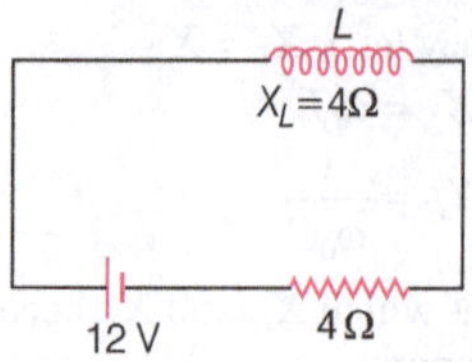

In DC circuit, inductor offers zero resistance,

$$\therefore \quad \text{Current, } I = \frac{12}{4+4} = 1.5\text{A}$$

NEET Close-up

Example Similar to PYQ Asked in NEET 2023 Manipur and NEET 2022

A coil of inductance 0.4 mH is connected to a capacitor of capacitance 400 pF. Resonant frequency of this circuit is

(a) 6×10^5 Hz (b) 4×10^5 Hz
(c) 3×10^6 Hz (d) 5×10^5 Hz

Sol. (*b*) Given, $L = 0.4\,\text{mH} = 0.4 \times 10^{-3}$ H,

$C = 400\,\text{pF} = 4 \times 10^{-10}\text{F}$

This is the condition of resonance.

∴ Resonant frequency,

$$f = \frac{1}{2\pi\sqrt{LC}} = \frac{1}{2 \times 3.14} \times \frac{1}{\sqrt{0.4 \times 10^{-3} \times 4 \times 10^{-10}}}$$

$$= \frac{10^7}{6.28 \times 4}\,\text{Hz} = 3.98 \times 10^5 \text{ Hz}$$

$$\simeq 4 \times 10^5 \text{ Hz}$$

Skill Builder

A series *L-C-R* circuit has inductance 5H, capacitance 20 μF and resistance 100 Ω. Resonant frequency will be

(a) 50 Hz (b) 100 Hz
(c) $\frac{100}{\pi}$ Hz (d) $\frac{50}{\pi}$ Hz

For more Practice Refer Q. No. 13, 22 of Gearing up for NEET.

STEP UP Practice 2

1. The reactance of a 25 μF capacitor at the AC frequency of 4000 Hz is
   (a) $\frac{5}{\pi}\Omega$ (b) $\sqrt{\frac{5}{\pi}}\Omega$
   (c) 10 Ω (d) $\sqrt{10}\,\Omega$
2. The capacity of a pure capacitor is 1 F. In DC circuits, its effective resistance will be
   (a) zero (b) infinite
   (c) 1 Ω (d) 1/2 Ω
3. **Statement I** When capacitive reactance is smaller than the inductive reactance in *L-C-R* series circuit, emf leads the current.

   Statement II The phase angle is the angle between the alternating emf and alternating current of the circuit.

   In the light of the above statements, choose the most appropriate answer from the options given below.
   (a) Both Statement I and Statement II are incorrect.
   (b) Statement I is correct but Statement II is incorrect.
   (c) Statement I is incorrect but Statement II is correct.
   (d) Both Statement I and Statement II are correct.
4. In an AC circuit, an alternating voltage $e = 200\sqrt{2}\sin 100t$ V is connected to a capacitor of capacity 1 μF. The rms value of the current in the circuit is
   (a) 100 mA (b) 200 mA (c) 20 mA (d) 10 mA
5. The reactance of a coil when used in the domestic AC power supply (220 V, 50 cycles per second) is 50 Ω. The inductance of the coil is nearly
   (a) 2.2 H (b) 1.6 H (c) 0.22 H (d) 0.16 H
6. An inductive coil has a resistance of 100 Ω. When an AC signal of frequency 1000 Hz is applied to the coil, the voltage leads the current by 45°. The inductance of the coil is
   (a) $\frac{1}{10\pi}$ (b) $\frac{1}{20\pi}$ (c) $\frac{1}{40\pi}$ (d) $\frac{1}{60\pi}$

7. Two inductors L_1 and L_2 are connected in parallel and a time varying current flows as shown in figure. Then, the ratio of currents I_1/I_2 at any time t is

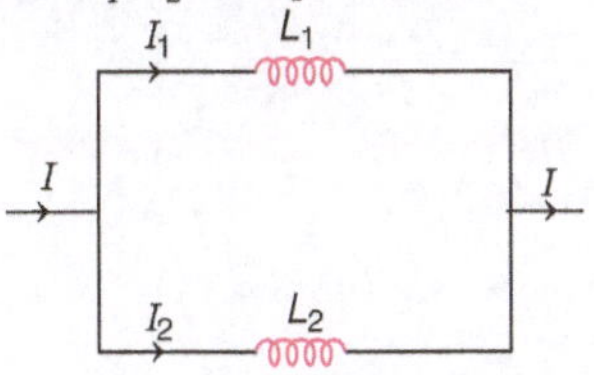

(a) L_1/L_2 (b) L_2/L_1
(c) $\frac{L_1}{(L_1+L_2)^2}$ (d) $\frac{L_2}{(L_1+L_2)^2}$

8. In L-R circuit, resistance is $8\,\Omega$ and inductive reactance is $6\,\Omega$, then impedance is
(a) $2\,\Omega$ (b) $14\,\Omega$ (c) $4\,\Omega$ (d) $10\,\Omega$

9. In an AC circuit, a resistance R is connected in series with an inductance L. If phase angle between voltage and current be 45°, the value of inductive reactance will be
(a) $R/4$
(b) $R/2$
(c) R
(d) cannot be found with the given data

10. **Statement I** The alternating current lags behind the emf by a phase angle of $\pi/2$, when AC flows through an inductor.
Statement II The inductive reactance increases as the frequency of AC source decreases.
In the light of the above statements, choose the most appropriate answer from the options given below.
(a) Both Statement I and Statement II are incorrect.
(b) Statement I is correct but Statement II is incorrect.
(c) Statement I is incorrect but Statement II is correct.
(d) Both Statement I and Statement II are correct.

11. In a circuit containing R and L, as the frequency of the impressed AC increases, the impedance of the circuit
(a) decreases
(b) increases
(c) remains unchanged
(d) first increases and then decreases

12. An AC voltage is applied to a resistance R and an inductor L in series. If R and the inductive reactance are both equal to 3Ω, the phase difference (in rad) between the applied voltage and the current in the circuit is
(a) $\pi/4$ (b) $\pi/2$ (c) zero (d) $\pi/6$

13. In an L-R circuit, the value of L is $\left(\frac{0.4}{\pi}\right)$ H and the value of R is $30\,\Omega$. If in the circuit, an alternating emf of 200 V at 50 cycle s^{-1} is connected, the impedance of the circuit and current will be
(a) $11.4\,\Omega$, 17.5 A (b) $30.7\,\Omega$, 6.5 A
(c) $40.4\,\Omega$, 5 A (d) $50\,\Omega$, 4 A

14. Which one of the following pair given below is incorrect about AC circuit?
(a) When $X_L = X_C$ $\rightarrow$ $\tan\phi = 0$
(b) When $X_L > X_C$ $\rightarrow$ $\tan\phi$ is negative
(c) In R-C circuit $\rightarrow$ $\tan\phi = \frac{X_C}{R}$
(d) In L-R circuit $\rightarrow$ $\tan\phi = \frac{X_L}{R}$

15. The instantaneous values of current and voltage in an AC circuit are given by
$$I = 6\sin\left(100\pi t + \frac{\pi}{4}\right)$$
$$V = 5\sin\left(100\pi t - \frac{\pi}{4}\right), \text{ then}$$
(a) current leads the voltage by 45°
(b) voltage leads the current by 90°
(c) current leads the voltage by 90°
(d) voltage leads the current by 45°

16. In an L-C-R series circuit the AC voltage across R, L and C come out as 10V, 10V and 20V, respectively. The voltage across the entire combination will be
(a) 30 V (b) $10\sqrt{3}$ V (c) 20 V (d) $10\sqrt{2}$ V

17. A sinusoidal voltage of peak value 300 V and an angular frequency $\omega = 400\,\text{rads}^{-1}$ is applied to series L-C-R circuit, in which $R = 3\Omega$, $L = 20$ mH and $C = 625\mu$F. The peak value of current in the circuit is
(a) $30\sqrt{2}$A (b) 60A (c) 100A (d) $60\sqrt{2}$A

18. **Statement I** An electric lamp connected in series with a variable capacitor and AC source, its brightness increases with increase in capacitance.
Statement II Capacitive reactance decreases with increase in capacitance of capacitor.
In the light of the above statements, choose the most appropriate answer from the options given below.
(a) Both Statement I and Statement II are incorrect.
(b) Statement I is correct but Statement II is incorrect.
(c) Statement I is incorrect but Statement II is correct.
(d) Both Statement I and Statement II are correct.

19. In an L-C-R series AC circuit, at resonance
(a) the capacitive reactance is more than the inductive
(b) the capacitive reactance equals the inductive reactance
(c) the capacitive reactance is less than the inductive reactance
(d) the current is minimum

20. An L-C-R series circuit connected to a source E, is at resonance. Then,
(a) the voltage across R is zero
(b) the voltage across R equals applied voltage
(c) the voltage across C is zero
(d) the voltage across C equals applied voltage

21. **Statement I** At resonance, LCR series circuit have a maximum current.
Statement II At resonance, in LCR series circuit, the current and emf are in phase with each other.
In the light of the above statements, choose the most appropriate answer from the options given below.
(a) Both Statement I and Statement II are incorrect.
(b) Statement I is correct but Statement II is incorrect.
(c) Statement I is incorrect but Statement II is correct.
(d) Both Statement I and Statement II are correct.

Module 3

Power in AC Circuits

- Power in AC Circuits
- Wattless Current

Power in AC Circuits

For electric circuits power is defined as the product of voltage and current.

In AC circuit, both emf and current changes continuously with respect to time, so in AC circuit, we have to calculate average power in complete cycle ($0 \to T$).

Hence, average power is defined as the average of instantaneous power in an AC circuit over a full cycle. Its SI unit is watt.

Instantaneous power, $P = VI$

$$[\because V = V_0 \sin\omega t, I = I_0 \sin(\omega t + \phi)]$$

Here, V and I are instantaneous voltage and current, respectively.

Total work done or energy spent in maintaining current over one full cycle is given by

$$W = \frac{V_0 I_0 T}{2} \cos\phi$$

Thus, average power associated in AC circuit is given by

$$P_{av} = \frac{W}{T} = \frac{V_0 I_0}{2} \cos\phi$$

$$P_{av} = \frac{V_0}{\sqrt{2}} \frac{I_0}{\sqrt{2}} \cos\phi$$

$$\boxed{P_{av} = V_{rms} I_{rms} \cos\phi}$$

Here, $\cos\phi$ is **power factor.**

Power factor is defined as cosine of the angle of lag or lead (*i.e.* $\cos\phi$). It is also defined as the ratio of resistance and impedance.

$$\boxed{\cos\phi = \frac{P_{av}}{V_{rms} I_{rms}} = \frac{\text{True power}}{\text{Apparent power}}}$$

It is said to be leading, if current leads voltage, lagging, if current lags voltage. Thus, a power factor of 0.5 lagging means current lags the voltage by 60° (as $\cos^{-1}(0.5) = 60°$).

Special cases

(i) **AC circuit containing R only**

Here, $\phi = 0°, P_{av} = V_{rms} I_{rms} \cos 0°$

$\Rightarrow P_{av} = V_{rms} I_{rms}$ [maximum]

Mentor's TIP

In Resistive (Pure) circuit, maximum power of an AC is dissipated.

(ii) **AC circuit containing L only**

$$\phi = \frac{\pi}{2} \text{ or } P_{av} = V_{rms} I_{rms} \cos\frac{\pi}{2} \Rightarrow P_{av} = 0$$

So, average power in L is zero.

(iii) **AC circuit containing C only**

$$\phi = \frac{\pi}{2} \text{ or } P_{av} = V_{rms} I_{rms} \cos\frac{\pi}{2} = 0$$

So, average power in C is zero.

(iv) **AC circuit containing L and R**

$$\tan\phi = \frac{\omega L}{R}$$

$$\Rightarrow \cos\phi = \frac{R}{\sqrt{R^2 + \omega^2 L^2}}$$

$$\Rightarrow P_{av} = V_{rms} I_{rms} \cdot \frac{R}{\sqrt{R^2 + \omega^2 L^2}}$$

(v) **AC circuit containing C and R**

$$\tan\phi = \frac{1/\omega C}{R}$$

$$\Rightarrow \cos\phi = \frac{R}{\sqrt{R^2 + 1/\omega^2 C^2}}$$

$$\Rightarrow P_{av} = V_{rms} I_{rms} \frac{R}{\sqrt{R^2 + 1/\omega^2 C^2}}$$

(vi) **AC circuit containing L, C and R**

$$\tan\phi = \frac{\omega L - 1/\omega C}{R}$$

$$\Rightarrow \cos\phi = \frac{R}{\sqrt{R^2 + (\omega L - 1/\omega C)^2}}$$

$$\Rightarrow P_{av} = V_{rms} I_{rms} \cdot \frac{R}{\sqrt{R^2 + \left(\omega L - \frac{1}{\omega C}\right)^2}}$$

The amplitude of the current falls by a factor of $\frac{1}{\sqrt{2}}$ and hence, the power ($P \propto I^2$) goes down by half.

The separation between these two half power points is $2\Delta\omega = \frac{\omega_0}{Q}$. This separation is called the full-width at half maximum and is $\frac{1}{Q}$ th fraction of the resonant frequency.

Example 19. *An iron cored coil is connected in series with an electric bulb, with an AC source, as shown in figure. As the iron piece is taken out of the coil, how will the brightness of bulb change?*

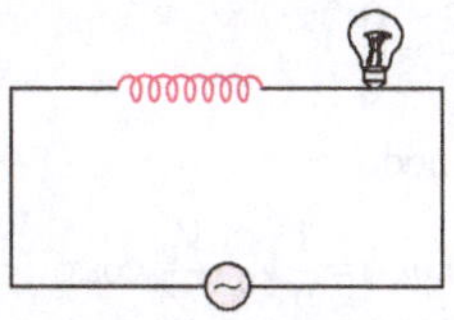

Sol. As the iron rod is taken out of the coil, the self-inductance of the coil decreases, the impedance of circuit decreases, hence current increases. So, power consumed (and hence brightness of bulb) by bulb increases.

Example 20. *A light bulb has the rating 200 W, 220 V. Find (i) resistance of the bulb filament and (ii) rms value of current flowing through the filament.*

Sol. (i) Resistance of the bulb,

$$R = \frac{V^2}{P} = \frac{220 \times 220}{200} = \frac{22 \times 22}{2} = 242\,\Omega$$

(ii) The rms value of current $= \frac{P}{V} = \frac{200}{220} = \frac{10}{11}\text{A} = 0.9\,\text{A}$

Example 21. *A series L-C-R circuit with $R = 20\,\Omega$, $L = 1.5$ H and $C = 35\,\mu F$ is connected to a variable frequency 200 V, AC supply. When the frequency of the supply equals the natural frequency of the circuit, what is the average power transferred to the circuit in one complete cycle?*

Sol. When the frequency of the supply equals the natural frequency of the circuit, the circuit is said to be in resonance. At resonance,

$$Z = R = 20\,\Omega$$

Since, the *L-C-R* circuit is resistive, so the phase angle between the current and voltage is zero.

i.e. $\phi = 0°$

and $I_{rms} = \frac{E_{rms}}{Z} = \frac{200}{20} = 10$ A

P = average power transferred per cycle.

$\therefore\ P = I_{rms} E_{rms} \cos 0°$

$= 10 \times 200 = 2000$ W

$= 2.0$ kW

NEET Close-up

Example Similar to PYQ Asked in NEET 2018

An inductor 11 mH, a capacitor 80 μF and a resistor 60 Ω are connected in series across a source of emf, $V = 15 \sin 314\, t$. The power loss in the circuit is

(a) 2.62 W (b) 1.53 W
(c) 1.37 W (d) 1 W

Sol. (c) Impedance Z in AC circuit is

$$Z = \sqrt{R^2 + (X_C - X_L)^2}$$

where, X_C = capacitive reactance and X_L = inductive reactance.

Also, $X_C = \frac{1}{\omega C}$ and $X_L = \omega L$

$$\therefore\quad Z = \sqrt{(60)^2 + \left(\frac{1}{314 \times 80 \times 10^{-6}} - 314 \times 11 \times 10^{-3}\right)^2}$$

or $Z = 70\,\Omega$

The power loss in the circuit is

$$P_{av} = \left(\frac{V_{rms}}{Z}\right)^2 R$$

$$\therefore\quad P_{av} = \left(\frac{15}{(\sqrt{2})70}\right)^2 \times 60 = 1.37\text{ W}$$

Skill Builder

An inductor of 51 mH, a capacitor 70 μF and a resistor 50Ω are connected in series across a source of emf $V = 20 \sin 314t$. The power loss in the circuit is

(a) 1.97 W (b) 2.52 W
(c) 3.62 W (d) 2.97 W

For more Practice Refer Q. No. 37, 43, 56 of Gearing up for NEET.

Example 22. *A series L-C-R circuit is connected across an AC source $E = 10 \sin\left[100\pi t - \frac{\pi}{6}\right]$. Current from the supply is $I = 2 \sin\left[100\pi t + \frac{\pi}{12}\right]$, what is the average power dissipated?*

Sol. Phase difference between voltage and current,

$$\phi = \frac{\pi}{12} - \left(-\frac{\pi}{6}\right) = \frac{\pi}{4}$$

$\Rightarrow$ Power factor $= \cos\phi = \cos\frac{\pi}{4} = \frac{1}{\sqrt{2}}$

Average power dissipated, $= \frac{V_m I_m}{2}\cos\phi$

$$= \frac{10 \times 2}{2} \times \frac{1}{\sqrt{2}} = 5\sqrt{2}\text{ W}$$

Example 23. *A 60 cycle per second AC circuit has a resistance of 200 Ω and inductor of 100 mH. What is the power factor? What capacitance placed in the circuit will make the power factor unity?*

Sol. $Z = \sqrt{R^2 + (\omega L)^2}$

$$= \sqrt{(200)^2 + (2\pi \times 60 \times 100 \times 10^{-3})^2} = 203.52\ \Omega$$

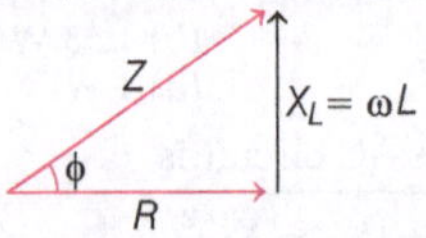

Power factor, $\cos\phi = \frac{R}{Z} = \frac{200}{203.52} = 0.983$

Now, for the power factor to be unity, $\phi = 0$ that means

$$X_L = X_C \text{ or } \omega L = \frac{1}{\omega C}$$

$\therefore$ $$C = \frac{1}{\omega^2 L} = \frac{1}{(2\pi \times 60)^2 \times 100 \times 10^{-3}}$$

$\therefore$ $$C = 70.36\ \mu F$$

Example 24. *An L-C-R series circuit with 100 Ω resistance is connected to an AC source of 200 V and angular frequency 300 rad s^{-1}. When only the capacitance is removed, the current lags behind the voltage by 60°. When only the inductance is removed, the current leads the voltage by 60°. Calculate the current and the power dissipated in the L-C-R circuit.*

Sol. When capacitance is removed,

$$\tan\phi = \frac{X_L}{R}$$

or $$\tan 60° = \frac{X_L}{R}$$

$\therefore$ $$X_L = \sqrt{3}R \qquad \text{...(i)}$$

When inductance is removed,

$$\tan\phi = \frac{X_C}{R} \text{ or } \tan 60° = \frac{X_C}{R}$$

$\therefore$ $$X_C = \sqrt{3}R \qquad \text{...(ii)}$$

From Eqs. (i) and (ii) we see that, $X_C = X_L$

So, the L-C-R circuit is in resonance.

Hence, $Z = R$

$\therefore$ $$I_{rms} = \frac{V_{rms}}{Z} = \frac{200}{100} = 2\text{ A}$$

Power dissipated $\langle P \rangle = V_{rms} I_{rms} \cos\phi$

At resonance, current and voltage are in phase or $\phi = 0°$

$\therefore$ $$\langle P \rangle = (200)(2)(1) = 400\text{ W}$$

Example 25. *Consider the following R-L-C circuit in which $R = 12\ \Omega$, $X_L = 24\ \Omega$, $X_C = 8\ \Omega$. The emf of source is given by $V = 10\sin(100\pi t)V$.*

(i) Find the energy dissipated in 10 min.

(ii) If resistance is removed from the circuit and value of inductance is doubled, express variation of current with time t in the new circuit.

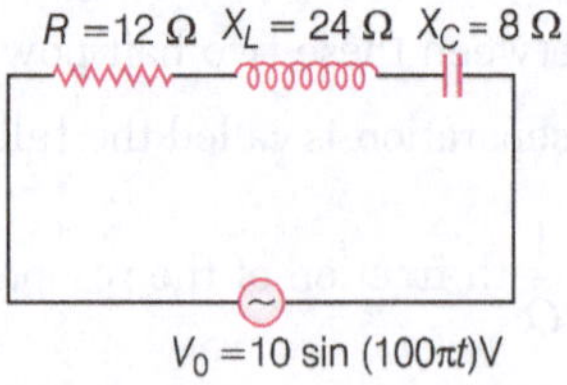

Sol. (i) Impedance,

$$Z = \sqrt{R^2 + (X_L - X_C)^2} = \sqrt{(12)^2 + (24-8)^2} = 20\ \Omega$$

$$\cos\phi = \frac{R}{Z} = \frac{12}{20} = \frac{3}{5}$$

Power consumed,

$$P = \frac{1}{2}V_0 I_0 \cos\phi = \frac{1}{2}V_0 \cdot \frac{V_0}{Z}\cos\phi$$

$$= \frac{1}{2}\frac{(10)^2}{(20)} \times \frac{3}{5} = 1.5\text{ W}$$

Energy dissipated, $E = Pt = (1.5)(10 \times 60) = 900\text{ J}$

(ii)

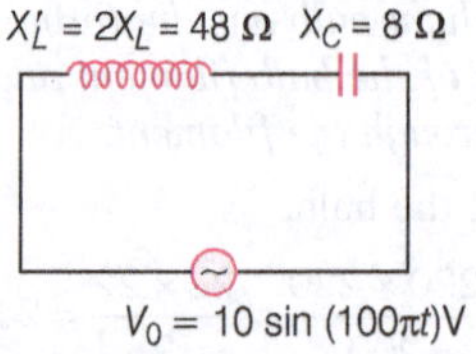

Impedance, $Z = X_L' - X_C = 48 - 8 = 40\Omega$

$\therefore$ Current, $I_0 = \frac{V_0}{Z} = \frac{10}{40} = \frac{1}{4}\text{ A}$

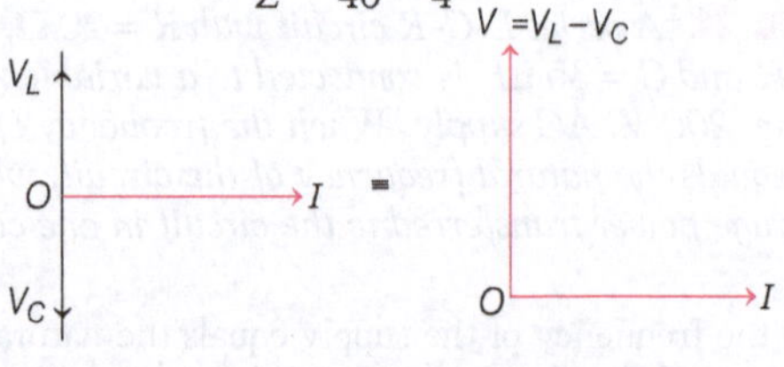

Current lags the voltage by π/2.

$$I = I_0 \sin(\omega t - \pi/2) = \frac{1}{4}\sin(100\pi t - \pi/2)\text{ A}$$

Wattless Current

The current which consumes no power for its maintainance in the circuit is called wattless current or idle current.

or

If the resistance in an AC circuit is zero, its power factor will be zero. Although the current flows in the circuit, yet the average power remains zero, *i.e.* there is no energy dissipation in the circuit. Such a circuit is called the wattless circuit and the current flowing is called the wattless current.

If the circuit contains either inductance or capacitance only, then phase difference between current and voltage is 90°, *i.e.* $\phi = 90°$. The average power in such a circuit is

$$P_{av} = V_{rms} \times I_{rms} \times \cos\phi$$

$$= V_{rms} \times I_{rms} \times \cos 90° = 0$$

The concept of wattless current is similar to that of a frictionless pendulum, where the total work done by gravity upon the pendulum in a cycle is zero.

STEP UP Practice 3

1. An electric heater rated 220 V and 550 W is connected to AC mains. The current drawn by it is
   (a) 0.8 A (b) 2.5 A
   (c) 0.4 A (d) 1.25 A
2. In an AC circuit, the power factor
   (a) is zero when the circuit contains an ideal resistance only
   (b) is unity when the circuit contains an ideal resistance only
   (c) is infinity when the circuit contains an ideal inductance only
   (d) None of the above
3. The average power dissipated in a pure capacitance C in an AC circuit is
   (a) CV (b) zero
   (c) $\frac{1}{CV^2}$ (d) $\frac{1}{4}CV^2$
4. **Assertion** (A) A capacitor of suitable capacitance can be used in an AC circuit in place of the choke coil.
   Reason (R) A capacitor block DC and allows AC only.
   In the light of the above statements, choose the correct answer from the options given below
   (a) Both A and R are true but R is not the correct explanation of A.
   (b) A is true but R is false.
   (c) A is false but R is true.
   (d) Both A and R are true and R is the correct explanation of A.
5. The impedance of a circuit consists of 3 Ω resistance and 4Ω reactance. The power factor of the circuit is
   (a) 0.4 (b) 0.6
   (c) 0.8 (d) 1.0
6. In an AC circuit, the potential difference V and current I are given respectively by
   $$V = 100\sin(100t)\text{V}$$
   and $$I = 100\sin\left(100t + \frac{\pi}{3}\right)\text{mA}$$
   The power dissipated in the circuit will be
   (a) 10^4 W (b) 10 W
   (c) 2.5 W (d) 5 W
7. The average power dissipated in a pure inductor of inductance L, when an AC current is passing through it, is
   (a) $\frac{1}{2}LI^2$ (b) $\frac{1}{4}LI^2$
   (c) $2LI^2$ (d) zero
8. **Assertion** (A) Choke coil is preferred over a resistor to adjust current in an AC circuit.
   Reason (R) Power factor for inductance is zero.
   In the light of the above statements, choose the correct answer from the options given below.
   (a) Both A and R are true but R is not the correct explanation of A.
   (b) A is true but R is false.
   (c) A is false but R is true.
   (d) Both A and R are true and R is the correct explanation of A.
9. Power dissipated in an L-C-R series circuit connected to an AC source of emf E is
   (a) $\frac{E^2R}{\left[R^2 + \left(L\omega - \frac{1}{C\omega}\right)^2\right]}$
   (b) $\frac{E^2\sqrt{R^2 + \left(L\omega - \frac{1}{C\omega}\right)^2}}{R}$
   (c) $\frac{E^2\left[R^2 + \left(L\omega - \frac{1}{C\omega}\right)^2\right]}{R}$
   (d) $\frac{E^2R}{\sqrt{R^2 + \left(L\omega + \frac{1}{C\omega}\right)^2}}$
10. A condenser of 250 pF is connected in series to a coil of inductance of 0.16 mH. Determine the resonant frequency.
    (a) 9×10^4 Hz (b) 16×10^7 Hz
    (c) 8×10^5 Hz (d) 9×10^3 Hz
11. Which one of the following pair given below is incorrect?
    (a) Power factor ($\cos\phi$) → $\frac{\text{True power}}{\text{Apparent power}}$
    (b) AC circuit containing L and R → $\tan\phi = \frac{\omega L}{R}$
    (c) AC circuit containing C and R → $\tan\phi = \frac{\omega C}{R}$
    (d) AC circuit containing L, C and R → $\tan\phi = \frac{\omega L - 1/\omega C}{R}$

12. A series *L-C-R* circuit contains inductance 5 mH, capacitance 2 μF and resistance 10 Ω. If the frequency of AC source is varied, then what is the frequency at which maximum power is dissipated?

(a) $\frac{10^5}{\pi}$ Hz (b) $\frac{10^{-5}}{\pi}$ Hz

(c) $\frac{2}{\pi}\times10^5$ Hz (d) $\frac{5}{\pi}\times10^3$ Hz

13. Assertion (A) The reactance of an circuit is zero. It is possible that the circuit contains a capacitor and an inductor.

Reason (R) In AC circuit, the average power delivered by the source never becomes zero.

In the light of the above statements, choose the correct answer from the options given below.

(a) Both A and R are true but R is not the correct explanation of A.

(b) A is true but R is false.

(c) A is false but R is true.

(d) Both A and R are true and R is the correct explanation of A.

14. The average power dissipated in AC circuit is 2 W. If a current flowing through a circuit is 2 A, impedance is 1 Ω, then what is the power factor of the circuit?

(a) 0.5 (b) 1

(c) Zero (d) $\frac{1}{\sqrt{2}}$

15. Assertion (A) No power loss associated with pure capacitor in AC circuit.

Reason (R) No current is flowing in this circuit.

In the light of the above statements, choose the correct answer from the options given below.

(a) Both A and R are true but R is not the correct explanation of A.

(b) A is true but R is false.

(c) A is false but R is true.

(d) Both A and R are true and R is the correct explanation of A.

Module 4

AC Based Devices

- Transformer • Electric Generator or Dynamo

Transformer

It is a device which is used to change the alternating voltage. The transformers are of the following types

Step-Up Transformer

It is used to increase the AC voltages.

Step-Down Transformer

It is used to decrease the AC voltages.

Principle

Transformer is based on the principle of mutual induction, *i.e.* whenever an amount of magnetic flux linked with a coil changes, an emf is induced in the neighbouring coil.

Construction

It consists of two coils, primary coil (*P*) and secondary coil (*S*), insulated from each other wounded on soft iron core. Often the primary coil is the input coil and secondary coil is the output coil. These soft iron cores are laminated to minimise eddy current loss.

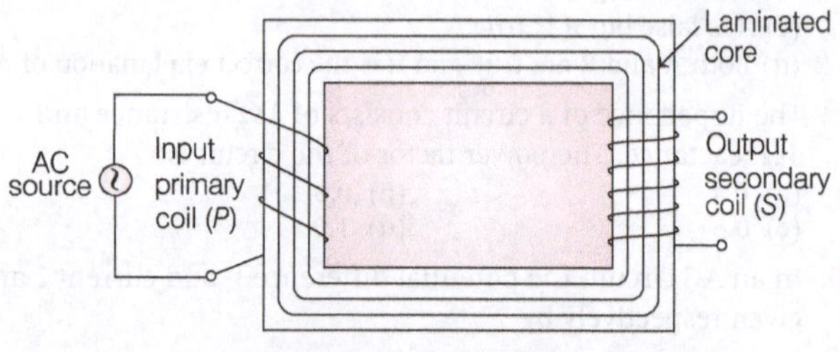

Construction of an transformer

Theory and Working

The value of the emf induced in secondary coil due to alternating voltage applied to primary depends on the number of turns in the secondary. We consider an **ideal transformer** in which the primary has negligible resistance and all the flux in the core links both primary and secondary windings.

Let ϕ be the flux in each turn in the core at time *t*, due to current in the primary, when a voltage V_P is applied to it.

Then, the induced emf or voltage ε_S, in the secondary having N_S turns is

$$\varepsilon_S = -N_S \frac{d\phi}{dt} \quad \text{...(i)}$$

The alternating flux ϕ also induces an emf, called back emf in the primary. This is

$$\varepsilon_P = -N_P \frac{d\phi}{dt} \quad \text{...(ii)}$$

But $\varepsilon_P = V_P$. If this were not so, the primary current would be infinite, since the primary has zero resistance (as considered). If the secondary is an open circuit or the current taken from it is small, then to a good approximation.

$$\varepsilon_S = V_S$$

where, V_S is the voltage across the secondary.

Therefore, Eqs. (i) and (ii) can be written as,

$$V_S = -N_S \frac{d\phi}{dt} \quad \text{...(iii)}$$

$$V_P = -N_P \frac{d\phi}{dt} \quad \text{...(iv)}$$

From Eqs. (iii) and (iv), we have

$$\frac{V_S}{V_P} = \frac{N_S}{N_P} \quad \text{...(v)}$$

The above relation is based on three assumptions

I. The primary resistance and current are small.

II. The same flux links both the primary and the secondary as there is very little leakage of magnetic flux.

III. The secondary current is small.

Efficiency of a transformer is defined as the ratio of output power to the input power.

i.e. $$\eta = \frac{\text{Output power}}{\text{Input power}} = \frac{V_S I_S}{V_P I_P}$$

If the transformer is assumed to be 100% efficient (no energy losses), the power input is equal to the power output, and since $P = IV$, $I_P V_P = I_S V_S$ ...(vi)

Although, some energy is always lost, still this is a good approximation, since a well designed transformer may have an efficiency of more than 95%.

Combining Eqs. (v) and (vi), we have

$$\frac{I_P}{I_S} = \frac{V_S}{V_P} = \frac{N_S}{N_P} \quad \text{...(vii)}$$

Since, I and V both oscillate with the same frequency as the AC source, Eq. (vii) also gives the ratio of the amplitudes or rms values of corresponding quantities.

Now, we can observe how a transformer affects the voltage and current. We have

$$V_S = \left(\frac{N_S}{N_P}\right) V_P \text{ and } I_S = \left(\frac{N_P}{N_S}\right) I_P \quad \text{...(viii)}$$

So, if the secondary coil has a greater number of turns than the primary (*i.e.* $N_S > N_P$), the voltage is stepped up ($V_S > V_P$). This type of arrangement is called a **step-up transformer**. However, in this arrangement, there is less current in the secondary than in the primary (*i.e.*, $N_P/N_S < 1$ and $I_S < I_P$). If the secondary coil has less turns than the primary (*i.e.* $N_S < N_P$), we have a **step-down transformer**. In this case, $V_S < V_P$ and $I_S > I_P$, *i.e.*, the voltage is stepped down (or reduced) and the current is increased. The equations obtained above apply to ideal transformers (*i.e.* which have zero energy losses).

NEET Close-up

Example Similar to PYQ Asked in NEET 2024

An ideal transformer having 100 turn in primary coil and 50 turns in secondary coil. The voltage across the secondary coil is 120 V. Then, the voltage across the primary coil will be

(a) 160 V (b) 220 V (c) 260 V (d) 240 V

Sol. (*d*) According to transformer ratio,

$$\frac{V_S}{V_P} = \frac{N_S}{N_P}$$

$$\Rightarrow \quad \frac{120}{V_P} = \frac{50}{100}$$

$$\Rightarrow \quad V_P = \frac{100}{50} \times 120$$

$$\Rightarrow \quad V_P = 240 \text{ V}$$

Skill Builder

An ideal transformer having 440 V across the primary coil and 260 V across the secondary coil. Its primary coil have 220 turn winding. Then, the number of turns in its secondary coil winding is

(a) 230 (b) 130
(c) 216 (d) 160

For more Practice Refer Q. No. 8, 11,13 of step-up practice 4 and Q. No. 77, 78, 79 of Gearing up for NEET.

Energy losses in transformers

In actual transformers, small energy losses do occur due to the following reasons.

(i) **Flux leakage** There is always some leakage of flux *i.e.*, not all of the flux that the primary passes through the secondary, due to poor design of the core or the air gaps in the core. It can be reduced by winding the primary and secondary coils one over the other.

(ii) **Resistance of the windings** The wire used for the windings has some resistance and so, energy is lost due to heat produced in the wire (I^2R). In high current, low voltage windings, this is minimised by using thick wire.

(iii) **Eddy currents** The alternating magnetic flux induces eddy currents in the iron core and causes heating. The effect is reduced by having a laminated core.

(iv) **Hysteresis** The magnetisation of the core is repeatedly reversed by an alternating magnetic field. The resulting expenditure of energy in the core appears as heat and is kept to a minimum by using a magnetic material which has a low hysteresis loss.

(v) **Magnetostriction** It is the humming noise of a transformer.

Uses of Transformers

Transformers are used in almost all AC operations. Some of them are given below

(i) In the induction furnaces.

(ii) In voltage regulators for TV, computer, refrigerator etc.

(iii) A step-down transformer is used for the purpose of weldings.

(iv) In the transmission of AC over long distances.

Example 26. *In a step-down transformer having primary to secondary turn ratio 10 : 1, the input voltage applied is 250V and output current is 10 A. Assuming 100% efficiency, calculate the*
(i) voltage across secondary coil,
(ii) current in primary coil
(iii) and power output.

Sol. Given, $\frac{N_S}{N_P}=\frac{1}{10}, V_P=250\,\text{V}$

and $I_S=10\,\text{A}$

(i) $\frac{V_S}{V_P}=\frac{N_S}{N_P}$

$$\Rightarrow V_S=\frac{N_S}{N_P}\times V_P=\frac{1}{10}\times 250=25\,\text{V}$$

(ii) $\frac{I_P}{I_S}=\frac{N_S}{N_P}$

$$\Rightarrow I_P=\frac{N_S}{N_P}I_S=\frac{1}{10}\times 10=1\text{A}$$

(iii) Power output $=V_S I_S=25\times 10=250\,\text{W}$

Example 27. *A 10 kW transformer has 20 turns in the primary and 100 turns in the secondary circuit. An AC voltage $V_1=600\sin 314\,t$ is applied to the primary. Find (i) the maximum value of flux and (ii) the maximum value of secondary voltage.*

Sol. (i) Flux linked with each turn of primary,

$$\phi=BA\cos\omega t=\phi_0\cos\omega t$$

Here, $\phi_0=BA=$ maximum value of flux linked with each turn

$$\therefore V_1=-N_1\frac{d\phi}{dt}=-N_1\frac{d}{dt}(\phi_0\cos\omega t)=\omega N_1\phi_0\sin\omega t$$

Peak value of $V_1=V_0=\omega N_1\phi_0$ or $\phi_0=\frac{V_0}{\omega N_1}$

Given, $V_1=600\sin 314\,t=V_0\sin\omega t$

$\therefore \quad V_0=600\,\text{V},\quad \omega=314\text{ rad s}^{-1}$

Hence, $\phi_0=\frac{600}{314\times 20}=0.0955\,\text{Wb}$

(ii) $\frac{V_2^0}{V_1^0}=\frac{N_2}{N_1}$

$\therefore$ Maximum value of secondary voltage is,

$$V_2^0=\frac{N_2}{N_1}V_1^0=\frac{100}{20}\times 600=3000\,\text{V}$$

Example 28. *(i) The primary of a transformer has 400 turns while the secondary has 2000 turns. If the power output from the secondary at 1100 V is 12.1 kW, calculate the primary voltage. (ii) If the resistance of the primary is 0.2 Ω and that of the secondary is 2.0 Ω and the efficiency of the transformer is 90 % calculate the heat losses in the primary and the secondary coils.*

Sol. (i) Given, $N_1=400, N_2=2000, V_2=1100\,\text{V}$

$$\text{As, } V_1=V_2\cdot\frac{N_1}{N_2}=1100\times\frac{400}{2000}=220\,\text{V}$$

(ii) Resistance of primary, $R_1=0.2\,\Omega$

Resistance of secondary, $R_2=2.0\,\Omega$

Output power, $P_2=V_2I_2=12.1\text{kW}=12100\,\text{W}$

$\therefore$ Current in the secondary,

$$I_2=\frac{P_2}{V_2}=\frac{12100}{1100}=11\text{A}$$

$$\text{As, efficiency}=\frac{\text{output power}}{\text{input power}}$$

$$\Rightarrow \frac{90}{100}=\frac{12100\,\text{W}}{\text{Input power}}$$

$$\text{Input power, } P_1=\frac{12100\times 100}{90}=13.44\times 10^3\,\text{W}$$

Also, input power, $P_1=V_1I_1$

$$\therefore \text{Current in the primary, } I_1=\frac{P_1}{V_1}=\frac{13.44\times 10^3}{220}=61.1\text{A}$$

Power loss in the primary,

$$=I_1^2R_1=(61.1)^2\times 0.2=746.64\,\text{W}$$

Power loss in the secondary,

$$=I_2^2R_2=(11)^2\times 2.0=242\,\text{W}$$

NEET Close-up

Example Similar to PYQ Asked in NEET 2023 and NEET 2021

A 6 V, 60 W lamp is connected to the secondary coil of a step down transformer whose primary coil is connected to 220 V AC. Assuming no power is loss. Current in primary coil is

(a) 0.27 A (b) 0.6 A
(c) 0.82 A (d) 0.12 A

Sol. (a) $P_P = P_S$

$$60 \text{ W} = 220 \text{ V} \times I_P$$

$$I_P = \frac{60}{220} = 0.27 \text{ A}$$

Skill Builder

A step down transformer connected to AC supply of 100 V is made to operate at 11 V, 50 W. Ignoring power loss, current in primary coil will be

(a) 1 A (b) 2 A (c) 0.2 A (d) 0.5 A

For more Practice Refer Q. No. 8, 11 of step-up practice 4 and Q. No. 77, 79 of Gearing up for NEET.

Electric Generator or Dynamo

Electric generator is a device which is used to convert mechanical energy to electrical energy. Generator provide nearly all of the power for electric power grids.

The reverse conversion of electrical energy to mechanical energy is done by electric motor.

Electric generators are of two types

1. AC generator 2. DC generator

AC generator or AC dynamo

It is used to produce alternating current energy from mechanical energy.

(i) Principle

It is based on the phenomenon of **electromagnetic induction,** *i.e.* whenever the amount of magnetic flux linked with a coil changes, an emf is induced in the coil. The direction of induced current is given by Fleming's right-hand rule.

(ii) Construction

AC generator has following parts

(a) **Armature** *ABCD* is a rectangular armature coil consisting of a large number of turns of insulated copper wire wound over a laminated soft iron core.

(b) **Field magnets** *N* and *S* are the pole pieces of a strong electromagnet in which the armature coil is rotated. Axis of rotation is perpendicular to the magnetic field lines.

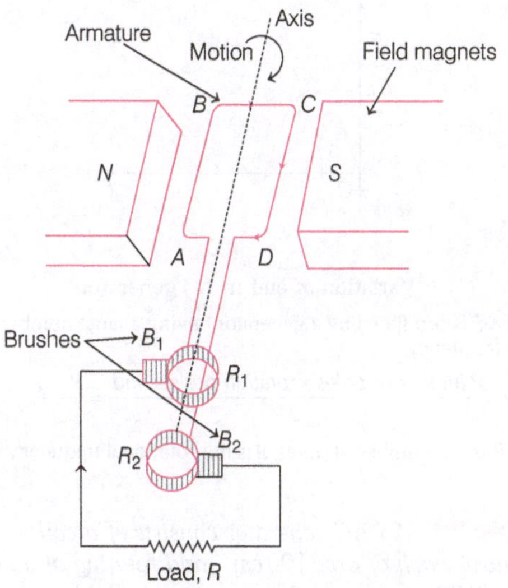

Construction of an AC generators

(c) **Slip rings** R_1 and R_2 are two hollow metallic rings which are connected by the two ends of armature coil. These rings rotate with the rotation of the coil.

(d) **Brushes** B_1 and B_2 are two flexible graphite contacts. They are fixed and are kept in light contact with R_1 and R_2, respectively. These are used to pass on current from the armature coil to the external load resistance R.

(e) **Source of energy** The armature coil is rotated with the help of turbine or any other device connected to it. The rotational kinetic energy of the turbine is converted into electrical energy by the AC generator.

(iii) Theory and working

As the armature coil is rotated in the magnetic field, angle θ between the field and normal to the coil changes continuously. Hence, magnetic flux linked with the coil also changes and therefore emf is induced in the coil. Induced current in the external circuit changes direction after every half rotation of the coil.

Hence, the induced current is of alternating in nature. The emf, so induced is given by the formula, $E = E_0 \sin\omega t$.

where, $E_0 = E_{max} = NAB\omega$,

ω = angular frequency of the coil,

N = number of turns in the coil,

A = area enclosed by each turn of the coil

and B = strength of magnetic field.

The variation of E with time in AC generator is shown in figure

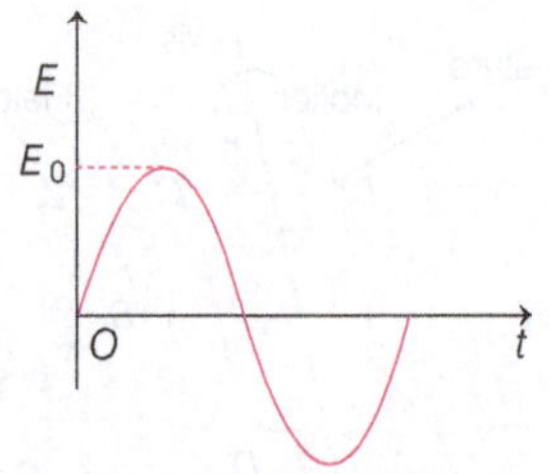

Variation of emf in AC generator

Note If AC is produced by a generator having a large number of poles, then its frequency

$$\nu = \frac{\text{Number of poles} \times \text{rotation per second}}{2} = \frac{P \times n}{2}$$

where, P is the number of poles, n is the rotational frequency of the coil.

Example 29. *An AC generator consists of a coil of 1000 turns each of area 100 cm^2 and rotating at an angular speed of 100 rpm in a uniform magnetic field of 3.6×10^{-2} T. Find the peak and rms value of emf induced in the coil.*

Sol. Given, number of turns, $N = 1000$,

Area, $A = 100\text{ cm}^2 = 100 \times 10^{-4}\text{ m}^2 = 10^{-2}\text{ m}^2$

Frequency, $\nu = 100$ rpm

$$= \frac{100}{60}\text{ rps} = \frac{5}{3}\text{ rps}$$

Magnetic field, $B = 3.6 \times 10^{-2}$ T

$\therefore$ Peak value of emf, $E_0 = NAB\omega$

$$= NAB(2\pi\nu)$$

$$= 1000 \times 10^{-2} \times 3.6 \times 10^{-2} \times 2 \times \pi \times \frac{5}{3}$$

$$= 3.77\text{ V}$$

$$E_{\text{rms}} \text{ or } E_V = \frac{E_0}{\sqrt{2}}$$

$$= 2.67\text{ V}$$

STEP UP Practice 4

1. What is increased in step-down transformer?
(a) Voltage (b) Current (c) Power (d) Current density

2. A transformer works on the principle of
(a) self-induction
(b) electrical inertia
(c) mutual induction
(d) magnetic effect of the electrical current

3. Quantity that remains unchanged in a transformer is
(a) voltage (b) current
(c) frequency (d) None of these

4. **Statement I** Transformers are used only in alternating current source not in direct current.
Statement II Only AC can be stepped up or down by means of transformers.
In the light of the above statements, choose the most appropriate answer from the options given below.
(a) Both Statement I and Statement II are incorrect.
(b) Statement I is correct but Statement II is incorrect.
(c) Statement I is incorrect but Statement II is correct.
(d) Both Statement I and Statement II are correct.

5. Choke coil is a device having
(a) low inductance and low resistance
(b) high inductance and high resistance
(c) low inductance and high resistance
(d) high inductance and low resistance

6. The transformation ratio in the step-up transformer is
(a) 1
(b) greater than one
(c) less than one
(d) the ratio greater or less than one depends on the other factors

7. The ratio of secondary to the primary turns in a transformer is 3 : 2. If the power output be P, then the input power neglecting all losses must be equal to
(a) $5P$ (b) $1.5P$ (c) P (d) $(2/5)P$

8. In a transformer, the number of turns in primary and secondary are 500 and 2000, respectively. If current in primary is 48 A, the current in the secondary is
(a) 12 A (b) 24 A (c) 48 A (d) 144 A

9. The core used in a transformer and other electromagnetic devices is laminated so that
(a) ratio of voltage in the primary and secondary may be increased
(b) energy loss due to eddy currents may be minimised
(c) the weight of the transformer may be reduced
(d) residual magnetism in the core may be reduced

10. **Statement I** Step-down transformer increases the current.
Statement II Transformer obeys the law of conservation of energy.
In the light of the above statements, choose the most appropriate answer from the options given below.
(a) Both Statement I and Statement II are incorrect.
(b) Statement I is correct but Statement II is incorrect.
(c) Statement I is incorrect but Statement II is correct.
(d) Both Statement I and Statement II are correct.

11. A step-down transformer has 50 turns on secondary and 1000 turns on primary winding. If a transformer is connected to 220 V, 1 A AC source, then what is output current of the transformer?
(a) $\frac{1}{20}$ A (b) 20 A (c) 100 A (d) 2 A

12. **Statement I** When a current flows in the coil of a transformer, then its core becomes hot.

Statement II The core of transformer is made of iron.

In the light of the above statements, choose the most appropriate answer from the options given below.

(a) Both Statement I and Statement II are incorrect.
(b) Statement I is correct but Statement II is incorrect.
(c) Statement I is incorrect but Statement II is correct.
(d) Both Statement I and Statement II are correct.

13. A step-up transformer operates on a 230 V line and supplies a current of 2 A. The ratio of primary and secondary winding is 1 : 25. The primary current is

(a) 12.5 A (b) 50 A (c) 8.8 A (d) 25 A

14. Which one of the following pair given below is correct about electric devices?

(a) Transformer → Electromagnetic Induction
(b) Electric generator → Mutual induction
(c) Eddy current loss → I^2R
(d) Efficiency of transformer → $\frac{V_S I_S}{V_P I_P}$

15. A dynamo converts

(a) mechanical energy into thermal energy
(b) electrical energy into thermal energy
(c) thermal energy into electrical energy
(d) mechanical energy into electrical energy

16. Transformer is used to

(a) convert AC to DC voltage
(b) convert DC to AC voltage
(c) obtain desired DC power
(d) obtain desired AC voltage and current

17. When speed of a DC generator decreases, the armature current

(a) increases
(b) decreases
(c) does not change
(d) increases and decreases continuously

18. Which of the following is constructed on the principle of electromagnetic induction?

(a) Galvanometer (b) Electric motor
(c) Generator (d) Voltmeter

19. **Statement I** There is always some flux leakage; i.e., not all of the flux due to primary passes through the secondary due to poor design of the core or the air gaps in the core.

Statement II Flux leakage can be reduced by winding the primary and secondary coils one over the other.

In the light of the above statements, choose the most appropriate answer from the options given below.

(a) Both Statement I and Statement II are incorrect.
(b) Statement I is correct but Statement II is incorrect.
(c) Statement I is incorrect but Statement II is correct.
(d) Both Statement I and Statement II are correct.

NEET Exclusive EXTRA BYTES

- The case of purely capacitive or inductive is similar to that of a frictionless pendulum, where the total work done by gravity on the pendulum in a cycle is zero.
- Phase difference between capacitive and inductive reactance is π.
- Energy stored in a capacitor resides in the region of its electric field.
- Voltage or current on L or C may be more than source voltage or current in LCR circuit.
- Resonance state's current is independent of L and C.
- Unit of $\sqrt{LC}$ is second.
- At resonance, the current through the supply and the voltage are in phase while the current through the capacitor leads the voltage by 90°.
- A series resonant L-C-R circuit is also used as a voltage amplification circuit.
- Power factor cannot be negative *i.e.*, its value is always between 0 and 1.
- The product of V_{rms} and i_{rms} gives the apparent power and true power = Apparent power × Power factor.

GEARING UP FOR NEET

Single Option Correct

1. A complex current wave is given by $i = (5 + 5 \sin 100\, \pi t)$ A. Its average value over one time period is given as
(a) 10 A (b) 5 A
(c) $\sqrt{50}$ A (d) 0

2. If the rms current in a 50 Hz AC circuit is 5 A, the value of the current 1/300 s after its value becomes zero is *[NCERT Exemplar]*
(a) $5\sqrt{2}$ A (b) $5\sqrt{3/2}$ A
(c) 5/6 A (d) $5/\sqrt{2}$ A

3. An alternating voltage is given by
$$e = e_1 \sin \omega t + e_2 \cos \omega t$$
Then, the root-mean-square value of voltage is given by
(a) $\sqrt{e_1^2 + e_2^2}$ (b) $\sqrt{e_2 e_2}$
(c) $\sqrt{\dfrac{e_1 e_2}{2}}$ (d) $\sqrt{\dfrac{e_1^2 + e_2^2}{2}}$

4. The output sinusoidal current *versus* time curve of a rectifier is shown in the figure. The average value of output current in this case is

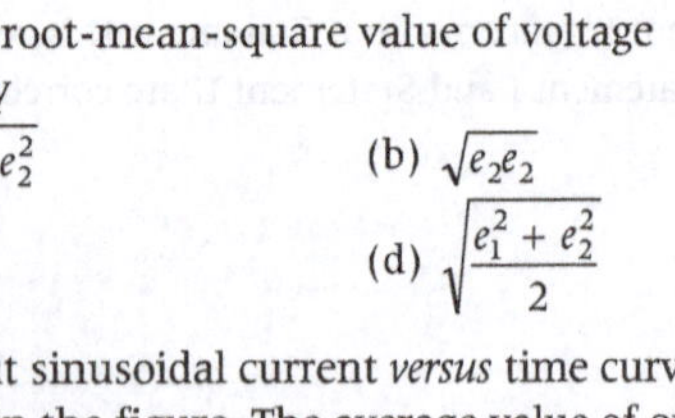

(a) 0 (b) $\dfrac{I_0}{2}$ (c) $\dfrac{2I_0}{\pi}$ (d) I_0

5. Voltage and current in an AC circuit are given by
$V = 5 \sin\left(100\pi t - \dfrac{\pi}{6}\right)$ and $I = 4 \sin\left(100\pi t + \dfrac{\pi}{6}\right)$
(a) voltage leads the current by 30°
(b) current leads the voltage by 30°
(c) current leads the voltage by 60°
(d) voltage leads the current by 60°

6. An electric current has both DC and AC components. DC component of 8A and AC component is given as $I = 6 \sin \omega t$. So, I_{rms} value of resultant current is
(a) 8.05 A (b) 9.05 A
(c) 11.58 A (d) 13.58 A

7. Two coils have a mutual inductance 0.005 H. The alternating current changes in the first coil according to equation $I = I_0 \sin \omega t$, where $I_0 = 10$ A and $\omega = 100\pi$ rads^{-1}. The maximum value of emf in the second coil is (in volt)
(a) 2π (b) 5π (c) π (d) 4π

8. Using an AC voltmeter, the potential difference in the electrical line in a house is found to be 234 V. If the line frequency is known to be 50 cycles per second, the equation for the line voltage is
(a) $165 \sin (200\pi t)$ (b) $234 \sin (100\pi t)$
(c) $331 \sin (100\pi t)$ (d) $440 \sin (200\pi t)$

9. In a certain circuit, current changes with time according to $i = 2\sqrt{t}$. Root mean square value of current between $t = 2$ to $t = 4$s will be
(a) 3 A (b) $3\sqrt{3}$ A
(c) $2\sqrt{3}$ A (d) $\sqrt{3}$ A

10. The resistance of a coil for DC is 5 Ω. In case of AC, the resistance will
(a) remain 5 Ω (b) decrease
(c) increase (d) be zero

11. The frequency for which a 5 μF capacitor has a reactance of $\dfrac{1}{1000}$ Ω is given by
(a) $\dfrac{100}{\pi}$ MHz (b) $\dfrac{100}{\pi}$ Hz
(c) $\dfrac{1}{1000}$ Hz (d) 1000 Hz

12. An *L-R* circuit has $R = 10\,\Omega$ and $L = 2$ H. If 120 V, 60 Hz AC voltage is applied, then current in the circuit will be
(a) 0.32 A (b) 0.16 A
(c) 0.48 A (d) 0.80 A

13. The resonant frequency of a circuit is f. If the capacitance is made 4 times the initial value, then the resonant frequency will become
(a) $f/2$ (b) $2f$
(c) f (d) $f/4$

14. An alternating emf is applied across a parallel combination of a resistance R, capacitance C and an inductance L. If I_R, I_L and I_C are the currents through R, L and C respectively, then the diagram which correctly represents, the phase relationship among I_R, I_L, I_C and source emf E, is given by

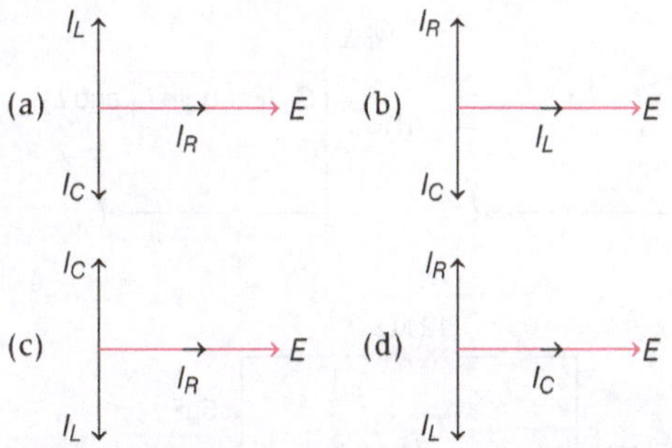

15. An alternating voltage $E = 200\sqrt{2}\sin(100t)$ is connected to a 1 μF capacitor through an AC ammeter. The reading of the ammeter shall be
(a) 10 mA (b) 20 mA (c) 40 mA (d) 80 mA

16. A resistor and a capacitor are connected in series with an AC source. If the potential drop across the capacitor is 5 V and that across resistor is 12 V, then applied voltage is
(a) 13 V (b) 17 V (c) 5 V (d) 12 V

17. An inductance of 1 mH, a condenser of 10 μF and a resistance of 50 Ω are connected in series. The reactances of inductor and condensers are same. The reactance of either of them will be
(a) 100 Ω (b) 30 Ω (c) 3.2 Ω (d) 10 Ω

18. An alternating voltage $V = 30\sin 50t + 40\cos 50t$ is applied to a resistor of resistance 10 Ω. The rms value of current through resistor is
(a) $\frac{5}{\sqrt{2}}$ A (b) $\frac{10}{\sqrt{2}}$ A
(c) 5 A (d) None of these

19. In the *L*-*C*-*R* circuit as shown in figure.

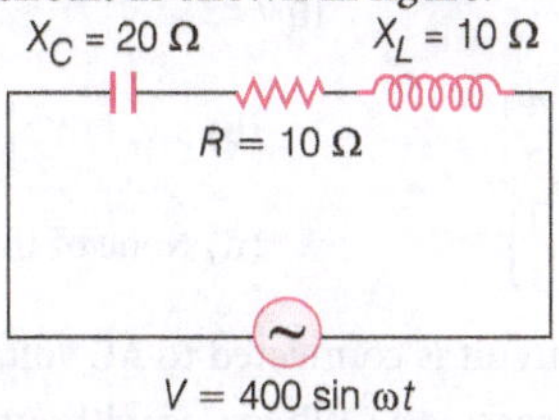

Choose the correct option from the following
(a) Current will lag the voltage
(b) Rms value of current is $20\sqrt{2}$ A
(c) Power factor of the circuit is $\frac{1}{2}$
(d) Voltage drop across resistance is 200 V

20. In the circuit shown, the AC source has voltage $V = 20\cos(\omega t)$ volt with $\omega = 2000\ \text{rad s}^{-1}$. The amplitude of the current will be nearest to

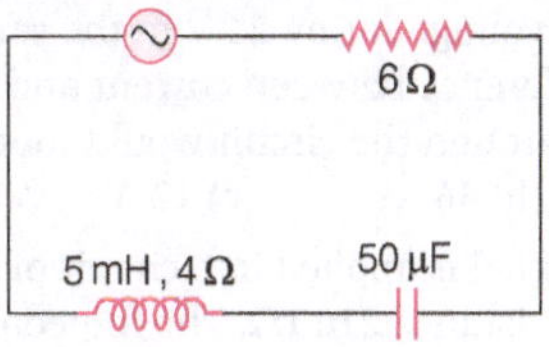

(a) 2 A (b) 3.3 A (c) $2/\sqrt{5}$ A (d) $\sqrt{5}$ A

21. An inductor *L*, a capacitor of 20 μF and a resistor of 10Ω are connected in series with an AC source of frequency 50 Hz. If the current is in phase with the voltage, then the inductance of the inductor is
(a) 2.00 H (b) 0.51 H
(c) 1.5 H (d) 0.99 H

22. An *L*-*C*-*R* series circuit consists of a resistance of 10 Ω, a capacitor of reactance 60 Ω and an inductor coil. The circuit is found to resonate when put across a 300 V, 100 Hz supply. The inductance of coil is (take, $\pi = 3$)
(a) 0.1 H (b) 0.01 H
(c) 0.2 H (d) 0.02 H

23. An AC voltage $V = V_0 \sin 100t$ is applied to the circuit, the phase difference between current and voltage is found to be $\frac{\pi}{4}$, then

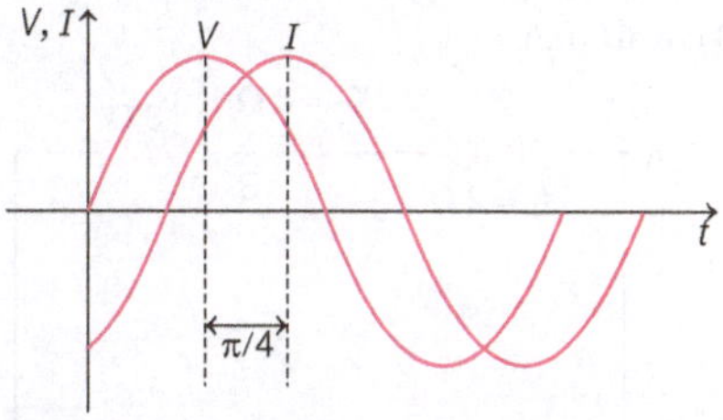

(a) $R = 100\ \Omega, C = 1\ \mu F$
(b) $R = 1\ k\Omega, C = 10\ \mu F$
(c) $R = 10\ k\Omega, L = 1\ H$
(d) $R = 1\ k\Omega, L = 10\ H$

24. In the given AC circuit, when switch *S* is at position 1, the source emf leads current by $\pi/6$. Now, if the switch is at position 2, then

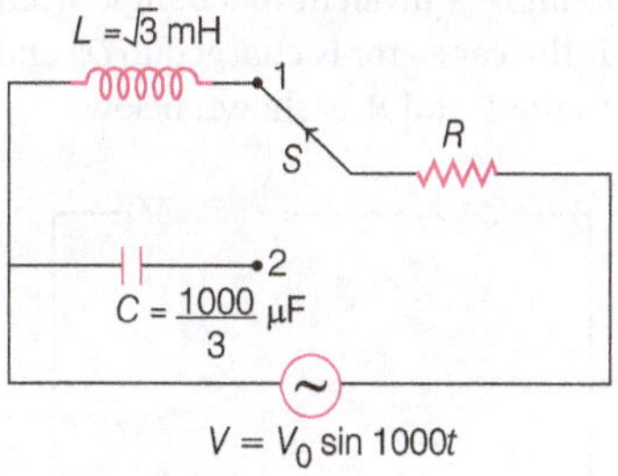

(a) current leads source emf by $\frac{\pi}{4}$
(b) current leads source emf by $\frac{\pi}{3}$
(c) source emf leads current by $\frac{\pi}{4}$
(d) source emf leads current by $\frac{\pi}{3}$

25. An arc lamp requires a direct current of 10 A at 80 V to function. If it is connected to a 220 V(rms), 50 Hz AC supply, the series inductor needed for it to work is close to
(a) 0.08 H (b) 0.044 H
(c) 0.064 H (d) 80 H

26. In the circuit shown in the figure, the ac source gives a voltage $V = 20\cos(2000t)$. Neglecting source resistance, the voltmeter and ammeter readings will be

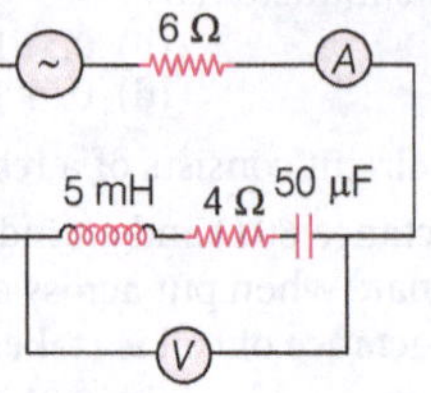

(a) 0 V, 0.47 A (b) 1.68 V, 0.47 A
(c) 0 V, 1.4 A (d) 5.6 V, 1.4 A

27. An inductor ($X_L = 2\ \Omega$), a capacitor ($X_C = 8\ \Omega$) and a resistance ($R = 8\ \Omega$) are connected in series with an AC source. The voltage output of AC source is given by $V = 10\cos(100\pi t)$.

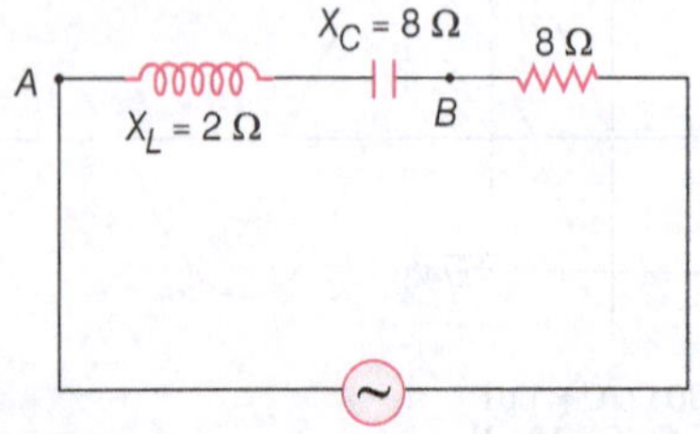

The instantaneous potential difference between points A and B, when the applied voltage is 3/5th of the maximum value of applied voltage is

(a) 0 V (b) 6 V
(c) 8 V (d) None of these

28. An L-C-R circuit is equivalent to a damped pendulum. In an L-C-R circuit the capacitor is charged to Q_0 and then connected to the L and R as shown below.

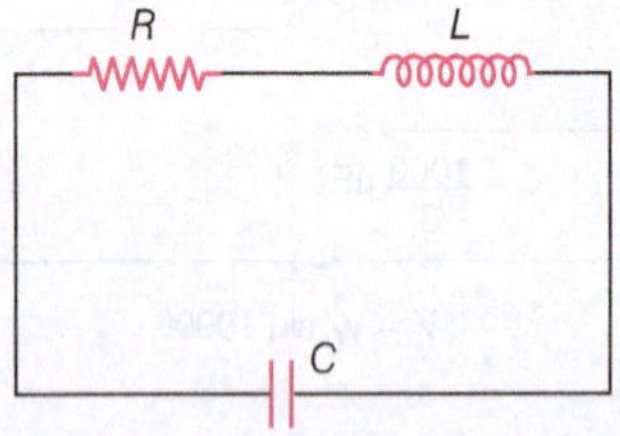

If a student plots graphs of the square of maximum charge (Q^2_{max}) on the capacitor with time (t) for two different values L_1 and $L_2 (L_1 > L_2)$ of L, then which of the following represents this graph correctly (plots are schematic and not drawn to scale)

(a)
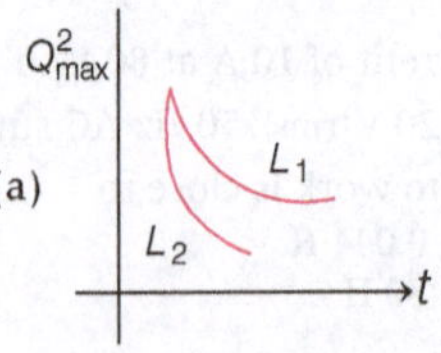

(b)
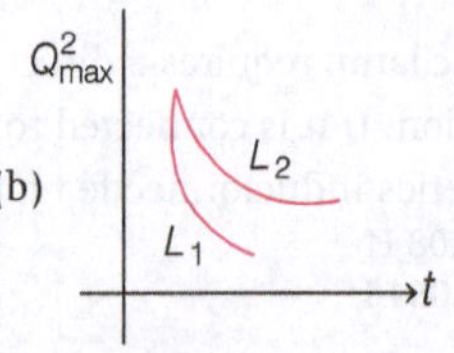

(c)
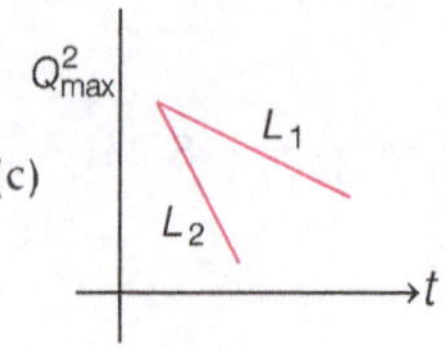

(d)
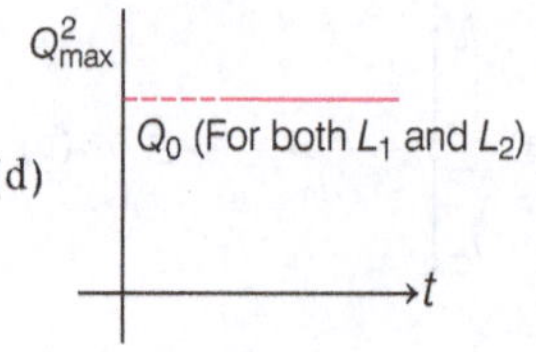

29.

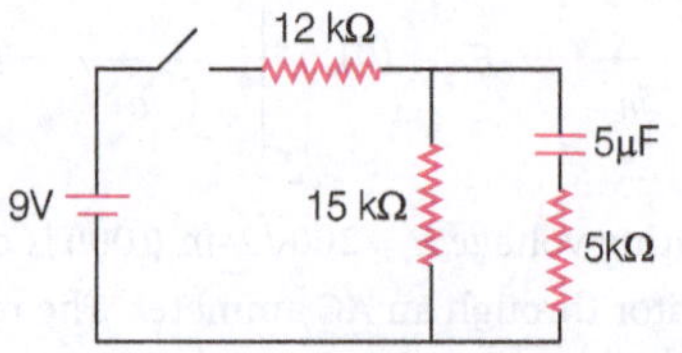

In the given circuit, find charge on capacitor after 1s of opening the switch at $t = \infty$.

(a) $20\,e^{-10}$ μC (b) $25\,e^{-10}$ μC
(c) $30\,e^{-10}$ μC (d) $35\,e^{-10}$ μC

30. In an L-C-R series circuit, source voltage is 120 V and voltage in inductor is 50 V and in resistance is 40 V, then determine voltage (in volt) in the capacitor.

(a) $V_C = 10(5 - 8\sqrt{2})$ (b) $V_C = 10(5 + 8\sqrt{2})$
(c) $V_C = 20(5 + 8\sqrt{2})$ (d) $V_C = 10(5 + 7\sqrt{2})$

31. In a series R-C circuit shown in figure, the applied voltage is 10 V and the voltage across capacitor is found to be 8V. Then, the voltage across R and the phase difference between current and the applied voltage will respectively be

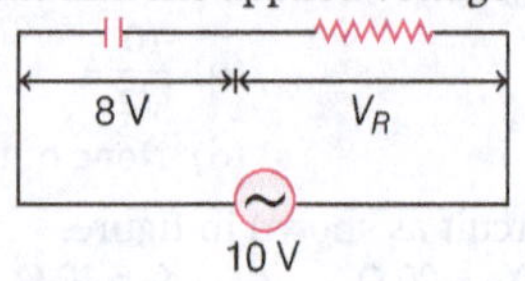

(a) 6 V, $\tan^{-1}\left(\frac{4}{3}\right)$ (b) 3 V, $\tan^{-1}\left(\frac{3}{4}\right)$
(c) 6 V, $\tan^{-1}\left(\frac{5}{3}\right)$ (d) None of these

32. A series R-C circuit is connected to AC voltage source. Consider two cases; (A) When C is without a dielectric medium and (B) When C is filled with dielectric of constant 4. The current I_R through the resistor and voltage V_C across the capacitor are compared in two cases. Which of the following is true?

(a) $I_R^A > I_R^B$ (b) $I_R^A < I_R^B$
(c) $V_C^A < V_C^B$ (d) None of these

33. An inductor coil is connected to a 12 V battery and drawing a current 24 A. This coil is connected to capacitor and an AC source of rms voltage rating 24 V in the series connection. The phase difference between current and emf is zero. The rms current through the circuit would found to be

(a) 48 A (b) 36 A (c) 12 A (d) 24 A

34. A 50 Hz AC signal is applied in a circuit of inductance of $(1/\pi)$ H and resistance 2100 Ω. The impedance offered by the circuit is

(a) 1500 Ω (b) 1700 Ω (c) 2102 Ω (d) 2500 Ω

35. In *R-L-C* series circuit, the potential difference across each element is 20 V. Now the value of the resistance alone is doubled, then PD across *R*, *L* and *C* respectively,
(a) 20 V, 10 V, 10 V (b) 20 V, 20 V, 20 V
(c) 20 V, 40 V, 40 V (d) 10 V, 20 V, 20 V

36. The self inductance of a choke coil is 10 mH. When it is connected with a 10 V DC source, then the loss of power is 20 W. When its is connected with 10 V AC source loss of power is 10 W. The frequency of AC source will be
(a) 80 Hz (b) 100 Hz (c) 120 Hz (d) 220 Hz

37. As given in the figure, a series circuit connected across a 200 V, 60 Hz line consists of a capacitor of capacitive reactance 30Ω, a non-inductive resistor of 44 Ω and a coil of inductive reactance 90Ω and resistance 36Ω. the power dissipated in the coil is

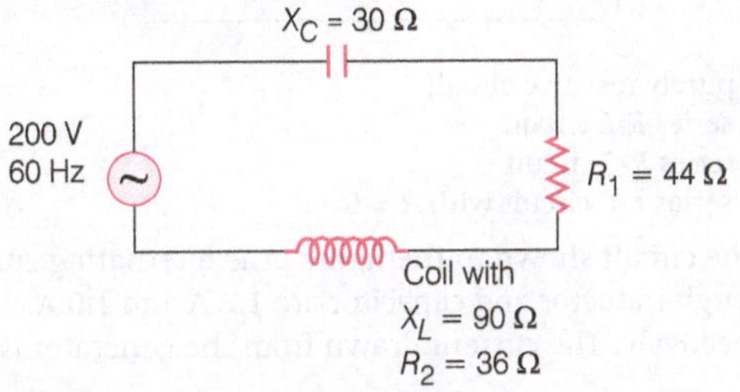

(a) 320 W (b) 176 W (c) 144 W (d) 0

38. A choke is preferred to a resistance for limiting current in AC circuit because
(a) choke is cheap
(b) there is no wastage of power
(c) choke is compact in size
(d) choke is a good absorber of heat

39. An AC supply gives 30 V which passes through a 10 Ω resistance. The power dissipated in it is
(a) $90\sqrt{2}$ W (b) 90 W
(c) $45\sqrt{2}$ W (d) 45 W

40. An alternating potential $V = V_0 \sin \omega t$ is applied across a circuit. As a result the current $I = I_0 \sin\left(\omega t - \frac{\pi}{2}\right)$ flows in it. The power consumed in the circuit per cycle is
(a) zero (b) $0.5\ V_0 I_0$
(c) $0.707\ V_0 I_0$ (d) $1.414\ V_0 I_0$

41. In a heating arrangement, an alternating current having a peak value of 28 A is used. To produce the same heat energy, if the constant current is used, its magnitude must be
(a) about 14 A (b) about 28 A
(c) about 20 A (d) Cannot say

42. A lamp consumes only 50% of peak power in an AC circuit. What is the phase difference between the applied voltage and circuit current?
(a) $\frac{\pi}{6}$ (b) $\frac{\pi}{3}$
(c) $\frac{\pi}{4}$ (d) $\frac{\pi}{2}$

43. 110 V is applied across a series circuit having resistance 11 Ω and impedance 22 Ω. The power consumed is
(a) 275 W (b) 366 W
(c) 550 W (d) 1100 W

44. To reduce the resonant frequency in an *L-C-R* series circuit with a generator ***[NCERT Exemplar]***
(a) the generator frequency should be reduced
(b) another capacitor should be added in parallel to the first
(c) the iron core of the inductor should be removed
(d) dielectric in the capacitor should be removed

45. In an *L-R* circuit, the inductive reactance is equal to the resistance *R* of the circuit. An emf $E = E_0 \cos(\omega t)$ is applied to the circuit. The power consumed in the circuit is
(a) $\frac{E_0^2}{\sqrt{2}R}$ (b) $\frac{E_0^2}{4R}$
(c) $\frac{E_0^2}{2R}$ (d) $\frac{E_0^2}{8R}$

46. In the series *L-C-R* circuit shown, the impedance is

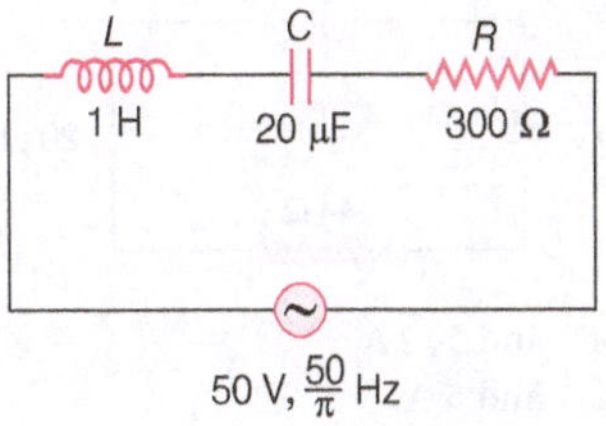

(a) 200 Ω (b) 100 Ω
(c) 300 Ω (d) 500 Ω

47. A group of electric lamps having a total power rating of 1000 W is supplied by an AC voltage, $E = 200 \sin(310\,t + 60°)$, then the rms value of the circuit current is
(a) 10 A (b) $5\sqrt{2}$ A
(c) 20 A (d) $10\sqrt{2}$ A

48. The power factor of an *R-L* circuit is $\frac{1}{\sqrt{2}}$. If the frequency of AC is doubled, what will be the power factor?
(a) $\frac{1}{\sqrt{3}}$ (b) $\frac{1}{\sqrt{5}}$
(c) $\frac{1}{\sqrt{7}}$ (d) $\frac{1}{\sqrt{11}}$

49. When a DC voltage of 200V is applied to a coil of self inductance $(2\sqrt{3}/\pi)$H, a current of 1A flows through it. But by replacing DC source with AC source of 200V, the current in the coil is reduced to 0.5A. Then, the frequency of AC supply is
(a) 30 Hz (b) 60 Hz
(c) 75 Hz (d) 50 Hz

50. One 10 V, 60 W bulb is to be connected to 100 V line. The required self-inductance of induction coil will be (f = 50 Hz)
(a) 0.052 H (b) 2.42 H
(c) 16.2 H (d) 162 mH

51. The reading of ammeter in the circuit shown will be

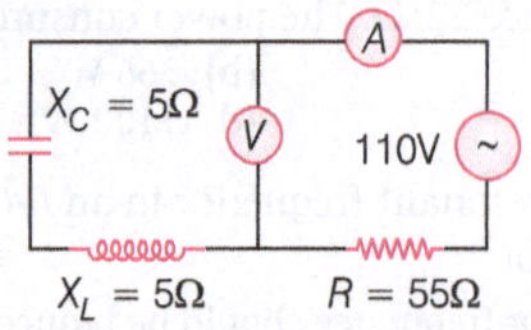

(a) 2A (b) 2.4 A (c) zero (d) 1.7 A

52. In series *L-C-R* circuit voltage drop across resistance is 8 V and across inductor is 6 V and across capacitor is 12 V. Then
(a) voltage of the source will be leading in the circuit
(b) voltage drop across each element will be less than the applied voltage
(c) power factor of the circuit will be 3/4
(d) None of the above

53. For the series *L-C-R* circuit shown in the figure, what is the resonance frequency and the current at the resonating frequency?

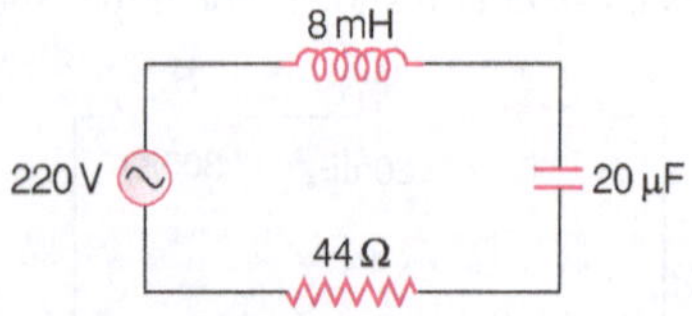

(a) 2500 rad s^{-1} and $5\sqrt{2}$ A
(b) 2500 rad s^{-1} and 5 A
(c) 2500 rad s^{-1} and $\frac{5}{\sqrt{2}}$ A
(d) 25 rad s^{-1} and $5\sqrt{2}$ A

54. In the given figure, a series *L-C-R* circuit is connected to a variable frequency source of 230 V. The impedance and amplitude of the current at the resonating frequency will be

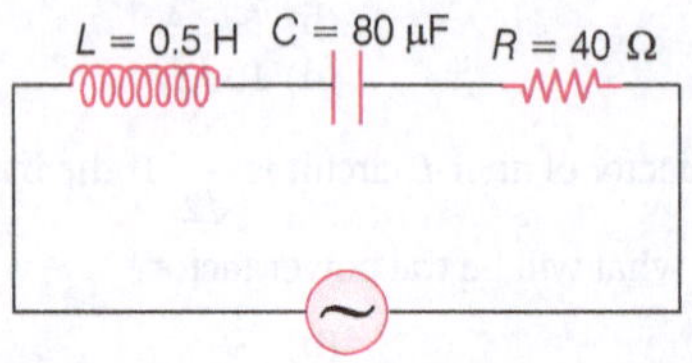

(a) 20 Ω and 4.2 A (b) 30 Ω and 6.9 A
(c) 25 Ω and 5.8 A (d) 40 Ω and 5.75 A

55. In figure, which voltmeter reads zero, when ω is equal to the resonant frequency of series *L-C-R* circuit?

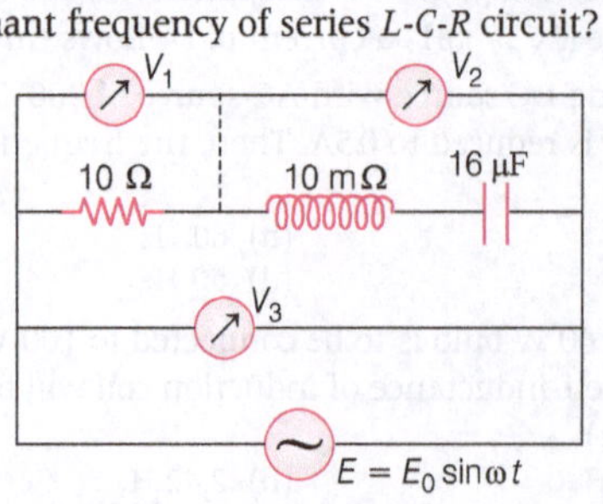

(a) V_1 (b) V_2
(c) V_3 (d) None of these

56. An *R-L-C* circuit containing a 52 Ω resistor, a 230 mH inductor, and a 8.8 μF capacitor is driven by an AC voltage source that has an amplitude of 150 V and frequency $f = 80$ Hz. How much average power is dissipated by this circuit?
(a) 78.6 W (b) Zero
(c) 19.6 W (d) 24.8 W

57. The following series *L-C-R* circuit, when driven by an emf source of angular frequency 70 kilo-radians per second, the circuit effectively behaves like

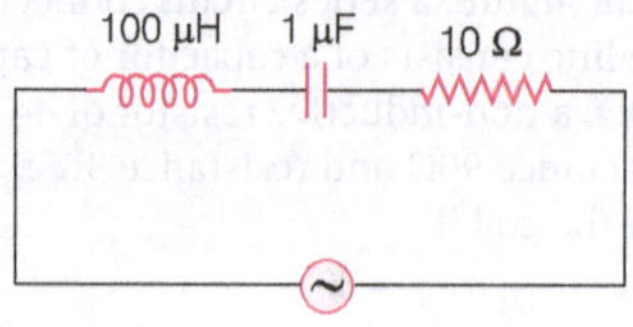

(a) purely resistive circuit
(b) series *R-L* circuit
(c) series *R-C* circuit
(d) series *L-C* circuit with $R = 0$

58. In the circuit shown in the figure , the alternating currents through inductor and capacitor are 1.2 A and 1.0 A, respectively. The current drawn from the generator is

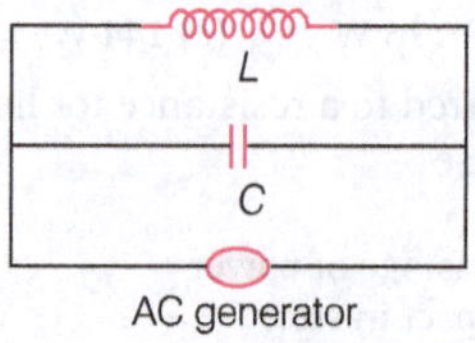

(a) 0.4 A (b) 0.2 A
(c) 1.0 A (d) 1.2 A

59. In the circuit shown in figure, the supply has a constant rms value *V* but variable frequency *f*. The frequency at which the voltage drop across *R* is maximum is

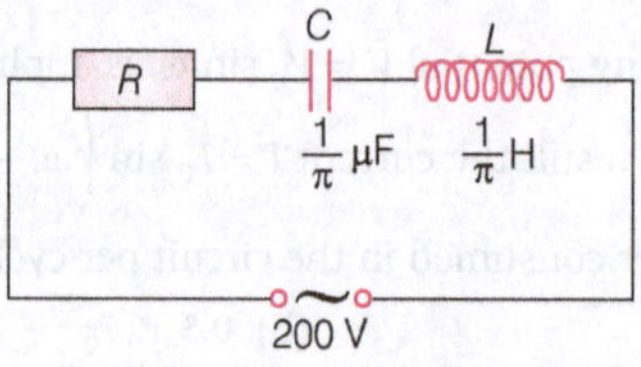

(a) 100 Hz (b) 500 Hz
(c) 300 Hz (d) None of these

60. An inductor of reactance 1 Ω and a resistor of 2 Ω are connected in series to the terminals of a 6V (rms) AC source. The power dissipated in the circuit is ***[NCERT Exemplar]***
(a) 8 W (b) 12 W
(c) 14.4 W (d) 18 W

61. An AC circuit consists of a resistance and a choke coil in series. The resistance is of 220 Ω and choke coils is of 0.7 H. The power absorbed from 220 V and 50 Hz, source connected with the circuit, is
(a) 55 W (b) 110 W
(c) 220 W (d) 440 W

62. In a series L-C-R circuit the voltage across resistance, capacitance and inductance is 10V each. If the capacitance is short circuited, the voltage across the inductance will be
(a) $\frac{10}{\sqrt{2}}$ V (b) 10 V (c) $10\sqrt{2}$ V (d) 20 V

63. An L-C-R series circuit with a resistance of 100 Ω is connected to an AC source of 200 V (rms) and angular frequency 300 rad s^{-1}. When only the capacitor is removed, the current lags behind the voltage by 60°. When only the inductor is removed the current leads the voltage by 60°. The average power dissipated in original L-C-R circuit is
(a) 50 W (b) 100 W
(c) 200 W (d) 400 W

64. A virtual current of 4 A and 50 Hz flows in an AC circuit containing a coil. The power consumed in the coil is 240 W. If the virtual voltage across the coil is 100 V, then its inductance will be
(a) $\frac{1}{3\pi}$ H (b) $\frac{1}{5\pi}$ H
(c) $\frac{1}{7\pi}$ H (d) $\frac{1}{9\pi}$ H

65. Which of the following options is correct with respect to the circuit diagram given below?

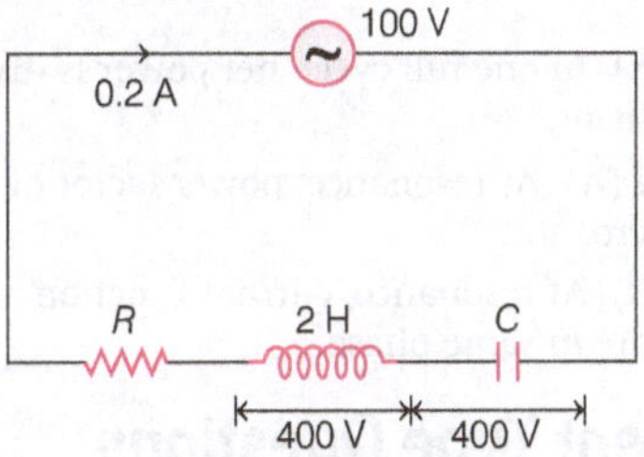

(a) $R = 400\,\Omega$, $C = 0.5\,\mu F$
(b) $R = 500\,\Omega$, $C = 0.5\,\mu F$
(c) $R = 500\,\Omega$, $C = 1\,\mu F$
(d) $R = 400\,\Omega$, $C = 0.1\,\mu F$

66. When 100 V DC is applied across a solenoid, a current of 1 A flows in it. When 100 V AC is applied across the same solenoid the current drops to 0.5 A. If the frequency of the AC source is 50 Hz, the impedance and inductance of the solenoid are
(a) 200 Ω and 0.55 H (b) 100 Ω and 0.86 H
(c) 200 Ω and 1.0 H (d) 1100 Ω and 0.93 H

67. Current through an AC series L-C-R circuit is 2 A if operated at resonant frequency, and 1 A if operated at 50% less than resonant frequency. The current (in A) if the frequency is 100% more than the resonant frequency, is
(a) $\sqrt{2}$ (b) 1
(c) $\sqrt{3}$ (d) Data insufficient

68. A circuit draws 330 W from a 110 V, 60 Hz AC line. The power factor is 0.6 and the current lags the voltage. The capacitance of a series capacitor that will result in a power factor of unity is equal to
(a) 31 μF (b) 54 μF
(c) 151 μF (d) 201 μF

69. Find resonance frequency in the given circuit

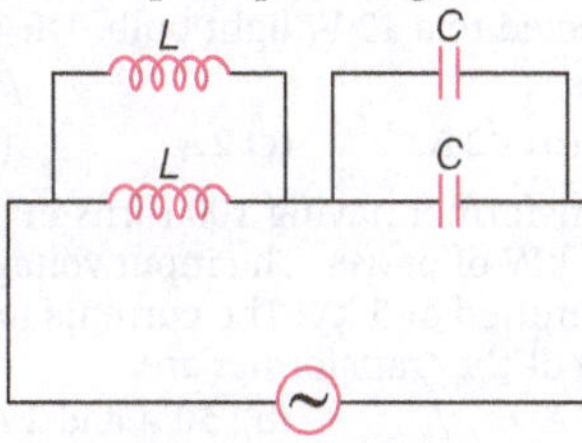

(a) $\frac{1}{\sqrt{LC}}$ (b) $\frac{2}{\sqrt{LC}}$ (c) $\frac{1}{2\sqrt{LC}}$ (d) $\frac{4}{\sqrt{LC}}$

70. An inductor 20 mH, a capacitor 100 μF and a resistor 50 Ω are connected in series across a source of emf $V = 10 \sin 314\,t$. The power loss in the circuit is
(a) 2.74 W (b) 0.43 W (c) 0.79 W (d) 1.13 W

71. In a circuit L, C and R are connected in series with an alternating voltage source of frequency f. The current leads the voltage by 45°. The value of C is
(a) $\frac{1}{2\pi f(2\pi fL + R)}$ (b) $\frac{1}{\pi f(2\pi fL + R)}$
(c) $\frac{1}{2\pi f(2\pi fL - R)}$ (d) $\frac{1}{\pi f(2\pi fL - R)}$

72. If in a L-R series circuit the power factor is $\frac{1}{2}$ and $R = 100\Omega$, then the value of L is, when AC mains is used
(a) π H (b) $\frac{\sqrt{3}}{\pi}$ H (c) $\frac{\pi}{\sqrt{3}}$ H (d) $\frac{\sqrt{2}}{\pi}$ H

73. The rms current in an AC circuit is 2 A. If the wattless current be $\sqrt{3}$A, what is the power factor of the circuit?
(a) $\frac{1}{2}$ (b) $\frac{1}{3}$ (c) $\frac{1}{\sqrt{3}}$ (d) $\frac{1}{\sqrt{2}}$

74. An AC ammeter is used to measure current in a circuit. When a given direct current passes through the circuit, the AC ammeter reads 3A. When another alternating current passes through the circuit, the AC ammeter reads 4A. Then, the reading of this ammeter, if DC and AC flow through the circuit simultaneously, is
(a) 3 A (b) 4 A (c) 7 A (d) 5 A

75. In an AC circuit, V and I are given by V=150 sin (150 t) volt and

$$I = 150 \sin\left[150\,t + \left(\frac{\pi}{3}\right)\right] \text{ ampere.}$$

The power dissipated in the circuit is
(a) 106 W (b) 150 W
(c) 5625 W (d) zero

76. In a series L-C-R circuit, resistance $R = 10\,\Omega$ and the impedance $Z = 10\Omega$. The phase difference between the current and the voltage is
(a) 0° (b) 30° (c) 45° (d) 60°

77. In a transformer, number of turns in the primary are 140 and that in the secondary are 280. If current in primary is 4 A, then that in the secondary is
(a) 4 A (b) 2 A (c) 6 A (d) 10 A

78. The output of a step-down transformer is measured to be 24 V when connected to a 12 W light bulb. The value of the peak current is *[NCERT Exemplar]*
(a) $(1/\sqrt{2})$ A (b) $\sqrt{2}$ A (c) 2A (d) $2\sqrt{2}$ A

79. A loss-free transformer having 100 turns in primary is used to transmit 10 kW of power. The input voltage is 200 V and power is transmitted at 5 kV. The currents in the primary and secondary of the transformer are
(a) 2 A and 50 A (b) 50 A and 2 A
(c) 25 A and 4 A (d) 12.5 A and 8 A

80. A transformer with turns ratio $\frac{N_1}{N_2} = \frac{50}{1}$ is connected to a 120 V AC supply. If primary and secondary circuit resistances are $1.5 k\Omega$ and 1Ω respectively, then find out power of output.
(a) 5.76 W (b) 11.4 W (c) 2.89 W (d) 756 W

81. A transformer is used to light 100 W-110 V lamp from 220 V mains. If the main current is 0.5 A, the efficiency of the transformer is
(a) 96% (b) 90% (c) 99% (d) 95%

82. A transformer of 100% efficiency has 200 turns in the primary coil and 40000 turns in secondary coil. It is connected to a 220 V main supply and secondary feeds to a 100 kΩ resistance. The potential difference per turn is
(a) 1.1 V (b) 25 V (c) 18 V (d) 11 V

83. A step down transformer is used on a 1000 V line to deliver 20 A at 120 V at the secondary coil. If the efficiency of the transformer is 80%, the current drawn from the line is
(a) 3 A (b) 30 A (c) 0.3 A (d) 2.4 A

84. An electric motor runs on DC source of emf 200 V and draws a current of 10 A. If the efficiency be 40%, then the resistance of armature is
(a) 2Ω (b) 8Ω (c) 12Ω (d) 16Ω

85. A generator at a utility company produces 100 A of current at 4000 V. The voltage is stepped up to 240000 V by a transformer before it is sent on a high voltage transmission line. The current in transmission line is
(a) 3.67 A (b) 2.67 A (c) 1.67 A (d) 2.40 A

86. A transformer has 500 primary turns and 10 secondary turns. If the secondary has a resistive load of 15 Ω, the currents in the primary and secondary respectively, are
(a) 0.16A, 3.2×10^{-3} A (b) 3.2×10^{-3}A, 0.16 A
(c) 0.16 A, 0.16 A (d) 3.2×10^{-3}A, 3.2×10^{-3}A

Assertion and Reason

Directions (Q. Nos. 1-6) *These questions consist of two statements each printed as Assertion (A) and Reason (R). While answering these questions, you are required to choose any one of the following four responses.*

(a) Both A and R are true but R is not the correct explanation of A.
(b) A is true but R is false.
(c) A is false but R is true.
(d) Both A and R are true and R is the correct explanation of A.

1. Assertion (A) If an inductor coil is connected to DC source, the current supplied by it is I_1. If the same coil is connected with an AC source of same voltage. Then current is I_2. Then $I_2 < I_1$.
Reason (R) In AC circuit, inductor coil offers more resistance.

2. Assertion (A) In an AC, only capacitor circuit has instantaneous power equals to zero at any instant of time.
Reason (R) Phase difference between current function and voltage function is 90°.

3. Assertion(A) When a ferromagnetic rod is inserted inside an inductor, then current in *L-C-R*, alternating circuit will decrease.
Reason (R) By inserting the ferromagnetic rod inside the inductor, coefficient of self induction and hence the inductive reactance will increase.

4. Assertion (A) In *L-C-R* series AC circuit, $X_L = X_C = R$ at a given frequency. When frequency is doubled, the impedance of the circuit is $\frac{\sqrt{13}}{2} R$.
Reason (R) The given frequency is resonance frequency.

5. Assertion (A) Average power in an AC circuit is given by $P = I^2_{\text{rms}} R$.
Reason (R) In one full cycle, net power is dissipated only along a resistor.

6. Assertion (A) At resonance, power factor of series *L-C-R* circuit is zero.
Reason (R) At resonance, current function and voltage functions are in same phase.

Statement Type Questions

Directions (Q. Nos. 1-6) *These questions consists of two statements, choose the most appropriate answer from the options given below.*

(a) Both Statement I and Statement II are incorrect.
(b) Statement I is correct but Statement II is incorrect.
(c) Statement I is incorrect but Statement II is correct.
(d) Both Statement I and Statement II are correct.

1. Statement I Charge amplitude of a capacitor of an *L-C-R* circuit is minimum at resonance.
Statement II At resonance circuit impedance is minimum and hence, current in circuit is maximum.

2. Statement I At resonance ratio of potential drop across inductor and of potential drop across resistor is more than 1.
Statement II At resonance, phase difference between current and voltage is zero.

3. Statement I Average power consumed by a circuit depends only on the total impedance of circuit.
Statement II Power $= I^2R$

4. Statement I Impedance of circuit is not treated as a phasor.
Statement II $Z = \sqrt{R^2 + X^2}$

5. **Statement I** Main characteristics of series resonant circuit is voltage magnification.

Statement II At resonance, potential drop across inductor or capacitor is Q times of applied voltage.

6. **Statement I** If half power point frequencies for an resonant L-C-R circuit are 2 s^{-1} and 8 s^{-1} respectively, then resonance occurs at 4 s^{-1}.

Statement II Bandwidth of circuit is $|f_2 - f_1|$, where f_1 and f_2 are half power point frequencies.

Match the Columns

1. Match the following two columns for L-C-R series AC circuit.

Column I	Column II
A. At resonance frequency	I. Power factor = 0
B. No resistance in the circuit	II. Power factor = 1
C. Frequency lower than the resonance frequency	III. Circuit is capacitive
D. Frequency greater than the resonance frequency	IV. Circuit is inductive

Choose the correct answer from the options given below.

(a) A-II, B-I, C-III, D-IV (b) A-IV, B-III, C-I, D-II
(c) A-III, B-IV, C-II, D-I (d) A-I, B-II, C-III, D-IV

2. Match the Column I with Column II.

Column I	Column II
A. Phase difference between current and voltage in a purely resistive AC circuit	I. $\frac{\pi}{2}$, current leads voltage
B. Phase difference between current and voltage in a pure inductive AC circuit	II. zero
C. Phase difference between current and voltage in a purely capacitive AC circuit	III. $\frac{\pi}{2}$, current lags voltage
D. Phase difference between current and voltage in an L-C-R circuit	IV. $\tan^{-1}\left(\frac{X_C - X_L}{R}\right)$

Choose the correct answer from the options given below.

(a) A-II, B-III, C-IV, D-I
(b) A-I, B-III, C-IV, D-II
(c) A-II, B-IV, C-III, D-I
(d) A-II, B-III, C-I, D-IV

3. In an AC series L-C-R circuit, applied voltage is

$$V = 100\sqrt{2}\sin(\omega t + 45°)\text{ V}$$

Given that, $R = 30\,\Omega$, $X_L = 50\,\Omega$ and $X_C = 10\,\Omega$

Now match the following two columns

Column I	Column II
A. Current in the circuit	I. 120 SI units
B. Power dissipated in the circuit	II. 60 SI units
C. Potential difference across resistance	III. 2 SI units
D. Potential difference across inductance	IV. None

Choose the correct answer from the options given below.

(a) A-IV, B-III, C-II, D-I (b) A-I, B-II, C-III, D-IV
(c) A-III, B-II, C-IV, D-I (d) A-III, B-I, C-II, D-IV

4. Match the following graphs in Column I with the correct entries in Column II. In Column II, first quantity listed is shown on Y-axis and second quantity listed is on X-axis of the graph.

Column I	Column II
A. 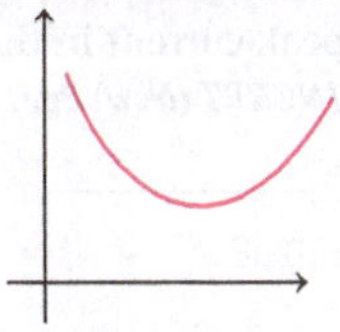	I. $\frac{1}{X_L}$ *versus* f for an inductor
B. 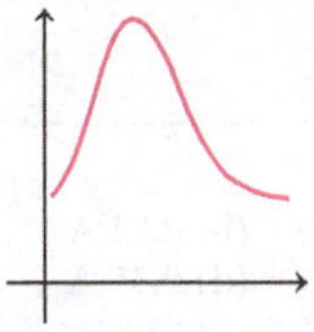	II. I *versus* f for a capacitor
C. 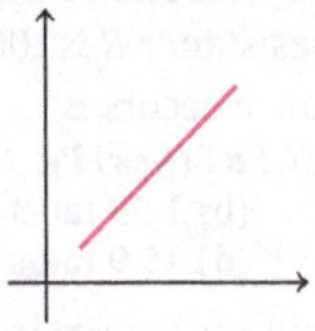	III. I *versus* f for L-C-R
D. 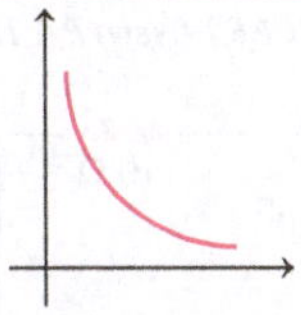	IV. Z *versus* f for an L-C-R

Choose the correct answer from the options given below.

(a) A-I, B-II, C-III, D-IV
(b) A-III, B-IV, C-II, D-I
(c) A-IV, B-III, C-II, D-I
(d) A-II, B-I, C-IV, D-III

Final Check Through PYQs

Module-I Introduction to AC

1. The peak voltage of the AC source is equal to **[NCERT (New) Pg. 180, NEET 2022]**
(a) the rms value of the AC source
(b) $\sqrt{2}$ times the rms value of the AC source
(c) $1/\sqrt{2}$ times the rms value of the AC source
(d) the value of voltage supplied to the circuit

Module-II AC Circuits

2. A 10 μF capacitor is connected to a 210 V, 50 Hz source as shown in figure. The peak current in the circuit is nearly ($\pi = 3.14$) **[NCERT (New) Pg. 184, NEET 2024]**

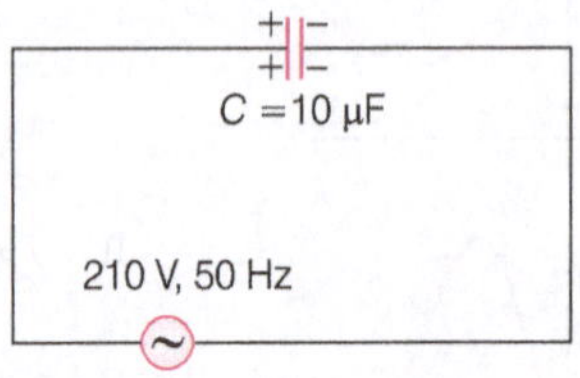

(a) 0.58 A
(b) 0.93 A
(c) 1.20 A
(d) 0.35 A

3. In a series *L-C-R* circuit, the inductance *L* is 10 mH, capacitance *C* is 1 μF and resistance *R* is 100 Ω. The frequency at which resonance occurs is **[NCERT (New) Pg. 186, NEET 2023]**
(a) 15.9 kHz
(b) 1.59 rad/s
(c) 1.59 kHz
(d) 15.9 rad/s

4. The net impedance of circuit (as shown in figure) will be **[NCERT (New) Pg. 186, NEET 2023]**

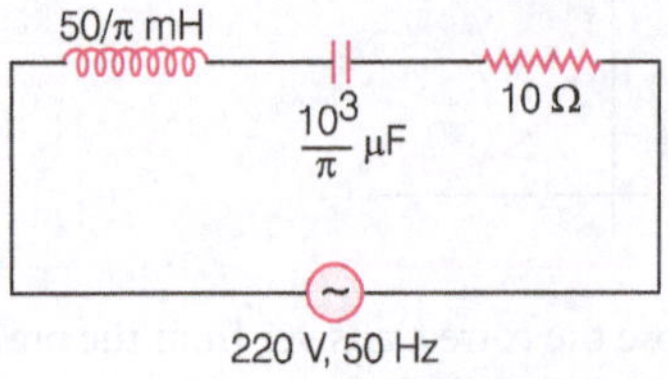

(a) 15 Ω
(b) $5\sqrt{5}\,\Omega$
(c) 25 Ω
(d) $10\sqrt{2}\,\Omega$

5. A series *L-C-R* circuit with inductance 10 H, capacitance 10 μF, resistance 50 Ω is connected to an AC source of voltage, $V = 200\sin(100\,t)$ volt. If the resonant frequency of the *L-C-R* circuit is ν_0 and the frequency of the AC source is ν, then **[NCERT (New) Pg. 186, NEET 2022]**
(a) $\nu_0 = \nu = \frac{50}{\pi}$ Hz
(b) $\nu_0 = \frac{50}{\pi}$ Hz, $\nu = 50$ Hz
(c) $\nu = 100$ Hz; $\nu_0 = \frac{100}{\pi}$ Hz
(d) $\nu_0 = \nu = 50$ Hz

6. An inductor of inductance *L*, a capacitor of capacitance *C* and a resistor of resistance *R* are connected in series to an AC source of potential difference *V* volts as shown in figure.

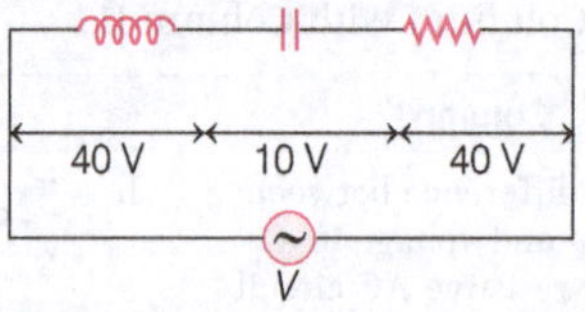

Potential difference across *L*, *C* and *R* is 40 V, 10 V and 40 V, respectively. The amplitude of current flowing through *L-C-R* series circuit is $10\sqrt{2}$ A. The impedance of the circuit is **[NCERT (New) Pg. 106, NEET 2021]**
(a) $4\sqrt{2}\,\Omega$
(b) $5/\sqrt{2}\,\Omega$
(c) 4 Ω
(d) 5 Ω

7. A 40 μF capacitor is connected to a 200 V, 50 Hz AC supply. The rms value of the current in the circuit is, nearly **[NCERT (New) Pg. 184, NEET (Sep.) 2020]**
(a) 2.05 A (b) 2.5 A (c) 25.1 A (d) 1.7 A

8. A circuit when connected to an AC source of 12 V gives a current of 0.2 A. The same circuit when connected to a DC source of 12 V, gives a current of 0.4 A. The circuit is **[NCERT (New) Pg. 186, NEET (Odisha) 2019]**
(a) series *LR*
(b) series *RC*
(c) series *LC*
(d) series *LCR*

9. Figure shows a circuit that contains three identical resistors with resistance $R = 9.0\,\Omega$ each, two identical inductors with inductance $L = 2.0$ mH each, and an ideal battery with emf $\varepsilon = 18$ V. The current *i* through the battery just after the switch closed is **[NCERT (New) Pg. 186, NEET 2017]**

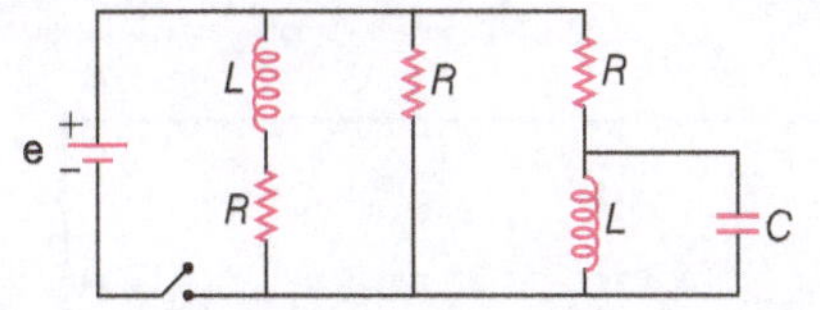

(a) 2 mA (b) 0.2 A (c) 4 A (d) 0 A

10. A 100 Ω resistance and a capacitor of 100 Ω reactance are connected in series across a 220 V source. When the capacitor is 50% charged, the peak value of the displacement current is

[NCERT (New) Pg. 186, NEET 2016]

(a) 2.2 A (b) 11 A
(c) 4.4 A (d) $11\sqrt{2}$A

11. A series *R-C* circuit is connected to an alternating voltage source. Consider two situations

[NCERT (Old) Pg. 244, AIPMT 2015]

(a) When capacitor is air filled.
(b) When capacitor is mica filled.

Current through resistor is i and voltage across capacitor is V, then

(a) $V_a < V_b$ (b) $V_a > V_b$
(c) $i_a > i_b$ (d) $V_a = V_b$

Module-III Power in AC Circuits

12. A series *L-C-R* circuit containing 5.0 H inductor, 80 μF capacitor and 40 Ω resistor is connected to 230 V variable frequency AC source. The angular frequencies of the source at which power transferred to the circuit is half the power at the resonant angular frequency are likely to be

[NCERT (New) Pg. 191, NEET 2021]

(a) 25 rad/s and 75 rad/s (b) 50 rad/s and 25 rad/s
(c) 46 rad/s and 54 rad/s (d) 42 rad/s and 58 rad/s

13. A series *L-C-R* circuit is connected to an AC voltage source. When L is removed from the circuit, the phase difference between current and voltage is $\pi/3$. If instead C is removed from the circuit, the phase difference is again $\pi/3$ between current and voltage. The power factor of the circuit is

[NCERT (New) Pg. 191, NEET (Sep.) 2020]

(a) 0.5 (b) 1.0 (c) −1.0 (d) zero

14. An inductor 20 mH, a capacitor 100 μF and a resistor 50 Ω are connected in series across a source of emf, $V = 10 \sin 314t$. The power loss in the circuit is

[NCERT (New) Pg. 191, NEET 2018]

(a) 0.79 W (b) 0.43 W (c) 2.74 W (d) 1.13 W

15. A small signal voltage $V(t) = V_0 \sin \omega t$ is applied across an ideal capacitor C ***[NCERT (New) Pg. 185, NEET 2016]***

(a) over a full cycle the capacitor C does not consume any energy from the voltage source
(b) current $I(t)$ is in phase with voltage $V(t)$
(c) current $I(t)$ leads voltage $V(t)$ by 180°
(d) current $I(t)$, lags voltage $V(t)$ by 90°

16. An inductor 20 mH, a capacitor 50 μF and a resistor 40Ω are connected in series across a source of emf $V = 10 \sin 340t$. The power loss in AC circuit is

[NCERT (New) Pg. 186, NEET 2016]

(a) 0.67 W (b) 0.76 W (c) 0.89 W (d) 0.51 W

17. The potential differences across the resistance, capacitance and inductance are 80 V, 40 V and 100 V respectively in an *L-C-R* circuit. The power factor of this circuit is ***[NCERT (New) Pg. 191, NEET 2016]***

(a) 0.4 (b) 0.5
(c) 0.8 (d) 1.0

18. A resistance R draws power P when connected to an AC source. If an inductance is now placed in series with the resistance, such that the impedance of the circuit becomes Z the power drawn will be

[NCERT (New) Pg. 186, AIPMT 2015]

(a) $P\left(\frac{R}{Z}\right)^2$ (b) $P\sqrt{\frac{R}{Z}}$ (c) $P\left(\frac{R}{Z}\right)$ (d) P

Module-IV AC Based Devices

19. In an ideal transformer, the turns ratio is $\frac{N_p}{N_s} = \frac{1}{2}$. The ratio $V_s : V_p$ is equal to (the symbols carry their usual meaning) ***[NCERT (New) Pg. 195, NEET 2024]***

(a) 1 : 2 (b) 2 : 1 (c) 1 : 1 (d) 1 : 4

20. A 12 V, 60 W lamp is connected to the secondary of a step down transformer, whose primary is connected to AC mains of 220 V. Assuming the transformer to be ideal, what is the current in the primary winding?

[NCERT (New) Pg. 195, NEET 2023]

(a) 2.7 A (b) 3.7 A
(c) 0.37 A (d) 0.27 A

21. A step down transformer connected to an AC mains supply of 220 V is made to operate at 11 V, 44 W lamp. Ignoring power losses in the transformer, what is the current in the primary circuit ?

[NCERT (New) Pg. 195, NEET 2021]

(a) 0.2 A (b) 0.4 A
(c) 2 A (d) 4 A

Answers

Step up Practice 1

1 (a)	2 (c)	3 (c)	4 (d)	5 (a)	6 (c)	7 (d)	8 (a)	9 (a)	10 (b)
11 (d)	12 (d)	13 (b)	14 (d)	15 (c)	16 (b)	17 (a)			

Step up Practice 2

1 (a)	2 (b)	3 (d)	4 (c)	5 (d)	6 (b)	7 (b)	8 (d)	9 (c)	10 (b)
11 (b)	12 (a)	13 (d)	14 (b)	15 (c)	16 (d)	17 (b)	18 (d)	19 (b)	20 (b)
21 (d)									

Step up Practice 3

1 (b)	2 (b)	3 (b)	4 (a)	5 (b)	6 (c)	7 (d)	8 (d)	9 (a)	10 (c)
11 (c)	12 (d)	13 (b)	14 (a)	15 (b)					

Step up Practice 4

1 (b)	2 (c)	3 (c)	4 (d)	5 (d)	6 (b)	7 (c)	8 (a)	9 (b)	10 (d)
11 (b)	12 (d)	13 (b)	14 (d)	15 (d)	16 (d)	17 (a)	18 (c)	19 (d)	

Gearing up for NEET

1 (b)	2 (b)	3 (d)	4 (c)	5 (c)	6 (b)	7 (b)	8 (c)	9 (c)	10 (c)
11 (a)	12 (b)	13 (a)	14 (c)	15 (b)	16 (a)	17 (d)	18 (a)	19 (d)	20 (a)
21 (b)	22 (a)	23 (b)	24 (a)	25 (c)	26 (d)	27 (b)	28 (a)	29 (b)	30 (a)
31 (a)	32 (b)	33 (a)	34 (c)	35 (a)	36 (a)	37 (a)	38 (b)	39 (b)	40 (a)
41 (c)	42 (b)	43 (a)	44 (b)	45 (b)	46 (d)	47 (b)	48 (b)	49 (d)	50 (a)
51 (a)	52 (d)	53 (b)	54 (d)	55 (b)	56 (a)	57 (b)	58 (b)	59 (b)	60 (c)
61 (b)	62 (a)	63 (d)	64 (b)	65 (b)	66 (a)	67 (b)	68 (b)	69 (a)	70 (c)
71 (c)	72 (b)	73 (a)	74 (d)	75 (c)	76 (a)	77 (b)	78 (a)	79 (b)	80 (a)
81 (b)	82 (a)	83 (a)	84 (c)	85 (c)	86 (b)				

Assertion and Reason

1 (d)	2 (c)	3 (c)	4 (a)	5 (a)	6 (c)

Statement Type Questions

1 (c)	2 (d)	3 (c)	4 (d)	5 (d)	6 (d)

Match the Columns

1 (a)	2 (d)	3 (d)	4 (c)

Final Check through PYQs : Module-I

1 (b)

Final Check through PYQs : Module-II

2 (b)	3 (c)	4 (b)	5 (a)	6 (d)	7 (b)	8 (a)	9 (c)	10 (a)	11 (b)

Final Check through PYQs : Module-III

12 (c)	13 (b)	14 (a)	15 (a)	16 (d)	17 (c)	18 (a)

Final Check through PYQs : Module-IV

19 (b)	20 (d)	21 (a)

Hints and Solutions

Step up Practice 1

1. (a) Alternating current is transmitted to take place at high voltage and low current.

2. (c) $I = 20\sin(100\pi t + 0.05\pi)$ A

$\therefore I_{rms} = \frac{20}{\sqrt{2}} = 10\sqrt{2}$ A

$\omega = 100\pi \Rightarrow f = 50\text{Hz}$

3. (c) $E = 141\sin(628t)$ V

$$E_{rms} = \frac{E_0}{\sqrt{2}} = \frac{141}{1.41} = 100\text{V}$$

and $2\pi f = 628$

$\Rightarrow f = 100\,\text{Hz}$

4. (d) Both A and R are true and R is the correct explanation of A.

The effect of AC on the body depends largely on the frequency. The usual frequency of 50 cps (or 60 cps) is extremely dangerous as it corresponds to the fibrillation frequency of the myocardium. This become cause of instant death.

5. (a) $I_{rms} = \frac{I_0}{\sqrt{2}} = \frac{5}{\sqrt{2}} = 3.536\,\text{A}$

Time taken, $T = \frac{1}{4 \times 60} = 4.167\text{ms}$

6. (c) Maximum potential difference, $V_0 = I_0 R$

$$= (I_{rms}\sqrt{2})R = (10\sqrt{2})(12) = 169.70 \text{ V}$$

7. (d) $I_{rms} = \frac{I_0}{\sqrt{2}} = \frac{\sqrt{2}}{\sqrt{2}} = 1\text{A}$

8. (a) Here, $V_{rms} = 220\text{V}$, $f = 50\,\text{Hz}$

Peak value of voltage, $V_0 = \sqrt{2}V_{rms} = 220\sqrt{2}$ V

The instantaneous value of voltage is

$$V = V_0 \sin 2\pi f t = 220\sqrt{2}\sin 2\pi \times 50t$$
$$= 220\sqrt{2}\sin 100\pi t$$

9. (a) Both A and R are true but R is not the correct explanation of A.

The mean average value of alternating current (or emf) during a half cycle is given by

$$I_m = 0.636\,I_0 \text{ (or } E_m = 0.636E_0)$$

During the next half cycle, the mean value of AC will be equal in magnitude but opposite in direction. For this reason the average value of AC over a complete cycle is always zero. So, the average value is always defined over a half cycle of AC.

10. (b) As we know that,

$$I_{mean} = \frac{2}{\pi}I_0 = 63.7\% \text{ of } I_0$$
$$E_{mean} = 63.7\% \text{ of } E_0$$
$$I_{rms} = \frac{I_0}{\sqrt{2}}$$
$$E_{rms} = \frac{E_0}{\sqrt{2}} = 70.7\% \text{ of } E_0$$

Hence, option (b) is correct.

11. (d) 220 V AC means the effective or virtual value of AC is 220 V, *i.e.*, $E_V = 220$ V. But 220 V DC has the same peak value (*i.e.*, 220 V only). Moreover, the shock of AC is attractive and that of DC is repulsive. Hence, 220 V AC is more dangerous than 220 V DC.

12. (d) Both A and R are true and R is the correct explanation of A.

When frequency of alternating current is increased, the effective resistance of the inductive coil increases. Current ($X_L = \omega L = 2\pi\nu L$) in the circuit containing inductor is given by $I = \frac{V}{X_L} = \frac{V}{2\pi\nu L}$

As inductive resistance of the inductor increases, current in the circuit decreases.

13. (b) Frequency of AC mains in India is 50 Hz.

14. (d) $2\pi f = 2000$

$\therefore f = \frac{1000}{\pi}$ Hz

15. (c) A is false but R is true.

Like direct current, an alternating current also produces magnetic field. But the magnitude and direction of the field goes on changing continuously with time.

16. (b) Given, $V = 100\sqrt{2}\sin 100t$ V

$C = 1\,\mu\text{F}$

The peak voltage, $V_0 = 100\sqrt{2}$ V and $\omega = 100$ rad/s

$\therefore$ rms voltage, $V_{rms} = \frac{V_0}{\sqrt{2}} = \frac{100\sqrt{2}}{\sqrt{2}} = 100$ V

$\therefore$ Current reading of the ammeter,

$$I = \frac{V_{rms}}{X_C} = \frac{V_{rms}}{\left(\frac{1}{\omega C}\right)} = \frac{100\text{ V}}{\frac{1}{100 \times 1 \times 10^{-6}}}$$
$$= 100 \times 100 \times 10^{-6} = 10^{-2}\text{ A}$$
$$= 10 \times 10^{-3}\text{ A} = 10\text{ mA}$$

17. (a) The current through the AC circuit is given by $i = 3\sin\omega t + 4\cos\omega t$

The maximum value of current is

$$I_{max} = \sqrt{3^2 + 4^2} = \sqrt{25} = 5\text{ A}$$

The rms value of current, $I_{rms} = \frac{I_{max}}{\sqrt{2}} = \frac{5}{\sqrt{2}}$ A

Step up Practice 2

1. (a) Capacitive reactance,

$$X_C = \frac{1}{2\pi f C} = \frac{1}{2\pi \times 4000 \times 25 \times 10^{-6}} = \frac{5}{\pi}\,\Omega$$

2. (b) In DC circuits, $f = 0$

$$\therefore \quad X_C = \frac{1}{2\pi(0)\,C} = \frac{1}{0} = \infty$$

3. (d) Both Statement I and Statement II are correct.

The phase angle for the L-C-R series circuit is given by

$$\tan\theta = \frac{X_L - X_C}{R} = \frac{\omega L - \omega C}{R}$$

where, X_L, X_C are inductive reactance and capacitive reactance respectively. When $X_L > X_C$ then $\tan\theta$ is positive i.e., θ is positive (between 0 and $\pi/2$).

Hence, emf leads the current.

4. (c) Given, $e = 200\sqrt{2}\sin 100t$

and $C = 1\,\mu\text{F}$

Here, $E_{rms} = \frac{200\sqrt{2}}{\sqrt{2}} = 200$ V

$$X_C = \frac{1}{\omega C} = \frac{1}{1 \times 10^{-6} \times 100} = 10^4\,\Omega$$

$$\therefore \quad i_{rms} = \frac{E_{rms}}{X_C} \Rightarrow i_{rms} = \frac{200}{10^4} = 2 \times 10^{-2}\text{ A}$$

$$= 20\text{ mA}$$

5. (d) $\because \quad X_L = (2\pi f L)$

$$\therefore \quad L = \frac{X_L}{2\pi f} = \frac{50}{(2\pi)(50)} = 0.16\text{ H}$$

6. (b) As, $\tan\phi = \frac{X_L}{R}$

$$\therefore \quad \tan 45^\circ = \frac{L\omega}{R}$$

$$\Rightarrow \quad L = \frac{R}{\omega} = \frac{100}{2\pi \times 1000} \qquad [\because \tan 45^\circ = 1]$$

$$\Rightarrow \quad L = \frac{1}{20\pi}$$

7. (b) As, $\quad I \propto \frac{1}{\omega L}$

$$\therefore \quad \frac{I_1}{I_2} = \frac{\omega L_2}{\omega L_1} = \frac{L_2}{L_1}$$

8. (d) $Z = \sqrt{R^2 + X_L^2} = \sqrt{8^2 + 6^2} = 10\,\Omega$

9. (c) $\tan 45^\circ = \frac{X_L}{R} \Rightarrow X_L = R$

10. (b) Statement I is correct but Statement II is incorrect.

When pure inductor is connected to source of an alternating emf, then instantaneous value of alternating emf is given by $E = E_0 \sin\omega t$, and corresponding alternating current is given by $I = I_0 \sin(\omega t - \pi/2)$. From these two equations it follows that alternating current lags behind emf by a phase angle of $\pi/2$. The inductive reactance, $X_L = \omega L = \pi \cdot 2\, f.L$, so when frequency increases correspondingly inductive.

11. (b) Impedance, $Z = \sqrt{R^2 + (2\pi f L)^2}$

As f increases, Z will increase.

12. (a) $\because \tan\phi = \frac{X_L}{R} = \frac{L\omega}{R}$

$$\therefore \quad \tan\phi = \frac{3}{3} \quad \Rightarrow \quad \tan\phi = 1$$

$$\phi = \tan^{-1}(1) \quad \Rightarrow \quad \phi = 45^\circ$$

$$\phi = \frac{\pi}{4}\text{ rad}$$

13. (d) Given, $X_L = \omega L = 2\pi f L = 2\pi \times 50 \times \frac{0.4}{\pi} = 40\,\Omega$

and $\quad R = 30\,\Omega$

$$\therefore \quad Z = \sqrt{R^2 + X_L^2} = \sqrt{(30)^2 + (40)^2} = 50\,\Omega$$

and $\quad I_{rms} = \frac{V_{rms}}{Z} = \frac{200}{50} = 4$ A

14. (b) As we know that, In case of impedance when $X_L > X_C$ then $\tan\phi$ is positive.

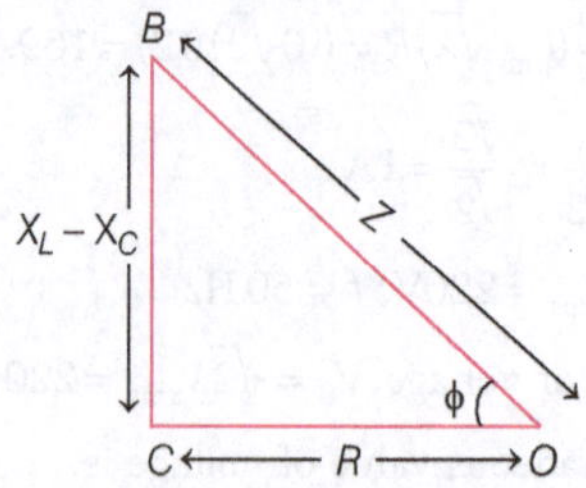

15. (c) The phase difference between instantaneous value of I and V is

$$\frac{\pi}{4} - \left(-\frac{\pi}{4}\right) = \frac{\pi}{2}$$

Hence, current leads the voltage by 90°.

16. (d) $V = \sqrt{V_R^2 + (V_L - V_C)^2} = 10\sqrt{2}$ V

17. (b) The impedance of the circuit is

$$Z = \sqrt{R^2 + (X_L - X_C)^2}$$

Here, $\quad X_L = \omega L = 400 \times 20 \times 10^{-3} = 8\,\Omega$

and $X_C = \frac{1}{\omega C} = \frac{1}{400 \times 625 \times 10^{-6}} = 4\,\Omega$

$\therefore \quad Z = \sqrt{(3)^2 + (8-4)^2} = 5\,\Omega$

$\therefore \quad I = \frac{E}{Z} = \frac{300}{5} = 60$ A

18. (*d*) Both Statement I and Statement II are correct.

Capacitive reactance $X_C = \frac{1}{\omega C}$, when capacitance C increases, the capacitive reactance decreases. Due to decreases in its value, the current in the circuit will increases $\left(I = \frac{E}{\sqrt{R^2 + X_C^2}}\right)$ and hence brightness of source (or electric lamp) will also increases.

19. (*b*) At resonance (series resonant circuit),

$$X_L = X_C \Rightarrow \quad Z_{min} = R$$

Impedance is minimum and current is maximum.

20. (*b*) Equation of voltage, $E = \sqrt{V_R^2 + (V_L - V_C)^2}$

At resonance (series circuit),

$$V_L = V_C \Rightarrow E = V_R$$

i.e. whole applied voltage appeared across the resistance.

21. (*d*) Both Statement I and Statement II are correct.

At resonance $X_L = X_C$ or $\omega L = \frac{1}{\omega C}$. Because of this impedance of *L-C-R* series circuit become equal to resistance of circuit ($Z = \sqrt{R^2 + (X_L - X_C)^2}$. Therefore from $I = \frac{E}{Z} = \frac{E}{R}$, at resonance, current in *L-C-R* series circuit is maximum correspondingly phase angle is also equal to zero. Therefore emf and current are in phase in *L-C-R* series circuit.

Step up Practice 3

1. (*b*) $P = VI$

$$I = \frac{P}{V} = \frac{550}{220} = 2.5 \text{ A}$$

2. (*b*) Power factor of an AC circuit is given by

$$\cos\phi = \frac{R}{Z}$$

For circuit containing an ideal resistance only, $Z = R$

$\therefore \quad \cos\phi = 1$

3. (*b*) As we know

Average power in AC circuit is given by

$$P = V_{rms}\, i_{rms} \cos\phi$$

For pure capacitive circuit $\phi = 90°$ So, $P = 0$.

4. (*a*) Both A and R are true and R is not the correct explanation of A.

We can use a capacitor of suitable capacitance as a choke coil, because average power consumed in an ideal capacitor is zero. Therefore, like a choke coil, a condenser can reduce AC without power dissipation.

5. (*b*) $Z = \sqrt{(3)^2 + (4)^2} = 5\,\Omega$

$$\cos\phi = \frac{R}{Z} = \frac{3}{5} = 0.6$$

6. (*c*) Voltage amplitude, $V_0 = 100$ V, current amplitude $I_0 = 100$ mA $= 100 \times 10^{-3}$ A and phase difference between I and V is $\phi = \frac{\pi}{3} = 60°$.

Now power dissipated is given by

$$P = \frac{V_0 I_0}{2} \cos\phi$$

$$= \frac{100 \times 100 \times 10^{-3}}{2} \times \cos 60° = 2.5 \text{ W}$$

7. (*d*) In case of a pure inductance, $R = 0$

$\therefore$ Power factor $= \cos\phi = \frac{R}{Z} = \frac{0}{X} = 0$

So, $\quad P_{av} = E_{rms} \cdot i_{rms} \times 0 = 0$

8. (*d*) Both A and R are true and R is the correct explanation of A.

If resistor is used in controlling AC supply, electrical energy will be wasted in the form of heat energy across the resistance wire. However, AC supply can be controlled with choke without any wastage energy. This is because, power factor (cos θ) for resistance is one and it is zero for an inductance.

9. (*a*) $P = I^2 R$

$$= \frac{E^2}{Z^2} R$$

$$= \frac{E^2 R}{[R^2] + \left(\omega L - \frac{1}{\omega C}\right)^2}$$

10. (*c*) $f_0 = \frac{1}{2\pi}\sqrt{\frac{1}{LC}}$

$$\Rightarrow f_0 = \frac{1}{2\pi}\sqrt{\frac{1}{250 \times 10^{-12} \times 0.16 \times 10^{-3}}}$$

$$\Rightarrow f_0 = 8 \times 10^5 \text{ Hz}$$

11. (*c*) As we know that,

AC circuit containing C and R

$$\tan\phi = \frac{1/\omega C}{R} = \frac{1}{RC\omega}$$

12. (*d*) We know that,

Resonant frequency is given by

$$f_0 = \frac{1}{2\pi\sqrt{LC}} = \frac{1}{2\pi\sqrt{5\times10^{-3}\times2\times10^{-6}}}$$

$$\Rightarrow \quad f_0 = \frac{1}{2\pi\sqrt{10^{-8}}} = \frac{1}{2\pi\times10^{-4}}$$

$$= \frac{10^4}{2\pi}\text{ Hz} = \frac{5}{\pi}\times10^3\text{ Hz}$$

13. (*b*) A is true but R is false.

If both L and C is there then, Impedance,

$$Z = \sqrt{X_L - X_C} = 0, \text{ if } X_L = X_C.$$

In case of *R*-*L* and *R*-*C* circuit, average power delivered by the source is zero.

14. (*a*) As average power, $\overline{P} = 2\text{ W}, I_{\text{rms}} = 2\text{ A}$,

impedance, $Z = 1\,\Omega$

Power factor $(\cos\phi) = ?$

We know that, $\overline{P} = V_{\text{rms}} \times I_{\text{rms}} \cdot \cos\phi$

$$\Rightarrow \quad \overline{P} = I_{\text{rms}}^2 Z \cdot \cos\phi \qquad [\because V_{\text{rms}} = I_{\text{rms}} \cdot Z]$$

$$\cos\phi = \frac{\overline{P}}{I_{\text{rms}}^2 \cdot Z} = \frac{2}{(2)^2\times1} = \frac{2}{4} = \frac{1}{2} = 0.5$$

15. (*b*) A is true but R is false.

When a capacitor is connected to an AC circuit, $E_{\text{rms}} = i_{\text{rms}}\left(\frac{1}{C\omega}\right)$ where $\frac{1}{C\omega}$ is the impedance due to capacitive resistance. The power consumed in this circuit is zero because the phase difference ϕ between emf and current in a pure capacitance AC circuit is power factor $\cos\phi = 0$. It is only for DC that a current does not flow.

Step up Practice 4

1. (*b*) In step-down transformer, $V_P > V_S$

but, $\frac{V_P}{V_S} = \frac{I_S}{I_P}$

$\therefore \quad I_S > I_P$

So, current increases in a step-down transformer.

2. (*c*) A transformer works on the principle of mutual induction.

3. (*c*) Frequency remains unchanged in a transformer.

4. (*d*) Both Statement I and Statement II are correct.

Transformers which convert low voltage into higher ones are called step-up transformers, while those which convert high voltage into lower ones are called step-down transformers. This is possible only for AC source and not for DC source.

5. (*d*) A choke coil must have high inductance and low resistance so that it can block high frequency alternating current.

6. (*b*) Transformation ratio,

$$k = \frac{N_S}{N_P} = \frac{V_S}{V_P}$$

For step-up transformer,

$$V_S > V_P, \text{ i.e. } N_S > N_P$$

Hence, $k > 1$.

7. (*c*) If we neglect all losses, then input power = output power.

8. (*a*) As, $\frac{N_1}{N_2} = \frac{I_2}{I_1} \Rightarrow I_2 = \left(\frac{N_1}{N_2}\right) I_1 = \left(\frac{500}{2000}\right)\times 48 = 12\text{ A}$

9. (*b*) The core is laminated to reduce eddy current to a minimum as they interfere with the efficient transfer of energy from the primary coil to secondary one.

10. (*d*) Both Statement I and Statement II are correct. If there is no loss of energy in transformer, then instantaneous output power is equal to instantaneous input power. From this we get,

$$\frac{e_S}{e_P} = \frac{I_P}{I_S}$$

So in step-up transformer voltage increases by decreasing the current. Similarly, step-down transformer decreases the voltage by increasing current. Therefore transformer simply transforms the voltage and current, obeying the law of conservation of energy.

11. (*b*) We know that,

$$V_S \times N_P = V_P \times N_S \quad \Rightarrow \quad \frac{N_S}{N_P} = \frac{V_S}{V_P}$$

where, V_S = voltage across secondary coil

V_P = voltage across primary coil = 220 V

N_P = number of turns is primary coil = 1000

and N_S = number of turns in secondary coil = 50

$$\Rightarrow \quad \frac{50}{1000} = \frac{V_S}{220}$$

$$\Rightarrow \quad V_S = \frac{50\times220}{1000} = 11\text{ V}$$

Power in the secondary coil = Power in the primary coil

$$V_S I_S = V_P I_P$$

$$\Rightarrow \quad 11\times I_S = 220\times1$$

$$\Rightarrow \quad I_S = \frac{220}{11} = 20\text{ A}$$

12. (*d*) Both Statement I and Statement II are correct.

When alternating current flows through the coil of a transformer, the core of transformer is magnetised and demagnetised repeatedly. The electrical energy taken by the core during magnetisation is not returned fully in demagnetisation. The energy remaining in the core appears in the form of heat.

13. (*b*) As we know that, for transformer, $\frac{V_1}{V_2} = \frac{I_2}{I_1} = \frac{N_1}{N_2}$

where all the symbols have their usual meanings. (Suffix 1 is for primary and 2 is for the secondary)

$$\Rightarrow \quad \frac{N_1}{N_2} = \frac{1}{25} = \frac{2}{I}$$

where, I = primary side current.

$$\therefore \quad I = 50\text{ A}$$

14. (*d*) As we know that,

Transformer works on the principle of mutual induction.

Electric generator work on the principle of electromagnetic induction.

I^2R is resistance of winding loss

$$\text{Efficiency } (\eta) = \frac{V_S I_S}{V_P I_P} = \frac{\text{Output Power}}{\text{Input Power}}$$

Hence, option (d) is correct.

15. (*d*) A dynamo converts mechanical energy into electrical energy.

16. (*d*) Transformer is used to obtain desired AC voltage and current because a transformer is a device based on the principle of mutual induction, which is used for converting large AC at low voltage into small current at high voltage.

17. (*a*) The armature current will increase if the speed of the DC generator start decreasing due to an increase in voltage drop at armature resistance.

18. (*c*) An electric generator is a type of machine that uses electromagnetic induction to generate electricity.

19. (*d*) Both Statement I and Statement II are correct.

Gearing up for NEET

1. (*b*) $< i >_T = < 5 >_R + < 5 \sin 100\,\pi t >_I$

$$= 5 + 0 = 5\text{ A}$$

2. (*b*) Given, $\nu = 50\text{ Hz}, I_{rms} = 5\text{A}$

$$t = \frac{1}{300}\text{ s}$$

We have to find $I(t)$,

$$I_0 = \text{Peak value} = \sqrt{2}\ I_{rms} = \sqrt{2} \times 5$$

$$= 5\sqrt{2}\text{ A}$$

$$I = I_0 \sin \omega t = 5\sqrt{2} \sin 2\pi\nu t$$

$$= 5\sqrt{2} \sin 2\pi \times 50 \times \frac{1}{300}$$

$$= 5\sqrt{2} \sin \frac{\pi}{3} = 5\sqrt{2} \times \frac{\sqrt{3}}{2}$$

$$= 5\sqrt{3/2}\text{ A}$$

3. (*d*) $e = \sqrt{e_1^2 + e_2^2} \sin(\omega t + \phi)$

where, $\cos\phi = \frac{e_1}{\sqrt{e_1^2 + e_2^2}}$

and $\sin\phi = \frac{e_2}{\sqrt{e_1^2 + e_2^2}}$

i.e., $\quad e_0 = \sqrt{e_1^2 + e_2^2}$

or $\quad e_{rms} = \frac{\sqrt{e_1^2 + e_2^2}}{\sqrt{2}}$

4. (*c*) Average value of output current is given by

$$I_{av} = \frac{\int_0^{T/2} I dt}{\int_0^{T/2} dt} = \frac{\int_0^{T/2} I_0 \sin \omega t\, dt}{T/2}$$

$$= \frac{2I_0}{T}\left[-\frac{\cos \omega t}{\omega}\right]_0^{T/2}$$

$$= \frac{2I_0}{T}\left[-\frac{\cos(\omega T/2)}{\omega} + \frac{\cos 0°}{\omega}\right]$$

$$= \frac{2I_0}{\omega T}[-\cos\pi + \cos 0°]$$

$$= \frac{2I_0}{2\pi}[1+1] = \frac{2I_0}{\pi}$$

5. (*c*) Phase difference between current and voltage,

$$\Delta\phi = \phi_2 - \phi_1 = \frac{\pi}{6} - \left(-\frac{\pi}{6}\right) = \frac{\pi}{3} \text{ or } 60°.$$

Hence, current leads voltage by 60°.

6. (*b*) $I_{rms} = \sqrt{(I^2)} = \sqrt{(8 + 6 \sin \omega t)^2}$

$$\Rightarrow \quad I_{rms} = \sqrt{((64 + 96 \sin \omega t + 36 \sin^2 \omega t))}$$

$$\Rightarrow \quad I_{rms} = \sqrt{(64) + 96 < \sin \omega t > + 36 < \sin^2 \omega t >}$$

$$\Rightarrow \quad I_{rms} = \sqrt{64 + 0 + 36 \times 0.5} = 9.05\text{ A}$$

Since, $< \sin^2 \omega t > = 0.5$

7. (*b*) Value of induced emf in coil,

$$e = M\frac{dI}{dt}$$

$$= 0.005 \times \frac{d}{dt}(I_0 \sin \omega t)$$

$$= 0.005 \times I_0\, \omega \cos \omega t$$

$$\therefore \quad e_{max} = 0.005 \times 10 \times 100\pi$$

$$= 5\pi\text{ V}$$

8. (c) Peak voltage, $V_0 = \sqrt{2}\, V_{rms} = 331\,\text{V}$

and $\quad \omega = 2\pi f = 100\,\pi$

$\Rightarrow \quad V_L = 331 \sin(100\,\pi t)$

where, V_L is line voltage.

9. (c) $$i_{rms}^2 = \frac{\int i^2\, dt}{\int dt}$$

$$= \frac{\int_2^4 (4t)\, dt}{\int_2^4 dt} = \frac{4\int_2^4 t\, dt}{2} = 2\left[\frac{t^2}{2}\right]_2^4 = 12\ \text{A}$$

$\Rightarrow \quad i_{rms} = 2\sqrt{3}\ \text{A}$

10. (c) In case of AC, $Z = \sqrt{R^2 + (\omega L)^2}$, while in case of DC, it is only R. So, in AC resistance increases.

11. (a) Capacitive reactance, $X_C = \dfrac{1}{2\pi \nu C}$

$$\Rightarrow \quad \frac{1}{1000} = \frac{1}{2\pi \times \nu \times 5 \times 10^{-6}}$$

$$\therefore \quad \nu = \frac{100}{\pi}\ \text{MHz}$$

12. (b) $$I = \frac{V}{Z} = \frac{V}{\sqrt{R^2 + (2\pi f L)^2}}$$

$$= \frac{120}{\sqrt{(10)^2 + (2\pi \times 60 \times 2)^2}} = 0.16\ \text{A}$$

13. (a) Resonant frequency, $f = \dfrac{1}{2\pi\sqrt{LC}}$

$$\therefore \quad f \propto \frac{1}{\sqrt{C}} \quad \text{or} \quad \frac{f_1}{f_2} = \sqrt{\frac{C_2}{C_1}}$$

$$\Rightarrow \quad \frac{f}{f_2} = \sqrt{\frac{4C}{C}} \Rightarrow f_2 = \frac{f}{2}$$

14. (c) Current in inductance I_L lags behind the voltage by $\pi/2$. Current in resistance I_R is in phase with voltage, while current in capacitance I_C leads the voltage by a phase of $\pi/2$.

15. (b) Reading of ammeter $= i_{rms}$

$$i_{rms} = \frac{V_{rms}}{X_C} = \frac{V_0}{\sqrt{2}} \times \omega C$$

$$= \frac{200\sqrt{2} \times 100 \times (1 \times 10^{-6})}{\sqrt{2}}$$

$$= 2 \times 10^{-2}\ \text{A} = 20\ \text{mA}$$

16. (a) Let the applied voltage be V volt

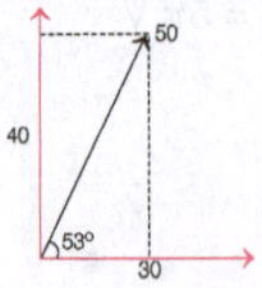

Here, $\quad V_R = 12\,\text{V}, V_C = 5\,\text{V}$

$$V = \sqrt{V_R^2 + V_C^2} = \sqrt{(12)^2 + (5)^2}$$

$$= \sqrt{144 + 25}$$

$$= \sqrt{169} = 13\ \text{V}$$

17. (d) According to problem, $X_L = X_C$

$$\omega L = \frac{1}{\omega C}$$

$$\therefore \quad \omega^2 = \frac{1}{LC} = \frac{1}{\sqrt{10^{-3} \times 10 \times 10^{-6}}}$$

$$\omega = \frac{1}{\sqrt{10^{-8}}} = 10^4$$

$$\therefore \quad X_L = \omega L = 10^4 \times 10^{-3} = 10\,\Omega$$

18. (a) $V = 30 \sin 50t + 40 \cos 50t = 50 \sin(50t + 53°)$

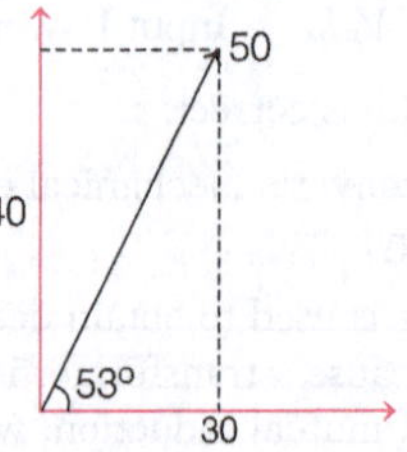

$$\therefore \quad I_{rms} = \frac{V_{rms}}{Z} = \frac{50/\sqrt{2}}{10} = \frac{5}{\sqrt{2}}\ \text{A}$$

19. (d) $X_C > X_L$. Hence, current will lead the voltage.

$$Z = \sqrt{R^2 + (X_C - X_L)^2} = 10\sqrt{2}\,\Omega$$

$$\therefore \quad I_{rms} = \frac{V_{rms}}{Z} = \frac{400/\sqrt{2}}{10\sqrt{2}} = 20\ \text{A}$$

$$\cos\phi = \frac{R}{Z} = \frac{1}{\sqrt{2}}$$

$$V_R = I_{rms} R = (20)(10) = 200\ \text{V}$$

20. (a) Total resistance of the circuit, $R = 6 + 4 = 10\,\Omega$

Capacitive reactance,

$$X_C = \frac{1}{\omega C} = \frac{1}{2000 \times 50 \times 10^{-6}} = 10\,\Omega$$

Inductive reactance,

$$X_L = \omega L = 2000 \times 5 \times 10^{-3} = 10\,\Omega$$

$$\therefore \quad Z = \sqrt{R^2 + (X_L - X_C)^2} = 10\,\Omega$$

Amplitude of current, $I_0 = \dfrac{V_0}{Z} = \dfrac{20}{10} = 2\text{A}$

21. (b) In an L-C-R circuit, the current and the voltage are in phase ($\phi = 0$), when

$$\tan\phi = \frac{\omega L - \dfrac{1}{\omega C}}{R} = 0 \quad \text{or} \quad \omega L = \frac{1}{\omega C}$$

or $$L = \frac{1}{\omega^2 C}$$

Here, $\quad \omega = 2\pi f = 2 \times 3.14 \times 50\ \text{s}^{-1} = 314\ \text{s}^{-1}$

and $C = 20\ \mu F = 20 \times 10^{-6}\ F$

$\therefore \quad L = \dfrac{1}{(314)^2 \times (20 \times 10^{-6})} = 0.51\ H$

22. (a) Angular velocity,

$$\omega_0 = 2\pi\nu = 2\pi \times 100$$
$$\omega_0 = 2 \times 3 \times 100$$
$$= 600\ \text{rads}^{-1} \qquad [\because \pi = 3]$$

Further, $\omega_0 = \dfrac{1}{\sqrt{LC}}$ ...(i)

Also, $X_C = \dfrac{1}{C\omega_0} = 60\ \Omega$

$\Rightarrow \quad C = \dfrac{1}{\omega_0 \times 60} = \dfrac{1}{600 \times 60}$

$\Rightarrow \quad C = \dfrac{1}{36 \times 10^3} F$

Putting values of C in Eq. (i), we get

$$600 = \frac{1}{\sqrt{L\left(\dfrac{1}{36\times10^3}\right)}}$$

$\Rightarrow \quad 36\times10^4 = \dfrac{36\times10^3}{L}$

$\Rightarrow \quad L = \dfrac{36\times10^3}{36\times10^4} = \dfrac{1}{10} = 0.1H$

23. (b) In the given graph current is leading the voltage by 45°. Therefore, circuit is C-R.

$$\tan\phi = \frac{X_C}{R} \text{ and } \phi = \frac{\pi}{4}$$

$\therefore \quad X_C = R$

$\Rightarrow \quad \omega CR = 1$

$\Rightarrow \quad CR = \dfrac{1}{\omega} = \dfrac{1}{100}$

When $R = 1k\Omega = 10^3\Omega$, then

$$C = \frac{1}{100 \times 10^3} = 10^{-5} F = 10\ \mu F$$

24. (a) In position-1,

$$\tan\frac{\pi}{6} = \frac{\omega L}{R} = \frac{(1000)(\sqrt{3}\times10^{-3})}{R}$$

or $\quad \dfrac{1}{\sqrt{3}} = \dfrac{\sqrt{3}}{R} \quad \therefore R = 3\Omega$

In position-2,

$$\tan\phi = \frac{X_C}{R} = \frac{(1/\omega C)}{R}$$

$$= \frac{1\Big/\left(1000 \times \dfrac{1000}{3} \times 10^{-6}\right)}{3} = 1$$

$\therefore \quad \phi = \dfrac{\pi}{4}$; so current leads source emf.

25. (c) $R = \dfrac{80}{10} = 8\Omega$

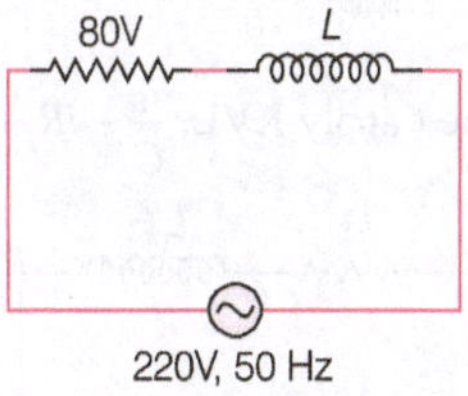

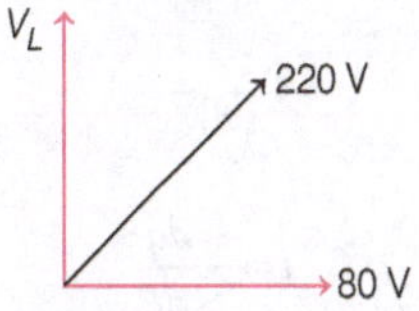

Also, $\quad V_L^2 + 80^2 = 220^2$

$$V_L^2 = (220 + 80)(220 - 80)$$
$$= 300 \times 140$$

$\Rightarrow \quad V_L = 204.9\ V$

$\Rightarrow \quad I_{rms}X_L = 204.9$

$\Rightarrow \quad \dfrac{220}{\sqrt{64 + X_L^2}} X_L = 204.9$

$\Rightarrow \quad X_L = 20 \Rightarrow L = \dfrac{20}{2\pi f} = 0.064\ H$

26. (d) $Z = \sqrt{(R)^2 + (X_L - X_C)^2}$

$$R = 10\Omega, X_L = \omega L = 2000 \times 5 \times 10^{-3} = 10\Omega$$

$$X_C = \frac{1}{\omega C} = \frac{1}{2000 \times 50 \times 10^{-6}}$$
$$= 10\Omega \Rightarrow Z = 10\Omega$$

Maximum current, $i_0 = \dfrac{V_0}{Z} = \dfrac{20}{10} = 2A$

Hence, $i_{rms} = \dfrac{2}{\sqrt{2}} = 1.4A$

and $\quad V_{rms} = 4 \times 1.4 = 5.6V$

27. (b) $Z = \sqrt{R^2 + (X_C - X_L)^2} = 10\Omega$

$$\cos\phi = \frac{R}{Z} = \frac{4}{5}$$

$\therefore \quad \phi = 37°$

$$I_0 = \frac{V_0}{Z} = \frac{10}{10} = 1A$$

$\therefore \quad I = 1\cos(100\pi t + 37°)$

Given, $\quad V = 10\cos(100\pi t)$

The applied voltage is $\dfrac{3}{5}$ th of the maximum applied voltage. Then, $100\ \pi t = \cos^{-1}(3/5) = 53°$

$\therefore \quad I = 1\cos(53° + 37°) = 0$

$\therefore \quad V_R = 0$

$\therefore \quad V_{AB} = V_{applied} = \frac{3}{5} \times 10 = 6\text{ V}$

28. (a) At any time t apply KVL, $\frac{q}{C} - iR - L\frac{di}{dt} = 0$

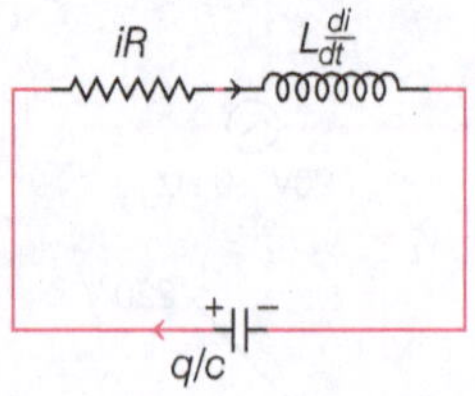

and $\quad i = -\frac{dq}{dt}$

$\Rightarrow \quad \frac{q}{C} + \frac{dq}{dt}R + \frac{Ld^2q}{dt^2} = 0$

$\Rightarrow \quad \frac{d^2q}{dt^2} + \frac{R}{L}\frac{dq}{dt} + \frac{q}{LC} = 0$

From damped harmonic oscillator, the amplitude is given by

$A = A_0 e^{-\frac{bt}{2m}}$, for general equation of double differential equation $\frac{d^2x}{dt^2} + \frac{b}{m}\frac{dx}{dt} + \frac{k}{m}x = 0$

$\Rightarrow \quad Q_{max} = Q_0 e^{-\frac{Rt}{2L}}$

$\Rightarrow \quad Q_{max}^2 = Q_0^2 e^{-\frac{Rt}{L}}$

Lesser the self-inductance, faster will be damping, hence correct graph is in option (a).

29. (b) At $t \to \infty$, capacitor works as an open circuit as shown in the figure.

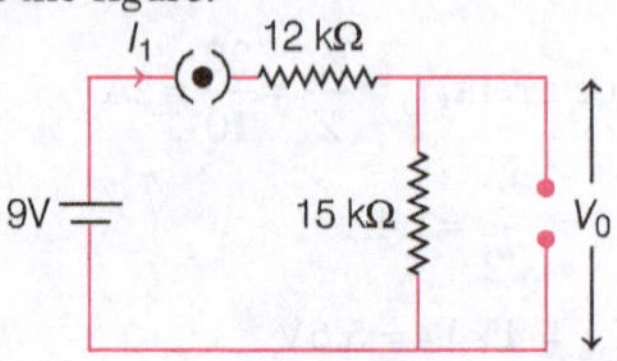

Therefore, current flow in the circuit,

$I_1 = \frac{9}{(12 + 15) \times 10^3} = \frac{1}{3} \times 10^{-3}\text{ A}$

$\therefore \quad V_0 = I_1 \times 15 \times 10^3$

$= \frac{1}{3} \times 10^{-3} \times 15 \times 10^3 = 5\text{ V}$

$\therefore$ Charge on capacitor of 5 μF,

$q_0 = CV_0 = 5 \times 10^{-6} \times 5$

$= 25 \times 10^{-6}\text{ C} = 25\ \mu\text{C}$

When switch is open, then capacitor starts discharging across $(5 + 15 = 20\text{ k}\Omega)$ and instantaneous charge on capacitor is given by

$q = q_0 e^{-t/RC}$

$= 25 e^{-\frac{1}{20\times10^3 \times 5\times10^{-6}}} \quad [\because t = 1\text{s}]$

$= 25 e^{-10}\ \mu\text{C}$

30. (a) Given, in L-C-R series circuit,

Source voltage (resultant voltage), $V = 120\text{ V}$

Voltage across inductor, $V_L = 50\text{ V}$

Voltage across resistor, $V_R = 40\text{ V}$

In L-C-R series circuit,

$V = \sqrt{V_R^2 + (V_L - V_C)^2}$

or $\quad 120 = \sqrt{40^2 + (50 - V_C)^2}$

$120^2 = 40^2 + (50 - V_C)^2$

$\Rightarrow \quad (50 - V_C)^2 = 12800$

$\Rightarrow \quad 50 - V_C = 80\sqrt{2}$

$\Rightarrow \quad V_C = 10(5 - 8\sqrt{2})\text{ V}$

31. (a) We know that, for series R-C circuit

$V^2 = V_C^2 + V_R^2$

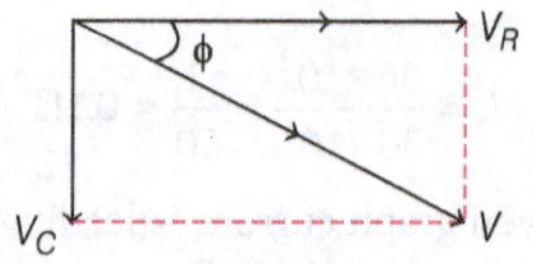

$100 = 64 + V_R^2$

$\Rightarrow \quad V_R^2 = 36$

$\Rightarrow \quad V_R = \sqrt{36} = 6\text{ V}$

Also, $\quad \tan\phi = \frac{V_C}{V_R} \Rightarrow \tan\phi = \frac{8}{6}$

$\tan\phi = \frac{4}{3}$

$\therefore \quad \phi = \tan^{-1}\left(\frac{4}{3}\right)$

32. (b) For circuit A,

Impedance, $Z_A = \sqrt{R^2 + \frac{1}{\omega^2 C^2}}$

Current in circuit, $I_R^A = \frac{V}{\sqrt{R^2 + (1/\omega^2 C^2)}}$ ...(i)

Potential difference across C,

$V_C^A = I_R^A \times \frac{1}{\omega C} = \frac{V}{\sqrt{(R\omega C)^2 + 1}}$

For circuit B,

Impedance, $Z_B = \sqrt{R^2 + \frac{1}{(4\omega)^2 C^2}}$

Current in circuit, $I_R^B = \dfrac{V}{\sqrt{R^2 + [1/(4\omega C)^2]}}$ ... (ii)

Potential difference across C,

$$V_C^B = I_R^B \times \frac{1}{4\omega C} = \frac{V}{\sqrt{(4R\omega C)^2 + 1}}$$

Hence, from above Eqs. (i) and (ii), we conclude that as numerator of I_R^B is increased from I_R^A.

So, $I_R^B > I_R^A$ and $V_C^A > V_C^B$.

33. (a) The resistance of inductor (coil), $R = \dfrac{12}{24} = 0.5\,\Omega$

If phase difference between current and emf is zero, then reactance of circuit must be zero.

The impedance of the circuit equals to resistance, *i.e.*

$Z = 0.5\,\Omega$

Now, rms current, $I_{rms} = \dfrac{V_{rms}}{Z} = \dfrac{24}{0.5} = 48$ A

34. (c) Impedance, $Z = \sqrt{R^2 + X_L^2}, X_L = \omega L = 2\pi f L$

Given, $R = 2100\,\Omega$, $f = 50$ Hz, $L = \dfrac{1}{\pi}$ H

$$\Rightarrow \quad Z = \sqrt{(2100)^2 + (2 \times 50)^2}$$
$$= \sqrt{(2100)^2 + (100)^2}$$
$$\Rightarrow \quad Z \approx 2102\,\Omega$$

35. (a) Given, the potential difference across each element is same, *i.e.* 20 V, so the circuit is at resonance.

We have, $V_R = V_L = V_C = 20$ V

If the value of R is doubled, then value of I reduced to half

$$\therefore \quad V_L = V_C = \frac{IX_L}{2} = \frac{IX_C}{2} = \frac{20}{2} = 10 \text{ V}$$

[$\because$ circuit is at resonance]

and $\quad V_R = I \times 2R = 20$ V

36. (a) With DC power, $P = \dfrac{V^2}{R}$

$$R = \frac{(10)^2}{20} = 5\,\Omega$$

With AC power, $P = \dfrac{V_{rms}^2 R}{Z^2}$

$$\Rightarrow \quad Z^2 = \frac{(10)^2 \times 5}{10} = 50\,\Omega$$

The impedance, $Z^2 = R^2 + 4\pi^2\nu^2L^2$

$$50 = (5)^2 + 4(3.14)^2 \times \nu^2 \times (10 \times 10^{-3})^2$$
$$\nu \simeq 80 \text{ Hz}$$

37. (a) We have, $X_L = 90\,\Omega, X_C = 30\,\Omega$

and $\quad R = R_1 + R_2 = 44 + 36 = 80\,\Omega$

Impedance, $Z = \sqrt{R^2 + (X_L - X_C)^2}$

$$= \sqrt{(80)^2 + (60)^2}$$
$$Z = \sqrt{6400 + 3600} = 100\,\Omega$$
$$I = \frac{V}{Z} = \frac{200}{100} = 2 \text{ A}$$
$$P_{av} = I^2R = (2)^2 \times 80 = 320 \text{ W}$$

38. (b) The power factor of choke coil is given by

$$\cos\phi = \frac{R}{\sqrt{R^2 + \omega^2L^2}} \approx \frac{R}{\omega L} \quad (\text{as } R << \omega L)$$

As $R << \omega L$, $\cos\phi$ is very small. Thus, the power absorbed by the coil is very small. The only loss of energy is due to hysteresis in the iron core, which is much less than the loss of energy in the resistance.

39. (b) Power dissipated in circuit, $P = \dfrac{V_{rms}^2}{R} = \dfrac{(30)^2}{10} = 90$ W

40. (a) As, $\phi = \pi/2$

$$P = V_{rms} I_{rms} \cos\phi$$
$$P = 0$$

41. (c) $\quad I_0 = 28$ A

$$\therefore \quad I_{rms} = \frac{I_0}{\sqrt{2}} \simeq 20 \text{ A}$$

42. (b) $\quad P = \dfrac{1}{2} V_0 I_0 \cos\phi$

$$\Rightarrow \quad P = P_{peak} \cos\phi$$
$$\Rightarrow \quad \frac{1}{2}(P_{peak}) = P_{peak} \cos\phi$$
$$\Rightarrow \quad \cos\phi = \frac{1}{2}$$
$$\Rightarrow \quad \phi = \frac{\pi}{3}$$

43. (a) $\quad P = V_{rms} I_{rms} \cos\phi$

$$= V_{rms}\left(\frac{V_{rms}}{Z}\right)\left(\frac{R}{Z}\right)$$
$$= \frac{(110)^2\,(11)}{(22)^2} = 275 \text{ W}$$

44. (b) We know that, resonant frequency in an L-C-R circuit is given by $\nu_0 = \dfrac{1}{2\pi\sqrt{LC}}$

Now to reduce ν_0 either we can increase L or we can increase C. To increase capacitance, we must connect another capacitor parallel to the first.

45. (b) $X_L = R \quad \therefore \; Z = \sqrt{2}R$

$$P = \left(\frac{V_{rms}}{Z}\right)^2 \cdot R = \left(\frac{E_0/\sqrt{2}}{\sqrt{2}R}\right)^2 \cdot R = \frac{E_0^2}{4R}$$

46. (d) $\quad X_L = 2\pi f L = 2\pi\left(\dfrac{50}{\pi}\right) \times 1 = 100\,\Omega$

$$X_C = \frac{1}{2\pi f C} = \frac{1}{2\pi\left(\dfrac{50}{\pi}\right) 20 \times 10^{-6}} = 500\,\Omega$$

Impedance, $Z = \sqrt{R^2 + (X_C - X_L)^2}$

$\Rightarrow \quad Z = \sqrt{(300)^2 + (400)^2} = 500\,\Omega$

47. (*b*) $P = V_{rms} I_{rms} = \frac{V_0}{\sqrt{2}} I_{rms}$

$\therefore \quad I_{rms} = \frac{1000\sqrt{2}}{200} = 5\sqrt{2}$ A

48. (*b*) Power factor, $\cos\phi = \frac{1}{\sqrt{2}} = \frac{R}{\sqrt{R^2 + \omega^2 L^2}}$

This gives, $\omega L = R$

When ω is doubled, we get

$$\cos\phi' = \frac{R}{\sqrt{R^2 + 4\omega^2 L^2}} = \frac{R}{\sqrt{R^2 + 4R^2}} = \frac{1}{\sqrt{5}}$$

49. (*d*) Resistance of coil $(R) = \frac{200}{1} = 200\,\Omega$

With AC source, $I = \frac{200}{\sqrt{R^2 + X_L^2}}$ or $0.5 = \frac{200}{\sqrt{R^2 + X_L^2}}$

$\Rightarrow \quad R^2 + (2\pi f L)^2 = (400)^2$

$\Rightarrow \quad \left(2\pi f \times \frac{2\sqrt{3}}{\pi}\right)^2 = (400)^2 - (200)^2 = 200 \times 600$

$\Rightarrow \quad 4\sqrt{3} f = \sqrt{12} \times 100 \Rightarrow f = 50$ Hz

50. (*a*) From, $P = VI = \frac{V^2}{R}$

$\Rightarrow \quad I = \frac{P}{V} = 6\text{A} \Rightarrow R = \frac{V^2}{P} = \frac{100}{60} = \frac{5}{3}\,\Omega$

Now, $I = \frac{V}{Z}$

$\Rightarrow \quad 6 = \frac{100}{\sqrt{\left(\frac{5}{3}\right)^2 + (2\pi f L)^2}}$

Solving this equation, we get

$L = 0.052$ H

51. (*a*) Given, $X_L = X_C = 5\Omega$, this is the condition of resonance.

So $V_L = V_C$, or net voltage across L and C combination will be zero.

$\therefore \quad Z = R = 55\Omega$

$I = \frac{V}{Z} = \frac{110}{55} = 2$ A

52. (*d*) Since, $V_C > V_L$

$\therefore \quad X_C > X_L$

Hence, current will lead the voltage.

$\therefore \quad V = \sqrt{V_R^2 + (V_C - V_L)^2} = 10\text{ V} < V_C$

$\cos\phi = \frac{R}{Z} = \frac{V_R}{V} = \frac{8}{10} = \frac{4}{5}$

53. (*b*) Resonance frequency, $\omega = \frac{1}{\sqrt{LC}}$

$= \frac{1}{\sqrt{8 \times 10^{-3} \times 20 \times 10^{-6}}}$

$= 2500 \text{ rads}^{-1}$

Resonance current, $I = \frac{V}{R} = \frac{220}{44} = 5$A

54. (*d*) At resonance, $X_L = X_C$

$\therefore \quad Z = R = 40\Omega$

and $I_{rms} = \frac{V_{rms}}{Z} = \frac{230}{40} = 5.75$ A

55. (*b*) At resonance,

$X_L = X_C$

$\therefore \quad V_1 = V_3$

Hence, V_2 will be zero.

56. (*a*)

$$Z = \sqrt{(52)^2 + \left[230 \times 10^{-3} \times 2\pi \times 80 - \frac{1}{2\pi \times 80 \times 8.8 \times 10^{-6}}\right]^2}$$

$= 122\,\Omega$

$$P = \left(\frac{V_{rms}}{Z}\right)^2 \cdot R = \left(\frac{150}{122}\right)^2 (52) = 78.6 \text{ W}$$

57. (*b*) Resonance frequency,

$$\omega_0 = \frac{1}{\sqrt{LC}} = \frac{1}{\sqrt{100 \times 10^{-6} \times 1 \times 10^{-6}}} = 10^5 \text{ rads}^{-1}$$

Now, given $\omega = 70$ kilo-rads^{-1} = 70000 rads^{-1}

$\Rightarrow \quad \omega_0 > \omega$

As $X_L \propto \omega$ and $X_C \propto \frac{1}{\omega}$

$\therefore \quad X_L > X_C$

The circuit will be series *R-L* circuit.

58. (*b*) $I_L = I_{0L} \sin\left(\omega t - \frac{\pi}{2}\right) = -1.2 \cos\omega t$

$I_C = I_{0C} \sin\left(\omega t + \frac{\pi}{2}\right) = 1.0 \cos\omega t$

$\therefore \quad I = I_L + I_C = -0.2 \cos\omega t \Rightarrow |I| = 0.2$ A

59. (*b*) Voltage drop across *R* is maximum at resonance, *i.e.* at

$$\omega = \frac{1}{\sqrt{LC}} \text{ or } f = \frac{\omega}{2\pi} = \frac{1}{2\pi\sqrt{LC}}$$

$$= \frac{1}{2\pi\sqrt{\left(\frac{1}{\pi}\right)\left(\frac{1}{\pi} \times 10^{-6}\right)}} = 500 \text{ Hz}$$

60. (*c*) Given, $X_L = 1\Omega, R = 2\Omega$

$V_{rms} = 6\text{ V}, P_{av} = ?$

Average power dissipated in the circuit,

$P_{av} = V_{rms} I_{rms} \cos\phi$ ...(i)

$$I_{rms}=\frac{I_0}{\sqrt{2}}=\frac{V_{rms}}{Z}$$

$$Z=\sqrt{R^2+X_L^2}=\sqrt{4+1}=\sqrt{5}\,\Omega$$

$$I_{rms}=\frac{6}{\sqrt{5}}\text{ A}$$

$$\cos\phi=\frac{R}{Z}=\frac{2}{\sqrt{5}}$$

$$P_{av}=6\times\frac{6}{\sqrt{5}}\times\frac{2}{\sqrt{5}} \quad \text{[from Eq. (i)]}$$

$$=\frac{72}{\sqrt{5}\sqrt{5}}=\frac{72}{5}=14.4\text{ W}$$

61. (*b*) $X_L=(2\pi fL)=2\pi\times 50\times 0.7=220\,\Omega$

$\therefore$ $Z=\sqrt{R^2+X_L^2}=220\sqrt{2}\,\Omega$

$$I_{rms}=\frac{V_{rms}}{Z}=\frac{220}{220\sqrt{2}}=\frac{1}{\sqrt{2}}\text{ A}$$

$\therefore$ Power, $P=I_{rms}^2\cdot R=\frac{1}{2}\times 220=110\text{ W}$

62. (*a*) $X_C=X_L=R$

$$V=\sqrt{V_R^2+(V_L-V_C)^2}$$

but $V_L=V_C$

$\therefore$ $V=V_R=10\text{ V}$

When capacitor is short circuited, $V_C=0$

and $V_R=V_L$ (as $R=X_L$)

$\therefore$ $V=\sqrt{V_R^2+V_L^2}$ or $10=\sqrt{2}\,V_L$

$\therefore$ $V_L=\frac{10}{\sqrt{2}}\text{ V}$

63. (*d*) Phase angle, $\tan\phi=\frac{X_L}{R}=\frac{X_C}{R}$

$\Rightarrow$ $\tan 60^\circ=\frac{X_L}{R}=\frac{X_C}{R}$

$\Rightarrow$ $X_L=X_C=\sqrt{3}R$

i.e., $Z=\sqrt{R^2+(\sqrt{3}R-\sqrt{3}R)^2}\Rightarrow Z=R$

So, average power, $P=\frac{V^2}{R}=\frac{200\times 200}{100}=400\text{ W}$

64. (*b*) Power consumed in the coil,

$$P=I_{rms}^2 R$$

$\therefore$ $R=\frac{P}{I_{rms}^2}=\frac{240}{16}=15\,\Omega$

Impedance, $Z=\frac{V}{I}=\frac{100}{4}=25\,\Omega$

Now, $X_L=\sqrt{Z^2-R^2}$

$$=\sqrt{(25)^2-(15)^2}=20\,\Omega$$

$\therefore$ $2\pi fL=20$

$$L=\frac{20}{2\pi\times 50}=\frac{1}{5\pi}\text{ H}$$

65. (*b*) Circuit is in resonance,

$\therefore$ $V=V_R=IR$

or $R=\frac{V}{I}=\frac{100}{0.2}=500\,\Omega$

$$X_L=\frac{V_L}{I}=\frac{400}{0.2}=2000\,\Omega=\omega L$$

$\therefore$ $\omega=1000\text{ rads}^{-1}$

Further, $X_L=X_C=2000\,\Omega=\frac{1}{\omega C}$

$\therefore$ $C=\frac{1}{2000\,\omega}=0.5\,\mu\text{F}$

66. (*a*) Impedance $=\frac{V_{AC}}{I_{AC}}=\frac{100}{0.5}=200\,\Omega=Z$

$$R=\frac{V_{DC}}{I_{DC}}=\frac{100}{1}=100\,\Omega$$

$$X_L=\sqrt{Z^2-R^2}=100\sqrt{3}\,\Omega=(2\pi fL)$$

$\therefore$ $L=\frac{100\sqrt{3}}{2\pi f}=\frac{100\times 1.732}{2\times 3.14\times 50}=0.55\text{ H}$

67. (*b*) At resonance, $X_C=X_L$

If ω is reduced to half,

$$X_C'=2X_C$$

$\left[\text{as } X_C\propto\frac{1}{\omega}\right]$

and $X_L'=\frac{X_L}{2}$

[as $X_L\propto\omega$]

If ω is made two times,

$$X_C'=\frac{X_C}{2}$$

and $X_L'=2X_L$

i.e. Value of Z will remain unchanged and current should be 1 A.

68. (*b*) Resistance of circuit,

$$R=\frac{V^2}{P}=\frac{110\times 110}{330}=\frac{110}{3}\,\Omega$$

Ist case Power factor, $\cos\phi=0.6$

Since, current lags the voltage, thus the circuit contains resistance and inductance.

$\therefore$ $\cos\phi=\frac{R}{\sqrt{R^2+X_L^2}}=0.6$

$\Rightarrow$ $R^2+X_L^2=\left(\frac{R}{0.6}\right)^2$

$\Rightarrow$ $X_L^2=\frac{R^2}{(0.6)^2}-R^2$

$$\Rightarrow \quad X_L^2 = \frac{R^2 \times 0.64}{0.36}$$

$$\therefore \quad X_L = \frac{0.8R}{0.6} = \frac{4R}{3} \quad \text{...(i)}$$

IInd case Now $\cos\phi = 1$ [given]

Therefore, circuit is purely resistive, *i.e.* it contains only resistance. This is the condition of resonance in which $X_L = X_C$

$$\therefore \quad X_C = \frac{4R}{3} = \frac{4}{3} \times \frac{110}{3} = \frac{440}{9}\Omega \quad \text{[from Eq. (i)]}$$

$$\Rightarrow \quad \frac{1}{2\pi fC} = \frac{440}{9}\Omega$$

$$\therefore \quad C = \frac{9}{2 \times 3.14 \times 60 \times 440} = 0.000054\,\text{F}$$

$$= 54\,\mu\text{F}$$

69. *(a)* In the given circuit diagram,

both inductors of inductance L are parallel to each other, hence

$$L_{eq} = \frac{L_1 L_2}{L_1 + L_2} = \frac{L.L}{L+L} = \frac{L}{2}$$

Similarly, $C_{eq} = C_1 + C_2 = C + C = 2C$

$\therefore$ Resonance frequency,

$$\omega_r = \frac{1}{\sqrt{L_{eq} \cdot C_{eq}}} = \sqrt{\frac{1}{\frac{L}{2} \cdot 2C}} = \sqrt{\frac{1}{LC}} = \frac{1}{\sqrt{LC}}$$

70. *(c)* Given, inductance, $L = 20$ mH

$$= 20 \times 10^{-3}\ \text{H}$$

Capacitance, $C = 100\ \mu\text{F} = 100 \times 10^{-6}\,\text{F}$

Resistance, $R = 50\,\Omega$ and emf, $V = 10 \sin 314t$ ...(i)

$\because$ The general equation of emf is given as $V = V_0 \sin \omega t$ ...(ii)

On comparing Eqs. (i) and (ii), we get

$$V_0 = 10\,\text{V}$$

$$\omega = 314\ \text{rad s}^{-1}$$

The power loss associated with the given AC circuit is given as

$$P = V_{rms} I_{rms} \cos\phi$$

$$= V_{rms}\left(\frac{V_{rms}}{Z}\right)\left(\frac{R}{Z}\right)$$

$$= \left(\frac{V_{rms}}{Z}\right)^2 R = \left(\frac{V_0}{\sqrt{2} \cdot Z}\right)^2 R \quad \text{...(iii)}$$

Impedance, $Z = \sqrt{R^2 + (X_L - X_C)^2}$

$$= \sqrt{R^2 + \left(\omega L - \frac{1}{\omega C}\right)^2}$$

Substituting the given values in the above equation, we get

$$Z = \sqrt{(50)^2 + \left[(314 \times 20 \times 10^{-3}) - \frac{1}{314 \times 10^{-4}}\right]^2}$$

$$= \sqrt{2500 + [6280 \times 10^{-3} - 0.00318 \times 10^4]^2}$$

$$= \sqrt{2500 + (-25.56)^2}$$

$$= 56.15\,\Omega \simeq 56\,\Omega$$

Now, substituting this values in Eq. (iii), we get

$$P = \left(\frac{10}{\sqrt{2} \times 56}\right)^2 \times 50 = \frac{100}{2 \times 3136} \times 50 = 0.79\ \text{W}$$

Thus, the power loss in the circuit is 0.79 W.

71. *(c)* In an L-C-R circuit,

$$\tan\phi = \frac{\omega L - \frac{1}{\omega C}}{R}$$

ϕ being the angle by which the current leads the voltage.

Given, $\phi = 45°$

$$\therefore \quad \tan 45° = \frac{\omega L - \frac{1}{\omega C}}{R}$$

$$\Rightarrow \quad 1 = \frac{\omega L - \frac{1}{\omega C}}{R}$$

$$\Rightarrow \quad R = \omega L - \frac{1}{\omega C}$$

$$\Rightarrow \quad \omega C = \frac{1}{\omega L - R}$$

$$\Rightarrow \quad C = \frac{1}{\omega(\omega L - R)}$$

$$= \frac{1}{2\pi f(2\pi fL - R)}$$

72. *(b)* Power factor, $\cos\phi = \frac{1}{2} \Rightarrow \phi = 60°$

$$\therefore \quad \tan 60° = \frac{\omega L}{R} \Rightarrow \sqrt{3} = \frac{2\pi\nu \times L}{100}$$

$$L = \frac{\sqrt{3} \times 100}{2\pi \times 50} = \frac{\sqrt{3}}{\pi}\,\text{H}$$

73. *(a)* We know that, $I_{WL} = I_{rms} \sin\phi$

$$\Rightarrow \sqrt{3} = 2\sin\phi \ \text{ or } \ \sin\phi = \frac{\sqrt{3}}{2} \Rightarrow \phi = 60°$$

So, power factor $= \cos\phi = \cos 60° = \frac{1}{2}$

74. *(d)* Quantity of heat liberated in the ammeter of resistance R

(i) due to direct current of 3 A $= (3)^2 R$ W

(ii) due to alternating current of 4 A $= (4)^2 R$ W

$\therefore$ Total heat produced per second

$= (3)^2 R + (4)^2 R = 25R$

Let the equivalent alternating current be I virtual ampere, then

$$I^2R = 25R \Rightarrow I = 5\text{ A}$$

75. (c) Given, $V = 150 \sin (150t)$ V

and $I = 150 \sin (150t + \pi/3)$ A

$\therefore \quad I_0 = 150$ A and $V_0 = 150$ V

Power, $P = \frac{1}{2} V_0 I_0 \cos \phi$

$= 0.5 \times 150 \times 150 \times \cos 60°$

$= 5625$ W

76. (a) Impedance, $Z = \sqrt{R^2 + (X_L - X_C)^2}$

$\therefore \quad 10 = \sqrt{(10)^2 + (X_L - X_C)^2}$

$\Rightarrow \quad 100 = 100 + (X_L - X_C)^2$

$\Rightarrow \quad X_L - X_C = 0 \quad$ ...(i)

Let ϕ is the phase difference between current and voltage,

$\therefore \quad \tan \phi = \frac{X_L - X_C}{R}$

$\therefore \quad \tan \phi = \frac{0}{R} \quad$ [from Eq. (i)]

$\phi = 0°$

77. (b) $\frac{N_P}{N_S} = \frac{V_P}{V_S} = \frac{i_S}{i_P}$

$\therefore \quad i_S = \frac{N_P i_P}{N_S} = \frac{4 \times 140}{280} = 2$A

78. (a) Secondary voltage, $V_S = 24$ V

Power associated with secondary, $P_S = 12$ W

$I_S = \frac{P_S}{V_S} = \frac{12}{24} = \frac{1}{2}$ A $= 0.5$ A

Peak value of the current in the secondary,

$I_0 = I_S\sqrt{2}$

$= (0.5)(1.414) = 0.707 = \frac{1}{\sqrt{2}}$ A

79. (b) $N_P = 100, P_i = 10$ kW, $V_i = 200$ V

$\therefore \quad I_P = \frac{P_i}{V_i} = \frac{10000}{200} = 50$ A

Input power = Output power (Neglecting all losses)

$\therefore \quad I_S = \frac{P_i}{V_o} = \frac{10000}{5000} = 2$A

80. (a) Given, turn ratio of a transformer,

$\frac{N_1}{N_2} = \frac{50}{1}$

$\Rightarrow \quad N_1 = 50N_2$

Since, $\quad \frac{N_1}{N_2} = \frac{V_1}{V_2}$

$50 = \frac{120}{V_2} \quad [V_1 = 120 \text{ V (given)}]$

$\Rightarrow \quad V_2 = \frac{12}{5}$ V

Output power at secondary coil,

$P_s = \frac{V_2^2}{R_2}$

$= \frac{\left(\frac{12}{5}\right)^2}{1} = \frac{144}{25} \quad [R_2 = 1\Omega \text{ (given)}]$

$= 5.76$ W

81. (b) Given, output power = 100 W

$V = 220$V, $I = 0.5$ A

We know that, efficiency $= \frac{\text{Output power}}{\text{Input power}} \times 100\%$

$= \frac{100}{220 \times 0.5} \times 100 = 90\%$

82. (a) From transformer ratio,

$\frac{V_S}{V_P} = \frac{N_S}{N_P}$

$\Rightarrow \quad V_S = \frac{V_P \times N_S}{N_P} = \frac{220 \times 40000}{200} = 44000$ V

Potential difference per turn is $\frac{V_S}{N_S} = \frac{44000}{40000} = 1.1$ V

83. (a) $\quad \eta = \frac{\text{Output power}}{\text{Input power}}$

$\Rightarrow \quad \frac{80}{100} = \frac{20 \times 120}{1000 \times I}$

$\Rightarrow \quad I = \frac{20 \times 120 \times 100}{1000 \times 80} = 3$ A

84. (c) Input power $= VI = 200 \times 10$

$= 2000$ W

Output power = Efficiency × Input power

$= \frac{40}{100} \times 2000 = 800$ W

Power loss in heating the armature

$= 2000 - 800 = 1200$ W

$\therefore \quad I^2R = 1200$

or $\quad R = \frac{1200}{I^2} = \frac{1200}{10 \times 10}$

or $\quad R = 12\Omega$

85. (c) For step-up transformer, $V_S > V_P$ and $I_S < I_P$

For an ideal transformer,

$V_S I_S = V_P I_P$

$\therefore \quad 240000\, I_S = 100 \times 4000$

or $\quad I_S = 1.67$ A

86. (b) We have, $\frac{N_s}{N_p} = \frac{i_p}{i_s} \Rightarrow \frac{10}{500} = \frac{i_p}{i_s}$

$$\Rightarrow \quad \frac{i_p}{i_s} = \frac{1}{50} \Rightarrow i_s = 50 i_p$$

This condition is satisfied only when current in primary is 3.2×10^{-3} A and in secondary is 0.16 A.

Assertion and Reason

1 (d) $Z_{DC} = r$

$$Z_{AC} = \sqrt{r^2 + X_L^2}$$

Here, r = internal resistance of the coil.

Also, $I \propto \frac{1}{Z} \therefore \quad I_1 > I_2$

2. (c) If $V = V_0 \sin \omega t$, then current function will lead the voltage function by 90°.

$\therefore \quad I = I_0 \cos \omega t$

$\therefore$ Instantaneous power,

$$P = VI = V_0 I_0 \sin \omega t \cos \omega t$$

or $\quad P \neq 0$ at all times

3. (c) $Z = \sqrt{R^2 + (X_L - X_C)^2}$

By inserting the ferromagnetic rod, L and therefore X_L will increase. But value of Z and therefore I may increase, decrease or remain same.

4. (a) At $X_L = X_C$, the given frequency is resonance frequency.

When frequency is doubled, $X_L = 2R$ [as $X_L \propto \omega$]

and $\quad X_C = \frac{R}{2}$ (as $X_C \propto 1/\omega$)

$$\therefore \quad Z = \sqrt{R^2 + \left(2R - \frac{R}{2}\right)^2} = \frac{\sqrt{13}}{2} R$$

5. (a) $P = V_{rms} I_{rms} \cos \phi = (I_{rms} Z)(I_{rms})\left(\frac{R}{Z}\right) = I_{rms}^2 R$

In one full cycle, the power is

$$P = P_R + P_L + P_C = P_R + 0 + 0 = P_R$$

i.e. Net power is dissipated only along resistor.

6. (c) At resonance, $\phi = 0°$

$\therefore \quad \cos \phi = 1$ or power factor = 1

Also, V and I are in same phase at resonance.

Statement Type Questions

1. (c) Statement I is incorrect but Statement II is correct.

Charge on capacitor of an L-C-R has an amplitude.

$$Q_0 = CV_0 = CI_0 X_C = C \frac{V_0}{Z} X_C$$

$$= \frac{CV_0}{\omega C \sqrt{R^2 + \left(\omega L - \frac{1}{\omega C}\right)^2}}$$

$$= \frac{V_0}{\sqrt{\omega^2 R^2 + \omega^2 (L_1 - 1/C)^2}}$$

$\frac{dQ_0}{d\omega} = 0$ when Q_0 is minimum.

$$\Rightarrow \quad \omega = \sqrt{\frac{1}{LC} - \frac{R^2}{2L^2}}$$

Statement II is correct.

2. (d) Both Statement I and Statement II are correct.

At resonance,

$$V_L = QV_R \quad \Rightarrow \quad \frac{V_L}{V_R} = Q > 1$$

3. (c) Statement I is incorrect but Statement II is correct.

Average power consumed depends also over the phase difference between voltage and current,

$$P_{av} = V_{rms} I_{rms} \cos \phi$$

4. (d) Both Statement I and Statement II are correct.

Impedance is not a sinusoidally varying quantity.

$\therefore$ It is not a phasor.

5. (d) Both Statement I and Statement II are correct.

At resonance

$$\omega_r = \frac{1}{\sqrt{LC}}$$

and $\quad X_L = L\omega = L\frac{1}{\sqrt{LC}} = \sqrt{\frac{L}{C}}$

Potential drop across inductor,

$$V_L = IX_L, \text{ where } I = \frac{V}{Z}$$

$$\frac{V_{rms}}{Z}\sqrt{\frac{L}{C}} = QV_{rms}$$

6. (d) Both Statement I and Statement II are correct.

If f_1 and f_2 are half power point frequencies, then

At f_1, $\quad X_C - X_L = R$

$$\Rightarrow \quad \frac{1}{2\pi f_1 C} - 2\pi f_1 L = R$$

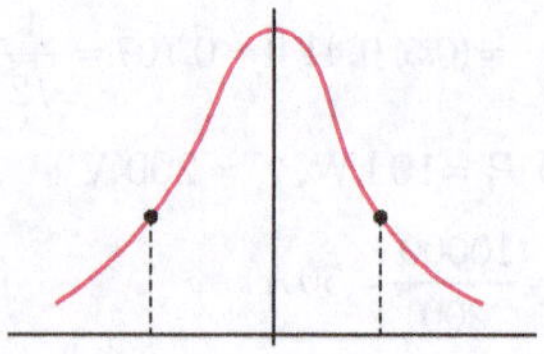

At f_2, $\quad X_L - X_C = R$

$$2\pi f_2 L - \frac{1}{2\pi f_1 C} = R$$

Subtracting, we get

$$\left(\frac{1}{2\pi f_1 C} - 2\pi f_1 L\right) - \left(2\pi f_2 L - \frac{1}{2\pi f_2 C}\right) = 0$$

$$\Rightarrow \quad \left(\frac{1}{\omega_1} + \frac{1}{\omega_2}\right)\frac{1}{C} = (\omega_1 + \omega_2) L_1$$

$$\Rightarrow \quad \frac{1}{\omega_1 \omega_2} = LC = \frac{1}{\omega_r^2}$$

$$\Rightarrow \quad \omega_r = \sqrt{\omega_1 \omega_2}$$

When $\omega_1 = 2$ and $\omega_2 = 8$, then $\omega_r = \sqrt{2 \times 8} = 4\ s^{-1}$

Match the Columns

1. (a) Power factor, $\cos\phi = \dfrac{R}{Z}$

At resonance frequency, $X_C = X_L \Rightarrow \phi = \dfrac{R}{R} = 1$

At frequency < resonance frequency, $X_L < X_C$ and $X_C \propto \dfrac{1}{\omega}$.

At frequency > resonance frequency, $X_L > X_C$ and $X_L \propto \omega$.

Hence, A-(II), B-(I), C-(III), D-(IV).

2. (d)
   A. Phase difference between current and voltage in purely resistive circuit is zero as current and voltage both are in phase so both will reach their maximum values at the same time.
   B. Phase difference between current and voltage in purely inductive circuit is $\dfrac{\pi}{2}$ and current lags voltage.
   C. Phase difference between current and voltage in purely capacitive circuit is $\dfrac{\pi}{2}$ and current leads voltage.
   D. Phase difference between current and voltage in L-C-R circuit is given by $\tan^{-1}\left(\dfrac{X_C - X_L}{R}\right)$.

   Hence, A-(II), B-(III), C-(I), D-(IV).

3. (d) As, $Z = \sqrt{R^2 + (X_L - X_C)^2} = 50\,\Omega$

$$\therefore \quad I = \frac{V_{rms}}{Z} = \frac{100\sqrt{2}/\sqrt{2}}{50} = \frac{100}{40} = 2\text{ A}$$

$$P = I^2 R = 120\text{ W}$$

$$V_R = IR = 60\text{ V}$$

$$V_L = IX_L = 100\text{ V}$$

Hence, A-(III), B-(I), C-(II), D-(IV).

4. (c) $Z = \sqrt{(X_L - X_C)^2 + R^2}$

$\because \; Z = R$ when $\omega_r = \dfrac{1}{\sqrt{LC}}$

Z is minimum at ω_r

Thus, **(A) → (IV)**

$$I = \frac{E}{Z}$$

When $f = f_r$, $Z = R$

and I reaches maximum.

Thus, **(B) → (III)**

$X_C = \dfrac{1}{\omega C}$, when $f \to \infty$, $X_C \to 0$

$$I = \frac{V}{X_C} = V\omega C = 2\pi fVC \;\Rightarrow\; I \propto f$$

Thus, **(C) → (II)**

As, $\quad X_L = \omega L \Rightarrow \dfrac{1}{X_L} \propto \dfrac{1}{f}$

Thus, **(D) → (I)**

Hence, A-(IV), B-(III), C-(II), D-(I).

Final Check Through PYQs

1. (b) We know that, peak voltage (V_0) and rms voltage (V_{rms}) are related as,

$$\therefore \quad V_0 = \sqrt{2}\,V_{rms}$$

2. (b) Given, $C = 10\mu F = 10 \times 10^{-6}$ F

Potential, $V = 210$ V

Frequency, $f = 50$ Hz

Reactance of circuit, $X_C = \dfrac{1}{\omega C}$

$$= \frac{1}{2\pi fC}$$

$$= \frac{1}{2 \times 3.14 \times 50 \times 10 \times 10^{-6}} = \frac{10^3}{3.14}$$

Peak current, $I_m = \dfrac{V\sqrt{2}}{X_C} = \dfrac{210 \times \sqrt{2}}{10^3}$

$$= \frac{3.14 \times 210 \times \sqrt{2}}{1000} = 0.93\text{ A}$$

3. (c) In series L-C-R circuit,

$$L = 10\text{ mH} = 10^{-2}\text{ H}$$

$$C = 1\,\mu F = 10^{-6}\text{ F}, R = 100\,\Omega$$

$\therefore$ Resonance frequency,

$$f = \frac{1}{2\pi\sqrt{LC}} = \frac{1}{2\pi\sqrt{10^{-2} \times 10^{-6}}}$$

$$= \frac{1}{2\pi \times 10^{-4}} = \frac{10^4}{2\pi} = 1.59 \times 10^3\text{ Hz}$$

$$= 1.59\text{ kHz}$$

4. (b) Given, $L = \dfrac{50}{\pi}$ mH $= \dfrac{5}{\pi} \times 10^{-2}$ H

$$C = \frac{10^3}{\pi}\,\mu F = \frac{1}{\pi} \times 10^{-3}\text{ F}$$

$$R = 10\,\Omega,\; f = 50\text{ Hz}, V = 220\text{ V}$$

$$\therefore \quad X_L = 2\pi fL$$

$$= 2\pi \times 50 \times \frac{5}{\pi} \times 10^{-2} = 5\,\Omega$$

$$X_C = \frac{1}{\omega C} = \frac{1}{2\pi fC}$$

$$= \frac{1}{2\pi \times 50 \times \frac{1}{\pi} \times 10^{-3}} = \frac{1}{10^{-1}} = 10\,\Omega$$

∴ Net impedance the circuit,

$$Z = \sqrt{R^2 + (X_C - X_L)^2}$$
$$= \sqrt{10^2 + (10-5)^2}$$
$$= \sqrt{125} = 5\sqrt{5}\ \Omega$$

5. (*a*) Given, In series *L-C-R* circuit,

$L = 10$ H, $C = 10\ \mu F = 10^{-5}$F

$R = 50\ \Omega$

Source voltage, $V = 200 \sin(100\, t)$ volt.

$\omega = 100$ rad/s

$$\therefore \quad 2\pi\nu = 100 \Rightarrow \nu = \frac{100}{2\pi} = \frac{50}{\pi}\ \text{Hz}$$

Resonance frequency,

$$\nu_0 = \frac{1}{2\pi\sqrt{LC}} = \frac{1}{2\pi\sqrt{10 \times 10^{-5}}}$$
$$= \frac{1}{2\,\pi \times 10^{-2}} = \frac{50}{\pi}\ \text{Hz}$$

Hence, $\nu = \nu_0 = \dfrac{50}{\pi}$ Hz

6. (*d*) The given circuit diagram as shown below

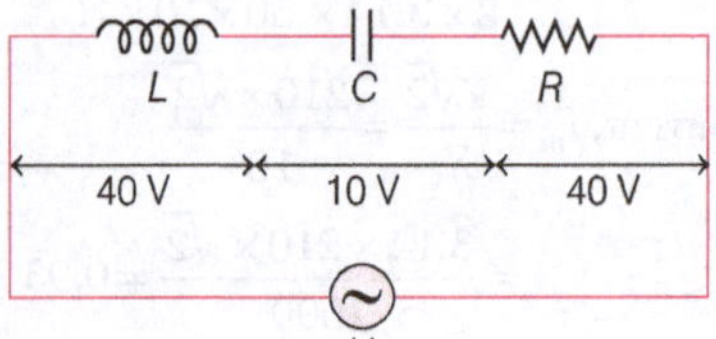

Given, $V_L = 40$ V, $V_C = 10$ V

and $V_R = 40$ V

$$I_0 = 10\sqrt{2}\ \text{A} \quad \text{...(i)}$$

$$\therefore \quad I_{rms} = \frac{I_0}{\sqrt{2}}$$

$$\Rightarrow \quad I_{rms} = \frac{10\sqrt{2}}{\sqrt{2}} \quad \text{[From Eq. (i)]}$$

$$\Rightarrow \quad I_{rms} = 10\ \text{A}$$

$$\therefore \quad V_{rms} = \sqrt{V_R^2 + (V_L - V_C)^2}$$

$$\Rightarrow \quad V_{rms} = \sqrt{(40)^2 + (40-10)^2}$$

$$\Rightarrow \quad V_{rms} = 50\ \text{V}$$

The impedance of the *L-C-R* series circuit,

$$Z = \frac{V_{rms}}{I_{rms}}$$

$$\Rightarrow \quad Z = \frac{50\ \text{V}}{10\ \text{A}}$$

or $\quad Z = 5\Omega$

7. (*b*) Given, $C = 40\ \mu F = 40 \times 10^{-6}$ F

$V_{rms} = 200$ V, $\nu = 50$ Hz

As, $\quad X_C = \dfrac{1}{2\pi\nu C}$

$$= \frac{1}{2\pi \times 50 \times 40 \times 10^{-6}} = \frac{250}{\pi}\ \Omega$$

$$\therefore I_{rms} = \frac{V_{rms}}{X_C} = \frac{200}{\left(\dfrac{250}{\pi}\right)} = 2.5\ \text{A}$$

8. (*a*) When the circuit is connected to AC source,

Voltage, $\quad V = 12$ V

Current, $\quad I = 0.2$ A

$$\Rightarrow \text{Impedance } Z = \frac{V}{I} = \frac{12}{0.2} = 60\ \Omega$$

When it is connected to DC source,

Voltage, $V = 12$ V, Current, $I = 0.4$ A

$$\Rightarrow \text{Resistance, } R = \frac{V}{I} = \frac{12}{0.4} = 30\Omega$$

As in case of DC supply, the capacitor act as an open circuit and no current flows through the circuit. So the given circuit will not have capacitor in series combination. Therefore the circuit should be a series *L-R* circuit.

9. (*c*) Just after switch is closed, given circuit is equivalent to the circuit shown below.

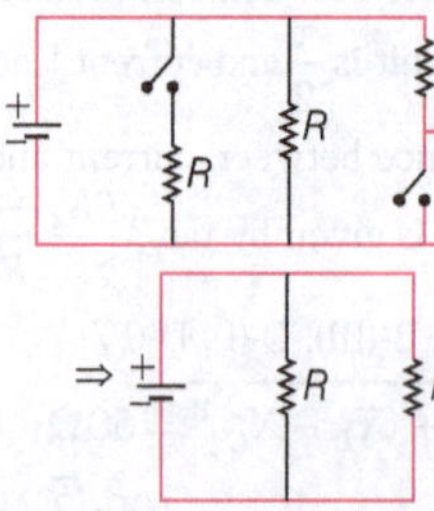

So, equivalent resistor $= \dfrac{R}{2} = \dfrac{9}{2}$ ohms

Battery emf, $V = 18$ volts

∴Current in circuit

$$= \frac{V}{R} = \frac{18 \times 2}{9} = 4\ \text{A}$$

10. (*a*) Impedance of the *R-C* circuit,

$$Z = \sqrt{R^2 + X_C^2}$$

where, $R = 100\ \Omega$ and $X_C = 100\ \Omega$

$$\Rightarrow \quad \tau = \sqrt{(100)^2 + (100)^2} = 100\sqrt{2}\ \Omega$$

Peak value of the current,

$$I_{max} = \frac{V_{max}}{Z} = \frac{220\sqrt{2}}{100\sqrt{2}} = 2.2\ \text{A}$$

11. (b) Net reactive capacitance,

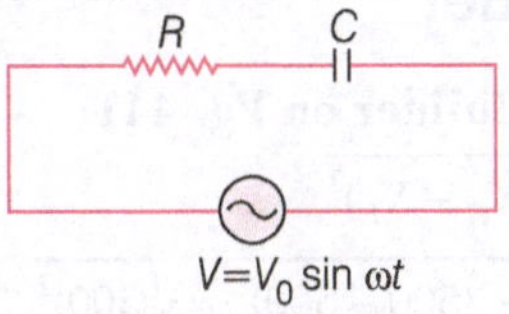

$$X_C = \frac{1}{2\pi fC} = \frac{V}{\sqrt{R^2 + \left(\frac{1}{2\pi fC}\right)^2}}$$

$$\Rightarrow \quad I = \frac{2\pi fC}{\sqrt{4\pi^2 f^2 C^2 R^2 + 1}} \times V$$

Voltage drop across capacitor,

$$V_C = I \times X_C$$

$$= \frac{2\pi fC}{\sqrt{4\pi^2 f^2 C^2 R^2 + 1}} \times \frac{1}{2\pi fC}$$

i.e. $$V_C = \frac{V}{\sqrt{4\pi^2 f^2 C^2 R^2 + 1}}$$

When mica is introduced, capacitance will increase hence, voltage across capacitor get decrease.

12. (c) Given, in the L-C-R series circuit,

$$L = 5\text{ H},$$

$$C = 80\,\mu\text{F}, R = 40\,\Omega$$

Supply voltage, $V = 230$ V

We know that, resonance frequency,

$$\omega_r = \frac{1}{\sqrt{LC}}$$

Substituting the values in the above equation, we get

$$\omega_r = \frac{1}{\sqrt{5 \times 80 \times 10^{-6}}} = 50 \text{ rad/s}$$

Therefore, the angular frequencies of the source at which power transferred to the circuit is half the power at the resonant angular frequency are

$$\omega = \omega_r \pm \Delta\omega \qquad \text{...(i)}$$

We know that,

$$\Delta\omega = \frac{R}{2L} \Rightarrow \Delta\omega = \frac{40}{2(5)}$$

$$\Rightarrow \quad \Delta\omega = 4$$

Using the Eq. (i), we get $\omega = \omega_r \pm \Delta\omega$

$$\omega = (50 \pm 4) \text{ rad / s}$$

So, the angular frequency is likely to be 46 rad/s and 54 rad/s.

13. (b) For L-C-R circuit, phase difference,

$$\phi = \tan^{-1}\left(\frac{X_L - X_C}{R}\right)$$

When L is removed, then $X_L = 0$

$$\therefore \quad \phi = \tan^{-1}\left(\frac{-X_C}{R}\right)$$

$$\Rightarrow \quad \tan\phi = \left|\frac{X_C}{R}\right| \qquad \text{...(i)}$$

When C is removed, then $X_C = 0$

$$\therefore \quad \phi = \tan^{-1}\left(\frac{X_L}{R}\right)$$

$$\Rightarrow \quad \tan\phi = \frac{X_L}{R} \qquad \text{...(ii)}$$

From Eqs. (i) and (ii), we get

$$X_L = X_C$$

∴ Impedance,

$$Z = \sqrt{R^2 + (X_L - X_C)^2} = R$$

Power factor,

$$\cos\phi = \frac{R}{Z} = \frac{R}{R} = 1$$

14. (a) Impedance Z in an AC circuit is

$$Z = \sqrt{R^2 + (X_C - X_L)^2}$$

where X_C = capacitive reactance and X_L = inductive reactance.

Also $X_C = \frac{1}{\omega C}$ and $X_L = \omega L$

$$\therefore \quad Z = \sqrt{(50)^2 + \left(\frac{1}{314 \times 100 \times 10^{-6}} - 314 \times 20 \times 10^{-3}\right)^2}$$

or $\quad Z = 56\,\Omega$

The power loss in the circuit is $P_{av} = \left(\frac{V_{rms}}{Z}\right)^2 R$

$$\therefore \quad P_{av} = \left(\frac{10}{(\sqrt{2})56}\right)^2 \times 50 = 0.79 \text{ W}$$

15. (a) For purely capacitive circuit, $\phi = \frac{\pi}{2}$ rad

In this case current is ahead of voltage by $\frac{\pi}{2}$. Hence, power in this case is given by $P = VI\cos\phi$

$$P = VI\cos 90° = 0$$

16. (d) Given,

Inductance $L = 20$ mH

Capacitance, $C = 50\,\mu$F

Resistance, $R = 40\,\Omega$

emf, $V = 10 \sin 340\,t$

∵ Power loss in AC circuit will be given as

$$P_{av} = I_V^2 R = \left[\frac{E_V}{Z}\right]^2 .R$$

$$= \left(\frac{10}{\sqrt{2}}\right)^2 .40 \frac{1}{40^2 + \left(340 \times 20 \times 10^{-3} - \frac{1}{340 \times 50 \times 10^{-6}}\right)^2}$$

$$\approx 0.46\text{W} \approx 0.51 \text{ W}$$

17. (c) Power factor of the L-C-R circuit

$$= \cos\phi = \frac{R}{Z}$$

$$= \frac{IR}{IZ} = \frac{80}{I\sqrt{(X_L - X_C)^2 + R^2}}$$

$$= \frac{80}{\sqrt{(IX_L - IX_C)^2 + (IR)^2}}$$

$$= \frac{80}{\sqrt{(100-40)^2 + (80)^2}} = 0.8$$

18. (a) When a resistor is connected to an AC source. The power drawn will be

$$P = V_{rms} \cdot I_{rms} = V_{rms} \cdot \frac{V_{rms}}{R}$$

$$\Rightarrow \quad V_{rms}^2 = PR$$

When an inductor is connected in series with the resistor, then the power drawn will be

$$P' = V_{rms} \cdot I_{rms} \cos\phi$$

where, ϕ = phase difference

$$\therefore \quad P' = \frac{V_{rms}^2}{R} \cdot \frac{R^2}{Z^2} = P \cdot R \cdot \frac{R}{Z^2}$$

$$\Rightarrow \quad P' = \frac{P \cdot R^2}{Z^2} = P\left(\frac{R}{Z}\right)^2$$

19. (b) We know that, transformation ratio,

$$r = \frac{N_s}{N_p} = \frac{V_s}{V_p}$$

$$\because \quad \frac{N_p}{N_s} = \frac{1}{2} = \frac{V_p}{V_s}$$

$$\Rightarrow \quad V_s : V_p = 2 : 1$$

20. (d) According to given situation,

$$V_S = 12\text{ V},$$

$$\therefore \quad I_S = \frac{P}{V_S} = \frac{60}{12} = 5\text{ A}$$

$\therefore$ Given, $V_P = 220$ V

For ideal transformer.

$$I_P V_P = I_S V_S$$

$$\Rightarrow \quad I_P = \frac{I_S V_S}{V_P} = \frac{5 \times 12}{220} = 0.27\text{ A}$$

21. (a) Given, the main supply line voltage in transformer,

$$V = 220\text{ V}$$

The rating of the lamp = 11 V, 44 W

We know that, $P = VI_P$ ...(i)

Here, P is the power that operates the lamp,

V is the supply line voltage,

I_P is the primary current in the transformer.

From Eq. (i), we get

$$\Rightarrow \quad 44 = I_P \times 220 \Rightarrow I_P = 0.2\text{ A}$$

Skill Builder

Sol. of Skill Builder on Pg. 441

(b) $Z = \sqrt{R^2 + (X_C - X_L)^2}$

$$= \sqrt{(300)^2 + (500-500)^2} = \sqrt{(300)^2}$$

$$Z = 300\,\Omega$$

Sol. of Skill Builder Pg. 442

(d) Given, $L = 5$ H

$C = 20\mu$F

$R = 100\Omega$

$\therefore$ Resonant frequency,

$$f = \frac{1}{2\pi\sqrt{LC}} = \frac{1}{2\pi} \times \frac{1}{\sqrt{5 \times 20 \times 10^{-6}}}$$

$$= \frac{1}{2\pi} \times \frac{10^2}{1} = \frac{50}{\pi}\text{ Hz}$$

Sol. of Skill Builder on Pg. 445

(d) Impedance Z in an AC circuit is

$$Z = \sqrt{R^2 + (X_C - X_L)^2}$$

where, X_C = capacitive reactance and X_L = inductive reactance.

Also, $X_C = \frac{1}{\omega C}$ and $X_L = \omega L$

$$\therefore \quad Z = \sqrt{(50)^2 + \left(\frac{1}{314 \times 70 \times 10^{-6}} - 314 \times 51 \times 10^{-3}\right)^2}$$

or $Z = 58\,\Omega$

The power loss in the circuit is $P_{av} = \left(\frac{V_{rms}}{Z}\right)^2 R$

$$\therefore \quad P_{av} = \left(\frac{20}{(\sqrt{2})58}\right)^2 \times 50 = 2.97\text{ W}$$

Sol. of Skill Builder on Pg. 449

(b) According to transformation ratio, $\frac{V_S}{V_P} = \frac{N_S}{N_P}$

$$\Rightarrow \quad N_S = \frac{V_S}{V_P} \times N_P$$

$$\Rightarrow \quad N_S = \frac{260}{440} \times 220$$

$$\Rightarrow \quad N_S = 130$$

Sol. of Skill Builder on Pg. 451

(d) $P_{primary} = P_{secondary}$

$$100 \times I_P = 50$$

$$I_P = \frac{50}{100}$$

$$I_P = 0.5\text{ A}$$

For deeper insight
Scan the QR Code

Chapter 9

Electromagnetic Waves

Learning Objectives

Module-I

- Displacement Current
- Maxwell's Equations
- Electromagnetic Waves
- Physical Quantities Associated with EM Waves

Module-II

- Electromagnetic Spectrum
- Radio Waves
- Microwaves
- Infrared Waves
- Visible Rays
- Ultraviolet Rays
- X-Rays
- Gamma(γ)-Rays

Chapter Overview with
NEET Connection

This chapter explains the wave nature of electromagnetic radiations like light and their propagation through the space . Without mastery over this chapter, it will be difficult to understand other chapters like Dual nature of matter & radiation and Atoms.

Special format questions can be easily framed on the following topics of this chapter

- Displacement Current
- Characteristics of EM Waves
- Electromagnetic Spectrum

For better understanding of this chapter

- Vector product of vectors will be helpful.
- Basic differentiation and integration will be helpful.
- Strong grip over concepts of electric field, magnetic field and electrostatic field potential is required.

Introduction

We have studied about electric and magnetic fields separately in the previous chapters. This chapter combines both of these fields. In this chapter, we will study about correction made by Maxwell in Ampere's circuital law, relation between electromagnetic waves and light and finally, we will study about the electromagnetic spectrum and their properties.

Module 1

Displacement Current and Properties of EM Waves

• Displacement Current • Maxwell's Equations • Electromagnetic Waves

After the discovery of electricity and magnetism Maxwell concluded that a variable electric and magnetic fields produces **electromagnetic waves.** Maxwell also concluded that electromagnetic waves are transverse in nature and that light is an electromagnetic wave.

While applying the Ampere's circuital law to find magnetic field at a point outside a capacitor connected to a time varying current, Maxwell noticed an inconsistency in Ampere's circuital law. So, he suggested the existence of an additional current and called it **displacement current**.

Displacement Current

It is defined as the, "current which is produced due to the rate of change of electric flux with respect to time". It is given by

$$I_d = \varepsilon_0 \frac{d}{dt}(\phi_E)$$

To evaluate this relation of displacement current, consider a parallel plate capacitor which is being charged as shown in the figure below.

According to Maxwell, contradiction in Ampere's circuital law is because of some missing term. This missing term must be such that one gets the same magnetic fields at point P, no matter what surface is used.

Also, this missing term must be related to changing electric field which passes through area A_1 between the plates of capacitor as shown in the figure.

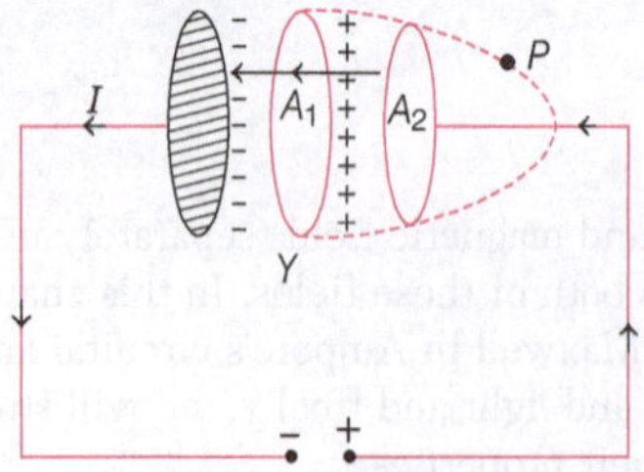

A parallel plate capacitor with an emf source

If at an instant, charge on the plates of capacitor is q, area of plate is A, then electric field between the plates is uniform, which is given by $E = \dfrac{q}{A\varepsilon_0}$ ...(i)

(this field is perpendicular to area A_1)

Electric field outside the plates is zero.

The electric flux through area A_1, $\phi_E = E \times A_1 = \dfrac{q}{A\varepsilon_0} \times A$

($A_1 = A$, because flux will pass through area A)

$$\therefore \quad \phi_E = \frac{q}{\varepsilon_0} \quad \text{...(ii)}$$

If charge on the capacitor plate changes with time, then

$$I = \frac{dq}{dt}$$

So,

$$\frac{d\phi_E}{dt} = \frac{1}{\varepsilon_0} \times \frac{dq}{dt}$$

This implies that, $\dfrac{dq}{dt} = \varepsilon_0 \dfrac{d\phi_E}{dt} \Rightarrow I_d = \varepsilon_0 \dfrac{d\phi_E}{dt}$

This current I_d (the missing term in the Ampere's circuital law) passes through the surface A_1 and is known as **Maxwell's displacement current.**

Hence, Ampere's circuital law $\left(\oint \mathbf{B} \cdot d\mathbf{l} = \mu_0 I\right)$ was modified to $\oint \mathbf{B} \cdot d\mathbf{l} = \mu_0 (I_c + I_d)$

$$\oint \mathbf{B} \cdot d\mathbf{l} = \mu_0 \left(I_c + \varepsilon_0 \frac{d\phi_E}{dt} \right)$$

It is called **modified Ampere's circuital law** or **Ampere-Maxwell's circuital law.**

where, I_c = conduction current,

$$I_d = \varepsilon_0 \frac{d\phi_E}{dt} = \text{displacement current}$$

and ϕ_E = flux of the electric field through the area bounded by closed surface.

Concept ladder

- The conduction and displacement currents are individually discontinuous but these together possess the property of continuity through any closed electric circuit.
- The displacement current is precisely equal to the conduction current when both are present in different parts of the circuit.
- The displacement current arises due to rate of change of electric flux (or electric field) between the two plates of the capacitor.
- Just as the conduction current, the displacement current is also the source of varying magnetic field.

Example 1. *Figure shows a capacitor made of two circular plates each of radius 12 cm and separated by 5.0 cm. The capacitor is being charged by an external source (not shown in the figure). The charging current is constant and equal to 0.15A.*

(i) Obtain the displacement current across the plates.

(ii) Is Kirchhoff's first rule (junction rule) valid at each plate of the capacitor? Explain.

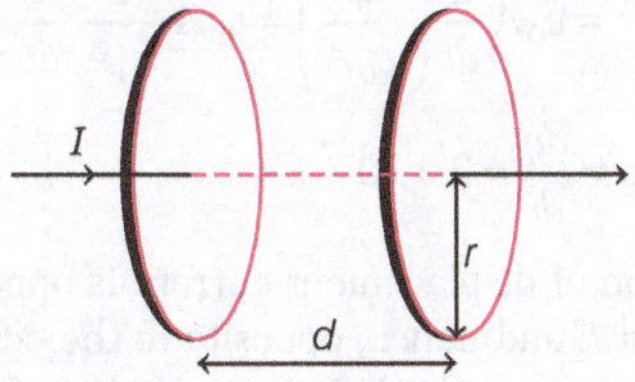

Sol. (i) As displacement current across the plates,

$$I_d = \varepsilon_0 \frac{d\phi_E}{dt}$$

where, ϕ_E = electric flux across the loop.

$$\phi_E = EA = \frac{q}{\varepsilon_0}$$

$$\therefore \quad I_d = \varepsilon_0 \frac{d}{dt}\left(\frac{q}{\varepsilon_0}\right) = \frac{\varepsilon_0}{\varepsilon_0} \cdot \frac{dq}{dt} = I = 0.15 \text{ A}$$

i.e. displacement current is equal to conduction current.

(ii) Yes, Kirchhoff's first rule is valid at each plate of the capacitor. As, net current is equal to the sum of the conduction current and the displacement current.

Example 2. *A parallel plate capacitor consists of two circular plates of radius R = 0.1 m. They are separated by a short distance. If electric field between the capacitor plates changes as* $\frac{dE}{dt} = 6 \times 10^{13} \frac{V}{m \times s}$. *Find displacement current between the plates.*

Sol. Given, area of plates, $A = \pi R^2 = 3.14 \times (0.1)^2 \text{m}^2$

and $\frac{dE}{dt} = 6 \times 10^{13} \frac{\text{V}}{\text{m} \times \text{s}}$

Displacement current between the plates,

$$I_d = \varepsilon_0 \frac{d\phi_E}{dt}$$

$$I_d = \varepsilon_0 A \frac{dE}{dt} \qquad \left(\because \frac{d\phi_E}{dt} = A\frac{dE}{dt}\right)$$

$$= 8.85 \times 10^{-12} \times 3.14 \times (0.1)^2 \times 6 \times 10^{13}$$

$$\Rightarrow \quad I_d = 16.67 \text{ A}$$

Mentor's TiP

- Since numerical value of displacement current is equal to that of conduction current, we can get its value by

$$i = C\frac{dV}{dt}$$

NEET Close-up

Example Similar to PYQ Asked in NEET 2024

A parallel plate capacitor is charged by a constant current 4 A, with plate area A and separation between the plate d. Consider a plane surface of area $A/2$ parallel to the plate and drawn symmetrically between the plates. Then, the displacement current is

(a) 4A (b) 2A
(c) 8A (d) 16A

Sol. (*b*) Charge on the capacitor plates at time t is given by,

$$q = tI$$

Electric field between the plates of the capacitor at this instant is,

$$E = \frac{q}{A\varepsilon_0} = \frac{tI}{A\varepsilon_0}$$

So, electric flux through the given area

$$\phi_E = \left(\frac{A}{2}\right) \cdot E = \frac{tI}{2\varepsilon_0}$$

Therefore, the displacement current,

$$I_d = \varepsilon_0 \frac{d\phi_E}{dt} = \varepsilon_0 \frac{d}{dt}\left(\frac{tI}{2\varepsilon_0}\right) = \frac{I}{2}$$

$$I_d = \frac{4}{2} = 2 \text{ A} \qquad [\text{current}, I = 4 \text{ A}]$$

Skill Builder

A parallel plate capacitor is charged by a constant current I, with plate area A and separation between the plates d. consider a plane surface of area $A/3$ parallel to the plates and drawn symmetrically between the plates. Then,

(a) The displacement current through this area is 3 times of conduction current.

(b) There is no change in displacement current

(c) The displacement current through this area is $\frac{1}{3}$rd times of conduction current.

(d) Data is not sufficient.

For more Practice Refer Q. No. 9, 11 of step up practice 1 and Q. No. 12 of Gearing up for NEET.

Maxwell's Equations

These equations give complete description of all electromagnetic interactions. Maxwell on the basis of his equations, predicted the existence of electromagnetic waves. These equations are as fundamental to electromagnetic phenomenon as Newton's law are for the study of mechanical phenomenon.

There are four Maxwell's equations which are explained as given below

1. Gauss's Law in Electrostatics

This law states that "the total electric flux through any closed surface is always equal to $\frac{1}{\varepsilon_0}$ times the net charge enclosed by that surface". This law relates electric field with a charge distribution.

It is given by $$\oint \mathbf{E} \cdot d\mathbf{S} = \frac{q}{\varepsilon_0}$$

This equation is called **Maxwell's first equation.**

2. Gauss's Law in Magnetism

This law states that "the net magnetic flux through any closed surface is always zero".

It is given by

$$\oint \mathbf{B} \cdot d\mathbf{S} = 0$$

This equation is called **Maxwell's second equation.**

3. Faraday's Law of Electromagnetic Induction

This law states that "the line integral of electric field along a closed path is equal to the rate of change of magnetic flux through the surface bounded by that closed path".

It is given by

$$\oint \mathbf{E} \cdot d\mathbf{l} = -\frac{d\phi_B}{dt}$$

This equation is called **Maxwell's third equation.**

4. Ampere-Maxwell's Circuital Law

This law states that "the line integral of the magnetic field along a closed path is equal to μ_0 times the total current (*i.e.* sum of conduction current and displacement current) threading the surface bounded by that closed path." It is given by

$$\oint \mathbf{B} \cdot d\mathbf{l} = \mu_0\left(I_c + \varepsilon_0 \frac{d\phi_E}{dt}\right)$$

This equation is called **Maxwell's** fourth equation.

Concept ladder

Maxwell's four equations in vacuum can also be written in differential form as follows

1. $\nabla \cdot \mathbf{E} = \frac{\rho}{\varepsilon_0}$
2. $\nabla \cdot \mathbf{B} = 0$
3. $\nabla \cdot \mathbf{E} = -\frac{\partial B}{\partial t}$
4. $\nabla \cdot \mathbf{B} = \mu_0\left(\mathbf{J} + \varepsilon_0 \frac{\partial \mathbf{E}}{\partial t}\right)$, where ρ is charge density and $\mathbf{J}$ is current density).

Example 3. *A parallel plate capacitor of area 40 cm^2 and plate separation 3.0 mm is charged initially to 80 μC. Due to radioactive source nearby, the medium between the plates gets slightly conducting and the plate loses charge initially at the rate of 2×10^{-7} Cs^{-1}. What is the magnitude and direction of displacement current? What is the magnetic field between the plates?*

Sol. Due to leaking, there is a flow of positive charge from the positive plate to the negative plate (or the flow of negative charge in the reverse direction). Thus, the conduction current within the plates is from the positive plate to the negative plate. Now, the displacement current,

$$I_d = \varepsilon_0 \frac{d\phi_E}{dt} = \varepsilon_0 A \frac{dE}{dt}$$

$$= \varepsilon_0 A \frac{d}{dt}\left(\frac{q}{\varepsilon_0 A}\right) = \varepsilon_0 A \frac{1}{\varepsilon_0 A}\frac{dq}{dt}$$

or $$I_d = \frac{dq}{dt} = 2 \times 10^{-7} \text{ Cs}^{-1}$$

The direction of displacement current is opposite to that of electric field E and hence, opposite to the conduction current. But its magnitude is same as that of the conduction current. The net current between the plates is zero.

Using Ampere-Maxwell's circuital law (I being replaced by $I = I_c + I_d = 0$),

$$\oint \mathbf{B} \cdot d\mathbf{l} = \mu_0 I = \mu_0 (I_c + I_d) = \mu_0 \times 0 = 0$$

So, the magnetic field within the plates is zero at all points.

Electromagnetic Waves

Electromagnetic waves (or EM waves) are the waves which are composed of changing electric field **E** and magnetic field **B**, sinusoidally and propagating through space such that, the two fields are perpendicular to each other and perpendicular to the direction of wave propagation.

Sources of Electromagnetic Waves

These waves are produced by accelerating charged particles which can be related with following physical phenomena

(i) A charge oscillating harmonically is a source of EM waves of same frequency.

A simple L-C oscillator and energy source as shown in figure can produce EM waves of desired frequency $\left(\nu = \frac{1}{2\pi\sqrt{LC}}\right)$.

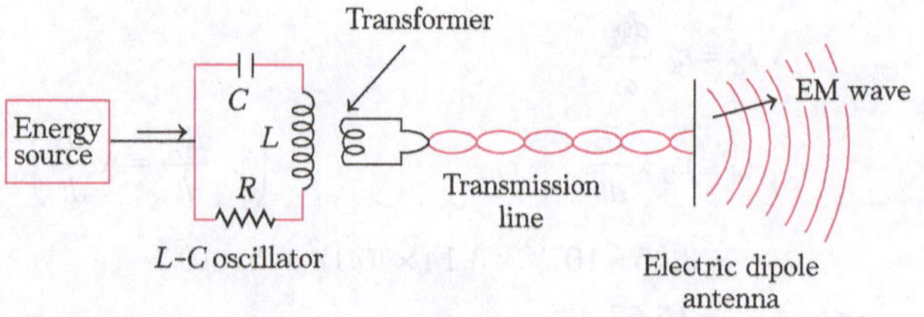

An arrangement for generating electromagnetic waves

Nature of EM Waves

1. Graphical Representation

During propagation of EM waves through a medium, electric field **E** and magnetic field **B** vary sinusoidally.

Electric field and magnetic field become maximum at same position and time.

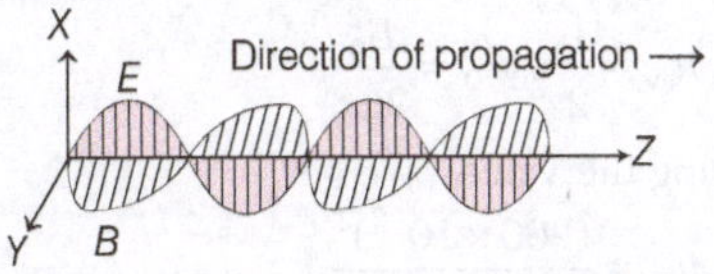

A plane EM wave travelling along Z-axis

Also, **E** and **B** are perpendicular to each other as well as to the direction of propagation of the wave ($\mathbf{E} \times \mathbf{B}$). In the given figure, electric field is along x-direction, magnetic field is along y-direction and the wave propagates along z-direction.

Therefore, $\mathbf{E}(x) \perp \mathbf{B}(y) \perp z$ (direction of propagation of the wave along z).

2. Equations of Electromagnetic Waves

The EM wave propagating in the positive z-direction may be represented by following equations

$$E = E_x = E_0 \sin(kz - \omega t)$$

$$B = B_y = B_0 \sin(kz - \omega t)$$

where, $k = 2\pi/\lambda$ (λ = wavelength),

$\omega = 2\pi\nu$ (ν = frequency),

E_0 = amplitude of varying electric field

and B_0 = amplitude of varying magnetic field.

If the EM wave propagates in negative z-direction, negative sign is replaced by positive sign and equations become

$$E = E_x = E_0 \sin(kz + \omega t)$$

$$B = B_y = B_0 \sin(kz + \omega t)$$

NEET Close-up

Example Similar to PYQ Asked in NEET 2020

The magnetic field in a plane electromagnetic wave is given by

$$B_y = (2 \times 10^{-7}\ \text{T}) \sin(0.5 \times 10^3 x + 1.5 \times 10^{11} t)$$

What is the wavelength and frequency of the wave?

(a) 1.26 cm, 2.4×10^{10} Hz (b) 1.7 cm, 2×10^{11} Hz
(c) 3.4 cm, 2.2×10^{10} Hz (d) 1.52 cm, 1.8×10^{11} Hz

Sol. (*a*) Comparing the given equation with the standard equation of electromagnetic wave,

$$B = B_0 \sin(kx + \omega t)$$

We have, $k = \dfrac{2\pi}{\lambda} = 0.5 \times 10^3$

$\Rightarrow$ $\lambda = \dfrac{2\pi}{0.5 \times 10^3}$ m $= 0.0126$ m $= 1.26$ cm

and $\omega = 2\pi\nu = 1.5 \times 10^{11}$

$\Rightarrow$ $\nu = \dfrac{1.5 \times 10^{11}}{2\pi} = 2.4 \times 10^{10}$ Hz

Skill Builder

For an EM wave, electric field is given by $E_x = (10\ \text{V/m}) \sin(100\pi t - 10\pi y)$. Its wavelength and direction of magnetic field respectively are.

(a) 0.2 m, $-\hat{\mathbf{k}}$ (b) 0.2 m, $\hat{\mathbf{k}}$
(c) 0.5m $-\hat{\mathbf{k}}$ (d) 5 m, $\hat{\mathbf{k}}$

For more Practice Refer, Q. No. 17,18 of Gearing up for NEET.

3. Characteristics of Electromagnetic Waves

(i) These waves do not require any material medium for propagation.

(ii) These waves travel in free space with the speed of light ($\cong 3.0 \times 10^8$ m/s).

(iii) Electromagnetic waves are transverse in nature.

(iv) The oscillating electric and magnetic field vectors of an EM wave are oriented along mutually perpendicular directions and are in phase.

(v) These waves are not deflected by electric field or magnetic field.

(vi) EM waves are polarised.

(vii) These waves carry energy and momentum.

(viii) EM waves exert pressure called radiation pressure.

(ix) Electric field vector of EM waves is responsible for its optical effects.

Physical Quantities Associated with EM Waves

Important physical quantities associated with EM waves are explained as given below

(i) Speed

In free space, it's speed,

$$c = \frac{1}{\sqrt{\mu_0 \varepsilon_0}} = \frac{E_0}{B_0}$$

$$= 3 \times 10^8\ \text{m/s}$$

In medium, $v = \dfrac{1}{\sqrt{\mu\varepsilon}}$

where, μ_0 = absolute permeability,

ε_0 = absolute permittivity,

μ = permeability of medium

and ε = permittivity of medium.

(ii) Energy

Electromagnetic energy can be termed electromagnetic radiation. Electromagnetic wave carry a significant amount of energy through a medium or vacuum from one place to another.

NEET Snapshot

The ratio of contributions made by the electric field and magnetic field components to the intensity of an electromagnetic wave is 1 : 1 [NEET 2020]

$$u_{av} = \frac{1}{2}\frac{B_0^2}{\mu_0} \quad \text{...(i)}$$

Intensity of electric field in EM waves, $u'_{av} = \frac{1}{2}\varepsilon_0 E_0^2$

or $u'_{av} = \frac{1}{2}\varepsilon_0 (cB_0)^2 \quad [\because E_0 = cB_0]$

or $u'_{av} = \frac{1}{2}\frac{B_0^2}{\mu_0} \quad \left[\because c = \frac{1}{\sqrt{\mu_0 \varepsilon_0}}\right]$

Now, taking ratio of Eqs. (i) and (ii), we get

$\therefore \frac{u'_{av}}{u_{av}}$

Scan for Video

(iii) Intensity

The energy crossing per unit area per unit time perpendicular to the direction of propagation of EM wave is called intensity of wave.

i.e. $$I = \frac{\text{Total EM wave energy } (u)}{\text{Surface area}(A) \times \text{Time}(t)}$$

$$= \frac{\text{Total energy density} \times \text{Volume}}{\text{Surface area} \times \text{Time}}$$

$$I = u_{av} \times c = \frac{1}{2}\varepsilon_0 E_0^2 c$$

$$= \frac{1}{2}\frac{B_0^2}{\mu_0} \cdot c \text{ Wm}^{-2}$$

Concept ladder

Intensity due to a point source Consider a point source S, emanating electromagnetic waves (light) in all directions.

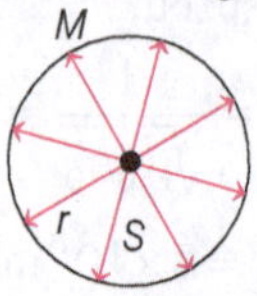

A point source emitting light in all directions

If power of the source is P, then intensity of light at any point M is $I = \frac{u}{A \times t} = \frac{P}{A} = \left(\frac{P}{4\pi r^2}\right) \text{W/m}^2$

In the same way, intensity of a line source, $I \propto 1/r$ and for a plane source, intensity is independent of r.

Example 4. *The magnetic field in a plane electromagnetic wave is given by* $B = (200\,\mu\text{ T})\sin\left[(4.0 \times 10^{15}\text{ s}^{-1})\left(t - \frac{x}{c}\right)\right]$. *Find the average energy density corresponding to the electric field.*

Sol. Average energy density corresponding to electric and magnetic field is equal and is given by

$$u_{av} = \frac{1}{2}\varepsilon_0 E_0^2 = \frac{B_0^2}{2\mu_0}$$

Substituting the values, we get

$$u_{av} = \frac{(200 \times 10^{-6})^2}{2(4\pi \times 10^{-7})}$$

$$= 15.9 \times 10^{-3} \simeq 16 \times 10^{-3}\text{ Jm}^{-3}$$

(iv) Momentum

EM waves also carry momentum. If a portion of EM wave of energy u propagating with speed c, then

linear momentum $= \frac{\text{energy } (u)}{\text{speed } (c)}$.

If wave is incident on a completely absorbing surface, then momentum delivered $p = \frac{u}{c}$. If wave is incident on a totally reflecting surface, then momentum delivered $p = \frac{2u}{c}$.

(v) Radiation Pressure

It is the mechanical pressure exerted upon any surface due to the exchange of momentum between the surface and the EM wave.

For a perfectly reflecting surface, $p_r = \frac{2S}{c}$,

where S = Poynting vector and c = speed of light.

For a perfectly absorbing surface, $p_a = \frac{S}{c}$

Example 5. *Electromagnetic waves travel in a medium with a speed of* $2 \times 10^8\text{ ms}^{-1}$. *The relative magnetic permeability of the medium is 1. Find the relative electrical permittivity.*

Sol. Given, $v = 2 \times 10^8\text{ms}^{-1}$ and $\mu_r = 1$

The speed of electromagnetic waves in a medium is given by $$v = \frac{1}{\sqrt{\mu\varepsilon}} \quad \text{...(i)}$$

where, μ and ε are permeability and permittivity of the medium, respectively.

Now, $\mu = \mu_0\mu_r$ and $\varepsilon = \varepsilon_0\varepsilon_r$

$\therefore$ Eq. (i) becomes, $$v = \frac{1}{\sqrt{\mu_0\mu_r\varepsilon_0\varepsilon_r}} = \frac{1}{\sqrt{\mu_0\varepsilon_0}} \times \frac{1}{\sqrt{\mu_r\varepsilon_r}}$$

$$\Rightarrow \quad v = \frac{c}{\sqrt{\mu_r\varepsilon_r}} \quad \left(\because c = \frac{1}{\sqrt{\mu_0\varepsilon_0}}\right)$$

On squaring both sides, we get

$$\varepsilon_r = \frac{c^2}{v^2\mu_r} = \frac{(3 \times 10^8)^2}{(2 \times 10^8)^2 \times 1} = 2.25$$

Example 6. *Find ratio of velocity of EM wave in medium of electric permittivity $A\varepsilon_0$ and $B\mu_0$ respectively with that of in vacuum.*

Sol. Velocity of EM wave in any medium

$$v = \frac{c}{\sqrt{\mu_r \varepsilon_r}}$$

$$\mu_r = \frac{B\mu_0}{\mu_0} = B$$

$$\varepsilon_r = \frac{A\varepsilon_0}{\varepsilon_0} = A \Rightarrow \frac{v}{c} = \frac{1}{\sqrt{AB}}$$

Example 7. *If both μ and ε of a medium are double than these value in vacuum, speed of EM wave in such medium will be*

(a) 1.5×10^8 m/s (b) 0.75×10^8 m/s
(c) 12×10^8 m/s (d) 1.8×10^8 m/s

Sol. (*a*) Velocity of EM wave in any medium

$$v = \frac{1}{\sqrt{\mu\varepsilon}} = \frac{1}{\sqrt{2\mu_0 2\varepsilon_0}} = \frac{1}{2}\frac{1}{\sqrt{\mu_0\,\varepsilon_0}} = \frac{c}{2}$$

$$= \frac{3 \times 10^8}{2} = 1.5 \times 10^8 \text{ m/s}$$

NEET Close-up

Example Similar to PYQ Asked in NEET 2023 and NEET 2018

A wave is traveling in $+y$ direction with its electric field component as 3 V/m $\hat{\mathbf{i}}$ at an instant. The magnetic field at this instant is

(a) $-10^8\,\hat{\mathbf{k}}$T (b) $-10^{-8}\,\hat{\mathbf{k}}$T (c) $10^8\,\hat{\mathbf{k}}$T (d) $10^{-8}\,\hat{\mathbf{k}}$T

Sol. (*d*) Magnitude of **B**

$$B_0 = \frac{E_0}{c} = \frac{3}{3 \times 10^8} = 10^{-8}\text{ T}$$

Direction can be found using poynting vector from question

$$\hat{\mathbf{i}} \times \hat{\mathbf{B}} = \hat{\mathbf{j}}$$

Clearly $\hat{\mathbf{B}} = -\hat{\mathbf{k}}$

So, $\mathbf{B} = B\hat{\mathbf{B}} = -10^{-8}\hat{\mathbf{k}}$ T

Skill Builder

For an EM wave $B_0 = 3 \times 10^3$ T, then the value of E_0 is

(a) 10^{-5} V/m (b) 10^5 V/m
(c) 9×10^{11} V/m (d) 9×10^5 V/m

For more practice Refer, Q. No. 16 of step up practice 1 and Q. No. 11, 20 of Gearing up for NEET.

STEP UP Practice 1

1. According to Maxwell's hypothesis, a changing electric field gives rise to
   (a) emf
   (b) electric current
   (c) magnetic field
   (d) pressure radiant

2. Maxwell in his famous equation of electromagnetism introduced the concept of
   (a) AC current
   (b) DC current
   (c) displacement current
   (d) impedance

3. Which of the following statement is incorrect about electromagnetic waves?
   (a) These are transverse in nature.
   (b) These are produced by accelerating charges.
   (c) They travel with the same speed in all media.
   (d) They travel in free space with the speed of light.

4. **Assertion** (A) When a charged particle moves in a circular path. It produces electromagnetic wave.
   Reason (R) Charged particle has acceleration.
   In the light of the above statements, choose the correct answer from the options given below
   (a) Both A and R are true but R is not the correct explanation of A.
   (b) A is true but R is false.
   (c) A is false but R is true.
   (d) Both A and R are true and R is the correct explanation of A.

5. Dimensions of $\varepsilon_0 \frac{d\phi_E}{dt}$ are same as that of
   (a) charge (b) potential
   (c) capacitance (d) current

6. According to Ampere-Maxwell's circuital law,
   (a) $\oint \mathbf{E} \cdot d\mathbf{S} = \frac{q}{\varepsilon_0}$ (b) $\oint \mathbf{E} \cdot d\mathbf{l} = -\frac{d\phi_B}{dt}$
   (c) $\oint \mathbf{B} \cdot d\mathbf{S} = 0$ (d) $\oint \mathbf{B} \cdot d\mathbf{l} = \mu_0\left(I_c + \varepsilon_0 \frac{d\phi_E}{dt}\right)$

7. **Assertion** (A) Dipole oscillations produce electromagnetic waves.
   Reason (R) Accelerated charge produces electromagnetic waves.

In the light of the above statements, choose the correct answer from the options given below

(a) Both A and R are true but R is not the correct explanation of A.
(b) A is true but R is false.
(c) A is false but R is true.
(d) Both A and R are true and R is the correct explanation of A.

8. The conduction current in ideal case through a circuit is zero when charge on capacitor is

(a) zero
(b) maximum
(c) any transient value
(d) depends on capacitor used

9. What is the displacement current between the square plate of side 1 cm of a capacitor, if electric field between the plates is changing at the rate of 3×10^6 $Vm^{-1}s^{-1}$?

(a) 2.7×10^{-9} A
(b) 3.2×10^{-5} A
(c) 4.2×10^{-6} A
(d) 4.0×10^{-5} A

10. **Assertion** (A) Static crashes are heard on radio, when lighting flash occurs in the sky.

Reason (R) Electromagnetic waves having frequency of radio wave range interfere with radio waves.

In the light of the above statements, choose the correct answer from the option given below.

(a) Both A and R are true but R is not the correct explanation of A.
(b) A is true but R is false.
(c) A is false but R is true.
(d) Both A and R are true and R is the correct explanation of A.

11. A parallel plate capacitor of plate separation 2 mm is connected in an electric circuit having source voltage 400 V. What is the value of the displacement current for 10^{-6} s, if the plate area is 60 cm^2?

(a) 1.062×10^{-2} A (b) 2.062×10^{-2} A
(c) 3.062×10^{-2} A (d) 5.062×10^{-2} A

12. The electric field of a plane electromagnetic wave varies with time of amplitude 2 Vm^{-1} propagating along Z-axis. The average density of the magnetic field is (in J m^{-3})

(a) 13.29×10^{-12} (b) 8.86×10^{-12}
(c) 17.71×10^{-12} (d) 4.43×10^{-12}

13. In an electromagnetic wave, the electric and magnetic fields are 100 Vm^{-1} and 0.265 T, respectively. The maximum rate of energy flow is

(a) 21×10^6 Wm^{-2} (b) 36.5×10^6 Wm^{-2}
(c) 46.7×10^6 Wm^{-2} (d) None of these

14. Which of the following pair given below is correct?

(a) Maxwell's First equation → $\oint \mathbf{E} \cdot d\mathbf{S} = 0$
(b) Maxwell's Second equation → $\oint \mathbf{B} \cdot d\mathbf{S} = \frac{q}{\varepsilon_0}$
(c) Faraday's law of Electromagnetic induction → $\oint \mathbf{E} \cdot dl = \frac{-d\phi_B}{dt}$
(d) Ampere-Maxwell's circuital law → $\oint \mathbf{B} \cdot dl = \mu_0(I_c + \varepsilon_0 ds)$

15. Radiations of intensity 0.5 Wm^{-2} are striking a metal plate. The pressure on the plate is

(a) 0.166×10^{-8} Nm^{-2} (b) 0.33×10^{-8} Nm^{-2}
(c) 0.111×10^{-8} Nm^{-2} (d) 0.083×10^{-8} Nm^{-2}

16. In an apparatus, the electric field was found to oscillate with amplitude of 18 Vm^{-1}. The magnitude of the oscillating magnetic field will be

(a) 4×10^{-6} T (b) 6×10^{-8} T
(c) 9×10^{-9} T (d) 11×10^{-11} T

17. The rms value of the electric field of the light coming from the sun is 720 NC^{-1}. The average total energy density of the electromagnetic wave is

(a) 6.37×10^{-9} J m^{-3}
(b) 81.35×10^{-12} J m^{-3}
(c) 3.5×10^{-3} J m^{-3}
(d) 4.58×10^{-6} J m^{-3}

18. Amongst the following relations, which is correct?

(a) $\sqrt{\varepsilon_0} E_0 = \sqrt{\mu_0} B_0$
(b) $\sqrt{\mu_0 \varepsilon_0} = B_0 / E_0$
(c) $E_0 = \sqrt{\mu_0 \varepsilon_0} B_0$
(d) $\sqrt{\mu_0} E_0 = \sqrt{\varepsilon_0} B_0$

19. **Assertion** (A) Light can travel in vacuum whereas sound cannot do so.

Reason (R) Light has an electromagnetic wave nature whereas sound is mechanical wave.

In the light of the above statements, choose the correct answer from the options given below.

(a) Both A and R are true but R is not the correct explanation of A.
(b) A is true but R is false.
(c) A is false but R is true.
(d) Both A and R are true and R is the correct explanation of A.

20. An electromagnetic wave going through vacuum is described by $E = E_0 \sin(kx - \omega t)$. Which of the following is independent of wavelength?

(a) k (b) ω (c) k/ω (d) $k\omega$

21. An L-C resonant circuit contains a 200 pF capacitor and a 100 μH inductor. It is set into oscillation coupled to an antenna. The wavelength of the radiated electromagnetic waves is

(a) 377 mm (b) 266 m
(c) 377 cm (d) 3.77 cm

Module 2

Electromagnetic Spectrum

- Electromagnetic Spectrum • Radio Waves • Microwaves • Infrared Waves
- Visible Rays • Ultraviolet Rays • X-Rays • Gamma (γ)-Rays

Electromagnetic Spectrum

The orderly arrangement of EM waves in increasing or decreasing order of wavelength λ or frequency ν is called **electromagnetic spectrum.** The range varies from 10^{-12} m to 10^{4} m, *i.e.* from γ-rays to radio waves as shown in the figure given below.

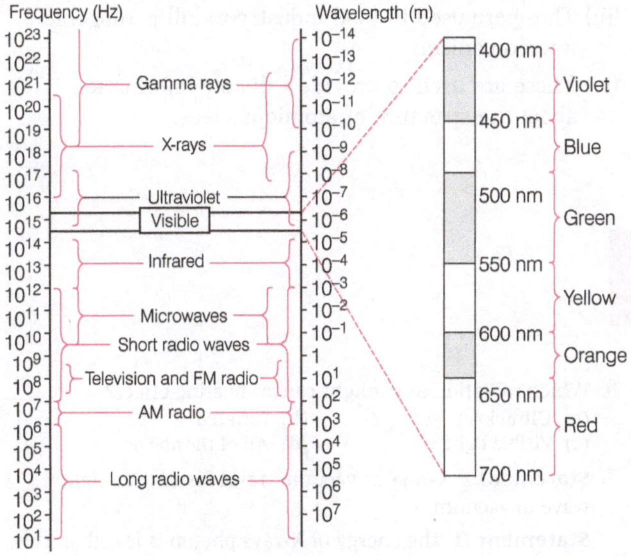

Electromagnetic spectrum

The wavelength ranges, frequency ranges and uses of the various regions of electromagnetic spectrum are summarised below

Radio Waves

These waves were first predicted by James Clerk Maxwell. Radio waves are produced due to oscillating charge particles between plates of capacitor in L-C circuit.

Uses of radio waves are given below

(i) These are used in AM (Amplitude Modulation) from 530 kHz to 1710 kHz. These are also used in ground wave propagation.

(ii) These are used in TV waves ranging from 54 MHz to 890 MHz.

(iii) These are used in FM (Frequency Modulation) ranging from 88 MHz to 108 MHz.

(iv) UHF (Ultra High Frequency) waves are used in cellular phones.

Microwaves

These waves were also predicted by James Clerk Maxwell. Microwaves are called **short wavelength radio waves** which are produced by vacuum tubes.

Uses of microwaves are given below

(i) These are used in RADAR systems for aircraft navigation.

(ii) These are used in microwave oven for cooking purpose.

(iii) These are used in the study of atomic and molecular structures.

(iv) These are used to measure the speed of vehicle, speed of cricket ball, etc.

Infrared Waves

These waves were discovered by Herschel. Infrared waves are also called **heat waves.** These waves are produced by heat radiating bodies and molecules. They have high penetration power.

Uses of infrared waves are given below

(i) These are used in heat therapy to heat muscular pain or sprain.

(ii) These are used in satellite for army purpose.

(iii) These are used in weather forecasting.

(iv) These are used for producing dehydrated fruits.

(v) These are used in solar water heater, solar cells and cooker.

(vi) These are used in TV remote as signal carrier.

(vii) These are used in night vision or infrared photography.

Visible Rays

These rays were discovered by Sir Isaac Newton. It is that part of spectrum which is visible by human eye.

Visible rays are used by the optical organs of humans and animals for three primary purposes given below

(i) To see things, avoid bumping from them and escape danger.
(ii) To find stuff to eat.
(iii) To find other living things with which to consort, so as to prolong the species.

Ultraviolet Rays

These rays were discovered by Johann Ritter in 1801. UV-rays are produced by special lamps and very hot bodies. The sun is an important source of UV-rays but fortunately these rays are absorbed by ozone layer.

Uses of ultraviolet rays are given below

(i) These are used in burglar alarm.
(ii) These are used to study molecular structure and in detection of invisible writing.
(iii) These are used to kill germs in minerals.
(iv) These are used to sterilise surgical instruments.

X-Rays

These rays were discovered by German professor Roentgen.

Uses of X-rays are given below

(i) These are used in surgery to detect the fracture, diseased organs, stones in the body.
(ii) These are used in engineering to detect fault, crack on bridges, testing of welds.
(iii) These are used at metro station to detect metal or explosive material.
(iv) These are used in scientific research.

Gamma (γ)-Rays

These rays were discovered by Rutherford. They have high penetration power.

Uses of gamma (γ)-rays are given below

(i) These are used to produce nuclear reaction.
(ii) These are used in radiotherapy for the treatment of tumour and cancer.
(iii) These are used in food industry to kill pathogenic microorganism.
(iv) These are used to provide valuable information about the structure of atomic nucleus.

STEP UP Practice 2

1. The frequency of visible light is of the order of
(a) 10^{15} Hz (b) 10^{10} Hz
(c) 10^6 Hz (d) 10^4 Hz

2. Which of the following wavelength falls in X-rays region?
(a) 1Å (b) 10^{-4}Å (c) 10^{-2}Å (d) 10^{-3}Å

3. **Statement I** X-rays, radio-waves, light waves and matter waves are all electromagnetic waves.
Statement II Electromagnetic waves are longitudinal in nature.
In the light of the above statements, choose the most appropriate answer from the options given below :
(a) Both Statement I and Statement II are incorrect.
(b) Statement I is correct but Statement II is incorrect.
(c) Statement I is incorrect but Statement II is correct.
(d) Both Statement I and Statement II are correct.

4. The percentage power of X-ray increases with the increases in its
(a) velocity (b) intensity
(c) frequency (d) wavelength

5. The range of wavelength of the visible light is
(a) 10 Å to 100 Å
(b) 4,000 Å to 8,000 Å
(c) 8,000 Å to 10,000 Å
(d) 10,000 Å to 15,000 Å

6. Which radiation in sunlight causes heating effect?
(a) Ultraviolet (b) Infrared
(c) Visible light (d) All of the above

7. **Statement I** X-rays in vacuum travel faster than light wave in vacuum.
Statement II The energy of X-rays photon is less than that of light photon.
In the light of the above statements, choose the most appropriate answer from the options given below :
(a) Both Statement I and Statement II are incorrect.
(b) Statement I is correct but Statement II is incorrect.
(c) Statement I is incorrect but Statement II is correct.
(d) Both Statement I and Statement II are correct.

8. Which of the following radiations has the least wavelength?
(a) γ-rays (b) β-rays (c) α-rays (d) X-rays

9. Which of the following is not electromagnetic waves?
(a) Cosmic rays (b) Gamma rays
(c) β-rays (d) X-rays

10. Which one of the following pair is correct?

	Type		Frequency
(a)	Radio wave	→	$< 10^7$ Hz
(b)	Microwave	→	10^9 to 10^{11} Hz
(c)	X-rays	→	10^{20} to 10^{22} Hz
(d)	UV rays	→	10^{12} to 10^{15} Hz

11. The ozone layer absorbs
(a) infrared radiations
(b) ultraviolet radiations
(c) X-rays
(d) γ-rays

12. Electromagnetic radiation of highest frequency is
(a) infrared radiations (b) visible radiation
(c) radio waves (d) γ-rays

13. Which of the following waves has the maximum wavelength?
(a) X-rays (b) IR-rays
(c) UV-rays (d) radio waves

14. Which of the following pairs is incorrect?
(a) Rays used in TV remote as signal carrier → Infrared
(b) Rays used in surgery to detect the fracture → X-rays
(c) Rays used to produce nuclear reaction → Ultraviolet
(d) Waves used in RADAR system → Microwaves

15. **Statement I** The electromagnetic waves are transverse in nature.
Statement II Waves of wavelength 10 mm are radiowave and microwave.
In the light of the above statements, choose the most appropriate answer from the options given below
(a) Both Statement I and Statement II are incorrect.
(b) Statement I is correct but Statement II is incorrect.
(c) Statement I is incorrect but Statement II is correct.
(d) Both Statement I and Statement II are correct.

16. The frequencies of X-rays, γ-rays and ultraviolet rays are respectively a, b and c. Then,
(a) $a < b, b > c$
(b) $a > b, b > c$
(c) $a > b, b < c$
(d) $a < b, b < c$

17. Radio waves and visible light in vacuum have
(a) same velocity but different wavelength
(b) continuous emission spectrum
(c) band absorption spectrum
(d) line emission spectrum

18. X-rays are not used for radar purposes because they are not
(a) reflected by target
(b) partly absorbed by target
(c) electromagnetic waves
(d) completely absorbed by target

19. **Statement I** Microwaves have more energy than the radio waves.
Statement II Energy of wave is directly proportional to the frequency.
In the light of the above statements, choose the most appropriate answer from the options given below
(a) Both Statement I and Statement II are incorrect.
(b) Statement I is correct but Statement II is incorrect.
(c) Statement I is incorrect but Statement II is correct.
(d) Both Statement I and Statement II are correct.

20. In which one of the following regions of the electromagnetic spectrum will the vibrational motion of molecules give rise to absorption?
(a) Ultraviolet (b) Microwaves
(c) Infrared (d) Radio waves

21. Which of the following electromagnetic waves is incorrectly paired with its frequency range?
(a) Radio wave → 10^4 Hz to 10^9 Hz
(b) Infrared wave → 10^{11} Hz to 10^{14} Hz
(c) Ultraviolet rays → 10^{14} Hz to 10^{17} Hz
(d) Gamma rays → 10^{18} Hz to 10^{26} Hz

NEET Exclusive EXTRA BYTES

- When a capacitor is connected with battery through wires, then conduction current (I_C) flows through wire and displacement current (I_D) flows between the gap of capacitor plates.
- Frequency is inherent property of EM waves and it does not change with change in medium during propagation.
- All electromagnetic waves are electrically neutral.
- **Poynting vector of an EM wave**
  The rate of flow of energy in an electromagnetic wave is described by the vector **S**. It is called the Poynting vector, which is defined by the expression,
  $$\mathbf{S} = \frac{1}{\mu_0}(\mathbf{E} \times \mathbf{B})$$
  Its magnitude **S** is related to the rate at which energy is transported by a wave across a unit area at any instant.
- Since, **E** and **B** are mutually perpendicular.
  Hence, $|\mathbf{E} \times \mathbf{B}| = E_0 B_0$
  Thus, $S = \dfrac{E_0 B_0}{\mu_0}$
- The SI unit of Poynting vector **S** is $Js^{-1}m^2$ or Wm^{-2}.
- The direction of the Poynting vector **S** of an EM wave at any point gives direction of the wave and the direction of energy transported at that point.
- Ultraviolet rays play an important role in the production of vitamin D in our skins.
- Microwave are used in operating a RADAR.
- Infrared waves are often knows as heat waves.

Production and detection of different types of electromagnetic waves

Type	Wavelength range	Frequency range	Production	Detection
Radio wave	> 0.1 m	$<10^9$ Hz	Rapid acceleration and deceleration of electrons in aerials.	Receiver's aerials
Microwave	0.1 m to 1 mm	10^9 to 10^{11} Hz	Klystron valve or magnetron valve.	Point contact diodes
Infrared wave	1 mm to 700 nm	10^{11} to 10^{14} Hz	Vibration of atoms and molecules.	Thermopiles, bolometer, infrared photographic film
Visible rays	700 nm to 400 nm	4×10^{14} to 8×10^{14} Hz	Electrons in atoms emit light when they move from higher energy level to a lower energy level.	The eye, photocells, photographic film
Ultraviolet rays	400 nm to 1 nm	10^{14} to 10^{17} Hz	Inner shell electrons in atoms moving from higher energy level to a lower energy level.	Photocells, photographic film
X-rays	1 nm to 10^{-3} nm	10^{16} to 10^{20} Hz	X-ray tubes or inner shell electrons.	Photographic film, Geiger tubes, ionisation chamber
Gamma rays	$<10^{-3}$ nm	$>10^{22}$ Hz	Radioactive decay of the nucleus.	Photographic film, Geiger tubes, ionisation chamber

GEARING UP FOR NEET

Single Option Correct

1. Energy of electromagnetic waves is due to their
(a) wavelength
(b) frequency
(c) electric and magnetic fields
(d) None of the above

2. Energy stored in electromagnetic oscillations is in the form of
(a) electrical energy
(b) magnetic energy
(c) Both (a) and (b)
(d) None of the above

3. Total energy density of electromagnetic waves in vacuum is given by the relation
(a) $\frac{1}{2} \cdot \frac{E^2}{\varepsilon_0} + \frac{B^2}{2\mu_0}$
(b) $\frac{1}{2}\varepsilon_0 E^2 + \frac{1}{2}\mu_0 B^2$
(c) $\frac{E^2 + B^2}{c}$
(d) $\frac{1}{4}\varepsilon_0 E^2 + \frac{B^2}{4\mu_0}$

4. For a medium with permittivity ε and permeability μ, the velocity of light is given by
(a) $\sqrt{\mu / \varepsilon}$ (b) $\sqrt{\mu\varepsilon}$
(c) $1/\sqrt{\mu\varepsilon}$ (d) $\sqrt{\varepsilon/\mu}$

5. The speed of electromagnetic wave in vacuum
(a) increases as we move from γ-rays to radio waves
(b) decreases as we move from γ-rays to radio waves
(c) is same for all of them
(d) None of the above

6. In a plane electromagnetic wave, the electric field oscillates sinusoidally at a frequency of 2×10^{10} Hz and amplitude 48 Vm^{-1}. The wavelength of the wave is
(a) 24×10^{-10} m
(b) 1.5×10^{-2} m
(c) 4.16×10^{8} m
(d) 3×10^{8} m

7. If **E** and **B** represent electric and magnetic field vectors of the electromagnetic wave, then the direction of propagation of electromagnetic wave is along *[NCERT Exemplar]*
(a) **E** (b) **B**
(c) **B** × **E** (d) **E** × **B**

8. An EM wave radiates outwards from a dipole antenna, with E_0 as the amplitude of its electric field vector. The electric field E_0 which transports significant energy from the source falls off as *[NCERT Exemplar]*
(a) $\frac{1}{r^3}$ (b) $\frac{1}{r^2}$
(c) $\frac{1}{r}$ (d) remains constant

9. The average electric field of electromagnetic waves in certain region of free space is 9×10^{-4} NC^{-1}. Then, the average magnetic field in the same region is of the order of
(a) 27×10^{-4} T (b) 3×10^{-12} T
(c) $\left(\frac{1}{3}\right) \times 10^{-12}$ T (d) 3×10^{12} T

10. The pressure exerted by an electromagnetic wave of intensity I Wm^{-2} on a non-reflecting surface is (c is the velocity of light)
(a) Ic (b) Ic^2
(c) I/c (d) I/c^2

11. The electric and the magnetic fields associated with an electromagnetic wave, propagating along the Z-axis, can be represented by
(a) $[E = E_0 \hat{k}, B = B_0 \hat{i}]$
(b) $[E = E_0 \hat{j}, B = B_0 \hat{j}]$
(c) $[E = E_0 \hat{j}, B = B_0 \hat{k}]$
(d) $[E = E_0 \hat{i}, B = B_0 \hat{j}]$

12. A parallel plate capacitor is charged to 60μC. Due to a radioactive source, the plate loses charge at the rate of $1.8 \times 10^{-8} Cs^{-1}$. The magnitude of displacement current is
(a) $1.8 \times 10^{-8} Cs^{-1}$
(b) $3.6 \times 10^{-8} Cs^{-1}$
(c) $4.1 \times 10^{-11} Cs^{-1}$
(d) $5.7 \times 10^{-12} Cs^{-1}$

13. Radiation of intensity $1 W/m^2$ are striking on a metal plate. The pressure on the plate is
(a) 0.66×10^{-8} N/m^2 (b) 0.25 N/m^2
(c) 2 N/m^2 (d) 4 N/m^2

14. An *L-C* resonant circuit contains a 200 pF capacitor and a 200 μH inductor. It is set into oscillation coupled to an antenna. The wavelength of the radiated electromagnetic waves is
(a) 377mm (b) 377 m
(c) 377 cm (d) 3.77 cm

15. An electromagnetic wave going through vacuum is described by $E = E_0 \sin(kx - \omega t)$, $B = B_0 \sin(kx - \omega t)$. Which of the following equations is true?
(a) $E_0 k = B_0 \omega$
(b) $E_0 \omega = B_0 k$
(c) $E_0 B_0 = \omega k$
(d) None of the above

16. A linearly polarised electromagnetic wave given as $\mathbf{E} = E_0 \hat{\mathbf{i}} \cos(\hat{\mathbf{k}}z - \omega t)$ is incident normally on a perfectly reflecting infinite wall at $z = a$. Assuming that the material of the wall is optically inactive, the reflected wave will be given as ***[NCERT Exemplar]***
(a) $\mathbf{E}_r = E_0 \hat{\mathbf{i}}(\hat{\mathbf{k}}z - \omega t)$
(b) $\mathbf{E}_r = E_0 \hat{\mathbf{i}} \cos(\hat{\mathbf{k}}z + \omega t)$
(c) $\mathbf{E}_r = -E_0 \hat{\mathbf{i}} \cos(\hat{\mathbf{k}}z + \omega t)$
(d) $\mathbf{E}_r = E_0 \hat{\mathbf{i}} \sin(\hat{\mathbf{k}}z - \omega t)$

17 A plane electromagnetic wave propagating in the *x*-direction has a wavelength 6.0 mm. The electric field is in the *y*-direction and its maximum magnitude is 33 Vm^{-1}. The equation for the electric field as a function of *x* and *t* is
(a) $11 \sin \pi (t - x/c)$
(b) $33 \sin \pi \times 10^{11} (t - x/c)$
(c) $33 \sin \pi (t - x/c)$
(d) $11 \sin \pi \times 10^{11} (t - x/c)$

18 An electromagnetic wave travels in vacuum along *z*-direction with $\mathbf{E} = (E_1 \hat{\mathbf{i}} + E_2 \hat{\mathbf{j}}) \cos(kz - \omega t)$. Choose the correct option from the following.
(a) The associated magnetic field is given as
$\mathbf{B} = \frac{1}{c}(E_1 \hat{\mathbf{i}} - E_2 \hat{\mathbf{j}}) \cos(kz + \omega t)$
(b) The associated magnetic field is given as
$\mathbf{B} = \frac{1}{c}(E_1 \hat{\mathbf{i}} + E_2 \hat{\mathbf{j}}) \cos(kz + \omega t)$
(c) The given electromagnetic field is circularly polarised
(d) The given electromagnetic wave is plane polarised

19 A perfectly reflecting mirror has an area of 1 cm^2. Light energy is allowed to fall on it for 1 h at the rate of 10 Wcm^{-2}. The force that acts on the mirror is
(a) 3.35×10^{-8} N (b) 6.67×10^{-8} N
(c) 1.34×10^{-7} N (d) 24×10^{-4} N

20 A plane electromagnetic wave is propagating along the *z*-direction. If the electric field component of this wave is in the direction $(\hat{\mathbf{i}} + \hat{\mathbf{j}})$, then which of the following is the direction of the magnetic field component?
(a) $(-\hat{\mathbf{i}} + \hat{\mathbf{j}})$ (b) $(\hat{\mathbf{i}} - \hat{\mathbf{j}})$
(c) $(-\hat{\mathbf{i}} - \hat{\mathbf{j}})$ (d) $(\hat{\mathbf{i}} + \hat{\mathbf{j}})$

21 The electric field intensity produced by the radiations coming from 100 W bulb at a 3 m distance is *E*. The electric field intensity produced by the radiations coming from 50 W bulb at the same distance is ***[NCERT Exemplar]***
(a) $\frac{E}{2}$ (b) $2E$
(c) $\frac{E}{\sqrt{2}}$ (d) $\sqrt{2}E$

22 Light with an energy flux of 20 W/cm^2 falls on a non-reflecting surface at normal incidence. If the surface has an area of 30 cm^2, then the total momentum delivered (for complete absorption) during 30 min is ***[NCERT Exemplar]***
(a) 36×10^{-5} kg-m/s
(b) 36×10^{-4} kg-m/s
(c) 108×10^{4} kg-m/s
(d) 1.08×10^{7} kg-m/s

23 Magnitude of the electric and magnetic fields in an electromagnetic wave radiated by a 200 W bulb at a distance 2 m from it is (Assuming efficiency of bulb is 5% and it behaves like a point source.)
(a) 12.27 N/C, 4.09×10^{-8} T
(b) 10 N/C, 10^{-5} T
(c) 11.7 N/C, 5×10^{-6} T
(d) 5 N/C, 10^{-4} T

24 A plane electromagnetic wave of frequency 20 MHz travels through a space along *x*-direction. If the electric field vector at a certain point in space is 6 Vm^{-1}, then what is the magnetic field vector at that point?
(a) 2×10^{-8} T (b) $\frac{1}{2} \times 10^{-8}$ T
(c) 2 T (d) $\frac{1}{2}$ T

25 The electric field associated with an electromagnetic wave in vacuum is given by $\mathbf{E} = \hat{\mathbf{i}}\, 40 \cos(kz - 6 \times 10^8 t)$, where *E*, *z* and *t* are in volt m^{-1}, metre and second, respectively. The value of wave vector *k* is
(a) 2 m^{-1} (b) 0.5 m^{-1} (c) 6 m^{-1} (d) 3 m^{-1}

26 The wave function (in SI unit) for a light wave is given as $\psi(x, t) = 10^3 \sin \pi (3 \times 10^6 x - 9 \times 10^{14} t)$.
The frequency of the wave is equal to
(a) 4.5×10^{14} Hz (b) 3.5×10^{14} Hz
(c) 3.5×10^{10} Hz (d) 2.5×10^{10} Hz

27 Which of the following wave cannot travel in vacuum?
(a) X-rays (b) Infrasonic waves
(c) Ultraviolet rays (d) Radio waves

28 Which of the following represents an infrared wavelength?
(a) 10^{-4} cm (b) 10^{-5} cm
(c) 10^{-6} cm (d) 10^{-7} cm

29 Which of the following electromagnetic waves have the longest wavelength?
(a) Heat waves (b) Light waves
(c) Radio waves (d) Microwaves

30 Radio waves diffract around building although light waves do not. The reason is that radio waves

(a) travel with speed larger than c
(b) have longer wavelength than light
(c) carry news
(d) are not electromagnetic waves

31 Frequency of wave is 6×10^{15} Hz. The wave is

(a) radio wave
(b) microwave
(c) X-ray
(d) ultraviolet rays

32 The frequency 1057 MHz of radiation arising from two close energy levels in hydrogen belongs to

(a) radio waves
(b) infrared waves
(c) microwaves
(d) γ-rays

33 The part of the spectrum of the electromagnetic radiation used to cook food is

(a) ultraviolet rays
(b) cosmic rays
(c) X-rays
(d) microwaves

34 Which of the following waves are used in RADAR systems for aircraft navigation?

(a) X-rays
(b) Infrared rays
(c) Ultraviolet rays
(d) Microwaves

35 The essential distinction between X-rays and γ-rays is that

(a) γ-rays have smaller wavelength than X-rays
(b) γ-rays emanate from nucleus while X-rays emanate from outer part of the atom
(c) γ-rays have greater ionising power than X-rays
(d) γ-rays are more penetrating than X-rays

36 The magnetic field in a plane electromagnetic wave is given by $B_y = 2\times10^{-7} \sin(0.5\times10^{3}x + 1.5\times10^{11}t)$.

This electromagnetic wave is

(a) a visible light (b) an infrared wave
(c) a microwave (d) a radio wave

37. One requires 11 eV of energy to dissociate a carbon monoxide molecule into carbon and oxygen atoms. The minimum frequency of the appropriate electromagnetic radiation to achieve the dissociation lies in ***[NCERT Exemplar]***

(a) visible region (b) infrared region
(c) ultraviolet region (d) microwave region

38. The electromagnetic waves detected using a thermopile and used in physical therapy are

(a) gamma radiations
(b) X-rays
(c) ultraviolet radiations
(d) infrared radiations

Assertion and Reason

Directions (Q. Nos. 1-5) *These questions consists of two statements each linked as Assertion (A) and Reason (R). While answering these questions you are required to choose anyone of the following four responses.*

(a) Both A and R are true but R is not the correct explanation of A.
(b) A is true but R is false.
(c) A is false but R is true.
(d) Both A and R are true and R is the correct explanation of A.

1. **Assertion** (A) In electromagnetic wave, the direction of variations of electric and magnetic field are perpendicular to each other and also perpendicular to the direction of wave propagation.

Reason (R) Electromagnetic waves are transverse in nature.

2. **Assertion** (A) Ultraviolet radiations of higher frequency wave are dangerous to human being.

Reason (R) Ultraviolet radiation are absorbed by the atmosphere.

3. **Assertion** (A) The frequency of the electromagnetic wave is equal to the frequency of accelerating charge.

Reason (R) The energy associated with the propagating wave comes at the expense of the energy of the source.

4. **Assertion**(A) In an electromagnetic wave, magnitude of magnetic field vector is much smaller than the magnitude of electric field vector.

Reason (R) Energy of electromagnetic waves is shared equally by the electric and magnetic field.

5. **Assertion** (A) The electric field and magnetic field have equal average values in linearly polarised plane electromagnetic wave.

Reason (R) The electric energy and magnetic energy have equal average values in linearly polarised plane electromagnetic wave.

Statement Type Questions

Directions (Q. Nos. 1-5) *These questions consists of two statements choose the most appropriate answer from the options gives below.*

(a) Both Statement I and Statement II are incorrect.
(b) Statement I is correct but Statement II is incorrect.
(c) Statement I is incorrect but Statement II is correct.
(d) Both Statement I and Statement II are correct.

1. **Statement I** Velocity of light is constant in all media.
   Statement II Light is an electromagnetic wave which has constant velocity in vacuum.
2. **Statement I** X-ray astronomy is possible only from satellites orbiting the earth.
   Statement II Efficiency of X-rays telescope is large as compared to any other telescope.
3. **Statement I** Only microwaves are used in radar.
   Statement II Microwaves have smaller wavelength than radio waves.
4. **Statement I** Infrared waves sometimes referred as heat waves.
   Statement II Infrared waves heat up the earth's surface.
5. **Statement I** When variable frequency AC source is connected to a capacitor, displacement current increase with increase in frequency.
   Statement II As frequency increases, conduction current also increases.

Match the Columns

1. Match the Column I with Column II

Column I	Column II
A. $\oint_S \mathbf{E}\cdot d\mathbf{S} = q/\varepsilon_0$	I. Faraday's law of EMI
B. $\oint_S \mathbf{B}\cdot d\mathbf{S} = 0$	II. Gauss's law in magnetism
C. $\oint \mathbf{E}\cdot d\mathbf{l} = -\dfrac{d\phi_B}{dt}$	III. Maxwell-Ampere's circuital law
D. $\oint \mathbf{B}\cdot d\mathbf{l} = \mu_0\left[I_c + \varepsilon_0 \dfrac{d\phi}{dt}\right]$	IV. Gauss's law in electrostatics

Choose the correct answer from the options given below.
(a) A-I, B-III, C-IV, D-II
(b) A-II , B-I, C-III, D-IV
(c) A-IV, B-II, C-I, D-III
(d) A-III, B-IV, C-II, D-I

2. Match the Column I (electromagnetic wave type) with Column II (its application).

Column I	Column II
A. Infrared waves	I. to treat muscular strain
B. Radio waves	II. for broadcasting
C. X-rays	III. to detect the fracture of bones
D. Ultraviolet rays	IV. absorbed by the ozone layer of the atmosphere

Choose the correct answer from the options given below.
(a) A-III, B-IV, C-II, D-I
(b) A-I , B-II, C-III, D-IV
(c) A-II, B-III, C-IV, D-I
(d) A-IV, B-I, C-II, D-III

Final Check Through PYQs

Module-I Displacement Current and Properties of EM Waves

1. A parallel plate capacitor is charged by connecting it to a battery through a resistor. If I is the current in the circuit, then in the gap between the plates **[NCERT (New) Pg. 202, NEET 2024]**
(a) There is no current
(b) Displacement current of magnitude equal to I flows in the same direction as I
(c) Displacement current of magnitude equal to I flows in a direction opposite to that of I
(d) Displacement current of magnitude greater than I flows but can be in any direction

2. The property which is not of an electromagnetic wave travelling in free space is that **[NCERT (New) Pg. 205, NEET 2024]**
(a) They are transverse in nature
(b) The energy density in electric field is equal to energy density in magnetic field
(c) They travel with a speed equal to $\frac{1}{\sqrt{\mu_0 \varepsilon_0}}$
(d) They originate from charges moving with uniform speed

3. In a plane electromagnetic wave travelling in free space, the electric field component oscillates sinusoidally at a frequency of 2.0×10^{10} Hz and amplitude 48 Vm^{-1}. Then, the amplitude of oscillating magnetic field is (Speed of light in free space $= 3 \times 10^8 \text{ ms}^{-1}$) **[NCERT (New) Pg. 206, NEET 2023]**
(a) 1.6×10^{-8} T (b) 1.6×10^{-7} T
(c) 1.6×10^{-6} T (d) 1.6×10^{-9} T

4. When light propagates through a material medium of relative permittivity ε_r and relative permeability μ_r, the velocity of light, v is given by (c-velocity of light in vacuum) **[NCERT (New) Pg. 207, NEET 2022]**
(a) $v = \sqrt{\frac{\mu_r}{\varepsilon_r}}$ (b) $v = \sqrt{\frac{\varepsilon_r}{\mu_r}}$ (c) $v = \frac{c}{\sqrt{\varepsilon_r \mu_r}}$ (d) $v = c$

5. A capacitor of capacitance C, is connected across an AC source of voltage V, given by $V = V_0 \sin \omega t$. The displacement current between the plates of the capacitor, would then be given by **[NCERT (New) Pg. 203, NEET 2021]**
(a) $I_d = V_0 \omega C \cos \omega t$ (b) $I_d = \frac{V_0}{\omega C} \cos \omega t$
(c) $I_d = \frac{V_0}{\omega C} \sin \omega t$ (d) $I_d = V_0 \omega C \sin \omega t$

6. For a plane electromagnetic wave propagating in x-direction, which one of the following combination gives the correct possible directions for electric field (E) and magnetic field (B), respectively? **[NCERT (New) Pg. 206, NEET 2021]**
(a) $\hat{j} + \hat{k}, \hat{j} + \hat{k}$ (b) $-\hat{j} + \hat{k}, -\hat{j} - \hat{k}$
(c) $\hat{j} + \hat{k}, -\hat{j} + \hat{k}$ (d) $-\hat{j} + \hat{k}, -\hat{j} + \hat{k}$

7. The magnetic field in a plane electromagnetic wave is given by $B_y = 2 \times 10^{-7} \sin(\pi \times 10^3 x + 3\pi \times 10^{11} t)T$
Calculate the wavelength. **[NCERT (New) Pg. 206, NEET (Oct.) 2020]**
(a) $\pi \times 10^3$ m (b) 2×10^{-3} m
(c) 2×10^3 m (d) $\pi \times 10^{-3}$ m

8. The ratio of contributions made by the electric field and magnetic field components, to the intensity of an electromagnetic wave is (where, c = speed of electromagnetic waves) **[NCERT (New) Pg. 203, NEET (Sep.) 2020]**
(a) 1 : 1 (b) $1 : c$ (c) $1 : c^2$ (d) $c : 1$

9. Light with an average flux of 20 W/cm^2 falls on a non-reflecting surface at normal incidence having surface area 20 cm^2. The energy received by the surface during time span of 1 min is **[NCERT (New) Pg. 203, NEET (Sep.) 2020]**
(a) 12×10^3 J (b) 24×10^3 J
(c) 48×10^3 J (d) 10×10^3 J

10. A parallel plate capacitor of capacitance 20μF is being charged by a voltage source whose potential is changing at the rate of 3 V/s. The conduction current through the connecting wires and the displacement current through the plates of the capacitor, would be, respectively. **[NCERT (New) Pg. 203, NEET 2019]**
(a) 60 μA, 60 μA (b) 60 μA, zero
(c) zero, zero (d) zero, 60 μA

11. For a transparent medium relative permeability and permittivity, μ_r and ε_r, are 1.0 and 1.44 respectively. The velocity of light in this medium would be **[NCERT (New) Pg. 207, NEET 2019]**
(a) 2.5×10^8 m/s (b) 3×10^8 m/s
(c) 2.08×10^8 m/s (d) 4.32×10^8 m/s

12. An EM wave is propagating in a medium with a velocity $v = v\hat{i}$. The instantaneous oscillating electric field of this EM wave is along $+Y$-axis. Then, the direction of oscillating magnetic field of EM wave will be along **[NCERT (New) Pg. 206, NEET 2018]**
(a) $-y$-direction (b) $+z$-direction
(c) $-z$-direction (d) $-x$-direction

13. In an electromagnetic wave in free space the root mean square value of the electric field is $E_{rms} = 6 \text{ Vm}^{-1}$. The peak value of the magnetic field is *[NCERT (New) Pg. 203, NEET 2017]*

(a) 2.83×10^{-8} T (b) 0.70×10^{-8} T
(c) 4.23×10^{-8} T (d) 1.41×10^{-8} T

14. A 100 Ω resistance and a capacitor of 100 Ω reactance are connected in series across a 220 V source. When the capacitor is 50% charged, the peak value of the displacement current is *[NCERT (New) Pg. 203, NEET 2016]*

(a) 2.2 A (b) 11 A
(c) 4.4 A (d) $11\sqrt{2}$ A

15. Out of the following options which one can be used to produce a propagating electromagnetic wave? *[NCERT (New) Pg. 205, NEET 2016]*

(a) A stationary charge
(b) A chargeless particle
(c) An accelerating charge
(d) A charge moving at constant velocity

16. A radiation of energy 'E' falls normally on a perfectly reflecting surface. The momentum transferred to the surface is (c = velocity of light) *[NCERT (Old) Pg. 277, AIPMT 2015]*

(a) $\frac{E}{c}$ (b) $\frac{2E}{c}$ (c) $\frac{2E}{c^2}$ (d) $\frac{E}{c^2}$

Module-II Electromagnetic Spectrum

17 Match Column-I with Column-II

Column-I (Electromagnetic waves)	Column-II (Wavelength)
A. AM radio waves	I. 10^{-10} m
B. Microwaves	II. 10^{2} m
C. Infrared radiations	III. 10^{-2} m
D. X-rays	IV. 10^{-4} m

[NCERT (New) Pg. 208, NEET 2022]

Choose the correct answer from the options given below.

(a) A-IV, B-III, C-II, D-I (b) A-III, B-II, C-I, D-IV
(c) A-III, B-IV, C-II, D-I (d) A-II, B-III, C-IV, D-I

18. The electromagnetic wave with shortest wavelength among the following is *[NCERT (New) Pg. 211, NEET (Oct.) 2020]*

(a) UV-rays (b) X-rays
(c) γ-rays (d) micro waves

19. The energy of the EM waves is of the order of 15 keV. To which part of the spectrum does it belong? *[NCERT (New) Pg. 211, AIPMT 2015]*

(a) X-rays (b) Infrared rays
(c) Ultraviolet rays (d) γ-rays

Answers

Step up Practice 1

1 (c)	2 (c)	3 (c)	4 (d)	5 (d)	6 (d)	7 (d)	8 (b)	9 (a)	10 (d)
11 (a)	12 (c)	13 (a)	14 (c)	15 (b)	16 (b)	17 (d)	18 (b)	19 (d)	20 (c)
21 (b)									

Step up Practice 2

1 (a)	2 (a)	3 (a)	4 (c)	5 (b)	6 (b)	7 (a)	8 (a)	9 (c)	10 (b)
11 (b)	12 (d)	13 (d)	14 (c)	15 (b)	16 (a)	17 (a)	18 (a)	19 (d)	20 (b)
21 (d)									

Gearing up for NEET

1 (c)	2 (c)	3 (d)	4 (c)	5 (c)	6 (b)	7 (d)	8 (c)	9 (b)	10 (c)
11 (d)	12 (a)	13 (a)	14 (b)	15 (a)	16 (b)	17 (b)	18 (d)	19 (b)	20 (a)
21 (c)	22 (b)	23 (a)	24 (a)	25 (a)	26 (a)	27 (b)	28 (a)	29 (c)	30 (b)
31 (d)	32 (a)	33 (d)	34 (d)	35 (b)	36 (c)	37 (c)	38 (d)		

Assertion and Reason

1 (d)	2 (a)	3 (a)	4 (a)	5 (a)

Statement Type Questions

1 (c)	2 (b)	3 (d)	4 (d)	5 (d)

Match the Columns

1 (c)	2 (b)

Final Check through PYQs : Module-I

1 (b)	2 (d)	3 (b)	4 (c)	5 (a)	6 (b)	7 (b)	8 (a)	9 (b)	10 (a)
11 (a)	12 (b)	13 (a)	14 (a)	15 (c)	16 (b)				

Final Check through PYQs : Module-II

17 (d)	18 (c)	19 (a)

Final Check

Hints and Solutions

Step up Practice 1

3. (*c*) Speed of electromagnetic wave depends on medium. Its highest speed is in vacuum.

4. (*d*) Both A and R are true and R is the correct explanation of A.

   Accelerated charges radiate electromagnetic waves.

5. (*d*) We have, displacement current, $I_d = \varepsilon_0 \frac{d\phi_E}{dt}$

   So, dimensions of $\varepsilon_0 \frac{d\phi_E}{dt}$ are same as that of current.

6. (*d*) Ampere-Maxwell's circuital law is given by

   $$\oint \mathbf{B} \cdot d\mathbf{l} = \mu_0 \cdot (I_c + I_d) = \mu_0 \left(I_c + \varepsilon_0 \frac{d\phi_E}{dt} \right)$$

7. (*d*) Both A and R are true and R is the correct explanation of A.

   According to the classical theory of Maxwell. The dipole oscillation gives radiation because the charges are accelerated.

8. (*b*) When capacitor is fully charged (*i.e.* charge on plates of capacitor is maximum) no current flows through the circuit. The potential of the plates became constant and there is no change in the electric field between the plates. So, both conduction current in the circuit and displacement current between the plates became zero.

9. (*a*) We know that, displacement current, $I_d = \varepsilon_0 A \frac{dE}{dt}$

   We have, $\varepsilon_0 = 8.85 \times 10^{-12} C^2 N^{-1} m^{-2}$

   Area, $A = 1 \text{ cm}^2 = 10^{-4} m^2$ and $\frac{dE}{dt} = 3 \times 10^6 Vm^{-1}s^{-1}$

   $\therefore \quad I_d = 8.85 \times 10^{-12} \times 10^{-4} \times 3 \times 10^6 \simeq 2.7 \times 10^{-9} A$

10. (*d*) Both A and R are true and R is the correct explanation of A.

11. (*a*) Displacement current, $I_d = \varepsilon_0 \frac{d\phi_E}{dt}$

    $$= \varepsilon_0 \frac{EA}{t} = \frac{\varepsilon_0 (V/d) \times A}{t} = \frac{\varepsilon_0 VA}{td}$$

    $$= \frac{8.85 \times 10^{-12} \times 400 \times (60 \times 10^{-4})}{10^{-6} \times (2 \times 10^{-3})}$$

    $$= 1.062 \times 10^{-2} A$$

12 (*c*) Amplitude of electric field and magnetic field are related by the relation, $\frac{E_0}{B_0} = c$

   Average energy density of the magnetic field,

   $$u_B = \frac{1}{2} \frac{B_0^2}{\mu_0} = \frac{1}{2} \frac{E_0^2}{\mu_0 c^2} \qquad \left(\because B_0 = \frac{E_0}{c} \right)$$

   $$= \frac{1}{2} \varepsilon_0 E_0^2 \qquad \left(\because c = \frac{1}{\sqrt{\mu_0 E_0}} \right)$$

   $$= \frac{1}{2} \times 8.85 \times 10^{-12} \times 2^2$$

   $$= 17.71 \times 10^{-12} \text{ Jm}^{-3}$$

13. (*a*) Here, $E_0 = 100 \text{ Vm}^{-1}$, $B_0 = 0.265$ T

    $\therefore$ Maximum rate of energy flow,

    $$S = \frac{E_0 \times B_0}{\mu_0} = \frac{100 \times 0.265}{4\pi \times 10^{-7}}$$

    $$= 21 \times 10^6 \text{ Wm}^{-2}$$

14. (*c*) As we know that,

    Maxwell's first equation $\longrightarrow \oint \mathbf{E} \cdot d\mathbf{S} = \frac{q}{\varepsilon_0}$, hence incorrect.

    Maxwell's second equation $\longrightarrow \oint \mathbf{B} \cdot d\mathbf{S} = 0$ (the net Magnetic flux through any closed surface is always zero), hence incorrect.

    Faraday's law of EMI $\longrightarrow \oint \mathbf{E} \cdot d\mathbf{l} = \frac{-d\phi_B}{dt}$ which is also called Maxwell's third equation, hence correct.

    Ampere-Maxwell's circuital law $\longrightarrow$

    $\oint \mathbf{B} \cdot d\mathbf{l} = \mu_0 \left(I_c + \varepsilon_0 \frac{d\phi_B}{dt} \right)$ is also called Maxwell's fourth equation, hence incorrect.

15. (*b*) As metal is reflecting surface and for this type of surface radiation pressure is given as

    $$p_r = \frac{2S}{c} = \frac{2 \times 0.5}{3 \times 10^8} = 0.33 \times 10^{-8} \text{ Nm}^{-2}$$

16. (*b*) As, $c = \frac{E_0}{B_0} \Rightarrow B_0 = \frac{E_0}{c} = \frac{18}{3 \times 10^8} = 6 \times 10^{-8}$ T

17. (*d*) Average energy density,

    $$u_{av} = \frac{1}{2} \varepsilon_0 E_0^2 = \frac{1}{2} \varepsilon_0 (\sqrt{2} E_{rms})^2 = \varepsilon_0 E_{rms}^2$$

    $$= 8.85 \times 10^{-12} \times (720)^2 = 4.58 \times 10^{-6} \text{ Jm}^{-3}$$

18. (*b*) As, $\frac{E_0}{B_0} = c = \frac{1}{\sqrt{\varepsilon_0 \mu_0}} \Rightarrow \sqrt{\mu_0 \varepsilon_0} = \frac{B_0}{E_0}$

    Here, $\quad c$ = speed of light

19. (*d*) Both A and R are true and R is the correct explanation of A.

Light being electromagnetic wave do not require any material medium for its propagation. Hence light can travel in vacuum. On the other hand sound is a mechanical wave and requires a material medium for its propagation. Hence, sound cannot travel in vacuum.

20. (*c*) The angular wave number, $k = \frac{2\pi}{\lambda}$, where λ is the wavelength. The angular frequency, $\omega = 2\pi\nu$

Ratio, $\frac{k}{\omega} = \frac{2\pi/\lambda}{2\pi\nu} = \frac{1}{\nu\lambda} = \frac{1}{c}$ = constant

21. (*b*) Frequency of *L-C* oscillations,

$$\nu = \frac{1}{2\pi\sqrt{LC}}$$

$$= \frac{1}{2 \times 3.14\sqrt{100 \times 10^{-6} \times 200 \times 10^{-12}}}$$

$$= 1.126 \times 10^{6} \text{ Hz}$$

So, wavelength, $\lambda = \frac{c}{\nu} = \frac{3 \times 10^{8}}{1.126 \times 10^{6}} = 266.4 \simeq 266$ m

Step up Practice 2

3. (*a*) Both Statement I and Statement II are incorrect.

Electromagnetic wave transverse in nature. X-rays, radio wave and light wave are transverse in nature and are part of the electromagnetic spectrum while matter waves are not transverse and they are not the part of electromagnetic wave.

4. (*c*) $E = h\nu$

$\therefore E \propto \nu$

5. (*b*) Wavelength of visible spectrum is 3900 Å - 7800 Å.

7. (*a*) Both Statement I and Statement II are incorrect.

All electromagnetic waves including X-rays travels with same velocity in vacuum. The energy of X-rays is greater than energy of light because energy is inversely proportional to wavelength ($E = hc/\lambda$) and wavelength of X-rays are smaller than light waves.

8. (*a*) $\lambda_{\gamma\text{-rays}} < \lambda_{\text{X-rays}} < \lambda_{\alpha\text{-rays}} < \lambda_{\beta\text{-rays}}$

9. (*c*) β-rays are beam of fast electrons.

10. (*b*) As we know that,

Frequency of Radiowave is $< 10^{9}$ Hz (incorrect)

Frequency of microwave is 10^{9} to 10^{11} Hz (correct)

Frequency of X-rays is 10^{16} to 10^{20} Hz (incorrect)

Frequency of UV-rays is 10^{14} to 10^{17} Hz (incorrect)

12. (*d*) $\nu_{\gamma\text{-rays}} > \nu_{\text{Visible radiation}} > \nu_{\text{Infrared}} > \nu_{\text{Radiowaves}}$

13. (*d*) $\lambda_{\text{Radiowaves}} > \lambda_{\text{UVrays}} > \lambda_{\text{IR rays}} > \lambda_{\text{X-rays}}$

14. (*c*) Gamma (γ) rays are useds to produce nuclear reaction.

15. (*b*) Statement I is correct but Statement II is incorrect. Wavelength of 10 mm lies in infrared region.

16. (*a*) $\nu_{\gamma\text{-rays}} > \nu_{\text{X-rays}} > \nu_{\text{UVrays}}$

17. (*a*) In vacuum velocity of all EM waves are same but their wavelengths are different.

18. (*a*) X-rays are not reflected from target. So cannot be used for radar.

19. (*d*) Both Statement I and Statement II are correct.

The frequency of microwave is much larger than the frequency of radio waves. Therefore equation $E = h\nu$ (where E = energy, h is Planck's constant and ν is frequency) shows that the energy of microwaves is much larger than the energy of radiowaves.

20. (*b*) Molecular spectra due to vibrational motion lie in the microwave region of EM-spectrum. Due to Kirchhoff's law in spectroscopy the same will be absorbed.

21. (*d*) Frequency range of Gamma rays is 10^{18} Hz to 10^{22} Hz.

Gearing up for NEET

3. (*d*) The energy in EM waves is divided equally between the electric and magnetic fields.

The total energy per unit volume, $u = u_e + u_m$

$$= \frac{1}{4}\varepsilon_0 E^2 + \frac{1}{4}\frac{B^2}{\mu_0}$$

4. (*c*) For a medium with permittivity ε and permeability μ, the velocity of light is given by $c = \frac{1}{\sqrt{\mu\varepsilon}}$.

5. (*c*) Speed of electromagnetic waves in vacuum

$$= \frac{1}{\sqrt{\mu_0 \varepsilon_0}} = \nu\lambda = \text{constant}$$

As, we go from γ-rays to radio waves frequency decreases and wavelength increases thereby maintaining the product constant.

6. (*b*) $\because$ Speed, $c = \nu\lambda$

$\therefore$ Wavelength, $\lambda = \frac{c}{\nu} = \frac{3 \times 10^{8}}{2 \times 10^{10}} = 1.5 \times 10^{-2}$ m

7. (*d*) The direction of propagation of electromagnetic wave is perpendicular to both electric field vector **E** and magnetic field vector **B**, *i.e.* in the direction of **E** × **B**.

This can be seen by the diagram given below

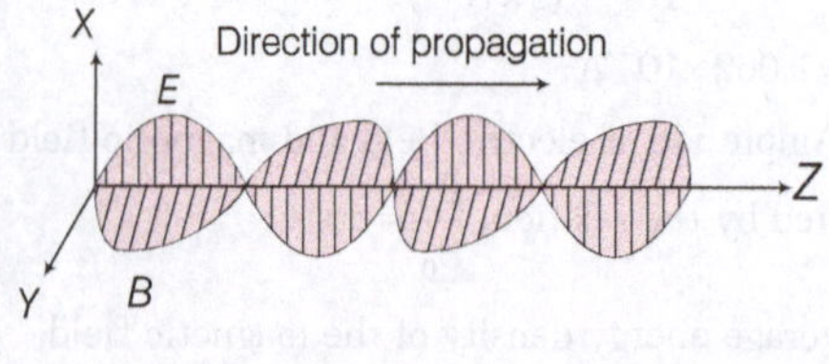

Here, electromagnetic wave is along the z-direction which is given by the cross product of **E** and **B**.

8 (c) From a dipole antenna, the electromagnetic waves are radiated outwards.

The amplitude of electric field vector E_0 which transports significant energy from the source falls off inversely as the distance r from the antenna, *i.e.* $E_0 \propto \frac{1}{r}$.

9. (b) Given, $E = 9 \times 10^{-4}\ NC^{-1}$

We know that, $c = \frac{E}{B}$

$$\Rightarrow \quad B = \frac{9 \times 10^{-4}}{3 \times 10^{8}} = 3 \times 10^{-12}\ T$$

10. (c) When a surface intercepts electromagnetic radiation, a force and a pressure are exerted on the surface. As the surface is non-reflecting, so it is completely absorbed and in such case, the force is

$$F = \frac{IA}{c}$$

The radiation pressure is the force per unit area,

$$p = \frac{F}{A} = \frac{I}{c}$$

12. (a) Displacement current is given by

$$I_d = \frac{dq}{dt} = 1.8 \times 10^{-8}\ Cs^{-1}$$

13. (a) As metal is a reflecting surface and for reflecting surface, radiation pressure,

$$p_r = \frac{2I}{c} = \frac{2 \times 1}{3 \times 10^{8}}$$

$$= 0.66 \times 10^{-8}\ Nm^{-2}$$

14. (b) Frequency of L-C oscillations,

$$\nu = \frac{1}{2\pi\sqrt{LC}} = \frac{1}{2 \times 3.14\sqrt{200 \times 10^{-6} \times 200 \times 10^{-12}}}$$

$$= 0.0796 \times 10^{7}\ Hz$$

So, wavelength, $\lambda = \frac{c}{\nu} = \frac{3 \times 10^{8}}{0.0796 \times 10^{7}} \simeq 377\ m$

15. (a) From $k = \frac{2\pi}{\lambda}$ and $\omega = 2\pi\nu$, we get

$$\frac{k}{\omega} = \frac{\frac{2\pi}{\lambda}}{2\pi\nu} = \frac{1}{\nu\lambda} = \frac{1}{c}$$

As, $\frac{E_0}{B_0} = c \Rightarrow \frac{k}{\omega} = \frac{B_0}{E_0}$

$$\Rightarrow \quad E_0 k = B_0 \omega$$

16. (b) When a wave is reflected from the denser medium, then the type of wave does not change but only its phase changes by 180° or π radian.

Thus, for the reflected wave $\mathbf{z} = -\mathbf{z}$, $\hat{\mathbf{i}} = -\hat{\mathbf{i}}$ and additional phase of π in the incident wave.

Here, the incident EM wave, $\mathbf{E} = E_0\hat{\mathbf{i}} \cos(\hat{\mathbf{k}}z - \omega t)$

Hence, the reflected EM wave,

$$\mathbf{E}_r = E_0(-\hat{\mathbf{i}})\cos[\hat{\mathbf{k}}(-z) - \omega t + \pi]$$

$$= -E_0\hat{\mathbf{i}} \cos[-(\hat{\mathbf{k}}z + \omega t) + \pi]$$

$$= E_0\hat{\mathbf{i}} \cos(\hat{\mathbf{k}}z + \omega t)$$

17. (b) Angular frequency, $\omega = 2\pi\nu = \frac{2\pi c}{\lambda}$ $\quad (\because \nu = c/\lambda)$

$$= \frac{2\pi \times 3 \times 10^{8}}{6 \times 10^{-3}} = \pi \times 10^{11}\ rads^{-1}$$

The equation for the electric field along Y-axis in the electromagnetic wave,

$$E_y = E_0 \sin \omega\left(t - \frac{x}{c}\right) = 33 \sin \pi \times 10^{11}(t - x/c)$$

18. (d) Here, in electromagnetic wave, the electric field vector is given as, $\mathbf{E} = (E_1\hat{\mathbf{i}} + E_2\hat{\mathbf{j}}) \cos(kz - \omega t)$

In electromagnetic wave, the associated magnetic field vector, $\mathbf{B} = \frac{\mathbf{E}}{c} = \frac{E_1\hat{\mathbf{i}} + E_2\hat{\mathbf{j}}}{c} \cos(kz - \omega t)$

Also, **E** and **B** are perpendicular to each other and the propagation of electromagnetic wave is perpendicular to **E** as well as **B**, so the given electromagnetic wave is plane polarised.

19. (b) Let E = energy falling on the surface per second $= 10\ W/cm^2$

Momentum of photons, $p = \frac{h}{\lambda} = \frac{h}{(c/\nu)} = \frac{h\nu}{c} = \frac{E}{c}$

On reflection, change in momentum per second

$$= 2p = \frac{2E}{c} = \frac{2 \times 10}{3 \times 10^{8}} = 6.67 \times 10^{-8}\ N$$

20. (a) The magnetic field component is perpendicular to the direction of propagation and the direction of electric field.

Using vector algebra $\mathbf{E} \times \mathbf{B}$ should be in z-direction.

i.e. the direction of propagation of electromagnetic wave.

$$\therefore \quad (\hat{\mathbf{i}} + \hat{\mathbf{j}}) \times (-\hat{\mathbf{i}} + \hat{\mathbf{j}}) = 2\hat{\mathbf{k}}$$

21. (c) We know that, $E_0 \propto \sqrt{P_{av}}$

$$\therefore \quad \frac{(E_0)_1}{(E_0)_2} = \sqrt{\frac{(P_{av})_1}{(P_{av})_2}}$$

$$\Rightarrow \quad \frac{E}{(E_0)_2} = \sqrt{\frac{100}{50}} \Rightarrow (E_0)_2 = E/\sqrt{2}$$

22. (*b*) Given, energy flux, $\phi = 20\,W/cm^2$

Area, $A = 30\ cm^2$

Time, $t = 30\ min = 30 \times 60\ s$

Now, total energy falling on the surface in time t,
$u = \phi At = 20 \times 30 \times (30 \times 60)\,J$

Momentum of the incident light $= \frac{u}{c}$

$$= \frac{20 \times 30 \times (30 \times 60)}{3 \times 10^8}$$

$$= 36 \times 10^{-4}\ kg\text{-}m/s$$

Momentum of the reflected light = 0

∴ Momentum delivered to the surface

$$= 36 \times 10^{-4} - 0$$

$$= 36 \times 10^{-4}\ kg\text{-}m/s$$

23. (*a*) Effective power of the bulb, $P = \frac{5}{100} \times 200 = 10\,W$

Intensity at distance r is given by

$$I = \frac{P}{4\pi r^2} = \frac{10}{4 \times 3.14 \times 2^2}$$

$$= \frac{10}{16 \times 3.14}$$

$$= 0.199 \simeq 0.2\ W/m^2$$

Also, $I = \frac{1}{2}\varepsilon_0 E_0^2 c$

$$\Rightarrow \quad E_0^2 = \frac{2I}{c \times \varepsilon_0}$$

Magnitude of electric field,

$$E_0 = \sqrt{\frac{2I}{c \times \varepsilon_0}}$$

$$= \sqrt{\frac{2 \times 0.2}{3 \times 10^8 \times 8.85 \times 10^{-12}}}$$

$$= 12.27\,N/C$$

∴ Magnitude of magnetic field, $B_0 = \frac{E_0}{c} = \frac{12.27}{3 \times 10^8}$

$$= \frac{12.27}{3} \times 10^{-8}\,T$$

$$= 4.09 \times 10^{-8}\,T$$

24. (*a*) The magnetic field, $B_0 = \frac{E_0}{c}$, where $c = 3 \times 10^8\ ms^{-1}$

$$\Rightarrow \quad B_0 = \frac{6}{3 \times 10^8} = 2 \times 10^{-8}\ T$$

25. (*a*) Electromagnetic wave equation,

$$E = E_0 \cos(kz - \omega t) \quad \text{...(i)}$$

Speed of electromagnetic wave,

$$v = \frac{\omega}{k}$$

Given, equation,

$$\mathbf{E} = \hat{\mathbf{i}}\,40 \cos(kz - 6 \times 10^8 t) \quad \text{...(ii)}$$

On comparing Eqs. (i) and (ii), we get

$$\omega = 6 \times 10^8$$

and $E_0 = 40$

Here, wave factor, $k = \frac{\omega}{v} = \frac{6 \times 10^8}{3 \times 10^8} = 2\ m^{-1}$

26. (*a*) The wave function

$$\psi(x, t) = 10^3 \sin \pi (3 \times 10^6 x - 9 \times 10^{14} t)$$

Here, angular frequency, $\omega = 9 \times 10^{14}\pi$

$$\omega = 2\pi\nu$$

$$\Rightarrow \quad \nu = \frac{\omega}{2\pi} = \frac{9 \times 10^{14}\pi}{2\pi}$$

$$= 4.5 \times 10^{14}\ Hz$$

27. (*b*) Infrasonic wave is not an electromagnetic wave. It is a mechanical wave which requires a material medium for propagation.

30. (*b*) Radio waves diffract around building although light waves do not. The reason is that radio waves have longer wavelength than light.

34. (*d*) $\lambda_{\text{Microwaves}} > \lambda_{\text{IR-rays}} >> \lambda_{\text{UV-rays}} > \lambda_{\text{X-rays}}$

Hence, microwaves are less energetic electromagnetic waves, which are used in RADAR system for aircraft navigation.

35. (*b*) The wavelength of the γ-rays is shorter. However, the essential distinction between them is the nature of emission.

36. (*c*) We have,

$$B_y = 2 \times 10^{-7} \sin(0.5 \times 10^3 x + 1.5 \times 10^{11} t)$$

Comparing with the standard equation, we get

$$B_y = B_0 \sin(kx + \omega t)$$

$$k = 0.5 \times 10^3$$

Wavelength, $\lambda = \frac{2\pi}{0.5 \times 10^3} = 0.01256\ m \quad \left(\because \lambda = \frac{2\pi}{k}\right)$

The wavelength range of microwaves is 10^{-3} m to 0.1 m. The wavelength of this wave lies between 10^{-3} m to 0.1 m, so the equation represents a microwave.

37. (*c*) Given, energy required to dissociate a carbon monoxide molecule into carbon and oxygen atoms, $E = 11\,eV$

We know that, $E = h\nu$

where, $h = 6.62 \times 10^{-34}$ J-s, ν = frequency

$\Rightarrow \quad 11\ eV = h\nu$

or $$\nu = \frac{11 \times 1.6 \times 10^{-19}}{h} \quad (\because 1\text{ eV} = 1.6 \times 10^{-19}\text{ J})$$

$$= \frac{11 \times 1.6 \times 10^{-19}}{6.62 \times 10^{-34}} = 2.65 \times 10^{15}\text{ Hz}$$

This frequency radiation belongs to ultraviolet region.

38. (*d*) The electromagnetic waves detected using a thermopile and used in physical therapy are infrared radiations for treating muscular strain.

Assertion and Reason

1. (*d*) As per Maxwell's equations, electric and magnetic fields in an electromagnetic waves are perpendicular to each other and to the direction of wave propagation. Because, electromagnetic waves are transverse in nature.
2. (*a*) The wavelength of ultraviolet waves is very small. Due to smaller wavelength and higher frequency, they are absorbed by atmosphere. They also cause skin diseases and are harmful to eye which may cause permanent blindness.
3. (*a*) The electromagnetic wave consists of oscillating electric and magnetic fields, thus these fields regenerate each other as the wave propagates through the space.

   The frequency of the electromagnetic wave is equals to the frequency of accelerating charge. The energy associated with the propagating wave comes at the expense of the energy of the source or the accelerated charge.
4. (*a*) Both A and R are true but R is not correct explanation of A.

   At every instant the ratio of the magnitudes of the electric field to the magnetic field of an EM wave is given by $E / B = c$.
5. (*a*) Both A and R are true and R is not correct explanation of A.

   In case of a linearly polarised plane electromagnetic wave, the average values of electric field and magnetic field are equal and average values of electric energy and magnetic energy are also equal.

Statement Type Questions

1. (*c*) Statement I is incorrect but statement II is correct. Velocity of light has different values in different media. It depends on the refractive index of the medium. Related by formula

$$v_{\text{medium}} = \frac{\text{Velocity of light in vacuum}}{\text{Refractive index of medium}}$$

2. (*b*) Statement I is correct but Statement II is incorrect.

   The earth's atmosphere is transparent to visible light and radio waves, but absorbs X-rays. Therefore, X-rays telescope cannot be used on earth surface.
3. (*d*) Both Statement I and Statement II are correct.

   In a radar, a beam signal is needed in particular direction which is possible if wavelength of wave is very small. Since the wavelength of microwaves is in the order of few millimeter, hence they are used in radar.
4. (*d*) Both Statement I and Statement II are correct.

   Infrared waves are sometimes called heat waves. This is because water molecules present in most materials readily absorb infrared waves. After absorption, their thermal motion increases, that is they heat up and heat their surroundings.
5. (*d*) Both Statement I and Statement II are correct.

   As frequency increase the capacitance of capacitor will decreases ($X_C = 1 / \omega C$) and correspondingly conduction current will increases since displacement current increases with increases in frequency of AC source.

Match the Columns

1. (*c*) A-IV, B-II, C-I, D-III
2. (*b*) A-I, B-II, C-III, D-IV

Final Check Through PYQs

1. (*b*) When a capacitor is charged through a battery, its opposite plates are charged to a maximum value.

   There is displacement current as the capacitor is being charged. *i.e.*, $I_C = 0$ and $I_D \neq 0$

$$I_d = \varepsilon_0 \frac{d\phi_E}{dt}$$

   Due to charging, ϕ_E changes and hence displacement current equal to conduction current arises while charging. *i.e.*, $I_C = I_D$.

   When capacitor gets fully charged, the displacement current becomes zero *i.e.*, $I_C \neq 0$ and $I_D = 0$.
2. (*d*) The EM waves originate from an accelerating charge. The charge moving with uniform velocity produces steady state magnetic field.
3. (*b*) Given, amplitude, of electric field, $E_0 = 48\text{ Vm}^{-1}$

   As we know, $\frac{|E|}{|B|} = c = \frac{E_0}{B_0}$

   where, E_0 = Amplitude of electric field.

   B_0 = Amplitude of magnetic field.

$$\therefore \quad B_0 = \frac{E_0}{c} = \frac{48\text{ Vm}^{-1}}{3 \times 10^8\text{ ms}^{-1}} = 1.6 \times 10^{-7}\text{ T}$$

4. (*c*) When light (EM wave) propagates through a material medium of relative permittivity ε_r and relative permeability μ_r, then velocity of light (EM wave) is given by $v = \frac{c}{\sqrt{\mu_r \varepsilon_r}}$

   where, c is speed of light in vacuum.

5. (a) Given, AC source voltage,

$$V = V_0 \sin \omega t \quad \text{...(i)}$$

We know that,

$$Q = CV \quad \text{...(ii)}$$

On differentiating Eq. (ii) w.r.t. time,

We get

$$\frac{dQ}{dt} = \frac{d(CV)}{dt} \Rightarrow \frac{dQ}{dt} = \frac{Cd(V_0 \sin \omega t)}{dt} \quad \text{[From Eq. (i)]}$$

$$\Rightarrow \frac{dQ}{dt} = C\omega V_0 \cos \omega t$$

As we know, the displacement current,

$$I_d = \frac{dQ}{dt} = V_0 \omega C \cos \omega t$$

6. (b) We know that, in electromagnetic wave, the electric field (E) and magnetic field (B) are perpendicular to each other, $\mathbf{E} \cdot \mathbf{B} = 0$

Consider the option (a):

$$(\hat{\mathbf{j}} + \hat{\mathbf{k}}) \cdot (\hat{\mathbf{j}} + \hat{\mathbf{k}}) = 1 + 1 = 2 \neq 0$$

So, it is incorrect option.

Consider the option (b);

$$(-\hat{\mathbf{j}} + \hat{\mathbf{k}}) \cdot (-\hat{\mathbf{j}} - \hat{\mathbf{k}}) = 1 - 1 = 0$$

Hence, it satisfies the condition $\mathbf{E} \cdot \mathbf{B} = 0$.

Similarly, options (c) and (d) are incorrect.

7. (b) Magnetic field in plane electromagnetic wave is given by

$$B_y = 2 \times 10^{-7} \sin (\pi \times 10^3 x + 3\pi \times 10^{11} t)\ \text{T}$$

Comparing with,

$$B_y = B_0 \sin (kx - \omega t), \text{ we get}$$

$$k = \pi \times 10^3$$

$$\Rightarrow \frac{2\pi}{\lambda} = \pi \times 10^3 \Rightarrow \lambda = \frac{2}{10^3}$$

$$= 2 \times 10^{-3}\ \text{m}$$

8. (a) Intensity of magnetic field in EM waves, $u_{av} = \frac{1}{2}\frac{B_0^2}{\mu_0}$

Intensity of electric field in EM waves,

$$u'_{av} = \frac{1}{2}\varepsilon_0 E_0^2$$

or $$u'_{av} = \frac{1}{2}\varepsilon_0 (cB_0)^2 \quad [\because E_0 = cB_0]$$

or $$u'_{av} = \frac{1}{2}\frac{B_0^2}{\mu_0} \quad \left[\because c = \frac{1}{\sqrt{\mu_0 \varepsilon_0}}\right]$$

$$\therefore \frac{u'_{av}}{u_{av}} = \frac{\frac{1}{2}\frac{B_0^2}{\mu_0}}{\frac{1}{2}\frac{B_0^2}{\mu_0}} = \frac{1}{1}$$

9. (b) Given, average flux = 20 W/cm^2

Surface area = 20 cm^2

Time = 1 min = 60 s

For non-reflecting surface,

energy received = average flux × surface area × time

$$= 20 \times 20 \times 60 = 24 \times 10^3\ \text{J}$$

10. (a) Given, $C = 20\ \mu\text{F} = 20 \times 10^{-6}$ F

and $$\frac{dV}{dt} = 3\ \text{V/s}$$

$$\therefore I_d = C\frac{dV}{dt}$$

Substituting the given values, we get

$$I_d = 20 \times 10^{-6} \times 3 = 60 \times 10^{-6}\ \text{A} = 60\ \mu\text{A}$$

As displacement current is in between the plates of capacitor and conduction current is in the connecting wires which are equal to each other. So, $I_c = I_d = 60\ \mu\text{A}$

11. (a) Given : $\varepsilon_r = 1.44, \mu_r = 1$

We know that, $\varepsilon_r = \frac{\varepsilon}{\varepsilon_0}$

$$\Rightarrow \varepsilon = \varepsilon_r \varepsilon_0 \text{ and } \mu_r = \frac{\mu}{\mu_0}$$

$$\Rightarrow \mu = \mu_r \mu_0$$

$\therefore$ Velocity of light in the medium will be

$$v = \frac{1}{\sqrt{\mu\varepsilon}} = \frac{1}{\sqrt{\mu_r \mu_0 \varepsilon_r \varepsilon_0}}$$

$$= \frac{c}{\sqrt{\mu_r \varepsilon_r}} = \frac{3 \times 10^8}{\sqrt{1 \times 1.44}} = 2.5 \times 10^8\ \text{m/s}$$

12. (b) Here, velocity of EM wave, $\mathbf{v} = v\hat{\mathbf{i}}$

Instantaneous oscillating electric field,

$$\mathbf{E} = E\hat{\mathbf{j}}$$

i.e. $$\mathbf{E} \times \mathbf{B} = v$$

$$\Rightarrow (E\hat{\mathbf{j}}) \times \mathbf{B} = v\hat{\mathbf{i}} \quad \text{...(i)}$$

As we know that from vector algebra,

$$\hat{\mathbf{j}} \times \hat{\mathbf{k}} = \hat{\mathbf{i}} \quad \text{...(ii)}$$

Comparing Eqs. (i) and (ii), we get

$$\mathbf{B} = B\hat{\mathbf{k}},$$

Where B (say) be the magnitude of magnetic field.

Thus, we can say that the direction of oscillating magnetic field of the EM wave will be along $+z$ direction.

13. (a) We know that,

$$\frac{E_{rms}}{B_{rms}} = c \text{ or } B_{rms} = \frac{E_{rms}}{c}$$

$$\Rightarrow B_{rms} = \frac{6}{3 \times 10^8} = 2 \times 10^{-8}\ \text{T}$$

Since, $\mathbf{B}_{rms} = \frac{B_0}{\sqrt{2}}$

$\therefore \quad B_0 = \mathbf{B}_{rms}\sqrt{2} = 2 \times 10^{-8} \times \sqrt{2}T$

$B_0 = 2.83 \times 10^{-8}$ T

14. (*a*) We know that, $Z = \sqrt{R^2 + X_C^2} = 100\sqrt{2}\ \Omega$

Peak value of displacement current

= Maximum conduction current in the circuit

$$= \frac{E_0}{Z} = \frac{220\sqrt{2}}{100\sqrt{2}} = 2.2 \text{ A}$$

15. (*c*) It is known that an electric charge at rest has electric field in the region around it, but no magnetic field. A moving charge produces both the electric and magnetic fields.

If a charge is moving with a constant velocity, the electric and magnetic fields will not change with time, hence no EM wave will be produced.

But if the charge is moving with a non-zero acceleration, both the electric and magnetic field will change with space and time, it then produces EM wave. This shows that an accelerated charge emits electromagnetic waves.

16. (*b*) The radiation energy is given by $E = \frac{hc}{\lambda}$

Initial momentum of the radiation is $P_i = \frac{h}{\lambda} = \frac{E}{c}$

The reflected momentum is $P_r = -\frac{h}{\lambda} = -\frac{E}{c}$

So, the change in momentum of light is

$$\Delta P_{light} = P_r - P_i = -\frac{2E}{c}$$

Thus, the momentum transferred to the surface is

$\Delta P_{light} = \frac{2E}{c}$.

17. (*d*) The wavelength of AM radio waves is 10^2 m. The wavelength of microwaves ranges between 10^{-3} m to 10^{-1} m.

Infrared radiations wavelength lies between 4×10^{-7} m to 7×10^{-3} m.

X-rays wavelength ranges from 10^{-8} m to 10^{-12} m.

18. (*c*) γ-rays has the shortest wavelength because it has higher frequency than UV-rays, microwaves and X-rays.

19. (*a*) Given, energy of EM waves is of the order of 15 keV

i.e. $\quad E = h\nu = h \times \frac{c}{\lambda}$

$\Rightarrow \quad \lambda = \frac{h \times c}{E}$

$$= \frac{6.624 \times 10^{-34} \times 3 \times 10^8}{15 \times 10^3 \times 1.6 \times 10^{-19}}$$

$$= \frac{1.3248 \times 10^{-29}}{1.6 \times 10^{-19}}$$

$= 0.828 \times 10^{-10}$ m

$= 0.828$ Å $\quad [\because 1 \text{Å} = 10^{-10} \text{ m}]$

$\lambda = 0.828$ Å

Thus, this spectrum is a part of X-rays.

Skill Builder

■ Sol. of Skill Builder on Pg. 485

(*c*) Charge on the capacitor plates at time *t* is

$$q = It$$

Electric field between the plates of the capacitor at this instant is,

$$E = \frac{q}{A\varepsilon_0} = \frac{It}{A\varepsilon_0}$$

So, electric flux through the given area,

$$\phi_E = \left(\frac{A}{3}\right) \cdot E = \frac{It}{3\varepsilon_0}$$

Therefore, the displacement current,

$$Id = \varepsilon_0 \frac{d\phi_E}{dt} = \varepsilon_0 \frac{d}{dt}\left(\frac{It}{3\varepsilon_0}\right) = \frac{I}{3}$$

■ Sol. of Skill Builder on Pg. 487

(*a*) Given, $E_x = (10 \text{ V/m}) \sin(100\pi t - 10\pi y)$

$= -(10 \text{ V/m}) \sin(10\pi y - 100\pi t) \quad$ ...(i)

On comparing Eq. i) with

$E_x = E_0 \sin(ky - \omega t)$

We have, $k = +10\pi$

we know, $\lambda = \frac{2\pi}{k} = \frac{2\pi}{10\pi} = 0.2$ m.

Direction can be found using poynting vectors,

$$\hat{\mathbf{i}} \times \hat{\mathbf{B}} = \hat{\mathbf{j}}$$

Clearly $\hat{\mathbf{B}} = -\hat{\mathbf{k}}$

■ Sol. of Skill Builder on Pg. 489

(*c*) Given, $B_0 = 3 \times 10^3$

$B_0 = \frac{E_0}{c}$

$\Rightarrow \quad E_0 = B_0 \times c$

$= 3 \times 10^3 \times 3 \times 10^8$

$= 9 \times 10^{11}$ V/m

For deeper insight
Scan the QR Code

Chapter 10

Ray Optics

Learning Objectives

Module-I

- Light Sources
- Reflection of Light
- Mirror
- Image Formation by Spherical Mirrors
- Mirror Formula
- Uses of Spherical Mirrors

Module-II

- Refraction of Light
- Image Formation due to Refraction at a Plane Surface
- Critical Angle and Total Internal Reflection (TIR)
- Applications of Total Internal Reflection
- Refraction at Spherical Surfaces

Module-III

- Lenses
- Image Formation by Lenses
- Lens Maker's Formula and Lens Formula
- Focal Length of Different Lenses
- Lens Immersed in a Liquid
- Magnification Produced by a Lens
- Power of a Lens
- Combination of Two or More Thin Lenses
- Prism
- Dispersion of Light by a Prism

Module-IV

- Microscope
- Telescope

Chapter Overview with *NEET Connection*

Concepts of this chapter are helpful for making many useful instruments like spectacles, lenses, microscope, telescope, camera, fibre optic cables etc. This chapter is also helpful for understanding other chapters like Wave Optics and Experimental Skills.

Special format questions can be easily framed on the following topics of this chapter.

- Reflection through spherical mirror, mirror formula.
- Refraction through plane surface, TIR.
- Refraction through spherical surface.
- Dispersion through prism.
- Working of microscope and telescope.

For better understanding of this chapter

- Concept and knowledge of measurement of angles is must.
- Laboratory exposure to optical devices will be helpful.
- Quick revision of Light chapter (Class 10th) will be helpful.

Introduction

Optics is a branch of Physics which deals with study of nature, properties, behaviour and effects of light. Optics is divided further into two branches namely Ray Optics and Wave Optics.

In this chapter, we will study about all the phenomenon that can be explained by ray nature of light. Ray optics concerns itself with image formation through reflection, and refraction, TIR, dispersion of light through prism and optical instruments (microscope and telescope).

Module 1

Reflection of Light

- Light Sources • Reflection of Light • Mirror • Image Formation by Spherical Mirrors
- Mirror Formula • Uses of Spherical Mirrors

Light Sources

We obtain light from different types of natural sources like sun, stars etc, and from artificial sources (man made) like-candle, electric bulb, etc. On the basis of this, light source can be categorised in two types as follows.

(i) **Luminous sources** These sources can produce their own light, *e.g.* sun, stars, electric bulb, etc.

(ii) **Non-luminous sources** These sources cannot produce their own light but return the light coming from a luminous source, *e.g.* moon, glass, etc.

Properties of Light

Following are the properties of light

(i) Light is itself invisible but in its presence we can see objects due to reflection of light.

(ii) Light is an electromagnetic wave which requires no medium for its propagation and its speed in vacuum is 3×10^8 m/s.

(iii) The wavelength of visible light ranges from 400 nm to 700 nm.

(iv) Light can be considered to propagate from one point to another, along a straight line joining them. The path is called a **ray of light** and a bundle of such rays constitutes a **beam of light**.

(v) Light can pass through transparent medium like glass, air, etc. However, it cannot pass through non-transparent mediums like wood, iron, etc.

(vi) Speed of light is different in different medium.

(vii) Light can reflect from polished surfaces.

(viii) When light travels from one medium to another medium, it deviates from the path.

Reflection of Light

When light is incident on a polished smooth surface, then most of the incident light returns to the same medium. This phenomenon of returning of light after striking a smooth polished surface is called **reflection of light**.

After reflection, velocity, wavelength and frequency of light remains same but intensity decreases.

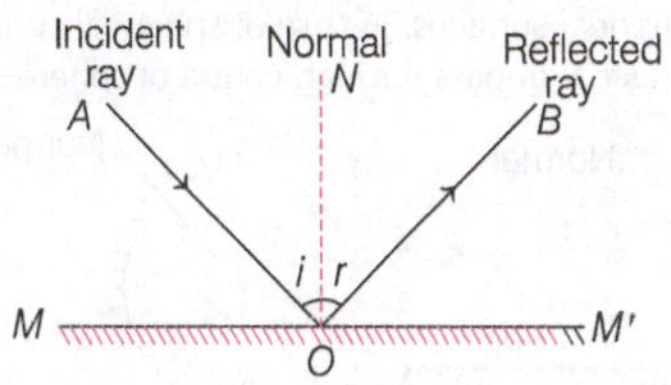

Reflection of light (plane surface)

Some Important Terms Related with Reflection of Light

(i) **Reflecting surface** The surface, after striking which, light reflects is called reflecting surface (MM').

(ii) **Incident ray** The incident ray (AO) on the reflecting surface is called incident ray.

(iii) **Reflected ray** The reflected ray (OB) after striking the reflecting surface is called reflected ray.

(iv) **Point of incidence** It is the point (O) on the reflecting surface at which incident light strikes.

(v) **Normal** It is the normal (ON) to the surface drawn from point of incidence (O) on the reflecting surface.

(vi) **Angle of incidence** It is the angle (i) between incident ray (AO) and the normal (ON). In the given figure, $\angle AON = i$.

(vii) **Angle of reflection** It is the angle (r) between reflected ray (OB) and the normal (ON). In the given figure, $\angle NOB = r$.

Laws of Reflection

There are two laws for reflection of light from a smooth reflecting surface.

(i) **First law** The angle of incidence is equal to the angle of reflection, *i.e.* $\angle i = \angle r$.

(ii) **Second law** The incident ray, the reflected ray and the normal at the point of incidence all lie in the same plane.

These laws are valid for plane as well as curved surfaces as shown in the figure given below.

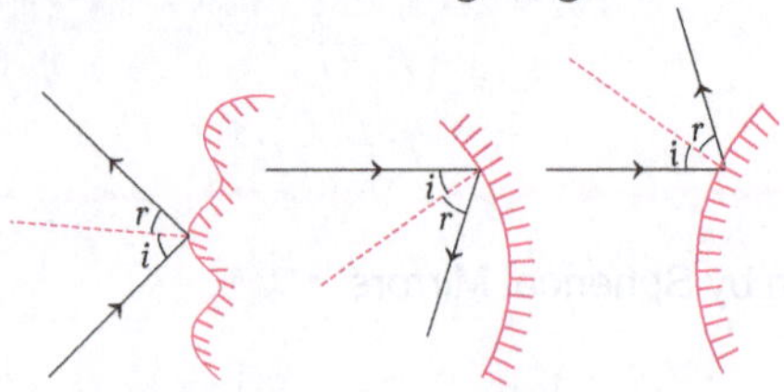

Reflection of light from curved surfaces

Concept ladder

- In geometrical optics, angles are measured with normal.
- Also in geometrical optics, we deal with plane and spherical surfaces. In case of spherical surface, normal to surface will pass through centre of sphere.

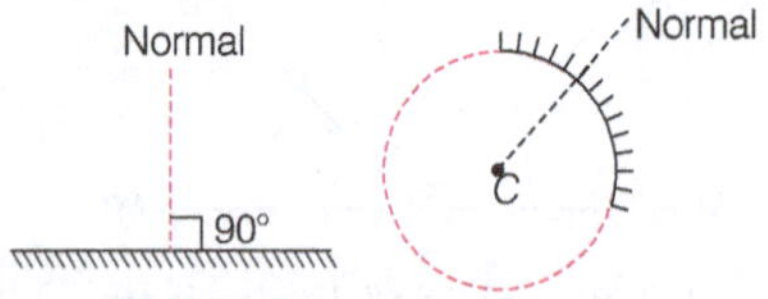

Image

Light rays emerging from an object (or a point) after reflection or refraction meets or appears to meet at a point is called image of object (or first point).

Images are of two types

(i) Real image

When light rays emerging from a point object really meets at a point, the later point is called real image of the first point. These types of images can be obtained on a screen.

(ii) Virtual image

When light rays emerging from a point object appears to meet at a point, the later point is called virtual image of the first point. These types of images cannot be obtained on a screen.

Mentor's Tip

- If the incident rays diverge from a point object, the object is **real object.**
- If rays are converging towards a mirror, the point where these rays would meet if there was no mirror is a **virtual object.**

Mirror

There are two types of Mirrors.

Plane Mirror

The mirror whose reflecting surface is plane is called plane mirror. It's one side is silvered and reflection takes place from other side as shown in the figure.

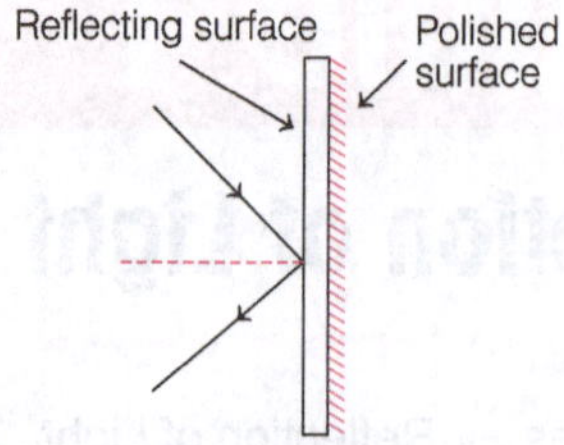

Plane mirror

Spherical Mirror

It is the part of a spherical transparent medium. One of the curved surfaces is polished and reflection takes place from other side.

Spherical mirrors are of two types

(a) **Concave mirror** A spherical mirror whose reflecting surface is towards the centre of the sphere is called concave mirror. In this mirror, outer curved surface is polished and reflection takes place from inner curved surface as shown in figure.

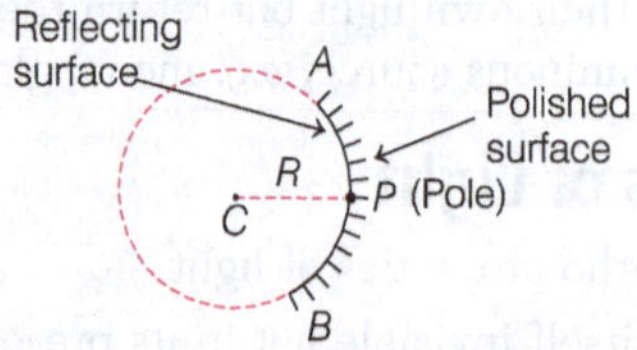

Concave mirror as a part of hollow sphere

(b) **Convex mirror** A spherical mirror whose reflecting surface is away from the centre of the sphere is called convex mirror. In this mirror, inner curved surface is polished and reflection takes place from outer curved surface as shown in figure.

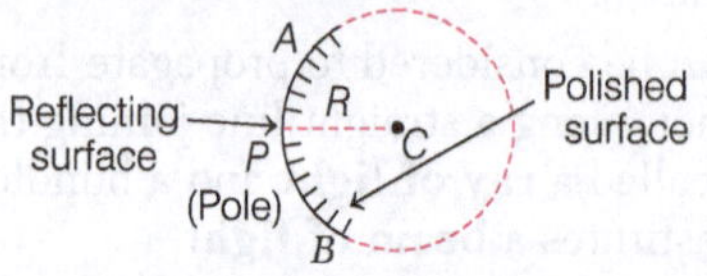

Convex mirror as a part of hollow sphere

Terms Related to Spherical Mirror

In case of these thin spherical mirrors important terms and their definitions are as follows

(i) **Pole** (P) It is the mid-point of the mirror.

(ii) **Centre of curvature** (C) It is the centre of the sphere of which the mirror is a part.

(iii) **Radius of curvature** (R) Distance between pole and centre of curvature is called radius of curvature. In the given figure, the distance CP is radius of curvature.

(iv) **Principal axis** The line joining the pole P and centre of curvature C when produced is called principal axis.

(v) **Aperture** (AB) Effective diameter of light reflecting area of the mirror is called aperture.

(vi) **Principal focus or focus** It is a point on the principal axis of the mirror at which the light rays coming parallel to principal axis actually meet after reflection (or appears to meet).

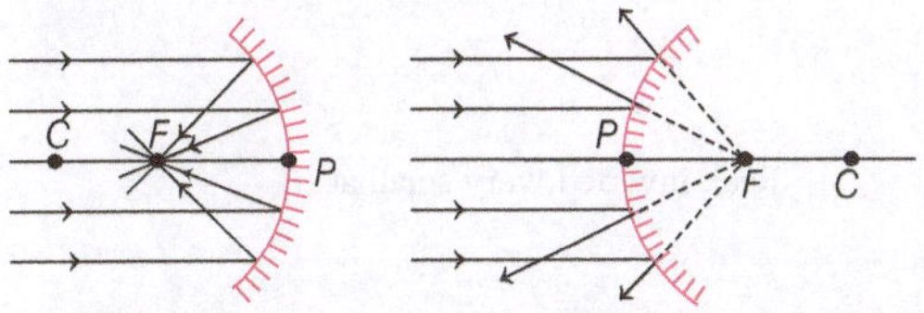

Principal focus of (a) concave mirror (a converging mirror) (b) convex mirror (a diverging mirror)

Focus of concave mirror is real, while focus of convex mirror is virtual.

(vii) **Focal length** The distance between pole and focus of a spherical mirror is called its focal length. It is represented by f. Focal length is independent of medium. i.e., if a spherical mirror is placed in water or any other mediums, its focal length remains unchanged.

Focal length of a mirror is equal to the half of radius of curvature of the mirror *i.e.*, $f = \dfrac{R}{2}$.

Mentor's TIP

- Focal length of a plane mirror is infinity and hence its power is zero.

Image Formation by Spherical Mirrors

By following some rules and sign conventions we can obtain the position and nature of image. These rules are given below.

Sign Convention

To derive the relevant formulae for reflection by spherical mirrors (concave or convex), we must first adopt a sign convention for measuring distances.

According to the Cartesian sign convention,

(i) All the distances are measured from pole (P) of the mirrors.

(ii) The principal axis of the mirror is taken as X-axis and the pole as origin.

(iii) Distances measured in the direction of the incident light are taken as positive and opposite to the direction of incident light as negative.

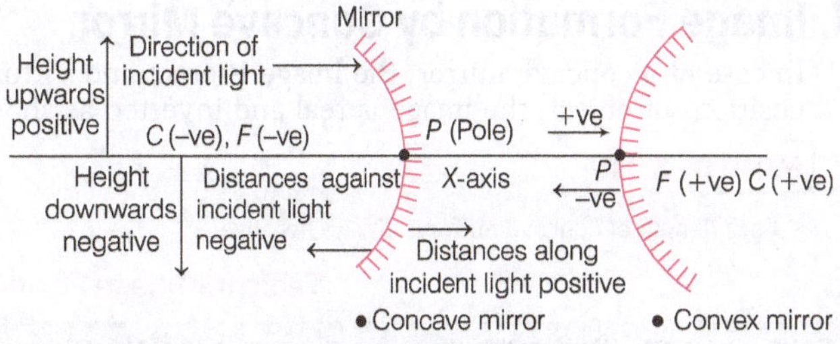

Cartesian sign convention

(iv) The heights measured upwards with respect to X-axis and normal to the principal axis of the mirror are taken as positive and the heights measured downwards are taken as negative.

Rules for Image Formation in Spherical Mirrors

In ray optics, to locate the image of an object, tracing of a ray as it reflects is very important. Following four types of rays are used for image formation.

Ray 1. A ray through the centre of curvature which strikes the mirror normally and is reflected back along the same path.

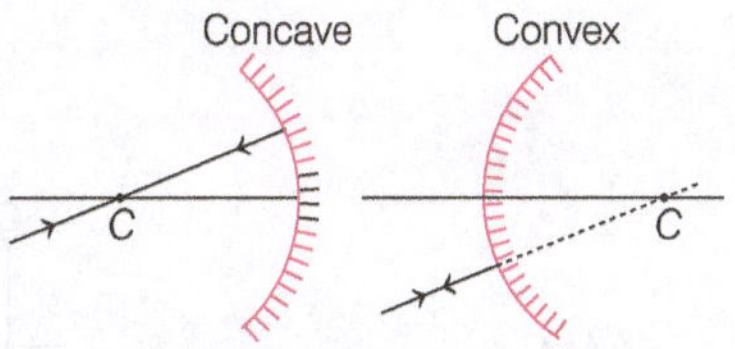

Ray 2. A ray parallel to principal axis after reflection either actually passes through the principal focus F or appears to diverge from it.

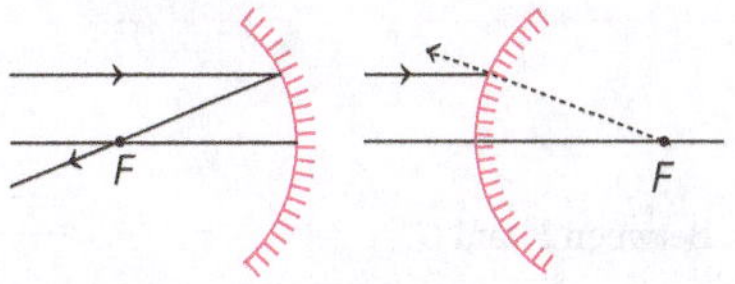

Ray 3. A ray passing through the principal focus F or a ray which appears to converge at F is reflected parallel to the principal axis.

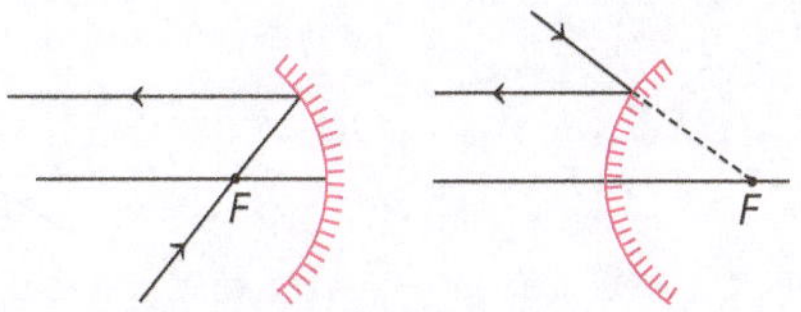

Ray 4. A ray striking at pole P is reflected symmetrically back in the opposite side following the laws of reflection.

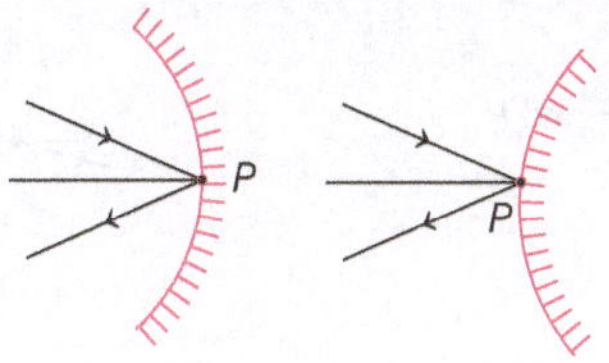

1. Image Formation by Concave Mirror

In case of a concave mirror, the image is erect and virtual when the object is placed between F and P. In all other positions of object, the image is real and inverted as shown in the table.

Mentor's TIP

- Focal length of concave mirror is always negative.

Table for Image Formation by Concave Mirror

S.No.	Position of Object	Ray Diagram	Properties of Image
(i)	At infinity	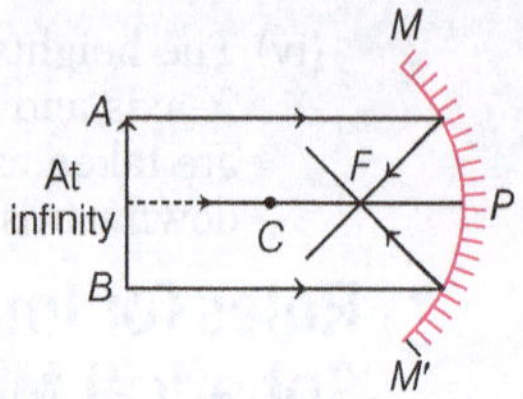	Real, inverted, very small at F
(ii)	Between infinity and C	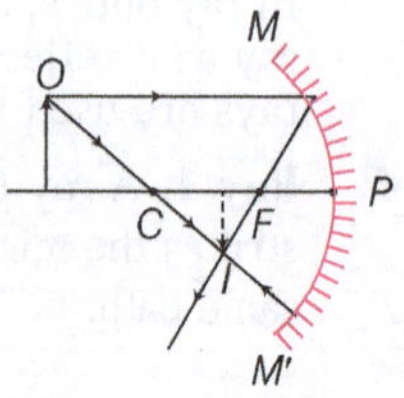	Real, inverted, diminished between F and C
(iii)	At C	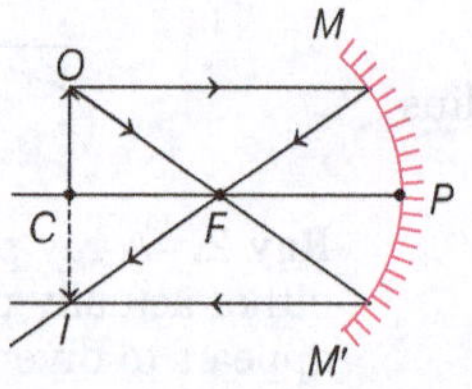	Real, inverted, equal in size at C
(iv)	Between F and C	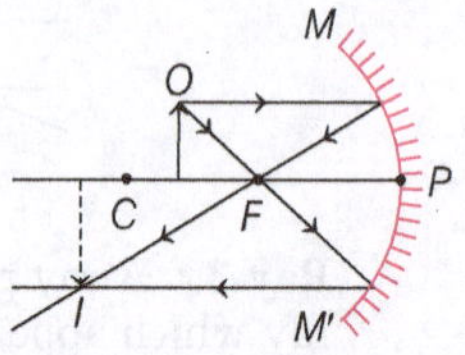	Real, inverted and very large between C and infinity
(v)	At F	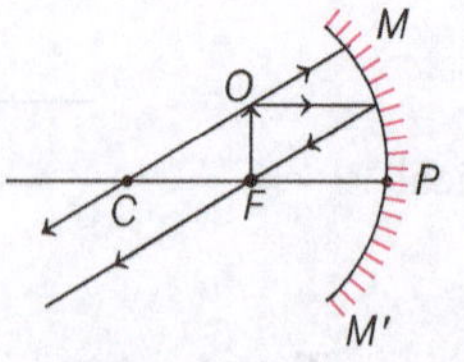	Real, inverted, very large at infinity
(vi)	Between F and P	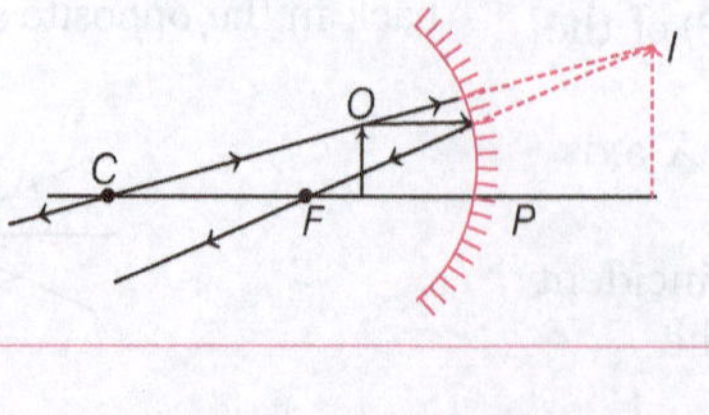	Virtual, erect, large in size behind the mirror

2. Image Formation by Convex Mirror

Image formed by convex mirror is always virtual, erect and diminished no matter where the object is placed. All the images formed by this mirror will be between pole and focus as shown in the table given below.

Table for Image Formation by Convex Mirror

S.No.	Position of Object	Ray Diagram	Properties of Image
(i)	At infinity	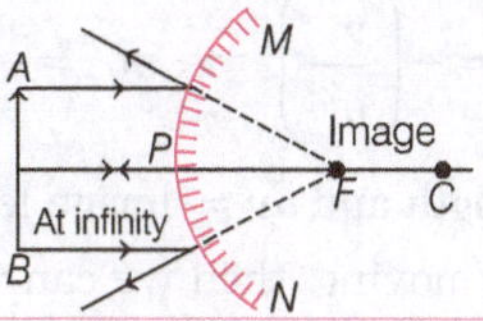	Virtual, erect, very small in size at F
(ii)	In front of mirror (at finite distance)	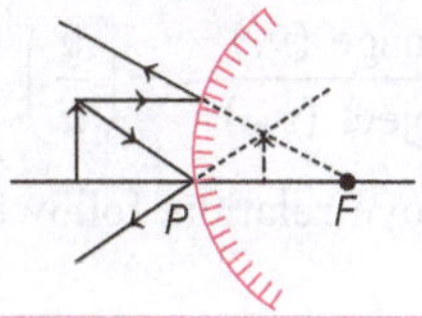	Virtual, erect, diminished between P and F

Mirror Formula

The relation among object distance (u), image distance (v) and focal length (f) of a mirror (concave or convex) can be established as $\frac{1}{v}+\frac{1}{u}=\frac{1}{f}$

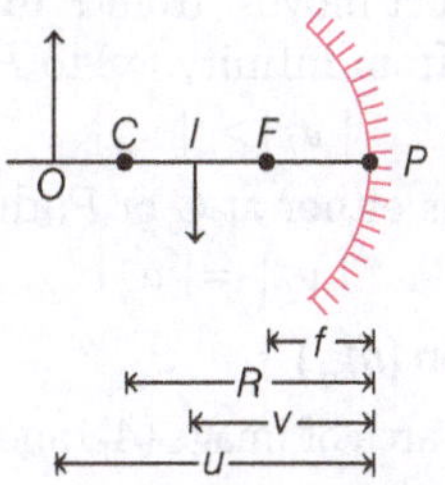

Image and object distances in a concave mirror

Here, f is positive for convex mirror and negative for concave mirror.

NEET Close-up

Example Similar to PYQ Asked in NEET 2020

An object is placed on the principal axis of a convex mirror at a distance $1.5f$ (f is focal length). The image will be formed at

(a) $\frac{3}{5}f$ (b) $\frac{5}{3}f$

(c) $\frac{1}{5}f$ (d) $\frac{2}{3}f$

Sol. (*a*) Given, $u=-1.5f=-\frac{3}{2}f \Rightarrow \frac{1}{v}+\frac{1}{u}=\frac{1}{f}$ (mirror formula)

$$\frac{1}{v}-\frac{2}{3f}=\frac{1}{f} \Rightarrow \frac{1}{v}=\frac{1}{f}\left(1+\frac{2}{3}\right)=\frac{5}{3f} \Rightarrow v=\frac{3f}{5}$$

Skill Builder

Distance of image from pole of a concave mirror with focal length 10 cm and object placed 25 cm away from pole is

(a) $-\frac{50}{3}$ cm (b) $-\frac{50}{7}$ cm

(c) $+\frac{50}{7}$ cm (d) $+\frac{50}{3}$ cm

For more Practice Refer Q. No. 17, 20 of step-up practice 1 and Q. No. 5 of Gearing up for NEET.

Important Informations Related to Mirror Formula

(i) Newton's Formula

In case of spherical mirrors, if object distance x_1 and image distance x_2 are measured from focus instead of pole, then $u=(f+x_1)$ and $v=(f+x_2)$. The mirror formula,

$\frac{1}{v}+\frac{1}{u}=\frac{1}{f}$ reduces to, $\frac{1}{f+x_2}+\frac{1}{f+x_1}=\frac{1}{f}$

which on simplification gives, $x_1x_2=f^2$

This formula is called **Newton's formula.**

(ii) *v versus u* Graph for a Plane Mirror

The focal length and the radius of curvature are infinite for a plane mirror.

$\therefore$ From mirror formula $\frac{1}{v}+\frac{1}{u}=0 \Rightarrow v=-u$

Thus, v *versus* u graph for a plane mirror is a straight line with slope equal to -1 as shown in figure.

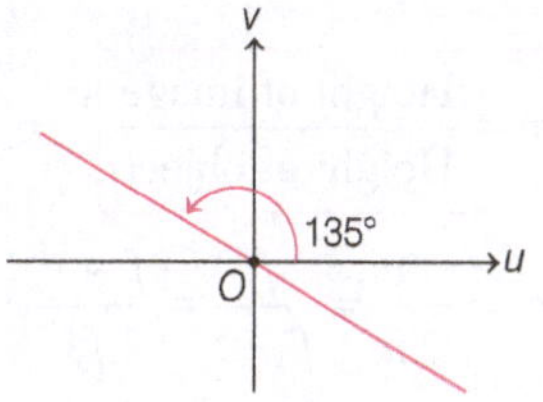

v *versus* u graph of a plane mirror

(iii) *v versus u* Graph for a Spherical Mirror

For a spherical mirror v *versus* u graph is a rectangular hyperbola as shown in figure.

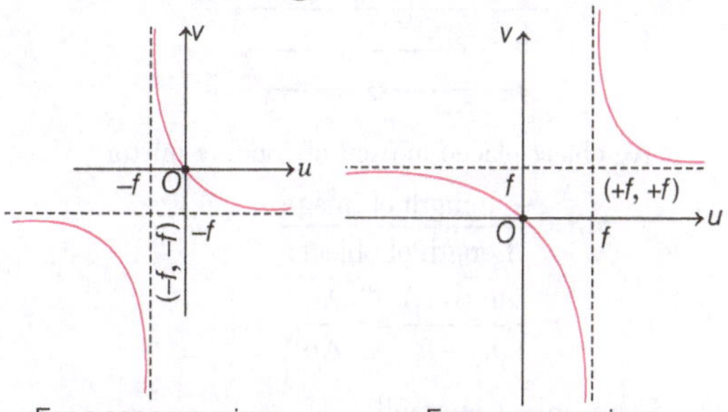

For a concave mirror For a convex mirror

v *versus* u graph for a spherical mirror

(iv) $\frac{1}{v}$ *versus* $\frac{1}{u}$ Graph for a Spherical Mirror

For a spherical mirror $\frac{1}{v}$ *versus* $\frac{1}{u}$ graph is a straight line as shown in figure.

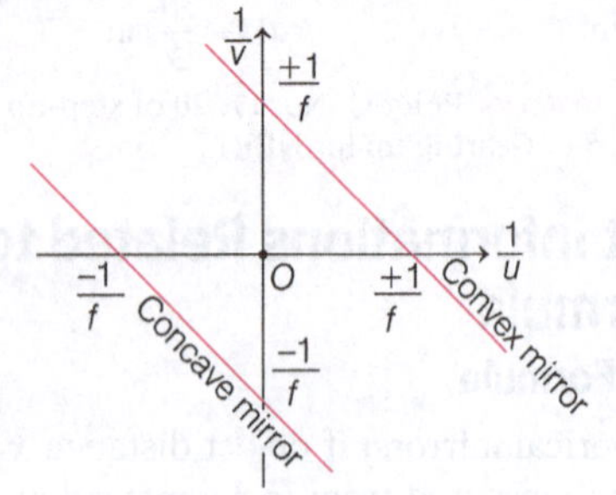

$\frac{1}{v}$ *versus* $\frac{1}{u}$ graph for a spherical mirror

Note *Coordinates of an object if given by* (x_0, y_0)*, then coordinates of image is*

$$(x_1, y_1) = \left(\frac{fx_0}{x_0 - f}, \frac{fy_0}{f - x_0}\right)$$

Magnification

The ratio of height of image formed by the mirror to height of object is called magnification produced by the mirror.

The Lateral, Transverse or Linear Magnification (m)

When an object is placed perpendicular to principal axis then the lateral, transverse or linear magnification is given as

$$m = \frac{\text{Height of image}}{\text{Height of object}}$$

Also, $\quad m = -\frac{v}{u} = \frac{f}{f - u} = \frac{f - v}{f}$

Axial or Longitudinal Magnification (m_L)

When an object is placed along principal axis, then

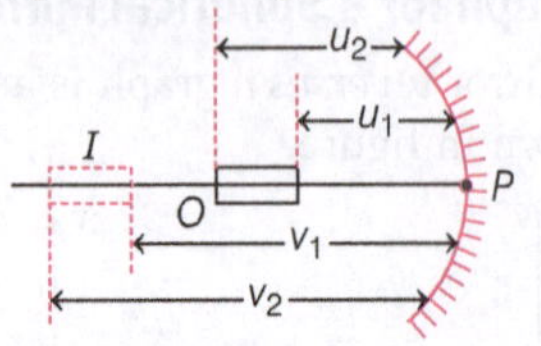

An object placed in front of concave mirror

$$m_L = \frac{-\text{ Length of image}}{\text{Length of object}}$$

$$= -\frac{(v_2 - v_1)}{u_2 - u_1} = -\frac{\Delta v}{\Delta u}$$

If length of the object is small,

$$m_L = \frac{dv}{du}$$

from mirror formula, $\frac{1}{v} + \frac{1}{u} = \frac{1}{f}$

By differentiation, we get

$$\frac{1}{v^2}\frac{dv}{du} - \frac{1}{u^2} = 0$$

or $\quad \frac{dv}{du} = -\left(\frac{v^2}{u^2}\right) \Rightarrow m_L = -m^2$

Here, du = object length and dv = image length

Also, when object is moving, then we can write

$$\frac{\text{Velocity of image } (v_I)}{\text{Velocity of object } (v_O)} = -\left(\frac{v}{u}\right)^2 = -\left(\frac{f}{u - f}\right)^2$$

On the basis of the above relation, following inferences can be given

(a) When object moves from $-\infty$ to F, the real image moves from F to $-\infty$ and when the object is placed between $-\infty$ to C, then

$$|v_I| < |v_o|$$

But, when the object is placed between C and F, then

$$|v_I| < |v_o|$$

(b) When the object moves from F to P, the virtual image moves from infinity (∞) to P, then

$$|v_I| > |v_o|$$

(c) When object is either at C or P, then

$$|v_I| = |v_o|$$

Areal Magnification (m_a)

It is given by ratio of area of image (A_I) and area of object (A_O)

$$\therefore \quad m_a = \frac{A_I}{A_O} = \left(\frac{v}{u}\right)^2 = \left(\frac{f}{f - u}\right)^2 = \left(\frac{f - v}{f}\right)^2$$

Concept ladder

- For real extended object, if the image is erect and virtual, then for,
  Concave mirror : $m > 1$,
  Plane mirror : $m = 1$ and
  Convex mirror : $m < 1$
- If the image is real, then the mirror is concave and for the object
  Beyond C : $m < -1$
  At C : $m = -1$ and Between C and F : $m > -1$

Example 1. An object is 30.0 *cm from a spherical mirror, along the central axis. The absolute value of lateral magnification is* 1/2. *The image produced is inverted. What is the focal length of the mirror?*

Sol. Image is inverted, so it is real, u and v both are negative.

Magnification is $\frac{1}{2}$, therefore, $v = \frac{u}{2}$.

Given, $u = -30$ cm and $v = -15$ cm

Using the mirror formula, $\frac{1}{v} + \frac{1}{u} = \frac{1}{f}$

we have, $$\frac{1}{f} = \frac{1}{-15} - \frac{1}{30} = -\frac{1}{10}$$

$\therefore$ Focal length $f = -10$ cm

Example 2. *A 4.5 cm needle is placed 12 cm away from a convex mirror of focal length 15 cm. Give the location of the image and the magnification. Describe what happens as the needle is moved farther from the mirror?*

Sol. Using the relation,

$$\frac{1}{f} = \frac{1}{u} + \frac{1}{v}, \text{ we get}$$

$$\frac{1}{v} = \frac{1}{f} - \frac{1}{u} = \frac{1}{15} - \left(\frac{1}{-12}\right)$$

$$\therefore \quad v = \frac{20}{3} \text{ cm} = +6.67 \text{ cm} \approx 6.7 \text{ cm}$$

The positive sign shows that the image is formed behind the mirror.

Using the relation, magnification $m = -\frac{v}{u}$, we get

$$m = -\frac{(20/3)}{-12} = +\frac{5}{9}$$

Hence, the image is virtual, erect and diminished.

As the needle is moved farther from the mirror, the image moves towards the focus (upto the focus only) and gets smaller and smaller in size.

Mentor's TIP

- Use sign convention explained in this session and carefully solve after that to avoid errors.

Example 3. *A small candle 2.5 cm in size is placed 27 cm in front of a concave mirror of radius of curvature 36 cm. At what distance from the mirror should a screen be placed in order to obtain a sharp image? Describe the nature and size of the image.*

Sol. (a) Using the relation, $\frac{1}{u} + \frac{1}{v} = \frac{1}{f}$

$$\frac{1}{v} = \frac{1}{f} - \frac{1}{u} = \frac{1}{-18} - \frac{1}{(-27)} \qquad \left(\because f = \frac{R}{2}\right)$$

$$\therefore \quad v = -54 \text{ cm}$$

The negative sign shows that the image is formed in front of the mirror, *i.e.*, on the side of the object itself. Thus, the screen must be placed at a distance of 54 cm in front of the mirror.

(b) Magnification, $m = -\frac{v}{u} = \frac{I}{O}$

we get, $$\frac{I}{2.5} = -\frac{(-54)}{(-27)}$$

or $$I = (2.5) \times (-2) = -5 \text{ cm}$$

Thus, clearly the image is real, inverted and magnified.

Example 4. *Find the distance of object from a concave mirror of focal length 10 cm, so that image size is four times the size of the object.*

Sol. Concave mirror can form real as well as virtual image. Here nature of image is not given in the question. So, we will consider two possible cases.

***Case I* (When image is real)** Real image is formed on the same side of the object, *i.e.* u, v and f all are negative. So let,

$$u = -x$$

then, $v = -4x$ as $\left|\frac{v}{u}\right| = |m| = 4$

and $f = -10$ cm

Substituting in, $\frac{1}{v} + \frac{1}{u} = \frac{1}{f}$

We have $$\frac{1}{-4x} - \frac{1}{x} = \frac{1}{-10}$$

or $$\frac{5}{4x} = \frac{1}{10}$$

$\therefore$ $x = 12.5$ cm

Note $|x| > |f|$ and we know that in case of a concave mirror, image is real when object lies beyond F.

Case II (When image is virtual) Mirror image is virtual when it is formed behind the mirror, *i.e.*, u and f are negative while v is positive. So let,

$$u = -y$$

then, $v = +4y$ and $f = -10$ cm

Substituting in, $\frac{1}{v} + \frac{1}{u} = \frac{1}{f}$

we have, $$\frac{1}{4y} - \frac{1}{y} = \frac{1}{-10}$$

or $$\frac{3}{4y} = \frac{1}{10}$$

or $$y = 7.5 \text{ cm}$$

Note Here $|y| < |f|$, as we know that image is virtual when the object lies between F and P.

Example 5. *A concave mirror has a radius of curvature of 24 cm. How far is an object from the mirror, if an image is formed that is*

(i) virtual and 3.0 times the size of the object,

(ii) real and 3.0 times the size of the object and

(iii) real and 1/3rd the size of the object?

Sol. Given, $R = -24$ cm (concave mirror)

Hence, $f = \frac{R}{2} = -12$ cm

(i) Image is virtual and 3 times larger. Hence, u is negative and v is positive. Simultaneously, $|v| = 3|u|$.

So let,

$$u = -x \text{ then, } v = +3x$$

Substituting values in the mirror formula $\frac{1}{v} + \frac{1}{u} = \frac{1}{f}$,

we have

$$\frac{1}{3x} - \frac{1}{x} = \frac{1}{-12}$$

$\therefore$ $x = 8$ cm

Therefore, object distance is 8 cm.

(ii) Image is real and three times larger. Hence, u and v both are negative and $|v| = 3|u|$.

So let,

$$u = -x$$

then, $v = -3x$

Substituting values in mirror formula, we have

$$\frac{1}{-3x} - \frac{1}{x} = -\frac{1}{12}$$

or $x = 16$ cm

$\therefore$ Object distance should be 16 cm.

(iii) Image is real and $\frac{1}{3}$rd the size of object. Hence, both u and v are negative and $|v| = \frac{|u|}{3}$.

So let,

$$u = -x$$

then, $v = -\frac{x}{3}$

Substituting values in the mirror formula, we have

$$-\frac{3}{x} - \frac{1}{x} = -\frac{1}{12}$$

or $x = 48$ cm

$\therefore$ Object distance should be 48 cm.

Example 6. *A thin stick of length f/5 is placed along the principal axis of a concave mirror of focal length f such that its image which is real and elongated just touches the stick. What is the magnification?*

Sol. One end of image coincides with one end of stick *i.e.*, either A or B is centre of curvature.

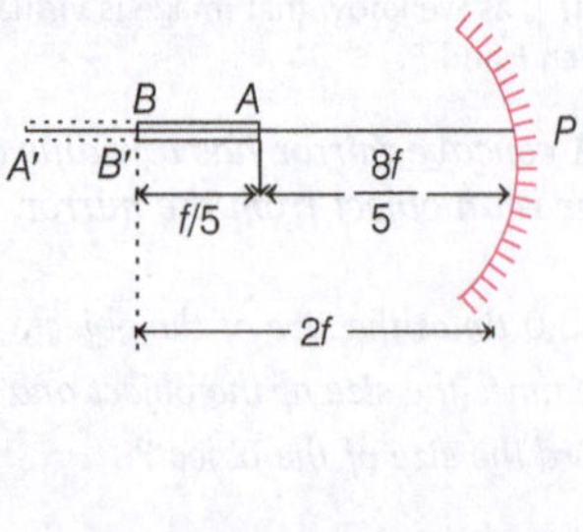

Since image is elongated, *i.e.* point B is centre of curvature. Image of B is formed on B itself as shown in the figure.

Image of A

$$u = -(2f - f/5) = \frac{-9f}{5}$$

$$f = -f, v = ?$$

$$\frac{1}{v} + \frac{1}{u} = \frac{1}{f}$$

$$\Rightarrow \frac{1}{v} + \frac{1}{-9f/5} = \frac{1}{-f}$$

$$\frac{1}{v} = -\frac{1}{f} + \frac{5}{9f} = \frac{-9+5}{9f} = \frac{-4}{9f} \Rightarrow v = -\frac{9f}{4}$$

Image length, $A'B' = -\frac{9f}{4} - (-2f) = -f/4$

Longitudinal magnification, $m_L = \frac{-A'B'}{AB} = \frac{f/4}{f/5} = \frac{5}{4}$

Uses of Spherical Mirrors

Uses of spherical mirrors (concave and convex mirrors) are given below

Concave Mirrors

(i) It is used as reflectors in search light, cinema projectors and headlights of vehicles, etc.

(ii) Concave mirror is also used as face looking or shaving mirror because it forms erect and magnified image.

(iii) These mirrors are used in dish antennas.

(iv) Concave mirrors are used by dentists and ENT specialists, in solar cookers, etc.

Convex Mirrors

(i) It is used as a reflector in street lamps to diverge the light over a large area.

(ii) Convex mirrors are used as rear view mirror (or driver's mirror) in vehicles, because it has a wider field of view than a plane mirror as shown in figure.

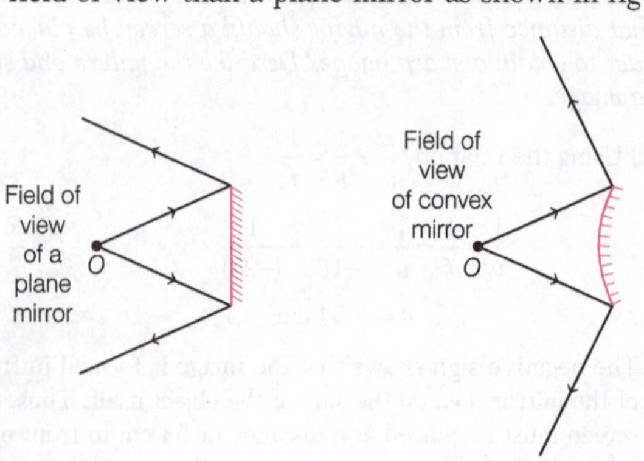

STEP UP Practice 1

1. Light falls on a plane reflecting surface. For what angle of incidence is the reflected ray normal to the incident ray?
(a) 60° (b) 45° (c) 90° (d) 30°

2. **Assertion** (A) A ray of light incident along the normal to the plane mirror retraces its path after reflection from the mirror.
Reason (R) A ray of light along the normal has angle of incidence as $\pi/2$ and hence, it retraces its own path after reflection from mirror.
In the light of the above statements, choose the correct answer from the options given below.
(a) Both A and R are true but R is not the correct explanation of A.
(b) A is true but R is false.
(c) A is false but R is true.
(d) Both A and R are true and R is the correct explanation of A.

3. A plane mirror reflects a pencil of light to form a real image, then the pencil of light incident on the mirror is
(a) parallel (b) convergent
(c) divergent (d) None of these

4. A man is 180 cm tall and his eyes are 10 cm below the top of his head. In order to see this entire height right from top to head, he uses a plane mirror kept at a distance of 1 m from him. The minimum length of the plane mirror is
(a) 180 cm (b) 90 cm (c) 85 cm (d) 170 cm

5. To get three images of a single object, one should have two plane mirrors at an angle of
(a) 30° (b) 60° (c) 90° (d) 150°

6. **Assertion** (A) Image formed by a spherical mirror of a point object is always lying on a straight line passing through point object and centre of curvature of mirror.
Reason (R) The ray which is incident on the spherical mirror, which is passing through centre of curvature return back on the same path.
In the light of the above statements, choose the correct answer from the options given below.
(a) Both A and R are true but R is not the correct explanation of A.
(b) A is true but R is false.
(c) A is false but R is true.
(d) Both A and R are true and R is the correct explanation of A.

7. An object (O) is placed between two parallel plane mirrors as shown in figure. Distance between 4th image is

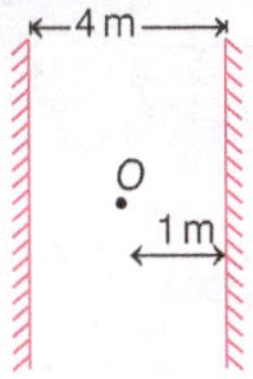

(a) 16 m (b) 32 m (c) 8 m (d) 64 m

8. A concave mirror of focal length f (in air) is immersed in water ($\mu = 4/3$). The focal length of the mirror in water will be
(a) f (b) $\frac{4}{3}f$
(c) $\frac{3}{4}f$ (d) $\frac{7}{3}f$

9. **Assertion** (A) In the case of concave mirror, the minimum distance between real object and its real image is zero.
Reason (R) If concave mirror forms virtual image of real object, the image is magnified.
In the light of the above statements, choose the correct answer from the options given below.
(a) Both A and R are true but R is not the correct explanation of A.
(b) A is true but R is false.
(c) A is false but R is true.
(d) Both A and R are true and R is the correct explanation of A.

10. An object is placed 40 cm from a concave mirror of focal length 20 cm. The image formed is
(a) real, inverted and same in size
(b) real, inverted and smaller in size
(c) virtual, erect and larger in size
(d) virtual, erect and smaller in size

11. A point object is placed at a distance of 30 cm from a convex mirror of focal length 30 cm. The image will form at
(a) infinity (b) pole
(c) focus (d) 15 cm behind the mirror

12. An object is placed at a distance of 30 cm from a concave mirror and its real image is formed at a distance of 30 cm from the mirror. The focal length of the mirror is
(a) -15 cm (b) -45 cm (c) -30 cm (d) -20 cm

13. A convex mirror of focal length f forms an image which is $1/n$ times the object. The distance of the object from the mirror is
(a) $(n-1)f$ (b) $\left[\frac{n-1}{n}\right]f$
(c) $\left[\frac{n+1}{n}\right]f$ (d) $(n+1)f$

14. **Assertion** (A) According to sign convention, radius of curvature is negative for convex mirror and positive for concave mirror.
Reason (R) All distances measured in direction of light are taken positive.
In the light of the above statements, choose the correct answer from the options given below
(a) Both A and R are true but R is not the correct explanation of A.
(b) A is true but R is false.
(c) A is false but R is true.
(d) Both A and R are true and R is the correct explanation of A.

15. Which one of the following pairs given below is correct regarding the image formation by a concave mirror?

	Object Position		Image Formed
(a)	At infinity	→	Real, inverted and very large at F.
(b)	At C	→	Virtual, inverted, equal in size at C.
(c)	At F	→	Real, inverted, very small at infinity.
(d)	Between F and C	→	Real, inverted, very large between C and infinity.

16. The focal length of a concave mirror is 50 cm. Where should be the object placed, so that its image is two times and inverted?
(a) 75 cm (b) 60 cm
(c) 125 cm (d) 50 cm

17. The image formed by a convex mirror of focal length 30 cm is a quarter of the size of the object. The distance of the object from the mirror is
(a) 30 cm (b) 90 cm (c) 120 cm (d) 60 cm

18. A concave mirror gives an image three times as large as the object placed at a distance of 20 cm from it. For the image to be real, the focal length should be
(a) 10 cm (b) 15 cm (c) 20 cm (d) 30 cm

19. **Assertion** (A) The focal length of the mirror is f and distance of the object from the focus is u. The magnification of the mirror is f/u.

Reason (R) Magnification $= \dfrac{\text{Size of image}}{\text{Size of object}}$

In the light of the above statements, choose the correct answer from the options given below
(a) Both A and R are true but R is not the correct explanation of A.
(b) A is true but R is false.
(c) A is false but R is true.
(d) Both A and R are true and R is the correct explanation of A.

20. An object of size 7.5 cm is placed infront of a convex mirror of radius of curvature 25 cm at a distance of 40 cm.The size of the image should be
(a) 2.3 cm (b) 1.78 cm
(c) 1 cm (d) 0.8 cm

21. A point object is placed at a distance of 10 cm and its real image is formed at a distance of 20 cm from a concave mirror. If the object is moved by 0.1 cm towards the mirror, the image will shift by about
(a) 0.4 cm away from the mirror
(b) 0.8 cm away from the mirror
(c) 0.4 cm towards the mirror
(d) 0.8 cm towards the mirror

Module 2
Refraction of Light

- Refraction of Light • Image Formation due to Refraction at a Plane Surface
- Critical Angle and Total Internal Reflection (TIR) • Applications of Total Internal Reflection
- Refraction at Spherical Surfaces

Refraction of Light

When a light passes from one medium to another medium, it deviates from its original path.

The phenomenon of change in path of light at the boundary of separation of two media, as it goes from one medium to another medium is called **refraction**.

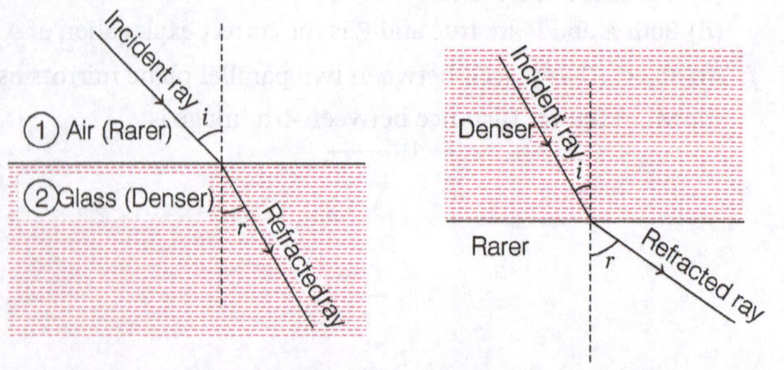

Refraction of light

- When a ray of light goes from a rarer medium to a denser medium, it bends towards the normal.
- When a ray of light goes from a denser medium to a rarer medium, it bends away from the normal.

Laws of Refraction

There are two laws of refraction as follows

(i) For two particular media, the ratio of the sine of the angle of incidence to the sine of the angle of refraction is constant, *i.e.* $\frac{\sin i}{\sin r} = \text{constant}$ ...(i)

This is known as **Snell's law.**

(ii) The incident ray, the normal and the refracted ray at the point of incidence all lie in the same plane.

Note The angle of deviation on refraction is $\delta = |i - r|$. If the incident ray is normal, refraction takes place without bending. In this case $i = r = 0$, *i.e.*, incident ray passes undeviated.

Refractive Index (μ or n)

The constant ratio $\frac{\sin i}{\sin r}$ is called the relative **refractive index**, for light passing from the first to the second medium.

Thus, $$\mu = \frac{\sin i}{\sin r} = \frac{\mu_2}{\mu_1} \quad ...(ii)$$

Refractive index is a dimensionless quantity and have no unit.

Absolute Refractive Index

When light travels from vacuum (or air) to any transparent medium, then refractive index of medium with respect to vacuum (or air) is called absolute refractive index *i.e.*,

$$\mu = \frac{\text{speed of light in vacuum}}{\text{speed of light in medium}} = \frac{c}{v}$$

Relative Refractive Index

When light travels from medium (1) to medium (2), then refractive index of medium (2) with respect to medium (1) is called relative refractive index *i.e.*, ${}_1\mu_2 = \frac{\mu_2}{\mu_1}$

Dependence of Refractive Index

The value of refractive index depends on

(i) The nature of the two media.

(ii) The temperature of the media.

(iii) The wavelength of the light.

(iv) It does not depend on the value of i (however refractive index $= \frac{\sin i}{\sin r}$) for a pair of media.

(v) According to Cauchy's formula,

$$\mu = A + \frac{B}{\lambda^2}$$

where, A and B are constants.

$\therefore$ As λ increases, μ decreases.

Important Points About Refractive Index

(i) Refractive index is a property of the medium.

(ii) A medium with higher value of μ is called denser medium and with the lower value of μ is called rarer medium.

(iii) The minimum value of refractive index (absolute) is 1 for vacuum. For air, it is 1.003 but practically, we will use $\mu = 1$ for air.

(iv) Maximum value of μ is 2.46 for diamond.

Concept ladder

- For more than two mediums (say n-mediums)

$${}_1\mu_2 \times {}_2\mu_3 \times {}_3\mu_4 \times \cdots {}_{n-1}\mu_n = {}_1\mu_n$$

- We can easily understand that

$${}_1\mu_2 = \frac{\mu_2}{\mu_1} = \frac{\sin i}{\sin r} = \frac{v_1}{v_2} = \frac{\lambda_1}{\lambda_2}$$

(v) Experiments show that, if the boundaries of the media are **parallel**, then the emergent ray CD, is parallel to the incident ray, however it is laterally displaced.

We can also directly apply the Snell's law in medium 1 and 5 *i.e.*, $\mu_1 \sin i_1 = \mu_5 \sin i_5$

$\Rightarrow \quad i_1 = i_5$ if $\mu_1 = \mu_5 \quad (\because \mu \sin i = \text{constant})$

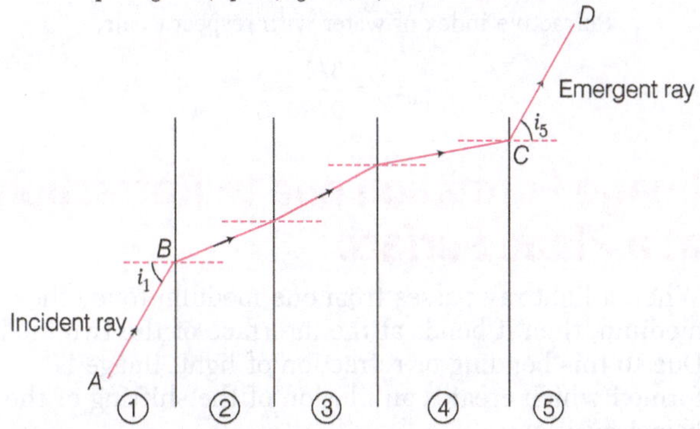

If any of the boundary is not parallel we cannot use this law directly by jumping the intervening media.

Example 7. *(i) Find the speed of light of wavelength $\lambda = 780\,nm$ (in air) in a medium of refractive index $\mu = 1.55$.*

(ii) What is the wavelength of this light in the given medium?

Sol. (i) Speed of light, $v = \frac{c}{\mu} = \frac{3.0 \times 10^8}{1.55}$

$= 1.94 \times 10^8$ m/s

(ii) Wavelength of light in the given medium,

$$\lambda_{medium} = \frac{\lambda_{air}}{\mu} = \frac{780}{1.55} \approx 503 \text{ nm}$$

Example 8. *Light of wavelength 300 nm in medium A enters into medium B through a plane surface. If frequency of light is 5×10^{14} Hz and $v_A / v_B = 4/5$, then find absolute refractive indices of media A and B.*

Sol. Speed, $v_A = \nu\lambda_A = 5 \times 10^{14} \times 300 \times 10^{-9} = 1.5 \times 10^8$ m/s

Absolute refractive index, $\mu_A = \frac{c}{v_A} = \frac{3 \times 10^8}{1.5 \times 10^8} = 2$

We have, $\mu \propto \frac{1}{v}$

$\therefore \quad \frac{\mu_A}{\mu_B} = \frac{v_B}{v_A} \Rightarrow \frac{2}{\mu_B} = \frac{5}{4}$

Refractive index, $\mu_B = \frac{2 \times 4}{5} = 1.6$

Mentor's TiP

- Light travels slower in medium of higher refractive index.

Example 9. *Refractive index of glass with respect to water is (9/8). Refractive index of glass with respect to air is (3/2). Find the refractive index of water with respect to air.*

Sol. Given, ${}_w\mu_g = 9/8$ and ${}_a\mu_g = 3/2$

As, ${}_a\mu_g \times {}_g\mu_w \times {}_w\mu_a = 1$

$\therefore \quad \frac{1}{{}_w\mu_a} = {}_a\mu_w = {}_a\mu_g \times {}_g\mu_w = \frac{{}_a\mu_g}{{}_w\mu_g}$

$\therefore$ Refractive index of water with respect to air,

$${}_a\mu_w = \frac{3/2}{9/8} = \frac{4}{3}$$

Image Formation due to Refraction at a Plane Surface

When a light ray passes from one medium to another medium, then it bends at the interface of the two media. Due to this bending or refraction of light, image is formed which creates an illusion of the shifting of the object position.

Following two types of shifts are possible after refraction from a plane surface

***Type* I The object (O) is in denser medium (glass, water, etc.) and is seen from rarer medium (air) normally through plane surface.**

In this condition, due to refraction of light, object in the denser medium as seen from rarer medium seems to be raised above as compared to its actual depth below the boundary of denser medium.

In the figure, $\angle AOB$ will be r and $\angle AIB$ is i. For normal incidence, (*i.e.* small angles of i and r)

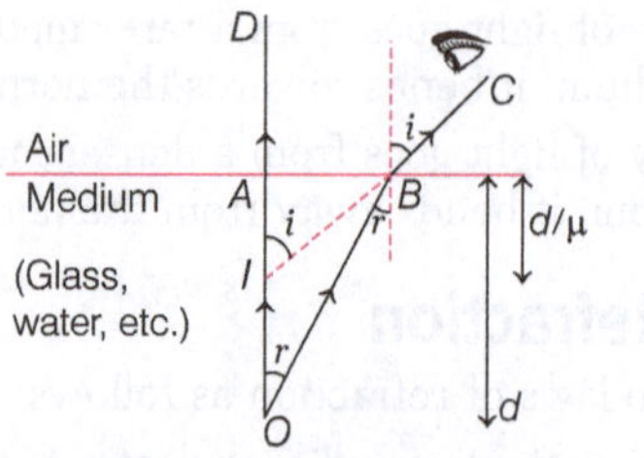

Object is in denser medium

$$\sin i \approx \tan i = \frac{AB}{AI} \quad \text{...(i)}$$

and $$\sin r \approx \tan r = \frac{AB}{AO} \quad \text{...(ii)}$$

On dividing Eq. (i) by Eq. (ii), we have

$$\frac{\sin i}{\sin r} = \frac{AO}{AI} \text{ or } \mu = \frac{AO}{AI} \quad \left(\because \frac{\sin i}{\sin r} = \mu\right)$$

$$\therefore \quad AI = \frac{AO}{\mu} = \frac{d}{\mu}$$

If point O is at a depth d from a water surface, then the above result is also written as

$$AI = d_{apparent} = \frac{AO (= d_{actual})}{\mu} = \frac{d}{\mu}$$

$$\therefore \quad \text{Shift} = OI = AO - AI = d\left(1 - \frac{1}{\mu}\right)$$

$$\boxed{\text{Apparent shift} = d\left(1 - \frac{1}{\mu}\right)}$$

where, d is actual depth of the object in the denser medium of refractive index μ.

Concept ladder

Lateral magnification due to immiscible liquids of refractive indices $\mu_1, \mu_2, \mu_3 \ldots\ldots \mu_n$ and their depths are $d_1, d_2, d_3 \ldots, d_n$, respectively.

- **Apparent depth** $d_{app} = \frac{d_1}{\mu_1} + \frac{d_2}{\mu_2} + \frac{d_3}{\mu_3} + \ldots + \frac{d_n}{\mu_n}$
- **Apparent shift**

$$= d_1\left[1 - \frac{1}{\mu_1}\right] + d_2\left[1 - \frac{1}{\mu_2}\right] + \ldots + d_n\left[1 - \frac{1}{\mu_n}\right]$$

***Type* II The object (O) is in rarer medium (air) and is seen from denser medium (glass, water, etc.) normally through plane surface.**

In this condition, due to refraction of light, object in the rarer medium as seen from denser medium seems to be raised above as compared to its actual height above the boundary of rarer medium. As the ray of light passes from rarer to denser medium, it bends towards the normal and hence the object will appear farther (at I) as shown in figure.

Proceeding as previous Eqs. (i) and (ii), we get

$$\mu = \frac{\sin i}{\sin r} = \frac{\tan i}{\tan r} = \frac{AB}{AO} \times \left(\frac{AI}{AB}\right)$$

$\Rightarrow \quad AI = \mu\,(AO) = \mu(h)$

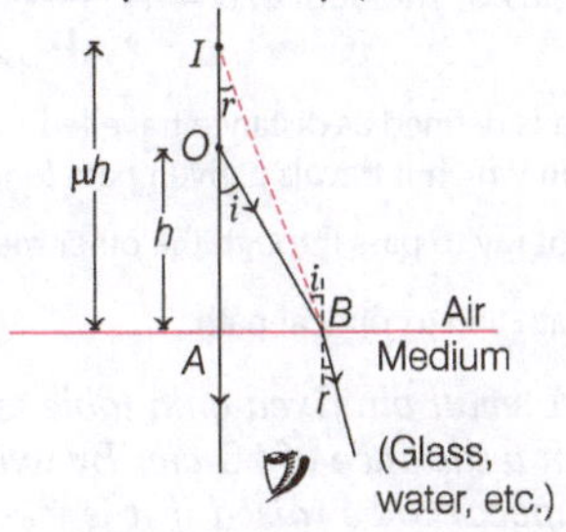

Object is in rarer medium

$\therefore$ Apparent height $(AI) = \mu$ (actual height)

and shift $= OI = AI - AO = (\mu - 1)h$

Mentor's Tip

- In all the above cases, the change in the value of x (depth or height) is μ times whether it is increasing or decreasing. All the relations can be derived for small angles of incidence as done in Type I.

Example 10. *A printed page is kept pressed by a glass cube ($\mu = 1.5$) of edge 9.0 cm. By what amount will the printed letters appear to be shifted when viewed from the top?*

Sol. The thickness of the cube $= t = 9.0$ cm. The shift in the position of the printed letters is

$$\Delta d = \left(1 - \frac{1}{\mu}\right)d = \left(1 - \frac{1}{1.5}\right) \times 9.0\text{ cm} = 3.0\text{ cm}$$

Example 11. *Consider the situation as shown in the diagram.*

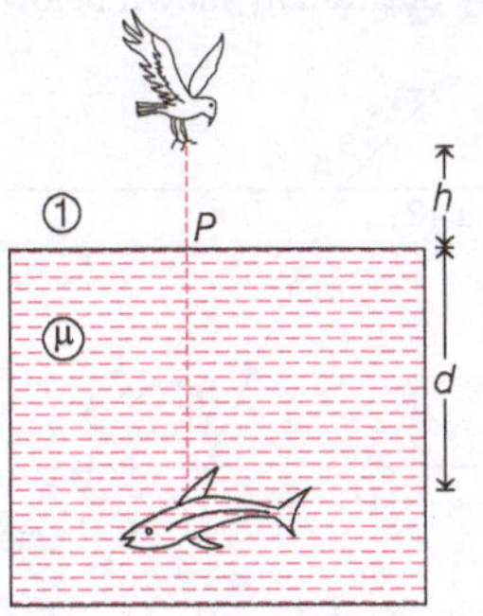

Find the distance between sparrow and fish as seen by (i) sparrow and (ii) fish.

Sol. (i) For sparrow, fish will appear nearer at distance d/μ from P,

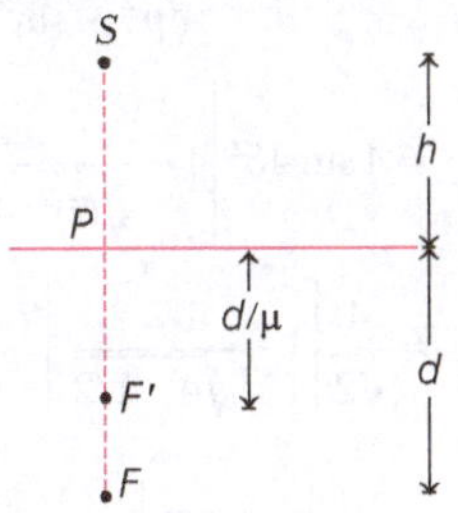

$$SF' = h + \frac{d}{\mu}$$

(ii) For fish, sparrow will appear farther at distance μh from P

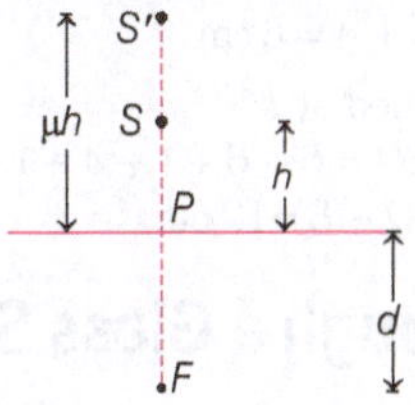

$$FS' = d + \mu h$$

Example 12. *A fish in an aquarium, approaches the left wall at a rate of 3 ms^{-1}, and observes a fly approaching it at 8 ms^{-1}. If the refractive index of water is (4/3), then find the actual velocity of the fly.*

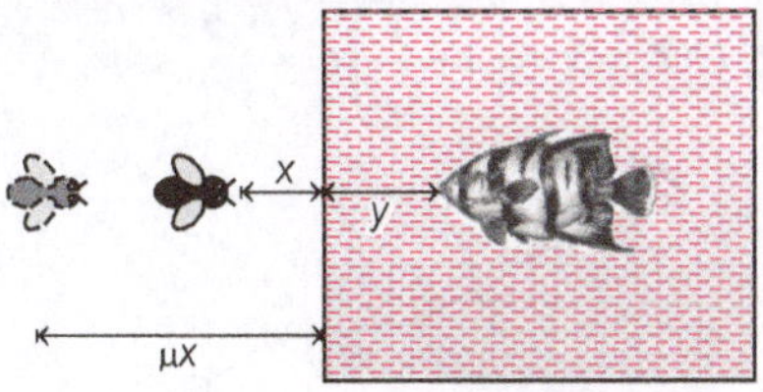

Sol. For the fish, apparent distance of the fly from the wall of the aquarium is μx.

If x is actual distance, then apparent velocity will be $= \dfrac{d\,(\mu x)}{dt}$

$$(v_{app})_{fly} = \mu\, v_{fly}$$

Now, the fish observes the velocity of the fly to be 8 ms^{-1}.

Therefore, apparent relative velocity = 8 ms^{-1}

$$\Rightarrow \quad v_{fish} + (v_{app})_{fly} = 8\text{ ms}^{-1}$$

$$\Rightarrow \quad 3 + \mu v_{fly} = 8$$

$$\therefore \text{Velocity of fly } v_{fly} = 5 \times \frac{3}{4} = 3.75\text{ ms}^{-1}$$

Example 13. *Consider the situation shown in figure.*

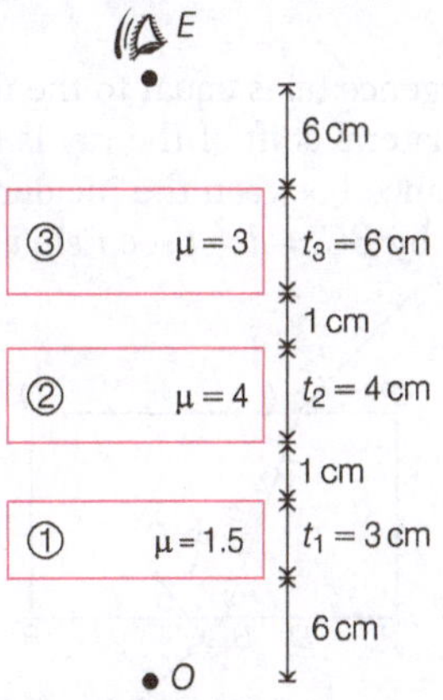

Find distance of image of O from eye E.

Sol. Shift by (1); $t_1(1 - 1/\mu_1) = 3(1 - 2/3) = 1$ cm

Shift by (2); $t_2(1 - 1/\mu_2) = 4(1 - 1/4) = 3$ cm

Shift by (3); $t_3(1 - 1/\mu_3) = 6(1 - 1/3) = 4$ cm

Total shift $= 1 + 3 + 4 = 8$ cm

Image of O is formed at I.

$OI = 8\text{ cm} \Rightarrow EO = 6 + 6 + 1 + 4 + 1 + 3 + 6 = 27\text{ cm}$

$EI = EO - OI = 27 - 8 = 19\text{ cm}$

Refraction through a Glass Slab

Normal shift

If a glass slab is placed in the path of a converging or diverging beam of light, then point of convergence or point of divergence appears to be shifted as shown in figure.

Normal shift, $OO' = x = \left(1 - \frac{1}{\mu}\right) t$

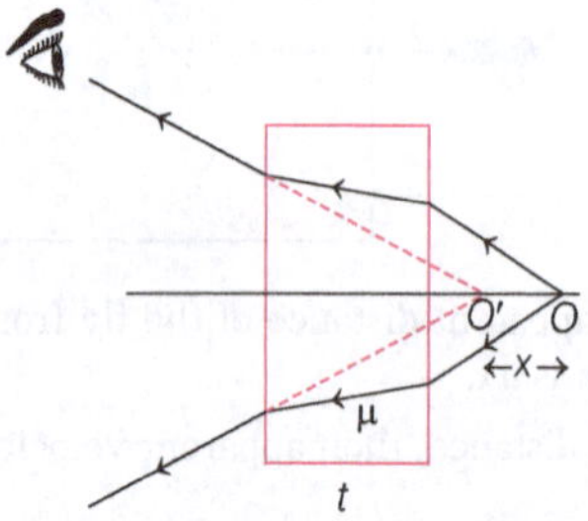

Normal shift by a glass slab

Mentor's TiP

Due to slab, if the $\mu_{slab} > \mu_{medium}$, then the shift is along the direction of incident ray and if, $\mu_{slab} < \mu_{medium}$, then the shift will be in opposite direction.

Lateral Shift

When a light ray passes through a glass slab it is refracted twice at the two parallel faces and finally emerges out parallel to it's incident direction *i.e.*, the ray undergoes no deviation $\delta = 0$.

The angle of emergence (e) is equal to the angle of incidence (i). The lateral shift of the ray is the perpendicular distance between the incident and emergent ray and it is given by $BC = d = t \sec r \sin(i - r)$.

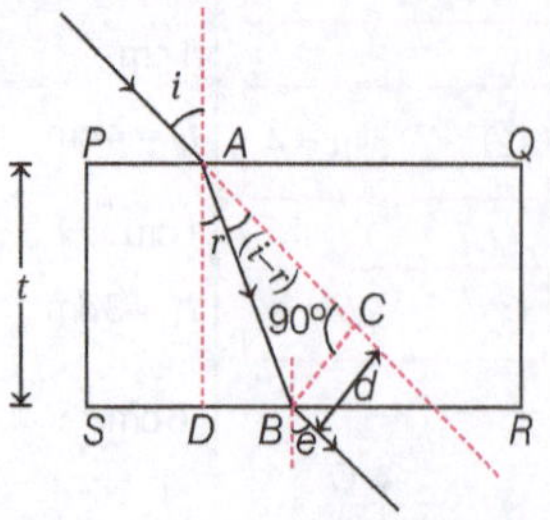

Lateral shift by a glass slab

or $\quad d = \left[1 - \frac{\cos i}{\sqrt{\mu^2 - \sin^2 i}}\right] t \sin i$

For small angles of incidence, $d = ti\left(\frac{\mu - 1}{\mu}\right)$

Note Optical path is defined as distance travelled by light in vacuum in the same time in which it travels a given path length in a medium. Time taken by light ray to pass through the other medium is $\frac{\mu x}{c}$, where x = geometrical path and μx optical path.

Example 14. *A small pin fixed on a table top is viewed from above from a distance of 50 cm. By what distance would the pin appear to be raised if it is viewed from the same point through a 15 cm thick glass slab held parallel to the table? Refractive index of glass = 1.5. Does the answer depend on the location of the slab?*

Sol. As we know, $d = \text{normal shift} = t - \frac{t}{\mu} = t\left(1 - \frac{1}{\mu}\right)$

$$= 15\left(1 - \frac{1}{1.5}\right) = 15\left(1 - \frac{2}{3}\right)$$

$$= 15 \times \frac{1}{3} = 5\text{ cm}$$

i.e., the pin appears to be raised by 5 cm.

No, the answer does not depend upon the location of the slab for small angles of incidence.

Example 15. *A light ray is incident at an angle of 45° with the normal on a 4 cm thick plate ($\mu = 2.0$). Find the shift in the path of the light as it emerges out from the plate.*

Sol. Consider the ray diagram as shown below

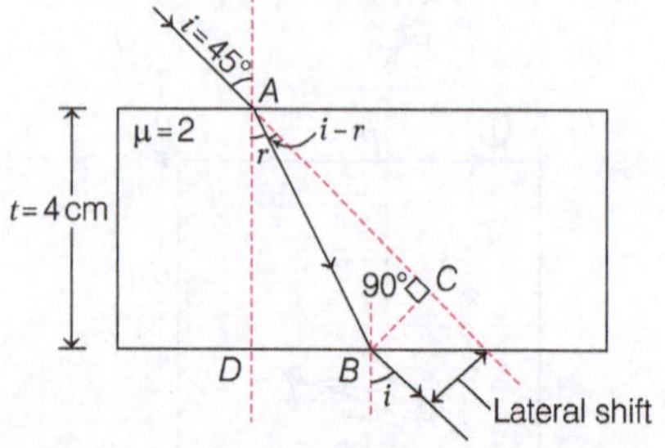

Lateral shift, $BC = \frac{t \sin(i - r)}{\cos r}$

$$= t \sin i\left[1 - \frac{\cos i}{\sqrt{\mu^2 - \sin^2 i}}\right]$$

$$= 4 \sin 45°\left[1 - \frac{\cos 45°}{\sqrt{(2)^2 - (\sin^2 45°)}}\right]$$

$$= \frac{4}{\sqrt{2}}\left[1 - \frac{1/\sqrt{2}}{\sqrt{4 - 1/2}}\right]$$

$$= 2\sqrt{2}\left(1 - \frac{1}{\sqrt{7}}\right)$$

$$= 1.76\text{ cm}$$

Example 16. *A point object O is placed in front of a concave mirror of focal length 10 cm. A glass slab of refractive index $\mu = 3/2$ and thickness 6 cm is inserted between object and mirror. Find the position of final image when the distance x shown in figure is*
(i) 5 cm and *(ii) 20 cm*

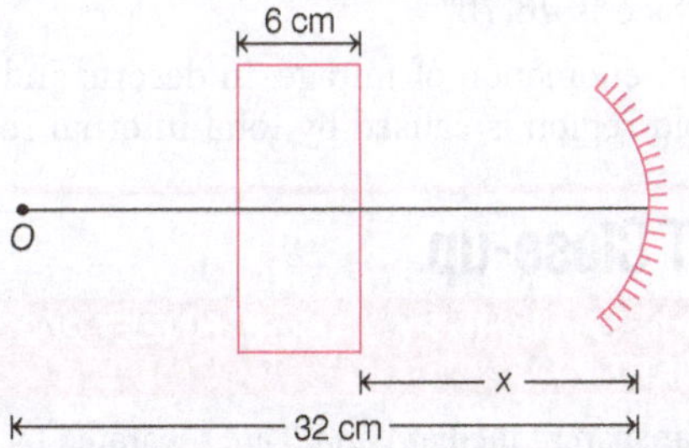

Sol. As we know, the normal shift produced by a glass slab,

$$\Delta x = \left(1 - \frac{1}{\mu}\right) t = \left(1 - \frac{2}{3}\right)(6) = 2 \text{ cm}$$

i.e., for the mirror the object is placed at a distance $(32 - \Delta x) = 32 - 2 = 30$ cm from it.

Applying mirror formula,

$$\frac{1}{v} + \frac{1}{u} = \frac{1}{f} \text{ or } \frac{1}{v} - \frac{1}{30} = -\frac{1}{10} \text{ or } v = -15 \text{ cm}$$

(i) **When x = 5 cm** The light falls on the slab on its return journey as shown. But the slab will again shift it by a distance, $\Delta x = 2$ cm. Hence, the final **real** image is formed at a distance $(15 + 2) = 17$ cm from the mirror.

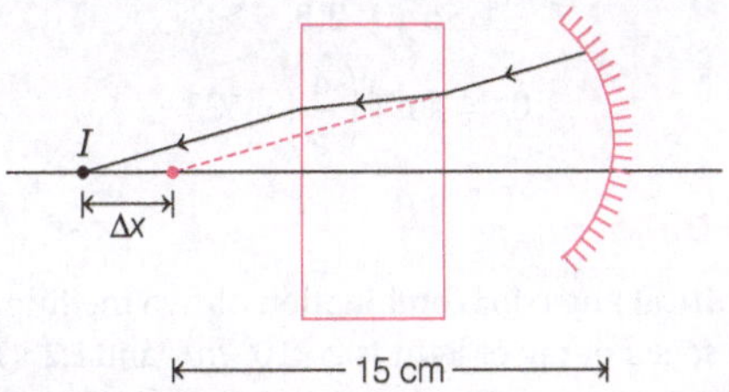

(ii) **When x = 20 cm** This time also the final image is at a distance 17 cm from the mirror but it is **virtual** as shown.

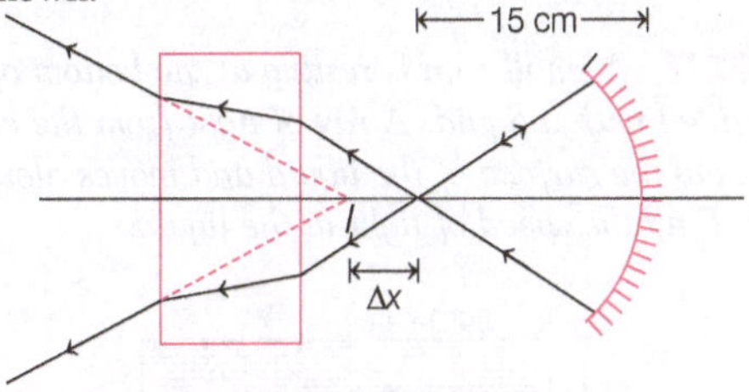

Critical Angle and Total Internal Reflection (TIR)

Whenever a ray of light goes from a denser medium to a rarer medium, it bends away from the normal. As angle of incidence in denser medium increases, angle of refraction also increases in rarer medium.

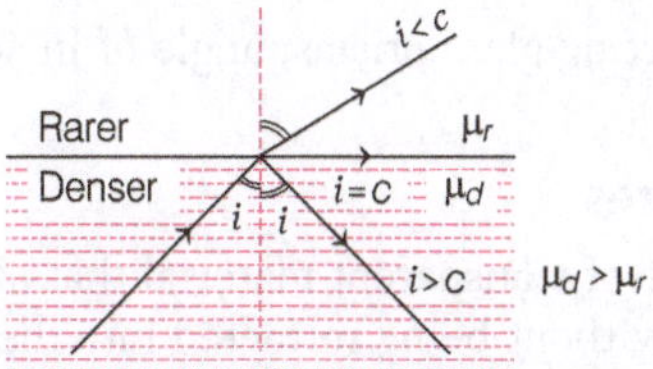

Total internal reflection

The angle of incidence ($\angle i$) in denser medium for which the angle of refraction ($\angle r$) in rarer medium is 90° is called the critical angle ($\angle C$ or $\angle \theta_C$).

$$\Rightarrow \quad \frac{\sin C}{\sin 90°} = \frac{\mu_{\text{rarer}}}{\mu_{\text{denser}}} = \frac{\mu_r}{\mu_d}$$

$$\Rightarrow \quad \sin C = \frac{\mu_r}{\mu_d} \Rightarrow C = \sin^{-1}\left(\frac{\mu_r}{\mu_d}\right)$$

Now, if the angle of incidence ($\angle i$) in the rarer medium is greater than the critical angle ($\angle C$), then the ray instead of suffering refraction is totally reflected back in the same (denser) medium.

This phenomenon is called total internal reflection. For total internal reflection to take place, following set of conditions must be obeyed.

(i) The ray must travel from denser medium to rarer medium.

(ii) The angle of incidence ($\angle i$) must be greater than the critical angle ($\angle C$).

Concept ladder When the rarer medium is air, $\mu_r = 1$ and $\mu_d = \mu$, then

Critical angle, $C = \sin^{-1}\left(\frac{1}{\mu}\right)$

Applications of Total Internal Reflection

TIR has following applications :

(i) Totally Reflecting Prisms

These prisms are right-angled isosceles triangle which turn light ray by 90° or 180°. They are based on the phenomenon of total internal reflection. Refractive index of crown glass is 3/2.

$$\text{Hence, } C = \sin^{-1}\left(\frac{1}{\mu}\right) = \sin^{-1}\left(\frac{2}{3}\right) \approx 42°$$

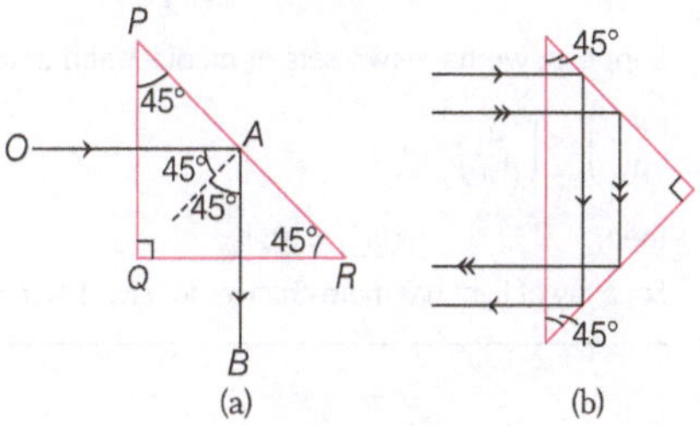

Prism reflectors

In totally reflecting glass prisms, angle of incidence is made 45° (> C).

(ii) Optical Fibres

It is a thin tube of transparent material that allows light to pass through, without being refracted into the air or another external medium. These fibres work on the principle of total internal reflection.

Optical fibres are fabricated with high quality composite glass/quartz fibres. The refractive index of core is higher than that of the cladding. When a signal in the form of light is directed at one end of the fibre at a suitable angle, it undergoes repeated total internal reflection along the length of the fibre and finally comes out from other end. Due to total internal reflection at each stage, no absorption of light takes places *i.e.*, there is no appreciable loss in the intensity of light.

Optical fibres are fabricated in such a way that light reflected at one side of the inner surface strikes the other surface at an angle larger than critical angle. Even, if fibre is bent, light can easily travel along the length.

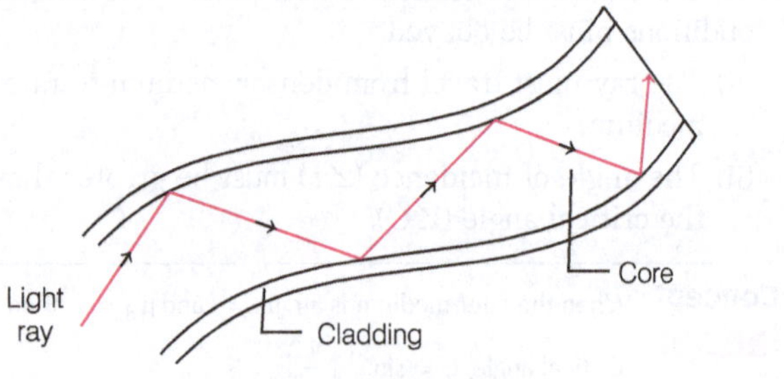

Typical structure of optical fibre

Uses

(i) In transmitting electrical and optical signals.
(ii) In visual examination of internal organs like esophagus, stomach and intestine.
(iii) In decorative lamps.

Concept ladder

- In optical fibres, $\mu_{core} > \mu_{cladding}$ and θ_c or $C = \sin^{-1}\left(\frac{\mu_{cladding}}{\mu_{core}}\right)$
- As, we have seen, $\theta_C = \sin^{-1}\left(\frac{\mu_r}{\mu_d}\right)$

Suppose, we have two sets of media 1 and 2 and $\left(\frac{\mu_r}{\mu_d}\right)_1 < \left(\frac{\mu_r}{\mu_d}\right)_2$

then, $(\theta_C)_1 < (\theta_C)_2$

So, a ray of light has more chances to have TIR in medium 1.

Some other Examples of Total Internal Reflection

(i) The sparkling of diamond is due to total internal reflection inside it.
(ii) Shining of air bubble in water is also due to total internal reflection. The critical angle of water-air interface is 48.75°.
(iii) The phenomenon of mirage in deserts and looming in cold region is caused by total internal reflection.

NEET Close-up

Example Similar to PYQ Asked in NEET 2022 and NEET 2023

Two transparent media A and B are separated by a plane boundary. The speed of light in those media is 1.2×10^8 m/s and 1.5×10^8 m/s respectively. Find critical angle of a ray of light for these two media.

(a) 53° (b) 67° (c) 48° (d) 57°

Sol. (*a*) $\mu_A = \frac{3 \times 10^8}{1.2 \times 10^8} = 2.5$

$$\mu_B = \frac{3 \times 10^8}{1.5 \times 10^8} = 2$$

For TIR, ray should travel from denser to rarer medium.

$$\mu_A \sin\theta_C = \mu_B \sin 90°$$

$$\sin\theta_C = \frac{\mu_B}{\mu_A} = \frac{2}{2.5} = \frac{4}{5}$$

$$\Rightarrow \quad \theta_C = \sin^{-1}\left(\frac{4}{5}\right) = 53°$$

Skill Builder

Find critical angle for combination of two mediums in which speed of ray of light is 2×10^8 m/s and 1.2×10^8 m/s.

(a) 30° (b) 37° (c) 45° (d) 60°

For more Practice Refer Q. No. 17 of step-up practice 2 and Q. No. 28, 33 of Gearing up for NEET.°

Example 17. *A small coin is resting at the bottom of a beaker filled with a liquid. A ray of light from the coin travels upto the surface of the liquid and moves along its surface. Find the speed of light in the liquid.*

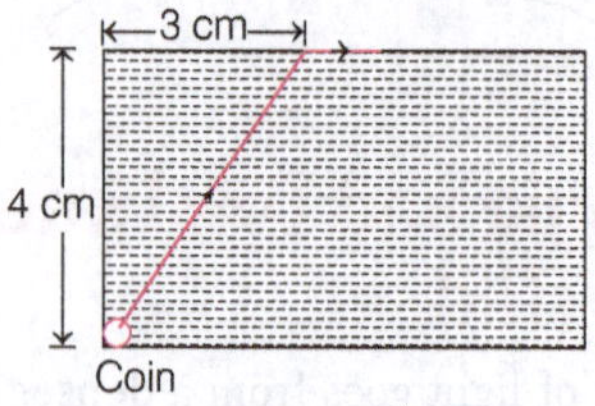

Sol. As shown in figure, a light ray from the coin will not emerge out of liquid, hence $i > C$.

Therefore, minimum radius R corresponds to, $i = C$

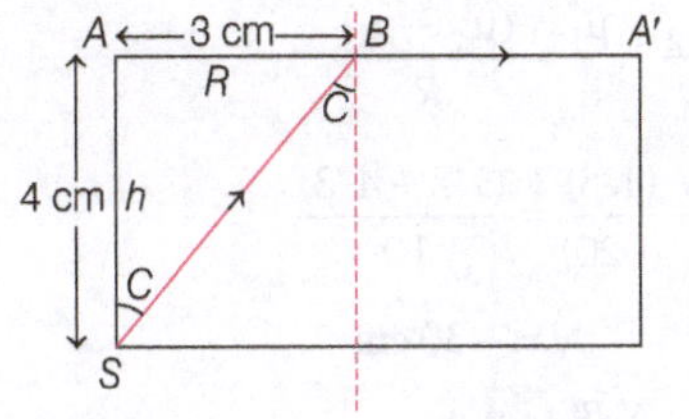

In ΔSAB, $\frac{R}{h} = \tan C$

$\Rightarrow \quad R = h \tan C$

$\Rightarrow \quad R = \frac{h}{\sqrt{\mu^2 - 1}} \qquad (\because \sin C = \mu)$

Given, $R = 3$ cm and $h = 4$ cm

$\therefore \quad \frac{3}{4} = \frac{1}{\sqrt{\mu^2 - 1}}$

$\Rightarrow \quad \mu^2 = \frac{25}{9}$

$\Rightarrow \quad \mu = \frac{5}{3}$

But, $\quad \mu = \frac{c}{v}$

$\Rightarrow$ Speed of light in liquid, $v = \frac{c}{\mu} = \frac{3 \times 10^8}{5/3}$

$= 1.8 \times 10^8 \text{ ms}^{-1}$

Refraction at Spherical Surfaces

When two transparent media are separated by a spherical surface, light incident on the surface from one side get refracted into the medium on the other side. Spherical surfaces are of two types as shown in figure.

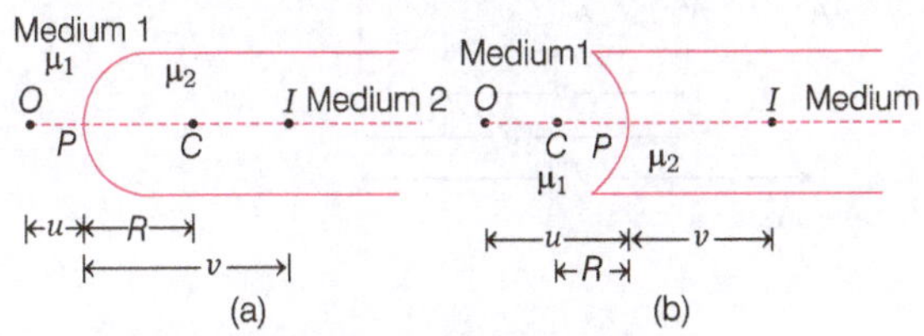

Spherical surface (a) convex (b) concave

For both surfaces, refraction formula is given by

$$\frac{\mu_2}{v} - \frac{\mu_1}{u} = \frac{\mu_2 - \mu_1}{R}$$

where μ_1 = refractive index of first medium,

μ_2 = refractive index of second medium,

R = radius of curvature of spherical surfaces,

u = object distance

and $\quad v$ = image distance.

Transverse magnification, $m = \frac{h_I}{h_O} = \frac{\mu_1 v}{\mu_2 u}$

Mentor's TiP

- For a plane surface, $R = \infty$, $\frac{\mu_2}{v} - \frac{\mu_1}{u} = 0$

Example 18. *Locate the image of the point object O. The point C is centre of curvature of the spherical surface.*

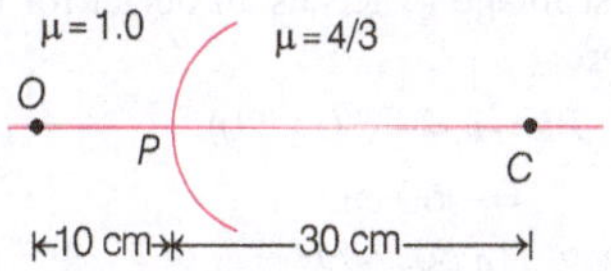

Sol. Here, $\mu_1 = 1$, $\mu_2 = 4/3$, $u = -10$ cm and $R = 30$ cm

Using the relation, $\frac{\mu_2}{v} - \frac{\mu_1}{u} = \frac{\mu_2 - \mu_1}{R}$

Substituting the values,

$\Rightarrow \quad \frac{4/3}{v} - \frac{1}{-10} = \frac{4/3 - 1}{30}$

$\Rightarrow \quad \frac{4}{3v} + \frac{1}{10} = \frac{1}{90}$

$\Rightarrow \quad \frac{4}{3v} = \frac{1}{90} - \frac{1}{10} = \frac{-8}{90}$

$\Rightarrow \quad v = -15$ cm

The image is formed 15 cm left of spherical surface and is virtual.

Example 19. *A glass sphere of radius $R = 10$ cm is kept inside water. A point object O is placed at 20 cm from A as shown in figure. Find the position and nature of the image when seen from other side of the sphere. Also draw the ray diagram. Given, $\mu_g = 3/2$ and $\mu_w = 4/3$.*

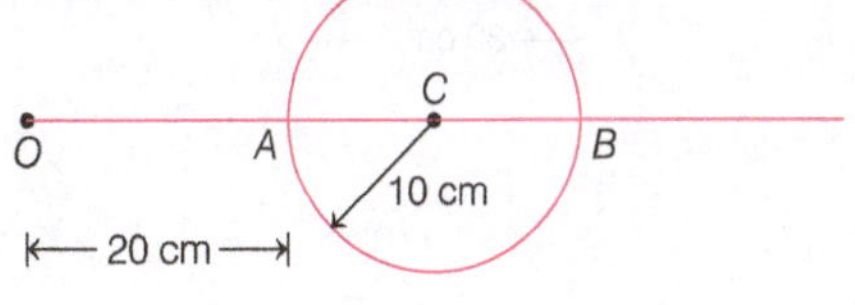

Sol. A ray of light starting from O gets refracted twice. The ray of light is travelling in a direction from left to right. Hence, the distances measured in this direction are taken positive.

Applying, $\frac{\mu_2}{v} - \frac{\mu_1}{u} = \frac{\mu_2 - \mu_1}{R}$, twice with proper signs.

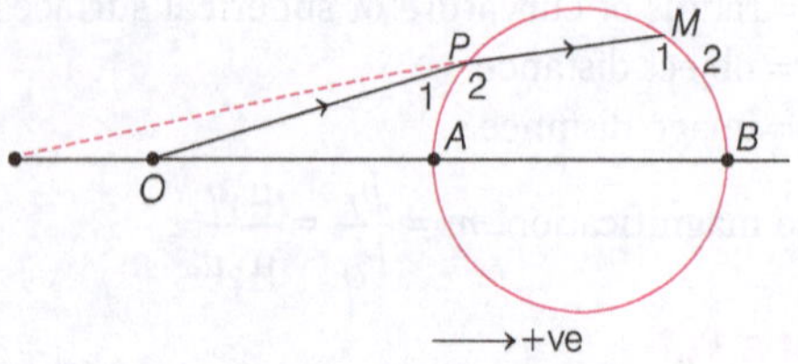

We have, $\frac{3/2}{AI_1} - \frac{4/3}{-20} = \frac{3/2 - 4/3}{10}$

or $AI_1 = -30$ cm

Now, the first image I_1, acts as an object for the second surface, where

$$BI_1 = u = -(30 + 20)$$
$$= -50 \text{ cm}$$

$\therefore \frac{4/3}{BI_2} - \frac{3/2}{-50} = \frac{4/3 - 3/2}{-10}$

$\therefore$ $BI_2 = -100$ cm, *i.e.* the final image I_2 is **virtual** and is formed at a distance 100 cm (towards left) from B. The ray diagram is as shown.

Following points should be noted while drawing the ray diagram.

(i) At point P, the ray travels from rarer to a denser medium. Hence, it will bend towards normal PC. At point M, it travels from a denser to a rarer medium, hence, moves away from the normal MC.

(ii) PM ray when extended backwards meets at I_1 and MN ray when extended meets at I_2.

Example 20. *A linear object of length 4 cm is placed at 30 cm from the plane surface of hemispherical glass of radius 10 cm. The hemispherical glass is surrounded by water. Find the final position and size of the image.*

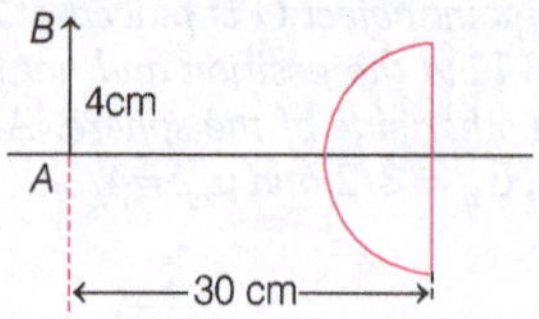

Sol. For 1st surface,

$$\mu_1 = \frac{4}{3}, \mu_2 = \frac{3}{2}, u = -20 \text{ cm and } R = +10 \text{ cm}$$

Using, $\frac{\mu_2}{v} - \frac{\mu_1}{\mu} = \frac{(\mu_2 - \mu_1)}{R}$

$\Rightarrow \frac{(3/2)}{v} - \frac{(4/3)}{(-20)} = \frac{(3/2 - 4/3)}{10}$

$\Rightarrow v = -30$ cm

Using, $\frac{A'B'}{AB} = \frac{\mu_1 v}{\mu_2 u}$

$\Rightarrow \frac{A'B'}{(4 \text{ cm})} = \frac{(4/3)(-30)}{(3/2)(-20)}$

$\Rightarrow A'B' = 5.3$ cm

$A'B'$ behaves as the object for plane surface,

$$\mu_1 = \frac{3}{2}, \mu_2 = \frac{4}{3}$$

and $R = \infty, u' = -40$

$\Rightarrow \frac{\mu_2}{v'} = \frac{\mu_1}{u'}$

$\Rightarrow \frac{(4/3)}{v'} = \frac{(3/2)}{(-40)}$

Solving it, we will get, $v' = -35.5$ cm

Now, using, $\frac{A''B''}{A'B'} = \frac{(\mu_1 v')}{(\mu_2 u')}$

$$\frac{A''B''}{(5.3)} = \frac{(3/2)(-35.5)}{(4/3)(-40)}$$

$\Rightarrow A''B'' \simeq 5.3$ cm

The final images in all the above cases are shown in figure.

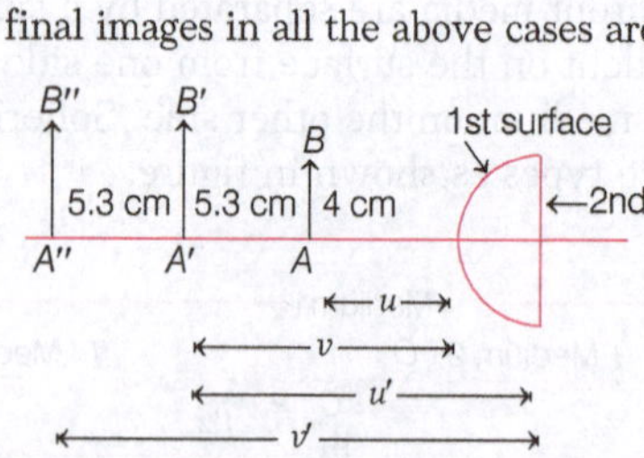

STEP UP Practice 2

1. When a ray of light falls on a given plate at an angle of incidence 60°, the reflected and refracted rays are found to be normal to each other. The refractive index of the material of the plate is
(a) $\frac{\sqrt{3}}{2}$ (b) 1.5
(c) 1.732 (d) 2

2. **Statement I** If $n_{21} > 1$, refracted ray bends towards the normal and when $n_{21} < 1$, refracted ray bends away from the normal.
Statement II $n_{21} = \frac{\sin i}{\sin r}$, angle i is in medium 1 and angle r is in medium 2.
In the light of the above statements, choose the most appropriate answer from the options given below.
(a) Both Statement I and Statement II are incorrect.
(b) Statement I is correct but Statement II is incorrect.
(c) Statement I is incorrect but Statement II is correct.
(d) Both Statement I and Statement II are correct.

3. A light wave has a frequency of 4×10^{14} Hz and a wavelength of 5×10^{-7} m in a medium. The refractive index of the medium is
(a) 1.5 (b) 1.33
(c) 1.25 (d) 1.75

4. If ${}_i\mu_j$ represents refractive index when a light ray goes from medium i to medium j, then the product ${}_2\mu_1 \times {}_3\mu_2 \times {}_4\mu_3$ is equal to
(a) ${}_3\mu_1$ (b) ${}_3\mu_2$
(c) $\frac{1}{{}_1\mu_4}$ (d) ${}_4\mu_2$

5. **Statement I** Refractive index of glass with respect to air is different for red light and violet light.
Statement II Refractive index of a pair of media depends on the wavelength of light used.
In the light of the above statements, choose the most appropriate answer from the options given below.
(a) Both Statement I and Statement II are incorrect.
(b) Statement I is correct but Statement II is incorrect.
(c) Statement I is incorrect but Statement II is correct.
(d) Both Statement I and Statement II are correct.

6. Absolute refractive indices of glass and water are $\frac{3}{2}$ and $\frac{4}{3}$. The ratio of velocities of light in glass and water will be
(a) 4 : 3 (b) 9 : 8
(c) 8 : 9 (d) 3 : 4

7. The refractive index of a certain glass is 1.5 for light whose wavelength in vacuum is 6000 Å. The wavelength of this light when it passes through glass is
(a) 4000 Å (b) 6000 Å
(c) 9000 Å (d) 15000 Å

8. The refractive indices of glass and water with respect to air are 3/2 and 4/3, respectively.The refractive index of glass with respect to water will be
(a) 8/9 (b) 9/8
(c) 7/6 (d) None of these

9. **Statement I** When a ray of light is refracted from water to glass, its wavelength decreases while frequency does not change.
Statement II When a ray of light is refracted from water of glass, it bends towards normal.
In the light of the above statements, choose the most appropriate answer from the options given below.
(a) Both Statement I and Statement II are incorrect.
(b) Statement I is correct but Statement II is incorrect.
(c) Statement I is incorrect but Statement II is correct.
(d) Both Statement I and Statement II are correct.

10. A spot is placed on the bottom of a slab made of transparent material of refractive index 1.5. The spot is viewed vertically from the top when it seems to be raised by 2 cm. Then, the height of the slab is
(a) 10 cm (b) 8 cm (c) 6 cm (d) 4 cm

11. An air bubble inside a glass slab ($\mu = 1.5$) appears 6 cm when viewed from one side and 4 cm when viewed from the opposite side. The thickness of the slab is
(a) 10 cm (b) 6.67 cm
(c) 15 cm (d) None of these

12. An under water swimmer is at a depth of 12 m below the surface of water. A bird is at a height of 18 m from the surface of water, directly above his eyes. For the swimmer the bird appears to be at a distance from the surface of water equal to (Refractive index of water is 4/3)
(a) 24 m (b) 12 m (c) 18 m (d) 9 m

13. A vessel of depth 2 d cm is half filled with a liquid of refractive index μ_1 and the upper half with a liquid of refractive index μ_2. The apparent depth of the vessel when seen perpendicularly from above is
(a) $d\left[\frac{\mu_1\mu_2}{\mu_1+\mu_2}\right]$ (b) $d\left[\frac{1}{\mu_1}+\frac{1}{\mu_2}\right]$
(c) $2d\left[\frac{1}{\mu_1}+\frac{1}{\mu_2}\right]$ (d) $2d\left[\frac{1}{\mu_1\mu_2}\right]$

14. Three immiscible transparent liquids with refractive indices 3/2, 4/3 and 6/5 are arranged one on top of another. The depths of the liquids are 3 cm, 4 cm and 6 cm, respectively. The apparent depth of the vessel is
(a) 10 cm (b) 9 cm (c) 8 cm (d) 7 cm

15. A glass slab is immersed in water. What will be the critical angle for a light ray at glass-water interface?
[Take, ${}_an_g = 1.50$, ${}_an_w = 1.33$ and $\sin^{-1}(0.887) = 62.5$]
(a) 48.8° (b) 72.8° (c) 62.5° (d) 64.5°

16. **Statement I** Critical angle of light while passing from glass to air is minimum for violet colour.
Statement II The wavelength of violet light is greater than the light of other colours.
In the light of the above statements, choose the most appropriate answer from the options given below :
(a) Both Statement I and Statement II are incorrect.
(b) Statement I is correct but Statement II is incorrect.
(c) Statement I is incorrect but Statement II is correct.
(d) Both Statement I and Statement II are correct.

17. The wavelength of light in two liquids x and y is 3500 Å and 7000 Å respectively, then the critical angle of x relative to y will be
(a) 60° (b) 45° (c) 30° (d) 15°

18. White light is incident on the interface of glass and air as shown in the figure. If green light is just totally internally reflected, then the emerging ray in air contains

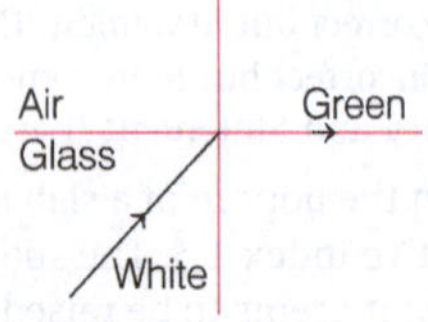

(a) yellow, orange, red
(b) violet, indigo, blue
(c) all colours
(d) all colours except green

19. **Statement I** Propagation of light through an optical fibre is due to total internal reflection taking place at the core-clade interface.
Statement II Refractive index of the material of the core of the optical fibre is greater than that of cladding.
In the light of the above statements, choose the most appropriate answer from the options given below :
(a) Both Statement I and Statement II are incorrect.
(b) Statement I is correct but Statement II is incorrect.
(c) Statement I is incorrect but Statement II is correct.
(d) Both Statement I and Statement II are correct.

20. A ray of light travelling in a transparent medium falls on a surface separating the medium from air at an angle of incidence of 45°. The ray undergoes total internal reflection. If n is the refractive index of the medium with respect to air, select the possible value of n from the following.
(a) 1.2 (b) 4/3 (c) 1.4 (d) 1.5

21. Which one of the following pairs given below is incorrect?
(a) Snell's law → $\frac{\sin i}{\sin r} = \text{constant}$
(b) Cauchy's formula → $\mu = A + \frac{B}{\lambda^2}$
(c) Apparent shift → $d(1-\mu)$
(d) Lateral shift (d) → $\left[1 - \frac{\cos i}{\sqrt{\mu^2 - \sin^2 i}}\right] t \sin i$

Module 3

Lens and Prism

• Lenses • Image Formation by Lenses • Lens Maker's Formula and Lens Formula
• Focal Length of Different Lenses • Lens Immersed in a Liquid • Magnification Produced by a Lens
• Power of a Lens • Combination of Two or More Thin Lenses • Prism • Dispersion of Light by a Prism

Lenses

Lens is a transparent medium (material) bounded by two surfaces atleast one of which should be spherical. Refractive index of the medium (material) should also be different from the surroundings.
Lenses are of two types.

(i) **Convex or converging lens** In this lens, a transparent medium is bounded by two surfaces such that it is thicker in the middle.

It is of four types (as shown)

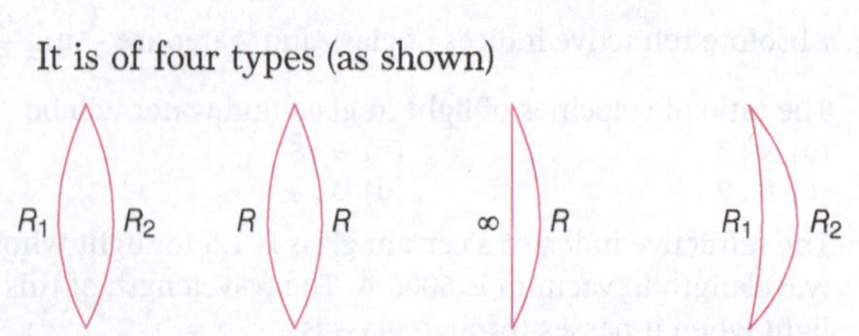

(a) Bi-convex or double-convex lens (b) Equi-convex or convex lens (c) Plano-convex lens (d) Concavo-convex lens

Types of convex lens

(ii) **Concave or diverging lens** In this lens, a transparent medium is bounded by two surfaces such that it is thinner in the middle. It is of four types (as shown)

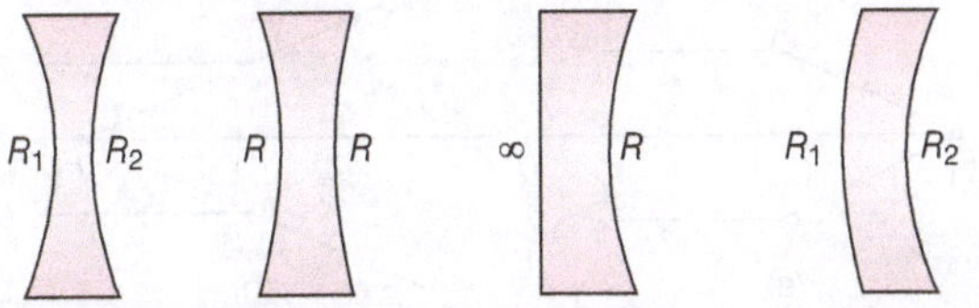

(a) Bi-concave or double-concave lens (b) Equi-concave or concave lens (c) Plano-concave lens (d) Convexo-concave lens

Types of concave lens

Some Definitions Related to Lenses

(i) **Optical centre** The optical centre is a point within or outside the lens, at which incident rays refract without deviation in its path.

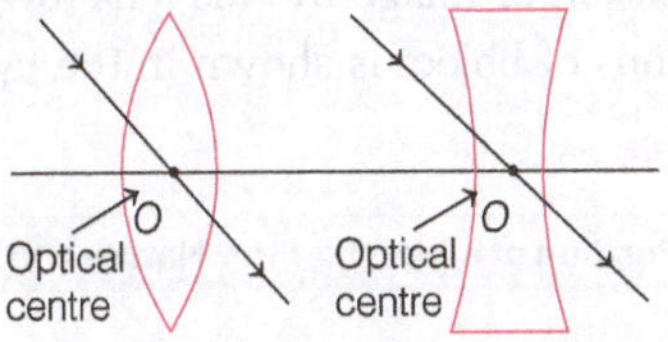

Optical centre

(ii) **Centre of curvature** The centres of the two imaginary spheres of which the lens is a part are called centres of curvature of the lens. A lens has two centres of curvature with respect to its two curved surfaces.

(iii) **Radii of curvature** The radii of the two imaginary spheres of which the lens is a part are called radii of curvature of the lens. A lens has two radii of curvature. These may or may not be equal.

(iv) **Principal axis** The straight line passing through the optical centre and centre of curvature of lens is called principal axis of lens.

(v) **Principal focus** Lens has two principal focus.

(a) **First principal focus** It is a point on the principal axis of lens, the rays starting from which (convex lens) or appear to converge at which (concave lens) become parallel to principal axis after refraction.

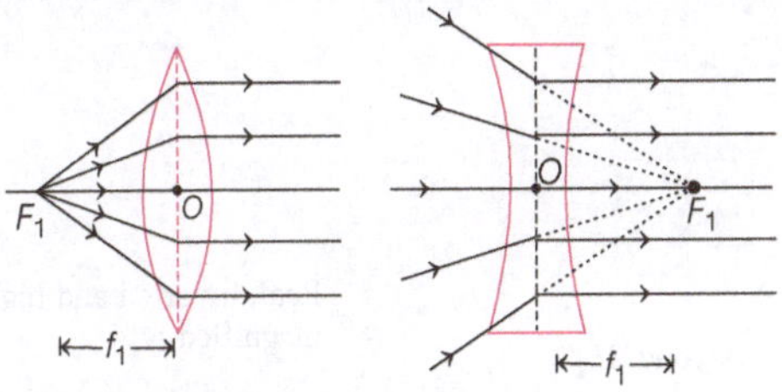

First principal focus

(b) **Second principal focus** It is the point on the principal axis at which the rays coming parallel to the principal axis converge (convex lens) or appear to diverge (concave lens) after refraction from the lens.

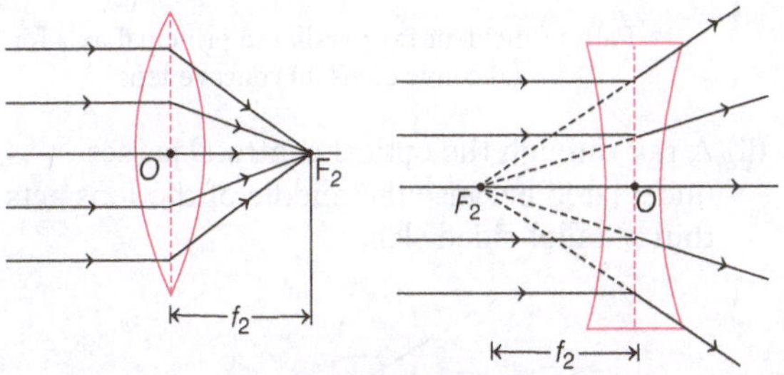

Second principal focus

Both the focuses of convex lens are real, while that of concave lens are virtual.

(vi) **Focal length** The distance between focus and optical centre of lens is called focal length of lens.

(vii) **Aperture** The effective diameter of circular boundary of the lens is called aperture.

Sign Convention for Lenses

(i) Sign convention for lenses are same as for spherical surfaces.

(ii) From the Figures, we can see that f_1 is negative for a convex lens and positive for a concave lens. But, f_2 is positive for convex lens and negative for concave lens.

(iii) $|f_1| = |f_2|$, if the media on the two sides of a thin lens have same refractive index.

(iv) We are mainly concerned with the second focus f_2. Thus, wherever we write the focal length f, it means the second principal focal length. Thus, $f = f_2$ and hence, f is positive for a convex lens and negative for a concave lens.

Law for Formation of Images by Lens

The position and nature of the image by lens, in any case can be obtained either from a ray diagram or by calculation.

Ray diagram

To construct the image of a small object perpendicular to the axis of a lens, two of the following three rays are drawn from the top of the object.

(i) A ray parallel to the principal axis after refraction passes through the principal focus or appears to diverge from it.

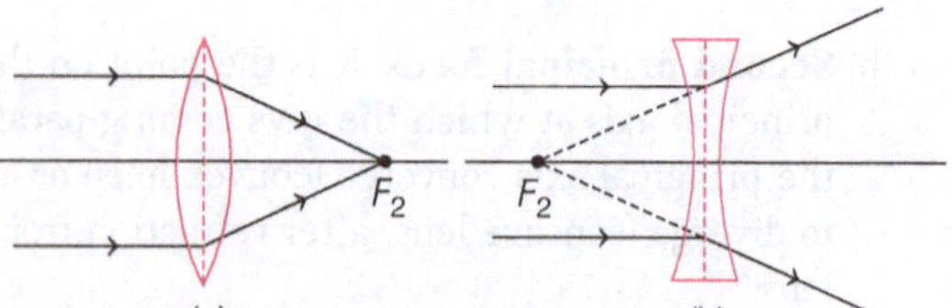

Path of incident ray parallel to principal axis for
(a) convex lens (b) concave lens

(ii) A ray through the optical centre O passes undeviated because the middle of the lens acts like a thin parallel-sided slab.

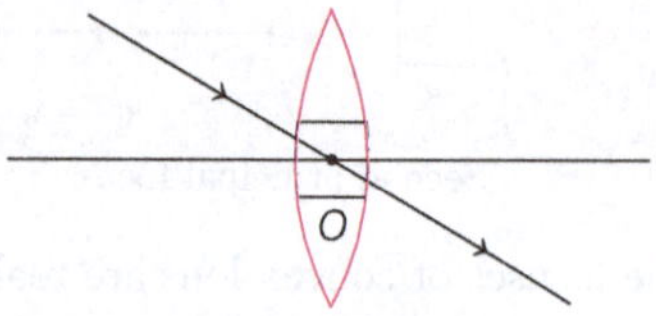

Path of incident ray passing through centre for convex lens

(iii) A ray passing through (incase of convex lens) or appears to pass through (incase of concave lens) the first focus F_1, becomes parallel to the principal axis after refraction.

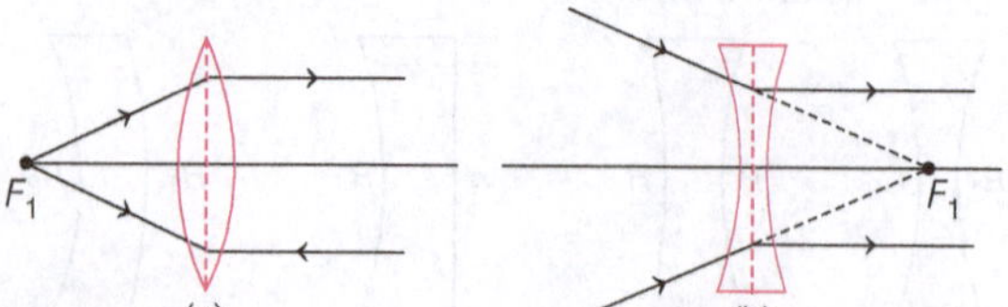

Path of incident ray passing through the focus for
(a) convex lens (b) concave lens

Image Formation by Lenses

Convex Lens

The image formed by convex lens depends on the position of object. Formation of image by this lens for different positions of object is shown in the table.

Formation of Image by Convex Lens

S.No.	Position of object	Ray diagram	Position of image	Nature and size of image
(i)	At infinity	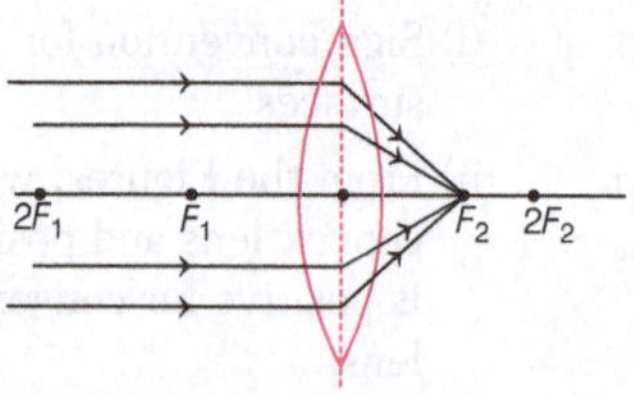	At the principal focus (F_2) or in the focal plane	Real, inverted and extremely diminished
(ii)	Beyond $2F_1$	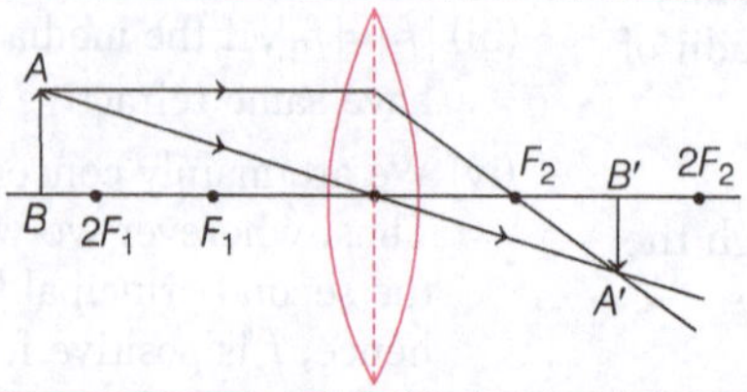	Between F_2 and $2F_2$	Real, inverted and diminished
(iii)	At $2F_1$	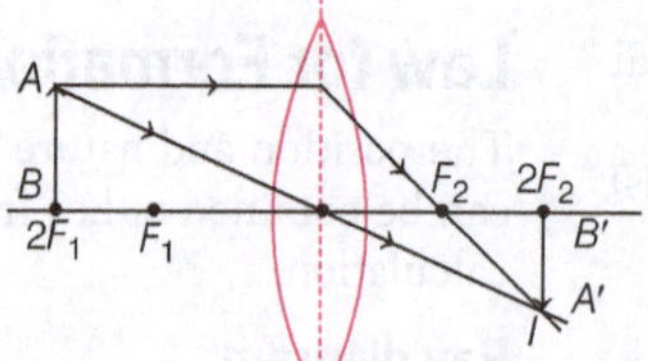	At $2F_2$	Real, inverted and of same size as the object
(iv)	Between F_1 and $2F_1$	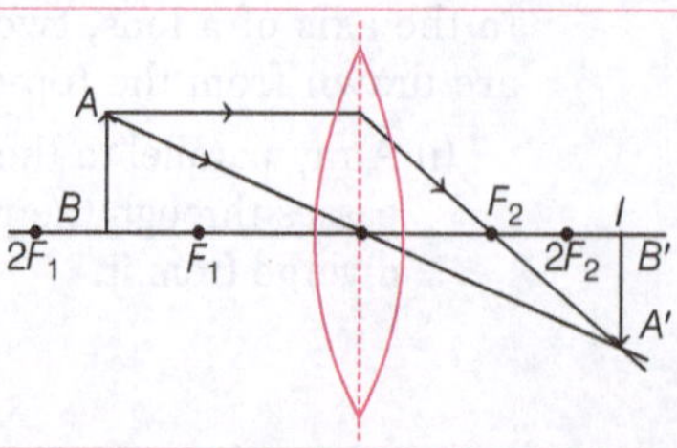	Beyond $2F_2$	Real, inverted and highly magnified

(v)	At F_1	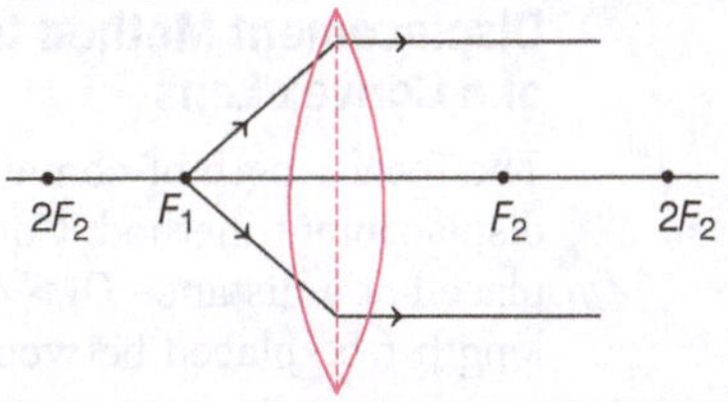	At infinity	Real, inverted and extremely magnified
(vi)	Between F_1 and optical centre	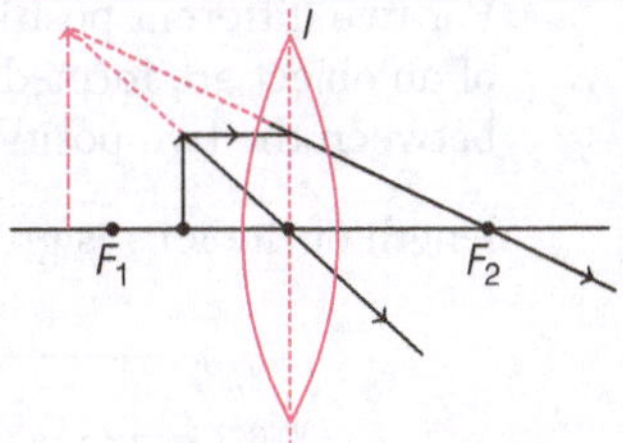	On the same side as the object	Virtual, erect and magnified

Concave Lens

The image formed by a concave lens is always virtual, erect and diminished. The image formation by this lens for different positions of object is shown in the table given below.

Image Formation by Concave Lens

S. No.	Position of object	Ray diagram	Position of image	Nature and size of image
(i)	At infinity	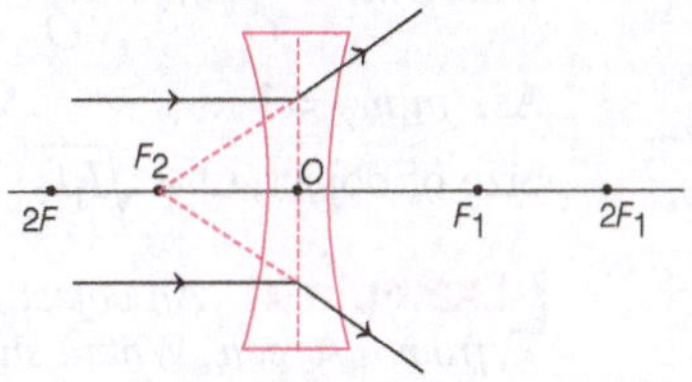	At the focus	Virtual, erect and point sized
(ii)	Anywhere on the principal axis	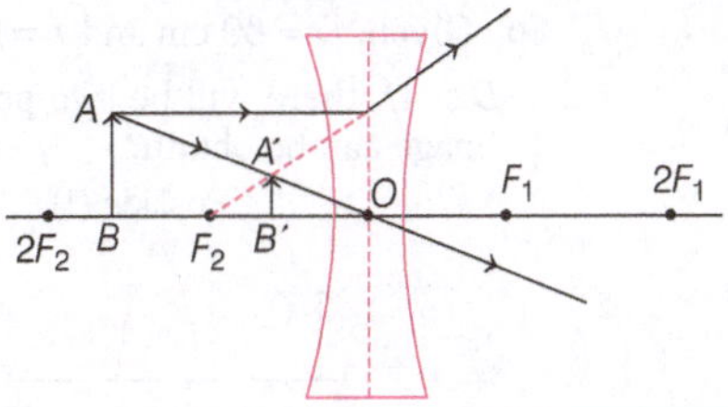	Between optical centre and F_2	Virtual, erect and diminished

Lens Maker's Formula and Lens Formula

Lens Maker's Formula

If R_1 and R_2 are the radii of curvature of first and second refracting surfaces of a thin lens of focal length f and refractive index μ (with respect to surrounding medium), the relation between f, μ, R_1 and R_2 is known as lens maker's formula and is given by,

$$\frac{1}{f} = (\mu - 1)\left(\frac{1}{R_1} - \frac{1}{R_2}\right)$$

Lens Formula

The expression which shows the relation between u, v and f is called lens formula and given by,

$$\frac{1}{v} - \frac{1}{u} = \frac{1}{f}$$

where, u is distance of object from the lens, v is distance of image from the lens and f is focal length of the lens.

Focal Length of Different Lenses

Focal lengths of different lenses are given below.

(i) **For equi-convex lens,** $R_1 = +R$ and $R_2 = -R$

$$f = \frac{R}{2(\mu - 1)}$$

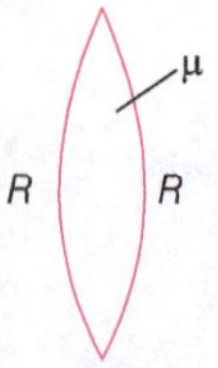

Equi-convex lens

(ii) **For equi-concave lens,** $R_1 = -R$ and $R_2 = +R$

$$f = -\frac{R}{2(\mu - 1)}$$

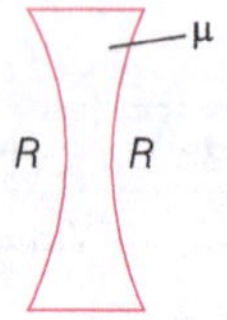

Equi-concave lens

(iii) **For plano-convex lens** $R_1 = R$ and $R_2 = \infty$

$$\therefore \quad f = \frac{R}{\mu - 1}$$

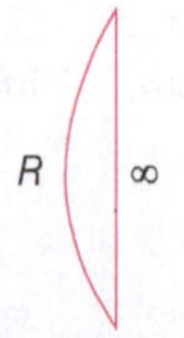

Plano-convex lens

(iv) **For plano-concave lens,**

$$R_1 = \infty, R_2 = R$$

$$\Rightarrow \quad f = \frac{-R}{(\mu - 1)}$$

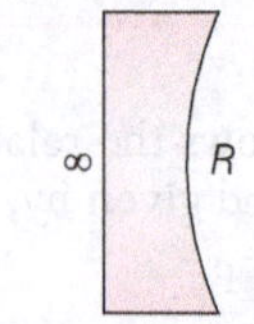

Plano-concave lens

Concept ladder
- In case of thin convex lens, if an object is placed at a distance x_1, from first focus and its image is formed at distance x_2, from the second focus, then $x_1 x_2 = f^2$.
- If some portion of a lens is covered with black paper, then full image will be formed but the brightness will be reduced.

Displacement Method to Determine the Focal Length of a Convex Lens

The focal length of convex lens can be determined by displacement method. Consider an object and a screen placed at a distance $D(> 4f)$ apart. Let a lens of focal length f be placed between the object and the screen. For two different positions of lens, two images (I_1 and I_2) of an object are formed at the screen. Let the distance between the two positions of the lens is x, then the focal length of the lens is given by $f = \dfrac{D^2 - x^2}{4D} = \dfrac{x}{m_1 - m_2}$

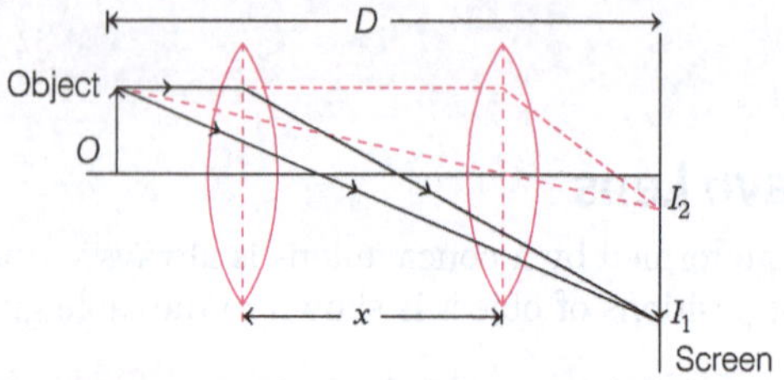

Two convex lenses separated by distance x

where $m_1 = \dfrac{I_1}{O}$, $m_2 = \dfrac{I_2}{O}$

As, $m_1 m_2 = 1$

Size of object, $O = \sqrt{I_1 I_2}$

Example 21. *An object is placed at a distance of 80 cm from a screen. Where should a convex lens of focal length 15 cm be placed so as to obtain a real image of the object?*

Sol. Given, $D = 80$ cm and $f = 15$ cm

$D > 4f$, there will be two positions of lens for which real image can be obtain.

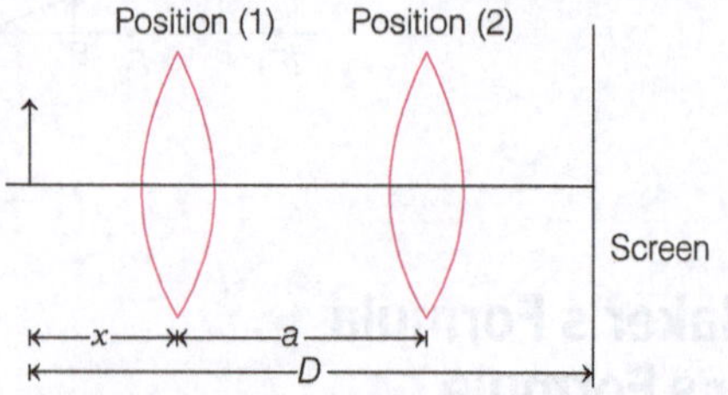

For lens in position (1), $u = -x$, $v = D - x = 80 - x$, $f = 15$ cm

As, $\dfrac{1}{v} - \dfrac{1}{u} = \dfrac{1}{f} \Rightarrow \dfrac{1}{80 - x} - \dfrac{1}{-x} = \dfrac{1}{15}$

$$\frac{80}{(80 - x)x} = \frac{1}{15} \Rightarrow x^2 - 80x + 1200 = 0$$

$$x^2 - 60x - 20x + 1200 = 0$$

$$\Rightarrow \quad x(x - 60) - 20(x - 60) = 0$$

$$\Rightarrow \quad (x - 20)(x - 60) = 0$$

$$\Rightarrow \quad x = 20 \text{ or } 60 \text{ cm}$$

Lens Immersed in a Liquid

If a lens (made of glass) of refractive index μ_g is immersed in a liquid of refractive μ_l, then its focal length f_l is given by

$$\frac{1}{f_l} = ({}_l\mu_g - 1)\left(\frac{1}{R_1} - \frac{1}{R_2}\right) \quad \text{...(i)}$$

If f_a is the focal length of lens in air, then

$$\frac{1}{f_a} = ({}_a\mu_g - 1)\left(\frac{1}{R_1} - \frac{1}{R_2}\right) \quad \text{...(ii)}$$

On dividing Eq. (ii) by Eq. (i), we get

$$\frac{f_l}{f_a} = \frac{({}_a\mu_g - 1)}{({}_l\mu_g - 1)} = \frac{({}_a\mu_g - 1)}{\left(\frac{{}_a\mu_g}{{}_a\mu_l} - 1\right)}$$

There are three cases based on this result.

(i) If $\mu_g > \mu_l$, *i.e.* lens is immersed in a liquid whose refractive index is less than that of material of lens.

Then, f_l and f_a are of same sign and $f_l > f_a$ that is the nature of lens remains unchanged, but its focal length increases and hence, power of lens decreases.

(ii) If $\mu_g = \mu_l$, *i.e.* lens is immersed in a liquid whose refractive index is same as that of material of lens.

Then, $f_l = \infty$. It means lens behaves as a plane glass plate and becomes invisible in the medium.

(iii) If $\mu_g < \mu_l$, *i.e.* lens is immersed in a liquid whose refractive index is greater than that of the material of lens.

Then, f_l and f_a have opposite signs and the nature of lens changes, *i.e.* a convex lens diverges the light rays and concave lens converges the light rays.

Example 22. *Find focal lengths of lenses made of glass ($\mu = 3/2$) and placed in air.*

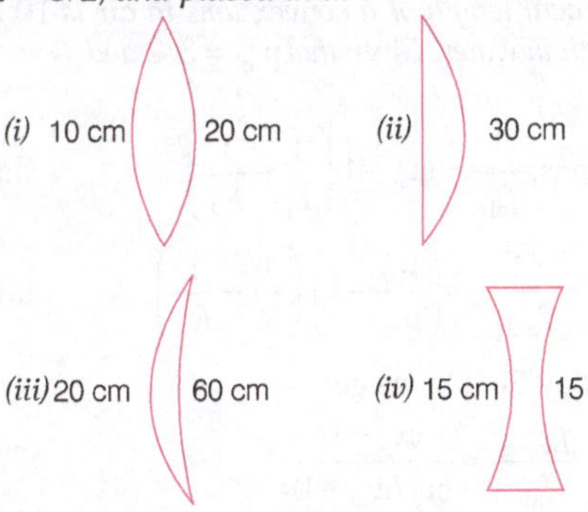

Sol. (i)

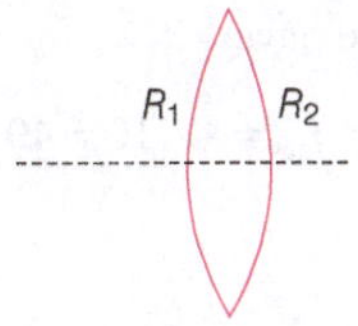

Given, $R_1 = 10$ cm, $R_2 = -20$ cm

On applying Lens maker's formula, we have

$$\frac{1}{f} = (\mu - 1)(1/R_1 - 1/R_2)$$

$$= \left(\frac{3}{2} - 1\right)\left(\frac{1}{10} - \frac{1}{(-20)}\right)$$

$$= \left(\frac{1}{2}\right)\left(\frac{3}{20}\right) = \frac{3}{40}$$

$\therefore$ Focal length of lens, $f = 40/3$ cm

(ii)

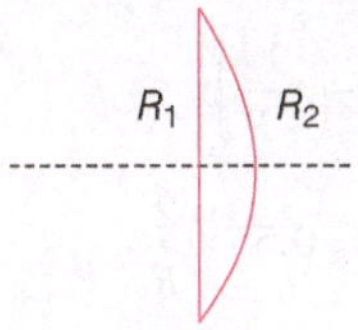

Given, $R_1 = \infty$, $R_2 = -30$ cm

From Lens maker's formula, we have

$$\frac{1}{f} = \left(\frac{3}{2} - 1\right)\left(\frac{1}{\infty} - \frac{1}{-30}\right) = \frac{1}{60}$$

$\therefore$ Focal length, $f = 60$ cm

(iii)

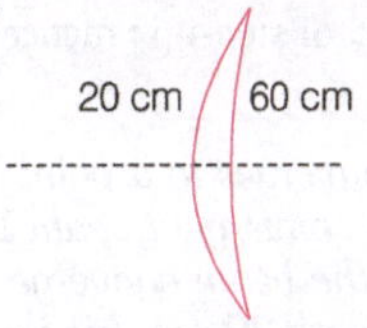

Given, $R_1 = 20$ cm, $R_2 = 30$ cm

From lens Maker's formula, we have

$$\frac{1}{f} = \left(\frac{3}{2} - 1\right)\left(\frac{1}{20} - \frac{1}{60}\right)$$

$$= \left(\frac{1}{2}\right)\left(\frac{2}{60}\right) = \frac{1}{30}$$

$\therefore$ Focal length, $f = 30$ cm

(iv)

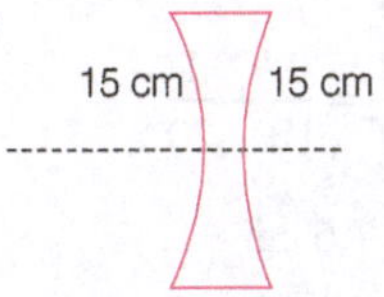

Given, $R_1 = -15$ cm, $R_2 = 15$ cm

From Lens maker's formula, we have

$$\frac{1}{f} = \left(\frac{3}{2} - 1\right)\left(\frac{1}{-15} - \frac{1}{15}\right)$$

$$= \left(\frac{1}{2}\right)\left(\frac{-2}{15}\right)$$

$\therefore$ Focal length, $f = -15$ cm

NEET Close-up

Example Similar to PYQ Asked in NEET 2019

Double-convex lenses are to be manufactured from a glass of refractive index 1.55, with both faces of the same radius of curvature. The radius of curvature required, if the focal length is to be 20 cm is

(a) 22 cm (b) 20 cm (c) 15 cm (d) 18 cm

Sol. (*a*) Using the relation,

$$\frac{1}{f} = (\mu - 1)\left(\frac{1}{R_1} - \frac{1}{R_2}\right), \text{ we get}$$

$$\frac{1}{20} = (1.55 - 1)\left[\frac{1}{R} - \left(\frac{1}{-R}\right)\right]$$

$$= 0.55\left[\frac{1}{R} + \frac{1}{R}\right] = 0.55 \times \frac{2}{R}$$

or $$R = 1.10 \times 20 = 22 \text{ cm}$$

Skill Builder

If the radius of curvature of the convex surface is 20 cm and focal length of the lens is 60 cm. Then, refractive index of the material of a plano-convex lens will be

(a) $\frac{4}{3}$ (b) $\frac{5}{3}$ (c) $\frac{5}{4}$ (d) $\frac{3}{2}$

For more Practice Refer Q. No. 15 of step-up practice 3 and Q. No. 74 of Gearing up for NEET.

Example 23. *A beam of light converges to a point P. Now a lens is placed on the path of the convergent beam 12 cm apart from P. At what point does the beam converge if the lens is (i) a convex lens of focal length 20 cm, (ii) a concave lens of focal length 16 cm?*

Sol. (i) For convex lens, $f = 20$ cm

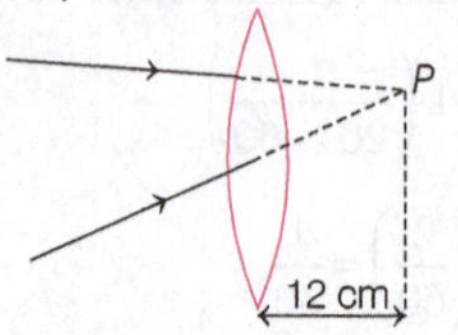

Using the formula, $\frac{1}{f} = \frac{1}{v} - \frac{1}{u}$, we get

$$\frac{1}{v} = \frac{1}{u} + \frac{1}{f} = \frac{1}{12} + \frac{1}{20}$$

$$\therefore \quad v = \frac{60}{8} = 7.5 \text{ cm}$$

i.e. the image is formed on the right of the lens and is real.

(ii) For concave lens, $f = -16$ cm

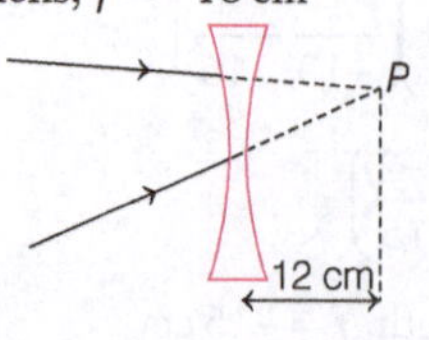

$\therefore$ Using the relation, $\frac{1}{f} = \frac{1}{v} - \frac{1}{u}$, we get

$$\frac{1}{v} = \frac{1}{f} + \frac{1}{u} = \frac{1}{-16} + \frac{1}{12}$$

$$\therefore \quad v = +48 \text{ cm}$$

The image is formed at 48 cm to the right of the lens where the beam would converge and is real.

Example 24. *The distance between two point sources of light is 24 cm. Find out where would you place a converging lens of focal length 9 cm, so that the images of both the sources are formed at the same point.*

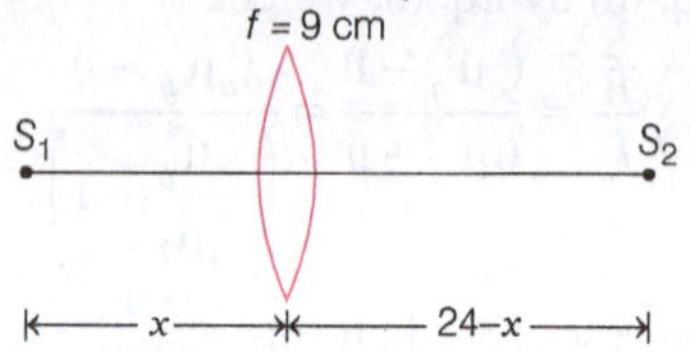

Sol. Using the relation, $\frac{1}{v} - \frac{1}{u} = \frac{1}{f}$

For S_1, $\frac{1}{v_1} - \frac{1}{-x} = \frac{1}{9} \Rightarrow \frac{1}{v_1} = \frac{1}{9} - \frac{1}{x}$ ...(i)

For S_2, $\frac{1}{v_2} - \frac{1}{-(24 - x)} = \frac{1}{9}$

$$\therefore \quad \frac{1}{v_2} = \frac{1}{9} - \frac{1}{24 - x} \quad \text{...(ii)}$$

Since, sign convention for S_1 and S_2 is just opposite. Hence,

$$v_1 = -v_2 \quad \text{or} \quad \frac{1}{v_1} = -\frac{1}{v_2}$$

$$\therefore \quad \frac{1}{9} - \frac{1}{x} = \frac{1}{24 - x} - \frac{1}{9}$$

Solving this equation we get, $x = 6$ cm. Therefore, the lens should be kept at a distance of 6 cm from either of the object.

Example 25. *Focal length of a convex lens in air is 10 cm. Find its focal length in water. Given that* $\mu_g = 3/2$ *and* $\mu_w = 4/3$.

Sol. Using the relations, $\frac{1}{f_{air}} = (\mu_g - 1)\left(\frac{1}{R_1} - \frac{1}{R_2}\right)$ ...(i)

and $\frac{1}{f_{water}} = \left(\frac{\mu_g}{\mu_w} - 1\right)\left(\frac{1}{R_1} - \frac{1}{R_2}\right)$ ...(ii)

Dividing Eq. (i) by Eq. (ii), we get

$$\frac{f_{water}}{f_{air}} = \frac{(\mu_g - 1)}{(\mu_g/\mu_w - 1)}$$

Substituting the values, we have

$$f_{water} = \frac{(3/2 - 1)}{\left(\frac{3/2}{4/3} - 1\right)} f_{air} = 4 f_{air} = 4 \times 10 = 40 \text{ cm}$$

Mentor's TIP

- Students can remember the result, $f_{water} = 4 f_{air}$, if $\mu_g = 3/2$ and $\mu_w = 4/3$.

Magnification Produced by a Lens

The ratio of the size of the image to the size of object is called magnification.

Transverse Magnification (m)

The lateral, transverse or linear magnification (m) produced by a lens is defined by,

$$m = \frac{\text{Height of image}}{\text{Height of object}}$$

$$= \frac{I}{O} = \frac{v}{u} = \frac{f}{f+u} = \frac{f-v}{f}$$

Note Use sign convention while solving the problems.

Longitudinal Magnification (m_L)

When an object is placed along the principal axis then

$$m_L = \frac{\text{Image length}}{\text{Object length}}$$

If length of the object is small,

$$m_L = \frac{dv}{du} = \left(\frac{v}{u}\right)^2 = \left(\frac{f}{u+f}\right)^2 = \left(\frac{f-v}{f}\right)^2$$

where, $du =$ object length, $dv =$ image length

Areal Magnification (M_S)

$$m_s = \frac{A_I}{A_O} = m^2 = \left(\frac{f}{f+u}\right)^2$$

(where, A_I = Area of image and A_O = area of object)

Example 26. *An object of size 3.0 cm is placed at 14 cm from concave lens of focal length 21 cm. Describe the image produced by the lens. What happens if the object is moved further away from the lens?*

Sol. Using the relation, $\frac{1}{f} = \frac{1}{v} - \frac{1}{u}$, we get

$$\frac{1}{v} = \frac{1}{f} + \frac{1}{u} = \frac{1}{-21} + \frac{1}{(-14)}$$

$\therefore \quad v = -8.4$ cm

$\therefore$ The image is virtual, erect and located at 8.4 cm from the lens on the same side as the object.

Also, we know that $m = \frac{I}{O} = \frac{v}{u}$

$$\therefore \quad I = \frac{v}{u} \times O = \frac{-8.4}{-14} \times 3 = 1.8 \text{ cm}$$

i.e. the image is of diminished size.

If the object is moved away from the lens, the virtual image moves towards the focus of the lens (but never beyond focus).

Example 27. *Find the distance of an object from a convex lens, if image is two times magnified and focal length of the lens is 10 cm.*

Sol. Convex lens forms both type of images real as well as virtual. Since, nature of the image is not mentioned in the question, we will have to consider both the cases.

When Image is Real Means v is positive and u is negative with $|v| = 2|u|$. Thus, if

$$u = -x \text{ then, } v = 2x \text{ and } f = 10 \text{ cm}$$

Substituting in, $\frac{1}{v} - \frac{1}{u} = \frac{1}{f}$

we have, $\frac{1}{2x} + \frac{1}{x} = \frac{1}{10}$ or $\frac{3}{2x} = \frac{1}{10}$

$\therefore \quad x = 15$ cm

This means object lies between F and $2F$.

When image is virtual Means v and u both are negative. So let,

$$u = -y \text{ then } v = -2y$$

and $\quad f = 10$ cm

Substituting in, $\frac{1}{v} - \frac{1}{u} = \frac{1}{f}$

we have, $\frac{1}{-2y} + \frac{1}{y} = \frac{1}{10}$ or $\frac{1}{2y} = \frac{1}{10}$

$\therefore \quad y = 5$ cm

This means object lies between F and P.

Power of a Lens

It is the ability of the lens to deviate the path of rays passing through it. If the lens converges the rays parallel to principal axis, its power is said positive and if it diverges the rays, its power is negative. It is given as

$$P(\text{in dioptre}) = \frac{1}{f(\text{in metre})}$$

Following table gives the sign of P and f for different type of lenses

Nature of lens	Focal length (f)	Power $P_L = \frac{1}{f}$	Converging /Diverging	Ray diagram
Convex lens	+ve	+ve	Converging	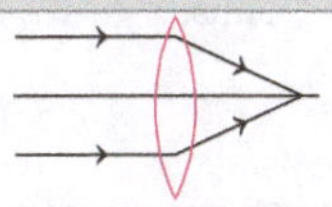
Concave lens	– ve	–ve	Diverging	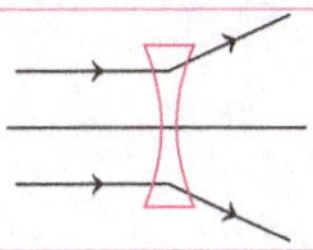

Example 28. *A spherical convex surface separates object and image space of refractive index 1.0 and 4/3. If radius of curvature of the surface is 10 cm, find its power.*

Sol. Let us see where does the parallel rays converge (or diverge) on the principal axis. Let us call it the focus and the corresponding length is the focal length f.

We have, $$\frac{\mu_2}{v}-\frac{\mu_1}{u}=\frac{\mu_2-\mu_1}{R}$$

$$\frac{4/3}{f}-\frac{1.0}{\infty}=\frac{4/3-1.0}{+10}$$

or focal length, $$f=40\text{ cm}=0.4\text{ m}$$

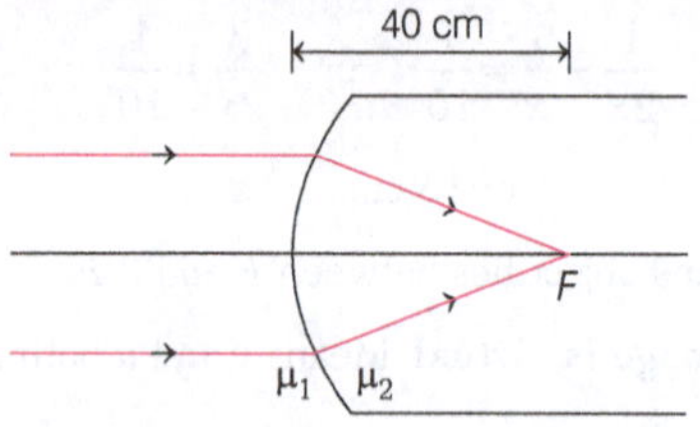

Since, the rays are converging, its power should be positive. Hence,

$$P\,(\text{in dioptre})=\frac{+1}{f\,(\text{in metre})}=\frac{1}{0.4}\quad\text{or}\quad P=2.5\text{ D}$$

Example 29. *A thin glass (refractive index 1.5) lens has optical power of −5 D in air. Calculate its optical power in a liquid medium with refractive index 1.6.*

Sol. From Lens Maker's formula we have,

$$\frac{1}{f_a}=(\mu-1)\left(\frac{1}{R_1}-\frac{1}{R_2}\right)$$

It is given that, $\mu=1.5$

$$\therefore\quad \frac{1}{f_a}=(1.5-1)\left(\frac{1}{R_1}-\frac{1}{R_2}\right)$$

and $$\frac{1}{f_m}=\left(\frac{\mu_g}{\mu_m}-1\right)\left(\frac{1}{R_1}-\frac{1}{R_2}\right)\quad\text{...(i)}$$

$$\Rightarrow\quad \frac{1}{f_m}=\left(\frac{1.5}{1.6}-1\right)\left(\frac{1}{R_1}-\frac{1}{R_2}\right)\quad\text{...(ii)}$$

Thus, $$\frac{f_m}{f_a}=\frac{(1.5-1)}{\left(\frac{1.5}{1.6}-1\right)}=-8$$

$$\Rightarrow\quad f_m=-8\times f_a$$

$$=-8\times\frac{-1}{5}=1.6\text{m}\left(\because\ f_a=\frac{1}{P}=-\frac{1}{5}\text{m}\right)$$

$\therefore$ Power of the lens, $$P_m=\frac{\mu}{f_m}=\frac{1.6}{1.6}=1\text{ D}$$

Combination of Two or More Thin Lenses

Combinations of lenses in contact are used in many optical instruments to improve their performance.

(i) **When two lenses are in contact,** combination will behave as a lens, which has lesser focal length.

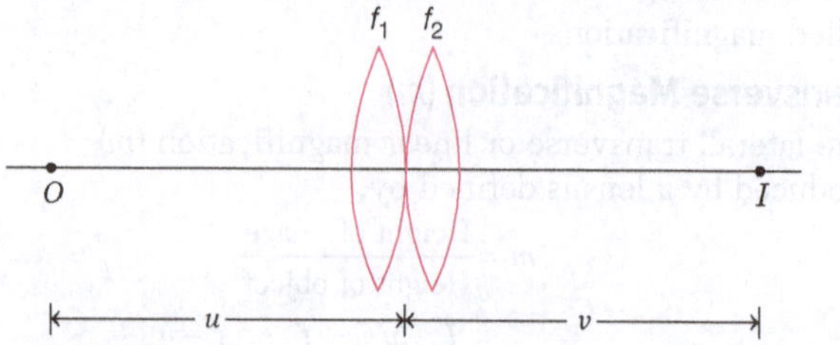

Combination of two convex lenses with zero separation

In this situation, combined focal length (F) is given as

$$\frac{1}{F}=\frac{1}{f_1}+\frac{1}{f_2}$$

Similarly, for more than two lenses in contact, the equivalent focal length is given by the formula,

$$\frac{1}{F}=\sum_{i=1}^{n}\frac{1}{f_i}=\frac{1}{f_1}+\frac{1}{f_2}+\ldots$$

Mentor's TiP

- Here f_1, f_2 etc., are to be substituted with their appropriate sign.

Similarly,

(a) Power of combination,

$$P=P_1+P_2+\ldots=\sum_{i=1}^{n}P_i$$

(b) Magnification of combination,

$$M=m_1\times m_2\times\ldots=\prod_{i=1}^{n}m_i$$

(ii) **Lenses separated by a distance**

If two lenses of focal lengths f_1 and f_2 are separated by a distance x, then its equivalent focal length

$$\frac{1}{F}=\frac{1}{f_1}+\frac{1}{f_2}-\frac{x}{f_1f_2}$$

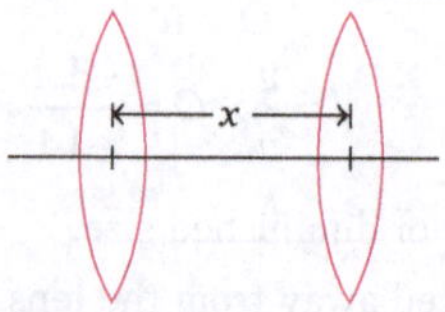

Combination of two convex lenses with x separation

(a) Power of combination,

$$P = P_1 + P_2 - xP_1P_2$$

(b) Total magnification remains unchanged *i.e.*,

$$m = m_1 \times m_2$$

Combination of two convex lenses behaves as

(i) convex lens, if $(f_1 + f_2) > 0$

(ii) glass plate, if $(f_1 + f_2) = 0$

(iii) concave lens, if $(f_1 + f_2) < 0$

NEET Close-up

Example Similar to PYQ Asked in NEET 2023

A converging lens of focal length 5.0 cm is placed in contact with a diverging lens of focal length 10.0 cm. The combined focal length of the system is

(a) 10 cm (b) 12 cm (c) 8 cm (d) 15 cm

Sol. (*a*) Here, $f_1 = +5.0$ cm and $f_2 = -10.0$ cm

Therefore, the combined focal length F is given by

$$\frac{1}{F} = \frac{1}{f_1} + \frac{1}{f_2} = \frac{1}{5.0} - \frac{1}{10.0} = +\frac{1}{10.0}$$

$\therefore \quad F = +10.0$ cm

i.e., the combination behaves as a converging lens of focal length 10.0 cm.

Skill Builder

Two convex lenses of same focal length, when placed in contact, the equivalent focal length of the combination will be

(a) doubled (b) unchanged
(c) halved (d) four times

For more Practice Refer Q. No. 11, 18 of step-up practice 3 and Q. No. 61, 66 of Gearing up for NEET.

Example 30. *Two thin equiconvex lenses each of focal length 0.2 m are placed coaxially with their optic centres 0.5m apart. Then find the focal length of the combination.*

Sol. Given, focal length of each lens, $f_1 = f_2 = 0.2$ m

Separation between the lenses, $d = 0.5$ m

$\therefore$ Focal length of the combination,

$$\frac{1}{F} = \frac{1}{f_1} + \frac{1}{f_2} - \frac{d}{f_1 f_2}$$

$$= \frac{1}{0.2} + \frac{1}{0.2} - \frac{0.5}{(0.2)(0.2)} = -2.5$$

$$\Rightarrow \quad F = -\frac{1}{2.5} = -0.4\,\text{m}$$

NEET Close-up

Example Similar to PYQ Asked in NEET 2023

Two plano-concave lenses of glass of refractive index 1.5 have radii of curvature of 20 and 30 cm. They are placed in contact with curved surface towards each other and the space between them is filled with a liquid of refractive index 2/3. The focal length of the system will be

(a) −15.5 cm (b) −14.4 cm (c) −11.2 cm (d) −16.3 cm

Sol. (*b*)

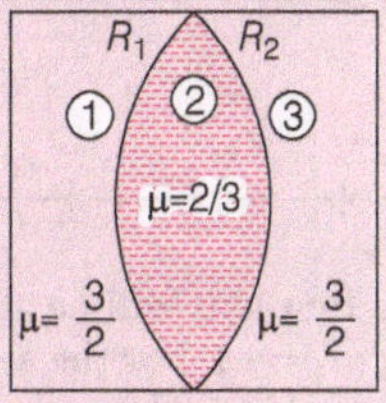

Lens 1,

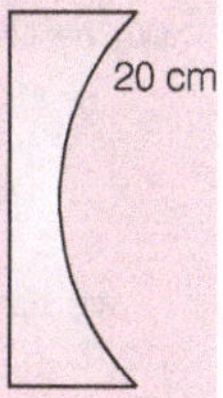

$$\frac{1}{f_1} = \left(\frac{3}{2} - 1\right)\left(\frac{1}{\infty} - \frac{1}{20}\right) = -\frac{1}{40}$$

Lens 2,

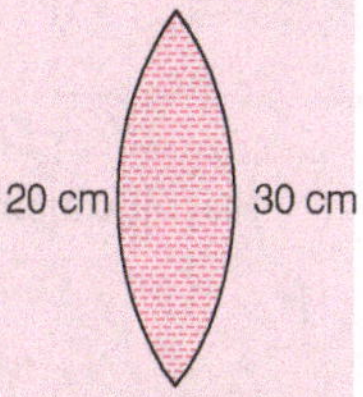

$$\frac{1}{f_2} = \left(\frac{2}{3} - 1\right)\left(\frac{1}{20} + \frac{1}{30}\right)$$

$$= -\left(\frac{1}{3}\right)\left(\frac{5}{60}\right) = -\frac{1}{36}$$

Lens 3,

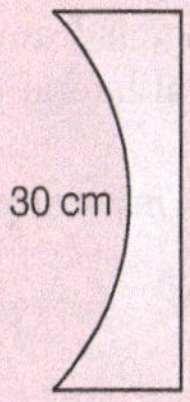

$$\frac{1}{f_3} = \left(\frac{3}{2} - 1\right)\left(\frac{1}{-30} - \frac{1}{\infty}\right) = \frac{-1}{60}$$

$$\therefore \quad \frac{1}{F} = \frac{1}{f_1} + \frac{1}{f_2} + \frac{1}{f_3} = \frac{-1}{40} - \frac{1}{36} - \frac{1}{60}$$

$$= \frac{-9 - 10 - 6}{360} = \frac{-25}{360} \quad \Rightarrow \quad F = -14.4 \text{ cm}$$

Skill Builder

Two plano-concave lenses of glass of refractive index 1.5 and both have radii of curvature of 10 cm. They are placed in contact with curved surface towards each other and the space between them is filled with a liquid of refractive index 2/3. The focal length of the system will be

(a) 6 cm (b) −6 cm (c) $\frac{60}{7}$ cm (d) $\frac{-60}{7}$ cm

For more Practice Refer Q. No. 14 of step-up practice 3.

Example 31. *Two thin converging lenses are placed on a common axis, so that the centre of one of them coincides with the focus of the other. An object is placed at a distance twice the focal length from the left-hand lens. Where will its image be? What is the lateral magnification? (The focal of each lens is f.)*

Sol.

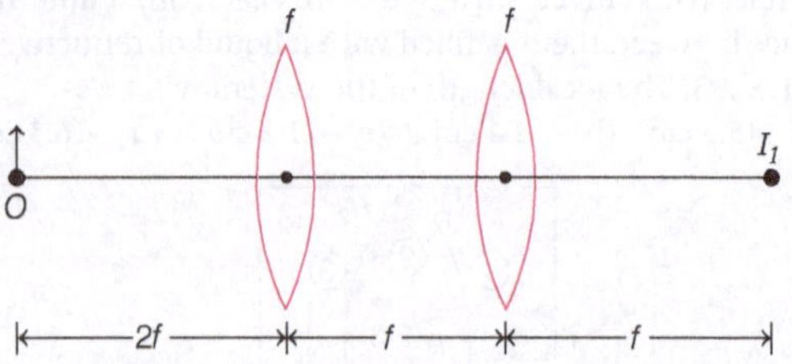

The image formed by first lens will be at a distance $2f$ with lateral magnification, $m_1 = -1$. For the second lens, this image will behave as a virtual object. Using the lens formula,

$$\frac{1}{v} - \frac{1}{u} = \frac{1}{f}$$

we have, $$\frac{1}{v} - \frac{1}{f} = \frac{1}{f}$$

$\therefore$ $$v = \frac{f}{2}$$

Magnification, $$m_2 = \frac{v_2}{u_2} = \frac{(f/2)}{f} = \frac{1}{2}$$

{since, $v_2 = v$ and $u_2 = f$}

Therefore, final image is formed at a distance $f/2$ from the second lens with total lateral magnification,

$$m = m_1 \times m_2 = (-1) \times \left(\frac{1}{2}\right) = -\frac{1}{2}$$

Cutting of Lens

(i) If a symmetrical convex lens of focal length f is cut into two parts along its optical axis, then focal length of each part (a plano-convex lens) is $2f$. However, if the two parts are joined as shown in figure, the focal length of combination is again f.

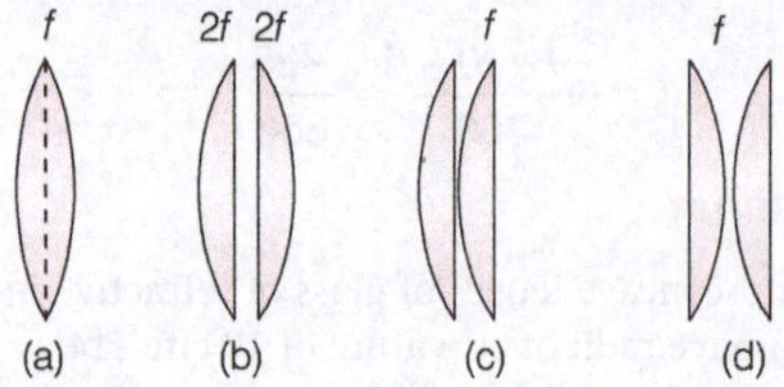

Convex lens cut along its optical axis

(ii) If a symmetrical convex lens of focal length f is cut into two parts along the principal axis, then focal length of each part remains unchanged to f. If these two parts are joined with curved ends on one side, then focal length of the combination is $f/2$. But on joining two parts in opposite sense the net focal length becomes ∞ (or net power = 0), *i.e.* it behaves like a plane glass.

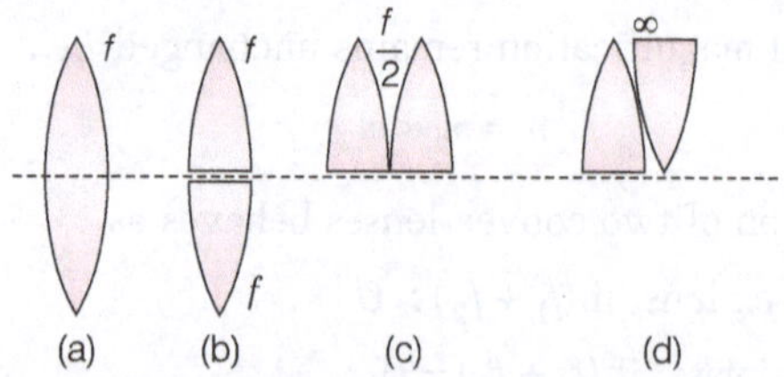

Convex lens cut along its principal axis

Prism

It is a portion of a transparent medium generally made of crown or flint glass and bounded by three planes intersecting by three parallel straight lines *AD*, *CF* and *BE* as shown in figure.

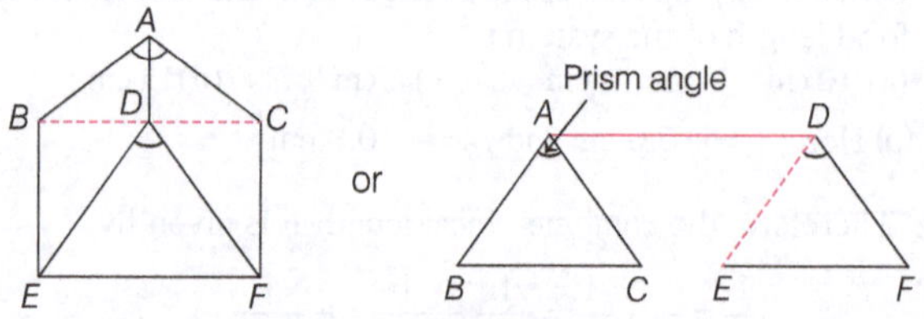

Prism

ABED and *ACFD* are two refracting faces as shown in the figure. $\angle A$ is called angle of prism or refracting angle.

Refraction of Light Through a Prism

The figure below shows the passage of light through a triangular prism *ABC*.

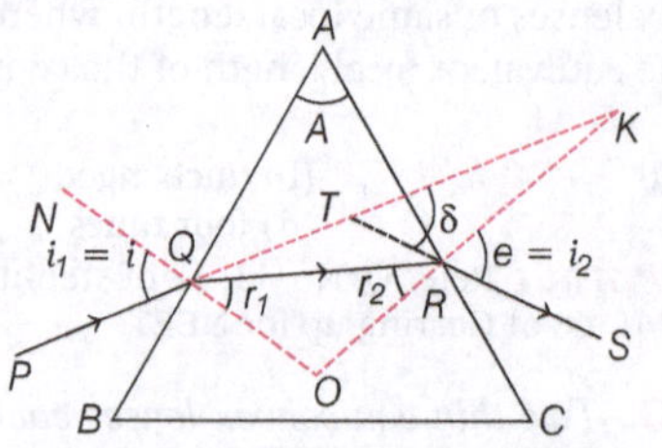

Cross-sectional view of a prism

The angles of incidence and refraction at first face *AB* are i and r_1, respectively.

The angle of refraction at the second face *AC* is r_2 and the angle of emergence is e.

The angle between the emergent ray *RS* and incident ray *PQ* is called angle of deviation (δ).

Here, angle of deviation is given by,

$$\delta = (i_1 + i_2) - A \quad \text{...(i)}$$

where, A is angle of prism and $\angle A = \angle r_1 + \angle r_2$, ... (ii)

or $\delta = (i + e) - A$, where e is angle of emergence which is equal to i_2.

If angle of incidence and refraction are small, then

$$\delta = (\mu - 1)A \qquad \text{...(iii)}$$

This expression shows that for a given angle A all rays entering a small angled prism at small angles of incidence suffer the same deviation.

Minimum Deviation

The angle of emergence of the ray from the second face equals the angle of incidence of the ray on the first face then deviation produced is minimum.

i.e. $$i_2 = i_1 = i \qquad \text{... (iv)}$$

and $$r_1 = r_2 = r \qquad \text{... (v)}$$

From Eqs. (ii) and (v), we get

$$r = \frac{A}{2}$$

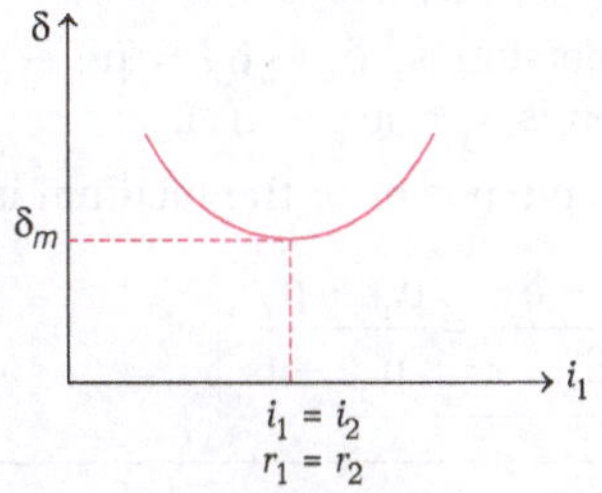

i_1 *versus* δ curve

Further at, $\delta = \delta_m = (i + i) - A$ or $i = \dfrac{A + \delta_m}{2}$

From Snell's law, $\mu = \dfrac{\sin i}{\sin r}$

or $$\mu = \frac{\sin\left(\dfrac{A + \delta_m}{2}\right)}{\sin\dfrac{A}{2}} \qquad \text{...(vi)}$$

Expression given as Eq. (vi) is also called **prism formula.**

For small angled prism, $\sin\left(\dfrac{A + \delta_m}{2}\right) \simeq \dfrac{A + \delta_m}{2}$ and

$\sin A/2 \simeq A/2$

From Eq. (vi), $\mu = \dfrac{(A + \delta_m)}{A} \Rightarrow \delta_m = (\mu - 1)A$

$$\Rightarrow \quad \delta_m = (\mu - 1)A \qquad \text{...(vii)}$$

Thus, Eq. (iii) has derived here.

Condition of no emergence

For no emergence of light, total internal reflections must take place at the second surface. For that, $r_2 > C$

So, $A > r_1 + C \qquad (\because A = r_1 + r_2)$

Maximum value of $r_1 = C$

So, $A \geq 2C$ for any angle of incidence.

If light ray is incident normally on first surface

i.e. $i = 0$, it means $\angle r = 0°$

So in this case, condition of no emergence from second surface is $A > C$

$$\therefore \quad \sin A > \sin C$$

$$\sin A > \frac{1}{\mu} \Rightarrow \mu > \operatorname{cosec} A$$

Example 32. *A ray of light is incident at an angle of 60° on the face of a prism having refracting angle 30°. The ray emerging out of the prism makes an angle 30° with the incident ray. Show that the emergent ray is perpendicular to the face through which, it emerges.*

Sol. Given, $i_1 = 60°, A = 30°$ and $\delta = 30°$.

From the relation, $\delta = (i_1 + i_2) - A$

we have, $i_2 = 0$

This means that the emergent ray is perpendicular to the face through which it emerges.

Example 33. *The angle of minimum deviation for a glass prism with $\mu = \sqrt{3}$ equals the refracting angle of the prism. What is the angle of the prism?*

Sol. Given, $A = \delta_m$

Using, $$\mu = \frac{\sin\left(\dfrac{A + \delta_m}{2}\right)}{\sin\left(\dfrac{A}{2}\right)}$$

we have, $$\sqrt{3} = \frac{\sin\left(\dfrac{A + A}{2}\right)}{\sin\left(\dfrac{A}{2}\right)}$$

or $$\sqrt{3} = \frac{\sin A}{\sin\left(\dfrac{A}{2}\right)} = \frac{2\sin\dfrac{A}{2}\cos\dfrac{A}{2}}{\sin\left(\dfrac{A}{2}\right)}$$

$$\therefore \quad \cos\frac{A}{2} = \frac{\sqrt{3}}{2}$$

$$\Rightarrow \quad \frac{A}{2} = 30° \text{ or } A = 60°$$

$$\Rightarrow \quad \delta_m = A = 60°$$

Example 34. *One face of a prism with a refractive angle of 30° is coated with silver. A ray incident on another face at an angle of 45° is refracted through first face and reflected from the silver coated face and retraces its path. What is the refractive index of the prism?*

Sol.

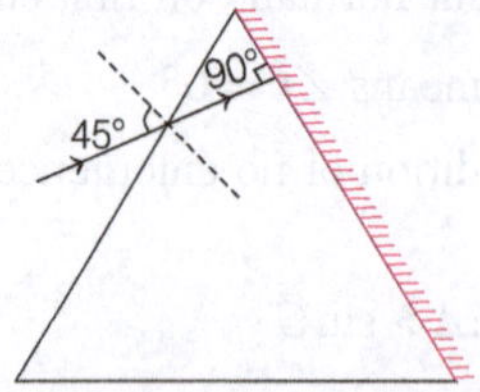

Given, $A = 30°$, $i_1 = 45°$ and $r_2 = 0$

Since, $r_1 + r_2 = A$

$\therefore$ $r_1 = A = 30°$

Now, refractive index of the prism,

$$\mu = \frac{\sin i_1}{\sin r_1} = \frac{\sin 45°}{\sin 30°} = \frac{1/\sqrt{2}}{1/2} = \sqrt{2}$$

Dispersion of Light by a Prism

If a beam of white light (contains all colours), is sent through the prism, it is then separated into a spectrum of its constituents colours. The spreading of white light into its colour components is called **dispersion.**

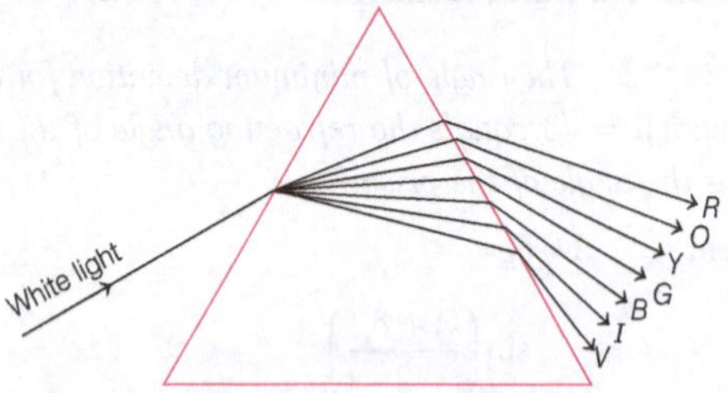

Dispersion of white light

If δ_r, δ_y and δ_v are the deviations for red, yellow and violet components, then average deviation is measured by δ_y as yellow light falls in between red and violet.
So, $\delta_v - \delta_r$ is called **angular dispersion.** The **dispersive power** of a material is defined as the ratio of angular dispersion to the average deviation when a white beam of light is passed through it. It is denoted by ω.

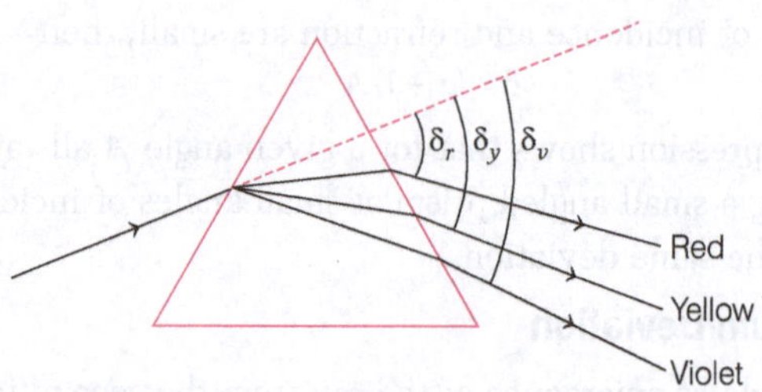

Deviation of rays of different colours in a prism

As we know, $\delta = (\mu - 1) A$

This equation is valid, when A and i are small. Suppose, a beam of white light is passed through such a prism, the deviation of red, yellow and violet light are given by,

$$\delta_r = (\mu_r - 1)A,$$
$$\delta_y = (\mu_y - 1)A,$$
and
$$\delta_v = (\mu_v - 1)A$$

The angular dispersion is, $\delta_v - \delta_r = (\mu_v - \mu_r) A$ and the average deviation is $\delta_y = (\mu_y - 1) A$.

Thus, the dispersive power of the medium is,

$$\omega = \frac{\delta_v - \delta_r}{\delta_y} = \frac{\mu_v - \mu_r}{\mu_y - 1} \quad \text{...(i)}$$

Concept ladder

- Deviation corresponding to yellow coloured light is average or mean deviation, $\mu_y = \frac{\mu_v + \mu_r}{2}$
- A single prism produces both deviation and dispersion simultaneously.

Example 35. *The refractive indices of flint glass for red and violet light are 1.613 and 1.632, respectively. Find the angular dispersion produced by the thin prism of flint glass having refracting angle 4°.*

Sol. Angular dispersion,

$$\theta = (\mu_v - \mu_r)A = (1.632 - 1.613) \times 4° = 0.076°$$

Example 36. *Evaluate the dispersive power of flint glass. The refractive indices of flint glass for red, yellow and violet light are 1.613, 1.620 and 1.632, respectively.*

Sol. Dispersive power is given by

$$\omega = \frac{\mu_v - \mu_r}{\mu_y - 1} = \frac{1.632 - 1.613}{1.620 - 1} = 0.031$$

STEP UP Practice 3

1. A convex lens has a focal length of 20 cm. It is used to form an image of an object placed 15 cm from lens. The image is
(a) virtual, inverted and enlarged
(b) real, inverted and diminished
(c) real, inverted and enlarged
(d) virtual, erect and enlarged

2. At what distance from a convex lens of focal length 30 cm an object should be placed, so that the size of image be (1/4)th of the object ?
(a) 30 cm (b) 60 cm
(c) 15 cm (d) 150 cm

3. **Assertion** (A) Converging property of a convergent lens remains same in all mediums.
Reason (R) Property of lens whether the ray is diverging or converging depends on the surrounding medium.
In the light of the above statements, choose the correct answer from the options given below.
(a) Both A and R are true but R is not the correct explanation of A.
(b) A is true but R is false.
(c) A is false but R is true.
(d) Both A and R are true and R is the correct explanation of A.

4. Distance of an object from a concave lens of focal length 20 cm is 40 cm. Then, linear magnification of the image is
(a) 1 (b) <1
(c) >1 (d) zero

5. In order to obtain a real image of magnification 2 using converging lens of focal length 20 cm, where should an object be placed?
(a) 50 cm (b) 30 cm
(c) –50 cm (d) –30 cm

6. The real image which is exactly equal to the size of an object is to be obtained on a screen with the help of a convex lens of focal length 15 cm. For this, what must be the distance between the object and screen?
(a) 15 cm (b) 30 cm
(c) 45 cm (d) 60 cm

7. **Assertion** (A) If a convex lens of glass is immersed in water its power decreases.
Reason (R) In water, convex lens behaves as concave lens.
In the light of the above statements, choose the correct answer from the options given below.
(a) Both A and R are true but R is not the correct explanation of A.
(b) A is true but R is false.
(c) A is false but R is true.
(d) Both A and R are true and R is the correct explanation of A.

8. A convex lens of refractive index 3/2 has a power of 2.5 D. If it is placed in a liquid of refractive index 2, the new power of the lens is
(a) 2.5 D (b) – 2.5 D
(c) 1.25 D (d) – 1.25 D

9. An object is placed at 10 cm from a lens and real image is formed with magnification of 0.5, then the lens is
(a) concave with focal length of (10/3) cm
(b) convex with focal length of (10/3) cm
(c) concave with focal length of 10 cm
(d) convex with focal length of 10 cm

10. **Assertion** (A) Power of a lens is defined as $P = 1/f$, f = focal length.
Reason (R) A lens of a high power has large focal length.
In the light of the above statements, choose the correct answer from the options given below :
(a) Both A and R are true but R is not the correct explanation of A.
(b) A is true but R is false.
(c) A is false but R is true.
(d) Both A and R are true and R is the correct explanation of A.

11. Two thin lenses, one of focal length +60 cm and the other of focal length –20 cm are put in contact. The combined focal length is
(a) +15 cm (b) –15 cm
(c) +30 cm (d) –30 cm

12. Two similar plano-convex lenses are combined together in three different ways as shown in the adjoining figure. The ratio of the focal lengths in three cases will be

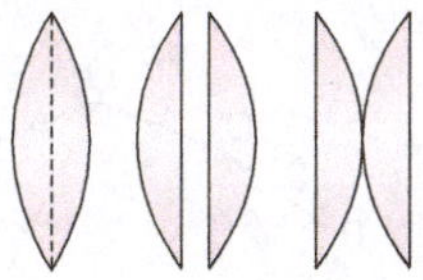

(a) 2 : 2 : 1
(b) 1 : 1 : 1
(c) 1 : 2 : 2
(d) 2 : 1 : 1

13. In the figure, an air lens of radii of curvature 10 cm ($R_1 = R_2$=10 cm) is cut in a cylinder of glass ($\mu = 2/3$). The focal length and the nature of the lens is

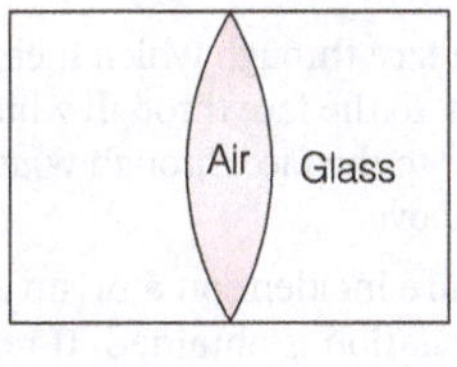

(a) 15 cm, concave
(b) 15 cm, convex
(c) ∞, neither concave nor convex
(d) 0, concave

14. A plano-convex lens is made of glass of refractive index 1.5. The radius of curvature of its convex surface is R. Its focal length is
(a) $R/2$ (b) R
(c) $2R$ (d) $1.5R$

15. Which one of the following pair given below is correct about focal length of various lenses?

(a) For equi-biconvex lens → $f = -\dfrac{R}{2(\mu - 1)}$

(b) For equi-biconcave lens → $f = \dfrac{R}{2(\mu - 1)}$

(c) For plano-convex lens → $f = \dfrac{R}{\mu - 1}$

(d) For plano-concave lens → $f = \dfrac{R}{\mu + 1}$

16. A plano-convex lens of curvature of 30 cm and refractive index 1.5 produces a real image of an object kept 90 cm from it. What is the magnification?

(a) 4 (b) 0.5 (c) 1.5 (d) 2

17. A convex lens of focal length 40 cm is in contact with a concave lens of focal length 25 cm. The power of combination is

(a) −1.5D (b) −6.5D
(c) +6.5D (d) +1.5D

18. The critical angle of a prism is 30°. The velocity of light in the medium is

(a) 1.5×10^8 m/s (b) 3×10^8 m/s
(c) 4.5×10^8 m/s (d) None of these

19. A ray of light is incident on an equilateral glass prism placed on a horizontal table. For minimum deviation which of the following is true?

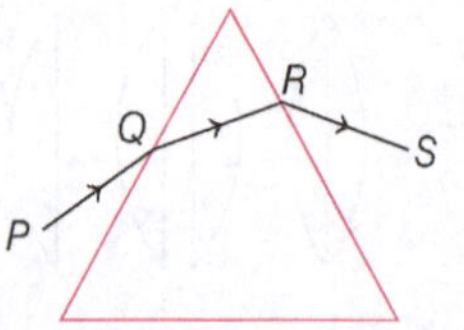

(a) *PQ* is horizontal (b) *QR* is horizontal
(c) *RS* is horizontal (d) Either *PQ* or *RS* is horizontal

20. A ray of light is incident at an angle of 60° on one face of a prism of angle 30°. The ray emerging out of the prism makes an angle of 30° with the incident ray. The emergent ray is

(a) normal to the face through which it emerges
(b) inclined at 30° to the face through which it emerges
(c) inclined at 60° to the face through which it emerges
(d) None of the above

21. When light rays are incident on a prism at an angle of 45°, the minimum deviation is obtained. If refractive index of the material of prism is $\sqrt{2}$, then the angle of prism will be

(a) 30° (b) 75°
(c) 90° (d) 60°

22. A ray of light passes through an equilateral glass prism in such a manner that the angle of incidence is equal to the angle of emergence and each of these angles is equal to 3/4 of the angle of the prism. The angle of deviation is

(a) 45° (b) 39°
(c) 20° (d) 30°

23. **Assertion** (A) Thin prisms do not deviate light much.
Reason (R) Thin prism have small angle *A* and hence, D_m (minimum deviation) is also very small is $D_m = [({}^1\mu_2 - 1)A]$, where ${}^1\mu_2$ is the refractive index of prism w.r.t. medium 1.

In the light of the above statements, choose the correct answer from the options given below.

(a) Both A and R are true but R is not the correct explanation of A.
(b) A is true but R is false.
(c) A is false but R is true.
(d) Both A and R are true and R is the correct explanation of A.

24. In a thin prism of glass (refractive index 1.5), which of the following relations between the angle of minimum deviations δ_m and angle of prism *r* will be correct?

(a) $\delta_m = r$ (b) $\delta_m = 1.5r$
(c) $\delta_m = 2r$ (d) $\delta_m = r/2$

25. The angle of minimum deviation for a prism of refractive index 1.5 is equal to the angle of the prism. The angle of prism is (Given, cos 41° = 0.75)

(a) 21° (b) 42°
(c) 60° (d) 82°

26. **Assertion** (A) A white light on passing through prism splits into its component colour such that the red light emerges nearest to the base of the prism.
Reason (R) Wavelength of red light is more than other component colours and hence, red light deviates least.

In the light of the above statements, choose the correct answer from the options given below.

(a) Both A and R are true but R is not the correct explanation of A.
(b) A is true but R is false.
(c) A is false but R is true.
(d) Both A and R are true and R is the correct explanation of A.

27. A thin prism P_1 with angle 6° and made from glass of refractive index 1.54 is combined with another thin prism P_2 of refractive index 1.72 to produce dispersion without deviation. The angle of prism P_2 will be

(a) 5°24′ (b) 4°30′
(c) 6° (d) 8°

Module 4

Optical Instruments

- Microscope
- Telescope

Microscope

It is an optical instrument used to see very small object.

Simple Microscope

It consists of a single convex lens (converging lens) of small focal length. The image formed by this microscope is erect, virtual, enlarged and on same side of object.

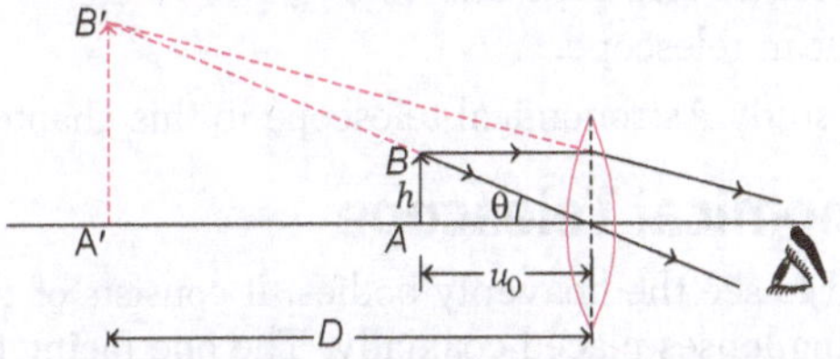

Image formation in a simple microscope

(i) When final image is formed at infinity.

Magnifying power, $M_\infty = \frac{D}{f}$

This is also called magnifying power for normal adjustment.

(ii) When final image is formed at D (near point).

Magnifying power, $M_D = 1 + \frac{D}{f}$

Concept ladder

- $M_D > M_\infty$, i.e. when final image is formed at 25 cm, angular magnification is increased but eye is most strained. On the other hand, when final image is at infinity, angular magnification is slightly less but eye is relaxed. So, the choice is yours, whether you want to see bigger size with strained eye or smaller size with relaxed eye.
- M can be increased by decreasing f, but due to several other aberrations the image becomes too defective at large magnification with a simple microscope. Roughly speaking a magnification power upto 4 is trouble free.

Example 37. *A 20 D lens is used as a magnifier. Where should the object be placed to obtain maximum angular magnification? (Given, D = 25 cm).*

Sol. Focal length of the lens, $f = \frac{1}{20}\ \text{m} = \frac{100}{20}\ \text{cm} = 5\ \text{cm}$

Maximum angular magnification is obtained when final image is formed at D. Hence, by using lens formula,

$$\frac{1}{-25} - \frac{1}{u_o} = \frac{1}{5} \Rightarrow u_o = -4.17\ \text{cm}$$

Compound Microscope

Simple microscope has a limited maximum magnification. So, for larger magnification, one can use compound microscope. It consists of two converging lenses arranged coaxially. The one facing the object is called **objective** and the one close to eye is called **eye-piece.** The objective has a smaller aperture and smaller focal length than those of the eye-piece.

The separation between the objective and the eye-piece (called the length of the microscope L) can be varied by appropriate screws fixed on the panel of microscope.

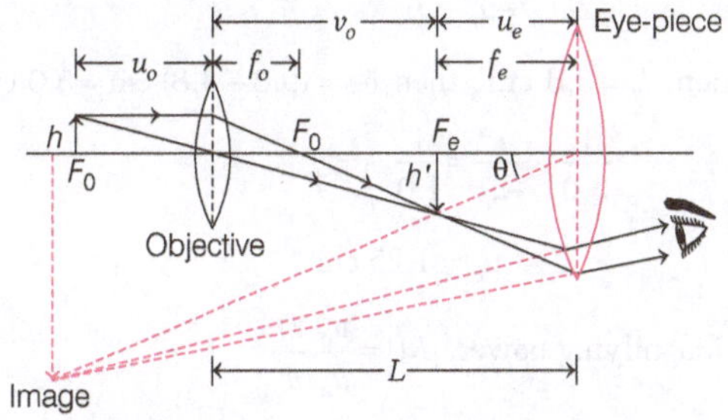

Image formation in a compound microscope

The object is placed beyond first focus of objective, so that an inverted and real image (intermediate image) is formed by the objective. This intermediate image acts as an object for the eye-piece and lies between first focus and pole of eye piece. The final magnified virtual image is formed by the eye-piece.

∴ Magnifying power of the compound microscope,

$$M = \frac{v_o}{u_o}\left(\frac{D}{u_e}\right)$$

or $M = M_o \times M_e$, where M_o is the magnifying power of objective and M_e is the magnifying power of eye-piece.

(i) When the final image is formed at infinity,

Magnifying power, $M_\infty = \frac{v_o}{u_o}\frac{D}{f_e}$

and $L_\infty = v_o + f_e \quad \left(\because M_\infty = \frac{(L_\infty - f_o - f_e)}{f_o f_e}\right)$

(ii) When the final image (by eye-piece) is formed at D.

Magnifying power, $M_D = \dfrac{v_o}{u_o}\left(1 + \dfrac{D}{f_e}\right)$

and $$L_D = v_o + |u_e| = v_o + \frac{Df_e}{D + f_e}$$

In general, object is placed very near to the principal focus of objective and f_0 is also very small, then

$$M_D = -\frac{L}{f_o}\left(1 + \frac{D}{f_e}\right)$$

Example 38. *The separation between the objective and the eye-piece of a compound microscope can be adjusted between 9.8 cm to 11.8 cm. If the focal lengths of the objective and the eye-piece are 1.0 cm and 6 cm respectively, find the range of the magnifying power, if the image is always needed at 24 cm from the eye.*

Sol. For eye-piece, it is given that

$$f_e = 6 \text{ cm}, \quad v_e = -24 \text{ cm}$$

$$\therefore \quad \frac{1}{-24} - \frac{1}{-u_e} = \frac{1}{6} \quad \text{or} \quad u_e = 4.8 \text{ cm}$$

When, $L = 9.8$ cm, then $v_o = (9.8 - 4.8)$ cm $= 5.0$ cm

$$\therefore \quad \frac{1}{5.0} - \frac{1}{-u_o} = \frac{1}{1.0}$$

or $$u_o = 1.25 \text{ cm}$$

or Magnifying power, $|M| = \dfrac{v_o}{u_o}\dfrac{D}{u_e}$

$$= \left(\frac{5.0}{1.25}\right)\left(\frac{25.0}{4.8}\right) = 20.83$$

When, $L = 11.8$ cm, then $v_o = (11.8 - 4.8)$ cm $= 7.0$ cm

$$\therefore \quad \frac{1}{7.0} - \frac{1}{-u_o} = \frac{1}{1.0} \quad \text{or} \quad u_o = 1.17 \text{ cm}$$

$$|M| = \frac{v_o}{u_o} \cdot \frac{D}{f_e} = \left(\frac{7.0}{1.17}\right)\left(\frac{25.0}{4.8}\right) = 31.16$$

Therefore, range of magnifying power is from 20.83 to 31.16.

Example 39. *A compound microscope has a magnifying power of 100 when the image is formed at infinity. The objective has a focal length of 0.5 cm and the tube length is 6.5 cm. Find the focal length of the eye-piece.*

Sol. When the final image is at infinity,

$$u_e = f_e = \text{tube length} - v_o$$

$$\therefore \quad f_e = 6.5 - v_o \quad \text{...(i)}$$

Since, $$|M_\infty| = \frac{v_o}{u_o} \cdot \frac{D}{f_e}$$

$$\therefore \quad 100 = \frac{v_o}{u_o} \cdot \frac{25}{f_e} \quad \text{or} \quad \frac{v_o}{u_o f_e} = 4 \quad \text{...(ii)}$$

For the objective,

$$\frac{1}{v_o} - \frac{1}{-u_o} = \frac{1}{f_o} = \frac{1}{0.5} \Rightarrow \frac{1}{v_o} + \frac{1}{u_o} = 2 \quad \text{...(iii)}$$

We have three unknowns v_o, u_o and f_e, solving these three equations, we get

$$f_e = 2 \text{ cm}$$

Telescope

A microscope is used to view the objects placed closed to it. To look at distant objects such as a star, a planet or a distant tree etc., we use telescopes. There are three types of refracting telescopes in use

(i) Astronomical telescope,

(ii) Terrestrial telescope and

(iii) Galilean telescope.

We will study Astronomical telescope in this chapter.

Astronomical Telescope

It is used to see the heavenly bodies. It consists of two converging lenses placed coaxially. The one facing the distant object is called the objective and has a large aperture and large focal length. The other is called the eye-piece, as the eye is placed closed to it.

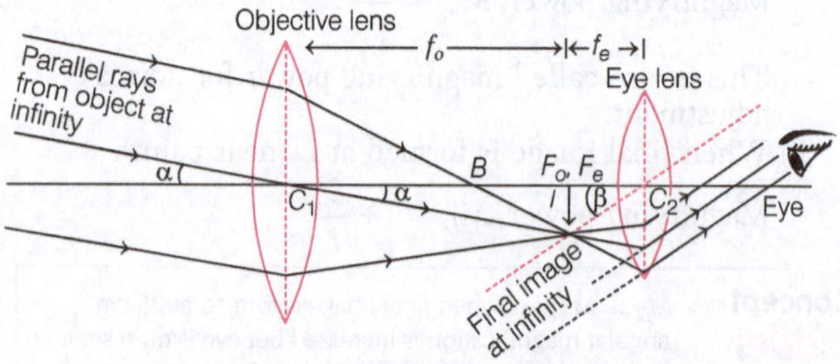

Image formation in an astronomical telescope

The intermediate image formed by objective is real, inverted and small and final image formed by eye-piece is real, inverted and highly magnified.

Magnifying Power

(i) **When object is at infinity**

Magnifying power, $$\boxed{M = \frac{\beta}{\alpha} = \frac{f_o}{u_e}}$$

where, α = angle subtended by object on objective and

β = angle subtended by final image at eye-piece.

$$\therefore \quad M_\infty = \frac{f_o}{f_e} \text{ and } L_\infty = f_o + f_e \quad (\because u_e = f_e)$$

(ii) **When the final image is at *D***

Magnifying power, $M_D = \frac{f_o}{f_e}\left(1+\frac{f_e}{D}\right)$

and $\boxed{L_D = f_o + \frac{Df_e}{D+f_e}}$

NEET Snapshot

A lens of large focal length is best suited as an objective of an astronomical telescope. ***[NEET 2021]***

The lens used in astronomical telescope is a convex lens. The magnification of an astronomical telescope is directly proportional to the focal length of the objective lenses.

Also, aperture size is large for a lens having large focal length which ensures better light gathering power.

Scan for Video

Summary of Formulae for Optical Instruments

Name of Optical Instruments	M	L	M_∞	M_D	L_∞	L_D
Simple microscope	$\frac{D}{u_o}$	—	$\frac{D}{f}$	$1+\frac{D}{f}$	—	—
Compound microscope	$\frac{v_o}{u_o}\frac{D}{u_e}$	$v_o + u_e$	$\frac{v_o}{u_o}\frac{D}{f_e}$	$\frac{v_o}{u_o}\left(1+\frac{D}{f_e}\right)$	$v_o + f_e$	$v_o + \frac{Df_e}{D+f_e}$
Astronomical telescope	$\frac{f_o}{u_e}$	$f_o + u_e$	$\frac{f_o}{f_e}$	$\frac{f_o}{f_e}\left(1+\frac{f_e}{D}\right)$	$f_o + f_e$	$f_o + \frac{Df_e}{D+f_e}$

Reflecting Telescope

This type of telescope is based upon the same principle at which the astronomical telescope works except that the formation of images takes place by reflection instead of by refraction. It consists of concave mirror of large aperture and large focal length (objective). A plane mirror is placed between the concave mirror and its focus. A small convex lens works as eye-piece.

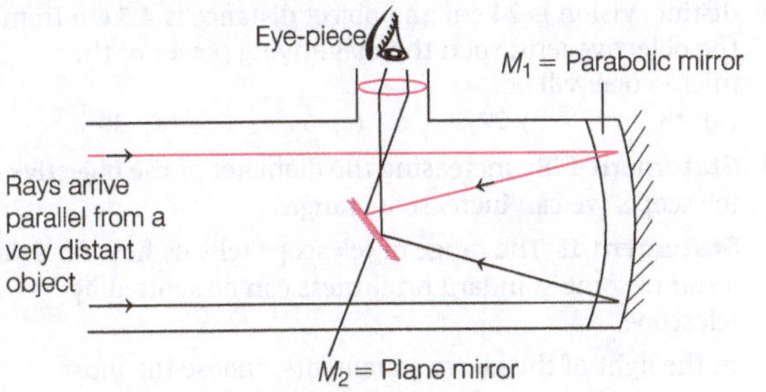

Reflecting telescope

If f_o is focal length of the concave spherical mirror and f_e the focal length of the eye-piece, then magnifying power of the reflecting telescope is given by $m = \frac{f_o}{f_e}$

Example 40. *A small telescope has an objective lens of focal length 140 cm and an eye-piece of focal length 5.0 cm. What is the magnifying power of the telescope for viewing distance objects when*

(i) the telescope is in normal adjustment (i.e., when the final image is at infinity)?

(ii) the final image is formed at the least distance of distinct vision 25 cm?

Sol. (i) When the telescope is in normal adjustment, the magnifying power is given by

$$M = \frac{f_o}{|f_e|} = +\frac{140}{5} = 28$$

(ii) When the final image is formed at the least distance of distinct vision, then M is given by

$$M = \frac{f_o}{|f_e|}\left(1+\frac{f_e}{D}\right) = \frac{140}{5}\left(1+\frac{5.0}{25}\right) = 33.6$$

NEET Close-up

Example Similar to PYQ Asked in NEET 2024

A small telescope has an objective lens of focal length 144 cm and an eye-piece of focal length 6.0 cm. Magnifying power of the telescope is

(a) 20 (b) 26 (c) 24 (d) 28

Sol. (c) M = magnifying power of telescope

L = separation between the objective and the eyepiece

In normal adjustment (*i.e.*, when the final image is formed at ∞),

$$M = \frac{f_o}{f_e} = -\frac{144}{6} = -24 \Rightarrow |M| = 24$$

Skill Builder

The eye-piece of an astronomical telescope has a focal length of 10 cm. The telescope is focused for normal vision of distant objects when the tube length is 1.0 *m*. The magnifying power of the telescope will be

(a) 10 (b) 9 (c) 6 (d) 12

For more Practice Refer Q. No. 14, 16 of step-up practice 4 and Q. No. 101, 108, 109 of Gearing up for NEET.

Example 41. *An astronomical telescope is to be designed to have a magnifying power of 50 in normal adjustment. If the length of the tube is 102 cm, find the powers of the objective and the eye-piece.*

Sol. Given, $M_\infty = 50$

$\therefore \quad \frac{f_o}{f_e} = 50$ ...(i)

Further, $L_\infty = 102$ cm

$\therefore \quad f_o + f_e = 102$ cm ...(ii)

Solving Eqs. (i) and (ii), we have

$f_o = 100$ cm and $f_e = 2$ cm

$\therefore$ Power of object, $P_o = \frac{1}{1.0} = 1$ D

and power of eye-piece, $P_e = \frac{1}{0.02} = 50$ D

STEP UP Practice 4

1. Magnifying power of a simple microscope is (when final image is formed at $D = 25$ cm from eye)

(a) $\frac{D}{f}$ (b) $1 + \frac{D}{f}$ (c) $1 + \frac{f}{D}$ (d) $1 - \frac{D}{f}$

2. A small object is placed at a distance of 4 cm from a simple microscope of focal length of 5 cm. Consider the given condition which of the following pair is incorrect.

(a) Nature of image → virtual image
(b) Image distance from the lens is → 20 cm
(c) The linear magnification is → 6
(d) The angular magnification is → 6.25

3. A compound microscope has two lenses. The magnifying power of one is 5 and the combined magnifying power is 100. The magnifying power of the other lens is

(a) 10 (b) 20 (c) 50 (d) 25

4. Which of the following statement is correct?

A. A simple magnifier or microscope is a converging lens of small focal length.
B. For microscope, the magnification in case of image formed at infinity is one more than the magnification when image is at the near point.
C. For larger magnifications, one uses two lenses, one compounding the effect of the other. This is known as a compound microscope.
D. The lens nearest the object is called objective and the lens near eye is called eyepiece.

(a) A, B and C only (b) A, C and D only
(c) A, B and D only (d) A and D only

5. A compound microscope has an objective with focal length $f_o = 1.0$ cm, an eyepiece with focal length, $f_e = 2.0$ cm and a tube length of 20 cm, then the magnification is

(a) 200 (b) 250
(c) 100 (d) 150

6. Which of the following statement(s) is/are correct?

A. In compound microscope, objective lens forms a real, inverted, magnified image of the object.
B. Eye-piece lens, produces the final image which is enlarged and virtual.
C. The final image is inverted with respect to the original object.

(a) A and B only (b) B and C only
(c) A and C only (d) A, B and C only

7. The length of the compound microscope is 14 cm. The magnifying power for relaxed eye is 25. If the focal length of eye lens is 5 cm, then the object distance for objective lens will be

(a) 1.8 cm (b) 1.5 cm (c) 2.1 cm (d) 2.4 cm

8. If the focal length of objective and eye lens are 1.2 cm and 3 cm respectively and the object is put 1.25 cm away from the objective lens and the final image is formed at infinity. The magnifying power of the microscope is

(a) 150 (b) 200 (c) 250 (d) 400

9. The focal length of objective and eye lens of a microscope are 4 cm and 8 cm, respectively. If the least distance of distinct vision is 24 cm and object distance is 4.5 cm from the objective lens, then the magnifying power of the microscope will be

(a) 18 (b) 32 (c) 64 (d) 20

10. **Statement I** By increasing the diameter of the objective of telescope, we can increase its range.

Statement II The range of telescope tells us how far away a star of some standard brightness can be spotted by telescope.

In the light of the above statements, choose the most appropriate answer from the options given below.

(a) Both Statement I and Statement II are incorrect.
(b) Statement I is correct but Statement II is incorrect.
(c) Statement I is incorrect but Statement II is correct.
(d) Both Statement I and Statement II are correct.

11. If the telescope is reversed, *i.e.* seen from the objective side, then

(a) object will appear very small
(b) object will appear very large
(c) there will be no effect on the image formed by the telescope
(d) image will be slightly greater than the earlier one

12. **Statement I** Focal length of the eye-piece of telescope is smaller as compared to the objective which has a large focal length and aperture.

Statement II For large focal length of objective than eye-piece, magnification is more in astronomical telescopes.

In the light of the above statements, choose the most appropriate answer from the options given below.

(a) Both Statement I and Statement II are incorrect.
(b) Statement I is correct but Statement II is incorrect.
(c) Statement I is incorrect but Statement II is correct.
(d) Both Statement I and Statement II are correct.

13. The aperture of a telescope is made large, because to
(a) increase the intensity of image
(b) decrease the intensity of image
(c) have greater magnification
(d) have lesser resolution

14. The focal lengths of the objective and eye lenses of a telescope are respectively, 200 cm and 5 cm. The maximum magnifying power of the telescope will be
(a) –40
(b) –48
(c) –60
(d) –100

15. An astronomical refractive telescope has an objective of focal length 20 m and an eyepiece of focal length 2 cm. Which of the following statement is/are correct?
A. The length of the telescope tube is 20.02 m.
B. The magnification is 1000.
C. The image formed is inverted.
D. An objective of a larger aperture will increase the brightness and reduce chromatic aberration of the image.

(a) A, C and D only (b) B, C and D only
(c) B and D only (d) A, B and C only

16. In an astronomical telescope, the focal length of the objective lens is 100 cm and of eyepiece is 2 cm. The magnifying power of the telescope for the normal eye is
(a) – 50 (b) –10 (c) 100 (d) $\frac{1}{50}$

17. The number of lenses in a terrestrial telescope is
(a) two (b) three (c) four (d) six

18. In Galilean telescope, the final image formed is
(a) real, erect and enlarged
(b) virtual, erect and enlarged
(c) real, inverted and enlarged
(d) virtual, inverted and enlarged

19. Reflecting telescope consists of
(a) convex mirror of large aperture
(b) concave mirror of large aperture
(c) concave lens of small aperture
(d) None of the above

20. A reflecting telescope has an objective lens of focal length 150 cm and an eyepiece of focal length 5.0 cm. What is the separation between the objective and the eyepiece?
(a) 1.25 m (b) 1.55 m (c) 1.3 m (d) 1.8 m

NEET Exclusive EXTRA BYTES

- Light travels in straight line in homogeneous mediums.
- In reflection, frequency, wavelength and speed of ray remains unchanged.
- Convex mirrors has large visibility region than plane mirrors and thereby used in vehicles for rear view.
- Concave mirrors are used to get larger images and thereby used in dental testing by doctors. Also, these are used as reflectors in headlights of vehicles and as street light.
- A sea diver can see outer world in a horizontal circle of radius $r = d \tan\theta_C$ at depth d in the water.
- If a lens made by multiple layers of different refractive indexes, the number of images is equal to types of layers.

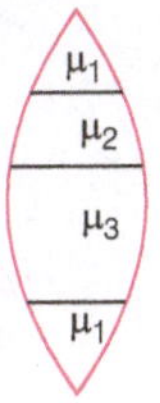

In given figure, types of layers = number of images = 3

- Radius of curvature of any spherical part of object can be measured by spherometer.
- Focal length of a lens depends on wavelengths

$$\frac{1}{f} \propto (\mu - 1) \propto \frac{1}{\lambda}$$

- Rainbow is a combined effect of refraction, reflection and dispersion of sunlight light passing through water drops.
- Creation of secondary rainbow is result of double internal reflection. It has reverse colour order than primary rainbow.

GEARING UP FOR NEET

Single Option Correct

1. The field of view is maximum for
(a) plane mirror (b) concave mirror
(c) convex mirror (d) cylindrical mirror

2. If object is placed 15 cm from a concave mirror of focal length 10 cm, then the nature of image formed will be
(a) magnified and inverted
(b) magnified and erect
(c) small in size and inverted
(d) small in size and erect

3. Two mirrors are placed at right angle to each other. A man is standing between them combing his hair. How many images will he see?
(a) 2 (b) 3
(c) 1 (d) zero

4. Two mirrors are kept at 60° to each other and a body is placed at the middle. The total number of images formed are
(a) six (b) four (c) five (d) three

5. A convex and a concave mirror of radii 10 cm each are placed facing each other and 15 cm apart. An object is placed exactly between them. If the reflection first takes place in concave and then in convex mirror, then the position of the final image will be
(a) 7 cm behind concave mirror
(b) at the pole of the concave mirror
(c) at the pole of the convex mirror
(d) 6.7 cm in front of concave mirror

6. An object of 5 cm height is placed 1m apart from a concave spherical mirror which has a radius of curvature of 20 cm. The size of the image is
(a) 0.11 cm (b) 0.5 cm (c) 0.55 cm (d) 0.60 cm

7. Where should a person stand straight from the pole of a convex mirror of focal length 2.0 m on its axis, so that the image formed become half of his original height?
(a) – 2.60 m (b) – 4.0 m (c) – 0.5 m (d) – 2.0 m

8. A ray of light is directed towards a corner reflector as shown in figure. The incident ray makes an angle of 22° with one of the mirrors. At what angle θ does the ray emerge?

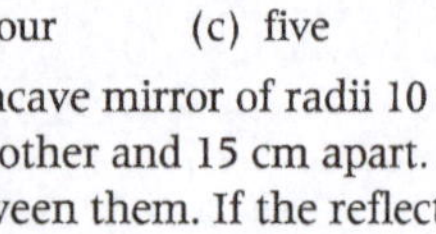

(a) 22° (b) 68° (c) 44° (d) 46°

9. The graph between u and v for a convex mirror is

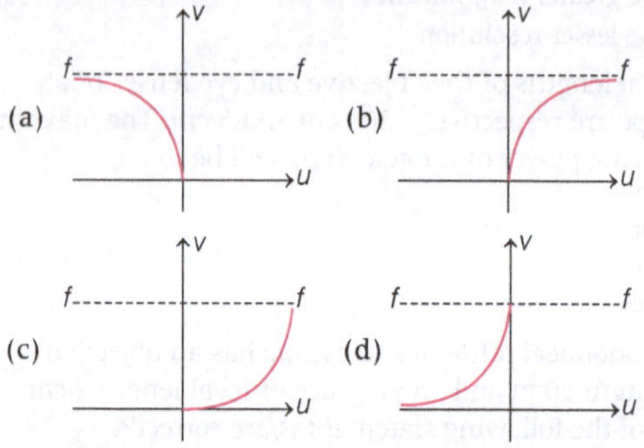

10. When a plane mirror is placed horizontally on ground at a distance of 60 m from the base of a tower, then the top of the tower and its image in the mirror subtend an angle of 90° at the corner of the mirror nearer to the base of tower. The height of the tower is
(a) 30 m (b) 60 m (c) 90 m (d) 120 m

11. A ray of light strikes a horizontal plane mirror at an angle of 45°. A second plane mirror is attached at an angle θ with it. If ray after reflection from second mirror runs parallel to the first mirror, then θ is
(a) 45° (b) 60° (c) 67.5° (d) 135°

12. A short linear object of length b lies along the axis of a concave mirror of focal length f at a distance u from the pole of the mirror, what is the size of image?
(a) $\left(\frac{f}{u-f}\right)b$ (b) $\left(\frac{f}{u-f}\right)^2 b$
(c) $\left(\frac{f}{u-f}\right)b^2$ (d) $\left(\frac{f}{u-f}\right)$

13. A mirror is inclined at an angle of θ with the horizontal. If a ray of light is incident at an angle of incidence θ, then the reflected ray makes the following angle with horizontal

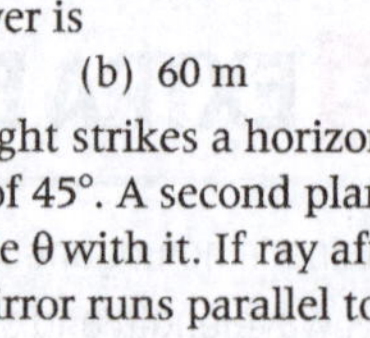

(a) (b) 2θ
(c) θ/2 (d) None of these

14. The graph shows part of variation of v with change in u for a concave mirror. Points plotted above the point P on the curve are for values of v

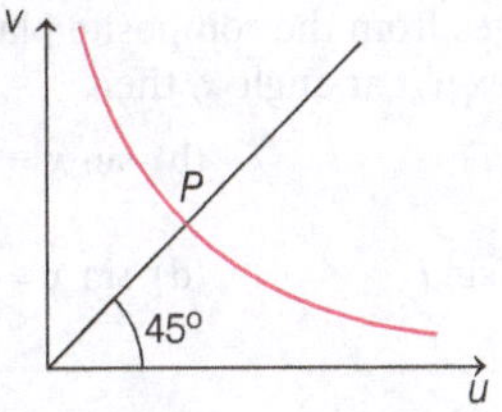

(a) smaller than f
(b) smaller than $2f$
(c) larger than $2f$
(d) larger than f but less than $2f$

15. An infinitely long rod lies along with the axis of a concave mirror of focal length f. The near end of the rod is at a distance $u > f$ from the mirror. Its image will have a length

(a) $\frac{f^2}{u-f}$ (b) $\frac{uf}{u-f}$ (c) $\frac{f^2}{u+f}$ (d) $\frac{uf}{u+f}$

16. The phenomena involved in the reflection of radiowaves by ionosphere is similar to ***[NCERT Exemplar]***

(a) reflection of light by a plane mirror
(b) total internal reflection of light in air during a mirage
(c) dispersion of light by water molecules during the formation of a rainbow
(d) scattering of light by the particles of air

17. When light wave suffers reflection at the interface from air to glass, then the change in phase of the reflected wave is equal to

(a) zero (b) $\frac{\pi}{2}$ (c) π (d) 2π

18. The direction of ray of light incident on a concave mirror is shown by PQ while directions in which the ray would travel after reflection is shown by four rays marked 1, 2, 3 and 4 (figure). Which of the four rays correctly shows the direction of reflected ray? ***[NCERT Exemplar]***

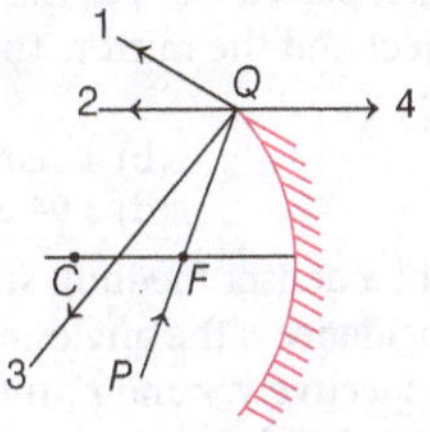

(a) 1 (b) 2 (c) 3 (d) 4

19. What should be the angle between two plane mirrors, so that whatever be the angle of incidence, the incident ray and the reflected ray from the two mirrors be parallel to each other?

(a) 60° (b) 90° (c) 120° (d) 45°

20. A thin rod of length $f/3$ lies along the axis of a concave mirror of focal length f. One end of its magnified image touches one end of the rod, the length of the image is

(a) f (b) $\frac{1}{2}f$
(c) $2f$ (d) $\frac{1}{4}f$

21. There are certain materials developed in laboratories which have a negative refractive index figure. A ray incident from air (medium 1) into such a medium (medium 2) shall follow a path given by ***[NCERT Exemplar]***

(a)
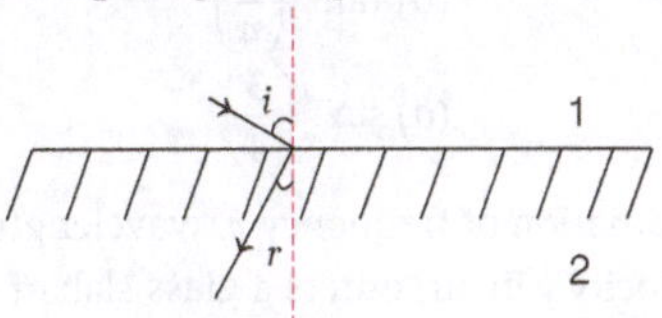

(b)
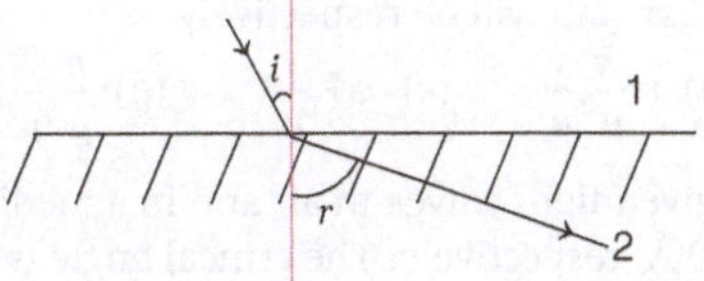

(c)
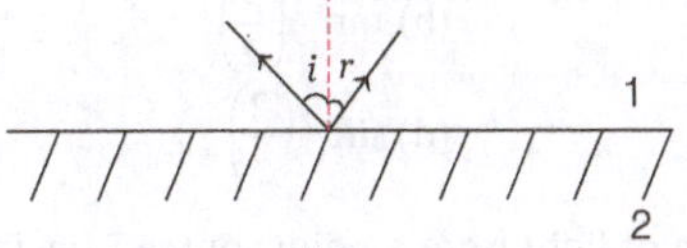

(d)
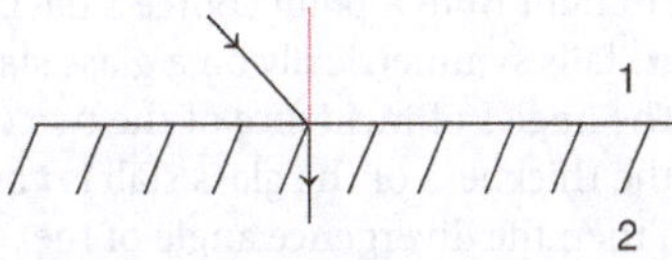

22. A point object is placed at the centre of a glass sphere of radius 6 cm and refractive index 1.5. The distance of the virtual image from the surface of the sphere is

(a) 2 cm (b) 4 cm (c) 6 cm (d) 12 cm

23. A ray of light is incident on the surface of separation of a medium at an angle of 45°and is refracted in the medium at an angle of 30°. What will be the velocity of light in the medium?

(a) 1.96×10^8 m/s (b) 2.12×10^8 m/s
(c) 265×10^8 m/s (d) 1.24×10^8 m/s

24. Wavelength of light in vacuum is 5890 Å, then its wavelength in glass ($\mu = 1.5$) will be

(a) 9372 Å (b) 7932 Å
(c) 7548 Å (d) 3927 Å

25. If refractive index of glass is 1.50 and of water is 1.33, then critical angle is

(a) $\sin^{-1}\left(\frac{8}{9}\right)$ (b) $\sin^{-1}\left(\frac{2}{3}\right)$
(c) $\cos^{-1}\left(\frac{8}{9}\right)$ (d) None of these

26. A mark at the bottom of a liquid appears to rise by 0.1 m and the depth of the liquid is 1 m. The refractive index of the liquid is

(a) 1.33 (b) 9/10 (c) 10/9 (d) 1.5

27. The time required for the light to pass through a glass slab (refractive index = 1.5) of thickness 4 mm is
(Take, speed of light in free space, $c = 3 \times 10^8$ ms^{-1})

(a) 10^{-11} s (b) 2×10^{-11} s
(c) 2×10^{11} s (d) 2×10^{-5} s

28. Light travels in two media A and B with speeds $1.8 \times 10^8 \text{ ms}^{-1}$ and $2.4 \times 10^8 \text{ ms}^{-1}$, respectively. Then, the critical angle between them is

(a) $\sin^{-1}\left(\frac{2}{3}\right)$ (b) $\tan^{-1}\left(\frac{3}{4}\right)$

(c) $\tan^{-1}\left(\frac{2}{3}\right)$ (d) $\sin^{-1}\left(\frac{3}{4}\right)$

29. Electromagnetic radiation of frequency n, wavelength λ, travelling with velocity v in air, enters a glass slab of refractive index μ. The frequency, wavelength and velocity of light in the glass slab will be respectively

(a) $\frac{n}{\mu}, \frac{\lambda}{\mu}, \frac{v}{\mu}$ (b) $n, \frac{\lambda}{\mu}, \frac{v}{\mu}$ (c) $n, \lambda, \frac{v}{\mu}$ (d) $\frac{n}{\mu}, \frac{\lambda}{\mu}, v$

30. Wavelength of given light waves in air and in a medium are 6000 Å and 3000 Å, respectively. The critical angle is

(a) $\tan^{-1}\left(\frac{2}{3}\right)$ (b) $\tan^{-1}\left(\frac{3}{2}\right)$

(c) $\sin^{-1}\left(\frac{1}{2}\right)$ (d) $\sin^{-1}\left(\frac{2}{3}\right)$

31. A diverging beam of light from a point source S having divergence angle α, falls symmetrically on a glass slab as shown in figure. The angles of incidence of the two extreme rays are equal. If the thickness of the glass slab is t and the refractive index n, then the divergence angle of the emergent beam is

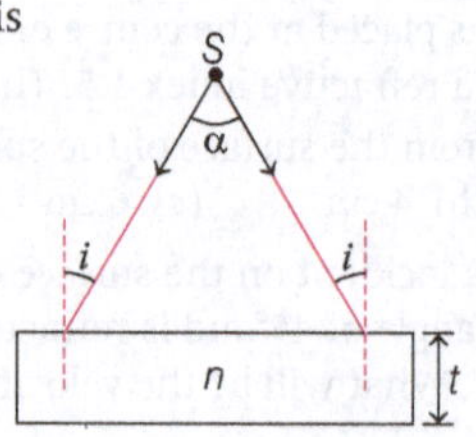

(a) zero (b) α

(c) $\sin^{-1}\frac{1}{n}$ (d) $2\sin^{-1}\left(\frac{1}{n}\right)$

32. If light travels a distance x in t_1 seconds in air and $10x$ distance in t_2 seconds in a medium, the critical angle of the medium, will be

(a) $\tan^{-1}\left(\frac{t_1}{t_2}\right)$ (b) $\sin^{-1}\left(\frac{t_1}{t_2}\right)$

(c) $\sin^{-1}\left(\frac{10t_1}{t_2}\right)$ (d) $\tan^{-1}\left(\frac{10t_1}{t_2}\right)$

33. The optical path of a monochromatic light is same whether, if it goes through 4.0 cm of glass or 4.5 cm of water. If the refractive index of glass is 1.53, then the refractive index of the water is

(a) 1.30 (b) 1.36

(c) 1.42 (d) 1.46

34. A ray of light travelling in transparent medium of refractive index μ falls on a surface separating the medium from air at an angle of incidence of 45°. For which of the following value of μ, the ray can undergo total internal reflection?

(a) $\mu = 1.33$ (b) $\mu = 1.41$

(c) $\mu = 1.50$ (d) $\mu = 1.25$

35. A ray of light, travelling in a medium of refractive index μ, is incident at an angle i on a composite transparent plate consisting of three plates of refractive indices μ_1, μ_2 and μ_3. The ray emerges from the composite plate into a medium of refractive index μ_4, at angle x, then

(a) $\sin x = \sin i$ (b) $\sin x = \frac{\mu}{\mu_4} \sin i$

(c) $\sin x = \frac{\mu_4}{\mu} \sin i$ (d) $\sin x = \frac{\mu_1}{\mu_2}\frac{\mu_3}{\mu_2}\frac{\mu}{\mu_4} \sin i$

36. How much water should be filled in a container of height 21 cm, so that it appears half filled to the observer when viewed from the top of the container? (Take, $\mu = 4/3$)

(a) 8 cm (b) 10.5 cm (c) 12 cm (d) 14 cm

37. A light ray going from air is incident (as shown in figure) at one end of a glass fibre (refractive index $\mu = 1.5$) making an incidence angle of 60° on the lateral surface,

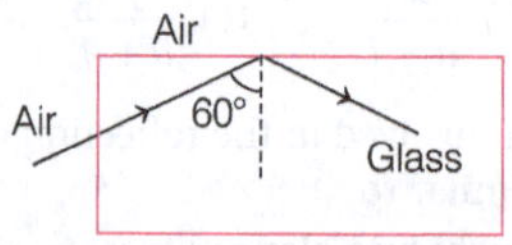

so that it undergoes a total internal reflection. How much time would it take to traverse the straight fibre of length 1 km?

(a) 3.3 μs (b) 6.6 μs

(c) 5.7 μs (d) 3.85 μs

38. A ray incident at a point as an angle of incidence of 60° enters a glass sphere of refractive index $n = \sqrt{3}$ and is reflected and refracted further at the surface of the sphere. The angle between the reflected and refracted rays at this surface is

(a) 50° (b) 60° (c) 90° (d) 40°

39. An object is placed at 21 cm infront of a concave mirror of radius of a curvature 10 cm. A glass slab of thickness 3 cm and $\mu = 1.5$ is then placed close to the mirror in the space between the object and the mirror. The position of final image formed is

(a) −3.94 cm (b) 4.3 cm

(c) −4.93 cm (d) 3.94 cm

40. If a ray of light in a denser medium strikes a rarer medium at an angle of incidence i, the angles of reflection and refraction are respectively, r and r'. If the reflected and refraction rays are at right angles to each other, the critical angle for the given pair of media is

(a) $\sin^{-1}(\tan r')$ (b) $\sin^{-1}(\tan r)$

(c) $\tan^{-1}(\sin i)$ (d) $\cot^{-1}(\tan i)$

41. The XZ-plane separates two media A and B with refractive indices μ_1 and μ_2, respectively. A ray of light travels from A and B. Its directions in the two media are given by the unit vectors $\mathbf{r}_A = a\hat{\mathbf{i}} + b\hat{\mathbf{j}}$ and $\mathbf{r}_B = \alpha\hat{\mathbf{i}} + \beta\hat{\mathbf{j}}$ respectively, where $\hat{\mathbf{i}}$ and $\hat{\mathbf{j}}$ are unit vectors in the x and y-directions. Then,

(a) $\mu_1 a = \mu_2 \alpha$ (b) $\mu_1 \alpha = \mu_2 a$

(c) $\mu_1 b = \mu_2 \beta$ (d) None of these

42. A ray of light is incident on surface of glass slab at an angle 45°. If the lateral shift produced per unit thickness is $\frac{1}{\sqrt{3}}$ m, the angle of refraction produced is

(a) $\tan^{-1}\left(\frac{\sqrt{3}}{2}\right)$ (b) $\tan^{-1}\left(1-\sqrt{\frac{2}{3}}\right)$

(c) $\sin^{-1}\left(1-\sqrt{\frac{2}{3}}\right)$ (d) $\tan^{-1}\left(\sqrt{\frac{2}{\sqrt{3}-1}}\right)$

43. In a lake, a fish rising vertically to the surface of water uniformly at the rate of 3 m/s, observes a bird diving vertically towards the water at the rate of 9 m/s. The actual velocity of the dive of the bird is
(Take, refractive index of water = 4/3)

(a) 3.6 m/s (b) 4.5 m/s
(c) 6.0 m/s (d) 12.0 m/s

44. Consider the situation as shown in figure. The point O is the centre and the light ray forms an angle of 60° with the normal.

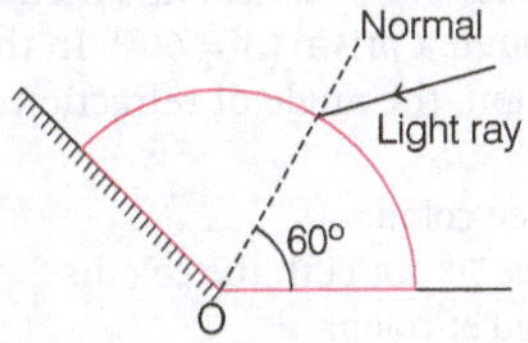

The normal makes an angle 60° with the horizontal and the mirror makes an angle 60° with the normal. The value of refractive index of that spherical portions, so that light ray retraces its path is

(a) $\sqrt{2}$ (b) $\frac{2}{\sqrt{3}}$

(c) $\frac{3}{2}$ (d) $\sqrt{3}$

45. A concave mirror is placed at the bottom of an empty tank with face upwards and axis vertical. When sunlight falls normally on the mirror, then it is focused at distance of 32 cm from the mirror. If the tank filled with water $\left(\mu=\frac{4}{3}\right)$ upto a height of 20 cm, then the sunlight will now get focused at

(a) 16 cm above water level (b) 9 cm above water level
(c) 24 cm below water level (d) 9 cm below water level

46. Given a slab with index $\mu = 1.33$ and incident light striking the top horizontal face at angle i as shown in figure. The maximum value of i for which total internal reflection occurs is

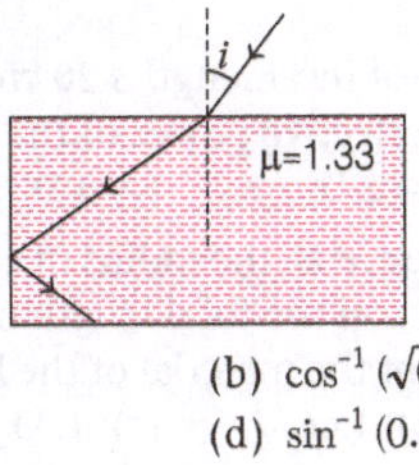

(a) $\sin^{-1}(\sqrt{0.77})$ (b) $\cos^{-1}(\sqrt{0.77})$
(c) $\sin^{-1}(0.77)$ (d) $\sin^{-1}(0.38)$

47. The apparent depth of water in cylindrical water tank of diameter $2R$ cm is reducing at the rate of x cm/min when water is being drained out at a constant rate. The amount of water drained (in cc/min) is (n_1 = refractive index of air, n_2 = refractive index of water)

(a) $\frac{x\pi R^2 n_1}{n_2}$ (b) $\frac{x\pi R^2 n_2}{n_1}$

(c) $\frac{2\pi R n_1}{n_2}$ (d) $\pi R^2 x$

48. In the figure shown, for an angle of incidence 45°, at the top surface, what is the minimum refractive index needed for total internal reflection at vertical face AD ?

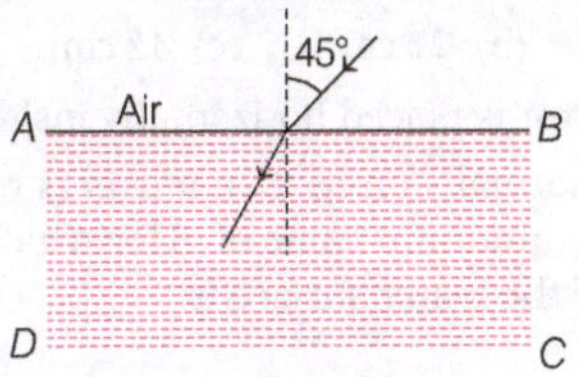

(a) $\frac{\sqrt{2}+1}{2}$ (b) $\sqrt{\frac{3}{2}}$ (c) $\sqrt{\frac{1}{2}}$ (d) $\sqrt{2}$

49. A ray of light passes from a medium A having refractive index 1.6 to the medium B having refractive index 1.5. The value of critical angle of medium A is

(a) $\sin^{-1}\sqrt{\frac{16}{15}}$ (b) $\sin^{-1}\left(\frac{16}{15}\right)$ (c) $\sin^{-1}\left(\frac{1}{2}\right)$ (d) $\sin^{-1}\left(\frac{15}{16}\right)$

50. In vacuum, to travel distance d, light takes time t and in medium to travel distance $5d$, it takes time T. The critical angle of the medium is

(a) $\sin^{-1}\left(\frac{5T}{t}\right)$ (b) $\sin^{-1}\left(\frac{5t}{3T}\right)$

(c) $\sin^{-1}\left(\frac{5t}{T}\right)$ (d) $\sin^{-1}\left(\frac{3t}{5T}\right)$

51. The speed of light in media M_1 and M_2 are 1.5×10^8 ms^{-1} and 2×10^8 ms^{-1}, respectively. A ray travels from medium M_1 to the medium M_2 with an angle of incidence θ. The ray suffers total internal reflection. Then, the value of the angle of incidence θ is

(a) $>\sin^{-1}\left(\frac{3}{4}\right)$ (b) $<\sin^{-1}\left(\frac{3}{4}\right)$

(c) $=\sin^{-1}\left(\frac{3}{4}\right)$ (d) $\leq\sin^{-1}\left(\frac{3}{4}\right)$

52. A hemispherical paper weight contains a small flower on its axis of symmetry at a distance of 4 cm from its flat surface. Where is the flower appears to an observer when he looks at it along the axis of symmetry from the top? (Take, refractive index of refraction of glass = 1.5)

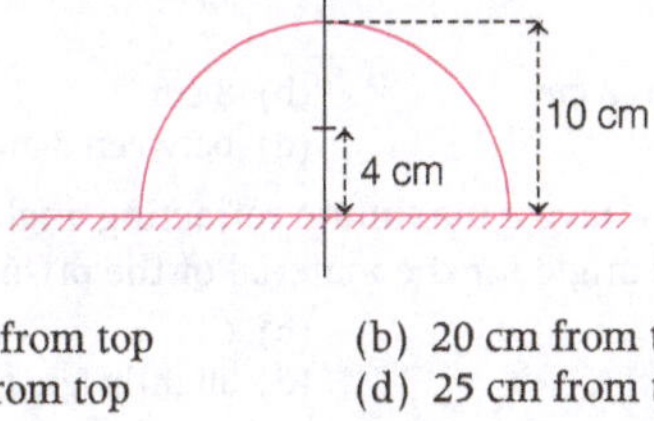

(a) 15 cm from top (b) 20 cm from top
(c) 5 cm from top (d) 25 cm from top

53. A slab of glass, of thickness 6 cm and refractive index $\mu = 1.5$ is placed infront of a concave mirror as shown in the figure. If the radius of curvature of the mirror is 40 cm and the reflected image coincides with the object, then the distance of the object from the mirror is

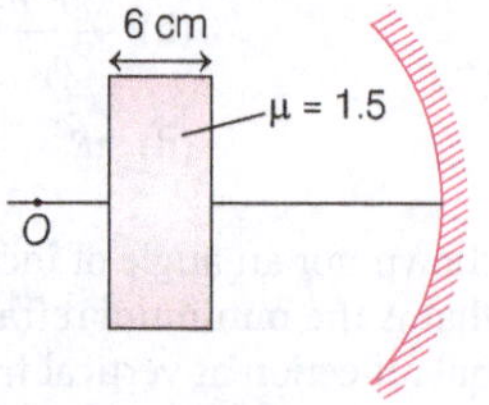

(a) 30 cm (b) 22 cm (c) 42 cm (d) 38 cm

54. A plane mirror is placed horizontally inside water ($\mu = 4/3$). A ray falls normally on it, then mirror is rotated through an angle θ, the minimum value of θ for which ray does not come out of the water surface is

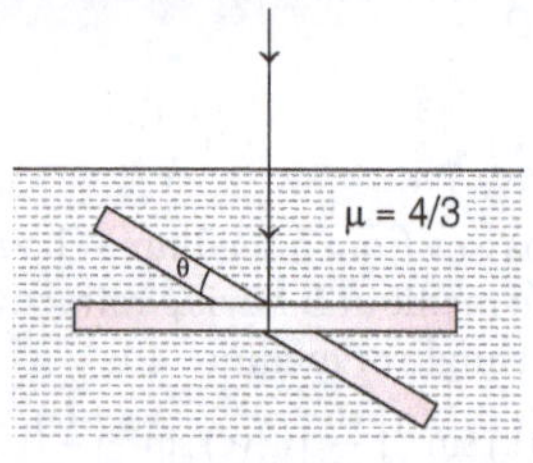

(a) $\pi/4$ (b) $\sin^{-1}\left(\frac{3}{4}\right)$
(c) $\frac{1}{2}\sin^{-1}\left(\frac{3}{4}\right)$ (d) $2\sin^{-1}\left(\frac{3}{4}\right)$

55. Which of the following quantities increases when wavelength of light is increased? Consider only the magnitudes.
(a) The power of a converging lens
(b) The focal length of a converging lens
(c) The power of a diverging lens
(d) None of the above

56. When an object is at distance x and y from a lens, a real image and a virtual image is formed respectively having same magnification. The focal length of the lens is
(a) $\frac{x+y}{2}$ (b) $x-y$ (c) $\sqrt{xy}$ (d) $x+y$

57. A plano-convex lens is made of refractive index of 1.6. The radius of curvature of the curved surface is 60 cm. The focal length of the lens is
(a) 400 cm (b) 200 cm
(c) 100 cm (d) 50 cm

58. An object has an image thrice of its original size when kept at 8 cm and 16 cm from a convex lens. Focal length of the lens is
(a) less than 8 cm (b) 8 cm
(c) 16 cm (d) between 8 and 16 cm

59. A prism can have a maximum refracting angle of (C = critical angle for the material of the prism)
(a) 60° (b) C
(c) $2C$ (d) slightly less than 180°

60. When a lens of refractive index n_1 is placed in a liquid of refractive index n_2, then the lens seems to be disappeared only, if
(a) $n_1 = n_2/2$ (b) $n_1 = 3n_2/2$
(c) $n_1 = n_2$ (d) $n_1 = 5n_2/2$

61. When a thin convex lens is put in contact with a thin concave lens of the same focal length f, then the resultant combination has focal length equal to
(a) $f/2$ (b) $2f$ (c) 0 (d) ∞

62. Under minimum deviation condition in a prism, if a ray is incident at an angle of 30°, then the angle between the emergent ray and the second refracting surface of the prism is
(a) 0° (b) 30° (c) 45° (d) 60°

63. If x_1 is the size of the magnified image and x_2 is the size of the diminished image in lens displacement method, then the size of the object is
(a) $\sqrt{x_1 x_2}$ (b) $x_1 x_2$ (c) $x_1^2 x_2$ (d) $x_1 x_2^2$

64. Two beams of red and violet colours made to pass separately through a prism ($A = 60°$). In the minimum deviation position, the angle of refraction inside the prism will be
(a) greater for red colour
(b) equal but not 30° for both the colours
(c) greater for violet colour
(d) 30° for both the colours

65. An object is placed at a distance u from an equiconvex lens such that the distance between the object and its real image is minimum. The focal length of the lens is f. The value of u is
(a) ∞ (b) $1.5f$ (c) $2f$ (d) $4f$

66. We have combined a convex lens of focal length f_1 and concave lens of focal length f_2 and their combined focal length was F. The combination of these lenses will behave like a concave lens, if
(a) $f_1 > f_2$ (b) $f_1 < f_2$
(c) $f_1 = f_2$ (d) $f_1 \le f_2$

67. The radius of curvature of the curved surface of a plano- convex lens is 20 cm. If the refractive index of the material of the lens be 1.5, then it will ***[NCERT Exemplar]***
(a) act as a convex lens only for the objects that lie on its curved side
(b) act as a concave lens for the objects that lie on its curved side
(c) act as a convex lens irrespective of the side on which the object lies
(d) act as a concave lens irrespective of side on which the object lies

68. Two thin lenses of focal lengths 20 cm and 25 cm are placed in contact. The effective power of the combination is
(a) 9 D (b) 2 D (c) 3 D (d) 7 D

69. In a plano-convex lens, the radius of curvature of convex surface is 10 cm and the focal length of the lens is 30 cm. The refractive index of the material of the lens will be
(a) 1.5 (b) 1.66 (c) 1.33 (d) 3

70. If the refractive index of a material of equilateral prism is $\sqrt{3}$, then angle of minimum deviation of the prism is
(a) 30° (b) 45° (c) 60° (d) 75°

71. A ray of light is incident at 60° on one face of a prism of angle 30° and the emergent ray makes 30° with the incident ray. The refractive index of the prism is
(a) 1.732 (b) 1.414 (c) 1.5 (d) 1.33

72. A convex lens forms an image of an object on a screen 30 cm from the lens. When the lens is moved 90 cm towards the object, then the image is again formed on the screen. Then, the focal length of the lens is
(a) 13 cm (b) 24 cm
(c) 33 cm (d) 40 cm

73. A double convex glass lens ($R_1 = R_2 = 10$ cm) having focal length equal to the focal length of a concave mirror. The radius of curvature of the concave mirror is ($\mu_g = 1.5$)
(a) 10 cm (b) 20 cm
(c) 40 cm (d) 15 cm

74. The radii of curvature of the two surfaces of a lens are 20 cm and 30 cm and the refractive index of the material of the lens is 1.5. If the lens is concave-convex, then the focal length of the lens is
(a) 24 cm (b) 10 cm (c) 15 cm (d) 120 cm

75. The power of a biconvex lens is 10 D and the radius of curvature of each surface is 10 cm. Then, the refractive index of the material of the lens is
(a) $\frac{3}{2}$ (b) $\frac{4}{3}$ (c) $\frac{9}{8}$ (d) $\frac{5}{3}$

76. Two lenses are placed in contact with each other and the focal length of combination is 80 cm. If the focal length of one is 20 cm, then the power of the other will be
(a) 1.66 D (b) 4.00 D
(c) −1.00 D (d) −3.75 D

77. A plano-convex lens of refractive index 1.5 and radius of curvature 30 cm is silvered at the curved surface. Now, the lens has been used to form the image of an object. What should be the distance of the object from the lens in order to have a real image of the size of the object?
(a) 20 cm (b) 30 cm
(c) 60 cm (d) 80 cm

78. A ray of light incident at an angle θ on a refracting face of a prism emerges from the other face normally. If the angle of the prism is 5° and the prism is made of a material of refractive index 1.5, then the angle of incidence is ***[NCERT Exemplar]***
(a) 7.5° (b) 5° (c) 15° (d) 2.5°

79. For a divergent lens, the object is at m times its focal length, where m is linear magnification produced by the lens having the value
(a) m (b) $\frac{1}{m}$
(c) $m+1$ (d) $\frac{1}{m+1}$

80. The figure shows an equiconvex lens of focal length f. If the lens is cut along PQ, the focal length of each half will be

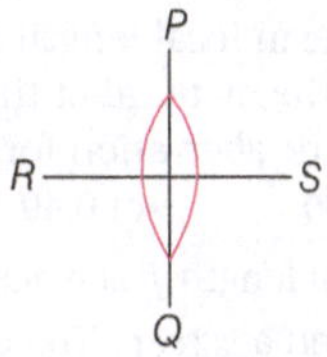

(a) $\frac{f}{2}$ (b) f (c) $2f$ (d) $4f$

81. A prism having refractive index 1.414 and refracting angle 30° has one of the refracting surfaces silvered. A beam of light incident on the other refracting surface will retrace its path, if the angle of incidence is
(a) 0° (b) 30° (c) 60° (d) 45°

82. Two thin lenses have a combined power of +9 D. When they are separated by a distance of 20 cm, then their equivalent power becomes $+\frac{27}{5}$ D. Their individual powers (in dioptre) are
(a) 1, 8 (b) 2, 7 (c) 3,6 (d) 4, 5

83. A convex lens of focal length 1.0 m and a concave lens of focal length 0.25 m are 0.75 m apart. A parallel beam of light is incident in the convex lens. The beam emerging after refraction from both lenses is
(a) parallel to principal axis (b) convergent
(c) divergent (d) None of these

84. For an angle of incidence θ on an equilateral prism of refractive index $\sqrt{3}$, the ray refracted is parallel to the base inside the prism. The value of θ is
(a) 30° (b) 45° (c) 60° (d) 75°

85. A thin prism of angle 6° made up of glass of refractive index 1.5 is combined with another prism made up of glass of refractive index 1.75 to produce dispersion without deviation. The angle of second prism is
(a) 7° (b) 9° (c) 4° (d) 5°

86. A double convex lens made of glass (refractive index n =1.5) has both radii of curvature of magnitude 20 cm. Incident light rays parallel to the axis of the lens will converge at a distance L such that
(a) $L = 20$ cm (b) $L = 10$ cm
(c) $L = 40$ cm (d) $L = \frac{20}{3}$ cm

87. A glass prism has a refractive angle of 90° and a refractive index of 1.5. A ray is incident at an angle of 30°. The ray emerges from an adjacent face at an angle of
(a) 60° (b) 30° (c) 45°
(d) the ray does not emerge from the prism

88. An equilateral prism deviates a ray through 45° for the two angles of incidence differing by 20°. The angle of incidence is
(a) 62.5° (b) 42.5°
(c) Both (a) and (b) (d) None of these

89. A thin plano-convex lens acts like a concave mirror of radius of curvature 20 cm when its plane surface is silvered. The radius of curvature of the curved surface, if index of refraction of its material is 1.5 will be
(a) 40 cm (b) 30 cm (c) 10 cm (d) 20 cm

90. A convex lens has mean focal length of 20 cm. The dispersive power of the material of the lens is 0.02. The longitudinal chromatic aberration for an object at infinity is
(a) 10^3 (b) 0.80 (c) 0.40 (d) 0.20

91. A convex lens of focal length f is placed somewhere in between an object and a screen. The distance between object and screen is x. If numerical value of magnification produced by lens is m, then focal length of lens is
(a) $\frac{mx}{(m+1)^2}$ (b) $\frac{mx}{(m-1)^2}$
(c) $\frac{(m+1)^2}{m}x$ (d) $\frac{(m-1)^2}{m}x$

92. A plano-convex lens has a maximum thickness of 6 cm. When placed on a horizontal table with the curved surface in contact with the table surface, then the apparent depth of the bottom most point of the lens is found to be 4 cm. If the lens is inverted such that the plane face of the lens is in contact with the surface of the table, then the apparent depth of the centre of the plane face is found to be $\frac{17}{3}$ cm. The radius of curvature of the lens is
(a) 68 cm (b) 75 cm (c) 128 cm (d) 34 cm

93. A ray falls on a prism ABC ($AB = BC$) and travels as shown in figure. The minimum refractive index of the prism material should be

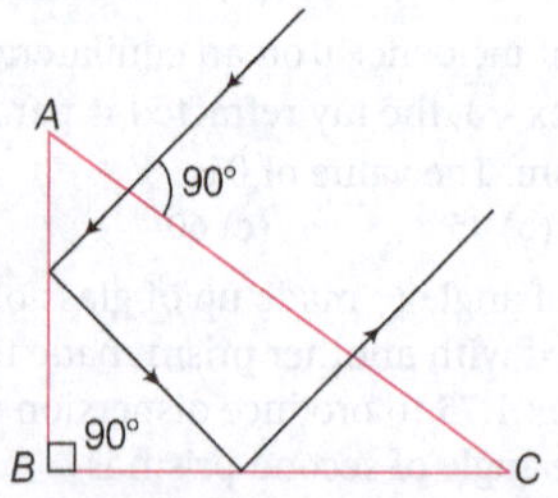

(a) 4/3 (b) $\sqrt{2}$ (c) 1.5 (d) $\sqrt{3}$

94. If the distances of an object and its virtual image from the focus of a convex lens of focal length f are 1 cm each, then f is
(a) 4 cm (b) $(\sqrt{2}+1)$ cm
(c) $2\sqrt{2}$ cm (d) $(2+\sqrt{2})$ cm

95. A thin convergent glass lens $\mu = 1.5$ has a power of + 5.0 D. When this lens is immersed in a liquid of refractive index μ_l it acts as diverging lens of focal length 100 cm. The value of μ_l should be
(a) $\frac{3}{2}$ (b) $\frac{4}{3}$ (c) $\frac{5}{3}$ (d) 2

96. The figure shows an equiconvex lens. What should be the condition on the refractive indices, so that the lens become diverging?

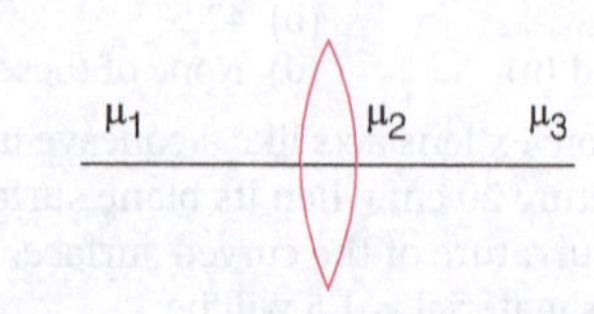

(a) $2\mu_3 > (\mu_1 - \mu_2)$ (b) $2\mu_2 < (\mu_1 + \mu_3)$
(c) $2\mu_2 > (2\mu_1 - \mu_3)$ (d) None of these

97. The graph shows, how the inverse of magnification $\frac{1}{m}$ produced by a convex thin lens, with variation in object distance u. What was the focal length of the lens used?

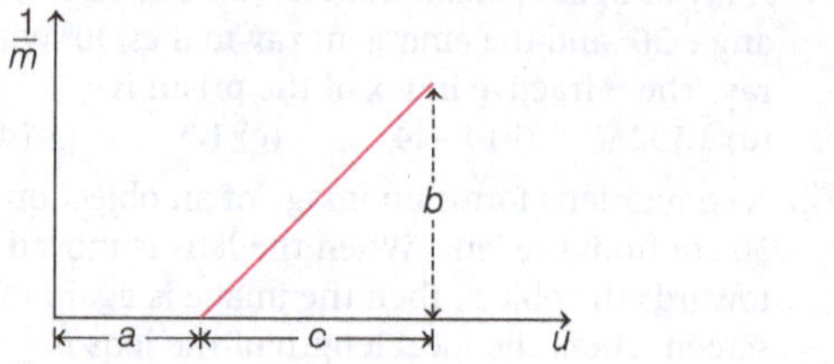

(a) $\frac{b}{c}$ (b) $\frac{b}{ca}$
(c) $\frac{bc}{a}$ (d) $\frac{c}{b}$

98. A convex lens of focal length 30 cm forms a real image three times larger than the object on a screen. Object and screen are moved until the image becomes twice the size of the object. If the shift of the object is 6 cm. The shift of screen is
(a) 28 cm (b) 14 cm
(c) 18 cm (d) 16 cm

99. A ray PQ incident on the refracting face BA is refracted in the prism BAC as shown in the figure and emerges from the other refracting face AC as RS, such that $AQ = AR$. If the angle of prism $A = 60°$ and the refractive index of the material of prism is $\sqrt{3}$, then the angle of deviation of the ray is

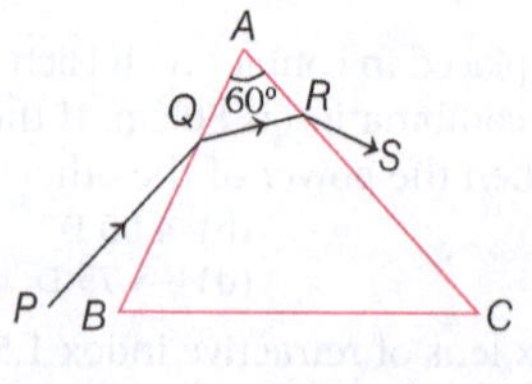

(a) 60° (b) 45°
(c) 30° (d) None of these

100 A thin symmetrical double convex lens of refractive index $\mu_2 = 1.5$ is placed between a medium of refractive index $\mu_1 = 1.4$ to the left and another medium of refractive index $\mu_3 = 1.6$ to the right. Then, the system behaves as
(a) a convex lens
(b) a concave lens
(c) a glass plate
(d) a convexo concave lens

101. An object is located 4 m from the first of two thin converging lenses of focal lengths 2 m and 1 m, respectively. The lenses are separated by 3 m. The final image formed by the second lens is located from the source at a distance of

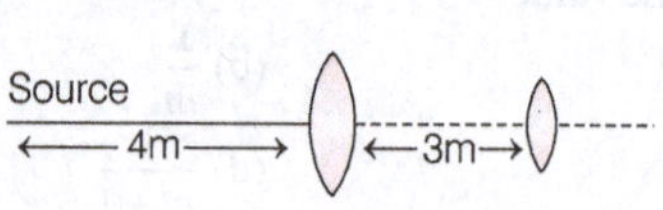

(a) 8 m (b) 5.5 m
(c) 6 m (d) 6.5 m

102. An object is placed 30 cm away from a convex lens of focal length 10 cm and a sharp image is formed on a screen. Now, a concave lens is placed in contact with the convex lens. The screen now has to be moved by 45 cm to get a sharp image again. The magnitude of focal length of the concave lens is (in cm)
(a) 72 (b) 60 (c) 36 (d) 20

103. A plano-convex lens fits exactly into a plano-concave lens. Their plane surfaces are parallel to each other. If lenses are made of different materials of refractive indices μ_1 and μ_2 and R is the radius of curvature of the curved surface of the lenses, then the focal length of the combination is
(a) $\frac{R}{2(\mu_1+\mu_2)}$ (b) $\frac{R}{2(\mu_1-\mu_2)}$
(c) $\frac{R}{(\mu_1-\mu_2)}$ (d) $\frac{2R}{(\mu_2-\mu_1)}$

104. A small angled prism of refractive index 1.4 is combined with another small angled prism of refractive index 1.6 to produce dispersion without deviation. If the angle of first prism is 6°, then the angle of the second prism is
(a) 8° (b) 6° (c) 4° (d) 2°

105. An object is placed at a distance of 10 cm from a co-axial combination of two lenses A and B in contact. The combination forms a real image three times the size of the object. If lens B is concave with a focal length of 30 cm, then the nature and focal length of lens A is
(a) convex, 12 cm (b) concave, 12 cm
(c) convex, 6 cm (d) convex, 18 cm

106. The minimum magnifying power of telescope is M. If the focal length of its eye lens is halved, the magnifying power will become
(a) $m/2$ (b) $2m$ (c) $3m$ (d) $4m$

107. A telescope has an objective of focal length 100 cm and an eyepiece of focal length 5 cm. What is the magnifying power of the telescope when it is in normal adjustment?
(a) 0.2 (b) 2.0 (c) 20 (d) 200

108. If the focal length of the eyepiece of a telescope is doubled, then its magnifying power (m) will be
(a) $2m$ (b) $3m$ (c) $m/2$ (d) $4m$

109. An astronomical telescope in normal adjustment receives light from a distance source S, the tube length is now decreased slightly, then
(a) no image will be formed
(b) a virtual image of S will be formed at a finite distance
(c) a large, real image of S will be formed behind the eye piece, far away from it
(d) a small, real image of S will be formed behind the eye-piece closes to it

110. An astronomical telescope has an angular magnification of magnitude 5 for distant objects. The separation between the objective and the eyepiece is 36 cm and the final image is formed at infinity. The focal length f_o of the objective and the focal length f_e of eyepiece are
(a) $f_o = 45$ cm and $f_e = -9$ cm
(b) $f_o = -7.2$ cm and $f_e = 5$ cm
(c) $f_o = 50$ cm and $f_e = 10$ cm
(d) $f_o = 30$ cm and $f_e = 6$ cm

111. The magnification produced by an astronomical telescope for normal adjustment is 10 and the length of the telescope is 1.1 m. The magnification, when the image is formed at least distance of distinct vision is
(a) 6 (b) 14 (c) 16 (d) 18

112. The focal lengths of the lenses of an astronomical telescope are 50 cm and 5 cm. The length of the telescope when the image is formed at the least distance of distinct vision is
(a) 45 cm (b) 55 cm
(c) $\frac{275}{6}$ cm (d) $\frac{325}{6}$ cm

113. If tube length of astronomical telescope is 105 cm and magnifying power is 20 for normal setting, then the focal length of objective is
(a) 100 cm (b) 10 cm (c) 20 cm (d) 25 cm

114. The focal lengths of the objective and eye lens of a microscope are 1 cm and 5 cm, respectively. If the magnifying power for the relaxed eye is 45, then the length of the tube is
(a) 30 cm (b) 25 cm (c) 15 cm (d) 12 cm

115. A telescope has a objective of focal length 50 cm and an eyepiece of focal length 5 cm. The least distance of distinct vision is 25 cm. The telescope is focused for distinct vision on a scale of 200 cm away. The separation between the objective and the eyepiece is
(a) 75 cm (b) 60 cm (c) 71 cm (d) 74 cm

116 The focal length of the objective of a terrestrial telescope is 80 cm and it is adjusted for parallel rays and its magnifying power is 20. If the focal length of erecting lens is 20 cm, then full length of telescope will be
(a) 84 cm (b) 100 cm (c) 124 cm (d) 164 cm

117. The magnifying power of a microscope with an objective of 5 mm focal length is 400. The length of its tube is 20 cm. Then, the focal length of the eye-piece is
(a) 200 cm (b) 160 cm (c) 2.5 cm (d) 0.1 cm

118. In a compound microscope, the focal length of the objective is 2.5 cm and of eye lens is 5 cm. If an object is placed at 3.75 cm before the objective and the image is formed at the least distance of distinct vision, then the distance between two lenses will be
(a) 11.67 cm (b) 12 cm
(c) 12.75 cm (d) 13 cm

Assertion and Reason

Directions (Q. Nos. 1-5) *These questions consist of two statements each printed as Assertion (A) and Reason (R). While answering these questions, you are required to choose any one of the following four responses.*
(a) Both A and R are true but R is not the correct explanation of A.
(b) A is true but R is false.
(c) A is false but R is true.
(d) Both A and R are true and R is the correct explanation of A.

1. **Assertion** (A) Infront of a concave mirror, a point object is placed between focus and centre of curvature. If a glass slab is placed between object and mirror, then image from mirror may become virtual.
   Reason (R) Glass slab always makes a virtual image of a real object.
2. **Assertion** (A) The refractive index of diamond is $\sqrt{6}$ and that of liquid is $\sqrt{3}$. If the light travels from diamond to the liquid, it will totally reflected when the angle of incidence is 30°.
   Reason (R) $\mu = \frac{1}{\sin C}$, where μ is the refractive index of diamond with respect to liquid.
3. **Assertion** (A) The images formed by total internal reflection are much brighter than those formed by mirrors or lenses.
   Reason (R) There is no loss of intensity in total internal reflection.
4. **Assertion** (A) A diverging lens (in air) cannot be made more diverging whatever be the medium we choose to completely immerse the lens.
   Reason (R) The minimum refractive index of any medium is 1.
5. **Assertion** (A) A hollow lens behaves like a thin glass plate.
   Reason (R) Power of this lens becomes zero.

Statement Type Questions

Directions (Q. Nos. 1-5) *These questions consists of two statements, choose the most appropriate answer from the options given below*

(a) Both Statement I and Statement II are incorrect.
(b) Statement I is correct but Statement II is incorrect.
(c) Statement I is incorrect but Statement II is correct.
(d) Both Statement I and Statement II are correct.

1. **Statement I** In the given figure, OO' is the principal axis of a spherical mirror. The image of point object S is S' $(h_2 < h_1)$. Then, the mirror is concave mirror placed right side of image S'.

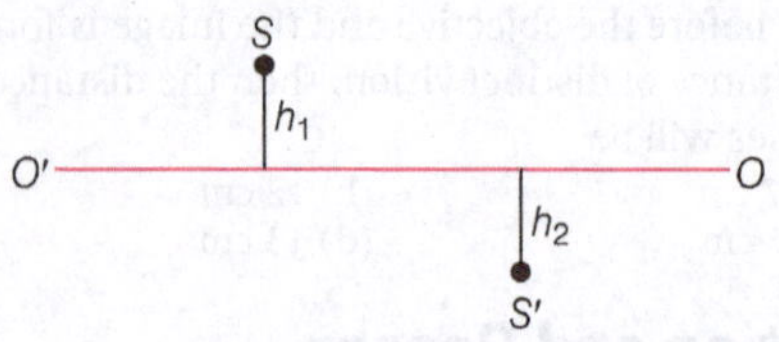

   Statement II If object and image both real, transverse magnification is negative.
2. **Statement I** The formula $\frac{\mu_2}{v} - \frac{\mu_1}{u} = \frac{\mu_2 - \mu_1}{r}$ is applicable for only paraxial rays.
   Statement II The laws of refraction is applicable for plane refractive surface as well as curved refractive surface.
3. **Statement I** The image of a virtual object formed by a thin converging lens is always real.
   Statement II In the case of thin lens, $\frac{1}{v} - \frac{1}{u} = \frac{1}{f}$.
4. **Statement I** If a diverging lens is placed in medium, whose refractive index is greater than that of lens, the lens behaves as converging lens.
   Statement II According to thin lens maker's formula.
   $$\frac{1}{f} = (\mu - 1)\left(\frac{1}{R_1} - \frac{1}{R_2}\right),$$
   where, $\mu = \frac{\text{Refractive index of lens}}{\text{Refractive index of surrounding}}$
5. **Statement I** When a thin prism is placed in a medium, whose refractive index is lesser than that of prism, deviation produced by prism decreases.
   Statement II Deviation produced by thin prism is same for any angle of incidence.

Match the Columns

1. Match the Column I with Column II.

	Column I		Column II
A.	$\frac{1}{f} = (\mu - 1)\left(\frac{1}{R_1} - \frac{1}{R_2}\right)$	I.	total internal reflection
B.	Light rays bend towards the normal when moving from a rarer to a denser medium.	II.	Refraction at a concave surface
C.	Light rays diverge when passing through and appear to originate from a point behind the surface	III.	Refraction at a convex surface
D.	$\sin i_e = \frac{\mu_2}{\mu_1}$, when $n_1 > n_2$	IV.	Lens maker's formula

Choose the correct answer from the options given below.
(a) A-(IV), B-(III), C-(II), D-(I)
(b) A-(III), B-(IV), C-(II) D-(I)
(c) A-(II), B-(III), C-(IV), D-(I)
(d) A-(I), B-(IV), C-(II), D, (III)

2. Consider a rectangular slab, whose refractive index varies as $\mu = 1 + \frac{y}{a}$, where $a = 1\ \text{m}^{-1}$.

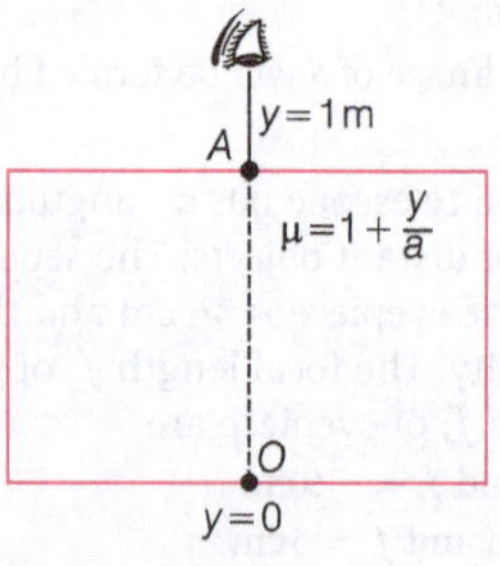

Match the Column I with Column II.

Column I	Column II
A. The equivalent refractive index of slab for normal incidence.	I. 5×10^{-9}
B. The apparent depth of point (in m).	II. 0.693
C. The optical path of a ray along (in m) .	III. 1.5
D. The time (in second) taken by light ray to go vertically from point to point .	IV. 1.44

Choose the correct answer from the options given below.

(a) A-(II), B-(IV), C-(I),D-(II)
(b) A-(III), B-(II), C-(IV) D, (I)
(c) A-(IV), B-(II), C-(III), D-(I)
(d) A-(I), B-(III), C-(II), D, (IV)

3. An equiconcave lens of refractive index μ_2 and focal length – 20 cm (in air) is kept in a medium of refractive index μ_1. Match the Column I with Column II.

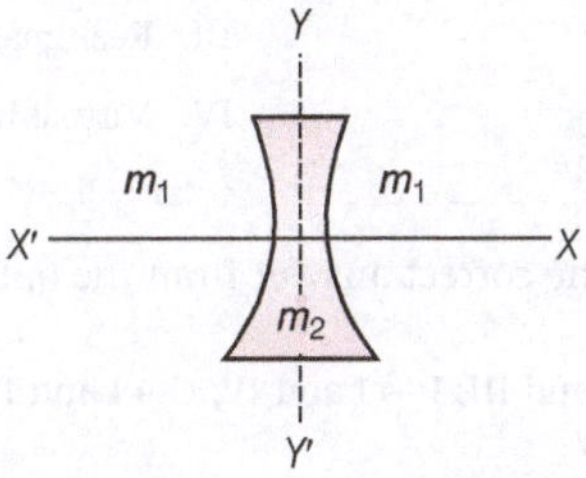

Column I	Column II
A. If lens is cut in two equal parts by a plane YY' (Take, $\mu_1 = 1$)	I. Lens will acts as glass slab
B. If lens is cut in two equal parts by a plane XX' (Take, $\mu_1 = 1$)	II. Lens will diverging and focal length will change
C. If $\mu_1 = \mu_2$	III. Lens will be diverging and focal length will remains same
D. If $\mu_1 > \mu_2$	IV. Lens will be converging and focal length will be change

Choose the correct answer from the options given below.

(a) A-(IV), B-(III), C-(II),D-(I)
(b) A-(II), B-(III), C-(I) D, (IV)
(c) A-(III), B-(IV), C-(II), D-(I)
(d) A-(I), B-(II), C-(III), D, (IV)

4. A compound microscope consists of two converging lenses of focal length 2 cm and 10 cm. The separation between lenses is 15 cm. Match the Column I with Column II.

Column I	Column II
A. Focal length of objective (in cm)	I. $-\frac{11}{4}$
B. For normal adjustment, object distance in (cm) from objective.	II. 3.75
C. For normal adjustment, numerical value of angular magnification	III. $\frac{10}{3}$
D. For clear vision, numerical value of angular magnification	IV. 2

Choose the correct answer from the options given below.

(a) A-(III), B-(II), C-(I), D-(IV)
(b) A-(II), B-(IV), C-(III) D, (I)
(c) A-(I), B-(II), C-(IV), D-(III)
(d) A-(IV), B-(III), C-(II), D, (I)

Final Check Through PYQs

Module-I Reflection of Light

1. An object is placed on the principal axis of a concave mirror at a distance of 1.5 f (f is the focal length). The image will be at ***[NCERT (New) Pg. 225, NEET (Oct.) 2020]***

(a) $-3f$ (b) $1.5f$ (c) $-1.5f$ (d) $3f$

2. An object is placed at a distance of 40 cm from a concave mirror of focal length 15 cm. If the object is displaced through a distance of 20 cm towards the mirror, the displacement of the image will be ***[NCERT (New) Pg. 225, NEET 2018]***

(a) 30 cm towards the mirror
(b) 36 cm away from the mirror
(c) 30 cm away from the mirror
(d) 36 cm towards the mirror

3. A beam of light from a source L is incident normally on a plane mirror fixed at a certain distance x from the source. The beam is reflected back as a spot on a scale placed just above the source L. When the mirror is rotated through a small angle θ, the spot of the light is found to move through a distance y on the scale. The angle θ is given by ***[NCERT (Old) Pg. 311, NEET 2017]***

(a) $\frac{y}{2x}$ (b) $\frac{y}{x}$ (c) $\frac{x}{2y}$ (d) $\frac{x}{y}$

4. Match the corresponding entries of Column-I with Column-II. [Where m is the magnification produced by the mirror] ***[NCERT (New) Pg. 225, NEET 2016]***

Column-I	Column-II
A. $m = -2$	I. Convex mirror
B. $m = -\frac{1}{2}$	II. Concave mirror
C. $m = +2$	III. Real image
D. $m = +\frac{1}{2}$	IV. Virtual image

Choose the correct answer from the options given below.

(a) A→I and III; B→I and IV; C→I and II; D→III and IV
(b) A→I and IV; B→II and III; C→II and IV; D→II and III
(c) A→III and IV; B→II and IV; C→II and III; D→I and IV
(d) A→II and III; B→II and III; C→II and IV; D→I and IV

Module-II Refraction of Light

5. Light travels a distance x in time t_1 in air and $10x$ in time t_2 in another denser medium. What is the critical angle for this medium? ***[NEET 2023]***

(a) $\sin^{-1}\left(\frac{10t_2}{t_1}\right)$ (b) $\sin^{-1}\left(\frac{t_1}{10t_2}\right)$

(c) $\sin^{-1}\left(\frac{10t_1}{t_2}\right)$ (d) $\sin^{-1}\left(\frac{t_2}{t_1}\right)$

6. Two transparent media A and B are separated by a plane boundary. The speed of light in those media are 1.5×10^8 m/s and 2.0×10^8 m/s, respectively. The critical angle for a ray of light for these two media is ***[NCERT (New) Pg. 230, NEET 2022]***

(a) $\sin^{-1}(0.750)$ (b) $\tan^{-1}(0.500)$

(c) $\tan^{-1}(0.750)$ (d) $\sin^{-1}(0.500)$

7. Find the value of the angle of emergence from the prism. Refractive index of the glass is $\sqrt{3}$. ***[NCERT (New) Pg. 230, NEET 2021]***

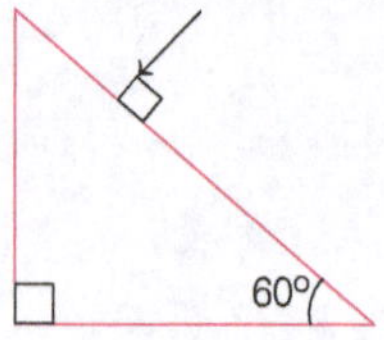

(a) 60° (b) 30°
(c) 45° (d) 90°

8. If the critical angle for total internal reflection from a medium to vacuum is 45°, then velocity of light in the medium is ***[NCERT (New) Pg. 230, NEET (Oct.) 2020]***

(a) 1.5×10^8 m/s (b) $\frac{3}{\sqrt{2}} \times 10^8$ m/s

(c) $\sqrt{2} \times 10^8$ m/s (d) 3×10^8 m/s

9. In total internal reflection when the angle of incidence is equal to the critical angle for the pair of media in contact, what will be angle of refraction? *[NCERT (New) Pg. 230, NEET (National) 2019]*
(a) 0°
(b) Equal to angle of incidence
(c) 90°
(d) 180°

10. An air bubble in a glass slab with refractive index 1.5 (near normal incidence) is 5 cm deep when viewed from one surface and 3 cm deep when viewed from the opposite face. The thickness (in cm) of the slab is *[NCERT (New) Pg. 233, NEET 2016]*
(a) 8 (b) 10
(c) 12 (d) 16

Module-III Lens and Prism

11. A light ray enters through a right angled prism at point P with the angle of incidence 30° as shown in figure. It travels through the prism parallel to its base BC and emerges along the face AC. The refractive index of the prism is *[NCERT (New) Pg. 240, NEET 2024]*

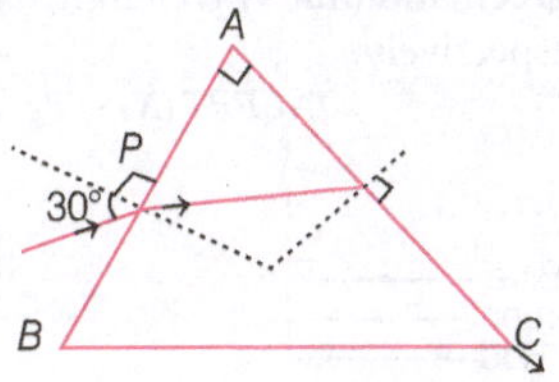

(a) $\frac{\sqrt{5}}{4}$ (b) $\frac{\sqrt{5}}{2}$ (c) $\frac{\sqrt{3}}{4}$ (d) $\frac{\sqrt{3}}{2}$

12. Two thin lenses are of same focal lengths (f), but one is convex and the other one is concave. When they are placed in contact with each other, the equivalent focal length of the combination will be *[NCERT (New) Pg. 238, NEET 2023]*
(a) $f/4$ (b) $f/2$
(c) infinite (d) Zero

13. In the figure shown here, what is the equivalent focal length of the combination of lenses (Assume that all layers are thin)? *[NCERT (New) Pg. 234, NEET 2023]*

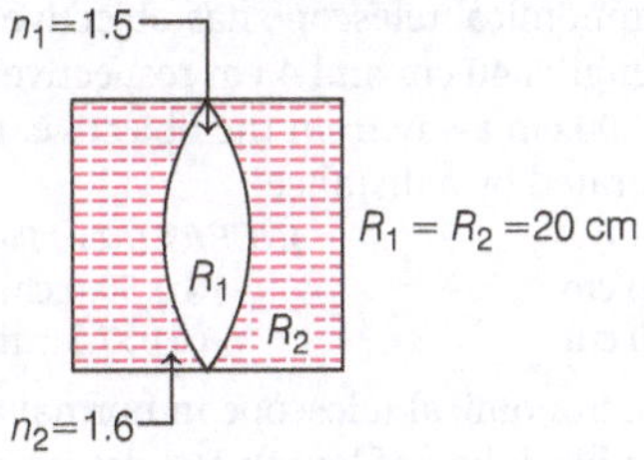

(a) – 40 cm (b) – 100 cm
(c) – 50 cm (d) 40 cm

14. A biconvex lens has radii of curvature, 20cm each. If the refractive index of the material of the lens is 1.5, the power of the lens is *[NCERT (New) Pg. 234, NEET 2022]*
(a) + 20 D (b) + 5D
(c) infinity (d) + 2D

15. A convex lens A of focal length 20 cm and a concave lens B of focal length 5 cm are kept along the same axis with a distance d between them. If a parallel beam of light falling on A leaves B as a parallel beam, then the distance d (in cm) will be *[NCERT (New) Pg. 238, NEET 2021]*
(a) 25 (b) 15
(c) 50 (d) 30

16. A ray is incident at an angle of incidence i on one surface of a small angle prism (with angle of prism A) and emerges normally from the opposite surface. If the refractive index of the material of the prism is μ, then the angle of incidence is nearly equal to *[NCERT (New) Pg. 240, NEET (Sep.) 2020]*
(a) $\frac{2A}{\mu}$ (b) μA (c) $\frac{\mu A}{2}$ (d) $\frac{A}{2\mu}$

17. The power of a biconvex lens is 10 D and the radius of curvature of each surface is 10 cm. Then, the refractive index of the material of the lens is *[NCERT (New) Pg. 234, NEET (Oct.) 2020]*
(a) $\frac{4}{3}$ (b) $\frac{9}{8}$ (c) $\frac{5}{3}$ (d) $\frac{3}{2}$

18. An equi-convex lens has power P it is cut into two symmetrical halves by a plane containing the principal axis. The power of one part will be *[NCERT (New) Pg. 234, NEET (Odisha) 2019]*
(a) 0 (b) $\frac{P}{2}$
(c) $\frac{P}{4}$ (d) P

19. A double convex lens has focal length 25 cm. The radius of curvature of one of the surfaces is doubled of the other. Find the radii, if the refractive index of the material of the lens is 1.5. *[NCERT (New) Pg. 234, NEET (Odisha) 2019]*
(a) 100 cm, 50 cm (b) 25 cm, 50 cm
(c) 18.75 cm, 37.5 cm (d) 50 cm, 100 cm

20. Two similar thin equi-convex lenses, of focal length f each, are kept co-axially in contact with each other such that the focal length of the combination is F_1. When the space between the two lenses is filled with glycerine (which has the same refractive index (μ = 1.5) as that of glass) then the equivalent focal length is F_2. The ratio $F_1 : F_2$ will be *[NCERT (New) Pg. 238, NEET (National) 2019]*
(a) 1 : 2 (b) 2 : 3
(c) 3 : 4 (d) 2 : 1

21. The refractive index of the material of a prism is $\sqrt{2}$ and the angle of the prism is 30°. One of the two refracting surfaces of the prism is made a mirror inwards, by silver coating. A beam of monochromatic light entering the prism from the other face will retrace its path (after reflection from the silvered surface) if its angle of incidence on the prism is *[NCERT (New) Pg. 240, NEET 2018]*

(a) 30° (b) 45° (c) 60° (d) zero

22. A thin prism having refracting angle 10° is made of glass of refractive index 1.42. This prism is combined with another thin prism of glass of refractive index 1.7. This combination produces dispersion without deviation. The refracting angle of second prism should be *[NCERT (New) Pg. 240, NEET 2017]*

(a) 4° (b) 6° (c) 8° (d) 10°

23. The angle of incidence for a ray of light at a refracting surface of a prism is 45°. The angle of prism is 60°. If the ray suffers minimum deviation through the prism, the angle of minimum deviation and refractive index of the material of the prism respectively, are *[NCERT (New) Pg. 240, NEET 2016]*

(a) 30°; $\sqrt{2}$ (b) 45°; $\sqrt{2}$ (c) 30°; $\frac{1}{\sqrt{2}}$ (d) 45°; $\frac{1}{\sqrt{2}}$

24. Two identical glass ($\mu_g = 3/2$) equi-convex lenses of focal length f each are kept in contact. The space between the two lenses is filled with water ($\mu_w = 4/3$). The focal length of the combination is *[NCERT (New) Pg. 234, NEET 2016]*

(a) $f/3$ (b) f (c) $\frac{4f}{3}$ (d) $\frac{3f}{4}$

25. Two identical thin plano-convex glass lenses (refractive index 1.5) each having radius of curvature of 20 cm are placed with their convex surfaces in contact at the centre. The intervening space is filled with oil of refractive index 1.7. The focal length of the combination is *[NCERT (New) Pg. 234, AIPMT 2015]*

(a) – 20 cm (b) – 25 cm (c) – 50 cm (d) 50 cm

26. The refracting angle of a prism is A, and refractive index of the material of the prism is cot ($A/2$). The angle of minimum deviation is *[NCERT (New) Pg. 240, AIPMT 2015]*

(a) $180° - 3A$ (b) $180° - 2A$ (c) $90° - A$ (d) $180° + 2A$

27. A beam of light consisting of red, green and blue colours is incident on a right angled prism. The refractive index of the material of the prism for the above red, green and blue wavelengths are 1.39, 1.44 and 1.47, respectively. *[NCERT (New) Pg. 240, AIPMT 2015]*

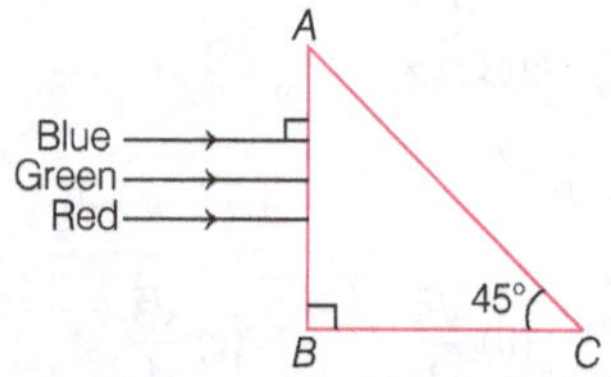

The prism will

(a) separate the blue colour part from the red and green colours
(b) separate all the three colours from one another
(c) not separate the three colours at all
(d) separate the red colour part from the green and blue colours

Module-IV Optical Instruments

28. A small telescope has an objective of focal length 140 cm and an eyepiece of focal length 5.0 cm. The magnifying power of telescope for viewing a distant object is *[NCERT (New) Pg. 242, NEET 2024]*

(a) 34 (b) 28 (c) 17 (d) 32

29. A lens of large focal length and large aperture is best suited as an objective of an astronomical telescope, since *[NCERT (New) Pg. 242, NEET 2021]*

(a) a large aperture contributes to the quality and visibility of the images
(b) a large area of the objective ensures better light gathering power
(c) a large aperture provides a better resolution
(d) All of the above

30. An astronomical telescope has objective and eyepiece of focal lengths 40 cm and 4 cm respectively. To view an object 200 cm away from the objective, the lenses must be separated by a distance *[NCERT (New) Pg. 242, NEET 2016]*

(a) 46.0 cm (b) 50.0 cm (c) 54.0 cm (d) 37.3 cm

31. In an astronomical telescope in normal adjustment a straight black line of length L is drawn on inside part of objective lens. The eye-piece forms a real image of this line. The length of this image is I. The magnification of the telescope is *[NCERT (New) Pg. 242, AIPMT 2015]*

(a) $\frac{L}{I} + 1$ (b) $\frac{L}{I} - 1$ (c) $\frac{L+1}{L-1}$ (d) $\frac{L}{I}$

Answers

Step up Practice 1

1 (b)	2 (b)	3 (b)	4 (b)	5 (c)	6 (d)	7 (b)	8 (a)	9 (a)	10 (a)
11 (d)	12 (a)	13 (a)	14 (c)	15 (d)	16 (a)	17 (b)	18 (b)	19 (c)	20 (b)
21 (a)									

Step up Practice 2

1 (c)	2 (d)	3 (a)	4 (c)	5 (d)	6 (c)	7 (a)	8 (b)	9 (d)	10 (c)
11 (c)	12 (a)	13 (b)	14 (a)	15 (c)	16 (b)	17 (c)	18 (a)	19 (d)	20 (c)
21 (c)									

Step up Practice 3

1 (d)	2 (d)	3 (c)	4 (b)	5 (d)	6 (b)	7 (b)	8 (d)	9 (b)	10 (b)
11 (d)	12 (b)	13 (a)	14 (c)	15 (c)	16 (d)	17 (a)	18 (a)	19 (b)	20 (a)
21 (d)	22 (d)	23 (d)	24 (a)	25 (d)	26 (c)	27 (b)			

Step up Practice 4

1 (b)	2 (c)	3 (b)	4 (b)	5 (b)	6 (d)	7 (a)	8 (b)	9 (b)	10 (d)
11 (a)	12 (d)	13 (a)	14 (b)	15 (d)	16 (a)	17 (b)	18 (b)	19 (b)	20 (b)

Gearing up for NEET

1 (c)	2 (a)	3 (b)	4 (c)	5 (c)	6 (c)	7 (d)	8 (b)	9 (a)	10 (b)
11 (c)	12 (b)	13 (d)	14 (c)	15 (a)	16 (b)	17 (c)	18 (b)	19 (b)	20 (b)
21 (a)	22 (c)	23 (b)	24 (d)	25 (a)	26 (c)	27 (b)	28 (d)	29 (b)	30 (c)
31 (b)	32 (c)	33 (b)	34 (c)	35 (b)	36 (d)	37 (d)	38 (c)	39 (c)	40 (b)
41 (a)	42 (b)	43 (b)	44 (d)	45 (b)	46 (a)	47 (b)	48 (b)	49 (d)	50 (c)
51 (a)	52 (c)	53 (c)	54 (c)	55 (b)	56 (a)	57 (c)	58 (d)	59 (c)	60 (c)
61 (d)	62 (d)	63 (a)	64 (d)	65 (c)	66 (a)	67 (c)	68 (a)	69 (c)	70 (c)
71 (a)	72 (b)	73 (b)	74 (d)	75 (a)	76 (d)	77 (a)	78 (a)	79 (d)	80 (c)
81 (d)	82 (c)	83 (a)	84 (c)	85 (c)	86 (a)	87 (d)	88 (c)	89 (c)	90 (c)
91 (a)	92 (d)	93 (b)	94 (b)	95 (c)	96 (b)	97 (d)	98 (a)	99 (a)	100 (c)
101 (b)	102 (d)	103 (c)	104 (c)	105 (c)	106 (b)	107 (c)	108 (c)	109 (b)	110 (d)
111 (b)	112 (d)	113 (a)	114 (c)	115 (c)	116 (d)	117 (c)	118 (a)		

Assertion and Reason

1 (b)	2 (c)	3 (d)	4 (d)	5 (d)

Statement Type Questions

1 (d)	2 (d)	3 (d)	4 (d)	5 (d)

Match the Columns

1 (a)	2 (c)	3 (b)	4 (d)

Final Check through PYQs : Module-I

1 (a)	2 (b)	3 (a)	4 (d)

Final Check through PYQs : Module-II

5 (c)	6 (a)	7 (a)	8 (b)	9 (c)	10 (c)

Final Check through PYQs : Module-III

11 (b)	12 (c)	13 (b)	14 (b)	15 (b)	16 (b)	17 (d)	18 (d)	19 (c)	20 (a)
21 (b)	22 (b)	23 (a)	24 (d)	25 (c)	26 (b)	27 (d)			

Final Check through PYQs : Module-IV

28 (b)	29 (d)	30 (c)	31 (d)

Hints and Solutions

Step up Practice 1

1. (*b*)

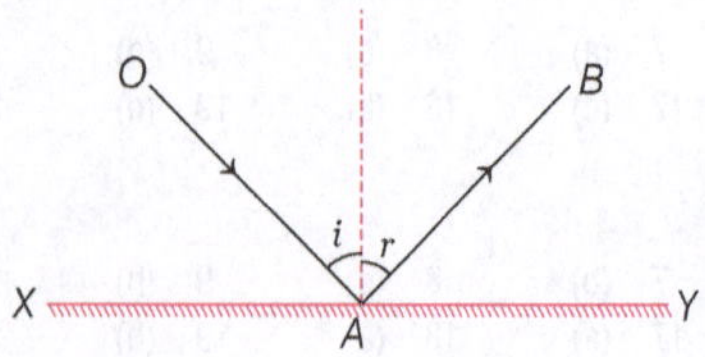

Here, XY is a plane reflecting surface,

OA and AB are the incident and reflected rays, respectively

i = angle of incidence

r = angle of reflection

As, $AB \perp OA$,

$\therefore$ $i + r = 90°$

Also, according to laws of reflection,

$r = i$

$\therefore$ $i + i = 90°$

$\Rightarrow$ $2i = 90°$

$\Rightarrow$ $i = \frac{90°}{2} = 45°$

2. (*b*) A is true but R is false.

Angle of incidence = Angle between incident ray and normal to the mirror = 0°

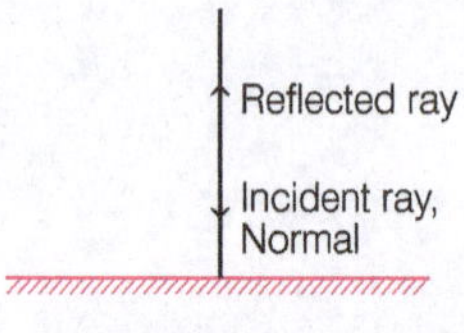

$\Rightarrow$ Angle of reflection = 0° (from laws of reflection)

Hence, the reflected ray retraces its path along the normal at an angle 0° with normal.

3. (*b*) When convergent beam is incident on a plane mirror, then mirror forms real image, for a virtual object.

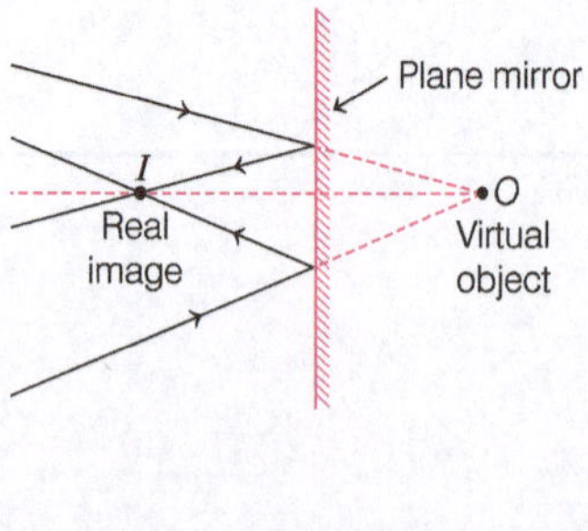

4. (*b*) According to ray diagram shown in figure

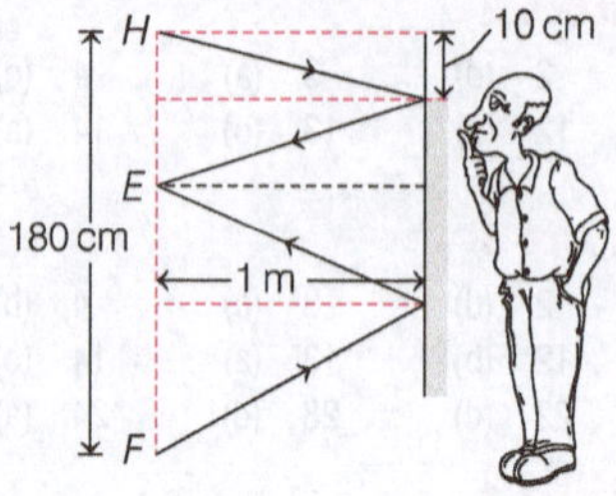

Length of mirror $= \frac{1}{2}(10 + 170) = 90$ cm

5. (*c*) As number of images, $n = 3$

So, $n = \frac{360}{\theta} - 1$

$\Rightarrow$ $3 = \frac{360}{\theta} - 1$

$\therefore$ $\theta = 90°$

6. (*d*) Both A and R are true and R is the correct explanation of A.

From figure, it is clear that object, centre of curvature and image are on a straight line. The ray which is passing through centre of curvature is normally incident on mirror.

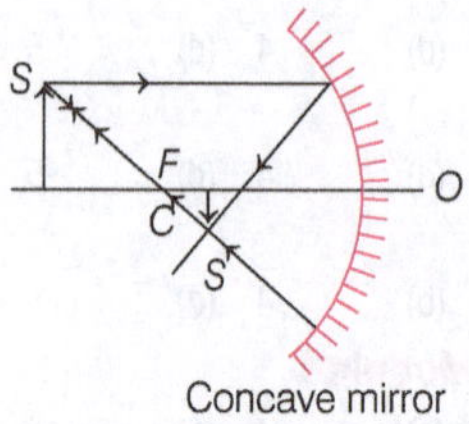

Concave mirror

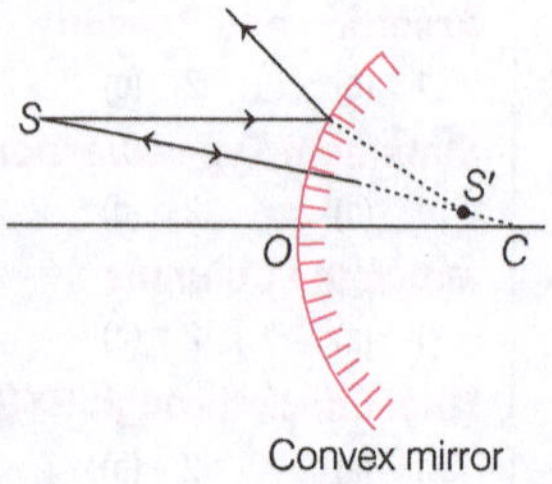

Convex mirror

So, it returns back on the same path.

7. (*b*) Distance between 4th images

$I_u I_u' = 2n(x + y) = 2 \times 4\,[3 + 1] = 32$ m

8. (*a*) On immersing a mirror in water, focal length of the mirror remains unchanged.

9. (*a*) Both A and R are true but R is not the correct explanation of A.

If object is placed at centre of curvature of concave mirror, its image is at the centre of curvature. Thus, minimum distance between object and its real image is zero. If object is between pole and focus of concave mirror, its image is virtual. If object is beyond focus, its image is real. Thus, concave mirror forms real as well as virtual image.

10. (*a*) Since, the object is at the centre of curvature of the mirror. So, image formed is real, inverted and same in size.

11. (*d*) Given, $u = -30$ cm and $f = 30$ cm

$$\frac{1}{v} + \frac{1}{-30} = \frac{1}{30} \Rightarrow \frac{1}{v} = \frac{1}{30} + \frac{1}{30} = \frac{1}{15}$$

$\therefore$ Distance from the mirror, $v = +15$ cm

The positive sign shows that the image is formed behind the mirror.

12. (*a*) Given, $u = -30$ cm

$v = -30$ cm

Using relation, $\frac{1}{f} = \frac{1}{v} + \frac{1}{u}$

$$\frac{1}{-30} + \frac{1}{-30} = \frac{1}{f}$$

$\therefore$ Focal length of the mirror, $f = -15$ cm

13. (*a*) Magnification, $m = +\frac{1}{n} = -\frac{v}{u}$

$\therefore \quad v = -\frac{u}{n}$

From mirror formula, $\frac{1}{f} = \frac{1}{\left(-\frac{u}{n}\right)} + \frac{1}{u}$

$\therefore$ The distance of the object from the mirror, $u = -(n-1)f$.

14. (*c*) According to sign convention, all distances are measured from the pole of the mirror or the optical centre of the lens.

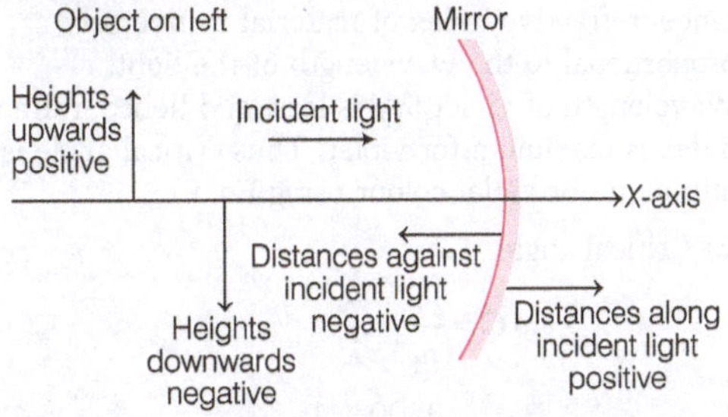

15. (*d*) In case of concave mirror when the object is at infinity, then the image formed will be real, inverted and very small in size at F. Hence, option (a) is incorrect.

At C then image should be real, inverted, equal in size at C. Hence, option (b) is incorrect.

At F then image should be real, inverted, very large at infinity. Hence, option (c) is incorrect.

Between F and C then image should be real, inverted, very large between C and infinity. Hence, option (d) is correct.

16. (*a*) In case of concave mirror, $m = -2$

Also, $m = \frac{f}{f-u}$

$$\Rightarrow \quad -2 = \frac{-50}{-50-u}$$

$\therefore$ Distance of the object from the mirror, $u = -75$ cm

17. (*b*) Magnification, $m = \frac{f}{f-u} \Rightarrow \left(+\frac{1}{4}\right) = \frac{+30}{+30-u}$

$\Rightarrow$ The distance of the object from the mirror,

$u = -90$ cm

18. (*b*) Magnification,

$$m = \frac{f}{f-u} \Rightarrow -3 = \frac{f}{f-(-20)}$$

$\Rightarrow$ The focal length of mirror, $f = -15$ cm

19. (*c*) A is false but R is true.

Magnification produced by mirror,

$$m = \frac{I}{O} = \frac{f}{f-u} = \frac{f}{x}.$$

where, x is distance from focus.

and $m = \frac{\text{Size of image } (I)}{\text{Size of object } (O)}$

20. (*b*) Magnification,

$$m = \frac{I}{O} = \frac{f}{f-u}$$

$$\Rightarrow \quad \frac{I}{7.5} = \frac{(R/2)}{(R/2)-u} = \frac{(25/2)}{(25/2)-(-40)}$$

$\therefore$ The size of the image, $I = 1.78$ cm

21. (*a*) From the relation,

$$\frac{1}{v} + \frac{1}{u} = \frac{1}{f}$$

We have, $\frac{-dv}{v^2} - \frac{du}{u^2} = 0$

$$\therefore dv = \frac{v^2}{u^2}(-du)$$

$$= -\left(\frac{20}{10}\right)^2 (0.1)$$

$= -0.4$ cm away from the mirror

Step up Practice 2

1. (*c*)

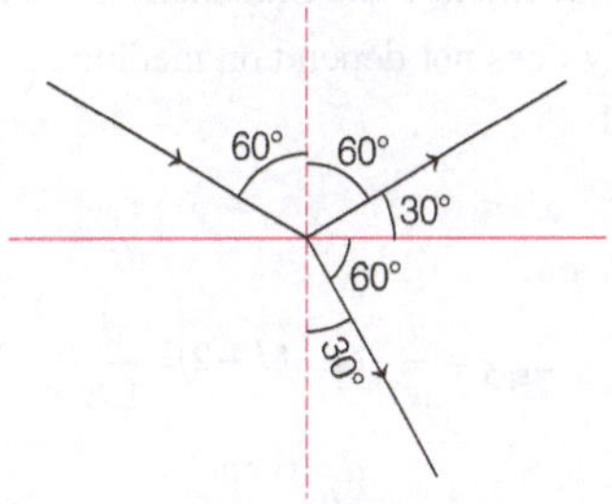

Refractive index of the material,

$$\mu = \frac{\sin i}{\sin r} = \frac{\sin 60°}{\sin 30°} = \sqrt{3} = 1.732$$

2. (*d*) Both Statement I and Statement II are correct.

If $n_{21} > 1, r < i$, *i.e.* the refracted ray bends towards the normal. In such a case medium 2 is said to be optically denser (or denser, in short) than medium 1.

On the other hand, if $n_{21} < 1, r > i$, the refracted ray bends away from the normal. This is the case when incident ray in a denser medium refracts into a rarer medium.

3. (*a*) Refractive index of the medium,

$$\mu = \frac{c}{v} = \frac{c}{n\lambda} = \frac{3 \times 10^8}{4 \times 10^{14} \times 5 \times 10^{-7}} = 1.5$$

4. (*c*) $_2\mu_1 \times {}_3\mu_2 \times {}_4\mu_3 = \frac{\mu_1}{\mu_2} \times \frac{\mu_2}{\mu_3} \times \frac{\mu_3}{\mu_4} = \frac{\mu_1}{\mu_4}$

$$= {}_4\mu_1 = \frac{1}{{}_1\mu_4}$$

5. (*d*) Both Statement I and Statement II are correct.

Refractive index of any pair of media is inversely proportional to wavelength of light.

Hence, $\lambda_v < \lambda_r$

$\Rightarrow$ $\mu_v > \mu_r$

where, λ_v and λ_r are the wavelengths of violet and red light and μ_r and μ_v are refractive index of violet and red light.

6. (*c*) As, $\mu = \frac{c}{v} \Rightarrow v \propto \frac{1}{\mu}$

$\therefore$ $\frac{v_1}{v_2} = \frac{\mu_2}{\mu_1}$

$\Rightarrow$ Ratio of velocities of light

$$\frac{v_g}{v_w} = \frac{\mu_w}{\mu_g} = \frac{4/3}{3/2} = \frac{8}{9}$$

7. (*a*) Wavelength of light, $\lambda' = \frac{\lambda}{\mu} = \frac{6000}{1.5} = 4000 \text{ Å}$

8. (*b*) Refractive index of glass with respect to water,

$$_w\mu_g = \frac{_a\mu_g}{_a\mu_w} = \frac{3/2}{4/3} = \frac{9}{8}$$

9. (*d*) Both Statement I and Statement II are correct.

Frequency does not depend on medium.

But $\lambda \propto \frac{1}{\mu}$.

10. (*c*) We have,

$$d_{app} = \frac{d}{\mu} \text{ or } (d-2) = \frac{d}{1.5}$$

$\therefore$ $d = 6$ cm

11. (*c*) $d_{actual} = (d_{app})\mu$

From one side, $d_1 = 6 \times 1.5 = 9$

From other side, $d_2 = 4 \times 1.5 = 6$

$\therefore$ $d = d_1 + d_2 = 15$ cm

12. (*a*) Distance from the surface of water,

$$h' = \mu h = \frac{4}{3} \times 18 = 24 \text{ m}$$

13. (*b*) Apparent depth, $h' = \frac{d_1}{\mu_1} + \frac{d_2}{\mu_2} = \frac{d}{\mu_1} + \frac{d}{\mu_2}$

$$= d\left(\frac{1}{\mu_1} + \frac{1}{\mu_2}\right)$$

14. (*a*) As, $d_{app} = \frac{d_1}{\mu_1} + \frac{d_2}{\mu_2} + \frac{d_3}{\mu_3} = \frac{3}{3/2} + \frac{4}{4/3} + \frac{6}{6/5}$

$$= 2 + 3 + 5$$
$$= 10 \text{ cm}$$

15. (*c*) The refractive index of glass relative to water is given by

$$_w n_g = \frac{_a n_g}{_a n_w} = \frac{1.50}{1.33}$$

If C be the critical angle at glass water interface, then

$$\sin C = \frac{1}{_w n_g} = \frac{1.33}{1.50} = 0.8867$$

$$C = \sin^{-1}(0.8867) = 62.5°$$

16. (*b*) Statement I is correct but Statement II is incorrect.

As, critical angle, $C = \sin^{-1}\left(\frac{\mu_r}{\mu_d}\right)$

In this case, $\left(\sin C = \frac{1}{\mu_d}\right)$ $\left[\because \mu = \frac{C}{\lambda}\right]$ ...(i)

Since, refractive index of material is inversely proportional to the wavelength of the light. Wavelength of violet (λ_v) is least and hence, refractive index is maximum for violet. Thus critical angle is minimum for violet colour using Eq. (i).

17. (*c*) Critical angle,

$$\sin C = \frac{n_2}{n_1} = \frac{\lambda_1}{\lambda_2}$$

$\Rightarrow$ $\sin C = \frac{3500}{7000} = \frac{1}{2}$

$\therefore$ $C = 30°$

18. (*a*) Critical angle, $\sin C = \frac{1}{\mu}$ or $C = \sin^{-1}\left(\frac{1}{\mu}\right)$

As μ decreases with increase in λ. Also, yellow, orange and red have higher wavelength than green, so μ will be less for these rays. Thus, critical angle for these rays will be high, hence if green is just totally internally reflected, then yellow, orange and red rays will emerge out.

19. (*d*) Both Statement I and Statement II are correct.

Optical fibre communication is based on the phenomenon of total internal reflection at core-clad interface.

The refractive index of the material of the core is greater than that of the cladding, hence, light striking at core-cladding interface gets totally internally reflected. The light undergoes and reaches the other end of the fibre.

20. (c) We have, $\sin i > \sin \theta_C$

$$\therefore \quad \sin 45° > \frac{1}{n} \text{ or } \frac{1}{\sqrt{2}} > \frac{1}{n}$$

$$\text{or} \quad n > \sqrt{2}$$

$$\text{or} \quad n > 1.414$$

21. (c) Apparent shift $= d\left(1 - \frac{1}{\mu}\right)$

Step up Practice 3

1. (d) When object lies between focus and pole of convex lens, image formed is virtual, erect and enlarged in size.

2. (d) Image is real, because virtual image always remains enlarged.

Magnification, $m = \frac{v}{u} = \frac{1}{4}$

Hence, consider $v = \frac{1}{4}x$ and $u = -x$

$$\text{Now,} \quad \frac{1}{v} - \frac{1}{u} = \frac{1}{f} \text{ or } \frac{1}{x/4} + \frac{1}{x} = \frac{1}{30}$$

$$\frac{5}{x} = \frac{1}{30}$$

$$\therefore \quad x = 150 \text{ cm}$$

3. (c) A is false but R is true.

In air or water a convex lens made of glass behaves as a convergent lens but when it is placed in carbon disulfide, it behaves as a divergent lens. Therefore, when a convergent lens is placed inside a transparent medium having refractive index greater than that of material of lens, it behaves as a divergent lens.

4. (b) For a concave lens, image is always smaller in size.

5. (d) For real image from converging lens, $m = -2$

$$\therefore \text{Magnification, } m = \frac{f}{f+u} \Rightarrow -2 = \frac{f}{u+f} = \frac{20}{u+20}$$

$$\Rightarrow \quad u = -30 \text{ cm}$$

6. (b) Keep the object at a distance $2f$ from the lens.

7. (b) A is true but R is false.

From lens Maker's formula,

$$\textbf{In air} \quad \frac{1}{f_1} = \left(\frac{\mu_{lens}}{\mu_{air}} - 1\right)\left[\frac{1}{R_1} - \frac{1}{R_2}\right]$$

$$\textbf{In water} \quad \frac{1}{f_2} = \left(\frac{\mu_{lens}}{\mu_{water}} - 1\right)\left[\frac{1}{R_1} - \frac{1}{R_2}\right]$$

$$\because \quad \frac{\mu_{lens}}{\mu_{water}} \frac{(3/2)}{(4/3)} < \frac{\mu_{lens}}{\mu_{air}} \frac{(3/2)}{(1)}$$

$\Rightarrow \frac{1}{f_2}$ or power is less in water but f_2 is positive, hence it behaves as convex lens and not as concave lens.

8. (d) We have, $P = (\mu - 1)\left[\frac{1}{R_1} - \frac{1}{R_2}\right]$

$$2.5 = \left(\frac{3}{2} - 1\right)\left(\frac{1}{R_1} - \frac{1}{R_2}\right) \quad \text{...(i)}$$

$$P' = \left(\frac{3/2}{2} - 1\right)\left(\frac{1}{R_1} - \frac{1}{R_2}\right) \quad \text{...(ii)}$$

Solving Eqs. (i) and (ii), we get

$$\therefore \quad P' = -1.25 \text{ D}$$

9. (b) We have $\frac{1}{f} = \frac{1}{v} - \frac{1}{u}$

$$\Rightarrow \quad \frac{1}{+5} - \frac{1}{-10} = \frac{1}{f} \quad \left(|v| = \frac{|u|}{2}\right)$$

$\therefore$ Focal length, $f = \frac{10}{3}$ cm

Positive sign implies that the lens is convex.

10. (b) A is true but R is false.

A lens with large focal length have less power.

i.e., $\quad P \propto \frac{1}{f}$ or $f \propto \frac{1}{P}$

11. (d) Focal length of combination,

$$\frac{1}{F} = \frac{1}{f_1} + \frac{1}{f_2} = \frac{1}{60} + \frac{1}{(-20)} \Rightarrow F = -30 \text{ cm}$$

12. (b) In each case, there is a combination of two plano-convex lenses placed close to each other. Focal length of combination $\frac{1}{F} = \frac{1}{2f} + \frac{1}{2f}$ is same in all cases, so ratio of focal length in three cases is 1 : 1 : 1.

13. (a) Focal length of air lens in glass is given as

$$\frac{1}{f} = ({}_g\mu_a - 1)\left(\frac{1}{R_1} - \frac{1}{R_2}\right)$$

$$= \left(\frac{2}{3} - 1\right)\left[\frac{1}{10} - \left(-\frac{1}{10}\right)\right]$$

$$\Rightarrow \quad f = -15 \text{ cm}$$

So, nature of lens is concave type.

14. (c) Focal length of plano-convex lens,

$$f = \frac{R}{\mu - 1} = \frac{R}{(1.5 - 1)} = 2R$$

15. (c) As we know that

For equi-biconvex lens, $f = \frac{R}{2(\mu - 1)}$

For equi-biconcave lens, $f = \frac{-R}{2(\mu - 1)}$

For plano-convex lens, $f = \frac{R}{\mu - 1}$

For plano-concave lens, $f = \frac{-R}{\mu + 1}$

Hence, option (c) is correct.

16. (*d*) We have, $\frac{1}{v} - \frac{1}{-90} = \frac{1}{f}$ and $(1.5 - 1)\left(\frac{1}{30}\right) = \frac{1}{f}$

$\therefore \quad v = 180$ cm

or $\quad |m| = \left|\frac{v}{u}\right| = \frac{180}{90} = 2.0$

17. (*a*) Focal length of the combination,

$$\frac{1}{F} = \frac{1}{f_1} + \frac{1}{f_2}$$

$$\Rightarrow \quad \frac{1}{F} = \frac{1}{(+40)} + \frac{1}{(-25)}$$

$$\Rightarrow \quad F = -\frac{200}{3} \text{ cm}$$

As, $\quad$ Power, $P = \frac{100}{F} = \frac{100}{(-200/3)} = -1.5$ D

18. (*a*) We have, $\sin \theta_C = \frac{1}{\mu}$

$$\therefore \quad \mu = \frac{1}{\sin 30^\circ} = 2$$

The velocity of light, $v = \frac{c}{\mu} = \frac{3.0 \times 10^8}{2}$

$$= 1.5 \times 10^8 \text{ m/s}$$

19. (*b*) In minimum deviation position, refracted ray inside an isosceles prism is parallel to the base of the prism.

20. (*a*) Deviation of ray in prism is given by

$$\delta = i + e - A$$

So, $\quad e = \delta + A - i = 30^\circ + 30^\circ - 60^\circ = 0^\circ$

So, emergent ray will make an angle of 90° with the face through which it emerges.

21. (*d*) Refractive index of prism, $\mu = \frac{\sin \frac{A + \delta_m}{2}}{\sin \frac{A}{2}}$

As, $\quad i = 45^\circ = \frac{A + \delta_m}{2}$

So, $\quad \frac{\sin 45^\circ}{\sin (A/2)} = \sqrt{2}$

$$\Rightarrow \quad \frac{1}{2} = \sin \frac{A}{2} \Rightarrow A = 60^\circ$$

22. (*d*) Given, $\quad i = e = \frac{3}{4} A = \frac{3}{4} \times 60^\circ = 45^\circ$

In the position of minimum deviation,

$$2i = A + \delta_m$$

or
$$\delta_m = 2i - A = 2 \times 45^\circ - 60 = 30^\circ$$

23. (*d*) Both A and R are true and R is the correct explanation of A.

For thin prisms, angle of prisms A is small.

For small A, $D_{\min}$ (minimum deviation) is also small.

So, $$\mu = \frac{\sin\left(\frac{A + D_{\min}}{2}\right)}{\sin (A/2)} \quad \text{...(i)}$$

$$\sin\left(\frac{A + D_{\min}}{2}\right) \approx \frac{A + D_{\min}}{2} \quad (\because \sin \theta \approx \theta \text{ for small } \theta)$$

and $\quad \sin \frac{A}{2} \approx \frac{A}{2}$

Using above approximations,

$$\mu = \frac{\frac{A + D_{\min}}{2}}{A/2} \Rightarrow D_{\min} = (\mu - 1)A$$

Hence, it can be seen that if A is small, $D_{\min}$ is also small.

24. (*a*) Angle of minimum deviation in prism,

$$\delta_m = (\mu - 1)A = (\mu - 1)(2r) \quad (\because r = A/2)$$
$$= (1.5 - 1)(2r) = 0.5 \times 2r = r$$

25. (*d*) Refractive index of prism, $\mu = \frac{\sin\left(\frac{A + \delta_m}{2}\right)}{\sin\left(\frac{A}{2}\right)}$

Substituting $A = \delta_m$ and $\mu = 1.5$, we get

$$\Rightarrow \quad 1.5 = \frac{\sin A}{\sin\left(\frac{A}{2}\right)} \Rightarrow \frac{1.5}{2} = \cos \frac{A}{2}$$

$$\Rightarrow \quad 0.75 = \cos \frac{A}{2}$$

We get, $\quad A = 82^\circ$

26. (*c*) A is false but R is true.

Dispersion takes place because the refractive index of medium for different wavelengths (colours) is different. The refractive index is inversely proportion to λ by Cauchy's expression as

$$\mu(\lambda) = r + \frac{b}{\lambda^2} + \frac{c}{\lambda^4}$$

Hence, deviation $(D) = (\mu - 1) A$

Since λ_{red} is more than other colours wavelength. So, deviation is least for red and have it appears farthest from the base of the prism.

27. (*b*) To produce dispersion without deviation,

$$\frac{A'}{A} = \frac{(\mu_y - 1)}{(\mu'_y - 1)}$$

$$\Rightarrow \quad \frac{A'}{6^\circ} = \frac{(1.54 - 1)}{(1.72 - 1)}$$

$$\Rightarrow \quad A' = 4.5^\circ = 4^\circ 30'$$

Step up Practice 4

1. (b) When final image is formed at $D = 25$ cm from eye.

In this situation, $v = -D$

From lens formula, $\frac{1}{v} - \frac{1}{u} = \frac{1}{f}$

We have $\frac{1}{-D} - \frac{1}{(-u)} = \frac{1}{f}$

i.e. $\frac{D}{u} = 1 + \frac{D}{f}$

So, magnifying power $= \frac{D}{u} = \left(1 + \frac{D}{f}\right)$

2. (c) Here, $u = -4$ cm, $f = 5$ cm

According to lens formula,

$\because \quad \frac{1}{v} - \frac{1}{u} = \frac{1}{f}$

or $\frac{1}{v} + \frac{1}{4} = \frac{1}{5}$

or $\frac{1}{v} = \frac{1}{5} - \frac{1}{4} = \frac{4-5}{20}$

$\therefore \quad v = -20$ cm

Thus, a virtual image is formed at distance 20 cm from the lens.

The linear magnification $= \frac{v}{u} = \frac{-20}{-4} = 5$

$m = \frac{\beta}{\alpha} = \frac{D}{u} = \frac{25}{4} = 6.25$

3. (b) Magnifying power, $m = m_o \times m_e$

$100 = 5 \times m_e$

$m_e = 20$

4. (b) The given statement (B) is incorrect and it can be corrected as,

For microscope, the magnification in case of image formed at infinity $\left(m = \frac{D}{f}\right)$ is one less than the magnification when the image is at the near point $\left[m = \left(1 + \frac{D}{f}\right)\right]$.

Rest statements are correct.

5. (b) Given, $f_o = 1.0$ cm, $f_e = 2.0$ cm and tube length, $L = 20$ cm.

The magnification due to objective is

$m_o = \frac{L}{f_o} = \frac{20}{1} = 20$

and due to eyepiece is $m_e = \frac{D}{f_e}$

where, D is the least distance of distinct vision = 25 cm

$\Rightarrow \quad m_e = \frac{25}{2} = 12.5$

The magnification of compound microscope is

$|m| = m_o m_e = \left(\frac{L}{f_o}\right)\left(\frac{D}{f_e}\right) = 20 \times 12.5 = 250$

6. (d) In compound microscope objective lens forms a real, inverted, magnified image of the object.

This serves as the object for the second lens, the eyepiece, which functions essentially like a simple microscope or magnifier, produces the final image, which is enlarged and virtual.

The first inverted image is thus meet (at or within) the focal plane of the eyepiece, at a distance appropriate for final image formation at infinity, or a little closer for image formation at the near point.

Clearly, the final image is inverted with respect to the original object.

Thus, none of the statement is incorrect.

7. (a) Length of compound microscope,

$L_\infty = v_o + f_e$

$\Rightarrow \quad 14 = v_o + 5$

$\therefore \quad v_o = 9$ cm

Magnifying power of microscope for relaxed eye,

$M = \frac{v_o}{u_o} \cdot \frac{D}{f_e}$

or $25 = \frac{9}{u_o} \cdot \frac{25}{5}$

or distance of object for objective, $u_o = \frac{9}{5} = 1.8$ cm

8. (b) When final image is formed at infinity,then magnifying power,

$M_\infty = -\frac{v_o}{u_o} \times \frac{D}{f_e}$

From $\frac{1}{f_o} = \frac{1}{v_o} - \frac{1}{u_o}$,

$\frac{1}{+1.2} = \frac{1}{v_o} - \frac{1}{(-1.25)}$

$\Rightarrow \quad v_o = 30$ cm

$\therefore \quad |M_\infty| = \frac{30}{1.25} \times \frac{25}{3} = 200$

9. (b) For objective lens, $\frac{1}{f_o} = \frac{1}{v_o} - \frac{1}{u_o}$

or $\frac{1}{4} = \frac{1}{v_o} - \frac{1}{(-4.5)} \Rightarrow |v_o| = 36$ cm

$\therefore$ Magnifying power, $|M| = \frac{v_o}{u_o}\left(1 + \frac{D}{f_e}\right)$

$= \frac{36}{4.5}\left(1 + \frac{24}{8}\right) = 32$

10. (*d*) Both Statement I and Statement II are correct.

The light gathering power (or brightness) of a telescope is directly proportional to the area of the objective lens.

Light gathering power $\propto \pi r^2 = \dfrac{\pi D^2}{4}$, where D is the diameter of the objective.

So, by increasing the objective diameter even far off stars may produce images of optimum brightness.

11. (*a*) If the telescope is reversed *i.e.*, seen from the objective side, then object will appear very small, because in this case magnification becomes reciprocal of initial magnification.

12. (*d*) Both Statement I and Statement II are correct.

For astronomical telescope, $|m| = \left|\dfrac{f_o}{f_e}\right|$.

So, magnification is inversely proportional to focal length of the eyepiece and directly proportional to focal length of objective. The larger f_o and smaller f_e will given better magnification.

13. (*a*) In a telescope, large aperture of objective helps in improving the brightness (image) by gathering more light from distant object.

14. (*b*) Magnifying power of astronomical telescope,

$$m = -\frac{f_o}{f_e}\left(1 + \frac{f_e}{D}\right) = -\frac{200}{5}\left(1 + \frac{5}{25}\right) = -48$$

15. (*d*) The given statement (D) is incorrect and it can be corrected as,

For objective, with large sized lenses the brightness increases and the chromatic aberration also increases.

Given, $f_o = 20$ m and $f_e = 2$ cm $= 0.02$ m.

In normal adjustment, length of telescope,

$$L = f_o + f_e = 20 + 0.02 = 20.02 \text{ m}$$

Magnification, $m = \dfrac{f_o}{f_e} = \dfrac{20}{0.02} = 1000$

Also, the image formed is inverted with respect to the object.

Rest statements are correct.

16. (*a*) Magnification of astronomical telescope for normal eye,

$$m = -\frac{f_o}{f_e} = -\frac{100}{2} = -50$$

17. (*b*) In terrestrial telescope, there are three lenses, objective, eye-piece and third is erecting lens, it is placed at $2f$ from intermediate image.

18. (*b*) If in an astronomical telescope, the convergent eyepiece is replaced by a divergent lens which is placed in such a way that rays from objective are directed towards its focus, final image will be erect, enlarged and virtual and hence, it is called Gallilean telescope.

19. (*b*) Reflecting telescope consists of concave mirror of large aperture.

20. (*b*) The separation between the objective and the eyepiece = length of the telescope tube

$\Rightarrow \quad L = f_o + f_e$

Given, $f_o = 150$ cm $= 1.5$ m, $f_e = 5$ cm $= 0.05$ m

$\Rightarrow \quad L = 1.5 + 0.05 = 1.55$ m

Gearing up for NEET

1. (*c*) The field of view in convex mirror is more as compared to plane or concave mirror. This is why it is used as rear view mirror in vehicles.

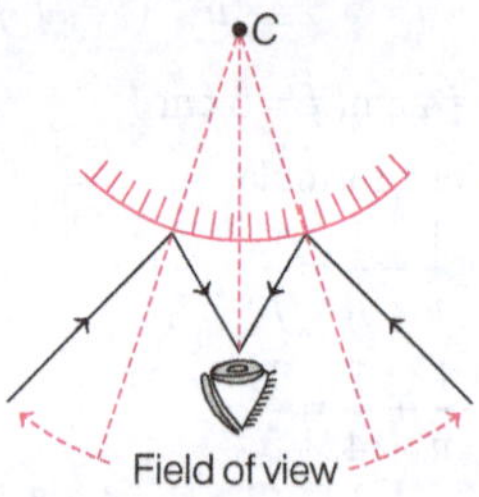

2. (*a*) When object is placed between centre of curvature and focus (*i.e.*, $f < u < 2f$), then image will be between $2f$ and ∞, real, inverted, large in size and $m > -1$

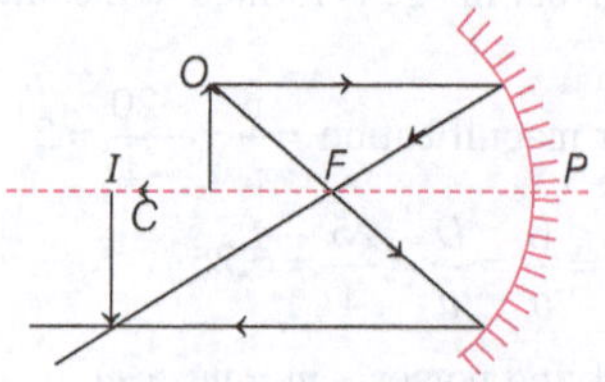

3. (*b*) The number of images formed depends upon the angle between the mirrors. If two mirrors make an angle θ with each other, then the number of images formed is

$$n = \frac{360^\circ}{\theta} - 1$$

When mirrors are kept mutually perpendicular to each other, then $\theta = 90^\circ$.

$$n = \frac{360}{90} - 1 = 3$$

4. (*c*) As, $n = \dfrac{360^\circ}{60^\circ} = 6$

Since, n is an even integer, so total number of images will be $(n-1)$ or 5.

5. (*c*) For concave mirror,

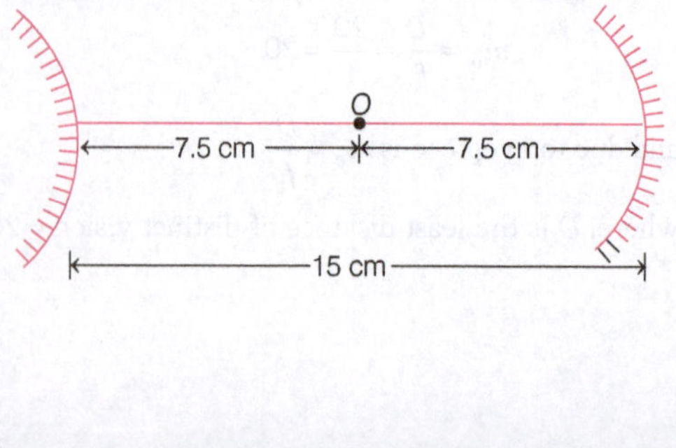

Using the relation, $\frac{1}{v} - \frac{1}{7.5} = -\frac{1}{5}$

$\therefore \quad v = -15$ cm

Therefore position of final Image will be at the pole of the convex mirror.

6. (c) We have, $\frac{I}{O} = \frac{f}{(f-u)}$

$\Rightarrow \quad \frac{I}{5} = \frac{-10}{-10-(-100)}$

$\Rightarrow \quad I = -0.55$

Size of the image, $I = 0.55$ cm

7. (d) Given, $m = +\frac{1}{2}, f = 2\text{ m} = 200\text{ cm}, u = ?$

$\therefore$ Magnification, $m = \frac{f}{(f-u)}$

$\Rightarrow \quad +\frac{1}{2} = \frac{200}{(200-u)}$

$\Rightarrow \quad 200 - u = 400$

$\Rightarrow \quad u = -200$ cm

or $\quad u = -2$ m

8. (b) From geometry of the figure,

Angle, $\theta = 90° - 22° = 68°$

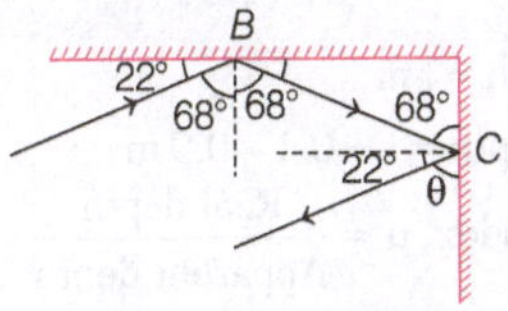

9. (a) u changes from 0 to $-\infty$, then v will change from 0 to $+f$.

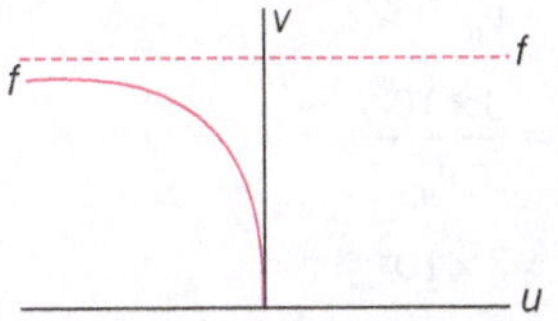

10. (b) Given, $AC = 60$ m and $\angle BCB' = 90°$

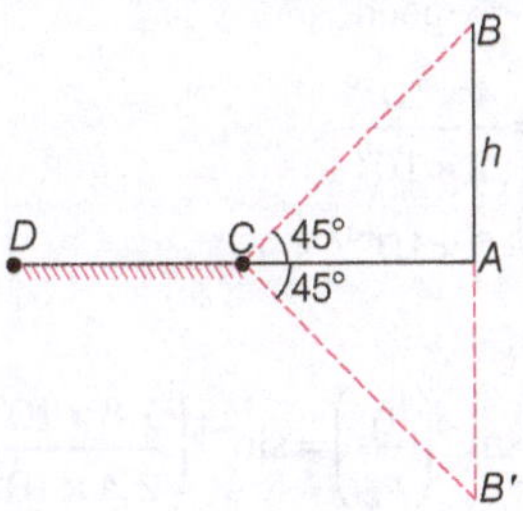

From the figure,

$\therefore$ Angle, $\angle BCA = \frac{\angle BCB'}{2} = 45°$

We have, $\tan 45° = \frac{h}{AC}$

$\Rightarrow \quad AC = h \Rightarrow h = 60$ m

11. (c) From the figure in ΔABC, $45° + 90° + 2\alpha = 180°$

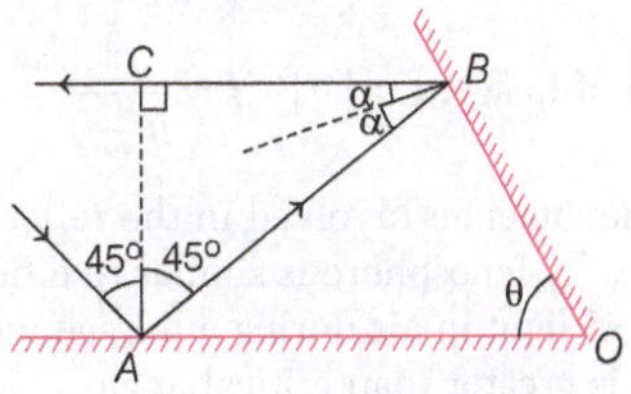

or $\quad \alpha = 22.5°$

$\angle OBA = 90° - \alpha$

In ΔOAB, $\theta + 45° + 90° - \alpha = 180° \Rightarrow \theta = 67.5°$

12. (b) Using mirror formula, $\frac{1}{v} + \frac{1}{(-u)} = \frac{1}{-f}$

Multiplying with u, $\frac{u}{v} = \frac{-u}{f} + 1 = \frac{f-u}{f}$

$\therefore$ Magnification, $m = -\frac{v}{u} = \left(\frac{f}{f-u}\right)$

Now, $\quad |dv| = m^2 |du|$

Size of image $= \left(\frac{f}{f-u}\right)^2 \cdot b = \left(\frac{f}{u-f}\right)^2 \cdot b$

13. (d) We have, $90° - \theta + 2\theta = 90°$

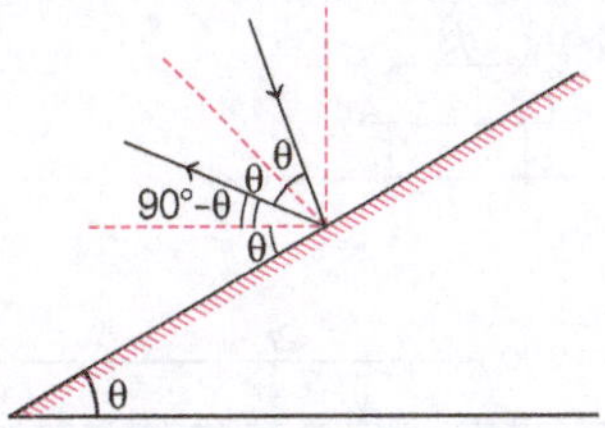

$\therefore \quad \theta = 0°$

Angle of reflected ray with horizontal $= 90° - \theta = 90°$

14. (c) At P, $u = v$ which is possible only when $u = 2f$

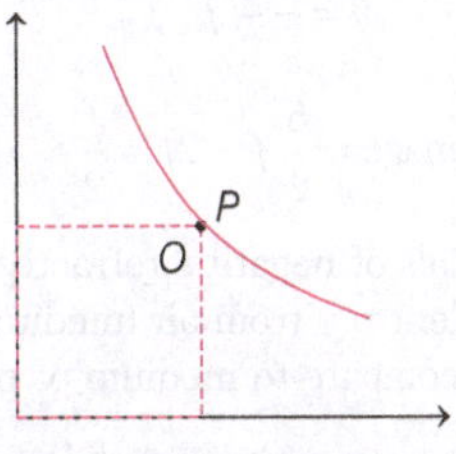

If we take another point Q just above P, then $v > 2f$.

15. (a) From the relation,

$\frac{1}{v} + \frac{1}{u} = \frac{1}{f}$ or $\frac{1}{v} - \frac{1}{u} = \frac{1}{-f}$

$\frac{1}{v} = \frac{1}{u} - \frac{1}{f}$ or $v = \left(\frac{uf}{f-u}\right)$

Since, $u > f$, v is negative

or $\quad |v| = \left(\frac{uf}{u-f}\right) > f$

The end which is at infinity will have its image at focus.

$\therefore$ Length of image, $L = |v| - f = \dfrac{f^2}{u-f}$

16. (b) The phenomenon involved in the reflection of radiowaves by ionosphere is similar to total internal reflection of light in air during a mirage when angle of incidence is greater than critical angle.

17. (c) On reflection from a rarer to denser medium, a phase difference of π occurs.

18. (b) The PQ ray of light passes through focus F and incident on the concave mirror, after reflection the ray should become parallel to the principal axis and shown by ray 2 in the figure.

19. (b) As, incident ray and reflected ray are parallel to each other it means, deviation, $\delta = 180°$

$\because \quad \delta = 360° - 2\theta$

$\therefore \quad 180° = 360° - 2\theta$

Angle between two plane mirrors,

$$\theta = 90°$$

20. (b) For end A of the rod, $u = 2f - \dfrac{f}{3} = \dfrac{5f}{3}$

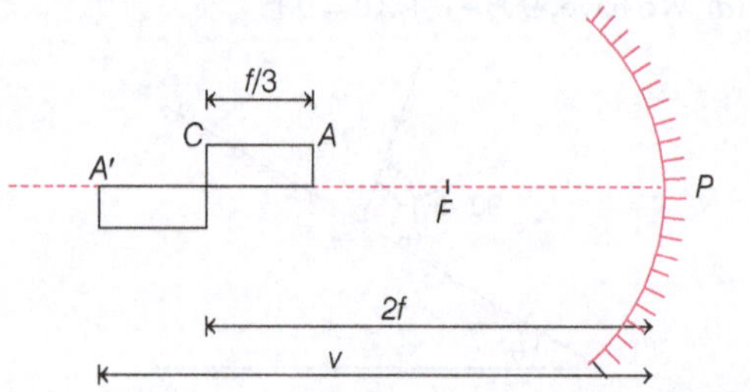

By using, $\dfrac{1}{f} = \dfrac{1}{v} + \dfrac{1}{u} \Rightarrow \dfrac{1}{-f} = \dfrac{1}{v} + \dfrac{1}{(-5f/3)}$

$\therefore \quad v = -\dfrac{5}{2}f$

So, length of image $= \dfrac{5}{2}f - 2f = \dfrac{f}{2}$

21. (a) The materials of negative refractive index are those in which incident ray from air (medium 1) bend differently as compare to medium of positive refractive index.

22. (c) All rays coming from object at centre are normal. So, no bending will take place. Hence, virtual image of point object will form at the centre of glass sphere. So, the distance of the virtual image from the surface of sphere is 6 cm.

23. (b) As, $\dfrac{c}{v} = \dfrac{\sin i}{\sin r}$

$\Rightarrow \quad v = \dfrac{c \times \sin r}{\sin i} = \dfrac{3 \times 10^8 \times \sin 30°}{\sin 45°}$

$= 2.12 \times 10^8$ m/s

24. (d) Given, wavelength in vacuum $= 5890$ Å

In a medium of refractive index, the wavelength of light decreases to $\dfrac{\lambda}{\mu} = \dfrac{5890}{1.5} \cong 3927$ Å.

25. (a) When a ray of light passes from a denser medium to a rarer medium, then it bends away from the normal at the interface of the two media.

The angle of incidence is measured with respect to the normal at the refractive boundary. It is given by

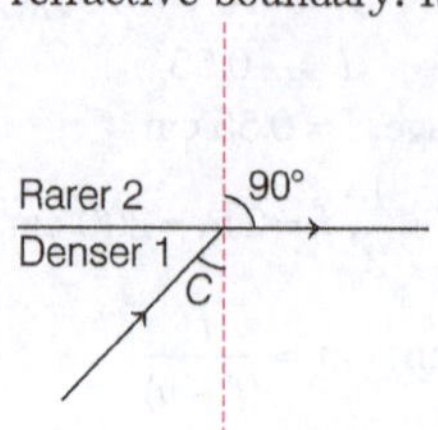

$$C = \sin^{-1}\left(\frac{n_2}{n_1}\right)$$

where, C is critical angle, n_2 is the refractive index of rarer medium and n_1 of the denser medium.

Given, $\quad n_2 = 1.33, n_1 = 1.50$

$$C = \sin^{-1}\left(\frac{1.33}{1.50}\right) \Rightarrow C = \sin^{-1}\left(\frac{8}{9}\right)$$

26. (c) Real depth $= 1$ m

Apparent depth $= 1 - 0.1 = 0.9$ m

Refractive index, $\mu = \dfrac{\text{Real depth}}{\text{Apparent depth}} = \dfrac{1}{0.9} = \dfrac{10}{9}$

27. (b) We have, $n_a v_a = n_g v_g$

$$\frac{n_g}{n_a} = \frac{v_a}{v_g}$$

$$\frac{3}{2} = \frac{3 \times 10^8}{v_g}$$

$$v_g = 2 \times 10^8$$

$$\text{Time} = \frac{\text{Distance}}{\text{Speed}}$$

$$t = \frac{4 \times 10^{-3}}{2 \times 10^8}$$

$$t = 2 \times 10^{-11} \text{ s}$$

28. (d) We have,

$$C = \sin^{-1}\left(\frac{v_1}{v_2}\right) = \sin^{-1}\left(\frac{1.8 \times 10^8}{2.4 \times 10^8}\right) = \sin^{-1}\left(\frac{3}{4}\right)$$

29. (b) In going from one medium to another, frequency remains same but wavelength and velocity decrease with the increase in refractive index *i.e.*, wavelength becomes $\lambda' = \lambda / \mu$ and velocity becomes,

$$c = \frac{v}{\mu}$$

30. (c) We have, $\frac{1}{\sin C} = \frac{\lambda_1}{\lambda_2}$

$\Rightarrow \frac{1}{\sin C} = \frac{6000}{3000}$

$\Rightarrow \frac{1}{\sin C} = \frac{6}{3} = 2 \Rightarrow \sin C = \frac{1}{2}$

$\Rightarrow$ Critical angle between two medium, $C = \sin^{-1}\left(\frac{1}{2}\right)$

31. (b) Since, rays after passing through the glass slab just suffer lateral displacement. So, angle between emergent ray is also α.

32. (c) From the formula,

$$\sin C = \frac{1}{_1\mu_2} \Rightarrow \sin C = {_2\mu_1}$$

$$\therefore \quad \frac{\mu_1}{\mu_2} = \frac{v_2}{v_1}$$

$$\Rightarrow \quad \sin C = \frac{10x/t_2}{x/t_1}$$

$$\sin C = \frac{10t_1}{t_2}$$

$$C = \sin^{-1}\left(\frac{10t_1}{t_2}\right)$$

33. (b) As optical paths are equal, hence

$$n_g x_g = n_w x_w$$

$$n_w = n_g \frac{x_g}{x_w}$$

Refractive index of the water,

$$n_w = 1.53 \times \frac{4.0}{4.5} = 1.36$$

34. (c) For total internal reflection, $i > C$

$$\Rightarrow \quad \sin i > \sin C \Rightarrow \sin 45° > \frac{1}{\mu}$$

$$\Rightarrow \quad \mu > \sqrt{2} \Rightarrow \mu > 1.414$$

35. (b) From Snell's law,

$$\mu \sin i = \text{constant}$$

$$\mu_4 \sin x = \mu \sin i$$

$$\therefore \quad \sin x = \frac{\mu}{\mu_4} \sin i$$

36. (d) According to the question, $\frac{h}{\mu} = \frac{21}{2} = 10.5$

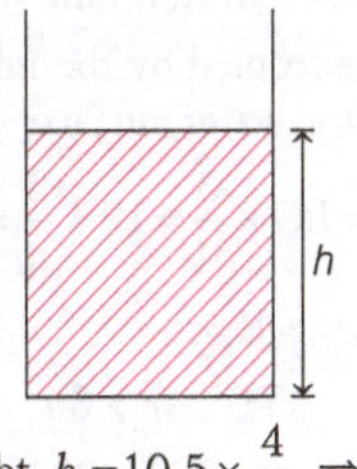

$\therefore$ Height, $h = 10.5 \times \frac{4}{3} \Rightarrow h = 14$ cm

37. (d) When total internal reflection just takes place from lateral surface, $i = C$, i.e. $60° = C$

$$\Rightarrow \quad \sin 60° = \sin C = \frac{1}{\mu} \Rightarrow \mu = \frac{2}{\sqrt{3}}$$

Time taken by light to traverse some distance in a medium,

$$t = \frac{\mu x}{c} = \frac{\frac{2}{\sqrt{3}} \times 10^3}{3 \times 10^8} = 3.85\,\mu s$$

38. (c) We have, refractive index, $\mu = \frac{\sin i}{\sin r} \Rightarrow \sqrt{3} = \frac{\sin 60°}{\sin r}$

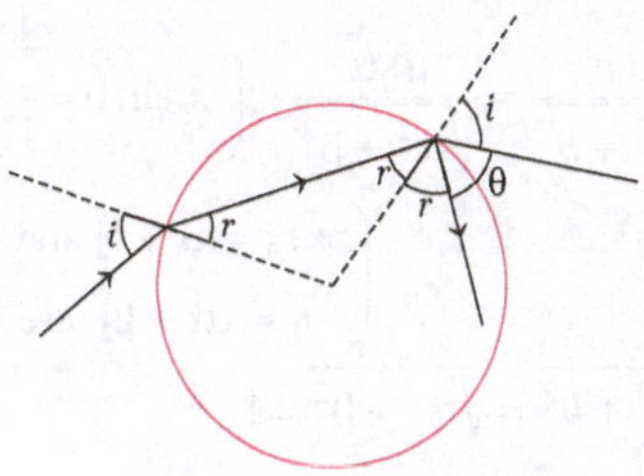

$$\sin r = \frac{1}{2}$$

Refracted angle, $r = 30°$

The angle between the reflected and refracted rays,

$$\theta = 180° - i - r = 90°$$

39. (c) Due to glass slab, increase in path

$$= (\mu - 1)t = (1.5 - 1)\,3 \text{ cm}$$
$$= 1.5 \text{ cm}$$

$\therefore \quad u' = -(21 + 1.5)$ cm

or $\quad u' = -22.5$ cm

Now, $\quad \frac{1}{-22.5} + \frac{1}{v} = \frac{1}{-5}$

or $\quad \frac{1}{v} = \frac{1}{22.5} - \frac{1}{5}$ or $\frac{1}{v} = \frac{5 - 22.5}{22.5 \times 5}$

or $\quad v = \frac{22.5 \times 5}{17.5}$ or $v = -6.43$ cm

The position of the final image $= -(6.43 - 1.5)$ cm $= -4.93$ cm

40. (b) We know that, $\frac{1}{\mu} = \frac{\sin i}{\sin r'}$ ...(i)

But $\quad r + r' = 90°$ or $r' = 90° - r$

$\sin r' = \sin(90° - r)$

$= \cos r$

or $\quad \sin r' = \cos i$ (since, $i = r$) ...(ii)

From Eqs. (i) and (ii), we get

$\therefore \quad \frac{1}{\mu} = \frac{\sin i}{\cos i}$

or $\quad \frac{1}{\mu} = \tan i$

or $\quad \sin i_C = \tan i = \tan r$

The critical angle for pair of media is,

$$i_C = \sin^{-1}(\tan r)$$

41. (a) From the Snell's law, $\mu_1 \sin i_1 = \mu_2 \sin i_2$

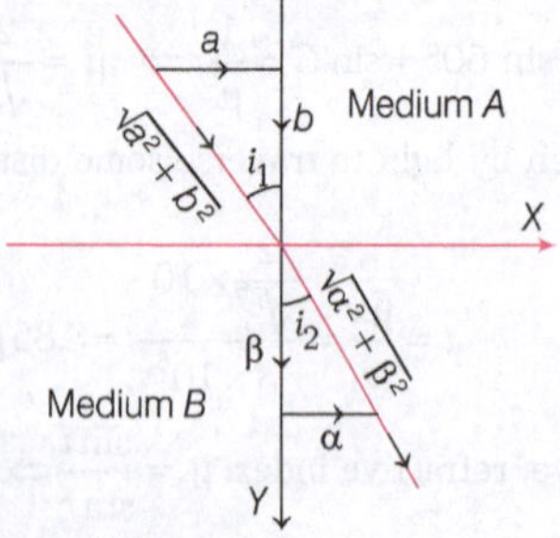

$$\therefore \quad \frac{\mu_1 a}{\sqrt{a^2+b^2}} = \frac{\mu_2 \alpha}{\sqrt{\alpha^2+\beta^2}} \quad \left(\because \sin\theta = \frac{\text{Height}}{\text{Hypotenuse}}\right)$$

$$\left(\because r_A = a\hat{\mathbf{i}} + b\hat{\mathbf{j}} \text{ and } r_B = \alpha\hat{\mathbf{i}} + \beta\hat{\mathbf{j}} \text{ are unit vectors}\right)$$

$$\sqrt{a^2+b^2} = \sqrt{\alpha^2+\beta^2} = 1$$

$$\therefore \quad \mu_1 a = \mu_2 \alpha$$

42. (b) Here, angle of incidence, $i = 45°$

$$\frac{\text{Lateral shift } (d)}{\text{Thickness of glass slab } (t)} = \frac{1}{\sqrt{3}}$$

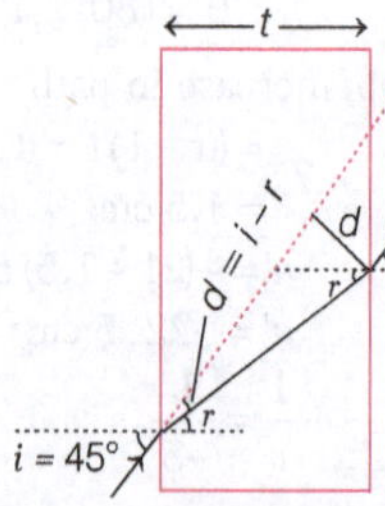

$$\text{Lateral shift, } d = \frac{t\sin\delta}{\cos r} = \frac{t\sin(i-r)}{\cos r}$$

$$\Rightarrow \quad \frac{d}{t} = \frac{\sin(i-r)}{\cos r}$$

$$\text{or} \quad \frac{d}{t} = \frac{\sin i\cos r - \cos i\sin r}{\cos r}$$

$$\text{or} \quad \frac{d}{t} = \frac{\sin 45°\cos r - \cos 45°\sin r}{\cos r}$$

$$= \frac{\cos r - \sin r}{\sqrt{2}\cos r}$$

$$\text{or} \quad \frac{d}{t} = \frac{1}{\sqrt{2}}(1-\tan r)$$

$$\text{or} \quad \frac{1}{\sqrt{3}} = \frac{1}{\sqrt{2}}(1-\tan r)$$

$$\text{or} \quad \tan r = 1 - \frac{\sqrt{2}}{\sqrt{3}}$$

or Angle of refraction,

$$r = \tan^{-1}\left(1 - \frac{\sqrt{2}}{\sqrt{3}}\right)$$

43. (b) Fish is observer and bird is object.

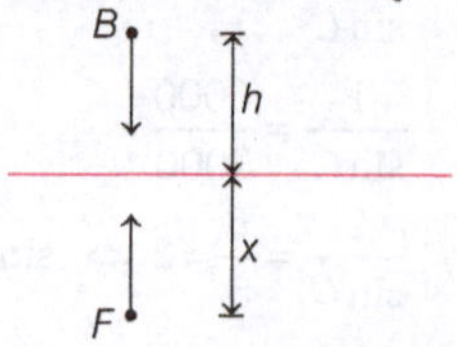

Apparent distance between F and B at some instant will be

$$y = (x + \mu h)$$

$$\left(-\frac{dy}{dt}\right) = \left(-\frac{dx}{dt}\right) + (\mu)\left(-\frac{dh}{dt}\right)$$

$$9 = 3 + \frac{4}{3}\left(-\frac{dh}{dt}\right)$$

$$\therefore \quad -\frac{dh}{dt} = 4.5 \text{ m/s}$$

44. (d) Refractive index, $\mu = \frac{\sin 60°}{\sin 30°}$

$$= \frac{\sqrt{3}/2}{1/2} = \sqrt{3}$$

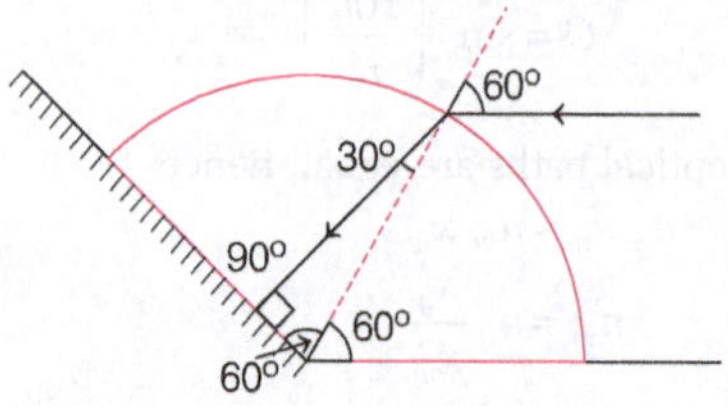

45. (b) In first case, when sun is at infinity, *i.e.*

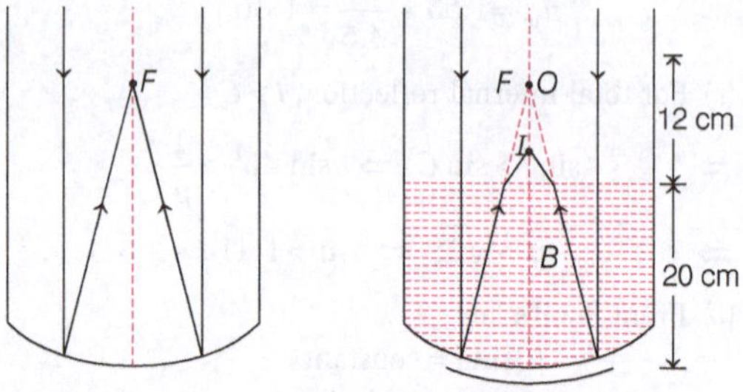

$$\therefore \quad u = \infty$$

$$\Rightarrow \quad \frac{1}{f} = \frac{1}{-32} + \frac{1}{(-\infty)}$$

$$\therefore \quad f = -32 \text{ cm}$$

When water is filled in that tank upto a height of 20 cm, the image formed by the mirror will act as virtual object O for water surface.

$$\therefore \quad BI = BO \times \frac{3}{4} = 12 \times \frac{3}{4} = 9 \text{ cm}$$

46. (a) For TIR to take place,

$$90° - r > \theta_C$$

$$\Rightarrow \quad r < 90° - \theta_C$$

From the relation,

$$\mu = \frac{\sin i}{\sin r}$$

$$\sin i = \mu \sin r$$

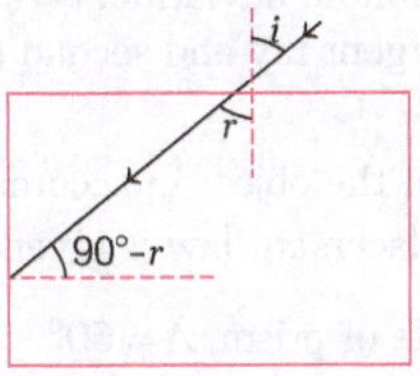

Since, for TIR to take place, $r < 90° - \theta_C$

$\therefore \quad i = \sin^{-1}\{\mu \sin r\}$

$i \le \sin^{-1}[\{n \sin (90° - \theta_C)\}]$

or $\quad i \le \sin^{-1}\{\mu \cos \theta_C\}$

or $\quad i \le \sin^{-1}\left\{\mu\sqrt{1 - \frac{1}{\mu^2}}\right\} \quad \left(\because \sin \theta_C = \frac{1}{\mu_C}\right)$

or $\quad i \le \sin^{-1}\left\{1.33\sqrt{1 - \frac{1}{(1.33)^2}}\right\}$

or $\quad i \le \sin^{-1}(\sqrt{0.77})$

Note For simplifying the calculation, take $1.33 = \frac{4}{3}$

47. (b) As, $y_a = \left(\frac{n_1}{n_2}\right) y$

Here, y = actual depth and y_a = apparent depth.

$$\therefore \quad y = \left(\frac{n_2}{n_1}\right) \cdot y_a \Rightarrow \left(-\frac{dy}{dt}\right) = \frac{n_2}{n_1}\left(-\frac{dy_a}{dt}\right) = \frac{n_2 x}{n_1}$$

The amount of water drained in cc/min

$$\therefore \quad \frac{dv}{dt} = A \cdot \left(-\frac{dy}{dt}\right) = \frac{\pi R^2 n_2 x}{n_1}$$

48. (b) At point P,

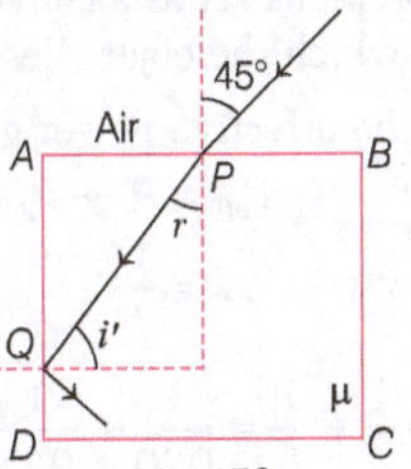

Refractive index, $\mu = \frac{\sin 45°}{\sin r} \Rightarrow \sin r = \frac{1}{\mu\sqrt{2}}$ ...(i)

At point Q, for total internal reflection, $\sin i' = \frac{1}{\mu}$

From figure, $\quad i' = 90° - r$

$\therefore \quad \sin(90° - r) = \frac{1}{\mu}$

$\Rightarrow \quad \cos r = \frac{1}{\mu}$ ...(ii)

Now, $\quad \cos r = \sqrt{1 - \sin^2 r}$

$$= \sqrt{\left(1 - \frac{1}{2\mu^2}\right)}$$

$$= \sqrt{\left(\frac{2\mu^2 - 1}{2\mu^2}\right)} \quad \text{...(iii)}$$

From Eqs. (ii) and (iii), we get

$$\frac{1}{\mu} = \sqrt{\frac{2\mu^2 - 1}{2\mu^2}}$$

Refractive index, $\mu = \sqrt{\frac{3}{2}}$

This is the minimum value of refractive index for total internal reflection at vertical face AD.

49. (d) As the law of refraction, we have

$$\frac{\sin i_C}{\sin 90°} = \frac{1.5}{1.6}$$

$\therefore \quad \sin i_C = \frac{15}{16}$

where, i_C = critical angle of medium.

or $\quad i_C = \sin^{-1}\left(\frac{15}{16}\right)$

50. (c) In vacuum, $c = d/t$

In medium, $v = \frac{5d}{T}$

As refractive index, $\mu = \frac{c}{v} = \frac{d/t}{5d/T} = \frac{T}{5t}$

Also, $\quad \sin C = \frac{1}{\mu}$ (where, C is critical angle)

$\therefore \quad C = \sin^{-1}\left[\frac{5t}{T}\right]$

51. (a) For total internal reflection, the angle of incidence of light in denser medium must be greater than the critical angle for the pair of media in contact, i.e. $i > C$.

We have, $\frac{1}{\sin C} = \frac{v_2}{v_1}$

Given, $\quad v_1 = 1.5 \times 10^8 \text{ ms}^{-1}$

$v_2 = 2 \times 10^8 \text{ ms}^{-1}$

Here, $\quad C = \sin^{-1}\left(\frac{v_1}{v_2}\right)$

For total internal reflection, $\theta > C$

$\therefore \quad \theta > \sin^{-1}\left(\frac{v_1}{v_2}\right)$

$\Rightarrow \quad \theta > \sin^{-1}\left(\frac{1.5 \times 10^8}{2 \times 10^8}\right)$

$\Rightarrow \quad \theta > \sin^{-1}\left(\frac{3}{4}\right)$

52. (c) We have, $\frac{\mu_2}{v} = \frac{\mu_1}{u} - \frac{\mu_2 - \mu_1}{R}$

$$\frac{1}{v} = \frac{1.5}{-6} - \frac{1-1.5}{-10}$$

$\therefore$ $v = -5$ cm

53. (c) Shift from the slab, $S = \left(1 - \frac{1}{\mu}\right)t = 2$ cm

Let x be the distance between object and mirror, then

$$x - 2 = 40 \quad \text{or} \quad x = 42 \text{ cm}$$

54. (c) The reflected ray will rotate by angle 2θ. For TIR to take place at water-air boundary,

$$\sin 2\theta > \sin\theta_C \quad \text{or} \quad \sin 2\theta > \frac{1}{\mu}$$

$$\therefore \quad \theta > \frac{1}{2}\sin^{-1}\left(\frac{3}{4}\right)$$

55. (b) With increase in wavelength, refractive index gets decreased. Therefore, focal length of lens will be increased.

56. (a) For real image,

$$u = -x$$
$$v = +mx$$

$$\therefore \quad \frac{1}{mx} - \frac{1}{-x} = \frac{1}{f} \quad \text{...(i)}$$

For virtual image, $u = -y$

Then, $v = -my$

$$\therefore \quad \frac{1}{-my} - \frac{1}{(-y)} = \frac{1}{f} \quad \text{...(ii)}$$

On solving Eqs. (i) and (ii), we get

$$f = \frac{x+y}{2}$$

57. (c) Here, $\frac{1}{f} = (\mu - 1)\left[\frac{1}{R_1} - \frac{1}{R_2}\right]$

$$\frac{1}{f} = (1.6 - 1)\left[\frac{1}{60} - \frac{1}{\infty}\right] = \frac{1}{100} \Rightarrow f = 100 \text{ cm}$$

58. (d) Magnification, $m = \pm 3$

We have, $m = \frac{f}{f+u}$

For virtual image, $3 = \frac{f}{f-8}$ ...(i)

For real image, $-3 = \frac{f}{f-16}$ ...(ii)

Solving Eqs. (i) and (ii), we get

$$f = 12 \text{ cm}$$

59. (c) For $A > 2C$, the ray of light does not emerge from the opposite face of the prism.

60. (c) If refractive index of lens n_1 is equal to refractive index of liquid n_2, then lens behaves as a plane glass plate and becomes invisible in the medium.

61. (d) Resultant focal length of combination,

$$F_{comb} = \frac{f_1 f_2}{f_1 + f_2} = \frac{f(-f)}{f + (-f)} = \infty$$

62. (d) Under minimum deviation, $i = e = 30°$, so angle between emergent ray and second refracting surface is $90° - 30° = 60°$.

63. (a) The size of the object in accordance with the Fresnel's displacement law is given by $\sqrt{x_1 x_2}$.

64. (d) Here, angle of prism, $A = 60°$

For minimum deviation, $A = 2r$

or $r = \frac{A}{2} = \frac{60°}{2} = 30°$ for both colours.

65. (c) For real image, object should be placed at distance $2f$ for minimum distance between object and its real image.

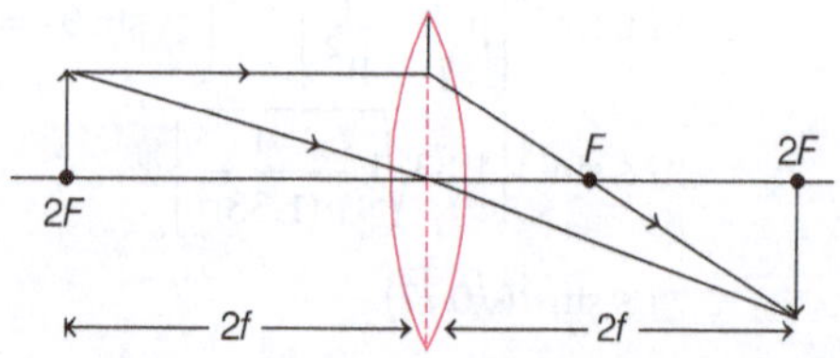

66. (a) For combination of one convex and one concave lens

$$\frac{1}{F} = \frac{1}{f_1} - \frac{1}{f_2}$$

$$\Rightarrow \quad F = \frac{f_1 f_2}{f_2 - f_1}$$

If $f_1 > f_2$, then F will be negative.

67. (c) Here, $R = 20$ cm, $\mu = 1.5$, on substituting the values in $f = \frac{R}{\mu - 1} = \frac{20}{1.5 - 1} = 40$ cm of converging nature as $f > 0$. Therefore, lens act as a convex lens irrespective of the side on which the object lies.

68. (a) We have, the effective power given by

$$P_{eff} = P_1 + P_2$$

Also, we know $P = \frac{1}{f}$

Hence, $P_{eff} = \frac{1}{f_1} + \frac{1}{f_2} = \frac{1}{0.20} + \frac{1}{0.25}$

$$= 5 + 4 = 9\text{ D}$$

69. (c) We have, $\frac{1}{f} = (\mu - 1)\left(\frac{1}{R_1} - \frac{1}{R_2}\right)$

$$\frac{1}{30} = (\mu - 1)\left(\frac{1}{10}\right)$$

The refractive index of the material of the lens,

$$\mu = \frac{4}{3} = 1.33$$

70. (c) Refractive index of the material of prism,

$$\mu = \frac{\sin\left(\frac{A+\delta_m}{2}\right)}{\sin\left(\frac{A}{2}\right)}$$

$$\Rightarrow \quad \sqrt{3} = \frac{\sin\left(\frac{60°+\delta_m}{2}\right)}{\sin\left(\frac{60°}{2}\right)}$$

$$\Rightarrow \quad \frac{\sqrt{3}}{2} = \sin\left(30° + \frac{\delta_m}{2}\right)$$

$\therefore$ Minimum deviation of the prism, $\delta_m = 60°$

71. (a) As, $A + \delta = i + e$ ...(i)

$\Rightarrow 30° + 30° = 60° + e$

Angle of emergence, $e = 60° - 60° = 0$

$r_1 = A = 30°$

$\therefore$ Refractive index, $\mu = \frac{\sin i}{\sin r} = \frac{\sin 60°}{\sin 30°} = \sqrt{3} = 1.732$

72. (b) We have, $\frac{1}{v} - \frac{1}{u} = \frac{1}{f}$

$$\because \quad \frac{1}{30} - \frac{1}{(-u)} = \frac{1}{f} \text{ or } \frac{1}{30} + \frac{1}{u} = \frac{1}{f} \quad ...(i)$$

Similarly, $\frac{1}{120} + \frac{1}{u-90} = \frac{1}{f}$ ...(ii)

On solving Eqs. (i) and (ii), we get

The focal length of the lens, $f = 24$ cm

73. (b) We have, $\frac{1}{f} = (1.5 - 1)\left(\frac{1}{10} + \frac{1}{10}\right)$

$\therefore$ Focal length, f = 10 cm

Radius of curvature, $R = 2f$ = 20 cm

74. (d) The focal length of the lens,

$$\frac{1}{f} = (\mu - 1)\left(\frac{1}{R_1} - \frac{1}{R_2}\right)$$

$$\frac{1}{f} = (1.5 - 1)\left(\frac{1}{20} - \frac{1}{30}\right)$$

$$\Rightarrow \quad \frac{1}{f} = 0.5\left(\frac{30-20}{600}\right)$$

$$\text{or} \quad \frac{1}{f} = \frac{1}{2} \times \frac{10}{600} = \frac{1}{120}$$

or focal length, f = 120 cm

75. (a) Power of a biconvex lens is 10 D and radius of curvature of each surface = 10 cm.

$$\Rightarrow \quad P = \frac{1}{f} = (\mu - 1)\left[\frac{1}{R_1} - \frac{1}{R_2}\right]$$

$$\Rightarrow \quad 10 = (\mu - 1)\left[\frac{100}{10} - \left(-\frac{100}{10}\right)\right]$$

$$\Rightarrow \quad 10 = (\mu - 1)[20]$$

$$\Rightarrow \quad (\mu - 1) = \frac{1}{2}$$

$\Rightarrow$ Refractive index of the material, $\mu = \frac{3}{2}$

76. (d) Focal length of the combination,

$$\frac{1}{F} = \frac{1}{f_1} + \frac{1}{f_2}$$

$$\Rightarrow \quad \frac{1}{80} = \frac{1}{20} + \frac{1}{f_2} \text{ or } f_2 = -\frac{80}{3} \text{ cm}$$

$\therefore$ Power of second lens, $P' = \frac{100}{f_2} = \frac{100}{(-80/3)} = -3.75$ D

77. (a) When plano-convex lens is silvered at curved surface, then it becomes concave mirror of focal length,

$$f = \frac{R}{2\mu} = \frac{30}{2 \times 1.5} = 10 \text{ cm}$$

If we have to find real image of same size of the object, then object must be placed at centre of curvature $u = 2f = 20$ cm.

78. (a) Since, deviation, $\delta = (\mu - 1)A = (1.5 - 1) \times 5° = 2.5°$

By geometry, angle of refraction by first surface is 5°.

But $\delta = \theta - r$, so we have $2.5° = \theta - 5°$

On solving, $\theta = 7.5°$

79. (d) Given, $u = mf$

$$\therefore \quad \frac{1}{v} - \frac{1}{(-mf)} = -\frac{1}{f} \Rightarrow \frac{1}{v} = -\frac{1}{f}\left(1 + \frac{1}{m}\right)$$

$$\Rightarrow \quad \frac{1}{v} = \frac{m+1}{-mf} \Rightarrow -\frac{v}{u} = \frac{1}{1+m}$$

80. (c) According to lens Maker's formula,

$$\frac{1}{f} = (\mu - 1)\left(\frac{1}{R} - \frac{1}{(-R)}\right)$$

$$\Rightarrow \quad \frac{1}{f} = (\mu - 1)\left(\frac{2}{R}\right) \quad ...(i)$$

On cutting, $\frac{1}{f'} = (\mu - 1)\left(\frac{1}{R} - \frac{1}{\infty}\right)$

$$\frac{1}{f'} = (\mu - 1)\left(\frac{1}{R}\right) \quad ...(ii)$$

From Eqs. (i) and (ii), we get $f' = 2f$.

81. (d) At second surface, there is no refraction, so

$$r_2 = 0$$

$$\therefore \quad r_1 = A = 30°$$

From Snell's law,

$$n = \frac{\sin i_1}{\sin r_1}$$

$$\Rightarrow \quad n = \frac{\sin i_1}{\sin 30°}$$

$$\Rightarrow \quad \sin i_1 = \sqrt{2} \times \frac{1}{2} = \frac{1}{\sqrt{2}}$$

$$\Rightarrow \quad \sin i_1 = \frac{1}{\sqrt{2}} \Rightarrow i_1 = 45^\circ$$

82. (c) Given, $P_1 + P_2 = 9$ ...(i)

We have, $P = P_1 + P_2 - dP_1 P_2$

$$\Rightarrow \quad \frac{27}{5} = 9 - \frac{20}{100} \times P_1 P_2$$

Again $(P_2 - P_1)^2 = (P_1 + P_2)^2 - 4P_1 P_2$

$$\Rightarrow \quad P_2 - P_1 = 3 \quad \text{...(ii)}$$

On solving Eqs. (i) and (ii), we get

$$P_1 = 3 \text{ and } P_2 = 6$$

83. (a) Power of system $= \frac{1}{f_1} + \frac{1}{f_2} - \frac{d}{f_1 f_2}$

$$= \frac{1}{1} + \left(\frac{1}{-0.25}\right) - \frac{0.75}{(1)(-0.25)}$$

$$= 1 - 4 + 3 = -3 + 3 = 0$$

Since, power of the system is zero, therefore the incident parallel beam of light will remain parallel after emerging from the system.

84. (c) Angle of incidence, $i = \theta$

Angle of equilateral prism,

$$A = 60^\circ$$

$$\mu = \sqrt{3}$$

In the case of minimum deviation, the refracted ray inside the prism is parallel to the base.

Hence, $r = \frac{A}{2} = \frac{60}{2} = 30^\circ$

$$\therefore \quad \mu = \frac{\sin i}{\sin r}$$

$$\Rightarrow \quad \mu = \frac{\sin \theta}{\sin r}$$

$$\Rightarrow \quad \sqrt{3} = \frac{\sin \theta}{\sin 30^\circ}$$

$$\Rightarrow \quad \sin \theta = \sqrt{3} \sin 30^\circ$$

$$\Rightarrow \quad \sin \theta = \sqrt{3} \times \frac{1}{2}$$

$$\Rightarrow \quad \sin \theta = \sin 60^\circ$$

$$\Rightarrow \quad \theta = 60^\circ$$

85. (c) For dispersion without deviation,

$$\frac{A}{A'} = \frac{(\mu' - 1)}{(\mu - 1)}$$

$$\frac{6^\circ}{A'} = \frac{0.75}{0.50}$$

$$A' = \frac{0.50 \times 6^\circ}{0.75}$$

$$A' = 4^\circ$$

86. (a) Here, $n = 1.5$, as per sign convention followed

$$R_1 = +20 \text{ cm and } R_2 = -20 \text{ cm}$$

$$\therefore \quad \frac{1}{f} = (n-1)\left(\frac{1}{R_1} - \frac{1}{R_2}\right)$$

$$= (1.5 - 1)\left[\frac{1}{(+20)} - \frac{1}{(-20)}\right] = 0.5 \times \frac{2}{20} = \frac{1}{20}$$

$$\Rightarrow \quad f = +20 \text{ cm}$$

Incident rays travelling parallel to the axis of lens will converge at its second principal focus, hence

$$L = +20 \text{ cm}$$

87. (d) Critical angle, $\theta_C = \sin^{-1}\left(\frac{1}{1.5}\right) = 41.8^\circ$

Incident angle, $i_1 = 30^\circ$

$$\therefore \quad \sin r_1 = \frac{\sin i_1}{\mu} = \frac{\sin(30^\circ)}{1.5}$$

$$r_1 = 19.5^\circ$$

or angle of emergence, $r_2 = A - r_1 = 90^\circ - 19.5^\circ = 70.5^\circ$

Since, $r_2 > \theta_C$

$\therefore$ The ray will not emerge from the prism.

88. (c) We have, $\delta = i_1 + i_2 - A$

$$45^\circ = (i_1 + i_2) - 60^\circ$$

$$\therefore \quad i_1 + i_2 = 105^\circ \quad \text{...(i)}$$

$$\text{and} \quad i_1 - i_2 = 20^\circ \quad \text{...(ii)}$$

On solving Eqs. (i) and (ii), we get

$$i_1 = 62.5^\circ \text{ and } i_2 = 42.5^\circ$$

89. (c) We have, $\frac{1}{f} = \frac{2\mu}{R_2} - \frac{2(\mu - 1)}{R_1}$

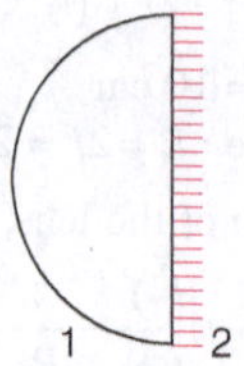

$$\frac{1}{-10} = \frac{2 \times 1.5}{\infty} - \frac{2(1.5 - 1)}{R}$$

$$\therefore \quad R = 10 \text{ cm}$$

90. (c) The separation between the images formed by extreme wavelengths of visible range is called the longitudinal chromatic aberration, given by

$$f_1 - f_2 = \omega \times f$$

where, ω is dispersive power.

Given, $\omega = 0.02$, $f = 20$ cm

$$\because \quad f_1 - f_2 = 0.02 \times 20 = 0.40$$

91. (a) Here, $x = u + v$ ...(i)

Magnification, $m = \frac{f}{f - u} = \frac{f - v}{f}$

Image is real, magnification is negative

$$-m = \frac{f}{f-u} \Rightarrow u = \frac{(m+1)}{m} f$$

From $\quad -m = \frac{f-v}{f} \Rightarrow v = (m+1)f$

Putting the value of v in Eq. (i), we get

$$x = \frac{(m+1)}{m} f + (m+1)f$$

$$\Rightarrow \quad f = \frac{mx}{(m+1)^2}$$

92. (*d*) As, $n = \dfrac{\text{Real depth}}{\text{Apparent depth}}$

$$\Rightarrow \quad n = \frac{6}{4} = \frac{3}{2}$$

Also, $\dfrac{n_1}{u} - \dfrac{n_2}{v} = \dfrac{n_1 - n_2}{R} \Rightarrow \dfrac{1.5}{6} - \dfrac{4}{17} = \dfrac{1.5-1}{R}$

Radius of curvature, $R = 34$ cm

93. (*b*) Angle i at both faces will be 45°. For TIR to take place,

$$i > \theta_C \quad \text{or} \quad \sin i > \sin \theta_C$$

$$\therefore \quad \frac{1}{\sqrt{2}} > \frac{1}{\mu} \quad \text{or} \quad \mu > \sqrt{2}$$

94. (*b*) As, per question,

$$\because \quad \frac{1}{-(f+1)} - \frac{1}{-(f-1)} = \frac{1}{f}$$

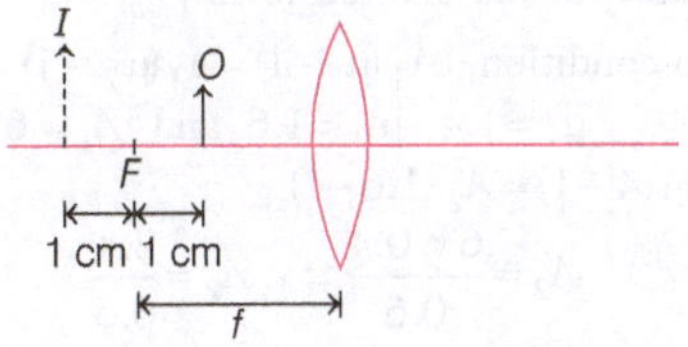

On solving, we get $f = (\sqrt{2}+1)$ cm

95. (*c*) When the lens in air, we have

$$P_a = \frac{1}{f_a} = \frac{\mu_g - \mu_a}{\mu_a}\left[\frac{1}{R_1} - \frac{1}{R_2}\right]$$

When the lens is in liquid, we have

$$P_l = \frac{1}{f_l} = \frac{\mu_g - \mu_l}{\mu_l}\left[\frac{1}{R_1} - \frac{1}{R_2}\right]$$

Given, $P_a = 5, P_l = -1, \mu_a = 1$ and $\mu_g = 1.5$

On solving, we get $\mu_l = \dfrac{5}{3}$

96. (*b*) We have, $\dfrac{\mu_2}{v_1} - \dfrac{\mu_1}{\infty} = \dfrac{\mu_2 - \mu_1}{R}$ ...(i)

and $\dfrac{\mu_3}{f} - \dfrac{\mu_2}{v_1} = \dfrac{\mu_3 - \mu_2}{-R}$ ...(ii)

From Eqs. (i) and (ii), we get

$$\frac{\mu_3}{f} = \frac{\mu_2 - \mu_1 - \mu_3 + \mu_2}{R} = \frac{2\mu_2 - (\mu_1 + \mu_3)}{R}$$

Lens will become diverging, if f is negative

i.e. $\quad 2\mu_2 < (\mu_1 + \mu_3)$

97. (*d*) Equation of straight line AB,

$$\frac{1}{m} = \tan\theta u - \frac{ba}{c}$$

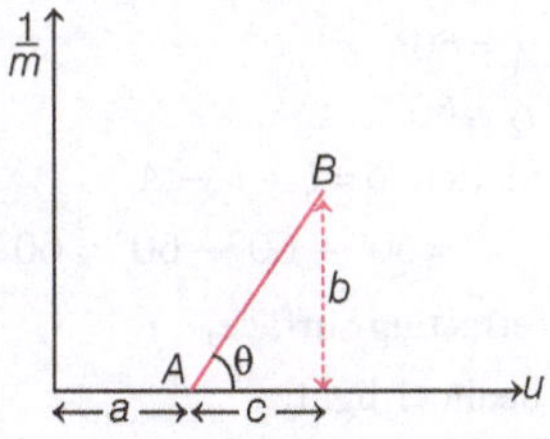

From, $\dfrac{1}{v} - \dfrac{1}{-u} = \dfrac{1}{+f}$

$$v = \frac{uf}{u-f} \quad \text{or} \quad \frac{v}{u} = m = \frac{f}{u-f} \Rightarrow \frac{1}{m} = \left(\frac{1}{f}\right)u - 1$$

Comparing this with equation of straight line, $1/f$ is the slope of line, which is b/c. So, the focal length of the lens used is $\dfrac{c}{b}$.

98. (*a*) We have, $\dfrac{1}{3x} - \dfrac{1}{(-x)} = \dfrac{1}{+30}$

$$\therefore \quad x = 40 \text{ cm} \quad \text{and} \quad 3x = 120 \text{ cm}$$

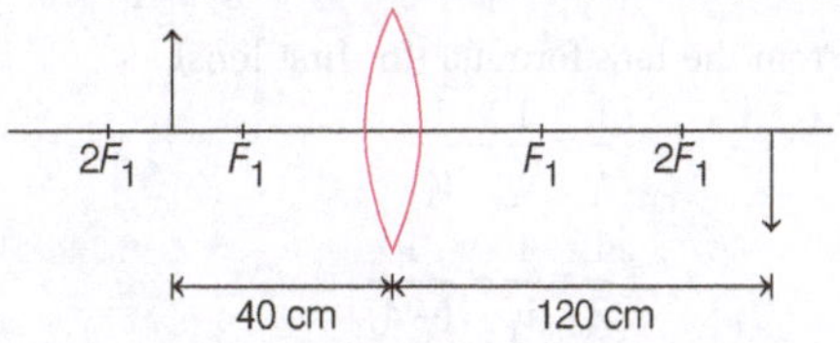

To decrease the magnification, object should be moved towards $2F_1$.

Hence, image will move towards $2F_2$. Let displacement is y, then

$$2(40+6) = (120-y) \quad \left(\because m = \frac{v}{u}\right)$$

$$\therefore \quad y = 28 \text{ cm}$$

99. (*a*) $AQ = AR$

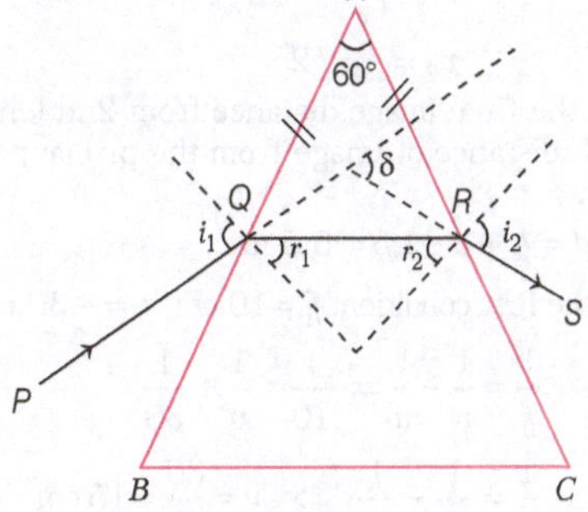

$$\Rightarrow \angle AQR = \angle ARQ = 60°$$

$\therefore \quad r_1 = r_2 = 30°$

$\sin i_1 = \mu \sin r_1$

$\Rightarrow \quad \sin i_1 = \sqrt{3} \sin 30°$

$= \sqrt{3} \times \frac{1}{2} = \frac{\sqrt{3}}{2}$

$\Rightarrow \quad i_1 = 60°$

Similarly, $i_2 = 60°$

In prism, deviation, $\delta = i_1 + i_2 - A$

$= 60° + 60° - 60° = 60°$

100. (*c*) For first refracting surface,

For parallel beam of light,

$$-\frac{\mu_1}{u} + \frac{\mu_2}{v} = \frac{\mu_2 - \mu_1}{R}$$

$$\Rightarrow \quad -\frac{1.4}{(-\infty)} + \frac{1.5}{v} = \frac{1.5 - 1.4}{R}$$

$$v = 15R$$

For second refracting surface,

$$\frac{\mu_2}{-15R} + \frac{\mu_3}{v'} = \frac{\mu_3 - \mu_2}{R}$$

$$\Rightarrow \quad \frac{1.5}{15R} + \frac{1.6}{v'} = \frac{1.6 - 1.5}{R}$$

$$\Rightarrow \quad v' = \infty$$

Hence, the combination behaves as glass plate.

101. (*b*) From the lens formula (for first lens),

$$\frac{1}{f_1} = \frac{1}{v_1} - \frac{1}{u_1}$$

$$\Rightarrow \quad \frac{1}{2} = \frac{1}{v_1} - \frac{1}{(-4)}$$

$$\Rightarrow \quad \frac{1}{2} - \frac{1}{4} = \frac{1}{v_1} = \frac{3}{4} \quad \text{...(i)}$$

$$\Rightarrow \quad v_1 = \frac{4}{3}, \; u_2 = 3 - \frac{4}{3} = 5/3$$

This image will be treated as the source for second lens, then again from lens formula, we have

$$\frac{1}{f_2} = \frac{1}{v_2} - \frac{1}{u_2} \Rightarrow \frac{1}{1} = \frac{1}{v_2} + 5/3 \quad \text{[by Eq. (i)]}$$

$$\Rightarrow \quad 1 - 5/3 = \frac{1}{v_2}$$

$$\Rightarrow \quad v_2 = -3/2$$

This is the final image distance from 2nd lens, so the overall distance of image from the primary source (or object).

Then, $d = 4 + 3 - 1.5 = 5.5$ m

102. (*d*) For the first condition, $f_1 = 10$ cm, $u = -30$ cm

then $\frac{1}{f_1} = \frac{1}{v} - \frac{1}{u} \Rightarrow \frac{1}{10} = \frac{1}{v} + \frac{1}{30}$

$$\frac{1}{v} = \frac{1}{10} - \frac{1}{30} \Rightarrow v = \frac{30}{2} = 15 \text{ cm}$$

For the second condition, when concave lens is placed,

$$v' = (15 + 45) = 60 \text{ cm} \Rightarrow \frac{1}{F} = \frac{1}{v'} - \frac{1}{u}$$

(where, F = focal length of combination)

$$\therefore \quad \frac{1}{F} = \frac{1}{60} + \frac{1}{30} \Rightarrow F = \frac{60}{3} = 20 \text{ cm}$$

The magnitude of focal length of concave lens,

$$\frac{1}{F} = \frac{1}{f_1} + \frac{1}{f_2} \Rightarrow \frac{1}{20} = \frac{1}{10} + \frac{1}{f_2}$$

$\Rightarrow \quad f_2 = -20$ cm (negative sign for concave lens)

103. (*c*) Focal length of the combination

$$\frac{1}{f} = \frac{1}{f_1} + \frac{1}{f_2} \quad \text{...(i)}$$

We have, $\frac{1}{f_1} = (\mu_1 - 1)\left(\frac{1}{\infty} - \frac{1}{-R}\right) = \frac{(\mu_1 - 1)}{R}$

and $\frac{1}{f_2} = (\mu_2 - 1)\left(\frac{1}{-R} - \frac{1}{\infty}\right) = -\frac{(\mu_2 - 1)}{R}$

Putting these values of $\frac{1}{f_1}$ and $\frac{1}{f_2}$ in Eq. (i), we get

$$\frac{1}{f} = \frac{(\mu_1 - 1)}{R} - \frac{(\mu_2 - 1)}{R}$$

$$= \frac{[\mu_1 - 1 - \mu_2 + 1]}{R} = \frac{\mu_1 - \mu_2}{R}$$

$$f = \frac{R}{\mu_1 - \mu_2}$$

104. (*c*) We know about the thin prism, $\delta_m = (\mu - 1)A$

In given condition, $A_1(\mu_1 - 1) = A_2(\mu_2 - 1)$

Given, $\mu_1 = 1.4$, $\mu_2 = 1.6$ and $A_1 = 6°$

Now, $6(1.4 - 1) = A_2(1.6 - 1)$

$$A_2 = \frac{6 \times 0.4}{0.6} \Rightarrow A_2 = \frac{2.4}{0.6}$$

$$A_2 = 4°$$

Hence, the angle of the second prism is 4°.

105. (*c*) $\therefore$ Magnification, $m = \frac{v}{-u} = -3$

$$v = 3u = 30 \text{ cm}$$

Focal length of co-axial combination,

$$\frac{1}{f_1} + \frac{1}{f_2} = \frac{1}{v} - \frac{1}{u}$$

$$-\frac{1}{30} + \frac{1}{f_2} = \frac{1}{30} + \frac{1}{10} = \frac{4}{30}$$

$$\frac{1}{f_2} = \frac{4}{30} + \frac{1}{30}$$

$$\frac{1}{f_2} = \frac{4 + 1}{30} = \frac{5}{30}$$

$$f_2 = \frac{30}{5} = 6 \text{ cm}$$

Hence, lens A is convex lens.

106. (b) $|m| = \frac{f_o}{f_e}$

When f_e is halved, so $m' = \frac{2 \times f_o}{f_e} = 2m$

107. (c) The magnifying power of the telescope in normal adjustment,

$$m = \frac{f_o}{f_e} = \frac{100}{5} = 20$$

108. (c) The magnifying power (m) of a telescope, $m = -\frac{f_o}{f_e}$.

Now, if the focal length of the eyepiece (f_e) is doubled, then the new magnification would be equal to

$m' = -\frac{f_o}{2f_e} = \frac{m}{2}$.

109. (b) In an astronomical telescope, $L = f_o + f_e$

When tube length is decreased, then the image formed by the objective lens will lie between principal focus and optical centre of eye lens instead of lying at the focus of eye lens. Therefore, a virtual image will be formed at a finite distance from the eye lens.

110. (d) In this case, $|m| = \frac{f_o}{f_e} = 5$ ...(i)

and length of telescope $= f_o + f_e = 36$ ...(ii)

On solving Eqs. (i) and (ii), we get

$f_e = 6$ cm, $f_o = 30$ cm

111. (b) Magnification, $|M| = \frac{f_o}{f_e} = 10$ or $f_o = 10 f_e$

Given,

$$f_e + f_o = 1.1 \text{ m}$$
$$f_e + 10 f_e = 1.1 \times 100 \text{ cm}$$
$$11 f_e = 110$$
$$f_e = 10$$

Magnification at least distance of distinct vision,

$$M_D = \frac{f_o}{f_e}\left(1 + \frac{f_e}{D}\right) = 10\left(1 + \frac{10}{25}\right)$$
$$= 10\left(\frac{35}{25}\right) = 14$$

112. (d) Length of the telescope when final image is formed at least distance of distinct vision,

$$L = f_o + u_e = f_o + \frac{f_e D}{f_e + D}$$
$$= 50 + \frac{5 \times 25}{(5 + 25)} = \frac{325}{6} \text{ cm}$$

113. (a) Given, $f_o + f_e = 105$

$$f_o + \frac{f_o}{20} = 105$$

$\Rightarrow$ $f_o = 100$ cm

114. (c) Magnifying power, $m_\infty = \frac{(L_\infty - f_o - f_e) \cdot D}{f_o f_e}$

$\Rightarrow$ $45 = \frac{(L_\infty - 1 - 5) \times 25}{1 \times 5}$

$\Rightarrow$ The length of the tube, $L_\infty = 15$ cm

115. (c) For objective, $\frac{1}{v_o} - \frac{1}{-200} = \frac{1}{50}$

$\therefore$ $v_o = \frac{200}{3}$ cm

For eyepiece, $\frac{1}{-25} - \frac{1}{(-u_e)} = \frac{1}{5}$

$\therefore$ $u_e = \frac{25}{6}$

Therefore, separation between objective and eye-piece,

$$L = v_o + u_e = \frac{200}{3} + \frac{25}{6} = \frac{425}{6} = 71 \text{ cm}$$

116. (d) For terrestrial telescope, magnification,

$$M = \frac{f_o}{f_e} = \frac{80}{f_e} = 20$$

$\Rightarrow$ $f_e = 4$ cm

Hence, length of terrestrial telescope

$$= f_o + f_e + 4f$$
$$= 80 + 4 + 4 \times 20$$
$$= 164 \text{ cm}$$

117. (c) We assume that, final image is formed at infinity and

$$M_\infty = \frac{(L_\infty - f_o - f_e) \cdot D}{f_o f_e} = \frac{LD}{f_o f_e}$$

or $400 = \frac{20 \times 25}{0.5 \times f_e}$

$\therefore$ $f_e = 2.5$ cm

118. (a) For objective lens, $\frac{1}{f_o} = \frac{1}{v_o} - \frac{1}{u_o}$

Using proper sign convention,

$$\frac{1}{+2.5} = \frac{1}{v_o} - \frac{1}{(-3.75)}$$

$\Rightarrow$ $v_o = 7.5$ cm

For eye lens, $\frac{1}{f_e} = \frac{1}{v_e} - \frac{1}{u_e}$

$$\frac{1}{+5} = \frac{1}{(-25)} - \frac{1}{u_e}$$

$\Rightarrow$ $u_e = -4.16$ cm or $|u_e| = 4.16$ cm

$\therefore$ Distance between the two lens $= 7.5 + 4.16$
$= 11.67$ cm

Assertion and Reason

1. (*b*) Glass slab will shift the object towards mirror. If it comes between pole and focus, the image will become virtual.

2. (*c*) For total internal reflection, the angle of incidence should be greater than the critical angle. As critical angle is 45°. Therefore, total internal reflection is not possible.

3. (*d*) In total internal reflection, 100% of incident light is reflected back into the same medium and there is no loss of intensity, while in reflection from mirrors and refraction from lenses, there is always same loss of intensity. Therefore, images formed by total internal reflection are much brighter than those formed by mirrors or lenses.

4. (*d*) When a diverging lens is immersed in a liquid, then its diverging power will either decrease or it will become converging.

5. (*d*) As, $\frac{1}{f_1} = (\mu - 1)\left(\frac{1}{R} - \frac{1}{R}\right) = 0$

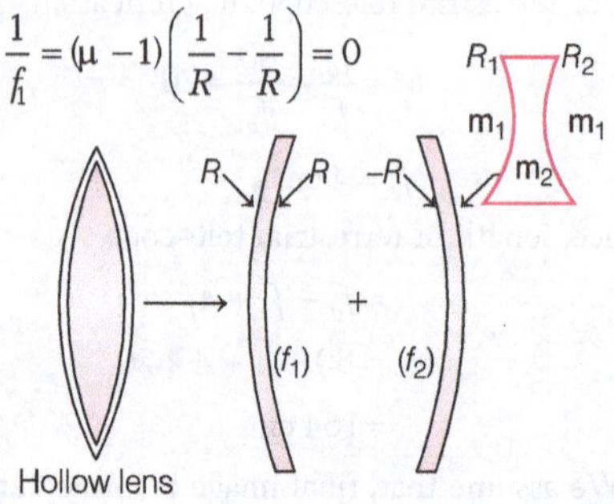

$$\therefore \quad P_1 = 0$$

$$\frac{1}{f_2} = (\mu - 1)\left(\frac{1}{-R} - \frac{1}{(-R)}\right) = 0$$

$$\therefore \quad P_2 = 0$$

Statement Type Questions

1. (*d*) Both Statement I and Statement II are correct.

From figure, Statement I is correct.

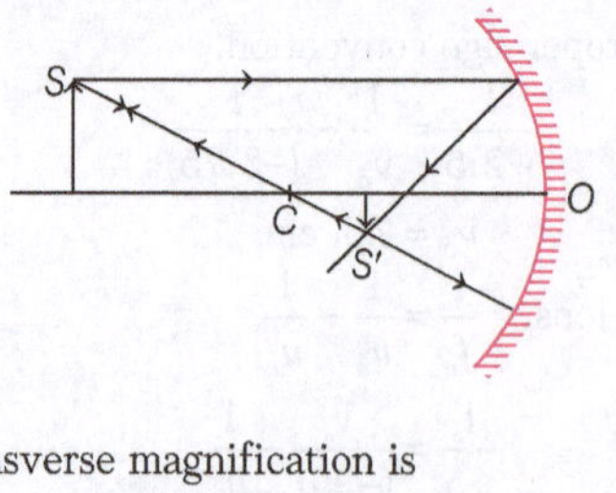

The transverse magnification is

$$m = \frac{\text{Image size}}{\text{Object size}} = \frac{-h_2}{h_1} \quad (\textit{i.e.}\text{ negative})$$

Hence, Statement I and Statement II are correct.

2. (*d*) Both Statement I and Statement II are correct.

Refractive surface formula is derived only for paraxial rays.

3. (*d*) Both Statement I and Statement II are correct.

For virtual object

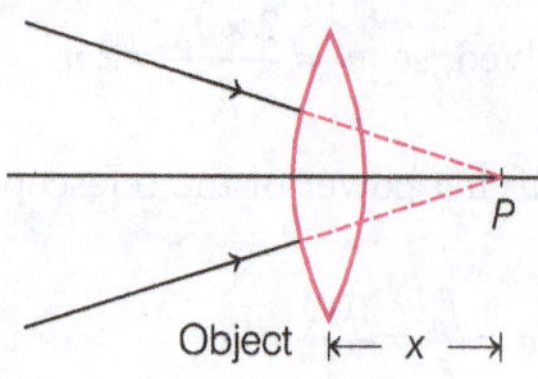

$$u = +x, F = +f$$

$$\because \quad \frac{1}{v} - \frac{1}{u} = \frac{1}{F}$$

$$\text{or} \quad \frac{1}{v} - \frac{1}{x} = \frac{1}{f}$$

$$\text{or} \quad \frac{1}{v} = \frac{1}{f} + \frac{1}{x}$$

$\therefore$ $v > 0$, it means image is real.

4. (*d*) Both Statement I and Statement II are correct.

$$\frac{1}{f} = \left(\frac{\mu_2}{\mu_1} - 1\right)\left(\frac{1}{R_1} - \frac{1}{R_2}\right)$$

$$= \left(\frac{\mu_2}{\mu_1} - 1\right)\left(-\frac{1}{R_1} - \frac{1}{R_2}\right)$$

Here, $\mu_2 < \mu_1$, the value of f is positive. Hence, lens behaves as converging lens.

5. (*d*) Both Statement I and Statement II are correct.

$\because$ $\delta = \left(\frac{\mu}{\mu_s} - 1\right)A$, Thus, the deviation decreases.

So, Statement I is correct. For thin prism the deviation is $\delta = (\mu - 1)A$. Thus the deviation produced by thin prism is independent of angle of incidence. Hence, Statement II is correct.

Match the Columns

1. (*a*) A. The lens Maker's formula is given by

$$\frac{1}{f} = (\mu - 1)\left(\frac{1}{R_1} - \frac{1}{R_2}\right)$$

B. At a convex surface, light rays travelling from a rarer medium to denser medium bend towards the normal, converging to a point. This makes convex lenses focus light to form real images.

C. At a concave surface, light rays travelling from a rarer to a denser medium bend towards the normal, diverging outward. This makes concave lenses spread out light rays, creating virtual images.

D. The critical angle is the angle of incidence in a denser medium beyond which light undergoes total internal reflection.

$$\left[\sin i_c = \frac{\mu_2}{\mu_1}\right]$$

Hence, A-(IV), B-(III), C-(II), D-(I).

2. (c) (A) $\mu_{eq} = \dfrac{\int_0^1 dy}{\int_0^1 \dfrac{dy}{\mu}} = \dfrac{[y]_0^1}{\int_0^1 \dfrac{dy}{1+\dfrac{y}{a}}} = \dfrac{1}{\ln 2}$ $(\because a = 1\,\text{m}^{-1})$

$= \dfrac{1}{0.693} = 1.44$

(B) Apparent depth $= \int \dfrac{dy}{\mu} = \int \dfrac{dy}{1+\dfrac{y}{a}} = \int_0^1 \dfrac{dy}{1+y}$ $(\because a = 1)$

$= [\ln(1+y)]_0^1 = \ln 2 = 0.693\ \text{m}$

(C) Optical path $= \int \mu\, dy = \int_0^1 \left(1+\dfrac{y}{a}\right) dy$

$= \int_0^1 (1+y)\, dy$ $(\because a = 1)$

$= \left[y + \dfrac{y^2}{2}\right]_0^1 = \dfrac{3}{2}\ \text{m} = 1.5\ \text{m}$

(D) Time $= \dfrac{\text{Optical path}}{3\times 10^8} = 5\times 10^{-9}\ \text{s}$

Hence, A-(IV), B-(II), C-(III), D-(I).

3. (b)

(A) $\because$ $P = P_1 + P_2$

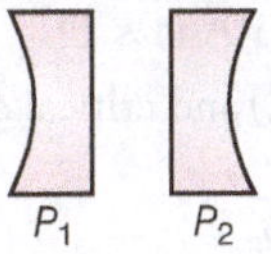

or $-\dfrac{1}{20} = 2P_1$

$\because$ $P_1 = -\dfrac{1}{40}$

(B) $\because$ $\dfrac{1}{f} = (\mu_2 - \mu_1)\left(\dfrac{1}{r_1} - \dfrac{1}{r_2}\right) = -\dfrac{1}{2.0}$

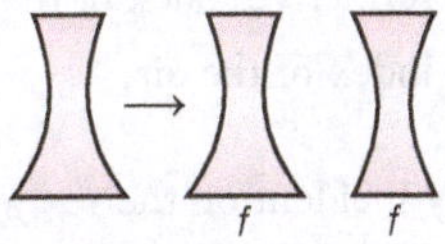

(C) $\because$ $\dfrac{1}{F} = \left(\dfrac{\mu_2}{\mu_1} - 1\right)\left(\dfrac{1}{r_1} - \dfrac{1}{r_2}\right) = 0$ $(\because \mu_2 = \mu_1)$

$\therefore$ $F = \infty$, So it acts as slab.

(D) $\dfrac{1}{F} = \left(\dfrac{\mu_2}{\mu_1} - 1\right)\left(\dfrac{1}{r_1} - \dfrac{1}{r_2}\right) > 0$

$\therefore$ It behaves as converging lens.

Hence, A-(II), B-(III), C-(I), D-(IV).

4. (d) (A) The focal length of objective is lesser than that of eyepiece.

$\therefore$ The focal length of objective = 2 cm

(B) Image due to objective should be at the focal plane of eyepiece.

$\therefore$ $v_o = 15 - 10 = 5\ \text{cm},\ f_o = 2\ \text{cm}$

$\dfrac{1}{v_o} - \dfrac{1}{u_o} = \dfrac{1}{f_o}$ or $\dfrac{1}{5} - \dfrac{1}{u_o} = \dfrac{1}{2}$

or $\dfrac{1}{u_o} = \dfrac{1}{5} - \dfrac{1}{2} = \dfrac{2-5}{10}$

$\therefore$ $u_o = -\dfrac{10}{3}\ \text{cm}$

(C) $m = \dfrac{v_o}{u_o}\dfrac{D}{f_e} = \dfrac{5}{\dfrac{-10}{3}} \times \dfrac{25}{10}$

$= -\dfrac{375}{100} = -3.75$

(D) For clear vision, $m = \dfrac{v_o}{u_o}\left(1 + \dfrac{D}{f_e}\right)$

Here, for eyepiece, $f_e = 10\ \text{cm}$, $v_e = -25\ \text{cm}$

$\therefore$ $\dfrac{1}{-25} - \dfrac{1}{u_e} = \dfrac{1}{10}$

or $-\dfrac{1}{10} - \dfrac{1}{25} = \dfrac{1}{u_e}$

or $\dfrac{-5-2}{50} = \dfrac{1}{u_e}$

$\therefore$ $u_e = \dfrac{-50}{7}$.

For objective, $v_o = 15 - \dfrac{50}{7} = \dfrac{25}{7}$

$\therefore$ $\dfrac{1}{v_o} - \dfrac{1}{u_o} = \dfrac{1}{2}$

or $1 - \dfrac{v_o}{u_o} = \dfrac{v_o}{2} = \dfrac{25}{14}$

$\therefore$ $\dfrac{v_o}{u_o} = 1 - \dfrac{25}{14} = -\dfrac{11}{14}$

$\therefore$ $m = -\dfrac{11}{14}\left(1 + \dfrac{25}{10}\right) = -\dfrac{11}{14} \times 3.5$

$= -\dfrac{11 \times 0.5}{2} = -\dfrac{11}{4}$.

Hence, A-(IV), B-(III), C-(II), D-(I).

Final Check Through PYQs

1. (a) Object distance, $u = -1.5f$

By mirror formula, $\dfrac{1}{v} + \dfrac{1}{u} = \dfrac{1}{f}$

$\Rightarrow$ $\dfrac{1}{v} + \dfrac{1}{-1.5f} = \dfrac{1}{-f}$

$\Rightarrow$ $\dfrac{1}{v} = -\dfrac{1}{f} + \dfrac{1}{1.5f} = \dfrac{1}{f}\left[-1 + \dfrac{1}{1.5}\right]$

$$= \frac{1}{f}\left[-1 + \frac{2}{3}\right]$$

$$\Rightarrow \quad \frac{1}{v} = \frac{1}{f}\left(-\frac{1}{3}\right) \Rightarrow v = -3f$$

2. (*b*) **Case I** When the object distance,

$u_1 = -40$ cm

Focal length of mirror, $f = -15$ cm

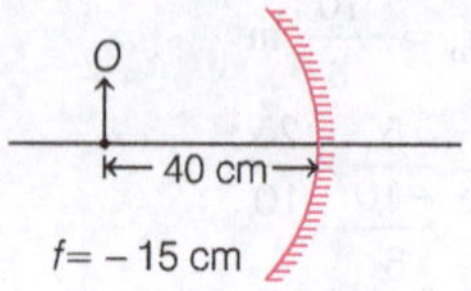

Using the mirror formula, we get

$$\frac{1}{f} = \frac{1}{v_1} + \frac{1}{u_1}$$

Substituting the given values, we get

$$-\frac{1}{15} = \frac{1}{v_1} + \left(\frac{-1}{40}\right)$$

$$\Rightarrow \quad \frac{1}{v_1} = \frac{1}{40} - \frac{1}{15} = \frac{3-8}{120} = \frac{-5}{120}$$

$$\Rightarrow \quad v_1 = \frac{-120}{5} = -24 \text{ cm}$$

Case II When the object distance,

$u_2 = 20$ cm

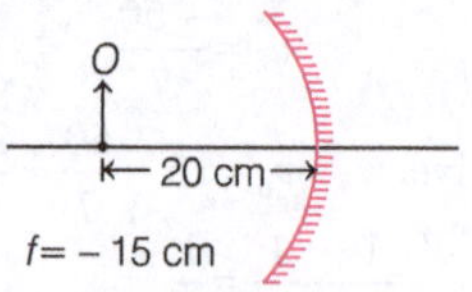

Using the mirror formula, we get

$$\frac{1}{f} = \frac{1}{v_2} + \frac{1}{u_2}$$

Substituting the given values, we get

$$-\frac{1}{15} = \frac{1}{v_2} + \left(-\frac{1}{20}\right)$$

$$\Rightarrow \quad \frac{1}{v_2} = \frac{1}{20} - \frac{1}{15} = \frac{3-4}{60} = \frac{-1}{60}$$

$$\Rightarrow \quad v_2 = -60 \text{ cm}$$

$\therefore$ The displacement of the image is

$$= v_2 - v_1$$
$$= -60 - (-24) = -60 + 24$$
$$= -36 \text{ cm} = 36 \text{ cm}$$

away from the mirror.

3. (*a*) According to the question

L = Light source

When the light beam is incident normally on the plane mirror, it is reflected back to the point from which it was coming. When the plane mirror is rotated by an angle θ, the reflected ray or beam of light must rotate by angle 2θ.

$$\tan 2\theta = y/x$$
$$2\theta = y/x$$
$$\theta = y/2x$$

4. (*d*) A concave mirror forms real and virtual images, whose magnification can be negative or positive depending upon the position of the object.

If object is placed between focus and pole the image obtained will be virtual and its magnification will be positive. In all other cases concave mirror forms real images whose magnification will be negative.

A convex mirror always forms a virtual image whose magnification will always be positive and magnitude less than 1. Hence, D $\rightarrow$ I and IV.

5. (*c*) According to given situation, $c = \frac{x}{t_1}$ and $v = \frac{10x}{t_2}$

$$\text{Since, } \sin i_c = \frac{1}{\mu} = \frac{1}{(c/v)} = \frac{v}{c} = \frac{\frac{10x}{t_2}}{\frac{x}{t_1}} = \frac{10t_1}{t_2}$$

$$\Rightarrow \quad i_c = \sin^{-1}\left(\frac{10t_1}{t_2}\right)$$

6. (*a*) Given, $v_A = 1.5 \times 10^8$ m/s

$v_B = 2 \times 10^8$ m/s

Refractive index (μ) and critical angle (i_c) are related as

$$\mu = \frac{1}{\sin i_c}$$

$$\Rightarrow \quad \sin i_c = \frac{1}{\mu} = \frac{1}{(v_B / v_A)} \qquad \left[\because \mu = \frac{v_B}{v_A}\right]$$

$$= \frac{v_A}{v_B} = \frac{1.5 \times 10^8}{2 \times 10^8} = 0.750$$

$$\Rightarrow \quad i_c = \sin^{-1}(0\cdot750)$$

7. (*a*) Given, the refractive index of the glass, $n_2 = \sqrt{3}$

The refractive index of the air,

$n_1 = 1$

The path of ray incident on the prism is as shown below

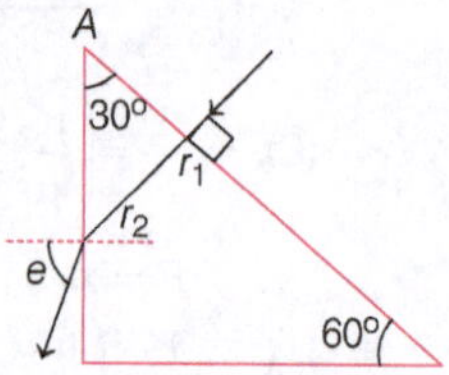

From the given figure, $r_1 = 0°$

As, $\quad A = r_1 + r_2$

where, A is the angle of prism.

$$30° = 0° + r_2$$

$$\Rightarrow \quad r_2 = 30°$$

Using the Snell's law, in glass and air interference,

$$n_2 \sin\theta_2 = n_1 \sin\theta_1$$

$$\Rightarrow \quad n_2 \sin r_2 = n_1 \sin e$$

$$\Rightarrow \sqrt{3} \sin 30° = 1 \times \sin e$$

$$\Rightarrow \quad \sin e = \frac{\sqrt{3}}{2}$$

$$\Rightarrow \quad \sin e = \sin 60° \Rightarrow e = 60°$$

8. (*b*) Critical angle, $i_C = 45°$

We know that, $\mu = \frac{1}{\sin i_C} = \frac{1}{\sin 45°} = \frac{1}{1/\sqrt{2}} = \sqrt{2}$

$\Rightarrow \quad \mu = \sqrt{2}$

$\Rightarrow \quad \frac{\text{Velocity of light in air}}{\text{Velocity of light in medium}} = \sqrt{2}$

$\Rightarrow \quad \frac{3 \times 10^8}{v_m} = \sqrt{2}$

$\Rightarrow \quad v_m = \frac{3}{\sqrt{2}} \times 10^8 \text{ m/s}$

9. (*c*) The total internal reflection is the phenomenon of reflection back of light in the denser medium when it travel from denser to rarer medium, when the angle of incidence is greater than the critical angle.

While the critical angle for a pair of given media in contact is the angle of incidence in denser medium for which the angle of refraction in rarer medium is 90°.

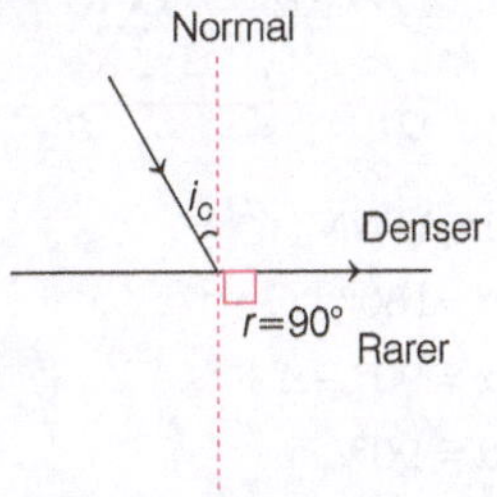

10. (*c*) Let thickness of the given slab is t. According to the question, when viewed from both the surfaces

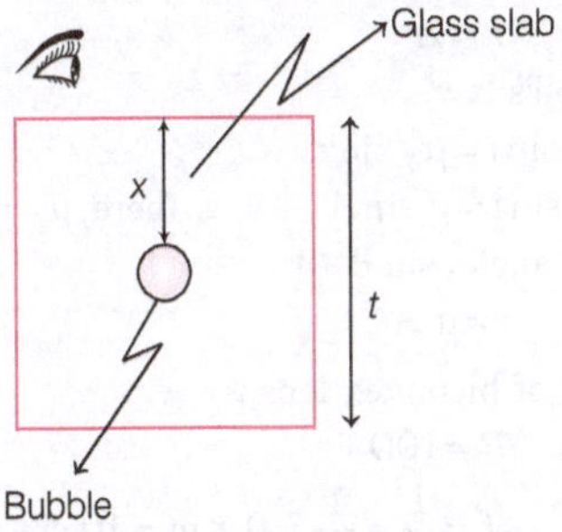

$$\frac{x}{\mu} + \frac{t-x}{\mu} = 3 + 5 \Rightarrow \frac{t}{\mu} = 8 \text{ cm}$$

$$\Rightarrow \quad t = 8 \times \mu \Rightarrow t = 8 \times \frac{3}{2} = 12 \text{ cm}$$

11. (*b*) Given, the rays in the prism is parallel to base

$$A = r_1 + r_2$$

i.e., $\quad r_2 = 90 - r_1 \quad$ ...(i)

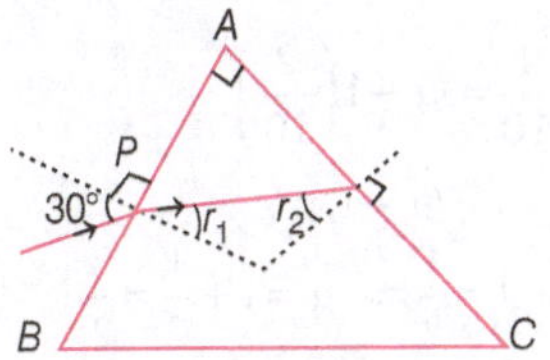

For AB interface,

$$\sin 30° = \mu \sin r_1$$

$\Rightarrow \quad \sin r_1 = \frac{1}{2\mu} \quad$ ...(ii)

For AC interface,

$$\mu \sin r_2 = 1 \sin 90°$$

$\Rightarrow \quad \sin r_2 = \frac{1}{\mu}$

$\Rightarrow \quad \sin (90 - r_1) = \frac{1}{\mu} \quad$ [from Eq. (i)]

$\quad \cos r_1 = \frac{1}{\mu} \quad$ ...(iii)

We know that, $\sin^2 \theta + \cos^2 \theta = 1$

From Eqs. (ii) and (iii), we get

$$\sin^2 r_1 + \cos^2 r_1 = 1$$

$\Rightarrow \quad \left(\frac{1}{2\mu}\right)^2 + \left(\frac{1}{\mu}\right)^2 = 1$

$\Rightarrow \quad \frac{1}{4\mu^2} + \frac{1}{\mu^2} = 1$

$\Rightarrow \quad \frac{1}{\mu^2}\left(\frac{1}{4} + \frac{1}{1}\right) = 1 \Rightarrow \mu^2 = \frac{5}{4} \Rightarrow \mu = \frac{\sqrt{5}}{2}$

12. (*c*) Focal length of convex lens,

$$f_1 = + f$$

Focal length of concave lens,

$$f_2 = - f$$

When both lenses are kept in contact, then equivalent focal length (F) is given by

$$\frac{1}{F} = \frac{1}{f_1} + \frac{1}{f_2} = \frac{1}{f} + \frac{1}{-f} = 0$$

$\Rightarrow \quad F = \infty$

13. (*b*) The given situation is shown below.

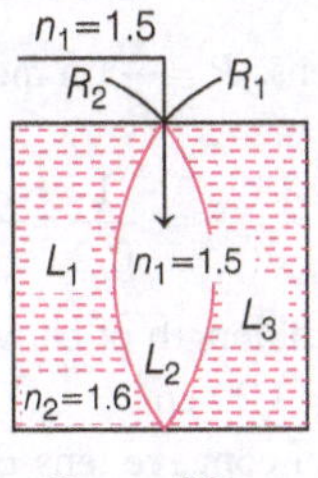

$\therefore \quad R_1 = 20$ cm, $R_2 = -20$ cm

Lens L_1 and L_3 are plano concave lens.

Focal length of lens L_1 is given as

$$\frac{1}{f_1} = (n_2 - 1)\left(\frac{1}{\infty} - \frac{1}{R_1}\right)$$

$$= (1.6 - 1)\left(-\frac{1}{20}\right) = -\frac{3}{100}$$

$\Rightarrow \quad \frac{1}{f_1} = \frac{-150}{3}$ cm

Similarly, focal length of lens L_3,

$$\frac{1}{f_3} = \frac{-100}{3}\text{ cm}$$

Now, focal length of convex lens L_2 is given as

$$\frac{1}{f_2} = (n_1 - 1)\left(\frac{1}{R_1} - \frac{1}{R_2}\right)$$

$$= (1.5-1)\left(\frac{1}{20} - \frac{1}{-20}\right) = \frac{1}{20}$$

$$\Rightarrow \quad \frac{1}{f_2} = 20\text{ cm}$$

If F be the focal length of combination, then

$$\frac{1}{F} = \frac{1}{f_1} + \frac{1}{f_2} + \frac{1}{f_3}$$

$$= \frac{-3}{100} + \frac{1}{20} + \frac{3}{100}$$

$$= \frac{-3+5-3}{100} = \frac{-1}{100}$$

$$\therefore \quad F = -100\text{ cm}$$

14. (*b*) For a biconvex lens,

$$R_1 = +20\text{ cm}$$
$$R_2 = -\ 20\text{cm}$$

and $\mu = 1.5$

By using lens Maker's formula, we have,

$$\frac{1}{f} = (\mu - 1)\left(\frac{1}{R_1} - \frac{1}{R_2}\right)$$

$$= (1.5-1)\left(\frac{1}{20} - \frac{1}{-20}\right)$$

$$= 0.5\left(\frac{2}{20}\right)$$

$$\Rightarrow \quad \frac{1}{f} = 0.5 \times \frac{1}{10} \Rightarrow f = \frac{10}{0.5}$$

$$\Rightarrow \quad f = 20\text{ cm} = 0.2\text{ m}$$

$\therefore$ Power of the lens, $P = \frac{1}{f}$ (in metre)

$$= \frac{1}{0.2} = +5\text{ D}$$

15. (*b*) Given, the focal length of convex lens A,

$$f_1 = +20\text{ cm}$$

The focal length of concave lens B,

$$f_2 = -\ 5\text{ cm}$$

The convex lens is the converging lens and the concave lens is the diverging lens.

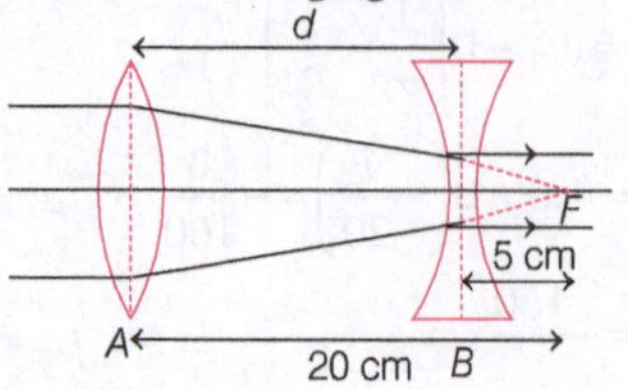

When the parallel beam of light passes through the convex lens, it converges at the focal point F and the distance between lens A to F point is 20 cm.

Now, after emerging from the lens B, the beam is still parallel in nature. So, the net focal length of the lens A and B will be infinite.

As we know, $\frac{1}{f} = \frac{1}{f_1} + \frac{1}{f} - \frac{d}{f_1 f_2}$

$$\Rightarrow \quad \frac{1}{\infty} = \frac{1}{20} - \frac{1}{5} + \frac{d}{20 \times 5}$$

$$\Rightarrow \quad \frac{3}{20} = \frac{d}{20 \times 5}$$

or $\quad d = 3 \times 5 = 15$ cm

16. (*b*) According to the question, the ray diagram can be shown as

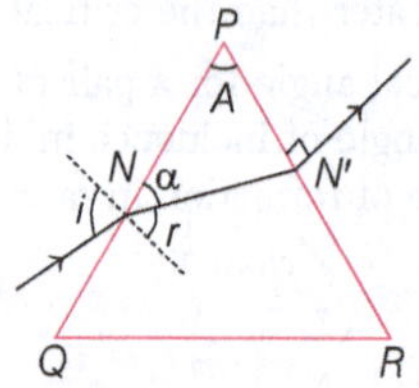

From figure in $\Delta PNN'$,

$$A + \alpha + 90° = 180°$$

$$\Rightarrow \quad \alpha = 90° - A \quad \text{...(i)}$$

Also, $\quad r + \alpha = 90°$

$$\Rightarrow \quad r = 90° - \alpha$$

$$= 90° - (90° - A) = A \quad [\because \text{ from Eq. (i)}]$$

$$\Rightarrow \quad r = A$$

From Snell's law,

$$\mu_1 \sin i = \mu_2 \sin r$$

$$\Rightarrow \quad \sin i = \mu \sin A \quad (\text{here, } \mu_1 = 1 \text{ and } \mu_2 = \mu)$$

For small angle, $\sin\theta \simeq \theta$

$$\Rightarrow \quad i = \mu A$$

17. (*d*) Power of biconvex lens,

$$P = 10\text{D}$$

$$\therefore \quad f = \frac{1}{P} = \frac{1}{10} = 0.1\text{ m} = 10\text{ cm}$$

$$R_1 = R_2 = 10\text{ cm}$$

By Lens Maker's formula,

$$\frac{1}{f} = (\mu - 1)\left(\frac{1}{R_1} - \frac{1}{R_2}\right)$$

$$\Rightarrow \quad \frac{1}{10} = (\mu - 1)\left(\frac{1}{10} - \frac{1}{-10}\right)$$

$$\Rightarrow \quad \frac{1}{10} = (\mu - 1)\left(\frac{2}{10}\right)$$

$$\Rightarrow \quad 1 = (\mu - 1) \times 2$$

$$\Rightarrow \quad \mu - 1 = \frac{1}{2} \Rightarrow \mu = 1 + \frac{1}{2} = \frac{3}{2}$$

18. (*d*) When the lens is cut along its principal axis, the focal length of the two halves will remain same because the radius of curvature of both the surfaces are still same. So, the power also remains same as

$$P = \frac{1}{f}$$

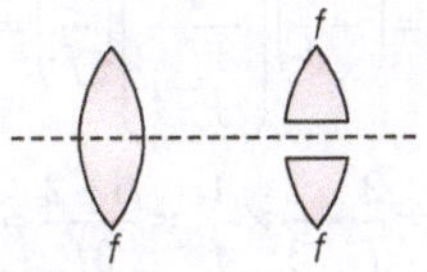

19. (*c*) Using the lens Maker's formula

$$\frac{1}{f} = \left(\frac{\mu_2 - \mu_1}{\mu_1}\right)\left(\frac{1}{R_1} - \frac{1}{R_2}\right)$$

Here, $f = 25$ cm, $\mu_2 = 1.5, \mu_1 = 1$ (for air)

let $R_1 = R$ and $R_2 = -2R$

$$\Rightarrow \quad \frac{1}{25} = \left(\frac{1.5-1}{1}\right)\left[\frac{1}{R} - \left(-\frac{1}{2R}\right)\right]$$

$$\frac{1}{25 \times 0.5} = \frac{1}{R} + \frac{1}{2R}$$

$$\Rightarrow \quad R = \frac{3}{2} \times 25 \times 0.5 = 18.75 \text{ cm}$$

$$\therefore \quad R_1 = 18.75 \text{ cm}$$

$$R_2 = 2 \times 18.75 = 37.5 \text{ cm}$$

20. (*a*) **Case I** When two equi-convex lens of focal length f_1 and f_2 respectively, are kept co-axially in contact, then the equivalent focal length of combination is

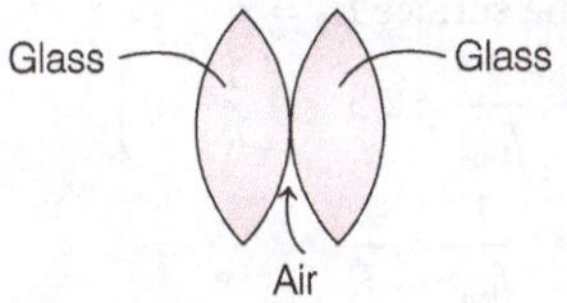

$$\frac{1}{F_1} = \frac{1}{f_1} + \frac{1}{f_2} = \frac{1}{f} + \frac{1}{f} \quad [\because \text{Here, } f_1 = f_2]$$

$$= \frac{2}{f}$$

$$\Rightarrow \quad F_1 = \frac{f}{2} \quad \text{...(i)}$$

Case II When glycerine of same refractive index as that of the glass is filled in the space between two lens, then the combination will now comprises of three lenses; first bi-convex, second bi-concave and third is bi-convex.

So, the focal length of the combination now is given as

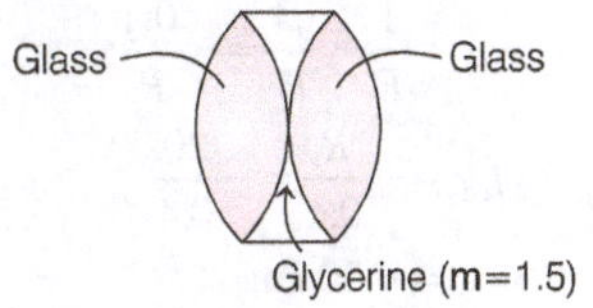

$$\frac{1}{F_2} = \frac{1}{f} + \frac{1}{(-f)} + \frac{1}{f} = \frac{1}{f}$$

$$\Rightarrow \quad F_2 = f \quad \text{... (ii)}$$

From Eqs. (i) and (ii), we get

$$F_1 : F_2 = 1 : 2$$

21. (*b*) According to the question, the figure of mentioned prism is given as

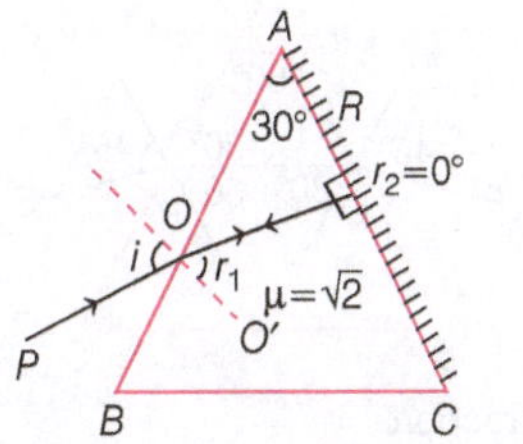

(since, there is no refraction at the face AC)

Given,

Refractive index of the material of prism, $\mu = \sqrt{2}$

Angle of prism, $A = 30°$

If the ray OR has to retrace its path after reflection (as per the given condition), then the ray has to fall normally on the surface AC.

This means $\angle ARO = \angle ORC = 90°$

In ΔAOR, $\angle AOR + \angle ARO + \angle OAR = 180°$

$$\Rightarrow \quad \angle AOR + 90° + 30° = 180°$$

$$\Rightarrow \quad \angle AOR = 180° - 120° = 60° \quad \text{...(i)}$$

As we know,

$$\angle AOR + \angle r_1 = 90°$$

$$\Rightarrow \quad \angle r_1 = 90° - 60° = 30° \quad \text{[From Eq. (i)]}$$

Applying Snell's law at the face AB, we get

$$\mu = \frac{\sin i}{\sin r_1}$$

Substituting the given values, we get

$$\sqrt{2} = \frac{\sin i}{\sin 30°}$$

$$\Rightarrow \quad \sin i = \sin 30° \times \sqrt{2} = \frac{1}{2} \times \sqrt{2} \quad \left(\because \sin 30° = \frac{1}{2}\right)$$

$$= \frac{1}{\sqrt{2}} \text{ or } i = \sin^{-1}\left(\frac{1}{\sqrt{2}}\right)$$

$$= 45° \quad \left(\because \sin 45° = \frac{1}{\sqrt{2}}\right)$$

22. (*b*) Let prism angle of the first and second prisms are A_1 and A_2 respectively.

Similarly, their refractive indices are μ_1 and μ_2.

Condition for dispersion without deviation is

$$\delta_1 - \delta_2 = 0$$

$$\Rightarrow \quad (\mu_1 - 1) A_1 - (\mu_2 - 1) A_2 = 0$$

$$\Rightarrow \quad A_2 = \left(\frac{\mu_1 - 1}{\mu_2 - 1}\right)$$

$$A_1 = \left(\frac{1.42 - 1}{1.7 - 1}\right)(10°)$$

$$\Rightarrow \quad A_2 = 6°$$

23. (*a*) The given situation is shown below.

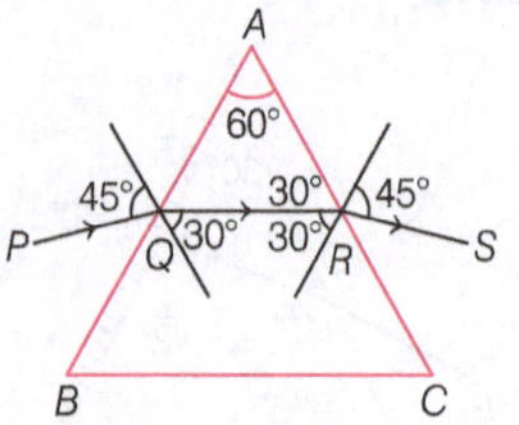

angle of refraction

$$r = r' = 30°$$

angle of emergence, $e = 45°$

Therefore, minimum deviation suffered by the ray is

$$\delta_{min} = i + e - (r + r')$$
$$= 90° - 60° = 30°$$

Also we know that

$$\mu = \frac{\sin\left(\frac{A + \delta_m}{2}\right)}{\sin \frac{A}{2}}$$

where, μ = refractive index of the material of the prism.

A = angle of prism = 60°

$$\therefore \quad \mu = \frac{\sin\left(\frac{60° + 30°}{2}\right)}{\sin \frac{60°}{2}} = \frac{\sin 45°}{\sin 30°}$$

$$= \frac{1/\sqrt{2}}{1/2} = \frac{2}{\sqrt{2}} = \sqrt{2}$$

24. (*d*) Consider the situation shown is figure. Let radius of curvature of lens surfaces is R. The combination is equivalent to three lenses in contact.

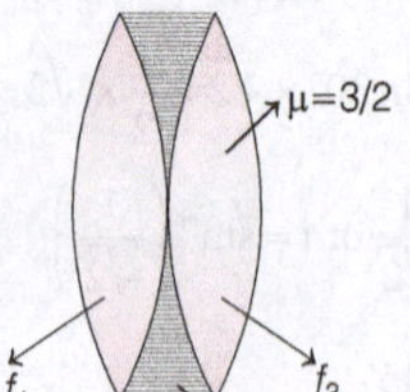

$$\therefore \quad \frac{1}{f_{eq}} = \frac{1}{f_1} + \frac{1}{f_2} + \frac{1}{f_3} = \frac{2}{f_1} + \frac{1}{f_2} \quad (\because f_1 = f_3)$$

Now $\quad \frac{1}{f_1} = \frac{1}{f_3} = (\mu - 1)\left(\frac{2}{R}\right) = \frac{1}{f}$

$$\frac{1}{f_2} = (\mu_w - 1)\left(-\frac{2}{R}\right)$$

$$= \left(\frac{4}{3} - 1\right)\left(\frac{-2}{R}\right)$$

$$= \left(\frac{1}{3}\right)\left(-\frac{2}{R}\right) = \left(\frac{-2}{3}\right)\left(\frac{1}{2(\mu - 1)}\right)$$

$$\Rightarrow \quad \frac{1}{f_2} = \left(-\frac{1}{3}\right)\left(\frac{1}{\frac{3}{2} - 1}\right)\left(\frac{1}{f}\right) = -\frac{2}{3} \times \frac{1}{f}$$

$$\therefore \quad \frac{1}{f_{eq}} = \frac{2}{f} - \frac{2}{3} \times \frac{1}{f} = \frac{6 - 2}{3f} = \frac{4}{3f}$$

$$\Rightarrow \quad f_{eq} = \frac{3f}{4}$$

25. (*c*) Given $\mu_g = 1.5$

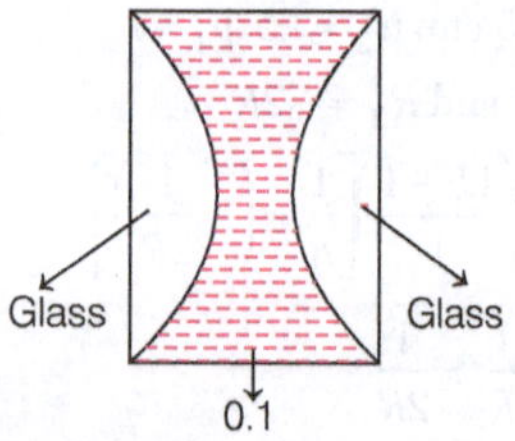

$$\mu_{oil} = 1.7$$

$$\Rightarrow \quad R = 20 \text{ cm}$$

From Lens Maker's formula for the plano convex lens

$$\frac{1}{f} = (\mu - 1)\left[\frac{1}{R_1} - \frac{1}{R_2}\right]$$

Here, $R_1 = R$

and for plane surface $R_2 = \infty$

$$\therefore \quad \frac{1}{f_{lens}} = (1.5 - 1)\left(\frac{1}{R} - 0\right)$$

$$\Rightarrow \quad \frac{1}{f_{lens}} = \frac{0.5}{R}$$

When the intervening medium is filled with oil, then focal length of the concave lens formed by the oil

$$\frac{1}{f_{concave}} = (1.7 - 1)\left(-\frac{1}{R} - \frac{1}{R}\right)$$

$$= -0.7 \times \frac{2}{R} = \frac{-1.4}{R}$$

Here, we have two concave surfaces

So, $\quad \frac{1}{f_{eq}} = 2 \times \frac{1}{f} + \frac{1}{f}$

$$= 2 \times \frac{0.5}{R} + \left(\frac{-1.4}{R}\right)$$

$$= \frac{1}{R} - \frac{1.4}{R} = -\frac{0.4}{R}$$

$$\therefore \quad f_{eq} = -\frac{R}{0.4} = -\frac{20}{0.4}$$

$$= -50 \text{ cm}$$

26. (*b*) As, we know that

$$\mu = \frac{\sin\left(\frac{A+D_m}{2}\right)}{\sin\frac{A}{2}}$$

$$\Rightarrow \quad \cot\frac{A}{2} = \frac{\sin\left(\frac{A+D_m}{2}\right)}{\sin\frac{A}{2}}$$

$$\Rightarrow \quad \frac{\cos\frac{A}{2}}{\sin\frac{A}{2}} = \frac{\sin\left(\frac{A+D_m}{2}\right)}{\sin\frac{A}{2}}$$

$$\sin\left(\frac{\pi}{2} - \frac{A}{2}\right) = \sin\left(\frac{A+D_m}{2}\right)$$

$$\Rightarrow \quad \frac{\pi}{2} - \frac{A}{2} = \frac{A}{2} + \frac{D_m}{2}$$

$$\Rightarrow \quad D_m = \pi - 2A$$

$$\Rightarrow \quad D_m = 180° - 2A$$

27. (*d*) For refractive index of a index,

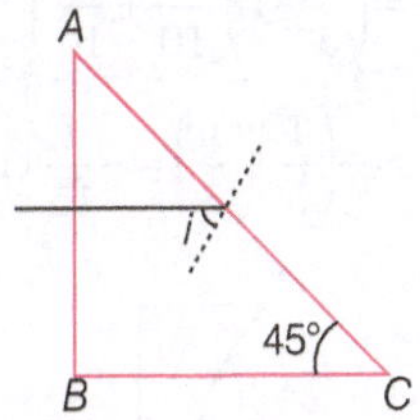

$$\mu = \frac{1}{\sin i_c} = \frac{1}{\sin 45°} = \sqrt{2}$$

As, $\mu_{red} = 1.39, \mu_{green} = 1.44$ and $\mu_{blue} = 1.47$

$\therefore (\mu_{red} = 1.39) < \mu, \mu_{green} > \mu, \mu_{blue} > \mu$

Thus, only red colour do not suffer total internal reflection.

28. (*b*) Given, focal length of objective, $f_o = 140$ cm

Focal length of eyepiece, $f_e = 5$ cm

Magnifying power, $m = \left[\frac{f_o}{f_e}\right]$

$$= \left[\frac{140}{5}\right] = 28$$

29. (*d*) The objective of an astronomical telescope has large focal length and large aperture. Because the lens used is a convex lens, the magnification of an astronomical telescope is directly proportional to the focal length of the objective lens.

This large aperture also contributes to the better quality and visibility of the images. Thus, it provides better resolution.

Due to large focal length of the objective, it covers large area which ensures better light gathering power.

Thus, all options (a), (b) and (c) are correct.

30. (*c*) According to question,

Focal length of objective lens, $(F_o) = +40$ cm

Focal length of eyepiece lens $(F_e) = 4$ cm

Object distance for objective lens $(u_o) = -200$ cm

Applying lens formula for objective lens

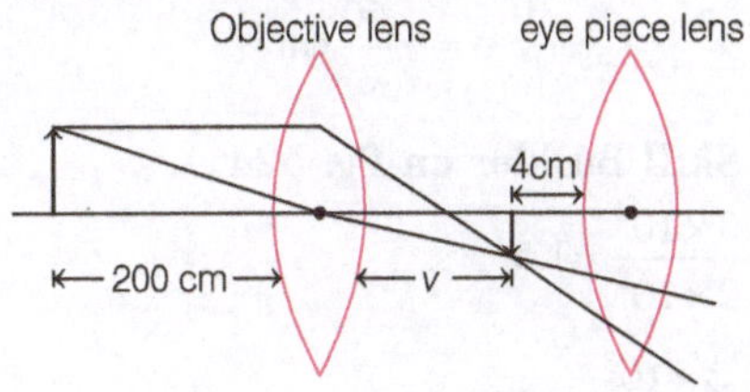

$$\frac{1}{v} - \frac{1}{u} = \frac{1}{f}$$

$$\Rightarrow \quad \frac{1}{v} - \frac{1}{-200} = \frac{1}{40}$$

$$\Rightarrow \quad \frac{1}{v} = \frac{1}{40} - \frac{1}{200} = \frac{5-1}{200} = \frac{4}{200}$$

$$\Rightarrow \quad v = 50 \text{ cm}$$

Image will be form at first focus of eyepiece lens.

So, for normal adjustment distance between objectives and eye piece lense (length of tube) will be

$$v + F_e \Rightarrow 50 + 4 \Rightarrow 54 \text{ cm}$$

31. (*d*)

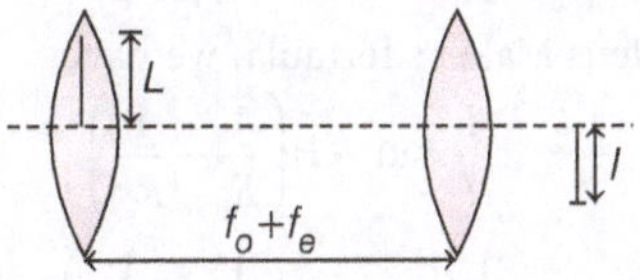

We know, magnification of telescope, we have

$$M = \frac{f_o}{f_e},$$

Here $\quad \frac{f_e}{f_e + u} = \frac{-I}{L}$

$$\Rightarrow \quad \frac{f_e}{f_e - (f_o + f_e)} = \frac{-I}{L} \Rightarrow \frac{f_e}{f_o} = \frac{I}{L}$$

i.e. $\quad M = \frac{L}{I}$

Skill Builder

■ Sol. of Skill Builder on Pg. 513

(*a*) Given, $u = -25$ cm

$\because \quad f = -10$ cm

Using mirror formula,

$$\frac{1}{f} = \frac{1}{v} + \frac{1}{u}$$

We have, $\frac{1}{-10} = \frac{1}{v} + \frac{1}{(-25)}$

$$\frac{-1}{10} = \frac{1}{v} - \frac{1}{25}$$

$$\Rightarrow \quad \frac{1}{v} = \frac{1}{25} - \frac{1}{10} = \frac{2-5}{50}$$

$$\frac{1}{v} = \frac{-3}{50}$$

$$v = -\frac{50}{3} \text{ cm}$$

■ Sol. of Skill Builder on Pg. 524

(*b*) $\mu_A = \frac{3 \times 10^8}{2 \times 10^8} = 1.5$

$$\mu_B = \frac{3 \times 10^8}{1.2 \times 10^8} = 2.5$$

For TIR, ray should travel from denser to rarer medium.

$$\mu_B \sin \theta_C = \mu_A \sin 90°$$

$$\sin \theta_C = \frac{\mu_A}{\mu_B} = \frac{1.5}{2.5} = \frac{3}{5}$$

$$\theta_C = \sin^{-1}\left(\frac{3}{5}\right)$$

$$\theta_C = 37°$$

■ Sol. of Skill Builder on Pg. 534

(*a*) Given, $R_1 = \infty$, $R_2 = -20$ cm, $f = 60$ cm

From lens Maker's formula, we have

$$\frac{1}{f} = (\mu - 1)\left(\frac{1}{R_1} - \frac{1}{R_2}\right)$$

$$\Rightarrow \quad \frac{1}{60} = (\mu - 1)\left(\frac{1}{\infty} - \frac{1}{-20}\right) = \frac{\mu - 1}{20}$$

$\therefore$ Refractive index, $\mu = 1 + \frac{1}{3} = \frac{4}{3}$.

■ Sol. of Skill Builder on Pg. 537

(*c*) Let focal length of both convex lenses is f.

Combination of two convex lenses with zero separation is given as

$$\frac{1}{F} = \frac{1}{f_1} + \frac{1}{f_2}$$

$$\frac{1}{F} = \frac{1}{f} + \frac{1}{f} \quad [\because f_1 = f_2 = f]$$

$$\frac{1}{F} = \frac{f + f}{f^2}$$

$$F = \frac{f^2}{2f}$$

$$F = \frac{f}{2}$$

$\therefore$ Equivalent focal length of combined lenses will be halved.

■ Sol. of Skill Builder on Pg. 537

(*b*) For lens 1,

$$\frac{1}{f_1} = \left(\frac{3}{2} - 1\right)\left(\frac{1}{\infty} - \frac{1}{10}\right) = -\frac{1}{20} \text{ cm}$$

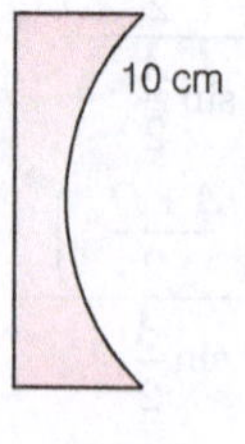

For lens 2,

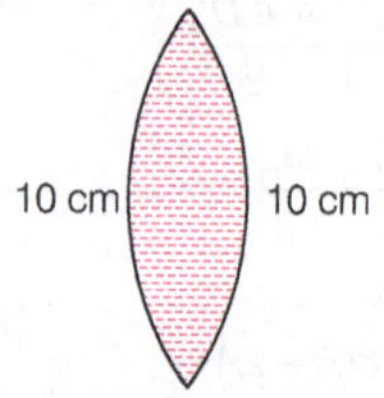

$$\frac{1}{f_2} = \left(\frac{2}{3} - 1\right)\left(\frac{1}{10} + \frac{1}{10}\right)$$

$$= -\left(\frac{1}{3}\right)\left(\frac{1}{5}\right) = -\frac{1}{15} \text{ cm}$$

For lens 3,

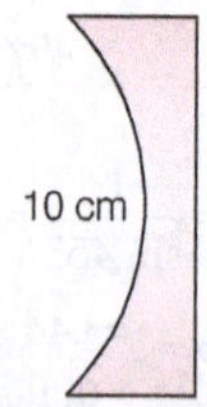

$$\frac{1}{f_3} = \left(\frac{3}{2} - 1\right)\left(\frac{1}{-10} - \frac{1}{\infty}\right) = \frac{-1}{20} \text{ cm}$$

$$\therefore \quad \frac{1}{F} = \frac{1}{f_1} + \frac{1}{f_2} + \frac{1}{f_3}$$

$$= \frac{-1}{20} - \frac{1}{15} - \frac{1}{20} = -\frac{1}{6} \text{ cm}$$

Hence, $F = -6$ cm

■ Sol. of Skill Builder on Pg. 545

(*b*) Given, $f_e = 10$ cm, $L_\infty = 1.0$ m $= 100$ cm

Since, $L_\infty = f_o + f_e$

$$\therefore \quad f_o = 100 - 10 = 90 \text{ cm}$$

Further, magnification $M_\infty = \frac{f_o}{f_e} = \frac{90}{10} = 9$

For deeper insight
Scan the QR Code

Chapter 11

Wave Optics

Learning Objectives

Module-I

- Huygens' Wave Theory of Light
- Wavefront
- Huygens' Principle of Secondary Wavelets
- Principle of Superposition of Waves
- Interference of Light Waves
- Coherent and Incoherent Sources

Module-II

- Young's Double Slit Experiment (YDSE)
- Distribution of Intensity

Module-III

- Diffraction of Light
- Fraunhofer Diffraction of Light due to a Single Slit
- Width of Central Maxima
- Polarisation of Light
- Malus' Law

Chapter Overview with NEET Connection

The study of wave optics is very important to learn and understand the wave nature of light. This chapter explains reflection and refraction on the basis of wave nature of light. Without having proper knowledge of this chapter, we cannot have a good hold on other chapter like Dual Nature of Matter and Radiation.

Special format questions can be easily framed on the following topics of this chapter

- Concept of interference and conditions of maxima and minima.
- Young's double slit experiment based numericals.
- Diffraction and numericals on Fraunhofer's diffraction.
- Polarisation and Brewster's law.

For better understanding of this chapter

- Basic idea about trigonometric functions is required.
- Connection between path difference, phase difference should be revisited from wave theory.
- Laboratory exposure of optics related experiments will be helpful.

Introduction

Phenomena of light such as reflection, refraction, dispersion can be easily explained using ray optics but there are certain other microscopic phenomena like interference, diffraction and polarisation which could not be explained by ray behaviour of light. For explanation of such concepts, wave nature of light was introduced. This study is explained under a new branch of physics named as Wave Optics.

In this chapter, we will study about Huygens' principle (which is the base of wave optics) and some interesting phenomenon of light : Interference, diffraction, polarisation.

Module 1

Huygens' Principle and Interference

• Huygens' Wave Theory of Light • Wavefront • Huygens' Principle of Secondary Wavelets
• Principle of Superposition of Waves • Interference of Light Waves • Coherent and Incoherent Sources

Huygens' Wave Theory of Light

In 1678, a Dutch scientist, Christian Huygens' propounded the wave theory of light. According to him,

(i) Light travels in the form of waves.
(ii) These waves travel in all the directions with the velocity of light.
(iii) The waves of light of different colours have different wavelengths.
(iv) Initially, the light waves were assumed to be longitudinal. But later on while explaining the phenomenon of polarisation, the light waves were considered to be transverse.
(v) The whole universe with all matter and space is filled with a luminiferous medium called **ether**, of very low density and very high elasticity.
(vi) Huygens' theory could explain reflection, refraction, interference, diffraction, polarisation but could not explain photoelectric effect and Compton's effect.
(vii) Wave theory introduced the concept of wavefront.

Wavefront

A wavefront is the locus of points (wavelets) having the same phase (a surface of constant phase) of oscillations. A wavelet is the point of disturbance due to propagation of light. A line perpendicular to a wavefront is called a **ray**.

Types of Wavefront

Depending on the shape of source of light, wavefronts can be of three types which are given below.

(i) Spherical wavefront

When light is emerging from a point source, wavefronts are spherical and concentric with point source at their centre as shown in figure by spheres 1, 2, 3 and 4. Rays are radial as shown by arrows.

In spherical wavefront, amplitude of light waves, $A \propto \frac{1}{r}$

and intensity of light waves, $I \propto \frac{1}{r^2}$.

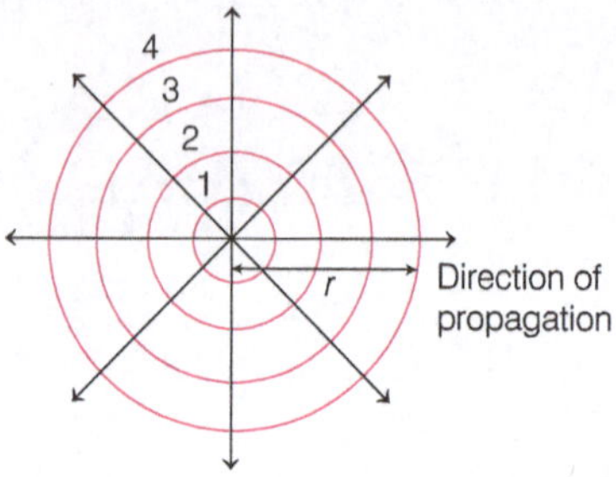

Spherical wavefront of a point source

(ii) Cylindrical wavefront

When the source of light is linear, *e.g.* a straight line source as shown in figure. All the points are equidistant from the source, therefore wavefronts 1, 2 and 3 are cylindrical and co-axial with the source as their common axis.

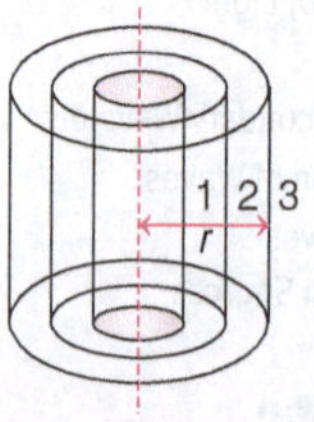

Cylindrical wavefront of a linear source

In this case, intensity of light waves, $I \propto \frac{1}{r}$

and amplitude of light waves, $A \propto \frac{1}{\sqrt{r}}$.

(iii) Plane wavefront

When light sources are emitting parallel rays or when the light is coming from a very far-off source, then wavefronts will be plane as shown in figure.

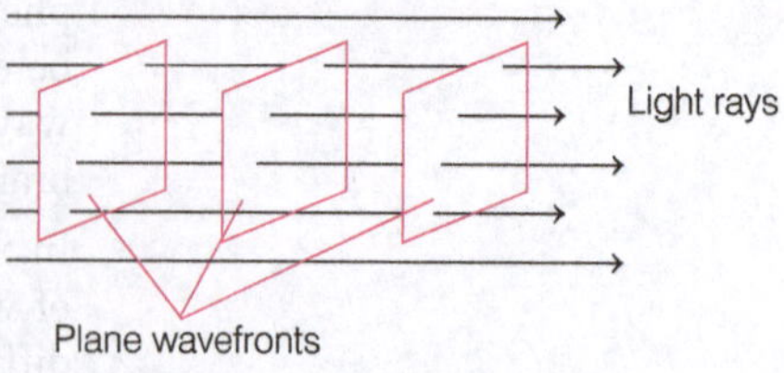

Plane wavefront of a distant source

In this case, intensity of light waves, $I \propto r^0$

and amplitude of light waves, $A \propto r^0$.

Mentor's TiP

Wavefronts parallel to *XY*-plane can be represented by z = constant. Similarly, wavefronts parallel to *YZ*-plane and *ZX*-plane are x = constant and y = constant, respectively.

Shapes of wavefronts of reflected and refracted waves

We have discussed the various types of wavefront. Keeping in mind those shapes, now we are going to see the shapes of wavefronts associated with reflected as well as refracted waves.

(i) Shapes of wavefronts before and after reflection from a plane and curved mirrors are as shown below.

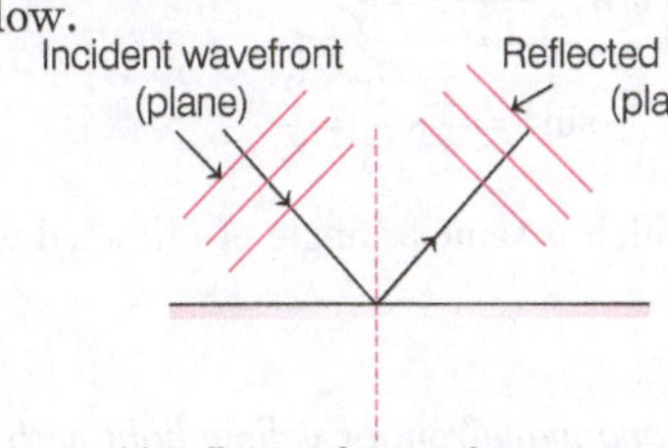

(a) Reflection from a plane mirror

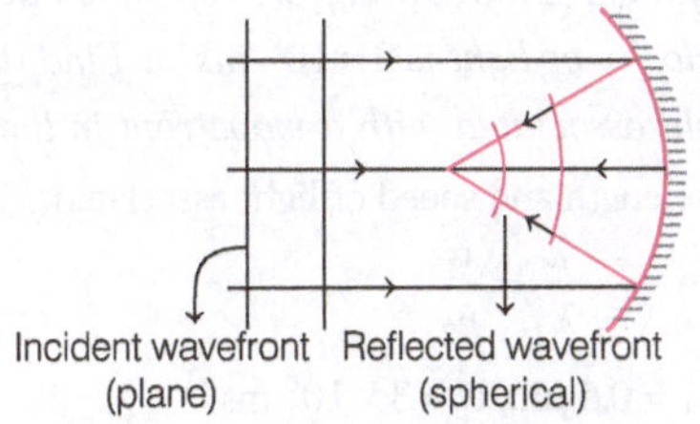

(b) Reflection from a concave mirror

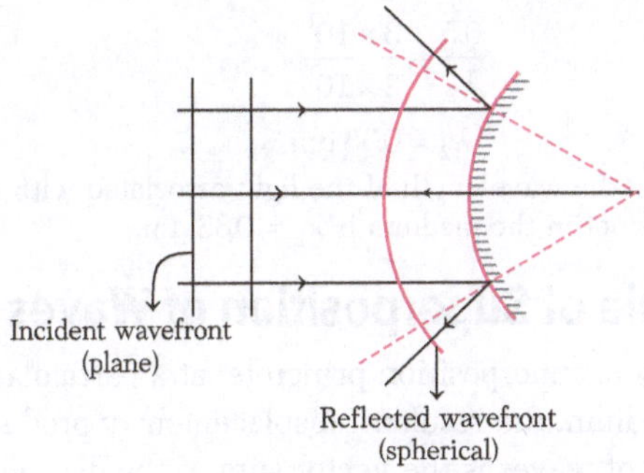

(c) Reflection from a convex mirror

Reflection from curved mirrors

(ii) Shapes of wavefronts before and after refraction from a plane and curved surfaces are as shown below.

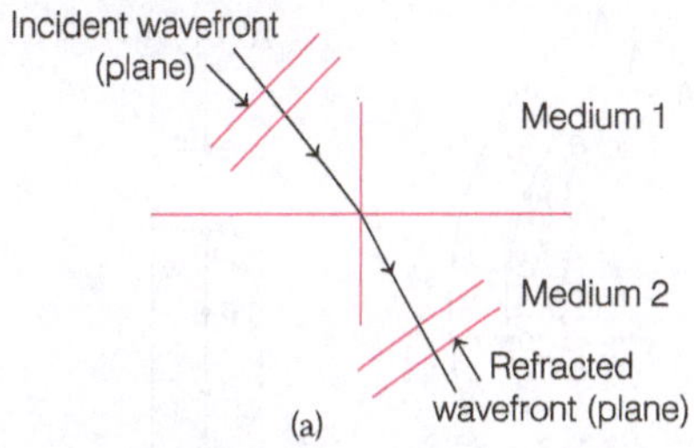

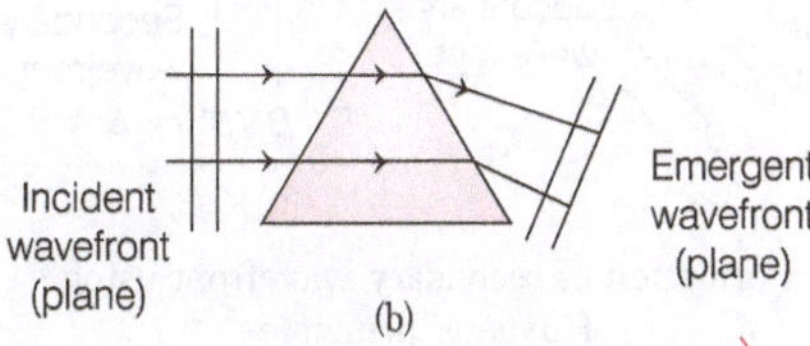

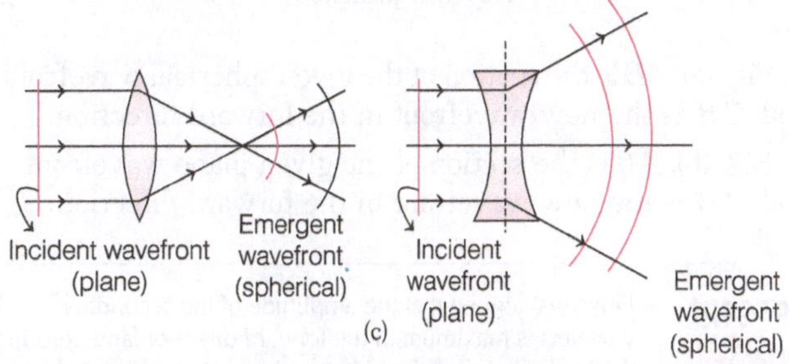

(a) Refraction from a plane surface
(b) Refraction from a prism
(c) Refraction through lenses

Huygens' Principle of Secondary Wavelets

In 1678, in order to explain the propagation of wave in a medium, Huygens' propounded a principle known as Huygens' principle of secondary wavelets by which at any instant, we can geometrically obtain the position of wavefront. He made following three assumptions.

(i) Every point on a given wavefront (called **primary wavefront**) can be regarded as fresh source of new disturbance and sends out its own spherical wavelets called **secondary wavelets.**

(ii) The secondary wavelets spread in all directions with the velocity of wave (*i.e.* velocity of light).

(iii) A surface touching these secondary wavelets, tangentially in the forward direction after an interval (Δt) gives the position and shape of the new wavefront. This is called **secondary wavefront.**

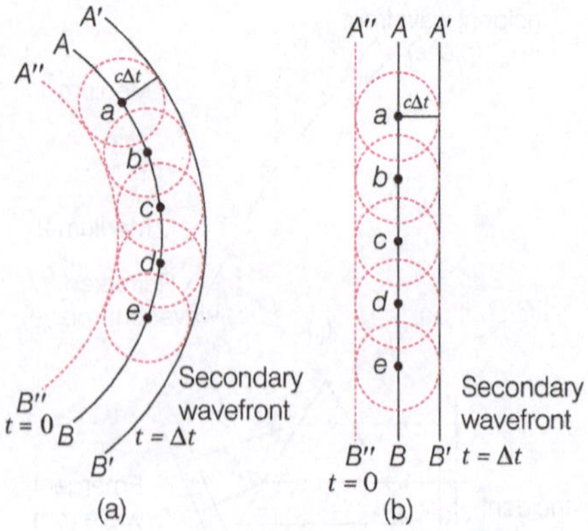

Formation of secondary wavefront using Huygens' principle

In Fig. (a), AB is the section of the given spherical wavefront and $A'B'$ is the new wavefront in the forward direction.

In Fig. (b), AB is the section of the given plane wavefront and $A'B'$ is the new wavefront in the forward direction.

Concept ladder
- Huygens' argued that the amplitude of the secondary wavelets is maximum in the forward direction and zero in the backward direction. Hence, the backward secondary wavelet is absent.

Merits

On the basis of Huygens' principle, many optical phenomena like interference, diffraction, reflection (or laws of reflection) as well as refraction (or Snell's law) could be explained.

Using Huygen's principle, laws of reflection ($\angle i = \angle r$) and law of refraction $\left(n_{21} = \frac{v_1}{v_2} = \frac{\lambda_1}{\lambda_2} = \frac{\sin i}{\sin r}\right)$ can be determined.

Demerits

Following are demerits of Huygens' principle

(i) This principle could not explain, why wavefronts of secondary wavelets are formed in forward direction and not in backward direction?

(ii) This theory assumes light waves as longitudinal waves, therefore could not explain polarisation of light.

(iii) Michelson-Morley does not assume the ether particle as a medium in his experiment.

(iv) This principle could not explain electromagnetic nature of light.

Example 1. *A plane wavefront is incident from air ($\mu = 1$) at an angle of 37° with a horizontal boundary of a refractive medium from air of refractive index $\mu = \frac{3}{2}$. Find the angle of refracted wavefront with the horizontal boundary.*

Sol. It has been given that incident wavefront makes 37° with horizontal. Hence, incident ray makes 37° with normal as the ray is perpendicular to the wavefront.

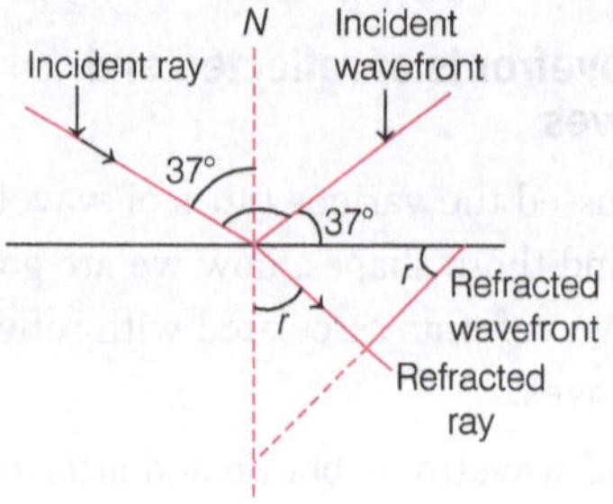

Now, by Snell's law, $\frac{\sin 37°}{\sin r} = \frac{3}{2}$

$\Rightarrow \quad \sin r = \frac{2}{3} \times \frac{3}{5} = \frac{2}{5}$

$\Rightarrow r = \sin^{-1}\left(\frac{2}{5}\right)$, which is same as angle of refracted wavefront with horizontal.

Example 2. *A plane wavefront of yellow light with wavelength 0.5 μm in air suffers refraction in a medium in which velocity of light is 2×10^8 ms^{-1}. Find the wavelength of the light associated with a wavefront in the medium.*

Sol. For wavelength and speed of light associated with a wavefront,

we have $\frac{\lambda_1}{\lambda_2} = \frac{v_1}{v_2}$

Here, $\lambda_1 = 0.5\ \mu\text{m}$, $v_1 = 3 \times 10^8\ \text{ms}^{-1}$

and $v_2 = 2 \times 10^8\ \text{ms}^{-1}$

$\therefore \quad \frac{0.5}{\lambda_2} = \frac{3 \times 10^8}{2 \times 10^8}$

$\Rightarrow \quad \lambda_2 = 0.33\ \mu\text{m}$

Hence, the wavelength of the light associated with a wavefront in the medium is $\lambda_2 = 0.33\ \mu\text{m}$.

Principle of Superposition of Waves

According to superposition principle, at a particular point in the medium, the resultant displacement y produced by a number of waves is the vector sum of the displacements produced by each of the waves ($y_1, y_2, \ldots$).

i.e. $\quad y = y_1 + y_2 + y_3 + y_4 + \ldots$

Clearly, each wave contributes as, if the other wave is not present. The superposition principle, which was stated first for mechanical waves is equally applicable to the electromagnetic (light) waves.

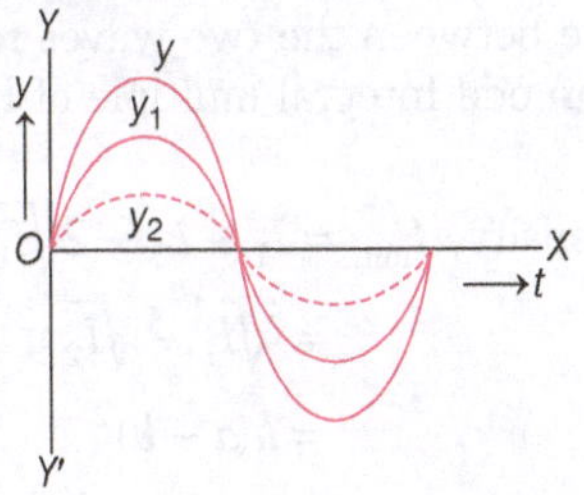

Superposition of waves

Interference of Light Waves

When two light waves of exactly equal frequency having constant phase difference with respect to time travelled in same direction and superimpose (overlap) with each other, then intensity of resultant wave does not remain uniform in space.

This phenomenon of formation of maximum intensity at some points and minimum intensity at some other points by the two identical light waves travelling in same direction is called the **interference of light**.

Types of Interference

Depending on phase difference in superimposing waves, interference is divided into two categories as follows

(i) Constructive Interference

When the two waves meet in same phase, *i.e.* the intensity of light is maximum, is called the constructive interference.

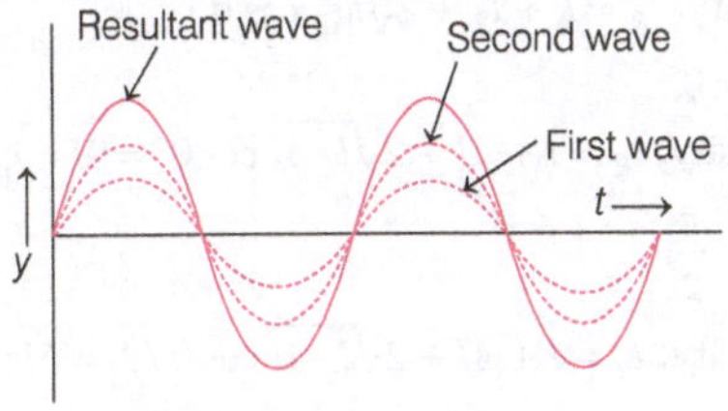

Constructive interference

(ii) Destructive interference

When the two waves meet in opposite phase, *i.e.* the intensity of light is minimum is called the destructive interference.

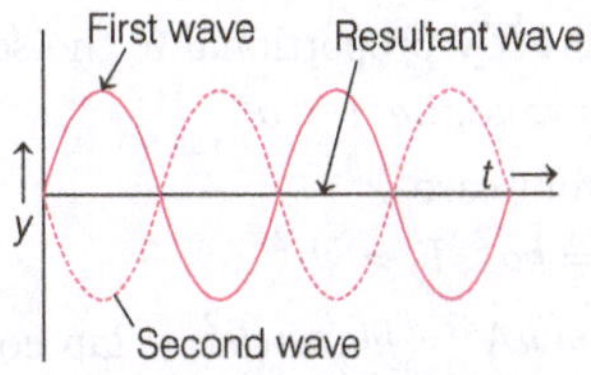

Destructive interference

Mentor's TiP

During interference of light, redistribution of energy (intensity) takes place but total energy remains conserved.

Expression for Resultant Intensity in Interference of Two Waves

Let the waves from two sources of light S_1 and S_2, interfere at the point P as shown in figure.

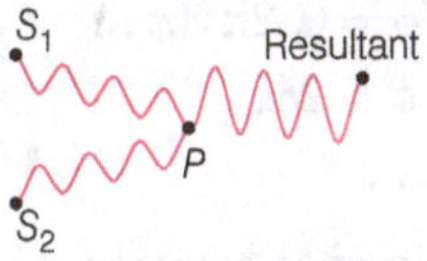

Interference of two waves

$$y_1 = a \sin \omega t$$

and $$y_2 = b \sin(\omega t + \phi)$$

where, a and b are the respective amplitudes of the two waves and ϕ is the constant phase angle by which second wave leads the first wave.

Applying superposition principle, the magnitude of the resultant displacement of the waves is

$$y = y_1 + y_2 \quad \text{or} \quad y = a \sin \omega t + b \sin(\omega t + \phi)$$

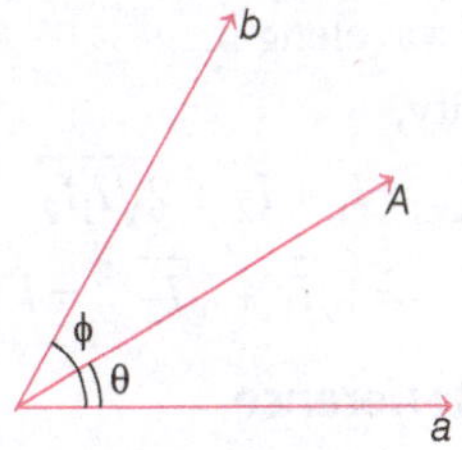

Resultant of amplitudes a and b

Therefore, we get

$$y = A \sin(\omega t + \theta)$$

where, A is the resultant amplitude and θ is the resultant phase difference as shown in figure.

$$\therefore \quad A = \sqrt{a^2 + b^2 + 2ab \cos \phi}$$

and $$\tan \theta = \frac{b \sin \phi}{a + b \cos \phi}$$

As, intensity is directly proportional to the square of the amplitude of the wave, *i.e.* $I \propto a^2$.

So, for two different cases,

$\therefore \quad I_1 = ka^2, I_2 = kb^2$

and $\quad I = kA^2 = k(a^2 + b^2 + 2ab\cos\phi)$

$$\therefore \quad I = I_1 + I_2 + 2\sqrt{I_1 I_2}\cos\phi$$

Mentor's TIP

Relation between path difference, phase difference and time difference, $\dfrac{2\pi}{\text{Phase diff.}} = \dfrac{\lambda}{\text{Path diff.}} = \dfrac{T}{\text{Time diff.}}$

For Constructive Interference

Intensity I should be maximum, for which

$\cos\phi = \text{maximum} = +1$

$\therefore$ Phase difference, $\phi = 0, 2\pi, 4\pi, \ldots$

i.e. $\quad \phi = 2n\pi$

where, $n = 0, 1, 2, 3, \ldots$

If Δx be the path difference between the two waves, then

$$\Delta x = \left(\frac{\lambda}{2\pi}\right)\phi = \left(\frac{\lambda}{2\pi}\right)(2n\pi) = n\lambda$$

$\therefore$ Path difference, $\Delta x = n\lambda$

where, $n = 0, 1, 2, 3, \ldots$

Hence, condition for constructive interference at a point is that, the phase difference between the two waves reaching the point should be zero or an even integral multiple of π. Equivalent path difference between the two waves reaching the point should be zero or an even integral multiple of wavelength.

$\therefore$ Maximum intensity,

$$I_{max} = I_1 + I_2 + 2\sqrt{I_1 I_2} = (\sqrt{I_1} + \sqrt{I_2})^2 = k(a+b)^2$$

For Destructive Interference

Intensity, I should be minimum, for which

$\cos\phi = \text{minimum} = -1$

$\therefore$ Phase difference, $\phi = \pi, 3\pi, 5\pi, \ldots$

i.e. $\quad \phi = (2n-1)\pi$

where, $n = 1, 2, 3, \ldots$

The corresponding path difference between the two waves is

$$\Delta x = \left(\frac{\lambda}{2\pi}\right)\phi = \left(\frac{\lambda}{2\pi}\right)(2n-1)\pi = (2n-1)\frac{\lambda}{2}$$

$\therefore$ Path difference, $\Delta x = (2n-1)\dfrac{\lambda}{2}$, where $n = 1, 2, 3\ldots$

Hence, condition for destructive interference at a point is that, the phase difference between the two waves reaching the point should be an odd integral multiple of π or path difference between the two waves reaching the point should be an odd integral multiple of half the wavelength.

$\therefore$ Minimum intensity, $I_{min} = I_1 + I_2 - 2\sqrt{I_1 I_2}$

$$= (\sqrt{I_1} - \sqrt{I_2})^2$$

$$= k(a-b)^2$$

Concept ladder

Comparison of Intensities of Maxima and Minima

As we know that,

$$I_{max} \propto (a+b)^2 \text{ and } I_{min} \propto (a-b)^2$$

$$\therefore \quad \frac{I_{max}}{I_{min}} = \frac{(a+b)^2}{(a-b)^2} = \frac{\left(\frac{a}{b}+1\right)^2}{\left(\frac{a}{b}-1\right)^2} = \frac{(r+1)^2}{(r-1)^2}$$

where, $r = \dfrac{a}{b}$ (ratio of amplitudes).

Also, we can write as

$$\frac{I_{max}}{I_{min}} = \left(\frac{\sqrt{I_1}+\sqrt{I_2}}{\sqrt{I_1}-\sqrt{I_2}}\right)^2 = \left(\frac{a+b}{a-b}\right)^2$$

Example 3. *Two sources of intensity I and 4I are used in an interference experiment. Find the intensity at a point, where the waves from two sources superimpose with a phase difference of (i) zero, (ii) $\pi/2$, (iii) π and (iv) ratio of maximum and minimum intensities.*

Sol. Given, $I_1 = I$ and $I_2 = 4I$

Intensity, $I_R = I_1 + I_2 + 2\sqrt{I_1 I_2}\cos\phi$

(i) At $\phi = 0$,

Intensity, $I_R = I + 4I + 2\sqrt{I \cdot 4I}\cos 0° = 9I = I_{max}$

(ii) At $\phi = \dfrac{\pi}{2}$,

Intensity, $I_R = I + 4I + 2\sqrt{I \cdot 4I}\cos(\pi/2) = 5I$

(iii) At $\phi = \pi$,

Intensity, $I_R = I + 4I + 2\sqrt{I \cdot 4I}\cos(\pi) = I = I_{min}$

(iv) Ratio of maximum and minimum intensities,

$$\frac{I_{max}}{I_{min}} = \frac{9I}{I} = 9:1$$

NEET Close-up

Example Similar to PYQ Asked in NEET 2016

The interference pattern is obtained with two coherent light sources with intensity ratio of 4. In the interference pattern, the ratio of $\frac{I_{max}-I_{min}}{I_{max}+I_{min}}$ will be

(a) $\frac{5}{3}$ (b) $\frac{4}{5}$ (c) $\frac{3}{5}$ (d) $\frac{7}{3}$

Sol. (*b*) Given, $\frac{I_2}{I_1}=4$

$\Rightarrow \quad I_2 = 4I_1$

$\therefore$ Ratio of intensities is given by

$$\frac{I_{max}-I_{min}}{I_{max}+I_{min}} = \frac{(\sqrt{I_2}+\sqrt{I_1})^2-(\sqrt{I_2}-\sqrt{I_1})^2}{(\sqrt{I_2}+\sqrt{I_1})^2+(\sqrt{I_2}-\sqrt{I_1})^2}$$

$$= \frac{\left(\sqrt{\frac{I_2}{I_1}}+1\right)^2-\left(\sqrt{\frac{I_2}{I_1}}-1\right)^2}{\left(\sqrt{\frac{I_2}{I_1}}+1\right)^2+\left(\sqrt{\frac{I_2}{I_1}}-1\right)^2}$$

$$= \frac{(\sqrt{4}+1)^2-(\sqrt{4}-1)^2}{(\sqrt{4}+1)^2+(\sqrt{4}-1)^2} = \frac{4}{5}$$

Skill Builder

The interference pattern is obtained with two coherent light sources of intensity 2. In the interference pattern, the ratio of $\frac{I_{max}+I_{min}}{I_{max}-I_{min}}$ will be

(a) $\frac{3\sqrt{2}}{4}$ (b) $\frac{2\sqrt{2}}{3}$ (c) $\frac{5\sqrt{2}}{2}$ (d) $\frac{3\sqrt{2}}{2}$

For more Practice Refer Q. No. 4 of Gearing up for NEET.

Example 4. *Two sources with intensity I_0 and $4I_0$ respectively, interfere at a point in a medium. Find the ratio of amplitudes.*

Sol. Since, $I \propto a^2$

$\therefore \quad ka_1^2 = I_1 = I_0$ and $ka_2^2 = I_2 = 4I_0$

$$\therefore \quad \frac{a_1^2}{a_2^2} = \frac{I_1}{I_2} = \frac{1}{4}$$

$$\Rightarrow \quad \frac{a_1}{a_2} = \frac{1}{2}$$

Coherent and Incoherent Sources

Light sources can be coherent or incoherent which are discussed below.

Coherent Sources

Two sources of light which continuously emit light waves of same frequency with a zero or constant phase difference between them are called coherent sources.

Incoherent Sources

Two sources of light which do not emit light waves with a constant phase difference are called incoherent sources.

Need of Coherent Sources for the Production of Interference Pattern

When two monochromatic waves of intensity I_1, I_2 and phase difference ϕ meet at a point, then the resultant intensity is given by

$$I = I_1 + I_2 + 2\sqrt{I_1 I_2}\cos\phi$$

Here, the term $2\sqrt{I_1 I_2}\cos\phi$ is called **interference term.**

There are two possibilities

(i) If $\cos\phi$ remains constant with time, then the total intensity at any point will be constant. The intensity will be maximum $(\sqrt{I_1}+\sqrt{I_2})^2$ at points, where $\cos\phi$ is 1 and minimum $(\sqrt{I_1}-\sqrt{I_2})^2$ at points, where $\cos\phi = -1$. The sources in this case are coherent.

(ii) If $\cos\phi$ varies continuously with time assumming both positive and negative values, then the average value of $\cos\phi$ will be zero over time interval of measurement. The interference term averages to zero. There will be same intensity $I = I_1 + I_2$ at every point. The two sources in this case are incoherent.

Mentor's Tip

Two different light sources are never coherent.

Example 5. *Two incoherent sources emitting lights of intensities I_0 and $3I_0$ interfere in a medium. Calculate the resultant intensity at any point.*

Sol. Since, the two sources are incoherent, so no sustained interference pattern is obtained.

We observe an average intensity,

$$I = I_1 + I_2 + 2\sqrt{I_1 I_2}\cos\phi$$

Now, $\cos\phi = 0$ in one complete cycle.

$$\therefore \quad I = I_1 + I_2 = 4I_0$$

Methods to Obtain Coherent Sources

By using following method, coherent sources can be obtained.

(i) Coherent sources of light should be obtained from a single source by some device.

(ii) The two sources should give monochromatic light.

(iii) Coherent sources are produced by

(a) division of wavefront (Young's double slit experiment).

(b) division of amplitude (partial reflection or refraction in thin films).

Necessary Conditions for Interference of Light

In order to obtain a sustained (permanent or stable) and observable interference pattern, the following conditions must be fulfilled

(i) **Sources must be coherent** In order to produce a stable interference pattern, the individual waves must maintain a constant phase relationship with one another, *i.e.* the two interfering sources must emit waves having a constant phase difference between them. If the phase difference between two sources does not remain constant, then the places of maxima and minima shift.

In case of mechanical waves, it is possible to keep a constant phase relationship between two different sources. But in case of light, two different light sources cannot be coherent.

(ii) **Same frequency or wavelength** Phase relationship between two waves can be kept constant only when their frequencies are same. Thus we can say that, two coherent sources must have the same frequency.

(iii) **Equality of amplitudes** The amplitudes of two interfering waves should be equal or approximately equal. Otherwise the difference between the intensities of maximas and minimas will be too small and the contrast will be poor. Maximum contrast is, however obtained when $A_1 = A_2$, because then minimum intensity will be zero.

STEP UP Practice 1

1. Monochromatic light of wavelength λ_1 travelling in medium of refractive index n_1 enters a denser medium of refractive index n_2. The wavelength in the second medium is

(a) $\lambda_1\left(\frac{n_1}{n_2}\right)$ (b) $\lambda_1\left(\frac{n_2}{n_1}\right)$ (c) λ_1 (d) $\lambda_1\left(\frac{n_2 - n_1}{n_1}\right)$

2. A light ray of frequency ν and wavelength λ enters a liquid of refractive index 3/2. The ray travels in the liquid with

(a) frequency ν and wavelength $\left(\frac{2}{3}\right)\lambda$

(b) frequency ν and wavelength $\left(\frac{3}{2}\right)\lambda$

(c) frequency ν and wavelength λ

(d) frequency $\left(\frac{3}{2}\right)$ν and wavelength λ

3. Choose the incorrect pair from the given below.

(a) In spherical wavefront, amplitude — of light wave $A \propto \frac{1}{r}$

(b) In spherical wavefront, intensity of — light wave $I \propto \frac{1}{r^2}$

(c) In cylindrical wavefront, amplitude — of light wave $A \propto \frac{1}{\sqrt{r}}$

(d) In cylindrical wavefront, intensity — of light wave $I \propto \frac{1}{\sqrt{r^3}}$

4. If two waves represented by $y_1 = 4 \sin \omega t$ and $y_2 = 3\sin\left(\omega t + \frac{\pi}{3}\right)$ interfere at a point, then the amplitude of the resulting wave will be about

(a) 7 m (b) 6 m
(c) 5 m (d) 3.5 m

5. Which of the following is not correct for a wavefront?

(a) It is a surface of constant phase.
(b) The path of ray of light is always parallel to wavefront.
(c) At wavefront, all particles vibrate in same phase.
(d) Spherical wavefront is obtained from point source.

6. If the amplitude ratio of two sources producing interference is 3 : 5, then the ratio of intensities at maxima and minima is

(a) 25 : 16 (b) 5 : 3
(c) 16 : 1 (d) 25 : 9

7. **Statement I** All bright interference bands have the same intensity.

Statement II In interference, all bands receive same light from two sources.

In the light of the above statements, choose the most appropriate answer from the options given below.

(a) Both Statement I and Statement II are incorrect.
(b) Statement I is correct but Statement II is incorrect.
(c) Statement I is incorrect but Statement II is correct.
(d) Both Statement I and Statement II are correct.

8. The ratio of intensities of two waves are given by 9 : 4. The ratio of the amplitudes of the two waves is
(a) 3 : 2 (b) 1 : 2
(c) 4 : 1 (d) 1 : 4

9. Among the two interfering monochromatic sources A and B, A is ahead of B in phase by 36°. If the observation be taken from point P, such that $PB - PA = \lambda/4$, then the phase difference between the waves from A and B reaching p is
(a) 156° (b) 140°
(c) 136° (d) 126°

10. Three waves of equal frequency having amplitudes 10 µm, 4 µm, 7 µ m arrive at a given point with successive phase difference of $\frac{\pi}{2}$, the amplitude of the resulting wave (in µm) is given by
(a) 4 (b) 5
(c) 6 (d) 7

11. Two sources of light of the same frequency produce intensities I and $4I$ at a point P when used individually. If they are used together such that the light from them reach P with a phase difference of $2\pi/3$, then the intensity at P will be
(a) $2I$ (b) $3I$ (c) $4I$ (d) $5I$

12. Statement I The maximum intensity in interference pattern is double the intensity due to each slit.
Statement II Intensity is directly proportional to square of amplitude.
In the light of the above statements, choose the most appropriate answer from the options given below.
(a) Both Statement I and Statement II are incorrect.
(b) Statement I is correct but Statement II is incorrect.
(c) Statement I is incorrect but Statement II is correct.
(d) Both Statement I and Statement II are correct.

13. To obtain sustained interference, the two light sources should be
(a) coherent
(b) narrow and placed close to each other
(c) non-coherent
(d) Both (a) and (b)

14. What is the path difference in case of destructive interference?
(a) $n\lambda$ (b) $n(\lambda + 1)$
(c) $\frac{(n+1)\lambda}{2}$ (d) $\frac{(2n+1)\lambda}{2}$

15. Statement I All points on a wavefront vibrate in same phase with same frequency.
Statement II Two sources are said to be coherent if they produce waves of same frequency with a constant phase difference.
In the light of the above statements, choose the most appropriate answer from the options given below.
(a) Both Statement I and Statement II are incorrect.
(b) Statement I is correct but Statement II is incorrect.
(c) Statement I is incorrect but Statement II is correct.
(d) Both Statement I and Statement II are correct.

16. Two light sources are said to be coherent if they are obtained from
(a) two independent point sources emitting light of the same wavelength
(b) a single point source
(c) a wide source
(d) two ordinary bulbs emitting light of different wavelengths

17. Statement I Only coherent light source produce sustained interference.
Statement II Coherent light sources emits of same wavelength and with a constant phase difference.
In the light of the above statements, choose the most appropriate answer from the options given below.
(a) Both Statement I and Statement II are incorrect.
(b) Statement I is correct but Statement II is incorrect.
(c) Statement I is incorrect but Statement II is correct.
(d) Both Statement I and Statement II are correct.

18. Two coherent sources of intensities I_1 and I_2 produce an interference pattern. The maximum intensity in the interference pattern will be
(a) $I_1 + I_2$ (b) $I_1^2 + I_2^2$
(c) $(I_1 + I_2)^2$ (d) $(\sqrt{I_1} + \sqrt{I_2})^2$

19. Let S_1 and S_2 are two sources and if wave from S_1 reaches some common point P be covering seven times of wavelength λ and from S_2 by covering nine times of wavelength λ.

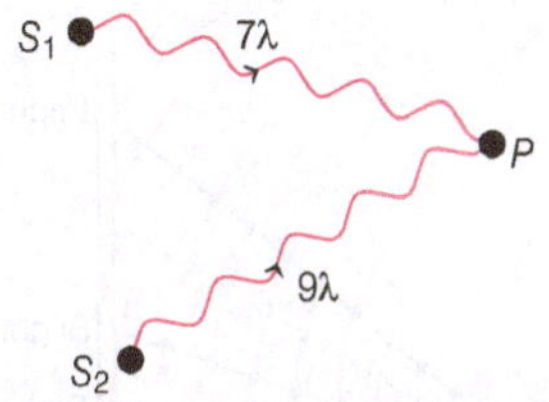

Which of the following statement(s) is/are correct?
(i) $S_2P - S_1P = 2\lambda$
(ii) Waves from S_1 arrives exactly two cycles earlier than waves from S_2.
(iii) At point P, waves from S_1 and S_2 are in phase.
(iv) At point P, waves from S_1 and S_2 are out of phase.
(a) only (iv) (b) (i), (ii) and (iii)
(c) (ii) and (iii) (d) (ii) and (iv)

20. Two coherent sources have intensity in the ratio of $\frac{100}{1}$.
Ratio of I_{max}/I_{min} is
(a) $\frac{1}{100}$ (b) $\frac{1}{10}$ (c) $\frac{10}{1}$ (d) $\frac{3}{2}$

Module 2

Young's Double Slit Experiment

- Young's Double Slit Experiment (YDSE)
- Distribution of Intensity

Young's Double Slit Experiment (YDSE)

One of the first to demonstrate the interference of light was Thomas Young in 1801.

In his experimental arrangement (as shown in figure), monochromatic light (single wavelength) from a narrow vertical slit S falls on two other narrow slits S_1 and S_2 which are very close together and equidistant from S. S_1 and S_2 act as two coherent sources (both being derived from S).

The emerging beams spread into the region beyond the slits. Superposition occurs in the shaded area, where the beams overlap.

Alternate bright and dark equally spaced vertical bands (interference fringes) can be observed on a screen placed at some distance from the slits.

If either of S_1 or S_2 is covered, then the fringes disappear.

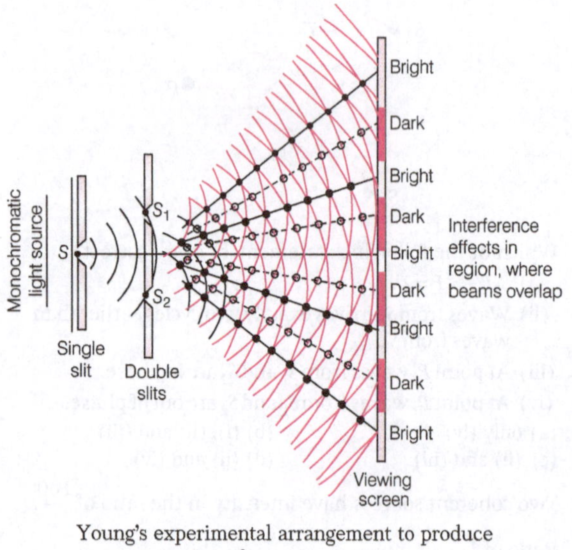

Young's experimental arrangement to produce interference pattern

Path Difference

Figure shows the light waves from S_1 and S_2 meeting at an arbitrary point P on the screen.

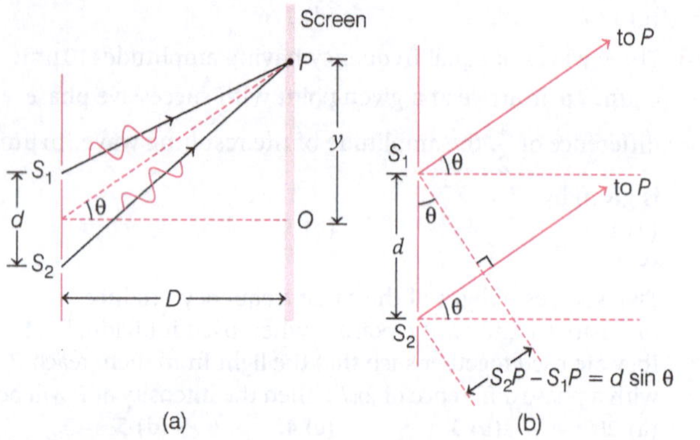

(a) To reach P, the light waves from S_1 and S_2 must travel different distances. (b) The path difference between the two rays is $d \sin\theta$.

Since $D >> d$, the two light rays are approximately parallel with a path difference,

$$\Delta x = S_2P - S_1P \approx d \sin\theta$$

In addition to our assumption that $D >> d$, we assume that $d >> \lambda$. These can be valid assumptions because in practice, D is often of the order of 1 m, d is a fraction of a millimetre and λ is a fraction of a micrometre for visible light. Under these conditions θ is small, thus we can use the approximation, $\sin\theta \approx \tan\theta = \dfrac{y}{D}$

$$\therefore \text{Path difference,} \qquad \Delta x = \frac{y}{D} d \qquad \text{...(i)}$$

This is the path difference between two waves meeting at a point on the screen. Due to this path difference, some points on the screen are bright and some points are dark. Now, we will discuss the position of these bright and dark fringes and fringe width under following points

Position of Bright Fringe

For maximum intensity at P,

$$\Delta x = n\lambda$$

or $\quad d \sin\theta = n\lambda \quad$ (where, $n = 0, \pm 1, \pm 2, \ldots$) $\quad$ ...(ii)

The bright fringe corresponding to the integer n is called the **nth order (or just nth) bright fringe.** The bright fringe for $n = 0$, is known as the central fringe and its centre (point O) is called the **central (or zero order) maximum.** Higher order bright fringes are situated symmetrically about the central fringe. It is useful to obtain expression for the position of the bright fringe measured vertical from O.

From Eqs. (i) and (ii), we get

Position of bright fringe,

$$y_{bright} = \frac{n\lambda}{d} D \quad ...(iii)$$

Example 6. *In a YDSE, green light of wavelength 500 nm is used. Where will be the second bright fringe formed for a set up in which separation between slits is 4 mm and the screen is placed 1 m from the slits?*

Sol. Position of second bright fringe,

$$y_2 = \frac{2\lambda D}{d} = \frac{2 \times 500 \times 10^{-9} \times 1}{4 \times 10^{-3}} = 0.25 \text{ mm}$$

Mentor's TIP

The second bright fringe will formed on both sides of the central bright fringe, hence, value of y_2 should be ± 25 mm.

Example 7. *Bichromatic light is used in YDSE having wavelengths $\lambda_1 = 400$ nm and $\lambda_2 = 700$ nm. Find minimum order of λ_1 which overlaps with λ_2.*

Sol. Let n_1 bright fringe of λ_1 overlaps with n_2 bright fringe of λ_2, then their position will be same. *i.e.*

$$\frac{n_1\lambda_1 D}{d} = \frac{n_2\lambda_2 D}{d} \quad \text{or} \quad \frac{n_1}{n_2} = \frac{\lambda_2}{\lambda_1} = \frac{700}{400} = \frac{7}{4}$$

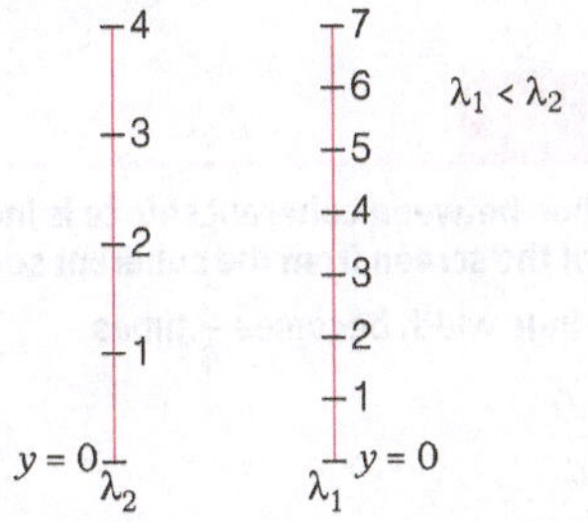

The ratio $\frac{n_1}{n_2} = \frac{7}{4}$ implies that 7th bright fringe of λ_1 will overlap with 4th bright fringe of λ_2.

Similarly, 14th bright fringe of λ_1 will overlap with 8th bright fringe of λ_2 and so on.

So, the minimum order of λ_1 which overlaps with λ_2 is 7.

Example 8. *Young's double slit experiment is carried out using microwaves of wavelength $\lambda = 3$ cm. Distance between the slits is $d = 5$ cm and the distance between the plane of slits and the screen is $D = 100$ cm. Find the number of maximas and their positions on the screen.*

Sol. For intensity maxima at P.

Path difference, $\Delta x = d \sin\theta = n\lambda$

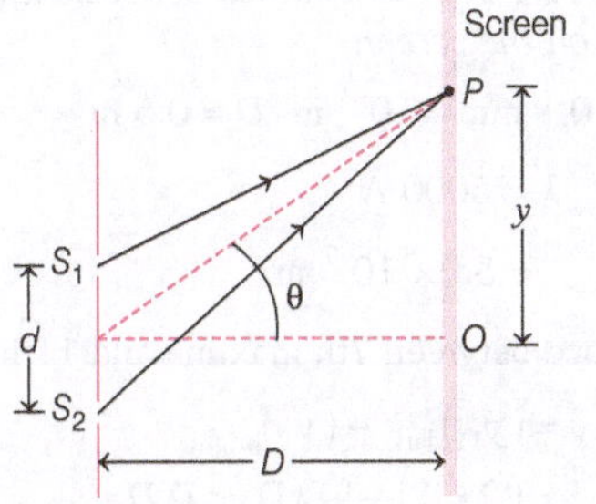

$$\Rightarrow \quad \sin\theta = n\frac{\lambda}{d} = n \times \frac{3}{5}$$

As $\sin\theta \le 1 \Rightarrow \frac{3n}{5} \le 1$ or $n \le \frac{5}{3}$

So, possible integral values of n are 0, ± 1

Hence $y = n\frac{\lambda D}{d}$ gives,

$$y = 0,\ y = \pm\frac{3}{5} \times 100 = \pm 60 \text{ cm}$$

So, there are 3 maximas on screen at $y = 0$ and $y = \pm 60$ cm

Position of Dark Fringe

In previous point, we obtained the position of bright fringe. In the similar way, we can obtain position of dark fringe as follows

For minimum intensity at P,

$$\Delta x = (2n-1)\frac{\lambda}{2}$$

or $$d \sin\theta = (2n-1)\frac{\lambda}{2} \text{ (where, } n = \pm 1, \pm 2, ...) \quad ...(iv)$$

The first minima ($n = \pm 1$) are adjacent to the central maximum on either side. We will obtain expression for position of dark fringe measured vertically from O.

From Eqs. (i) and (iv), we get

Position of dark fringe,

$$y_{dark} = \frac{(2n-1)\lambda}{2d} D \quad ...(v)$$

NEET Snapshot

If the monochromatic source in Young's double slit experiment is replaced by white light, then a central bright white fringe surrounded by a few coloured fringes will observe. ***[NEET 2024]***

When YDSE is performed in white light instead of monochromatic light, all wavelengths show their maxima and minima in orders of their wavelength. At central point on screen, path difference is zero for all wavelength. Thus a central bright fringe is observed along with few fringes that will be of different colours.

Example 9. *In YDSE, the two slits are separated by 0.1 mm and they are 0.5 m from the screen. The wavelength of light used is 5000 Å. Find the distance between 7th maxima and 11th minima on the screen.*

Sol. Given, $d = 0.1\text{ mm} = 10^{-4}\text{ m}$, $D = 0.5\text{ m}$

and $\lambda = 5000\text{ Å}$

$$= 5.0 \times 10^{-7}\text{ m}$$

The distance between 7th maxima and 11th minima is

$$\Delta y = (y_{11})_{\text{dark}} - (y_7)_{\text{bright}}$$

$$= \frac{(2 \times 11 - 1)\lambda D}{2d} - \frac{7\lambda D}{d}$$

or $$\Delta y = \frac{7\lambda D}{2d}$$

$$= \frac{7 \times 5.0 \times 10^{-7} \times 0.5}{2 \times 10^{-4}}$$

$$= 8.75 \times 10^{-3}\text{ m}$$

$$= 8.75\text{ mm}$$

Fringe Width

Distance between two adjacent bright (or dark) fringes is called the fringe width. It is denoted by β.

Thus,

$$\beta = \frac{n\lambda D}{d} - \frac{(n-1)\lambda D}{d} = \frac{\lambda D}{d}$$

or $$\beta = \frac{\lambda D}{d} \quad \text{...(vi)}$$

Alternatively, we can show that distance between two successive dark fringes is also $\frac{\lambda D}{d}$.

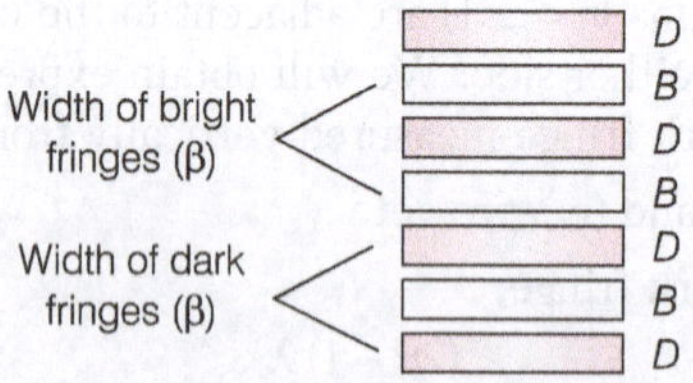

Width of bright and dark fringes

Important Points Related with Fringe Width

As we know that, fringe width (β) is the distance between two successive maxima or minima. It is given by

$$\beta = \frac{\lambda D}{d} \quad \text{or} \quad \beta \propto \lambda$$

Two conclusions can be drawn from this relation

(i) If Young's double slit experiment apparatus is immersed in a liquid of refractive index μ, then wavelength of light and hence fringe width decreases μ times.

(ii) If white light is used in place of a monochromatic light, then coloured fringes are obtained on the screen with red fringes of larger size than that of violet because $\lambda_{\text{red}} > \lambda_{\text{violet}}$.

But note that centre is still white because there, path difference is zero for all colours. Hence, all the wavelengths interfere constructively. At other places, light will interfere destructively for those wavelengths for whom path difference is $\lambda/2$, $3\lambda/2$, ..., etc., and they will interfere constructively for the wavelengths for whom path difference is λ, 2λ, ..., etc.

Example 10. *In YDSE, two slits are placed 2 mm from each other. Interference pattern is observed on a screen placed 2 m from the plane of slits. What is the fringe width for a light of wavelength 400 nm?*

Sol. Given, $d = 2\text{ mm} = 2 \times 10^{-3}\text{ m}$, $D = 2\text{ m}$

and $\lambda = 400\text{ nm} = 400 \times 10^{-9}\text{ m}$

$\therefore$ Fringe width, $$\beta = \frac{\lambda D}{d} = \frac{400 \times 10^{-9} \times 2}{2 \times 10^{-3}}$$

$$= 400 \times 10^{-6}\text{m}$$

NEET Snapshot

In YDSE if separation between coherent source is increased to double and the distance of the screen from the coherent source is decreased to half, then the fringe width becomes $\frac{1}{4}$ times. *[NEET 2020]*

Fringe width, $\beta = \frac{\lambda D}{d}$

$$\therefore \quad \frac{\beta_2}{\beta_1} = \frac{\frac{\lambda_2 D_2}{d_2}}{\frac{\lambda_1 D_1}{d_1}} \quad \left[\text{as } \lambda_1 = \lambda_2, D_2 = \frac{1}{2}D, d_2 = 2d\right]$$

$$\frac{\beta_2}{\beta_1} = \frac{\frac{1}{2}D_1}{2d_1} \times \frac{d_1}{D_1} = \frac{1}{4}$$

$$\therefore \quad \beta_2 = \frac{1}{4}\beta_1$$

Example 11. *In Young's double slit experiment with monochromatic light, fringes are obtained on a screen placed at some distance from the plane of slits. If the screen is moved by 5 cm towards the slits, then the change in fringe width is 30 μm. If the distance between the slits is 1 mm, then calculate wavelength of the light used.*

Sol. Fringe width, $\beta = \frac{D\lambda}{d}$ ...(i)

When D decreases, then fringe width decreases,

$$\beta - 30 \times 10^{-6} = \frac{(D - 5 \times 10^{-2})\lambda}{d} \quad \text{...(ii)}$$

Subtracting Eq. (ii) from Eq. (i), we get

$$30 \times 10^{-6} = \frac{5 \times 10^{-2}\lambda}{d} = \frac{5 \times 10^{-2}\lambda}{1 \times 10^{-3}}$$

Wavelength of the light,

$$\lambda = \frac{30 \times 10^{-6} \times 10^{-3}}{5 \times 10^{-2}}$$

$$= 6 \times 10^{-7} = 600 \times 10^{-9} \text{m}$$

$$= 600 \text{ nm}$$

NEET Close-up

Example Similar to PYQ Asked in NEET 2022

In YDSE, 10 fringes are observed at screen with $\lambda = 500$ nm. If light of wavelength $\lambda = 400$ nm is used, then number of fringes on the screen will be

(a) 14 (b) 12 (c) 11 (d) 16

Sol. (*b*) Since D and d are same in both cases

$$\beta = \frac{n_1\lambda_1 D}{d} = \frac{n_2\lambda_2 D}{d}$$

$$\Rightarrow \quad n_1\lambda_1 = n_2\lambda_2$$

$$\Rightarrow \quad n_2 = n_1\frac{\lambda_1}{\lambda_2} = 10 \times \frac{500}{400}$$

or $\quad n_2 = 12.5$

or 12 fringes will be obtained on the screen.

Skill Builder

A screen is visible with 10 fringes when $\lambda = 6000$ Å is used in YDSE. If distance between screen and slits is doubled and Wavelength of source is changed to 4000 Å, then number of fringes on screen will be

(a) 7 (b) 8 (c) 9 (d) 10

For more Practice Refer Q. No. 1 of Step-up practice 2 and Q. No. 24 of Gearing up for NEET.

Angular Width of Fringes

Let angular position of nth bright fringe is θ_n and because of its small value $\tan\theta_n \approx \theta_n$

$$\therefore \quad \theta_n = \frac{Y_n}{D} = \frac{nD\lambda/d}{D} = \frac{n\lambda}{d}$$

Similarly, if angular position of $(n+1)$th bright fringe is θ_{n+1}, then $\theta_{n+1} = \frac{Y_{n+1}}{D} = \frac{(n+1)\,D\lambda/d}{D} = \frac{(n+1)\lambda}{d}$

∴ Angular width of a fringe,

$$\theta = \theta_{n+1} - \theta_n = \frac{(n+1)\lambda}{d} - \frac{n\lambda}{d} = \frac{\lambda}{d}$$

Also, $\quad \beta = \frac{D}{d}\lambda$

$$\therefore \quad \boxed{\theta = \frac{\lambda}{d} = \frac{\beta}{D}}$$

It is independent of n, *i.e.* angular width of all fringes are same.

Example 12. *Two slits in YDSE are placed 1 mm from each other. Interference pattern is observed on a screen placed 1 m from the plane of slits. What is the angular fringe width for a light of wavelength 400 nm.*

Sol. Given, $d = 1 \text{ mm} = 10^{-3}$ m

$$D = 1 \text{ m}, \lambda = 400 \text{ nm} = 400 \times 10^{-9} \text{m}$$

$$\text{Angular fringe width, } \theta = \frac{\lambda}{d} = \frac{400 \times 10^{-9}}{10^{-3}}$$

$$= 400 \times 10^{-6} \text{ rad}$$

NEET Snapshot

Any relative movement between sources and screen does not affect angular separation, however it changes with change in λ. *[NEET 2023]*

Angular separation of fringe, $\theta = \frac{\lambda}{d}$

i.e., Angular separation does not depend on the distance between screen and plane of slits but it depends on the wavelength of light.

Scan for Video

Example 13. *In Young's double slit experiment, separation between slits is 1 mm, distance of screen from slits is 2 m. If wavelength of incident light is 500 nm, determine*

(i) fringe width

(ii) angular fringe width

(iii) distance between 4th bright fringe and 3rd dark fringe.

(iv) if whole arrangement is immersed in water ($\mu_w = 4/3$), new angular fringe width.

Sol. Given, $d = 1 \text{ mm} = 1 \times 10^{-3}$ m $D = 2$ m,

$$\lambda = 500 \text{ nm} = 500 \times 10^{-9} \text{m}$$

(i) Fringe width,

$$\beta = \frac{D\lambda}{d} = \frac{2 \times 500 \times 10^{-9}}{1 \times 10^{-3}} = 10^{-3} \text{ m} = 1 \text{mm}$$

(ii) Angular fringe width,

$$\theta = \frac{\lambda}{d} = \frac{500 \times 10^{-9}}{1 \times 10^{-3}} = 5 \times 10^{-4} \text{rad}$$

(iii) Distance of 4th bright fringe from centre,

$$y_4 = \frac{nD\lambda}{d} = \frac{4D\lambda}{d}$$

Distance of 3rd dark fringe from centre,

$$y_3' = \frac{(2n-1)D\lambda}{2d} = \frac{(2\times 3-1)D\lambda}{2d} = \frac{5D\lambda}{2d}$$

Distance between 4th bright fringe and 3rd dark fringe is

$$y_4 - y_3' = \frac{4D\lambda}{d} - \frac{5D\lambda}{2d} = \frac{3D\lambda}{2d} = \frac{3}{2}\beta = \frac{3}{2}\times 1 = \frac{3}{2}\text{mm}$$

(iv) New angular fringe width,

$$\theta_w = \frac{\theta}{\mu_w} = \frac{5\times 10^{-4}}{4/3} = \frac{15}{4}\times 10^{-4}\ \text{rad}$$

Concept ladder Intensity of the fringes in YDSE can be explained exactly same as intensity in case of any other interference.

Distribution of Intensity

The distribution of intensity in Young's double slit experiment is shown below

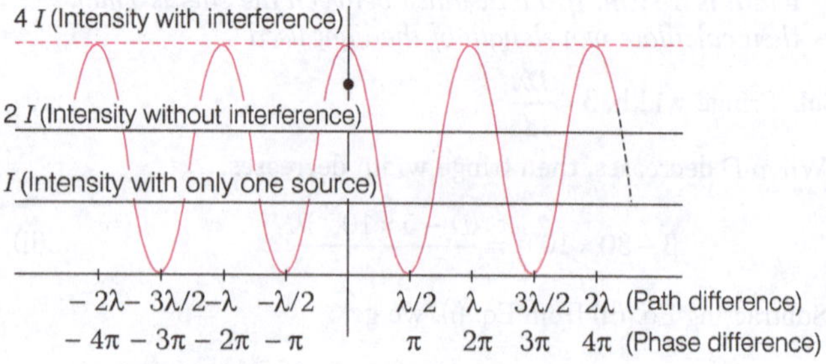

Distribution of intensity in YDSE

STEP UP Practice 2

1. In Young's double slit experiment, green light (λ = 5461 Å) is used and 60 fringes were seen in the field view. Now, sodium light is used (λ = 5890 Å), then number of fringes observed are

(a) 40 (b) 60 (c) 50 (d) 55

2. In Young's double slit experiment, the ratio of intensities of bright and dark fringes is 9.This means that

(a) the intensities of individual sources are 5 and 4 units respectively

(b) the intensities of individual sources are 4 and 1 units respectively

(c) the ratio of their amplitudes is 3

(d) the ratio of their amplitudes is 4

3. In Young's double slit experiment, instead of taking slits of equal widths, one slit is made twice as wide as the other. Then, in the interference pattern

(a) the intensities of both the maxima and the minima increase

(b) the intensity of maxima increases and the minima has zero intensity

(c) the intensity of maxima decreases and that of the minima increases

(d) the intensity of maxima decreases and the minima has zero intensity

4. **Assertion (A)** If the whole apparatus of Young's experiment is immersed in liquid, the fringe width will decrease.

Reason (R) The wavelength of light in water is more than that of air.

In the light of the above statements, choose the correct answer from the options given below.

(a) Both A and R are true but R is not the correct explanation of A.

(b) A is true but R is false.

(c) A is false but R is true.

(d) Both A and R are true and R is the correct explanation of A.

5. In Young's double slit experiment, the aperture screen distance is 2 m. The fringe width is 1 mm. Light of 600 nm is used. If a thin plate of glass (μ = 1.5) of thickness 0.06 mm is placed over one of the slits, then there will be a lateral displacement of the fringes by

(a) zero (b) 5 cm

(c) 10 cm (d) 15 cm

6. In Young's double slit experiment, when two light waves form third minimum intensity, they have

(a) phase difference of 3π (b) phase difference of $\frac{5\pi}{2}$

(c) path difference of 3λ (d) path difference of $\frac{5\lambda}{2}$

7. In Young's double slit experiment, an interference pattern is obtained for λ = 6000 Å, coming from two coherent sources S_1 and S_2. At certain point P on the screen third dark fringe is formed, then the path difference $S_1P - S_2P$ (in micron) is

(a) 0.75 (b) 1.5 (c) 3.0 (d) 4.5

8. The light of wavelength 6328 Å is incident on a slit of width 0.2 mm perpendicularly, the angular fringe width will be

(a) 0.36° (b) 0.18°

(c) 0.72° (d) 0.09°

9. In Young's double slit experiment, if the widths of the slits are in the ratio 9 : 4, the ratio of the intensity at maxima to the intensity at minima will be

(a) 169 : 25 (b) 81 : 16
(c) 25 : 1 (d) 9 : 4

10. In Young's double slit experiment, an interference pattern is obtained on a screen by a light of wavelength 12000 Å coming from the coherent sources S_1 and S_2. At certain point P on the screen third dark fringe is formed, then the path differences $S_1P - S_2P$ in microns is

(a) 0.75 (b) 1.5
(c) 3.0 (d) 4.5

11. Assertion (A) Young's double slit experiment can be performed using a source of white light.

Reason (R) The wavelength of red light is less than the wavelength of other colour in white light.

In the light of the above statements, choose the correct answer from the options given below.

(a) Both A and R are true but R is not the correct explanation of A.
(b) A is true but R is false.
(c) A is false but R is true.
(d) Both A and R are true and R is the correct explanation of A.

12. In Young's double slit experiment, the intensity on the screen at a point where path difference is λ is Q. What will be the intensity at the point where path difference is $\lambda/4$?

(a) $\frac{Q}{4}$ (b) $\frac{Q}{2}$ (c) Q (d) Zero

13. A Young's double slit experiment is performed with white light, then choose incorrect option.

(a) the fringe next to the central will be red
(b) the central fringe will be white
(c) the fringe next to the central will be violet
(d) there will not be a completely dark fringe

14. In a Young's double slit experiment, the slit separation is 1 mm and the screen is 1 m from the slit. For a monochromatic light of wavelength 300 nm, the distance of 3rd minima from the central maxima is

(a) 0.50 mm (b) 0.75 mm
(c) 1.50 mm (d) 1.75 mm

15. Consider the following statements in case of Young's double slit experiment.

I. A slit S is necessary, if we use an ordinary extended source of light.
II. A slit S is not needed, if we use an ordinary but well collimated beam of light.
III. A slit S is not needed, if we use a spatially coherent source of light.

(a) I, II and III (b) Both I and II
(c) Both II and III (d) Both I and III

16. Two slits are separated by a distance of 0.5 mm and illuminated with light of $\lambda = 6000$ Å. If the screen is placed 2.5 m from the slits, the distance of the third bright image from the centre will be

(a) 1.5 mm (b) 3 mm
(c) 6 mm (d) 9 mm

17. If one of the slit of a standard Young's double slit experiment is covered by a thin parallel sided glass slab so that it transmits only one-half the light intensity of the other, then choose the incorrect option.

(a) The fringe pattern will get shifted towards the covered slit
(b) The fringe pattern will get shifted away from the covered slit
(c) The bright fringes will be less bright and the dark ones will be more bright
(d) The fringe width will remain unchanged

18. Assertion (A) In interference, all the fringes are of same width.

Reason (R) In interference, fringe width is independent of position of the fringe.

In the light of the above statements, choose the correct answer from the options given below :

(a) Both A and R are true but R is not the correct explanation of A.
(b) A is true but R is false.
(c) A is false but is R true.
(d) Both A and R are true and R is the correct explanation of A.

19. Bichromatic light of wavelengths $\lambda_1 = 5000$ Å and $\lambda_2 = 7000$ Å are used in Young's double slit experiment. Then,

(a) 14th order maxima of λ_1 will coincide with 10th order maxima of λ_2
(b) 21st order maxima of λ_2 will coincide with 15th order maxima of λ_1
(c) 14th order minima of λ_1 will coincide with 8th order minima of λ_2
(d) 3rd order minima of λ_1 will coincide with 4th order minima of λ_2

20. For light diverging from a point source,

(a) the wavefront is spherical
(b) the intensity increases in proportion to the distance squared
(c) the wavefront is parabolic
(d) the intensity at the wavefront does not depend on the distance

21. In a Young's double slit experiment, the slit separation is 1 mm and the screen is 1m from the slit. For a monochromatic light of wavelength 500 nm, the distance of 3rd minima from the central maxima is

(a) 4.75 mm (b) 3.36 mm
(c) 1.25 mm (d) 2.25 mm

22. Assertion (A) If phase difference between the light waves emerging from the slits of the Young's experiment is π radian, the central fringe will be dark.

Reason (R) Phase difference is equal to $(2\pi/\lambda)$ times of path difference.

In the light of the above statements, choose the correct answer from the options given below

(a) Both A and R are true but R is not the correct explanation of A.
(b) A is true but R is false.
(c) A is false but R is true.
(d) Both A and R are true and R is the correct explanation of A.

23. Two slits at a distance of 1 mm are illuminated by a light of wavelength 6.5×10^{-7} m. The interference fringes are observed on a screen placed at a distance of 1 m. The distance between third dark fringe and fifth bright fringe will be
(a) 0.65 mm (b) 1.63 mm (c) 3.25 mm (d) 4.88 mm

24. Which of the following pair is incorrect?
(a) Position of bright fringe — $Y_{\text{bright}} = \dfrac{n\lambda}{d}D$
(b) Position of dark fringe — $Y_{\text{dark}} = \dfrac{(2n-1)\lambda}{2d}D$
(c) Distance between two adjacent bright (or dark) fringes — $\beta = \dfrac{2\lambda D}{d}$
(d) Angular width of fringes — $\theta = \dfrac{\beta}{D}$

Module 3
Diffraction and Polarisation

- Diffraction of Light • Fraunhofer diffraction of Light Due to a Single Slit • Width of Central Maxima
- Polarisation of Light • Malus' Law

Diffraction of Light

The phenomenon of bending of light around the corners of an obstacle/aperture of the size of the wavelength is called **diffraction.** Other waves, such as sound waves and water waves, also have this property of spreading when passing through apertures or by sharp edges.

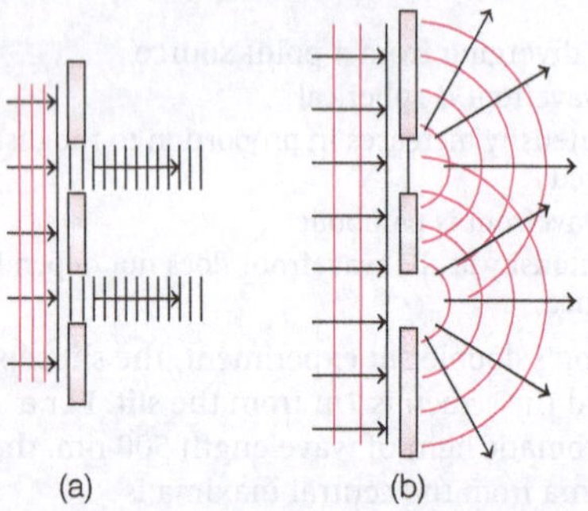

(a) If light waves did not spread out after passing through the slits, no interference would occurs. (b) The light waves from the two slits overlap as they spread out, filling the shadowed regions with light and producing interference fringes.

Diffraction Pattern

In general, diffraction occurs when waves pass through small openings, around obstacles or pass through sharp edges, as shown in figure. When an opaque object is placed between a point source of light and a screen, no sharp boundary exists on the screen between a shadowed region and an illuminated region. The illuminated region above the shadow of the object contains alternating light and dark fringes. Such a display is called a diffraction pattern.

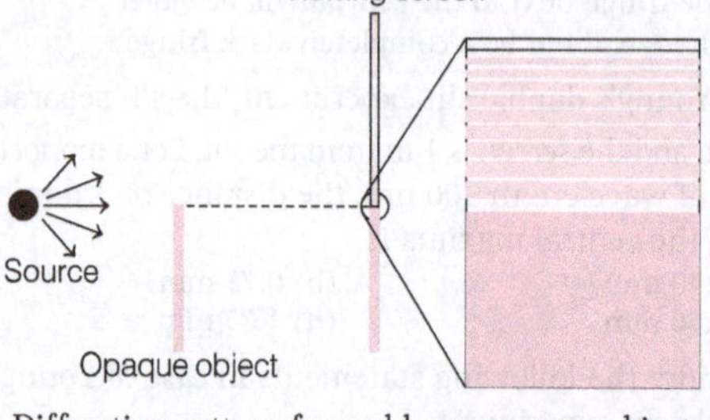

Diffraction pattern formed by an opaque object

In reality, light bends around the top edge of the object and enter this region. Because of these effects, a diffraction pattern consisting of bright and dark fringes appears in the region above.

Types of Diffraction of Light

The phenomenon of diffraction is divided mainly in the following two classes

(i) Fresnel diffraction

If source and screen are at finite distance from the obstacle or aperture, then diffraction observed is known as Fresnel diffraction (as shown in the figure).

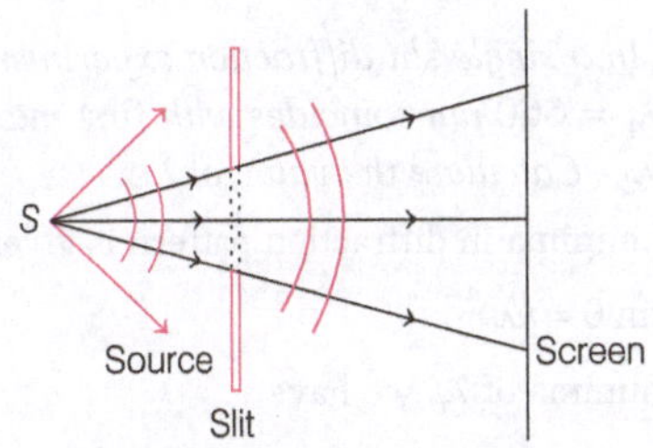

Fresnel diffraction through a slit

(ii) Fraunhofer Diffraction

When all the rays passing through a narrow slit are approximately parallel to one another, this can be achieved experimentally either by placing the screen far from the opening used to create the diffraction or by using a converging lens to focus the rays once they pass through the opening, as shown in figure.

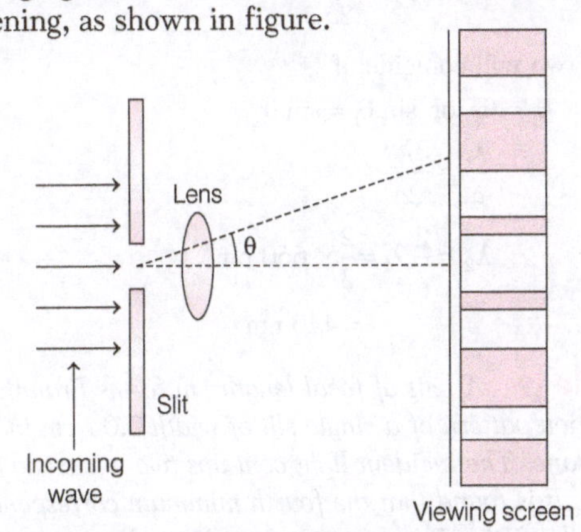

Fraunhofer diffraction pattern of a single slit. The pattern consists of a central bright fringe flanked by much weaker maxima alternating with dark fringes.

The diffraction produced in such an arrangement is called Fraunhofer diffraction.

Fraunhofer Diffraction of Light due to a Single Slit

Suppose a plane wavefront is incident on a slit AB (of width a). Each and every part of the exposed part of the plane wavefront (*i.e.* every part of the slit) acts as a source of secondary wavelets spreading in all directions.

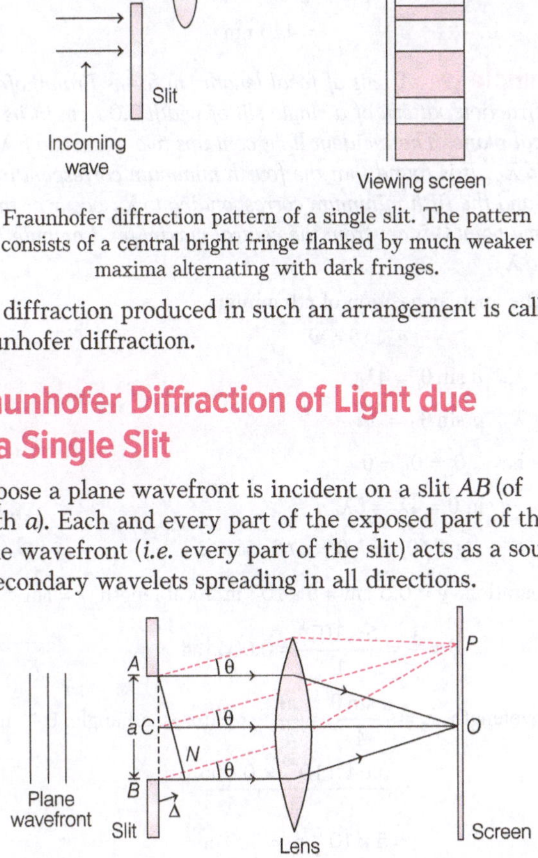

A plane wavefront is incident on the slit AB, which forms a diffraction pattern on the screen

The diffraction is obtained on a screen placed at a large distance. (In practice, this condition is achieved by placing the screen at the focal plane of a converging lens placed just after the slit).

The diffraction pattern consists of a central bright fringe (central maxima) surrounded by dark and bright lines (called **secondary minima** and **maxima**).

At point O on the screen, the central maxima is obtained. The wavelets originating from points A and B meet in the same phase at this point, hence at point O, intensity is maximum.

Secondary minima For obtaining nth secondary minima at point P on the screen, path difference between the diffracted waves $a\sin\theta = \pm n\lambda$, where $n = 1, 2, 3, \ldots$.

(i) Angular position of nth secondary minima,

$$\sin\theta \approx \theta = \frac{n\lambda}{a}$$

(ii) Distance of nth secondary minima from central maxima,

$$y_n = D\cdot\theta \Rightarrow \frac{n\lambda D}{a}$$

$$\boxed{y_n = \frac{n\lambda f}{a}}$$

where, D = distance between slit and screen,
$f \approx D$ = focal length of converging lens.

Secondary maxima For obtaining nth secondary maxima at point P on the screen, path difference $= a\sin\theta = (2n+1)\frac{\lambda}{2}$,

where $n = 1, 2, 3, \ldots$

(i) Angular position of nth secondary maxima,

$$\sin\theta \approx \theta = \frac{(2n+1)\lambda}{2a}$$

(ii) Distance of nth secondary maxima from central maxima,

$$y_n = D\cdot\theta = \frac{(2n+1)\lambda D}{2a}$$

$$\boxed{y_n = \frac{(2n+1)\lambda f}{2a}}$$

Example 14. *A screen is placed 50 cm from a single slit, which is illuminated with 6000 Å light. If distance between first and third minima in the diffraction pattern is 3 mm, what is the width of the slit?*

Sol. Given, $D = 50$ cm and $\lambda = 6000\text{ Å} = 6000 \times 10^{-10}$m

Distance between first and third minima,

$$y_3 - y_1 = \frac{3D\lambda}{a} - \frac{D\lambda}{a} = \frac{2D\lambda}{a}$$

$$\Rightarrow \quad 3\times 10^{-3} = \frac{2\times 0.5\times 6000\times 10^{-10}}{a}$$

Therefore, width of the slit, $a = 200\times 10^{-6}\text{m} = 0.2\text{ mm}$

Example 15. *A beam of light of wavelength 400 nm falls on a narrow slit and the resulting diffraction pattern is observed on a screen 2 m away from the slit. It is observed that 2nd order minima occurs at a distance of 2 mm from the position of central maxima. Find the width of the slit.*

Sol. Given, $\lambda = 400\text{nm} = 400 \times 10^{-9}\text{m}$,
$D = 2\text{m},\ y = 2\text{mm} = 2 \times 10^{-3}\text{m}$

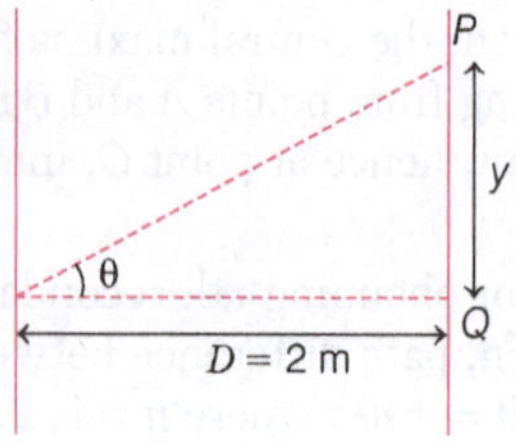

Let point P is the point of second order minima.

Now, $\sin\theta = \tan\theta \approx \theta = \dfrac{2 \times 10^{-3}}{2} = 10^{-3}$

Let the slit separation be a.

Now, for second order minima,

$$\theta = \frac{2\lambda}{a} = 10^{-3}$$

$$\Rightarrow \quad \frac{2 \times 400 \times 10^{-9}}{a} = 10^{-3}$$

Thus, we obtain $a = 0.8$ mm.

Example 16. *A beam of light of wavelength 600 nm from a distant source falls on a single slit 2 mm wide and the resulting diffraction pattern is observed on a screen 2m away. What is the distance between the first dark fringe on either side of central bright fringe?*

Sol. Given, $\lambda = 600$ nm, $a = 2 \times 10^{-3}\text{m}$ and $D = 2\text{m}$

Distance of first dark fringe from centre, $y_1 = \dfrac{D\lambda}{a}$

Distance between the first dark fringe on either side of the central bright fringe,

$$2y_1 = \frac{2D\lambda}{a} = \frac{2 \times 2 \times 600 \times 10^{-9}}{2 \times 10^{-3}} = 1200 \times 10^{-6}\text{m}$$

$$= 1.2 \times 10^{-3}\text{m} = 1.2\text{mm}$$

Example 17. *A slit of width d is illuminated by red light of wavelength 6500Å. For what value of d will the first maximum fall at angle of diffraction of 30°?*

Sol. For first secondary maximum of the diffraction pattern,

$$d\sin\theta = \frac{3\lambda}{2}$$

$$\therefore \quad d = \frac{3\lambda}{2\sin\theta} = \frac{3 \times 6500 \times 10^{-10}}{2 \times \sin 30°}$$

$$= 1.95 \times 10^{-6}\text{ m}$$

Example 18. *In a single slit diffraction experiment, first minima for $\lambda_1 = 660$ nm coincides with first maxima for wavelength λ_2. Calculate the value of λ_2.*

Sol. Position of minima in diffraction pattern is given by

$$a\sin\theta = n\lambda$$

For first minima of λ_1, we have

$$a\sin\theta_1 = (1)\lambda_1 \quad \text{or} \quad \sin\theta_1 = \frac{\lambda_1}{a} \qquad \text{...(i)}$$

The first maxima approximately lies between first and second minima. For wavelength λ_2, its position will be

$$a\sin\theta_2 = \frac{3}{2}\lambda_2$$

$$\therefore \quad \sin\theta_2 = \frac{3\lambda_2}{2a} \qquad \text{...(ii)}$$

The two will coincide, if

$$\theta_1 = \theta_2 \quad \text{or} \quad \sin\theta_1 = \sin\theta_2$$

$$\therefore \quad \frac{\lambda_1}{a} = \frac{3\lambda_2}{2a}$$

$$\text{or} \quad \lambda_2 = \frac{2}{3}\lambda_1 = \frac{2}{3} \times 660 \text{ nm}$$

$$= 440 \text{ nm}$$

Example 19. *A lens of focal length 1m forms Fraunhofer diffraction pattern of a single slit of width 0.04 cm in its focal plane. The incident light contains two wavelength λ_1 and λ_2. It is found that the fourth minimum corresponding to λ_1 and the fifth minimum corresponding to λ_2 occur at the same point 0.5 cm from the central maximum. Compute λ_1 and λ_2.*

Sol. The angular position of nth minima,

$$a\sin\theta = n\lambda$$

For λ_1, $a\sin\theta_1 = 4\lambda_1$ ...(i)

For λ_2, $a\sin\theta_2 = 5\lambda_2$ ...(ii)

We have, $\theta_1 = \theta_2 = \theta$

$$\therefore \quad a\sin\theta = 4\lambda_1 = 5\lambda_2 \qquad \text{...(iii)}$$

$$y = f\theta \Rightarrow \theta = y/f \qquad [\because D = f]$$

Separation, $y = 0.5 \text{ cm} = 5 \times 10^{-3}\text{m}$, focal length, $f = 1\text{m}$

$$\theta = \frac{y}{f} = \frac{5 \times 10^{-3}}{1} = 0.005 \text{ rad}$$

$$\text{Wavelength, } \lambda_1 = \frac{a\sin\theta}{4} = \frac{a\theta}{4} \quad (\text{for small angle, } \theta \simeq \sin\theta)$$

$$= \frac{0.04 \times 10^{-2} \times 0.005}{4}$$

$$= 5 \times 10^{-7}\text{ m} = 500\text{ nm}$$

$$\text{Wavelength, } \lambda_2 = \frac{4\lambda_1}{5} = \frac{4 \times 500}{5} = 400\text{ nm}$$

Width of Central Maxima

Diffraction pattern can be graphically shown as below

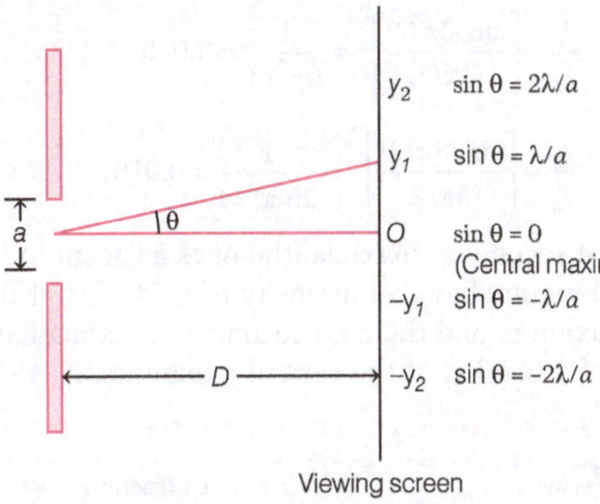

Fraunhofer diffraction pattern from a single slit of width *a*. The positions of two minima on each side of the central maximum are labelled.

The point *O* corresponds to the position of central maxima and the position $-3\lambda, -2\lambda, -\lambda, \lambda, 2\lambda, 3\lambda, \ldots$ are secondary minima. The above conditions for diffraction maxima and minima are exactly reverse of mathematical conditions for interference maxima and minima. The width of central maximum is the distance between first secondary minimum on either side of the central bright fringe at point *O*.

For first secondary minimum,

$$a \sin\theta = \lambda \quad \text{or} \quad \sin\theta = \frac{\lambda}{a} \qquad \ldots\text{(i)}$$

If θ is small, $\sin\theta \approx \theta = \frac{y}{D}$. ...(ii)

From Eqs. (i) and (ii), we get

$$\frac{y}{D} = \frac{\lambda}{a}$$

or

$$y = \frac{D\lambda}{a}$$

Width of central maximum $= 2y = \frac{2D\lambda}{a}$

As the slit width *a* increases, width of central maximum decreases.

Angular width of central maxima, $2\theta = \frac{2\lambda}{a}$.

Example 20. *Light of wavelength 580 nm is incident on a slit having a width of 0.300 mm. The viewing screen is 2.00 m from the slit. Find the position of the first dark fringe and the width of the central bright fringe.*

Sol. The two dark fringes that flank the central bright fringe correspond to $n = \pm 1$, hence we find that

$$\sin\theta = \pm\frac{\lambda}{a} = \pm\frac{5.80\times 10^{-7}\ \text{m}}{0.300\times 10^{-3}\ \text{m}} = \pm 1.93\times 10^{-3}$$

Therefore, the position of the first minima measured from the central axis are given by

$$y_1 \approx D\sin\theta = \pm D\frac{\lambda}{a} = \pm 2\times 1.93\times 10^{-3}$$

$$= \pm 3.86\times 10^{-3}\ \text{m}$$

The positive and negative signs correspond to the dark fringes on either side of the central bright fringe. Hence, the width of the central bright fringe is equal to

$$2|y_1| = 7.72\times 10^{-3}\ \text{m} = 7.72\ \text{mm}$$

Note that this value is much greater than the width of the slit. However, as the slit width is increased, the diffraction pattern narrows, corresponding to smaller values of θ. In fact, for large values of *a*, the various maxima and minima are so closely spaced that only a large central bright area resembling the geometric image of the slit is observed.

Example 21. *Angular width of central maximum in the Fraunhofer diffraction pattern of a slit is measured. The slit is illuminated by light of wavelength 6000 Å. When the slit is illuminated by light of another wavelength, then the angular width decreases by 30%. Calculate the wavelength of this light. The same decrease in the angular width of central maximum is obtained when the original apparatus is immersed in a liquid. Find the refractive index of the liquid.*

Sol. Angular width of central maximum $= \frac{2\lambda}{a}$

$$\Rightarrow \quad \theta_1 = \frac{2\lambda_1}{a} \qquad \ldots\text{(i)}$$

$$\theta_2 = \theta_1 \times 0.7 = \frac{2\lambda_2}{a} \qquad \ldots\text{(ii)}$$

On dividing Eq. (i) by Eq. (ii), we get

$$\frac{1}{0.7} = \frac{\lambda_1}{\lambda_2} = \frac{600}{\lambda_2} \qquad (\because \lambda_1 = 6000\,\text{Å} = 600\,\text{nm})$$

Wavelength, $\lambda_2 = 420\,\text{nm}$

When immersed in liquid, $\lambda_2 = \lambda_1/\mu$

Using Eqs. (i) and (ii), we get

$$\Rightarrow \quad \frac{2\lambda_1/\mu}{a} = \frac{2\lambda_1}{a}\times 0.7 \Rightarrow \frac{1}{0.7} = \mu$$

Refractive index of the liquid, $\mu = \frac{10}{7} = 1.42$

Intensity of Single Slit Diffraction Pattern

We can use phasors to determine the light intensity distribution for a single slit diffraction pattern. The proof is beyond our syllabus, we are just writing here the intensity at angle θ.

$$I = I_0\left[\frac{\sin\beta/2}{\beta/2}\right]^2$$

Here, $\frac{\beta}{2} = \frac{\pi a \sin\theta}{\lambda}$

or $I = I_0 \left[\frac{\sin(\pi a \sin\theta)/\lambda}{(\pi a \sin\theta)/\lambda}\right]^2$ (at angle θ)

Here, I_0 is the intensity at $\theta = 0°$ (the central maximum). From this result we see that minima occurs, when

$$\frac{\pi a \sin\theta}{\lambda} = m\pi \text{ or } \sin\theta = m\frac{\lambda}{a}$$

where, $m = \pm 1, \pm 2, \ldots$ (not zero)

Intensity Distribution Curve

The equation of minima gives the values of θ for which the diffraction pattern has zero light intensity, *i.e.* when a dark fringe is formed.

However, it tells us nothing about the variation in light intensity along the screen. The general features of the intensity distribution are shown in figure. A broad central bright fringe is observed, this fringe is flanked by much weaker bright fringes alternating with dark fringes. The various dark fringes occur at the values of θ. Each bright fringe peak lies approximately half-way between its bordering dark fringe minima.

Note that the central bright maximum is twice as wide as the secondary maxima.

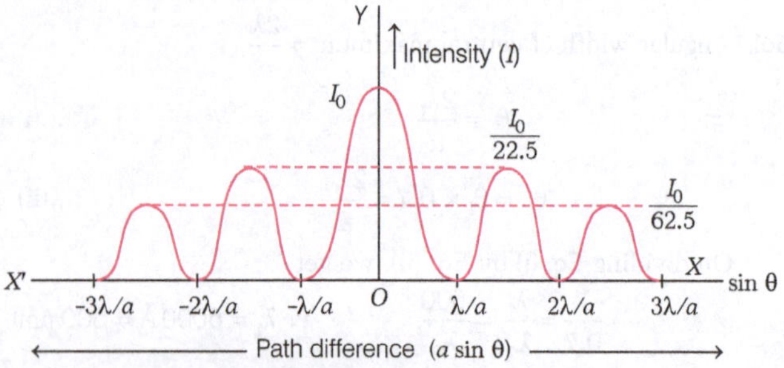

Intensity distribution curve on the screen in diffraction pattern with sin θ

Example 23. *Find the ratio of the intensities of the secondary maxima to the intensity of the central maximum for the single-slit Fraunhofer diffraction pattern.*

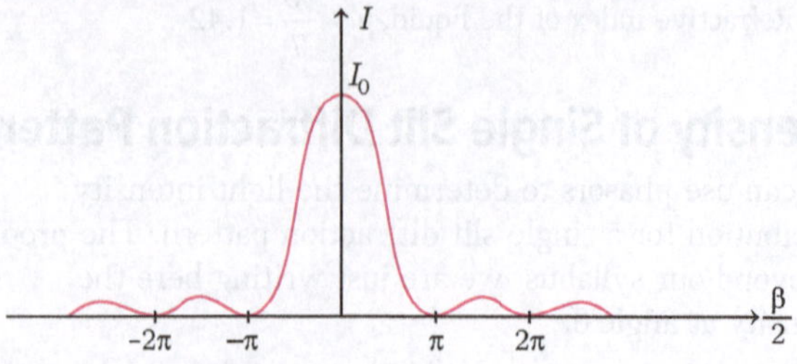

Sol. To a good approximation, the secondary maxima lie mid-way between the zero points. From figure, we see that this corresponds to β/2 values of 3π/2, 5π/2, 7π/2, ...

$$\therefore \quad \frac{I_1}{I_0} = \left[\frac{\sin(3\pi/2)}{(3\pi/2)}\right]^2 = \frac{1}{9\pi^2/4} = 0.045$$

$$\frac{I_2}{I_0} = \left[\frac{\sin(5\pi/2)}{5\pi/2}\right]^2 = \frac{1}{25\pi^2/4} = 0.016$$

i.e. the first secondary maxima (the ones adjacent to the central maximum) have an intensity of 4.5% that of the central maximum and the next secondary maxima have an intensity of 1.6% that of the central maximum.

Difference between Interference and Diffraction

Interference	Diffraction
It is due to superposition of waves from two coherent sources.	It is due to superposition of wavelets from same wavefronts.
All bright fringes are of same intensity.	Intensity decreases with the increase in the order of maxima.
The dark fringes are almost black.	Dark fringes are not perfectly black.
Fringes are of same width $\frac{\lambda D}{d}$.	The central maximum is of double the width of the secondary maxima, so width is not equal.
The number of bands is large.	The number of bands is small.
Bands are equally spaced.	Bands are unequally spaced.

Polarisation of Light

Light is an electromagnetic wave in which electric and magnetic field vectors vary sinusoidally perpendicular to each other as well as perpendicular to the direction of propagation of wave of light.

"The phenomenon of limiting the vibration of electric field vector in one direction in a plane perpendicular to the direction of propagation of light wave is called polarisation of light".

The plane perpendicular to the plane of oscillation is called **plane of polarisation.**

Note *In ordinary light (sunlight, bulb light, etc.), the electric field vectors are distributed in all directions is called* ***unpolarised light.***

Polaroids

These are thin film of ultramicroscopic crystals of herapathite or iodoquinine sulphate with their optic axis parallel to each other and it is used to produce the plane polarised light. It is based on the principle of selective absorption and is more effective than the tourmaline crystal.

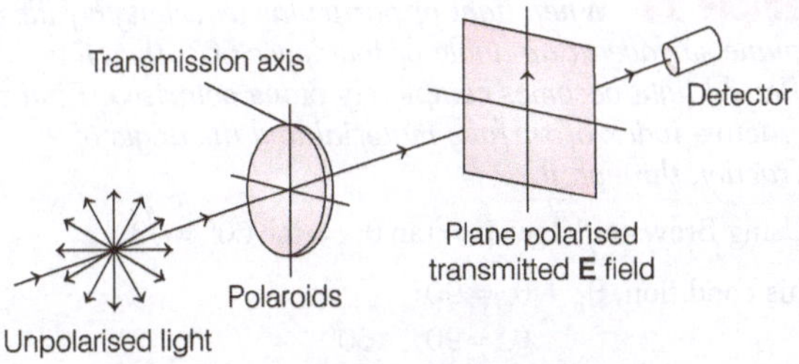

Unpolarised light passes through polaroids

(i) Polaroids allow the light oscillations parallel to the transmission axis to pass through them.

(ii) The crystal or polaroid on which unpolarised light is incident is called **polariser.** Crystal or polaroid on which polarised light is incident is called **analyser.**

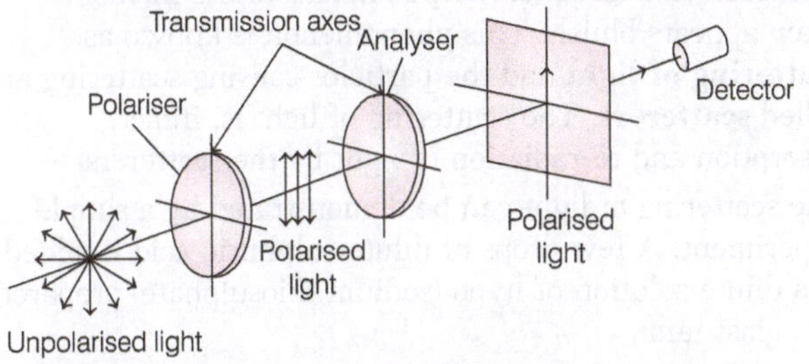

Transmission axis of the polariser and analyser are parallel to each other, so whole of the polarised light passes through analyser

(iii) If the transmission axis of analyser is perpendicular to that of the polariser, then no light passes through the analyser.

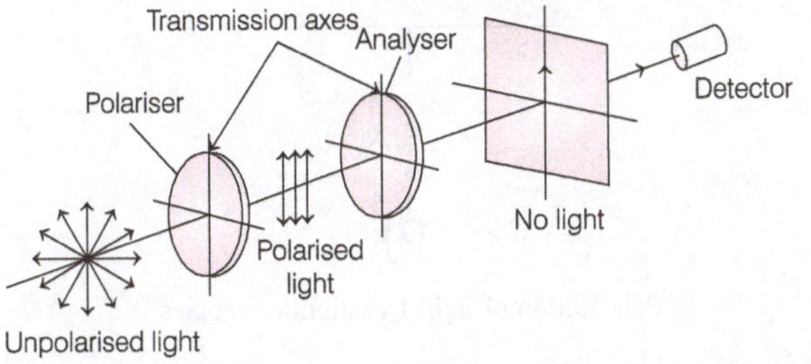

Transmission axis of the analyser is perpendicular to the polariser, hence no light passes through the analyser

Uses of Polaroids

Polaroids are used

(i) in sunglasses.

(ii) to prepare filters.

(iii) for laboratory purpose.

(iv) in head light of automobiles.

(v) in three-dimensional motion pictures.

(vi) to improve colour contrast in old paintings.

Malus' Law

This law states that "the intensity of the polarised light transmitted through the analyser varies as the square of the cosine of the angle between the plane of transmission of the analyser and the plane of the polariser".

If I_0 be the intensity of the polarised light incident on the analyser and θ be the angle between the transmission axes of the polariser and the analyser, the intensity of the light transmitted through the analyser is given by $I = I_0 \cos^2 \theta$.

NEET Close-up

Example Similar to PYQ Asked in NEET 2017

A linearly polarised light of intensity I_0 passes through an analyser making angle of 45° with polarised light.

Intensity of emitted light is

(a) I_0^2 (b) $2I$ (c) $I_0 / 2$ (d) $\sqrt{2}I_0$

Sol. (c) $I = I_0 \cos^2 \theta = I_0 \cos^2 45°$

$\Rightarrow$ $I = I_0/2$

Skill Builder

A linearly polarised light of intensity 20 lumen is incident on a polariser. Angle between polarised light and polariser, so that intensity of outgoing light becomes 15 lumen will be

(a) 30° (b) 45°
(c) 60° (d) 75°

For more Practice Refer Q.No. 13, 16 of Step-up practice 3 and Q.No. 74 of Gearing up for NEET.

Example 23. *Two polaroids are oriented with their planes perpendicular to incident light and transmission axis making an angle of 30° with each other. What fraction of incident unpolarised light is transmitted?*

Sol.

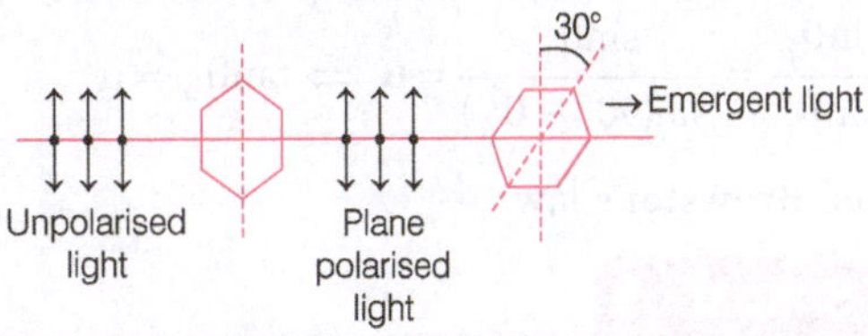

Suppose intensity of unpolarised light $= I'$

$\therefore$ Intensity of polarised light

$$= \frac{I'}{2}$$

Intensity of emergent light is $I = \frac{I'}{2} \cos^2 30° = \frac{I'}{2} \times \frac{3}{4} = \frac{3I'}{8}$

$\therefore$ Fraction of incident unpolarised light transmitted,

$$\frac{I}{I'} = \frac{3}{8}$$

or $$\frac{I}{I'} \times 100 = \frac{300}{8} = 37.5\%$$

Mentor's TiP

If an unpolarised light is converted into plane polarised light (say by passing it through a polaroid), then its intensity becomes half. *i.e.*

$I_0 = \frac{I_i}{2}$.

So, $I = \frac{I_i}{2}\cos^2\theta$

where, I_i = intensity of unpolarised light.

Polarisation by Reflection

When a beam of unpolarised light is reflected from a transparent medium (refractive index = μ), then the reflected light is completely plane polarised at a certain angle of incidence (called the **angle of polarisation** θ_p).

In this case, reflected and refracted waves are perpendicular to each other.

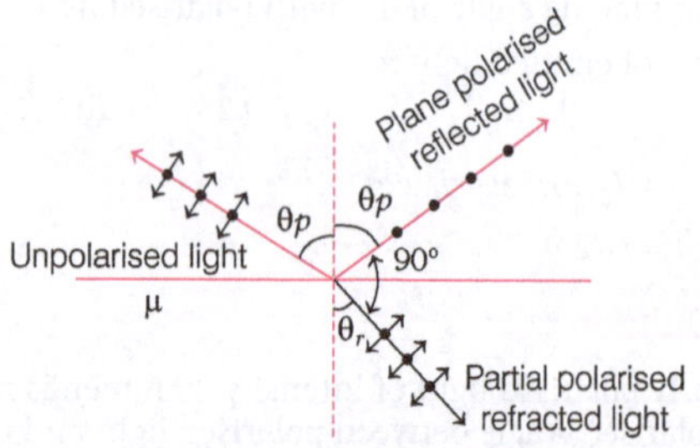

Polarisation of light by reflection

By Snell's law, $\frac{\sin\theta_p}{\sin\theta_r} = \mu$

Now, since reflected ray is perpendicular to refracted ray

$$90° + \theta_p + \theta_r = 180°$$

$$\Rightarrow \quad \theta_p + \theta_r = 90°$$

$$\Rightarrow \quad \theta_r = 90° - \theta_p$$

Now, $\frac{\sin\theta_p}{\sin\theta_r} = \frac{\sin\theta_p}{\sin(90° - \theta_p)} = \mu \Rightarrow \tan\theta_p = \mu$

It is called **Brewster's** law.

NEET Snapshot

The Brewster's angle θ_p for an interface should lies between 45° to 90°. *[NEET 2020]*

Since $\mu \geq 1$, so $\tan\theta_p \geq 1$

or $45° \leq \theta_p \leq 90°$

Example 24. *When light of particular wavelength falls on a plane surface at an angle of incidence 60°, then the reflected light becomes completely plane polarised. Find the refractive index of surface material and the angle of refraction through it.*

Sol. Using Brewster's law, $\mu = \tan\theta_p = \tan 60° = \sqrt{3}$

At this condition, $\theta_p + \theta_r = 90°$

$\therefore \quad \theta_r = 90° - 60°$

Angle of refraction, $\theta_r = 30°$

Polarisation of Light by Scattering

When a beam of white light passes through a medium consisting of small particles of size of the order of the wavelength of light (dust, smoke, air molecules), then the light seen in a direction perpendicular to the incident beam appears bluish. This phenomenon is known as **scattering of light** and the particles causing scattering are called **scatterers**. The scattering of light is, infact, absorption and re-radiation of light by the scatterers.

The scattering of light can be demonstrated by a simple experiment. A few drops of dilute sulphuric acid is added to a dilute solution of hypo (sodium thiosulphate) prepared in a glass tank.

A precipitate of fine sulphur particles is formed, the particles grow in size with time. Now, a beam of light from a bright source is sent through the tank. The light scattered by the sulphur particles in a direction at right angles to the incident light appears bluish as shown in figure below.

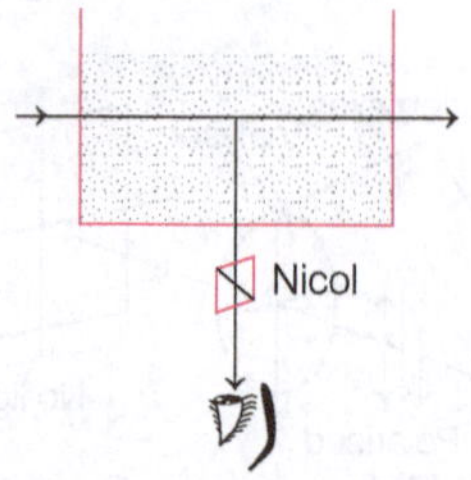

Polarisation of light by sulphur particles

When the scattered bluish light is seen through an analyser (*e.g.* a rotating Nicol) a variation in intensity with minimum intensity zero is found. This shows that the light scattered in a direction perpendicular to the incident light is plane polarised.

STEP UP Practice 3

1. In Fresnel's class of diffraction, the
   (a) obstacle screen distance is finite
   (b) the diffracted wavefront is considered as spherical
   (c) no convex lens is used to focus the diffraction fringes on the screen
   (d) All of the above

2. Angular width of central maxima in the Fraunhofer diffraction pattern of a slit is measured. The slit is illuminated by light of wavelength 5000 Å. When the slit is illuminated by light of another wavelength, the angular width decreases by 40%. The wavelength of this light will be
   (a) 6000 Å (b) 4200Å
   (c) 3000 Å (d) 1800 Å

3. In a single slit diffraction experiment, first minimum for red light (660 nm) coincides with first maximum of some other wavelength λ'. The value of λ' is
   (a) 4400 Å (b) 6600 Å
   (c) 2000 Å (d) 3500 Å

4. Direction of the first secondary maxima in the Fraunhofer diffraction pattern at a single slit is given by (*a* is the width of the slit)
   (a) $a \sin \theta = \frac{\lambda}{2}$
   (b) $a \cos \theta = \frac{3\lambda}{2}$
   (c) $a \sin \theta = \lambda$
   (d) $a \sin \theta = \frac{3\lambda}{2}$

5. **Statement I** We cannot get diffraction pattern from a wide slit illuminated by monochromatic light.
   Statement II In diffraction pattern, all the bright bands are not of the same intensity.
   In the light of the above statements, choose the most appropriate answer from the options given below.
   (a) Both Statement I and Statement II are incorrect.
   (b) Statement I is correct but Statement II is incorrect.
   (c) Statement I is incorrect but Statement II is correct.
   (d) Both Statement I and Statement II are correct.

6. A parallel monochromatic beam of light is incident normally on a narrow slit. A diffraction pattern is formed on a screen placed perpendicular to the direction of incident beam. At the first maximum of the diffraction pattern the phase difference between the rays coming from the edges of the slit is
   (a) 0 (b) $\frac{\pi}{2}$ (c) π (d) 2π

7. The angle of polarisation for any medium is 60°, what will be critical angle for this
   (a) $\sin^{-1}\sqrt{3}$ (b) $\tan^{-1}\sqrt{3}$
   (c) $\cos^{-1}\sqrt{3}$ (d) $\sin^{-1}\left(\frac{1}{\sqrt{3}}\right)$

8. When the angle of incidence on a material is 60°, then the reflected light is completely polarised. The velocity (in ms^{-1}) of the refracted ray inside the material is
   (a) 3×10^8 (b) $\left(\frac{3}{\sqrt{2}}\right) \times 10^8$
   (c) $\sqrt{3} \times 10^8$ (d) 0.5×10^8

9. **Statement I** Coloured spectrum is seen when we look through a muslin cloth.
   Statement II The coloured spectrum is due to diffraction of white light on passing through fine slits made by fine threads in the muslin cloth.
   In the light of the above statements, choose the most appropriate answer from the options given below.
   (a) Both Statement I and Statement II are incorrect.
   (b) Statement I is correct but Statement II is incorrect.
   (c) Statement I is incorrect but Statement II is correct.
   (d) Both Statement I and Statement II are correct.

10. When unpolarised light beam is incident from air onto glass ($n = 1.5$) at the polarising angle,
    (a) reflected beam is polarised 100 percent
    (b) reflected and refracted beams are partially polarised
    (c) the reason for option (a) is that almost all the light is reflected
    (d) All of the above

11. Light is incident on a glass surface at polarising angle of 57.5°. Then, the angle between the incident ray and the refracted ray is
    (a) 57.5° (b) 115°
    (c) 65° (d) 205°

12. I. For diffraction through a single slit, the wavelength of wave must be comparable to the size of slit.
    II. The diffraction is very common in sound waves but not so common in light waves.
    III. Diffraction is only observed in electromagnetic waves.
    Which of the given statement(s) is/are correct for phenomenon of diffraction?
    (a) Only I
    (b) Both II and III
    (c) Both I and II
    (d) I, II and III

13. A beam of natural light falls on a system of 6 polaroids, which are arranged in succession such that each polaroid is turned through 30° with respect to the preceding one. The percentage of incident intensity that passes through the system will be
(a) 100% (b) 50% (c) 30% (d) 12%

14. In the visible region of the spectrum the rotation of the plane of polarisation is given by $\theta = x + \frac{y}{\lambda^2}$. The optical rotation produced by a particular material is found to be 30° per mm at $\lambda = 5000$ Å and 50° per mm at $\lambda = 4000$ Å. The value of constant x will be
(a) $+\frac{50^\circ}{9}$ per mm (b) $-\frac{50^\circ}{9}$ per mm
(c) $+\frac{9^\circ}{50}$ per mm (d) $-\frac{9^\circ}{50}$ per mm

15. **Statement I** When tiny circular obstacle is placed in the path of light from some distance, a bright spot is seen at the centre of the shadow of the obstacle.
Statement II Destructive interference occurs at the centre of the shadow.
In the light of the above statements, choose the most appropriate answer from the options given below.
(a) Both Statement I and Statement II are incorrect.
(b) Statement I is correct but Statement II is incorrect.
(c) Statement I is incorrect but Statement II is correct.
(d) Both Statement I and Statement II are correct.

16. Two Nicols are oriented with their principal planes making an angle of 30°. The percentage of incident unpolarised light which passes through the system is
(a) 50% (b) 100%
(c) 12.5% (d) 37.5%

17. **Statement I** Radio waves can be polarised.
Statement II Sound waves in air are longitudinal in nature.
In the light of the above statements, choose the most appropriate answer from the options given below.
(a) Both Statement I and Statement II are incorrect.
(b) Statement I is correct but Statement II is incorrect.
(c) Statement I is incorrect but Statement II is correct.
(d) Both Statement I and Statement II are correct.

18. The angle of polarisation for any medium is 30°. What will be critical angle for this?
(a) $\sin^{-1}\sqrt{3}$
(b) $\tan^{-1}\sqrt{3}$
(c) $\cos^{-1}\sqrt{3}$
(d) $\sin^{-1}\frac{1}{\sqrt{3}}$

19. The reflected ray is found to be completely polarised when sunlight is incident on water surface at an angle of incident 53° and 45°. Now choose the correct pair from the given below.
(a) The angle of refraction when angle of incident ray is 53° → 45°
(b) The refractive index of water when angle of incident ray is 53° → $\frac{4}{3}$
(c) The angle of refraction when angle of incident ray is 45° → 30°
(d) The refractive index of water when angle of incident ray is 45° → $\frac{1}{\sqrt{2}}$

20. I. Dots and arrows indicates that both polarisations are present in the incident and refracted waves.
II. The reflected light is not linearly polarised.
III. Transmitted intensity will be zero when the axis of the analyser is in the plane of the figure.

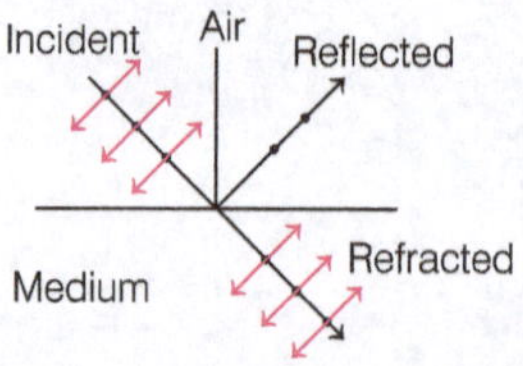

Which of the following statement(s) is/are correct with reference to the figure given?
(a) Only I
(b) Only II
(c) Both I and III
(d) Both I and II

NEET Exclusive EXTRA BYTES

- In interference, energy is redistributed from dark to fright fringes but no energy is created or destroyed. Thus, energy conservation law remains valid in interference.
- In interference,

  Intensity $\propto$ Slit width $\propto$ (Amplitude)^2
- If Young's double slit experiment is performed in any medium of refractive index μ, then λ fringe width and angular width all will decrease.
- Shape of fringes on the screen in YDSE is hyperbolic but if the screen is placed at very large distance from slits, then the hyperbola nearly looks straight line in shape.
- **Interference in thin films** Interference effects are commonly observed in thin films, such as thin layers of oil on water or the thin surface of a soap bubble.
- The varied colour's are observed when white light is incident on such films result from the interference of waves reflected from the two surfaces of the film.
- In diffraction,

  (i) Width of central maxima $\propto \lambda$.

  (ii) Width of central maxima is higher for narrower slit.
- Polarisation can occur only for transverse waves, which shows EM waves (optical waves) are transverse in nature.
- If a transverse mechanical wave is passed through a narrow slit, so that the plane of vibration of the wave is parallel to the slit, then the wave passes through the slit with its vibrations being unaffected and the wave is said to be plane polarised.

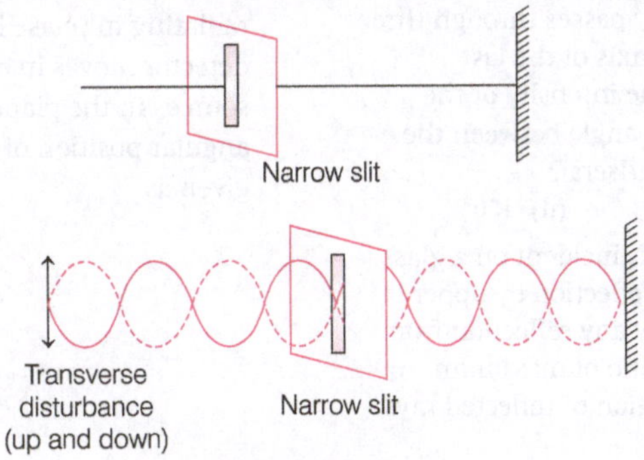

Polarisation of transverse wave

GEARING UP FOR NEET

Single Correct Option

1. Two waves of same frequency and same amplitude from two monochromatic sources are allowed to superpose at a certain point. If in one case, the phase difference is 0 and in other case it is $\pi/2$, then the ratio of the intensities in the two cases will be

(a) 1 : 1 (b) 2 : 1
(c) 4 : 1 (d) None of the above

2. In Young's double slit experiment, fringes of width β are produced on a screen kept at a distance of 1 m from the slit. When the screen is moved away by 5×10^{-2}m, fringe width changes by 3×10^{-5}m. The separation between the slits is 1×10^{-3}m. The wavelength of the light used is

(a) 500 nm (b) 400 nm (c) 600 nm (d) 800 nm

3. Unpolarised light of intensity 32 Wm^{-2} passes through three polarisers such that the transmission axis of the last polariser is crossed with the first. If the intensity of the emerging light is 3 Wm^{-2}. What is the angle between the transmission axes of the first two polarisers ?

(a) 60° (b) 45° (c) 90° (d) 120°

4. A parallel beam of light of intensity I is incident on a glass plate. 25% of light is reflected in any reflection by upper surface and 50% of light is reflected by any reflection from lower surface. Rest is refracted. The ratio of maximum to minimum intensity in interference region of reflected rays is

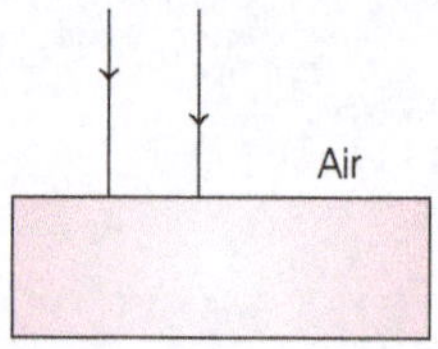

(a) $\left(\frac{\frac{1}{2}+\sqrt{\frac{3}{8}}}{\frac{1}{2}-\sqrt{\frac{3}{8}}}\right)^2$ (b) $\left(\frac{\frac{1}{4}+\sqrt{\frac{3}{8}}}{\frac{1}{2}-\sqrt{\frac{3}{8}}}\right)^2$

(c) $\frac{5}{8}$ (d) None of these

5. An interference is observed due to two coherent sources separated by a distance 5λ along Y-axis, where λ is the wavelength of light. A detector D is moved along the positive X-axis. The number of point on the X-axis excluding the points $x = 0$ and $x = \infty$ at which resultant intensity will be maximum, are

(a) 4 (b) 5
(c) ∞ (d) zero

6. Two coherent light sources A and B are at a distance 3λ from each other (λ = wavelength). The distance from A on the X-axis at which the interference is constructive, is

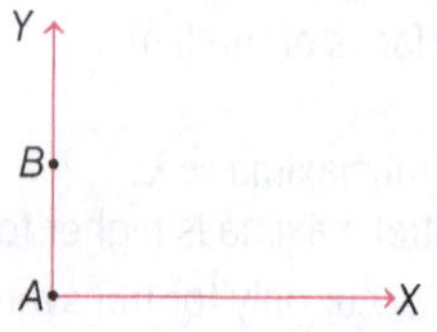

(a) 3λ (b) 8λ (c) $5\lambda/4$ (d) 8.75λ

7. Two coherent sources separated by distance d are radiating in phase having wavelength λ. A detector moves in a big circle around the two sources in the plane of the two sources. The angular position of $n = 4$ interference maxima is given as

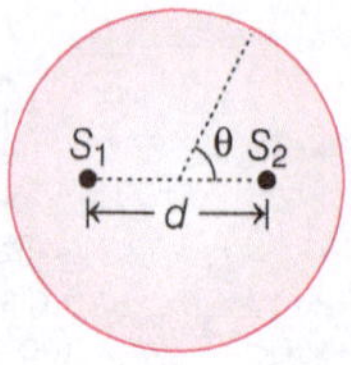

(a) $\sin^{-1}\frac{n\lambda}{d}$ (b) $\cos^{-1}\frac{4\lambda}{d}$

(c) $\tan^{-1}\frac{d}{4\lambda}$ (d) $\cos^{-1}\frac{\lambda}{4d}$

8. Consider a ray of light incident from air onto a slab of glass (refractive index n) of width d, at an angle θ. The phase difference between the ray reflected by the top surface of the glass and the bottom surface is **[NCERT Exemplar]**

(a) $\frac{4\pi nd}{\lambda}\left(1-\frac{1}{n^2}\sin^2\theta\right)^{-1/2}+\pi$

(b) $\frac{4\pi nd}{\lambda}\left(1-\frac{1}{n^2}\sin^2\theta\right)^{1/2}$

(c) $\frac{4\pi nd}{\lambda}\left(1-\frac{1}{n^2}\sin^2\theta\right)^{1/2}+\frac{\pi}{2}$

(d) $\frac{4\pi nd}{\lambda}\left(1-\frac{1}{n^2}\sin^2\theta\right)^{1/2}+2\pi$

9. In the diagram below, CP represents a wavefront and AO and BP, the corresponding incident rays. Find the condition of θ for constructive interference at point P between the rays BP and reflected ray OP

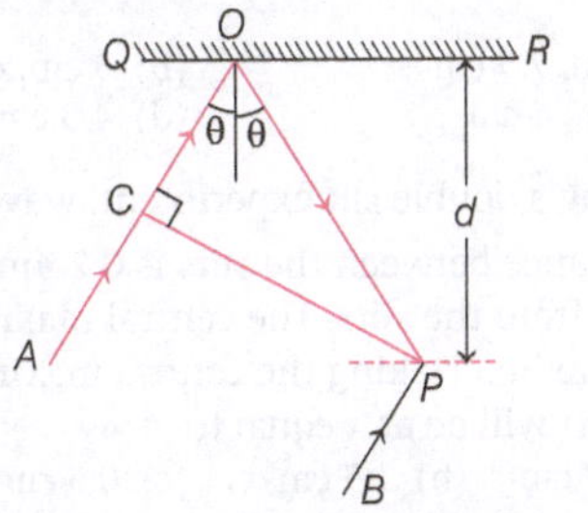

(a) $\cos\theta = 3\lambda/2d$ (b) $\cos\theta = \lambda/4d$
(c) $\sec\theta - \cos\theta = \lambda/d$ (d) $\sec\theta - \cos\theta = 4\lambda/d$

10. Wavefront is the locus of all points, where the particles of the medium vibrate with the same
(a) phase (b) amplitude
(c) frequency (d) period

11. To observe diffraction, the size of the obstacle
(a) should be much larger than the wavelength
(b) has no relation to wavelength
(c) should be of the order of wavelength
(d) should be $\lambda/2$, where λ is the wavelength

12. A beam of light of wavelength 590 nm is focussed by a converging lens of diameter 10 cm at a distance of 20 cm from it. Find the diameter of the disc image formed
(a) 2.9×10^{-4} cm (b) 7.51×10^{-4} cm
(c) 8.72×10^{-4} cm (d) 9.80×10^{-4} cm

13. Two coherent monochromatic beams of intensities I and $4I$ respectively, are superposed. Then, the maximum and minimum intensities in the resulting pattern are
(a) $5I$ and $3I$ (b) $9I$ and $3I$
(c) $4I$ and I (d) $9I$ and I

14. The condition for obtaining secondary maxima in the diffraction pattern due to single slit is
(a) $a\sin\theta = \frac{n\lambda}{2}$ (b) $a\sin\theta = (2n-1)\lambda/2$
(c) $a\sin\theta = n\lambda$ (d) $a\sin\theta = (2n-1)\lambda$

15. A fringe width of a certain interference pattern is $\beta = 0.002$ cm. What is the distance of 5th dark fringe from centre?
(a) 1×10^{-2} cm (b) 11×10^{-2} cm
(c) 1.1×10^{-2} cm (d) 3.28×10^{6} cm

16. A parallel beam of fast moving electrons is incident normally on a narrow slit. A fluorescent screen is placed at a large distance from the slit. If the speed of the electrons is increased, then which of the following statement is correct?
(a) Diffraction pattern is not observed on the screen in the case of electrons.
(b) The angular width of the central maximum of the diffraction pattern will increase.
(c) The angular width of the central maximum will decrease.
(d) The angular width of the central maximum will be unaffected.

17. In the case of light waves from two coherent sources S_1 and S_2, there will be constructive interference at an arbitrary point P, if the path difference, $S_1P - S_2P$ is
(a) $\left(n + \frac{1}{2}\right)\lambda$ (b) $n\lambda$
(c) $\left(n - \frac{1}{2}\right)\lambda$ (d) $\frac{\lambda}{2}$

18. In a single slit diffraction of light of wavelengths by a slit of width e, the size of the central maximum on a screen at a distance b is
(a) $2b\lambda + e$ (b) $\frac{2b\lambda}{e}$
(c) $\frac{2b\lambda}{e} + e$ (d) $\frac{2b\lambda}{e} - e$

19. In Young's double slit experiment, the fringe width is β. If entire arrangement is placed in a liquid of refractive index n, then the fringe width becomes
(a) $\frac{\beta}{n+1}$ (b) $n\beta$ (c) $\frac{\beta}{n}$ (d) $\frac{\beta}{n-1}$

20. Consider the sunlight incident on a slit of width 10^4 Å. The image seen through the slit shall ***[NCERT Exemplar]***
(a) be a fine sharp slit white in colour at the centre
(b) a bright slit white at the centre diffusing to zero intensities at the edges
(c) a bright slit white at the centre diffusing to regions of different colours
(d) only be a diffused slit white in colour

21. In Young's double slit experiment, the angular width of a fringe formed on a distant screen is 1°, the wavelength of light used is 6000 Å. The spacing between the slits is
(a) 6×10^{-7} m (b) 6.8×10^{-5} m (c) 3.4×10^{-5} m (d) 3.4×10^{-4} m

22. Monochromatic light from a narrow slit illuminates two parallel narrow slits producing an interference pattern on a screen. The separation between the two slits is now doubled and the distance between the screen and the slits is reduced to half. The fringe width
(a) is doubled (b) becomes four times
(c) becomes one-fourth (d) remains the same

23. Two slits separated by a distance of 1 mm, are illuminated with red light of wavelength 6.5×10^{-7} m. The interference fringes are observed on a screen placed 1 m from the slits. The distance between the third dark fringe and the fifth bright fringe is equal to
(a) 0.65 mm (b) 1.63 mm (c) 3.25 mm (d) 4.88 mm

24. In Young's double slit experiment, 12 fringes are observed to be formed in a certain segment of the screen, when light of wavelength 600 nm is used. If the wavelength of light is changed to 400 nm, number of fringes observed in the same segment of the screen is given by
(a) 12 (b) 18 (c) 24 (d) 30

25. A parallel beam of monochromatic light of wavelength 5000 Å is incident normally on a single narrow slit of width 0.001 mm. The light is focused by a convex lens on a screen placed on the focal plane. The first minima will be formed for the angle of diffraction equal to

(a) 0° (b) 15° (c) 30° (d) 60°

26. In Young's double slit experiment, the 10th maxima of wavelength λ_1 is at a distance of y_1 from the central maximum. When the wavelength of the source is changed to λ_2, 5th maxima is at a distance of y_2 from its central maximum. The ratio $\left(\frac{y_1}{y_2}\right)$ is

(a) $\frac{2\lambda_1}{\lambda_2}$ (b) $\frac{2\lambda_2}{\lambda_1}$ (c) $\frac{\lambda_1}{2\lambda_2}$ (d) $\frac{\lambda_2}{2\lambda_1}$

27. It is found that when waves of same intensity from two coherent sources superpose at a certain point, then the resultant intensity is equal to the intensity of one wave only. This means that the phase difference between the two waves at that point is

(a) zero (b) $\frac{\pi}{3}$ (c) $\frac{2\pi}{3}$ (d) π

28. Young's double slit experiment is performed in a liquid. The 10th bright fringe in liquid lies on screen where 6th dark fringe lies in vacuum. The refractive index of the liquid is approximately

(a) 1.8 (b) 1.54 (c) 1.67 (d) 1.2

29. In a Young's double slit experiment using red and blue lights of wavelengths 600 nm and 480 nm respectively, the value of n for which the nth red fringe coincides with $(n+1)$th blue fringe is

(a) 5 (b) 4 (c) 3 (d) 2

30. In Young's double slit experiment, how many maximas can be obtained on a screen (including the central maximum) on both sides of the central fringes, if $\lambda = 2000$ Å and $d = 7000$ Å?

(a) 12 (b) 7 (c) 18 (d) 4

31. A beam of light parallel to central line AB is incident on the plane of slits. The number of minima obtained on the large screen is n_1. Now, if the beam is tilted by some angle ($\neq 90°$) as shown in figure, then the number of minima obtained is n_2. Then,

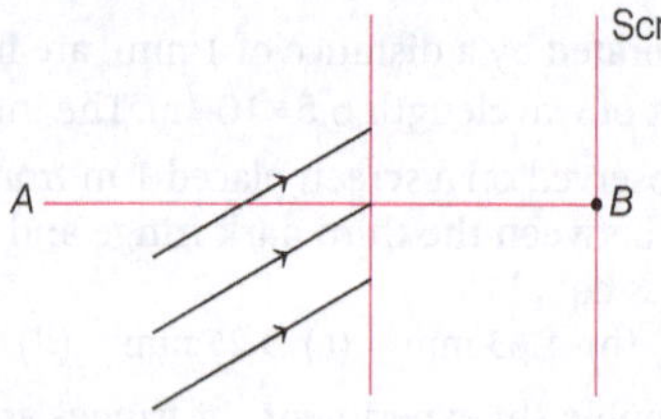

(a) $n_1 = n_2$ (b) $n_1 > n_2$
(c) $n_2 > n_1$ (d) n_2 will be zero

32. In a Young's double slit experiment, one of the slits is covered with a transparent sheet of thickness 3.6×10^{-3} cm due to which position of central fringe shifts to a position originally occupied by 30th bright fringe. The refractive index of the sheet, if $\lambda = 6000$ Å is

(a) 1.5 (b) 1.2
(c) 1.4 (d) 1.6

33. In Young's double slit experiment, the y-coordinates of central maximum and 10th maxima are 2 cm and 5 cm, respectively. When the YDSE apparatus is immersed in a liquid of refractive index 1.5. The corresponding y-coordinates will be

(a) 2 cm, 7.5 cm (b) 3 cm, 6 cm
(c) 2 cm, 4 cm (d) 4/3 cm, 10/3 cm

34. In Young's double slit experiment, wavelength $\lambda = 5000$ Å, the distance between the slits is 0.2 mm and the screen is at 200 cm from the slits. The central maxima is at $x = 0$. The third maxima (taking the central maxima as zeroth maxima) will be at x equal to

(a) 1.67 cm (b) 1.5 cm (c) 0.5 cm (d) 5.0 cm

35. In the Young's double slit experiment, the intensities at two points P_1 and P_2 on the screen are respectively I_1 and I_2. If P_1 is located at the centre of a bright fringe and P_2 is located at a distance equal to a quarter of fringe width from P_1, then $\frac{I_1}{I_2}$ is

(a) 2 (b) 3
(c) 4 (d) None of these

36. Figure shows a standard two slit arrangement with slits S_1, S_2. P_1, P_2 are the two minima points on either side of P (figure).

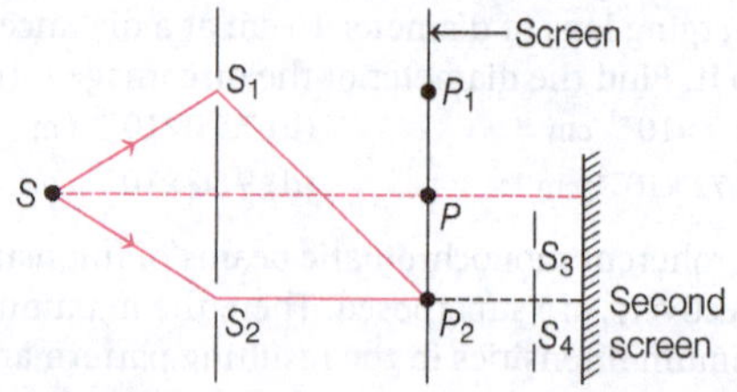

At point P_2 on the screen, there is a hole and behind P_2 is a second 2-slit arrangement with slits S_3, S_4 and a second screen behind them. ***[NCERT Exemplar]***

(a) There would be no interference pattern on the second screen but it would be lighted
(b) The second screen would be totally dark
(c) There would be a single bright point on the second screen
(d) There would be a regular two slit pattern on the second screen

37. In Young's double slit experiment, the two slits acts as coherent sources of equal amplitude A and wavelength λ. In another experiment with the same set up the two slits are sources of equal amplitude A and wavelength λ but are incoherent. The ratio of the intensity of light at the mid-point of the screen in the first case to that in the second case is

(a) 4 : 1 (b) 1 : 1 (c) 2 : 1 (d) 1 : 4

38. At two points P and Q on screen in Young's double slit experiment. Waves from slits S_1 and S_2 have a path difference of 0 and $\frac{\lambda}{4}$, respectively. The ratio of intensities at P and Q will be $m:1$. What is m here?

(a) 2 (b) 3 (c) 1 (d) 4

39. In the standard Young's double slit experiment, the intensity on the screen at a point distant 1.25 fringe widths from the central maximum is (assuming slits to be identical)
(a) $\frac{1}{2}I_{max}$ (b) $\frac{1}{4}I_{max}$ (c) $\frac{1}{3}I_{max}$ (d) I_{max}

40. In a Young's double slit experiment, D equals the distance of screen and d is the separation between the slits. The distance of the nearest point to the central maximum, where the intensity is same as that due to a single slit, is equal to
(a) $\frac{D\lambda}{d}$ (b) $\frac{D\lambda}{2d}$
(c) $\frac{D\lambda}{3d}$ (d) $\frac{2D\lambda}{d}$

41. The intensity of each of the two slits in Young's double slit experiment is I_0. Calculate the minimum separation between the two points on the screen where intensities are $2I_0$ and I_0. (Given, fringe width = α)
(a) $\frac{\alpha}{4}$ (b) $\frac{\alpha}{3}$ (c) $\frac{\alpha}{12}$ (d) None of these

42. The critical angle of a certain medium is $\sin^{-1}\left(\frac{3}{5}\right)$. The polarising angle of the medium is $\tan^{-1}\left(\frac{5}{n}\right)$. Find the value of n.
(a) 2 (b) 5
(c) 3 (d) 1

43. In a Young's double slit experiment, using unequal slit widths, the intensity at a point mid-way between a bright and dark fringes is $4I$. If one slit is covered by an opaque film, intensity at that point becomes $2I$. If the other is covered instead, then the intensity at that point is
(a) $2I$ (b) $5I$
(c) $(5+2\sqrt{2})\,I$ (d) $(5+4\sqrt{2})\,I$

44. Two ideal slits S_1 and S_2 are at a distance d apart and illuminated by light of wavelength λ passing through an ideal source slit S placed on the line through S_2 as shown below. The distance between the plane of slits and the source slit is D.

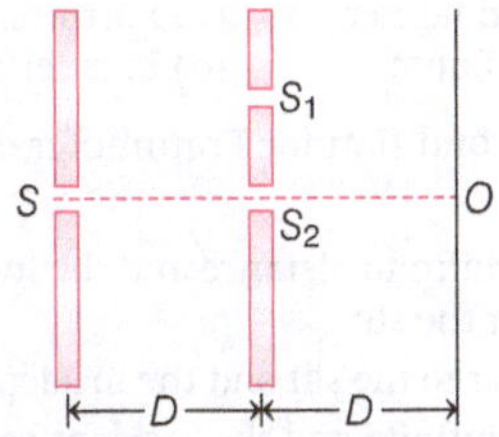

A screen is held at a distance D from the plane of the slits. The minimum value of d for which there is darkness at O is
(a) $\sqrt{\frac{3\lambda D}{2}}$ (b) $\sqrt{\lambda D}$
(c) $\sqrt{\frac{\lambda D}{2}}$ (d) $\sqrt{3\lambda D}$

45. The maximum numbers of possible interference maxima for slit separation equal to twice the wavelength in Young's double slit experiment, is
(a) infinite (b) five (c) three (d) zero

46. Light of wavelength λ is incident on slit of width d. The resulting diffraction pattern is observed on a screen placed at distance D. The linear width of central maxima is equal to width of the slit, then D is
(a) $\frac{2\lambda^2}{d}$ (b) $\frac{d^2}{2\lambda}$ (c) $\frac{d}{\lambda}$ (d) $\frac{2\lambda}{d}$

47. A beam of light contains two wavelengths 6500 Å and 5200 Å. They form interference fringes in Young's double slit experiment. What is the least distance (approx) from central maxima, where the bright fringes due to both wavelength coincide? The distance between the slits is 2 mm and distance between the screen and slit is 120 cm.
(a) 0.16 cm (b) 0.32 cm (c) 0.48 cm (d) 1.92 cm

48. The parallel beams of monochromatic light of wavelength 4.5×10^{-7} m passes through a long slit with width 0.2×10^{-3} m. The angular divergence in which most of the light is
(a) 4.5×10^{-3} rad (b) $4.5\,\pi$ rad
(c) 2.25×10^{-3} rad (d) 9×10^{-3} rad

49. In Young's double slit experiment, when wavelength used is 6000 Å and the screen is 40 cm from the slits, the fringes are 0.012 cm wide. What is the distance between the slits?
(a) 0.24 cm (b) 0.2 cm (c) 2.4 cm (d) 0.024 cm

50. A plane wave of wavelength 6250 Å is incident normally on a slit of width 2×10^{-2} cm. The width of the principal maximum of diffraction pattern on a screen at a distance of 50 cm will be
(a) 312.5×10^{-3} cm (b) 312.5×10^{-4} cm
(c) 312 cm (d) 312.5×10^{-5} cm

51. A plane polarised light is incident normally on a tourmaline plate. Its **E** vector make an angle of 60° with the optic axis of the plate. Find the percentage difference between initial and final intensities.
(a) 50% (b) 25%
(c) 75% (d) 90%

52. In Young's double slit experiment, the locus of the point P lying in a plane with a constant path difference between two interfering waves is
(a) a hyperbola (b) a straight line
(c) an ellipse (d) a parabola

53. In the Young's double slit experiment, the intensity of light at a point on the screen (where the path difference is λ) is K, (λ being the wavelength of light used). The intensity at a point where the path difference is $\lambda/4$, will be
(a) K (b) $K/4$
(c) $K/2$ (d) zero

54. In Young's double slit experiment, the ratio of maximum and minimum intensities in the fringe system is 9 : 1. The ratio of amplitudes of coherent sources is
(a) 9 : 1 (b) 3 : 1
(c) 2 : 1 (d) 1 : 1

55. In Young's double slit interference experiment, using two coherent waves of different amplitudes, the intensities ratio between bright and dark fringes is 3. Then, the value of the wave amplitudes ratio that arrive there is

(a) $\left(\frac{\sqrt{3}+1}{\sqrt{3}-1}\right)$ (b) $\left(\frac{\sqrt{3}-1}{\sqrt{3}+1}\right)$

(c) $\sqrt{3}:1$ (d) $1:\sqrt{3}$

56. In Young's double slit experiment, the slits are 2 mm apart and are illuminated by photons of two wavelengths $\lambda_1 = 12000$ Å and $\lambda_2 = 10000$ Å. At what minimum distance from the common central bright fringe on the screen 2 m from the slit will a bright fringe from one interference pattern coincide with a bright fringe from the other?

(a) 8 mm (b) 6 mm
(c) 4 mm (d) 3 mm

57. If two slits in Young's experiment are 0.4 mm apart and fringe width on a screen 200 cm away is 2 mm, the wavelength of light illuminating the slits is

(a) 500 nm (b) 600 nm
(c) 400 nm (d) 300 nm

58. Light of wavelength λ from a point source falls on a small circular obstacle of diameter d. Dark and bright circular rings around a central bright spot are formed on a screen beyond the obstacle. The distance between the screen and obstacle is D. Then, the condition for the formation of rings is

(a) $\sqrt{\lambda} \approx \frac{d}{4D}$ (b) $\lambda \approx \frac{d^2}{4D}$

(c) $d \approx \frac{\lambda^2}{D}$ (d) $\lambda \approx \frac{D}{4}$

59. A narrow slit of width 2 mm is illuminated by monochromatic light of wavelength 500 nm. The distance between the first minima on either side on a screen at a distance of 1 m is

(a) 5 mm (b) 6 mm
(c) 2 mm (d) 12 mm

60. When we close one slit in the Young's double slit experiment, then

(a) the bandwidth increased
(b) the bandwidth is decreased
(c) the bandwidth remains unchanged
(d) the diffraction pattern is observed

61. In Young's double slit experiment, the phase difference between the two waves reaching at the location of the third dark fringe is

(a) π (b) $\frac{3\pi}{2}$

(c) 5π (d) 3π

62. In Young's double slit experiment, the fringe width is 1×10^{-4} m. If the distance between the slit and screen is doubled and the distance between two slits is reduced to half and the wavelength is changed from 6.4×10^{-7} m to 4.0×10^{-7} m, then the value of new fringe width will be

(a) 2.5×10^{-4} m (b) 2.0×10^{-4} m
(c) 1×10^{-4} m (d) 0.5×10^{-4} m

63. In a Young's double slit interference experiment, the fringe width obtained with a light of wavelength 5900 Å was 1.2 mm for parallel narrow slits placed 2 mm apart. In this arrangement, if the slit separation is increased by one-and-half times the previous value, then the fringe width is

(a) 0.9 mm (b) 0.8 mm (c) 1.8 mm (d) 1.6 mm

64. In Young's double slit experiment, the angular width of the fringes is 0.20° for the sodium light ($\lambda = 5890$ Å). In order to increase the angular width of the fringes by 10%, the necessary change in wavelength is

(a) zero (b) increased by 6479 Å
(c) decreased by 589 Å (d) increased by 589 Å

65. In Young's double slit experiment, the intensity of light coming from one of the slits is doubled the intensity from the other slit. The ratio of the maximum intensity to the minimum intensity in the interference fringe pattern observed is

(a) 34 (b) 40 (c) 25 (d) 38

66. In Young's double slit experiment, if d, D and λ represents, the distance between the slits, the distance of the screen from the slits and wavelength of light used respectively, then the bandwidth is inversely proportional to

(a) λ (b) d (c) D (d) λ^2

67. In Young's double slit experiment, the two slits are separated by 1 mm and the screen is placed 1m away. The fringe separation for blue light of wavelength 500 nm is

(a) 10 mm (b) 0.5 mm (c) 20 mm (d) 15 mm

68. The slit width, when a light of wavelength 6500 Å is incident on a slit, if first minima for red light is at 30°, is

(a) 1×10^{-6} m (b) 5.2×10^{-6} m
(c) 1.3×10^{-6} m (d) 2.6×10^{-6} m

69. A grating which would be most suitable for constructing a spectrometer for the visible and ultraviolet region, should have

(a) 100 lines cm^{-1} (b) 1000 lines cm^{-1}
(c) 10000 lines cm^{-1} (d) 1000000 lines cm^{-1}

70. In a single slit diffraction experiment, the width of the slit is made double its original width. Then, the central maximum on the diffraction pattern will become

(a) narrower and fainter (b) narrower and brighter
(c) broader and fainter (d) broader and brighter

71. Find the right condition for Fraunhofer diffraction due to a single slit.

(a) Source is at infinite distance and the incident beam has converged at the slit.
(b) Source is near to the slit and the incident beam is parallel.
(c) Source is at infinity and the incident beam is parallel.
(d) Source is near to the slit and the incident beam has converged at the slit.

72. The polarising angle of glass is 57°. A ray of light which is incident at this angle will have an angle of refraction as

(a) 43° (b) 25°
(c) 38° (d) 33°

73. The angle of incidence at which reflected light is totally polarised for refraction from air to glass (refractive index μ) is

(a) $\sin^{-1}\mu$ (b) $\sin^{-1}\left(\frac{1}{\mu}\right)$ (c) $\tan^{-1}\left(\frac{1}{\mu}\right)$ (d) $\tan^{-1}(\mu)$

74. A polarised light of intensity I_0 is passed through another polariser whose pass axis makes an angle of 60° with the pass axis of the former. What is the intensity of emergent polarised light from second polariser?

(a) $I = I_0$ (b) $I = I_0/6$
(c) $I = I_0/5$ (d) $I = I_0/4$

75. Which of the following phenomena support the wave theory of light?

1. Scattering
2. Interference
3. Diffraction
4. Velocity of light in a denser medium is less than the velocity of light in the rarer medium.

(a) 1, 2 and 3 (b) 1, 2 and 4 (c) 2, 3 and 4 (d) 1, 3 and 4

76. The critical angle of a certain medium is $\sin^{-1}\left(\frac{3}{5}\right)$. The polarising angle of the medium is

(a) $\sin^{-1}\left(\frac{4}{5}\right)$ (b) $\tan^{-1}\left(\frac{5}{3}\right)$
(c) $\tan^{-1}\left(\frac{3}{4}\right)$ (d) $\tan^{-1}\left(\frac{4}{3}\right)$

Assertion and Reason

Directions (Q. Nos. 1-5) *These questions consist of two statements each linked as Assertion and Reason. While answering these questions you are required to choose any one of the following four responses.*

(a) Both A and R are true but R is not the correct explanation of A.
(b) A is true but R is false.
(c) A is false but R is true.
(d) Both A and R are true and R is the correct explanation of A.

1. **Assertion** (A) Two coherent sources transmit waves of equal intensity I_0. Resultant intensity at a point where path difference is $\frac{\lambda}{3}$ is also I_0.

Reason (R) In interference, resultant intensity at any point is the average intensity of two individual intensities.

2. **Assertion** (A) In Young's double slit experiment, ratio of $\frac{I_{max}}{I_{min}}$ is infinite.

Reason (R) If width of any one of the slits is slightly increased, then this ratio will decrease.

3. **Assertion** (A) When the screen is moved closed to the plane of slits, then fringe width increases.

Reason (R) Fringe width is directly proportional to the distance between the screen and plane of slits.

4. **Assertion** (A) When monochromatic light source is replaced by source of white light, then central fringe will be white.

Reason (R) Fringe width does not depend on the wavelength of light used.

5. **Assertion** (A) The unpolarised light and polarised light can be distinguished from each other by using polaroid.

Reason (R) A polaroid is capable of producing plane polarised beam of light.

Statement Type Questions

Directions (Q. Nos. 1-5) *These questions consist of two statements, choose the most appropriate answer from the options given below.*

(a) Both Statement I and Statement II are incorrect.
(b) Statement I is correct but Statement II is incorrect.
(c) Statement I is incorrect but Statement II is correct.
(d) Both Statement I and Statement II are correct.

1. **Statement I** Two coherent sources always have constant phase relationship.

Statement II White light from two coherent sources is reaching the screen. If the path difference at a point on the screen for yellow light is $\frac{3\lambda}{2}$, then the fringe at that point will be coloured.

2. **Statement I** When Young's double slit experiment performed with a source of white light, only black and white fringes are observed.

Statement II White light does not disperse in different colours in case of interference.

3. **Statement I** In interference of two waves, all bright fringes are of same intensity.

Statement II In diffraction, bands are unequally spaced.

4. **Statement I** In YDSE, bright and dark fringe are equally spaced.

Statement II Fringe width only depends upon phase difference.

5. **Statement I** In Young's double slit experiment, interference pattern disappears when one of the slit is closed.

Statement II Interference occurs due to superposition of light waves from two coherent sources.

Match the Columns

1. Two waves from coherent sources meet at a point in a phase difference of ϕ. Both the waves have some intensities. Match the following columns.

Column I	Column II
A. If $\phi = 60°$	I. Resultant intensity will become four times.
B. If $\phi = 90°$	II. Resultant intensity will become two times.
C. If $\phi = 0°$	III. Resultant intensity will remain unchanged.
D. If $\phi = 120°$	IV. Resultant intensity will become three times.

Choose the correct answer from the options given below.

(a) A-IV, B-II, C-I, D-III
(b) A-I, B-II, C-IV, D-III
(c) A-II, B-III, C-I, D-IV
(d) A-I, B-III, C-II, D-IV

2. Match the Column I (location of the dark fringe) to Column II (phase difference between two waves in YDSE).

Column I	Column II
A. $n = 4$	I. 11π
B. $n = 2$	II. 9π
C. $n = 5$	III. 7π
D. $n = 6$	IV. 3π

Choose the correct answer from the options given below.

(a) A-I, B-II, C-III, D-IV
(b) A-III, B-IV, C-II, D-I
(c) A-IV, B-III, C-I, D-II
(d) A-III, B-IV, C-I, D-II

3. In the Young's double slit experiment as shown in the figure, Δx is the path difference between waves at a point on screen. Now, a thin transparent glass sheet is introduced infront of S_1 which absorbed 75% of light incident on it.

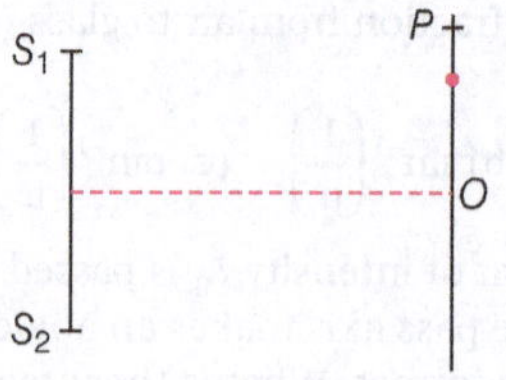

Match the Column I with Column II .

Column I	Column II
A. Intensity of maxima will	I. Increase
B. Intensity of minima will	II. Decrease
C. Fringe width will	III. Remains same
D. Fringe pattern will	IV. Shift downward

Choose the correct answer from the options given below.

(a) A-I, B-II, C-IV, D-III
(b) A-II, B-I, C-III, D-IV
(c) A-IV, B-III, C-II, D-I
(d) A-III, B-IV, C-I, D-II

4. Match the Column I (critical angle of certain medium) with with Column II (polarising angle of medium).

Column I	Column II
A. $\sin^{-1}\left(\frac{1}{\sqrt{3}}\right)$	I. 30°
B. $\sin^{-1}\left(\frac{4}{3}\right)$	II. 45°
C. $\sin^{-1}(1)$	III. 37°
D. $\sin^{-1}(\sqrt{3})$	IV. 60°

Choose the correct answer from the options given below.

(a) A-IV, B-III, C-II, D-I
(b) A-III, B-IV, C-I, D-II
(c) A-I B-II, C-III, D-IV
(d) A-II, B-I, C-III, D-IV

Final Check Through PYQs

Module-I Huygens' Principle and Interference

1. The interference pattern is obtained with two coherent light sources of intensity ratio n. In the interference pattern, the ratio $\frac{I_{max}-I_{min}}{I_{max}+I_{min}}$ will be ***[NCERT (New) Pg. 265, NEET 2016]***

(a) $\frac{\sqrt{n}}{n+1}$ (b) $\frac{2\sqrt{n}}{n+1}$
(c) $\frac{\sqrt{n}}{(n+1)^2}$ (d) $\frac{2\sqrt{n}}{(n+1)^2}$

Module-II Young's Double Slit Experiment

2. If the monochromatic source in Young's double slit experiment is replaced by white light, then ***[NCERT (New) Pg. 266, NEET 2024]***
(a) interference pattern will disappear
(b) there will be a central dark fringe surrounded by a few coloured fringes
(c) there will be a central bright white fringe surrounded by a few coloured fringes
(d) all bright fringes will be of equal width

3. For Young's double slit experiment, two statements are given below ***[NCERT (New) Pg. 266, NEET 2023]***
Statement I If screen is moved away from the plane of slits, angular separation of the fringes remains constant.
Statement II If the monochromatic source is replaced by another monochromatic source of larger wavelength, the angular separation of fringes decreases.
In the light of the above statements, choose the correct answer from the options given below
(a) Both Statement I and Statement II are incorrect.
(b) Statement I is correct but Statement II is incorrect.
(c) Statement I is incorrect but Statement II is correct.
(d) Both Statement I and Statement II are correct.

4. In a Young's double slit experiment, a student observes 8 fringes in a certain segment of screen when a monochromatic light of 600 nm wavelength is used. If the wavelength of light is changed to 400 nm, then the number of fringes he would observe in the same region of the screen is ***[NCERT (New) Pg. 266, NEET 2022]***
(a) 8 (b) 9 (c) 12 (d) 6

5. Two coherent sources of light interfere and produce fringe pattern on a screen. For central maximum, the phase difference between the two waves will be ***[NCERT (New) Pg. 264, NEET (Oct.) 2020]***
(a) zero (b) π
(c) $3\pi/2$ (d) $\pi/2$

6. In Young's double slit experiment, if the separation between coherent sources is halved and the distance of the screen from the coherent sources is doubled, then the fringe width becomes ***[NCERT (New) Pg. 266, NEET (Sep.) 2020]***
(a) half (b) four times
(c) one-fourth (d) double

7. In a Young's double slit experiment, if there is no initial phase difference between the light from the two slits, a point on the screen corresponding to the fifth minimum has path difference is ***[NCERT (New) Pg. 266, NEET (Odisha) 2020, 19]***
(a) $5\frac{\lambda}{2}$ (b) $10\frac{\lambda}{2}$
(c) $9\frac{\lambda}{2}$ (d) $11\frac{\lambda}{2}$

8. In a double slit experiment, when light of wavelength 400 nm was used, the angular width of the first minima formed on a screen placed 1 m away, was found to be 0.2°. What will be the angular width of the first minima, if the entire experimental apparatus is immersed in water? ($\mu_{water} = 4/3$) ***[NCERT (New) Pg. 266, NEET (National) 2019]***
(a) 0.15° (b) 0.051° (c) 0.1° (d) 0.266°

9. In Young's double slit experiment the separation d between the slits is 2 mm, the wavelength λ of the light used is 5896 Å and distance D between the screen and slits is 100 cm. It is found that the angular width of the fringes is 0.20°. To increase the fringe angular width to 0.21° (with same λ and D) the separation between the slits needs to be changed to ***[NCERT (New) Pg. 266, NEET 2018]***
(a) 1.8 mm (b) 1.9 mm
(c) 2.1 mm (d) 1.7 mm

10. Young's double slit experiment is first performed in air and then in a medium other than air. It is found that 8th bright fringe in the medium lies where 5th dark fringe lies in air. The refractive index of the medium is nearly *[NCERT (New) Pg. 266, NEET 2017]*
(a) 1.25 (b) 1.59
(c) 1.69 (d) 1.78

11. The intensity at the maximum in a Young's double slit experiment is I_0. Distance between two slits is $d = 5\lambda$, where λ is the wavelength of light used in the experiment. What will be the intensity infront of one of the slits on the screen placed at a distance $D = 10\,d$? *[NCERT (New) Pg. 266, NEET 2016]*
(a) $\frac{I_0}{4}$ (b) $\frac{3}{4}I_0$ (c) $\frac{I_0}{2}$ (d) I_0

12. In a double slit experiment, the two slits are 1 mm apart and the screen is placed 1 m away. A monochromatic light of wavelength 500 nm is used. What will be the width of each slit for obtaining ten maxima of double slit within the central maxima of single slit pattern? *[NCERT (New) Pg. 266, AIPMT 2015]*
(a) 0.2 mm (b) 0.1 mm
(c) 0.5 mm (d) 0.02 mm

13. Two slits in Young's experiment have widths in the ratio 1 : 25. The ratio of intensity at the maxima and minima in the interference pattern $\frac{I_{max}}{I_{min}}$ is *[NCERT (New) Pg. 266, AIPMT 2015]*
(a) $\frac{9}{4}$ (b) $\frac{121}{49}$ (c) $\frac{49}{121}$ (d) $\frac{4}{9}$

Module-III Diffraction and Polarisation

14. An unpolarised light beam strikes a glass surface at Brewster's angle, then *[NCERT (Old) Pg. 379, NEET 2024]*
(a) the reflected light will be partially polarised
(b) the refracted light will be completely polarised
(c) both the reflected and refracted light will be completely polarised
(d) the reflected light will be completely polarised but the refracted light will be partially polarised

15. A light ray falls on a glass surface of refractive index $\sqrt{3}$ at an angle 60°. The angle between the refracted and reflected rays would be *[NCERT (Old) Pg. 379, NEET 2022]*
(a) 60° (b) 90°
(c) 120° (d) 30°

16. The Brewster's angle I_B for an interface should be *[NCERT (Old) Pg. 379, NEET (Sep.) 2020]*
(a) $30° < I_B < 45°$ (b) $45° < I_B < 90°$
(c) $I_B = 90°$ (d) $0° < I_B < 30°$

17. Angular width of the central maxima in the Fraunhofer diffraction for $\lambda = 6000$ Å is θ_0. When the same slit is illuminated by another monochromatic light, the angular width decreases by 30%. The wavelength of this light is *[NCERT (Old) Pg. 369, NEET (Odisha) 2019]*
(a) 1800 Å (b) 4200 Å (c) 6000 Å (d) 420 Å

18. Unpolarised light is incident from air on a plane surface of a material of refractive index μ. At a particular angle of incidence i, it is found that the reflected and refracted rays are perpendicular to each other. Which of the following options is correct for this situation? *[NCERT (Old) Pg. 380, NEET 2018]*
(a) $i = \sin^{-1}\left(\frac{1}{\mu}\right)$
(b) Reflected light is polarised with its electric vector perpendicular to the plane of incidence
(c) Reflected light is polarised with its electric vector parallel to the plane of incidence
(d) $i = \tan^{-1}\left(\frac{1}{\mu}\right)$

19. Two polaroids P_1 and P_2 are placed with their axis perpendicular to each other. Unpolarised light I_0 is incident on P_1. A third polaroid P_3 is kept in between P_1 and P_2 such that its axis makes an angle 45° with that of P_1. The intensity of transmitted light through P_2 is *[NCERT (Old) Pg. 271, NEET 2017]*
(a) $\frac{I_0}{2}$ (b) $\frac{I_0}{4}$ (c) $\frac{I_0}{8}$ (d) $\frac{I_0}{16}$

20. In a diffraction pattern due to a single slit of width a, the first minimum is observed at an angle 30° when light of wavelength 5000 Å is incident on the slit. The first secondary maximum is observed at an angle of *[NCERT (Old) Pg. 369, NEET 2016]*
(a) $\sin^{-1}\left(\frac{2}{3}\right)$ (b) $\sin^{-1}\left(\frac{1}{2}\right)$ (c) $\sin^{-1}\left(\frac{3}{4}\right)$ (d) $\sin^{-1}\left(\frac{1}{4}\right)$

21. A linear aperture whose width is 0.02 cm is placed immediately in front of a lens of focal length 60 cm. The aperture is illuminated normally by a parallel beam of wavelength 5×10^{-5} cm. The distance of the first dark band of the diffraction pattern from the centre of the screen is *[NCERT (Old) Pg. 369, NEET 2016]*
(a) 0.10 cm (b) 0.25 cm
(c) 0.20 cm (d) 0.15 cm

22. For a parallel beam of monochromatic light of wavelength λ diffraction is produced by a single slit whose width a is of the order of the wavelength of the light. If D is the distance of the screen from the slit, the width of the central maxima will be *[NCERT (Old) Pg. 369, AIPMT 2015]*
(a) $\frac{2D\lambda}{a}$ (b) $\frac{D\lambda}{a}$ (c) $\frac{Da}{\lambda}$ (d) $\frac{2Da}{\lambda}$

23. At the first minimum adjacent to the central maximum of a single slit diffraction pattern, the phase difference between the Huygens' wavelet from the edge of the slit and the wavelet from the mid-point of the slit is *[NCERT (Old) Pg. 369, AIPMT 2015]*

(a) $\frac{\pi}{4}$ radian (b) $\frac{\pi}{2}$ radian
(c) π radian (d) $\frac{\pi}{8}$ radian

Answers

Step up Practice 1

1 (a)	2 (a)	3 (d)	4 (b)	5 (b)	6 (c)	7 (b)	8 (a)	9 (d)	10 (b)
11 (b)	12 (c)	13 (d)	14 (d)	15 (c)	16 (b)	17 (d)	18 (d)	19 (b)	20 (d)

Step up Practice 2

1 (d)	2 (b)	3 (a)	4 (b)	5 (b)	6 (d)	7 (b)	8 (b)	9 (c)	10 (c)
11 (b)	12 (b)	13 (a)	14 (b)	15 (d)	16 (d)	17 (b)	18 (d)	19 (a)	20 (a)
21 (c)	22 (a)	23 (b)	24 (c)						

Step up Practice 3

1 (d)	2 (c)	3 (a)	4 (d)	5 (d)	6 (d)	7 (d)	8 (c)	9 (d)	10 (a)
11 (d)	12 (c)	13 (d)	14 (b)	15 (b)	16 (c)	17 (d)	18 (a)	19 (b)	20 (c)

Gearing up for NEET

1 (b)	2 (c)	3 (a)	4 (d)	5 (b)	6 (c)	7 (b)	8 (a)	9 (b)	10 (a)
11 (c)	12 (a)	13 (d)	14 (b)	15 (c)	16 (c)	17 (b)	18 (c)	19 (c)	20 (a)
21 (c)	22 (c)	23 (b)	24 (b)	25 (c)	26 (a)	27 (c)	28 (a)	29 (b)	30 (b)
31 (a)	32 (a)	33 (c)	34 (b)	35 (a)	36 (d)	37 (c)	38 (a)	39 (a)	40 (c)
41 (c)	42 (c)	43 (a)	44 (c)	45 (b)	46 (b)	47 (a)	48 (a)	49 (b)	50 (a)
51 (c)	52 (a)	53 (c)	54 (c)	55 (c)	56 (b)	57 (c)	58 (b)	59 (a)	60 (d)
61 (c)	62 (a)	63 (b)	64 (d)	65 (a)	66 (b)	67 (b)	68 (c)	69 (d)	70 (a)
71 (c)	72 (d)	73 (d)	74 (d)	75 (c)	76 (b)				

Assertion and Reason

1 (b)	2 (a)	3 (c)	4 (b)	5 (d)

Statement Type Questions

1 (d)	2 (a)	3 (d)	4 (b)	5 (a)

Match the Columns

1 (a)	2 (b)	3 (b)	4 (a)

Final Check through PYQs : Module-I

1 (b)

Final Check through PYQs : Module-II

2 (c)	3 (b)	4 (c)	5 (a)	6 (b)	7 (c)	8 (a)	9 (b)	10 (d)	11 (c)
12 (a)	13 (a)								

Final Check through PYQs : Module-III

14 (d)	15 (b)	16 (b)	17 (b)	18 (b)	19 (c)	20 (c)	21 (d)	22 (a)	23 (c)

Hints and Solutions

Step up Practice 1

1. (*a*) As we know that,

$$n_1 = \frac{c}{v_1} = \frac{v\lambda}{v\lambda_1} = \frac{\lambda}{\lambda_1}$$

and $$n_2 = \frac{c}{v_2} = \frac{v\lambda}{v\lambda_2} = \frac{\lambda}{\lambda_2}$$

Now, $$\frac{n_1}{n_2} = \frac{\lambda_2}{\lambda_1}$$

or $$\lambda_2 = \left(\frac{n_1}{n_2}\right)\lambda_1$$

Hence, wavelength is the second medium is $\lambda_1\left(\frac{n_1}{n_2}\right)$.

2. (*a*) We know that,

$$\mu = \frac{c}{v} = \frac{v\lambda}{v\lambda'}$$

$$\frac{3}{2} = \frac{\lambda}{\lambda'} \quad \text{or} \quad \lambda' = \frac{2\lambda}{3}$$

Note that the frequency remains unchanged.

Hence, frequency ν and wavelength $\left(\frac{2}{3}\right)\lambda$.

3. (*d*) In cylindrical wavefront, intensity of light wave, $I \propto \frac{1}{r}$.

4. (*b*) Here, phase difference, $\phi = \pi/3$

So, amplitude of resulting wave,

$$A = \sqrt{a_1^2 + a_2^2 + 2a_1a_2 \cos\phi}$$

$$= \sqrt{4^2 + 3^2 + 2 \times 4 \times 3 \times \cos(\pi/3)} \approx 6 \text{ m}$$

5. (*b*) The path of ray of light is always perpendicular to wavefront.

6. (*c*) In interference,

$$\frac{I_{max}}{I_{min}} = \frac{(\sqrt{I_1} + \sqrt{I_2})^2}{(\sqrt{I_1} - \sqrt{I_2})^2} = \frac{(A_1 + A_2)^2}{(A_1 - A_2)^2}$$

Given, $$\frac{A_1}{A_2} = \frac{3}{5}$$

$\therefore$ $$\frac{I_{max}}{I_{min}} = \frac{(3+5)^2}{(3-5)^2} = \frac{16}{1}$$

7. (*b*) Statement I is correct but Statement II is incorrect.

Bright interference bands have the same intensity because they result from constructive interference where the wave from two slits reinforce each other.

$I_{max} \propto (a_1 + a_2)^2$, which is constant.

All bands do not receive same light because each band is at different distance from the two sources.

8. (*a*) $I \propto a^2 \Rightarrow \frac{a_1}{a_2} = \left(\frac{9}{4}\right)^{1/2} = \frac{3}{2}$

Hence, ratio of amplitude is 3 : 2.

9. (*d*) Total phase difference

= Initial phase difference + Phase difference due to path

$$= 36° + \frac{360°}{\lambda} \times \Delta x$$

$$= 36° + \frac{360°}{\lambda} \times \frac{\lambda}{4} = 36° + 90° = 126°$$

10. (*b*) Given, the amplitudes of the waves are $a_1 = 10\ \mu\text{m}$, $a_2 = 4\ \mu\text{m}$ and $a_3 = 7\ \mu\text{m}$ and the phase difference between 1st and 2nd wave is $\frac{\pi}{2}$ and that between 2nd and 3rd wave is $\frac{\pi}{2}$.

Therefore, phase difference between 1st and 3rd is π. Combining 1st with 3rd, their resultant amplitude is given by

$$A_1^2 = a_1^2 + a_3^2 + 2a_1a_3 \cos\phi$$

or $$A_1 = \sqrt{10^2 + 7^2 + 2 \times 10 \times 7 \cos\pi}$$

$$= \sqrt{100 + 49 - 140}$$

$$= \sqrt{9} = 3\ \mu\text{m in the direction of first.}$$

Now combining this with 2nd wave we have the resultant amplitude

$$A^2 = A_1^2 + a_2^2 + 2A_1a_2 \cos\frac{\pi}{2}$$

or $$A = \sqrt{3^2 + 4^2 + 2 \times 3 \cos 90°}$$

$$= \sqrt{9 + 16} = 5\ \mu\text{m}$$

Hence, amplitude of resulting wave is 5 μm.

11. (*b*) $I = I_1 + I_2 + 2\sqrt{I_1I_2} \cos\phi$

$$= I + 4I + 2\sqrt{I \times 4I} \times \cos\frac{2\pi}{3}$$

$$= 5I + 4I \times \left(-\frac{1}{2}\right) = 5I - 2I = 3I$$

12. (*c*) Statement I is incorrect but Statement II is correct.

Let the amplitude of waves from each slit be a, therefore intensity due to each slit $= a^2$.

If interference is destructive, the resultant amplitude $= a - a = 0$

$\therefore$ Minimum intensity = 0

In case when interference is constructive, the resultant amplitude $= a + a = 2a$

$\therefore$ Maximum intensity $= (2a)^2 = 4a^2$

which is four times the intensity due to each slit.

14. (*d*) For destructive interference,

$$\cos\phi = \text{minimum} = -1$$

i.e. $\phi = \pi, 3\pi, 5\pi$

or $\phi = (2n+1)\pi$

where, $n = 0, 1, 2, 3, \ldots$

or $$\Delta x = \frac{\lambda}{2\pi} \times \phi = \frac{(2n+1)\lambda}{2}$$

15. (*c*) Statement I is incorrect but Statement II is correct.

All points on the wavefront have same displacement but they don't need to be oscillate with same frequency and constant phase difference.

16. (*b*) When two sources are obtained from a single source, the wavefront is divided into two parts. These two wavefronts acts as if they emanated from two sources having a fixed phase relationship.

17. (*d*) Both Statement I and Statement II are correct.

18. (*d*) Resultant intensity for two interfering waves is given by

$$I_R = I_1 + I_2 + 2\sqrt{I_1 I_2}\cos\phi$$

For maximum, $\cos\phi = \text{maximum} = 1$

$$\therefore \quad I_{max} = I_1 + I_2 + 2\sqrt{I_1 I_2} = (\sqrt{I_1} + \sqrt{I_2})^2$$

19. (*b*) Given, $S_1P = 7\lambda$ and $S_2P = 9\lambda$

For constructive interference at any point, the path difference between waves should be 2λ.

Now, we have, $S_2P - S_1P = 9\lambda - 7\lambda$

$\Rightarrow$ $S_2P - S_1P = 2\lambda$

Therefore, the sources S_1 and S_2 are said to interfere constructively.

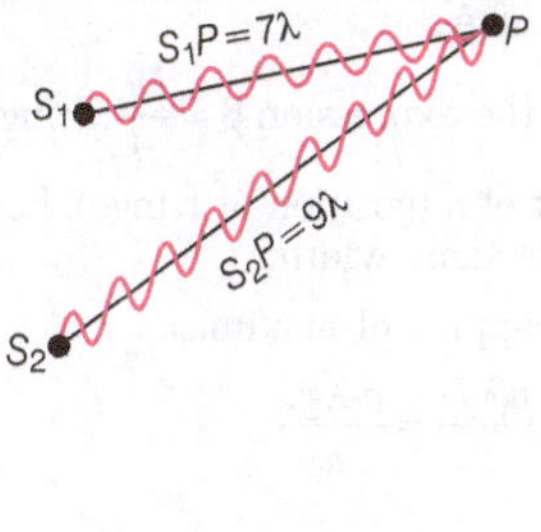

The waves emanating from S_1 will arrive exactly two cycles earlier than the waves from S_2 as $S_2P - S_1P = 2\lambda$ and will again be in phase.

Thus, the statements given in option (b) are incorrect, rest are correct.

20. (*d*) Given, $I_1 = 100, I_2 = 1$

$$\frac{I_1}{I_2} = \frac{100}{1}$$

Now, $$\frac{I_{max}}{I_{min}} = \left(\frac{\sqrt{\frac{I_1}{I_2}}+1}{\sqrt{\frac{I_1}{I_2}}-1}\right)^2 = \left(\frac{\sqrt{100}+1}{\sqrt{100}-1}\right)^2 = \frac{121}{81} \approx \frac{3}{2}$$

Step up Practice 2

1. (*d*) We have, $n_1\lambda_1 = n_2\lambda_2$

Number of fringes, $$n_2 = \frac{n_1\lambda_1}{\lambda_2} = \frac{60 \times 5461 \times 10^{-10}}{5890 \times 10^{-10}} = 55$$

2. (*b*) Given, $$\frac{I_{bright}}{I_{dark}} = \frac{I_{max}}{I_{min}} = 9$$

or $$\left(\frac{a_1 + a_2}{a_1 - a_2}\right)^2 = 9 \quad \text{or} \quad \frac{a_1 + a_2}{a_1 - a_2} = 3$$

$$\Rightarrow \quad \frac{a_1}{a_2} = \frac{3+1}{3-1} \Rightarrow \frac{a_1}{a_2} = 2$$

So, $$\frac{I_1}{I_2} = \frac{a_1^2}{a_2^2} = \frac{4}{1}$$

3. (*a*) In interference between waves of equal amplitudes a, the minimum intensity is zero and the maximum intensity is proportional to $4a^2$ (because slit width $\propto$ amplitude). For waves of unequal amplitudes a and $A (A > a)$, the minimum intensity is non-zero and the maximum intensity is proportional to $(a + A)^2$, which is greater than $4a^2$.

So, the intensities of both the maxima and the minima increase.

4. (*b*) A is true but R is false.

On immersing the apparatus in water, the wavelength of light decrease $\left(\lambda' = \frac{\lambda}{\mu}\right)$. Hence, it follows from the expression of fringe width $\left(\beta = \frac{D\lambda}{d}\right)$, that when apparatus is immersed in liquid, the fringe width will decrease.

The wavelength of light in water is smaller than wavelength in air because refractive index of water is greater than air and as we know $\mu \propto \frac{1}{\lambda}$.

5. (b) When thin plate of glass is introduced, then lateral displacement of fringes

$$=\frac{\beta}{\lambda}(\mu-1)t$$

$$=\frac{1\times10^{-3}}{600\times10^{-9}}(1.5-1)\times0.06\times10^{-3}$$

$$=\frac{1}{20}\text{m}=5\text{ cm}$$

6. (d) For minima, path difference should be an odd multiple of half wavelength.

i.e. $\Delta x=(2n-1)\frac{\lambda}{2}$

For third minima ($n=3$), $\Delta x=(2\times3-1)\frac{\lambda}{2}=\frac{5\lambda}{2}$

7. (b) For dark fringe at point P,

$$S_1P-S_2P=\frac{5\lambda}{2}$$

$$=5\times\frac{6000}{2}=15000\text{ Å}$$

$$=1.5\text{ micron}$$

8. (b) Angular fringe width, $\theta=\frac{\lambda}{d}$

$$=\frac{6328\times10^{-10}}{2\times10^{-4}}\times\frac{180}{\pi}=0.18°$$

9. (c) Slit width ratio = 9 : 4, hence $I_1:I_2=9:4$.

$$\therefore\quad\frac{a_1^2}{a_2^2}=\frac{9}{4}$$

$$\Rightarrow\quad\frac{a_1}{a_2}=\frac{3}{2}$$

$$\therefore\quad\frac{I_{max}}{I_{min}}=\frac{(a_1+a_2)^2}{(a_1-a_2)^2}=\frac{25}{1}$$

Hence, ratio of the intensity at maxima to the intensity at minima will be 25 : 1.

10. (c) For dark fringe at P

$$S_1P-S_2P=\Delta x=(2n-1)\lambda/2$$

Here $n=3$ and $\lambda=12000$ Å

So, $\Delta x=\frac{5\lambda}{2}=5\times\frac{12000}{2}=30000$ Å

$=3$ micron

11. (b) A is true but R is false.

When source in Young's double slit experiment is of white light, the central fringe is white as all colours meet there in phase.

Red light has a longer wavelength than other colours on the visible light spectrum.

12. (b) By using phase difference $\phi=\frac{2\pi}{\lambda}(\Delta x)$

For path difference λ, phase difference $\phi_1=2\pi$ and for path difference $\lambda/4$, phase difference $\phi_2=\pi/2$.

Also by using $I=4I_0\cos^2\frac{\phi}{2}\Rightarrow\frac{I_1}{I_2}=\frac{\cos^2(\phi_1/2)}{\cos^2(\phi_2/2)}$

$$\Rightarrow\frac{Q}{I_2}=\frac{\cos^2(2\pi/2)}{\cos^2\left(\frac{\pi/2}{2}\right)}=\frac{1}{1/2}\Rightarrow I_2=\frac{Q}{2}$$

13. (a) λ_V is least 5, therefore ω is minimum (as $\omega\propto\lambda$). Hence, the fringe next to centre will be violet.

14. (b) Distance of nth minima from central bright fringe,

$$x_n=\frac{(2n-1)\lambda D}{2d}$$

For $n=3$ or 3rd minima,

$$x_3=\frac{(2\times3-1)\times300\times10^{-9}\times1}{2\times1\times10^{-3}}$$

$$=\frac{5\times300\times10^{-6}}{2}=0.75\times10^{-3}\text{ m}$$

$$=0.75\text{ mm}$$

15. (d) In case of Young's double slit experiment, a slit S is necessary, if we use an ordinary extended source of light while it is not needed, if we use a spatially coherent source of light.

16. (d) Distance of nth bright fringe from the centre,

$$y_n=\frac{n\lambda D}{d}$$

So, $y_3=\frac{3\times6000\times10^{-10}\times2.5}{0.5\times10^{-3}}$

$$=9\times10^{-3}\text{ m}=9\text{ mm}$$

17. (b) At centre, $\Delta x=0$ for all wavelengths. Hence, all wavelengths interfere constructively at centre. So, it is white.

$$I_{max}=(\sqrt{I_1}+\sqrt{I_2})^2,$$

$$I_{min}=(\sqrt{I_1}-\sqrt{I_2})^2$$

when $I_1=I_2=I_0$

$I_{max}=4I_0$ and $I_{min}=0$

when $I_2=\frac{I_0}{2}$,

then $I_{max}<4I_0$

and $I_{min}>0$

18. (d) Both A and R are true and R is the correct explanation of A.

As given in the expression $\beta=\frac{D\lambda}{d}$, fringe width β is independent of n (position of fringe), hence all the fringes are of same width.

19. (a) For overlapping of maximas,

$$\frac{n_1\lambda_1D}{d}=\frac{n_2\lambda_2D}{d}$$

or $\frac{n_1}{n_2} = \frac{\lambda_2}{\lambda_1} = \frac{7}{5}, \frac{14}{10} \ldots$

$\Rightarrow$ 14th order maxima of λ_1 will coincide with 10th order maxima of λ_2.

For overlapping of minimas

$$\frac{(2n_1 - 1)\lambda_1 D}{2d} = \frac{(2n_2 - 1)\lambda_2 D}{2d}$$

$$\therefore \quad \frac{2n_1 - 1}{2n_2 - 1} = \frac{\lambda_2}{\lambda_1} = \frac{7}{5}$$

20. (*a*) Consider the diagram in which light diverges from a point source (*O*).

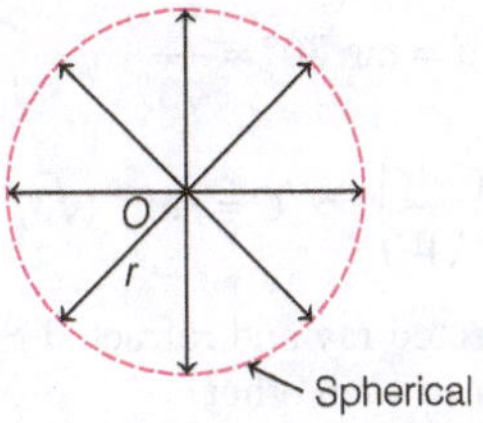

Due to the point source, light propagates in all directions symmetrically and hence, wavefront will be spherical as shown in the above diagram.

If power of the source is *P*, then intensity of the source will be

$$I = \frac{P}{4\pi r^2}$$

where, *r* is radius of the wavefront at any time.

21. (*c*) Given, $d = 1\text{ mm} = 1 \times 10^{-3}\text{ m}, D = 1\text{ m}$

$\lambda = 500\text{ mm} = 500 \times 10^{-9}\text{ m}$

Distance of *n*th minima from central maxima,

$$x_n = \frac{(2n-1)\lambda}{2} \frac{D}{d}$$

$$= \frac{(2 \times 3 - 1) \times 500 \times 10^{-9}}{2} \times \frac{1}{1 \times 10^{-3}}$$

$$= 2.5 \times 500 \times 10^{-6} = 12.5 \times 10^{-4}\text{ m}$$

$$= 1.25\text{ mm}$$

22. (*a*) Both A and R are true but R is not the correct explanation of A.

The central fringe is bright when there is no path difference between the waves reaching there. But if there is initial phase difference of π between two waves, then the central fringe will be dark.

23. (*b*) Given, wavelength $= 6.5 \times 10^{-7}$ m

Slit distance $(d) = 1$ mm, Screen distance $= 1$ m

Distance between *n*th bright fringe and *m*th dark fringe $(n > m)$

$$\Delta x = \left(n - m + \frac{1}{2}\right)\beta$$

$$= \left(5 - 3 + \frac{1}{2}\right) \times \frac{6.5 \times 10^{-7} \times 1}{1 \times 10^{-3}}$$

$$= 1.63\text{ mm}$$

24. (*c*) Distance between two adjacent fringes is $\frac{\lambda D}{d}$.

Step up Practice 3

1. (*d*) In Fresnel's class of diffraction, the source of light and the screen on which the diffraction pattern is observed are at finite distance from diffracting obstacle. In this no lenses are used and the incident waveform is either spherical or cylindrical.

2. (*c*) Angular width $\beta = \frac{2\lambda}{d}$

$$\Rightarrow \quad \frac{\beta_1}{\beta_2} = \frac{\lambda_1}{\lambda_2} \Rightarrow \frac{\beta}{\frac{60}{100}\beta} = \frac{5000}{\lambda_2}$$

$$\Rightarrow \quad \lambda_2 = 3000\text{ Å}$$

3. (*a*) Given, first maximum for red light is 660 nm

In a single slit diffraction experiment, position of minima is given by $d \sin\theta = n\lambda$.

So, for first minima of red light, $\sin\theta = 1 \times \left(\frac{\lambda_R}{d}\right)$

and as first maxima is mid-way between first and second minima, for wavelength λ', its position will be

$$d \sin\theta' = \frac{\lambda' + 2\lambda'}{2} \Rightarrow \sin\theta' = \frac{3\lambda'}{2d}$$

According to given condition, $\sin\theta = \sin\theta'$

$$\Rightarrow \quad \lambda' = \frac{2}{3}\lambda_R$$

So, $\lambda' = \frac{2}{3} \times 660 = 440\text{ nm} = 4400\text{ Å}$

Hence, value of λ' is 4400 Å.

4. (*d*) In single slit, for *n*th secondary maxima path difference

$$a \sin\theta = (2n + 1)\frac{\lambda}{2}$$

For first secondary maximum, $n = 1$

$$\therefore \quad a \sin\theta = \frac{3\lambda}{2}$$

5. (*d*) Both Statement I and Statement II are correct.

When slit is wide (*i.e.*, $a >> \lambda$), bending of light becomes so small that it cannot be detected upto a certain distance of screen from the slit. Hence, practically, no diffraction occurs.

6. (*d*) The phase difference ϕ between the wavelets from the top edge and the bottom edge of the slit is $\phi = \frac{2\pi}{\lambda}(d \sin\theta)$, where *d* is the slit width. The first minima of the diffraction pattern occurs at $\sin\theta = \frac{\lambda}{d}$

So, $\phi = \frac{2\pi}{\lambda}\left(d \times \frac{\lambda}{d}\right) = 2\pi$.

7. (d) By using $\mu = \tan \theta_P \Rightarrow \mu = \tan 60° = \sqrt{3}$

Also, $C = \sin^{-1}\left(\frac{1}{\mu}\right) \Rightarrow C = \sin^{-1}\left(\frac{1}{\sqrt{3}}\right)$

8. (c) From Brewster's law, $\mu = \tan i_p$

$\Rightarrow \frac{c}{v} = \tan 60° = \sqrt{3}$

$\Rightarrow v = \frac{c}{\sqrt{3}} = \frac{3 \times 10^8}{\sqrt{3}} = \sqrt{3} \times 10^8 \text{ ms}^{-1}$

9. (d) Both Statement I and Statement II are correct.
Since the diffraction occur when size of the obstacle is comparable to the wavelength of the light. So, the gap in the threads of muslin cloth fulfil this condition. Thus, coloured spectrum is seen on it.

10. (a) According to Brewster's law, when a beam of ordinary light (*i.e.* unpolarised) is reflected from a transparent medium (like glass), the reflected light is completely plane polarised at certain angle of incidence called the angle of polarisation.

11. (d) Required angle $= 2i_p + 90° = 2 \times 57.5° + 90° = 205°$

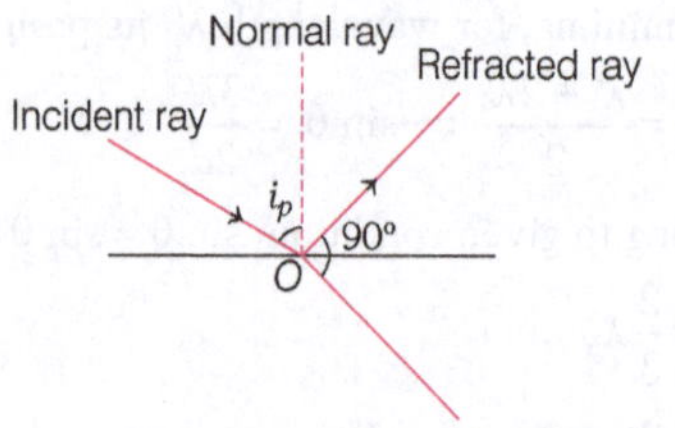

12. (c) The statements I and II are correct but III is incorrect and it can be corrected as,
Diffraction is a wave phenomenon. It is observed in electromagnetic and longitudinal waves as well.

13. (d) If I is the final intensity and I_0 is the initial intensity then

$$I = \frac{I_0}{2}(\cos^2 30°)^5 \text{ or } \frac{I}{I_0} = \frac{1}{2} \times \left(\frac{\sqrt{3}}{2}\right)^{10} = 0.12$$

Hence, required percentage is 12%.

14. (b) $\theta = x + \frac{y}{\lambda^2}$

$$30° = x + \frac{y}{(5000)^2} \text{ and } 50° = x + \frac{y}{(4000)^2}$$

Solving for x, we get $x = -\frac{50°}{9}$ per mm

15. (b) Statement I is correct but Statement II is incorrect.
The wave diffracted from the edges of circular obstacle, placed in the path of light, interfere constructively at the centre of the shadow resulting in the formation of a bright spot.

16. (c) Intensity of polarised light from first polariser

$= \frac{100}{2} = 50$

$I = 50 \cos^2 30°$

$= \frac{50}{4} = 12.5$

17. (d) Both Statement I and Statement II are correct.
Radio waves can be polarised because they are transverse in nature.

18. (a) By using, $\mu = \tan \theta_p$

$\Rightarrow \mu = \tan 30° = \frac{1}{\sqrt{3}}$

also $C = \sin^{-1}\left(\frac{1}{\mu}\right) \Rightarrow C = \sin^{-1}(\sqrt{3})$

19. (b) Here, reflected ray and refracted ray are mutually perpendicular to each other.
When angle of incident ray is 53°

$i + r = 90°$

$\therefore r = 90° - 53° = 37°$

According to Brewster's law refractive index, $\mu = \tan i_p$

$\therefore \tan 53° = \frac{4}{3}$

when angle of incident ray is 45°

$i + r = 90°$

$\therefore r = 90° - 45° = 45°$

and refractive index, $\mu = \tan 45° = 1$

20. (c) The statements I and III are correct but II is incorrect and it can be corrected as,
As the figure shows, the reflected light is linearly polarised perpendicular to the plane of the figure (represented by dots). This can be checked by looking at the reflected light through an analyser.

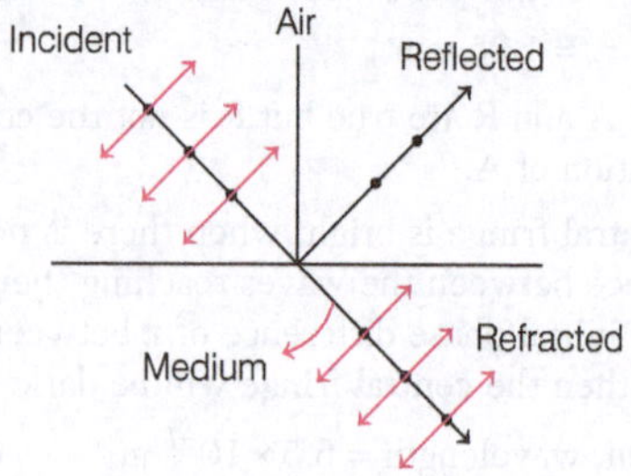

Gearing up for NEET

1. (b) When phase difference is 0, intensity is maximum, *i.e.*, I_{max}.

When $\phi = \frac{\pi}{2}$ or $\frac{\phi}{2} = \frac{\pi}{4}$,

The intensity will be $I = I_{max} \cos^2 \frac{\phi}{2} = \frac{I_{max}}{2}$

$\therefore$ The desired ratio is 2 : 1.

2. (c) In Young's double slit experiment, we have

$$\beta = \frac{\lambda D}{d}$$

$$\Delta\beta = \frac{\lambda \Delta D}{d} \Rightarrow \lambda = \frac{\Delta\beta d}{\Delta D}$$

$$\lambda = \frac{3\times10^{-5}\times1\times10^{-3}}{5\times10^{-2}}$$

$$= 6\times10^{-7} \text{ m}$$

or $\lambda = 600$ nm

3. (a) $I_2 = I_1 \cos^2(90° - \theta) = \frac{I'}{2}\cos^2\theta \sin^2\theta = \frac{I'}{8}(\sin 2\theta)^2$

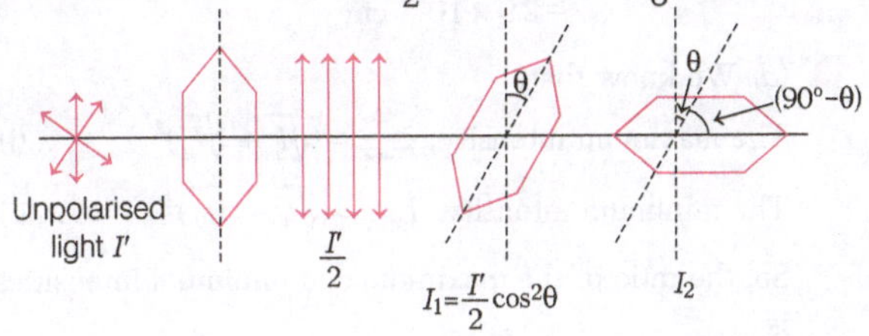

$$3 = \frac{32}{8}(\sin 2\theta)^2$$

$$\sin 2\theta = \frac{\sqrt{3}}{2} = \sin 60° \text{ or } \sin 120°$$

$$\theta = 30° \text{ or } 60°$$

4. (d) $I_1 = \frac{I}{4}$ and $I_2 = \frac{9I}{32}$

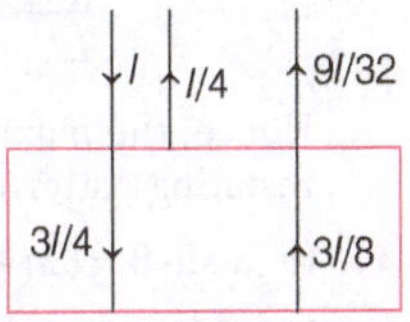

$$\therefore \frac{I_1}{I_2} = \frac{8}{9}$$

or $\sqrt{\frac{I_1}{I_2}} = \frac{2\sqrt{2}}{3}$

$$\therefore \frac{I_{max}}{I_{min}} = \left(\frac{\sqrt{I_1/I_2}+1}{\sqrt{I_1/I_2}-1}\right)^2 = \left(\frac{2\sqrt{2}+3}{2\sqrt{2}-3}\right)^2$$

5. (b) At $x = 0$, $\Delta x = 5\lambda$

which corresponds to a maximum.

At $x = \infty$, $\Delta x = 0$, this also corresponds to a maximum.

$\therefore$ Other possible maxima between $x = 0$ and $x = \infty$ are $\Delta x = \lambda, 2\lambda, 3\lambda, 4\lambda, 5\lambda$.

Since, $d = n\lambda \Rightarrow n = 5$ on each side.

6. (c) Say P be the point on X-axis, where constructive interference is obtained.

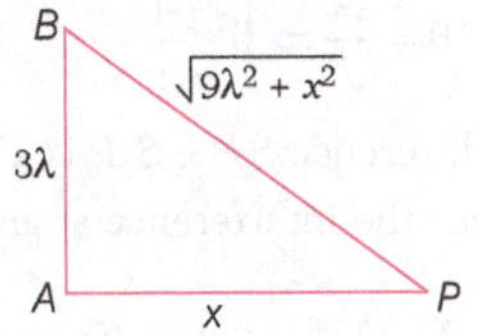

$$BP - AP = 2\lambda \text{ or } \lambda$$

$$\therefore \sqrt{9\lambda^2 + x^2} - x = 2\lambda$$

$$\therefore 9\lambda^2 + x^2 = x^2 + 4\lambda^2 + 4x\lambda$$

$$\Rightarrow x = \frac{5\lambda}{4}$$

Further, $\sqrt{9\lambda^2 + x^2} - x = \lambda$

$$\therefore 9\lambda^2 + x^2 = x^2 + \lambda^2 + 2x\lambda$$

$$\therefore x = 4\lambda$$

Hence, the distance from A on the X-axis at which the interference is constructive is $5\lambda/4$.

7. (b) Path difference at a point Q on the circle is

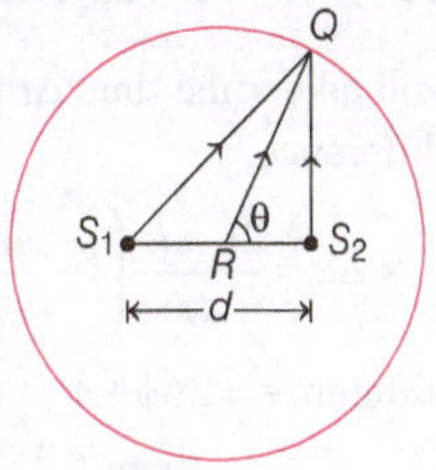

$$\Delta y = d \cos\theta \quad \text{...(i)}$$

For maxima at Q, path difference should be integer multiple of wavelength

$$\Delta y = n\lambda \quad \text{...(ii)}$$

From Eqs. (i) and (ii), we get

$$n\lambda = d\cos\theta$$

$$\therefore \theta = \cos^{-1}\left(\frac{n\lambda}{d}\right)$$

For $n = 4$

Angular position, $\theta = \cos^{-1}\left(\frac{4\lambda}{d}\right)$

8. (a) Consider the diagram, the ray P is incident at an angle θ and gets reflected in the direction P' and refracted in the direction P''. Due to reflection from the glass medium, there is a phase change of π.

Time taken to travel along OP''

$$\Delta t = \frac{OP''}{v} = \frac{d/\cos r}{c/n} = \frac{nd}{c\cos r}$$

From Snell's law, $n = \frac{\sin\theta}{\sin r}$

$$\Rightarrow \sin r = \frac{\sin\theta}{n}$$

$$\cos r = \sqrt{1-\sin^2 r} = \sqrt{1-\frac{\sin^2\theta}{n^2}}$$

$$\therefore \Delta t = \frac{nd}{c\left(1-\frac{\sin^2\theta}{n^2}\right)^{1/2}}$$

$$= \frac{nd}{c}\left(1 - \frac{\sin^2\theta}{n^2}\right)^{-1/2}$$

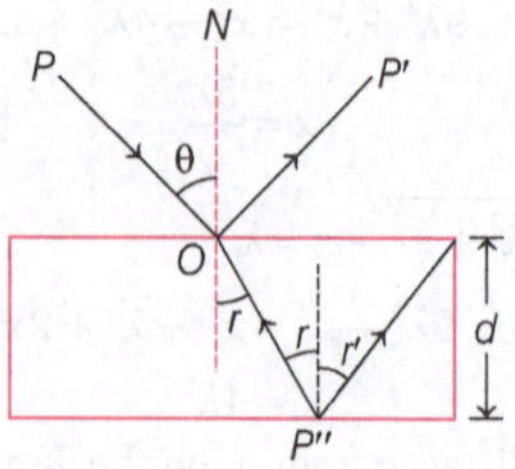

Path difference, $\Delta x = c\Delta t$

As, we know $\Delta\phi = \frac{2\pi}{\lambda} \times$ Path difference

The right ray will take same time Δt to cover $P''Q$.

Hence, phase difference,

$$\Delta\phi = \frac{2\pi}{\lambda} \times \Delta x = \frac{2\pi\, ndc}{\lambda c}\left(1 - \frac{\sin^2\theta}{n^2}\right)^{-1/2}$$

So, net phase difference $= 2\Delta\phi + \pi$

$$= \frac{4n\pi d}{\lambda}\left(1 - \frac{1}{n^2}\sin^2\theta\right)^{-1/2} + \pi$$

$[\because cT = \lambda]$

9. (*b*) Path difference between the two rays is given by

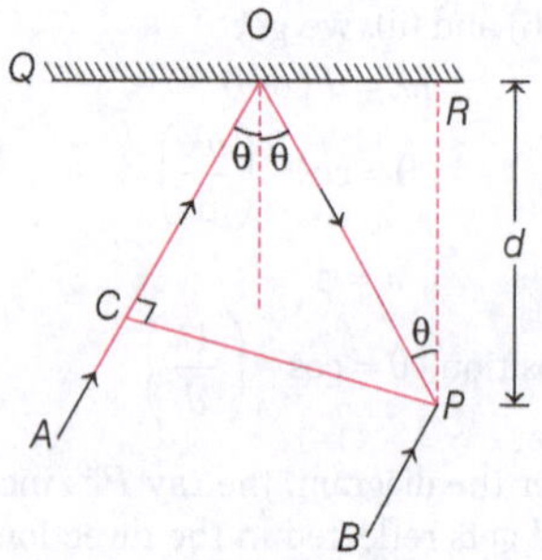

$$\Delta = CO + PO$$

$\because \quad PR = d$

So, $\quad PO = d\sec\theta$

and $\quad CO = PO\cos 2\theta = d\sec\theta\cos 2\theta$

So, $\quad \Delta = (d\sec\theta + d\sec\theta\cos 2\theta)$

Phase difference between two rays is $\phi = \pi$ (as one ray is reflected one and another is direct).

Now, for constructive interference, path difference should be even multiple of half-wavelength.

i.e. $\quad \Delta = \lambda/2, 3\lambda/2, \ldots$

So, $d\sec\theta + d\sec\theta\cos 2\theta = \frac{\lambda}{2}$

or $\quad d\sec\theta\,(1 + \cos 2\theta) = \frac{\lambda}{2}$

or $\quad d\sec\theta(2\cos^2\theta) = \frac{\lambda}{2}$

$\therefore \quad \cos\theta = \lambda/4d$

10. (*a*) On the wavefront, all the points are in the same phase.

11. (*c*) To observe diffraction, the size of the obstacle should be of the order of wavelength, *i.e.*, $\lambda \approx d$.

12 (*a*) Given, wavelength, $\lambda = 590$ nm $= 590 \times 10^{-9}$ m

Diameter of lens $= 10 \times 10^{-2}$ m

Focal length of lens $= 20 \times 10^{-2}$ m

Now, the diameter of image disc

$$D = 2R = 2\left(1.22\frac{\lambda D}{b}\right)$$

$$= \left(\frac{1.22 \times 590 \times 10^{-9} \times 20 \times 10^{-2}}{10 \times 10^{-2}}\right) \times 2$$

$$\simeq 2.9 \times 10^{-4} \text{ cm}$$

13. (*d*) We know that,

The maximum intensity, $I_{max} = (\sqrt{I_1} + \sqrt{I_2})^2$ ...(i)

The minimum intensity, $I_{min} = (\sqrt{I_1} - \sqrt{I_2})^2$ ...(ii)

So, the ratio of the maximum and minimum intensities is

$$\frac{I_{max}}{I_{min}} = \frac{(\sqrt{I_1} + \sqrt{I_2})^2}{(\sqrt{I_1} - \sqrt{I_2})^2}$$

$$= \frac{(\sqrt{4I} + \sqrt{I})^2}{(\sqrt{4I} - \sqrt{I})^2}$$

$$\Rightarrow \quad \frac{I_{max}}{I_{min}} = \left(\frac{3\sqrt{I}}{\sqrt{I}}\right)^2 = \frac{9}{1} = 9:1$$

Hence, the maximum and minimum intensities in the resulting pattern are $9I$ and I.

14. (*b*) $a\sin\theta = (2n-1)\lambda/2$ is the condition for obtaining secondary maxima in the diffraction pattern due to single slit.

15. (*c*) The distance of dark fringe from centre is given by

$$x_n = (2n+1)\frac{\lambda D}{2d}$$

As, $n = 5$ for 5th dark fringe.

So, $\quad x_5 = \frac{11}{2}\frac{\lambda D}{d} = \frac{11}{2}\beta \quad \left(\because \frac{\lambda D}{d} = \beta\right)$

$= 11/2 \times 0.002 = 0.011$ cm

$= 1.1 \times 10^{-2}$ cm

16. (*c*) We know, $\lambda = \frac{h}{mv}$

and $\quad \theta = \frac{2\lambda}{d} \Rightarrow \theta \propto \frac{1}{v}$

17. (*b*) The path difference $S_1P - S_2P$ is a whole number of wavelength, for the interference at an arbitrary point P.

So, $S_1P - S_2P = n\lambda$ (for maximum intensity)

18. (c) The direction in which the first minima occurs is θ (say), then $e \sin\theta = \lambda$

or $e\theta = \lambda$ or $\theta = \frac{\lambda}{e}$ ($\because \theta \simeq \sin\theta$, when θ is small)

Width of the central maximum $= 2b\theta + e = \frac{2b\lambda}{e} + e$

19. (c) We have, $\beta = \frac{\lambda D}{d}$

$\because$ The arrangement is placed in a liquid of refractive index n.

$\therefore \quad \lambda' = \frac{\lambda}{n}$

Therefore, fringe width, $\beta' = \frac{\lambda D}{dn}$ or $\beta' = \frac{\beta}{n}$

20. (a) Given, width of the slit $= 10^4$ Å

$= 10^4 \times 10^{-10}$ m

$= 10^{-6}$ m $= 1$ μm

Wavelength of (visible) sunlight varies from 4000 Å to 7000 Å.

As the width of slit is comparable to that of wavelength, hence diffraction occurs with maxima at centre. So, at the centre all colours appear, *i.e.*, mixing of colours form white colour at the centre.

21. (c) θ (in radian) $= \frac{\lambda}{d}$

$\therefore \quad d = \frac{\lambda}{\theta} = \frac{6\times10^{-7}}{\pi/180^\circ} = 3.4\times10^{-5}$m

22. (c) Fringe width, $\beta = \frac{\lambda D}{d} \Rightarrow \beta \propto \frac{D}{d}$

$$\frac{\beta_2}{\beta_1} = \frac{D_2}{d_2} \times \frac{d_1}{D_1} = \frac{\frac{1}{2}D_1}{2d_1} \times \frac{d_1}{D_1} = \frac{1}{4} \Rightarrow \beta_2 = \frac{\beta_1}{4}$$

23. (b) $\Delta y = \frac{5\lambda D}{d} - \frac{5\lambda D}{2d} = \frac{5\lambda D}{2d}$

$= \frac{5\times 6.5\times 10^{-7}\times 1}{2\times 10^{-3}}$ m $= 1.63$ mm

24. (b) $n_1\lambda_1 = n_2\lambda_2 \Rightarrow n_2 = \frac{n_1\lambda_1}{\lambda_2} = 12\times\frac{600}{400} = 18$

25. (c) In single narrow slit, for first minima,

$d\sin\theta = \lambda \Rightarrow \sin\theta = \frac{\lambda}{d}$

$\therefore \quad \theta = \sin^{-1}\left(\frac{5000\times10^{-10}}{0.001\times10^{-3}}\right) = 30^\circ$

26. (a) We have, $y_1 = \frac{10\lambda_1 D}{d}$, $y_2 = \frac{5\lambda_2 D}{d}$

$\therefore \quad \frac{y_1}{y_2} = \frac{2\lambda_1}{\lambda_2}$

27. (c) Intensity, $I = 4I_0 \cos^2\frac{\phi}{2}$

$\because \quad I = I_0 \Rightarrow \cos^2\frac{\phi}{2} = \frac{1}{4}$

$\therefore \quad \phi = \frac{2\pi}{3}$

28. (a) We have, $\frac{2(6)-1}{2}\beta = 10\beta'$

$\therefore \quad \frac{\beta}{\beta'} = \frac{10}{5.5} = 1.8 = \mu$

29. (b) Let nth red fringe coincides with mth blue fringe, then

$\frac{n\lambda_R D}{d} = \frac{m\lambda_B D}{d}$

$\therefore \quad \frac{n}{m} = \frac{\lambda_B}{\lambda_R} = \frac{480}{600} = \frac{4}{5}$

i.e., 4th red fringe coincides with 5th blue fringe. Next 8th red fringe will coincide with 10th blue fringe and so on. Thus, $n = 4$

and $m = n + 1 = 5$

30. (b) For maximum (brightness) intensity on the screen, path difference should be integer multiple of wavelength, *i.e.*,

$d\sin\theta = n\lambda$

$\sin\theta = \frac{n\lambda}{d} = \frac{n(2000)}{7000} = \frac{n}{3.5}$

As, $(\sin\theta)_{max} = 1 \Rightarrow n = 3.5$

So, number of maximas $= 0, \pm1, \pm2, \pm3$

Thus, only seven maximas can be obtained on both sides of the screen.

31. (a) Fringe size will not change, *i.e.*, $n_1 = n_2$.

32. (a) Number of fringes shifted, $N = \frac{(\mu-1)t}{\lambda}$

$\therefore$ Refractive index of the sheet,

$$\mu = \frac{N\lambda}{t} + 1 = \frac{30\times6000\times10^{-10}}{3.6\times10^{-5}} + 1 = 1.5$$

33. (c) Fringe width, $\beta = \frac{D\lambda}{d}$

i.e. $\beta \propto \lambda$

So, wavelength λ and hence fringe width β decreases 1.5 or $\frac{3}{2}$ times when immersed in liquid. The distance between central maximum and 10th maxima is 3 cm in vacuum. When immersed in liquid it will reduce to 2 cm. Position of central maximum will not change while 10th maxima will be obtained at $y = 4$ cm.

34. (b) Position of third maxima,

$$x_3 = \frac{3\lambda D}{d} = \frac{3(5\times10^{-5})(200)}{0.02} = 1.5 \text{ cm}$$

35. (a) According to the question,

$$y = \frac{\omega}{4} = \frac{\lambda D}{4d} \Rightarrow \Delta x = \frac{yd}{D} = \frac{\lambda}{4}$$

Phase difference, $\phi = \frac{2\pi}{\lambda} \cdot \Delta x = \frac{\pi}{2}$

$\therefore \quad \frac{\phi}{2} = \frac{\pi}{4}$

Now, intensity, $I_2 = I_1 \cos^2 \frac{\phi}{2}$

or $\quad \frac{I_1}{I_2} = \frac{1}{\cos^2 \phi/2} = 2$

36. (d) According to question, there is a hole at point P_2. From Huygens' principle, wave will propagates from the sources S_1 and S_2. Each point on the screen will acts as secondary sources of wavelets.

Now, there is a hole at point P_2 (minima). The hole will act as a source of fresh light for the slits S_3 and S_4.

Therefore, there will be a regular two slit pattern on the second screen.

37. (c) Intensity in the first case, $I_1 = (\sqrt{I_0} + \sqrt{I_0})^2 = 4I_0$

where, I_0 = intensity due to each source.

Intensity in second case, $I_2 = I_0 + I_0 = 2I_0$

$\therefore \quad \frac{I_1}{I_2} = \frac{4I_0}{2I_0} = \frac{2}{1}$

38. (a) Let I_0 be the intensity of light emitted from the source, then

Resultant intensity, $I = 4I_0 \cos^2 \frac{\phi}{2}$

$$I_1 = 4I_0 \cos^2 \frac{\phi}{2} = 4I_0$$

Now, $\quad \Delta x = \frac{\lambda}{4}$

$$\phi = \frac{2\pi}{\lambda} \times \Delta x = \frac{2\pi}{\lambda} \times \frac{\lambda}{4}$$

$\Rightarrow \quad \phi = \frac{\pi}{2}$

and $\quad I_2 = 4I_0 \cos^2 \frac{\pi}{4} = 2I_0$

$$I_1 : I_2 = 2 : 1$$

39. (a) Path difference, $\Delta x = \frac{yd}{D} = \left(\frac{1.25\lambda D}{d}\right)\left(\frac{d}{D}\right)$

$$= 1.25\lambda = \frac{5}{4}\lambda$$

Phase difference, $\phi = \frac{2\pi}{\lambda} \cdot \Delta x$

$$= \frac{2\pi}{\lambda} \times \frac{5}{4}\lambda = \frac{5}{2}\pi$$

$\therefore \quad \frac{\phi}{2} = \frac{5}{4}\pi = 225°$

$\therefore$ Intensity, $I = I_{max} \cos^2 \frac{\phi}{2} = \frac{1}{2} I_{max}$

40. (c) Intensity, $I = 4I_0 \cos^2 \frac{\phi}{2}$

$\Rightarrow \quad \frac{\cos^2 \phi}{2} = \frac{1}{4}$

$\Rightarrow \quad I = I_0$

$\therefore \quad \phi = \frac{2\pi}{3} = \frac{2\pi}{\lambda} \cdot \Delta x = \frac{2\pi}{\lambda}\left(\frac{yd}{D}\right)$

$\therefore \quad y = \frac{\lambda D}{3d}$

41. (c) $2I_0 = 4I_0 \cos^2 \frac{\phi}{2}$

$$\phi = \frac{\pi}{2} = \frac{2\pi}{\lambda} \cdot \Delta x = \frac{2\pi}{\lambda} \cdot \left(\frac{y_1 d}{D}\right)$$

$\therefore \quad y_1 = \frac{\lambda D}{4d}$

Further, $I_0 = 4I_0 \cos^2 \frac{\phi}{2}$

$\Rightarrow \quad \phi = \frac{2\pi}{3} = \frac{2\pi}{\lambda} \Delta x = \frac{2\pi}{\lambda}\left(\frac{y_2 d}{D}\right)$

$\therefore \quad y_2 = \frac{\lambda D}{3d}$

Minimum separation, $\Delta y = y_2 - y_1 = \frac{1}{12}\left(\frac{\lambda D}{d}\right) = \frac{\alpha}{12}$

42 (c) We know that, $\tan i = \frac{1}{\sin C}$

$$\cot i = \sin\left[\sin^{-1}\left(\frac{3}{5}\right)\right]$$

$\Rightarrow \quad \tan i = \frac{5}{3}$

$\Rightarrow \quad i = \tan^{-1}\left(\frac{5}{3}\right)$

$\therefore \quad n = 3$

43. (a) Location of the point, $y = \frac{\omega}{4} = \frac{\lambda D}{4d}$

$\Rightarrow \quad \Delta x = \frac{yd}{D} = \frac{\lambda}{4}$

$\Rightarrow \quad \phi = \frac{2\pi}{\lambda} \cdot \Delta x = \frac{\pi}{2}$

$\because \quad I_R = I_1 + I_2 + 2\sqrt{I_1 I_2} \cos \phi$

$\therefore \quad 4I = 2I + I_2 + 0$

$\Rightarrow \quad I_2 = 2I$

44. (c) Path difference between the waves reaching at O,

$$\Delta = \Delta_1 + \Delta_2$$

where, Δ_1 = initial path difference and Δ_2 = path difference between the waves after emerging from slits.

Now, $\Delta_1 = SS_1 - SS_2 = \sqrt{(D^2 + d^2)} - D$

and $\Delta_2 = S_1O - S_2O = \sqrt{(D^2 + d^2)} - D$

$\therefore$ $\Delta = 2\{\sqrt{(D^2 + d^2)} - D\} = 2\{(D^2 + d^2)^{1/2} - D\}$

$$= 2\left\{\left(D + \frac{d^2}{2D}\right) - D\right\}$$

(from binomial expansion)

$$= \frac{d^2}{D}$$

For obtaining dark at O, Δ must be equals to $(2n-1)\frac{\lambda}{2}$.

i.e. $\frac{d^2}{D} = (2n-1)\frac{\lambda}{2}$

$\therefore$ $d^2 = \frac{(2n-1)\lambda D}{2}$ or $d = \sqrt{\frac{(2n-1)\lambda D}{2}}$

For minimum distance $(n = 1)$,

So, $d = \sqrt{\frac{\lambda D}{2}}$

45. (b) The condition of interference maxima is

$d \sin\theta = n\lambda$, $\sin\theta = \frac{n\lambda}{d}$

Given, $d = 2\lambda$ and $\sin\theta = \frac{n\lambda}{2\lambda} = \frac{n}{2}$

The magnitude of $\sin\theta$ lies between 0 and 1.

When $n = 0$, $\sin\theta = 0 \Rightarrow \theta = 0°$

When $n = 1$, $\sin\theta = 1/2 \Rightarrow \theta = 30°$

When $n = 2$, $\sin\theta = 1 \Rightarrow \theta = 90°$

Thus, there is central maximum at $\theta = 0°$, on either side of it maxima lie at $\theta = 30°$ and $\theta = 90°$, so maximum number of possible interference maxima is five.

46. (b) In diffraction, fringe width, $\beta = \frac{\lambda D}{d}$

When $\frac{d}{2} = \beta$, then $\frac{d}{2} = \frac{\lambda D}{d} \Rightarrow D = \frac{d^2}{2\lambda}$

47. (a) To find the point of coincidence of bright fringes, we can equate the distance of bright fringes from the central maximum, made by both the wavelengths of light.

Given, distance between the screen and slit,

$D = 120 \text{ cm} = 120 \times 10^{-2}$ m

Slit width, $d = 2 \text{ mm} = 2 \times 10^{-3}$ m

$\lambda_1 = 6500$ Å and $\lambda_2 = 5200$ Å

Let nth fringe due to $\lambda_2 = 5200$ Å coincide with $(n-1)$th bright fringe due to $\lambda_1 = 6500$ Å.

$\therefore$ $\frac{Dn\lambda_2}{d} = \frac{D(n-1)\lambda_1}{d}$

or $n \times 5200 = (n-1)\, 6500$

or $4n = 5n - 5$

$\Rightarrow$ $n = 5$

So, the least distance required, $y_n = \frac{n\lambda_2 D}{d}$

$$= \frac{5 \times 5200 \times 10^{-10} \times 120 \times 10^{-2}}{2 \times 10^{-3}}$$

$$= 0.16 \times 10^{-2} \text{m} = 0.16 \text{ cm}$$

48. (a) Most of the light is diffracted between the two first order minima. These minima occur at angles given by $b \sin\theta = \pm\lambda$.

$\Rightarrow$ $\sin\theta = \pm\frac{\lambda}{b} = \pm\frac{4.5 \times 10^{-7}}{0.2 \times 10^{-3}} = \pm 2.25 \times 10^{-3}$

$\Rightarrow$ $\theta \simeq 2.25 \times 10^{-3}$ rad (angle is very small)

The angular divergence, $2\theta = 4.5 \times 10^{-3}$ rad

49. (b) Fringe width, $\beta = \frac{D\lambda}{d}$

$\Rightarrow$ $d = \frac{D\lambda}{\beta} = \frac{6000 \times 10^{-10} \times 40 \times 10^{-2}}{0.012 \times 10^{-2}} = 0.2$ cm

50. (a) According to the question,

$\lambda = 6250 \text{ Å} = 6250 \times 10^{-10} \times 10^2$ cm

$= 6250 \times 10^{-8}$ cm

Width of the slit, $a = 2 \times 10^{-2}$ cm

The angular width of central maximum, $\beta = 2\theta = 2\frac{\lambda}{a}$

Thus, linear width is

$$L = \beta \times D = \frac{2\lambda}{a} \times D$$

$$= \frac{2 \times 6250 \times 10^{-8}}{2 \times 10^{-2}} \times 50$$

$$= 6250 \times 10^{-6} \times 50 = 3125 \times 10^{-4}$$

$$= 312.5 \times 10^{-3} \text{ cm}$$

51. (c) According to law of Malus, when a beam of completely plane polarised light is incident on an analyser, the resultant intensity of light I transmitted from an analyser varies directly as the square of cosine angle between plane of analyser and polariser.

Let initial intensity is I and final intensity is I', then

$$I' = I\cos^2 60° = I\left(\frac{1}{2}\right)^2 = \frac{I}{4}$$

Now, % difference between initial and final intensities,

$$= \frac{I - (I/4)}{I} \times 100 = \frac{3I}{4} \times \frac{1}{I} \times 100$$

$$= \frac{3}{4} \times 100 = 75\,\%$$

52. (a) In Young's double slit experiment, the locus of the point P lying in a plane with a constant path difference between the two interfering waves is a hyperbola.

53. (c) For net intensity, $I' = 4I_0 \cos^2 \frac{\phi}{2}$

Case I $K = 4I_0 \cos^2\left(\frac{2\pi}{2}\right) \quad \left(\because \phi = \frac{2\pi}{\lambda} \times \lambda\right)$

$$K = 4I_0 \cos^2 (\pi) \Rightarrow K = 4I_0 \quad \text{...(i)}$$

Case II $K' = 4I_0 \cos^2\left(\frac{\pi/2}{2}\right) \quad \left(\because \phi = \frac{2\pi}{\lambda} \times \frac{\lambda}{4}\right)$

$$K' = 4I_0 \cos^2 (\pi/4)$$

$$\Rightarrow K' = 2I_0 \quad \text{...(ii)}$$

Comparing Eqs. (i) and (ii), we get

$$K' = K/2$$

54. (c) $\frac{I_{max}}{I_{min}} = \left(\frac{a_{max}}{a_{min}}\right)^2 = \left(\frac{a_1 + a_2}{a_1 - a_2}\right)^2$

According to given question, $\frac{I_{max}}{I_{min}} = \frac{9}{1}$

$$\Rightarrow 9 = \left(\frac{a_1/a_2 + 1}{a_1/a_2 - 1}\right)^2$$

$$\Rightarrow (3)^2 = \left(\frac{a_1/a_2 + 1}{a_1/a_2 - 1}\right)^2$$

$$\Rightarrow 3 = \frac{a_1/a_2 + 1}{a_1/a_2 - 1}$$

$$\Rightarrow 3\left(\frac{a_1}{a_2}\right) - 3 = \frac{a_1}{a_2} + 1$$

$$\Rightarrow 2\left(\frac{a_1}{a_2}\right) = 4$$

$$\Rightarrow \frac{a_1}{a_2} = \frac{4}{2} = \frac{2}{1}$$

$$\Rightarrow a_1 : a_2 = 2 : 1$$

55. (c) According to given question,

$$I_1 : I_2 = 3 : 1, \; a_1 : a_2 = ?$$

The intensity of light due to an illuminated slit is directly proportional to the width of the slit, if ω_1 and ω_2 be the width of two silts and I_1 and I_2 are the intensities of light on the screen due to the respective slits, then

$$\frac{w_1}{w_2} = \frac{I_1}{I_2} = \left(\frac{a_1}{a_2}\right)^2$$

where, a_1 and a_2 are the amplitudes of the corresponding light wave.

Here, $\frac{w_1}{w_2} = \frac{3}{1}$

$$\Rightarrow \left(\frac{a_1}{a_2}\right)^2 = \frac{3}{1} \text{ or } a_1 : a_2 = \sqrt{3} : 1$$

56. (b) Given, $\lambda_1 = 12000$ Å and $\lambda_2 = 10000$ Å, $D = 2$ m and $d = 2$ mm $= 2 \times 10^{-3}$ m

We have, $\frac{\lambda_1}{\lambda_2} = \frac{12000}{10000} = \frac{6}{5} = \frac{n_2}{n_1}$

As, $x = \frac{n_1 \lambda_1 D}{d} = \frac{5 \times 12000 \times 10^{-10} \times 2}{2 \times 10^{-3}}$

$$= 5 \times 1.2 \times 10^4 \times 10^{-10} \times 10^3 = 6 \text{ mm}$$

57. (c) Fringe width, $\beta = \frac{D\lambda}{d}$

Given, $d = 0.4$ mm, $D = 200$ cm $= 2000$ mm

$\beta = 2$ mm

$$\therefore \quad 2 = \frac{2000 \times \lambda}{0.4} \Rightarrow \lambda = 400 \text{ nm}$$

58. (b) Here, the condition for the formation of rings is $\lambda \approx \frac{d^2}{4D}$.

59. (a) We know that,

$$\text{Distance} = \frac{2\lambda}{b} \times d$$

$$= \frac{2 \times 0.5 \times 10^{-4}}{2} \times 100 = 5 \text{ mm}$$

60. (d) When we close one slit in the Young's double slit experiment, then the single slit diffraction pattern is observed.

61. (c) $\Delta\phi = (2n - 1)\pi$

For $n = 3$, $\Delta\phi = 5\pi$

62. (a) Fringe width, $\beta = \frac{D\lambda}{d}$

According to question, $\frac{\beta_2}{\beta_1} = \frac{\lambda_2 D_2 d_1}{\lambda_1 D_1 d_2}$

Here, $D_2 = 2D_1$ and $d_2 = \frac{d_1}{2}$

$$\Rightarrow \frac{\beta_2}{\beta_1} = \frac{\lambda_2 (2D_1) \times d_1}{\lambda_1 (D_1) \times \left(\frac{d_1}{2}\right)} = 4\frac{\lambda_2}{\lambda_1} = \frac{4 \times 4 \times 10^{-7}}{6.4 \times 10^{-7}}$$

$$\Rightarrow \beta_2 = \frac{4 \times 4 \times 10^{-7} \times 1 \times 10^{-4}}{6.4 \times 10^{-7}} = 2.5 \times 10^{-4} \text{ m}$$

63. (b) By Young's double slit interference experiment,

$$\beta = \frac{\lambda D}{d}$$

Given, $\beta_1 = 1.2$ mm, $\frac{d_2}{d_1} = 1\frac{1}{2} = 1.5$

So, $\beta \propto \frac{1}{d} \Rightarrow \frac{\beta_1}{\beta_2} = \frac{1/d_1}{1/d_2}$

$\Rightarrow \frac{\beta_1}{\beta_2} = \frac{d_2}{d_1} = 1.5 \Rightarrow \frac{1.2}{\beta_2} = 1.5$

$\Rightarrow \beta_2 = \frac{1.2}{1.5} = \frac{4}{5} = 0.8\text{ mm}$

64. (*d*) Let λ be the wavelength of monochromatic light incident on slit *S*, then the angular distance between two consecutive fringes, *i.e.*, the angular fringe width is $\theta = \lambda/d$ ...(i)

where, d = distance between coherent sources.

Given, $\frac{\Delta\theta}{\theta} = \frac{10}{100}$

So, from Eq. (i), $\frac{\Delta\lambda}{\lambda} = \frac{\Delta\theta}{\theta} = \frac{10}{100} = 0.1$

$\Rightarrow \Delta\lambda = 0.1\lambda = 0.1 \times 5890\text{ Å} = 589\text{ Å}$ (increases)

65. (*a*) $\frac{I_{max}}{I_{min}} = \frac{(\sqrt{2I}+\sqrt{I})^2}{(\sqrt{2I}-\sqrt{I})^2} = \left(\frac{\sqrt{2}+1}{\sqrt{2}-1}\right)^2$ (given)

$\Rightarrow \frac{I_{max}}{I_{min}} = \left[\frac{(\sqrt{2}+1)(\sqrt{2}+1)}{(\sqrt{2}-1)(\sqrt{2}+1)}\right]^2$

$= \left(\frac{2+1+2\sqrt{2}}{2-1}\right)^2$

$= \frac{9+8+12\sqrt{2}}{1} = 34$

66. (*b*) The bandwidth is inversely proportional to the distance between the slits *d*.

As, $\beta = \frac{\lambda D}{d} \Rightarrow \beta \propto \frac{1}{d}$

67. (*b*) Given,

$d = 1\text{mm} = 1 \times 10^{-3}\text{ m}, \lambda = 500\text{ nm} = 500 \times 10^{-9}\text{ m}$

and $D = 1\text{m}$

Fringe separation, $\beta = \frac{\lambda D}{d} = \frac{500 \times 10^{-9} \times 1}{1 \times 10^{-3}}$

$= 500 \times 10^{-6}$

$= 0.5 \times 10^{-3}\text{ m} = 0.5\text{ mm}$

68. (*c*) Given, $n = 1, \lambda = 6500\text{ Å} = 6500 \times 10^{-10}\text{ m}$

and $\sin 30° = \frac{1}{2}$

$\Rightarrow d = \frac{n\lambda}{\sin 30°} = \frac{6500 \times 10^{-10}}{(1/2)}$

$\Rightarrow d = 1.3 \times 10^{-6}\text{ m}$

69. (*d*) Grating with 10^6 lines/cm is suitable for constructing spectrometer for visible and ultraviolet region because this corresponds to the wavelength, equivalent to the wavelengths of visible and ultraviolet region.

70. (*a*) Width of central maximum, $\beta = \frac{2D\lambda}{d}$

As, we increase d to $2d$, β becomes $\frac{\beta}{2}$.

So, it becomes narrower and fainter.

71. (*c*) The source is at infinity and incident beam is parallel.

72. (*d*) Given, $\theta_p = 57°$

According to Brewster's law, we have

$\theta_p + r = 90° \Rightarrow r = 90° - \theta_p = 90° - 57°$

Angle of refraction, $r = 33°$

73. (*d*) Suppose, i_p is the Brewster's angle, when unpolarised light is incident at an polarising angle, the reflected component along *OB* and refracted component along *OC* in the following figure.

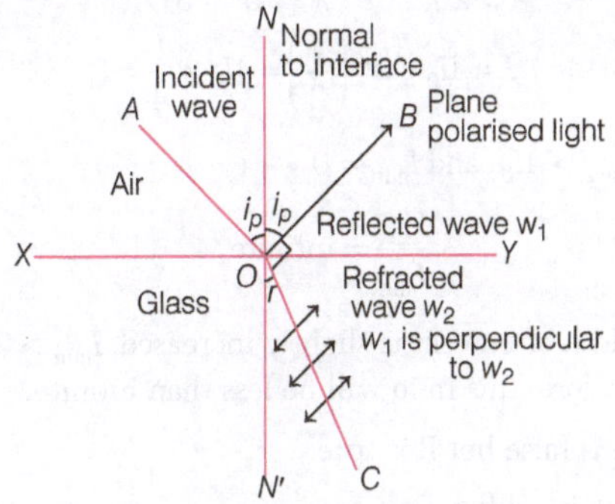

Now, $\angle BOY + \angle YOC = 90°$

$(90° - i_p) + (90° - r) = 90°$

Here, r is the angle of refraction.

$\Rightarrow 90° - i_p = r$

According to Snell's law, $\mu = \frac{\sin i}{\sin r}$

When $i = i_p$, $r = 90° - i_p$, then

$\mu = \frac{\sin i_p}{\sin(90° - i_p)} = \frac{\sin i_p}{\cos i_p} = \tan i_p$

$\therefore i_p = \tan^{-1}(\mu)$

where, i_p is polarised angle.

74. (*d*) By Malus' law, $I = I_0 \cos^2\theta$

(where, I = intensity of emergent polarised light, I_0 = intensity passed through polariser)

Given, $\theta = 60°, I = ?$

$\Rightarrow I = I_0 \times \cos^2 60° = I_0 \times \left(\frac{1}{2}\right)^2 = \frac{I_0}{4}$

75. (*c*) Wave theory of light explains the phenomenon of interference, diffraction and velocity of light in a denser medium or rarer medium, but this theory fails to explain the scattering of light.

76. (*b*) For polarising angle,

$$\mu = \tan i_p \text{ and } \mu = \frac{1}{\sin C}$$

$$\tan i_p = \frac{1}{\sin C}$$

where, C = critical angle.

$$\therefore \quad \cot i_p = \sin\left(\sin^{-1}\left(\frac{3}{5}\right)\right)$$

$$\Rightarrow \quad \cot i_p = \frac{3}{5} \text{ or } \tan i = \frac{5}{3}$$

$$\text{or} \quad i_p = \tan^{-1}\left(\frac{5}{3}\right)$$

Assertion and Reason

1. (b) $$\phi = \frac{2\pi}{\lambda} \cdot \Delta x = \frac{2\pi}{\lambda} \times \frac{\lambda}{3} = \frac{2\pi}{3}$$

and $$I = 4I_0 \cos^2\left(\frac{\phi}{2}\right) = 4I_0 \times \frac{1}{4} = I_0$$

2. (a) $I_{max} > 4I_0$ and $I_{min} = 0$

$$\therefore \quad \frac{I_{max}}{I_{min}} = \text{infinite}$$

If width of one slit is slightly increased, $I_{min} > 0$. Therefore, this ratio will be less than infinite.

3. (c) A is false but R is true

$$\beta \propto D$$

4. (b) When white light is used, then path difference for all components of white light is zero at the central position, hence central fringe will be white.

Since, $\beta = \frac{D\lambda}{d}$

$\therefore \quad \beta \propto \lambda$

5. (d) When a polaroid is rotated in the path of unpolarised light, the intensity of light transmitted from polaroid remain undiminished (because unpolarised light contains waves vibrating in all possible planes with equal probability).

However, when the polaroid is rotated in path of plane polarised light, its intensity will vary from maximum (when the vibrations of the plane polarised light are parallel to the axis of the polaroid) to minimum (when the direction of the vibrations becomes perpendicular to the axis of the crystal). Thus, using polaroid, we can easily identify that whether the light is polarised or not.

Statement Type Questions

1. (d) Both statements I and II are correct.

When the source is emitting yellow light, then there will be a dark fringe at a point where path difference is $\frac{3\lambda}{2}$ [from condition for dark fringe $x = (2n+1)\lambda/2$].

If the light is white, then the fringe will be coloured, the yellow and neighbouring colours being absent.

2. (a) Both Statement I and Statement II are incorrect.

When Young's double slit experiment is performed by a source of white light, the central fringe will be white, there will not be a completely dark fringe and the fringe next to the central fringe will be violet.

3. (d) Both Statement I and Statement II are correct.

In a interference pattern, the light waves from two coherent, monochromatic sources will interfere constructively and destructively to produce a pattern of antinodes and nodes, *i.e.* maxima of light patterns are of same intensity.

In diffraction, as order increase, the spacing between consecutive bands decreases.

4. (b) Statement I is correct but Statement II is incorrect.

Fringe width is given by $\beta = \frac{D\lambda}{d}$

where, D = distance between slit and screen, d = distance between coherent sources of light and λ = wavelength of incident light.

It is independent of the phase difference and same for both bright and dark fringes.

5. (a) Both Statement I and Statement II are correct.

Interference occurs only due to superposition of light waves from two sources. When one of the slit is closed, then it acts as general illumination from a single source. Interference does not take place.

Match the Columns

1. (a) Resultant intensity of two waves from coherent sources is given by

$$I_R = I_1 + I_2 + 2\sqrt{I_1 I_2} \cos\phi$$

Here, $I_1 = I_2 = I$

So, $I_R = 2I + 2I\cos\phi$

(A) If $\phi = 60°$,

$$I_R = 2I + 2I\cos 60°$$
$$= 2I + 2I \times \frac{1}{2} = 3I$$

(B) If $\phi = 90°$,

$$I_R = 2I + 2I\cos 90° = 2I$$

(C) If $\phi = 0°$,

$$I_R = 2I + 2I\cos 0° = 4I$$

(D) If $\phi = 120°$,

$$I_R = 2I + 2I\cos 120° = 2I + 2I \times \left(-\frac{1}{2}\right) = I$$

Hence, A-(IV), B-(II), C-(I), D-(III).

2. (*b*) For dark fringe, $\Delta\phi = (2n - 1)\pi$

(A) For $n = 4$,

$$\Delta\phi = (2 \times 4 - 1)\pi = 7\pi$$

(B) For $n = 2$,

$$\Delta\phi = (2 \times 2 - 1)\pi = 3\pi$$

(C) For $n = 5$,

$$\Delta\phi = (2 \times 5 - 1)\pi = 9\pi$$

(D) For $n = 6$,

$$\Delta\phi = (2 \times 6 - 1)\pi = 11\pi$$

Hence, A-(III), B-(IV), C-(II), D-(I).

3. (*b*)

A. Before introducing transparent sheet, intensity of maxima is $4I_0$. After introducing transparent sheet, intensity of maxima is

$$\left(\sqrt{I_0} + \sqrt{\frac{I_0}{4}}\right)^2 = I_0\left(1 + \frac{1}{2}\right)^2 = \frac{9}{4}I_0$$

Thus, intensity of maxima will decrease.

B. Before introducing transparent sheet, intensity of minima is zero. After introducing transparent sheet, intensity of minima is

$$(\sqrt{I_0} - \sqrt{I_0/4})^2 = \frac{I_0}{4}$$

C. Fringe width, $\beta = \frac{D}{d}\lambda$. Hence, it remains unchanged.

D. Since, transparent sheet is used infront S_1, so fringe pattern will shift downward.

Hence, A-(II), B-(I), C-(III), D-(IV).

4. (*a*) For polarising angle, $\mu = \tan i_p$

and $$\mu = \frac{1}{\sin C}$$

$$\tan i_p = \frac{1}{\sin C}$$

where, C is critical angle,

(A) ∴ $$\cot i_p = \sin\left(\sin^{-1}\left(\frac{1}{\sqrt{3}}\right)\right)$$

$$\cot i_p = \frac{1}{\sqrt{3}} \text{ or } \tan i_p = \sqrt{3}$$

or $$i_p = \tan^{-1}(\sqrt{3}) = 60°$$

(B) ∴ $$\cot i_p = \sin\left(\sin^{-1}\left(\frac{4}{3}\right)\right)$$

$$\cot i_p = \frac{4}{3} \text{ or } \tan i_p = \frac{3}{4}$$

or $$i_p = \tan^{-1}\left(\frac{3}{4}\right) = 37°$$

(C) ∴ $$\cot i_p = \sin(\sin^{-1}(1))$$

$$\cot i_p = 1 \text{ or } \tan i_p = 1$$

or $$i_p = \tan^{-1}(1) = 45°$$

(D) ∴ $$\cot i_p = \sin(\sin^{-1}(\sqrt{3}))$$

$$\cot i_p = \sqrt{3}$$

or $$\tan i_p = \frac{1}{\sqrt{3}}$$

or $$i_p = \tan^{-1}\left(\frac{1}{\sqrt{3}}\right) = 30°$$

Hence, A-(IV), B-(III), C-(II), D-(I).

Final Check Through PYQs

1. (*b*) It is given that, $\frac{I_2}{I_1} = n \Rightarrow I_2 = nI_1$

∴ Ratio of intensities is given by

$$\frac{I_{max} - I_{min}}{I_{max} + I_{min}} = \frac{(\sqrt{I_2} + \sqrt{I_1})^2 - (\sqrt{I_2} - \sqrt{I_1})^2}{(\sqrt{I_1} + \sqrt{I_2})^2 + (\sqrt{I_2} - \sqrt{I_1})^2)}$$

$$= \frac{\left(\sqrt{\frac{I_2}{I_1}} + 1\right)^2 - \left(\sqrt{\frac{I_2}{I_1}} - 1\right)^2}{\left(\sqrt{\frac{I_2}{I_1}} + 1\right)^2 + \left(\sqrt{\frac{I_2}{I_1}} - 1\right)^2}$$

$$= \frac{(\sqrt{n} + 1)^2 - (\sqrt{n} - 1)^2}{(\sqrt{n} + 1)^2 + (\sqrt{n} - 1)^2} = \frac{2\sqrt{n}}{n + 1}$$

2. (*c*) When YDSE is performed in white light instead of monochromatic light, all wavelengths show their maxima and minima in orders of their wavelength. At central point on screen, path difference is zero for all wavelengths. Thus a central bright fringe is observed along with few fringes that will be different colours.

3. (*b*) Angular separation of fringes, $\theta = \frac{\lambda}{d}$

i.e. Angular separation does not depend on the distance between screen and plane of slits. Thus, Statement I is correct.

Since, $\theta \propto \lambda$

Thus, if the monochromatic source is replaced by another monochromatic source of larger wavelength, then angular separation of fringes increases. Hence, Statement II is incorrect.

4. (c) In Young's double slit experiment, wavelength of light used is inversely proportional to the number of fringes observed.

i.e. $\lambda_1 n_1 = \lambda_2 n_2$

$$n_2 = \frac{n_1 \lambda_1}{\lambda_2}$$

Here, $\lambda_1 = 600 \text{ nm} = 6 \times 10^{-7} \text{ m}$

$\lambda_2 = 400 \text{ nm} = 4 \times 10^{-7} \text{ m}$

$n_1 = 8$

$$\therefore \quad n_2 = \frac{8 \times 6 \times 10^{-7}}{4 \times 10^{-7}} = 12$$

5. (a) For central maximum, path difference is zero for both coherent sources in interference.

Hence, phase difference

$$= \frac{2\pi}{\lambda} \times \text{path difference}$$

$$= \frac{2\pi}{\lambda} \times 0 = 0$$

6. (b) Fringe width, $\beta = \frac{\lambda D}{d}$

$$\therefore \quad \frac{\beta_2}{\beta_1} = \frac{\frac{\lambda_2 D_2}{d_2}}{\frac{\lambda_1 D_1}{d_1}} \quad \left[\text{As } \lambda_1 = \lambda_2, D_2 = 2D_1 \text{ and } d_2 = \frac{d_1}{2}\right]$$

$$\therefore \quad \frac{\beta_2}{\beta_1} = \frac{2D_1}{\left(\frac{d_1}{2}\right)} \times \frac{d_1}{D_1} = 4 \Rightarrow \beta_2 = 4\beta_1$$

i.e. Fringe width becomes four times.

7. (c) In a YDSE, the path difference for nth minima is given by $\Delta y = (2n-1)\frac{\lambda}{2}$

For 5th minima, $n = 5$

$$\therefore \quad \Delta y = [2(5) - 1]\frac{\lambda}{2} = \frac{9\lambda}{2}$$

8. (a) The angular width in YDSE is given by $\theta = \frac{\beta}{D}$

If YDSE apparatus is immersed in a liquid of refractive index μ, then the wavelength of light and hence the angular width decreases by μ times.

i.e. $\theta' = \frac{\beta}{\mu D} = \frac{\theta}{\mu}$

Here, μ (for water) $= 4/3$ and $\theta = 0.2°$

$$\Rightarrow \quad \theta' = \frac{0.2}{4/3} = 0.15°$$

9. (b) Here, $\theta_1 = 0.20°, \theta_2 = 0.21°$

$d_1 = 2 \text{ mm}$

We know that

Angular width, $\theta = \frac{\lambda}{d}$

$$\Rightarrow \quad \theta \propto \frac{1}{d} \quad [\because \lambda \text{ same for both}]$$

$$\therefore \quad \frac{\theta_1}{\theta_2} = \frac{d_2}{d_1}$$

$$d_2 = \frac{\theta_1}{\theta_2} \times d_1 = \frac{0.20}{0.21} \times 2$$

$$= 1.9 \text{ mm}$$

10. (d) According to question,

5th dark fringe in air = 8 bright fringe in the medium

$$(2 \times 5 - 1)\frac{\lambda D}{2d} = 8\frac{\lambda D}{\mu d}$$

$$\Rightarrow \quad 9\frac{\lambda D}{2d} = 8\frac{\lambda D}{\mu d}$$

$$\Rightarrow \quad \frac{9}{2} = \frac{8}{\mu} \Rightarrow \mu = \frac{8 \times 2}{9}$$

$$\mu = \frac{16}{9} = 1.7777 \approx 1.78$$

11. (c)

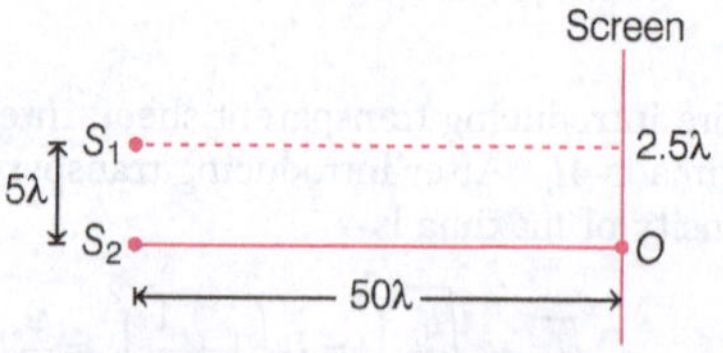

In the above figure, S_1 and S_2 are the two different slits.

Given, distance between slits S_1 and S_2, $d = 5\lambda$

distance between screen and slits,

$$D = 10d = 50\lambda$$

Here, λ is the wavelength of light used in the experiment.

According to question, the intensity at maximum in this Young's double slit experiment is I_0.

$\Rightarrow I_{max} = I_0$

$$\because \text{Path difference} = \frac{dY_n}{D} = \frac{d \times \frac{d}{2}}{10d} = \frac{d}{20} = \frac{\lambda}{4} \quad \{\because d = 5\lambda\}$$

A path difference of λ corresponds to phase difference 2π, so for path difference $\lambda/4$, phase difference

$$\phi = \frac{2\pi}{\lambda} \times \frac{\lambda}{4}$$

$$= \pi/2 = 90°$$

As we know, $I = I_0 \cos^2 \frac{\phi}{2}$

$$\Rightarrow \quad I = I_0 \cos^2 \frac{90^\circ}{2}$$

$$\Rightarrow \quad I = I_0 \times \left(\frac{1}{\sqrt{2}}\right)^2 \Rightarrow I = \frac{I_0}{2}$$

12. (*a*) Given, $d = 1 \text{ mm} = 1 \times 10^{-3}$ m

$D = 1$ m, $\lambda = 500$ nm

$= 5 \times 10^{-7}$ m

As, width of central maxima = width of 10 maxima

$$\therefore \quad \frac{2D\lambda}{a} = 10\left(\frac{\lambda D}{d}\right)$$

$$\Rightarrow \quad a = \frac{d}{5} = \frac{10^{-3}}{5} = 0.2 \times 10^{-3} \text{m}$$

$= 0.2$ mm

13. (*a*) Given, YDSE experiment, having two slits of width are in the ratio of 1 : 25.

So, ratio of intensity,

$$\frac{I_1}{I_2} = \frac{\beta_1}{\beta_2} = \frac{1}{25} \Rightarrow \frac{I_2}{I_1} = \frac{25}{1}$$

$$\therefore \quad \frac{I_{max}}{I_{min}} = \frac{(\sqrt{I_2} + \sqrt{I_1})^2}{(\sqrt{I_2} - \sqrt{I_1})^2} = \left[\frac{\sqrt{\frac{I_2}{I_1}} + 1}{\sqrt{\frac{I_2}{I_1}} - 1}\right]^2$$

$$\Rightarrow \quad \left[\frac{5+1}{5-1}\right]^2 = \left(\frac{6}{4}\right)^2 = \frac{36}{16} = \frac{9}{4}$$

Thus, $\dfrac{I_{max}}{I_{min}} = \dfrac{9}{4}$

14. (*d*) At Brewster's law, the angle between refracted and reflected rays is 90°.

Therefore the reflected ray is completely linearly polarised and the refracted ray is partially polarised.

15. (*b*) Given, refractive index of glass surface

$\mu = \sqrt{3}$

Angle of incidence, $i = 60°$

Since, above situation follows Brewster's law because,

$\mu = \tan i$

$= \tan 60° = \sqrt{3}$

Hence, angle i is equal to polarising angle i_p.

i.e. $\quad i_p = i = 60°$

By Snell's law $\mu = \dfrac{\sin i_p}{\sin r}$

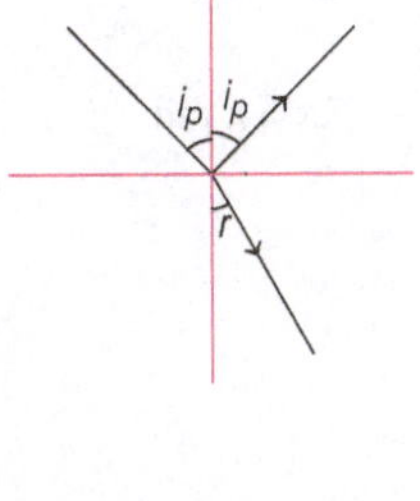

$$\Rightarrow \quad \tan i_p = \frac{\sin i_p}{\sin r} \qquad [\text{Since, } \mu = \tan i_p]$$

$$\Rightarrow \quad \frac{\sin i_p}{\cos i_p} = \frac{\sin i_p}{\sin r}$$

$$\Rightarrow \quad \cos i_p = \sin r$$

$$\Rightarrow \quad \cos i_p = \cos(90° - r)$$

$$\Rightarrow \quad i_p = 90° - r$$

$$\Rightarrow \quad r + i_p = 90°$$

Hence, angle between the refracted and reflected rays

$= 180° - (r + i_p)$

$= 180° - (90°) = 90°$

It is also called Brewster's law.

16. (*b*) The Brewster's angle i_b for an interface should lies between 45° to 90°, i.e. $45° < i_B < 90°$.

17. (*b*) The angular width of central maxima is given by

$$2\theta = \frac{2\lambda}{a} \qquad \text{...(i)}$$

where, λ = wavelength of light used

a = width of the slit

For $\quad \lambda_1 = 6000$ Å, $2\theta = \theta_0$ (given)

For another light of wavelength λ_2 (says), the angular width decreases by 30%, so

$$2\theta = \left(\frac{100 - 30}{100}\right)\theta_0 = \frac{70}{100}\theta_0 = 0.7\theta_0$$

As slit width is constant, so using Eq. (i) for these values, we get

$$\frac{\theta_0}{0.7\theta_0} = \frac{\lambda_1}{\lambda_2}$$

$$\Rightarrow \quad \lambda_2 = \lambda_1 \times 0.7 = 6000 \times 0.7 = 4200 \text{ Å}$$

18. (*b*) The figure shown below represents the course of path an unpolarised light follows when it is incident from air on plane surface of material of refractive index μ.

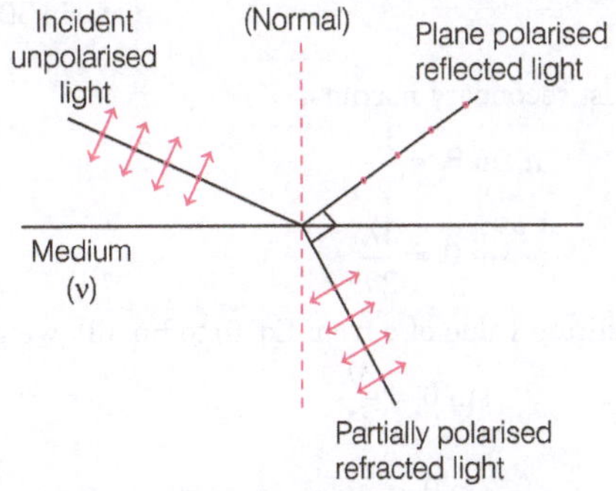

When the beam of unpolarised light is reflected from a medium (refractive index = μ) and if reflected and refracted light are perpendicular to each other, then the reflected light is completely plane polarised at a certain angle of incidence. This means, the reflected light has electric vector perpendicular to incidence plane.

19. (c) According to the question,

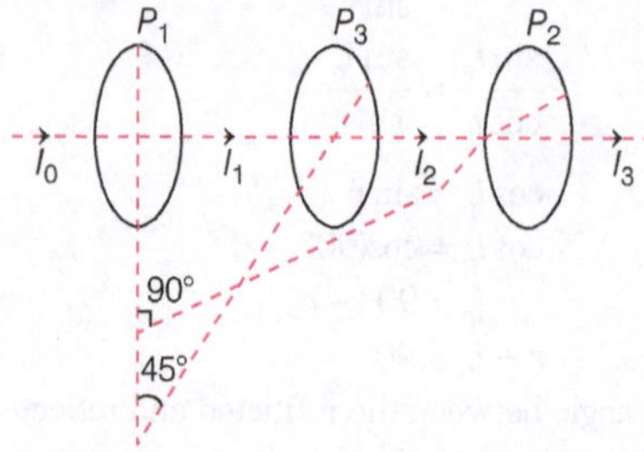

From the above diagram, intensity transmitted through P_3,

$$I_2 = \frac{I_0}{2}\cos^2 45°$$

$$\Rightarrow \quad I_2 = \frac{I_0}{2} \times \left(\frac{1}{\sqrt{2}}\right)^2$$

$$\Rightarrow \quad I_2 = \frac{I_0}{4}$$

Similarly, intensity transmitted through P_2,

$$I_3 = \frac{I_0}{4}\cos^2 45°$$

$$\Rightarrow \quad I_3 = \frac{I_0}{4} \times \left(\frac{1}{\sqrt{2}}\right)^2$$

$$\Rightarrow \quad I_3 = \frac{I_0}{4} \times \frac{1}{2} \Rightarrow I_3 = \frac{I_0}{8}$$

20. (c) As the first minimum is observed at an angle of 30° in a diffraction pattern due to a single slit of width a.

i.e. $\quad n = 1, \; \theta = 30°$

$\because$ According to Bragg's law of diffraction,

$$a \sin \theta = n\lambda$$

$$\Rightarrow \quad a \sin 30° = (1)\,\lambda \qquad (n = 1)$$

$$\Rightarrow \quad a = 2\lambda \qquad \text{...(i)}$$

$$\left\{\because \sin 30° = \frac{1}{2}\right\}$$

For Ist secondary maxima,

$$a \sin \theta_1 = \frac{3\lambda}{2}$$

$$\Rightarrow \quad \sin \theta_1 = \frac{3\lambda}{2a} \qquad \text{...(ii)}$$

Substitute value of a from Eq. (i) to Eq. (ii), we get

$$\sin \theta_1 = \frac{3\lambda}{4\lambda}$$

$$\Rightarrow \quad \sin \theta_1 = \frac{3}{4}$$

$$\Rightarrow \quad \theta_1 = \sin^{-1}\left(\frac{3}{4}\right)$$

21. (d) For the distance of the first dark band of the diffraction pattern from the centre of the screen is given by positon of Ist minima.

i.e. $\quad Y = \frac{\lambda D}{a}$

where, λ = wavelength of parallel beams

D = focal length

a = width of linear aperture.

$$\Rightarrow \quad Y = \frac{(5 \times 10^{-5})\,(0.6)}{0.02 \times 10^{-2}} \qquad \text{(given)}$$

$$\Rightarrow \quad Y = 0.15 \text{ cm}$$

22. (a) For the condition of maxima

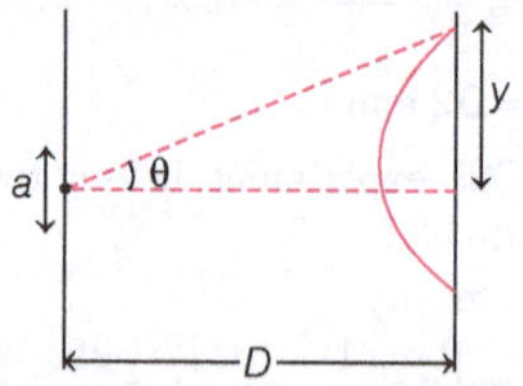

$$\sin \theta = \frac{\lambda}{a}$$

From the geometry,

$$\sin \theta = \theta = \frac{Y}{D} \text{ (for small angle)}$$

So, $\quad \frac{Y}{D} = \frac{\lambda}{a} \Rightarrow Y = \frac{\lambda D}{a}$

Hence, width of central maxima

$$= 2Y = \frac{2\lambda D}{a}$$

23. (c) For first minima at P,

$$a \sin \theta = n\lambda$$

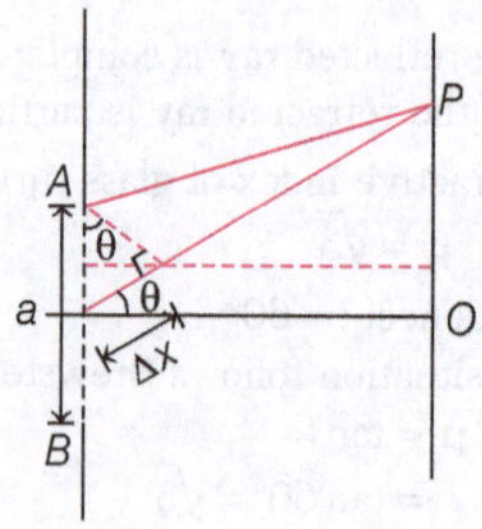

where, $n = 1$

$\Rightarrow a \sin \theta = \lambda$

So, phase difference,

$$\Delta\phi_1 = \frac{\Delta x_1}{\lambda} \times 2\pi = \frac{(a/2)\sin\theta}{\lambda} \times 2\pi$$

$$= \frac{\lambda}{2\lambda} \times 2\pi = \pi \text{ rad}$$

Skill Builder

■ Sol. of Skill Builder on Pg. 595

(*a*) It is given that, $\frac{I_2}{I_1} = 2$

$\therefore$ Ratio of intensities is given by

$$\frac{I_{max} + I_{min}}{I_{max} - I_{min}} = \frac{(\sqrt{I_1} + \sqrt{I_2})^2 + (\sqrt{I_2} - \sqrt{I_1})^2}{(\sqrt{I_2} + \sqrt{I_1})^2 - (\sqrt{I_2} - \sqrt{I_1})^2}$$

$$= \frac{\left(\sqrt{\frac{I_2}{I_1}} + 1\right)^2 + \left(\sqrt{\frac{I_2}{I_1}} - 1\right)^2}{\left(\sqrt{\frac{I_2}{I_1}} + 1\right)^2 - \left(\sqrt{\frac{I_2}{I_1}} - 1\right)^2}$$

$$= \frac{(\sqrt{2}+1)^2 + (\sqrt{2}-1)^2}{(\sqrt{2}+1)^2 - (\sqrt{2}-1)^2}$$

$$= \frac{(2+1)}{2\sqrt{2}} = \frac{3}{2\sqrt{2}} = \frac{3\sqrt{2}}{4}$$

■ Sol. of Skill Builder on Pg. 601

(*a*) Given, $n_1 = 10$

$\lambda_1 = 6000$ Å

$D_1 = D$

$\lambda_2 = 4000$ Å

$D_2 = 2D$

Using, $\frac{\lambda_1 n_1 D_1}{d} = \frac{\lambda_2 n_2 D_2}{d}$

$$\frac{6000 \times 10 \times D}{d} = \frac{4000 \times n_2 \times 2D}{d}$$

$$n_2 = 7.5$$

or 7 fringes will be obtained on the screen.

■ Sol. of Skill Builder on Pg. 609

(*a*) Given, $I_0 = 20$ lumen

$I = 15$ lumen

We know that, $I = I_0 \cos^2\theta$

$$15 = 20\cos^2\theta$$

$$\frac{15}{20} = \cos^2\theta$$

$$\frac{3}{4} = \cos^2\theta$$

$$\frac{\sqrt{3}}{2} = \cos\theta$$

$\Rightarrow$ $\theta = 30°$ $\left[\because \cos 30° = \frac{\sqrt{3}}{2}\right]$

For deeper insight
Scan the QR Code

Chapter 12

Dual Nature of Radiation and Matter

Learning Objectives

Module-I

- Electron Emission
- Photoelectric Effect
- Experimental Study of Photoelectric Effect
- Laws of Photoelectric Emission

Module-II

- Planck's Quantum Theory (Particle Nature of Light : the Photon)
- Einstein's Photoelectric Equation

Module-III

- Matter Waves : de-Broglie Waves
- Characteristics of Matter Waves

Chapter Overview with *NEET Connection*

This chapter is useful for the learning of complete quantum Physics. Without having strong hold on this chapter, it will be difficult to understand the chapter like atoms.

Special format questions can be easily framed on the following topics of this chapter :

- Graphs in photoelectric effect.
- Einstein's equation of photoelectric effect.
- Special terms such as threshold frequency, stopping potential, etc., and factors affecting those parameters.
- de-Broglie equation and its different form forms different particles.

For better understanding of this chapter

- Proper understanding of wave optics is required.
- Knowledge of graphs formation from equations will be helpful.

Introduction

In previous chapter, we studied about wave nature and its related phenomena. But there are some other phenomena such as photoelectric effect, which could not be explained on the basis of wave nature. According to these phenomena light show particle nature. Thus, to explain the wave nature and particle nature of light. Concept of dual nature of radiation introduce.

In this chapter, we will study about Planck's quantum theory, photoelectric effect and its explanation by Einstein, de-Broglie hypothesis and explanation of dual nature of radiations as well as matter.

Module 1

Photoelectric Effect

- Electron Emission • Photoelectric Effect • Experimental Study of Photoelectric Effect
- Laws of Photoelectric Emission

Electron Emission

In metals, the electrons in the outer shells (valence electrons) are loosely bound to the atoms, hence they are free to move easily within the metal surface but cannot leave their own surface. Such electrons are called **free electrons.**

These free electrons can be emitted or ejected from the metals, if they have sufficient energy to overcome the attractive pull of metal surface. The phenomenon of emission of these electrons from the surface of a metal is called electron emission.

The minimum required energy for the electron emission from the metal surface can be supplied to the free electrons by any of the following physical processes

(i) **Thermionic emission** The energy to the free electrons can be given by heating the metal. This process of emission of electrons is known as thermionic emission. The electrons, so emitted, are known as **thermions.**

(ii) **Field emission** When a conductor is put under strong electric field ($\approx 10^8$ V/m), the free electrons on it experience an electric force in the opposite direction of field. Beyond a certain limit, electrons start coming out of the metal surface. Emission of electrons from a metal surface by this method is called the field emission.

Mentor's TIP

- Field emission is also known as **cold emission** or **cold cathode emission.** One of the example of cold emission is spark plug.

(iii) **Photoelectric emission** It is the phenomenon of emission of electrons from the surface of metal when light radiations of suitable frequency fall on it. Here, the energy to free electrons is supplied by light photons.

Work Function

To pull out electrons from the surface of the metal, a certain minimum amount of energy is required. This minimum energy required by the electrons is called the work function of the metal. It is denoted by ϕ_0 or W.

It is measured in eV (electron-volt). 1 eV is defined as the energy gained by an electron when it has been accelerated by a potential difference of one volt (1 V), so that

$$1 \text{ eV} = 1.602 \times 10^{-19} \text{J}$$

Amongst metals, caesium is regarded as the best photosensitive material as it has lowest work function ($\phi_0 = 2.14$ eV), whereas work function for platinum is highest ($\phi_0 = 5.65$ eV).

Mentor's TIP

- Work function depends on the properties of the metal and the nature of its surface. It decreases with increase in temperature.

Photoelectric Effect

The phenomenon of emission of electrons from the surface of metal, when radiations of suitable frequency fall on it, is known as photoelectric effect.

The emitted electrons (as shown in figure) are called **photoelectrons** and the current, so produced is called **photoelectric current.**

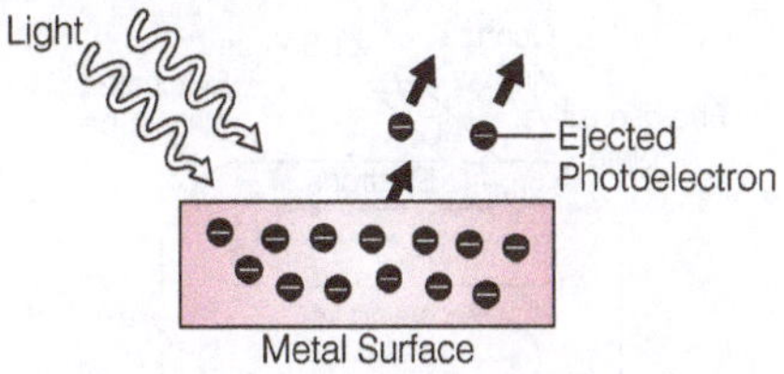

Emission of photoelectrons from the metal surface

Alkali metals like lithium, sodium, potassium, caesium, etc., show photoelectric effect with visible light, whereas the metals like zinc, cadmium, magnesium, etc., are sensitive only to ultraviolet light. Such materials are known as photosensitive materials.

The phenomenon of photoelectric effect was discovered by Heinrich Hertz in 1887, while detailed investigation on photoelectric emission was done by Wilhelm Hallwachs and Philipp Lenard.

NEET Snapshot

Caesium cannot emit photoelectron, if incident radiation has an energy of 1.9 eV. *[NEET 2023]*

The work function of caesium is 2.14 eV and for photoelectric emission, energy of incident radiation must be greater than or equal to work function of photosensitive surface.

Scan for Video

Hertz's Observation

- Hertz experimentally investigated on production of electromagnetic waves using spark discharge method.
- He found high voltage sparks (electrons) across metal when illuminated by UV light.
- Electrons escape from the surface into the surrounding environment are findings of Hertz's observations.

Lenard's Observation

- UV radiations incidented on metal plate (emitter) placed inside an evacuated glass tube which had two electrodes.
- It is found that current flows through the electrodes in the closed circuit (see experimental study of photoelectric effect).
- Lenard established that current flows confirmly due to incident light.
- Lenard studied how this current varies with collector plates' potential difference with frequency and with intensity of incident light.

Experimental Study of Photoelectric Effect

An extensive study of photoelectric effect was made by Lenard and RA Millikan. Given figure shows the experimental arrangement for the study of photoelectric effect.

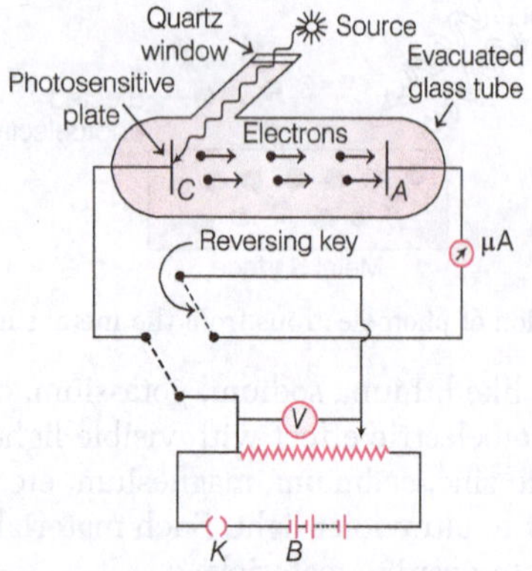

Experimental arrangement for the study of photoelectric effect

It consists of an evacuated glass or quartz tube which encloses a photosensitive plate C (called **emitter**) and a metal plate A (called **collector**). A transparent quartz window is sealed onto the glass tube which permits ultraviolet radiation to pass through it and fall on photosensitive plate C. The electrons are emitted by the plate C and are collected by the plate A. When the collector plate A is positive with respect to the emitter plate C, the electrons are attracted towards it and hence photoelectric current is constituted.

The experimental arrangement given above is used to study the variation of photoelectric current with intensity of radiation, frequency of radiation and the potential difference between the plates A and C.

These variations are described below

Effect of Intensity of Light on Photocurrent

For a fixed frequency of incident radiation and accelerating potential, the photoelectric current increases linearly with increase in intensity of incident light as shown in graph.

As the photoelectric current is directly proportional to the number of photoelectrons emitted per second.

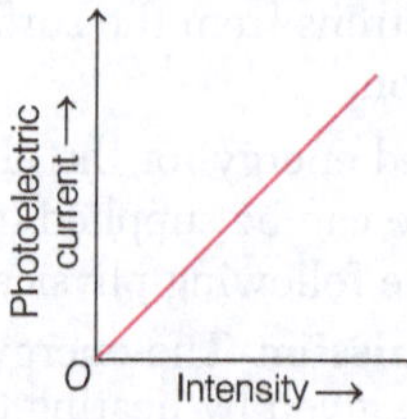

Variation of photoelectric current with intensity of light

So, for constant frequency of incident radiation, the number of photoelectrons emitted per second is directly proportional to the intensity of the incident radiations, *i.e.*

intensity ∝ photoelectric current

$$\propto \text{number of photoelectrons emitted/second} \propto \frac{1}{(\text{distance})^2}$$

Effect of Potential on Photoelectric Current

For a fixed frequency and intensity of incident light, photoelectric current increases with increase in potential applied to the collector, as shown in the graph below.

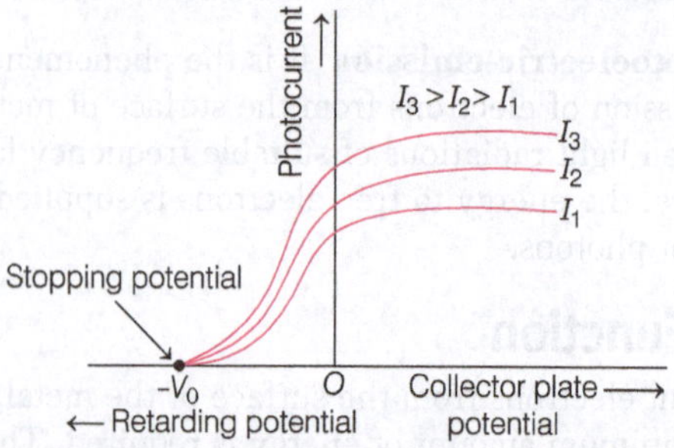

Variation of photoelectric current with collector plate potential for different intensities but constant frequency of incident radiation

From the above graph, we observe that

(i) At some stage, for a certain positive potential of plate *A*, all the emitted electrons are collected by the plate *A*, and the photoelectric current becomes maximum or saturates. If we further increase the accelerating potential of plate *A*, the photocurrent does not increase. This maximum value of photoelectric current is called **saturation current.**

Mentor's TiP

- Saturation current corresponds to the case when all the photoelectrons emitted by the plate *C* reaches plate *A*.

(ii) When the potential is decreased, the current decreases but does not become zero at zero potential. This shows that, even in the absence of accelerating potential, few photoelectrons manage to reach the plate *A* on their own due to their kinetic energy.

(iii) For a particular frequency of incident radiation, the minimum negative (retarding) potential V_0 given to plate *A* for which the photoelectric current stops or becomes zero is called **cut-off** or **stopping potential.**

In this condition, no electron (even the most energetic electron) reaches to plate *A*, *i.e.* the stopping potential is sufficient to repel even the most energetic photoelectron with maximum kinetic energy K_{max}. Hence, maximum kinetic energy of emitted electrons is given as

$$K_{max} = eV_0 = \frac{1}{2}mv_{max}^2$$

where, m is the mass of photoelectron and v_{max} is the maximum velocity of emitted photoelectron.

Concept ladder

For the radiation of a given frequency and material of plate C, the value of stopping potential V_0 is independent of the intensity of the incident radiation. It means that, the maximum kinetic energy of emitted photoelectron depends on the light source and the emitter plate material but is independent of intensity of incident radiation.

Example 1. *The photoelectric cut-off voltage in a certain experiment is 1.5 V. What is the maximum kinetic energy of photoelectrons emitted?*

Sol. Maximum kinetic energy of photoelectrons, $K_{max} = eV_0$

where, $e = 1.6 \times 10^{-19}$ C, $V_0 = 1.5$ V

$$\therefore \quad K_{max} = 1.6 \times 10^{-19} \times 1.5 = 2.4 \times 10^{-19} \text{ J}$$

Example 2. *In an experimental study of photoelectric effect, the stopping potential for a metallic surface is 5.68 V. What will be the maximum velocity of the electrons?*

Sol. Stopping potential, $V_0 = 5.68$ V,

$$m_e = 9.1 \times 10^{-31} \text{ kg}$$

$$\text{Maximum KE, } K_{max} = \frac{1}{2}mv_{max}^2 = eV_0$$

$$\Rightarrow v_{max} = \sqrt{\frac{2eV_0}{m}} = \sqrt{\frac{2 \times 1.6 \times 10^{-19} \times 5.68}{9.1 \times 10^{-31}}}$$

$$= 1.414 \times 10^6 \text{ ms}^{-1}$$

Effect of Frequency of Incident Radiation on Stopping Potential

Let us take radiations of different frequencies but of same intensity. For each radiation, the variation of photoelectric current against the potential difference between the plates is as shown in the graph below

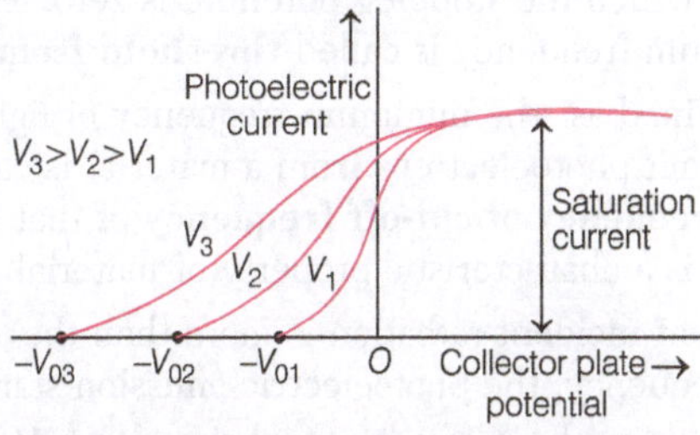

Variation of photoelectric current with collector plate potential for different frequencies but same intensity of incident radiation

From the above graph, we observe that

(i) The value of stopping potential is different for radiation of different frequencies but value of saturation current (for given intensity) remains same for all incident radiations as intensity remains constant.

(ii) The value of stopping potential is more negative for radiation of higher incident frequency. That means, the energy of the emitted electrons depends on the frequency of incident radiations. Greater the frequency of incident radiation, greater is the maximum kinetic energy of photoelectrons, consequently greater retarding potential or stopping potential is required to stop them completely.

(iii) The value of saturation current depends on the intensity of incident radiation but is independent of the frequency of the incident radiation.

Stopping Potential *versus* Frequency Graph

If we plot a graph between stopping potential and the frequency of the incident radiation for two different metals *A* and *B*, we get the graph as shown in the figure.

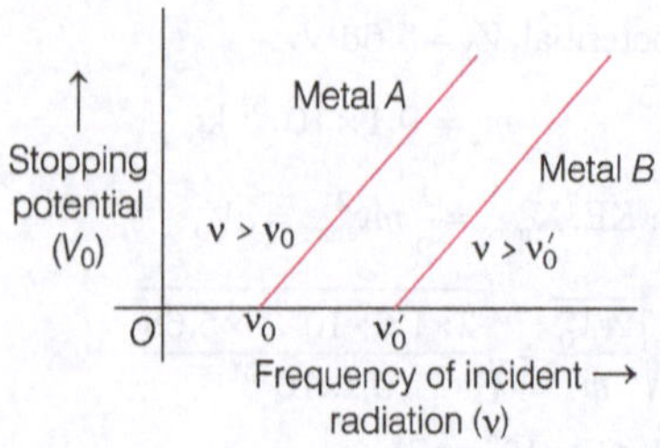

Variation of stopping potential with frequency of incident light for a given photosensitive material

From the above graph, we observe that

(i) The stopping potential V_0 varies linearly with the frequency of incident radiation for a given photosensitive material.

(ii) There exists a certain minimum cut-off frequency ν_0 for which the stopping potential is zero. This minimum frequency is called **threshold frequency**.

It can be defined as "the minimum frequency of light which can emit photoelectrons from a material is called **threshold frequency** or **cut-off frequency** of that material". It is a characteristic property of material.

If frequency of incident radiation is more than the threshold frequency, the photoelectric emission starts instantaneously without any apparent time lag ($\sim 10^{-9}$ s or less), even when the incident radiation has low intensity.

Laws of Photoelectric Emission

On the basis of the experimental results on photoelectric effect, Lenard and Millikan gave the following laws of photoelectric emission

(i) For a given photosensitive material and frequency of incident radiation, the photoelectric current or number of photoelectrons ejected per second is directly proportional to the intensity of the incident light.

(ii) For a given material and frequency of incident radiation, saturation current is found to be proportional to the intensity of incident radiation, whereas the stopping potential is independent of its intensity.

(iii) For a given material, there exists a certain minimum frequency of the incident radiation below which no emissions of photoelectrons take place. This frequency is called threshold frequency.

Above the threshold frequency, the maximum kinetic energy of the emitted photoelectrons or equivalent stopping potential is independent of the intensity of the incident light but depends only upon the frequency (or wavelength) of the incident light.

(iv) The photoelectric emission is an instantaneous process. The time lag between the incidence of radiations and emission of photoelectrons is very small, less than 10^{-9} s, even when incident radiation is made exceedingly dim.

Failure of Wave Theory in Explaining Photoelectric Effect

The wave theory of light given by Huygens' could not explain the photoelectric emission due to the following main reasons.

(i) According to the wave picture of light, the free electrons at the surface of the metal absorb the radiant energy continuously.

The greater the intensity of radiation, the greater should be the energy absorbed by each electron. The maximum kinetic energy of the photoelectrons on the surface is then expected to increase with increase in intensity.

But according to experimental facts, the maximum kinetic energy of ejected photoelectrons is independent of intensity of incident radiation.

(ii) According to wave theory of light, no matter what the frequency of radiation is, a sufficiently intense beam of radiation should be able to impart enough energy to the electrons, so that they exceed the minimum energy needed to escape from metal surface.

A threshold frequency, therefore should not exist which contradicts the experimental fact that no photoelectric emission takes place below that threshold frequency, no matter whatsoever may be its intensity.

(iii) According to the wave theory of light, the absorption of energy by electron takes place continuously over the entire wavefront of the radiation. Since a large number of electrons absorb energy, the energy absorbed per electron per unit time turns out to be small.

Hence, it will take hours or more for a single electron to come out of the metal which contradicts the experimental fact that photoelectron emission is instantaneous ($\sim 10^{-9}$ s).

STEP UP Practice 1

1. The number of photoelectrons emitted per second from a metal surface increases when
   (a) the energy of incident photons increases
   (b) the frequency of incident light increases
   (c) the wavelength of the incident light increases
   (d) the intensity of the incident light increases
2. When stopping potential is applied in an experiment on photoelectric effect, no photocurrent is observed. This means that
   (a) the emission of photoelectrons is stopped
   (b) the photoelectrons are emitted but are reabsorbed by the emitter metal
   (c) the photoelectrons are accumulated near the collector plate
   (d) the photoelectrons are dispersed from the sides of the apparat us
3. If intensity of incident light is increased in photoelectric effect, then which of the following is true?
   (a) Maximum KE of ejected electron will increase.
   (b) Work function will remain unchanged.
   (c) Stopping potential will decrease.
   (d) Maximum KE of ejected electron will decrease.
4. **Assertion** (A) The process of photoelectric emission is different to that of thermionic emission.
   Reason (R) The process of thermionic emission is temperature dependent, but photoelectric emission is independent of temperature.
   In the light of the above statements, choose the correct answer from the options given below.
   (a) Both A and R are true but R is not the correct explanation of A.
   (b) A is true but R is false.
   (c) A is false but R is true.
   (d) Both A and R are true and R is the correct explanation of A.
5. Which of the following statement is correct?
   (a) The current in a photocell increases with increasing frequency of light.
   (b) The photocurrent is proportional to applied voltage.
   (c) The photocurrent increases with increasing intensity of light.
   (d) The stopping potential increases with increasing intensity of incident light.
6. Photoelectric effect involves conversion of
   (a) nuclear energy into electrical energy
   (b) atomic energy into electrical energy
   (c) electronic energy into electrical energy
   (d) light energy into electrical energy
7. **Assertion** (A) Photoelectric emission is an instantaneous process.
   Reason (R) There is no time lag between incidence of light and emission of photoelectrons.
   In the light of the above statements, choose the correct answer from the options given below.
   (a) Both A and R are true but R is not the correct explanation of A.
   (b) A is true but R is false.
   (c) A is false but R is true.
   (d) Both A and R are true and R is the correct explanation of A.
8. The stopping potential (V_0)
   (a) depends upon the angle of incident light
   (b) depends upon the intensity of incident light
   (c) does not depend on nature of surface
   (d) is independent of the intensity of the incident light
9. The retarding potential for having zero photoelectric current
   (a) is directly proportional to the wavelength of incident light.
   (b) increases uniformly with the increase in the wavelength of incident light.
   (c) is directly proportional to the frequency of incident light.
   (d) increases uniformly with the increase in the intensity of incident light wave.
10. **Assertion** (A) Work function of aluminium is 4.2 eV. Emission of electrons will not be possible if two photons each of energy 2.5 eV strike an electron of aluminium.
    Reason (R) For photoelectric emission, the energy of each photon should be greater than the work function of aluminium.
    In the light of the above statements, choose the correct answer from the options given below.
    (a) Both A and R are true but R is not the correct explanation of A.
    (b) A is true but R is false.
    (c) A is false but R is true.
    (d) Both A and R are true and R is the correct explanation of A.
11. A point source of light is used in an experiment on photoelectric effect. Which of the following curves best represents the variation of photoelectric current i with distance x of the source from the emitter?

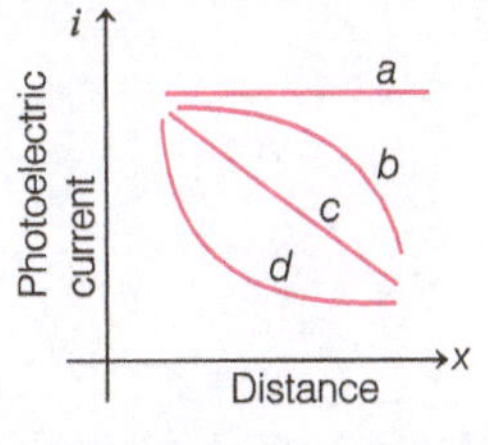

    (a) a (b) b (c) c (d) d
12. I. In the experimental set-up used for studying the photoelectric effect, a monochromatic light from the source of sufficiently short wavelength is used.
    II. The intensity of the light incident on the emitter plate is independent of the distance of the light source from the emitter.
    Which of the following statement(s) is/are incorrect?
    (a) Only I (b) Only II
    (c) Both I and II (d) Neither I nor II

13. Maximum kinetic energy of emitted electron from the surface of a metal is K. When frequency of incident light is doubled, then maximum kinetic energy of emitted electrons is K', then

(a) $K' > 2K$ (b) $K' < 2K$
(c) $K' = 2K$ (d) Data is insufficient

14. For the graph as shown below

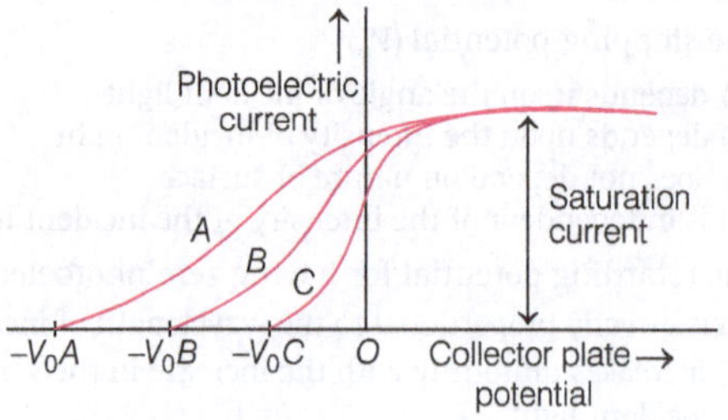

Which of the following statement(s) is/are correct?

I. Stopping potential are in the order $V_{OA} > V_{OB} > V_{OC}$, if the frequencies are in the order $\nu_A > \nu_B > \nu_C$.

II. Greater the frequency of incident radiation, lesser would be the maximum kinetic energy of photoelectrons.

(a) Only I
(b) Only II
(c) Both I and II
(d) Neither I nor II

15. The work function of aluminium is 4.2 eV. If two photons, each of energy 3.5 eV strike on an electron of aluminium, then emission of electrons will be

(a) possible
(b) not possible
(c) Data is incomplete
(d) depend upon the area of the surface

16. Which one of the following pair given below is correct?

(a) Intensity of light $\rightarrow \propto \frac{1}{\text{(Photoelectric current)}}$

(b) Photoelectric current $\rightarrow \propto \frac{1}{\text{(Distance)}^3}$

(c) Number of photoelectrons emitted/second $\rightarrow \propto \text{(Distance)}^2$

(d) $KE_{max} \rightarrow eV_0$

17. Variation of stopping potential V_0 with frequency ν of incident radiation for photosensitive materials A and B are as shown below

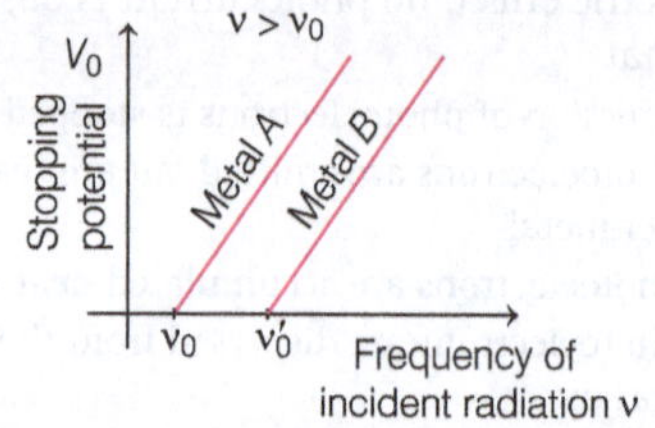

Which of the following statement(s) is/are correct?

I. Stopping potential varies linearly with frequency of incident radiation.

II. There exists a maximum frequency, only above which the photoemission could takes place.

(a) Only I (b) Only II
(c) Both I and II (d) Neither I nor II

18. When yellow light is incident on a surface, no electrons are emitted while green light can emit. If red light is incident on the surface, then

(a) no electrons are emitted
(b) photons are emitted
(c) electrons of higher energy are emitted
(d) electrons of lower energy are emitted

Module 2

Quantum Theory and Einstein's Photoelectric Equations

• Planck's Quantum Theory (Particle Nature of Light : The Photon) • Einstein's Photoelectric Equation

Planck's Quantum Theory

(Particle Nature of Light : The Photon)

In 1990, Max Planck proposed his quantum theory of radiation. According to this theory, the energy of an electromagnetic wave is not continuously distributed over the wavefront, instead it travels in the form of discrete packets or bundles of energy called **quanta**. One quantum of light radiation is called a **photon**, which travels with the speed of light. Photoelectric effect, thus gave evidence that light consists of packets of energy.

Energy of a photon is given by

$$E = h\nu = \frac{hc}{\lambda}$$

where, h ($\simeq 6.63 \times 10^{-34}$ Js) is the Planck's constant, ν is the frequency of radiation or photon, c is the speed of light and λ is the wavelength of photon. The energy E is expressed in electron-volt (eV).

The momentum of photon is given by

$$p = \frac{E}{c} = \frac{h\nu}{c} = \frac{h}{\lambda} \text{ kg-ms}^{-1}$$

Characteristic Properties of Photons

Different characteristic properties of photons are given below

(i) In interaction of radiation with matter, radiation behaves as if it is made up of particles called **photons**.

(ii) A photon in vacuum travels with a speed of light c (i.e. 3×10^8 ms^{-1}) in straight line.

(iii) According to the theory of relativity, the mass m of a particle moving with velocity v, comparable with the velocity of light c is given by

$$m = \frac{m_0}{\sqrt{1 - \frac{v^2}{c^2}}} \Rightarrow m_0 = m\sqrt{1 - \frac{v^2}{c^2}}$$

where, m_0 is the mass of the particle at rest.

As a photon moves with the speed of light, i.e. $v = c$, hence $m_0 = 0$. So, rest mass of photon is zero, *i.e.* the photon cannot exist at rest.

(iv) The inertial mass of a photon is given by

$$m = \frac{E}{c^2} = \frac{h}{c\lambda} = \frac{h\nu}{c^2}$$

(v) Irrespective of the intensity of radiation, all the photons of a particular frequency ν or wavelength λ have the same energy $E\left(= h\nu = \frac{hc}{\lambda}\right)$ and momentum $p\left(= \frac{h\nu}{c} = \frac{h}{\lambda}\right)$.

(vi) Energy of a photon depends upon frequency of the photon, so the energy of the photon does not change when photon travels from one medium to another.

(vii) As, velocity of a photon is different in different media, so wavelength of the photon also changes in different media.

(viii) Photons are not deflected by electric and magnetic fields. This shows that photons are electrically neutral.

(ix) Total energy and total momentum are conserved in photon-particle collision. However, the number of photons may not be conserved in collision. As, the photon may be absorbed or a new photon may be created during a collision.

Single electron absorbs energy of a single photon.

Example 3. *What is the energy (in joule) associated with a photon of wavelength 4000 Å?*

Sol. Energy of a photon, $E = \frac{hc}{\lambda} = \frac{6.6 \times 10^{-34} \times 3 \times 10^8}{4 \times 10^{-7}}$

$$= 4.95 \times 10^{-19} \text{ J}$$

Example 4. *The momentum of photon of electromagnetic radiation is 3.3×10^{-29} kg-ms^{-1}. Find out the frequency and wavelength of the wave associated with it.*

Sol. Given, $h = 6.63 \times 10^{-34}$ J-s, $c = 3 \times 10^8$ ms^{-1},

$$p = 3.3 \times 10^{-29} \text{ kg-ms}^{-1}$$

(i) Momentum, $p = \frac{h\nu}{c}$

$$\Rightarrow \quad \nu = \frac{pc}{h} = \frac{3.3 \times 10^{-29} \times 3 \times 10^{8}}{6.63 \times 10^{-34}}$$

$$= 1.5 \times 10^{13} \text{ Hz}$$

(ii) $\lambda = \frac{c}{\nu} = \frac{3 \times 10^{8}}{1.5 \times 10^{13}} = 2 \times 10^{-5} \text{ m}$

NEET Close-up

Example Similar to PYQ Asked in NEET 2024

Choose the correct statements about photon among the following.

A. Photons have zero resting mass.

B. Energy of photons (in eV) is $\frac{12375}{\lambda(\text{in Å})}$.

C. All photons of light of a particular wave length have the same energy.

D. Photons can be destroyed or created when radiation is absorbed or emitted, respectively.

Choose the correct answer from the options given below

(a) A, B and C only (b) A and B only
(c) B and C only (d) All of the above

Sol. (*d*) (A) Photons have no rest mass.

(B) $E = \frac{hc}{\lambda}$

where, $h = 6.26 \times 10^{-34}$ J-s

$c = 3 \times 10^{8}$ m/s

$$E = \frac{19.878 \times 10^{-26}}{\lambda} \text{ J}$$

$$E \text{ (in eV)} = \frac{19.878 \times 10^{-26}}{1.602 \times 10^{-19}\,\lambda} = \frac{12375}{\lambda \text{ (in Å)}}$$

(C) Energy of all photons will remain same for particular wavelength.

(D) Destruction of photon occurs when photons are absorbed by electrons and creation occurs when a photon is emitted by an electron.

Skill Builder

Energy of photons in free space depends on

(A) frequency of photons
(B) intensity of photons
(C) both frequency and intensity of photons
(D) velocity of photons

Choose the correct answer from the options given below.

(a) A and D only (b) B and D only
(c) C only (d) D only

For more Practice Refer Q. No. 6 of step up practice-2 and Q. No. 5, 6 of Gearing up for NEET.

Intensity of Photons

A moving photon carries momentum with it. Therefore, pressure and intensity are also associated with photons. Consider an area A through which light (photons) emitted by a source of total energy E and intensity I is passing normally as shown in the figure.

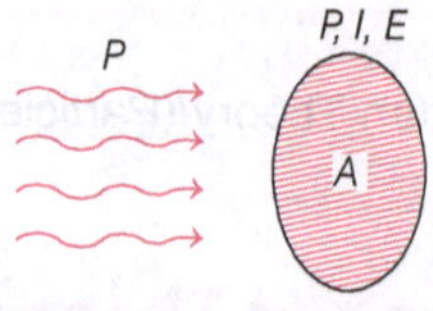

Photon of energy E passing normally through an area A

If power of the source is P, then we can write,

Total energy of photons, $E = Nh\nu = N\left(\frac{hc}{\lambda}\right)$

$\therefore$ Power of source, $P = \frac{E}{t} = \frac{Nh\nu}{t} = nh\nu = \frac{nhc}{\lambda} \quad \left(\because n = \frac{N}{t}\right)$

Also, we can write

$$n = P/E = \frac{P}{h\nu} = \frac{P\lambda}{hc}$$

As, intensity or energy flux is defined as the energy crossing per unit area normally per second.

$$\Rightarrow \quad \text{Intensity, } I = \frac{P}{A} = \frac{E}{tA} = \frac{nh\nu}{A} = n\frac{hc}{A\lambda}$$

where, A = area normal to incident light,

N = number of photons

and n = number of photons/s.

Concept ladder

- At a distance r from a point source of power P, intensity of photons is given by $I = \frac{P}{4\pi r^2} \Rightarrow I \propto \frac{1}{r^2}$.
- For a line source of power P, intensity of photons is given by $I \propto \frac{P}{2\pi r l} \Rightarrow I \propto \frac{1}{r}$

Example 5. *The intensity of sunlight reaching the surface of the earth is* 1.388×10^{3} *W/m*^{2}*. How many photons (nearly) per square metre are incident on the earth per second? Assume that, the photons in the sunlight have an average wavelength of 550 nm.*

Sol. Let, n = number of photons incident on earth per second per m^2

and E' = energy of each photon $= \frac{hc}{\lambda}$.

If E be the energy of all photons reaching the surface of earth per second per unit area, then

$$E = nE' = \frac{nhc}{\lambda}$$

Intensity = Energy of photons reaching the earth per second per unit area

Given, $I = 1.388 \times 10^3\ \text{W/m}^2$

$= 1.388 \times 10^3\ \text{Js}^{-1}\ \text{m}^{-2}$

$$\therefore \quad \frac{nhc}{\lambda} = I$$

or $$n = \frac{I}{\left(\frac{hc}{\lambda}\right)} = \frac{1.388 \times 10^3}{hc} \times \lambda$$

$$= \frac{1.388 \times 10^3 \times 550 \times 10^{-9}}{6.62 \times 10^{-34} \times 3 \times 10^8}$$

$$= 3.84 \times 10^{21}$$

NEET Close-up

Example Similar to PYQ Asked in NEET 2021

The number of photons per second on an average emitted by the source of monochromatic light of wavelength 5000 Å, when it delivers the power of 2.2×10^{-3} W is

(a) $\frac{5}{9} \times 10^{16}$ (b) $\frac{4}{9} \times 10^{16}$ (c) $\frac{4}{18} \times 10^{15}$ (d) $\frac{2}{9} \times 10^{17}$

Sol. (*a*) Power $= \frac{\text{Energy}}{\text{Time}} = \frac{nh\nu}{t}$

$$\Rightarrow \quad \frac{n}{t} = \frac{\text{Power}}{h\nu} = \frac{P\lambda}{hc}$$

$$\Rightarrow \quad \frac{n}{t} = \frac{2.2 \times 10^{-3} \times 5000 \times 10^{-10}}{6.6 \times 10^{-34} \times 3 \times 10^8}$$

$$= \frac{5}{9} \times 10^{16} \text{ photons per second}$$

Skill Builder

A source emits 10^{16} photons per second with frequency of 10^{20} Hz. Power of source is

(a) 662 W (b) 66.2 W
(c) 6.62 kW (d) 66.2 kW

For more Practice Refer Q. No. 4, 8 of step up practice-2

Einstein's Photoelectric Equation

In 1905, Albert Einstein explained the various laws of photoelectric emission on the basis of Planck's quantum theory. According to Planck's quantum theory, light radiations consist of tiny packets of energy called **quanta.** One quantum of light radiation is called a **photon** which travels with the speed of light.

The energy of a photon is given by

$$\boxed{E = h\nu}$$

where, h is Planck's constant and ν is the frequency of light radiation.

When a photon of energy $h\nu$ falls on a metal surface, the energy of the photon is absorbed by the electron and is used in following two ways.

(i) A part of energy is utilised to overcome the surface barrier and come out of the metal surface. This part of energy is called **work function.**
It is expressed as $\boxed{\phi_0 = h\nu_0}$

(ii) The remaining part of the energy is used in giving a velocity v to the emitted photoelectron. This is equal to the maximum kinetic energy of the photoelectrons $\left(\frac{1}{2} mv_{max}^2\right)$, where m is the mass of the photoelectron. This can be seen in the figure given below

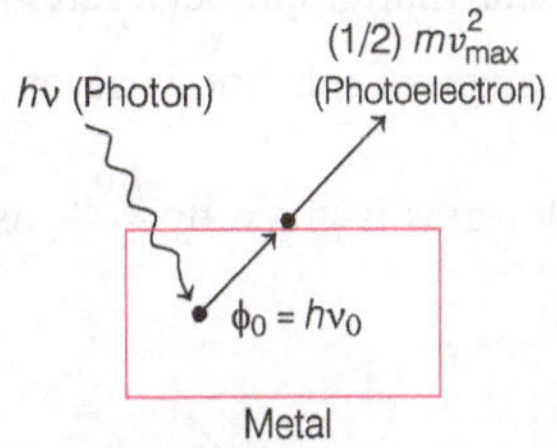

Emission of photoelectron by a metal when a photon is absorbed by it

According to the law of conservation of energy,

$$h\nu = \phi_0 + \frac{1}{2} mv_{max}^2 = h\nu_0 + \frac{1}{2} mv_{max}^2$$

$$\therefore \quad \frac{1}{2} mv_{max}^2 = K_{max} = h(\nu - \nu_0) = h\nu - \phi_0$$

or $$\boxed{K_{max} = h\nu - \phi_0}$$

This equation is called **Einstein's photoelectric equation.**

From Einstein's equation, it is clear that K_{max} does not depend on intensity of incident light.

Relation between Stopping Potential (V_0), Frequency (ν) and Wavelength (λ) of Incident Light

Maximum kinetic energy is given by

$$K_{max} = h(\nu - \nu_0)$$

If stopping potential is V_0, then

$$K_{max} = eV_0$$

$$\therefore \quad eV_0 = h(\nu - \nu_0) \quad \text{...(i)}$$

If λ = wavelength of the incident radiation,
λ_0 = threshold wavelength for the metal surface
and c = velocity of light.

Then, $\nu = \frac{c}{\lambda}$ and $\nu_0 = \frac{c}{\lambda_0}$

Putting these values in Eq. (i), we get

$$eV_0 = h\left(\frac{c}{\lambda} - \frac{c}{\lambda_0}\right) \Rightarrow eV_0 = hc\left(\frac{1}{\lambda} - \frac{1}{\lambda_0}\right) \quad ...(ii)$$

Slope of the Graph between V_0 and ν_0

Consider the equation,

$$eV_0 = hc\left(\frac{1}{\lambda} - \frac{1}{\lambda_0}\right) \Rightarrow V_0 = \frac{h}{e}\left(\frac{c}{\lambda} - \frac{c}{\lambda_0}\right)$$

or

$$V_0 = \frac{h}{e}\nu - \frac{h\nu_0}{e} \quad ...(iii)$$

Comparing Eq. (iii) with the straight line equation, *i.e.* $y = mx + c$, it is clear that graph between V_0 and ν_0 is a straight line. The slope of this line is given by $\tan\theta = \frac{h}{e}$ and intercept on V_0-axis is given by $\frac{h\nu_0}{e}$, as shown in the graph

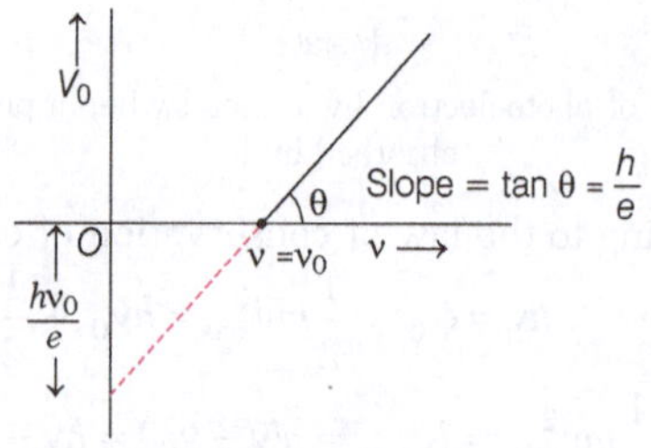

Graph of V_0 *versus* ν

In terms of wavelength, we can write

$$V_0 = \frac{hc}{\lambda e} - \frac{hc}{\lambda_0 e} \quad ...(iv)$$

From the Eq. (iv), it is clear that graph between V_0 and $\frac{1}{\lambda}$ is also a straight line. The slope of this line is given by $\tan\theta = \frac{hc}{e}$ and intercept on V_0-axis is given by $\frac{hc}{\lambda_0 e}$, as shown in the graph.

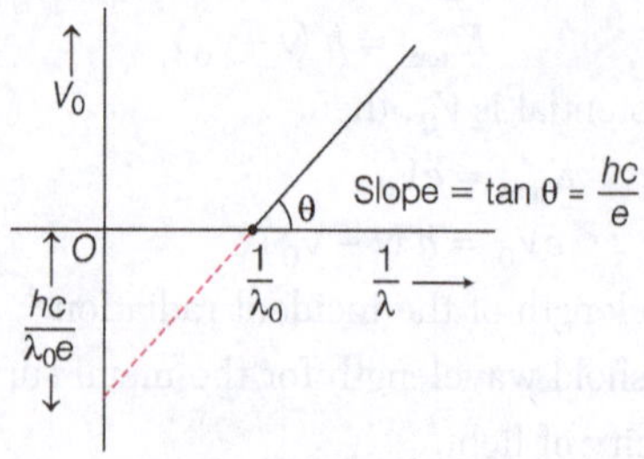

Graph of V_0 *versus* $1/\lambda$

Explanation of Photoelectric Effect from Einstein's Equation

Einstein explained all the observations of photoelectric effect using Einstein's photoelectric equation.

These are as follow

(i) From photoelectric equation, it is clear that K_{max} is independent of intensity of radiation but depends linearly on ν.

(ii) Photoelectric emission is possible only, if $h\nu > \phi_0$.

or $\quad h\nu > h\nu_0 \quad (\because \phi_0 = h\nu_0)$

$\Rightarrow \quad \nu > \nu_0$

where, ν_0 is threshold frequency. If $\nu < \nu_0$, then kinetic energy of electron comes out to be negative, which is not possible, so no photoelectric emission is possible below ν_0, even if the incident radiation is of high intensity and falls on the surface for long duration.

(iii) Intensity of radiation (I) is proportional to the number of energy quanta per unit area per unit time (n). Higher the value of n, higher the number of electrons emitted (for $\nu > \nu_0$).

That is the reason (for $\nu > \nu_0$),

photocurrent ∝ intensity

(iv) The absorption of photon by electron is instantaneous process, hence emission of electrons is instantaneous.

Note Practically only one electron is ejected by 1 million photons.

$$\text{Quantum efficiency} = \frac{\text{Number of electrons ejected / sec}}{\text{Number of photons incident / sec}}$$

$$\Rightarrow \quad \eta = \frac{n'}{n} \times 100\%$$

Example 6. *The work function for a certain metal is 4.2 eV. Will this metal give photoelectric emission for incident radiation of wavelength 330 nm?*

Sol. Here, W = work function of certain metal = 4.2 eV

$$= (4.2 \times 1.6 \times 10^{-19})\text{ J} = 6.72 \times 10^{-19}\text{ J}$$

$$(\because 1\text{ eV} = 1.6 \times 10^{-19}\text{ J})$$

If E be the energy of the photon of incident light, then

$$E = h\nu = \frac{hc}{\lambda} = \frac{6.62 \times 10^{-34} \times 3 \times 10^8}{330 \times 10^{-9}}\text{ J}$$

$$= 6.01 \times 10^{-19}\text{ J}$$

The photoelectric emission is possible only if $E = h\nu > \phi$, where ϕ is work function of metal. Here, $E < \phi$, so this metal will not give photoelectric emission for incident radiation of wavelength 330 nm.

Example 7. *The threshold frequency for a certain metal is 3.3×10^{14} Hz. If light of frequency 8.2×10^{14} Hz is incident on the metal, predict the cut-off voltage for the photoelectric emission.*

Sol. Using the relation, $h\nu - h\nu_0 = eV_0$

We get, $V_0 = h\left(\frac{\nu-\nu_0}{e}\right)$

Here, $\nu_0 = 3.3\times 10^{14}$ Hz, $\nu = 8.2\times 10^{14}$ Hz

$$= 6.62\times 10^{-34}\times\left(\frac{8.2\times 10^{14} - 3.3\times 10^{14}}{1.6\times 10^{-19}}\right)$$

$$= 2.03 \text{ V}$$

NEET Close-up

Example Similar to PYQ Asked in NEET 2019

Work function of a metal is 6.62 eV. The minimum frequency of incident ray required to produce photocurrent from this metal is

(a) 1.6×10^{15} Hz (b) 2×10^{15} Hz

(c) 2.5×10^{15} Hz (d) 2×10^{16} Hz

Sol. (*a*) Work function, $W = h\nu_0$

$$\Rightarrow \quad \nu_0 = \frac{W}{h} = \frac{6.62\times 1.6\times 10^{-19}}{6.62\times 10^{-34}}$$

$$\Rightarrow \quad \nu_0 = 1.6\times 10^{15} \text{ Hz}$$

Skill Builder

Work function of a photosensitive material is 2 eV. The largest wavelength that can cause photoelectric effect from this material (approximately) is

(a) 6100 nm (b) 6200 nm

(c) 620 nm (d) 610 nm

For more Practice Refer Q. No. 11 of step up practice 2 and Q. No. 9, 16 of Gearing up for NEET.

Example 8. *Light of frequency 7.21×10^{14} Hz is incident on a metal surface. Electrons with a maximum speed of 6.0×10^5 m/s are ejected from the surface. What is the threshold frequency for photoemission of electrons?*

Sol. Using Einstein's photoelectric equation, $h\nu - h\nu_0 = \frac{1}{2}mv_{max}^2$,

We get $h\nu_0 = h\nu - \frac{1}{2}mv_{max}^2$

$$\therefore \quad \nu_0 = \nu - \frac{mv_{max}^2}{2h}$$

Here, $\nu = 7.21\times 10^{14}$ Hz

$v_{max} = 6.0\times 10^5$ m/s

and m = mass of electron $= 91\times 10^{-31}$ kg

$\therefore$ Threshold frequency, ν_0

$$= 7.21\times 10^{14} - \frac{9.1\times 10^{-31}\times(6.0\times 10^5)^2}{2\times 6.62\times 10^{-34}}$$

$$= 7.21\times 10^{14} - 2.47\times 10^{14} = 4.74\times 10^{14} \text{ Hz}$$

Example 9. *The work function of caesium is 2.14 eV. Calculate*

(i) the threshold frequency for caesium and

(ii) the wavelength of the incident light, if the photocurrent is brought to zero by a stopping potential of 0.60 V.

(Given, $h = 6.63\times 10^{-34}$ J-s.)

Sol. Here, $V_0 = 0.60$ V

$$\phi_0 = 2.14 \text{ eV} = 2.14\times 1.6\times 10^{-19} \text{ J}$$

(i) Threshold frequency, $\nu_0 = \frac{\phi_0}{h}$ $(\because \phi_0 = h\nu_0)$

$$= \frac{2.14\times 1.6\times 10^{-19}}{6.63\times 10^{-34}} = 5.16\times 10^{14} \text{ Hz}$$

(ii) As, $eV_0 = \frac{hc}{\lambda} - \phi_0$ or $\lambda = \frac{hc}{(eV_0 + \phi_0)}$

$$= \frac{6.63\times 10^{-34}\times 3\times 10^8}{(1.6\times 10^{-19}\times 0.60 + 2.14\times 1.6\times 10^{-19})}$$

$$\approx 454\times 10^{-9} \text{m}$$

$$= 454 \text{ nm}$$

Example 10. *In an experiment on photoelectric effect, the slope of the cut-off voltage versus frequency of incident light is found to be 4.12×10^{-15} Vs. Calculate the value of Planck's constant.*

Sol. We know, $eV_0 = h\nu - W$

$$\therefore \quad V_0 = \left(\frac{h}{e}\right)\nu - \frac{W}{e}$$

Given, slope $= 4.12\times 10^{-15}$ Vs $= \frac{h}{e}$

$$\therefore \quad h = 4.12\times 10^{-15}\times e$$

$$= 4.12\times 10^{-15}\times 1.6\times 10^{-19}$$

$$= 6.592\times 10^{-34} \text{ Js}^{-1}$$

STEP UP Practice 2

1. The momentum of the photon of wavelength 5000 Å will be
(a) 1.3×10^{-27} kg-ms^{-1} (b) 1.3×10^{-28} kg-ms^{-1}
(c) 4×10^{-29} kg-ms^{-1} (d) 4×10^{-18} kg-ms^{-1}

2. The momentum of a photon is 2×10^{-16} g-cms^{-1}. Its energy is
(a) 0.61×10^{-26} erg (b) 2.0×10^{-26} erg
(c) 6×10^{-6} erg (d) 6×10^{-8} erg

3. Amongst the following relation, which of one is correct?
(a) $E^2 = p^2c^2$ (b) $E^2 = p^2c$
(c) $E^2 = pc^2$ (d) $E^2 = p^2/c^2$

4. The number of photons of wavelength 540 nm emitted per second by an electric bulb of power 100 W is (Take, $h = 6 \times 10^{-34}$ J-s)
(a) 100 (b) 1000 (c) 3×10^{20} (d) 3×10^{18}

5. **Statement I** Stopping potential depends upon the frequency of incident light but it is independent of the intensity of the light.
Statement II The maximum kinetic energy of the photoelectrons is proportional to stopping potential.
In the light of the above statements, choose the most appropriate answer from the options given below.
(a) Both Statement I and Statement II are incorrect.
(b) Statement I is correct but Statement II is incorrect.
(c) Statement I is incorrect but Statement II is correct.
(d) Both Statement I and Statement II are correct.

6. All photons present in a light beam of single frequency have
(a) same frequency but different momentum
(b) same momentum but different frequency
(c) different frequency and different momentum
(d) same frequency and same momentum

7. The wavelength of light in the visible region is about 760 nm for red colour. The energy of photon (in eV) at the red end of the visible spectrum is
(a) 6.63 (b) 3.62 (c) 7.61 (d) 1.64

8. The energy flux of sunlight reaching the surface of the earth is 1.52×10^3 Wm^{-2}. The photons in the sunlight have an average wavelength of 520 nm. How many photons per square metre are incident on the earth per second?
(a) 4×10^{21} (b) 4×10^{34} (c) 4×10^{31} (d) 4×10^{28}

9. **Statement I** Photoelectric effect demonstrates the wave nature of light.
Statement II The number of photoelectrons is proportional to the frequency of light.
In the light of the above statements, choose the most appropriate answer from the options given below.
(a) Both Statement I and Statement II are incorrect.
(b) Statement I is correct but Statement II is incorrect.
(c) Statement I is incorrect but Statement II is correct.
(d) Both Statement I and Statement II are correct.

10. When radiation is incident on a photoelectrons emitter, the stopping potential is found to be 9 V. If e/m for the electron is 1.8×10^{11} C kg^{-1}, the maximum velocity of the ejected electrons is
(a) 6×10^5 ms^{-1} (b) 8×10^5 ms^{-1}
(c) 1.8×10^6 ms^{-1} (d) 1.8×10^5 ms^{-1}

11. Work function of caesium is 2.14 eV. Threshold frequency of caesium is
(a) 5.14×10^{14} Hz (b) 6×10^{14} Hz
(c) 3×10^{14} Hz (d) 5.16×10^{14} Hz

12. The work function of metal is 1 eV. Light of wavelength 3000 Å is incident on this metal surface. The velocity of emitted photoelectrons will be
(a) 10 m/s (b) 1×10^3 m/s
(c) 1×10^4 m/s (d) 1×10^6 m/s

13. **Statement I** Photosensitivity of a metal is high, if its work function is small.
Statement II Work function $= h\nu_0$, where ν_0 is the threshold frequency.
In the light of the above statements, choose the most appropriate answer from the options given below.
(a) Both Statement I and Statement II are incorrect.
(b) Statement I is correct but Statement II is incorrect.
(c) Statement I is incorrect but Statement II is correct.
(d) Both Statement I and Statement II are correct.

14. A radio transmitter radiates 1 kW power at a wavelength 198.6 m. How many photons does it emit per second?
(a) 10^{10} (b) 10^{20} (c) 10^{30} (d) 10^{40}

15. If the energy of a photon corresponding to a wavelength of 6000 Å is 3.32×10^{-19} J, the photon energy for a wavelength of 4000 Å will be
(a) 1.4 eV (b) 4.9 eV (c) 3.1 eV (d) 1.6 eV

16. **Statement I** Some photographic plates are not affected by red light but are immediately blackened by white light.
Statement II The wavelength of red light is less than the wavelength of many components of white light.
In the light of the above statements, choose the most appropriate answer from the options given below.
(a) Both Statement I and Statement II are incorrect.
(b) Statement I is correct but Statement II is incorrect.
(c) Statement I is incorrect but Statement II is correct.
(d) Both Statement I and Statement II are correct.

17. A photon of wavelength 4400 Å is passing through vacuum. The effective mass and momentum of the photon are respectively
(a) 5×10^{-36} kg, 1.5×10^{-27} kg-m/s
(b) 5×10^{-35} kg, 1.5×10^{-26} kg-m/s
(c) zero, 1.5×10^{-26} kg-m/s
(d) 5×10^{-36} kg, 1.67×10^{-43} kg-m/s

18. If we express the energy of a photon in keV and the wavelength in angstroms, then energy of a photon can be calculated from the relation

(a) $E = 12.4\,h\nu$ (b) $E = 12.4\,h/\lambda$
(c) $E = 12.4/\lambda$ (d) $E = h\nu$

19. Which of the following pair given below is incorrect?

(a) Einstein's photoelectric equation $\rightarrow K_{max} = h\nu - \phi_0$

(b) Quantum efficiency $\rightarrow \dfrac{\text{No. of electron ejected/second}}{\text{No. of photons incident/second}}$

(c) Momentum of photon $\rightarrow \dfrac{h}{\lambda}\,\text{kg-ms}^{-1}$

(d) m_0 $\rightarrow m\sqrt{1-\dfrac{c^2}{v^2}}$

20. The energy of a photon of light with wavelength 5000 Å is approximately 3.5 eV. This way the energy of an X-ray photon with wavelength 1 Å would be

(a) 3.5/5000 eV (b) $2.5/(5000)^2$ eV
(c) 3.5×5000 eV (d) $3.5 \times (5000)^2$ eV

Module 3

Dual Nature of Matter

- Matter Waves : de-Broglie Waves
- Characteristics of Matter Waves

In 1924, the French physicist Louis de-Broglie put forward the bold hypothesis that moving particles of matter should also display wave like properties under suitable condition, *i.e.* the particles like electrons, protons, neutrons, etc., can have particle as well as wave nature.

Matter Waves : de-Broglie Waves

According to de-Broglie, a wave is associated with moving material particle which controls the particle in every respect. The wave associated with moving particle is called matter waves or de-Broglie wave and it propagates in the form of wave packets with group velocity. Wavelength associated with de-Broglie wave is called **de-Broglie wavelength** and is given by

$$\lambda = \frac{h}{mv} = \frac{h}{p}$$

where, m, v and p are the mass, velocity and momentum of particle respectively and h is Planck's constant.

According to Planck's quantum theory, the energy of the photon is given by

$$E = h\nu = \frac{hc}{\lambda} \quad \text{...(i)}$$

According to Einstein's theory, the energy of the photon is given by

$$E = mc^2 \quad \text{...(ii)}$$

From Eqs. (i) and (ii), we get

$$\lambda = \frac{h}{mc} = \frac{h}{p}$$

where, $p = mc$ is momentum of a photon.

Calculation of de-Broglie Wavelength of an Accelerating Electron

Let an electron of charge e having mass m be accelerated from rest through a potential difference V, then gain in kinetic energy of electron is given by

$$K = \frac{1}{2}m_e v^2$$

Work done on electron $= eV$

$$\therefore \quad \frac{1}{2}m_e v^2 = eV$$

$$\Rightarrow \quad v = \sqrt{\frac{2eV}{m_e}}$$

Momentum is given by $p = m_e v = \sqrt{2eV\,m_e}$

The wavelength associated with moving electron is given by

$$\lambda = \frac{h}{\sqrt{2eVm_e}}$$

Substituting the value of h, e and m_e in above equation,

we get $$\lambda = \frac{6.63\times 10^{-34}}{\sqrt{2\times 9.1\times 10^{-31}\times 1.6\times 10^{-19}\,V}}$$

$$\Rightarrow \quad \lambda = \frac{12.27}{\sqrt{V}}\,\text{Å}$$

Similarly, de-Broglie wavelength for other charged particles can be given by $\lambda = \frac{h}{p}$

where, $p = \sqrt{2m(\text{KE})} = \sqrt{2mqV}$

Concept ladder

- **For proton** $\lambda = \frac{h}{\sqrt{2m_p q}}$

  On putting the values of h, m_p and q, we get

  $$\lambda = \frac{0.286}{\sqrt{V}}\,\text{Å}$$

- **For deuteron,** $\lambda = \frac{0.202}{\sqrt{V}}\,\text{Å}$
- **For α-particle,** $\lambda = \frac{0.101}{\sqrt{V}}\,\text{Å}$

Example 11. *A particle of mass 1 mg has the same wavelength as an electron moving with a velocity of $3\times 10^6\,ms^{-1}$. What is the velocity of the particle?*

Sol. de-Broglie wavelength, $\lambda = \frac{h}{mv}$

As both particle and electron are having same wavelength, therefore their momentum will be equal.

$$m_p v_p = m_e v_e$$

$$\Rightarrow \quad v_p = \frac{m_e v_e}{m_p}$$

$$= \frac{9.1\times 10^{-31}\times 3\times 10^6}{10^{-6}}$$

$$\Rightarrow \quad v_p = 2.7\times 10^{-18}\ \text{ms}^{-1}$$

Example 12. *When the momentum of a proton is changed by an amount p_0, the corresponding change in the de-Broglie wavelength is found to be 0.25%. Find the original momentum of the photon.*

Sol. As $\lambda \propto \frac{1}{p}$

$$\Rightarrow \quad \frac{\Delta p}{p} = -\frac{\Delta\lambda}{\lambda}$$

$$\Rightarrow \quad \frac{p_0}{p} = \frac{0.25}{100}$$

$$\Rightarrow \quad p = 400p_0$$

NEET Close-up

Example Similar to PYQ Asked in NEET 2020 and NEET 2019

An electron is accelerated through a potential difference of 16 V. Its de-Broglie wavelength is

(a) 3.675 Å (b) 3.236 Å (c) 2.225 Å (d) 1.326 Å

Sol. (*a*) For electron,

$$\lambda = \frac{12.27}{\sqrt{V}}\,\text{Å} = \frac{12.27}{\sqrt{16}}\,\text{Å} = \frac{12.27}{4}\,\text{Å} \Rightarrow \lambda = 3.675\,\text{Å}$$

Skill Builder

The de-Broglie wavelength associated with an electron, accelerated by a potential difference of 100 V is given by

(a) 12.27 Å (b) 12.27 nm
(c) 0.1227 nm (d) 1.227 nm

For more Practice Refer Q. No. 8 of step up practice 3 and Q. No. 40, 47, 49 of Gearing up for NEET.

Example 13. *The kinetic energy of an electron is 5 eV. Calculate the de-Broglie wavelength associated with it (Take, $h = 6.6\times 10^{-34}$ Js and $m_e = 9.1\times 10^{-31}$ kg)*

Sol. de-Broglie wavelength associated with the electron,

$$\lambda = \frac{h}{\sqrt{2m\,(\text{KE})}} = \frac{6.6\times 10^{-34}}{\sqrt{2\times 9.1\times 10^{-31}\times 5\times 1.6\times 10^{-19}}}$$

$$= 5.469\times 10^{-10}\,\text{m} = 5.47\,\text{Å}$$

Example 14. *Find out the energy that should be added to an electron in terms of initial energy to reduce its de-Broglie wavelengths from 10^{-10} m to 0.5×10^{-10} m.*

Sol. de-Broglie wavelength is given by

$$\lambda = \frac{h}{\sqrt{2mE}} \Rightarrow \lambda \propto \frac{1}{\sqrt{E}}$$

$$\because \quad \frac{\lambda_1}{\lambda_2} = \sqrt{\frac{E_2}{E_1}} \Rightarrow \frac{10^{-10}}{0.5\times 10^{-10}} = \sqrt{\frac{E_1}{E_2}}$$

$$\Rightarrow \quad E_2 = 4E_1$$

Hence, added energy $= E_2 - E_1 = 4E_1 - E_1 = 3E_1$

Example 15. *What is the*

(a) momentum,

(b) speed and

(c) de-Broglie wavelength of an electron with kinetic energy of 120 eV?

Sol. (a) Using the relation, $E = \frac{p^2}{2m}$, we get

$$p = \sqrt{2mE}$$

$$= \sqrt{2\times 9.1\times 10^{-31}\times 120\times 1.6\times 10^{-19}}$$

$$= 5.91\times 10^{-24}\ \text{kg-ms}^{-1}$$

(b) Speed, $v = \frac{p}{m} = \frac{5.91 \times 10^{-24}}{9.1 \times 10^{-31}} = 6.5 \times 10^6 \text{ ms}^{-1}$

(c) de-Broglie wavelength is given by

$$\lambda = \frac{h}{p} = \frac{6.62 \times 10^{-34}}{5.91 \times 10^{-24}} = 1.12 \times 10^{-10} \text{ m}$$

Example 16. *What is the de-Broglie wavelength of a nitrogen molecule in air at 300 K? Assume that, the molecule is moving with the root-mean-square speed of molecules at this temperature. (Atomic mass of nitrogen = 14.0076 u)*

Sol. Let v = rms speed of N_2 molecule at 300 K

or $$v = \sqrt{\frac{3kT}{m}}$$

where, k = Boltzmann constant $= 1.38 \times 10^{-23} \text{ JK}^{-1}$

or $$v = \sqrt{\frac{3 \times 1.38 \times 10^{-23} \times 300}{28.0152 \times 1.67 \times 10^{-27}}}$$
$$= 5.15 \times 10^2 \text{ ms}^{-1}$$

Using the formula, $\lambda = \frac{h}{mv}$, we get

$$\lambda = \frac{6.62 \times 10^{-34}}{28.0152 \times 1.67 \times 10^{-27} \times 5.15 \times 10^2}$$
$$= 2.75 \times 10^{-11} \text{ m}$$

Example 17. *The wavelength of light from the spectral emission line of sodium is 589 nm. Find the kinetic energy at which*

(a) an electron and

(b) a neutron, would have the same de-Broglie wavelength?

Sol. (a) Let E_1 = KE of electron

Using the relation, $\lambda = \frac{h}{\sqrt{2m_e E}}$, we get

$$\Rightarrow \quad \lambda^2 = \frac{h^2}{2m_e E}$$

$$\therefore \quad E_1 = \frac{h^2}{2m_e\lambda^2} = \frac{(6.62 \times 10^{-34})^2}{2 \times 9.1 \times 10^{-31} \times (589 \times 10^{-9})^2}$$
$$= 6.94 \times 10^{-25} \text{ J}$$
$$= \frac{6.94 \times 10^{-25}}{1.6 \times 10^{-19}} \text{ eV} = 4.34 \times 10^{-6} \text{ eV}$$

(b) E_2 = KE of neutron

$$\therefore \quad E_2 = \frac{h^2}{2m_n\lambda^2} = \frac{(6.62 \times 10^{-34})^2}{2 \times 1.67 \times 10^{-27} \times (589 \times 10^{-9})^2}$$
$$= 3.782 \times 10^{-28} \text{ J}$$
$$= \frac{3.782 \times 10^{-28}}{1.6 \times 10^{-19}} \text{ eV}$$
$$= 2.36 \times 10^{-9} \text{ eV}$$

Example 18.

(a) For which value of kinetic energy of a neutron will the associated de-Broglie wavelength be 1.40×10^{-10} m?

(b) Also, find the de-Broglie wavelength of a neutron, in thermal equilibrium with matter, having an average kinetic energy of $\frac{3}{2}kT$ at 300 K.

Sol. (a) Using the formula $\lambda = \frac{h}{\sqrt{2mE}}$, we get

$$\Rightarrow \quad \lambda^2 = \frac{h^2}{2mE}$$

or $$E = \frac{h^2}{2m\lambda^2} = \frac{(6.62 \times 10^{-34})^2}{2 \times 1.67 \times 10^{-27} \times (1.40 \times 10^{-10})^2}$$
$$= 6.69 \times 10^{-21} \text{ J}$$
$$= \frac{6.69 \times 10^{-21}}{1.6 \times 10^{-19}} \text{ eV} = 4.184 \times 10^{-2} \text{ eV}$$

(b) Here, T = absolute temperature = 300 K

k = Boltzmann constant

$= 1.38 \times 10^{-23} \text{ JK}^{-1}$

E = kinetic energy of neutron

$$= \frac{3}{2}kT = \frac{3}{2} \times 1.38 \times 10^{-23} \times 300$$
$$= 6.21 \times 10^{-21} \text{ J}$$

Using the relation, $\lambda = \frac{h}{\sqrt{2mE}}$, we get

$$\lambda = \frac{6.62 \times 10^{-34}}{\sqrt{2 \times 1.67 \times 10^{-27} \times 6.21 \times 10^{-21}}}$$
$$= 1.455 \times 10^{-10} \text{ m} = 0.1455 \text{ m}$$

de-Broglie Wavelength Associated with Uncharged Particles

For neutron, de-Broglie wavelength is given as

$$\lambda_{\text{neutron}} = \frac{0.286 \times 10^{-10}}{\sqrt{E \text{ (in eV)}}} \text{ m} = \frac{0.286}{\sqrt{E \text{ (in eV)}}} \text{ Å}$$

Energy of thermal neutrons or gas molecules at ordinary temperature is given by

$$E = \frac{3}{2}kT \Rightarrow \boxed{\lambda = \frac{h}{\sqrt{3mkT}}}$$

where, T = absolute temperature

and k = Boltzmann's constant

$= 1.38 \times 10^{-23}$ J/K.

Also, $$\lambda_{\text{thermal neutrons}} = \frac{25.17}{\sqrt{T}} \text{ Å}$$

Characteristics of Matter Waves

Characteristics of matter waves are given below

(i) Matter waves are not electromagnetic waves in nature.

(ii) These waves are non-mechanical waves, *i.e.* they can travel in vacuum.

(iii) Matter waves are independent of charge, *i.e.* they are associated with every moving particle (whether charged or uncharged).

(iv) Observation of matter waves is possible only when the de-Broglie wavelength is of the order of size of the particle (*i.e.* the waves are diffracted).

(v) The phase velocity of the matter waves can be greater than the speed of the light.

(vi) The number of de-Broglie waves associated with *n*th orbital electron is *n*.

STEP UP Practice 3

1. The wavelength of the matter wave is independent of which amongst the given associated variable/physical quantity?
(a) Mass (b) Velocity (c) Momentum (d) Charge

2. If the velocity of an electron is doubled, its de-Broglie frequency will
(a) be halved (b) remain same
(c) be doubled (d) become four times

3. Proton and α-particles have the same de-Broglie wavelength. Which quantity will remain same for both of them?
(a) Charge (b) Energy
(c) Speed (d) Momentum

4. **Assertion** (A) There is a physical significance of matter waves.
Reason (R) Both interference and diffraction occurs in it.
In the light of the above statements, choose the correct answer from the options given below.
(a) Both A and R are true but R is not the correct explanation of A.
(b) A is true but R is false.
(c) A is false but R is true.
(d) Both A and R are true and R is the correct explanation of A.

5. A photon, an electron and a very small unknown particle have the same wavelength. The one with the most energy is
(a) photon
(b) electron
(c) unknown particle
(d) depends upon the wavelength and the properties of the particle

6. If λ_p and λ_e denote the de-Broglie wavelength of proton and electron after they are accelerated from rest through the same potential difference, then
(a) $\lambda_e = \lambda_p$ (b) $\lambda_e < \lambda_p$
(c) $\lambda_e > \lambda_p$ (d) $\lambda_e = \lambda_p/2$

7. When the kinetic energy of an electron is increased, the wavelength of the associated wave will
(a) increase
(b) decrease
(c) not depend on the kinetic energy
(d) None of the above

8. The de-Broglie wavelength associated with an electron, accelerated through a potential difference of 100 V is
(a) 0.12 nm (b) 0.15 nm
(c) 0.20 nm (d) 0.25 nm

9. **Assertion** (A) de-Broglie wavelength of a gas molecule is inversely proportional to the square root of temperature.
Reason (R) The root mean square velocity of gas molecules depends on temperature.
In the light of the above statements, choose the correct answer from the options given below.
(a) Both A and R are true but R is not the correct explanation of A.
(b) A is true but R is false.
(c) A is false but R is true.
(d) Both A and R are true and R is the correct explanation of A.

10. The de-Broglie wavelength of a neutron at 27°C is λ. What will be its wavelength at 927°C?
(a) $\frac{\lambda}{2}$ (b) $\frac{\lambda}{3}$ (c) $\frac{\lambda}{4}$ (d) $\frac{\lambda}{9}$

11. Which one of the following pair is incorrect?
(a) $\lambda_{\text{neutron}} \rightarrow \frac{0.286}{\sqrt{E(\text{in eV})}}$ Å
(b) $\lambda_{\text{thermal neutron}} \rightarrow \frac{25.17}{\sqrt{T}}$ Å
(c) Matter wave → Electromagnetic wave in nature
(d) $\lambda_{\text{de-Broglie}} \rightarrow \frac{h}{mv}$

12. The speed of an electron having a wavelength 10^{-12} m is
(a) 7.25×10^8 m/s (b) 6.25×10^6 m/s
(c) 5.25×10^6 m/s (d) 4.24×10^6 m/s

13. Photon and electron are given same energy (10^{-20} J). Wavelength associated with photon and electron are λ_{Ph} and λ_{el} then correct statement will be
(a) $\lambda_{\text{Ph}} > \lambda_{\text{el}}$ (b) $\lambda_{\text{Ph}} < \lambda_{\text{el}}$
(c) $\lambda_{\text{Ph}} = \lambda_{\text{el}}$ (d) $\frac{\lambda_{\text{el}}}{\lambda_{\text{Ph}}} = c$

14. **Assertion (A)** de-Broglie equation is significant for microscopic particles.

Reason (R) de-Broglie wavelength is inversely proportional to the mass of a particle when velocity is kept constant.

In the light of the above statements, choose the correct answer from the options given below.

(a) Both A and R are true but R is not the correct explanation of A.
(b) A is true but R is false.
(c) A is false but R is true.
(d) Both A and R are true and R is the correct explanation of A.

15. The log-log graph between the energy E of an electron and its de-Broglie wavelength λ will be

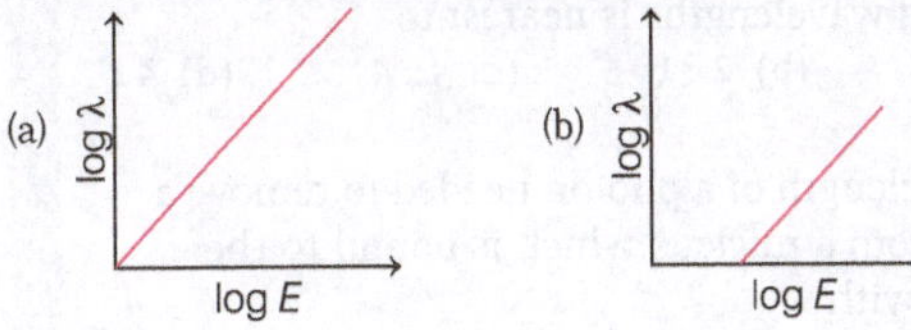

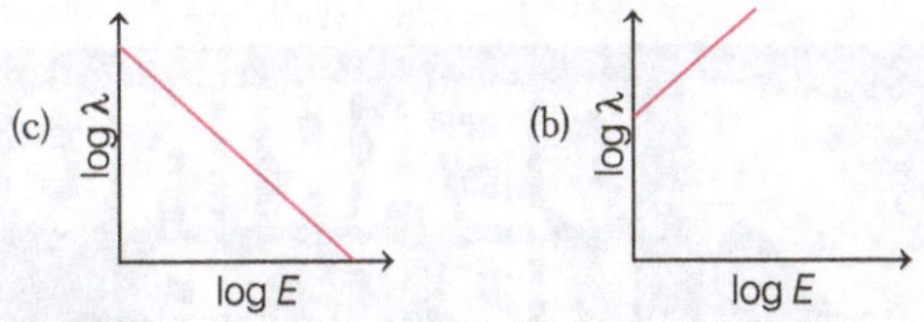

16. **Assertion** (A) Resolving power of electron microscope increases as electron is accelerated through higher voltage.

Reason (R) de-Broglie wavelength of electron decreases as accelerating voltage of electron increases.

In the light of the above statements, choose the correct answer from the options given below.

(a) Both A and R are true but R is not the correct explanation of A.
(b) A is true but R is false.
(c) A is false but R is true.
(d) Both A and R are true and R is the correct explanation of A

NEET Exclusive EXTRA BYTES

- All the free electrons present in metal do not have same energy. At constant temperature, these electrons have a certain energy distribution. Due to this energy distribution of free electrons, energy required to eject an electron is different for different electrons.
- Work function only indicates the minimum energy required for the electrons in the highest level of the conduction band to get out from the metal. All the electrons in the metal do not belong to this energy level. They occupy a continuous band of levels. Consequently, for the same incident radiation, electron knocked off from different energy levels come out with different energies.
- Light of lower wavelength is more effective than higher wavelength in photoelectric effect.
- For a frequency lower than cut-off frequency, no photoelectric emission is possible even if the intensity is large.
- Stopping potential is independent of distance between collector and emitter.
- UV light for metals and visible light for alkyl metal produces photocurrent.
- Work function depends only on nature of metal.
- Einstein's photoelectric equation is based on energy conservation law.
- Interaction between electron and photon is one to one.
- When light energy photon (X-rays or γ-rays) strikes with any free electron, then energy of photon (and hence its frequency) decreases. This phenomena explains particle nature of light and known as Compton's effect.
- Macroscopic objects in our daily life do not show wave like properties.
- de-Broglie wavelength is independent of the charge and nature of the material particles.

GEARING UP FOR NEET

Single Correct Option

1. In a photoemissive cell with exciting wavelength λ, the fastest electron has speed v. If the exciting wavelength is changed to $\frac{\lambda}{4}$, the speed of the fastest emitted electron will be
(a) $2v$ (b) $\frac{v}{2}$ (c) $< 2v$ (d) $> 2v$

2. Light of wavelength λ, strikes a photoelectric surface and electrons are ejected with an energy E. If E is to be increased to exactly twice its original value, the wavelength changes to λ', where
(a) λ' is less than $\lambda/2$
(b) λ' is greater than $\lambda/2$
(c) λ' is greater than $\lambda/2$ but less than λ
(d) λ' is exactly equal to $\lambda/2$

3. Let p and E denote the linear momentum and energy of a photon. If the wavelength is decreased, then
(a) Both p and E increase
(b) p increases and E decreases
(c) p decreases and E increases
(d) Both p and E decrease

4. The energy of incident photons corresponding to maximum wavelength of visible light is
(a) 3.2 eV (b) 7 eV (c) 1.76 eV (d) 1 eV

5. The momentum of a photon is 6.6×10^{-29} kg-ms^{-1}. The frequency of the radiation (in Hz) is
(a) 3×10^{13} (b) 3×10^{8} (c) 3×10^{15} (d) 3×10^{6}

6. The frequency of a photon having energy 100 eV is (Take, $h = 6.62 \times 10^{-34}$ Js; 1 eV $= 1.6 \times 10^{-19}$ J)
(a) 2417×10^{-16} Hz (b) 2.417×10^{16} Hz
(c) 2417×10^{17} Hz (d) 10.54×10^{17} Hz

7. According to Einstein's photoelectric equation, the graph of KE of the photoelectron emitted from the metal *versus* the frequency of the incident radiation gives a straight line graph, whose slope
(a) depends on the intensity of the incident radiation
(b) depends on the nature of the metal and also on the intensity of incident radiation
(c) is same for all metals and independent of the intensity of the incident radiation
(d) depends on the nature of the metal

8. Sodium and copper have work functions 2.3 eV and 4.5 eV respectively, then the ratio of their threshold wavelengths is nearest to
(a) 1 : 2 (b) 2 : 1 (c) 1 : 4 (d) 4 : 1

9. The wavelength of a photon needed to remove a proton from a nucleus which is bound to the nucleus with 1 MeV energy is nearly *[NCERT Exemplar]*
(a) 1.2 nm (b) 1.2×10^{-3} nm
(c) 1.2×10^{-6} nm (d) 1.2×10 nm

10. The retarding potential necessary to stop the emission of photoelectron, when a target material of work function 1.24 eV is irradiated with light of wavelength 4.36×10^{-7} m is
(a) 0.36 V (b) 1.60 V (c) 2.84 V (d) 4.08 V

11. The surface of some material is radiated, by waves of $\lambda_1 = 3.5 \times 10^{-7}$ m and $\lambda_2 = 5.4 \times 10^{-7}$ m, respectively. The ratio of the stopping potential in two cases is 2 : 1. The work function of the material is
(a) 0.86 eV (b) 1.345 eV
(c) 1.05 eV (d) 2.20 eV

12. Mercury violet light ($\lambda = 4558$ Å) is falling on a photosensitive material ($\phi = 2.5$ eV). The speed of the ejected electrons is in ms^{-1}, about
(a) 3×10^{5} (b) 2.65×10^{5}
(c) 4×10^{4} (d) 3.65×10^{7}

13. Consider a beam of electrons (each electron with energy E_0) incident on a metal surface kept in an evacuated chamber. Then, *[NCERT Exemplar]*
(a) no electrons will be emitted as only photons can emit electrons
(b) electrons can be emitted but all with an energy E_0
(c) electrons can be emitted with any energy, with a maximum of $E_0 - \phi$ (ϕ is the work function)
(d) electrons can be emitted with any energy, with a maximum of E_0

14. In a photoelectric experiment, the relation between applied potential difference between cathode and anode (V) and the photoelectric current (I) was found to be as shown in graph below. If Planck's constant $h = 6.6 \times 10^{-34}$ J-s and

work function $\phi_0 = 4\,\text{eV}$, the frequency of incident radiation would be nearly (in s^{-1})

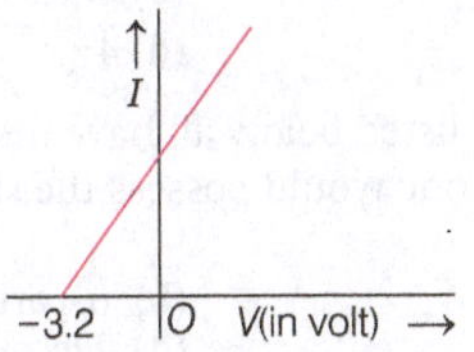

(a) 0.436×10^{18} (b) 1.436×10^{17}
(c) 1.939×10^{14} (d) 0.775×10^{16}

15. Maximum KE of a photoelectron is E when the wavelength of incident light is λ. If energy becomes four times when wavelength is reduced to one-third, then work function of the metal is
(a) $\frac{3hc}{\lambda}$ (b) $\frac{hc}{3\lambda}$ (c) $\frac{hc}{\lambda}$ (d) $\frac{hc}{2\lambda}$

16. The work function for tungsten and sodium are 4.5 eV and 2.3 eV, respectively. If the threshold wavelength λ for sodium is 5600 Å, then the value of λ for tungsten is
(a) 5893 Å (b) 10683 Å
(c) 2862 Å (d) 528 Å

17. The threshold frequency of the metal of the cathode in a photoelectric cell is 1×10^{15} Hz. When a certain beam of light is incident on the cathode, it is found that a stopping potential 4.144 V is required to reduce the current to zero. The frequency of the incident radiation is
(a) 2.5×10^{15} Hz (b) 2×10^{15} Hz
(c) 4.144×10^{15} Hz (d) 3×10^{16} Hz

18. If maximum velocity with which an electron can be emitted from a photocell is 4×10^8 cm/s, the stopping potential is (Take, mass of electron $= 9 \times 10^{-31}$ kg)
(a) 30 V (b) 45 V (c) 59 V (d) 49 V

19. In an experiment on photoelectric effect, the frequency ν of the incident light is plotted against the stopping potential V_0. The work function of the photoelectric surface is given by (e is electronic charge)

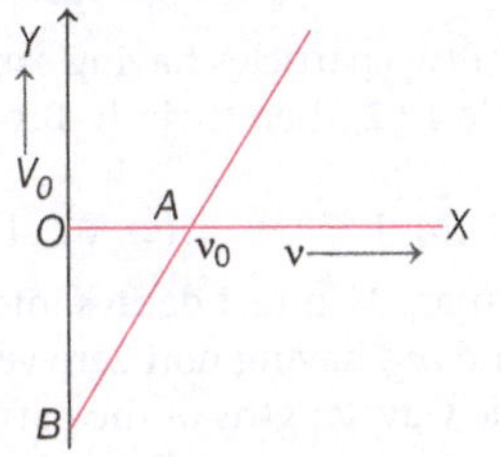

(a) $OB \times e$ in eV (b) OB in volt
(c) OA in eV (d) the slope of the line AB

20. When ultraviolet light of wavelength 100 nm is incident upon silver plate, a potential of 7.7 V is required to stop the photoelectrons from reaching the collector plate. How much potential will be required to stop the photoelectrons when light of wavelength 200 nm is incident upon silver?
(a) 1.5 V (b) 3.85 V
(c) 2.35 V (d) 15.4 V

21. When 1 cm thick surface is illuminated with light of wavelength λ, the stopping potential is V. When the same surface is illuminated by light of wavelength 2λ, the stopping potential is $V/3$. Threshold wavelength for metallic surface is
(a) $4\lambda/3$ (b) 4λ
(c) 6λ (d) $8\lambda/3$

22. If 5% of the energy supplied to a bulb is irradiated as visible light, how many quanta are emitted per second by a 100 W lamp? (Assume, wavelength of visible light as 5.6×10^{-5} cm)
(a) 1.4×10^{19} (b) 3×10^{3}
(c) 1.4×10^{-19} (d) 3×10^{4}

23. Minimum light intensity that can be perceived by normal human eye is about 10^{-10} Wbm^{-2}. What is the minimum number of photons of wavelength 660 nm that must enter the pupil in 1 s for one to see the object? (Area of cross-section of the pupil is 10^{-4} m^2)
(a) 3.3×10^2 (b) 3.3×10^3
(c) 3.3×10^4 (d) 3.3×10^5

24. Radiations of two photon having energies twice and five times the work function of metal are incident successively on the metal surface. The ratio of the maximum velocity of the photoelectrons emitted in the two cases will be
(a) 1 : 1 (b) 1 : 2
(c) 1 : 3 (d) 1 : 4

25. Work function of nickel is 5.01 eV. When ultraviolet radiation of wavelength 2000 Å is incident on the surface of nickel, electrons are emitted. What will be the maximum velocity of emitted electrons?
(a) 3×10^8 ms^{-1}
(b) 6.46×10^5 ms^{-1}
(c) 10.36×10^5 ms^{-1}
(d) 8.54×10^6 ms^{-1}

26. When radiation of wavelength λ is incident on a metallic surface, the stopping potential is 4.8 V. If the same surface is illuminated with radiation of double the wavelength, then the stopping potential becomes 1.6 V. Then, the threshold wavelength for the surface is
(a) 2λ (b) 4λ (c) 6λ (d) 8λ

27. A 1100 W light bulb is placed at the centre of a spherical chamber of radius 20 cm. Assume that, 60% the energy supplied to the bulb is converted into light and that the surface of the chamber is perfectly absorbing. The force and pressure exerted by the light on the surface of chamber is
(a) 3.6×10^{-6} N, 4.4×10^{-6} N/m^2
(b) 7.3×10^{-6} N, 8.8×10^{-6} N/m^2
(c) 3.6×10^{-6} N, 8.8×10^{-6} N/m^2
(d) 7.3×10^{-6} N, 4.4×10^{-6} N/m^2

28. A parallel beam of monochromatic light of wavelength 663 nm is incident on a totally reflecting plane mirror. The angle of incidence is 60° and the number of photons striking the mirror per second is 1.0×10^{19}. The value of the force exerted by it on the surface is
(a) 10^{-6} N (b) 10^{-7} N
(c) 10^{-8} N (d) 10^{-9} N

29. Light of wavelength 330 nm falling on a piece of metal ejects electrons with sufficient energy which requires voltage V_0 to prevent them from reaching a collector. In the same set up, light of wavelength 220 nm, ejects electrons which require twice the voltage V_0 to stop them in reaching a collector. The numerical value of voltage V_0 is

(a) $\frac{16}{15}$ V (b) $\frac{15}{16}$ V

(c) $\frac{15}{8}$ V (d) $\frac{8}{15}$

30. When a light beam of frequency ν is incident on a metal surface, photoelectrons are emitted. If these electrons describe a circle of radius r in a magnetic field of strength B, then the work function of the metal is

(a) $h\nu + \frac{Ber}{2m_e}$ (b) $h\nu - \frac{(Ber)^2}{2m_e}$

(c) $h\nu + \frac{(Ber)^2}{2m_e}$ (d) $h\nu - \frac{Ber}{2m_e}$

31. The work function of metals is in the range of 2 eV to 5 eV. Find which of the following wavelength of light cannot be used for photoelectric effect. (Consider, Planck's constant $= 4 \times 10^{-15}$ eV-s and velocity of light $= 3 \times 10^8 \text{ ms}^{-1}$)

(a) 510 nm (b) 650 nm

(c) 400 nm (d) 570 nm

32. When the energy of the incident radiation is increased by 20%, the kinetic energy of the photoelectrons emitted from a metal surface increased from 0.5 eV to 0.8 eV. The work function of the metal is

(a) 0.65 eV (b) 1 eV

(c) 1.3 eV (d) 1.5 eV

33. Light of wavelength λ_A and λ_B falls on two identical metal plates A and B, respectively. The maximum kinetic energy of photoelectrons is K_A and K_B respectively, then which one of the following relations is true? ($\lambda_A = 2\lambda_B$)

(a) $K_A < \frac{K_B}{2}$ (b) $2K_A = K_B$

(c) $K_A = 2K_B$ (d) $K_A > 2K_B$

34. A light of wavelength 5000 Å falls on a sensitive plate with photoelectric work function 1.90 eV. Kinetic energy of the emitted photoelectrons will be

(Take, $h = 6.62 \times 10^{-34}$ Js)

(a) 0.1 eV (b) 2 eV

(c) 0.58 eV (d) 1.581 eV

35. When monochromatic light falls on a photosensitive material, the number of photoelectron emitted per second is n and their maximum kinetic energy is K_{max}. If the intensity of incident light is doubled, then

(a) n is doubled but K_{max} remains same

(b) K_{max} is double but n remains same

(c) Both n and K_{max} are doubled

(d) Both n and K_{max} are halved

36. The threshold frequency for a certain photosensitive metal is ν_0. When it is illuminated by light of frequency $\nu = 2\nu_0$, the maximum velocity of photoelectrons is v_0. What will be the maximum velocity of the photoelectrons when the same metal is illuminated by light of frequency $\nu = 5\nu_0$?

(a) $\sqrt{2}v_0$ (b) $2v_0$

(c) $2\sqrt{2}v_0$ (d) $4v_0$

37. If the particles listed below all have the same kinetic energy, which one would possess the shortest de-Broglie wavelength?

(a) Deuteron (b) α-particle

(c) Proton (d) Electron

38. An electron and proton are accelerated through the same potential difference. The ratio of their de-Broglie wavelength will be

(a) $(m_p/m_e)^{1/2}$ (b) m_e/m_p

(c) m_p/m_e (d) 1

39. If the de-Broglie wavelengths for a proton and for α-particle are equal, then their velocities will be in the ratio

(a) 4 : 1 (b) 2 : 1 (c) 1 : 2 (d) 1 : 4

40. The de-Broglie wavelength of an electron having 80 eV of energy is nearly (Take, 1eV $= 1.6 \times 10^{-19}$ J, mass of electron $= 9.1 \times 10^{-31}$ kg and Planck's constant $= 6.6 \times 10^{-34}$ Js)

(a) 140 Å (b) 0.14 Å

(c) 14 Å (d) 1.4 Å

41. The de-Broglie wavelength of neutrons in thermal equilibrium is

(a) $\frac{30.8}{\sqrt{T}}$ Å (b) $\frac{308}{\sqrt{T}}$ Å

(c) $\frac{0.308}{\sqrt{T}}$ Å (d) $\frac{0.0308}{\sqrt{T}}$ Å

42. The de-Broglie wavelength of an electron in a metal at 27°C is

(a) 3.5×10^{-9} m (b) 4.2×10^{-9} m

(c) 5.6×10^{-9} m (d) 6.2×10^{-9} m

43. An electron of mass m_e and a proton of mass m_p are moving with the same speed. The ratio of their de-Broglie wavelengths λ_e/λ_p is

(a) 1 (b) 1836 (c) $\frac{1}{1836}$ (d) 918

44. The masses of two particles having same kinetic energies are in the ratio 1 : 2, then their de-Broglie wavelengths are in the ratio

(a) 2 : 1 (b) 1 : 2 (c) $\sqrt{2}$: 1 (d) $\sqrt{3}$: 1

45. A particle of mass M at rest decays into two particles of masses m_1 and m_2, having non-zero velocities. The ratio of the de-Broglie wavelengths of the particles, λ_1/λ_2 is

(a) m_1/m_2 (b) m_2/m_1

(c) 1 : 1 (d) $\sqrt{m_2}/\sqrt{m_1}$

46. The de-Broglie wavelength associated with an electron moving with a velocity 0.5 cms^{-1} and rest mass $= 9.1 \times 10^{-31}$ kg is

(a) 4.2×10^{-12} m (b) 3.6×10^{-12} m

(c) 5.0×10^{-12} m (d) 4.2×10^{-10} m

47. A proton accelerated through a potential difference of 100 V, has de-Broglie wavelength λ_0. The de-Broglie wavelength of an α-particle, accelerated through 800 V is

(a) $\frac{\lambda_0}{\sqrt{2}}$ (b) $\frac{\lambda_0}{2}$
(c) $\frac{\lambda_0}{4}$ (d) $\frac{\lambda_0}{8}$

48. An electron and a photon possess the same de-Broglie wavelength. If E_e and E_p respectively are the energies of electron and photon and v and c are their respective velocities, then $\frac{E_e}{E_p}$ is equal to

(a) $\frac{v}{c}$ (b) $\frac{v}{2c}$
(c) $\frac{v}{3c}$ (d) $\frac{v}{4c}$

49. An electron of mass m when accelerated through a potential difference V has de-Broglie wavelength λ. The de-Broglie wavelength associated with a proton of mass M accelerated through the same potential difference will be

(a) $\lambda\frac{m}{M}$ (b) $\lambda\sqrt{\frac{m}{M}}$
(c) $\lambda\frac{M}{m}$ (d) $\lambda\sqrt{\frac{M}{m}}$

50. A particle is dropped from a height H. The de-Broglie wavelength of the particle as a function of height is proportional to *[NCERT Exemplar]*

(a) H (b) $H^{1/2}$ (c) H^0 (d) $H^{-1/2}$

51. If the momentum of an electron is changed by Δp, then the de-Broglie wavelength associated with it changes by 0.50%. The initial momentum of electron will be

(a) $\frac{\Delta p}{200}$ (b) $\frac{\Delta p}{199}$ (c) $199\,\Delta p$ (d) $400\,\Delta p$

52. A proton, a neutron, an electron and an α-particle have same energy, then their de-Broglie wavelengths compare as *[NCERT Exemplar]*

(a) $\lambda_p = \lambda_n > \lambda_e > \lambda_\alpha$ (b) $\lambda_\alpha < \lambda_p = \lambda_n < \lambda_e$
(c) $\lambda_e < \lambda_p = \lambda_n > \lambda_\alpha$ (d) $\lambda_e = \lambda_p = \lambda_n = \lambda_\alpha$

53. An electron (mass m) with an initial velocity $\mathbf{v} = v_0\hat{\mathbf{i}}$ is in an electric field $\mathbf{E} = E_0\hat{\mathbf{j}}$. If $\lambda_0 = h/mv_0$, its de-Broglie wavelength at time t is given by *[NCERT Exemplar]*

(a) λ_0 (b) $\lambda_0\sqrt{1+\frac{e^2E_0^2t^2}{m^2v_0^2}}$

(c) $\frac{\lambda_0}{\sqrt{1+\frac{e^2E_0^2t^2}{m^2v_0^2}}}$ (d) $\frac{\lambda_0}{\left(1+\frac{e^2E_0^2t^2}{m^2v_0^2}\right)}$

54. When photons of energy 4.25 eV strike the surface of a metal A, the ejected photoelectrons have maximum kinetic energy T_A expressed in eV and de-Broglie wavelength λ_A. The maximum kinetic energy of photoelectron liberated from another metal B by photons of energy 4.70 eV is $T_B = (T_A - 1.50)$ eV. If the de-Broglie wavelength of these photoelectrons is $\lambda_B = 2\lambda_A$, then choose the wrong option.

(a) The work function of A is 2.25 eV
(b) The work function of B is 4.20 eV
(c) $T_A = 2.00$ eV
(d) $T_B = 2.75$ eV

55. The wavelength λ of a photon and the de-Broglie wavelength of an electron have the same value. Find the ratio of energy of photon to the kinetic energy of electron in terms of mass m, speed of light c and Planck's constant (h).

(a) $\lambda mc/h$ (b) hmc/λ
(c) $2hmc/\lambda$ (d) $2\lambda mc/h$

56. The de-Broglie wavelength of an electron is the same as that of a 50 keV X-ray photon. The ratio of the energy of the photon to the kinetic energy of the electron is (the energy equivalent of electron mass of 0.5 MeV)

(a) 1 : 50 (b) 1 : 20
(c) 20 : 1 (d) 50 : 1

Assertion and Reason

Directions (Q. Nos. 1-5) *These questions consist of two statements each printed as Assertion (A) and Reason (R). While answering these questions, you are required to choose any one of the following four responses.*

(a) Both A and R are true but R is not the correct explanation of A.
(b) A is true but R is false.
(c) A is false but R is true.
(d) Both A and R are true and R is the correct explanation of A.

1. Assertion (A) Electromagnetic theory of light failed to explain photoelectric effect.

Reason (R) Photoelectric effect can only be explained by assuming particle nature of light.

2. Assertion (A) Photoelectric emission is an instantaneous process.

Reason (R) There is very small time lag ($\sim 10^{-9}$s) between incidence of light and emission of photoelectron.

3. Assertion (A) When wavelength of incident radiation in a photoelectric experiment is decreased, then the stopping potential will decrease.

Reason (R) With decrease in wavelength, energy of incident light increases.

4. Assertion (A) Work function of different metals is different.

Reason (R) Work function is the minimum energy required by an electron to just escape from the metal surface. It will be different for different metals depending on their structure.

5. Assertion (A) In photoelectric effect, if the intensity of light is doubled, then maximum kinetic energy of photoelectrons will become double.

Reason (R) The maximum kinetic energy of emitted photoelectrons depends on nature of material of the plate.

Statement Type Questions

Directions (Q. Nos. 1-5) *These questions consists of two statements, choose the most appropriate answer from the options given below.*

(a) Both Statement I and Statement II are incorrect.
(b) Statement I is correct but Statement II is incorrect.
(c) Statement I is incorrect but Statement II is correct.
(d) Both Statement I and Statement II are correct.

1. **Statement I** When photoemission occurs in a gaseous target, photoemission can occurs at all frequencies of incident photons.
Statement II In a gas sample, speed of an atom may be different from other atoms.

2. **Statement I** Work function for every emitted electron is same in case of photoemission.
Statement II Work function is minimum energy required by an electron to come out of metal surface with zero speed.

3. **Statement I** Though light of a single frequency (monochromatic) is incident on a metal, the energies of emitted photoelectrons are different.
Statement II The energy of electrons emitted from inside the metal surface is lost in collision with the other atoms in the metal.

4. **Statement I** The de-Broglie wavelength of a neutron when its kinetic energy (K) is λ. Its wavelength is 2λ when its kinetic energy is $4K$.
Statement II The de-Broglie wavelength λ is directly proportional to square root of the kinetic energy.

5. **Statement I** The energy (E) and momentum (p) of a photon are related $p = E / c$.
Statement II The photon behaves like a particle.

Match the Columns

1. Match the Column I (the photoelectric cut-off voltage) with Column II (to the highest kinetic energy released respectively).

Column I	Column II
A. 1.5 V	I. 0.8×10^{-19} J
B. 2.4 V	II. 2.4×10^{-19} J
C. 0.5 V	III. 3.8×10^{-19} J
D. 1.8 V	IV. 2.9×10^{-19} J

Choose the correct answer from the options given below.
(a) A-I, B-II, C-III, D-IV
(b) A-II, B-I, C-III, D-IV
(c) A-II, B-III, C-IV- D-I
(d) A-II, B-III, C-I, D-IV

2. Match the Column I with Column II when wavelength of light is 660 nm.

Column I	Column II
A. Momentum of photon (in kg-m/s)	I. 2.2×10^{20}
B. Number of photons emitted per second by a 66 W source of monochromatic light	II. 6.67×10^{17}
C. Number of photons emitted per second by a one watt bulb, if its efficiency is 20%.	III. 6.7×10^{13}
D. The rate at which photons striking the surface, if the intensity of light is 100 mW/m^2 and surface area is 2 cm^2 (in per second)	IV. 1.00×10^{-27}

Choose the correct answer from the options given below.
(a) A-IV, B-I, C-II, D-III
(b) A-IV, B-I, C-III, D-II
(c) A-II, B-I, C-III, D-IV
(d) A-I, B-II, C-IV, D-III

3. Match the Column I with Column II when KE of an electron is 100 eV

Column I	Column II
A. Momentum (in kg-ms^{-1})	I. 1.22×10^{-10}
B. Speed (in ms^{-1})	II. 5.9×10^{6}
C. de-Broglie wavelength (in m)	III. 5.4×10^{-24}
D. frequency (in s^{-1})	IV. 2.46×10^{18}

Choose the correct answer from the given options.
(a) A-II, B-I, C-III, D-IV
(b) A-III, B-II, C-I, D-IV
(c) A-I, B-II, C-III, D-IV
(d) A-II, B-I, C-IV, D-III

Final Check Through PYQs

Module-I Photoelectric Effect

1. The work functions of caesium (Cs), potassium (K) and sodium (Na) are 2.14 eV, 2.30 eV and 2.75 eV, respectively. If incident electromagnetic radiation has an incident energy of 2.20 eV. Which of these photosensitive surfaces may emit photoelectrons? *[NCERT (New) Pg. 277, NEET 2023]*
(a) Both Na and K (b) K only
(c) Na only (d) Cs only

2. Light of frequency 1.5 times the threshold frequency is incident on a photosensitive material. What will be the photoelectric current, if the frequency is halved and intensity is doubled? *[NCERT (New) Pg. 278, NEET (Sep.) 2020]*
(a) Four times (b) One-fourth
(c) Zero (d) Doubled

Module-II Quantum Theory and Einstein's Photoelectric Equations

3. If c is the velocity of light in free space, the correct statements about photon among the following are
A. The energy of a photon is $E = h\nu$.
B. The velocity of a photon in space is c.
C. The momentum of a photon, $p = \frac{h\nu}{c}$
D. In a photon-electron collision, both total energy and total momentum are conserved.
E. Photon possesses positive charge.
Choose the correct answer from the options given below. *[NCERT (New) Pg. 283, NEET 2024]*
(a) A and B only (b) A, B, C and D only
(c) A, C and D only (d) A, B, D and E only

4. When two monochromatic lights of frequency ν and $\nu/2$ are incident on a photoelectric metal, their stopping potential becomes $V_s/2$ and V_s, respectively. The threshold frequency for this metal is *[NCERT (New) Pg. 281, NEET 2022]*
(a) 3ν (b) $\frac{2}{3}\nu$
(c) $\frac{3}{2}\nu$ (d) 2ν

5. The number of photons per second on average emitted by the source of monochromatic light of wavelength 600 nm, when it delivers the power of 3.3×10^{-3} W will be ($h = 6.6 \times 10^{-34}$ J-s) *[NCERT (New) Pg. 283, NEET 2021]*
(a) 10^{18} (b) 10^{17} (c) 10^{16} (d) 10^{15}

6. The work function of a photosensitive material is 4.0 eV. This longest wavelength of light that can cause photon emission from the substance is (approximately) *[NCERT (New) Pg. 281, NEET (Odisha) 2019]*
(a) 3100 nm (b) 966 nm
(c) 31 nm (d) 310 nm

7. When the light of frequency $2\nu_0$ (where, ν_0 is threshold frequency), is incident on a metal plate, the maximum velocity of electrons emitted is v_1. When the frequency of the incident radiation is increased to $5\nu_0$, the maximum velocity of electrons emitted from the same plate is v_2. The ratio of v_1 to v_2 is *[NCERT (New) Pg. 281, NEET 2018]*
(a) 4 : 1 (b) 1 : 4
(c) 1 : 2 (d) 2 : 1

8. The photoelectric threshold wavelength of silver is 3250×10^{-10} m. The velocity of the electron ejected from a silver surface by ultraviolet light of wavelength 2536×10^{-10} m is (Given, $h = 4.14 \times 10^{-15}$ eV-s and $c = 3 \times 10^8$ ms^{-1}) *[NCERT (New) Pg. 281, NEET 2017]*
(a) $\approx 6 \times 10^5$ ms^{-1} (b) $\approx 0.6 \times 10^7$ ms^{-1}
(c) $\approx 61 \times 10^3$ ms^{-1} (d) $\approx 0.3 \times 10^6$ ms^{-1}

9. When a metallic surface is illuminated with radiation of wavelength λ, the stopping potential is V. If the same surface is illuminated with radiation of wavelength 2λ, the stopping potential is $V/4$. The threshold wavelength for the metallic surface is *[NCERT (New) Pg. 281, NEET 2016]*
(a) 5λ (b) $\frac{5}{2}\lambda$
(c) 3λ (d) 4λ

10. Photons with energy 5 eV are incident on a cathode C in a photoelectric cell. The maximum energy of emitted photoelectrons is 2 eV. When photons of energy 6 eV are incident on C, no photoelectrons will reach the anode A, if the stopping potential of A relative to C is *[NCERT (New) Pg. 281, NEET 2016]*
(a) + 3 V (b) + 4 V
(c) − 1 V (d) − 3 V

11. A certain metallic surface is illuminated with monochromatic light of wavelength λ. The stopping potential for photoelectric current for this light is $3V_0$. If the same surface is illuminated with light of wavelength 2λ, the stopping potential is V_0. The threshold wavelength for this surface for photoelectric effect is *[NCERT (New) Pg. 281, AIPMT 2015]*

(a) 6λ (b) 4λ
(c) $\lambda/4$ (d) $\lambda/6$

12. A photoelectric surface is illuminated successively by monochromatic light of wavelength λ and $\lambda/2$. If the maximum kinetic energy of the emitted photoelectrons in the second case is 3 times that in the first case, the work function of the surface of the material is (h = Planck's constant, c = speed of light) *[NCERT (New) Pg. 281, AIPMT 2015]*

(a) $\frac{hc}{2\lambda}$ (b) $\frac{hc}{\lambda}$ (c) $\frac{2hc}{\lambda}$ (d) $\frac{hc}{3\lambda}$

Module-III Dual Nature of Matter

13. The graph which shows the variation of $\frac{1}{\lambda^2}$ and its kinetic energy, E is (where, λ is de-Broglie wavelength of a free particle) *[NCERT (New) Pg. 285, NEET 2024]*

(a) 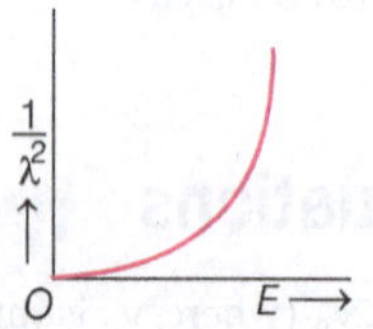

(b) 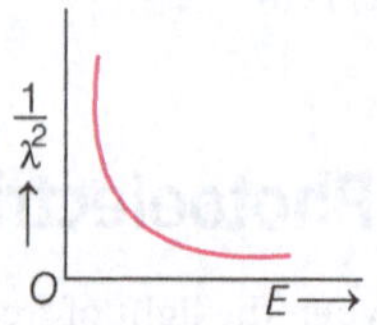

(c) 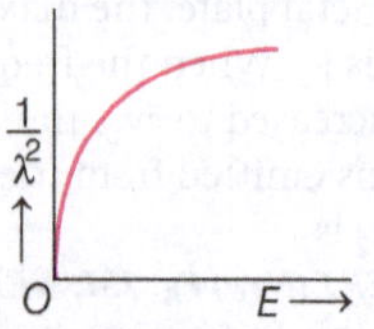

(d) 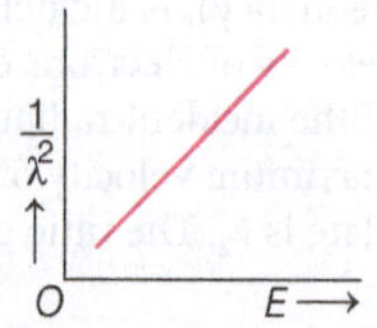

14. The graph which shows the variation of the de-Broglie wavelength (λ) of a particle and its associated momentum (p) is *[NCERT (New) Pg. 285, NEET 2022]*

(a) 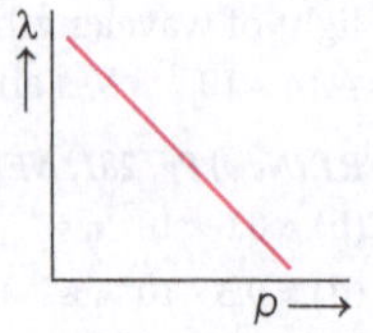

(b) 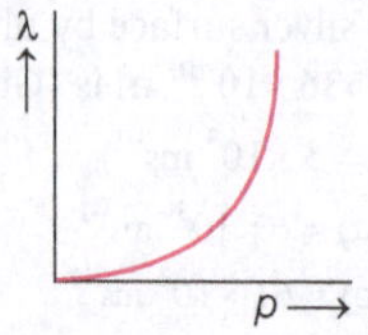

(c) 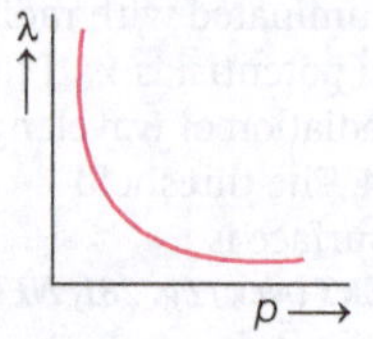

(d) 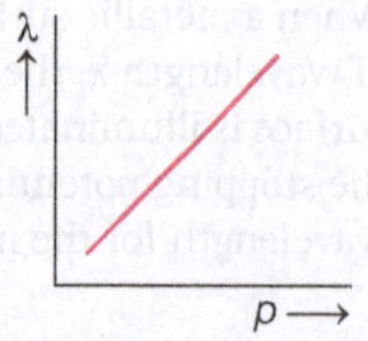

15. An electromagnetic wave of wavelength λ is incident on a photosensitive surface of negligible work function. If m mass of photoelectron emitted from the surface has de-Broglie wavelength λ_d, then *[NCERT (New) Pg. 285, NEET 2021]*

(a) $\lambda = \left(\frac{2h}{mc}\right)\lambda_d^2$ (b) $\lambda = \left(\frac{2m}{hc}\right)\lambda_d^2$
(c) $\lambda = \left(\frac{2mc}{h}\right)\lambda^2$ (d) $\lambda = \left(\frac{2mc}{h}\right)\lambda_d^2$

16. The de-Broglie wavelength of an electron moving with kinetic energy of 144 eV is nearly *[NCERT (New) Pg. 285, NEET (Oct.) 2020]*

(a) 102×10^{-3} nm
(b) 102×10^{-4} nm
(c) 102×10^{-5} nm
(d) 102×10^{-2} nm

17. The wave nature of electrons was experimentally verified by *[NCERT (New) Pg. 285, NEET (Oct.) 2020]*

(a) de-Broglie
(b) Hertz
(c) Einstein
(d) Davisson and Germer

18. An electron is accelerated from rest through a potential difference of V volt. If the de-Broglie wavelength of the electron is 1.227×10^{-2} nm, the potential difference is *[NCERT (New) Pg. 285, NEET (Sep.) 2020]*

(a) 10^2 V (b) 10^3 V
(c) 10^4 V (d) 10 V

19. A proton and an α-particle are accelerated from rest to the same energy. The de-Broglie wavelengths λ_p and λ_α are in the ratio *[NCERT (New) Pg. 285, NEET (Odisha) 2019]*

(a) 2 : 1 (b) 1 : 1
(c) $\sqrt{2}$: 1 (d) 4 : 1

20. An electron is accelerated through a potential difference of 10000 V. Its de-Broglie wavelength is nearly ($m_e = 9 \times 10^{-31}$ kg) *[NCERT (New) Pg. 285, NEET (National) 2019]*

(a) 12.2×10^{-12} m (b) 12.2×10^{-14} m
(c) 12.2 nm (d) 12.2×10^{-13} m

21. An electron of mass m with a velocity $\mathbf{v} = v_0\hat{\mathbf{i}}$ $(v_0 > 0)$ enters an electric field $\mathbf{E} = -E_0\hat{\mathbf{i}}$ (E_0 = constant > 0) at $t = 0$. If λ_0 is its de-Broglie wavelength initially, then its de-Broglie wavelength at time t is *[NCERT (New) Pg. 285, NEET 2018]*

(a) $\lambda_0 t$ (b) $\lambda_0\left(1 + \frac{eE_0}{mv_0}t\right)$
(c) $\frac{\lambda_0}{\left(1 + \frac{eE_0}{mv_0}t\right)}$ (d) λ_0

Final Check

22. The de-Broglie wavelength of a neutron in thermal equilibrium with heavy water at a temperature T (kelvin) and mass m, is *[NCERT (New) Pg. 285, NEET 2017]*

(a) $\frac{h}{\sqrt{mkT}}$ (b) $\frac{h}{\sqrt{3mkT}}$ (c) $\frac{2h}{\sqrt{3mkT}}$ (d) $\frac{2h}{\sqrt{mkT}}$

23. An electron of mass m and a photon have same energy E. The ratio of de-Broglie wavelengths associated with them is *[NCERT (New) Pg. 285, NEET 2016]*

(a) $\left(\frac{E}{2m}\right)^{1/2}$ (b) $c(2mE)^{1/2}$

(c) $\frac{1}{c}\left(\frac{2m}{E}\right)^{1/2}$ (d) $\frac{1}{c}\left(\frac{E}{2m}\right)^{1/2}$

24. Electrons of mass m with de-Broglie wavelength λ fall on the target in an X-ray tube. The cut-off wavelength (λ_0) of the emitted X-ray is *[NCERT (New) Pg. 285, NEET 2016]*

(a) $\lambda_0 = \frac{2mc\lambda^2}{h}$ (b) $\lambda_0 = \frac{2h}{mc}$

(c) $\lambda_0 = \frac{2m^2c^2\lambda^3}{h^2}$ (d) $\lambda_0 = \lambda$

25. Which of the following figures represent the variation of particle momentum and the associated de-Broglie wavelength? *[NCERT (New) Pg. 285, AIPMT 2015]*

(a) 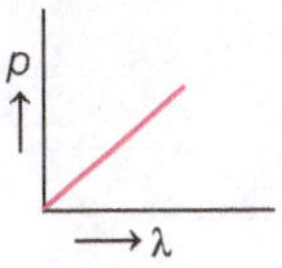

(b) 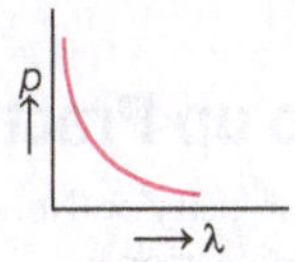

(c) 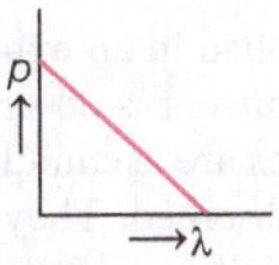

(d) 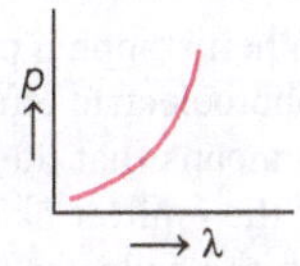

26. Light of wavelength 500 nm is incident on a metal with work function 2.28 eV. The de-Broglie wavelength of the emitted electron is *[NCERT (New) Pg. 285, AIPMT 2015]*

(a) $\geq 2.8 \times 10^{-9}$ m (b) $\leq 2.8 \times 10^{-12}$ m

(c) $< 2.8 \times 10^{-10}$ m (d) $< 2.8 \times 10^{-9}$ m

Answers

Step up Practice 1

1 (d)	2 (b)	3 (b)	4 (d)	5 (c)	6 (d)	7 (d)	8 (d)	9 (c)	10 (d)
11 (d)	12 (b)	13 (a)	14 (a)	15 (b)	16 (d)	17 (c)	18 (a)		

Step up Practice 2

1 (a)	2 (c)	3 (a)	4 (c)	5 (d)	6 (d)	7 (d)	8 (a)	9 (a)	10 (c)
11 (d)	12 (d)	13 (d)	14 (c)	15 (c)	16 (d)	17 (a)	18 (c)	19 (d)	20 (c)

Step up Practice 3

1 (d)	2 (c)	3 (d)	4 (d)	5 (a)	6 (c)	7 (b)	8 (a)	9 (d)	10 (a)
11 (c)	12 (a)	13 (a)	14 (d)	15 (c)	16 (d)				

Gearing up for NEET

1 (d)	2 (c)	3 (a)	4 (c)	5 (a)	6 (b)	7 (c)	8 (b)	9 (b)	10 (b)
11 (c)	12 (b)	13 (d)	14 (c)	15 (b)	16 (c)	17 (b)	18 (b)	19 (a)	20 (a)
21 (b)	22 (a)	23 (c)	24 (b)	25 (b)	26 (b)	27 (a)	28 (c)	29 (c)	30 (b)
31 (b)	32 (b)	33 (a)	34 (c)	35 (a)	36 (a)	37 (b)	38 (a)	39 (a)	40 (d)
41 (a)	42 (d)	43 (b)	44 (c)	45 (c)	46 (a)	47 (d)	48 (b)	49 (b)	50 (d)
51 (c)	52 (b)	53 (c)	54 (d)	55 (d)	56 (c)				

Assertion and Reason

1 (a)	2 (d)	3 (c)	4 (d)	5 (c)

Statement Type Questions

1 (c)	2 (c)	3 (d)	4 (a)	5 (d)

Match the Columns

1 (d)	2 (a)	3 (b)

Final Check through PYQs : Module-I

1 (d)	2 (c)

Final Check through PYQs : Module-II

3 (b)	4 (c)	5 (c)	6 (d)	7 (c)	8 (a)	9 (c)	10 (d)	11 (b)	12 (a)

Final Check through PYQs : Module-III

13 (d)	14 (c)	15 (d)	16 (d)	17 (a)	18 (c)	19 (a)	20 (a)	21 (c)	22 (b)
23 (d)	24 (a)	25 (b)	26 (a)						

Hints and Solutions

Step up Practice 1

1. (*d*) Intensity ∝ (No. of photons) ∝ (No. of photoelectrons).

2. (*b*) When stopping potential is applied in an experiment on photoelectric effect, no photocurrent is observed. This means that the photoelectrons are accumulated near the emitter plate and are reabsorbed. They can't reach the collector plate.

3. (*b*) With the increase in intensity of light, photoelectric current increases, but kinetic energy of ejected electron, stopping potential and work function remains unchanged.

4. (*d*) Both A and R are true and R is the correct explanation of A.

   In photoelectric emission, the free electrons in the metal absorb the photons, acquire energy and come out of the metal. In thermionic emission, electrons acquire energy by heat. Hence, this effect is temperature dependent.

5. (*c*) Photoelectric current ∝ Intensity of light.

6. (*d*) Photoelectric effect involves emission of electrons known as photoelectrons from the metal surface when light of suitable frequency illuminates this metal's surface. These emitted photoelectrons, when ejected from an emitter plate inside a glass tube by UV-radiations which are then attracted towards the collector plate by the electric field.

   Thus, this electron flow through the glass tube results in flow of current.

   This means, this effect involves conversion of light energy into electrical energy.

7. (*d*) Both A and R are true and R is the correct explanation of A.

8. (*d*) Stopping potential depends upon the energy of photon.

9. (*c*) Retarding potential, $V_0 = \frac{h}{e}(\nu - \nu_0)$.

10. (*d*) Both A and R are true and R is the correct explanation of A.

    This is because the probability is very low for two photons of energy 2.5 eV making a collision with the same electron in the metal simultaneously.

11. (*d*) As the distance of source from the surface increases, intensity of radiation decreases.

    $\because$ Intensity $I \propto \frac{1}{(\text{distance } x)^2}$ and

    Since, photoelectric current (i) ∝ intensity (I)

    Thus, the variation of i *versus* x is correctly depicted by the curve *d* in the given figure.

12. (*b*) The statement II is incorrect and it can be corrected as,

    In the experimental set-up used for studying the photoelectric effect,

    the intensity of light can be varied by changing the distance of the light source from the emitter. As,

    $$\text{Intensity} \propto \frac{1}{(\text{Distance})^2}$$

    Rest statement is correct.

13. (*a*) As $K_{max} = E - W$

    $$\Rightarrow \quad K = E - W \quad \text{...(i)}$$

    and $K' = 2E - W$

    $= 2(E) - (E - K)$ [using Eq. (i)]

    $= E + K = K + W + K = W + 2K$

    $$\Rightarrow \quad K' > 2K \quad (\because W > 0)$$

14. (*a*) The statement I is correct but rest is incorrect and it can be corrected as,

    From the given graph, we can say that we have obtained different values of stopping potential but the same value of the saturation current for incident radiation of different frequencies. Since, the energy of emitted electron depends on the frequency of the incident radiations. This means, stopping potential is more negative for higher frequencies of incident radiation. Thus, we can conclude that,

    I. stopping potential are in the order $V_{OA} > V_{OB} > V_{OC}$, if the frequencies are in the order $\nu_A > \nu_B > \nu_C$.

    II. This further implies that greater the frequency of incident radiation, greater is the maximum kinetic energy of the photoelectrons. Consequently we need greater retarding potential to stop them completely.

15. (*b*) For photoemission to take place, $h\nu > \phi_0$.

    Here, $E < \phi_0$, so it is not possible.

16. (*d*) As we know that,

    intensity of light ∝ photoelectric current

    $\Rightarrow$ photoelectric current $\propto \frac{1}{(\text{distance})^2}$, hence incorrect.

    No. of photoelectrons emitted/second $\propto \frac{1}{(\text{Distance})^2}$

    Hence, incorrect.

    $KE_{max} = eV_0$ Hence, correct.

17. (c) Both statements I & II are correct.

We know that, there exists a certain minimum cut-off frequency ν_0 for which the stopping potential is zero. This means, for a frequency ν of incident radiation lower than the cut-off frequency ν_0, no photoelectric emission is possible even, if the intensity is large.

18. (a) We know, $\lambda_r > \lambda_y > \lambda_g$.

Here, threshold wavelength $< \lambda_y$.

Step up Practice 2

1. (a) Momentum,

$$p = \frac{h}{\lambda} = \frac{6.6 \times 10^{-34}}{(5000 \times 10^{-10})}$$
$$= 1.3 \times 10^{-27} \text{ kg-ms}^{-1}$$

2. (c) Momentum, $p = \frac{E}{c}$

$$\Rightarrow \quad E = pc = 2 \times 10^{-16} \times (3 \times 10^{10}) = 6 \times 10^{-6} \text{ erg}$$

3. (a) Momentum, $p = \frac{E}{c}$

$$\Rightarrow \quad E = pc \Rightarrow E^2 = p^2c^2$$

4. (c) Power, $P = \frac{nhc}{\lambda}$

$$\therefore \quad 100 = \frac{n \times 6 \times 10^{-34} \times 3 \times 10^8}{540 \times 10^{-9}} \Rightarrow n = 3 \times 10^{20}$$

5. (d) Both Statement I and Statement II are correct.

Stopping potential is measure of maximum kinetic energy of emitted photoelectron ($eV_0 = K_{max}$) and K_{max} depends upon the frequency of incident light but it is independent of intensity of light.

6. (d) Momentum of a photon $= \frac{h}{\lambda} = \frac{h\nu}{c}$

So, all have same momentum.

7. (d) For red light, $\lambda = 760$ nm

Energy, $E = h\nu = \frac{hc}{\lambda}$

Hence, $E = \frac{6.63 \times 10^{-34} \times 3 \times 10^8}{760 \times 10^{-9}}$

$$= 2.62 \times 10^{-19} \text{ J}$$
$$= \frac{2.62 \times 10^{-19}}{1.6 \times 10^{-19}} \text{ eV} = 1.64 \text{ eV}$$

8. (a) Here, $I = 1.52 \times 10^3 \text{ Wm}^{-2}$

$\lambda = 520 \times 10^{-9}$ m, $h = 6.63 \times 10^{-34}$ Js

Number of photons incident on earth's surface per second per square metre is

$$n = \frac{I}{E} = \frac{I}{hc}\lambda \qquad \left[\because E = \frac{hc}{\lambda}\right]$$

$$\Rightarrow \quad n = \frac{1.52 \times 10^3 \times 520 \times 10^{-9}}{6.63 \times 10^{-34} \times 3 \times 10^8}$$
$$= 4 \times 10^{21} \text{ photons per metre}^2 \text{ per second}$$

9. (a) Both Statement I and Statement II are incorrect.

Photoelectric effect can be explained on the basis of quantum theory or particle nature of light, where wave nature of light fails to explain the photoelectric effect. The number of photoelectrons is proportional to the intensity of incident light.

$I = nh\nu$, where n is the number of photon emitted/absorbed per unit area per second, n and $\lambda\nu$ are independent factors.

10. (c) $\frac{1}{2} mv_{max}^2 = eV_0 \Rightarrow v_{max} = \sqrt{2\left(\frac{e}{m}\right)V_0}$

$$= \sqrt{2 \times 1.8 \times 10^{11} \times 9} = 1.8 \times 10^6 \text{ m/s}$$

Hence, the maximum velocity of the ejected electrons is 1.8×10^6 m/s.

11. (d) Work function, $\phi_0 = h\nu_0$

$\therefore$ Threshold frequency,

$$\nu_0 = \frac{\phi_0}{h} = \frac{2.14 \times 1.6 \times 10^{-19}}{6.62 \times 10^{-34}} = 5.16 \times 10^{14} \text{ Hz}$$

12. (d) $E = W_0 + K_{max}$; $E = \frac{12375}{3000} = 4.125$ eV

$$\Rightarrow \quad K_{max} = E - W_0 = 4.125 \text{ eV} - 1 \text{ eV} = 3.125 \text{ eV}$$
$$\Rightarrow \quad \frac{1}{2} mv_{max}^2 = 3.125 \times 1.6 \times 10^{-19} \text{ J}$$
$$\Rightarrow \quad v_{max} = \sqrt{\frac{2 \times 3.125 \times 1.6 \times 10^{-19}}{9.1 \times 10^{-31}}} = 1 \times 10^6 \text{ m/s}$$

Hence, the velocity of emitted photoelectrons is 1×10^6 m/s.

13. (d) Both Statement I and Statement II are correct.

Less work function means less energy is required for ejecting out the electrons.

14. (c) We know that, $P = \frac{W}{t} = \frac{nhc}{\lambda t}$

$$\Rightarrow 10^3 = \frac{n \times 6.6 \times 10^{-34} \times 3 \times 10^8}{198.6 \times 7} \Rightarrow n = 10^{30}$$

15. (c) Given, $\lambda_2 = 6000$ Å,

$E_1 = 3.32 \times 10^{-19}$ J,

$\lambda_1 = 4000$ Å

$$\therefore \quad E = \frac{hc}{\lambda} \Rightarrow \frac{E_1}{E_2} = \frac{\lambda_1}{\lambda_2}$$
$$\Rightarrow \quad \frac{3.32 \times 10^{-19}}{E_2} = \frac{4000}{6000}$$
$$\Rightarrow \quad E_2 = 4.98 \times 10^{-19} \text{ J} = 3.1 \text{ eV}$$

16. (b) Statement I is correct but Statement II is incorrect. The energy of red light photon is less than the work function of photographic plate, while the energies of many components of white light such as blue, violet etc., are more than the work function of photographic plate. Infact different photographic plates are used for different regions of spectra.

17. (a) Given, $\lambda = 4400$ Å

$$\therefore \quad p = \frac{h}{\lambda} = \frac{6.6 \times 10^{-34}}{4400 \times 10^{-10}} = 1.5 \times 10^{-27} \text{ kg-m/s}$$

and mass, $m = \frac{p}{c} = \frac{1.5 \times 10^{-27}}{3 \times 10^{8}} = 5 \times 10^{-36}$ kg

18. (c) We know that, energy of photon,

$$E = \frac{hc}{\lambda} \text{ J} = \frac{hc}{e\lambda} \text{ (eV)}$$

$$\Rightarrow E(\text{eV}) = \frac{6.6 \times 10^{-34} \times 3 \times 10^{8}}{1.6 \times 10^{-19} \times \lambda(\text{Å})} = \frac{12375}{\lambda(\text{Å})}$$

$$\Rightarrow E(\text{keV}) = \frac{12.37}{\lambda(\text{Å})} \approx \frac{12.4}{\lambda}$$

19. (d) We know that, $m_0 = m\sqrt{1 - \frac{v^2}{c^2}}$, hence incorrect.

20. (c) We know that,

$$E \propto \frac{1}{\lambda} \Rightarrow \frac{3.5}{E'} = \frac{1}{5000} \Rightarrow E' = 3.5 \times 5000 \text{ eV}$$

Step up Practice 3

1. (d) The wavelength of matter wave is independent of charge.

2. (c) As, $\lambda = \frac{h}{mv}$

where, v = velocity of an electron

and λ = de-Broglie wavelength.

Also, $\lambda \propto 1/\nu$ (de-Broglie frequency)

When v is doubled, λ gets halved and ν (de-Broglie frequency) gets doubled.

3. (d) As, $\lambda = \frac{h}{p}$, so for $\lambda_p = \lambda_\alpha$, we get

$$p_p = p_\alpha$$

4. (d) Both A and R are true and R is the correct explanation of A.

Matter waves are central part of the theory of quantum mechanics, being an example of wave particle duality. All matter can exhibit wave like behaviour.

For example, a beam of electrons can be diffracted just like a beam of light of a water wave. It is an example of diffraction.

5. (a) All the three particles have same wavelength, therefore they will have same momentum say p. Energy of photon $E = pc$. Therefore, energy of photon is maximum.

6. (c) $\lambda = \frac{h}{\sqrt{2qVm}}$ or $\lambda \propto \frac{1}{\sqrt{m}}$

As $m_e < m_p$

$\therefore \quad \lambda_e > \lambda_p$

7. (b) Wavelength, $\lambda = \frac{h}{p} = \frac{h}{\sqrt{2mE}}$

$$\therefore \quad \lambda \propto \frac{1}{\sqrt{E}} \quad (h \text{ and } m \text{ are constants})$$

So, when the KE of an electron is increased, the wavelength of the associated wave will decrease.

8. (a) The de-Broglie wavelength, $\lambda = \frac{1.227}{\sqrt{V}}$ nm

Here, $V = 100$ V

$$\Rightarrow \quad \lambda = \frac{1.227}{\sqrt{100}} \text{ nm} \simeq 0.123 \text{ nm}$$

9. (d) Both A and R are true and R is the correct explanation of A.

$$v_{\text{rms}} = \sqrt{\frac{3RT}{M}}$$

So, $\quad v_{\text{rms}} \propto \sqrt{T}$

Again de-Broglie wavelength, $\lambda = \frac{h}{mv}$

So, $\quad \lambda \propto \frac{1}{\sqrt{T}}$

10. (a) As $\lambda \propto \frac{1}{\sqrt{T}} \Rightarrow \frac{\lambda_1}{\lambda_2} = \sqrt{\frac{T_2}{T_1}}$

Here, $T_2 = 927°\text{C} = (927 + 273) \text{ K} = 1200 \text{ K}$

$T_1 = 27°\text{C} = (27 + 273)\text{K} = 300 \text{ K}$

$\lambda_1 = \lambda$

$$\therefore \quad \frac{\lambda}{\lambda_2} = \sqrt{\frac{1200}{300}} \Rightarrow \lambda_2 = \frac{\lambda}{2}$$

11. (c) As we know that, matter waves are non-mechanical waves and not electromagnetic wave in nature.

12. (a) By using $\lambda_{\text{electron}} = \frac{h}{m_e v} \Rightarrow v = \frac{h}{m_e \lambda_e}$

$$= \frac{6.6 \times 10^{-34}}{9.1 \times 10^{-31} \times 10^{-12}} = 7.25 \times 10^{8} \text{ m/s}$$

13. (a) We know that, wavelength of photon will be greater than that of electron because mass of photon is less than that of electron $\Rightarrow \lambda_{\text{ph}} > \lambda_{\text{el}}$

14. (d) Both A and R are true and R is the correct explanation of A.

de-Broglie wavelength, $\lambda = \frac{h}{mv}$

where, λ and v remaining constant, $\lambda \propto \frac{1}{m}$

So, as the mass of the particle becomes smaller and smaller the de-Broglie wavelength of the particle becomes more and more significant.

15. (c) $\lambda = \frac{h}{\sqrt{2mE}} = \frac{h}{\sqrt{2m}} \cdot \frac{1}{\sqrt{E}}$

Multiplying log on both sides,

$$\log \lambda = \log \frac{h}{\sqrt{2m}} + \log \frac{1}{\sqrt{E}}$$

$$\Rightarrow \quad \log \lambda = \log \frac{h}{\sqrt{2m}} - \frac{1}{2}\log E$$

$$\Rightarrow \quad \log \lambda = -\frac{1}{2}\log E + \log \frac{h}{\sqrt{2m}}$$

This is the equation of straight line having slope (–1/2) and positive intercept on log λ-axis.

16. (d) Both A and R are true and R is the correct explanation of A.

de-Broglie wavelength is given $\lambda = \frac{h}{\sqrt{2meV}}$

So, as accelerating potential V increases, the wavelength decreases.

Resolving power of microscope $= \frac{2\mu \sin\beta}{1.22\lambda}$

So, as wavelength λ decreases, resolving power increases.

Gearing up for NEET

1. (d) As, $\frac{1}{2}mv_{max}^2 = \frac{hc}{\lambda} - \phi_0$

$$v_{max} = \sqrt{\frac{2}{m}\left(\frac{hc}{\lambda} - \phi_0\right)} = v$$

and $$v'_{max} = \sqrt{\frac{2}{m}\left(\frac{hc}{\lambda/4} - \phi_0\right)}$$

$$= 2\sqrt{\frac{2}{m}\left(\frac{hc}{\lambda} - \phi_0\right) + \frac{6}{m}\phi_0}$$

$$> 2v$$

2. (c) Energy of photoelectron, $E = \frac{hc}{\lambda} - \phi_0$

$$\Rightarrow \quad \frac{hc}{\lambda} = E + \phi_0 \quad \text{...(i)}$$

where, ϕ_0 is the work function for the metal surface (constant).

When $E' = 2E$, then

$$2E = \frac{hc}{\lambda'} - \phi_0$$

$$\Rightarrow \quad \frac{hc}{\lambda'} = 2E + \phi_0 \quad \text{...(ii)}$$

Dividing Eq. (i) by Eq. (ii), we get

$$\frac{\lambda'}{\lambda} = \frac{E + \phi_0}{2E + \phi_0}$$

$$\Rightarrow \quad \frac{\lambda'}{\lambda} = \frac{(E + \phi_0)}{2\left(E + \frac{\phi_0}{2}\right)}$$

$$\therefore \quad \frac{\lambda'}{\lambda} > \frac{1}{2} \text{ or } \lambda' > \frac{\lambda}{2}$$

or $$\lambda > \lambda' > \frac{\lambda}{2}$$

3. (a) As, $\lambda = \frac{h}{p}$

and $\lambda = \frac{h}{\sqrt{2mE}}$

$$\Rightarrow \quad \lambda \propto \frac{1}{p} \propto \frac{1}{E}$$

So, when wavelength is decreased, both p and E increase.

4. (c) $E \text{ (in eV)} = \frac{12375}{\lambda \text{ (in Å)}} = \frac{12375}{7000} = 1.76 \text{ eV}$

5. (a) As, $p = \frac{h\nu}{c}$

$$\therefore \quad \nu = \frac{pc}{h} = \frac{(6.6 \times 10^{-29})(3 \times 10^{8})}{(6.6 \times 10^{-34})}$$

$$= 3 \times 10^{13} \text{ Hz}$$

6. (b) Given, $E = 100 \text{ eV} = (100 \times 1.6 \times 10^{-19}) \text{ J}$

and $h = 6.62 \times 10^{-34}$ Js

$$E = h\nu$$

or $$\nu = \frac{E}{h} = \frac{100 \times 1.6 \times 10^{-19}}{6.62 \times 10^{-34}}$$

$$= 0.2417 \times 10^{17} = 2.417 \times 10^{16} \text{ Hz}$$

7. (c) According to Einstein's photoelectric equation,

$$KE_{max} = h\nu - \phi_0$$

Comparing with the equation of straight line

$$y = mx + c$$

We get, slope of graph between KE and $\nu = h$ (i.e. same for all metals)

8. (b) Work function, $W_0 = h\nu_0$

For sodium, $W_{01} = h\nu_{01} = \frac{hc}{\lambda_{01}} \Rightarrow \frac{2.3 \text{ eV}}{h} = \nu_{01} = \frac{c}{\lambda_{01}}$

For copper, $W_{02} = h\nu_{02}$

$$\Rightarrow \quad \frac{4.5 \text{ eV}}{h} = \nu_{02} = \frac{c}{\lambda_{02}}$$

$$\therefore \quad \frac{\lambda_{01}}{\lambda_{02}} = \frac{ch}{2.3} \times \frac{4.5}{ch} \simeq \frac{2}{1} \Rightarrow \lambda_{01} : \lambda_{02} = 2:1$$

9. (b) Given in the question,

Energy of photon, $E = 1 \text{ MeV} = 10^6$ eV

$$\therefore \quad hc = 1243 \text{ eV-nm}$$

Now, $E = \frac{hc}{\lambda}$

$\Rightarrow \quad \lambda = \frac{hc}{E} = \frac{1243 \text{ eV-nm}}{10^6 \text{ eV}}$

$= 1.2 \times 10^{-3}$ nm

10. (b) $E = \frac{12375}{\lambda \text{ (in Å)}} = \frac{12375}{4360} = 2.84$ eV

$\therefore \quad K_{max} = E - W = 1.60$ eV

Thus, the retarding potential is 1.60 V.

11. (c) $E_1 = \frac{12375}{3500}$ eV $= 3.54$ eV

and $E_2 = \frac{12375}{5400}$ eV $= 2.29$ eV

Now, $\frac{2}{1} = \frac{3.54 - W}{2.29 - W}$

Solving this equation, we get $W = 1.05$ eV.

12. (b) By using $E = W_0 + \frac{1}{2} m v_{max}^2$; where

$E = \frac{12375}{4558} = 2.71$ eV

$\Rightarrow \quad 2.71 \text{ eV} = 2.5 \text{ eV} + \frac{1}{2} \times 9.1 \times 10^{-31} \times v_{max}^2$

$\Rightarrow \quad 0.21 \times 1.6 \times 10^{-19} = \frac{1}{2} \times 9.1 \times 10^{-31} \times v_{max}^2$

$\Rightarrow \quad v_{max} = 2.65 \times 10^5$ m/s

Hence, speed of the ejected electrons is 2.65×10^5 m/s.

13. (d) When a beam of electrons of energy E_0 is incident on a metal surface kept in an evacuated chamber, electrons can be emitted with maximum energy E_0 (due to elastic collision) and with any energy less than E_0, when a part of incident energy of electron is used in liberating the electrons from the surface of metal.

14. (c) From the given graph, we get

$V_0 = -3.2$ V

As, $eV_0 = h\nu - \phi_0$

$\Rightarrow \quad \nu = \frac{eV_0 + \phi_0}{h}$

$= \frac{-3.2 \times 1.6 \times 10^{-19} + 4 \times 1.6 \times 10^{-19}}{6.6 \times 10^{-34}}$

$= 1.939 \times 10^{14}$ s^{-1}

15. (b) As, $E = \frac{hc}{\lambda} - \phi_0$ ...(i)

$4E = \frac{hc}{\lambda / 3} - \phi_0$ ...(ii)

Solving these equations, we get

$\phi_0 = \frac{hc}{3\lambda}$

16. (c) Work function, $\phi_0 = \frac{hc}{\lambda_0}$

$\therefore \quad \frac{(\phi_0)_T}{(\phi_0)_{Na}} = \frac{\lambda_{Na}}{\lambda_T}$

or $\lambda_T = \frac{\lambda_{Na} \times (\phi_0)_{Na}}{(\phi_0)_T} = \frac{5600 \times 2.3}{4.5} = 2862$ Å

17. (b) Stopping potential, $V_0 = \frac{h}{e}(\nu - \nu_0)$

or $(\nu - \nu_0) = \frac{V_0 \times e}{h} = \frac{4.144 \times 1.6 \times 10^{-19}}{6.63 \times 10^{-34}}$

$\Rightarrow \quad \nu - 1 \times 10^{15} = 10^{15}$

Frequency $= 10^{15} + 1 \times 10^{15} = 2 \times 10^{15}$ Hz

18. (b) Given, $v_{max} = 4 \times 10^8$ cm/s $= 4 \times 10^6$ m/s

$\therefore \quad K_{max} = \frac{1}{2} m v_{max}^2 = \frac{1}{2} \times 9 \times 10^{-31} \times (4 \times 10^6)^2$

$= 7.2 \times 10^{-18}$ J $= 45$ eV

Hence, stopping potential,

$V_0 = \frac{K_{max}}{e} = \frac{45 \text{ eV}}{e} = 45$ V

19. (a) According to Einstein's equation,

$h\nu = \phi_0 + K_{max}$

where, ϕ_0 is the work function.

$\Rightarrow \quad h\nu = \phi_0 + eV_0 \Rightarrow V_0 = \frac{h\nu}{e} - \frac{\phi_0}{e}$

Comparing with equation, $y = mx + c$

$\phi_0 = -(\text{intercept}) \times e = OB \times e$ in eV

20. (a) Here, $\lambda_1 = \frac{12375}{E_1 \text{ (eV)}}$ Å $= 1000$ Å

$\therefore \quad E_1 = 12.375$ eV

Similarly, $E_2(\text{eV}) = \frac{12375}{\lambda_2(\text{Å})}$ eV $= \frac{12375}{2000} = 6.1875$ eV

Now, $E_1 - W_0 = eV_1$

and $E_2 - W_0 = eV_2$

Hence, $12.375 - W_0 = 7.7\,eV$

and $6.1875 - W_0 = eV_2$

Solving, we get $V_2 = 1.5$ V

21. (b) According to the question,

$eV = hc\left(\frac{1}{\lambda} - \frac{1}{\lambda_0}\right)$ ...(i)

and $\frac{eV}{3} = hc\left(\frac{1}{2\lambda} - \frac{1}{\lambda_0}\right)$ ...(ii)

Dividing Eq. (i) by Eq. (ii), we get

$$3 = \frac{\left(\frac{1}{\lambda} - \frac{1}{\lambda_0}\right)}{\left(\frac{1}{2\lambda} - \frac{1}{\lambda_0}\right)}$$

or $3\left(\frac{1}{2\lambda}-\frac{1}{\lambda_0}\right)=\frac{1}{\lambda}-\frac{1}{\lambda_0}$

or $\frac{3}{2\lambda}-\frac{1}{\lambda}=\frac{3}{\lambda_0}-\frac{1}{\lambda_0}$

or $\frac{1}{2\lambda}=\frac{2}{\lambda_0}$

Threshold wavelength for metallic surface, $\lambda_0 = 4\lambda$

22. (a) Energy radiated as visible light $=\frac{5}{100}\times 100 = 5$ J/s

Let n be the number of photons emitted per second, then

$$nh\nu = E = 5$$

$$\therefore \quad n = \frac{5\lambda}{hc} = \frac{5\times 5.6\times 10^{-7}}{(6.62\times 10^{-34})(3\times 10^{8})}$$

$$\approx 1.4\times 10^{19}$$

23. (c) Intensity, $I = 10^{-10}$ Wbm^{-2} $= 10^{-10}$ Js^{-1} m^{-2}.

Let the number of photons required be n, then

$$I = \frac{nh\nu}{A} = \frac{nh\nu}{10^{-4}} = 10^{-10}$$

Hence, $$n = \frac{10^{-10}\times 10^{-4}}{h\nu} = 10^{-14}\frac{\lambda}{hc}$$

$$= \frac{10^{-14}\times 660\times 10^{-9}}{6.6\times 10^{-34}\times 3\times 10^{8}} = 3.3\times 10^{4}$$

24. (b) As, $E - W_0 = \frac{1}{2}mv^2$

First case, $2W_0 - W_0 = \frac{1}{2}mv_1^2$ ...(i)

Second case, $5W_0 - W_0 = \frac{1}{2}mv_2^2$ ...(ii)

On dividing Eq. (i) by Eq. (ii), we get

$$\frac{2W_0 - W_0}{5W_0 - W_0} = \frac{v_1^2}{v_2^2} \text{ or } \frac{v_1}{v_2} = \frac{1}{2}$$

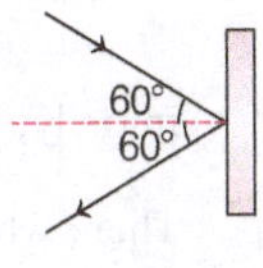

25. (b) Energy corresponding to 2000 Å,

$$E = \frac{12375}{\lambda(\text{in Å})} = \frac{12375}{2000}\text{ eV} = 6.2\text{ eV}$$

Maximum kinetic energy,

$$K = h\nu - h\nu_0$$
$$K = E - W$$
$$= (6.2 - 5.01)\text{ eV} = 1.19\text{ eV}$$

Now, $$K = \frac{1}{2}mv_{max}^2$$

$$\Rightarrow \frac{1}{2}\times 9.1\times 10^{-31}\times v_{max}^2 = 1.19\times 1.6\times 10^{-19}$$

or $$v_{max}^2 = \frac{1.19\times 1.6\times 10^{-19}\times 2}{9.1\times 10^{-31}}$$

or $$v_{max}^2 = 0.418\times 10^{12} = 41.8\times 10^{10}$$

or $$v_{max} = 6.46\times 10^{5}\text{ m/s}$$

26. (b) From equation,

$$eV_0 = hc\left(\frac{1}{\lambda}-\frac{1}{\lambda_0}\right)$$

$$4.8 = \frac{hc}{e}\left(\frac{1}{\lambda}-\frac{1}{\lambda_0}\right) \quad \text{...(i)}$$

and $$1.6 = \frac{hc}{e}\left(\frac{1}{2\lambda}-\frac{1}{\lambda_0}\right) \quad \text{...(ii)}$$

On dividing Eq. (i) by Eq. (ii), we get

$$\frac{\left(\frac{1}{\lambda}-\frac{1}{\lambda_0}\right)}{\left(\frac{1}{2\lambda}-\frac{1}{\lambda_0}\right)} = \frac{4.8}{1.6} \Rightarrow \lambda_0 = 4\lambda$$

27. (a) Consider a spherical chamber of radius 20 cm. Bulb is placed at point S as shown in figure.

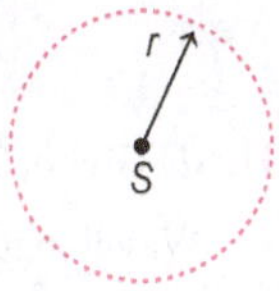

Intensity of light at surface,

$$I = \frac{0.6P}{4\pi r^2}$$

Force exerted on the surface, $F = \frac{P}{c}$

where, P is power of bulb.

$$\therefore \quad F = \frac{1100}{3\times 10^{8}} = 3.6\times 10^{-6}\text{ N}$$

Pressure exerted by light

$$= \frac{I}{c} = \frac{0.6P}{4\pi r^2 c}$$

$$= \frac{0.6\times 1100}{4\pi(0.2)^2\times 3\times 10^{8}}$$

$$= 4.4\times 10^{-6}\text{ N/m}^2$$

28. (c) Force totally reflecting surface,

$$F = \frac{2P\cos 60°}{c}$$

$$= \frac{2\times\frac{nhc}{\lambda}\cos 60°}{c} = \frac{10^{19}\times 6.6\times 10^{-34}}{663\times 10^{-9}}$$

$$= 10^{-8}\text{ N}$$

29. (c) Let W be the work function of metal, then

$$eV_0 = \frac{hc}{330\times 10^{-9}} - W \quad \text{...(i)}$$

$$e(2V_0) = \frac{hc}{220\times 10^{-9}} - W \quad \text{...(ii)}$$

Solving these two equations, we get

$$V_0 = \frac{10^{9}\times h\times c}{110\times e\times 6}$$

$$= \frac{10^{9}\times 6.6\times 10^{-34}\times 3\times 10^{8}}{110\times 1.6\times 10^{-19}\times 6} = \frac{15}{8}\text{ V}$$

30. (b) When charged particle is moving on a circular path in a uniform magnetic field B, then

$$\frac{mv^2}{r} = qvB \Rightarrow \frac{mv}{r} = qB \Rightarrow v = \frac{qBr}{m}$$

Thus, kinetic energy $= \frac{1}{2}mv^2 = \frac{1}{2}m \times \left(\frac{qBr}{m}\right)^2$

$$= \frac{1}{2m}(qBr)^2$$

Now for photoelectric effect, Einstein's equation is

$$hv = W + (\text{KE})$$

where, W = work function

$$\Rightarrow \quad hv - \text{KE} = W \Rightarrow W = hv - \frac{(qBr)^2}{2m}$$

Here, charged particle is a photoelectron denoted by e

$$\therefore \quad W = hv - \frac{(eBr)^2}{2m_e}$$

31. (b) Given, $2\text{ eV} \le \phi \le 5\text{ eV}$

Wavelength corresponding to minimum and maximum values of work function are

$$\lambda_{max} = \frac{hc}{E} = \frac{4 \times 10^{-15} \times 3 \times 10^8}{2}$$

$$= 6 \times 10^{-7}\text{m} = 600\text{ nm}$$

and $$\lambda_{min} = \frac{hc}{E} = \frac{4 \times 10^{-15} \times 3 \times 10^8}{5}$$

$$= 2.4 \times 10^{-7}\text{m} = 240\text{ nm}$$

Clearly, wavelength range would be

$$240\text{ nm} \le \lambda \le 600\text{ nm}$$

Thus, wavelength 650 nm is not suitable for photoelectric effect.

32. (b) From Einstein's photoelectric equation,

$$(\text{KE})_{max} = hv - \phi_0$$

For first condition, $0.5 = E - \phi_0$ ...(i)

For second condition,

$$0.8 = \left(E + \frac{E \times 20}{100}\right) - \phi_0$$

$$\Rightarrow \quad 0.8 = 1.2E - \phi_0 \quad \text{...(ii)}$$

From Eqs. (i) and (ii), we get

$$0.3 = 0.2\,E$$

$$\Rightarrow \quad E = \frac{3}{2} = 1.5\text{ eV}$$

From Eq. (i), $\phi_0 = E - 0.5 = 1.5 - 0.5 = 1\text{ eV}$

33. (a) According to Einstein's photoelectric equation,

$$K_A = \frac{hc}{\lambda_A} - \phi \Rightarrow K_A + \phi = \frac{hc}{\lambda_A}$$

and $$K_B = \frac{hc}{\lambda_B} - \phi = \frac{hc}{(\lambda_A/2)} - \phi$$

or $$K_B = \frac{2hc}{\lambda_A} - \phi = 2(K_A + \phi) - \phi = 2K_A + \phi$$

$$\Rightarrow \quad K_A < \frac{K_B}{2}$$

34. (c) From photoelectric equation, $E_K = E - W$

where, E_K is kinetic energy of emitted photoelectrons, W is the work function and E is the energy supplied.

$$E = hv = \frac{hc}{\lambda}$$

where, h is Planck's constant, c is the speed of light and λ is the wavelength.

$$\therefore \quad E = \frac{6.6 \times 10^{-34} \times 3 \times 10^8}{5000 \times 10^{-10}}$$

$$= 3.96 \times 10^{-19}\text{ J}$$

Also, $1\text{ eV} = 1.6 \times 10^{-19}\text{ J}$

$$\therefore \quad E = \frac{3.96 \times 10^{-19}}{1.6 \times 10^{-19}} = 2.48\text{ eV}$$

Hence, $E_K = 2.48 - 1.90 = 0.58\text{ eV}$

35. (a) We know that, $K_{max} = eV_0$

where, e is the charge in the electron. Since, at the stopping potential, the photoelectric current cannot be obtained by increasing the intensity of the incident light. Thus, stopping potential or maximum kinetic energy of the photoelectrons, does not depend upon the intensity of the incident light. If the intensity of light be doubled, then the number of photoelectrons emitted per second is doubled.

So, n is doubled but K_{max} remains same.

36. (a) According to Einstein's photoelectric equation,

$$K_{max} = hv - hv_0$$

Initially, $\frac{1}{2}mv_0^2 = h(2v_0) - (v_0) = hv_0$ ...(i)

Then, when, $v = 5v_0$

$$\frac{1}{2}mv^2 = 5hv_0 - hv_0 = 4hv_0$$

$$\Rightarrow \quad \frac{1}{2}mv^2 = 4(1/2\, mv_0^2) \quad \text{[from Eq. (i)]}$$

$$\Rightarrow \quad v^2 = 4v_0^2 \text{ or } v = \sqrt{2}\,v_0$$

37. (b) As, $\lambda = \frac{h}{\sqrt{2mK}} \Rightarrow \lambda \propto \frac{1}{\sqrt{m}}$

Since, mass of α-particle is largest as compare to all the particles given. So, λ is shortest for α-particle.

38. (a) As, $\lambda = \frac{h}{\sqrt{2mE}} = \frac{h}{\sqrt{2qVm}}$

So, $\lambda \propto \frac{1}{\sqrt{m}} \quad \therefore \quad \frac{\lambda_e}{\lambda_p} = \left(\frac{m_p}{m_e}\right)^{1/2}$

39. (a) As, $\lambda = \frac{h}{p} = \frac{h}{mv}$

So, $\frac{h}{m_1 v_1} = \frac{h}{m_2 v_2}$

$\therefore \quad \frac{v_1}{v_2} = \frac{m_2}{m_1} = \frac{4}{1} \quad (\because m_\alpha = 4m_p)$

40. (d) As, $\lambda = \frac{h}{\sqrt{2mE}} = \frac{6.6 \times 10^{-34}}{\sqrt{2 \times 9.1 \times 10^{-31} \times 80 \times 1.6 \times 10^{-19}}}$

$= 1.4$ Å

41. (a) de-Broglie wavelength,

$$\lambda = \frac{h}{\sqrt{2mkT}} = \frac{6.62 \times 10^{-34}}{\sqrt{2 \times 1.67 \times 10^{-27} \times 1.38 \times 10^{-23} T}}$$

$$= \frac{6.62 \times 10^{-34}}{2.15 \times 10^{-25} \sqrt{T}} \text{ m}$$

$$= \frac{3.079}{\sqrt{T}} \times 10^{-9} \text{ m} = \frac{30.79}{\sqrt{T}} \text{ Å}$$

$$\approx \frac{30.8}{\sqrt{T}} \text{ Å}$$

42. (d) Mass of an electron, $m = 9.11 \times 10^{-31}$ kg

$T = 27 + 273 = 300$ K

de-Broglie wavelength of electron, $\lambda = \frac{h}{\sqrt{3mkT}}$

$$= \frac{6.6 \times 10^{-34}}{\sqrt{3 \times 9.11 \times 10^{-31} \times 1.38 \times 10^{-23} \times 300}} \text{ m}$$

$= 6.2 \times 10^{-9}$ m

43. (b) de-Broglie wavelength, $\lambda = \frac{h}{mv}$

For electron, $\lambda_e = \frac{h}{m_e v}$ ...(i)

For proton, $\lambda_p = \frac{h}{m_p v}$ ...(ii)

On dividing Eq. (i) by Eq. (ii), we get

$$\frac{\lambda_e}{\lambda_p} = \frac{\frac{h}{m_e v}}{\frac{h}{m_p v}}$$

$\Rightarrow \quad \frac{\lambda_e}{\lambda_p} = \frac{m_p}{m_e}$

$\Rightarrow \quad \frac{\lambda_e}{\lambda_p} = \frac{1.67 \times 10^{-27}}{9.1 \times 10^{-31}}$

$= 0.183516 \times 10^4 \simeq 1836$

44. (c) $\frac{E_1}{E_2} = \frac{1}{2}$ (given)

We know that, $\lambda = \frac{h}{\sqrt{2mK}} \Rightarrow \lambda \propto \frac{1}{\sqrt{K}}$

$\Rightarrow \quad \frac{\lambda_1}{\lambda_2} = \frac{\sqrt{K_2}}{\sqrt{K_1}} \Rightarrow \frac{\lambda_1^2}{\lambda_2^2} = \frac{K_2}{K_1}$

$\Rightarrow \quad \frac{\lambda_1^2}{\lambda_2^2} = \frac{2}{1} \Rightarrow \lambda_1 : \lambda_2 = \sqrt{2} : 1$

45. (c) By law of conservation of momentum,

$$0 = m_1 v_1 + m_2 v_2$$
$$m_1 v_1 = - m_2 v_2$$

Negative sign indicates that both the particles are moving in opposite directions. Now, de-Broglie wavelengths,

$$\lambda_1 = \frac{h}{m_1 v_1} \text{ and } \lambda_2 = \frac{h}{m_2 v_2}$$

$\therefore \quad \frac{\lambda_1}{\lambda_2} = \frac{m_2 v_2}{m_1 v_1} = 1 : 1$

46. (a) Mass of electron in motion is

$$m = \frac{m_0}{\sqrt{1 - \frac{v^2}{c^2}}} = \frac{m_0}{\sqrt{1 - \frac{(0.5c)^2}{c^2}}} = \frac{m_0}{\sqrt{0.75}}$$

$\therefore \quad \lambda = \frac{h}{mv} = \frac{6.6 \times 10^{-34} \times \sqrt{0.75}}{m_0 v}$

$$= \frac{6.6 \times 10^{-34} \times \sqrt{0.75}}{9.1 \times 10^{-31} \times 1.5 \times 10^8} = 4.2 \times 10^{-12} \text{ m}$$

47. (d) As, $\lambda = \frac{h}{\sqrt{2qVm}}$ or $\lambda \propto \frac{1}{\sqrt{qVm}}$

$\therefore \quad \frac{\lambda_\alpha}{\lambda_p} = \frac{\sqrt{q_p V_p m_p}}{\sqrt{q_\alpha V_\alpha m_\alpha}} = \sqrt{\frac{1 \times 100 \times 1}{2 \times 800 \times 4}} = \frac{1}{8}$

$\therefore \quad \lambda_\alpha = \frac{\lambda_p}{8} = \frac{\lambda_0}{8}$

48. (b) de-Broglie wavelength,

$$\lambda = \frac{h}{\sqrt{2mE_e}} = \frac{hc}{E_p}$$

or $\quad 2mE_e = \frac{E_p^2}{c^2}$ ...(i)

But $\quad E_e = \frac{1}{2} mv^2$ or $m = \frac{2E_e}{v^2}$

From Eq. (i), we get

$$2\left[\frac{2E_e}{v^2}\right] E_e = \frac{E_p^2}{c^2} \text{ or } \frac{4E_e^2}{v^2} = \frac{E_p^2}{c^2}$$

or $\quad \frac{E_e^2}{E_p^2} = \frac{v^2}{4c^2}$ or $\frac{E_e}{E_p} = \frac{v}{2c}$

49. (b) As, $\lambda = \frac{h}{\sqrt{2mE}} \Rightarrow \lambda \propto \frac{1}{\sqrt{m}}$

$\because \quad \frac{\lambda_1}{\lambda_2} = \sqrt{\frac{m_2}{m_1}}$

So, $\frac{\lambda}{\lambda_2} = \sqrt{\frac{M}{m}}$

$\therefore \quad \lambda_2 = \lambda\sqrt{\left(\frac{m}{M}\right)}$

50. (*d*) Velocity of a body falling from a height H is given by

$$v = \sqrt{2gH}$$

We know that, de-Broglie wavelength,

$$\lambda = \frac{h}{mv} = \frac{h}{m\sqrt{2gH}} = \frac{h}{m\sqrt{2g}\sqrt{H}}$$

Here, $\frac{h}{m\sqrt{2g}}$ is a constant (say K).

So, $\lambda = K\frac{1}{\sqrt{H}} \Rightarrow \lambda \propto \frac{1}{\sqrt{H}}$

$\Rightarrow \quad \lambda \propto H^{-1/2}$

51. (*c*) de-Broglie wavelength, $\lambda = \frac{h}{p}$

$\Rightarrow \quad \lambda - \frac{0.5\lambda}{100} = \frac{h}{p + \Delta p}$

$\Rightarrow \quad \frac{199\lambda}{200} = \frac{h}{p + \Delta p} = \frac{199h}{200p}$

$\Rightarrow \quad p + \Delta p = \frac{200}{199}p \Rightarrow p = 199\,\Delta p$

52. (*b*) We know that, the relation between λ and K is given by

$$\lambda = \frac{h}{\sqrt{2mK}}$$

Here, for the given value of energy K, $\frac{h}{\sqrt{2K}}$ is a constant.

Thus, $\lambda \propto \frac{1}{\sqrt{m}}$

$\therefore \quad \lambda_p : \lambda_n : \lambda_e : \lambda_\alpha$

$$= \frac{1}{\sqrt{m_p}} : \frac{1}{\sqrt{m_n}} : \frac{1}{\sqrt{m_e}} : \frac{1}{\sqrt{m_\alpha}}$$

Since, $m_p = m_n$, hence $\lambda_p = \lambda_n$

As, $m_\alpha > m_p$, therefore $\lambda_\alpha < \lambda_p$

As, $m_e < m_n$, therefore $\lambda_e > \lambda_n$

Hence, $\lambda_\alpha < \lambda_p = \lambda_n < \lambda_e$

53. (*c*) Initial de-Broglie wavelength of electron, $\lambda_0 = \frac{h}{mv_0}$

Force on electron in electric field, $\mathbf{F} = -e\mathbf{E} = -eE_0\hat{\mathbf{j}}$

Acceleration of electron, $\mathbf{a} = \frac{\mathbf{F}}{m} = -\frac{eE_0\hat{\mathbf{j}}}{m}$

It is acting along negative Y-axis.

The initial velocity of electron along X-axis, $\mathbf{v}_{x_0} = v_0\hat{\mathbf{i}}$.

Initial velocity of electron along Y-axis, $\mathbf{v}_{y_0} = 0$.

Velocity of electron after time t along X-axis, $\mathbf{v}_x = v_0\hat{\mathbf{i}}$

Velocity of electron after time t along Y-axis,

$$\mathbf{v}_y = 0 + \left(-\frac{eE_0}{m}\hat{\mathbf{j}}\right)t = -\frac{eE_0}{m}t\hat{\mathbf{j}}$$

Magnitude of velocity of electron after time t,

$$\mathbf{v} = \sqrt{v_x^2 + v_y^2} = \sqrt{v_0^2 + \left(\frac{-eE_0}{m}t\right)^2}$$

$$= v_0\sqrt{1 + \frac{e^2E_0^2t^2}{m^2v_0^2}}$$

de-Broglie wavelength, $\lambda' = \frac{h}{mv}$

$$= \frac{h}{mv_0\sqrt{1 + e^2E_0^2t^2/(m^2v_0^2)}}$$

$$= \frac{\lambda_0}{\sqrt{1 + e^2E_0^2t^2/m^2v_0^2}}$$

54. (*d*) We know that, $K_{max} = E - W$

$\therefore \quad T_A = 4.25 - W_A$ ...(i)

$T_B = (T_A - 1.50) = 4.70 - W_B$ ...(ii)

From these two equations, we have

$W_B - W_A = 1.95$ eV ...(iii)

de-Broglie wavelength is given by

$$\lambda = \frac{h}{\sqrt{2Km}}$$

or $\quad \lambda \propto \frac{1}{\sqrt{K}}$

$\therefore \quad \frac{\lambda_B}{\lambda_A} = \sqrt{\frac{K_A}{K_B}} \Rightarrow 2 = \sqrt{\frac{T_A}{T_A - 1.5}}$

$\Rightarrow \quad T_A = 2$ eV, $W_A = 2.25$ eV, $W_B = 4.20$ eV

and $\quad T_B = 0.5$ eV

55. (*d*) The de-Broglie wavelength of an electron,

$$\lambda = \frac{h}{mv} \Rightarrow v = \frac{h}{m\lambda} \quad \text{...(i)}$$

Energy of photon,

$E_p = \frac{hc}{\lambda}$ (since, λ is same for electron and photon) ... (ii)

Kinetic energy of photon to kinetic energy of electron

$$= \frac{E_p}{E_e} = \frac{\frac{hc}{\lambda}}{\left(\frac{1}{2}\right)mv^2} = \frac{2hc}{\lambda mv^2}$$

Substituting the value of v from Eq. (i), we get

$$\frac{E_p}{E_e} = \frac{2hc}{\lambda m\left(\frac{h}{m\lambda}\right)^2} = \frac{2\lambda mc}{h}$$

56. (c) de-Broglie wavelength, $\lambda = \frac{h}{\sqrt{2mK}}$

The kinetic energy of the electron,

$$K_{electron} = \frac{h^2}{2m \cdot \lambda^2} \quad ...(i)$$

where, h = Planck's constant, λ = wavelength

The photon energy, $E_{photon} = \frac{ch}{\lambda} \quad ...(ii)$

On dividing Eq. (ii) by Eq. (i), we get

$$\frac{E_{photon}}{K_{electron}} = \frac{ch/\lambda}{h^2/2m \cdot \lambda^2} = \frac{hc \cdot \lambda^2 2m}{h^2 \cdot \lambda} = \frac{2m\lambda c}{h}$$

$$= \frac{2(mc^2)}{hc/\lambda} = \frac{2 \times (5 \times 10^5)}{50 \times 10^3} = 20$$

$F_{photon} : K_{electron} = 20:1$

Assertion and Reason

1. (a) The electromagnetic theory of light failed to explain photoelectric effect. It cannot be explained by assuming wave nature of radiation. If wave nature of radiation is assumed, then it will take quite a long time (about one year) for electron to come out of the metal surface which contradicts the experimental observations. Thus, photoelectric effect can only be explained by assuming particle nature of light.
2. (d) There is a very small time lag between the instants, the photon of light falls on the metal surface and emission of photoelectrons from the metal surface. Thus, photoelectric effect is an instantaneous process.
3. (c) Decreasing the λ of incident photon means energy of incident light is increased, so E_k increases and hence stopping potential increases.
4. (d) Both A and R are true and R is the correct explanation of A.
5. (c) The maximum kinetic energy of emitted photoelectrons depends on the radiation source and nature of material of plate but is independent of the intensity.

   So, it will remain unchanged.

Statement Type Questions

1. (c) Statement I is incorrect as photoemission in a gas sample occurs only when incident photon has energy greater than ionisation energy of electron of gas atom. Statement II is correct.
2. (c) Statement I is incorrect as work function is energy, required for emission of an electron.

   Work function is more for an electron deep inside metal surface, whereas it is least for a surface electron. Also, work function increases with number of electrons emitted Statement II is correct.
3. (d) Both Statement I and Statement II are correct.

   When a light of single frequency falls on the electron of inner layer of metal, then this electron comes out of the metal surface after a large number of collisions with atom of its upper layer.
4. (a) Both Statement I and Statement II are incorrect.

$$\lambda = \frac{h}{\sqrt{2mK}},$$

i.e. $\lambda \propto \frac{1}{\sqrt{K}}$

$$\therefore \quad \frac{\lambda'}{\lambda} = \sqrt{\frac{K}{K'}} = \sqrt{\frac{K}{4K}} = \frac{1}{2}$$

$$\Rightarrow \quad \lambda' = \frac{\lambda}{2}$$

5. (d) Both Statement I and Statement II are correct.

   Momentum of a photons is given by $p = h\nu / c$

   Also, the photon is a form of energy, photon behaves as a particle having energy $E = \frac{hc}{\lambda}$, so $p = \frac{E}{c}$.

Match the Columns

1. (d) $KE_{max} = eV_0$

A. $V_0 = 1.5$ V

$KE_{max} = 1.6 \times 10^{-19} \times 1.5$

$= 2.4 \times 10^{-19}$ J

B. $V_0 = 2.4$ V

$KE_{max} = 1.6 \times 10^{-19} \times 2.4$

$= 3.8 \times 10^{-19}$ J

C. $V_0 = 0.5$ V

$KE_{max} = eV_0$

$= 1.6 \times 10^{-19} \times 0.5$

$= 0.8 \times 10^{-19}$ J

D. $V_0 = 1.8$ V

$KE_{max} = 1.6 \times 10^{-19} \times 1.8$

$= 2.9 \times 10^{-19}$ J

Hence, A-(II), B-(III), C-(I), D-(IV).

2. (a) A. Momentum of photon,

$$p = \frac{h}{\lambda} = \frac{6.6 \times 10^{-34}}{660 \times 10^{-9}}$$

$$= 1.00 \times 10^{-27} \text{ kg-m/s}$$

B. Power of the source, $P = \frac{nhc}{\lambda}$

$$n = \frac{P\lambda}{hc} = \frac{66 \times 660 \times 10^{-9}}{6.6 \times 10^{-34} \times 3 \times 10^8}$$

$$= 2.2 \times 10^{20}$$

C. Efficiency $= \frac{\text{Output power}}{\text{Input power}}$

$\Rightarrow \quad \frac{20}{100} = \frac{P}{1}$

$\Rightarrow \quad P = \frac{1}{5}$ W

$\therefore$ No. of photons emitted,

$$n = \frac{P\lambda}{hc} = \frac{1}{5} \times \frac{660 \times 10^{-9}}{6.6 \times 10^{-34} \times 3 \times 10^{8}}$$

$$= 6.67 \times 10^{17}$$

D. Rate at which photons strike the surface,

$$n = \frac{p\lambda}{hc} = \frac{IA\lambda}{hc} = \frac{100 \times 10^{-3} \times 2 \times 10^{-4} \times 660 \times 10^{-9}}{6.6 \times 10^{-34} \times 3 \times 10^{8}}$$

$$= 6.7 \times 10^{13} \text{ per second}$$

Hence, A-(IV), B-(I), C-(II), D-III.

3. (*b*) Using relation, $E = \frac{p^2}{2m}$ ...(i)

(A) From Eq. (i), we get

$$p = \sqrt{2mE}$$

$$= \sqrt{2 \times 9.1 \times 10^{-31} \times 100 \times 1.6 \times 10^{-19}}$$

$$= 5.4 \times 10^{-24} \text{ kg-ms}^{-1}$$

(B) Speed, $v = \frac{p}{m} = \frac{5.4 \times 10^{-24}}{9.1 \times 10^{-31}} = 5.9 \times 10^{6}$ ms^{-1}

(C) de-Broglie wavelength is given by

$$\lambda = \frac{h}{p} = \frac{6.62 \times 10^{-34}}{5.4 \times 10^{-24}}$$

$$= 1.22 \times 10^{-10} \text{ m}$$

(D) Frequency, $\nu = \frac{c}{\lambda} = \frac{3.0 \times 10^{8}}{1.22 \times 10^{-10}}$

$$= 2.46 \times 10^{18} \text{s}^{-1}$$

Hence, A-(III), B-(II), C-(I), D-(IV).

Final Check Through PYQs

1. (*d*) For photoelectric emission, energy of incident electromagnetic radiation must be greater than or equal to work function of photosensitive surface. Thus, only Cs can emit photoelectron.

2. (*c*) Initially, frequency of light,

$$\nu = 1.5\nu_0$$

But when the frequency of incident light is halved, then $\nu' = \frac{\nu}{2} = 0.75\nu_0$. Thus, it becomes less than the threshold frequency. In that case, no photoelectric effect takes place.

Hence, photoelectric current becomes zero.

3. (*b*) Photon is quanta of energy. It is a massless and chargeless particle. The rest mass of photon is zero. In free space, it moves with velocity *c* and energy of photon is equal to $h\nu$. The momentum of the photon is given as $p = \frac{E}{c} = \frac{h\nu}{c}$.

4. (*c*) Using Einstein's photoelectric equation,

$$eV' = h\nu' - h\nu_0$$

When $\nu' = \nu$

and $V' = \frac{V_s}{2}$, then

$$\frac{eV_s}{2} = h\nu - h\nu_0 \quad \text{...(i)}$$

Again, when $\nu' = \frac{\nu}{2}$ and $V' = V_s$, then

$$\therefore \quad eV_s = \frac{h\nu}{2} - h\nu_0 \quad \text{...(ii)}$$

Dividing Eq. (i) by Eq. (ii), we get

$$\frac{eV_s/2}{eV_s} = \frac{h\nu - h\nu_0}{\frac{h\nu}{2} - h\nu_0}$$

$$\Rightarrow \quad \frac{1}{2} = \frac{(\nu - \nu_0)}{\frac{\nu}{2} - \nu_0}$$

$$\Rightarrow \quad \frac{\nu}{2} - \nu_0 = 2\nu - 2\nu_0$$

$$\Rightarrow \quad \nu_0 = \frac{3}{2}\nu$$

5. (*c*) Given, the monochromatic light of the wavelength,

$$\lambda = 600 \text{ nm}$$

The power of the source,

$$P = 3.3 \times 10^{-3} \text{ W}$$

We know that, $P = \frac{nhc}{\lambda}$

Substituting the values in the above equation, we get

$$3.3 \times 10^{-3} = \frac{n \times 6.6 \times 10^{-34} \times 3 \times 10^{8}}{600 \times 10^{-9}}$$

$$\Rightarrow \quad n = 10^{16}$$

6. (*d*) The work function of material is given by

$$\phi = h\nu$$

$$\Rightarrow \quad \phi = \frac{hc}{\lambda} \quad \text{...(i)} \left[\because \nu = \frac{c}{\lambda}\right]$$

where, h = Planck's constant

$= 6.63 \times 10^{-34}$ J-s

c = speed of light

$= 3 \times 10^{8}$ ms^{-1}

and λ = wavelength of light

Here, $\phi = 4 \text{ eV} = 4 \times 1.6 \times 10^{-19}$ J

Substituting the given values in Eq. (i), we get

$$4 \times 1.6 \times 10^{-19} = \frac{6.63 \times 10^{-34} \times 3 \times 10^{8}}{\lambda}$$

or $$\lambda = \frac{6.63\times10^{-34}\times3\times10^{8}}{4\times1.6\times10^{-19}}$$

$$= 3.108\times10^{-7}\text{ m} \simeq 310\text{ nm}$$

7. (c) According to the Einstein's photoelectric equation,

$$K_{max} = \frac{1}{2}mv_2^2 = h\nu - \phi_0$$

$$= h\nu - h\nu_0 \quad \text{...(i)}$$

When incident frequency of light,

$$\nu = 2\nu_0$$

Substituting the value of ν in Eq. (i), we get

$$\frac{1}{2}m\,v_1^2 = h(2\nu_0) - h\nu_0$$

$$= 2h\nu_0 - h\nu_0 = h\nu_0 \quad \text{...(ii)}$$

If incident frequency of radiation,

$$\nu = 5\nu_0$$

Substituting the value of ν in Eq. (i), we get

$$\frac{1}{2}mv_2^2 = h(5\nu_0) - h\nu_0$$

$$= 5h\nu_0 - h\nu_0 = 4h\nu_0 \quad \text{...(iii)}$$

On dividing Eq. (ii) by Eq (iii), we get

$$\frac{\frac{1}{2}mv_1^2}{\frac{1}{2}mv_2^2} = \frac{h\nu_0}{4h\nu_0}$$

$$\Rightarrow \quad \frac{v_1^2}{v_2^2} = \frac{1}{4} \text{ or } \frac{v_1}{v_2} = \frac{1}{2}$$

$$\therefore \quad v_1 : v_2 = 1:2$$

8. (a) $K = \frac{1}{2}mv^2 = h\nu - h\nu_0 = \frac{hc}{\lambda} - \frac{hc}{\lambda_0}$

Given, $\lambda_0 = 3250\times10^{-10}$ m

$\lambda = 2536\times10^{-10}$ m

Let velocity of ejected electron be v.

Now, applying Einstein's photoelectric equation, we have

$$E = K + \phi_0$$

$$\Rightarrow \quad h\nu = \frac{1}{2}m_e v^2 + h\nu_0$$

$$\Rightarrow \quad \frac{1}{2}m_e v^2 = h\nu - h\nu_0$$

$$= hc\left(\frac{1}{\lambda} - \frac{1}{\lambda_0}\right)$$

⇒ Velocity of electron,

$$v = \sqrt{\frac{2hc}{m_e}\left(\frac{1}{\lambda} - \frac{1}{\lambda_0}\right)}$$

$$= \sqrt{\frac{2\times4.14\times10^{-15}\times1.6\times10^{-19}\times3\times10^{8}}{9.1\times10^{-31}}\left(\frac{3250-2536}{3250\times2536}\right)\times\frac{1}{10^{-10}}}$$

$$= 0.6\times10^{6}\text{ ms}^{-1} = 6\times10^{5}\text{ ms}^{-1}$$

9. (c) In Ist case, when a metallic surface is illuminated with radiation of wavelength λ, the stopping potential is V.

So, photoelectric equation can be written as

$$eV = \frac{hc}{\lambda} - \frac{hc}{\lambda_0} \quad \text{...(i)}$$

In IInd case, when the same surface is illuminated with radiation of wavelength 2λ, the stopping potential is $\frac{V}{4}$.

So, photoelectric equation can be written as

$$\frac{eV}{4} = \frac{hc}{2\lambda} - \frac{hc}{\lambda_0}$$

$$\Rightarrow \quad eV = \frac{4hc}{2\lambda} - \frac{4hc}{\lambda_0} \quad \text{...(ii)}$$

From Eqs. (i) and (ii), we get

$$\Rightarrow \quad \frac{hc}{\lambda} - \frac{hc}{\lambda_0} = \frac{4hc}{2\lambda} - \frac{4hc}{\lambda_0}$$

$$\Rightarrow \quad \frac{1}{\lambda} - \frac{1}{\lambda_0} = \frac{2}{\lambda} - \frac{4}{\lambda_0}$$

$$\Rightarrow \quad \lambda_0 = 3\lambda$$

10. (d) We know that, $E = (\text{KE})_{max}$ + Work function (ϕ)

where, $\phi = h\nu_0, E = h\nu$

$$(\text{KE})_{max} = \frac{1}{2}mv_0^2$$

$$\Rightarrow \quad (\text{KE})_{max} = h\nu - \phi$$

$$\Rightarrow \quad 2\text{eV} = 5\text{ eV} - \phi \quad \text{(given)}$$

$$\Rightarrow \quad \phi = 3\text{ eV}$$

Thus, $V_{cathode} - V_{anode} = 3$ V

$$\Rightarrow \quad V_{anode} - V_{cathode} = -3\text{ V}$$

11. (b) From photoelectric equation,

$$h\nu = W + eV_0$$

(where, W = work function)

So, $$\frac{hc}{\lambda} = W + 3eV_0 \quad \text{...(i)}$$

Also, $$\frac{hc}{2\lambda} = W + eV_0$$

$$\Rightarrow \quad \frac{hc}{\lambda} = 2W + 2eV_0 \quad \text{...(ii)}$$

Subtracting Eq. (i) from Eq. (ii), we get

$$0 = W - eV_0$$

$$\Rightarrow \quad W = eV_0$$

From Eq. (i), $\frac{hc}{\lambda} = eV_0 + 3eV_0 = 4eV_0$

The threshold wavelength is given by

$$\lambda_{th} = \frac{hc}{W} = \frac{4eV_0\lambda}{eV_0} = 4\lambda$$

12. (a) According to Einstein's photoelectric equation,

$$E = K_{max} + W$$

$$\Rightarrow \quad K_{max} = E - W = h\nu - W$$

$$K_{max} = \frac{hc}{\lambda} - W \quad \text{...(i)}$$

Similarly, in second case, maximum kinetic energy of emitted electron is 3 times that in first case, we get

$$3K_{max} = \frac{hc}{\frac{\lambda}{2}} - W \quad \text{...(ii)}$$

Solving Eqs. (i) and (ii), we get work function of an emitted electron from a metal surface.

$$W = \frac{hc}{2\lambda}$$

13. (d) We know that $\lambda = \frac{h}{p} = \frac{h}{\sqrt{2mE}}$

Here, E = kinetic energy

Thus, $\lambda^2 = \frac{h^2}{2mE} \Rightarrow \frac{1}{\lambda^2} = \frac{2mE}{h^2}$

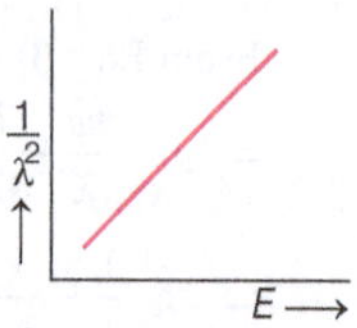

Hence, option (d) is correct.

14. (c) de-Broglie wavelength (λ) of a moving particle is given as

$$\lambda = \frac{h}{p} \qquad \therefore \quad \lambda \propto \frac{1}{p}$$

Hence, the graph showing the variation of de-Broglie wavelength (λ) of a moving particle with its momentum (p) is shown below.

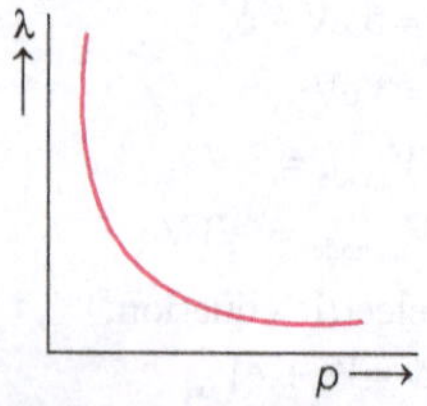

15. (d) Since, work function is negligible. Therefore, kinetic energy of emitted electron = Energy of incident photon i.e.,

$$\frac{1}{2}mv^2 = h\nu$$

$$\Rightarrow \quad \frac{p^2}{2m} = \frac{hc}{\lambda}$$

$$\Rightarrow \quad p = \sqrt{\frac{2mhc}{\lambda}}$$

de-Broglie wavelength of emitted electrons is

$$\lambda_d = \frac{h}{p} = \frac{h}{\sqrt{\frac{2mhc}{\lambda}}} \Rightarrow \lambda_d = \sqrt{\frac{h\lambda}{2mc}}$$

$$\Rightarrow \quad \lambda = \left(\frac{2mc}{h}\right)\lambda_d^2$$

16. (d) Kinetic energy of electron,

$$K = 144 \text{ eV}$$

$$\Rightarrow \quad eV = 144 \text{ eV}$$

$$\Rightarrow \quad V = 144 \text{ V}$$

$\therefore$ de-Broglie wavelength

$$\lambda = \frac{1.227}{\sqrt{V}}\text{Å} = \frac{1.227}{\sqrt{144}}\text{Å} = \frac{1.227}{12}\text{Å}$$

$$= 0.102\text{Å} = 1.02 \text{ nm}$$

$$= 102 \times 10^{-2} \text{ nm}$$

17. (a) The wave nature of electrons was experimentally verified by de-Broglie.

18. (c) Given, $\lambda = 1.227 \times 10^{-2}$ nm

$$= 1.227 \times 10^{-11} \text{ m}$$

Relation for de-Broglie wavelength for moving electron is

$$\lambda = \frac{12.27}{\sqrt{V}}\text{Å}$$

$$\Rightarrow \quad \sqrt{V} = \frac{12.27}{\lambda} \times 10^{-10} \text{ m}$$

$$= \frac{12.27 \times 10^{-10}}{1.227 \times 10^{-11}} = 10^2$$

$$\Rightarrow \quad V = 10^4 \text{ V}$$

19. (a) The de-Broglie wavelength associated with a charged particle is given by

$$\lambda = \frac{h}{p}$$

where, h = Planck's constant and

p = momentum = $\sqrt{2m\text{KE}}$ (here, KE is the kinetic energy of the charged particle)

$$\Rightarrow \quad \lambda = \frac{h}{\sqrt{2m\text{KE}}}$$

For proton and α-particle, the wavelengths are respectively given as

$$\lambda_\alpha = \frac{h}{\sqrt{2m_p\text{KE}_p}}$$

and $$\lambda_p = \frac{h}{\sqrt{2m_\alpha\text{KE}_\alpha}}$$

$$\therefore \quad \frac{\lambda_p}{\lambda_\alpha} = \frac{\sqrt{2m_\alpha\text{KE}_\alpha}}{\sqrt{2m_p\text{KE}_p}} \quad \text{...(i)}$$

Here, $\text{KE}_\alpha = \text{KE}_p$

and $m_\alpha = 4m_p$

Substituting these above mentioned relations in Eq. (i), we get

$$\Rightarrow \quad \frac{\lambda_p}{\lambda_\alpha} = \sqrt{\frac{4m_p}{m_p}} = \frac{2}{1}$$

or $$\lambda_p : \lambda_\alpha = 2:1$$

20. (*a*) Given, potential difference, $V = 10000$ V

If electron is accelerated through a potential of V volt, then the wavelength associated with it is given by

$$\lambda = \frac{12.27}{\sqrt{V}} \text{Å} = \frac{12.27}{\sqrt{10000}} \times 10^{-10}$$

$$= \frac{12.27 \times 10^{-10}}{100}$$

$$= 12.27 \times 10^{-12} \text{ m}$$

21. (*c*) According to the question,

$$\mathbf{v} = v_0 \hat{\mathbf{i}}, \quad \mathbf{E} = -E_0 \hat{\mathbf{i}}$$

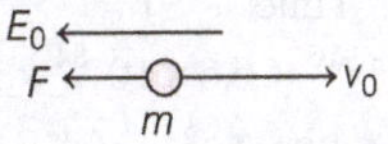

Thus, magnitude of force on the electron due to the electric field,

$$|\mathbf{F}| = q|\mathbf{E}| \Rightarrow F = eE_0$$

From Newton's second law of motion,

$$F = ma$$

$$\therefore \quad F = ma = eE_0$$

$$\Rightarrow \quad a = \frac{eE_0}{m} \quad \text{...(i)}$$

$$\text{or} \quad \mathbf{a} = \frac{(-e)(-E_0\hat{\mathbf{i}})}{m} = \frac{eE_0}{m}\hat{\mathbf{i}}$$

From first equation of motion, $v = u + at$

Here, u (initial velocity) $= v_0$

$$\Rightarrow \quad v = v_0 + \frac{eE_0}{m}t \quad \text{[From Eq. (i)] ...(ii)}$$

Initial de-Broglie wavelength of the electron is given as

$$\lambda_0 = h / mv_0$$

$$\Rightarrow \quad h = \lambda_0 m v_0 \quad \text{...(iii)}$$

After time t, de-Broglie wavelength is given as

$$\lambda = h / mv$$

Substituting the value of v from Eq. (ii), we get

$$\lambda = \frac{h}{m\left(v_0 + \frac{eE_0}{m}t\right)} = \frac{h}{mv_0\left[1 + \frac{eE_0}{mv_0}t\right]}$$

$$= \frac{\lambda_0 m v_0}{mv_0\left[1 + \frac{eE_0}{mv_0}t\right]} \quad \text{[from Eq. (iii)]}$$

$$= \frac{\lambda_0}{\left[1 + \frac{eE_0}{mv_0}t\right]}$$

$$\therefore \quad \lambda = \frac{\lambda_0}{1 + \frac{eE_0}{mv_0}t}$$

22. (*b*) de-Broglie wavelength associated with a moving particle can be given as

$$\lambda = \frac{h}{p} = \frac{h}{\sqrt{2m((\text{KE})}}$$

At thermal equilibrium, temperature of neutron and heavy water will be same.

This common temperature is given as, T.

Kinetic energy of the neutron is

$$\text{KE} = \frac{3}{2}kT$$

$\therefore$ de-Broglie wavelength of the neutron,

$$\lambda = \frac{h}{p} = \frac{h}{\sqrt{2m(\text{KE})}}$$

$$= \frac{h}{\sqrt{2m \times \frac{3}{2}kT}} = \frac{h}{\sqrt{3mkT}}$$

23. (*d*) Since, it is given that electron has mass m. de-Broglie's wavelength for an electron will be given as

$$\lambda_e = \frac{h}{p} \quad \text{...(i)}$$

As kinetic energy of electron

$$E = \frac{p^2}{2m}$$

$$\Rightarrow \quad p = \sqrt{2mE} \quad \text{...(ii)}$$

From Eqs. (i) and (ii), we get

$$\lambda_e = \frac{h}{\sqrt{2mE}} \quad \text{...(iii)}$$

Energy of a photon can be given as

$$E = h\nu$$

$$\Rightarrow \quad E = \frac{hc}{\lambda_p}$$

$$\Rightarrow \quad \lambda_p = \frac{hc}{E} \quad \text{...(iv)}$$

Now, divide Eq. (iii) by Eq. (iv), we get

$$\frac{\lambda_e}{\lambda_p} = \frac{h}{\sqrt{2mE}} \cdot \frac{E}{hc}$$

$$\Rightarrow \quad \frac{\lambda_e}{\lambda_p} = \frac{1}{c} \cdot \sqrt{\frac{E}{2m}}$$

24. (*a*) Given, mass of electrons $= m$

de-Broglie wavelength $= \lambda$

So, kinetic energy of electron $= \frac{p^2}{2m}$

$$= \frac{\left(\frac{h}{\lambda}\right)^2}{2m} = \frac{h^2}{2m\lambda^2}$$

Now, maximum energy of photon can be given by

$$E = \frac{hc}{\lambda_0} = \frac{h^2}{2m\lambda^2}$$

$$\Rightarrow \quad \lambda_0 = \frac{hc \times 2\lambda^2 \cdot m}{h^2} = \frac{2mc\lambda^2}{h}$$

25. (*b*) The de-Broglie wavelength is given by

$$\lambda = \frac{h}{p}$$

$$\Rightarrow \quad p\lambda = h$$

This equation is in the form of $yx = c$, which is the equation of a rectangular hyperbola.
Hence, the graph given in option (b) is the correct one.

26. (*a*) According to Einstein's photoelectric equation,

$$K_{max} = \frac{hc}{\lambda} - \phi_0$$

Given, $\lambda = 500$ nm,

$$hc = 1240 \text{ eV-nm}$$

and $\phi = 2.28$ eV

$$\therefore \quad K_{max} = \frac{1240 \text{ eV-nm}}{500 \text{ nm}} - 2.28 \text{ eV}$$

$$= 2.48 \text{ eV} - 2.28 = 0.2 \text{ eV}$$

The de-Broglie wavelength,

$$\lambda_{emin} = \frac{12.27}{\sqrt{KE_{max}(eV)}} = \frac{12.27}{\sqrt{0.2}}$$

$$= 27.436 \text{ Å}$$

$$= 27.436 \times 10^{-10} \text{ m}$$

Thus, minimum wavelength of the emitted electron is

$$\lambda_{min} = 2.7436 \times 10^{-9} \text{ m}$$

$$\simeq 2.8 \times 10^{-9} \text{ m}$$

So, $\lambda \geq 2.8 \times 10^{-9}$ m

Skill Builder

Sol. to Skill Builder on Pg. 650

(*d*) The energy of photon is given by

$$E = h\nu$$

where, h is Planck's constant and ν is the frequency of electromagnetic wave associated with the photon.
Velocity of photon is equal to speed of light

$$\therefore \quad E = h\nu$$

$$= \frac{hc}{\lambda}$$

$E \propto$ velocity of photon.

Sol. to Skill Builder on Pg. 651

(*a*) We know that,

$$\text{Power} = \frac{\text{Energy}}{\text{Time}} = \frac{nh\nu}{t}$$

$$= 10^{16} \times 6.6 \times 10^{-34} \times 10^{20}$$

$$= 6.62 \times 10^{2}$$

$$= 662 \text{ W}$$

Sol. to Skill Builder on Pg. 653

(*c*) Work function, $W = h\nu$

$$W = \frac{hc}{\lambda} \Rightarrow \lambda = \frac{hc}{W}$$

$$= \frac{6.62 \times 10^{-34} \times 3.0 \times 10^{8}}{2 \times 1.6 \times 10^{-19}}$$

$$= 6.20 \times 10^{-7} \text{ m}$$

$$= 620 \text{ nm}$$

Sol. to Skill Builder on Pg. 656

(*c*) For electron, $\lambda = \frac{12.27}{\sqrt{V}}$ Å

$$= \frac{12.27}{\sqrt{100}} \text{ Å} = \frac{12.27}{10} \text{ Å}$$

$$= 1.227 \text{ Å} = 0.1227 \text{ nm}$$

For deeper insight
Scan the QR Code

Chapter 13

Atoms

Learning Objectives

Module-I

- Rutherford's α-Particle Scattering Experiment
- Electron Orbits

Module-II

- Bohr's Atomic Model
- de-Broglie Explanation of Bohr's Second Postulate of Quantisation

Module-III

- Absorption and Emission Spectrum
- Hydrogen Spectrum

Chapter Overview with NEET Connection

This chapter provides visualisation of structure of atom, process of absorption and generation of photons. It also explains the quantum nature of atom and its connectivity with mechanics. Without this chapter, it will be difficult to understanding other chapters like Nuclei and Dual Nature of Matter and Radiation.

Special Format questions can be easily framed on the following topics of this chapter

- Distance of closest approach in Rutherford model
- Trajectory of α-particle and energy of electron
- Numericals based on Bohr's model
- Different spectral lines of H-atom.

For better understanding of this chapter

- Basic knowledge of electrostatic force will be helpful.
- Knowledge of circular motion from class 11th is required.

Introduction

The basic unit of matter and defining structure of any element is atom. In 1898, JJ Thomson for the first time proposed the physical structure of an atom and named it as **Plum-Pudding model**. Then, Rutherford performed an experiment on α-particle scattering in early 90's to investigate the atomic structure.

In this chapter, we will study Bohr's model, energy levels, hydrogen spectrum and X-rays followed by Rutherford α-particle scattering experiment.

Module 1

Rutherford's Model

- Rutherford's α-Particle Scattering Experiment • Electron Orbits

Rutherford's α-Particle Scattering Experiment

Rutherford with his two assistants, Geiger and Marsden did an experiment in 1911, in which they directed a narrow beam of α-particle on a gold foil of about 10^{-8} m thickness. α-particles were emitted by a radioactive material, $^{214}_{83}Bi$ kept inside a thick lead box. These α-particles were collimated into narrow beam by their passage through lead bricks. This well collimated beam was then allowed to fall on a thin gold foil. While passing through the gold foil, α-particles scattered through different angles. A zinc sulphide (ZnS) screen and a microscope was placed on the other side of the gold foil. This screen was movable, so as to receive the α-particles, scattered from the gold foil at angles varying from 0° to 180°.

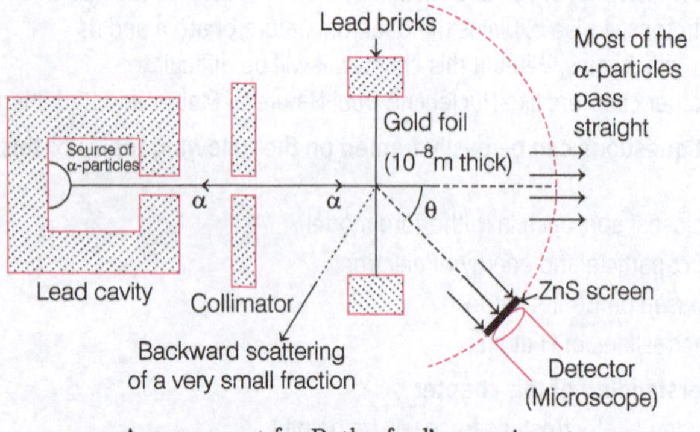

Arrangement for Rutherford's experiment

When an α-particle strikes the screen, it produces a flash of light which were observed by the microscope.

Observations

Rutherford made following observations from the experiment

(i) Most of the α-particles pass through the foil remains undeflected.

(ii) Some of them are deflected through small angles.

(iii) Few α-particles (about 1 in 8000) are deflected through an angle more than 90°.

(iv) A very few α-particles return back, *i.e.* deflected by 180°. Thus, few α-particles reverse their motion without actually touching the gold foil.

(v) The scattering of α-particles is proportional to the thickness of target for thin targets.

(vi) The number of α-particles scattered per unit area $N(\theta)$ at scattering angle θ varies inversely as $\sin^4(\theta/2)$,

i.e., $$N(\theta) \propto \frac{1}{\sin^4(\theta/2)}$$

This number $[N(\theta)]$ as a function of θ can be represented by following graph.

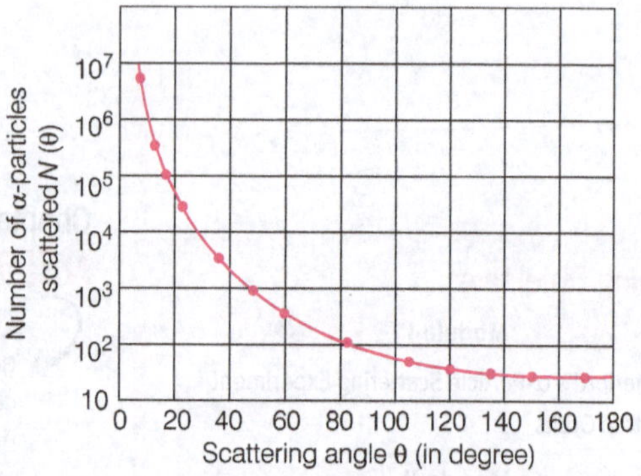

Number of α-particles scattered *versus* scattering angle θ

Mentor's TIP

- Electrons of atoms are light weight as compared to α-particles, hence deviation occurs when α-particles comes in vicinity of nucleus. Due to Coulomb's force of repulsion, the path of the α-particles after deflection becomes hyperbolic but the nucleus remains at rest.

Example 1. *In Rutherford's α-particle experiment with thin gold foil, 8100 scattered α-particles per unit area per minute were observed at an angle of 60°. Find the number of scattered α-particles per unit area per minute at an angle of 120°.*

Sol. It is given that, $\theta_1 = 60°, \theta_2 = 120°, N_1 = 8100, N_2 = ?$

Number of α-particles scattered at an angle θ,

$$N \propto \frac{1}{\sin^4\left(\frac{\theta}{2}\right)} \Rightarrow \frac{N_1}{N_2} = \frac{\left(\sin^4\frac{\theta_2}{2}\right)}{\left(\sin^4\frac{\theta_1}{2}\right)}$$

$$\Rightarrow \frac{8100}{N_2} = \frac{\left(\sin^4\frac{120°}{2}\right)}{\left(\sin^4\frac{60°}{2}\right)}$$

$$\Rightarrow \quad \frac{8100}{N_2} = \frac{\sin^4 60°}{\sin^4 30°}$$

$$\Rightarrow \quad N_2 = \frac{8100 \times \frac{1}{16}}{\frac{9}{16}} = 900$$

Rutherford's Atomic Model

The essential features of Rutherford's model of the atom or planetary model of the atom are as follows

(i) Most of the mass (at least 99.95%) and all of the charge of an atom is concentrated in a very small region of atom called **atomic nucleus.**

(ii) Nucleus is positively charged and its size is of the order of 10^{-15} m $\approx$ 1 fermi. The nucleus occupies only about 10^{-12} of the total volume of the atom or less.

(iii) In an atom, maximum space is empty and the electrons revolve around the nucleus in the same way as the planets revolve around the sun (*i.e.* in elliptical orbits).

Distance of Closest Approach

The minimum distance from the nucleus upto which the α-particle approaches is called the distance of closest approach (r_0). At this distance (when particle deflect by 180°), whole of the KE of α-particle converts into electrostatic potential energy,

i.e. $$\frac{1}{2}mv^2 = \frac{1}{4\pi\varepsilon_0}\frac{(Ze)\,2e}{r_0}$$

[$\because$ charge on α-particle is $+2e$ and charge on target nucleus is Ze, where Z is atomic number]

$$\Rightarrow \quad r_0 = \frac{1}{4\pi\varepsilon_0}\frac{2Ze^2}{\left[\frac{1}{2}mv^2\right]} = \frac{4kZe^2}{mv^2} \qquad \left(\because k = \frac{1}{4\pi\varepsilon_0}\right)$$

where, m is mass and v is velocity of α-particle.

This distance of closest approach (r_0) can be seen in the figure below.

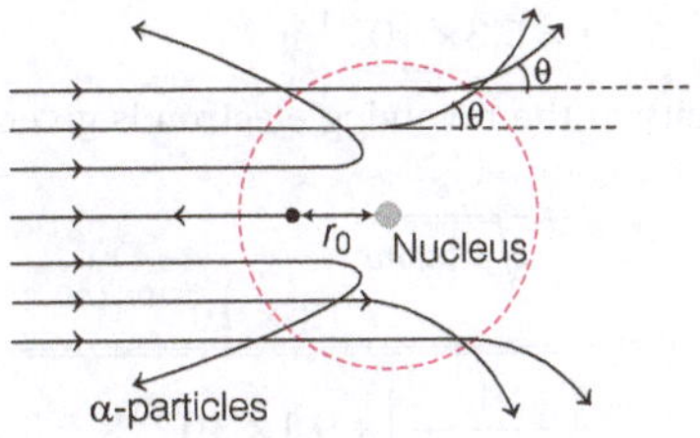

Distance of closest approach (r_0)

Example 2. *An α-particle of energy 5 MeV is scattered through 180° by a fixed uranium nucleus. Determine the distance of the closest approach.*

Sol. According to law of conservation of energy,

Kinetic energy of α-particle = Potential energy of α-particle at the distance of closest approach

i.e. $$\frac{1}{2}mv^2 = \frac{1}{4\pi\varepsilon_0}\frac{q_1q_2}{r_0}$$

Given, atomic number of uranium, $Z = 92$

Charge of electron, $e = 1.6 \times 10^{-19}$C

Charge of α-particle, $q_1 = 2e$

Charge of uranium nucleus, $q_2 = 92e$

$$\therefore 5\text{ MeV} = \frac{9 \times 10^9 \times (2e) \times (92e)}{r_0} \qquad \left(\because \text{given, } \frac{1}{2}mv^2 = 5\text{ MeV}\right)$$

$$\Rightarrow \quad r_0 = \frac{9\times 10^9 \times 2\times 92\times (1.6\times 10^{-19})^2}{5\times 10^6 \times 1.6\times 10^{-19}}$$

$$(\because 1\text{ eV} = 1.6 \times 10^{-19}\text{ J})$$

$$\therefore \quad r_0 = 5.3\times 10^{-14}\text{ m} = 5.3\times 10^{-12}\text{ cm}$$

Example 3. *Atomic number of silver metal is 47. Calculate the speed at which a beam of protons has to be fired at a sheet of silver foil, if the protons were able to approach within 2.5×10^{-14} m of the silver nucleus.*

Sol. The distance between protons and silver nucleus,

$$r = 2.5 \times 10^{-14}\text{m}$$

Mass of proton, $m = 1.67 \times 10^{-27}$ kg

Charge of protons, $q_1 = 1.6 \times 10^{-19}$C

Atomic number of silver, $Z = 47$

Charge of silver nucleus, $q_2 = Ze = (47)(1.6 \times 10^{-19})$C

By the law of conservation of energy, at distance of closest approach, the kinetic energy of proton must be equal to the potential energy of proton at that point. Therefore, we get

$$K = U \Rightarrow \frac{1}{2}mv^2 = \frac{kq_1q_2}{r}$$

Therefore, $$v = \sqrt{\frac{2kq_1q_2}{mr}}$$

$$= \sqrt{\frac{2\times (9\times 10^9)(1.6\times 10^{-19})(47)(1.6\times 10^{-19})}{(1.67\times 10^{-27})(2.5\times 10^{-14})}}$$

$$= 2.26 \times 10^7\text{ ms}^{-1}$$

Impact Parameter (*b*)

Perpendicular distance of the velocity vector of α-particle from the central line of the nucleus of the atom is called impact parameter (as shown in figure).

Mathematically, it is expressed as

$$b = \frac{1}{4\pi\varepsilon_0} \cdot \frac{Ze^2 \cot\frac{\theta}{2}}{K}$$

Thus, smaller the impact parameter b, greater the scattering angle θ and greater the kinetic energy of α-particle.

Example 4. *In Rutherford scattering experiment, what will be the correct angle for α-particles scattering for an impact parameter, $b = 0$?*

Sol. We know that, impact parameter, $b \propto \cot\frac{\theta}{2}$

$$\Rightarrow \quad b = K \cot\frac{\theta}{2}$$

where, K is a constant.

Here, if $b = 0$

$$\Rightarrow \quad K\cot(\theta/2) = 0 \Rightarrow \cot(\theta/2) = 0 \Rightarrow \frac{\theta}{2} = \frac{\pi}{2}$$

Hence, $\quad \theta = \pi = 180°$

α-Particle Trajectory

The α-particles which passes through the atom at a large distance from the nucleus experience a small electrostatic force of repulsion due to the nucleus and hence, undergoes a very small deflection. However, the α-particles which passes through the atom at a smaller distance from the nucleus suffer a large deflection. On the other hand, α-particles which travel towards the nucleus directly, slow down and ultimately comes to rest and then after being deflected through 180° retrace their path.

The trajectory of the α-particles at various scattering angles, is shown in the figure below.

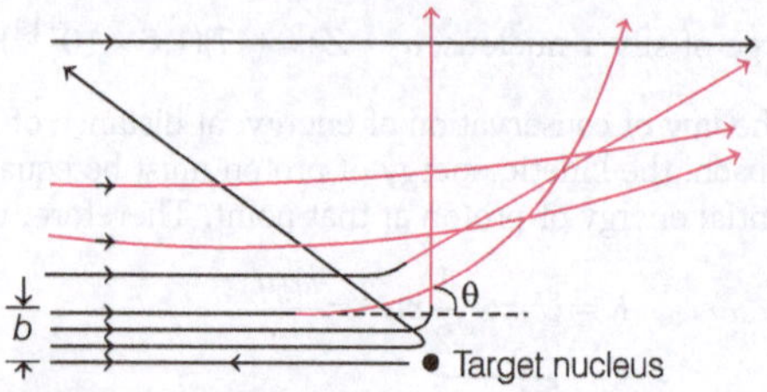

Trajectory of α-particles and impact parameter b.

Electron Orbits

In the Rutherford's nuclear model of the atom, the atom as an electrically neutral sphere consisting of a very small, massive and positively charged nucleus at the centre surrounded by the revolving electrons in their respective dynamically stable orbits. The electrostatic force of attraction F_e between the revolving electrons and the nucleus provides the requisite centripetal force F_c to keep them in their orbits. Thus, for a dynamically stable orbit in a H-atom,

$$F_c = F_e \Rightarrow \frac{mv^2}{r} = \frac{1}{4\pi\varepsilon_0} \cdot \frac{e^2}{r^2} \qquad (\because Z = 1)$$

Thus, the relation between the orbit radius and the electron velocity, $r = \dfrac{e^2}{4\pi\varepsilon_0 mv^2}$.

The kinetic energy K and electrostatic potential energy U of the electron in H-atom are

$$K = \frac{1}{2}mv^2 = \frac{e^2}{8\pi\varepsilon_0 r} \qquad \left(\because mv^2 = \frac{e^2}{4\pi\varepsilon_0 r}\right)$$

and
$$U = -2K = -\frac{e^2}{4\pi\varepsilon_0 r}$$

(the negative sign in U signifies that the electrostatic force is in the $-r$ direction or attractive in nature.) Thus, the total mechanical energy E of the electron in a H-atom is

$$E = K + U = \frac{e^2}{8\pi\varepsilon_0 r} - \frac{e^2}{4\pi\varepsilon_0 r} = -\frac{e^2}{8\pi\varepsilon_0 r}$$

Mentor's Tip

- The total energy within the atom is negative, the negative sign here implies that the electrostatic force between nucleus and electron is attractive in nature. If the total energy is considered to be positive, then the electrostatic force between the nucleus and electron becomes repulsive and electron will not follow a closed path around the nucleus and it will leave the atom.

Example 5. *It is found experimentally that 13.6 eV energy is required to separate a hydrogen atom into a proton and an electron. Calculate the velocity of the electron in hydrogen atom.*

Sol. Total energy of the electron in hydrogen atom

$$= -13.6 \text{ eV} = -13.6 \times 1.6 \times 10^{-19} \text{ J} = -2.2 \times 10^{-18} \text{ J}$$

Total energy of the electron in hydrogen atom,

$$\therefore \quad -\frac{e^2}{8\pi\varepsilon_0 r} = -2.2 \times 10^{-18}$$

Orbital radius, $r = \dfrac{(9 \times 10^9)(1.6 \times 10^{-19})^2}{(2)(2.2 \times 10^{-18})}$

$$\left(\because \frac{1}{4\pi\varepsilon_0} = 9 \times 10^9 \text{ Nm}^2\text{C}^{-2}\right)$$

or $\quad r = 5.3 \times 10^{-11}$ m

The velocity of the revolving electron is given by

$$\Rightarrow \quad v = \frac{e}{\sqrt{4\pi\varepsilon_0 mr}}$$

We have $v = \dfrac{1.6 \times 10^{-19}}{\sqrt{\left(\dfrac{1}{9 \times 10^9}\right) \times 9.1 \times 10^{-31} \times 5.3 \times 10^{-11}}}$

or $\quad v = 2.2 \times 10^6$ m/s

STEP UP Practice 1

1. For scattering of α-particles, Rutherford's suggested that
   (a) mass of atom and its positive charge were concentrated at centre of atom
   (b) only mass of atom is concentrated at centre of atom
   (c) only positive charge of atom is concentrated at centre of atom
   (d) mass of atom is uniformly distributed throughout its volume

2. **Assertion** (A) Atom as a whole is electrically neutral.
   Reason (R) Atom contains equal amount of positive and negative charges.
   In the light of the above statements, choose the correct answer from the options given below.
   (a) Both A and R are true but R is not the correct explanation of A.
   (b) A is true but R is false.
   (c) A is false but R is true.
   (d) Both A and R are true and R is the correct explanation of A.

3. Order of ratio of e/m ratio of proton, α-particles and electrons is
   (a) $\left(\frac{e}{m}\right)_p > \left(\frac{e}{m}\right)_\alpha > \left(\frac{e}{m}\right)_e$
   (b) $\left(\frac{e}{m}\right)_e > \left(\frac{e}{m}\right)_p > \left(\frac{e}{m}\right)_\alpha$
   (c) $\left(\frac{e}{m}\right)_\alpha > \left(\frac{e}{m}\right)_e > \left(\frac{e}{m}\right)_p$
   (d) All are equal

4. Rutherford's atomic model can be visualised as

(a) 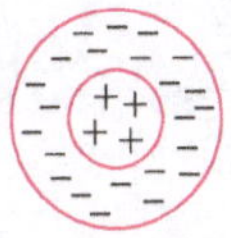
(b) 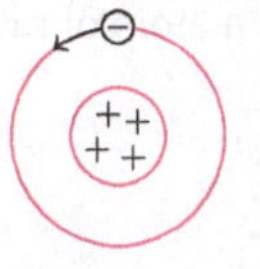
(c) 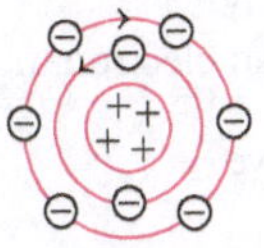
(d) 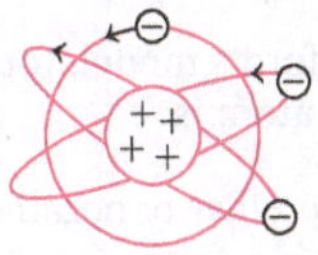

5. **Assertion** (A) Rutherford's atomic model is not stable.
   Reason (R) According to classical electromagnetic theory, an accelerating charged particle emits radiation in form of electromagnetic radiation.
   In the light of the above statements, choose the correct answer from the options given below.
   (a) Both A and R are true but R is not the correct explanation of A.
   (b) A is true but R is false.
   (c) A is false but R is true.
   (d) Both A and R are true and R is the correct explanation of A.

6. In Geiger-Marsden experiment, in a head-on collision between an α-particle and a gold nucleus, the minimum separation is 4×10^{-14} m. The energy of α-particle is (Take, atomic number of gold = 79)
   (a) 5.68 MeV (b) 8 MeV
   (c) 4.47 MeV (d) 7.24 MeV

7. In Geiger-Marsden experiment detection of α-particles scattered at a particular angle is done by
   (a) counting flashes produced by α-particles on a ZnS coated screen
   (b) counting spots produced on a photographic film
   (c) using a galvanometer detector
   (d) using a Geiger-counter

8. Gold foil used in Geiger-Marsden experiment as about 10^{-8} m thick. This ensures
   (a) gold foil's gravitational pull is small as possible
   (b) gold foil is deflected when α-particle stream is not incident centrally over it
   (c) gold foil provides no resistance to passage of α-particles
   (d) most α-particle will not suffer more than 1° scattering during passage through gold foil

9. Correct figure of Geiger-Marsden experiment is

(a) 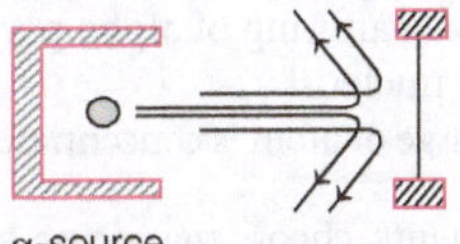

(b) 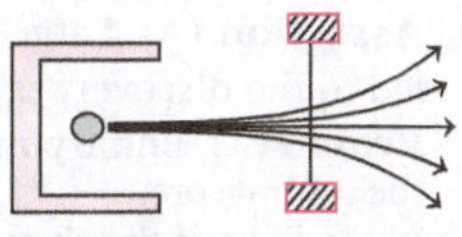

(c) 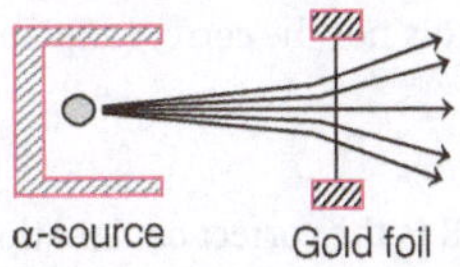

(d) 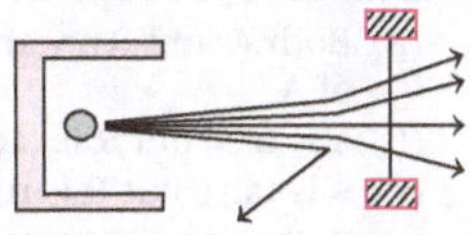

10. **Assertion** (A) The positively charged nucleus of an atom has radius of almost 10^{-15} m.
    Reason (R) In an α-particle scattering experiment, the distance of closest approach for α-particles is 10^{-15} m.
    In the light of the above statements, choose the correct answer from the options given below.
    (a) Both A and R are true but R is not the correct explanation of A.
    (b) A is true but R is false.
    (c) A is false but R is true.
    (d) Both A and R are true and R is the correct explanation of A.

11. An alpha nucleus of energy $\frac{1}{2}mv^2$ bombards a heavy nuclear target of charge Ze. Then, the distance of closest approach for the alpha nucleus will be proportional to
    (a) v^2 (b) $1/m$
    (c) $1/v^4$ (d) $1/Ze$

12. Trajectory of an α-particle is shown in figure below. Then, impact parameter is

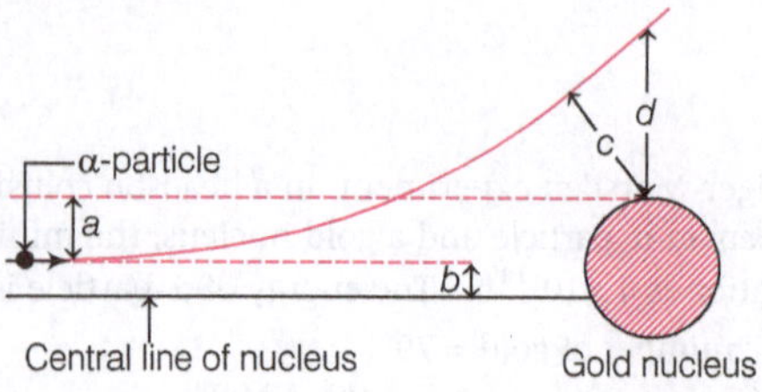

(a) a (b) b
(c) c (d) d

13. If impact parameter is very small, then scattering angle is around
(a) zero (b) 90°
(c) 180° (d) 360°

14. In Rutherford scattering experiment for scattering angle of 360°, what will be the value of impact parameter?
(a) 0 (b) ∞
(c) 1 (d) Data insufficient

15. The number of α-particles scattered per unit area $N(\theta)$ at scattering angle θ varies inversely as
(a) $\cos^4\left(\frac{\theta}{2}\right)$ (b) $\sin^4\left(\frac{\theta}{2}\right)$
(c) $\tan^4\left(\frac{\theta}{2}\right)$ (d) $\cot^4\left(\frac{\theta}{2}\right)$

16. **Assertion** (A) Large angle of scattering of alpha particles led to the discovery of atomic nucleus.
Reason (R) Entire positive charge of atom is concentrated in the central core.
In the light of the above statements, choose the correct answer from the options given below.
(a) Both A and R are true but R is not the correct explanation of A.
(b) A is true but R is false.
(c) A is false but R is true.
(d) Both A and R are true and R is the correct explanation of A.

17. Which of the following pair is incorrect?
(a) Centripetal force (F_c) of electron → $\frac{mv^2}{r}$
(b) Electrostatic force of attraction between electron and nucleus → $\frac{1}{4\pi\varepsilon_0}\cdot\frac{e^3}{r^3}$
(c) Impact parameter (b) → $\frac{1}{4\pi\varepsilon_0}\cdot\frac{Ze^2\cot\frac{\theta}{2}}{K}$
(d) Scattering of α-particle $N(\theta)$ → $\frac{1}{\sin^4\left(\frac{\theta}{2}\right)}$

18. **Assertion** (A) The force of repulsion between atomic nucleus and α-particle *varies* with distance according to inverse square law.
Reason (R) Rutherford did α-particle scattering experiment.
In the light of the above statements, choose the correct answer from the options given below.
(a) Both A and R are true but R is not the correct explanation of A.
(b) A is true but R is false.
(c) A is false but R is true.
(d) Both A and R are true and R is the correct explanation of A.

19. For separation r between gold nucleus and an α-particle, the magnitude of repulsive force is given by
(a) $F = \frac{1}{4\pi\varepsilon_0}\cdot\frac{2e^2}{r^2}$ (b) $F = \frac{1}{4\pi\varepsilon_0}\cdot\frac{e^2}{r^2}$
(c) $F = \frac{158\cdot e^2}{4\pi\varepsilon_0 r^2}$ (d) $F = \frac{56e^2}{4\pi\varepsilon_0 r^2}$

20. In Rutherford's model, if F_e indicates electrostatic force between electron and nucleus and F_c indicates the centripetal force on revolving electron, then
(a) $F_e = F_c$ (b) $F_e > F_c$
(c) $F_e < F_c$ (d) None of these

21. In Rutherford's model, if v is velocity of electron and r is its orbital radius, then in case of a hydrogen atom
(a) $r = \frac{e^2}{8\pi\varepsilon_0 mv^2}$ (b) $r = \frac{e^2}{8\pi\varepsilon_0 v}$
(c) $r = \frac{e^2}{4\pi\varepsilon_0 mv^2}$ (d) $r = \frac{e^2}{4\pi\varepsilon_0 v}$

22. In Rutherford's model, kinetic energy of revolving electron into hydrogen atom of radius r is given by
(a) $K = \frac{e^2}{4\pi\varepsilon_0 r}$ (b) $K = \frac{e^2}{8\pi\varepsilon_0 r^2}$
(c) $K = \frac{-e^2}{8\pi\varepsilon_0 r}$ (d) $K = \frac{e^2}{8\pi\varepsilon_0 r}$

23. In Rutherford's model, total energy of an electron in a hydrogen atom is
(a) positive (b) negative
(c) either positive or negative (d) zero

24. In which of the following systems will the radius of the first orbit ($n = 1$) be minimum?
(a) Hydrogen atom (b) Deuterium atom
(c) Singly ionised helium (d) Doubly ionised lithium

Module 2

Bohr's Model

- Bohr's Atomic Model
- de-Broglie Explanation of Bohr's Second Postulate of Quantisation

Bohr's Atomic Model

The work of Rutherford was rejected on the basis of classical theory (any accelerating charge produces electromagnetic wave and loses energy, hence atom should be unstable). This shortcoming was rectified by Neil Bohr through his atomic model.

Bohr proposed a model for hydrogen atom which is applicable for some lighter atoms in which a single electron revolves around a stationary nucleus of positive charge which are usually known as **hydrogen like atom**, *e.g.* ${}_1H^1$, ${}_1H^2$, He^+, Li^{++}, etc.

Bohr's model is based on the following three postulates

(i) Bohr postulated that an electron in an atom can move around nucleus in certain circular **stable orbits** without emitting radiations.

(ii) Electrons can revolve only in those orbits in which their angular momentum is an integral multiple of $h/2\pi$, where h is Planck's constant. If the mass of the electron be m and it is revolving with velocity v in an orbit of radius r, then its angular momentum will be mvr.

According to Bohr's postulate, we have angular momentum, $L = mvr = nh/2\pi$

where, n is an integer ($n = 1, 2, 3, \ldots$) and is called the **principal quantum number** of the orbit. This equation is called **Bohr's quantisation condition.**

(iii) When the atom receives energy from outside, then one (or more) of its outer electrons leaves its orbit and goes to some higher orbit. This state of the atom is called **excited state.**

The electron in the higher orbit stays only for 10^{-8} s and returns back to lower orbit. While returning back, the electron radiates energy in the form of electromagnetic waves.

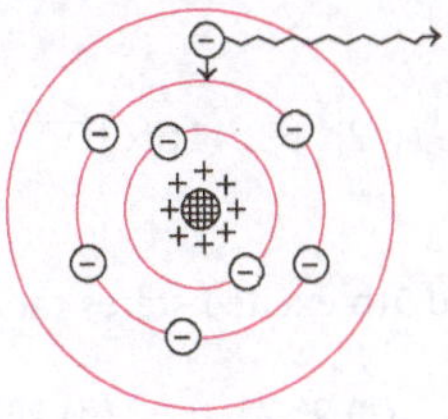

Electron falls down to lower orbit and emits energy

If the energy of electron in the higher orbit be E_2 and that in the lower orbit be E_1, then the frequency ν of the radiated waves is given by

$$h\nu = E_2 - E_1$$

or $$\nu = \frac{E_2 - E_1}{h}$$

This equation is called **Bohr's frequency condition.**

NEET Snapshot

Bohr's Model is not valid for Ne^+ (Neon +). ***[NEET 2020]***

Bohr's model is valid for atoms having only electron. Ne^+ ion have more than one electron, hence Bohr's model is not valid for this ion.

Example 6. *Compute the angular momentum in 4th orbit, if L is the angular momentum of the electron in the 2nd orbit of hydrogen atom.*

(a) 0 (b) L
(c) $2L$ (d) $3L$

Sol. (c) We know that, the angular momentum of the electron of hydrogen atom in nth orbit,

$$L_n = \frac{nh}{2\pi} \quad \ldots(i)$$

But according to question, the angular momentum in 2nd orbit ($n = 2$) is L.

So, $$L = \frac{2h}{2\pi} = \frac{h}{\pi} \quad \ldots(ii)$$

Hence, the angular momentum in 4th orbit is

$$L_4 = \frac{4h}{2\pi} = \frac{2h}{\pi} = 2L \quad \text{[from Eq. (ii)]}$$

Mathematical Analysis of Bohr's Atomic Model of Hydrogen like Atoms

A hydrogen like atom consists of a tiny positively charged nucleus and an electron revolving in a stable circular orbit around it as shown in the figure below.

Let e, m and v be respectively, the charge, mass and velocity of the revolving electron and r be the radius of the orbit. The positive charge of the nucleus is Ze, where Z is the atomic number (in case of hydrogen atom, $Z = 1$). As the centripetal force is provided by the electrostatic force of attraction, we have

$$\frac{mv^2}{r} = \frac{1}{4\pi\varepsilon_0}\frac{(Ze)\times e}{r^2} \quad \text{or} \quad \boxed{mv^2 = \frac{Ze^2}{4\pi\varepsilon_0 r}} \quad ...(i)$$

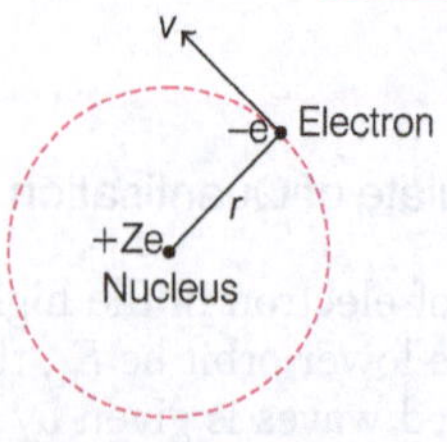

An electron is revolving around a nucleus of hydrogen like atoms

From the first postulate, the angular momentum of the electron,

$$\boxed{mvr = n\frac{h}{2\pi}} \quad ...(ii)$$

Radius of Electron in *n*th Orbit

Squaring Eq. (ii) and dividing by Eq. (i), we get

$$\boxed{r_n = n^2\frac{h^2\varepsilon_0}{\pi m Ze^2}} \; (\because r = r_n) \quad ...(iii)$$

This is the equation for the radii of the permitted orbits. According to this equation, $r_n \propto n^2$.

Since, $n = 1, 2, 3, \ldots$, and so on, it follows that the radii of the permitted orbits increase in the ratio $1:4:9:16\ldots:$ and so on, from the first orbit.

Bohr's Radius

The radius of the first orbit ($n = 1$) of H-atom ($Z = 1$) will be

$$\boxed{r_1 = \frac{h^2\varepsilon_0}{\pi m e^2}} \quad ...(iv)$$

Substituting the value of constants, we get $r_1 = 0.53$ Å. This is called Bohr's radius. From Eqs. (iii) and (iv), we get

Radius of *n*th orbit is, $r_n = 0.53\frac{n^2}{Z}$ Å $= \frac{n^2}{Z}r_1$

Variations of r_n

Using the relation, $r_n = \frac{n^2}{Z}r_1$, we can plot the following graphs

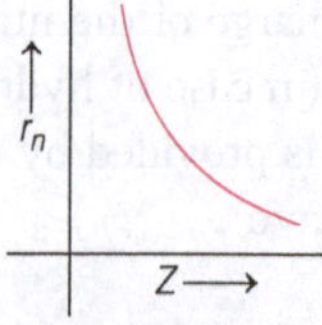

r_n *versus Z* graph

Here, $r_n \propto 1/Z$

Nature of graph will be rectangular hyperbola.

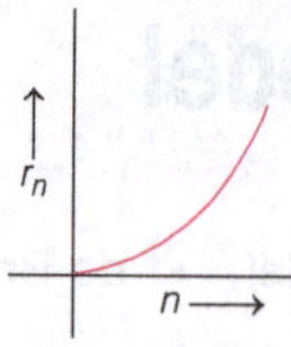

r_n *versus n* graph

Here, $\sqrt{r_n} \propto n$

Nature of graph will be parabola.

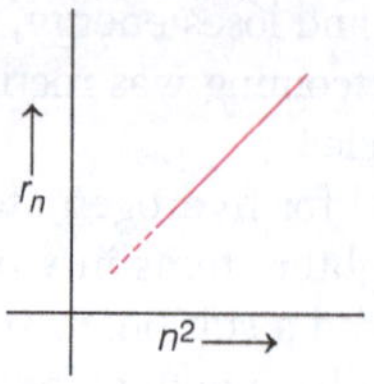

r_n *versus* n^2 graph

Here, $r_n \propto n^2$

Nature of graph will be straight line.

Example 7. *Using known values for hydrogen atom, calculate radius of third orbit for* Li^{2+}.

Sol. As, for Li^{2+} ($Z = 3$),

Further we know that, $r_n = \frac{n^2}{Z}r_1$

Substituting, $n = 3$, $Z = 3$ and $r_1 = 0.529$ Å

We have, $r_3 = \frac{(3)^2}{(3)}(0.529)\text{Å} = 1.587\text{Å}$

NEET Close-up

Example Similar to PYQ Asked in NEET 2023

The radius of 2nd orbit of hydrogen atom ($r_0 = 5.29\times10^{-11}$ m) will be

(a) 2.1×10^{-10} m
(b) 5.29×10^{-11} m
(c) 1.1×10^{-10} m
(d) 1.8×10^{-10} m

Sol. (*a*) We know that, radius of *n*th orbit of hydrogen atom,

$$r_n = r_0 \times n^2$$

So, radius of 2nd orbit, r_2

$$= 5.29\times10^{-11}\times(2)^2 = 2.116\times10^{-10} \text{ m}$$

Skill Builder

The ratio of 3rd excited and 5th excited states radii for hydrogen atom is

(a) 4 : 9 (b) 9 : 4 (c) 9 : 25 (d) 25 : 9

For more Practice Refer Q. No. 1 of step up practice-2 and Q. No. 19 of Gearing up for NEET.

Speed of Electron in *n*th Orbit

From Eq. (ii), we have $v_n = n\dfrac{h}{2\pi mr}$

Putting the value of r from Eq. (iii), we get

$$v_n = \frac{Ze^2}{2h\varepsilon_0}\frac{1}{n} \quad ...(v)$$

where, principal quantum number,

$$n = 1, 2, 3, ..., \text{and so on.}$$

Thus, $v_n \propto \dfrac{1}{n}$

This shows that the velocity of electron is maximum in the lowest orbit ($n = 1$) and goes on decreasing in higher orbits. The velocity of electron in the first orbit ($n = 1$) of H-atom ($Z = 1$) is

$$v_1 = \frac{e^2}{2h\varepsilon_0} = \frac{c}{137} \simeq 2.2\times 10^6 \text{ ms}^{-1} \quad ...(vi)$$

Thus, from Eqs. (v) and (vi), we get
Velocity of electron in *n*th orbit is,

$$v_n = 2.2\times 10^6 \frac{Z}{n}\text{ms}^{-1} = \frac{Z}{n}v_1$$

Variations of v_n

Using the relation, $v_n = \dfrac{Z}{n}v_1$, we can plot the following graph

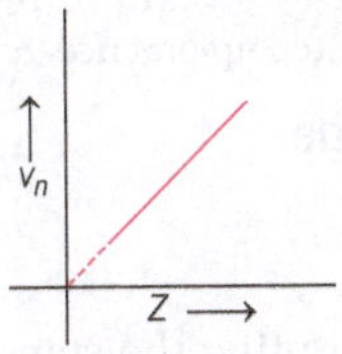

v_n *versus* Z *graph*

Here, $v_n \propto Z$
Nature of graph will be straight line.

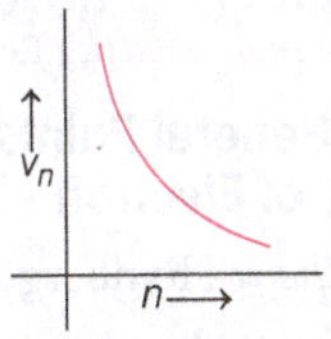

v_n *versus* n *graph*

Here, $v_n \propto 1/n$
Nature of graph will be rectangular hyperbola.

Example 8. *Using known values for hydrogen atom, calculate speed of electron in fourth orbit of* He^+.

Sol. As, for He^+ ($Z = 2$),

Also, we know that, $v_n = \dfrac{Z}{n}v_1$

Substituting $n = 4$, $Z = 2$ and $v_1 = 2.2\times 10^6$ ms^{-1}, we get

$$v_4 = \left(\frac{2}{4}\right)(2.2\times 10^6)$$
$$= 1.1\times 10^6 \text{ ms}^{-1}$$

Time Period and Frequency of Revolution of Electron in *n*th Orbit

Number of revolutions completed per second by the electron in a stationary orbit, around the nucleus is known as its **frequency**. It is represented by ν.

From $v_n = r\omega_n = r_n(2\pi\nu_n)$ $\quad (\because \omega_n = 2\pi\nu_n)$

$$\therefore \quad \nu_n = \frac{v_n}{2\pi r_n}$$

Putting the value of v_n in above equation, we get

$$\nu_n = \frac{1}{2\pi r_n}\frac{Ze^2}{2h\varepsilon_0}\frac{1}{n} \quad \text{[from Eq. (v)]}$$

$$\Rightarrow \quad \nu_n = \frac{1}{4\pi\varepsilon_0}\cdot\frac{Ze^2}{nhr_n} \Rightarrow \nu_n = \frac{kZe^2}{nhr_n} \quad \left(\because k = \frac{1}{4\pi\varepsilon_0}\right)$$

$\therefore$ Time period of revolution of electron in *n*th orbit,

$$T_n = \frac{1}{\nu_n} = \frac{nhr_n}{kZe^2}$$

Since, $r_n \propto \dfrac{n^2}{Z}$

$$\therefore \quad T_n \propto \frac{n^3}{Z^2} \text{ and } \nu_n \propto \frac{Z^2}{n^3}$$

Also, $\omega_n = 2\pi\nu_n$

$$\Rightarrow \quad \omega_n \propto \frac{Z^2}{n^3}$$

Example 9. *Find the ratio of product of velocity and time period of electron orbiting in 2nd and 3rd stable orbits for an hydrogen like atom.*

Sol. We know that, time period $T_n \propto n^3$ and velocity $v_n \propto 1/n$.

$\Rightarrow$ Time period $(T_n)\times$ velocity $(v_n) \propto n^2$

$$\therefore \quad \frac{T_2 v_2}{T_3 v_3} = \frac{2^2}{3^2} = \frac{4}{9}$$

Example 10. *In the Bohr model of hydrogen atom, the electron is pictured to rotate in a circular orbit of radius* 5×10^{-11} *m at a speed* 2.2×10^6 *ms*$^{-1}$. *Calculate the current associated with electron motion?*

Sol. Frequency of revolution of electron can be written as,

$$\nu = \frac{v}{2\pi r} = \frac{2.2\times 10^6}{2\pi(5\times 10^{-11})} = 7\times 10^{15} \text{ Hz}$$

$\therefore$ Current associated, $I = q/t = q\nu$ $\quad \left(\because \dfrac{1}{t} = \nu\right)$

$$= (1.6\times 10^{-19})(7\times 10^{15})$$
$$= 11.2\times 10^{-4}\text{A} = 1.12 \text{ mA}$$

Energy of Electron in nth Orbit

The energy E of an electron in an orbit is the sum of kinetic and potential energies.

Kinetic Energy

Electron possess kinetic energy because of its motion. Inner orbits have greater kinetic energy than outer ones.

Mathematically, $KE_n = \frac{1}{2} m v_n^2$

Substituting the value of v_n from Eq. (v), we get

i.e. $$v_n = \frac{Ze^2}{2h\varepsilon_0}\left(\frac{1}{n}\right)$$

we get $$KE_n = \frac{mZ^2e^4}{8\varepsilon_0^2 n^2 h^2}$$

or $$KE_n = \frac{mZ^2e^4}{8\varepsilon_0^2 h^2}\left(\frac{1}{n^2}\right) \quad ...(vii)$$

In simplified form,

$$\boxed{KE_n = \frac{RhcZ^2}{n^2}}$$

where, $$R = \frac{me^4}{8\varepsilon_0^2 ch^3} = \text{Rydberg's constant}$$

$$= 1.09 \times 10^7 \text{ m}^{-1}$$

Potential Energy

The potential energy of the electron in an orbit is due to the electrostatic attraction by nucleus.

Mathematically, $$U_n = \frac{1}{4\pi\varepsilon_0} \frac{(Ze)(-e)}{r_n}$$

$$= -\frac{1}{4\pi\varepsilon_0} \frac{Ze^2}{r_n}$$

Substituting the value of r_n from Eq. (iii), we get

i.e. $$r_n = \frac{n^2h^2\varepsilon_0}{\pi m Z e^2}$$

we get $$U_n = \frac{-mZ^2e^4}{4\varepsilon_0^2 n^2 h^2} \quad ...(viii)$$

In simplified form,

$$\boxed{U_n = -\frac{2RhcZ^2}{n^2}}$$

Total Energy

The total energy of the electron,

$$E_n = KE_n + U_n = \frac{Ze^2}{8\pi\varepsilon_0 r_n} - \frac{Ze^2}{4\pi\varepsilon_0 r_n} = -\frac{Ze^2}{8\pi\varepsilon_0 r_n}$$

Substituting for r_n from Eq. (iii), we get

$$E_n = \frac{-mZ^2e^4}{8\varepsilon_0^2 h^2}\left(\frac{1}{n^2}\right) \quad ...(ix)$$

This is the expression for the total energy of the electron in the nth orbit

or $$\boxed{E_n = \frac{-RhcZ^2}{n^2}}$$

Also, from the above equations, we can write

$$U_n = -2KE_n \Rightarrow |U_n| = 2|KE_n|$$

$$\therefore \quad E_n = KE_n - 2KE_n = -KE_n$$

NEET Close-up

Example Similar to PYQ Asked in NEET 2019

The ground state energy of hydrogen atom is – 13.6 eV. What is the kinetic and potential energies of the electron in this state?

(a) –13.6 eV, 27.2 eV (b) 6.3 eV, – 13.6 eV
(c) 27.2 eV, – 27.2 eV (d) 13.6 eV, – 27.2 eV

Sol. (*d*) As, we know that, kinetic energy = – total energy

$$= -(-13.6)\text{ eV} = 13.6 \text{ eV}$$

and potential energy = + 2 (total energy)

$$= 2(-13.6)\text{ eV} = -27.2 \text{ eV}$$

Skill Builder

Kinetic Energy of an electron in ground state of H-atom is 10eV, then its total ground state energy will be

(a) 10 eV (b) 20 eV (c) –10 eV (d) –20 eV

For more Practice Refer Q. No. 19 of step up practice-2.

Some General Points Related to the Energy of Electron

(i) $Rhc = 1 \text{ Rydberg} = 13.6 \text{ eV}$.

(ii) For hydrogen atom $Z = 1$, substituting the standard values, we get $E_n = \frac{-13.6}{n^2}$ eV.

(iii) Negative energy of the electron shows that the electron is bound to the nucleus and is not free to leave it.

(iv) For $n = 1$, $E_1 = -13.6$ eV. Substituting $n = 2, 3, 4, ...$ etc, we get energies of electron in different orbits.

i.e. $E_2 = -3.40 \text{ eV}, E_3 = -1.51 \text{ eV} ... E_\infty = 0.$

Energy of absorbed photon, $\Delta E = h\nu = \frac{hc}{\lambda}$

where, ν = frequency of absorbed photon,
λ = wavelength of absorbed photon
and c = speed of light.

So, we can write

$$\Delta E = h\nu = \frac{hc}{\lambda} = E_{n_2} - E_{n_1} = \frac{Z^2me^4}{8\varepsilon_0^2 h^2}\left(\frac{1}{n_1^2} - \frac{1}{n_2^2}\right)$$

$$\Rightarrow \quad \frac{1}{\lambda} = \frac{Z^2 me^4}{8h^3 \varepsilon_0^2 c}\left(\frac{1}{n_1^2} - \frac{1}{n_2^2}\right)$$

or
$$\frac{1}{\lambda} = Z^2 R\left(\frac{1}{n_1^2} - \frac{1}{n_2^2}\right)$$

where, R is Rydberg's constant.

Note The reciprocal of the wavelength is called **wave number**.

$$\Rightarrow \quad \bar{\nu} = 1/\lambda$$

Concept ladder

In hydrogen like atom, if an electron jumps from n_1 to n_2 then energy required to jump

$$\Delta E = 13.6 Z^2\left(\frac{1}{n_1^2} - \frac{1}{n_2^2}\right)$$

Energy levels of H-Atom

$E_1 = -13.6$ eV, $E_2 = -3.4$ eV, $E_3 = -1.51$ eV and so on

Energy required to move from E_1 to E_2

$$\Delta E = E_2 - E_1 = 10.2 \text{ eV}$$

Similarly $\quad E_3 - E_1 = 12.09$ eV and so on.

Energy level diagram for H-atom is as follows

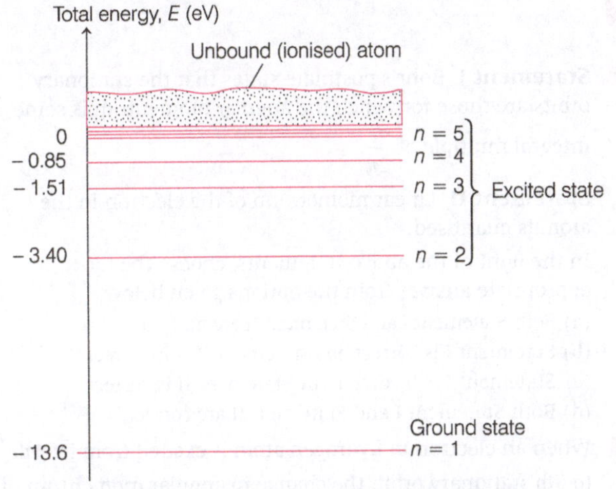

The energy level diagram for the hydrogen atom.

Example 11. *A difference of 2.3 eV separates two energy levels in an atom. What is the frequency of radiation emitted when the atom make a transition from the upper level to the lower level?*

Sol. Here, difference of energy,

$$\Delta E = 2.3 \text{ eV} = 2.3 \times 1.6 \times 10^{-19} \text{ J}$$

$$(\because 1 \text{ eV} = 1.6 \times 10^{-19} \text{ J})$$

Using the relation, $h\nu = \Delta E = E_2 - E_1$

or
$$\nu = \frac{\Delta E}{h} = \frac{2.3 \times 1.6 \times 10^{-19}}{6.62 \times 10^{-34}}$$

$$= 0.5559 \times 10^{15} \approx 5.6 \times 10^{14} \text{ Hz}$$

Example 12. *Determine the wavelength of the radiation required to excite the electron in Li^{++} from the first to the third Bohr orbit.*

Sol. Given, for Li^{++}, $Z = 3$ and as the excitation is from first to third Bohr orbit, so $n_1 = 1, n_2 = 3$

Using the relation,

$$\frac{1}{\lambda} = Z^2 R\left(\frac{1}{n_1^2} - \frac{1}{n_2^2}\right) = (3)^2 R\left(\frac{1}{1^2} - \frac{1}{3^2}\right) = 8R$$

$$\Rightarrow \text{Wavelength, } \lambda = \frac{1}{8R} = \frac{1}{8 \times 1.097 \times 10^7} = 0.114 \times 10^{-7}$$

$$= 11.4 \text{ nm}$$

Mentor's Tip

- Excitation Energy (from $n = 1$ to $n = 2$) $= E_2 - E_1$
- Excitation Potential $= \dfrac{(E_2 - E_1) \text{ in eV}}{e}$
- Ionisation Energy = – Energy of given state
- Ionisation Potential $= \dfrac{\text{Ionisation Energy (in eV)}}{e}$
- Binding Energy = – Energy of given state

Limitations of Bohr's Model

The limitation of Bohr's model are as follows

(i) Bohr's model is applicable only to a single electron atoms/ions.

(ii) It does not explain the fine structure of spectral lines. Application of external magnetic field (Zeeman effect) and external electric field (Stark effect) to radiating atoms could not be explained.

(iii) Bohr's assumption regarding stationary orbits is against Heisenberg uncertainty principle.

(iv) No explanation is given regarding principle of quantisation of angular momentum.

(v) This model does not explain why orbits of electrons are taken as circular whereas elliptical orbits are also possible.

de-Broglie Explanation of Bohr's Second Postulate of Quantisation

According to de-Broglie, a stationary orbit is that which contains an integral number of de-Broglie standing waves associated with the revolving electron.

For an electron revolving in nth circular orbit of radius r_n,

Total distance covered = Circumference of the orbit = $2\pi r_n$

$\therefore$ For the permissible orbit, $2\pi r_n = n\lambda$

According to de-Broglie wavelength, $\lambda = \dfrac{h}{mv_n}$

where, v_n = speed of electron revolving in nth orbit.

$$\therefore \quad 2\pi r_n = \frac{nh}{mv_n} \text{ or } mv_n r_n = \frac{nh}{2\pi} = n(h/2\pi)$$

i.e. angular momentum of electron revolving in nth orbit must be an integral multiple of $h/2\pi$, which is the quantum condition proposed by Bohr in second postulate.

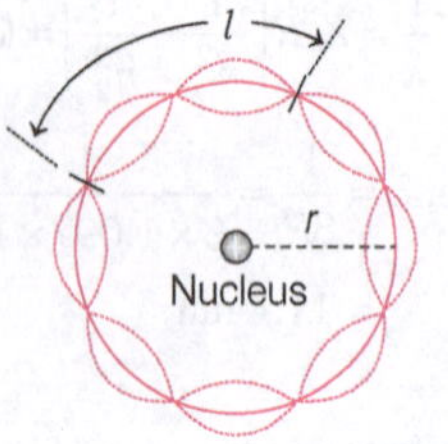

A standing wave is shown on a circular orbit for $n = 4$

Example 13. *An electron of a hydrogen like atom is in excited state. If total energy of the electron is –4.6 eV, then evaluate*

(i) the kinetic energy and

(ii) the de-Broglie wavelength of the electron.

Sol. Given, total energy of electron, $E = -4.6$ eV

(i) Kinetic energy of electron, $K = -$(Total energy, E)

$$\Rightarrow \quad K = -E = -(-4.6) = 4.6 \text{ eV}$$

(ii) de-Broglie wavelength,

$$\lambda_d = \frac{h}{\sqrt{2mK}} = \frac{6.6 \times 10^{-34}}{\sqrt{2 \times 9.1 \times 10^{-31} \times 4.6 \times 1.6 \times 10^{-19}}}$$

$$= 0.57 \times 10^{-9} \text{ m}$$

$$= 0.57 \text{ nm}$$

STEP UP Practice 2

1. In Bohr's model, the atomic radius of the first orbit is r_0, then the radius of the third orbit is
(a) $r_0/9$ (b) r_0
(c) $9r_0$ (d) $3r_0$

2. **Statement I** Bohr had to postulate that the electrons in stationary orbits around the nucleus do not radiate.
Statement II According to classical physics all moving electrons radiate.
In the light of the above statements, choose the most appropriate answer from the options given below.
(a) Both Statement I and Statement II are incorrect.
(b) Statement I is correct but Statement II is incorrect.
(c) Statement I is incorrect but Statement II is correct.
(d) Both Statement I and Statement II are correct.

3. **Statement I** Electrons in the atom are held due to coulomb forces.
Statement II The atom is stable only because the centripetal force due to coulomb's law is balanced by the centrifugal force.
In the light of the above statements, choose the most appropriate answer from the options given below.
(a) Both Statement I and Statement II are incorrect.
(b) Statement I is correct but Statement II is incorrect.
(c) Statement I is incorrect but Statement II is correct.
(d) Both Statement I and Statement II are correct.

4. Energy of an electron in an excited state of hydrogen atom is – 3.4 eV. Its angular momentum will be
(a) 1.11×10^{34} Js (b) 1.51×10^{-31} Js
(c) 2.11×10^{-34} Js (d) 3.72×10^{-34} Js

5. **Statement I** Bohr's postulate states that the stationary orbits are those for which the angular momentum is some integral multiple of $\frac{h}{2\pi}$.
Statement II Linear momentum of the electron in the atom is quantised.
In the light of the above statements, choose the most appropriate answer from the options given below.
(a) Both Statement I and Statement II are incorrect.
(b) Statement I is correct but Statement II is incorrect.
(c) Statement I is incorrect but Statement II is correct.
(d) Both Statement I and Statement II are correct.

6. When an electron in hydrogen atom is excited from its 4th to 5th stationary orbit, the change in angular momentum of electron is
(a) 4.6×10^{-34} Js (b) 3.32×10^{-34} Js
(c) 1.05×10^{-34} Js (d) 2.08×10^{-34} Js

7. The ratio of speed of an electron in ground state in Bohr's first orbit of hydrogen atom to the velocity of light in air is
(a) $\frac{e^2}{2\pi hc}$ (b) $\frac{2e\pi}{hc}$ (c) $\frac{e^3}{2\pi hc}$ (d) $\frac{2\pi e^2}{hc}$

8. According to classical electromagnetic theory, the electron revolving around a proton in hydrogen atom in an orbit of radius 5.3×10^{-11} m with velocity $2.2 \times 10^6 \text{ ms}^{-1}$
(a) does not emit any radiation
(b) emits radiation of any frequency
(c) emits frequency of light of 6.6×10^{15} Hz
(d) emits frequency of light of 2.2×10^{15} Hz

9. In Bohr's atomic model, speed and time period of revolution of an electron in $n = 3$ level are respectively
(a) $v = 1.09 \times 10^6\ ms^{-1}$, $T = 1.52 \times 10^{-16} s$
(b) $v = 2.19 \times 10^6\ ms^{-1}$, $T = 1.52 \times 10^{-16} s$
(c) $v = 7.29 \times 10^6\ ms^{-1}$, $T = 1.22 \times 10^{-16} s$
(d) $v = 7.29 \times 10^5\ ms^{-1}$, $T = 4.10 \times 10^{-15} s$

10. Which of the following pair is correct?

(a)	Bohr's frequency condition	→	$\frac{E_1 - E_2}{h}$
(b)	Angular momentum (mvr)	→	$\frac{nh}{\pi}$
(c)	Bohr's radius (r_n)	→	$n^2 \frac{h^2 \varepsilon_0}{\pi m Z e^2}$
(d)	Wave number $(\bar{v})$	→	λ

11. The speed of electron in ground state energy level is $2.6 \times 10^6 ms^{-1}$, then its speed in fourth excited state will be
(a) $5.6 \times 10^6\ ms^{-1}$
(b) $6 \times 10^5\ ms^{-1}$
(c) $5.5 \times 10^5\ ms^{-1}$
(d) $4.3 \times 10^6\ ms^{-1}$

12. The orbital frequency of an electron in hydrogen like atom is proportional to
(a) n^3 (b) n^{-3}
(c) n (d) n^0

13. In the nth orbit, the energy of an electron, $E_n = -\frac{13.6}{n^2}$ eV for hydrogen atom. The energy required to take the electron from first orbit to second orbit will be
(a) 10.2 eV (b) 12.1 eV
(c) 13.6 eV (d) 3.4 eV

14. In hydrogen atom, if the difference in the energy of the electron in $n = 2$ and $n = 3$ orbits is E, the ionisation energy of hydrogen atom is
(a) $13.2E$ (b) $7.2E$
(c) $5.6E$ (d) $3.2E$

15. In which of the following transitions will the wavelength be minimum?
(a) $n = 5$ to $n = 4$ (b) $n = 4$ to $n = 3$
(c) $n = 3$ to $n = 2$ (d) $n = 2$ to $n = 1$

16. In which of the following systems will the wavelength corresponding to $n = 2$ to $n = 1$ be minimum?
(a) Hydrogen atom
(b) Deuterium atom
(c) Singly ionised helium
(d) Doubly ionised lithium

17. Ratio of wavelengths emitted for transition $2 \to 1$ in Li^{2+}, He^+ and H is
(a) 1 : 2 : 3 (b) 1 : 4 : 9
(c) 4 : 9 : 36 (d) 3 : 2 : 1

18. Which of the following statements is true for hydrogen atom?
(a) Angular momentum $\propto \frac{1}{n}$
(b) Linear momentum $\propto \frac{1}{n}$
(c) Radius $\propto \frac{1}{n}$
(d) Energy $\propto \frac{1}{n}$

19. If the orbital radius of the electron in a hydrogen atom is 4.7×10^{-11} m. Compute the kinetic energy of the electron in hydrogen atom.
(a) 15.3 eV (b) – 15.3 eV
(c) 13.6 eV (d) –13.6 eV

20. As the electron in Bohr orbit of hydrogen atom passes from state $n = 2$ to $n = 1$, the kinetic energy (K) and potential energy (U) changes as
(a) K becomes twice, U becomes four times
(b) K becomes four times, U becomes twice
(c) K becomes four times, U also four times
(d) K becomes twice, U also two times

21. **Statement I** The total energy of an electron revolving in any stationary orbit is negative.
Statement II Energy can have positive or negative values.
In the light of the above statements, choose the most appropriate answer from the options given below.
(a) Both Statement I and Statement II are incorrect.
(b) Statement I is correct but Statement II is incorrect.
(c) Statement I is incorrect but Statement II is correct.
(d) Both Statement I and Statement II are correct.

22. If energy of a hydrogen atom in nth orbit is E_n, then energy of a singly ionised helium (He^+) atom in nth orbit will be
(a) $4E_n$ (b) $E_n/4$
(c) $2E_n$ (d) $E_n/2$

23. For the Bohr's first orbit of circumference $2\pi r$, the de-Broglie wavelength of revolving electron will be
(a) $2\pi r$ (b) πr
(c) $\frac{1}{2\pi r}$ (d) $\frac{1}{4\pi r}$

Module 3

Hydrogen Spectrum

- Absorption and Emission Spectrum
- Hydrogen Spectrum

Absorption and Emission Spectrum

An atom can be excited by incident photon or by collision. If an atom absorbs a photon, it goes to higher orbits/state and remains, there for a time of 10^{-8} s and returns back to ground state by different ways.

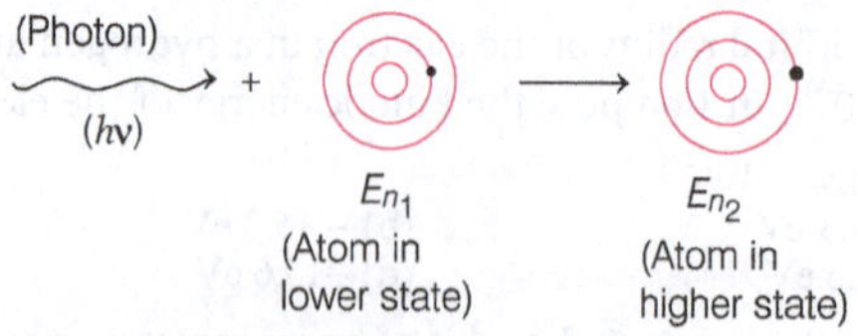

Absorption of photon by an atom

From the above diagram, it is clear that

$$E_{n_1} + h\nu = E_{n_2}$$

Let us now consider an example in which a photon of energy 12.09 eV is incident on hydrogen atom in ground state.

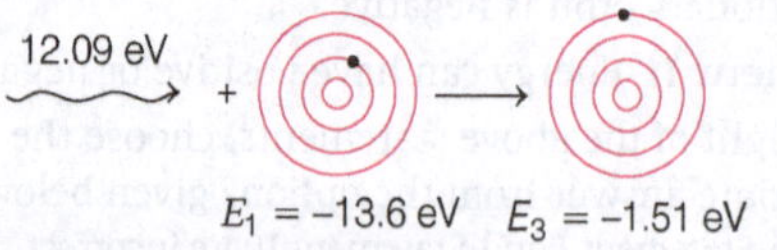

Absorption of photon of energy 12.09 eV by an atom

Energy of the atom after absorption

$$= 12.09 + (-13.6) = -1.51 \text{ eV}$$
$$= E_3$$

After absorbing photon, the atom goes to state $n = 3$, hence in this absorption spectrum, we have single line as shown below

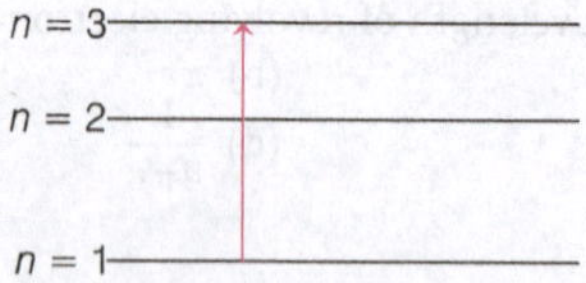

Absorption spectrum

Now, in this state $n = 3$, the atom remains for the time 10^{-8}s and then returns to ground state by emitting photon(s). This atom can come directly to $n = 1$ by emitting one photon or by emitting two photons from $n = 3 \to 2$, $2 \to 1$. Therefore, possible transitions are $3 \to 2$, $2 \to 1$, $3 \to 1$, as shown in the figure.

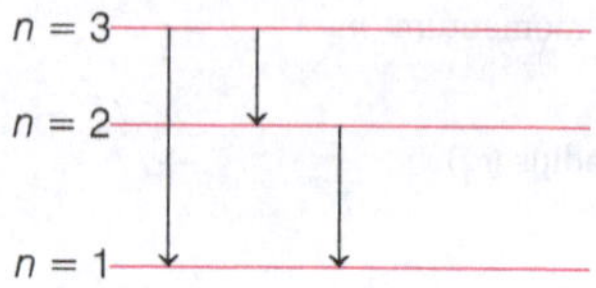

Emission spectrum

Concept ladder

- Emission/absorption of photons only takes place when the energy of the photon is exactly equal to the difference of energy level.
- For an atom to makes transition from $n = n_1$ to $n = n_2$, number of lines in emission spectrum,

$$N = \frac{(n_1 - n_2)(n_1 - n_2 + 1)}{2}$$

Putting $n_1 = n$ and $n_2 = 1$, this reduces to $N = \frac{n(n-1)}{2}$

Example 14. *Monochromatic radiation of wavelength λ is incident on a hydrogen sample in ground state. Hydrogen atoms absorb a fraction of light and subsequently emit radiation of ten different wavelengths. Find the value of λ.*

Sol. From nth energy state a total of $\frac{n(n-1)}{2}$ lines are emitted.

$$\therefore \quad \frac{n(n-1)}{2} = 10 \quad \text{or} \quad n = 5$$

Further, $\quad E_n = \frac{E_1}{n^2}$

$$\therefore \quad E_5 = \frac{-13.6}{(5)^2} = -0.54 \text{ eV}$$

The energy needed to take a hydrogen atom from its ground state to $n = 5$ is,

$$\Delta E = E_5 - E_1 = -0.54 - (-13.6)$$
$$= 13.06 \text{ eV}$$

The corresponding wavelength of light,

$$\lambda = \frac{12375}{\Delta E} \text{ Å} = \frac{12375}{13.06} = 947.5 \text{ Å}$$

Example 15. *Ionisation potential of hydrogen atom is 13.6 V. Hydrogen atoms in the ground state are excited by monochromatic radiation of photon energy is 12.1 eV. According to Bohr's theory, find the possible spectral lines emitted by hydrogen.*

Sol. Ionisation energy corresponding to ionisation potential

$$= -13.6 \text{ eV}$$

Energy of incident photon $= 12.1$ eV

So, the energy of electron in excited state

$$= -13.6 + 12.1 = -1.5 \text{ eV}$$

As, $\quad E_n = -\dfrac{13.6}{n^2}$ eV

$$\Rightarrow \quad -1.5 = \frac{-13.6}{n^2} \Rightarrow n^2 = \frac{-13.6}{-1.5} = 9 \Rightarrow n = 3$$

i.e. the energy of electron in excited state corresponds to third orbit.

The possible spectral lines are when electron jumps from orbit 3rd to 2nd, 3rd to 1st and 2nd to 1st. Thus, three spectral lines are emitted.

Example 16. *An electron is moving in an orbit of a hydrogen atom from which there can be a maximum of six transition. An electron is moving in an orbit of another hydrogen atom from which there can be a maximum of three transition. Find ratio of the velocities of the electron in these two orbits.*

Sol. Number of spectral lines obtained due to transition of electrons from nth orbit to lower orbit is given by

$$N = \frac{n(n-1)}{2}$$

Case I $\quad 6 = \dfrac{n_1(n_1 - 1)}{2}$

$$\Rightarrow \quad n_1^2 - n_1 - 12 = 0$$

$$\Rightarrow \quad (n_1 - 4)(n_1 + 3) = 0 \Rightarrow n_1 = 4$$

because n_1 cannot be negative, *i.e.* -3.

Case II $\quad 3 = \dfrac{n_2(n_2 - 1)}{2}$

$$\Rightarrow \quad n_2^2 - n_2 - 6 = 0 \Rightarrow (n_2 + 2)(n_2 - 3) = 0$$

$$\Rightarrow \quad n_2 = 3$$

because n_2 cannot be negative, *i.e.* -2.

Velocity of electron in hydrogen atom in nth orbit,

$$v_n \propto \frac{1}{n} \Rightarrow \frac{v_n}{v'_n} = \frac{n_2}{n_1} \Rightarrow \frac{v_6}{v_3} = \frac{3}{4}$$

Hydrogen Spectrum

Hydrogen spectrum or the line spectra of hydrogen atom consists of discrete bright lines in a dark background and it is specifically known as **hydrogen emission spectrum.**

There is one more type of hydrogen spectrum that exists where we get dark lines on the bright background, it is known as **absorption spectrum.**

Hydrogen being the simplest atom, has the simplest spectrum. In its observed spectrum, spacing between lines within certain sets of the spectrum decreases in a regular way. Each of these sets is called a **spectral series.** The very first of such series is the Balmer series.

Balmer find an empirical formula by the observation of a small part of this spectrum and it is represented by

$$\frac{1}{\lambda} = R\left(\frac{1}{2^2} - \frac{1}{n^2}\right), \text{ where } n = 3, 4, 5, \ldots$$

where, R is a constant called **Rydberg's constant** and its value is 1.097×10^7 m^{-1}.

Balmer series in the emission spectrum of H-atom is shown below.

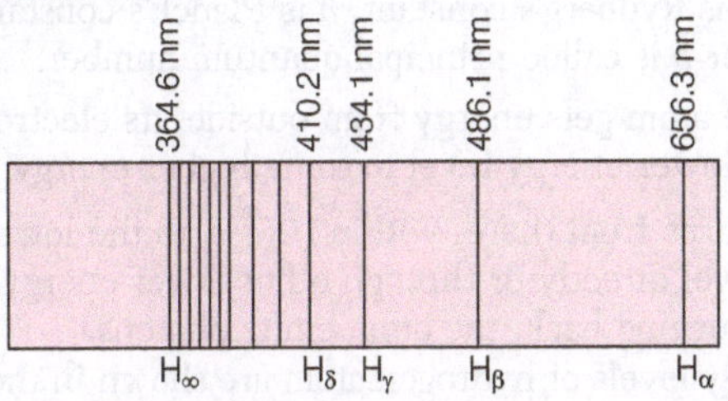

Balmer series in the emission spectrum of hydrogen

The line with the longest wavelength 656.3 nm in the red is called $\mathbf{H_\alpha}$ and the next line with wavelength 486.1 nm in blue-green is called $\mathbf{H_\beta}$ and so on.

Other series of spectra for hydrogen were subsequently discovered and known by the name of their discoverers. The lines of Balmer series are found in the visible part of the spectrum.

Other series were found in the invisible parts of the spectrum *e.g.* Lyman series in the ultraviolet region and Paschen, Brackett and Pfund series in the infrared region. The wavelengths of line in these series can be expressed by the following formulae

(i) For Lyman series

$$\frac{1}{\lambda} = R\left(\frac{1}{1^2} - \frac{1}{n^2}\right), \text{ where } n = 2, 3, 4, \ldots$$

(ii) For Balmer series

$$\frac{1}{\lambda} = R\left(\frac{1}{2^2} - \frac{1}{n^2}\right), \text{ where } n = 3, 4, 5, \ldots$$

(iii) For Paschen series

$$\frac{1}{\lambda} = R\left(\frac{1}{3^2} - \frac{1}{n^2}\right), \text{ where } n = 4, 5, 6, \ldots$$

(iv) For Brackett series

$$\frac{1}{\lambda} = R\left(\frac{1}{4^2} - \frac{1}{n^2}\right), \text{ where } n = 5, 6, 7, \ldots$$

(v) For Pfund series

$$\frac{1}{\lambda} = R\left(\frac{1}{5^2} - \frac{1}{n^2}\right), \text{ where } n = 6, 7, 8, \ldots$$

Explanation

Different series of hydrogen spectrum can be explained by Bohr's theory.

According to Bohr's theory, if the ionised state of hydrogen atom be taken as zero energy level (at ∞), then the energies of the different energy levels of the atom can be expressed by the following formula

$$E_n = -\frac{Rhc}{n^2}, \text{ where } n = 1, 2, 3, \ldots$$

where, R is Rydberg's constant, h is Planck's constant and the integer n is called principal quantum number.

When the atom gets energy from outside, its electron goes from the lower energy level to some higher energy level. But it returns from there, within 10^{-8} s, to the lower energy level directly or through other lower energy levels. While returning back, the atom emits photons.

The energy levels of hydrogen atom are shown in the figure

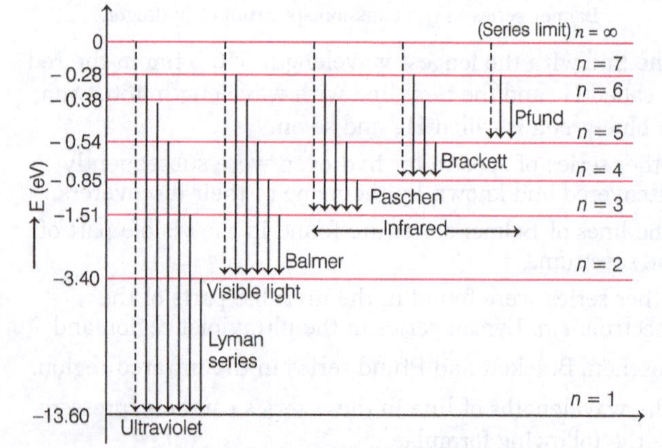

Emission spectrum of H-atom

Series Limit

The transitions corresponding to maximum energy or smallest wavelength of a given series of hydrogen spectrum is called series limit.

To calculate wavelength corresponding to series limit, we use $n_2 = \infty$.

For Lyman series, $\frac{1}{\lambda} = R\left(\frac{1}{1^2} - \frac{1}{\infty}\right) \Rightarrow \lambda = \frac{1}{R}$

For Balmer series, $\frac{1}{\lambda} = \frac{R}{4}$

In general, series limit $\frac{1}{\lambda} = \frac{R}{n^2}$

where, $n = 1, 2, 3, 4, \ldots$.

NEET Snapshot

Atom of each element have their characteristics spectrum. *[NEET 2024]*

Atoms have different energy levels, so emission and absorption spectrum of every atom is unique.

Scan for Video

Example 17. *A 12.5 eV electron beam is used to bombard gaseous hydrogen at room temperature. Which series of wavelengths will be emitted?*

Sol. Energy of electron beam, $E = 12.5$ eV

Planck's constant, $h = 6.62 \times 10^{-34}$ J-s

So, using the relation,

$E = \frac{hc}{\lambda}$, we get

$$\lambda = \frac{hc}{E} = \frac{6.62 \times 10^{-34} \times 3 \times 10^8}{12.5 \times 1.6 \times 10^{-19}}$$

$$= 0.993 \times 10^{-7} = 993 \times 10^{-10} \text{ m}$$

$$= 993 \text{ Å}$$

This wavelength falls in the range of Lyman series (912 Å to 1216 Å), thus we conclude that Lyman series is emitted.

Example 18. *In H-atom, a transition takes place from $n = 3$ to $n = 2$ orbit. Calculate the wavelength of the emitted photon and will the photon be visible? To which spectral series will this photon belong? (Take, $R = 1.097 \times 10^7 m^{-1}$)*

Sol. The wavelength of the emitted photon is given by

$$\frac{1}{\lambda} = R\left(\frac{1}{n_1^2} - \frac{1}{n_2^2}\right)$$

When the transition takes place from $n = 3$ to $n = 2$, then

$$\frac{1}{\lambda} = (1.097 \times 10^7)\left(\frac{1}{2^2} - \frac{1}{3^2}\right) = 1.097 \times 10^7 \times \frac{5}{36}$$

$$\therefore \quad \lambda = \frac{36}{1.097 \times 10^7 \times 5} = 6.563 \times 10^{-7} \text{m}$$

$$= 6563 \text{ Å}$$

λ falls in the visible (red) part of the spectrum, hence the photon will be visible. This photon is the first member of the Balmer series.

Example 19. *What is the shortest wavelength present in the Paschen series of spectral lines?*

Sol. For the shortest wavelength of Paschen series of spectral lines, $n_1 = 3, n_2 = \infty$. If λ_{min} be the minimum wavelength in this series of spectral lines, then

$$\frac{1}{\lambda_{min}} = R\left(\frac{1}{(3)^2} - \frac{1}{(\infty)^2}\right) = \frac{R}{9}$$

or $\lambda_{min} = \frac{9}{R} = \frac{9}{1.097\times 10^7}$ $(\because R = 1.097\times 10^7 m^{-1})$

$= 8204.2\times 10^{-10}$ m $= 8204.2$ Å

NEET Close-up

Example Similar to PYQ Asked in NEET 2023

In hydrogen spectrum, the shortest wavelength in Balmer series is λ. Then, what is the shortest wavelength in the Pfund series?

(a) $\frac{16\lambda}{3}$ (b) $\frac{9\lambda}{4}$
(c) $\frac{25\lambda}{4}$ (d) $\frac{12\lambda}{5}$

Sol. (c) In hydrogen spectrum,

$$\frac{1}{\lambda} = R\left(\frac{1}{n_1^2} - \frac{1}{n_2^2}\right)$$

For shortest wavelength in the Balmer series,

$n_1 = 2$ and $n_2 = \infty$

$$\therefore \frac{1}{\lambda_B} = R\left(\frac{1}{2^2} - \frac{1}{\infty^2}\right)$$

$$\Rightarrow \frac{1}{\lambda} = \frac{R}{4} \quad \{\because \lambda_B = \lambda\}$$

$$\Rightarrow R = \frac{4}{\lambda} \quad \ldots (i)$$

For the shortest wavelength of Pfund series,

$n_1 = 5$ and $n_2 = \infty$

$$\therefore \frac{1}{\lambda_P} = R\left(\frac{1}{5^2} - \frac{1}{\infty^2}\right)$$

$$= \frac{R}{25} = \frac{4/\lambda}{25} \quad \text{[from Eq. (i)]}$$

$$\Rightarrow \frac{1}{\lambda_P} = \frac{4}{25\lambda}$$

$$\Rightarrow \lambda_P = \frac{25\lambda}{4}$$

Skill Builder

In hydrogen spectrum, the shortest wavelength in the lyman series is λ. The shortest wavelength in the Paschen series is

(a) 7λ (b) 8λ
(c) 9λ (d) 10λ

For More Practice Refer Q. No. 8, 9, 12, 15 of step up practice-3 and Q. No. 77 of Gearing up for NEET.

Example 20. *Find the largest and shortest wavelengths in the Brackett series for hydrogen. In what region of the electromagnetic spectrum does each series lie?*

Sol. The wavelength relation for Bracket series is given by

$$\frac{1}{\lambda} = R\left(\frac{1}{4^2} - \frac{1}{n^2}\right), \text{ where } n = 5, 6, \ldots$$

The largest wavelength is corresponding to $n = 5$.

$$\therefore \frac{1}{\lambda_{max}} = 1.097\times 10^7\left(\frac{1}{16} - \frac{1}{25}\right)$$

or $\lambda_{max} = 40.650\times 10^{-7}$ m $= 40650$ Å

The shortest wavelength corresponds to $n = \infty$.

$$\therefore \frac{1}{\lambda_{min}} = 1.097\times 10^7\left(\frac{1}{16} - \frac{1}{\infty}\right)$$

or $\lambda_{min} = 14.58\times 10^{-7}$ m $= 14585$ Å

Both of these wavelengths lie in infrared region of electromagnetic spectrum.

Example 21. *If the series limit wavelength of the Lyman series for hydrogen atom is 912 Å, then find the series limit wavelength for the Balmer series for the hydrogen atom.*

Sol. For series limit wavelength of Lyman series,

$n_1 = 1, n_2 = \infty$

$$\Rightarrow \frac{1}{\lambda} = R\left(\frac{1}{n_1^2} - \frac{1}{n_2^2}\right) = R$$

or $\lambda = \frac{1}{R} = 912\text{Å} = 912\times 10^{-10}$m ...(i)

For series limit of Balmer series, we can write $n_1 = 2, n_2 = \infty$

$$\Rightarrow \frac{1}{\lambda} = R\left(\frac{1}{n_1^2} - \frac{1}{n_2^2}\right)$$

$$= R\left[\frac{1}{(2)^2} - \frac{1}{(\infty)^2}\right] = \frac{R}{4}$$

$$\therefore \lambda = \frac{4}{R} = 4\times 912\times 10^{-10}\text{m} \quad \text{[from Eq. (i)]}$$

$$= 4\times 912 \text{ Å} = 3648 \text{ Å}$$

Example 22. *Calculate (i) the wavelength and (ii) the frequency of the H_β line of the Balmer series for hydrogen.*

Sol. (i) H_β line of Balmer series corresponds to the transition from $n = 4$ to $n = 2$ level. So, the corresponding wavelength for H_β line is

$$\frac{1}{\lambda} = (1.097\times 10^7)\left(\frac{1}{2^2} - \frac{1}{4^2}\right)$$

or $\lambda = 4.9\times 10^{-7}$ m

(ii) Further, $f = \frac{c}{\lambda} = \frac{3\times 10^8}{4.9\times 10^{-7}}$

STEP UP Practice 3

1. When an electron de-excites from level n to level $n-1$ in an hydrogen atom, frequency of emitted radiation is
(a) n times of frequency of revolution of electron in the orbit
(b) $(n-1)$ times of frequency of revolution of electron in orbit
(c) same as that of frequency of revolution of electron in the orbit only for large values of n
(d) same as that of frequency of revolution of electron in the orbit only for small values of n

2. The ionisation energy of hydrogen is 13.6 eV. The energy of the photon released when an electron jumps from the first excited state ($n = 2$) to the ground state of hydrogen atom is
(a) 3.4 eV (b) 4.53 eV (c) 10.2 eV (d) 13.6 eV

3. If an electron in hydrogen atom jumps from an orbit of level $n = 3$ to an orbit of level $n = 2$, emitted radiation has a frequency (R = Rydberg's constant, c = velocity of light)
(a) $\frac{3Rc}{27}$ (b) $\frac{Rc}{25}$ (c) $\frac{8Rc}{9}$ (d) $\frac{5Rc}{36}$

4. **Assertion** (A) Energy required to excite an electron in hydrogen atom to its first excited state is 10.2 eV.
Reason (R) Energy of an electron of hydrogen atom is $-\frac{13.6}{n^2}$ eV.
In the light of the above statements, choose the correct answer from the options given below.
(a) Both A and R are true but R is not the correct explanation of A.
(b) A is true but R is false.
(c) A is false but R is true.
(d) Both A and R are true and R is the correct explanation of A.

5. **Assertion** (A) It is essential that all the lines available in the emission spectrum will not be available in the absorption spectrum.
Reason (R) The spectrum of hydrogen atom is only absorption spectrum.
In the light of the above statements, choose the correct answer from the options given below.
(a) Both A and R are true but R is not the correct explanation of A.
(b) A is true but R is false.
(c) A is false but R is true.
(d) Both A and R are true and R is the correct explanation of A.

6. **Assertion** (A) Between any two given energy levels, the number of absorption transitions is always less than the number of emission transition.
Reason (R) Absorption transition is a one step process it starts always from the ground level, whereas an emission transition may start from any higher energy level and end at any lower energy level.
In the light of the above statements, choose the correct answer from the options given below.
(a) Both A and R are true but R is not the correct explanation of A.
(b) A is true but R is false.
(c) A is false but R is true.
(d) Both A and R are true and R is the correct explanation of A.

7. Which one of the series of hydrogen spectrum is in the visible region?
(a) Lyman series (b) Balmer series
(c) Paschen series (d) Brackett series

8. The ratio of the largest to shortest wavelengths in Balmer series of hydrogen spectrum is
(a) $\frac{25}{9}$ (b) $\frac{17}{6}$ (c) $\frac{9}{5}$ (d) $\frac{5}{4}$

9. If wavelength of the first line of the Balmer series of hydrogen is 6561Å, the wavelength of the second line of the series should be
(a) 13122Å (b) 3280Å (c) 4860Å (d) 2187Å

10. **Assertion** (A) For Balmer series of hydrogen spectrum, the value $n_1 = 2$ and $n_2 = 3, 4, 5$.
Reason (R) The value of n for a line in Balmer series of hydrogen spectrum having the highest wavelengths is 4 and 6.
In the light of the above statements, choose the correct answer from the options given below.
(a) Both A and R are true but R is not the correct explanation of A.
(b) A is true but R is false.
(c) A is false but R is true.
(d) Both A and R are true and R is the correct explanation of A.

11. The ionisation energy of the electron in the hydrogen atom in its ground state is 13.6 eV. The atoms are excited to higher energy levels to emit radiations of 6 wavelengths. Maximum wavelength of emitted radiation corresponds to the transition between
(a) $n = 3$ to $n = 1$ states (b) $n = 4$ to $n = 3$ states
(c) $n = 3$ to $n = 2$ states (d) $n = 2$ to $n = 1$ states

12. Ratio of longest wavelengths corresponding to Lyman and Balmer series in hydrogen spectrum is
(a) $\frac{5}{27}$ (b) $\frac{3}{23}$ (c) $\frac{7}{29}$ (d) $\frac{9}{31}$

13. Which series of hydrogen spectrum corresponds to ultraviolet region?
(a) Balmer series (b) Brackett series
(c) Paschen series (d) Lyman series

14. If the series limit of Lyman series for hydrogen atom is equal to the series limit of Balmer series for a hydrogen like atom, then atomic number of this hydrogen like atom is
(a) 1 (b) 2 (c) 3 (d) 4

15. The wavelength of first line of Balmer series is 6563 Å. The wavelength of first line of Lyman series will be
(a) 1215.4 Å (b) 2500 Å (c) 7500 Å (d) 600 Å

16. If ν_1 is the frequency of the series limit of Lyman series, ν_2 is the frequency of the first line of Lyman series and ν_3 is the frequency of the series limit of the Balmer series. Then,
(a) $\nu_1 - \nu_2 = \nu_3$ (b) $\nu_1 = \nu_2 - \nu_3$
(c) $\frac{1}{\nu_2} = \frac{1}{\nu_1} + \frac{1}{\nu_3}$ (d) $\frac{1}{\nu_1} = \frac{1}{\nu_2} + \frac{1}{\nu_3}$

17. Electron in hydrogen atom first jumps from third excited state to second excited state and then from second excited to the first excited state. The ratio of the wavelengths $\lambda_1:\lambda_2$ emitted in the two cases is

(a) $\frac{7}{5}$ (b) $\frac{27}{20}$

(c) $\frac{27}{5}$ (d) $\frac{20}{7}$

18. Which one of the following pair is incorrect?

(a) According to Bohr's theory, $E_n \rightarrow \frac{-Rhc}{n^2}$

(b) $\lambda_{Lyman} : \lambda_{Balmer} \rightarrow 1:4$

(c) $\frac{1}{\lambda} \rightarrow n^2R$(for series limit)

(d) Ionisation potential $\rightarrow \frac{\text{Ionisation energy}}{e}$ (in eV

NEET Exclusive EXTRA BYTES

- In Hydrogen atom, both electrons and Nucleus revolves about the axis passing through their common COM.
- Recoil energy of atom is given by $\frac{p^2}{2m}$.
- Reduced mass of two particle system of H-atom is given by $\mu = \frac{m_e m_H}{m_e + m_H}$.
- Results of Bohr's Model

Physical Quantity	Proportional to
Radius (r_n)	n^2/Z
Speed (v_n)	Z/n
Frequency (f), angular speed (ω_n)	Z^2/n^3
Time period (T_n)	n^3/Z^2
Orbital Current	Z^2/n^3
Energy	Z^2/n^2

- Total number of emission lines from some excited state n_1 to another energy state $n_2 (< n_1)$ is given by $\frac{(n_1 - n_2)(n_1 - n_2 + 1)}{2}$.
- As the principal quantum number n is increased in hydrogen and hydrogen like atoms, some quantities are decreased and some are increased. The quantities which are increased and decreased are shown below

  Increased $\rightarrow$ Radius, potential energy, total energy, time period and angular momentum.

  Decreased $\rightarrow$ Speed, kinetic energy and angular speed.

GEARING UP FOR NEET

Single Correct Option

1. In Rutherford scattering experiment, what will be the ratio of impact parameter for scattering angles $\theta_1 = 90°$ and $\theta_2 = 120°$.
(a) 1 (b) $\sqrt{2}$ (c) 2 (d) $\sqrt{3}$

2. The velocity of an electron in the first orbit of H-atom is v. The velocity of an electron in the 2nd orbit of He^+ is
(a) $2v$ (b) v (c) $v/2$ (d) $v/4$

3. If the number of scattering particles are 56 for 90° angle, then at an angle 60°, number of scattered particles will be
(a) 224 (b) 256 (c) 98 (d) 108

4. The diagram shows the path of four α-particles of the same energy being scattered by the nucleus of an atom simultaneously. Which of these are/is not physically possible?

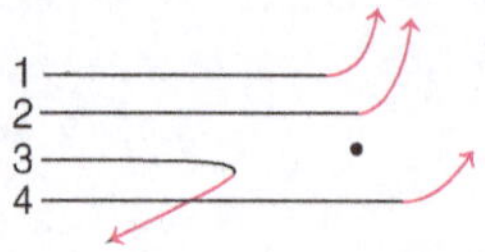

(a) Both 3 and 4 (b) Both 2 and 3
(c) Both 1 and 4 (d) Only 4

5. If ω is the speed of electron in the nth orbit hydrogen atom, then
(a) $\omega \propto n^{1/2}$ (b) $\omega \propto \frac{1}{n}$
(c) $\omega \propto \frac{1}{n^2}$ (d) $\omega \propto \frac{1}{n^3}$

6. The wavelength of the first spectral line of sodium 5896 Å. The first excitation potential of sodium atom will be (Planck's constant, $h = 6.63 \times 10^{-34}$ J-s)
(a) 4.2 eV (b) 3.5 eV
(c) 2.1 eV (d) None of these

7. A beam of fast moving α-particles were directed towards a thin film of gold. The parts A', B' and C' of the transmitted and reflected beams corresponding to the incident parts A, B and C of the beam, are shown in the adjoining diagram. The number of α-particles in

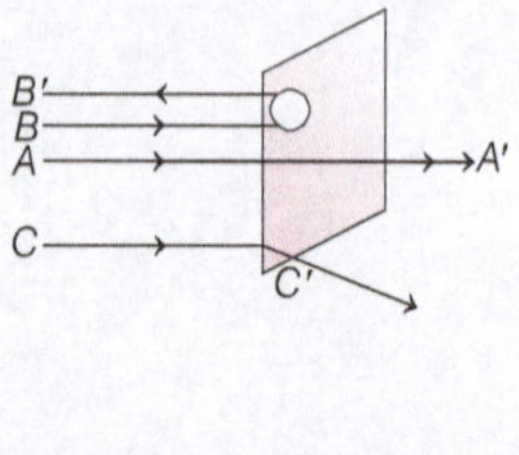

(a) B' will be minimum and in C' maximum
(b) A' will be maximum and in B' minimum
(c) A' will be minimum and in B' maximum
(d) C' will be minimum and in B' maximum

8. The Rutherford scattering experiment proves that an atom consists of
(a) a sphere of positive charge in which electrons are embedded like seeds of water-melon
(b) a sphere of negative charge in which protons are embedded like seeds of water-melon
(c) a sphere of electron cloud in which the positive charge is placed at the centre of the sphere
(d) a sphere of neutral charge

9. If an α-particle of mass m, charge q and velocity v is incident on a nucleus of charge Q and mass m, then the distance of closest approach is
(a) $\frac{Qq}{4\pi\varepsilon_0 m^2}$ (b) $\frac{Qq}{2\pi\varepsilon_0 mv^2}$
(c) $\frac{Qq\, mv^2}{2}$ (d) $\frac{Qq}{mv^2}$

10. Excitation energy of a hydrogen like ion in its first excitation state is 40.8 eV. Energy needed to remove the electron from the ion in ground state is
(a) 54.4 eV (b) 13.6 eV
(c) 40.8 eV (d) 27.2 eV

11. The simple Bohr model cannot be directly applied to calculate the energy levels of an atom with many electrons. This is because ***[NCERT Exemplar]***
(a) of the electrons not being subject to a central force
(b) of the electrons colliding with each other
(c) of screening effects
(d) the force between the nucleus and an electron will not longer be given by Coulomb's law

12. An electron moves in a circular orbit at a distance from a proton with kinetic energy E. To escape to infinity, the minimum energy which must be supplied to the electron is
(a) E (b) $2E$ (c) $0.5E$ (d) $E\sqrt{2}$

13. The minimum energy required to ionise an atom is the energy equal to
(a) add one electron to the gaseous state of atom
(b) excite the atom from its ground state to its first excited state

(c) remove one outermost electron from the gaseous state of atom
(d) remove one innermost electron from the gaseous state of atom

14. The orbital angular momentum of electron in the n_1th shell of element of atomic number Z_1 is L_1 and the same in the n_2th shell of element of atomic number Z_2 is L_2. If $L_2 > L_1$, then
(a) $n_2 > n_1$ (b) $Z_2 > Z_1$
(c) $n_2 Z_2 > n_1 Z_1$ (d) Both (a) and (b)

15. The difference in angular momentum associated with the electron in the two successive orbits of hydrogen atom is
(a) $\frac{h}{\pi}$ (b) $\frac{h}{2\pi}$ (c) $\frac{h}{2}$ (d) $(n-1)\frac{h}{2\pi}$

16. In a hypothetical Bohr hydrogen, the mass of the electron is doubled. The energy E_0 and radius r_0 of the first orbit will be (a_0 is the Bohr radius)
(a) $E_0 = -27.2$ eV, $r_0 = a_0/2$ (b) $E_0 = -27.2$ eV, $r_0 = a_0$
(c) $E_0 = -13.6$ eV $r_0 = a_0/2$ (d) $E_0 = -13.6$ eV, $r_0 = a_0$

17. An electron makes a transition from 4th orbit to 2nd orbit of a hydrogen atom. The wave number of the emitted radiations will be (R = Rydberg's constant)
(a) $\frac{16}{3R}$ (b) $\frac{2R}{16}$ (c) $\frac{3R}{16}$ (d) $\frac{4R}{16}$

18. If the radius of first Bohr's orbit is x, then de-Broglie wavelength of electron in 3rd orbit is nearly
(a) $2\pi x$ (b) $6\pi x$ (c) $9x$ (d) $\frac{x}{3}$

19. Taking the Bohr radius as $a_0 = 53$ pm, the radius of Li^{++} ion in its ground state, on the basis of Bohr's model, will be about ***[NCERT Exemplar]***
(a) 53 pm (b) 27 pm (c) 18 pm (d) 13 pm

20. When an electron in hydrogen atom is excited, from its 4th to 5th stationary orbit, the change in angular momentum of electron is (take, Planck's constant, $h = 6.6 \times 10^{-34}$ J-s)
(a) 4.16×10^{-34} J-s (b) 3.32×10^{-34} J-s
(c) 1.05×10^{-34} J-s (d) 5.25×10^{-34} J-s

21. An electron revolves around a nucleus of charge Ze. In order to excite the electron from the state $n = 2$ to $n = 3$, the energy required is 47.2 eV. Z is equal to
(a) 3 (b) 4 (c) 5 (d) 2

22. Ionisation potential of hydrogen atom is 13.6 V. Hydrogen atoms in the ground state are excited by monochromatic radiation of photon energy 12.1 eV. The spectral lines emitted by hydrogen atoms according to Bohr's theory will be
(a) one (b) two (c) three (d) four

23. The acceleration of electron in the first orbit of hydrogen atom is
(a) $\frac{4\pi^2 m}{h^3}$ (b) $\frac{h^2}{4\pi^2 mr}$ (c) $\frac{h^2}{4\pi^2 m^2 r^3}$ (d) $\frac{m^2 h^2}{4\pi^2 r^3}$

24. The magnetic moment (μ) of a revolving electron around the nucleus varies with principal quantum number n as
(a) $\mu \propto n$ (b) $\mu \propto 1/n$ (c) $\mu \propto n^2$ (d) $\mu \propto 1/n^2$

25. The ratio between acceleration of the electron in singly ionised helium atom and doubly ionised lithium atom (both in ground state) is
(a) $\frac{4}{9}$ (b) $\frac{27}{8}$ (c) $\frac{8}{27}$ (d) $\frac{9}{4}$

26. An electron with kinetic energy 5 eV is incident on a H-atom in its ground state. The collision
(a) must be elastic
(b) may be partially elastic
(c) must be completely inelastic
(d) may be completely inelastic

27. The energy of an electron in excited hydrogen atom is -3.4 eV. Then, according to Bohr's theory, the angular momentum of the electron is
(a) 2.1×10^{-34} J-s (b) 3×10^{-34} J-s
(c) 2×10^{-34} J-s (d) 0.5×10^{-34} J-s

28. The shortest wavelength which can be obtained in hydrogen spectrum is ($R = 10^7$ m^{-1})
(a) 1000 Å (b) 800 Å (c) 1300 Å (d) 2100 Å

29. Energy of 24.6 eV is required to remove one of the electron from a neutral helium atom. The energy (in eV) required to remove both the electrons from a neutral helium atom is
(a) 38.2 (b) 49.2 (c) 51.8 (d) 79.0

30. According to Moseley's law the ratio of the slope of graph between $\sqrt{f}$ and Z for K_β and K_α is
(a) $\sqrt{\frac{32}{27}}$ (b) $\sqrt{\frac{27}{32}}$ (c) $\sqrt{\frac{5}{36}}$ (d) $\sqrt{\frac{36}{5}}$

31. de-Broglie wavelength of an electron in the nth Bohr orbit of hydrogen atom is λ_n and the angular momentum is J_n, then
(a) $J_n \propto \lambda_n$ (b) $\lambda_n \propto \frac{1}{J_n}$
(c) $\lambda_n \propto J_n^2$ (d) None of these

32. An α-particle accelerated through V volt is fired towards a nucleus. Its distance of closest approach is r. If a proton accelerated through the same potential is fired towards the same nucleus, the distance of closest approach of proton will be
(a) r (b) $2r$ (c) $\frac{r}{2}$ (d) $\frac{r}{4}$

33. The radius of hydrogen atom in its ground state is 5.3×10^{-11} m. After collision with an electron it is found to have a radius of 21.2×10^{-11} m. What is the principal quantum number n of the final state of the atom?
(a) $n = 4$ (b) $n = 2$
(c) $n = 16$ (d) $n = 3$

34. In a Rutherford scattering experiment, when a projectile of charge Z_1 and mass M_1 approaches a target nucleus of charge Z_2 and mass M_2, the distance to closest approach is r_0. The energy of the projectile is
(a) directly proportional to $M_1 \times M_2$
(b) directly proportional to $Z_1 Z_2$
(c) directly proportional to Z_1
(d) directly proportional to mass M_1

35. In the Bohr's model of a hydrogen atom, the centripetal force is furnished by the Coulomb attraction between the proton and the electron. If a_0 is the radius of the ground state orbit, m is the mass, e is the charge on electron and ε_0 is the permittivity of free space, the speed of the electron is

(a) $\frac{e}{\sqrt{\varepsilon_0 a_0 m}}$ (b) zero (c) $\frac{e}{\sqrt{4\pi\varepsilon_0 a_0 m}}$ (d) $\frac{\sqrt{4\,\varepsilon_0 a_0 m}}{e}$

36. In a hydrogen atom, the binding energy of the electron in the ground state is E_1. Then the frequency of revolution of the electron in the nth orbit is

(a) $\frac{2E_1}{n^3 h}$ (b) $\frac{2E_1 n^3}{h}$ (c) $\sqrt{\frac{2mE_1}{n^3 h}}$ (d) $\frac{E_1 n^2}{h}$

37. The electron in a hydrogen atom makes transition from M shell to L-shell. The ratio of magnitude of initial to final acceleration of the electron is

(a) 9 : 4 (b) 81 : 16
(c) 4 : 9 (d) 16 : 81

38. For the ground state, the electron in the H-atom has an angular momentum = h, according to the simple Bohr model. Angular momentum is a vector and hence there will be infinitely many orbits with the vector pointing in all possible directions. In actuality, this is not true, *[NCERT Exemplar]*

(a) because Bohr model gives incorrect values of angular momentum
(b) because only one of these would have a minimum energy
(c) angular momentum must be in the direction of spin of electron
(d) because electrons go around only in horizontal orbits

39. A H-atom moving with speed v makes a head on collision with a H-atom at rest. Both atoms are in ground state. The minimum value of velocity v for which one of the atom may excite is($m_H = 1.67 \times 10^{-27}$ kg)

(a) 6.25×10^4 ms^{-1} (b) 8×10^4 ms^{-1}
(c) 7.25×10^4 ms^{-1} (d) 13.6×10^4 ms^{-1}

40. In an inelastic collision an electron excites a hydrogen atom from its ground state to a M-shell state. A second electron collides instantaneously with the excited hydrogen atom in the M-shell state and ionizes it. At least how much energy the second electron transfers to the atom in the M-shell state?

(a) + 3.4 eV (b) + 1.51 eV
(c) − 3.4 eV (d) − 1.51 eV

41. A hydrogen-like atom emits radiations of frequency 2.7×10^{15} Hz when it makes a transition from $n = 2$ to $n = 1$. The frequency emitted in a transition from $n = 3$ to $n = 1$ will be

(a) 1.8×10^{15} Hz (b) 3.2×10^{15} Hz
(c) 4.7×10^5 Hz (d) 6.9×10^{15} Hz

42. Two H-atoms in the ground state collide inelastically. The maximum amount by which their combined kinetic energy is reduced is *[NCERT Exemplar]*

(a) 10.2 eV (b) 20.40 eV
(c) 13.6 eV (d) 27.2 eV

43. Figure shows the energy levels P, Q, R, S and G of an atom where G is the ground state. A red line in the emission spectrum of the atom can be obtained by an energy level change from Q to S. A blue line can be obtained by following energy level change

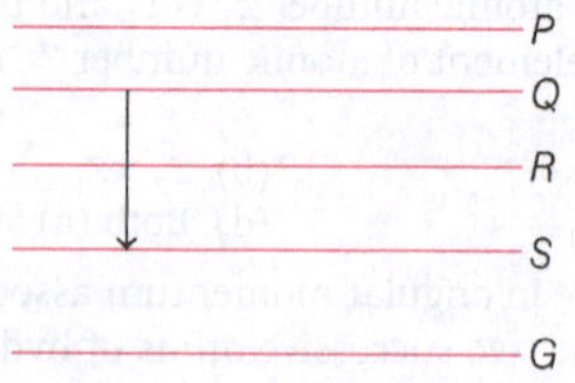

(a) P to Q (b) Q to P (c) R to S (d) R to G

44. The binding energy of a H-atom, considering an electron moving around a fixed nuclei (proton), is

$$B = -\frac{me^4}{8n^2\varepsilon_0^2h^2} \quad (m = \text{electron mass})$$

If one decides to work in a frame of reference where the electron is at rest, the proton would be moving around it. By similar arguments, the binding energy would be

$$B = -\frac{Me^4}{8n^2\varepsilon_0^2h^2} \quad (M = \text{proton mass})$$

This last expression is not correct, because *[NCERT Exemplar]*

(a) n would not be integral
(b) Bohr-quantisation applies only two electron
(c) the frame in which the electron is at rest, is non-inertial
(d) the motion of the proton would not be in circular orbits, even approximately.

45. The distance of closest approach of an α-particle fired towards a nucleus with momentum p, is r. If the momentum of the α-particle is $2p$, then the corresponding distance of closest approach is

(a) $r/2$ (b) $2r$
(c) $4r$ (d) $r/4$

46. The first excited state of hydrogen atom is 10.2 eV above its ground state. The temperature is needed to excite hydrogen atoms to first excited level, is

(a) 7.9×10^4 K (b) 3.5×10^4 K
(c) 5.8×10^4 K (d) 14×10^4 K

47. Hydrogen ($_1H^1$), deuterium ($_1H^2$), singly ionised helium ($_2He^4$)$^+$ and doubly ionised lithium ($_3Li^6$)$^{++}$ all have one electron around the nucleus. Consider an electron transition from $n = 2$ to $n = 1$. If the wave lengths of emitted radiation are λ_1, λ_2, λ_3 and λ_4 respectively, then approximately which one of the following is correct?

(a) $4\lambda_1 = 2\lambda_2 = 2\lambda_3 = \lambda_4$ (b) $\lambda_1 = 2\lambda_2 = 2\lambda_3 = \lambda_4$
(c) $\lambda_1 = \lambda_2 = 4\lambda_3 = 9\lambda_4$ (d) $\lambda_1 = 2\lambda_2 = 3\lambda_3 = 4\lambda_4$

48. Suppose an electron is attracted towards the origin by a force $\frac{k}{r}$, where k is a constant and r is the distance of the electron from the origin. By applying Bohr model to this system, the radius of the nth orbital of the electron is found to be r_n and the kinetic energy of the electron to be T_n.

Then, which of the following is true?

(a) T_n independent of $n, r_n \propto n$

(b) $T_n \propto \frac{1}{n}, r_n \propto n$

(c) $T_n \propto \frac{1}{n}, r_n \propto n^2$

(d) $T_n \propto \frac{1}{n^2}, r_n \propto n^2$

49. A photon of wavelength 300 nm interacts with a stationary hydrogen atom in ground state. During the interaction, whole energy of the photon is transferred to the electron of the atom. State which possibility is correct. (Take, Planck's constant $= 4 \times 10^{-15}$ eVs, velocity of light $= 3 \times 10^8 \text{ ms}^{-1}$, ionisation energy of hydrogen = 13.6 eV)

(a) Electron will be knocked out of the atom.
(b) Electron will go to any excited state of the atom.
(c) Electron will go only to first excited state of the atom.
(d) Electron will keep orbiting in the ground state of the atom.

50. The ionisation potential of hydrogen atom is −13.6 eV. An electron in the ground state of a hydrogen atom absorbs a photon of energy 12.75 eV. How many different spectral lines can one expect when the electron make a downward transition

(a) 1 (b) 4 (c) 2 (d) 6

51. Hydrogen atom in ground state is excited by a monochromatic radiation of $\lambda = 975$ Å. Number of spectral lines in the resulting spectrum emitted will be

(a) 3 (b) 2 (c) 6 (d) 10

52. The de-Broglie wavelength of an electron in 4th orbit is (where, r = radius of 1st orbit)

(a) $2\pi r$ (b) $4\pi r$
(c) $8\pi r$ (d) $16\pi r$

53. According to Bohr model of hydrogen atom, only those orbits are permissible which satisfy the condition

(a) $mv = nh$ (b) $\frac{mv^2}{r} = n\left(\frac{h}{2\pi}\right)$

(c) $mvr = n\left(\frac{h}{2\pi}\right)$ (d) $mvr^2 = n\left(\frac{h}{2\pi}\right)$

54. If ground state energy of hydrogen atom is −13.6 eV, then potential energy of electron in 3rd excited state is

(a) 2.70 eV (b) − 2.70 eV
(c) − 1.70 eV (d) 1.70 eV

55. The K_α X-ray of molybdenum has a wavelength of 71×10^{-12} m. If the energy of a molybdenum atom with K-electron removed is 23.32 keV, then the energy of molybdenum atom when an L-electron removed is $(hc = 12.42 \times 10^{-7} \text{ eV})$

(a) 17.5 keV (b) 40.82 keV
(c) 23.32 keV (d) 5.82 keV

56. The ionisation energy of an electron in the ground state of helium atom is 24.6 eV. The energy required to remove both the electron is

(a) 51.8 eV (b) 79 eV
(c) 38.2 eV (d) 49.2 eV

57. The figure shows the energy level of certain atom. When the electron de-excites from $3E$ to E, an electromagentic wave of wavelength λ is emitted. What is the wavelength of the electromagnetic wave emitted when the electron de-excites from $\frac{5E}{3}$ to E?

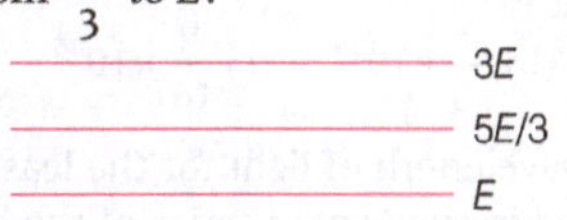

(a) 3λ (b) 2λ (c) 5λ (d) $\frac{3\lambda}{5}$

58. As per Bohr model, the minimum energy (in eV) required to remove an electron from the ground state of doubly ionised Li-atom ($Z = 3$) is

(a) 151 (b) 28.7 (c) 53.9 (d) 122.4

59. An electron of a stationary hydrogen atom passes from the fifth energy level to the ground level. The velocity that the atom acquired as a result of photon emission will be (m is the mass of the electron, R is Rydberg constant and h is Planck's constant)

(a) $\frac{24hR}{25m}$ (b) $\frac{25hR}{24m}$ (c) $\frac{25m}{24hR}$ (d) $\frac{24m}{25hR}$

60. In Bohr model of hydrogen atom, the force on the electron depends on the principal quantum number (n) as

(a) independent of n (b) $F \propto \frac{1}{n^5}$

(c) $F \propto \frac{1}{n^4}$ (d) $F \propto \frac{1}{n^3}$

61. The wavelength of K_α line in copper is 1.5 Å. The ionisation energy of K electron in copper is

(a) 11.2×10^{-17} J (b) 13.2×10^{-16} J
(c) 1.7×10^{-15} J (d) 10×10^{-16} J

62. The electron of a hydrogen atom revolves round the proton in a circular nth orbit of radius $r_n = \varepsilon_0 n^2 h^2 / (\pi m e^2)$ with a speed, $v_n = \frac{e^2}{2\varepsilon_0 nh}$.

The current due to the circulating charge is proportional to

(a) e^2 (b) e^3 (c) e^5 (d) e^6

63. Consider a hydrogen like atom whose energy in nth excited state is given by $E_n = -\frac{13.6Z^2}{n^2}$, when this excited atom makes a transition from excited state to ground state, most energetic photons have energy $E_{max} = 52.224$ eV and least energetic photons have energy $E_{min} = 1.224$ eV. The atomic number of atom is

(a) 2 (b) 4 (c) 5 (d) None of these

64. Hydrogen atom is excited from ground state to another excited state with principal quantum number ($n = 4$). Then, the number of spectral lines in the emission spectra will be

(a) 2 (b) 3
(c) 5 (d) 6

65. In which of the following systems will the radius of the first orbit ($n = 1$) be minimum?

(a) Hydrogen atom (b) Deuterium atom
(c) Singly ionised helium (d) Doubly ionised lithium

66. An electron jumps from the 4th orbit to 2nd orbit of the hydrogen atom. Given, Rydberg's constant $R = 10^5 \text{cm}^{-1}$, the frequency (in Hz) of the emitted radiations will be

(a) $\frac{3}{16} \times 10^5$ (b) $\frac{3}{16} \times 10^{15}$ (c) $\frac{9}{16} \times 10^{15}$ (d) $\frac{3}{4} \times 10^{15}$

67. What is the wavelength of light for the least energetic photon emitted in the Lyman series of the hydrogen spectrum? (Take, hc = 1240 eV-nm)

(a) 122 nm (b) 82 nm (c) 150 nm (d) 102 nm

68. Hydrogen atom emits blue light when it jumps from $n = 4$ energy level to the $n = 2$ level. Which colour of light would the atom emit when it changes from the $n = 5$ level to the $n = 2$ level?

(a) Red (b) Yellow (c) Green (d) Violet

69. The electron in a hydrogen atom makes a transition from $n = n_1$ to $n = n_2$ state. The time period of the electron in the initial state (n_1) is eight times that in the final state (n_2). The possible values of n_1 and n_2 are

(a) $n_1 = 8, n_2 = 1$ (b) $n_1 = 2, n_2 = 1$
(c) $n_1 = 2, n_2 = 4$ (d) $n_1 = 1, n_2 = 8$

70. The wavelength of K_α line for an element of atomic number 43 is λ. Then the wavelength of K_α line for an element of atomic number 29 is

(a) $\frac{43}{29}\lambda$ (b) $\frac{42}{28}\lambda$ (c) $\frac{9}{4}\lambda$ (d) $\frac{4}{9}\lambda$

71. The wavelength of radiation emitted is λ_0 when an electron jumps from the third to the second orbit of hydrogen atom. For the electron jump from the fourth to the second orbit of the hydrogen atom, the wavelength of radiation emitted will be

(a) $\frac{16}{25}\lambda_0$ (b) $\frac{20}{27}\lambda_0$ (c) $\frac{27}{20}\lambda_0$ (d) $\frac{25}{16}\lambda_0$

72. When an electron jumps from the orbit $n = 2$ to $n = 4$, then wavelength of the radiations absorbed will be (R is Rydberg's constant)

(a) $\frac{16}{3R}$ (b) $\frac{16}{5R}$ (c) $\frac{5R}{16}$ (d) $\frac{3R}{16}$

73. The given diagram indicates, the energy levels of a certain atom. When the system moves from $2E$ level to E, a photon of wavelength λ is emitted. The wavelength of photon produced during its transition from $4E/3$ level to E is

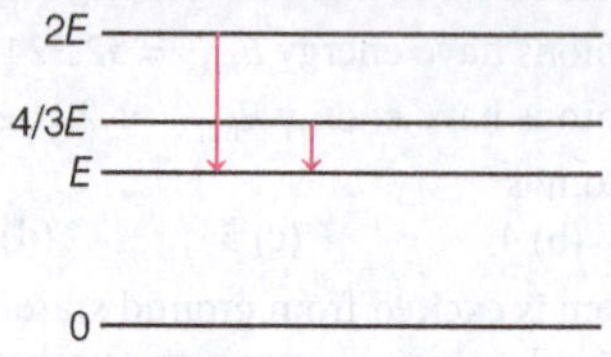

(a) $\lambda/3$ (b) $3\lambda/4$ (c) $4\lambda/3$ (d) 3λ

74. The shortest wavelength in Lyman series is 91.2 nm. The longest wavelength of the series is

(a) 121.6 nm (b) 182.4 nm (c) 243.4 nm (d) 364.8 nm

75. An excited hydrogen atom emits a photon of wavelength λ in returning to the ground state. The quantum number n of the excited state is given by (R = Rydberg constant)

(a) $\sqrt{\lambda R(\lambda R - 1)}$ (b) $\sqrt{\frac{\lambda R}{(\lambda R - 1)}}$

(c) $\sqrt{\frac{(\lambda R - 1)}{\lambda R}}$ (d) $\sqrt{\frac{1}{\lambda R(\lambda R - 1)}}$

76. The recoil momentum of H-atom due to the transition of an electron from $n = 4$ state to $n = 1$ state is

(a) 13.6×10^{-19} kg ms^{-1} (b) 6.8×10^{-27} kg ms^{-1}
(c) 12.75×10^{-24} kg ms^{-1} (d) 9.86×10^{-18} kg ms^{-1}

77. The first member of the Balmer's series of the hydrogen has a wavelength λ, the wavelength of the second member of its series is

(a) $\frac{27}{20}\lambda$ (b) $\frac{20}{27}\lambda$ (c) $\frac{27}{10}\lambda$ (d) $\frac{10}{9}\lambda$

78. In figure the energy levels of the hydrogen atom have been shown along with some transitions marking A, B, C. The transitions A, B, and C respectively, represents

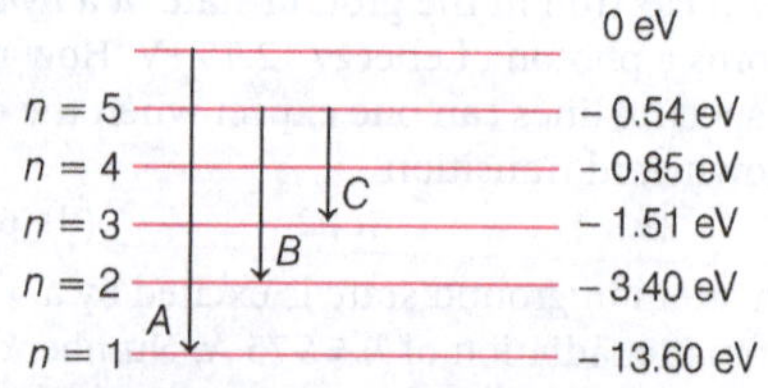

(a) the first member of the Lyman series, third member of Balmer series and second member of Paschen series
(b) the ionisation potential of H, second member of Balmer series and third member of Paschen series
(c) the series limit of Lyman series, second member of Balmer series and second member of Paschen series
(d) the series limit of Lyman series, third member of Balmer series and second member of Paschen series

79. Imagine an atom made up of a proton and a hypothetical particle of double the mass of the electron but having the same charge as the electron. Apply the Bohr atomic model and consider all possible transitions of this hypothetical particle to the first excited level. The longest wavelength of photon in the Balmer series has wavelength λ (given in terms of the Rydberg constant R for hydrogen atom) equal to

(a) $\frac{9}{5R}$ (b) $\frac{36}{5R}$ (c) $\frac{18}{5R}$ (d) $\frac{4}{5R}$

80. Energy levels A, B and C of a certain atom corresponding to increasing values of energy, i.e. $E_A < E_B < E_C$. If λ_1, λ_2 and λ_3 are the wavelengths of radiations corresponding to the transitions C to B, B to A and C to A respectively, which of the following option is correct?

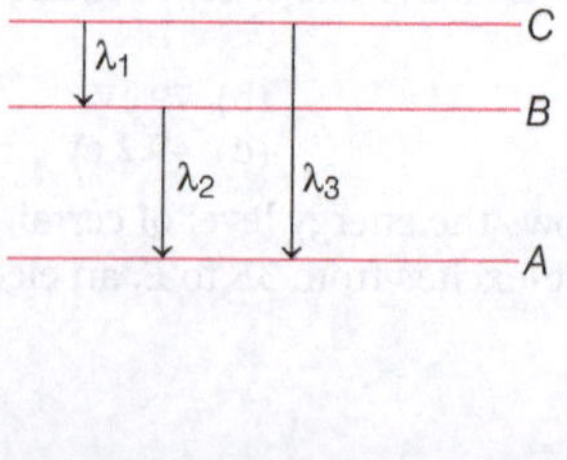

(a) $\lambda_3 = \lambda_1 + \lambda_2$ (b) $\lambda_3 = \dfrac{\lambda_1 \lambda_2}{\lambda_1 + \lambda_2}$

(c) $\lambda_1 + \lambda_2 + \lambda_3 = 0$ (d) $\lambda_3^2 = \lambda_1^2 + \lambda_2^2$

81. The following diagram indicates the energy levels of a certain atom when the system moves from $4E$ level to E. A photon of wavelength λ_1 is emitted. The wavelength of photon produced during its transition from $7/3\,E$ level to E is λ_2. The ratio λ_1/λ_2 will be

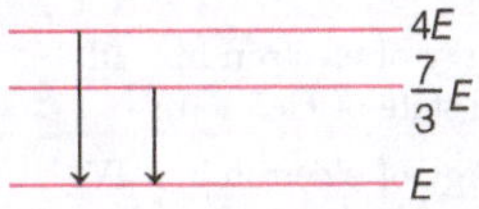

(a) $\dfrac{4}{9}$ (b) $\dfrac{4}{8}$ (c) $\dfrac{3}{8}$ (d) $\dfrac{5}{9}$

82. The diagram shows the energy levels for an electron in a certain atom. Which transition shown represents the emission of a photon with the most energy?

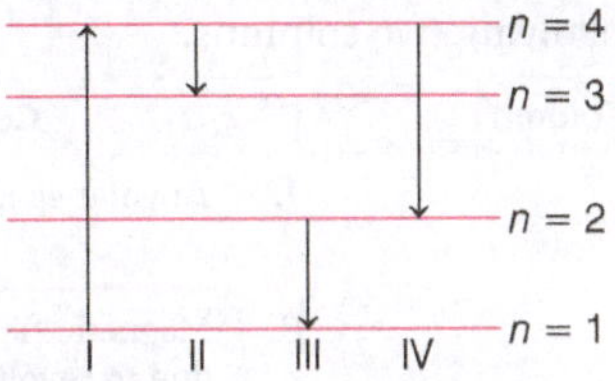

(a) III (b) IV (c) I (d) II

83. Light emitted during the de excitation of electron from $n = 3$ to $n = 2$, when incident on a metal, photoelectrons are just emitted from that metal. In which of the following de excitations photoelectric effect is not possible?

(a) From $n = 2$ to $n = 1$ (b) From $n = 3$ to $n = 1$

(c) From $n = 5$ to $n = 2$ (d) From $n = 4$ to $n = 3$

Assertion and Reason

Directions (Q. Nos. 1-5) *These questions consist of two statements each linked as Assertion (A) and Reason (R). While answering these questions you are required to choose any one of the following four responses.*

(a) Both A and R are true but R is not the correct explanation of A.
(b) A is true but R is false.
(c) A is false but R is true.
(d) Both A and R are true and R is the correct explanation of A.

1. **Assertion** (A) The radius of second orbit of hydrogen atom is 2.1Å.

Reason (R) Radius of nth orbit of hydrogen atom is $r_n \propto n^2$.

2. **Assertion** (A) Angular momentum of single electron in any orbit of hydrogen type atoms is independent of the atomic number of the element.

Reason (R) In ground state, angular momentum is minimum.

3. **Assertion** (A) Second orbit circumference of hydrogen atom is two times the de-Broglie wavelength of electrons in that orbit.

Reason (R) de-Broglie wavelength of electron in ground state is minimum.

4. **Assertion** (A) The first excitation energy of hydrogen atom is 10.2 eV.

Reason (R) Ionisation energy is equal to energy required to knock an electron completly out of the atom.

5. **Assertion** (A) Balmer series lies in the visible region of electromagnetic spectrum.

Reason (R) $\dfrac{1}{\lambda} = R\left(\dfrac{1}{2^2} - \dfrac{1}{n^2}\right)$, where $n = 3, 4, 5, \ldots$.

Statement Type Questions

Directions (Q. Nos. 1-5) *These questions consists of two statements, choose the most appropriate answer from the options given below.*

(a) Both Statement I and Statement II are incorrect.
(b) Statement I is correct but Statement II is incorrect.
(c) Statement I is incorrect but Statement II is correct.
(d) Both Statement I and Statement II are correct.

1. **Statement I** Rutherford's model cannot explain line emission spectrum of hydrogen atom.

Statement II Practically, a line emission spectrum is obtained but according to Rutherford's model, emission spectrum must be a continuous spectrum.

2. **Statement I** In Rutherford's model, there is not a continuous emission of energy by electron.

Statement II A negative total energy is necessary for a stationary stable orbit.

3. **Statement I** Considering Bohr's atom, graph of $\log_e\left(\dfrac{r_n}{r_1}\right)$ and $\log_e n$ has a slope of 2.

Statement II In case of Bohr's atom, $r_n = 0.53\left(\dfrac{n^2}{Z}\right)$ Å.

4. **Statement I** A hypothetical one electron atom (hydrogen like) with energy levels defined by $E_n = \dfrac{-18.0}{n^2}$ eV, shows only three distinct wavelengths in its emission spectrum, when bombarded by electrons accelerated by a potential difference of 16.2 V.

Statement II Maximum possible number of emission lines produced by an electron, when it makes transition from nth stationary state is $\dfrac{n}{2}(n-1)$.

5. **Statement I** Atoms of each element are stable and emit characteristic spectrum.

Statement II The spectrum provides useful information about the atomic structure.

Match the Columns

1. On the basis of Bohr's atomic model match the Column I and Column II for a hydrogen like atom, which have atomic number Z.

Column I		Column II
A.	Radius of orbit	I. proportional to Z
B.	Current due to motion of electron	II. inversely proportional to Z
C.	Magnetic field at centre of atom	III. proportional to Z^2
D.	Velocity of electron	IV. proportional to Z^3

Choose the correct answer from the options given below.

(a) A-IV, B-II, C-III, D-I
(b) A-I, B-IV, C-II, D-III
(c) A-II, B-III, C-IV, D-I
(d) A-III, B-I, C-II, D-IV

2. In Column I physical quantities corresponding to hydrogen and hydrogen like atoms are given. In Column II, powers of principal quantum number n are given on which, those physical quantities depend. Match the two columns.

Column I		Column II	
A.	Centripetal acceleration in circular motion of electron	I.	-4
B.	Angular momentum of electron	II.	1
C.	Moment of inertia of electron about centroidal axis	III.	4
D.	Energy of electron	IV.	-2

Choose the correct answer from the options given below.

(a) A-IV, B-I, C-III, D-II
(b) A-I, B-II, C-III, D-IV
(c) A-IV, B-II, C-I, D-III
(d) A-II, B-III, C-I, D-IV

3. Ground state energy of hydrogen atom is E_0. Match the following two columns.

Column I		Column II	
A.	Electrostatic potential energy in ground state of hydrogen atom	I.	$4E_0$
B.	Total energy in first excited state of He^+ ion	II.	$-2E_0$
C.	Kinetic energy of electron in first excited state of He^+ ion	III.	$2E_0$
D.	Kinetic energy of electron in ground state of hydrogen atom	IV.	$\frac{-E_0}{2}$

Choose the correct answer from the options given below.

(a) A-I, B-II, C-III, D-IV
(b) A-II, B-IV, C-III, D-I
(c) A-IV, B-III, C-I, D-II
(d) A-III, B-I, C-II, D-IV

4. Match the following two columns.

Column I		Column II	
A.	$\frac{Z^3}{n^5}$	I.	Angular speed
B.	$\frac{Z^2}{n^2}$	II.	Magnetic field at the centre due to revolution of electron
C.	$\frac{Z^2}{n^3}$	III.	Potential energy of an electron in nth orbit
D.	$\frac{Z}{n}$	IV.	Speed of electron in nth orbit

Choose the correct answer from the options given below.

(a) A-II, B-III, C-I, D-IV
(b) A-III, B-II, C-IV, D-I
(c) A-I, B-II, C-III, D-IV
(d) A-IV, B-III, C-II, D-IV

Final Check Through PYQs

Module-I Rutherford Model

1. When an α-particle of mass m moving with velocity v bombards on a heavy nucleus of charge Ze, its distance of closest approach from the nucleus depends on m as *[NCERT (New) Pg. 295, NEET 2016]*
(a) $\frac{1}{\sqrt{m}}$ (b) $\frac{1}{m^2}$
(c) m (d) $\frac{1}{m}$

Module-II Bohr's Model

2. The radius of inner most orbit of hydrogen atom is 5.3×10^{-11} m. What is the radius of third allowed orbit of hydrogen atom? *[NCERT (New) Pg. 296, NEET 2023]*
(a) 1.06 Å (b) 1.59 Å
(c) 4.77 Å (d) 0.53 Å

3. Let T_1 and T_2 be the energy of an electron in the first and second excited states of hydrogen atom, respectively. According to the Bohr's model of an atom, the ratio of $T_1 : T_2$ is *[NCERT (New) Pg. 299, NEET 2022]*
(a) 4 : 1 (b) 4 : 9
(c) 9 : 4 (d) 1 : 4

4. The total energy of an electron in the nth stationary orbit of the hydrogen atom can be obtained by *[NCERT (New) Pg. 299, NEET (Oct.) 2020]*
(a) $E_n = \frac{13.6}{n^2}$ eV (b) $E_n = -\frac{13.6}{n^2}$ eV
(c) $E_n = -\frac{1.36}{n^2}$ eV (d) $E_n = -13.6 \times n^2$ eV

5. For which one of the following, Bohr model is not valid? *[NCERT (New) Pg. 300, NEET (Sep.) 2020]*
(a) Singly ionised helium atom (He^+)
(b) Deuteron atom
(c) Singly ionised neon atom (Ne^+)
(d) Hydrogen atom

6. The radius of the first permitted Bohr orbit for the electron, in a hydrogen atom equals 0.51 Å and its ground state energy equals – 13.6 eV. If the electron in the hydrogen atom is replaced by muon (μ^{-1}) [Charge same as electron and mass 207 m_e], the first Bohr radius and ground state energy will be *[NCERT (New) Pg. 296, NEET (Odisha) 2019]*
(a) 0.53×10^{-13} m, – 3.6 eV
(b) 25.6×10^{-13} m, – 2.8 eV
(c) 2.56×10^{-13} m, – 2.8 keV
(d) 2.56×10^{-13} m, – 13.6 eV

7. The total energy of an electron in an atom in an orbit is –3.4 eV. Its kinetic and potential energies are, respectively *[NCERT (New) Pg. 299, NEET (National) 2019]*
(a) –3.4 eV, –6.8 eV (b) 3.4 eV, –6.8 eV
(c) 3.4 eV, 3.4 eV (d) –3.4 eV, –3.4 eV

8. The ratio of kinetic energy to the total energy of an electron in a Bohr orbit of the hydrogen atom, is *[NCERT (New) Pg. 299, NEET 2018]*
(a) 2 : –1 (b) 1 : –1
(c) 1 : 1 (d) 1 : – 2

9. If an electron in a hydrogen atom jumps from the 3rd orbit to the 2nd orbit, it emits a photon of wavelength λ. When it jumps from the 4th orbit to the 3rd orbit, the corresponding wavelength of the photon will be *[NCERT (New) Pg. 296, NEET 2016]*
(a) $\frac{16}{25}\lambda$ (b) $\frac{9}{16}\lambda$
(c) $\frac{20}{7}\lambda$ (d) $\frac{20}{13}\lambda$

10. Consider 3rd orbit of He^+ (Helium), using non-relativistic approach, the speed of electron in this orbit will be (given $K = 9 \times 10^9$ constant, $Z = 2$ and h (Planck's constant) $= 6.6 \times 10^{-34}$ J-s) *[NCERT (New) Pg. 296, AIPMT 2015]*
(a) 2.92×10^6 m/s (b) 1.46×10^6 m/s
(c) 0.73×10^6 m/s (d) 3.0×10^8 m/s

Module-III Hydrogen Spectrum

11. Match the following two columns.

Column I (Spectral lines of Hydrogen for transitions from)		Column II (Wavelengths (nm))
A. $n_2 = 3$ to $n_1 = 2$	I.	410.2
B. $n_2 = 4$ to $n_1 = 2$	II.	434.1
C. $n_2 = 5$ to $n_1 = 2$	III.	656.3
D. $n_2 = 6$ to $n_1 = 2$	IV.	486.1

[NCERT (New) Pg. 296, NEET 2024]

Choose the correct answer from the options given below.
(a) A-II, B-I, C-IV, D-III
(b) A-III, B-IV, C-II, D-I
(c) A-IV, B-III, C-I, D-II
(d) A-I, B-II, C-III, D-IV

12. Given below are two statements.

Statement I Atoms are electrically neutral as they contain equal number of positive and negative charges.

Statement II Atoms of each element are stable and emit their characteristic spectrum.

[NCERT (New) Pg. 296, NEET 2024]

In the light of the above statements, choose the most appropriate answer from the options given below.
(a) Both Statement I and Statement II are correct.
(b) Both Statement I and Statement II are incorrect.
(c) Statement I is correct but Statement II is incorrect.
(d) Statement I is incorrect but Statement II is correct.

13. In hydrogen spectrum, the shortest wavelength in the Balmer series is λ. The shortest wavelength in the Brackett series is *[NCERT (New) Pg. 296, NEET 2023]*
(a) 4λ (b) 9λ
(c) 16λ (d) 2λ

14. The ratio of wavelengths of the last line of Balmer series and the last line of Lyman series is *[NCERT (New) Pg. 296, NEET 2017]*
(a) 2 (b) 1
(c) 4 (d) 0.5

15. In the spectrum of hydrogen, the ratio of the longest wavelength in the Lyman series to the longest wavelength in the Balmer series is *[NCERT (New) Pg. 296, AIPMT 2015]*
(a) $\frac{4}{9}$ (b) $\frac{9}{4}$
(c) $\frac{27}{5}$ (d) $\frac{5}{27}$

Answers

Step up Practice 1

1 (a)	2 (d)	3 (b)	4 (d)	5 (d)	6 (a)	7 (a)	8 (d)	9 (d)	10 (d)
11 (b)	12 (b)	13 (c)	14 (b)	15 (b)	16 (d)	17 (b)	18 (a)	19 (c)	20 (a)
21 (c)	22 (d)	23 (b)	24 (d)						

Step up Practice 2

1 (c)	2 (b)	3 (b)	4 (c)	5 (b)	6 (c)	7 (d)	8 (c)	9 (d)	10 (c)
11 (b)	12 (b)	13 (a)	14 (b)	15 (d)	16 (d)	17 (c)	18 (b)	19 (a)	20 (c)
21 (d)	22 (a)	23 (a)							

Step up Practice 3

1 (c)	2 (c)	3 (d)	4 (d)	5 (b)	6 (c)	7 (b)	8 (c)	9 (c)	10 (b)
11 (b)	12 (a)	13 (d)	14 (b)	15 (a)	16 (a)	17 (d)	18 (c)		

Gearing up for NEET

1 (d)	2 (b)	3 (a)	4 (d)	5 (d)	6 (c)	7 (b)	8 (c)	9 (b)	10 (a)
11 (d)	12 (a)	13 (c)	14 (a)	15 (b)	16 (a)	17 (c)	18 (b)	19 (c)	20 (c)
21 (c)	22 (c)	23 (c)	24 (a)	25 (c)	26 (a)	27 (a)	28 (a)	29 (d)	30 (a)
31 (a)	32 (a)	33 (b)	34 (b)	35 (c)	36 (a)	37 (d)	38 (a)	39 (a)	40 (d)
41 (b)	42 (a)	43 (d)	44 (c)	45 (d)	46 (a)	47 (c)	48 (a)	49 (d)	50 (d)
51 (a)	52 (c)	53 (c)	54 (c)	55 (b)	56 (b)	57 (a)	58 (d)	59 (a)	60 (c)
61 (b)	62 (c)	63 (a)	64 (d)	65 (d)	66 (c)	67 (a)	68 (d)	69 (b)	70 (c)
71 (b)	72 (a)	73 (d)	74 (a)	75 (b)	76 (b)	77 (b)	78 (d)	79 (c)	80 (b)
81 (a)	82 (a)	83 (d)							

Assertion and Reason

1 (d)	2 (a)	3 (a)	4 (a)	5 (d)

Statement Type Questions

1 (d)	2 (c)	3 (d)	4 (d)	5 (d)

Match the Columns

1 (c)	2 (b)	3 (d)	4 (a)

Final Check through PYQs : Module-I

1 (d)

Final Check through PYQs : Module-II

2 (c)	3 (c)	4 (b)	5 (c)	6 (c)	7 (b)	8 (b)	9 (c)	10 (b)

Final Check through PYQs : Module-III

11 (b)	12 (c)	13 (a)	14 (c)	15 (d)

Hints and Solutions

Step up Practice 1

1. (*a*) In Rutherford's nuclear model of the atom, the entire positive charge and most of the mass of the atom are concentrated in the nucleus with the electrons some distance away.

2. (*d*) Both A and R are true and R is the correct explanation of A.

   Atom is electrically neutral. The atom contains positively charged protons and negatively charged electrons in equal numbers which make the atom neutral.

3. (*b*) For an electron,

   $e = 1.6\times 10^{-19}$ C, $m_e = 9.1\times 10^{-31}$ kg

   For a proton, $e = 1.6\times 10^{-19}$ C, $m_p = 1.6\times 10^{-27}$ kg

   For an α-particle,

   $e = 2\times 1.6\times 10^{-19}$ C, $m_\alpha \approx 4\times 1.6\times 10^{-27}$ kg

   Clearly, $\left(\frac{e}{m}\right)_e > \left(\frac{e}{m}\right)_p > \left(\frac{e}{m}\right)_\alpha$

4. (*d*) Rutherford's atom had a positively charged centre and electrons were revolving around it. It is also called the planetary model of the atom.

5. (*d*) Both A and R are true and R is the correct explanation of A.

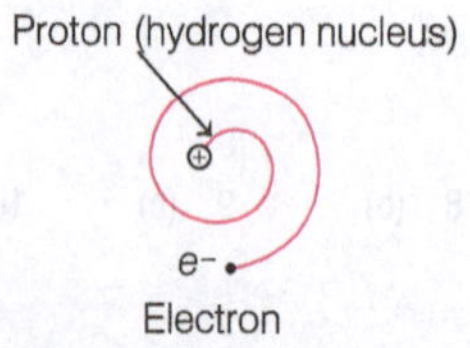

   According to classical electromagnetic theory, an accelerating charged particle emits radiation in the form of electromagnetic waves. The energy of an accelerating electron should, therefore continuously decrease. The electron would spiral inward and eventually fall into the nucleus as shown in figure. Thus, such an atom cannot be stable.

6. (*a*) At distance of minimum separation, KE = PE.

   $$\Rightarrow \quad KE = \frac{k\,Ze\cdot 2e}{r}$$

   $$\text{or} \quad KE = \frac{9\times 10^9 \times 79\times 2\times (1.6\times 10^{-19})^2}{4\times 10^{-14}}\ \text{J}$$

   $$= \frac{9\times 10^9 \times 79\times 2\,(1.6\times 10^{-19})^2}{4\times 10^{-14}\times 1.6\times 10^{-19}}\ \text{eV}$$

   $$= 5.688 \text{ MeV} \quad (\because 1 \text{ MeV} = 1.6\times 10^{-19}\text{ J})$$

7. (*a*) The scattered α-particles were observed through a rotatable detector consisting of zinc sulphide screen and a microscope. The scattered α-particles on striking the screen produced brief light flashes or scintillations. These flashes may be viewed through a microscope and the distribution of the number of scattered particles may be studied as a function of angle of scattering.

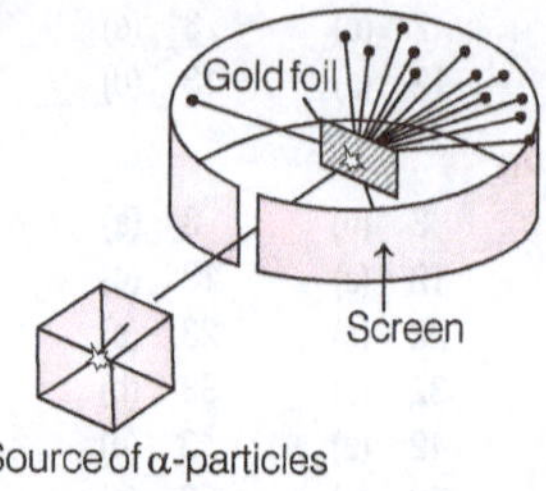

8. (*d*) As the gold foil is very thin, it can be assumed that α-particles will suffer not more than 1° scattering during their passage through it. Therefore, computation of the trajectory of an α-particle scattered by a single nucleus is enough.

9. (*d*) Most of α-particles pass straight through, few are deflected at small angles and very few are deflected by larger angles.

10. (*d*) Both A and R are true and R is the correct explanation of A.

    In α-particle scattering experiment, Rutherford found a small number of α-particles scattered back through an angle approaching to 180°. This is possible only if the positive charges are concentrated at the centre or nucleus of the atom.

11. (*b*) For the distance of closest approach, we can write

    $$\frac{1}{2}mv^2 = \frac{k\times (Ze)(2e)}{r_0} \quad \Rightarrow \quad r_0 \propto \frac{1}{m}$$

12. (*b*) The impact parameter is the perpendicular distance of the initial velocity vector of the α-particle from the centre line of the nucleus of atom.

13. (*c*) α-particle close to the nucleus (small impact parameter) suffers large scattering. In case of head-on collision, the impact parameter is minimum and the α-particle rebounds back ($\theta \simeq \pi$). For a large impact parameter, the α-particle goes nearly undeviated and has a small deflection ($\theta \simeq 0$).

14. (*b*) We know that, impact parameter, $b = K\cot\frac{\theta}{2}$

    Given, $\theta = 360°$

    $\therefore \quad b = K\times \cot 180° = \infty$

15. (b) $\sin^4\left(\frac{\theta}{2}\right)$

16. (d) Both A and R are true and R is the correct explanation of A.

α-particle is positively charged, so is the nucleus, so the large angle of scattering of α-particle shows that the nucleus is positively charged and concentrated in the central core.

17. (b) As we know that electrostatic force of attraction between electron and nucleus is $\frac{1}{4\pi\varepsilon_0}\frac{e^2}{r^2}$, hence, incorrect.

18. (a) Both A and R are true but R is not the correct explanation of A.

Rutherford confirmed that the repulsive force of α-particle due to nucleus varies with distance according to inverse square law and that the positive charges are concentrated at the centre and not distributed throughout the atom.

19. (c) For separation r, force between α-particle (charge $2e$) and gold nucleus (charge Ze) is

$$F = \frac{1}{4\pi\varepsilon_0} \times \frac{2e\,(Ze)}{r^2}$$

For gold, $Z = 79$

$$\therefore \quad F = \frac{1}{4\pi\varepsilon_0}\cdot\frac{158\,e^2}{r^2}$$

20. (a) The electrostatic force of attraction, F_e between the revolving electrons and the nucleus provides the centripetal force (F_c) to keep them in their orbits. Thus, for a dynamically stable orbit in a hydrogen atom $F_e = F_c$.

21. (c) $\frac{ke \times e}{r^2} = \frac{mv^2}{r}$

i.e., $r = \frac{e^2}{4\pi\varepsilon_0 mv^2}$

22. (d) The kinetic energy (K) of the electron in hydrogen atom is

$$K = \frac{1}{2}mv^2 = \frac{e^2}{8\pi\varepsilon_0 r}$$

23. (b) The total energy E of the electron in a hydrogen atom is

$$E = K + U = \frac{e^2}{8\pi\varepsilon_0 r} - \frac{e^2}{4\pi\varepsilon_0 r} = -\frac{e^2}{8\pi\varepsilon_0 r}$$

The total energy of the electron is negative. This implies the fact that the electron is bound to the nucleus. If E is positive, an electron will not follow a closed orbit around the nucleus.

24. (d) $r_n \propto \frac{n^2}{Z}$ or $r_n \propto \frac{1}{Z}$ (when n is constant)

Since, Z is minimum for hydrogen atom and maximum for doubly ionised lithium. so, r is minimum for option (d).

Step up Practice 2

1. (c) As, $r \propto n^2$

$$\frac{r_3}{r_1} = \frac{3^2}{1^2} = 9$$

$$\Rightarrow \quad r_3 = 9r_1 = 9r_0 \quad (\because r_1 = r_0)$$

2. (b) Statement I is correct but Statement II is incorrect.

Bohr postulated that electrons in stationary orbits around the nucleus do not radiate. This is the one of Bohr's postulate, according to this, the electrons radiates only when they go from one orbit to the next lower orbit.

According to classical physics only accelerated charge particles can radiate.

3. (b) Statement I is correct but Statement II is incorrect.

According to postulates of Bohr's atom model the electron revolves around the nucleus in fixed orbit of definite radii. Electrons revolve around the nucleus in fixed orbit due to centripetal force obtained from coulomb force.

4. (c) Using $E_n = -\frac{13.6}{n^2} = -3.4$ eV, we get $n = 2$

∴ Angular momentum

$$L = \frac{nh}{2\pi} = \frac{2\times 6.6\times 10^{-34}}{2\times 3.14} = 2.11\times 10^{-34} \text{ J-s}$$

5. (b) Statement I is correct but Statement II is incorrect.

Bohr's postulate states that the stationary orbits are those for which the angular momentum is some integral multiple of $\frac{h}{2\pi}$. i.e., $L = n\frac{h}{2\pi}$, where n is an integer called a quantum number. But linear momentum is not quantised.

6. (c) Change in angular momentum

$$\Delta L = L_2 - L_1 = \frac{n_2 h}{2\pi} - \frac{n_1 h}{2\pi} = \frac{6.6\times 10^{-34}}{2\times 3.14}\times(5-4)$$

$$= 1.05\times 10^{-34} \text{ J-s}$$

7. (d) In hydrogen atom, speed of an electron $v_n = \frac{2\pi Ze^2}{nh}$

and $v = \frac{2\pi e^2}{h} \Rightarrow \frac{v}{c} = \frac{2\pi e^2}{hc}$ $(\because Z = 1, n = 1)$

8. (c) The frequency of the electron moving around the proton is

$$\nu = \frac{v}{2\pi r} = \frac{2.2\times 10^6 \text{ m s}^{-1}}{2\pi\,(5.3\times 10^{-11} \text{ m})}$$

$$\approx 6.6\times 10^{15} \text{ Hz}$$

According to the classical electromagnetic theory, we know that the frequency of the electromagnetic waves emitted by the revolving electrons is equal to the frequency of its revolution around the nucleus. Thus, the initial frequency of the light emitted is 6.6×10^{15} Hz.

9. (d) Using, $v_n = \frac{1}{137}\frac{c}{n}$, we get

$$v_3 = \frac{1}{137}\times\frac{3\times10^8}{3} = 7.29\times10^5\ \text{ms}^{-1}$$

Also, $T_n = \frac{2\pi r_n}{v_n}$

$$\therefore\quad T_3 = \frac{2\pi r_3}{v_3} = \frac{2\pi\,(3^2\times0.53\times10^{-10})}{7.29\times10^5} = 4.10\times10^{-15}\ \text{s}$$

10. (c) As we know that,

Bohr's frequency condition $= \frac{E_2 - E_1}{h}$, hence, incorrect

Angular momentum $(mvr) = \frac{nh}{2\pi}$, hence, incorrect

Bohr's radius $(r_n) = n^2\frac{h^2\varepsilon_0}{\pi m Ze^2}$, hence, correct

Wave number (is reciprocal of wavelength.

$\therefore\quad \bar{v} = \frac{1}{\lambda}$, hence, incorrect.

11. (b) According to Bohr's model

$$v = \frac{2\pi Ke^2 Z}{nh}\quad\text{or}\quad v\propto\frac{1}{n}$$

$$\therefore\quad \frac{v_A}{v_B} = \frac{n_B}{n_A}$$

$$\therefore\quad v_B = v_A\times\frac{n_A}{n_B} = 2.6\times10^6\times\frac{1}{4} = 6\times10^5\ \text{ms}^{-1}$$

12. (b) Time period of revolution of electron in nth orbit,

$$T_n = \frac{nhr_n}{kZe^2}\quad\left(\text{where, } k = \frac{1}{4\pi\varepsilon_0}\right)$$

Since, $r_n \propto \frac{n^2}{Z}$

$$\therefore\quad T_n \propto n^3 \Rightarrow \frac{1}{v_n}\propto n^3\ \text{ or } v_n\propto n^{-3}$$

13. (a) For $n = 2$, using, $E_n = \frac{-13.6\text{eV}}{n^2}$,

$$E_2 = -\frac{13.6}{(2)^2} = -3.4\ \text{eV}$$

For $n = 1$, $E_1 = -13.6$ eV

$$\therefore\quad E_{1\to2} = E_2 - E_1 = -3.4 - (-13.6) = 10.2\ \text{eV}$$

14. (b) $E_3 - E_2 = E$ or $E = -13.6\left(\frac{1}{n_1^2} - \frac{1}{n_2^2}\right) = E_1\left(\frac{1}{9} - \frac{1}{4}\right)$

$$\Rightarrow\quad E = \frac{E_1}{9} - \frac{E_1}{4}\quad\text{or}\quad E_1 = -7.2E$$

$\therefore$ Ionisation energy of hydrogen atom is $7.2E$.

15. (d) The wavelength will be minimum for which $\left(\frac{1}{n_f^2} - \frac{1}{n_i^2}\right)$ is maximum. Hence, option (d) is correct.

16. (d) Wavelength is minimum for which Z is maximum $\left(\text{Since, } \lambda\propto\frac{1}{Z^2}\right)$

$\therefore$ Here, $Z_{max} = 3$ for lithium.

17. (c) According to Rydberg's formula,

$$\frac{1}{\lambda} = RZ^2\left(\frac{1}{n_1^2} - \frac{1}{n_2^2}\right) \Rightarrow \lambda\propto\frac{1}{Z^2}$$

$$\frac{1}{3^2}:\frac{1}{2^2}:\frac{1}{1^2} = \frac{1}{9}:\frac{1}{4}:\frac{1}{1} = 4:9:36$$

Hence, $\lambda_{Li^{2+}} : \lambda_{He^+} : \lambda_H = 4:9:36.$

18. (b) Angular momentum,

$$L = mvr = \frac{nh}{2\pi}\quad\text{or}\quad mv = \frac{nh}{2\pi r}$$

Now, $r\propto n^2$

Also, $E\propto\frac{1}{n^2}$

$$\therefore\quad mv = p\propto\frac{nh}{2\pi n^2}$$

$$p\propto\frac{h}{2\pi n}\Rightarrow p\propto\frac{1}{n}$$

19. (a) $K = \frac{e^2}{8\pi\varepsilon_0 r} = \frac{(9\times10^9\ \text{Nm}^2/\text{C}^2)(1.6\times10^{-19}\text{C})^2}{(2)(4.7\times10^{-11}\text{m})}$

$$= 2.45\times10^{-18}\ \text{J}$$
$$= 15.3\ \text{eV}$$

20. (c) As we know, potential energy $U = 2E, K = -E$

and $E = -\frac{13.6}{n^2}$

For state $n = 1$, $E_1 = \frac{-13.6}{(1)^2} = -13.6$

For state $n = 2$, $E_2 = \frac{-13.6}{(2)^2} = \frac{E_1}{4} \Rightarrow E_1 = 4E_2$

But, $K = -E$, so, $K_1 = 4K_2$

Similarly, for state $n = 1$, potential energy

$$(U_1) = 2E_1 = 2\times\frac{-13.6}{(1)^2} = -2\times13.6$$

For state $n = 2$, potential energy

$$(U_2) = 2E_2 = 2\times\frac{-13.6}{(2)^2} = \frac{-2\times13.6}{4}$$

$$U_2 = \frac{U_1}{4}\Rightarrow U_1 = 4U_2$$

21. (*d*) Both Statement I and Statement II are correct.

Energy can have positive or negative values. In the atom the electrons are bound. The negative energy of the revolving electrons does not allow the electrons to leave the atom. That the electrons are bound within the atom is indicated by the energy being negative.

22. (*a*) $$E_n = -\frac{13.6}{n^2} Z^2 \cdot \text{eV}$$

So, for a singly ionised helium atom $(Z = 2)$;

$$E_{\text{He}_n} = E_{\text{H}_n} 2^2 = 4E_n$$

23. (*a*) According to Bohr's first postulate,

$$mvr = \frac{nh}{2\pi}$$

$$\therefore \quad 2\pi r = n\left(\frac{h}{mv}\right) = n\lambda$$

For $n = 1, \lambda = 2\pi r$

Step up Practice 3

1. (*c*) When an electron de-excites from level n to level $(n-1)$ in an hydrogen atom, then frequency of emitted radiation is always equals to classical frequency of revolution of electron in nth orbit.

2. (*c*) The energy of the photon $= Rhc\left(\frac{1}{1^2} - \frac{1}{n^2}\right)$

$$\Rightarrow \quad 13.6\left(\frac{1}{1} - \frac{1}{4}\right) = 13.6\left(\frac{4-1}{4}\right)$$

$$= 13.6 \times \frac{3}{4} = \frac{40.8}{4} = 10.2 \text{ eV}$$

3. (*d*) When an electron jumps from orbit n_i to orbit n_f $(n_i > n_f)$, the frequency of emitted photon is given by

$$\nu = cR\left(\frac{1}{n_f^2} - \frac{1}{n_i^2}\right)$$

$$\Rightarrow \quad \nu = cR\left(\frac{1}{2^2} - \frac{1}{3^2}\right)$$

$$\nu = cR\left(\frac{5}{36}\right) \Rightarrow \nu = \frac{5cR}{36}$$

4. (*d*) Both A and R are true and R is the correct explanation of A.

The energy required to excite an electron in hydrogen atom to its first excited state, is an energy equal to $E_2 - E_1 = -3.40 \text{ eV} - -(13.6) \text{ eV} = 10.2 \text{eV}$.

5. (*b*) A is true but R is false.

Emission transitions can take place between any higher energy level and any energy level below it while absorption transition start from the lowest energy level only and may end at any higher energy level. Hence, number of absorptions transitions between two given energy levels is always less than the number of emission transitions between same two levels.

6. (*c*) A is false but R is true.

For the given atom, energy levels are

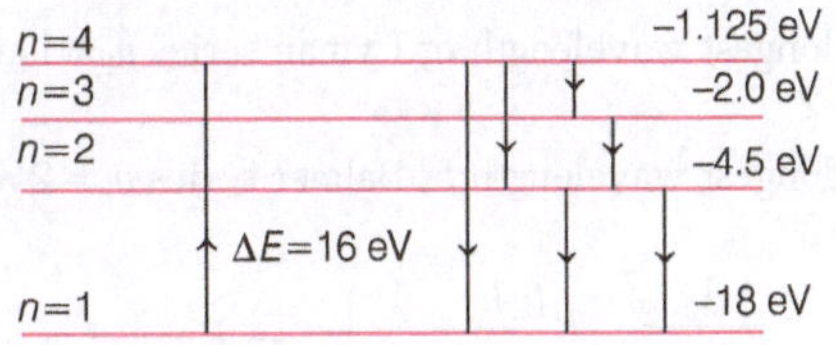

So, atom is excited to $n = 3$ state (atmost)

Clearly emission lines contains $= \frac{n}{2}(n-1)$

$$= \frac{3(3-1)}{2} = 6 \text{ spectral lines.}$$

7. (*b*) Balmer series lies in the visible region.

8. (*c*) $$\lambda \propto \frac{1}{\left(\frac{1}{n_f^2} - \frac{1}{n_i^2}\right)}$$

$$\therefore \quad \frac{\lambda_{\text{largest}}}{\lambda_{\text{shortest}}} = \frac{\left(\frac{1}{4} - \frac{1}{\infty}\right)}{\left(\frac{1}{4} - \frac{1}{9}\right)} = \frac{(1/4)}{(5/36)} = \frac{9}{5}$$

9. (*c*) Wavelength of spectral line in Balmer series is given by

$$\frac{1}{\lambda} = R\left(\frac{1}{2^2} - \frac{1}{n^2}\right)$$

For first line of Balmer series, $n = 3$

$$\Rightarrow \quad \frac{1}{\lambda_1} = R\left(\frac{1}{2^2} - \frac{1}{3^2}\right) = \frac{5R}{36}$$

For second line, $n = 4$

$$\Rightarrow \quad \frac{1}{\lambda_2} = R\left(\frac{1}{2^2} - \frac{1}{4^2}\right) = \frac{3R}{16}$$

$$\therefore \quad \frac{\lambda_2}{\lambda_1} = \frac{20}{27} \Rightarrow \lambda_2 = \frac{20}{27} \times \lambda_1$$

$$\Rightarrow \quad \lambda_2 = \frac{20}{27} \times 6561 = 4860 \text{ Å}$$

10. (*b*) A is true and R is false.

The value of n for a line in Balmer series of hydrogen spectrum having the highest wavelength will be $n_1 = 2$ and $n_2 = 3$ because this transition will have lowest energy and so highest wavelength.

11. (*b*) Number of lines emitted $= \frac{n(n-1)}{2}$

where, $n =$ number of orbit from which transition takes place.

$$\Rightarrow \quad 6 = \frac{n(n-1)}{2} \text{ or } n = 4$$

$\therefore$ The wavelength of emitted radiations will be maximum for transition $n = 4$ to $n = 3$.

12. (a) As, $\frac{1}{\lambda} = R\left[\frac{1}{n_1^2} - \frac{1}{n_2^2}\right]$

For longest wavelength of Lyman series $n_1 = 1$ and $n_2 = 2$

For longest wavelength of Balmer series $n_1 = 2$ and $n_2 = 3$

$$\frac{\frac{1}{\lambda_{Balmer}}}{\frac{1}{\lambda_{Lyman}}} = \frac{R\left(\frac{1}{2^2} - \frac{1}{3^2}\right)}{R\left(\frac{1}{1^2} - \frac{1}{2^2}\right)} = \frac{\frac{5}{36}R}{\frac{3}{4}R}$$

So, $\frac{\lambda_{Lyman}}{\lambda_{Balmer}} = \frac{5}{27}$

13. (d) The Lyman Series of Hydrogen spectrum lies in the ultraviolet region.

14. (b) By using, $\frac{1}{\lambda} = RZ^2\left[\frac{1}{n_1^2} - \frac{1}{n_2^2}\right]$

Lyman series for hydrogen atom, $\frac{1}{\lambda_{min}} = R\left[\frac{1}{1^2} - \frac{1}{\infty}\right] = R$

$$\frac{1}{\lambda_{min}} = R \text{ or } (\lambda_{min})_H = \frac{1}{R} \quad ...(i)$$

Balmer series for another atom,

$$\frac{1}{\lambda_{min}} = RZ^2\left(\frac{1}{2^2} - \frac{1}{\infty}\right) = \frac{RZ^2}{4}$$

$$\Rightarrow \quad \lambda_{min} = \frac{4}{RZ^2} \quad ...(ii)$$

From Eqs. (i) and (ii), we get

$$\frac{1}{R} = \frac{4}{RZ^2} \Rightarrow Z = 2$$

15. (a) $\frac{\lambda_{Lyman}}{\lambda_{Balmer}} = \frac{\left(\frac{1}{2^2} - \frac{1}{3^2}\right)}{\left(\frac{1}{1^2} - \frac{1}{2^2}\right)} = \frac{5}{27}$

$$\left[\because \frac{1}{\lambda} = R\left(\frac{1}{n_f^2} - \frac{1}{n_i^2}\right)\right]$$

$$\Rightarrow \quad \lambda_{Lyman} = \frac{5}{27} \times \lambda_{Balmer} = \frac{5}{27} \times 6563 = 1215.4 \text{ Å}$$

16. (a) We know that frequency, $\nu_1 = Rc\left(\frac{1}{n_1^2} - \frac{1}{n_2^2}\right)$

This gives,

$$\nu_1 = Rc\left(1 - \frac{1}{\infty}\right) = Rc \Rightarrow \nu_2 = Rc\left(1 - \frac{1}{4}\right) = \frac{3}{4}Rc$$

$$\nu_3 = Rc\left(\frac{1}{4} - \frac{1}{\infty}\right) = \frac{Rc}{4} \Rightarrow \nu_1 - \nu_2 = \nu_3$$

17. (d) Here, for wavelength λ_1, $n_1 = 4$ and $n_2 = 3$ and for λ_2, $n_1 = 3$ and $n_2 = 2$

We have, $\frac{1}{\lambda} = -R\left[\frac{1}{n_2^2} - \frac{1}{n_1^2}\right]$

So, for λ_1

$$\Rightarrow \quad \frac{1}{\lambda_1} = -R\left[\frac{1}{(4)^2} - \frac{1}{(3)^2}\right]$$

$$\frac{1}{\lambda_1} = R\left[\frac{7}{144}\right] \quad ...(i)$$

Similarly, for λ_2

$$\Rightarrow \quad \frac{1}{\lambda_2} = -R\left[\frac{1}{(3)^2} - \frac{1}{(2)^2}\right]$$

$$\frac{1}{\lambda_2} = R\left[\frac{5}{36}\right] \quad ...(ii)$$

Hence, from Eqs. (i) and (ii), we get

$$\frac{\lambda_1}{\lambda_2} = \frac{20}{7}$$

18. (c) As we know that, to calculate wavelength in series limit

$$\lambda \propto \frac{1}{R}$$

$$\therefore \quad \frac{1}{\lambda} = \frac{R}{n^2} \text{ (in general)}$$

Hence, option (c) is incorrect.

Gearing up for NEET

1. (d) Impact parameter, $b \propto \cot\frac{\theta}{2} \Rightarrow \frac{b_1}{b_2} = \frac{\cot 45°}{\cot 60°} = \sqrt{3}$

2. (b) $v \propto \frac{Z}{n}$, since Z and n both have become twice.

Thus,

Velocity of electron in second orbit of He^+ will be v.

3. (a) According to scattering formula,

$$N \propto \frac{1}{\sin^4(\theta/2)} \Rightarrow \frac{N_2}{N_1} = \left[\frac{\sin(\theta_1/2)}{\sin(\theta_2/2)}\right]^4$$

$$\Rightarrow \quad \frac{N_2}{N_1} = \left[\frac{\sin\frac{90°}{2}}{\sin\frac{60°}{2}}\right]^4 = \left[\frac{\sin 45°}{\sin 30°}\right]^4$$

$$\Rightarrow \quad N_2 = (\sqrt{2})^4 \times N_1 = 4 \times 56 = 224$$

4. (d) α-particles cannot be attracted by the nucleus.

5. (d) $L_n = \frac{nh}{2\pi} \Rightarrow I\omega = \frac{nh}{2\pi}$

$$\Rightarrow (mr^2)\,\omega = \frac{nh}{2\pi}$$

As, $\quad r \propto n^2$

$$\therefore \quad \omega \propto \frac{1}{n^3}$$

6. (c) The energy of first excitation of sodium is

$$E = h\nu = \frac{hc}{\lambda}$$

$$\therefore \quad E = \frac{6.63\times 10^{-34} \times 3\times 10^{8}}{5896\times 10^{-10}} \text{ J}$$

$$E = 3.37\times 10^{-19} \text{ J}$$

Also, since 1.6×10^{-19} J = 1 eV

$$\therefore \quad E = \frac{3.37\times 10^{-19}}{1.6\times 10^{-19}}$$

$$\Rightarrow \quad E = 2.1 \text{ eV}$$

Hence, corresponding first excitation potential is 2.1 V.

7. (b) Because atom is hollow and whole mass of atom is concentrated in a small centre called nucleus. So, A' will be maximum while B' minimum.

8. (c) Rutherford's model states that an atom is a sphere of diameter about 10^{-10} m with whole of its positive charge concentrated at the centre and electron revolves around this centre.

9. (b) According to the question,

For the distance of closest approach kinetic energy will totally be converted to potential energy.

Hence, $\frac{1}{2}mv^2 = \frac{1}{4\pi\varepsilon_0}\frac{Qq}{r_0} \Rightarrow r_0 = \frac{Qq}{2\pi\varepsilon_0 mv^2}$

10. (a) Excitation energy, $\Delta E = E_2 - E_1 = 13.6\, Z^2\left[\frac{1}{1^2} - \frac{1}{2^2}\right]$

$$40.8 = 13.6\, Z^2 \times \frac{3}{4}$$

$$\therefore \quad Z = 2$$

So, required energy to remove the electron from ground state

$$= + \frac{13.6\, Z^2}{(1)^2} = 13.6\,(2)^2 = 54.4 \text{ eV}$$

11. (d) In case of many electron atom, there is a repulsive force due to other electrons. Due to which the Coulomb force is no more a central force and Bohr model cannot be applied.

12. (a) If kinetic energy is E, then total energy will be $-E$, *i.e.* energy E must be supplied to the electron to escape to infinity.

13. (c) The minimum energy required to ionise an atom is equal to the energy to excite an electron in the atom from its ground state corresponding to $n = 1$, to its ionisation level corresponding to $n = \infty$. If the amount of energy given to atom is equal to the ionisation energy, then the electron is just able to become a free electron and the atom is about to be ionised.

When this occurs, one outermost electron from the atom is just to be removed from the atom. Much higher energy is necessary to free an innermost electron from the atom because this will occur only after the outermost electrons are all removed.

14. (a) $L = \frac{nh}{2\pi}$, it does not depend on Z. $[\because n_2 > n_1]$

15. (b) $\Delta L = \frac{nh}{2\pi} - \frac{(n-1)h}{2\pi} = \frac{h}{2\pi}$

16. (a) $E \propto m$ and $r \propto \frac{1}{m}$

i.e. energy will become two times and radius will become half.

Hence, $E_0 = 2(-13.6) = -27.2$ eV and $r_0 = a_0/2$

17. (c) Wave number is reciprocal of wavelength,

$$\nu = \frac{1}{\lambda} = R\left[\frac{1}{n_1^2} - \frac{1}{n_2^2}\right] = R\left[\frac{1}{2^2} - \frac{1}{4^2}\right]$$

$$= R\left[\frac{1}{4} - \frac{1}{16}\right] = \frac{3R}{16}$$

18. (b) $r_3 = (3)^2 \cdot r_1 = 9x$

Now, $3\lambda_3 = (2\pi r_3) = 18\pi x$

$$\therefore \quad \lambda_3 = 6\pi x$$

19. (c) The atomic number of lithium is 3, therefore the radius of Li^{++} ion in its ground state, on the basis of Bohr's model, will be about $\frac{1}{3}$ times to that of Bohr radius.

Therefore, the radius of lithium ion is near $\frac{53}{3} \approx 18$ pm.

20. (c) Change in the angular momentum,

$$\Delta L = L_{n_2} - L_{n_1} = \frac{n_2 h}{2\pi} - \frac{n_1 h}{2\pi}$$

$$\Delta L = \frac{h}{2\pi}(n_2 - n_1) = \frac{6.6\times 10^{-34}}{2\times 3.14}(5-4)$$

$$= 1.05\times 10^{-34} \text{ J-s}$$

21. (c) $Z^2\left[\frac{13.6}{4} - \frac{13.6}{9}\right] = 47.2$

$$\therefore \quad Z = 5$$

22. (c) Final energy of electron $= -13.6 + 12.1 = -1.51$ eV

This energy corresponds to third level, *i.e.* $n = 3$

Hence, number of spectral lines emitted

$$= \frac{n(n-1)}{2} = \frac{3(3-1)}{2} = 3$$

23. (c) As, $mvr = \frac{h}{2\pi}$ (in first orbit)

$$\therefore \quad v = \frac{h}{2\pi mr} \Rightarrow a = \frac{v^2}{r} = \frac{h^2}{4\pi^2 m^2 r^3}$$

24. (a) Magnetic moment μ of a revolving electron is given by

$$\mu = \frac{e}{2m}L = \frac{e}{2m}\cdot\frac{nh}{2\pi} = \left(\frac{eh}{2m}\right)\cdot\frac{n}{2\pi} = \frac{n}{2\pi}\mu_B$$

where, $\mu_B = \frac{eh}{2m}$ is Bohr magneton.

$\therefore \quad \mu \propto n$

25. (c) $a = \frac{v^2}{r}$ or $a \propto \frac{(Z^2)}{(1/Z)}$

$\therefore \quad a \propto Z^3$

For singly ionised helium atom, $Z = 2$ and doubly ionised lithium atom, $Z = 3$

$$\Rightarrow \quad \frac{a_{He^+}}{a_{Li^{++}}} = \frac{(2)^3}{(3)^3} = \frac{8}{27}$$

26. (a) In hydrogen atom, $E_2 - E_1 = 10.2$ eV

Since, 5 eV < 10.2 eV

The electron cannot excite the hydrogen atom, therefore the collision must be elastic.

27. (a) According to the question,

Energy, $E = -3.4$ eV

$$\Rightarrow \quad -\frac{13.6}{n^2} = -3.4$$

$$\Rightarrow \quad n^2 = 4 \Rightarrow n = 2$$

So, the angular momentum of the electron, $mvr = \frac{nh}{2\pi}$

$$L = mvr = \frac{2\times 6.626\times 10^{-34}}{2\times 3.14}$$

$$= \frac{6.626\times 10^{-34}}{3.14} = 2.1\times 10^{-34} \text{ J-s}$$

28. (a) The wavelength can be given as

$$\frac{1}{\lambda} = Z^2R\left(\frac{1}{n_1^2} - \frac{1}{n_2^2}\right) \quad \text{...(i)}$$

For λ to be shortest, $\left(\frac{1}{n_1^2} - \frac{1}{n_2^2}\right)$ should be maximum.

So, $n_2 = \infty$ and $n_1 = 1$

Now, from Eq. (i), we get

$$\frac{1}{\lambda} = R\left(\frac{1}{1}\right) \Rightarrow \lambda = \frac{1}{R} = \frac{1}{10^7} \text{ m} \simeq 1000 \text{ Å}$$

29. (d) After removing one electron from helium atom it will become hydrogen like atom.

$$\therefore \quad E = 24.6 + (13.6)(2)^2 = 79 \text{ eV}$$

30. (a) As, $\sqrt{f} \propto (Z-1)\sqrt{\frac{1}{n_1^2} - \frac{1}{n_2^2}}$

$$\therefore \quad \text{Slope} \propto \sqrt{\frac{1}{n_1^2} - \frac{1}{n_2^2}}$$

$$\therefore \quad \frac{(\text{Slope})_{K_\beta}}{(\text{Slope})_{K_\alpha}} = \frac{\sqrt{1-\frac{1}{9}}}{\sqrt{1-\frac{1}{4}}} = \sqrt{\frac{8}{9}\times\frac{4}{3}} = \sqrt{\frac{32}{27}}$$

31. (a) $\lambda = \frac{h}{p} = \frac{h}{mv}$ or $\lambda \propto \frac{1}{v}$

$$\left(\because v \propto \frac{1}{n}\right)$$

$$\therefore \quad \lambda_n \propto n \quad J_n = n\frac{h}{2\pi}, \quad i.e. \quad J_n \propto n$$

Hence, $J_n \propto \lambda_n$

32. (a) For α-particle, at distance of closest approach, then

Decrease in KE = Increase in PE

$$2 \text{ eV} = \frac{1}{4\pi\varepsilon_0}\cdot\frac{2e\cdot Ze}{r^2}$$

$$\Rightarrow \quad Ze = 4\pi\varepsilon_0 r^2 \text{ V} \quad \text{...(i)}$$

For proton, if r_1 be the distance of closest approach

Decrease in KE = Increase in PE

$$R_1^2 = \frac{1}{4\pi\varepsilon_0 V}(Ze)$$

$$= \frac{1}{4\pi\varepsilon_0 V}\cdot 4\pi\varepsilon_0 r^2 V \quad \text{[from Eq. (i)]}$$

$$\Rightarrow \quad r_1^2 = r^2$$

$$\Rightarrow \quad r_1 = r$$

33. (b) Since, $r \propto n^2$ i.e. $\frac{r_f}{r_i} = \left(\frac{n_f}{n_i}\right)^2$

$$\Rightarrow \quad \frac{21.2\times 10^{-11}}{5.3\times 10^{-11}} = \left(\frac{n}{1}\right)^2$$

$$\Rightarrow \quad n^2 = 4 \Rightarrow n = 2$$

34. (b) The energy of the projectile will be equivalent to potential energy of the charge system,

$$E = \frac{1}{4\pi\varepsilon_0}\frac{Z_1Z_2}{r_0} \Rightarrow \text{Energy, } E \propto Z_1Z_2$$

35. (c) $\frac{mv^2}{a_0} = \frac{1}{4\pi\varepsilon_0}\frac{e^2}{a_0^2}$

$$\Rightarrow \quad v = \frac{e}{\sqrt{4\pi\varepsilon_0 m a_0}}$$

36. (a) Here, $E_1 = \frac{me^4}{8\varepsilon_0^2h^2} \Rightarrow me^4 = 8\varepsilon_0^2h^2E_1$

$$f_n = \frac{v_n}{2\pi r_n} = \frac{(e^2/2\,\varepsilon_0 nh)}{(2\pi)\,\varepsilon_0 n^2h^2/\pi me^2}$$

$$= \frac{me^4}{4\varepsilon_0^2n^3h^3} = \frac{8E_1\varepsilon_0^2h^2}{4\varepsilon_0^2n^3h^3} = \frac{2E_1}{n^3h}$$

37. (d) As, $a = v^2/r$

$$r \propto n^2 \text{ and } v \propto \frac{1}{n}$$

$$\therefore \quad a \propto \frac{1}{n^4}$$

$$\Rightarrow \frac{a_M}{a_L} = \left(\frac{2}{3}\right)^4 = \frac{16}{81}$$

38. (a) In the simple Bohr model, only the magnitude of angular momentum is kept equal to some integral multiple of $\frac{h}{2\pi}$, where h is Planck's constant and thus, the Bohr model gives incorrect values of angular momentum.

39. (a) Minimum 10.2 eV energy is required to excite a hydrogen atom. In perfectly inelastic collision maximum energy is lost.

$$\therefore \text{ Energy lost } = \frac{1}{2}(2m)\left(\frac{v}{2}\right)^2 = 10.2 \times 1.6 \times 10^{-19}$$

$$\frac{1}{4}mv^2 = 1.632 \times 10^{-18}$$

$$\therefore \text{ Velocity, } v = \sqrt{\frac{1.632 \times 4 \times 10^{-18}}{1.67 \times 10^{-27}}}$$

$$= 6.25 \times 10^4 \text{ ms}^{-1}$$

40. (d) The ground state of hydrogen ($n = 1$) is represented by K, the first excited state ($n = 2$) is represented by L, the second excited state ($n = 3$) is represent by M. So, the energy transferred by the second electron can be given by

$$E = -13.6\left(\frac{1}{n_1^2} - \frac{1}{n_2^2}\right)$$

$$= -13.6\left(\frac{1}{3^2} - \frac{1}{\infty^2}\right)$$

$$\simeq -1.51 \text{ eV}$$

41. (b) According to Bohr's theory, the wavelength of the radiation

$$\frac{1}{\lambda} = Z^2R\left(\frac{1}{n_1^2} - \frac{1}{n_2^2}\right) \Rightarrow \frac{\nu}{c} = Z^2R\left(\frac{1}{n_1^2} - \frac{1}{n_2^2}\right)$$

$$\nu = cZ^2R\left(\frac{1}{n_1^2} - \frac{1}{n_2^2}\right)$$

$$\Rightarrow 2.7 \times 10^{15} = cZ^2R\left(\frac{1}{1^2} - \frac{1}{2^2}\right) \Rightarrow Z^2R = \frac{32}{27}$$

$$\nu = cZ^2R\left(\frac{1}{1^2} - \frac{1}{3^2}\right) \Rightarrow \nu = \frac{32}{27} \times 2.7 \times 10^{15}$$

$$= 3.2 \times 10^{15} \text{ Hz}$$

42. (a) The total energy associated with the two H-atoms in the ground state collide inelastically
$= 2 \times (13.6 \text{ eV}) = 27.2$ eV.
The maximum amount by which their combined kinetic energy is reduced when any one of them goes into first excited state after the inelastic collision.
The total energy associated with the two H-atoms after the collision

$$= \left(\frac{13.6}{2^2}\right) + (13.6) = 17.0 \text{ eV}$$

Therefore, maximum loss of their combined kinetic energy

$$= 27.2 - 17.0 = 10.2 \text{ eV}$$

43. (d) If E is the energy radiated in transition, then from figure

$$E_{R \to G} > E_{Q \to S} > E_{R \to S} > E_{Q \to R} > E_{P \to Q}$$

For obtaining blue line, energy radiated should be more.
Hence, correct option is (d).

44. (c) When one decides to work in a frame of reference where the electron is at rest, the given expression is not true as it forms the non-inertial frame of reference.

45. (d) At the distance of closed approach r,

$$K = \frac{1}{4\pi\varepsilon_0}\frac{(2e)(Ze)}{r} \Rightarrow r = \frac{2Ze^2}{4\pi\varepsilon_0 K}$$

where, Ze = charge of the nucleus,
$2e$ = charge of the alpha particle
and K = kinetic energy of the alpha particle.

$$\because \quad K = \frac{p^2}{2m}$$

where, p is the momentum of the α-particle and m is the mass of the electron.

$$\therefore \quad r = \frac{2Ze^2 2m}{4\pi\varepsilon_0 p^2} \text{ or } r \propto \frac{1}{p^2}$$

$$\frac{r'}{r} = \left(\frac{p}{p'}\right)^2 = \left(\frac{p}{2p}\right)^2 = \frac{1}{4} \Rightarrow r' = \frac{r}{4}$$

46. (a) According to kinetic interpretation of temperature,

$$\text{KE} = \left(\frac{1}{2}mv^2\right) = \frac{3}{2}kT$$

$$\Rightarrow 10.2 \times 1.6 \times 10^{-19} = \frac{3}{2} \times (1.38 \times 10^{-23})T$$

$$\Rightarrow \quad T = 7.9 \times 10^4 \text{ K}$$

47. (c) $\frac{1}{\lambda} = RZ^2\left(\frac{1}{1^2} - \frac{1}{2^2}\right)$

$$\frac{1}{\lambda_1} = R(1)^2(3/4), \frac{1}{\lambda_2} = R(1)^2(3/4)$$

$$\frac{1}{\lambda_3} = R(2)^2(3/4), \frac{1}{\lambda_4} = R3^2(3/4)$$

$$\frac{1}{\lambda_1} = \frac{1}{\lambda_2} = \frac{1}{4\lambda_3} = \frac{1}{9\lambda_4}$$

$$\Rightarrow \lambda_1 = \lambda_2 = 4\lambda_3 = 9\lambda_4$$

So, option (c) is correct.

48. (*a*) According to Bohr theory,

$$mvr = n\frac{h}{2\pi} \Rightarrow v = \frac{nh}{2\pi mr}$$

and $$\frac{mv^2}{r} \propto \frac{k}{r}$$

$$\Rightarrow \frac{m}{r}\left(\frac{n^2h^2}{4\pi^2m^2r^2}\right) \propto \frac{k}{r}$$

$$\Rightarrow r_n \propto n$$

Kinetic energy of the electron,

$$T = \frac{1}{2}mv^2 = \frac{1}{2}m\left(\frac{n^2h^2}{4\pi^2m^2r^2}\right)$$

$$\Rightarrow T_n \propto \frac{n^2}{r^2}$$

But as $r \propto n$, therefore $T \propto n^0$

49. (*d*) The energy of the photon,

$$E = \frac{hc}{\lambda} = \frac{4\times 10^{-15} \times 3\times 10^8}{300\times 10^{-9}} = 4\text{eV}$$

The ionisation energy is 13.6 eV which is greater than the energy of photon, so electron cannot be knocked out or into excited state. Thus, it will keep orbiting in ground state of the atom.

50. (*d*) $E = E_1 / n^2$

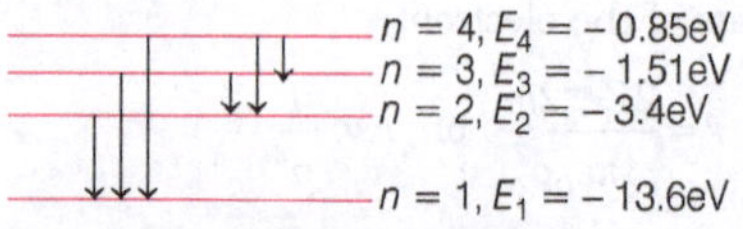

Energy levels of H-atom

Energy used for excitation is 12.75 eV,

i.e. $(-13.6 + 12.75)$ eV $= -0.85$eV

The photons of energy 12.75 eV can excite the fourth level of H-atom. As spectral lines emitted is $= \frac{n(n-1)}{2}$

$$= \frac{4(3)}{2} = 6$$

Therefore, six lines will be emitted.

51. (*a*) Energy provided to the ground state electron

$$= \frac{hc}{\lambda} = \frac{6.6\times 10^{-34} \times 3\times 10^8}{975\times 10^{-10}}$$

$$= \frac{6.6\times 3}{975} \times 10^{-16}$$

$$= 0.020\times 10^{-16} = 2\times 10^{-18}\text{ J}$$

$$= \frac{20\times 10^{-19}}{1.6\times 10^{-19}}\text{ eV}$$

$$= \frac{20}{1.6} = 12.5\text{ eV}$$

It means the electron is jump to $n = 3$ from $n = 1$. The number of possible spectral lines from $n = 3$ to $n = 1$ is 3.

i.e. $(n = 3) \longrightarrow (n = 1)$

$(n = 3) \longrightarrow (n = 2)$

and $(n = 2) \longrightarrow (n = 1)$

52. (*c*) de-Broglie wavelength, $\lambda = \frac{h}{p}$ ...(i)

According to Bohr's quantisation condition,

$$mvr_n = \frac{nh}{2\pi} \Rightarrow pr_n = \frac{nh}{2\pi} \quad \text{...(ii)}$$

From Eqs. (i) and (ii), we get

$$\lambda = \frac{h \times 2\pi r_n}{nh} \Rightarrow \lambda = \frac{2\pi r_n}{n}$$

For fourth orbit $(n = 4) \Rightarrow \lambda = \frac{2\pi r_4}{4}$ ...(iii)

Moreover, $r \propto n^2 \Rightarrow \frac{r_1}{r_4} = \frac{(1)^2}{(4)^2} \Rightarrow r_4 = 16r$

Substituting the value of r_4 in Eq. (iii), we get

$$\lambda = \frac{2\pi[16r_1]}{4} = 8\pi r_1 = 8\pi r (\because \text{ given, } r_1 = r)$$

53. (*c*) According to Bohr's model, electrons can revolve those orbits in which their angular momentum is an integral multiple of $h/2\pi$. *i.e.* $mvr = \frac{nh}{2\pi}$

54. (*c*) Potential energy of an electron in 3rd excited state

$$= 2E_4 = 2\left(\frac{E_1}{4^2}\right)$$

$$= 2\left(\frac{-13.6}{16}\right) = -1.70\text{ eV}$$

55. (*b*) Given, $E_K = 23.32$ keV

$$= 23.32 \times 10^3 \text{ eV}$$

$$hc = 12.42\times 10^{-7} \text{ eV}$$

and $$\lambda_{K_\alpha} = 71\times 10^{-12}\text{ m}$$

Now, $$E_L - E_K = \frac{hc}{\lambda_{K_\alpha}}$$

$$E_L - 23.32\times 10^3 = \frac{12.42\times 10^{-7}}{71\times 10^{-12}}$$

$$\Rightarrow E_L = 40812.9$$

$$= 40.82\text{ keV}$$

56. (b) Ionisation energy in ground state = 24.6 eV

Energy required to remove 2nd electron from He^{2+}

$$= Z^2 \ (13.6) \text{ eV}$$
$$= (2)^2 \ (13.6) = 54.4 \text{ eV}$$

So, total energy required = 24.6 + 54.4 = 79 eV

57. (a) As, electron de-excites from $3E \to E$

$$\therefore \quad h\nu = 3E - E \text{ or } \frac{hc}{\lambda} = 2E \quad \text{...(i)}$$

When electron de-excites from $\frac{5E}{3} \to E$

$$\frac{hc}{\lambda'} = \frac{5E}{3} - E = \frac{2E}{3} \quad \text{...(ii)}$$

Substituting the value of E from Eq. (i) in above equation

$$\frac{hc}{\lambda'} = \frac{2}{3}\left(\frac{hc}{2\lambda}\right) \Rightarrow \lambda' = 3\lambda$$

58. (d) Minimum energy,

$$E = 13.6 Z^2 \text{ eV}$$
$$= 13.6\,(3)^2 = 122.4 \text{ eV}$$

59. (a) Here, $E_5 - E_1 = \frac{hc}{\lambda}$

and $\frac{Rhc}{25} - Rhc = \frac{hc}{\lambda}$

$$\Rightarrow \quad \frac{24}{25}R = \frac{1}{\lambda}$$

But $p = \frac{h}{\lambda}$ and $v = \frac{h}{m\lambda} = \frac{24\,Rh}{25\,m}$

60. (c) We have, $F \propto \frac{v^2}{r}$

Also, $\quad v \propto \frac{1}{n}$ and $r \propto n^2$

$$\Rightarrow \quad F \propto \frac{1}{n^4}$$

61. (b) Required ionisation energy,

$$E = \frac{hc}{\lambda} = \frac{6.6 \times 10^{-34} \times 3 \times 10^8}{1.5 \times 10^{-10}}$$
$$= 13.2 \times 10^{-16} \text{ J}$$

62. (c) Time period of electron,

$$T = \frac{2\pi r}{v} = \frac{\dfrac{2\pi \times \varepsilon_0 n^2 h^2}{\pi m e^2}}{\dfrac{e^2}{2\varepsilon_0 n h}}$$

$$T = \frac{4\varepsilon_0^2 n^3 h^3}{me^4}$$

Current, $\quad i = \frac{e}{T} = \frac{e}{\dfrac{4\varepsilon_0^2 n^3 h^3}{me^4}}$

$$\Rightarrow \quad i = \frac{me^5}{4\varepsilon_0^2 n^3 h^3}$$

i.e. $\quad i \propto e^5$

63. (a) Maximum energy is liberated for transition $E_n \to E_1$ and minimum energy for $E_n \to E_{n-1}$.

Hence, $\quad \frac{E_1}{n^2} - E_1 = 52.224 \text{ eV} \quad \text{...(i)}$

and $\quad \frac{E_1}{n^2} - \frac{E_1}{(n-1)^2} = 1.224 \text{ eV} \quad \text{...(ii)}$

Solving Eqs. (i) and (ii), we get

$$E_1 = -54.4 \text{eV and } n = 5$$

But $\quad E_1 = -\frac{13.6 Z^2}{1^2}$

$$\therefore \quad -54.4 = -\frac{13.6}{1^2} Z^2 \Rightarrow Z = 2$$

64. (d) If $n = 4$, then spectral lines emitted $= \frac{n(n-1)}{2} = 6$

65. (d) $r_n \propto \frac{n^2}{Z}$ or $r_n \propto \frac{1}{Z}$

where, Z is maximum for doubly ionised lithium. Therefore, for doubly ionised lithium radius of the first orbit will be minimum.

66. (c) $\frac{1}{\lambda} = R\left(\frac{1}{2^2} - \frac{1}{4^2}\right) = R\left(\frac{16-4}{16 \times 4}\right) = \frac{12R}{16 \times 4} = \frac{3}{16}R$

or $\quad \lambda = \frac{16}{3R}$

$$\nu = \frac{c}{\lambda} = \frac{3 \times 10^8 \times 10^7 \times 3}{16}$$

$(\because R = 10^5 \text{cm}^{-1}, = 10^7 \text{ m}^{-1} \text{ given})$

$$= \frac{9}{16} \times 10^{15} \text{ Hz}$$

67. (a) Given, $\quad hc = 1240$ eV-nm

For least energetic photon, $E = E_2 - E_1 = 10.2$ eV

We know that, $E = \frac{hc}{\lambda}$ or

$$\lambda = \frac{hc}{E} \Rightarrow \lambda = \frac{1240}{10.2}$$
$$\lambda = 121.57 \approx 122 \text{ nm}$$

68. (d) $\Delta E \propto \left(\frac{1}{n_1^2} - \frac{1}{n_2^2}\right)$

Also, $\Delta E \propto \frac{1}{\lambda}$

Since, λ is less for transition from $n = 5$ to $n = 2$ than for $n = 4$ to $n = 2$.

From the given option, only $\lambda_{\text{violet}} < \lambda_{\text{blue}}$. Thus, light of violet colour would have been emitted.

69. (*b*) In a hydrogen atom the time period is given by $T \propto n^3$

$$\frac{T_1}{T_2} = \left(\frac{n_1}{n_2}\right)^3 \Rightarrow \frac{8}{1} = \left(\frac{n_1}{n_2}\right)^3 \Rightarrow \frac{n_1}{n_2} = \frac{2}{1}$$

Thus, the values must be $n_1 = 2$ and $n_2 = 1$.

70. (*c*) For K_α line, $\lambda_{K_\alpha} \propto \frac{1}{(Z-1)^2}$

So, $$\frac{\lambda_2}{\lambda_1} = \left(\frac{Z_1 - 1}{Z_2 - 1}\right)^2 \quad (\because \lambda_1 = \lambda)$$

$$\Rightarrow \frac{\lambda_2}{\lambda} = \left(\frac{43-1}{29-1}\right)^2 = \left(\frac{42}{28}\right)^2$$

$$\Rightarrow \lambda_2 = \frac{9}{4}\lambda$$

71. (*b*) For transition $n = 3$ to $n = 2$,

$$\frac{1}{\lambda_1} = R\left[\frac{1}{2^2} - \frac{1}{3^2}\right] = \frac{5R}{36} \quad ...(i)$$

For transition $n = 4$ to $n = 2$,

$$\frac{1}{\lambda_2} = R\left[\frac{1}{2^2} - \frac{1}{4^2}\right] = \frac{3R}{16} \quad ...(ii)$$

Now, dividing Eq. (i) by Eq. (ii), we get

$$\frac{\lambda_2}{\lambda_1} = \frac{20}{27} \text{ or } \lambda_2 = \frac{20}{27}\lambda_1 = \frac{20}{27}\lambda_0 \quad (\because \lambda_1 = \lambda_0)$$

72. (*a*) Wavelength is given by $\frac{1}{\lambda} = R\left(\frac{1}{n_1^2} - \frac{1}{n_2^2}\right)$

$$\Rightarrow \frac{1}{\lambda} = R\left[\frac{1}{(2)^2} - \frac{1}{(4)^2}\right]$$

$$\Rightarrow \frac{1}{\lambda} = R\left(\frac{1}{4} - \frac{1}{16}\right) \Rightarrow \frac{1}{\lambda} = R\left(\frac{4-1}{16}\right)$$

$$\Rightarrow \frac{1}{\lambda} = \frac{3R}{16} \Rightarrow \lambda = \frac{16}{3R}$$

73. (*d*) $\lambda \propto \frac{1}{\Delta E}$

$$\therefore \frac{\lambda'}{\lambda} = \frac{(2E - E)}{(4E/3 - E)} = \frac{1}{1/3} = 3$$

$$\therefore \lambda' = 3\lambda$$

74. (*a*) The wavelength of lines is given by

$$\frac{1}{\lambda} = R\left(\frac{1}{1^2} - \frac{1}{n^2}\right)$$

For Lyman series, the shortest wavelength is for $n = \infty$ and longest is for $n = 2$.

$$\therefore \frac{1}{\lambda_S} = R\left(\frac{1}{1^2}\right) \quad ...(i)$$

$$\frac{1}{\lambda_L} = R\left(\frac{1}{1^2} - \frac{1}{2^2}\right) = \frac{3}{4}R \quad ...(ii)$$

On dividing Eq. (i) by Eq. (ii), we get

$$\frac{\lambda_L}{\lambda_S} = \frac{4}{3}$$

Given, $\lambda_S = 91.2$ nm $\Rightarrow \lambda_L = 91.2 \times \frac{4}{3} = 121.6$ nm

75. (*b*) As, $\frac{1}{\lambda} = R\left(\frac{1}{1^2} - \frac{1}{n^2}\right)$

$$\therefore \frac{R}{n^2} = R - \frac{1}{\lambda} = \frac{\lambda R - 1}{\lambda}$$

or $$n = \sqrt{\frac{\lambda R}{\lambda R - 1}}$$

76. (*b*) $\Delta E_{4\to 1} = \left(\frac{13.6}{1^2} - \frac{13.6}{16}\right)$ eV $= 12.75$ eV

Momentum of hydrogen atom = Momentum of photon

$$= \frac{E}{c} = \frac{12.75 \times 1.6 \times 10^{-19}}{3.0 \times 10^8} = 6.8 \times 10^{-27} \text{ kg-ms}^{-1}$$

77. (*b*) For the wavelength of Balmer's series,

$$\frac{1}{\lambda} = R\left(\frac{1}{2^2} - \frac{1}{n^2}\right)$$

where, R is Rydberg's constant.

For Balmer series, $n = 3$ gives the first member of series and $n = 4$ gives the second member of series.

Hence, $$\frac{1}{\lambda_1} = R\left(\frac{1}{2^2} - \frac{1}{3^2}\right) = R\left(\frac{5}{36}\right) \quad ...(i)$$

$$\Rightarrow \frac{1}{\lambda_2} = R\left(\frac{1}{2^2} - \frac{1}{4^2}\right) = R\left(\frac{12}{16 \times 4}\right) = \frac{3R}{16} \quad ...(ii)$$

$$\Rightarrow \frac{\lambda_2}{\lambda_1} = \frac{16}{3} \times \frac{5}{36} = \frac{20}{27}$$

Given, $$\lambda_1 = \lambda \Rightarrow \lambda_2 = \frac{20}{27}\lambda$$

78. (*d*) The transition marked as A represents series limit of Lyman series, B represents third member of Balmer series and C represents second member of Paschen series.

79. (*c*) $E \propto m \quad \therefore \lambda \propto \frac{1}{m}$

In case of hydrogen atom for longest wavelength of photon in the Balmer series,

$$\frac{1}{\lambda} = R\left(\frac{1}{4} - \frac{1}{9}\right) \text{ or } \lambda = \frac{36}{5R}$$

For this atom, $$\lambda' = \frac{\lambda}{2} = \frac{18}{5R} \quad (\because m = 2m)$$

80. (*b*) Let energy corresponding to state A, B and C be E_A, E_B and E_C, respectively.

So, from energy level diagram,

$$(E_C - E_B) + (E_B - E_A) = (E_C - E_A)$$

or $$\frac{hc}{\lambda_1}+\frac{hc}{\lambda_2}=\frac{hc}{\lambda_3}$$

$$\Rightarrow \quad \lambda_3=\frac{\lambda_1\lambda_2}{\lambda_1+\lambda_2}$$

81. (a) For transition from 4E to E,

$$(4E-E)=\frac{hc}{\lambda_1} \Rightarrow \lambda_1=\frac{hc}{3E} \quad \text{...(i)}$$

For transition from $\frac{7}{3}E$ to E,

$$\left(\frac{7}{3}E-E\right)=\frac{hc}{\lambda_2} \Rightarrow \lambda_2=\frac{3hc}{4E} \quad \text{...(ii)}$$

From Eqs. (i) and (ii), we get $\frac{\lambda_1}{\lambda_2}=\frac{4}{9}$

82. (a) Energy of emitted photon, $E=Rhc\left(\frac{1}{n_1^2}-\frac{1}{n_2^2}\right)$

$$\Rightarrow R_{(4\to 3)}=Rhc\left(\frac{1}{3^2}-\frac{1}{4^2}\right)=Rhc\left(\frac{7}{9\times 16}\right)=0.05\,Rhc$$

$$E_{(4\to 2)}=Rhc\left(\frac{1}{2^2}-\frac{1}{4^2}\right)=Rhc\left(\frac{3}{16}\right)=0.2Rhc$$

$$E_{(2\to 1)}=Rhc\left[\frac{1}{(1)^2}-\frac{1}{(2)^2}\right]=Rhc\left(\frac{3}{4}\right)=0.75Rhc$$

and $$E_{(1\to 4)}=Rhc\left[\frac{1}{(4)^2}-\frac{1}{(1)^2}\right]=-\frac{8}{9}Rhc=-0.9Rhc$$

Thus, transition III gives largest amount of energy.

83. (d) The photoelectric effect is possible when light of sufficient energy incident on metal surface. When electron de-excites from $n=3$ to $n=2$, the light produces photoelectric effect. So, for the given options, the photoelectric effect is not possible for that level in which energy of emitted light is less than that for $n=3$ to $n=2$. Since, $(h\nu)_{4\to 3}<(h\nu)_{3\to 2}$

Hence, photoelectric effect is not possible from $n=4$ to $n=3$.

Assertion and Reason

1. (d) Both A and R are true and R is the correct explanation of A.

Radius of Bohr's orbit $r \propto n^2$

$$\Rightarrow \frac{r_1}{r_2}=\left(\frac{n_1}{n_2}\right)^2 \Rightarrow \frac{5.29\times 10^{-11}}{r_2}=\left(\frac{1}{2}\right)^2$$

$$\Rightarrow r_2=5.29\times 10^{-11}\times 4=21.16\times 10^{-11}\text{ m}$$

$$=2.116\times 10^{-10}\text{ m}$$

$$\simeq=2.1\text{ Å}$$

2. (a) Both A and R are true but R is not the correct explanation of A.

$$L=n\left(\frac{h}{2\pi}\right),\ \text{i.e. } L\propto n.$$

In ground state $n=1$,

so $L=$ minimum.

3. (a) Both A and R are true but R is not the correct explanation of A.

For second orbit, $mv_2r_2=2\left(\frac{h}{2\pi}\right)$

$$\therefore\ 2\pi r_2=2\left(\frac{h}{mv_2}\right)=2\lambda_2$$

Further, $\lambda=\frac{h}{p}$

Speed or momentum is maximum in ground state. Hence, wavelength is minimum.

4. (a) Both A and R are correct but R is not the correct explanation of A.

First excitation energy $=E_2-E_1$

$$=\frac{-13.6}{2^2}-(-13.6)=10.2\text{ eV}$$

5. (d) Both A and R are true and R is the correct explanation of A.

The wavelength in Balmer series is given by

$$\frac{1}{\lambda}=R\left(\frac{1}{2^2}-\frac{1}{n^2}\right),\ \text{where } n=3,4,5$$

$$\frac{1}{\lambda_{max}}=R\left(\frac{1}{2^2}-\frac{1}{3^2}\right)$$

$$\Rightarrow \lambda_{max}=\frac{36}{5R}=\frac{36}{5\times 1.097\times 10^7}=6563\text{ Å}$$

and $$\frac{1}{\lambda_{min}}=R\left(\frac{1}{2^2}-\frac{1}{\infty^2}\right)$$

$$\Rightarrow \lambda_{max}=\frac{4}{R}=\frac{4}{1.097\times 10^7}=3646\text{ Å}$$

The wavelength 6563Å and 3646Å lie in visible region. Therefore, Balmer series lies in visible region.

Statement Type Questions

1. (d) Both Statement I and Statement II are correct.

2. (c) Statement I is incorrect but Statement II is correct.

Statement I is incorrect as in Rutherford's model there is a continuous emission of energy by rotating electron.

Statement II is correct, a negative energy means a stable orbit.

3. (d) Both Statement I and Statement II are correct.

$$r_n\propto n^2$$

$$r_1=\frac{0.53}{Z}$$

$$r_n = \frac{0.53}{Z} n^2 \Rightarrow \frac{r_n}{r_1} = n^2$$

$$\Rightarrow \quad \log_e\left(\frac{r_n}{r_1}\right) = 2\log_e n$$

This is a graph through origin with slope 2.

4. (d) Both Statement I and Statement II are correct.

Energy of electron accelerated by a potential difference of 16.2 V is 16.2 eV with this energy, the electron can excited the atom $n = 1$ to $n = 3$ as

$E_4 - E_1 = -1.125 - (-18.0) = 16.875 \text{ eV} > 16.2 \text{ eV}$

$E_3 - E_1 = -2.0 - (-18.0) = 16.0 \text{ eV} > 16.2 \text{ eV}$

Hence, only λ_{32}, λ_{31} and λ_{21} is in its emission spectrum.

5. (d) Both Statement I and Statement II are correct.

Atoms of each element are stable and emit characteristics spectrum. The spectrum consists of a set of isolated parallel lines is termed as line spectrum. It provides useful information about the atomic structure.

Match the Columns

1. (c) Radius $= 0.53 \cdot \frac{n^2}{Z}$ (Å)

$$\text{Speed} = 2.2 \times 10^6 \frac{Z}{n} \text{ms}^{-1}$$

$$\text{Current} = ef = \frac{me^5}{4\pi\varepsilon_0^2 h^3} \cdot \frac{Z^2}{n^3}$$

$$\text{Magnetic field, } B = \frac{\mu_0 i_n}{2r_n} = \frac{\pi m^2 e^7 \mu_0}{8\varepsilon_0^3 h^5} \cdot \frac{Z^3}{n^5}$$

Hence, A-II, B-III, C-IV, D-I.

2. (b) (A) $a = r\omega^2 \propto (n^2)(n^{-3})^2 \propto n^{-4}$

(B) $L = \frac{nh}{2\pi}$ or $L \propto n$

(C) $I = mr^2$ or $I \propto r^2 \propto (n^2)^2 \propto n^4$

(D) $E \propto \frac{Z^2}{n^2}$

Hence, A-(I), B-(II), C-(III), D-(IV).

3. (d) A. Ground state energy = Total energy of atom Hence, total energy of hydrogen atom is E_0. Also potential energy is 2 times of total energy i.e. $\text{PE} = 2E_0$ of hydrogen $= 2E_0$

B. Since $E \propto \frac{Z^2}{n^2}$

$\Rightarrow$ Total energy of first excited state of He^+ is $4E_0$.

C. Kinetic energy is half of –ve value of total energy i.e. $\quad KE_{He^+} = -2E_0$

D. Kinetic energy of hydrogen atom will be $\frac{-E_0}{2}$

Hence, A-(III), B-(I), C-(II), D-(IV).

4. (a) Angular speed, $\omega = 2\pi n = 2\pi \frac{v}{2\pi r} = \frac{v}{r}$

As, $\quad v \propto \frac{Z}{n}$ and $r \propto \frac{n^2}{Z} \Rightarrow \omega \propto \frac{Z^2}{n^3}$

$$E_n \propto \frac{Z^2}{n^2}$$

$$B_{\text{centre}} = \mu_0 \frac{\frac{eV}{2\pi r}}{2r} = \frac{\mu_0 eV}{4\pi r^2} \propto \frac{Z^3}{n^5}$$

Hence, A-(II), B-(III), C-(I), D-(IV).

Final Check Through PYQs

1. (d) When an α-particle of mass m moving with velocity v bombards on a heavy nucleus of charge Ze, then there will be no loss of energy as in this case, initial kinetic energy of α-particle = potential energy of α-particle at closest approach.

$$\Rightarrow \quad \frac{1}{2} mv^2 = \frac{2Ze^2}{4\pi\varepsilon_0 r_0}$$

$$\Rightarrow \quad r_0 \propto \frac{1}{m}$$

2. (c) Radius of innermost orbit of H-atom

$$r_0 = 5.3 \times 10^{-11} \text{ m}$$

∴ Radius of third allowed orbit of H-atom.

$$r_3 = r_0 n^2 = r_0 (3)^2$$
$$= 9r_0 = 9 \times 5.3 \times 10^{-11}$$
$$= 47.7 \times 10^{-11} = 4.77 \times 10^{-10} \text{ m}$$
$$= 4.77 \text{ Å}$$

3. (c) According to Bohr's model of H-atom, energy of an electron revolving in nth orbit.

$$E = \frac{-13 \cdot 6}{n^2} \text{ eV}$$

Here, for the first excited state.

$$T_1 = E_1 = \frac{-13 \cdot 6}{n_1^2} = \frac{-13 \cdot 6}{2^2} \quad [\because n_1 = 2]$$

For the second excited state,

$$T_2 = E_2 = \frac{-13 \cdot 6}{n_2^2} = \frac{-13 \cdot 6}{3^2} \text{ eV} \quad [\because n_2 = 3]$$

$$\therefore \quad \frac{T_1}{T_2} = \frac{-13 \cdot 6 / 2^2}{-13 \cdot 6 / 3^2} = \frac{3^2}{2^2} = \frac{9}{4}$$

$$\Rightarrow \quad T_1 : T_2 = 9 : 4$$

4. (b) Total energy of an electron in the nth stationary orbit of hydrogen atom is given by

$$E_n = \frac{-Rhc}{n^2} = \frac{-13.6}{n^2} \text{ eV} \quad [\because Rhc = 13.6 \text{ eV}]$$

5. (c) Since, Bohr's model is valid for hydrogen and hydrogen like atoms He^+, deuteron, etc. So, it is not valid for singly ionised neon atom (Ne^+).

6. (c) Hydrogen atom can be considered to be the system of two charges, positive charged nucleus and negative charged electron. A system of this kind is equivalent to a single particle of mass m' that revolves around the position of the heavier particle. Then, the reduced mass of electron is $m' = \frac{mM}{m+M}$

Its values is less than m.

Given, radius of first orbit for electron

$$r_1 = 0.51 \text{ Å},$$

ground state energy of electron,

$$E_1 = -13.6 \text{ eV},$$

mass of electron $= m_e$

mass of muon, $m_\mu = 207 m_e$ and

mass of nucleus, $M = 1836\, m_e$

When electron in hydrogen atom is replaced by muon, the reduced mass of muon is

$$m_\mu' = \frac{m_\mu M}{m_\mu + M} \quad \text{...(i)}$$

Substituting the given values in Eq. (i), we get

$$m_\mu' = \frac{207 m_e \times 1836 m_e}{207 m_e + 1836 m_e}$$

$$\approx 186\, m_e \quad \text{...(ii)}$$

The radius of first orbit in hydrogen atom for electron is given by,

$$r_1 = \frac{h^2 \varepsilon_0}{\pi m_e e^2} \quad \text{...(iii)}$$

The radius of first orbit for muon is

$$r_1' = \frac{h^2 \varepsilon_0}{\pi m_\mu' e^2} \quad [\because \text{charge of } \mu = \text{charge of } e^-]$$

$$= \frac{h^2 \varepsilon_0}{\pi \times 186 m_e e^2} \quad \text{[From Eq. (ii)]}$$

$$= \left(\frac{h^2 \varepsilon_0}{\pi m_e e^2}\right)\frac{1}{186} = \frac{r_1}{186} \quad \text{[From Eq. (iii)]}$$

$$= \frac{0.51}{186} \text{ Å} \quad [\because r_1 = 0.51 \text{ Å}]$$

$$= 2.74 \times 10^{-13} \text{ m}$$

$$\simeq 2.56 \times 10^{-13} \text{ m} \quad [\because 1 \text{ Å} = 10^{-10} \text{ m}]$$

The total energy of electron is given by

$$E_n = \frac{-mZ^2 e^4}{8\varepsilon_0^2 h^2}\left(\frac{1}{n^2}\right)$$

$$\Rightarrow \quad E_n \propto m$$

For electron in first orbit of hydrogen atom,

$$E_1 = k m_e \quad \text{...(iv)}$$

where, $k = \frac{e^4}{8\varepsilon_0^2 h^2}$ = constant.

For muon in first orbit

$$E_1' = k m_\mu'$$

$$= k \times 186 m_e \quad \text{[from Eq. (i)]}$$

$$= 186 k m_e$$

$$= 186 E_1 \quad \text{[from Eq. (iv)]}$$

$$= 186(-13.6) \text{ eV} \quad \text{[Given]}$$

$$= -2529.6 \text{ eV}$$

$$= -2.5 \text{ keV}$$

$$\simeq -2.8 \text{ keV}$$

7. (b) According to Bohr's model,

$$\text{KE} = \frac{Rhc}{n^2} \quad \text{...(i)}$$

Similarly, potential energy is given by,

$$\text{PE} = -\frac{2Rhc}{n^2} \quad \text{...(ii)}$$

$\therefore$ Total energy, $E = \text{PE} + \text{KE}$

$$= -\frac{Rhc}{n^2} \quad \text{[From Eqs. (i) and (ii)]}$$

$\Rightarrow$ KE $= -E$ and PE $= 2E$

Given, $E = -3.4$ eV

$\therefore$ KE $= -(-3.4) = 3.4$ eV

and PE $= 2(-3.4) = -6.8$ eV

8. (b) Kinetic energy, $\text{KE}_n = \frac{Rhc}{n^2}$ ...(i)

Total energy, $\text{TE}_n = \frac{-Rhc}{n^2}$ ...(ii)

Dividing Eq. (i) by Eq. (ii), we get

$$\frac{\text{KE}_n}{\text{TE}_n} = \frac{\left(\frac{Rhc}{n^2}\right)}{-\left(\frac{Rhc}{n^2}\right)}$$

$\Rightarrow$ $\text{KE}_n : \text{TE}_n = 1 : -1$

9. (c) From Rydberg's formula,

$$\frac{1}{\lambda} = R\left(\frac{1}{n_f^2} - \frac{1}{n_i^2}\right)$$

$$= R\left(\frac{1}{2^2} - \frac{1}{3^2}\right) = \frac{5R}{36}$$

$$\frac{1}{\lambda'} = R\left(\frac{1}{3^2} - \frac{1}{4^2}\right) = \frac{7R}{144}$$

$$\frac{1}{\lambda} / \frac{1}{\lambda'} = \frac{5R}{36} \div \frac{7R}{144}$$

$$\Rightarrow \quad \frac{\lambda'}{\lambda} = \frac{5R}{36} \times \frac{144}{7R} = \frac{20}{7}$$

$$\Rightarrow \quad \lambda' = \frac{20}{7}\lambda$$

10. (*b*) Energy of electron in the 3rd orbit of He^+ is

$$E_3 = -13.6 \times \frac{Z^2}{n^2} \text{ eV} = -13.6 \times \frac{4}{3^2} \text{ eV}$$

$$= -13.6 \times \frac{4}{9} \times 1.6 \times 10^{-19} \text{ J}$$

From Bohr's model, $E_3 = -KE_3 = -\frac{1}{2} m_e v^2$

$$\Rightarrow \frac{1}{2} \times 9.1 \times 10^{-31} \times v^2$$

$$= -13.6 \times \frac{4}{9} \times 1.6 \times 10^{-19}$$

$$\Rightarrow v^2 = \frac{136 \times 16 \times 4 \times 2 \times 10^{-11}}{9 \times 91}$$

or, $v = 1.46 \times 10^6$ m/s

11. (*b*) The wavelength of spectral line is given by

$$\frac{1}{\lambda} = R\left[\frac{1}{n_1^2} - \frac{1}{n_2^2}\right]$$

A. $$\frac{1}{\lambda} = 1.09737 \times 10^7 \left[\frac{1}{2^2} - \frac{1}{3^2}\right]$$

$$\Rightarrow \lambda = \frac{36 \times 10^{-7}}{5 \times 1.09737} = 6.56114 \times 10^{-7} \text{m}$$

$$\simeq 656.3 \text{ nm}$$

B. $$\lambda = \frac{10^{-7}}{1.09737\left[\frac{1}{2^2} - \frac{1}{4^2}\right]} = 4.8601 \times 10^{-7} \text{ m}$$

$$\simeq 486.1 \text{ nm}$$

C. $$\lambda = \frac{10^{-7}}{1.09737 \times \left[\frac{1}{2^2} - \frac{1}{5^2}\right]}$$

$$= \frac{10^{-7} \times 100}{1.09737 \times 21} = 4.3393 \times 10^{-7} \text{ m}$$

$$\simeq 434.1 \text{ nm}$$

D. $$\lambda = \frac{10^{-7}}{1.09737 \times \left[\frac{1}{2^2} - \frac{1}{6^2}\right]}$$

$$= \frac{10^{-7} \times 144}{1.09737 \times 32} \simeq 410.2 \text{ nm}$$

Hence, A-III, B-IV, C-II, D-I.

12. (*c*) Atoms are electrically neutral as they contain equal number of protons and electrons. Statement II is incorrect because atom of radioactive elements are not stable.

13. (*a*) In hydrogen spectrum,

$$\frac{1}{\lambda} = R\left(\frac{1}{n_1^2} - \frac{1}{n_2^2}\right)$$

For shortest wavelength in the Balmer series,

$$n_1 = 2 \text{ and } n_2 = \infty$$

$$\therefore \frac{1}{\lambda} = R\left(\frac{1}{2^2} - \frac{1}{\infty^2}\right)$$

$$\Rightarrow \frac{1}{\lambda} = \frac{R}{4}$$

$$\Rightarrow R = \frac{4}{\lambda} \quad \text{...(i)}$$

For the shortest wavelength of Brackett series, $n_1 = 4$ and $n_2 = \infty$

$$\therefore \frac{1}{\lambda_B} = R\left(\frac{1}{4^2} - \frac{1}{\infty^2}\right)$$

$$= \frac{R}{16} = \frac{4/\lambda}{16}$$

$$\Rightarrow \frac{1}{\lambda_B} = \frac{1}{4\lambda} \Rightarrow \lambda_B = 4\lambda$$

14. (*c*) Wavelength of spectral lines are given by

$$\frac{1}{\lambda} = z^2 R\left(\frac{1}{n_1^2} - \frac{1}{n_2^2}\right)$$

For last line of Balmer series,

$$n_1 = 2 \text{ and } n_2 = \infty$$

$$\Rightarrow \frac{1}{\lambda_B} = z^2 R\left(\frac{1}{2^2} - \frac{1}{\infty^2}\right)$$

$$= \frac{R}{4} \quad [\because z = 1]$$

Similarly, for last line of Lyman series,

$$n_1 = 1 \text{ and } n_2 = \infty$$

$$\Rightarrow \frac{1}{\lambda_2} = z^2 R\left(\frac{1}{1^2} - \frac{1}{\infty^2}\right) = R$$

$$\therefore \frac{\frac{1}{\lambda_B}}{\frac{1}{\lambda_L}} = \frac{\frac{R}{4}}{R} = \frac{1}{4}$$

$$\Rightarrow \frac{\lambda_L}{\lambda_B} = \frac{1}{4} \Rightarrow \frac{\lambda_B}{\lambda_L} = 4$$

15. (*d*) In hydrogen atom, wavelength of characteristic spectrum

$$\frac{1}{\lambda} = Rz^2\left[\frac{1}{n_1^2} - \frac{1}{n_2^2}\right]$$

For Lyman series $n_1 = 1, n_2 = 2$

$$\frac{1}{\lambda_1} = Rz^2\left[\frac{1}{(1)^2} - \frac{1}{(2)^2}\right] \quad \text{...(i)}$$

For Balmer series $n_1 = 2, n_2 = 3$

$$\frac{1}{\lambda_2} = Rz^2\left[\frac{1}{(2)^2} - \frac{1}{(3)^2}\right] \quad \text{...(ii)}$$

Dividing Eq. (ii) by Eq. (i) we get

$$\frac{\lambda_1}{\lambda_2}=\frac{Rz^2\left[\frac{1}{4}-\frac{1}{9}\right]}{Rz^2\left[1-\frac{1}{4}\right]}=\frac{\frac{5}{36}}{\frac{3}{4}}$$

$$\frac{\lambda_1}{\lambda_2}=\frac{5}{36}\times\frac{4}{3}=\frac{5}{27}$$

Skill Builder

■ Sol. of Skill Builder on Pg. 690

(c) we have, $r_n = r_0 n^2$

Now, $\frac{r_3}{r_5}=\frac{r_0(3)^2}{r_5(5)^2}=9:25$

■ Sol. of Skill Builder on Pg. 692

(c) Total energy in ground state = – Kinetic energy

$\Rightarrow$ Total energy = –10 eV

■ Sol. of Skill Builder on Pg. 699

(c) In hydrogen spectrum, $\frac{1}{\lambda}=R\left(\frac{1}{n_1^2}-\frac{1}{n_2^2}\right)$

For shortest wavelength in Lyman series,

$n_1 = 1$ and $n_2 = \infty$

$$\therefore \quad \frac{1}{\lambda_L}=R\left(\frac{1}{1^2}-\frac{1}{\infty^2}\right)$$

$$\frac{1}{\lambda}=R \qquad \{\because \lambda_L=\lambda\}$$

$$\lambda=\frac{1}{R} \qquad \text{... (i)}$$

For shortest wavelength of Paschen series,

$n_1 = 3$ and $n_2 = \infty$

$$\therefore \quad \frac{1}{\lambda_P}=R\left(\frac{1}{3^2}-\frac{1}{\infty^2}\right)$$

$$\lambda_P=\frac{9}{R}$$

From Eq. (i), $\lambda_P=\frac{9}{1/\lambda}=9\lambda$

For deeper insight
Scan the QR Code

Chapter 14

Nuclei

Chapter Overview with
NEET Connection

This chapter contains the concept of nuclear physics. It will be difficult to learn and understand whole nuclear reactions without the deep understanding of concepts and their applications belonging to this chapter.

Special format questions can easily be framed on the following topics of this chapter

- Properties of nuclei
- Mass-energy relation and binding energy of nucleon
- Nuclear reaction

For better understanding of this chapter

- Basic idea and visualisation of atom are required
- Numerical calculation part should be strong.

Learning Objectives

Module-I

- Nucleus
- Mass-Energy Relation
- Binding Energy of Nucleus
- Binding Energy Curve
- Nuclear Forces
- Nuclear Stability

Module-II

- Nuclear Reaction
- Nuclear Energy

Introduction

In the previous chapter, we have learnt fundamental structure of the atoms and discovery of nucleus which was done by Rutherford during his α-scattering experiment. Just like atoms nucleons is also composed of tiny particles (proton and neutron). Different combinations of these protons and neutrons produces nucleus of all visible and invisible matter. Out of these nucleus, some are stable and other are radioactive.

In this chapter, we will study properties of nuclei on microscale such as its size, mass, density, etc., nuclear stability and nuclear reactions.

Module 1

Nucleus, Mass Defect and Binding Energy

- Nucleus • Mass-Energy Relation • Binding Energy of Nucleus
- Binding Energy Curve • Nuclear Forces • Nuclear Stability

Nucleus

As per the Rutherford's experiment, it was concluded that the entire positive charge and mass of an atom was present at its very tiny centre known as nucleus.

Composition of Nucleus

Nucleus is composed of two types of particles

(i) **Protons** Positively charged particles

(ii) **Neutrons** Neutral particles

Mass of neutron is slightly greater than the mass of the proton.

$$\text{Mass of proton, } m_p = 16726231 \times 10^{-27}\,\text{kg}$$

$$\text{Mass of neutron, } m_n = 1.6749286 \times 10^{-27}\,\text{kg}$$

$$m_p \simeq 1840\, m_e$$

where, m_e = mass of electron.

Atomic Number

Atomic number of an element is the number of proton present inside the nucleus. It is also equal to the number of electrons revolving in various orbits around the nucleus of an uncharged atom. It is represented by Z.

Atomic number (Z) = Number of proton

= Number of electron

Mass Number

The total number of neutrons and protons, *i.e.* number of nucleons present inside the nucleus of an element is called its mass number A. Number of neutrons is represented by N.

So, mass number $(A) = Z + N$

A chemical element is represented by

$_Z(\text{chemical symbol})^A$ or $_ZX^A$.

Total charge of the nucleus is equal to the total charge on all protons Z in it, *i.e.* Ze, where $e = 1.6 \times 10^{-19}$ C.

Size of Nucleus

From various experiments, it was found that the volume of the nucleus is directly proportional to the number of nucleons (mass number) constituting the nucleus.

Let R is the radius of the nucleus having mass number A, then volume, $V = \frac{4}{3}\pi R^3 \propto A \Rightarrow R \propto A^{1/3}$

$$\Rightarrow \boxed{R = R_0 A^{1/3}}$$

where, $R_0 = 1.2 \times 10^{-15}$ m, is the range of nuclear size.

It is also known as **nuclear unit radius.**

Owing to the small size of the nucleus, fermi (fm) is found to be a convenient unit of length in nuclear physics.

It is defined as, 1 fermi (fm) $= 10^{-15}$ m.

NEET Close-up

Example Similar to PYQ Asked in NEET 2015

If nuclear radius of Al is 6.4 fm, then the nuclear radius of ^{125}Fe will be

(a) 10 fm (b) 12 fm (c) 15 fm (d) 7 fm

Sol. (*a*) Radius of the nucleus, $R = R_0 A^{1/3}$

$$\frac{R_{Fe}}{R_{Al}} = \left(\frac{A_{Fe}}{A_{Al}}\right)^{1/3} = \left(\frac{125}{27}\right)^{1/3} = \frac{5}{3}$$

$$\text{Radius, } R_{Fe} = \frac{5}{3} R_{Al} = \frac{5}{3} \times 6.4 \approx 10\,\text{fm}$$

Skill Builder

If a nuclei splits into two nuclei having mass numbers A and B, then ratio of radius of two daughter nuclei respectively is

(a) $\frac{A}{B}$ (b) $\frac{B}{A}$ (c) $\left(\frac{A}{B}\right)^{1/3}$ (d) $\left(\frac{B}{A}\right)^{1/3}$

For more Practice Refer Q. No. 5 of Step up practice 1 and Q. No. 11 of Gearing up for NEET.

Nuclear Density

Density of nuclear matter is the ratio of mass of nucleus to its volume.

If m is the average mass of a nucleon ($\simeq 1.67 \times 10^{-27}$ kg) and A is the mass number of element, then the mass of nucleus = mA. If R is the nuclear radius, then

$$\text{Volume of nucleus} = \frac{4}{3}\pi R^3 = \frac{4}{3}\pi(R_0 A^{1/3})^3 = \frac{4}{3}\pi R_0^3 A$$

$$\text{As, density of nuclear matter} = \frac{\text{mass of nucleus}}{\text{volume of nucleus}}$$

$$\therefore \quad \rho = \frac{mA}{\frac{4}{3}\pi R_0^3 A} \quad \text{or} \quad \boxed{\rho = \frac{3m}{4\pi R_0^3}}$$

Thus, the density of nucleus is constant and independent of A for all nuclei. Different nuclei are like a drop of liquid of constant density. The density of nuclear matter is approximately $2.3 \times 10^{17}\,\text{kgm}^{-3}$. This density is very large as compared to ordinary matter.

Mentor's Tip

$$\text{Number of nucleon per unit volume} = \frac{\text{Density}}{\text{Mass of one nucleon}}$$

Density of nucleus is constant i.e. 2.3×10^{17} kg hence

$$\text{Number of nucleons per unit volume} = \frac{2.3 \times 10^{17}}{1.67 \times 10^{-27}} \text{ per m}^3 \cong 10^{44} \text{ per m}^3$$

Example 1. *Assuming that protons and neutrons have equal masses, calculate how many times nuclear matter is denser than water. (Take, mass of nucleon = 1.67×10^{-27} kg and $R_0 = 1.2 \times 10^{-15}$ m)*

Sol. Density of nucleus ,

$$\rho = \frac{3m}{4\pi R_0^3} = \frac{3 \times 1.67 \times 10^{-27}}{4 \times \frac{22}{7} \times (1.2 \times 10^{-15})^3}$$

$$= \frac{7 \times 3 \times 1.67 \times 10^{18}}{88 \times 1.2 \times 1.2 \times 1.2} = 2.307 \times 10^{17}\ \text{kg/m}^3$$

Density of water, $\rho' = 10^3\ \text{kg/m}^3$

$$\therefore \quad \frac{\rho}{\rho'} = \frac{2.307 \times 10^{17}}{10^3} = 2.307 \times 10^{14}$$

Mass-Energy Relation

According to Einstein, mass and energy are interconvertible. He predicted that, if the energy of a body changes by an amount E, its mass changes by an amount Δm given by the equation, $\quad E = \Delta mc^2$

where, c is the speed of light.

Everyday examples of energy gain are too small to produce detectable changes of mass. But in nuclear physics, this plays an important role. Mass appears as energy and the two can be regarded as equivalent.

NEET Snapshot

Energy equivalent of a substance does not change, if its mass does not change. ***[NEET 2020]***

Relation for energy equivalent of mass, $E = mc^2$

where, c is speed of light and it is constant.

If mass does not change, then it is also constant. Therefore, energy equivalent of a mass does not change.

Scan for Video

Example 2. *Calculate energy equivalent of 2g of a substance.*

Sol. Mass-energy relation, $E = mc^2$

$$= 2 \times 10^{-3} \times (3 \times 10^8)^2 = 18 \times 10^{13}$$

$$\Rightarrow \quad E = 1.8 \times 10^{14}\ \text{J}$$

Mass Defect of Nucleus

It has been found that, the rest mass of the nucleus of a stable atom is always less than the sum of the masses of its constituents nucleons (protons and neutrons) in the free state. The difference between the sum of the masses of the nucleons constituting a nucleus and the rest mass of the nucleus is called mass defect (Δm).

Mass defect, Δm = (Mass of protons + Mass of neutrons) − Mass of the nucleus

Let us consider an atom of element $_ZX^A$, its atomic number is Z and mass number is A. Thus, its nucleus has Z protons and $(A - Z)$ neutrons. If m_p is the mass of a proton, m_n is the mass of a neutrons and m_N is the mass of the nucleus, then the mass defect,

$$\boxed{\Delta m = Zm_p + (A - Z)m_n - m_N}$$

Atomic Mass Unit or amu

In nuclear physics, mass is measured in unified atomic mass units abbreviated amu or u as mass of an atom is very small.

(i) The amu is defined as $\frac{1}{12}$ th mass of a $_6C^{12}$ atom.

(ii) 1 amu (or 1u) = 1.66×10^{-27} kg.

(iii) It can be shown using relation ($\Delta E = \Delta mc^2$) that, 1u mass has energy of 931.5 MeV.

For 1u, $\quad \Delta m = 1.66 \times 10^{-27}$ kg

$$c = 3 \times 10^8\ \text{ms}^{-1}$$

$$\therefore \quad \Delta E = \Delta mc^2 = 1.66 \times 10^{-27}\,(3 \times 10^8)^2$$

$$= 1.494 \times 10^{-10}\ \text{J}$$

$$= \frac{1.494 \times 10^{-10}}{1.6 \times 10^{-19}}\ \text{eV} = 931.5\ \text{MeV}$$

$$\therefore \quad \boxed{\mathbf{1\,u = 931.5\ MeV}}$$

Example 3. *Calculate the mass defect of helium ($_2He^4$).* *(Take, mass of proton = 1.007276 u, mass of neutron = 1.008665 u and mass of $_2He^4$ = 4.001506 u)*

Sol. Mass defect = Mass of nucleons – Mass of nucleus

[Here, A(mass number) = 4

and Z(atomic number) = 2

∴ Number of protons = 2

and number of neutrons = $A - Z = 4 - 2 = 2$]

Δm = Mass of 2 protons + Mass of 2 neutrons – Mass of nucleus

$= [2 \times 1.007276 + 2 \times 1.008665 - 4.001506]$

$= 0.030376$ u

Example 4. *Calculate the energy required to remove the least tightly bound neutron in $_{20}Ca^{40}$. (Given, mass of $_{20}Ca^{40}$ = 39.962589 amu, mass of $_{20}Ca^{39}$ = 38.970691 amu and mass of neutron = 1.008665 amu)*

Sol. Here in order to remove a neutron, energy has to be supplied.

Mass defect, $\Delta m = M(^{39}_{20}\text{Ca}) + M(^1_0 n) - M(^{40}_{20}\text{Ca})$

$= 38.970691 + 1.008665 - 39.962589$

$= 0.016767$ amu

Equivalent energy $= 0.016767 \times 931$ ($\because$ 1 amu = 931 MeV)

$= 15.6$ MeV

Example 5. *A neutron breaks into a proton and an electron. Calculate the energy produced in this reaction. (Take, $m_e = 9 \times 10^{-31}$ kg, $m_p = 1.6725 \times 10^{-27}$ kg, $m_n = 1.6747 \times 10^{-27}$ kg and $c = 3 \times 10^8$ m/s)*

Sol. We have, $^1_0 n \rightarrow {}^1_1 p + {}^0_{-1} e$

Mass defect, $\Delta m = m_n - m_p - m_e$

$= [1.6747 \times 10^{-27} - 1.6725 \times 10^{-27} - 0.0009 \times 10^{-27}]$

$= 1.3 \times 10^{-30}$ kg

Energy produced $= \Delta mc^2 = 1.3 \times 10^{-30} \times (3 \times 10^8)^2$

$= 11.7 \times 10^{-14}$ J

$= \dfrac{11.7 \times 10^{-14}}{1.6 \times 10^{-13}}$ ($\because$ 1 MeV $= 1.6 \times 10^{-13}$ J)

$= 0.73$ MeV

Binding Energy of Nucleus

The binding energy (E_b) of a nucleus is defined as the minimum energy required to separate its nucleons and place them at rest at infinite distance apart.

Or

The binding energy of a nucleus may be defined as the energy equivalent to the mass defect of the nucleus.

If Δm is mass defect, then according to Einstein's mass-energy relation,

Binding energy $= \Delta mc^2 = [\{Zm_p + (A - Z)m_n\} - m_N] \cdot c^2$

This binding energy is expressed in joule, if Δm is measured in kg.

If Δm is measured in amu, then binding energy,

$$E_b = \Delta m \times 931 \text{ MeV}$$

where, $\Delta m = [\{Zm_p + (A - Z)m_n\} - m_N]$ amu

Mentor's Tip

Binding energy can also be written as

$E_b = [Zm_H + (A - Z)m_N - m_A]c^2$

where, m_H is the mass of H-atom and m_A the atomic mass. By using the masses of H-atoms rather than protons, masses of the electrons in the atom cancel out. We do this because it is atomic masses that are measured directly by mass spectrometer. A slight error made by doing so, but that is negligible.

Example 6. *Find the binding energy of an α-particle from the following data.*

[Take, mass of the helium nucleus, m ($_2He^4$) = 4.001265 u, mass of proton, m_p = 1.007277 u, mass of neutron, m_n = 1.008666 u and 1 u = 931.4813 MeV]

Sol. α-particle consists of 2 protons and 2 neutrons.

Mass defect, $\Delta m = [Zm_p + Nm_n - m(^4_2\text{He})]$

$= 2 \times 1.007277 + 2 \times 1.008666 - 4.001265$

$= 0.03062$ u

Binding energy $= \Delta m \times 931.4813$ MeV

$= 0.03062 \times 931.48 = 28.52$ MeV

Binding Energy per Nucleon

The average energy required to release a nucleon from the nucleus is called binding energy per nucleon.

Binding energy per nucleon

$$= \frac{\text{Total binding energy}}{\text{Mass number (i.e. total number of nucleons)}}$$

$$= \frac{\Delta m \times 931 \text{MeV}}{A}$$

$$\Rightarrow \quad E_{bn} = \frac{E_b}{A}$$

Binding energy per nucleon ∝ Stability of nucleus.

Example 7. *Binding energy of $_{17}Cl^{35}$ and $_{15}P^{31}$ are 287.67 MeV and 262.48 MeV. Which of the two nuclei is more stable?*

Sol. Binding energy per nucleon of $_{17}\text{Cl}^{35} = \dfrac{\text{Binding energy}}{\text{Mass number}}$

$= \dfrac{287.67}{35} = 8.22$ MeV

Binding energy per nucleon of $_{15}P^{31} = \frac{262.48}{31} = 8.47\,\text{MeV}$

BE of $_{15}P^{31}$ is more than BE of $_{17}Cl^{35}$.

Hence, $_{15}P^{31}$ is more stable.

Example 8 *If the binding energy per nucleon of deuteron is 1.115 MeV, find its mass defect in atomic mass unit.*

Sol. Binding energy per nucleon, $E_{bn} = \frac{E_b}{A}$

For deuteron, atomic mass, $A = 2$

Substituting the values in above equation, we get

$$1.115\ \text{MeV} = \frac{E_b}{2} \Rightarrow E_b = 2 \times 1.115\ \text{MeV}$$

Since, $E_b = 931.5 \times \Delta m$

$$\Rightarrow \Delta m = \frac{E_b}{931.5} \Rightarrow \Delta m = \frac{2 \times 1.115}{931.5} = 0.0024\ \text{u}$$

NEET Close-up

Example Similar to PYQ Asked in NEET 2021

A nucleus of mass number A breaks into two nuclei of equal mass number $A/2$. If unfragmented nucleus has energy E_1 per nucleon and fragmented nuclei have energies $E_2 (E_2 > E_1)$ per nucleon, then total binding energies gain in this process is

(a) $\frac{(E_1 - E_2)}{A}$ (b) $(E_2 - E_1)A$

(c) $\frac{E_1 E_2}{A}$ (d) $\frac{(E_1 + E_2)}{A}$

Sol. (*b*) Gain in BE =

BE of products − BE of reactants

$$= \left(E_2 \times \frac{A}{2} \times 2\right) - (E_1 \times A)$$

$$= (E_2 - E_1)A$$

Skill Builder

A nucleus ($A = 270$) breaks into two nuclei of mass numbers $A_1 = 130$ and $A_2 = 140$. If binding energy of the three nuclei are (respectively 6.5 MeV, 7 MeV and 7.5 MeV, then binding energy gain will be

(a) 205 MeV (b) 200 MeV (c) 5 MeV (d) 105 MeV

For more Practice Refer Q. No. 13 of Step up practice 1 and Q. No. 6 of Gearing up for NEET.

Binding Energy Curve

It is the graph between binding energy per nucleon and total number of nucleons (*i.e.* mass number *A*).

Some features of this curve are given below.

(i) The curve has almost a flat maximum roughly from $A = 50$ to $A = 80$ corresponding to an average BE/nucleon of about 8.5 MeV, so the nuclei having mass number between 50 to 80 are most stable. Iron (Fe^{56}) ($A = 56$), having a BE/nucleon of about 8.8 MeV has maximum stability.

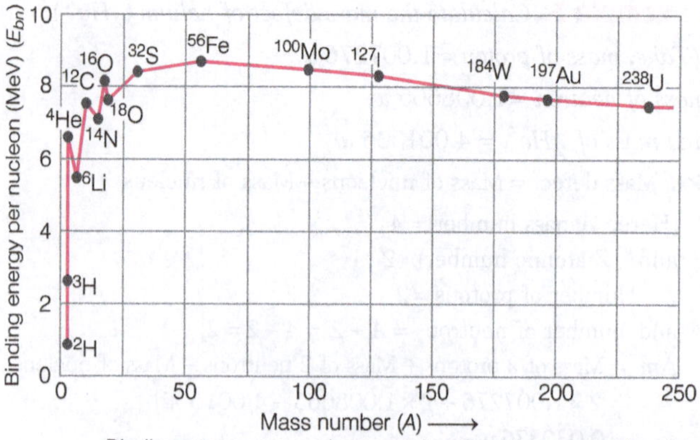

Binding energy per nucleon as a function of mass number *A*

(ii) For nuclei having mass number more than 80, the average binding energy per nucleon decreases slowly and drop to about 7.6 MeV for uranium ($A = 238$).

The lower value of binding energy per nucleon fails to overcome the repulsion among protons in nuclei having large number of protons, *i.e.* the nuclei of heavier atoms, beyond $_{83}Bi^{209}$ are radioactive.

(iii) For nuclei having mass number below 20, it decreases sharply. e.g., for heavy hydrogen (H^2), it is only about 1.1 MeV. This shows that the nuclei having mass number below 20 are comparatively less stable.

(iv) Below $A = 50$, the curve does not fall continuously but has subsidiary peaks at $_8O^{16}$, $_6C^{12}$ and $_2He^4$. This shows that these (even-even) nuclei are more stable than their immediate neighbours.

Conclusions from the Graph

(i) The curve shows that very heavy and very light nuclei have a lower average BE/nucleon than the nuclei of intermediate masses. So, if a very heavy nucleus (such as U^{238}) be split into two lighter nuclei near the flat maximum of the curve, the BE/nucleon will increase. Hence, energy will be released in the process. This method of releasing nuclear energy by breaking up a heavy nucleus into two lighter nuclei of comparable masses is called **nuclear fission.** It is the basis of nuclear bombs and nuclear reactors.

(ii) Alternatively, if two or more very light nuclei (such as H^2) be combined to form a heavier nucleus (such as He^4), the BE/nucleon will again increase and now by a much greater amount than in the fission process. This will result in much larger release of energy. This method of releasing nuclear energy is called **nuclear fusion.** It occurs inside sun and other stars and is the source of their energy.

(iii) Force between nucleons is attractive and very strong, so that it can produce binding energy per nucleon in MeV.

(iv) The nuclear force is constant for $30 < A < 170$, this implies that the force is short-ranged.

Nuclear Forces

As we know that, nucleus consists of positively charged proton and neutral particle neutron. The protons due to their positive charge repel each other, so there must be a strong force inside the nucleus which overcome the repulsive force of protons and bind them together inside the nucleus. This force is called nuclear force.

Therefore, the forces that holds the nucleons together inside the nucleus of an atom are called nuclear forces.

Some important properties of nuclear forces are given below.

(i) Nuclear forces are charge independent.

(ii) Nuclear forces are short range forces. These do not exist at large distances greater than 10^{-15} m.

(iii) These are attractive force and cause stability of the nucleus.

(iv) Nuclear forces are non-central force.

(v) Nuclear forces are the strongest force in nature.

(vi) Nuclear forces depends on the direction of the spins of the nucleons. The force is stronger, if the spin of nucleons is parallel and is weak, if it is anti-parallel.

(vii) Electrical and gravitational forces follow inverse square law (*i.e.* $F \propto 1/r^2$) but nuclear forces are complicated in nature and does not follow it.

Concept ladder

- A Japanese scientist Yukawa in 1935 suggested that the nuclear forces are **exchange forces** which are produced by the exchange of new particles called **π-mesons between nucleons.** These particles were later on actually discovered in cosmic radiation.
- There are three types of π-mesons. π^+, π^- and π^0. There is a continuous exchange of π-mesons between protons and neutrons due to which they continue to be converted into one another.

$$p \to \pi^+ + n \text{ and } n \to p + \pi^-$$

- The forces between a pair of neutrons or a pair of protons are the result of the exchange of neutral meson (π^0) between them. *i.e.* $p \to p' + \pi^0$ and $n \to n' + \pi^0$

  Thus, exchange of π meson between nucleons keeps the nucleons bound together. It is responsible for the nuclear force.

Nuclear Stability

The stability of a nucleus is determined by the value of its binding energy per nucleon. Higher the binding energy of nucleon, more stable is the nucleus. The stability of nucleus is also determined by its neutron to proton ratio.

A plot of number of neutrons and number of protons is shown in the figure below.

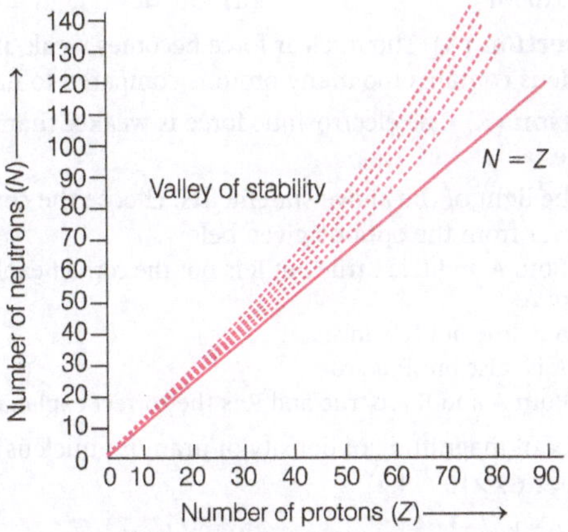

Graphical representation of number of neutrons *versus* number of protons

In the figure, the solid line shows the nuclei with equal number of protons and neutrons ($N = Z$). Only light nuclei are on this line, *i.e.* they are stable if they contain approximately same number of protons and neutrons.

Heavy nuclei are stable, only when they have more neutrons than protons.

The long narrow region shown in the figure, which contains the cluster of short lines representing stable nuclei is referred to as the valley of stability.

The nuclide $^{209}_{83}$Bi is the heaviest stable nucleus.

Experimental study shows that the stable nuclei contain even number of protons or neutrons or both.

STEP UP Practice 1

1. If a proton and anti-proton come close to each other and annihilate, how much energy will be released?
(a) 1.5×10^{-10} J (b) 3×10^{-10} J
(c) 4.5×10^{-10} J (d) 4×10^{-10} J

2. The rest energy of an electron is
(a) 510 keV (b) 652 keV
(c) 510 MeV (d) 736 MeV

3. **Assertion** (A) The nuclear force becomes weak, if the nucleus contains too many protons compared to neutrons.
Reason (R) The electrostatic force is weaker than nuclear force.
In the light of the above statements, choose the correct answer from the options given below.
(a) Both A and R are true but R is not the correct explanation of A.
(b) A is true but R is false.
(c) A is false but is R true.
(d) Both A and R are true and R is the correct explanation of A.

4. Order of magnitude of density of uranium nucleus is ($m_p = 1.67 \times 10^{-27}$ kg)
(a) 10^{20} kg/m^3 (b) 10^{17} kg/m^3
(c) 10^{14} kg/m^3 (d) 10^{11} kg/m^3

5. Radius of ${}_2^4$He nucleus is 4 fm. The radius of ${}_{82}^{206}$Pb nucleus will be
(a) 5 fm (b) 6 fm (c) 14.88 fm (d) 8 fm

6. **Assertion** (A) Nuclei having mass number about 60 are most stable.
Reason (R) When two or more light nuclei are combined into a heavier nucleus, then the binding energy per nucleon will increase.
In the light of the above statements, choose the correct answer from the options given below
(a) Both A and R are true but R is not the correct explanation of A.
(b) A is true but R is false.
(c) A is false but is R true.
(d) Both A and R are true and R is the correct explanation of A.

7. If an electron and a positron annihilate, then the energy released is
(a) 3.2×10^{-13} J (b) 1.6×10^{-13} J
(c) 4.8×10^{-13} J (d) 6.4×10^{-13} J

8. The mass defect in a particular nuclear reaction is 0.3 g. The amount of energy liberated in (kilowatt hours) is (velocity of light = 3×10^8 ms^{-1})
(a) 1.5×10^6 (b) 2.5×10^6
(c) 3×10^6 (d) 7.5×10^6

9. **Assertion** (A) Generally heavy nuclei are unstable.
Reason (R) It has more neutrons and protons.
In the light of the above statements, choose the correct answer from the options given below.
(a) Both A and R are true but R is not the correct explanation of A.
(b) A is true but R is false.
(c) A is false but is R true.
(d) Both A and R are true and R is the correct explanation of A.

10. If m, m_n and m_p are the masses of ${}_ZX^A$ nucleus, neutron and proton respectively, then
(a) $m < (A-Z)m_n + Zm_p$ (b) $m = (A-Z)m_n + Zm_p$
(c) $m = (A-Z)m_p + Zm_n$ (d) $m > (A-Z)m_n + Zm_p$

11. The masses of neutron and proton are 1.0087 amu and 1.0073 amu, respectively. If the neutrons and protons combine to form a helium nucleus (alpha particles) of mass 4.0015 amu, the binding energy of the helium nucleus will be (1 amu = 931 MeV)
(a) 28.4 MeV (b) 20.8 MeV (c) 27.3 MeV (d) 14.2 MeV

12. Assume that protons and neutrons have equal masses. Given that nuclear radius is given by $R = 1.2 \times 10^{-15} A^{1/3}$ metre and mass of nucleon $= 1.67 \times 10^{-27}$ kg on the basis of above condition, which of the following pair is not correctly paired?
(a) Nuclear mass → $1.67 \times 10^{-27} A$ kg
(b) Nuclear volume → 7.24×10^{-45} Am^3
(c) Nuclear density → 7.59×10^{40} m^{-3}
(d) Ratio of nuclear density to density of water → 2.307×10^{14}

13. In a fission reaction ${}_{92}^{236}\text{U} \rightarrow {}^{117}X + {}^{117}Y + n + n$, the binding energy per nucleon of X and Y is 8.5 MeV, whereas of ^{236}U is 7.6 MeV. The total energy liberated will be about
(a) 200 keV (b) 2 MeV (c) 200 MeV (d) 2000 MeV

14. The mass number of a nucleus is
(a) always less than its atomic number
(b) always more than its atomic number
(c) always equal to its atomic number
(d) sometimes more than and sometimes equal to its atomic number

15. In comparison to ^{12}C atom, ^{14}C atom have
(a) two extra protons and two extra electrons
(b) two extra protons but no extra electrons
(c) two extra neutrons but no extra electrons
(d) two extra neutrons and two extra electrons

16. In ${}_{88}\text{Ra}^{226}$ nucleus, there are
(a) 138 protons and 88 neutrons
(b) 138 neutrons and 88 protons
(c) 226 neutrons and 88 electrons
(d) 226 neutrons and 138 electrons

17. In helium nucleus, there are
(a) 2 protons and 2 electrons
(b) 2 neutrons, 12 protons and 2 electrons
(c) 2 protons and 2 neutrons
(d) 2 positrons and 2 protons

18. Assertion (A) $^{14}_{7}N$ is stable.

Reason (R) Nuclei having an odd number of protons and odd number of neutrons are generally less stable than the one having even number of protons and even number of neutrons.

In the light of the above statements, choose the correct answer from the options given below.

(a) Both A and R are true but R is not the correct explanation of A.
(b) A is true but R is false.
(c) A is false but is true.
(d) Both A and R are true and R is the correct explanation of A.

19. Assertion (A) Mass defect in nuclear reaction is less than 1%.

Reason (R) In nuclear reaction, change in BE per nucleon is generally less than 1%.

In the light of the above statements, choose the correct answer from the options given below.

(a) Both A and R are true but R is not the correct explanation of A.
(b) A is true but R is false.
(c) A is false but R is true.
(d) Both A and R are true and R is the correct explanation of A.

Module 2

Nuclear Energy

- Nuclear Reaction
- Nuclear Energy

Nuclear Reaction

The process by which the identity of a nucleus is changed when it is bombarded by an energetic particle is called nuclear reaction. The general expression for the nuclear reaction is a follows.

$$\underset{\text{(Parent nucleus)}}{X} + \underset{\text{(Incident particle)}}{a} \longrightarrow \underset{\text{(Compound nucleus)}}{C} \longrightarrow \underset{\text{(Product nucleus)}}{Y} + \underset{\text{(Daughter nucleus)}}{b} + \underset{\text{Energy}}{Q}$$

Here, X & a are the reactants, Y & b are the products and Q is the kinetic energy released in the nuclear reaction.

Conservation laws obeyed by nuclear reaction are,

(i) Mass number and electric charge is conserved.

i.e. $\Sigma Z_{\text{initial}} = \Sigma Z_{\text{final}}, \ \Sigma A_{\text{initial}} = \Sigma A_{\text{final}}$

(ii) Linear momentum and angular momentum are conserved.

(iii) Total energy of the reaction remains conserved, here the term Q helps to balance the total energy of reaction.

Q-value

Q-value means the difference between the rest mass energy of initial constituents and the rest mass energy of final constituents of a nuclear reaction.

Q-value of nuclear reaction

As considered, $X + a \longrightarrow Y + b + Q$

where, $Q = U_i - U_f$

Here, U_i = rest mass energy of initial constituents

and U_f = rest mass energy of final constituents

$$= (M_X + M_a - M_Y - M_b) \cdot c^2$$

If $Q = +$ve, reaction is exothermic

and $Q = -$ve, reaction is endothermic.

e.g. **For α-decay,** ${}_Z X^A \rightarrow {}_{Z-2}Y^{A-4} + {}_2\text{He}^4$ (alpha particle)

So, Q-value will be

$$Q = [m({}_Z X^A) - m({}_{Z-2}Y^{A-4}) - m({}_2\text{He}^4)] \cdot c^2$$

which represents the kinetic energy available to the products.

For β⁻-decay, ${}_Z X^A \rightarrow {}_{Z+1}Y^A + e^- + \bar{\nu}$

$$U_i = [m({}_Z X^A) - Zm_e] \cdot c^2$$

$$U_f = [m({}_{Z+1}Y^A) - (Z+1)m_e + m_e] \cdot c^2$$

Kinetic energy available to the products,

$$Q = U_i - U_f = [m({}_Z X^A) - m({}_{Z+1}Y^A)] \cdot c^2$$

For β⁺-decay, ${}_Z X^A \rightarrow {}_{Z-1}Y^A + e^+ + \nu$

$$U_i = [m({}_Z X^A) - Zm_e] \cdot c^2$$

$$U_f = [m({}_{Z-1}Y^A) - (Z-1)m_e + m_e] \cdot c^2$$

Kinetic energy available to the products,

$$Q = [m({}_Z X^A) - m({}_{Z-1}Y^A) - 2m_e] \cdot c^2$$

For electron capture, ${}_Z X^A \rightarrow {}_{Z-1}Y^A$

$$Q = [m({}_Z X^A) - m({}_{Z-1}Y^A)] \cdot c^2$$

NEET Close-up

Example Similar to PYQ Asked in NEET 2024

$${}^{235}_{92}P \xrightarrow{\alpha} Q \xrightarrow{e^+} R \xrightarrow{\beta^-} S \xrightarrow{e^-} T$$

In the nuclear emission stated above, the mass number and atomic number of the product *T* respectively, are

(a) 231, 90 (b) 231, 91 (c) 238, 91 (d) 238, 90

Sol. (*b*) ${}^{235}_{92}P \xrightarrow{\alpha} {}^{231}_{90}Q \xrightarrow{e^+} {}^{231}_{89}R \xrightarrow{\beta^-} {}^{231}_{90}S \xrightarrow{e^-} {}^{231}_{91}T$

$A = 231$ and $Z = 91$

Skill Builder

An element *X*-decays, first by positron emission and then α-particles are emitted in successive radioactive decay. If the product nucleus has a mass number 235 and atomic number 87, the mass number and atomic number of element *X* are

(a) 239, 91 (b) 243, 91
(c) 239, 90 (d) 239, 89

For more Practice Refer Q. No. 2 of Step up practice 1.

Nuclear Energy

The energy released during nuclear reaction is called nuclear energy. Generally, there is loss of mass in nuclear reaction, which results (according to Einstein's equation) into release of energy.

Consequently, if nuclei with less total binding energy transform to nuclei with greater binding energy, there will be a net energy release. This happens when a heavy nucleus decays into two or more intermediate mass fragments (fission) or when light nuclei fuse into a heavier nucleus (fusion).

In a nuclear reaction, the energy released is of the order of MeV. For same quantity of matter, nuclear sources produces a million times more energy than a chemical source.

Two distinct ways of obtaining energy from nucleus are as

(i) Nuclear fission (ii) Nuclear fusion

Nuclear Fission

The process of splitting of a heavy nucleus into two lighter nuclei of comparable masses (after bombardment with a energetic particle) with liberation of energy is called nuclear fission.

Fission reaction resulting from the absorption of neutron is known as **induced fission.**

One of the common example of fission is when uranium isotope ${}_{92}U^{235}$ bombarded with a neutron breaks into two intermediate mass nuclear fragments.

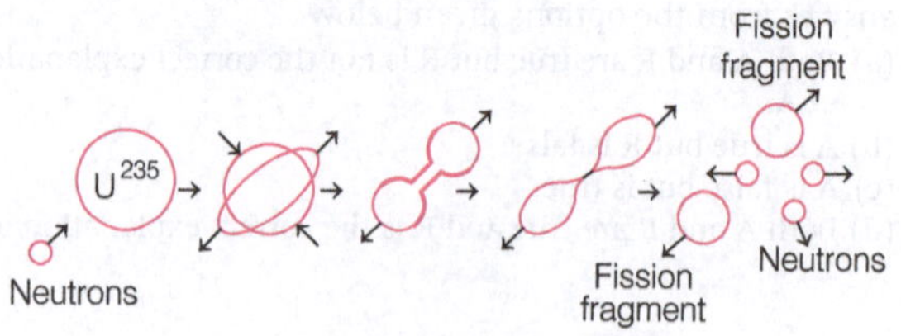

Nuclear fission in U^{235}

$${}_{92}U^{235} + {}_0n^1 \rightarrow \underset{\text{Unstable nucleus}}{{}_{92}U^{236}} \rightarrow {}_{56}Ba^{144} + {}_{36}Kr^{89} + 3\,{}_0n^1 + Q$$

This is one of the type into which the fission of ${}_{92}U^{235}$ takes place, there can be other combinations also.

In general, fission nuclei contains excess of neutrons, therefore are highly unstable. Hence, undergo beta decay until they reaches a stable end product.

The energy released in U^{235} fission is about 200 MeV or 0.8 MeV per nucleon and on an average 2.5 neutrons are liberated. These neutrons are called **fast neutrons** and their energy is about 2 MeV (each). These fast neutrons can escape from the reaction. So, in order to proceed the reaction, they are needed to slow down. Fission of U^{235} occurs by slow neutrons only of energy about 1 eV or even by thermal neutrons of energy about 0.025 eV.

Concept ladder

- The mass of the compound nucleus must be greater than the sum of masses of fission products.
- The $\frac{\text{binding energy}}{A}$ of compound nucleus must be less than that of the fission products. Hence, mass difference, *i.e.* mass defect, is converted into energy ($E = mc^2$). Thus, tremendous amount of energy is released, first appears as kinetic energy of the fragments and neutrons, then it is transferred to the surrounding appearing as heat.

Chain Reaction

In nuclear fission, many neutrons are produced along with the release of large energy. Under favourable conditions, these neutrons can cause further fission of other nuclei, producing large number of neutrons.

Thus, a chain of nuclear fissions is established which continues until the whole of the uranium is consumed.

In the chain reaction, the number of nuclei undergoing fission increases very fast, so the energy produced takes a tremendous magnitude very soon.

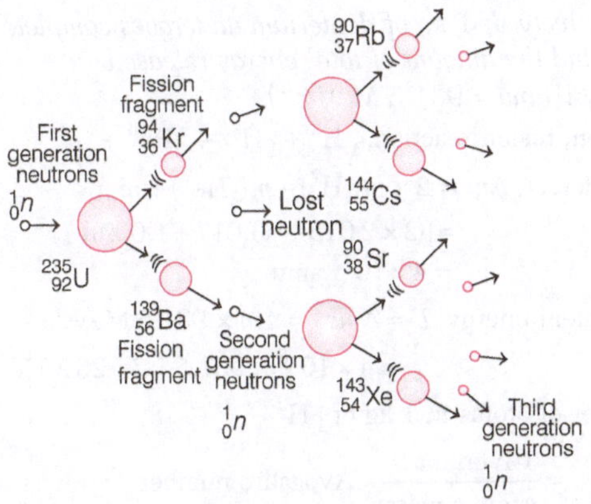

Fission reaction

Important Points Related to Chain Reaction

A chain reaction once started will remain steady, accelerate or retard depends upon neutron reproduction factor or multiplication factor (K) which is defined as

$$K = \frac{\text{Rate of production of neutrons}}{\text{Rate of loss of neutrons}}$$

Concept ladder

- If $K = 1$, then chain reaction will be steady. The size of the fissionable sample used is said to be the **critical size** and its mass, the **critical mass.**
- If $K > 1$, then chain reaction grows faster. Size of the material is said to be **supercritical.**
- If $K < 1$, then chain reaction comes to hault. Size of the material is said as **sub-critical.**

There are two types of chain reaction.

(i) **Controlled chain reaction** The reaction which can be controlled by absorbing suitable number of neutrons at each stage of the reaction, so that all neutrons are absorbed except one, which is available for further fission. This type of reaction is called controlled chain reaction. The rate of this reaction is slow and the energy liberated is always less than the explosive energy. The reproduction factor is $K = 1$. Nuclear reactor works on this principle.

(ii) **Uncontrolled chain reaction** The reaction which cannot be controlled externally because there are more than one neutron taking part in reaction. So, the reaction will accelerate at such a rapid rate that the whole material will explode within few micro-seconds, liberating tremendous amount of energy. The reproduction factor is $K > 1$. Atom bomb works on this principle.

Nuclear Fusion

When two light nuclei combine to form a heavier nucleus, then this process is called nuclear fusion.

In order to fuse two nuclei, they must come together in the range of nuclear force and to do this, they must overcome electrical repulsion of their positive charges. Hence, the kinetic energy required for fusion depends on the Coulomb barrier height $\approx 400\,\text{keV}$ for two protons. This energy is only achieved at high temperature. Hence, for fusion, high pressure $\approx 10^{16}$ atm and high temperature of the order of 10^7K to 10^8K is required and so the reaction is called **thermonuclear reaction.**

e.g. Two deuterons (heavy-hydrogen nuclei) can be fused to form a triton (tritium) according to following reaction

$$_1H^2 + {_1H^2} \rightarrow {_1H^3} + {_1H^1} + 4.0\text{ MeV (energy)}$$

The triton, so formed can further fuse with a third deuteron to form an α-particle.

$$_1H^3 + {_1H^2} \rightarrow {_2He^4} + {_0n^1} + 17.6\text{ MeV (energy)}$$

The net result of the two reactions is the fusion of three deuterons and the formation of α-particle ($_2He^4$), a neutron ($_0n^1$) and a proton ($_1H^1$). The total energy released is 21.6 MeV.

Solar energy is due to fusion in the interior of the sun which has a temperature of 1.5×10^7 K ($<< 3\times10^8$ K). The fusion in star and sun involves protons whose energies are much above the average energy.

The fusion reaction in the sun is a multi-step process in which hydrogen is fused into helium, which is as follows

$$_1H^1 + {_1H^1} \longrightarrow {_1H^2} + e^+ + \nu + 0.42\text{ MeV} \quad \text{...(i)}$$

$$e^+ + e^- \longrightarrow \gamma + \gamma + 1.02\text{ MeV} \quad \text{...(ii)}$$

$$_1H^2 + {_1H^1} \longrightarrow {_2He^3} + \gamma + 5.49\text{ MeV} \quad \text{...(iii)}$$

$$_2He^3 + {_2He^3} \longrightarrow {_2He^4} + {_1H^1} + {_1H^1} + 12.86\text{ MeV} \quad \text{...(iv)}$$

First three reactions occurs twice to react to fourth reaction.

$\Rightarrow \quad 2(\text{i}) + 2(\text{ii}) + 2(\text{iii}) + (\text{iv})$

$\Rightarrow \quad 4\,{_1H^1} + 2e^- \longrightarrow {_2He^4} + 2\nu + 6\gamma + 26.7\,\text{MeV}$

Thus, four hydrogen atoms combine to form an $_2He^4$ atom with a release of 26.7MeV of energy.

As the hydrogen in the core gets depleted and becomes helium, the core start to cool. The star begins to collapse under its own gravity, which decreases the temperature of the core.

Note Hydrogen bomb is due to nuclear fusion.

Controlled Thermonuclear Fusion

The aim of thermonuclear fusion is to generate steady power by heating the nuclear fuel to the temperature in the range of 10^8K. At these temperature, the fuel is a mixture of positive ions and electrons (plasma). The challenge is to confine this plasma, since no container can stand such a high temperature. Several countries around the world including India are developing techniques for this.

If a controlled fusion reaction can be achieved, then an almost unlimited supply of energy will become available from deuterium in the water of oceans.

Example 9. *The binding energy per nucleon of deuterium and helium atom is 1.1 MeV and 7.0 MeV, respectively. If two deuterium nuclei fuse to form helium atom, find the energy released.*

Sol. Given, fusion reaction,

$${}_1H^2 + {}_1H^2 \longrightarrow {}_2He^4 + \text{Energy}$$

Binding energy of a $({}_1H^2)$ deuterium nuclei

$$= 2 \times 1.1 = 2.2 \text{ MeV}$$

Total binding energy of two deuterium nuclei

$$= 2.2 \times 2 = 4.4 \text{ MeV}$$

Binding energy of a $({}_2He^4)$ nuclei $= 4 \times 7 = 28$ MeV

So, energy released in fusion = Final BE − Initial BE

$$= 28 - 4.4 = 23.6 \text{ MeV}$$

Example 10. *In the fusion reaction ${}_1H^2 + {}_1H^2 \rightarrow {}_2He^3 + {}_0n^1$, the masses of deuteron, helium and neutron expressed in amu are 2.015, 3.017 and 1.009, respectively. If 1 kg of deuterium undergoes complete fusion, then find the amount of total energy released.*

(Take, 1 amu = 931.5 MeV/c^2)

Sol. Given, fusion reaction, ${}_1H^2 + {}_1H^2 \rightarrow {}_2He^3 + {}_0n^1$

Mass defect, $\Delta m = [2 \times m({}_1H^2) - m({}_2He^4) + m_n]$

$$= [(2 \times 2.015) - (3.017 + 1.009)]$$

$$= 4 \times 10^{-3} \text{ amu}$$

Equivalent energy, $E = \Delta mc^2 = \Delta m \times 931.5 \text{ MeV}/c^2$

$$= 4 \times 10^{-3} \times 931.5 = 3.726 \text{ MeV}$$

Number of atoms in 1 kg of ${}_1H^2$

$$= \frac{\text{Given mass}}{\text{Atomic mass}} \times \text{Avogadro number}$$

$$= \frac{1000}{2} \times 6.023 \times 10^{23}$$

In one reaction, two atoms of ${}_1^2H$ are used.

So, total energy released

$$= \frac{1}{2}\left(\frac{1000}{2} \times 6.023 \times 10^{23}\right) \times 3.726 \times 1.6 \times 10^{-13}$$

$$= 8.98 \times 10^{13} \simeq 9 \times 10^{13} \text{ J}$$

STEP UP Practice 2

1. In the nuclear reaction ${}_2He^4 + {}_ZX^A \rightarrow {}_{Z+2}Y^{A+3} + B$, where, B denotes
   (a) electron (b) positron
   (c) proton (d) neutron

2. In the given nuclear reaction A, B, C, D and E represents

$${}_{92}U^{238} \xrightarrow{\alpha} {}_BTh^A \xrightarrow{\beta^-} {}_DPa^C \xrightarrow{E} {}_{92}U^{234}$$

   (a) $A = 234, B = 90, C = 234, D = 91$ and $E = \beta^-$
   (b) $A = 234, B = 90, C = 238, D = 94$ and $E = \alpha$
   (c) $A = 238, B = 93, C = 234, D = 91$ and $E = \beta^-$
   (d) $A = 234, B = 90, C = 234, D = 93$ and $E = \alpha$

3. A reaction between a proton and ${}_8O^{18}$ that produces ${}_9F^{18}$ must also liberate
   (a) ${}_0n^1$ (b) ${}_1e^0$ (c) ${}_1n^0$ (d) ${}_0e^1$

4. **Statement I** There is a chain reaction when uranium is bombarded with slow neutrons.
   Statement II When uranium is bombarded with slow neutrons, more neutrons are produced.
   In the light of the above statements, choose the most appropriate answer from the options given below.
   (a) Both Statement I and Statement II are incorrect.
   (b) Statement I is correct but Statement II is incorrect.
   (c) Statement I is incorrect but Statement II is correct.
   (d) Both Statement I and Statement II are correct.

5. 1 g of hydrogen is converted into 0.993 g of helium in a thermonuclear reaction. The energy released in
   (a) 6.3×10^7 J (b) 6.3×10^{11} J
   (c) 6.3×10^{14} J (d) 6.3×10^{20} J

6. An atomic power station has a generating capacity of 200 MW. The energy generated in a day by this station is
   (a) 200 MJ (b) 200 J
   (c) 4.8×10^6 J (d) 1.728×10^{13} J

7. **Statement I** A fusion reaction can be more easily controlled than a fission reaction.
   Statement II The percentage of mass converted to energy in a fission reaction is 0.1% whereas in a fusion reaction it, is 0.4%.
   In the light of the above statements, choose the most appropriate answer from the options given below.
   (a) Both Statement I and Statement II are incorrect.
   (b) Statement I is correct but Statement II is incorrect.
   (c) Statement I is incorrect but Statement II is correct.
   (d) Both Statement I and Statement II are correct.

8. If 200 MeV energy is released in the fission of a single U^{235} nucleus,the number of fissions required per second to produce 1 kilowatt power shall be (Given, 1 eV $= 1.6 \times 10^{-19}$ J)
   (a) 3.125×10^{13} (b) 3.125×10^{14}
   (c) 3.125×10^{15} (d) 3.125×10^{16}

9. Statement I The ratio for time taken for light emission from an atom to that for release of nuclear energy in fission is 1 : 100.

Statement II Time taken for the light emission from an atom is of the order of 10^{-8} s.

In the light of the above statements, choose the most appropriate answer from the options given below.
(a) Both Statement I and Statement II are incorrect.
(b) Statement I is correct but Statement II is incorrect.
(c) Statement I is incorrect but Statement II is correct.
(d) Both Statement I and Statement II are correct.

10. If the energy released in the fission of one nucleus is 200 MeV, then the number of nuclei required per second in a power plant of 16 kW will be
(a) 0.5×10^{15}
(b) 0.5×10^{12}
(c) 5×10^{12}
(d) 5×10^{11}

11. To generate a power of 3.2 MW, the number of fissions of U^{235} per second is (Energy released per fission = 200 MeV, $1 \text{eV} = 1.6 \times 10^{-19}$ J)
(a) 1×10^{17} (b) 6×10^{17}
(c) 3.6×10^{16} (d) 6×10^{16}

12. The nuclear reaction ${}_1^1\text{H} + {}_1^1\text{H} = {}_2^4\text{He}$ (mass of deuteron = 2.0141 amu and mass of He = 4.0024 amu) is
(a) fusion reaction releasing 24 MeV energy
(b) fusion reaction absorbing 24 MeV energy
(c) fission reaction releasing 0.0258 MeV energy
(d) fission reaction absorbing 0.0258 MeV energy

13. For fusion reaction,
(a) extremely low pressure is required
(b) extremely high temperature is required
(c) a heavy nucleus splits into two smaller nuclei
(d) released energy is very small

14. The sun radiates energy in all directions. The average radiations received on the earth surface from the sun is 1.4 kW/m^2. The average earth-sun distance is 1.5×10^{11} m. The mass lost by the sun per day is
(1 day = 86400 s)
(a) 4.4×10^9 kg
(b) 76×10^{14} kg
(c) 38×10^{12} kg
(d) 38×10^{13} kg

15. An atomic power nuclear reactor can deliver 300 MW. The energy released due to fission of each nucleus of uranium atom U^{238} is 170 MeV. The number of uranium atoms fissioned per hour will be
(a) 30×10^{25} (b) 39.6×10^{21}
(c) 10×10^{20} (d) 5×10^{15}

16. Statement I Energy is released in a nuclear reaction.

Statement II In any nuclear reaction, the reactants and resultant products obey the law of conservation of charge and mass only.

In the light of the above statements, choose the most appropriate answer from the options given below.
(a) Both Statement I and Statement II are incorrect.
(b) Statement I is correct but Statement II is incorrect.
(c) Statement I is incorrect but Statement II is correct.
(d) Both Statement I and Statement II are correct.

17. Assuming that about 20 MeV of energy is released per fusion reaction

$${}_1\text{H}^2 + {}_1\text{H}^2 \rightarrow {}_0n^1 + {}_2\text{He}^4$$

Then, the number of ${}_1\text{H}^2$ atoms consumed per day in a fusion reactor of power 1 MW will approximately be
(a) 26×10^{20} (b) 27×10^{21}
(c) 24×10^{19} (d) 23×10^{26}

18. Fission of nuclei is possible because the binding energy per nucleon in them
(a) increases with mass number at high mass number
(b) decreases with mass number at high mass number
(c) increases with mass number at low mass number
(d) decreases with mass number at low mass number

19. Which of these is a fusion reaction?
(a) ${}^3\text{H}_1 + {}^2\text{H}_1 \rightarrow {}^4\text{He}_2 + {}^1n_0$
(b) ${}^{238}\text{U}_{92} \rightarrow {}^{206}\text{Pb}_{82} + 8\,({}^4\text{He}_2) + 6\,({}^0\text{B}_1)$
(c) ${}^{12}\text{C}_7 \rightarrow {}^{12}\text{C}_6 + \beta + \gamma$
(d) None of the above

20. Statement I For the fission of heavy nuclei, neutrons are more effective than protons.

Statement II Neutrons are heavier than protons.

In the light of the above statements, choose the most appropriate answer from the options given below.
(a) Both Statement I and Statement II are incorrect.
(b) Statement I is correct but Statement II is incorrect.
(c) Statement I is incorrect but Statement II is correct.
(d) Both Statement I and Statement II are correct.

NEET Exclusive EXTRA BYTES

- When an energetic γ-ray photon falls on a heavy substance, it is absorbed by nucleus of the substance and an electron and a positron are produced.

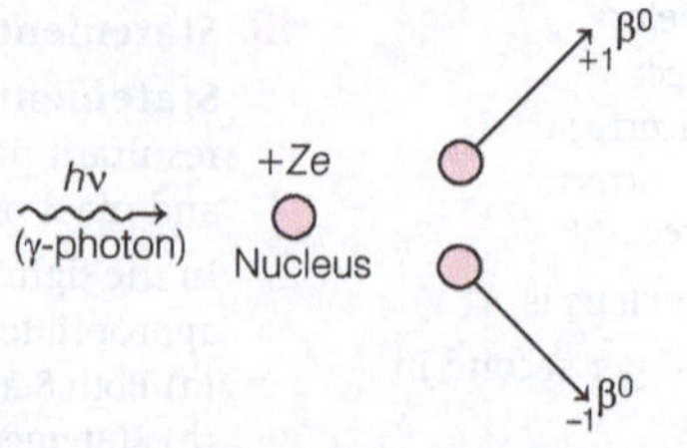

This phenomenon is called **pair production** and can be represented by the following equation

$$h\nu \longrightarrow {}_{+1}\beta^0 + {}_{-1}\beta^0$$

- The converse phenomenon of pair production is called **pair annihilation**. When an electron and a positron come very close to each other, they annihilate each other by combining together and two γ-photons are produced. This phenomenon can be represented by the following equation

$$_{+1}\beta^0 + {}_{-1}\beta^0 \longrightarrow h\nu + h\nu$$

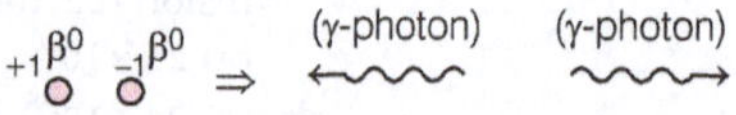

- **Various Decay Pathways**

Alpha decay	${}^{A}_{Z}X \longrightarrow {}^{A-4}_{Z-2}Y + {}^{4}_{2}\text{He}$
Beta decay (β^-)	${}^{A}_{Z}X \longrightarrow {}_{Z+1}^{A}Y + e^- + \overline{\nu}$
Beta decay (β^+)	${}^{A}_{Z}X \longrightarrow {}_{Z-1}^{A}Y + e^+ + \nu$
Electron capture	${}^{A}_{Z}X + e^- \longrightarrow {}_{Z-1}^{A}Y + \nu$
Gamma decay	${}^{A}_{Z}X^* \longrightarrow {}^{A}_{Z}X + \gamma$

Here, ν and $\overline{\nu}$ indicate the particles neutrino and antinutrino.

- A nuclear reactor is a device in which nuclear fission can be carried out through a sustained and controlled chain reaction. It is also called an **atomic pile**. It is thus a source of controlled energy which is utilised for many useful purposes. Nuclear reactor's energy is used to generate steam, which operates on a turbine and turns an electric generator.
- Key components of nuclear reactor
  - (i) **Fuel** The fissionable material used in the reactor is called fuel of the reactor. *e.g.* Uranium isotope, thorium isotope, etc.
  - (ii) **Moderator** It is used to slow down the fast moving neutrons. Heavy water (D_2O) is the best moderator.
  - (iii) **Control rods** The neutrons available for fusion are controlled by moving the cadmium rods in or out of the core of reactor.
  - (iv) **Shielding** It is the protective covering made of concrete wall to protect from the harmful radiations.

GEARING UP FOR NEET

Single Correct Option

1. Heavy stable nuclei have more neutrons than protons. This is because of the fact that *[NCERT Exemplar]*

(a) neutrons are heavier than protons
(b) electrostatic force between protons are repulsive
(c) neutrons decay into protons through beta decay
(d) nuclear forces between neutrons are weaker than that between protons

2. When the number of nucleons in nuclei increases, then the binding energy per nucleon

(a) increases continuously with mass number
(b) decreases continuously with mass number
(c) remains constant with mass number
(d) first increases and then decreases with increase in mass number

3. The binding energy per nucleon is maximum in the case of

(a) ${}_{2}^{4}He$ (b) ${}_{26}^{56}Fe$ (c) ${}_{56}^{141}Ba$ (d) ${}_{92}^{235}U$

4. The curve of binding energy per nucleon as a function of atomic mass number has a sharp peak for helium nucleus.
This implies that helium

(a) can easily be broken up
(b) is very stable
(c) can be used as fissionable material
(d) is radioactive

5. The binding energies of the nuclei A and B are E_a and E_b, respectively. Three atoms of the element B fuse to give one atom of element A and an energy Q is released, then E_a, E_b and Q are related as

(a) $E_a - 3E_b = Q$ (b) $3E_b - E_a = Q$
(c) $E_a + 3E_b = Q$ (d) $E_b + 3E_a = Q$

6. In the reaction ${}_{1}^{2}H + {}_{1}^{3}H \rightarrow {}_{2}^{4}He + {}_{0}n^{1}$, if the binding energies of ${}_{1}^{2}H$, ${}_{1}^{3}H$ and ${}_{2}^{4}He$ are respectively a, b and c (in MeV), then the energy (in MeV) released in this reaction is

(a) $c + a - b$ (b) $c - a - b$ (c) $a + b + c$ (d) $a + b - c$

7. What is the binding energy per nucleon of ${}_{6}C^{12}$ nucleus?
Given, mass of C^{12} $(m_C) = 12.000$ u
Mass of proton $(m_p) = 1.0078$ u
Mass of neutron $(m_n) = 1.0087$ u
and 1 amu $= 931.4 \frac{\text{MeV}}{c^2}$.

(a) 5.26 MeV (b) 6.2 MeV
(c) 4.65 MeV (d) 7.68 MeV

8. Binding energy per nucleon *versus* mass number curve for nuclei is shown in the figure. W, X, Y and Z are four nuclei indicated on the curve. The process that would release energy is

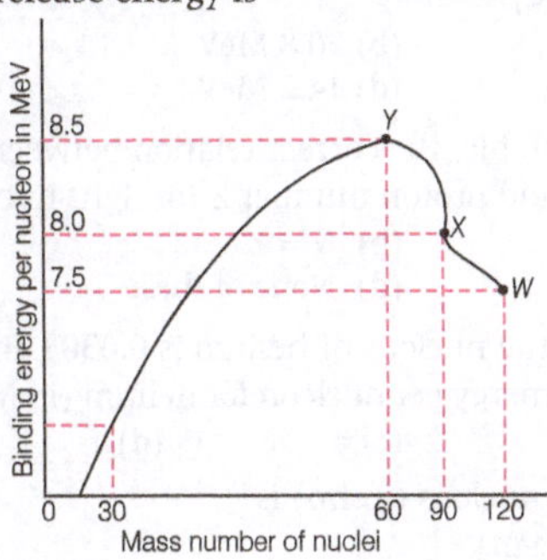

(a) $Y \rightarrow 2Z$ (b) $W \rightarrow X + Y$
(c) $W \rightarrow 2Y$ (d) $X \rightarrow Y + Z$

9. The gravitational force between H-atom of mass M and another particle of mass m will be given by Newton's law $F = G\frac{M \cdot m}{r^2}$, where r is in metre and *[NCERT Exemplar]*

(a) $M = m_{\text{proton}} + m_{\text{electron}}$
(b) $M = m_{\text{proton}} + m_{\text{electron}} - \frac{B}{c^2}$ $(B = 13.6 \text{ eV})$
(c) M is not relate to the mass of the hydrogen atom
(d) $M = m_{\text{proton}} + m_{\text{electron}} - \frac{|V|}{c^2}$ ($|V|$ = magnitude of the potential energy of electron in the H-atom)

10. A star initially has 10^{40} deuterons. It produces energy *via* the processes ${}_{1}^{2}H + {}_{1}^{2}H \rightarrow {}_{1}^{3}H + p$ and ${}_{1}^{2}H + {}_{1}^{3}H \rightarrow {}_{2}^{4}He + n$, where the masses of the nuclei are $m({}^{2}H) = 2.014$ amu, $m(p) = 1.007$ amu, $m(n) = 1.008$ amu and $m({}^{4}He) = 4.001$ amu. If the average power radiated by the star is 10^{16} W, then the deuteron supply of the star is exhausted in a time of the order of

(a) 10^{18} s (b) 10^{28} s (c) 10^{12} s (d) 10^{16} s

11. Two spherical nuclei have mass numbers 216 and 64 with their radii R_1 and R_2, respectively. The ratio $\frac{R_1}{R_2}$ is equal to

(a) 3 : 2 (b) 1 : 3 (c) 1 : 2 (d) 2 : 3

12. The binding energy per nucleon of ${}^7_3Li$ and ${}^4_2He$ nuclei are 5.60 MeV and 7.06 MeV, respectively. In the nuclear reaction ${}^7_3Li + {}^1_1H \rightarrow {}^4_2He + {}^4_2He + Q$, the value of energy Q released is
(a) 19.6 MeV (b) – 2.4 MeV
(c) 8.4 MeV (d) 17.3 MeV

13. The mass defect in a particular nuclear reaction is 0.3 g. The amount of energy liberated (in kwh) is
(Velocity of light = 3×10^8 m/s)
(a) 1.5×10^6 (b) 2.5×10^6
(c) 3×10^6 (d) 7.5×10^6

14. The masses of neutron and proton are 1.0087 amu and 1.0073 amu respectively. If the neutrons and protons combine to form a helium nucleus (alpha particles) of mass 4.0015 amu, the binding energy of the helium nucleus will be (1 amu = 931 MeV)
(a) 28.4 MeV (b) 20.8 MeV
(c) 27.3 MeV (d) 14.2 MeV

15. For a nucleus to be stable, the correct relation between neutron number N and proton number Z for light nuclei is
(a) $N > Z$ (b) $N = Z$
(c) $N < Z$ (d) None of these

16. The mass defect for the nucleus of helium is 0.0303 amu, What is the binding energy per nucleon for helium (in MeV)?
(a) 28 (b) 7 (c) 4 (d) 1

17. The radius of ${}_{29}Cu^{64}$ nucleus (in fm) is
(Take, $R_0 = 1.2 \times 10^{-15}$ m)
(a) 4.8 (b) 1.2 (c) 7.7 (d) 9.6

18. Density of a nucleus is
(a) more for lighter elements and less for heavier elements
(b) more for heavier elements and less for lighter elements
(c) very less compared to ordinary matter
(d) a constant

19. If a nucleus with mass number $A = 240$ with $E_{bn} = 7.6$ MeV breaks into two fragments of $A = 120$ and $E_{bn} = 8.5$ MeV, then released energy is around
(a) 216 MeV
(b) 200 MeV
(c) 100 MeV
(d) Cannot be estimated from given data

20. If the nuclear radius of ${}^{27}Al$ is 3.6 fm, the approximate nuclear radius of ${}^{64}Cu$ (in fm) is
(a) 2.4 (b) 1.2 (c) 4.8 (d) 3.6

21. Mass of iron nucleus is 55.85 u and $A = 56$. Its nuclear density will be (Take, $R_0 = 1.2 \times 10^{-15}$ m)
(a) 4.28×10^{17} kg m^{-3} (b) 2×10^{10} kg m^{-3}
(c) 2.29×10^{17} kg m^{-3} (d) 9×10^{10} kg m^{-3}

22. Consider the binding energy of ${}_{17}Cl^{35}$ and ${}_{15}P^{31}$ are 287.67 MeV and 262.48 MeV, respectively. Then,
(a) ${}_{17}Cl^{35}$ is more stable than ${}_{15}P^{31}$
(b) ${}_{15}P^{31}$ is more stable than ${}_{17}Cl^{35}$
(c) stability of both the elements is equivalent
(d) cannot be estimated from the given data

23. If the binding energy per nucleon of deuteron is 2.115 MeV, then its mass of defect in atomic mass unit is
(a) 0.0024 u (b) 25.62 u (c) 96.24 u (d) 0.0045 u

24. Given, $m({}^{56}_{26}Fe) = 55.934939$ u, $m_{proton} = 1.007825$ u and $m_{neutron} = 1.008665$ u, then BE per nucleon of Fe is
(a) 8.790 MeV (b) 7.75 MeV
(c) 7.5 MeV (d) 9.28 MeV

25. Given, mass of neutron = 1.00866 u, mass of a proton = 1.00727 u and mass of ${}^{16}_8O = 15.99053$ u. Then, the energy required to separate ${}^{16}_8O$ into its constituents is
(a) 12.7 MeV (b) 931.5 MeV
(c) 1.49×10^{-19} J (d) 127.5 MeV

26. Mass defect of helium (${}_2He^4$) is [Take, mass of proton, $m_p = 1.0072676$ u, mass of neutrons, $m_n = 1.008665$ u and mass of ${}_2He^4 = 4.001506$ u]
(a) 0.016767 u (b) 1.00726 u
(c) 2.00686 u (d) 0.0303592 u

27. How much mass has to be converted into energy to produce electric power of 200 MW for one hour?
(a) 2×10^{-6} kg (b) 8×10^{-6} kg
(c) 1×10^{-6} kg (d) 3×10^{-6} kg

28. Energy equivalent of 2 g of a substance is
(a) 18×10^{13} mJ (b) 18×10^{13} J
(c) 9×10^{13} mJ (d) 9×10^{13} J

29. On bombarding U^{235} by slow neutron, 200 MeV energy is released. If the power output of atomic reactor is 1.6 MW, then the rate of fission will be
(a) 5×10^{22} s^{-1} (b) 5×10^{16} s^{-1}
(c) 8×10^{16} s^{-1} (d) 20×10^{16} s^{-1}

30. In a nuclear reactor, the fuel is consumed at the rate of 1 mgs^{-1}. The power generated (in kW) is
(a) 9×10^{14} (b) 9×10^7
(c) 9×10^8 (d) 9×10^{12}

31. An atomic power nuclear reactor can deliver 300 MW. The energy released due to fission of each nucleus of uranium atoms U^{238} is 170 MeV. The number of uranium atoms fissioned per hour will be
(a) 30×10^{25} (b) 4×10^{22}
(c) 10×10^{20} (d) 5×10^{15}

32. Suppose that a reactor using U-235 has an output of 700 MW and is 20% efficient.An atom of U^{235} undergoes fission in a reactor liberating 200 MeV energy, then, energy generated from the reactor per fission and mass of uranium it consume in 24 h are
(a) 3.2×10^{-11} J, 3.7 kg (b) 6.4×10^{-11} J, 2.5 kg
(c) 3.2×10^{-12} J, 2.5 kg (d) 6.4×10^{-12} J, 3.7 kg

33. Fusion reaction takes place at high temperature as
(a) molecules break at higher temperature
(b) nuclei break at high temperature
(c) atoms get ionised at high temperature
(d) kinetic energy is enough to overcome the Coulomb repulsive force between nuclei

34. In the fusion reaction, ${}_1^2H + {}_1^2H \longrightarrow {}_2^3He + {}_0^1n$ the masses of deuteron, helium and neutron expressed in amu are 2.015, 3.017 and 1.009, respectively. If 1 kg of deuterium undergoes complete fusion, find the amount of total energy released. (1 amu = 931.5 MeV)
(a) 9.0×10^{13} J (b) 20×10^5 J
(c) 5×10^{15} J (d) 8×10^5 J

35. Which of the following process will result into fission reaction?
(a) ${}_{92}U^{235}$ is bombarded with fast moving neutrons
(b) ${}_{92}U^{235}$ is bombarded with thermal neutrons
(c) U^{238} is bombarded with slow moving neutrons
(d) U^{235} being unstable breaks into smaller fragments

36. In an atomic bomb, the energy is released due to
(a) chain reaction of neutrons and ${}_{92}U^{235}$
(b) chain reaction of neutrons and ${}_{92}U^{238}$
(c) chain reaction of neutrons and ${}_{92}U^{240}$
(d) chain reaction of neutrons and ${}_{92}U^{236}$

37. Boron rods are used in nuclear reactors because
(a) boron can absorb neutrons
(b) strength is given to the plant
(c) boron speeds up neutrons
(d) the reactors look good

38. A nuclear reaction along with the masses of the particle taking part in it is as follows

A	+	B	$\rightarrow$	C	+	D	+ QMeV
1.002 amu		1.004 amu		1.001 amu		1.003 amu	

The energy Q liberated in the reaction is
(a) 1.234 MeV (b) 0.931 MeV
(c) 0.465 MeV (d) 1.863 MeV

39. If the energy released in the fission of one nucleus is 200 MeV, then the number of nuclei required per second in a power plant of 16 kW will be
(a) 0.5×10^{14} (b) 0.5×10^{22} (c) 5×10^{12} (d) 5×10^{14}

40. In the nuclear fusion reaction ${}_1^2H + {}_1^3H \rightarrow {}_2^4He + {}_0^1n$, given that the repulsive potential energy between the two nuclei is -7.7×10^{-14} J. The temperature at which the gases must be heated to initiate the reaction is of the order of [Boltzmann's constant, $k = 1.38 \times 10^{-23}$ J/K]
(a) 10^9K (b) 10^7K (c) 10^5K (d) 10^3K

41. Assuming that about 200 MeV energy is released per fission of ${}_{92}U^{235}$ nuclei. What would be the mass of U^{235} consumed per day in the fission of reactor of power 1 MW approximately?
(a) 10 kg (b) 1 kg (c) 1 g (d) 10 g

42. The number of neutrons released when ${}_{92}^{235}U$ undergoes fission by absorbing ${}_0^1n$ and (${}_{56}^{144}Ba + {}_{36}^{89}Kr$) are formed
(a) 0 (b) 1 (c) 2 (d) 3

43. To generate a power of 3.2 MW, the number of fission of U^{235} per minute is (Energy released per fission = 200 MeV, 1 eV = 1.6×10^{-19} J)
(a) 6×10^{18} (b) 6×10^{17} (c) 6×10^{15} (d) 6×10^{16}

44. The kinetic energy of α-particle emitted in the α-decay of ${}_{88}Ra^{226}$ is
[Take, m(Ra) = 226.02540 u,
m(Rn) = 222.01750 u
and m(He) = 4.002603 u]
(a) 5.201 MeV (b) 3.301 MeV
(c) 6.023 MeV (d) 4.871 MeV

45. In a nuclear reactor, the number of U^{235} nuclei undergoing fissions per second is 4×10^{20}. If the energy released per fission is 250 MeV, then the total energy released in 10 h is (1 eV = 1.6×10^{-19} J)
(a) 576×10^6J (b) 576×10^{12}J
(c) 576×10^{15}J (d) 576×10^{18}J

46. The energy released by the fission of one uranium atom is 200 MeV. The number of fission per second required to produce 6.4W power is
(a) 2×10^{11} (b) 10^{11}
(c) 10^{10} (d) 2×10^{10}

47. What is the energy released by fission of 1 g of U^{235}? (Assume 200 MeV energy is liberated on fission of 1 nucleus)
(a) 2.26×10^4 kWh (b) 1.2×10^4 kWh
(c) 4.5×10^2 kWh (d) 2.5×10^2 kWh

48. The fusion reaction in the sun is a multi-step process in which the
(a) helium is burned into deuterons
(b) helium is burned into hydrogen
(c) deuteron is burned into hydrogen
(d) hydrogen is burned into helium

49. An atom bomb weighing 1 kg explodes releasing 9×10^{13} J of energy. What percentage of mass is converted into energy?
(a) 0.1% (b) 1%
(c) 2% (d) 10%

50. A luminous body radiates energy at a rate 3.6×10^{28} J/s, then loss of the mass of the body per second is
(a) 2×10^3 kg/s (b) 3×10^4 kg/s
(c) 4×10^{11} kg/s (d) 5×10^5 kg/s

Assertion and Reason

Directions (Q. Nos. 1-5) *These questions consist of two statements each printed as Assertion and Reason. While answering these questions you are required to choose anyone of the following four responses.*
(a) Both A and R are true but R is not the correct explanation of A.
(b) A is true but R is false.
(c) A is false but R is true.
(d) Both A and R are true and R is the correct explanation of A.

1. **Assertion** (A) Ratio of mass of nucleus of H-atom and proton is approximately 1 : 2.
Reason (R) Nucleus of the lightest atom of H-atom of hydrogen is usually known as proton.

2. **Assertion** (A) Mass is not conserved, but mass and energy are conserved as a single entity is called mass energy.

Reason (R) Mass and energy are inter-convertible in accordance with Einstein's relation, $E = mc^2$.

3. **Assertion** (A) Lighter nuclei tend to fuse to attain a unstable structure.

Reason (R) When lighter nuclei fuse together, they form heavier nuclei with greater binding energy per nucleon.

4. **Assertion** (A) Nuclear fusion is possible in laboratory.

Reason (R) Extremely high temperature to carry out nuclear fusion is attained by causing explosion due to fission process.

5. **Assertion** (A) Density of all nuclei is same.

Reason (R) Radius of nucleus is directly proportional to the cube root of mass number.

Statement Type Questions

Directions (Q. Nos. 1-5) *These questions consist of two statements, choose the most appropriate answer from the options given below.*

(a) Both Statement I and Statement II are incorrect.
(b) Statement I is correct but Statement II is incorrect.
(c) Statement I is incorrect but Statement II is correct.
(d) Both Statement I and Statement II are correct.

1. **Statement I** It is not possible to use ^{35}Cl as the fuel for fusion energy.

Statement II The binding energy of ^{35}Cl is too small.

2. **Statement I** Sum of masses of nucleons is always greater than the mass of their nucleus.

Statement II A system is most stable in a configuration, when it has lowest possible energy.

3. **Statement I** The binding energy per nucleon, for nuclei with atomic mass number $A > 100$ decreases with A.

Statement II The nuclear forces are weak for heavier nuclei.

4. **Statement I** Energy is released when heavy nuclei undergo fission or light nuclei undergo fusion.

Statement II For heavy nuclei, binding energy per nucleon increases with increasing Z while for light nuclei it decreases with increasing Z.

5. **Statement I** Sun is constantly loosing mass due to thermonuclear fusion.

Statement II A fusion reaction is more energetic than a fission reaction.

Match the Columns

1. Match the Column I (mass number) with the Column II (radius of nucleus).

Column I	Column II
A. 216	I. 2.4×10^{-15} m
B. 64	II. 6.0×10^{-15} m
C. 125	III. 4.8×10^{-15} m
D. 8	IV. 7.2×10^{-15} m

Choose the correct answer from the options given below.
(a) A-II, B-III, C-I, D-IV
(b) A-I, B-IV, C-I, D-II
(c) A-III, B-I, C-IV, D-II
(d) A-IV, B-III, C-II, D-I

2. In Column I, the mass of defect in a particular reaction is given and in Column II, amount of energy liberated in kilowatt hour is given. Match the Column I to the appropriate value from Column II.

Column I (in g)	Column II (in kWh)
A. 0.3	I. 1.5×10^7
B. 0.5	II. 7.5×10^6
C. 0.1	III. 1.25×10^7
D. 0.6	IV. 2.5×10^6

Choose the correct answer from the options given below.
(a) A-II, B-III, C-IV, D-I
(b) A-II , B-I, C-IV, D-III
(c) A-I, B-II, C-III, D-IV
(d) A-I, B-IV, C-III, D-II

3. Match the nuclear reactions given in Column I with the energy involved in these reactions in Column II

Column I	Column II
A. $^2_1\text{H} + ^2_1\text{H} \longrightarrow ^3_1\text{H} + ^1_1\text{H} + E_1$	I. 17.6 MeV
B. $^3_1\text{H} + ^2_1\text{H} \longrightarrow ^4_1\text{He} + ^1_0n + E_2$	II. 18.3 MeV
C. $^2_1\text{H} + ^2_1\text{H} \longrightarrow ^3_2\text{He} + ^1_0n + E_3$	III. 4 MeV
D. $^3_2\text{H} + ^2_1\text{H} \longrightarrow ^4_2\text{He} + E_4$	IV. 13.3MeV

Choose the correct answer from the options given below
(a) A-I, B-IV, C-III, D-II
(b) A-III , B-I, C-IV, D-II
(c) A-I, B-II, C-III, D-IV
(d) A-III, B-IV, C-II, D-I

4 A heavy nucleus P of mass number 240 and binding energy 7.6 MeV per nucleon splits into two nuclei Q and R of mass number 110, 130 and binding energy per nucleon 8.5 MeV and 8.4 MeV, respectively.

On the basis on above condition match Column I (energies) with Column II (values)

Column I	Column II
A. Binding energy of nucleus P (in MeV)	I. 935
B. Binding energy of nucleus Q (in MeV)	II. 1092
C. Binding energy of nucleus R (in MeV)	III. 203
D. Energy released per fission (in MeV)	IV. 1824

Choose the correct answer from the options given below.
(a) A-IV, B-II, C-I, D-III
(b) A-IV, B-II, C-III, D-I
(c) A-IV, B-I, C-II, D-III
(d) A-II, B-IV, C-I, D-III

Final Check Through PYQs

Module-I Nucleus, Mass Defect and Binding Energy

1. A nucleus of mass number 189 splits into two nuclei having mass number 125 and 64. The ratio of radius of two daughter nuclei, respectively is:
[NCERT (New) Pg. 309, NEET 2022]
(a) 4 : 5 (b) 5 : 4 (c) 25 : 16 (d) 1 : 1

2. A nucleus with mass number 240 breaks into two fragments each of mass number 120, the binding energy per nucleon of unfragmented nuclei is 7.6 MeV while that of fragments is 8.5 MeV. The total gain in the binding energy in the process is
[NCERT (New) Pg. 315, NEET 2021]
(a) 0.9 MeV (b) 9.4 MeV (c) 804 MeV (d) 216 MeV

3. The energy equivalent of 0.5 g of a substance is
[NCERT (New) Pg. 311, NEET (Sep.) 2020]
(a) 4.5×10^{13} J (b) 1.5×10^{13} J
(c) 0.5×10^{13} J (d) 4.5×10^{16}

4. If radius of the $^{27}_{13}Al$ nucleus is taken to be R_{Al}, then the radius of $^{125}_{53}Te$ nucleus is nearly
[NCERT (New) Pg. 309, AIPMT 2015]
(a) $\left(\frac{53}{13}\right)^{\frac{1}{3}} R_{Al}$ (b) $\frac{5}{3} R_{Al}$ (c) $\frac{3}{5} R_{Al}$ (d) $\left(\frac{13}{53}\right)^{\frac{1}{3}} R_{Al}$

Module-II Nuclear Energy

5. $^{290}_{82}X \xrightarrow{\alpha} {}^{286}_{80}Y \xrightarrow{e^+} Z \xrightarrow{\beta^-} P \xrightarrow{e^-} Q$

In the nuclear emission stated above, the mass number and atomic number of the product Q respectively are
[NCERT (Old) Pg. 449, NEET 2024]
(a) 280, 81 (b) 286, 80 (c) 288, 82 (d) 286, 81

6. In the given nuclear reaction, the element X is
[NCERT (Old) Pg. 449, NEET 2022]

$$^{22}_{11}Na \longrightarrow X + e^+ + \nu$$

(a) $^{23}_{10}Ne$ (b) $^{22}_{10}Ne$ (c) $^{22}_{12}Mg$ (d) $^{23}_{11}Na$

7. When a uranium isotope $^{235}_{92}U$ is bombarded with a neutron, it generates $^{89}_{36}Kr$, three neutrons and
[NCERT (New) Pg. 315, NEET (Sep.) 2020]
(a) $^{91}_{40}Zr$ (b) $^{101}_{36}Kr$ (c) $^{103}_{36}Kr$ (d) $^{144}_{56}Ba$

Answers

Step up Practice 1

1 (b)	2 (a)	3 (a)	4 (b)	5 (c)	6 (a)	7 (b)	8 (d)	9 (a)	10 (a)
11 (a)	12 (c)	13 (c)	14 (d)	15 (c)	16 (b)	17 (c)	18 (a)	19 (d)	

Step up Practice 2

1 (d)	2 (a)	3 (a)	4 (d)	5 (b)	6 (d)	7 (c)	8 (a)	9 (d)	10 (a)
11 (a)	12 (a)	13 (b)	14 (d)	15 (b)	16 (d)	17 (b)	18 (b)	19 (a)	20 (d)

Gearing up for NEET

1 (b)	2 (d)	3 (b)	4 (b)	5 (a)	6 (b)	7 (d)	8 (c)	9 (b)	10 (c)
11 (a)	12 (d)	13 (d)	14 (a)	15 (b)	16 (b)	17 (a)	18 (d)	19 (a)	20 (c)
21 (c)	22 (b)	23 (d)	24 (a)	25 (d)	26 (d)	27 (b)	28 (b)	29 (b)	30 (b)
31 (b)	32 (d)	33 (d)	34 (a)	35 (b)	36 (a)	37 (a)	38 (d)	39 (d)	40 (a)
41 (c)	42 (d)	43 (a)	44 (d)	45 (b)	46 (a)	47 (a)	48 (d)	49 (a)	50 (c)

Assertion and Reason

1 (c)	2 (d)	3 (c)	4 (c)	5 (a)

Statement Type Questions

1 (b)	2 (d)	3 (b)	4 (b)	5 (d)

Match the Columns

1 (d)	2 (a)	3 (b)	4 (c)

Final Check through PYQs : Module-I

1 (b)	2 (d)	3 (a)	4 (b)

Final Check through PYQs : Module-II

5 (d)	6 (b)	7 (d)

Hints and Solutions

Step up Practice 1

1. (b) According to question,
Mass of proton = Mass of anti-proton
$= 1.67 \times 10^{-27}$ kg $= 1$ amu
Energy equivalent to 1 amu = 931 MeV
So, energy equivalent to 2 amu $= 2 \times 931$ MeV
$= 1862 \times 10^6 \times 1.6 \times 10^{-19} = 2.97 \times 10^{-10}$ J
$= 3 \times 10^{-10}$ J

2. (a) Rest energy of an electron $= m_e c^2$
Here, $m_e = 9.1 \times 10^{-31}$ kg
and $c = 3 \times 10^8$ m/s
$\therefore$ Rest energy of an electron
$$= 9.1 \times 10^{-31} \times (3 \times 10^8)^2 \text{ J}$$
$$= \frac{9.1 \times 10^{-31} \times (3 \times 10^8)^2}{1.6 \times 10^{-19}} \text{ eV}$$
$$= 510 \text{ keV}$$

3. (a) Both A and R are true but R is not the correct explanation of A.
Nuclear forces are strongest when the number of proton equals the number of neutrons. An excess of protons compared to neutrons weakens the nuclear force.

4. (b) $\therefore$ Mass, $m \approx A \times 1.67 \times 10^{-27}$
where, A is the mass number.
Volume of uranium nucleus will be
$$V = \frac{4}{3}\pi r^3 = \frac{4}{3}\pi[(1.25 \times 10^{-15})A^{1/3}]^3$$
$$\simeq (8.2 \times 10^{-45} \text{ m}^3)A$$
Hence, density of uranium nucleus,
$$\rho = \frac{m}{V} = \frac{A(1.67 \times 10^{-27})}{(8.2 \times 10^{-45})A}$$
$$= 2.0 \times 10^{17} \text{ kg/m}^3$$

5. (c) We have, $r \propto A^{1/3} \Rightarrow \frac{r_2}{r_1} = \left(\frac{A_2}{A_1}\right)^{1/3} = \left(\frac{206}{4}\right)^{1/3}$
$$\therefore \quad r_2 = 4\left(\frac{206}{4}\right)^{1/3} = 14.88 \text{ fm}$$

6. (a) Both A and R are true but R is not the correct explanation of A.
The nuclei having mass number $A = 56$ have maximum binding energy per nucleon (about 8.7 MeV).
So,the nuclei are most stable.

7. (b) Mass of electron = Mass of positron $= 9.1 \times 10^{-31}$ kg
Energy released, $E = (2m) \cdot c^2$
$$= 2 \times 9.1 \times 10^{-31} \times (3 \times 10^8)^2$$
$$= 1.6 \times 10^{-13} \text{ J}$$

8. (d) $E = \Delta mc^2$; $\Delta m = 0.3$ g $= 0.3 \times 10^{-3}$ kg (given)
$\Rightarrow$ Amount of energy, $E = \frac{0.3}{1000} \times (3 \times 10^8)^2$
$$= 2.7 \times 10^{13} \text{ J}$$
$$= \frac{2.7 \times 10^{13}}{3.6 \times 10^6} = 7.5 \times 10^6 \text{ kWh}$$
$(\because 1 \text{ kWh} = 3.6 \times 10^6 \text{ J})$

9. (a) Both A and R are true but R is not the correct explanation of A.
In heavy nuclei, the repulsive forces between the protons are more effective than the nuclear attractive forces and these forces reduce the stability of the nucleus.

10. (a) The mass of nucleus formed is always less than the sum of the masses of the constituent proton and neutrons.
i.e. $\quad m < (A - Z)m_n + Zm_p$

11. (a) BE $= \Delta mc^2 = \Delta m \times 931$ MeV
$\Rightarrow$ BE $= [Zm_p + (A - Z)m_n - m_N] \times 931$
$$= [2(1.0087 + 1.0073) - 4.0015] \times 931$$
$$= 28.4 \text{ MeV}$$

12. (c) Here, $R = 1.2 \times 10^{-15} A^{1/3}$ m
Mass of nucleon, $m = 1.67 \times 10^{-27}$ kg
Nuclear mass $= mA = 1.67 \times 10^{-27} \times A$ kg
Nuclear volume $= \frac{4}{3}\pi R^3$
$$= \frac{4}{3}\pi(1.2 \times 10^{-15} A^{1/3})^3 \text{m}^3$$
Nuclear density, $\rho_{nu} = \frac{1.67 \times 10^{-27} \times A}{\frac{4}{3}\pi(1.2 \times 10^{-15} A^{1/3})^3}$
$$= 2.307 \times 10^{17} \text{ kg m}^{-3}$$
Now, density of water,
$$\rho_{water} = 10^3 \text{ kg m}^{-3}$$
Ratio of nuclear density and density of water,
$$\therefore \quad \frac{\rho_{nu}}{\rho_{water}} = \frac{2.307 \times 10^{17}}{10^3} = 2.307 \times 10^{14}$$

13. (c) Energy released = Products energy − Reactants energy

$$= 8.5 \times 234 - 7.6 \times 236$$
$$= 195.4 \text{ MeV} \approx 200 \text{ MeV}$$

14. (d) The mass number of a nucleus is more than its atomic number, but in hydrogen, atomic number and mass number are equal.

15. (c) For ${}_6C^{12}$

Proton = 6, electron = 6 and neutron = 6

For ${}_6C^{14}$

Proton = 6, electron = 6 and neutron = 8

16. (b) ${}_ZX^A = {}_{88}Ra^{226}$

Number of protons, $Z = 88$

Number of neutrons, $N = A - Z = 226 - 88 = 138$

17. (c) Helium nucleus = ${}_2He^4$

Number of protons = $Z = 2$

Number of neutrons = $A - Z = 4 - 2 = 2$

18. (a) Both A and R are true but R is not the correct explanation of A.

Nitrogen is a stable element. Those elements which have an odd number of protons and an odd number of neutrons are generally unstable. ${}^{14}_{4}N$ has 7 protons and 7 neutrons, *i.e.* odd number of both protons and neutrons but it is an exception. It is stable element.

19. (d) Both A and R are true and R is the correct explanation of A.

Step up Practice 2

1. (d) The given equation is ${}_2He^4 + {}_ZX^A \rightarrow {}_{Z+2}Y^{A+3} + B$

Applying mass conservation,

$4 + A = A + 3 + x \Rightarrow x = 1$

Applying charge conservation,

$2 + Z = Z + 2 + n \Rightarrow n = 0$

Hence, B is a neutron.

2. (a) ${}_{92}U^{238} \xrightarrow{\alpha} {}_{90}Th^{234} \xrightarrow{\beta^-} {}_{91}Pa^{234} \xrightarrow{{}_{-1}\beta^0} {}_{92}U^{234}$

So, $A = 234$, $B = 90$, $C = 234$, $D = 91$ and $E = \beta^-$

3. (a) ${}_8O^{18} + {}_1H^1 \rightarrow {}_9F^{18} + {}_0n^1$

4. (d) Both Statement I and Statement II are correct.

When uranium is bombarded by slow neutrons, the reaction is represented as

$${}^{235}_{92}U + {}^{1}_{0}n \rightarrow {}^{144}_{56}Ba + {}^{89}_{36}Kr + 3{}_0n^1 + \text{Energy}$$

As more neutrons are produced, the Statement II is correct. These are additional neutrons strike other uranium nuclei to produce even more neutrons. Thus, a chain reaction is established.

5. (b) $\Delta m = 1 - 0.993 = 0.007$ g

$$\therefore \quad E = (\Delta m)c^2 = (0.007 \times 10^{-3})(3 \times 10^8)^2$$
$$= 63 \times 10^{10} \text{ J} = 6.3 \times 10^{11} \text{ J}$$

6. (d) Energy/day $= 200 \times 10^6 \times 24 \times 3600$

$$= 2 \times 2.4 \times 3.6 \times 10^{12}$$
$$= 1728 \times 10^{10}$$
$$= 1.728 \times 10^{13} \text{ J}$$

7. (c) Statement I is incorrect but Statement II is correct.

Percentage of mass converted to energy in a fission reaction is 0.1%, whereas in a fusion reaction, it is 0.4%. Consequently the amount of energy released in more in a fusion than in a fission reaction.

It is not easy to control a fusion reaction. Number of fusions taking place is larger.

8. (a) Power, $P = n\left(\frac{E}{t}\right)$

$$\Rightarrow \quad 1000 = \frac{n \times 200 \times 10^6 \times 1.6 \times 10^{-19}}{t}$$

$$\Rightarrow \quad \frac{n}{t} = 3.125 \times 10^{13}$$

9. (d) Both Statement I and Statement II are correct.

Time taken for the light emission from an atom $\approx 10^{-8}$s.

Time taken for release of energy in fission $\approx 10^{-6}$s.

$$\text{Required ratio} = \frac{10^{-8}}{10^{-6}} = \frac{1}{100} = 1:100$$

10. (a) Energy released in the fission of one nucleus

$$= 200 \text{ MeV}$$
$$= 200 \times 10^6 \times 1.6 \times 10^{-19} \text{ J}$$
$$= 3.2 \times 10^{-11} \text{ J}$$
$$P = 16 \text{ kW} = 16 \times 10^3 \text{ W}$$

Now, number of nuclei required per second,

$$n = \frac{P}{E} = \frac{16 \times 10^3}{3.2 \times 10^{-11}} = 0.5 \times 10^{15}$$

11. (a) Number of fissions per second

$$= \frac{\text{Power output}}{\text{Energy released per fission}}$$

$$= \frac{3.2 \times 10^6}{200 \times 10^6 \times 1.6 \times 10^{-19}} = 1 \times 10^{17}$$

12. (a) In nuclear reaction, total mass of reactants

$$= (2.0141) \times 2 = 4.0282 \text{ amu}$$

Total mass of products = 4.0024 amu

$$\text{Mass defect} = 4.0282 \text{ amu} - 4.0024 \text{ amu}$$
$$= 0.0258 \text{ amu}$$

$$\therefore \quad \text{Energy release, } E = 931 \times 0.0258 = 24 \text{ MeV}$$

13. (b) Fusion reaction takes place at very high temperature and pressure.

Released energy is very large in fusion reaction.

14. (*d*) Energy radiated $= 1.4\ \text{kW/m}^2$

$$= 1.4\ \text{kJ/sm}^2$$

$$= \frac{1.4\ \text{kJ}}{\frac{1}{86400}\ \text{day m}^2}$$

$$= \frac{1.4 \times 86400}{\text{day m}^2}$$

Total energy radiated/day

$$= \frac{4\pi(1.5 \times 10^{11})^2 \times 1.4 \times 86400}{1}\ \frac{\text{kJ}}{\text{day}} = E$$

$\therefore \quad E = mc^2$

$\Rightarrow \quad m = \frac{E}{c^2}$

$\therefore$ Mass lost by the sun per day

$$= \frac{4\pi(1.5 \times 10^{11})^2 \times 1.4 \times 86400}{(3 \times 10^8)^2} = 38 \times 10^{13}\ \text{kg}$$

15. (*b*) $P = \frac{nE}{t} \Rightarrow 300 \times 10^6$

$$= \frac{n \times 170 \times 10^6 \times 1.6 \times 10^{-19}}{t}$$

$\therefore$ Number of atoms per second $\frac{n}{t} = 1.102 \times 10^{19}$

Number of atoms per hour $= 1.102 \times 10^{19} \times 3600$

$$= 39.6 \times 10^{21}$$

16. (*d*) Statement I is correct but Statement II is incorrect.

In both fission and fusion, large amount of energy is released. The Statement II is also correct because charge, mass, momentum and energy all are conserved.

17. (*b*) $P = 10^6$ W

Time $= 1$ day $= 24 \times 36 \times 10^2$ s

Energy produced, in fusion reaction,

$$U = Pt = 10^6 \times 24 \times 36 \times 10^2$$

$$= 24 \times 36 \times 10^8\ \text{J}$$

Energy released per fusion reaction

$$= 20\ \text{MeV} = 32 \times 10^{-13}\ \text{J}$$

Energy released per atom of ${}_1\text{H}^2 = 32 \times 10^{-13}$ J

Number of ${}_1\text{H}^2$ atoms used

$$= \frac{24 \times 36 \times 10^8}{32 \times 10^{-13}} = 27 \times 10^{21}$$

18. (*b*) As we can see in the graph, that for high atomic masses nuclei, the binding energy per nucleon decreases with increase in mass number.

Fission leads to decrease in mass number. Decrease in mass number will increase stability of nuclei, making fission of nuclei possible for heavier nuclei.

19. (*a*) In fusion reaction, two lighter nuclei combine to form a heavy nucleus.

20. (*d*) Both Statement I and Statement II are correct.

A neutron is slightly heavier than a proton. As neutrons are chargeless particles, they penetrate matter more than protons. Therefore, they are more effective than protons in fission reactions.

Gearing up for NEET

1 (*b*) Heavy stable nuclei have more neutrons than protons. This is because electrostatic force between protons is repulsive which may reduce stability.

2. (*d*) In binding energy per nucleon *versus* mass number curve, the binding energy per nucleon first increases and then decreases with increase in mass number.

3. (*b*) Binding energy per nucleon increases with atomic number and it is maximum for iron. After it, binding energy per nucleon of iron decreases.

4. (*b*) The elements high on the BE *versus* mass number plot are very tightly bound and hence are stable. And the elements those are lower on this plot, are less tightly bound and hence are unstable.

Since, helium nucleus shown a peak on this plot, so it is very stable.

5. (*a*) Three atoms of $B \longrightarrow$ One atom of A

$$\therefore \quad Q = E_a - 3E_b$$

6. (*b*) During fusion, BE of daughter nucleus is always greater than the total energy of the parent nuclei, so energy released

$$= c - (a + b) = c - a - b$$

7. (*d*) Binding energy per nucleon

$$= \frac{[\{Zm_p + (A - Z)m_n\} - M] \times 931.4}{\text{Mass number } (A)}$$

$$= \left(\frac{6 \times 1.0078 + 6 \times 1.0087 - 12}{12}\right) \times 931.4$$

$$= 7.68\ \text{MeV}$$

8. (*c*) Energy is released in a process when total binding energy (BE) of the nucleus is increased or we can say when total BE of products is more than the reactants. By calculation, we can see that only in case of option (c), this happens.

Given, $W \to 2Y$

BE of reactants $= 120 \times 7.5$

$$= 900\ \text{MeV}$$

and BE of products $= 2 \times 60 \times 8.5$

$$= 1020\ \text{MeV}$$

i.e. BE of products > BE of reactants.

Hence, energy is released in the process of option (c).

9. (b) Given, $F = \frac{GMm}{r^2}$

where, M = effective mass of hydrogen atom
= mass of electron + mass of proton − (B/c^2)

where, B is BE of hydrogen atom = 13.6 eV

10. (c) Net process is, $3\,_1H^2 \rightarrow {}_2He^4 + p + n$

Mass defect, $\Delta m = (3 \times 2.014) - 4.001 - 1.007 - 1.008 = 0.026$ amu

Energy released by the fusion of three deuterons

$= \Delta m \times 931.48$
$= 0.026 \times 931.48$ MeV
$= 0.026 \times 931.48 \times 1.6 \times 10^{-13}$ J
$= 3.87 \times 10^{-12}$ J

$\therefore$ Total energy released $= \frac{10^{40}}{3} \times 3.87 \times 10^{-12}$ J
$= 1.29 \times 10^{28}$ J

Total time $= \frac{1.29 \times 10^{28}}{10^{16}} = 1.29 \times 10^{12}$ s

$\left(\because \text{Power} = \frac{\text{Energy}}{\text{Time}}\right)$

$\therefore$ The order of time is 10^{12} s.

11. (a) Radius of nuclei having mass number A is determined as

$R = R_0 A^{1/3}$ (where, R_0 = constant)

where, $R_0 = 1.2 \times 10^{-15}$m

This implies, $\frac{R_1}{R_2} = \left(\frac{A_1}{A_2}\right)^{1/3} = \left(\frac{216}{64}\right)^{1/3} = \frac{6}{4}$

$\Rightarrow R_1 : R_2 = 3 : 2$

12. (d) The binding energy for $_1H^1$ is zero and also not given in the question, so we can ignore it.

$Q = 2(4 \times 7.06) - (7 \times 5.60)$
$= (8 \times 7.06) - (7 \times 5.60)$
$= 56.48 - 39.2$
$= 17.28$ MeV
$\simeq 17.3$ MeV

13. (d) $E = \Delta mc^2 \Rightarrow E = \frac{0.3}{1000} \times (3 \times 10^8)^2 = 2.7 \times 10^{13}$ J

$= \frac{2.7 \times 10^{13}}{3.6 \times 10^6} = 7.5 \times 10^6$ kWh

$\therefore$ The amount of energy liberated is 7.5×10^6 kWh.

14. (a) BE $= \Delta mc^2 = [2(1.0087 + 1.0073) - 4.0015] \times 931$
$= 28.4$ MeV

15. (b) For stability, in case of lighter nuclei $\frac{N}{Z} = 1$

and for stability of heavier nuclei, $\frac{N}{Z} > 1$.

16. (b) Mass defect of helium nucleus, $\Delta m = 0.0303$ amu

Binding energy $= \Delta mc^2$
$= 0.0303$ (amu) $\times$ 931.5 (MeV/amu)
≈ 28 MeV

Number of nucleon in helium nucleus = 4

Thus, binding energy per nucleon $= \frac{28}{4} = 7$ MeV

17. (a) Radius of nucleus, $R = R_0 A^{1/3}$.

where, R_0 is a constant and A is the mass number.

$R_{Cu} = (1.2 \times 10^{-15})(64)^{1/3} = (1.2 \times 10^{-15}) \times (4^3)^{1/3}$
$= 4.8 \times 10^{-15}$ m $= 4.8$ fm

18. (d) Density of a nucleus, $\rho = \frac{\text{Mass}}{\text{Volume}} = \frac{mA}{\frac{4}{3}\pi R_0^3 A} = \frac{3m}{4\pi R_0^3}$ ...(i)

As, mass of nucleon, $m = m_p = m_n = 1.67 \times 10^{-27}$ kg

and $R_0 = 1.2 \times 10^{-15}$ m.

Substituting these values in Eq. (i), we get

$$\rho = \frac{3 \times 1.67 \times 10^{-27}}{4 \times 3.14 \times (1.2 \times 10^{-15})^3} \approx 2.3 \times 10^{17} \text{ kgm}^{-3}$$

which is a constant and independent of A, for all nuclei. Also, density of nuclear matter is very large as compared to ordinary matter.

19. (a) Given,

E_{bn} for $A = 240$ nucleus is about 7.6 MeV.

E_{bn} for the two $A = 120$ fragments nuclei is about 8.5 MeV.

So, gain in binding energy of nucleon is about $(8.5 - 7.6) = 0.9$ MeV

Hence, the total gain in binding energy $= 240 \times 0.9 = 216$ MeV

20. (c) Nuclear radius, $R \propto A^{1/3}$, where A is mass number.

For ^{27}Al,

$R = R_0 A^{1/3} = R_0 (27)^{1/3} = 3R_0$

$R_0 = \frac{3.6}{3} = 1.2$ fm [$\because R = 3.6$ fm, for Al]

For ^{64}Cu, $R = R_0 A^{1/3} = 1.2(64)^{1/3} = 4.8$ fm

21. (c) Given, $m_{Fe} = 55.85$u,
$= 55.85 \times 1.66 \times 10^{-27}$ kg
$= 9.27 \times 10^{-26}$ kg,

$A = 56$ and $R_0 = 1.2 \times 10^{-15}$ m

Nuclear density $= \frac{\text{Mass}}{\text{Volume}} = \frac{m_{Fe}}{(4/3)\pi R_0^3 A}$

$= \frac{9.27 \times 10^{-26}}{(4\pi/3)(1.2 \times 10^{-15})^3} \times \frac{1}{56}$
$= 2.29 \times 10^{17}$ kg m^{-3}

22. (b) Given, E_{bn} of chlorine = 278.67 MeV

and E_{bn} of phosphorus = 262.48 MeV

Binding energy per nucleon of $_{17}Cl^{35}$

$$= \frac{\text{Binding energy}}{\text{Mass number}} = \frac{287.67}{35} = 8.22 \text{ MeV}$$

Similarly,

Binding energy per nucleon of $_{15}P^{31} = \frac{262.48}{31}$

$$= 8.47 \text{ MeV}$$

Since, BE of $_{15}P^{31}$ is more than BE of $_{17}Cl^{35}$, hence $_{15}P^{31}$ is more stable.

23. (d) Binding energy per nucleon is $E_{bn} = \frac{E_b}{A}$ ...(i)

For deuteron, atomic mass, $A = 2$ and $E_{bn} = 2.115$ MeV

$$2.115 = \frac{E_b}{2}$$

$\Rightarrow$ $E_b = 2 \times 2.115 \text{ MeV} = 4.23$

$\therefore$ Mass number, $\Delta m = \frac{4.23}{931}$

$\Rightarrow$ $\Delta m = 0.0045 \text{u}$

24. (a) Given, $m(^{56}_{26}\text{Fe}) = 55.934939$ u,

$m_p = 1.007825$ u

and $m_n = 1.008665$ u

Also, $A = 56$ and $Z = 26$

$^{56}_{26}$Fe nucleus has 26 protons and $(56 - 26) = 30$ neutrons.

$\therefore$ Mass defect $= [Zm_p + (A - Z)m_n] - M$

$= (26m_p + 30m_n) - m(^{56}_{26}\text{Fe})$

$= [26(1.007825) + 30(1.008665)] - 55.934939$

$= 56.46340 - 55.934939$

$= 0.528461$ u

Total BE $= \Delta m \times 931$ MeV

$= 0.528461 \times 931.5$

$= 492.26$ MeV

$\therefore$ Binding energy per nucleon

$$= \frac{\text{Total BE}}{A} = \frac{492.26}{56} = 8.790 \text{ MeV}$$

25. (d) Given, mass of neutron = 1.00866 u,

mass of a proton = 1.00727 u, mass of $^{16}_{8}\text{O} = 15.99053$ u

Mass number, $A = 16$,

Atomic number, $Z = 8$

Number of protons = 8

Number of neutrons $= (A - Z) = 8$

Therefore, mass of 8 neutrons $= 8 \times 1.00866$ u

Mass of 8 protons $= 8 \times 1.00727$ u

So, the expected mass of $^{16}_{8}$O nucleus,

$= 8\,(1.00866 + 1.00727)$

$= 8 \times 2.01593 \text{ u} = 16.12744$ u

Thus, mass defect,

$\Delta m = 16.12744 \text{u} - 15.99053$ u

$= 0.13691$ u

Since, 1u = 931.5 MeV

For $^{16}_{8}$O, $\Delta m = 0.13691$ u

$= 0.13691 \times 931.5$

$= 127.5$ MeV

Thus, the energy required to separate $^{16}_{8}$O into its constituents is 127.5 MeV.

26. (d) Mass defect, Δm

= Mass of nucleons - Mass of nucleus

$= [Zm_p + (A - Z)m_n] - M_n$

Here, mass number, $A = 4$

Atomic number, $Z = 2$

Number of protons = 2

Number of neutrons $= A - Z = 4 - 2 = 2$

$m_p = 1.0072676$ u

$m_n = 1.008665$ u and $M_n = 4.001506$ u

Mass of nucleon in $_2He^4$ =

Mass of 2 protons + Mass of 2 neutrons

So, mass of nucleons $= 2 \times 1.0072676 + 2 \times 1.008665$

$\therefore$ $\Delta m = 2 \times 1.0072676 + 2 \times 1.008665 - 4.001506$

$= 0.0303592$ u

27. (b) We have,

$P = 200 \text{ MW} = 200 \times 10^6 \text{ W} = 2 \times 10^8$ W,

$t = 1 \text{ h} = 3600$ s

As, energy, $E = P \times t = 2 \times 10^8 \times 3600$

Also, $E = mc^2$

$$\Rightarrow \quad m = \frac{E}{c^2} = \frac{2 \times 10^8 \times 3600}{(3 \times 10^8)^2}$$

$= 8 \times 10^{-6}$ kg

28. (b) According to mass-energy equivalence relation,

Energy, $E = mc^2$

By substituting,

$m = 2 \text{ g} = 2 \times 10^{-3} \text{ kg}, c = 3 \times 10^8 \text{ ms}^{-1}$

We have, $E = 2 \times 10^{-3} \times (3 \times 10^8)^2$

$\Rightarrow$ $E = 2 \times 10^{-3} \times 9 \times 10^{16} = 18 \times 10^{13}$ J

29. (b) Energy released on bombarding U^{235} by neutron

= 200 MeV

$= 200 \times 10^6 \times 1.6 \times 10^{-19}$ J

Power output of atomic reactor = 1.6 MW

$= 1.6 \times 10^6$ W

$$\therefore \quad \text{Rate of fission} = \frac{1.6 \times 10^6}{200 \times 10^6 \times 1.6 \times 10^{-19}}$$

$= 5 \times 10^{16} \text{ s}^{-1}$

30. (*b*) From Einstein's mass-energy relation, the energy released is $\Delta E = \Delta mc^2$

where, Δm is mass and c is speed of light.

Given, $\Delta m = 1 \text{ mg} = 1 \times 10^{-6}$ kg, $c = 3 \times 10^8 \text{ ms}^{-1}$

$\therefore \quad \Delta E = 1 \times 10^{-6} \times (3 \times 10^8)^2 = 9 \times 10^{10}$ J

The rate at which energy is dissipated is known as power,

$$P = \frac{\Delta E}{t} = \frac{9 \times 10^{10}}{1} = 9 \times 10^{10} \text{ W}$$

$\therefore \quad P = 9 \times 10^7$ kW

31. (*b*) Power $= \frac{\text{Energy}}{\text{Time}} = 300$ MW

$= 300 \times 10^6 \text{ W} = 3 \times 10^8 \text{ Js}^{-1}$

Energy released due to fission,

$= 170 \text{ MeV} = 170 \times 10^6 \times 1.6 \times 10^{-19}$

$= 27.2 \times 10^{-12}$ J

Number of atoms fissioned per second

$$= \frac{\text{Energy released per second}}{\text{Energy released per fission}}$$

$$= \frac{3 \times 10^8}{27.2 \times 10^{-12}} = \frac{3 \times 10^{20}}{27.2}$$

Number of atoms fissioned per hour

$$= \frac{3 \times 10^{20} \times 3600}{27.2} = \frac{3 \times 36}{27.2} \times 10^{22} \approx 4 \times 10^{22}$$

32. (*d*) Energy released in each fission of $U^{235} = 200$ MeV

$= 200 \times 10^6 \times 1.6 \times 10^{-19} \text{ J} = 3.2 \times 10^{-11}$ J

Since, only 20% of this is utilised efficiently, therefore energy generated from the reactor per fission

$= 3.2 \times 10^{-11} \times 0.20 = 6.4 \times 10^{-12}$ J

As, the output of the reactor is 700 MW, the number of fission required per second

$$= \frac{700 \times 10^6}{6.4 \times 10^{-12}} = 1.1 \times 10^{20} \text{ s}^{-1}$$

The number of U^{-235} atoms consumed in 24 h

$= 24 \times 60 \times 60 \times 1.1 \times 10^{20} = 9.5 \times 10^{24}$

There are 6.02×10^{26} atoms in 235 kg of U-235.

Therefore, the mass of U-235 consumed during 24 h

$$= \frac{9.5 \times 10^{24}}{6.02 \times 10^{26}} \times 235 \text{ kg} = 3.7 \text{ kg}$$

Thus, energy generated from the reactor per fission and mass of uranium are 6.4×10^{-12} J and 3.7 kg.

33. (*d*) For fusion reaction to take place, the two nuclei must come close enough, so that the attractive short range nuclear force is able to affect them. Also, they must have suitable energy, enough to overcome the Coulomb repulsive force barrier.

This could only be achieved, if the reaction is taking place at high temperature, which could make the particles of the system to have enough kinetic energy to overcome Coulomb repulsive force between nuclei.

34. (*a*) Given, fusion reaction,

$${}^2_1\text{H} + {}^2_1\text{H} \longrightarrow {}^3_2\text{He} + {}^1_0n$$

Mass of deuteron $({}^2_1\text{H}) = 2.015$ amu

Mass of helium $({}^3_2\text{He}) = 3.017$ amu

and mass of neutron $({}^1_0n) = 1.009$ amu

Mass defect, $\Delta m = $ Mass of $({}^2_1\text{H})$ − Mass of $({}^3_2\text{He} + {}^1_0n)$

$\Rightarrow \quad \Delta m = 2(2.015) - (3.017 + 1.009)$

$= 0.004$ amu

$\therefore$ Energy released $= (0.004 \times 931.5)$ MeV

$= 3.726$ MeV

Energy released per deuteron $= \frac{3.726}{2} = 1.863$ MeV

Number of deutrons in 1 kg $= \frac{6.02 \times 10^{26}}{2}$

$= 3.01 \times 10^{26}$

$\therefore$ Energy released per kg of deuterium fusion

$= (3.01 \times 10^{26} \times 1.863)$

$= 5.6 \times 10^{26}$ MeV

$= 5.6 \times 10^{26} \times 10^6 \times 1.6 \times 10^{-19}$ J

$\approx 9.0 \times 10^{13}$ J

35. (*b*) U^{235} is to be bombarded by slow moving neutron or thermal neutron, but U^{238} is to be bombarded by fast moving neutron for fission.

36. (*a*) To sustain a chain reaction in atom bomb one of the neutrons emitted in the fission of ^{235}U must be captured by another ^{235}U nucleus and causes its fission.

37. (*a*) When a neutron collides with uranium atom, then energy is released along with three more neutrons which further collide with another uranium atom and, so the chain reaction continues. Thus boron rods in nuclear reactor are used to absorb excess neutrons, so that the reaction rate remains under control.

38. (*d*) $Q = (1.002 + 1.004 - 1.001 - 1.003)(931.5)$ MeV

$= 1.863$ MeV

39. (*d*) Energy released in the fission of one nucleus

$= 200$ MeV

$= 200 \times 10^6 \times 1.6 \times 10^{-19}$

$= 3.2 \times 10^{-11}$ J

$P = 16 \text{ kW} = 16 \times 10^3$ W

Now, number of nuclei required per second

$$n = \frac{P}{E} = \frac{16 \times 10^3}{3.2 \times 10^{-11}} = 5 \times 10^{14}$$

40. (*a*) Kinetic energy of the molecules of a gas at a temperature T is $\frac{3}{2}kT$.

$\therefore$ To initiate the reaction $\frac{3}{2}kT = 7.7 \times 10^{-14}$ J

$$\Rightarrow \quad \frac{3}{2} \times 1.38 \times 10^{-23}\, T = 7.7 \times 10^{-14}$$

$$\Rightarrow \quad T = 3.7 \times 10^9 \text{K}$$

Thus, the order of temperature is 10^9 K.

41. (*c*) As, $n = \frac{m}{A} N_A \Rightarrow E = \left(\frac{m}{A} N_A \times 200 \times 1.6 \times 10^{-13}\right)$ J

For 1 day $= 24 \times 3600$

$$\text{Power} = \frac{E}{t} = \frac{mN_A \times 3.2 \times 10^{-11}}{235 \times 24 \times 3600} = 10^6$$

($\because$ given, $P = 10^6$ W)

$$\therefore \text{Mass, } m = \frac{1 \times 10^6 \times 24 \times 3600 \times 235}{3.2 \times 10^{-11} \times 6.02 \times 10^{23}} \approx 1 \text{ g}$$

42. (*d*) Fission reaction can be written as

$${}^{235}_{92}\text{U} + {}^{1}_{0}n \rightarrow {}^{144}_{56}\text{Ba} + {}^{89}_{36}\text{Kr} + {}^{X}_{0}n + Q$$

Due to mass conservation,

$$235 + 1 = 144 + 89 + X$$

$$\therefore \quad X = 3$$

43. (*a*) Number of fission per second

$$= \frac{\text{Power output}}{\text{Energy released per fission}}$$

$$= \frac{3.2 \times 10^6}{200 \times 10^6 \times 1.6 \times 10^{-19}} = 1 \times 10^{17}$$

The number of fission of U^{235} per minute

$$= 60 \times 1 \times 10^{17} = 6 \times 10^{18}$$

44. (*d*) The reaction should be

$${}_{88}\text{Ra}^{226} \longrightarrow {}_{86}\text{Rn}^{222} + {}_{2}\text{He}^4$$

$$Q\text{-value} = \begin{bmatrix} \text{(mass number of Ra)} \\ -\text{(mass number of Rn)} \\ -m\,(\text{He}^4) \end{bmatrix} \text{u} \times 931.5 \text{ MeV}$$

$$= 0.005297 \times 931.5 = 4.934 \text{ MeV}$$

Kinetic energy of α-particle

$$= \frac{m\,(\text{Rn})}{m\,(\text{Ra})} \times Q\text{-value} \simeq 4.871 \text{ MeV}$$

45. (*b*) The fission per second $= 4 \times 10^{20}$

So, the energy released per second

$$= (4 \times 10^{20} \times 250) \text{ MeV}$$

$$= (4 \times 10^{20} \times 250 \times 10^6 \times 1.6 \times 10^{-19}) \text{ J}$$

Therefore, energy released in 10 h $= 36 \times 10^3$ s,

$$E = (36 \times 10^3 \times 4 \times 10^{20} \times 250 \times 10^6 \times 1.6 \times 10^{-19}) \text{ J}$$

$$= (36 \times 4 \times 250 \times 1.6 \times 10^{10}) \text{ J}$$

$$= (57600 \times 10^{10}) \text{ J}$$

$$= 576 \times 10^{12} \text{ J}$$

46. (*a*) Let there is n number of fission per second produces a power of 6.4 W, then

$$n \times 200 \times 10^6 \times 1.6 \times 10^{-19} = 6.4$$

$$\Rightarrow \quad n = \frac{6.4}{200 \times 10^{-13} \times 1.6} = \frac{4}{2 \times 10^{-11}} = 2 \times 10^{11}$$

47. (*a*) Energy released in one fission of ${}^{235}_{92}$U nucleus

$$= 200 \text{ MeV}$$

Mass of uranium $= 1$ g

We know that, 235 g of ^{235}U has 6.023×10^{23} atoms or nuclei.

$\therefore$ Energy released in fission of 1 g of U^{235},

$$E = \frac{6.023 \times 10^{23} \times 1 \times 200}{235} = 5.1 \times 10^{23} \text{ MeV}$$

$$= (5.1 \times 10^{23} \times 1.6 \times 10^{-13}) \text{ J}$$

$$= \frac{5.1 \times 10^{23} \times 1.6 \times 10^{-13}}{3.6 \times 10^6} \text{ kWh}$$

$$= 2.26 \times 10^4 \text{ kWh}$$

48. (*d*) The fusion reaction in the sun is a multi-step process in which the hydrogen is burned into helium. Because in fusion, lighter nuclei combine to form heavier nucleus.

49. (*a*) From $E = (\Delta m)c^2$,

$$\Delta m = \frac{E}{c^2} = \frac{9 \times 10^{13}}{(3 \times 10^8)^2} = 10^{-3} \text{kg}$$

$$\therefore \quad \frac{\Delta m}{m} \times 100 = \frac{10^{-3}}{1} \times 100 = 0.1\ \%$$

50. (*c*) Energy and mass are related by the relation, $E = mc^2$

Differentiating, we get

$$\frac{dE}{dt} = m \times [0] + c^2 \frac{dm}{dt}$$

$$\Rightarrow \quad 3.6 \times 10^{28} = 9 \times 10^{16} \frac{dm}{dt}$$

$$\Rightarrow \quad \frac{dm}{dt} = 4 \times 10^{11} \text{ kg/s}$$

Assertion and Reason

1. (*c*) A is false but R is true.

The nucleus of the lightest atom of hydrogen which has a relative abundance of 99.985% is called proton. Thus, we conclude that ratio of the mass of nucleus of H-atom and the proton is unity.

2. (*d*) Both A and R are true and R is the correct explanation of A.

3. (c) A is false but R is true.

Lighter nuclei tend to fuse to attain a stable structure.

4. (c) A is false but R is true.

Nuclear fusion is not possible in laboratory.

Nuclear fusion requires very high temperature of 10^6 and 10^7 K.

5. (a) Both A and R are true but R is not the correct explanation of A.

Statement Type Questions

1. (b) Statement I is correct but Statement II is incorrect.

The process of nuclear fusion can be explained with the help of concept of binding energy per nucleon of very light nuclei and the intermediate nuclei. Binding energy per nucleon of very light nuclei are less than that of intermediate nuclei. It means light nuclei are less stable than that of intermediate nuclei. As ^{35}Cl has a large binding energy, therefore it cannot be used as fuel for fusion energy.

2. (d) Both Statement I and Statement II are correct.

Σ(mass of nucleons) > M (mass of nucleus)

A higher mass means a higher energy state or configuration, a lower mass means a lower energy state which is stable.

3. (b) Statement I is correct but Statement II is incorrect.

The decrease in binding energy per nucleon for heavy nuclei ($A > 100$) due to increase in Coulomb repulsion between the protons inside the nucleus.

4. (b) Statement I is correct but Statement II is incorrect.

We know that, energy is released when heavy nuclei undergo fission or light nuclei undergo fusion. Therefore Statement I is correct.

Statement II is incorrect because for heavy nuclei, the binding energy per nucleon decreases with increasing Z and for light nuclei, BE/nucleon increases with increasing Z.

5. (d) Both Statement I and Statement II are correct.

Match the Columns

1. (d) Radius of nucleus,

$$R = R_0 A^{1/3}$$

where, $R_0 = 1.2 \times 10^{-15}$ m, A = mass number

(A) $A = 216$

$R = 1.2 \times 10^{-15} \times (216)^{1/3} = 7.2 \times 10^{-15}$ m

(B) $A = 64$

$R = 1.2 \times 10^{-15} \times (64)^{1/3} = 4.8 \times 10^{-15}$ m

(C) $A = 125$

$R = 1.2 \times 10^{-15} \times (125)^{1/3} = 6.0 \times 10^{-15}$ m

(D) $A = 8$

$R = 1.2 \times 10^{-15} \times (8)^{1/3} = 2.4 \times 10^{-15}$ m

2. (a) (A) $E = \Delta m \cdot c^2$

$$\Rightarrow \quad E = \frac{0.3}{1000} \times (3 \times 10^8)^2 = 2.7 \times 10^{13} \text{ J}$$

$$= \frac{2.7 \times 10^{13}}{3.6 \times 10^6} = 7.5 \times 10^6$$

(B) $$E = \frac{0.5}{1000}(3 \times 10^8)^2 = 4.5 \times 10^{13} \text{ J}$$

$$= \frac{4.5 \times 10^{13}}{3.6 \times 10^6} = 1.25 \times 10^7$$

(C) $$E = \frac{0.1}{1000}(3 \times 10^8)^2 = 0.9 \times 10^{13}$$

$$= \frac{0.9 \times 10^{13}}{3.6 \times 10^6} = 2.5 \times 10^6$$

(D) $$E = \frac{0.6}{1000}(3 \times 10^8)^2 = 5.4 \times 10^{13}$$

$$= \frac{5.4 \times 10^{13}}{3.6 \times 10^6} = 1.5 \times 10^7$$

3. (b) $E_1 = [2m(_1H^2) - m(_1H^3) - m(_1H^1)]$

$\times$ 931.5 MeV = 4 MeV

$E_2 = [-m(_1He^4) - m(_0n^1) + m(_1H^3) + m(_1H^2)]$

$\times$ 931.5 meV = 17.6 MeV

$E_3 = [-m(_2He^3) - m(_0n^1) + 2m(_1H^2)]$

$\times$ 931.5 MeV = 13.3 MeV

$E_4 = [m(_2He^3) + m(_1H^2) - m(_2He^4)] \times 931.5$ MeV

$= 18.3$ MeV

Hence, A-(III), B-(I), C-(IV), D-(II).

4. (c) BE of nucleus

$P = 7.6 \times 240 = 1824$ MeV

BE of nucleus

$Q = 8.5 \times 110 = 935$ MeV

BE of nucleus

$R = 8.4 \times 130 = 1092$ MeV

Energy released per fission

= BE of R + BE of Q − BE of P

$= 1092 + 935 - 1824 = 203$ MeV.

Hence, A-(IV), B-(I), C-(II), D-(III).

Final Check Through PYQs

1. (b) Given, mass number of parent nucleus, $A = 189$

Mass number of daughters nuclei,

$A_1 = 125$ and $A_2 = 64$

We know that, $R = R_0(A^{1/3})$

$$\therefore \quad \frac{R_1}{R_2} = \left(\frac{A_1}{A_2}\right)^{1/3} = \left(\frac{125}{64}\right)^{1/3}$$

$$= \left[\left(\frac{5}{4}\right)^3\right]^{1/3} = \frac{5}{4}$$

$\therefore \quad R_1 : R_2 = 5 : 4$

2. (*d*) A nucleus with mass number 240 breaks into two fragments each of mass number 120.

$$X^{240} \longrightarrow Y^{120} + Z^{120}$$

Given, the binding energy per nucleon of unfragmented nuclei, $X = 7.6$ MeV

The binding energy per nucleon of fragmented nuclei, $Y = Z = 8.5$ MeV

Now, we shall determine the total gain in binding energy.

Gain in binding energy = Binding energy of products − Binding energy of reactants

Gain in binding energy

$$= 2 \times 120 \times 8.5 - 240 \times 7.6$$
$$= 216 \text{ MeV}$$

3. (*a*) Given,

$$m = 0.5 \text{ g} = 0.5 \times 10^{-3} \text{ kg}$$

Relation for energy equivalent of mass is

$$E = mc^2$$

where, c is speed of light.

$$= 0.5 \times 10^{-3} \times (3 \times 10^8)^2 \quad (\because c = 3 \times 10^8)$$
$$= 4.5 \times 10^{13} \text{ J}$$

4. (*b*) Radius of the nucleus is given by

$$R = R_0 A^{1/3} \Rightarrow R \propto A^{1/3}$$

$$\frac{R_{\text{Al}}}{R_{\text{Te}}} = \left(\frac{A_{\text{Al}}}{A_{\text{Te}}}\right)^{1/3} = \left(\frac{27}{125}\right)^{1/3} = \frac{3}{5} \quad R_{\text{Te}} = \frac{5}{3} R_{\text{Al}}$$

5. (*d*) Given,

$$^{290}_{82}X \xrightarrow{\alpha} Y \xrightarrow{e^+} Z \xrightarrow{\beta^-} P \xrightarrow{e^-} Q$$

From $X \to Y$, α-particle is emitted, thus $^{286}_{80}Y$.

From $X \to Y$, e^+ is emitted, thus $^{286}_{79}Z$.

Again $Z \to P$, β^- is emitted, thus $^{286}_{80}P$.

From $P \to Q$, e^- is emitted, thus $^{286}_{81}Q$.

6. (*b*) The given nuclear reaction is represented as

$$^{22}_{11}\text{Na} \longrightarrow {}^{M}_{Z}X + e^+ + \nu$$

Since, atomic number and mass number are same for both side of reaction.

Hence, for atomic number,

$$11 = Z + 1 \Rightarrow Z = 10$$

For mass number,

$$22 = M \Rightarrow M = 22$$

$$\therefore \quad {}^{M}_{Z}X = {}^{22}_{10}\text{Ne}$$

7. (*d*) Here,

$$^{235}_{92}\text{U} + {}^{1}_{0}n \longrightarrow {}^{89}_{36}\text{Kr} + {}^{A}_{Z}X + 3\,({}^{1}_{0}n)$$

According to the law of conservation,

$$(\text{Atomic number})_{\text{Reactant}} = (\text{Atomic number})_{\text{Product}}$$
$$92 + 0 = 36 + Z$$
$$\Rightarrow \quad Z = 92 - 36 = 56$$

Similarly,

$$(\text{Atomic masses})_{\text{Reactant}} = (\text{Atomic masses})_{\text{Product}}$$
$$235 + 1 = 89 + A + 3 \times 1$$
$$\Rightarrow \quad A = 144$$

$\therefore$ Other element is $^{144}_{56}$Ba.

Skill Builder

Sol. of Skill Builder on Pg. 729

(*c*) Radius of the nucleus, $R = R_0 A^{1/3}$

$$R_A = R_0 A^{1/3}$$
$$R_B = R_0 B^{1/3}$$
$$\frac{R_A}{R_B} = \left(\frac{A}{B}\right)^{1/3}$$

Sol. of Skill Builder on Pg. 732

(*a*) Gain in BE = BE of products − BE of reactants

$$= (A_1 \times 7 + A_2 \times 7.5) - (A \times 6.5)$$
$$= (130 \times 7 + 140 \times 7.5) - (270 \times 6.5)$$
$$= (910 + 1050) - (1755)$$
$$= (1960 - 1755) = 205 \text{ MeV}$$

Sol. of Skill Builder on Pg. 736

(*c*) $^{A}_{Z}X \xrightarrow{\beta^+} {}^{A}_{Z-1}X \xrightarrow{\alpha} {}^{A-4}_{Z-3}X$

$$A - 4 = 235$$
$$A = 235 + 4$$
$$= 239$$
$$Z - 3 = 87$$
$$Z = 87 + 3 = 90$$

The mass number and atomic number of element are 239 and 90, respectively.

For deeper insight
Scan the QR Code

Chapter 15

Semiconductor Electronics : Materials, Devices and Simple Circuits

Learning Objectives

Module-I

- Classification of Solids
- Semiconductors
- Electrical Conduction Through Semiconductors
- Effect of Temperature on Conductivity of Semiconductor

Module-II

- *p-n* Junction
- Semiconductor Diode or *p-n* Junction Diode
- Biasing of *p-n* Junction Diode
- *V-I* Characteristic Curve of a *p-n* Junction Diode
- *p-n* Junction Diode as a Rectifier
- Special Types of *p-n* Junction Diode

Module-III

- Logic Gates
- Combination of Logic Gates
- NAND and NOR Gates as Digital Building Blocks

Chapter Overview with NEET Connection

This chapter is the base of smart devices like phone, TV, LED bulb etc. This chapter contains the basic concepts of semiconductor physics and logic gates. Without mastery over this chapter, it will be difficult to understand semiconductor devices and their applications.

Special format questions can easily be framed on the following topics of this chapter

- Electric properties of semiconductor.
- Formation of *p-n* junction diode.
- Biasing of *p-n* junction diode.
- Diodes as rectifiers.
- Logic gates

For better understanding of this Chapter

- Basic concepts of electric current should be memorised.
- Knowledge of binary number system is required.
- Experimental exposure in lab will be helpful.

Introduction

Solid is a state of matter which has a definite shape and a definite volume. Most of the solids can be classified in three types as per their electrical conductivity, *i.e.* conductors, insulators and semiconductors.

Conductors are those materials through which electric charge can flow easily, while insulators are those through which electric charge is difficult to flow. There are, however, certain solids whose electrical conductivity is intermediate between conductors and insulators. They are called **semiconductors**. Silicon and germanium are a few examples of semiconductors. In this chapter, we will study about semiconductors, diodes and use of these diodes to form different types of logic gates.

Module 1

Semiconductors and its Types

- Classification of Solids • Semiconductors • Electrical Conduction Through Semiconductors
- Effect of Temperature on Conductivity of Semiconductor

Classification of Solids

On the basis of the relative values of electrical conductivity (σ) or resistivity ($\rho = 1/\sigma$), the solids are broadly classified as

(i) **Conductors or Metals** They possess very low resistivity (or high conductivity).

$$\rho \sim 10^{-2} - 10^{-8}\ \Omega\text{-m}$$

$$\sigma \sim 10^{2} - 10^{8}\ \text{Sm}^{-1}$$

(ii) **Semiconductors** They have resistivity or conductivity intermediate to metals and insulators.

$$\rho \sim 10^{-5} - 10^{6}\ \Omega\text{-m}$$

$$\sigma \sim 10^{5} - 10^{-6}\ \text{Sm}^{-1}$$

(iii) **Insulators** They have high resistivity (or low conductivity).

$$\rho \sim 10^{11} - 10^{19}\ \Omega\text{-m}$$

$$\sigma \sim 10^{-11} - 10^{-19}\ \text{Sm}^{-1}$$

The values of ρ and σ given above are indicative of magnitude and could well go outside the ranges as well.

Semiconductors

The energy band structure of a semiconductor is shown in figure. It is similar to that of an insulator but with a comparatively small energy gap (E_g < 3eV). At absolute zero temperature, the conduction band of semiconductors is totally empty and valence band is completely filled. Therefore, they behave as a insulators at low temperatures. However, at room temperature, some electrons in the valence band acquire thermal energy greater than energy band gap and jump over to the conduction band where they are free to move under the influence of a small electric field and acquire small conductivity.

Hence, the resistance of semiconductor is not as high as that of insulators.

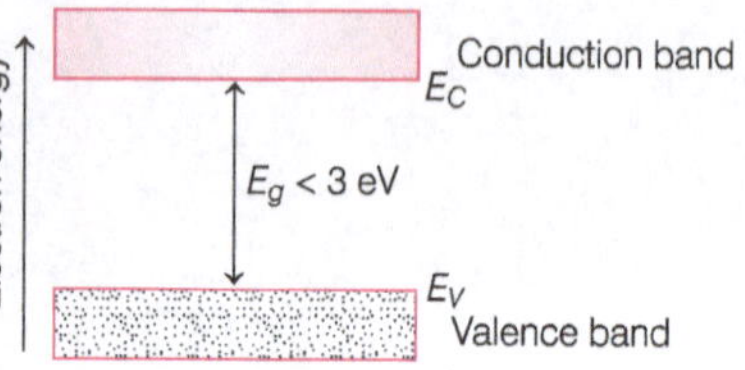

Energy band gap for semiconductors

Types of Semiconductors

As discussed above, in semiconductors, the conduction band and the valence band are separated by a relatively small energy gap. For silicon, this gap is 1.1 eV and for germanium it is 0.7 eV. However at 0 K, they behave as an insulator. On the basis of purity, semiconductors are divided in two groups.

1. Intrinsic Semiconductors

A pure (free from impurity) semiconductor which has a valency 4 is called an intrinsic semiconductor. Pure germanium and silicon in their natural state are intrinsic semiconductors.

Si and Ge both have 4 valence electrons. In crystalline structure, each Si or Ge atom share each of its four valence electrons with four nearest neighbouring atoms and forms covalent bond.

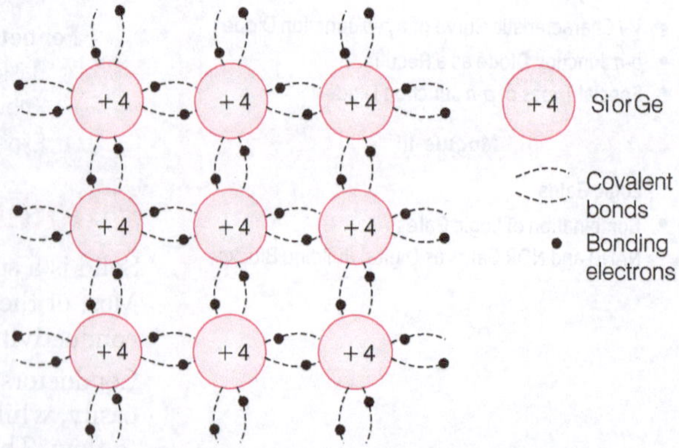

Schematic two-dimensional representation of Si or Ge structure showing covalent bonds at low temperature (all bonds intact). +4 symbol indicates inner cores of Si or Ge.

At temperature close to zero, all shared electrons are tightly bound and so no free electrons are available to conduct electricity through the crystal.

At room temperature, however a few of the covalent bonds are broken due to thermal agitation and thus some of the valence electrons become free. Thus, we can say that, a valence electrons is shifted to conduction band leaving a vacancy of electron in valence band. This vacancy is known as **hole** and carries a positive charge *e*.

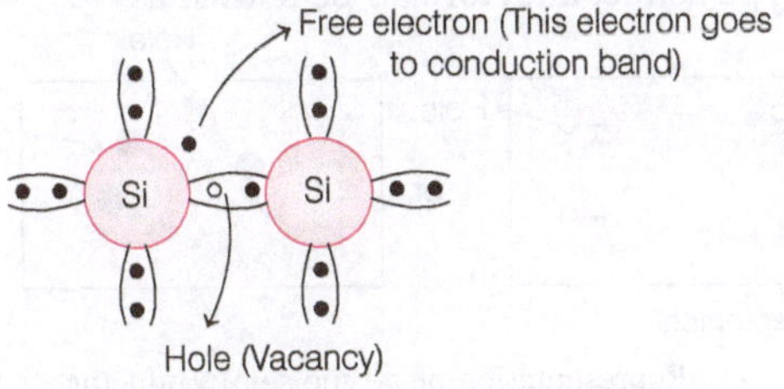

Generation of hole due to thermal agitation

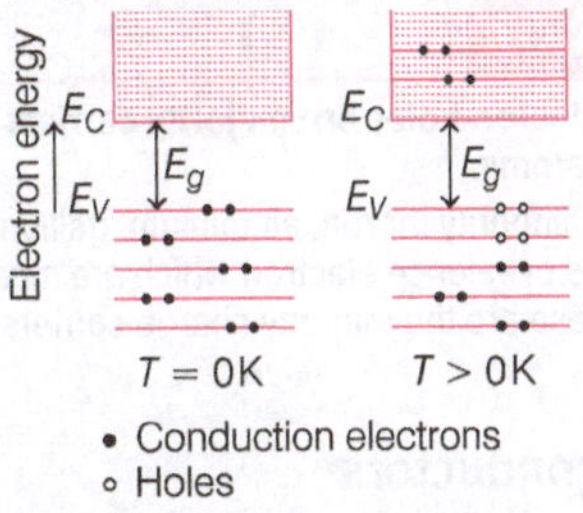

Energy band diagram for an intrinsic semiconductor at $T = 0\,K$ and $T > 0\,K$

In intrinsic (or pure) semiconductors, the number of free electrons per unit volume (n_e) is equal to the number of holes per unit volume (n_h) and it is also equal to the number of intrinsic charge carriers per unit volume (n_i).

Mathematically, we have the relation

$$n_e = n_h = n_i$$

Here, (n_i) is also called **intrinsic carrier concentration.**

At equilibrium, $\boxed{n_e n_h = n_i^2}$

This is known as **mass-action law.**

Under the action of an electric field, holes move towards negative potential giving hole current I_h and electron move towards positive potential giving electron current I_e. The total current is the sum of the electron current I_e and the hole current I_h.

i.e. $\boxed{I = I_e + I_h}$

Example 1. *In an intrinsic (pure) semiconductor, the number of conduction electrons is 7×10^{19} per cubic metre. Find the total number of current carriers (electrons and holes) in the same semiconductor of size 1 cm × 1 cm × 1 mm.*

Sol. In an intrinsic semiconductor, $n_e = n_h$

where, n_e = number of conduction electrons per unit volume

and n_h = number of holes per unit volume.

Given, $n_e = 7 \times 10^{19}$ per m^3

$\therefore$ $n_h = n_e = 7 \times 10^{19}$ per m^3

So, total current carrier density

$$n_e + n_h = 7 \times 10^{19} + 7 \times 10^{19} = 14 \times 10^{19} \text{ per m}^3$$

Now, total number of current carrier

$$= \text{Number density} \times \text{Volume}$$
$$= (14 \times 10^{19}) \times (10^{-2} \times 10^{-2} \times 10^{-3})$$
$$= 1.4 \times 10^{13}$$

Example 2. *Pure Si at 300 K has equal electron (n_e) and hole (n_h) concentration of $1.5 \times 10^{16}\ m^{-3}$. By some means hole concentration increases to $3 \times 10^{22}\ m^{-3}$. Now, calculate n_e in the Si.*

Sol. Given, $n_i = 1.5 \times 10^{16}$ m^{-3}, $n_h = 3 \times 10^{22}$ m^{-3}

For the semiconductor in thermal equilibrium,

$n_e n_h = n_i^2$ (Law of mass action)

$$\Rightarrow \quad n_e = \frac{n_i^2}{n_h} = \frac{(1.5 \times 10^{16})^2}{3 \times 10^{22}} = 7.5 \times 10^9 \text{m}^{-3}$$

Example 3. *The number of conduction electrons (in per cubic metre) present in a pure semiconductor is 6.5×10^{19}. Calculate the number of holes in a sample having dimensions 1 cm × 1 cm × 2 mm.*

Sol. Here, number of conduction electrons, $n_e = 6.5 \times 10^{19}$ m^{-3}

Volume of the sample, $V = 1$ cm × 1 cm × 2 mm $= 2 \times 10^{-7}$ m^3

Number of holes in the sample (N_h) = Number of electrons in the sample (N_e)

$$= N_e \times V$$
$$= 6.5 \times 10^{19} \times 2 \times 10^{-7}$$
$$= 1.3 \times 10^{13}$$

2. Extrinsic Semiconductors

The conductivity of an intrinsic semiconductor is very poor (unless the temperature is very high). At ordinary temperature, only one covalent bond breaks in 10^9 atoms of Ge. It means that, only 1 atom in 10^9 atoms is available for conduction. Conductivity of an intrinsic (pure) semiconductor is significantly increased, if some pentavalent or trivalent impurity is mixed with it. Such impure semiconductors are called **extrinsic or doped semiconductors.**

Mentor's TIP

When some desirable impurity is added to intrinsic semiconductor deliberately, then this process is called **doping** and the impurity atoms are called **dopants**.

There are two types of dopants used in doping in the tetravalent Si or Ge

(i) Trivalent (valency 3) atoms: *e.g.* Indium (In), Boron (B), Aluminium (Al), etc.

(ii) Pentavalent (valency 5) atoms: *e.g.* Arsenic (As), Antimony (Sb), phosphorus (P), etc.

Depending upon the nature of impurity added in intrinsic semiconductor, the extrinsic semiconductors are of two types

(i) *p*-type semiconductor (ii) *n*-type semiconductor

(i) *p*-type semiconductors

It is obtained when a trivalent impurity (*e.g.* boron, aluminium, gallium or indium) is added to a germanium or silicon crystal.

The impurity atom has one valence electron less than Si or Ge, therefore its three valence electrons form covalent bonds with neighbouring three Ge (or Si) atoms while the fourth valence electron of Ge (or Si) is not able to form the bond.

So, the bond between the fourth neighbouring Ge (or Si) and the trivalent impurity has a vacancy or hole as shown in figure.

This vacancy can be filled by an electron in outer orbit in the atom (it may jump to fill the vacancy), leaving a vacancy or hole at its own site.

With this electron, the trivalent impurity atom becomes negatively charged.

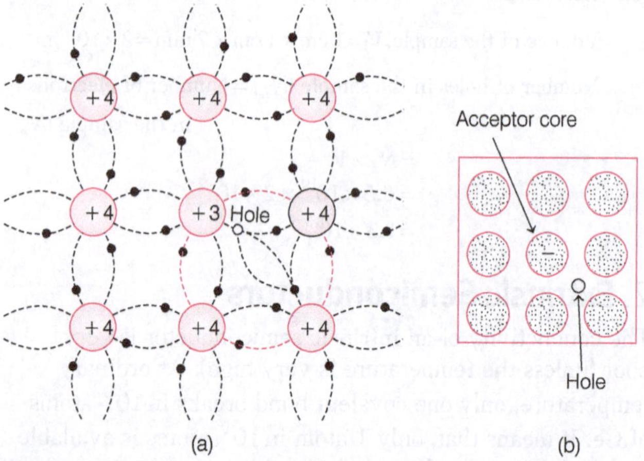

(a) Trivalent acceptor atom (In, Al, B, etc.) doped in tetravalent Si or Ge lattice giving *p*-type semiconductor.
(b) Commonly used schematic representation of *p*-type material which shows only the fixed core of the substituent acceptor with one effective additional negative charge and its associated hole.

So, the dopant atom of *p*-type semiconductor can be considered as core of the negative charge along with its associated hole.

The trivalent impurity atoms are called **acceptor atoms** because they create holes which accept electrons.

Following points are worthnoting regarding to *p*-type semiconductors

(a) Holes are the majority charge carriers and electrons are minority charge carriers in case of *p*-type semiconductors or number of holes are much greater than the number of electrons. *i.e.* $n_h >> n_e$; $i_h > i_e$.

(b) *p*-type semiconductor is electrically neutral.

(c) Conductivity, $\sigma = n_h \mu_h e$

(d) *p*-type semiconductor can be shown as

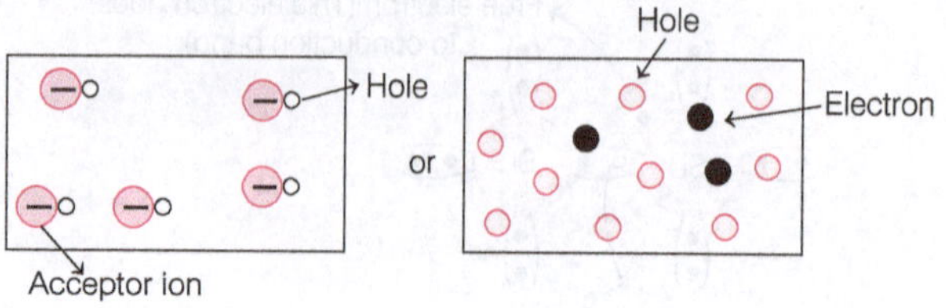

Representation of *p*-type semiconductor

NEET Snapshot

In *p*-type semiconductor, holes are majority carriers and doping is made by trivalent atoms. *[NEET 2019]*

Addition of trivalent impurity (boron, aluminium, gallium or indum) creates defficiencies of valence electron which are most commonly known as holes. These are the majority charge carriers in this type of semiconductor.

(ii) *n*-type Semiconductors

It is obtained, when a pentavalent impurity atom (*e.g.* antimony, phosphorus or arsenic) is added to a Ge (or Si) crystal. Here, the impurity atom has one valence electron more than Si or Ge, therefore four of the five valence electrons of the impurity atom form covalent bonds with four neighbouring Ge (or Si) atoms and the fifth valence electron becomes free to move inside the crystal lattice.

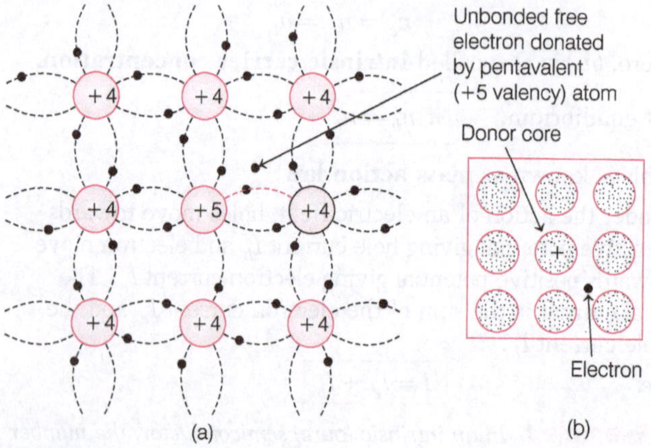

(a) Pentavalent donor atom (As, Sb, P, etc.) doped in tetravalent Si or Ge giving *n*-type semiconductor and (b) Commonly used schematic representation of *n*-type material which shows only the fixed cores of the substituent donors with one additional effective positive charge and its associated extra electron.

Thus, by doping pentavalent impurity, number of free electrons increases.

The impurity (pentavalent) atoms are called **donor atoms** because they donate conduction electrons to the crystal.

The number of electrons made available for conduction (by dopant atoms) depend strongly upon the dopant level and is independent of increase in temperature.

Following points are noteworthy regarding *n*-type semiconductors.

(a) Electrons are the majority charge carriers and holes are minority charge carriers or number of electrons are much greater than the number of holes.

i.e. $n_e >> n_h;\ i_e >> i_h$

(b) *n*-type semiconductor is also electrically neutral.

(c) Conductivity, $\sigma = n_e \mu_e e$

(d) *n*-type semiconductor can be shown as

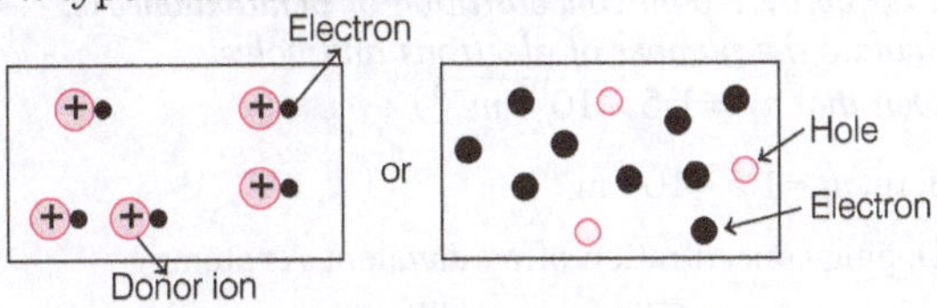

Representation of *n*-type semiconductor

Energy Band in Extrinsic Semiconductors

Energy band structure of semiconductor is affected due to doping. In extrinsic semiconductors, additional energy states due to donor impurities (donor energy level E_D) and acceptor impurities (acceptor energy level E_A) also exist.

In the energy band diagram of *n*-type semiconductor, the donor energy level E_D is slightly below the bottom E_C of conduction band and the electrons from this level move into conduction band with very small supply of energy. So, the conduction band have most of the electrons coming from donor impurities.

In *p*-type semiconductors, the acceptor energy level E_A is slightly above the top energy level E_V of the valence band. With very small supply of energy, an electron from the valence band can jump to the energy level E_A and ionise the acceptor negatively. At room temperature, most of the acceptor atoms get ionised leaving hole in valence band. Thus, at room temperature, the density of holes in valence band is mainly due to impurity.

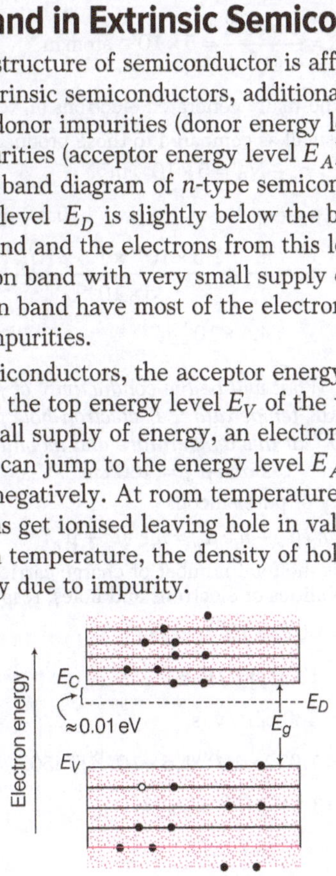

(a) $T > 0$ K

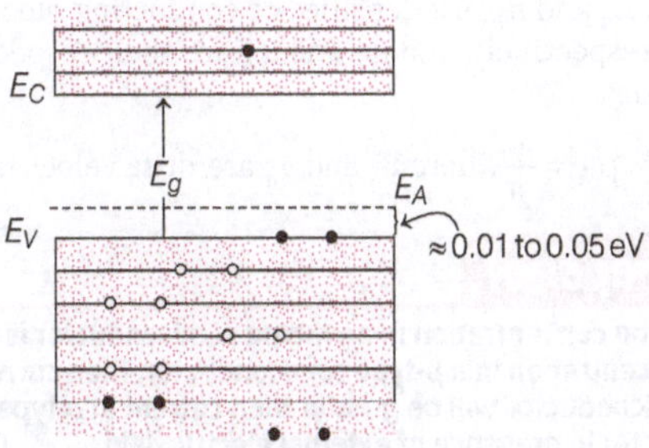

(b) $T > 0$ K

Energy bands of (a) *n*-type semiconductor at $T > 0$ K and (b) *p*-type semiconductor at $T > 0$ K

Electrical Conduction through Semiconductors

When a battery is connected across a semiconductor (whether intrinsic or extrinsic), a potential difference is developed across its ends. Due to the potential difference, an electric field is produced inside the semiconductors. A current (although very small) starts flowing through the semiconductor. This current may be due to the motion of (i) free electrons (i_e) and (ii) holes (i_h). Electrons move in opposite direction of electric field while holes move in the same direction.

The motion of holes towards right (in the figure) take place because electrons from right hand side come to fill this hole creating a new hole in their own position. Thus, we can say that holes are moving from left to right. So, current in a semiconductor can be written as

$$i = i_e + i_h$$

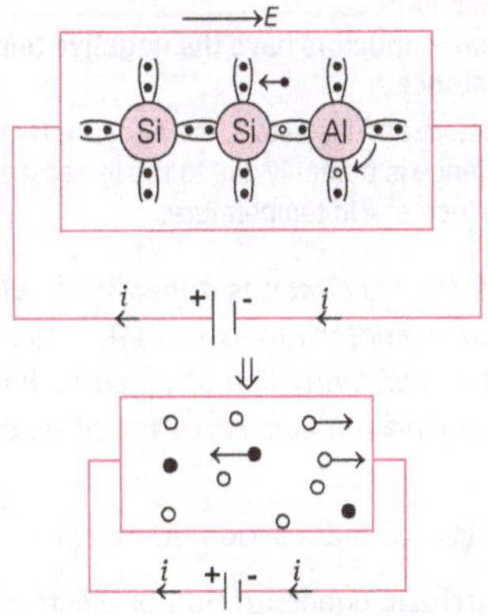

Conduction through semiconductors

But it should be noted that, mobility of holes is less than the mobility of electrons.

Conductivity of semiconductors is given by

$$\sigma = n_e e \mu_e + n_h e \mu_h$$

where, n_e and n_h are densities of conducting electrons and holes, respectively and μ_e and μ_h are their respective mobilities,

$\mu_e = \frac{v_e}{E}, \mu_h = \frac{v_h}{E}$, here v_e and v_h are drift velocities.

NEET Snapshot

If the electron concentration in an *n*-type semiconductor is the same as hole concentration in a *p*-type semiconductor, then current in *n*-type semiconductor will be greater than current in *p*-type semiconductor in presence of external electric field. *[NEET 2021]*

The mobility of charge carriers in *n*-type semiconductor is greater than mobility of charge carriers in *p*-type semiconductor.

Effect of Temperature on Conductivity of Semiconductor

The conductivity of a semiconductor increases (or the resistivity decreases) with rise in temperature. This is because, as the temperature rises, more and more of the covalent bonds in the crystal lattice break, thus creating more and more charge carriers (electron-hole pairs). This results in increasing conductivity.

The temperature dependence of charge carrier density is given by

$$n_i \propto e^{-E_g/2kT}$$

where, n_i is number of electron-hole pair, E_g is the energy gap of the semiconductor and k is Boltzmann's constant. Thus, the charge carrier density and hence the conductivity of the semiconductor increases exponentially with rise in temperature.

NEET Snapshot

Insulators and semiconductors have the negative temperature coefficient of resistance. *[NEET 2020]*

In both semiconductors and insulators, the negative temperature coefficient of resistance is primarily due to the increase in charge carrier concentration with increase in temperature.

Example 4. *A Ge specimen is doped with Al. The concentration of acceptor atoms is ~ 10^{21} atoms/m^3. Given that, the intrinsic concentration of electron-hole pairs is ~ 10^{19} /m^3, then find the concentration of electrons in the specimen.*

Sol. According to law of mass action, $n_i^2 = n_h n_e$

Here, n_i = intrinsic concentration of electron hole pair

$= 10^{19} /\text{m}^3$

and n_h = concentration of acceptor atoms $= 10^{21}$ atoms/m^3.

$$\therefore \quad n_e = \frac{n_i^2}{n_h} = \frac{(10^{19})^2}{(10^{21})} = 10^{17} /\text{m}^3$$

Example 5. *A semiconductor has equal electron-hole concentration of 6×10^8 m^{-3}. On doping with certain impurity, electron concentration increases to 9×10^{12} m^{-3}.*
(i) Identify the new semiconductor obtained after doping.
(ii) Calculate the new hole concentration.
(iii) How does the energy gap vary with doping?

Sol. (i) As, the electron concentration increases after doping, so the new semiconductor obtained is of *n*-type.

(ii) As, $n_e n_h = n_i^2$ (Law of mass action)

Here, $n_i = 6 \times 10^8$ m^{-3}, $n_e = 9 \times 10^{12}$ m^{-3}

$$\therefore \quad n_h = \frac{n_i^2}{n_e} = \frac{(6 \times 10^8)^2}{9 \times 10^{12}} = 4 \times 10^4 \text{ m}^{-3}$$

(iii) The energy gap decreases with doping.

Example 6. *Suppose a pure Si crystal has 5×10^{28} atoms m^{-3}. It is doped by 1 ppm concentration of pentavalent As. Calculate the number of electrons and holes. (Given that $n_i = 1.5 \times 10^{16}$ m^{-3})*

Sol. Here, $n_i = 1.5 \times 10^{16}$ m^{-3}

Doping concentration of pentavalent As atoms

= 1 ppm = 1 part per million

$\therefore$ Number density of pentavalent as atoms,

$$N_D = \frac{5 \times 10^{28}}{10^6} = 5 \times 10^{22} \text{ atom m}^{-3}$$

Now, the thermally generated electrons ($n_i \propto 10^{16}$ m^{-3}) are negligibly small as compared to those produced by doping, so $\quad n_e \simeq N_D = 5 \times 10^{22}$ m^{-3}

Also, $\quad n_e n_h = n_i^2$ (Law of mass action)

$$\therefore \quad n_h = \frac{n_i^2}{n_e} = \frac{1.5 \times 10^{16} \times 1.5 \times 10^{16}}{5 \times 10^{22}} = 4.5 \times 10^9 \text{ m}^{-3}$$

Example 7. *What will be the conductivity of pure silicon crystal at 300K temperature? If electron-hole pairs per cm^3 is 1.072×10^{10} at this temperature and mobilities are $\mu_h = 1350$ cm^2/V-s and $\mu_e = 480$ cm^2/V-s.*

Sol. Conductivity of pure silicon,

$$\sigma = n_i e \mu_e + n_i e \mu_h = n_i e (\mu_e + \mu_h)$$

where, n_i is the total number of charge carrier, μ_e and μ_h are the mobilities of electrons and holes, respectively.

Here, $n_i = 1.072 \times 10^{10}$ per cm^3

$\mu_h = 1350$ cm^2/V-s

$\mu_e = 480$ cm^2/V-s

$$\Rightarrow \quad \sigma = (1.072 \times 10^{10})(1.6 \times 10^{-19})(1350 + 480)$$

$$= 3.14 \times 10^{-6} \text{ mho/cm}$$

Example 8. *An intrinsic germanium semiconductor is to be made n-type semiconductor of conductivity 6 mho/cm. Calculate the number density of donor atoms required, if the mobility of electrons in n-type semiconductor is 3850 cm^2/V-s.*

Sol. In n-type semiconductor, $n_e >> n_h$

Let number density of donor atoms, $N_D = n_e$

Conductivity of semiconductor is given by $\sigma = n_e e \mu_e$

On putting the values, we get

$$6 \times 10^2 = n_e \times 1.6 \times 10^{-19} \times 3850 \times 10^{-4}$$

$$\Rightarrow \quad n_e = 9.7 \times 10^{21}/\text{m}^3$$

Example 9. *The concentration of hole-electron pairs in pure germanium at $T = 300$ K is 7×10^{15} per cubic metre. Antimony is doped into germanium in a proportion of 1 atom per 10^7 Ge atoms. Assuming that, half of the impurity atoms contribute electron in the conduction band, calculate the factor by which the number of charge carriers increases due to doping. The number of germanium atoms per cubic metre is 5×10^{28}.*

Sol. In pure semiconductor, electron-hole pair concentration,

$$n_h = n_e = 7 \times 10^{15} \text{m}^{-3}$$

Total charge carrier,

$$n_{\text{total initial}} = n_h + n_e = 7 \times 10^{15} + 7 \times 10^{15} = 14 \times 10^{15}$$

After doping, donor impurity,

$$N_D = \frac{5 \times 10^{28}}{10^7} = 5 \times 10^{21}$$

and $$n'_e = \frac{N_D}{2} = 2.5 \times 10^{21}$$

So, $$n_{\text{final}} = n_h + n'_e$$

$$\Rightarrow \quad n_{\text{final}} \approx n'_e \approx 2.5 \times 10^{21} \quad (\because n'_e >> n_h)$$

$$\text{Factor} = \frac{n_{\text{final}} - n_{\text{initial}}}{n_{\text{initial}}} = \frac{2.5 \times 10^{21} - 14 \times 10^{15}}{14 \times 10^{15}} \approx \frac{2.5 \times 10^{21}}{14 \times 10^{15}} = 1.8 \times 10^5$$

Example 10. *Find the resistivity of a sample in which 10^{19} atoms of phosphorus are added per m^3. Take the resistivity of pure silicon as 3000 Ω-m and the mobilities of electrons and holes as 0.15 m^2/V-s and 0.030 m^2/V-s, respectively.*

Sol. The conductivity of a pure silicon is given by

$$\sigma_i = n_i e (\mu_e + \mu_h)$$

Also, the resistivity is reciprocal of conductivity.

$$\therefore \quad \rho_i = \frac{1}{\sigma_i} = \frac{1}{n_i e (\mu_e + \mu_h)}$$

$$\Rightarrow \quad n_i = \frac{1}{\rho_i e(\mu_e + \mu_h)} = \frac{1}{3000 \times 1.6 \times 10^{-19} (0.15 + 0.030)} = 1.157 \times 10^{16}/\text{m}^3$$

When 10^{19} atoms of phosphorus (donor atoms) are added per m^3, we have

$$n_e >> n_i$$

or $$n_e >> n_h$$

$$\Rightarrow \quad n_e = 10^{19}$$

$$\therefore \quad \rho = \frac{1}{n_e e \mu_e} = \frac{1}{10^{19} \times 1.6 \times 10^{-19} \times 0.15} = 4.17 \Omega\text{-m}$$

Example 11. *A pure germanium plate of area 3.5×10^{-4} m^2 and of thickness 1.5×10^{-3} m is connected across a battery of potential 5 V. Find the amount of current produced at room temperature in the germanium sample. Also, find the amount of heat generated in the plate in 120 s. Given that the concentration of carriers in germanium at room temperature is 1.6×10^6 per cubic metre. The mobilities of electrons and holes are 0.4 $m^2 V^{-1} s^{-1}$ and 0.2 $m^2 V^{-1} s^{-1}$, respectively.*

Sol. Conductivity of semiconductor is given by

$$\sigma = n_e e \mu_e + n_h e \mu_h$$

Since semiconductor is intrinsic, so $n_e = n_h = n_i$

Conductivity, $$\sigma = n_i e (\mu_e + \mu_h)$$

$$= 1.6 \times 10^6 \times 1.6 \times 10^{-19} (0.4 + 0.2)$$

$$= 1.536 \times 10^{-13} \Omega^{-1}\text{m}^{-1}$$

Current flowing, $I = JA$

where, J = current density $= \sigma E = \sigma \left(\frac{V}{d}\right)$

$$\therefore \quad I = JA = \sigma \left(\frac{V}{d}\right) \cdot A$$

$$= 1.536 \times 10^{-13} \left(\frac{5}{1.5 \times 10^{-3}}\right) (3.5 \times 10^{-4})$$

$$= 1.79 \times 10^{-13} \text{ A}$$

Heat produced, $H = VIt = 5 \times 1.79 \times 10^{-13} \times 120$

$$= 10.74 \times 10^{-11} \text{ J}$$

STEP UP Practice 1

1. To obtain p-type semiconductor, we need to dope pure Si with
(a) aluminium (b) phosphorus
(c) oxygen (d) germanium

2. The charge on a hole is equal to the charge of
(a) atom (b) proton (c) neutron (d) electron

3. If n_e and n_h represent the number of free electrons density and holes density respectively in a semiconducting material, then for n-type semiconducting material
(a) $n_e << n_h$ (b) $n_e >> n_h$
(c) $n_e = n_h$ (d) $n_e = n_h = 0$

4. **Assertion** (A) Electron has higher mobility than hole in a semiconductor.
Reason (R) Mass of electron is less than the mass of hole.
In the light of the above statements, choose the correct answer from the options given below.
(a) Both A and R are true but R is not the correct explanation of A.
(b) A is true but R is false.
(c) A is false but is R true.
(d) Both A and R are true and R is the correct explanation of A.

5. Which of the following has negative temperature coefficient of resistance?
(a) Copper (b) Aluminium
(c) Iron (d) Germanium

6. An n-type and p-type silicon can be obtained by doping pure silicon with
(a) arsenic and phosphorus
(b) indium and aluminium
(c) phosphorus and indium
(d) aluminium and boron

7. Let n_h and n_e be the number of holes and conduction electrons respectively in a semiconductor, then
(a) $n_h > n_e$ in an intrinsic semiconductor
(b) $n_h = n_e$ in an extrinsic semiconductor
(c) $n_h = n_e$ in an intrinsic semiconductor
(d) $n_h > n_p$ in an intrinsic semiconductor

8. **Assertion** (A) Conductivity of a semiconductor increases with temperature.
Reason (R) When temperature of a semiconductor is increased, energy gap between valence band and conduction band decreases.
In the light of the above statements, choose the correct answer from the options given below.
(a) Both A and R are true but R is not the correct explanation of A.
(b) A is true but R is false.
(c) A is false but is R true.
(d) Both A and R are true and R is the correct explanation of A.

9. In p-type semiconductor, the majority and minority charge carriers are respectively
(a) protons and electrons (b) electrons and protons
(c) electrons and holes (d) holes and electrons

10. The electrical resistance of which of the following decreases with rise in temperature?
(a) Metals (b) Semiconductors
(c) Gold (d) Constantan

11. Iron and silicon wires are heated from 30°C to 50°C. The correct statement is that
(a) Resistance of both wires increases.
(b) Resistance of both wires decreases.
(c) Resistance of iron wire increases and that of silicon wire decreases.
(d) Resistance of iron wire increases and that of silicon wire increases.

12. Which of the following pair given below is correct?
(a) p-type semiconductor → Pentavalent impurity
(b) n-type semiconductor → Pentavalent impurity
(c) Trivalent impurity → Arsenic, phosphorus
(d) Pentavalent impurity → Indium, boron

13. A pure semiconductor has equal electron and hole concentration of $10^{16}\ m^{-3}$. Doping by indium increases n_h to $4.5 \times 10^{22}\ m^{-3}$, what is n_e in the doped semiconductor?
(a) $10^6\ m^{-3}$ (b) $10^{22}\ m^{-3}$
(c) $\dfrac{10^{32}}{4.5 \times 10^{22}}\ m^{-3}$ (d) $4.5 \times 10^{22}\ m^{-3}$

14. The valency of an impurity atom added to germanium crystal in order to convert it into a p-type semiconductor is
(a) 6 (b) 5 (c) 4 (d) 3

15. **Assertion** (A) Rate of recombination for both intrinsic and extrinsic semiconductors are equal.
Reason (R) For an extrinsic semiconductor, $n_e n_h = n_i^2$.
In the light of the above statements, choose the correct answer from the options given below.
(a) Both A and R are true but R is not the correct explanation of A.
(b) A is true but R is false.
(c) A is false but is R true.
(d) Both A and R are true and R is the correct explanation of A.

16. A silicon specimen is made into a p-type semiconductor by doping, on an average, one indium atom per 5×10^8 silicon atoms. If the number density of atoms in the silicon specimen is 5×10^{28} atoms/m^3, then the number of acceptor atoms in silicon per cubic centimetre will be
(a) 2.5×10^{30} (b) 1.0×10^{13}
(c) 1.0×10^{14} (d) 2.5×10^{36}

17. In a pure silicon ($n_i = 10^{16}/\text{m}^3$) crystal at 300 K, 10^{21} atoms of phosphorus are added per cubic meter. The new hole concentration will be

(a) 10^{21} per m^3
(b) 10^{19} per m^3
(c) 10^{11} per m^3
(d) 10^{5} per m^3

18. Assertion (A) When a light beam of wavelength 600 nm is incident over a semiconductor with 2.8 eV energy gap, conductivity of semiconductor increases.

Reason (R) If an electron absorbs a photon of energy hf such that $hf > E_g$, then it is transferred to the conduction band.

In the light of the above statements, choose the correct answer from the options given below.

(a) Both A and R are true but R is not the correct explanation of A.
(b) A is true but R is false.
(c) A is false but R is true.
(d) Both A and R are true and R is the correct explanation of A.

Module 2

Semiconductors Diode and Rectifiers

- *p-n* Junction • Semiconductor Diode or *p-n* Junction Diode • Biasing of *p-n* Junction Diode
- *V-I* Characteristic Curve of a *p-n* Junction Diode • *p-n* Junction Diode as a Rectifier
- Special Types of *p-n* Junction Diode

p-n Junction

A *p*-type or *n*-type silicon crystal can be made by adding appropriate impurity as discussed above. Separately *p*- and *n*-type semiconductors have limited use. When the two types are combined, a number of new characteristic appears, which makes the combination a very useful device. So, when a *p*-type semiconductor is suitably joined to an *n*-type semiconductor, then resulting arrangement is called *p-n* junction.

A *p-n* junction is formed either when a *p*-type semiconductor is grown on *n*-type semiconductor or *n*-type is grown on *p*-type semiconductor as given below.

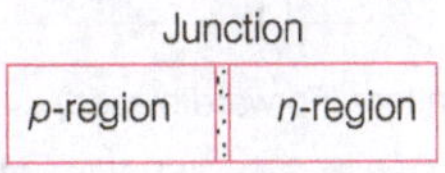

A *p-n* junction

Formation of Depletion Region in *p-n* Junction

In an *n*-type semiconductor, the concentration of electrons is more than the concentration of holes. Similarly, in a *p*-type semiconductor, the concentration of holes is more than the concentration of electrons.

During formation of *p-n* junction and due to the concentration gradient across *p* and *n*-sides, holes diffuse from *p*-side to *n*-side ($p \rightarrow n$) and electrons diffuse from *n*-side to *p*-side ($n \rightarrow p$). The diffused charge carriers combine with their counterparts in the immediate vicinity of the junction and neutralise each other.

Thus, near the junction positive charge is built on *n*-side and negative charge on *p*-side as shown in the figure.

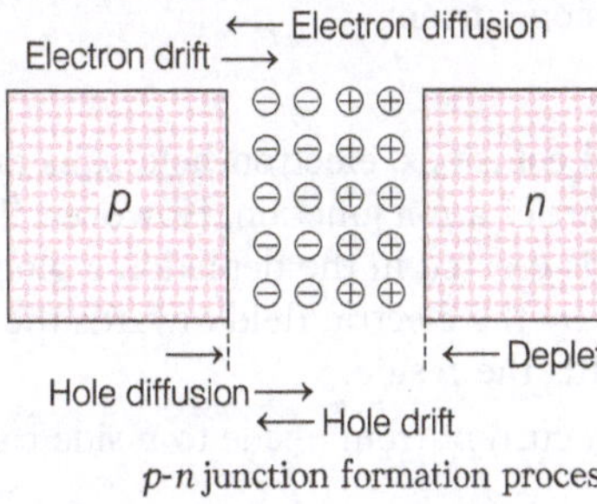

p-n junction formation process

This set up a potential difference across the junction and an internal electric field E_i directed from *n*-side to *p*-side. The equilibrium is established when the field E_i becomes strong enough to stop further diffusion of the majority charge carriers (however it helps the minority charge carriers to diffuse across the junction).

The region on either side of the junction which becomes depleted (free) from the mobile charge carriers is called

depletion region or **depletion layer.** The width of depletion region is of the order of 10^{-6} m or 1 μm.

The potential difference developed across the depletion region is called the **potential barrier**. Potential barrier depends on dopant concentration in the semiconductor and temperature of the junction.

On the average, the potential barrier in *p-n* junction is ~ 0.5 V and is given by $E_B = \frac{V_B}{d} \Rightarrow \boxed{V_B = E_B\, d}$

where, E_B = barrier electric field

and d = width of depletion region.

For Ge, V_B = 0.3 V and for silicon, V_B = 0.7 V.

Given below are the graphs of potential *versus* distance, charge density *versus* distance and electric field *versus* distance across the depletion region.

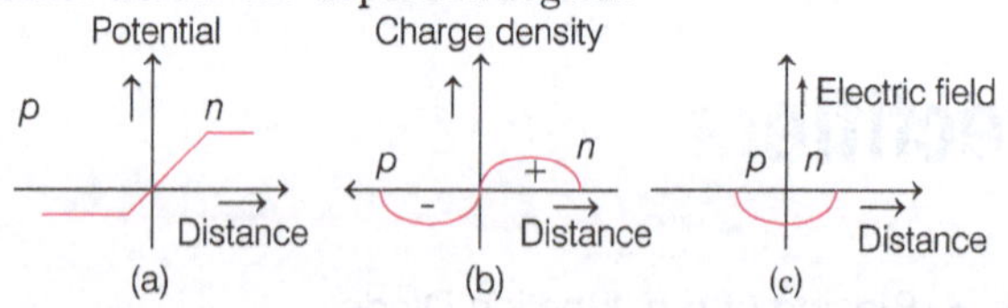

(a) Potential *versus* distance, (b) Charge density *versus* distance, (c) Electric field *versus* distance across the depletion region

Current Flow across a *p-n* Junction

There are two types of current flow across a *p-n* junction, which are discussed below

1. Diffusion Current

Because of concentration difference, holes try to diffuse from the *p*-side to the *n*-side and electrons from *n*-side to *p*-side at the *p-n* junction. However, only those holes/ electrons cross the junction which have high kinetic energy. The diffusion give rise to a current from *p*-side to *n*-side called diffusion current.

2. Drift Current

Because of thermal collisions, electron-hole pairs are created at every part of a *p-n* junction. However, if an electron-hole pair is created in the depletion region, the electron is pushed by the electric field towards the *n*-side and the hole towards the *p*-side.

This gives rise to a current from *n*-side to *p*-side called the drift current.

Thus, we have, diffusion current,

$I_{df} \longrightarrow$ from *p*-side to *n*-side

and drift current, $I_{dr} \longrightarrow$ from *n*-side to *p*-side

Mentor's TIP

In steady state, diffusion current (I_{df}) is equal to the drift current (I_{dr}). Thus, net current across a *p-n* junction is zero.

Semiconductor Diode or *p-n* Junction Diode

A semiconductor diode [Fig. (a)] is basically a *p-n* junction with metallic contacts provided at the ends for the application of an external voltage. It is a two terminal device. A *p-n* junction diode is represented by the symbol as shown in Fig. (b).

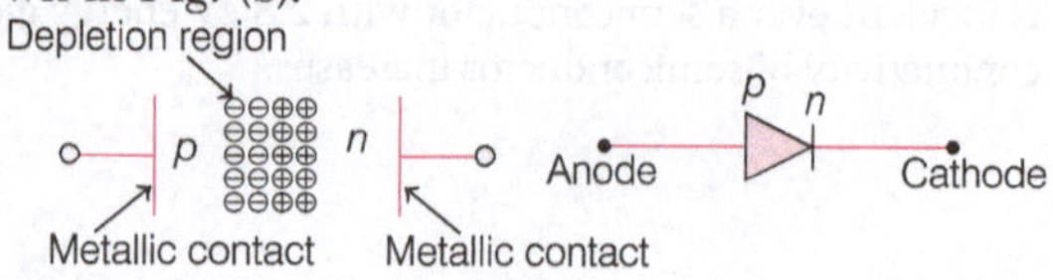

(a) Semiconductor diode (b) Symbol for *p-n* junction diode

The direction of arrow indicates the conventional direction of current.

Biasing of *p-n* Junction Diode

Biasing is the method of connecting external battery or emf source to a *p-n* junction diode. The junction diode can be connected to an external battery in following two ways.

1. Forward Biasing

A junction is said to be forward biased when the positive terminal of the external battery is connected to the *p*-side and negative terminal to the *n*-side of the diode.

Flow of Current in Forward Biasing

In this situation, the forward voltage opposes the potential barrier, due to which the potential barrier decreases and hence width of depletion layer decreases. Under the effect of external electric field, holes in the *p*-region and electrons in *n*-region, both move towards the junction.

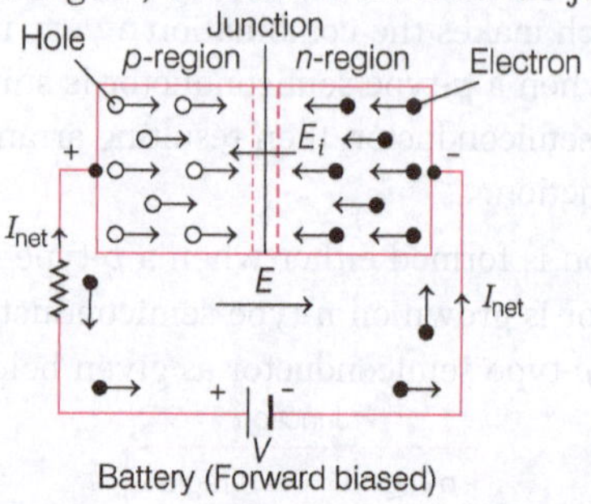

These holes and electrons mutually combine just near the junction and cease to exist. For each electron-hole combination, a covalent bond breaks up in the *p*-region near the positive terminal of the battery.

Of the hole and electron so produced, the hole moves towards the junction, while the electron enters the positive terminal of the battery through the connecting wire. Just at this moment, an electron is released from the negative terminal of the battery which enters the *n*-region to replace the electron lost by combining with a hole at the junction.

Thus, a current called **forward current**, is constituted by the motion of majority charge carriers across the junction. In forward bias, the junction diode offers low resistance (ideally zero). Also, $I_{df} > I_{dr}$ or I_{net} is from p-side to n-side.

2. Reverse Biasing

A junction diode is said to be reverse biased when the positive terminal of the external battery is connected to the n-side and negative terminal to the p-side of the diode.

NEET Snapshot

Width of depletion region of a *p-n* junction diode increased in reverse bias. *[NEET 2020]*

Under reverse bias condition, the holes of p-side are attracted towards the negative terminal of the battery and electrons of the n-sides are attracted towards the positive terminal of the battery. This increases the width of the depletion layer.

Scan for Video

Flow of Current in Reverse Biasing

In this situation, the reverse voltage supports the potential barrier, due to which the potential barrier increases and hence width of depletion layer increases. Under the effect of external electric field, holes in the p-region and electrons in the n-region are pushed away from the junction, *i.e.* they cannot be combined at the junction.

So, there is almost no flow of current due to majority charge carriers.

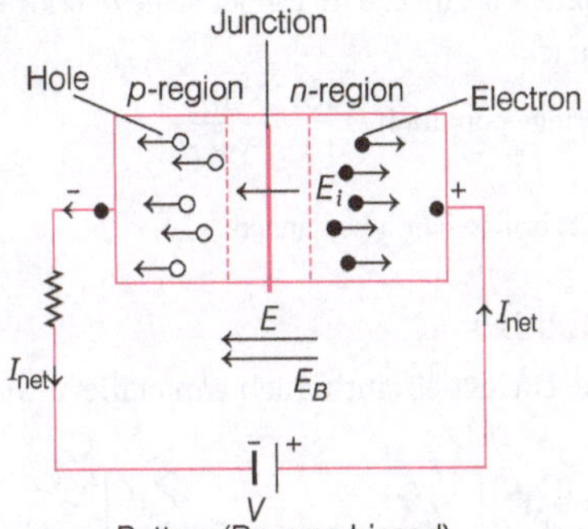

Battery (Reverse biased)

However, a very small current due to minority charge carriers, flows across the junction. This current is called **reverse saturation current.** Here, $I_{dr} > I_{df}$ or I_{net} is from n-side to p-side.

Concept ladder

- The *p-n* junction allows a much larger current flow in forward biasing than in reverse biasing. This is crudely, the basis of the action of a *p-n* junction as a rectifier.
- In forward bias, diode current is majorly due to diffusion while in reverse bias, it is due to drift current.

Example 12. *Find the net resistance of the network shown in the figure between the points P and Q, if (i) $V_P > V_Q$, (ii) $V_P < V_Q$.*

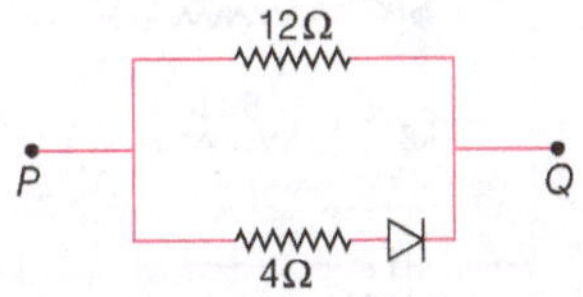

Sol. (i) When $V_P > V_Q$, the diode is in forward biased. Let, the resistance of diode will be taken as zero. So, the net resistance is $\frac{4 \times 12}{4+12} = 3\Omega$.

(ii) When $V_P < V_Q$, the diode is reverse biased. Let, there will be no current in the diode branch, hence $4\,\Omega$ resistance is ineffective. So, the net resistance is $12\,\Omega$.

NEET Close-up

Example Similar to PYQ Asked in NEET 2020

Which of the following diode forward biased?

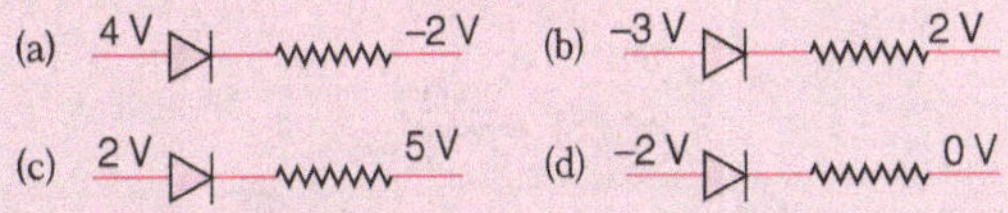

Sol. (a) For forward biasing, p-part of diode must be at higher potential than n-part of diode.

Skill Builder

Which of the following diode forward biased?

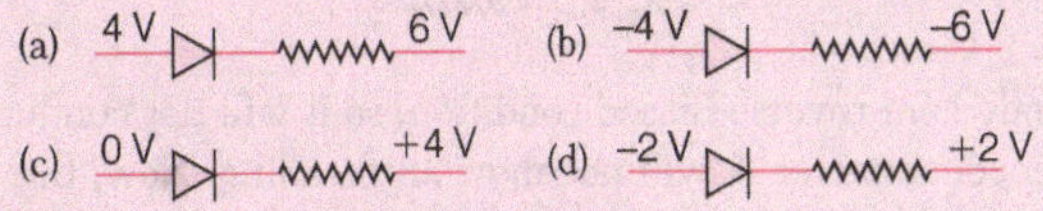

For more Practice Refer Q. No. 6 of step up practice-2 and Q.No. 39, 43, 60 of Gearing up for NEET.

Example 13. *The diode used in the circuit shown in the figure has a constant voltage drop of 0.5 V at all currents and a maximum power rating of 200 mW. What should be the value of the resistor R, connected in series with the diode, for obtaining maximum current?*

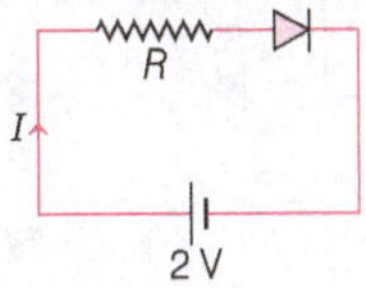

Sol. Current through diode (or circuit), $I = \frac{\text{Power}}{\text{Voltage}}$

$$\therefore \quad I = \frac{200 \times 10^{-3}\,\text{W}}{0.5\,\text{V}} = 0.4\,\text{A}$$

and resistance, $R = \frac{\text{net voltage}}{\text{current}} = \frac{2-0.5}{0.4} = 3.75\Omega$

Example 14. *Find current passing through 4 Ω and 8 Ω resistance in the circuit shown in figure.*

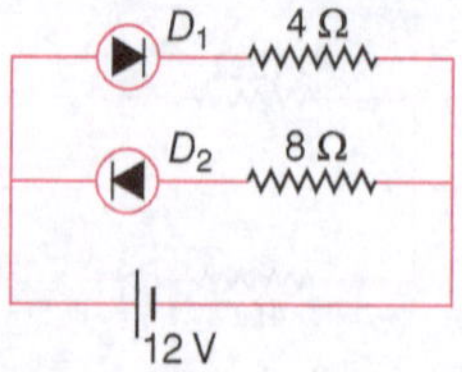

Sol. In the given circuit, diode D_1 is in forward biased and D_2 is in reverse biased. Hence, D_1 will conduct but D_2 will not. Therefore, current through 8 Ω resistance will be zero while through 4 Ω resistance will be $\frac{12}{4} = 3$ A.

Example 15. *Consider the circuit diagram shown below. Two ammeters A_1 and A_2 are connected across a diode and resistor, respectively. Find the amount of current flowing through these two ammeters. Neglect the resistances of the ammeters.*

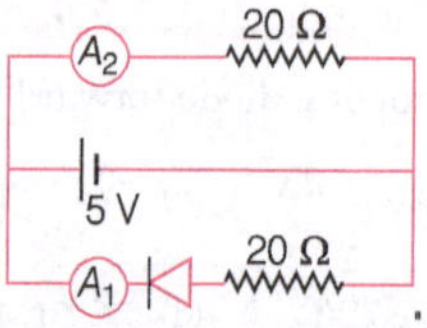

Sol. Let the current I_1 flows across diode and I_2 flows across A_2 as shown below

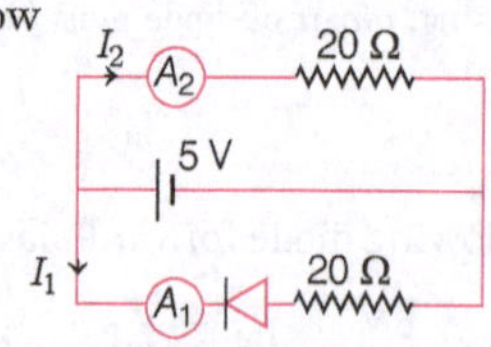

Diode is in reverse biased condition, so it will not conduct. Hence, ammeter A_1 will not show any reading. Now, the value of I_2 will be

$$I_2 = \frac{V}{R} = \frac{5}{20} = 0.25 \text{ A}$$

Example 16. *(i) Calculate the value of V_0 and i, if the silicon and germanium diode start conducting at 0.7 V and 0.3 V, respectively.*

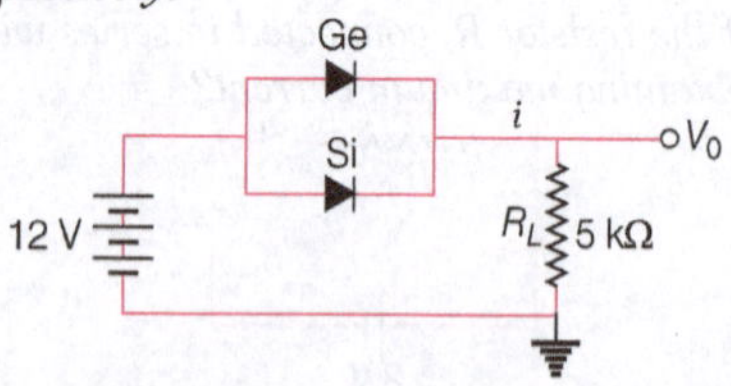

(ii) If the Ge diode connection is now reversed, what will be the new values of V_0 and i?

Sol. (i) Ge diode will start conducting before the silicon diode does so. The effective forward voltage across Ge diode is $(12 - 0.3)\ V = 11.7$ V. This will appear as the output voltage across the load,

i.e. $\quad V_o = 11.7 \text{ V}$

Current through R_L, $i = \frac{11.7}{5 \times 10^3}$ A $= 2.34$ mA

(ii) On reversing the connection of Ge diode, it will be reverse biased and conduct no current. Only Si diode will conduct, therefore

$$V_o = (12 - 0.7) \text{ V} = 11.3 \text{ V}$$

and current, $i = \frac{11.3}{5 \times 10^3}$ A $= 2.26$ mA

NEET Close-up

Example Similar to PYQ Asked in NEET 2024

Choose the correct circuit which can achieve the bridge balance.

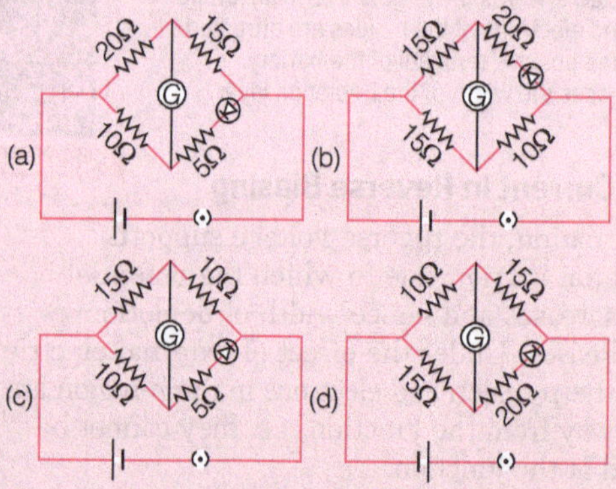

Sol. (c) For a diode to be active, it must be forward biased. In options (a), (b) and (d), diodes are reverse biased.

Hence, options (a), (b) and (d) cannot achieve bridge balance.

For option (c),

balance bridge condition is $\frac{15}{10} = \frac{10}{5 + r_d}$

If $r_d = \frac{5}{3}$ Ω, bridge can be balanced.

Skill Builder

Choose the correct circuit which can achieve the bridge balance.

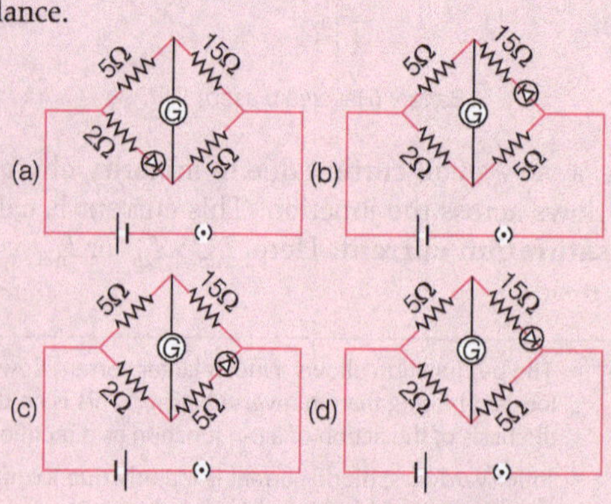

For more practice Refer Q. No. 72, 75, 88, 89 of NEET Gearing up.

V-I Characteristic Curve of a *p-n* Junction Diode

The voltage-current characteristic curves of a *p-n* junction diode are graphs showing the change in current flowing through the junction with change in a applied voltage, when the junction is in forward biased and in reverse biased.

1. Forward Biased Characteristics

When the diode is in forward biased, *i.e.* *p*-side is kept at higher potential, the current in the diode changes with the voltage applied across the diode.

A graph is plotted between voltage and current. The curve so obtained is the forward characteristic of the diode. At the start when applied voltage is low, the current through diode is almost zero. It is because of potential barrier, which opposes the applied voltage.

Till the applied voltage exceeds the potential barrier, the current increases very slowly with increase in applied voltage (*OA* portion of the graph).

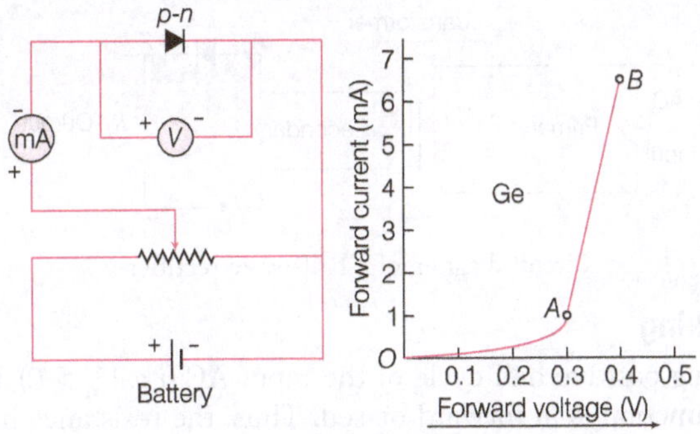

Forward biased characteristics of a diode

After this voltage, the diode current increases rapidly (*AB* portion of the graph), even for very small increase in the diode voltage.

In this situation, the diode behaves like a conductor. The forward voltage beyond which the current through the junction starts increasing rapidly with voltage is called the **threshold voltage** or **cut-off voltage** or **knee voltage.**

If line *AB* is extended back, it cuts the voltage axis at potential barrier voltage.

The value of the cut-in voltage is about 0.3 V for a germanium diode and 0.7 V for a silicon diode.

2. Reverse Biased Characteristics

The circuit diagram for studying reverse biased characteristics is shown in the figure

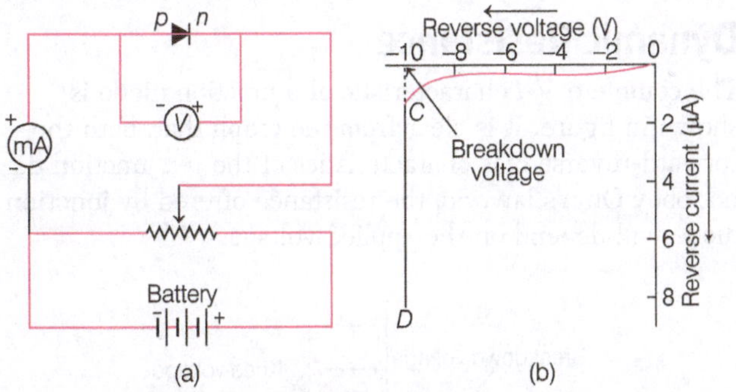

Reverse biased characteristics of a diode

In reverse biased, the applied voltage supports the flow of minority charge carriers across the junction. So, a very small current flows across the junction due to minority charge carriers.

Motion of minority charge carriers is also supported by internal potential barrier, so all the minority carriers cross over the junction.

Therefore, the small reverse current remains almost constant over a sufficiently long range of reverse bias voltage, increasing very little with increasing voltage (*OC* portion of the graph).

This reverse current is voltage independent upto certain voltage known as **breakdown voltage** and this voltage independent current is called **reverse saturation current.**

This reverse saturation current depends only on temperature of the junction. If is found that for every 1° rise in temperature, the reverse saturation current increases by about 7%. So for every 10°C rise, the I_0 becomes nearly double. If the reverse biased voltage is too high, then *p-n* junction breaks.

It is of following two types

(a) Zener Breakdown

When reverse bias voltage is increased, the electric field across the junction also increases. At some stage, the electric field becomes so high, that it breaks the covalent bonds creating electron-hole pairs. Thus, a large number of carriers are generated. So, this causes a large current to flow. This mechanism is known as zener breakdown.

(b) Avalanche Breakdown

At high reverse voltage, due to high electric field, the minority charge carriers, while crossing the junction acquire very high velocities. These by collision breaks down the covalent bonds generating more carriers. A chain reaction is established giving rise to high current. This mechanism is called Avalanche breakdown.

Mentor's TiP

- Zener breakdown occurs in a highly doped *p-n* junction whereas Avalanche breakdown occurs in a lightly doped *p-n* junction.

Dynamic Resistance

The complete V-I characteristic of a junction diode is shown in figure. It is clear from the graph that, both the forward-reverse bias characteristics of the p-n junction do not obey Ohm's law. So, the resistance offered by junction diode will depend on the applied voltage.

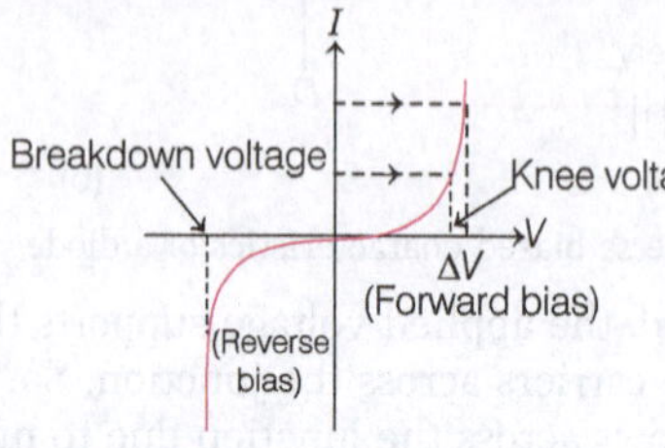

Complete V-I characteristic of a junction diode

Here, we will take the dynamic resistance which is defined as the ratio of small change in voltage to the small change in current produced. It is also called dynamic resistance of the junction diode and is denoted by r_d.

Thus, $$r_d = \frac{\Delta V}{\Delta I}$$

The region of the characteristic curve, where dynamic resistance is almost independent of the applied voltage is called the **linear region of junction diode.**

Example 17. *A silicon diode is connected to a load resistance R_L as shown in the figure. Let $V_{in} = 10$ V and $R_L = 10\,k\Omega$.*

(i) If barrier voltage, $V_B = 0.7$ V, then calculate

(a) output voltage across R_L, (b) current in diode

(c) and forward resistance.

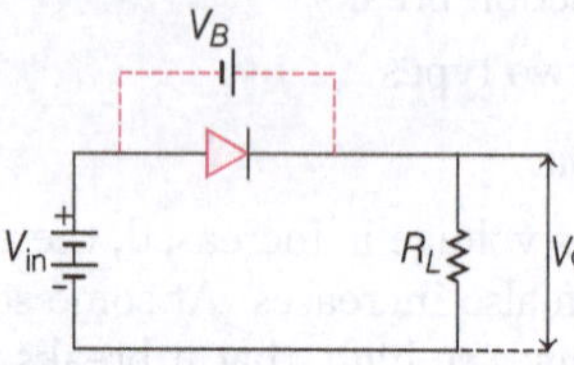

(ii) If diode is assumed ideal, then what will be

(a) output voltage

(b) and output current in diode?

Sol. (i) (a) As, $V_{out} = V_{in} - V_B$

where, V_B = barrier voltage

$\therefore \quad V_{out} = 10 - 0.7 = 9.3$ V

(b) As diode is in forward biased state, so it will conduct

$$\therefore \quad I = \frac{V_{out}}{R_L} = \frac{9.3}{10 \times 10^3} = 0.9 \text{ mA}$$

(c) Forward resistance, $$r_f = \frac{V_B}{I} = \frac{0.7}{0.9 \times 10^{-3}} = 777\Omega$$

(ii) For ideal diode, $r_f = 0, V_B = 0$

(a) $V_{out} = V_{in} = 10$ V (b) $I = \frac{V_{out}}{R_L} = \frac{10}{10 \times 10^3} = 1$ mA

p-n Junction Diode as a Rectifier

A rectifier is a device which converts an alternating current (or voltage) into a direct (or unidirectional) current (or voltage).

Principle A p-n junction diode can works as an excellent rectifier because it permits current in one direction only. It offers a low resistance for the current to flow when it is forward biased, but a very high resistance when reverse biased.

Thus, it allows current to flow through it in only one direction and acts as a rectifier.

The junction diode can be used either as a half-wave rectifier or as a full wave rectifier.

1. p-n Junction Diode as Half-Wave Rectifier

A simple rectifier circuit called the half-wave rectifier, using only one diode is shown in figure. The AC voltage to be rectified is connected to the primary coil of a step-down transformer. Secondary coil is connected to the diode through resistor R_L across which, output is obtained.

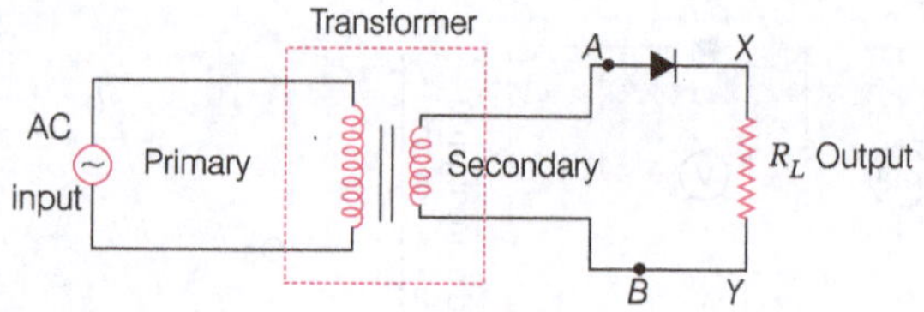

Circuit diagram of a half-wave rectifier

Working

During positive half cycle of the input AC (*i.e.* $V_A > 0$), the p-n junction is in forward biased. Thus, the resistance in p-n junction becomes low and current flows. Hence, we get output in the load.

During negative half cycle of the input AC (*i.e.* $V_A < 0$), the p-n junction is in reverse biased. Thus, the resistance of p-n junction is high and current does not flow. Hence, no output is obtained across the load.

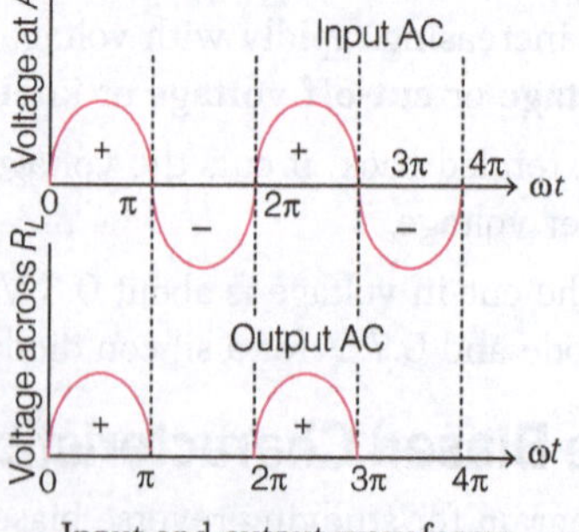

Input and output waveforms

Important Points Related to Half-wave Rectifier

(i) **Average output** in one cycle

$$I_{DC} = \frac{I_0}{\pi} \text{ and } V_{DC} = \frac{V_0}{\pi}; I_0 = \frac{V_0}{r_f + R_L},$$

$$V_{DC} = \frac{V_0}{\pi\left(1 + \frac{r_f}{R_L}\right)} \quad \left(\begin{array}{l}\text{where, } r_f = \text{forward biased resistance.}\\ \text{and } R_L = \text{load resistance.}\end{array}\right)$$

(ii) **rms output** $I_{rms} = \frac{I_0}{2}, V_{rms} = \frac{V_0}{2}$

(iii) The ratio of the effective alternating component of the output voltage (or current) to the DC component is known as **ripple factor**.

$$r = \frac{I_{AC}}{I_{DC}} = \left[\left(\frac{I_{rms}}{I_{DC}}\right)^2 - 1\right]^{1/2} = 1.21$$

The smaller the ripple factor, more effective will be rectifier.

(iv) **Peak inverse voltage** (PIV) The maximum reverse biased voltage that can be applied before commencement of breakdown region is called the peak inverse voltage. When diode is not conducting, then PIV across it will be V_0.

(v) **Efficiency** It is given by

$$\eta = \frac{P_{out}}{P_{in}} \times 100\% = \frac{40.6\%}{1 + r_f / R_L}$$

If $R_L >> r_f$, then $\eta = 40.6\%$ and if $R_L = r_f$, then $\eta = 20.3\%$.

(vi) The ratio of i_{rms} and i_{DC} is known as **form factor.**

$$\text{Form factor} = \frac{I_{rms}}{I_{DC}} = \frac{\pi}{2} = 1.57$$

NEET Snapshot

Frequency of output voltage obtained from the half-wave rectifier is same as frequency of input AC voltage. *[NEET 2022]*

The half-wave rectifier only allows one half cycle of an AC voltage waveform to pass through. The output waveform completes one cycle at the same time as the input waveform. So, the output frequency is equal to the input frequency.

Example 18. *The applied input AC to a half wave rectifier is 60 W and the DC output is 20 W. Find the rectification efficiency. Also, calculate the value of power efficiency.*

Sol. Rectification efficiency is the ratio of DC output power to the AC input power, *i.e.*

$$\eta = \frac{\text{DC output power}}{\text{AC input power}} \times 100$$

Here, DC output power = 20 W

AC input power = 60 W

$$\therefore \text{ Rectification efficiency, } \eta = \frac{20}{60} \times 100 = 33.3\%$$

Also, power efficiency is given by

$$PE = \frac{\text{DC output power}}{\text{AC input power for half cycle}} \times 100\,\%$$

$$= \frac{20}{30} \times 100\,\% = 66.67\%$$

2. *p-n* Junction Diode as Full Wave Rectifier

The full wave rectifiers are of two types

(i) Centre tap full wave rectifier

(ii) Full wave bridge rectifier

These are described in detail below.

(i) Centre Tap Full Wave Rectifier

Figure shows a circuit which is used in full wave rectification. Two diodes are used for this purpose.

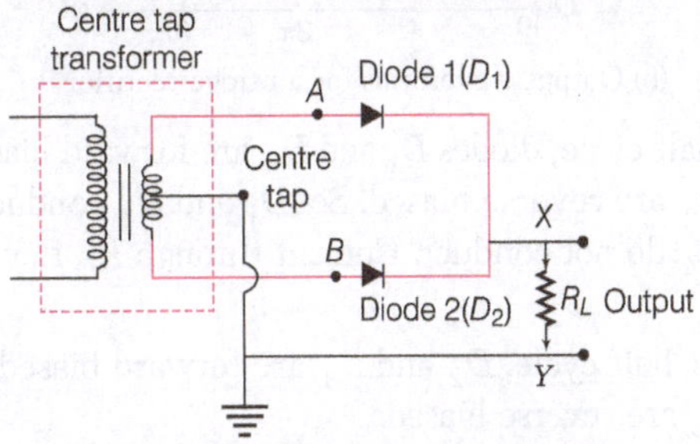

Circuit diagram of full wave rectifier

Working

During the positive half cycle of the input AC, the diode D_1 is in forward biased and the diode D_2 is in reverse biased. The forward current flows through diode D_1. During the negative half cycle, the diode D_1 is reverse biased and diode D_2 is forward biased. Thus, current flows through diode D_2.

Thus, we find that during both the halves, current flows in the same direction.

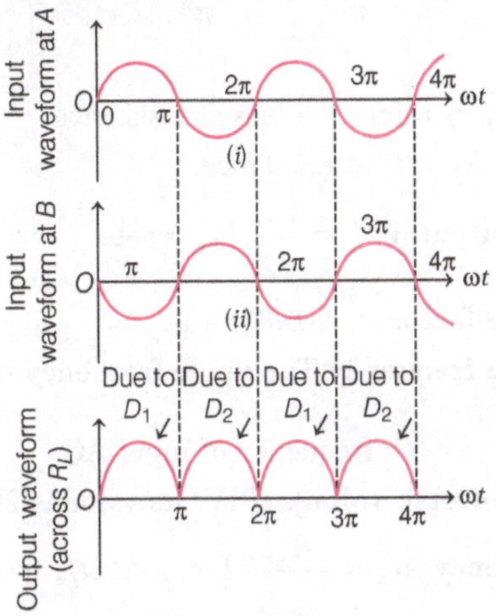

Input and output waveforms of a full-wave rectifier

(ii) Full Wave Bridge Rectifier

Another full wave rectifier called the bridge rectifier uses four diodes as shown in figure.

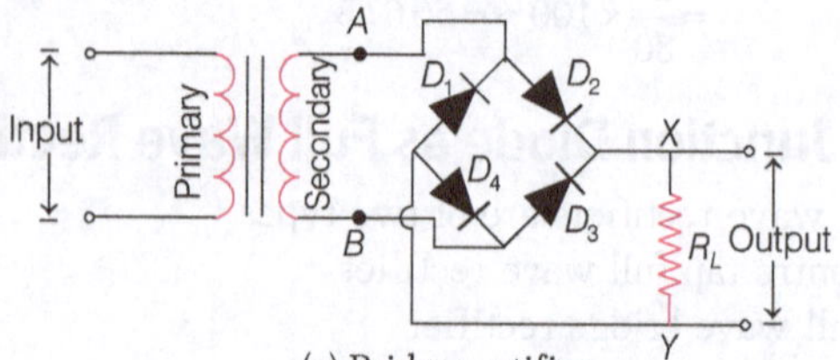

(a) Bridge rectifier

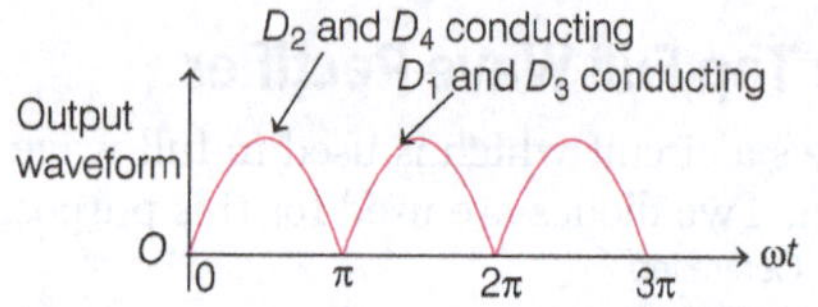

(b) Output waveforms for a bridge rectifier

For one-half cycle, diodes D_1 and D_3 are forward biased and D_2 and D_4 are reverse biased. So, D_1 and D_3 conduct but D_2 and D_4 do not conduct. Current through R_L flows from X to Y.

In another half cycle, D_2 and D_4 are forward biased and D_1 and D_3 are reverse biased.

So, in this half cycle, D_2 and D_4 conduct but D_1 and D_3 do not. Current again flows from X to Y through R_L. Thus, we see that current through R_L always flows in one direction from X to Y.

Important Points Related to Full Wave Rectifier

(i) Output voltage is obtained across the load resistance R_L. It is not constant but pulsating in nature.

(ii) **Average output**

$$V_{av} = \frac{2V_0}{\pi}, I_{av} = \frac{2I_0}{\pi}, V_{DC} = \frac{2V_0}{\pi\left(1+\dfrac{r_f}{R_L}\right)}$$

where, r_f = forward biased resistance

and R_L = load resistance.

(iii) **rms output** $V_{rms} = \dfrac{V_0}{\sqrt{2}}, I_{rms} = \dfrac{I_0}{\sqrt{2}}$

(iv) **Ripple factor** $r = 0.48 = 48\%$

(v) **Ripple frequency** The ripple frequency of full wave rectifier

= 2 × frequency of input AC

(vi) **Peak inverse voltage (PIV)** Its value is $2V_0$.

(vii) **Efficiency** $\eta_\% = \dfrac{81.2}{1+\dfrac{r_f}{R_L}}$ for $r_f << R_L$, $\eta = 81.2\%$

(viii) **Form factor,** $f = \dfrac{I_{rms}}{I_{DC}} = \dfrac{\pi}{2\sqrt{2}}$

Concept ladder

- The output frequency in full wave rectification is double that of input frequency but in half-wave rectification, the input and output frequency remains the same.
- Output of a rectifier contains AC ripples. These ripples are removed by filter circuits.

Example 19. *In a full wave rectifier circuit operating from 100 Hz mains frequency, what is the fundamental frequency in the ripple?*

Sol. In full wave rectification, output signal (ripple) frequency is double that of input frequency. So, output frequency is 200 Hz.

Example 20. *In a centre tap full wave rectifier, the value of the load resistance is $2\,k\Omega$. The voltage applied across the half of the secondary winding is given by $V = 220 \sin 314t$. Assume that, the each diode has a forward bias dynamic resistance of $20\,\Omega$. Calculate (i) the peak value of current, (ii) the DC value of current (iii) and the rms value of current.*

Sol. Comparing $V = 220 \sin 314t$ with general equation

$V = V_0 \sin \omega t$, we get

$V_0 = 220\,V$ and $\omega = 314\text{ rads}^{-1}$

Also, it is given that $R_L = 2\,k\Omega = 2000\,\Omega$, $r_f = 20\,\Omega$

(i) Peak value of current,

$$I_0 = \frac{V_0}{(r_f + R_L)} = \frac{220}{20+2000} \approx 109\text{ mA}$$

(ii) DC value of current, $I_{DC} = \dfrac{2I_0}{\pi} = \dfrac{2\times 109}{3.14} = 69.4\text{ mA}$

(iii) rms value of current, $I_{rms} = \dfrac{I_0}{\sqrt{2}} = 0.707 \times 109$

$= 77.06\text{ mA}$

Special Types of *p-n* Junction Diode

The junction diodes are of many types

1. Light Emitting Diode (LED)

It is an important light source used in optical communication and it converts electrical energy into light energy. It is a forward biased p-n junction which emits light spontaneously.

(i) Symbol

It is represented by the symbol shown below. In actual, it has two leads, the shorter lead represents n or cathode side while the longer lead represents p or anode side.

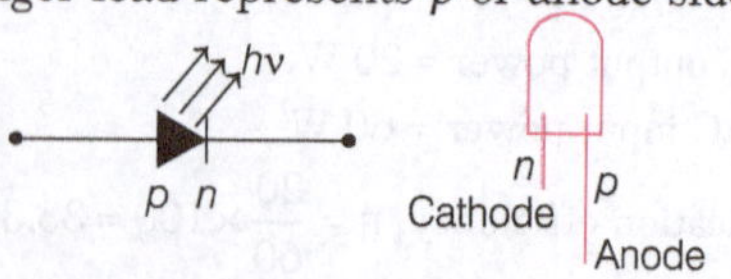

(ii) Working

When p-n junction is forward biased, electrons and holes move towards opposite sides of junction through it. Therefore, there are excess minority carriers on the either side of the junction boundary, which recombines with majority carriers near the junction.

On recombination of electron and hole, the energy is given out in the form of heat and light.

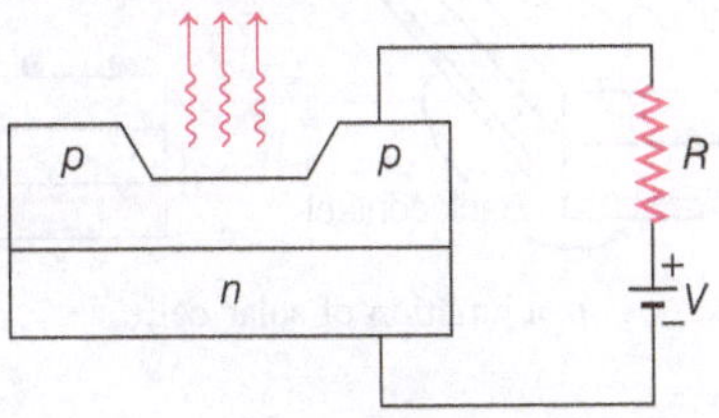

A forward biased LED

(iii) *V-I* Characteristics

V-I characteristics of LED are given below, which is similar to that of a simple junction diode. But the threshold voltages are much higher and slightly different for each colour. The reverse breakdown voltages of LEDs are very low. The colour of light emitted by a given LED, depends on its band gap energy. The photon emitted by an LED is of energy equal to or slightly less than the band gap energy. Forward current conducted by the junction determines the intensity of light emitted by LED.

A low voltage DC supply is required to operate an LED.

Current drawn by LED is of the order of milliampere. So, in practice, a resistor of suitable value is joined in series with the LED to limit the current upto the safe value required.

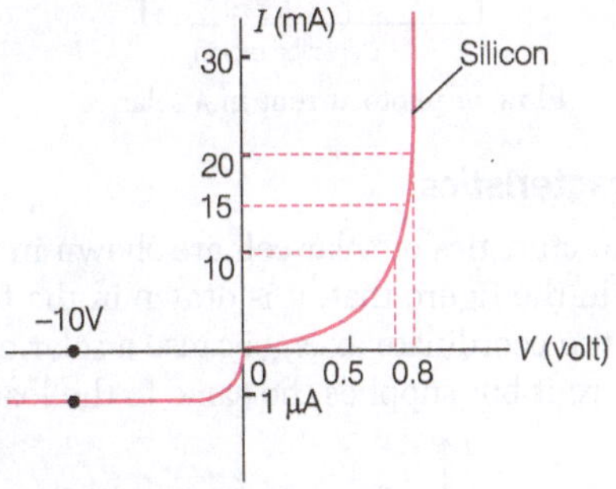

V-I characteristics of LED

(iv) Advantages

(a) Fast action and no warm up time is required.

(b) The bandwidth of emitted light is 100 Å to 500 Å, so its nearly (not exactly) monochromatic.

(c) Long-life and ruggedness.

(d) Low operational voltage and less power consumed.

(e) Fast ON-OFF switching capability.

Example 21. *A voltage drop of 2 V occurs across a light emitting diode (LED) and a current of 10 μA is passed through it when it is operated with a 6 V battery having a limiting resistor R. What is the value of R?*

Sol. Current, $I = \frac{V}{R}$ or $R = \frac{V}{I}$

Resistance of limiting resistor,

$$R = \frac{(6-2)\text{V}}{10 \times 10^{-6}\text{A}} = 400\ \text{k}\Omega$$

2. Photodiode

A photodiode is a special type of junction diode used for detecting optical signals. It is a reverse biased p-n junction made from photosensitive material. In photodiode, current carriers are generated by photons through photo-excitation.

(i) Symbol

The symbol of a photodiode is shown below.

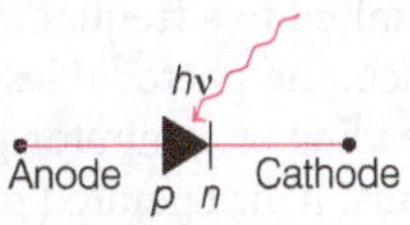

(ii) Construction

A photodiode is fabricated with a transparent cover to allow light to fall on the diode and is operated under reverse bias.

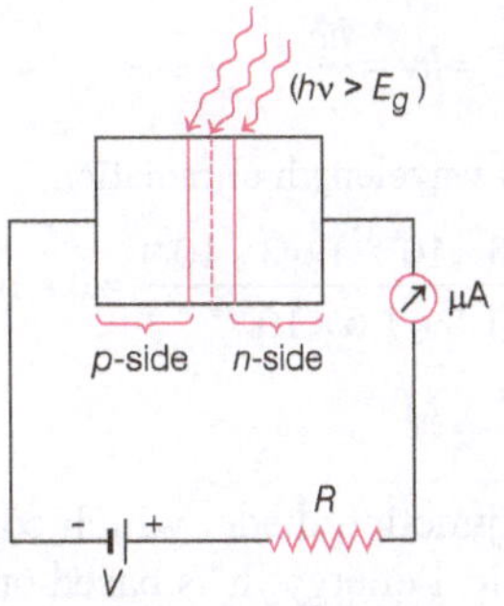

A reverse biased photodiode illuminated with light

(iii) Working

When the photodiode is illuminated with light (photons), having energy greater than the energy gap of the semiconductor, then electron-hole pairs are generated due to the absorption of photons. These charge carriers contribute to the reverse current. They increase the conductivity of the semiconductor.

Larger the intensity of the incident light, larger will be the conductivity of the semiconductor. The value of reverse saturation current increases with the increase in intensity of incident light.

Hence, a measurement of the change in the reverse saturation current on illumination can give the values of light intensity.

(iv) *V-I* Characteristics

Its *V-I* characteristics are shown in the figure given below. We observe from the figure that, current in photodiode changes with the change in light intensity (*I*) when reverse bias is applied.

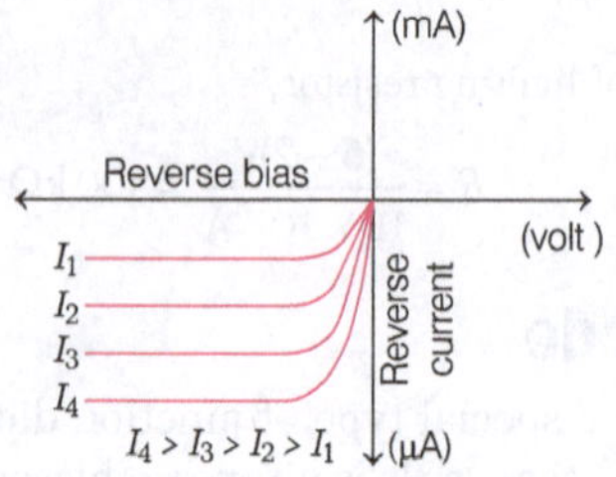

Characteristics of photodiode at different intensites

(v) Uses

The *p-n* photodiode can operate at frequencies of the order of 1MHz, in contrast to the slow and bulk type photo-conductor which is limited to a frequency range from 100 to 5000 Hz. Hence, the photodiodes are extensively used in high speed reading of computer punched cards, light- detection systems, light-operated switches, counting of objects interrupting a light-beam, etc.

Example 22. *A p-n photodiode is made of a material with a band gap of* 1.5 eV. *What is the minimum wavelength of radiation that can be absorbed by the material?*

Sol Use, energy, $E = h\nu = \dfrac{hc}{\lambda}$

The minimum wavelength of radiation,

$$\lambda = \frac{hc}{E} = \frac{(6.6 \times 10^{-34}) \times (3 \times 10^{8})}{1.5 \times 1.6 \times 10^{-19}} = 8 \times 10^{-7} \text{ m} = 800 \text{ nm}$$

3. Solar cell

Solar cell is a *p-n* junction diode, which converts solar energy into electrical energy. It is based on photovoltaic effect.

(i) Symbol

Its symbol is

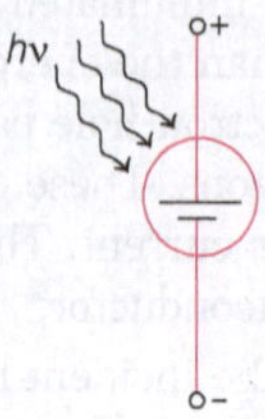

(ii) Construction

It consists of a silicon or gallium-arsenide *p-n* junction diode packed in a can with glass window on the top. Here, a thin layer of *n*-type is grown on a *p*-type semiconductor. The top of the *n*-layer has few finger electrodes for the light to reach it. The bottom of the *p*-layer is provided with a current collecting electrode.

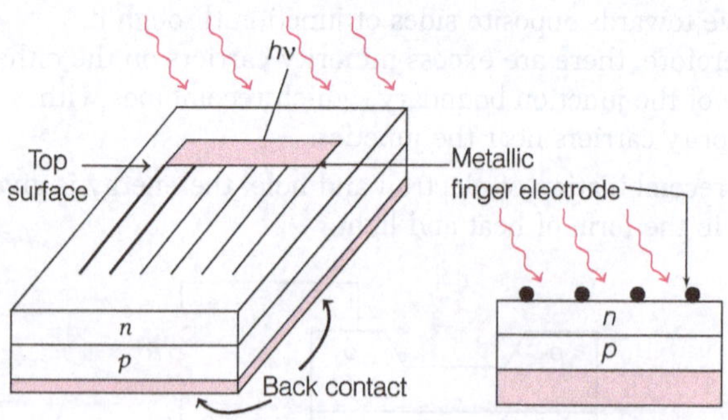

p-n junction of solar cell

(iii) Working

When photons of light (of energy $h\nu > E_g$) falls at the junction, electron-hole pairs are generated near the junction and they move in opposite directions due to junction field. They will be collected at the two sides of the junction, giving rise to a photo voltage between the top and bottom metal electrodes.

The top metal contact acts as negative electrode and bottom metal contact acts as positive electrode. When an external load is connected across metal electrodes, a photocurrent flows.

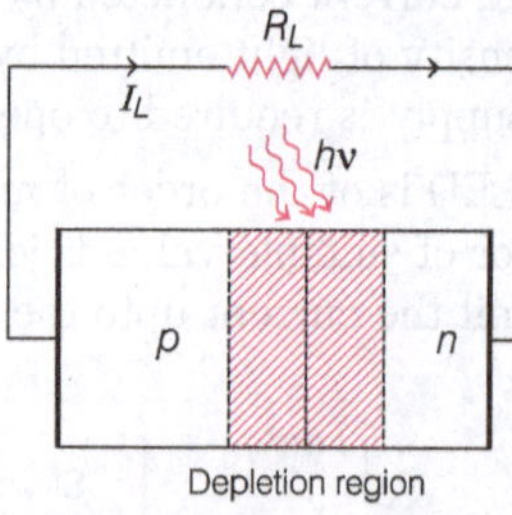

Flow of photocurrent in a solar cell

(iv) *I-V* characteristics

The *I-V* characteristics of solar cell are shown in the figure. We can see in the figure that, it is drawn in the fourth quadrant of the coordinate axes, because a solar cell does not draw current but supplies the same to the load.

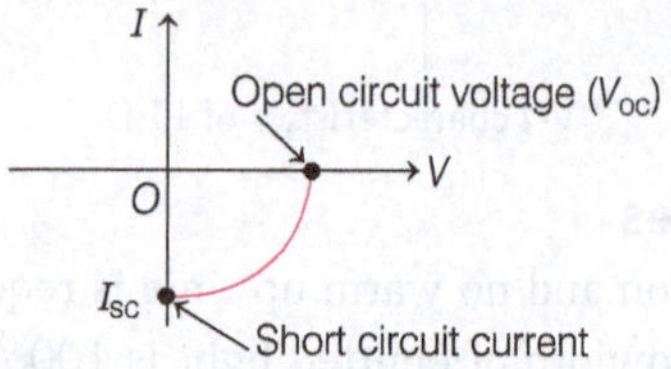

(v) Uses

Solar cells are used in space vehicles for charging batteries in day time and then taking electrical power from them during night.

4. Zener Diode

It is a reverse biased heavily doped *p-n* junction diode. It is operated in breakdown region.

Zener diode is designed to operate in the reverse breakdown voltage continuously without being damaged. This can be achieved by changing the thickness of the depletion layer to which the voltage is applied. Current through the zener diode is controlled by an external resistance. Zener diode is represented by the symbol shown below

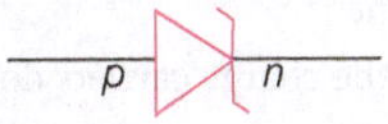

(i) *V-I* Characteristics

The *V-I* characteristics of zener diode is shown below and we observe that when the applied reverse voltage (V) reaches the breakdown voltage (V_Z) of the zener diode, there is a large change in the current.

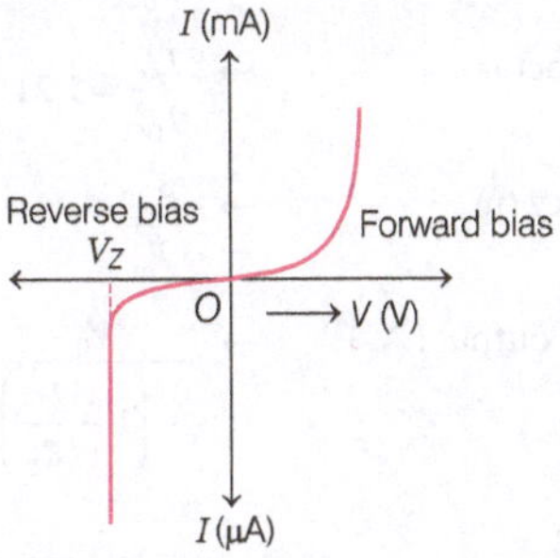

But after the breakdown voltage V_Z, a large change in the current can be produced by almost insignificant change in the reverse bias voltage.

(ii) Uses

Though zener diode finds numerous applications in electronics but mainly it is used as a voltage stabiliser (voltage regulator) and as a fixed reference voltage for calibrating voltmeters.

Zener Diode as a Voltage Regulator

This is the most important application of a zener diode.

(a) Principle

When the applied reverse voltage V reaches the breakdown voltage V_Z of the zener diode, there is a large change in the current. So, after the breakdown voltage V_Z, a large change in the current can be produced by almost insignificant change in the reverse bias voltage, *i.e.* zener voltage remains constant even though the current through the zener diode varies over a wide range.

Zener diode is joined in reverse bias to the fluctuating DC input voltage through a resistance R.

The constant output voltage is taken across a load resistance connected in parallel with zener diode.

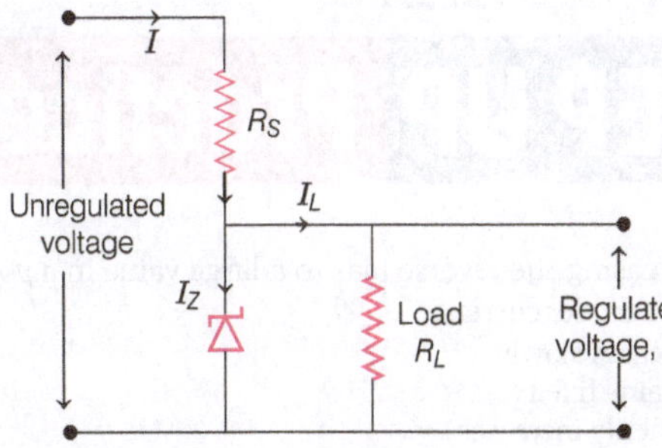

Circuit diagram of zener diode as a voltage regulator

(b) Working

Here, when input DC voltage increases beyond a certain limit, the current through the circuit rises sharply, causing a sufficient increase in the voltage drop across the resistor R_S.

Thus, the voltage across the zener diode remains constant and also the output voltage remains constant at V_Z. When the input DC voltage decreases, the current through the circuit goes down sharply causing sufficient decrease in the voltage drop across the resistance.

Thus, the voltage across the zener diode remains constant and also the output voltage across R_L remains constant at V_Z.

Hence, the output voltage remains constant in both conditions. Figure shows the graph of output voltage V_o *versus* input voltage V_{in} of a zener diode. Clearly, the output voltage remains constant after the reverse breakdown voltage V_Z.

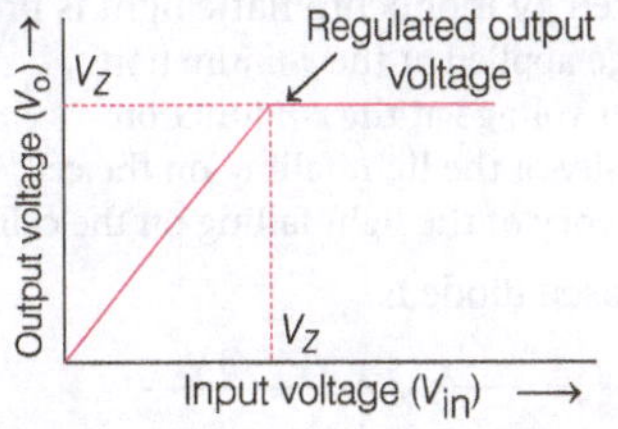

Graph of V_o *versus* V_{in} for a zener diode

Example 23. *The breakdown voltage of a zener diode is 12 V. It is used in a voltage regulator circuit shown in figure. Find the current through the diode.*

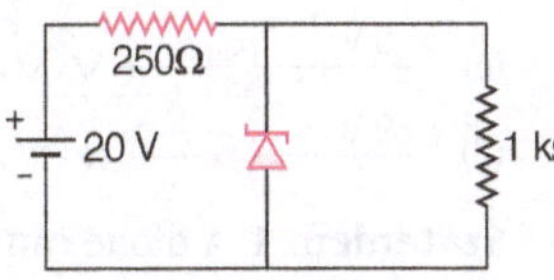

Sol. Current through 250 Ω resistor, $I_1 = \dfrac{\text{Net voltage}}{\text{Resistance}} = \dfrac{(20-12)}{250}$

$$= 32 \times 10^{-3} \text{ A} = 32 \text{ mA}$$

Current through 1 kΩ resistor,

$$I_2 = \frac{12}{1 \times 10^3} = 12 \times 10^{-3} \text{ A} = 12 \text{ mA}$$

So, current through the zener diode,

$$I_Z = I_1 - I_2 = 32 \text{ mA} - 12 \text{ mA} = 20 \text{ mA}$$

STEP UP Practice 2

1. On increasing the reverse bias to a large value in a *p-n* junction diode, current
(a) increases slowly
(b) remains fixed
(c) suddenly increases
(d) decreases slowly

2. In *p-n* junction, avalanche current flows in circuit when biasing is
(a) forward (b) reverse
(c) zero (d) excess

3. **Statement I** In a *p-n* junction with open ends, there is no motion of charge carriers.
Statement II In a *p-n* junction with open ends, the electric field is varying.
In the light of the above statements, choose the most appropriate answer from the options given below.
(a) Both Statement I and Statement II are incorrect.
(b) Statement I is correct but Statement II is incorrect.
(c) Statement I is incorrect but Statement II is correct.
(d) Both Statement I and Statement II are correct.

4. The *p-n* junction diode is used as
(a) an amplifier
(b) a rectifier
(c) an oscillator
(d) a modulator

5. In a *p-n* junction photocell, the value of photo-electromotive force produced by monochromatic light is proportional to
(a) the voltage applied at the *p-n* junction
(b) the barrier voltage at the *p-n* junction
(c) the intensity of the light falling on the cell
(d) the frequency of the light falling on the cell

6. A reverse-biased diode is

(a) 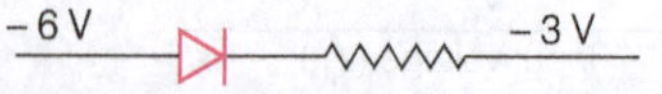

(b) 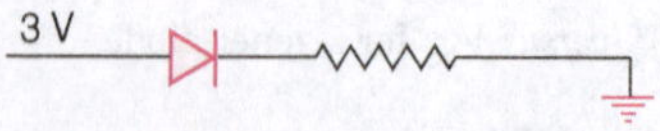

(c) 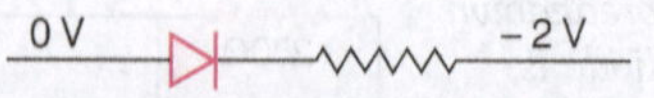

(d) 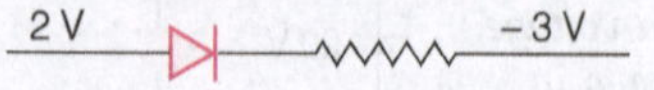

7. **Statement I** A diode can be used to rectify alternating voltages.
Statement II A *p-n* junction allows current to pass only when it is in reverse bias.
In the light of the above statements, choose the most appropriate answer from the options given below.
(a) Both Statement I and Statement II are incorrect.
(b) Statement I is correct but Statement II is incorrect.
(c) Statement I is incorrect but Statement II is correct.
(d) Both Statement I and Statement II are correct.

8. The maximum efficiency of full wave rectifier is
(a) 100% (b) 25.20%
(c) 40.2% (d) 81.2%

9. No bias is applied to *p-n* junction, then the current
(a) is zero because the number of charge carriers flowing on both sides is same
(b) is zero because the charge carriers do not move
(c) is non-zero
(d) None of the above

10. Which one of the following pair given below is incorrect about the half-wave rectifier?
(a) Form factor $\rightarrow \frac{I_{rms}}{I_{DC}} = 1.57$
(b) Ripple factor $\rightarrow \frac{I_{AC}}{I_{DC}} = 1.21$
(c) Efficiency (η) $\rightarrow \frac{P_{out}}{P_{in}}$
(d) Average output (V_{DC}) $\rightarrow \frac{V_0}{\pi\left(1 - \frac{r_f}{R_L}\right)}$

11. A 4 V battery is connected across the points *A* and *B* as shown in the figure given below. Assuming that the resistance of each diode is zero in forward bias and infinity in reverse bias, the current supplied by the battery when its positive terminal is connected to *A* is

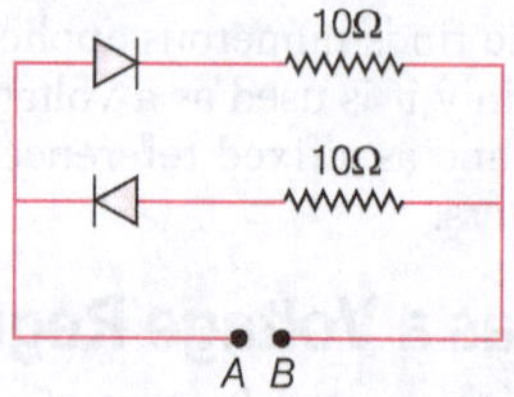

(a) 0.2 A (b) 0.4 A
(c) zero (d) 0.1 A

12. **Statement I** The depletion layer in the *p-n* junction is free from mobile charge carriers.
Statement II There is no electric field across the barrier junction.
In the light of the above statements, choose the most appropriate answer from the options given below.
(a) Both Statement I and Statement II are incorrect.
(b) Statement I is correct but Statement II is incorrect.
(c) Statement I is incorrect but Statement II is correct.
(d) Both Statement I and Statement II are correct.

13. A diode is connected to 220 V (rms) AC in series with a capacitor as shown in figure. The voltage across the capacitor is

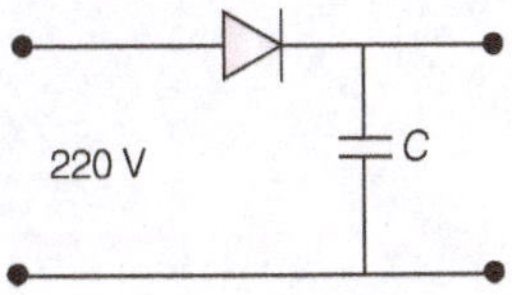

(a) 220 V (b) 110 V

(c) 311.1 V (d) $\frac{220}{\sqrt{2}}$ V

14. In the circuit shown in figure, the maximum output voltage V_0 is

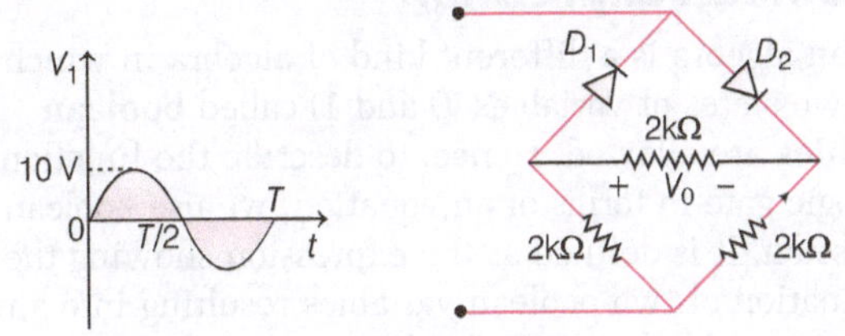

(a) 0 (b) 5 V

(c) 10 V (d) $\frac{5}{\sqrt{2}}$ V

15. In the middle of the depletion layer of a reverse-biased *p-n* junction, the
(a) potential is zero
(b) electrical field is zero
(c) potential is maximum
(d) electric field is maximum

16. **Statement I** An electron on *p*-side of a *p-n* junction moves to *n*-side just an instant after drifting of charge carriers occurs across junction plane.
Statement II Drifting of charge carriers reduces the concentration gradient across junction plane.
In the light of the above statements, choose the most appropriate answer from the options given below.
(a) Both Statement I and Statement II are incorrect.
(b) Statement I is correct but Statement II is incorrect.
(c) Statement I is incorrect but Statement II is correct.
(d) Both Statement I and Statement II are correct.

17. When a *p-n* junction diode is made from gallium arsenide, energy is released at the junction due to the recombination of electrons and holes. This energy is in
(a) visible region
(b) infrared region
(c) UV region
(d) X-ray region

18. *p-n* junction diode,
(a) the current in the reverse biased condition is generally very small
(b) the current in the reverse biased condition is small but the forward biased current is independent of the bias voltage
(c) the reverse biased current in strongly dependent on the applied bias voltage
(d) the forward biased current is very small in comparison to reverse biased current

19. **Statement I** In a semiconductor diode, the reverse biased current is due to drift of free electrons and holes.
Statement II The drift of electrons and holes is due to thermal excitations.
In the light of the above statements, choose the most appropriate answer from the options given below.
(a) Both Statement I and Statement II are incorrect.
(b) Statement I is correct but Statement II is incorrect.
(c) Statement I is incorrect but Statement II is correct.
(d) Both Statement I and Statement II are correct.

20. Different voltages are applied across a *p-n* junction and the currents are measured for each value. Which of the following graphs is obtained between voltage and current?

(a)
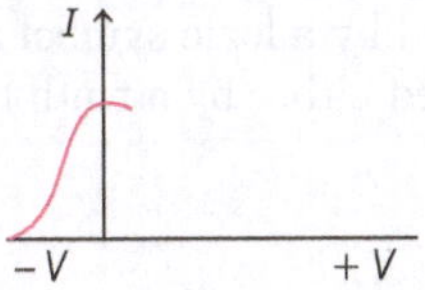

(b)
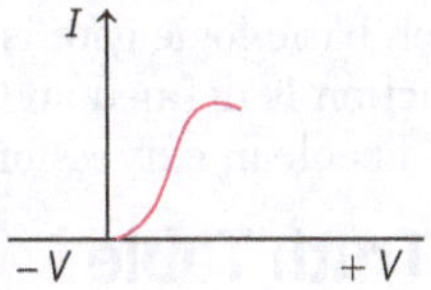

(c)
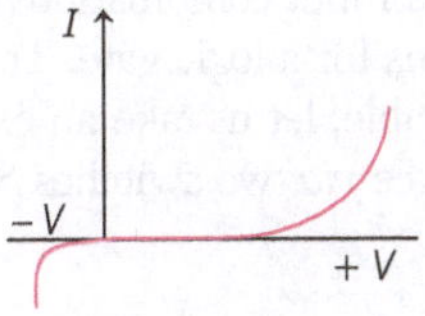

(d)
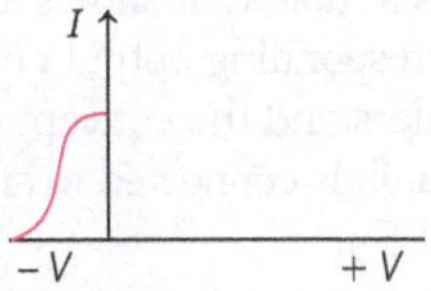

21. A waveform shown when applied to the following circuit will produce which of the following output waveform? [Assume, ideal diode configuration]

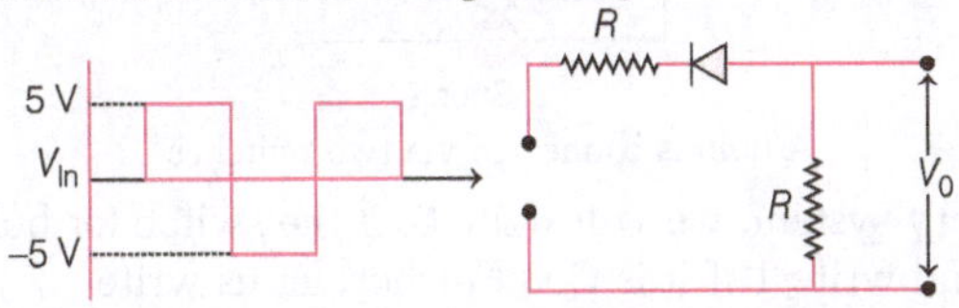

(a)

(b)

(c)

(d)

Module 3
Logic Gates

- Logic Gates
- Combination of Logic Gates
- NAND and NOR Gates as Digital Building Blocks

Logic Gates

Logic gates are the building blocks of digital circuit that makes use of diodes and transistors to perform switching function. It is used for performing a particular logical operation. In other words, a gate is a digital circuit that follows certain logical relationship between the input and output voltages.

A logic gate has one output but one or more inputs. There are three basic gates named as OR gate, AND gate and NOT gate.

Each basic logic gate is indicated by a logic symbol and its function is defined and described either by a truth table or by a boolean expression.

1. Truth Table

It is a table that shows all possible input combinations and the corresponding output combinations for a logic gate. To understand the concept of truth table, let us take an example. A bulb is connected to an AC source *via* two switches S_1 and S_2.

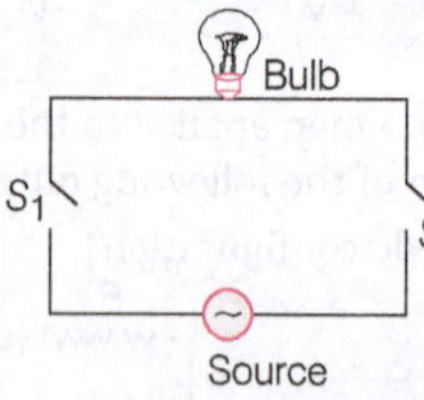

A bulb is connected via two switches

In binary system, we will write 0, if the switch (or bulb) is OFF and write 1 if it is ON. Further, let us write

A for state of switch S_1,
B for state of switch S_2
and C for state of the bulb.

Now, let us make a table (called truth table).

Switch S_1	Switch S_2	Bulb	A	B	C
OFF	ON	OFF	0	1	0
ON	OFF	OFF	1	0	0
OFF	OFF	OFF	0	0	0
ON	ON	ON	1	1	1

Here, A and B represent the input combination and C represents the output for this particular circuit. This table is called **truth table** and is used to define or describe the function of a particular logic gate.

2. Boolean Expression

Boolean algebra is a different kind of algebra in which only two states of variables (0 and 1) called **boolean variables** are allowed. Hence, to describe the functioning of a logic gate in terms of an equation, we use boolean expression. It is defined as the expression showing the combination of two boolean variables resulting into a new boolean variable known as boolean expression.

Some Useful Postulates and Laws of Boolean Algebra

(i) **Boolean postulates**

(a) $0 + A = A$ (b) $1 + A = 1$

(c) $0 \cdot A = 0$ (d) $1 \cdot A = A$

(e) $A + \overline{A} = 1$

(ii) **Identity law**

(a) $A + A = A$

(b) $A \cdot A = A$

(iii) **Negation law** $\overline{\overline{A}} = A$

(iv) **De-Morgan's theorem** It states that, the complement of the whole sum is equal to the product of individual complements and *vice-versa. i.e.*

(a) $\overline{A + B} = \overline{A} \cdot \overline{B}$ (b) $\overline{A \cdot B} = \overline{A} + \overline{B}$

De-Morgan's theorem also states that

(a) $\overline{\overline{A} + \overline{B}} = \overline{\overline{A}} \cdot \overline{\overline{B}} = A \cdot B$

(b) $\overline{\overline{A} \cdot \overline{B}} = \overline{\overline{A}} + \overline{\overline{B}} = A + B$

(v) **Commutative laws**

(a) $A + B = B + A$ (b) $A \cdot B = B \cdot A$

(vi) **Associative laws**

(a) $A + (B + C) = (A + B) + C$

(b) $A \cdot (B \cdot C) = (A \cdot B) \cdot C$

(vii) **Distributive laws**

(a) $A \cdot (B + C) = A \cdot B + A \cdot C$

(b) $(A + B) \cdot (A + C) = A + BC$

(viii) **Absorption laws**

(a) $A + A \cdot B = A$ (b) $A \cdot (A + B) = A$

(c) $A \cdot (A + \overline{A}) = A$ (d) $\overline{A} \cdot (A + B) = \overline{A} \cdot B$

(ix) **Boolean identities**

(a) $A + \overline{A}B = A + B$ (b) $A(\overline{A} + B) = AB$

(c) $A + BC = (A + B)(A + C)$

Types of Logic Gates

Logic gates are classified as

1. OR Gate

An OR gate has two or more inputs and one output. In this gate, if any of the input or all the inputs are 1, then output is 1.

OR operation Consider the circuit given below.

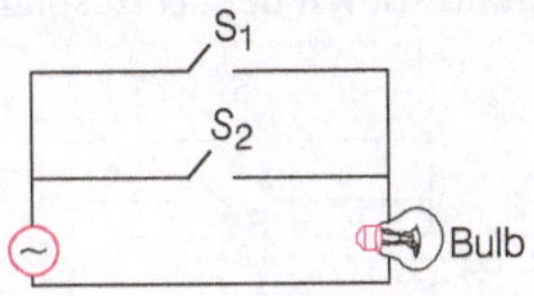

Circuit of OR operation

The two switches are connected in parallel, so when S_1 or S_2 is closed, the bulb is ON, *i.e.* it glows. So, it represents OR operation.

Boolean Expression

Let the two input of OR gate be A and B respectively and its output be Y.

$$Y = A + B$$

Logic Symbol

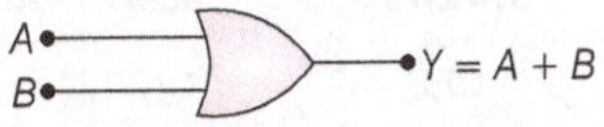

Truth Table

Input		Output
A	B	Y = A + B
0	0	0
0	1	1
1	0	1
1	1	1

Mentor's TiP

- OR gate can be formed by *p-n* junction diodes. Its circuit diagram is shown below.

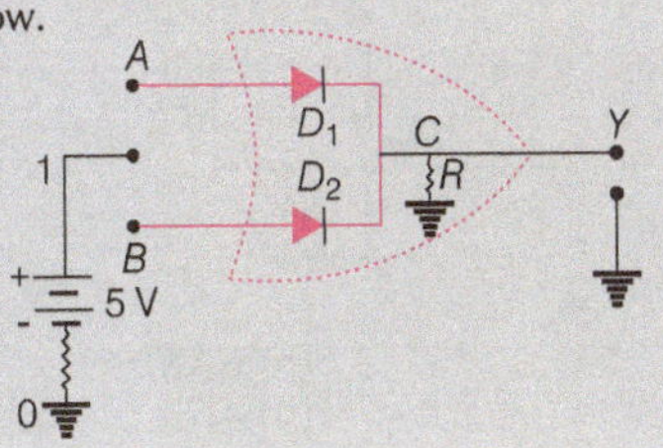

Input and Output Waveforms for an OR Gate

The output of an OR gate is high when either A or B or both the inputs are high. Therefore, the output waveform Y will be as shown in figure.

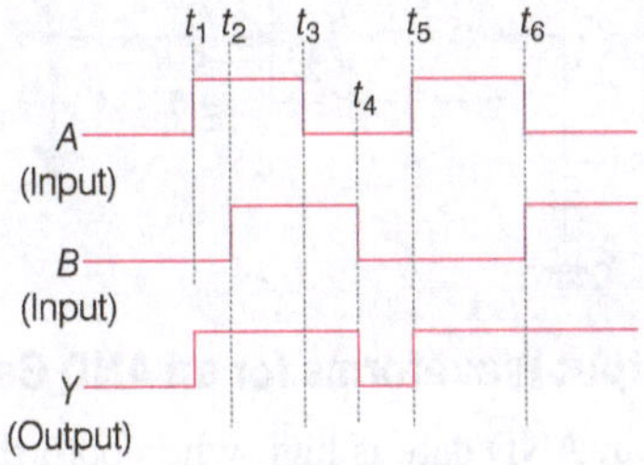

2. AND Gate

It has two or more inputs and one output. In AND gate, output is 1 only when all the inputs are 1.

AND Operation

Consider the circuit given below.

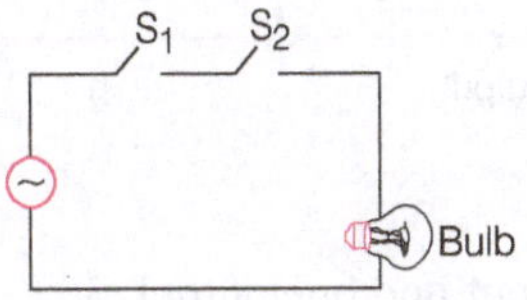

Circuit of AND operation

Now, the two switches are connected in series. If any one switch is open, the current will not flow and hence, bulb will not glow. So, when S_1 and S_2 are closed, bulb is ON, *i.e.* it glow. So, it represents AND operation.

Boolean Expression

Let the inputs of AND gate be A and B respectively and its output be Y.

$$Y = A \cdot B$$

Logic Symbol

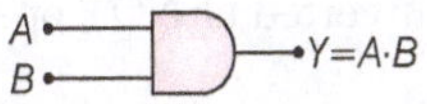

Truth Table

Input		Output
A	B	Y = A·B
0	0	0
0	1	0
1	0	0
1	1	1

Mentor's Tip

- The simplest circuit of AND gate can be made by combination of two diodes which is given below.

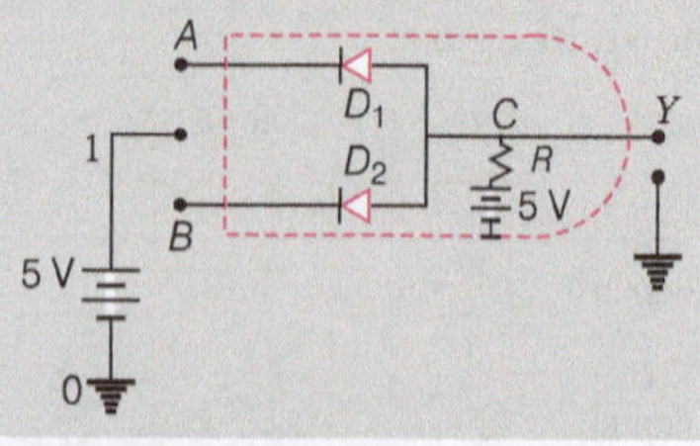

Input and Output Waveforms for an AND Gate

The output of an AND gate is high when both the inputs are high, otherwise the output is low. Therefore, the output waveform Y for AND gate will be as shown in figure.

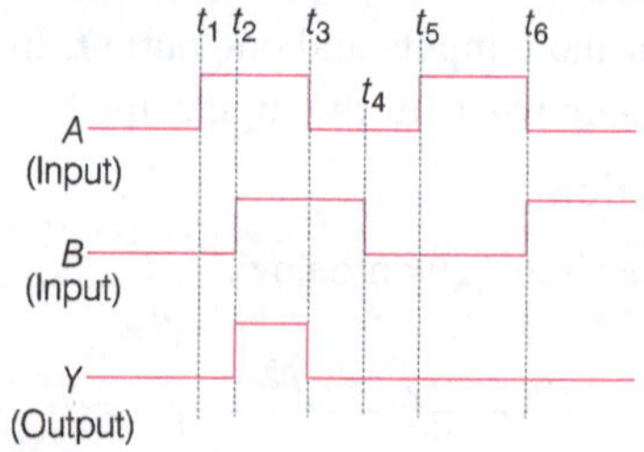

3. NOT Gate

It has only one input and one output.

It gives an inverted version of its input, *i.e.* if input is 1, then output is 0 and *vice-versa*.

NOT Operation

Consider the circuit given below

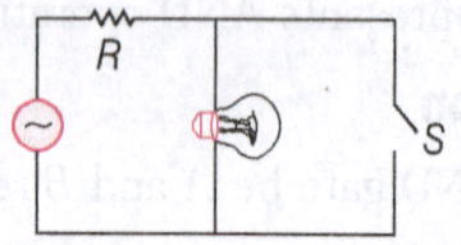

Circuit of NOT operation

Here, only one switch is used and it is connected in parallel with bulb. So, when S is open, bulb is ON, *i.e.* it glows. It represents inverted or NOT operation.

Boolean Expression

Let the input of NOT gate be A and its output be Y.

$$Y = \overline{A}$$

Logic Symbol

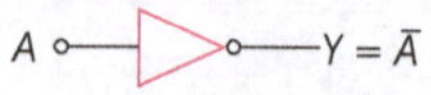

Truth Table

Input	Output
A	$Y = \overline{A}$
0	1
1	0

Input and Output Waveforms for NOT gate

The output of a NOT gate is high when the input is low and *vice-versa*. Therefore, the output waveform Y for NOT gate is as shown in figure.

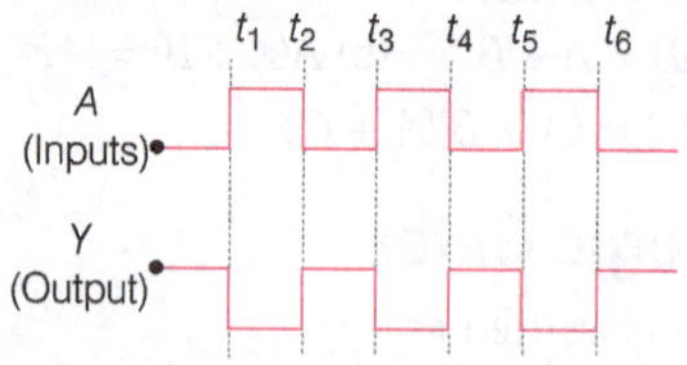

NEET Close-up

Example Similar to PYQ Asked in NEET 2019

The circuit diagram shown here corresponds to the logic gate.

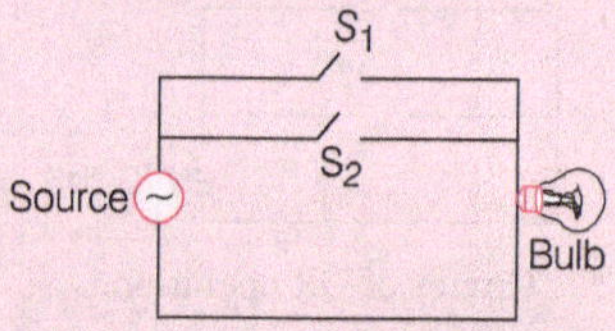

(a) OR (b) AND
(c) NAND (d) NOT

Sol. (*a*) Here, the two switches can be operated in different combinations. Note that the two switches are connected in parallel. So, if one switch is OFF, the bulb will still glow. We will write 0, if the switch is OFF and write 1 if it is ON. Further, A stands for state of switch S_1 and B stands for state of switch S_2 and C for state of bulb. Now, let us make a truth table based on this.

Switch S_1	Switch S_2	Bulb	A	B	C
ON	OFF	ON	1	0	1
OFF	ON	ON	0	1	1
OFF	OFF	OFF	0	0	0
ON	ON	ON	1	1	1

Hence, given circuit is equal to OR gate.

Skill Builder

The circuit diagram shown here corresponds to the logic gate,

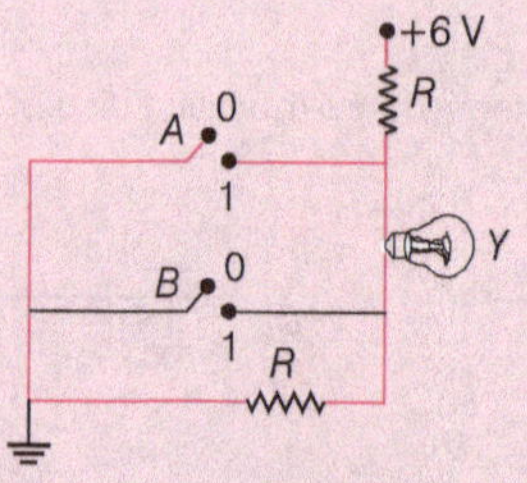

(a) OR (b) NAND
(c) NOT (d) AND

For more Practice Refer Q. No. 1, 6 of step up practice -3.

Combination of Logic Gates

Various combinations of three basic gates (*i.e.* OR, AND and NOT) give rise to complicated digital circuits. Let us now discuss a few combinations of these basic gates using their symbols.

1. NAND Gate

It has two or more inputs and one output. This is an AND gate followed by a NOT gate. In this gate, if all the inputs are 1, then output will be 0. Let the two inputs of NAND gate be A and B respectively and its output be Y.

Boolean Expression

$$Y = \overline{A \cdot B} \text{ or } Y = \overline{AB}$$

Logic Symbol

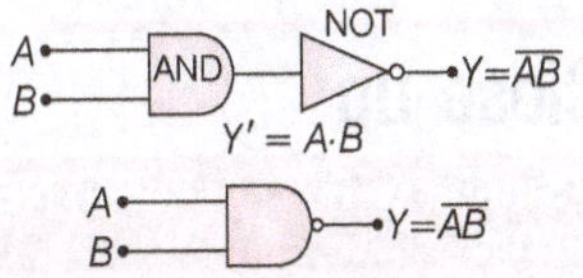

Truth Table

Input			Output
A	B	$Y' = A \cdot B$	$Y = \overline{AB}$
0	0	0	1
0	1	0	1
1	0	0	1
1	1	1	0

Input and Output Waveforms for NAND Gate

The output waveform for NAND gate will be as shown in figure.

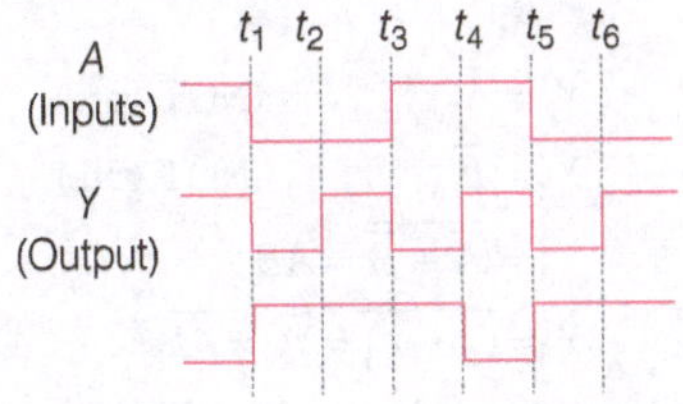

2. NOR Gate

It has two or more inputs and one output. When a NOT operation is applied after OR gate, then it is called NOR gate.

In this gate, if all the inputs are 0, then only output will be 1, otherwise it is 0. Let the two inputs be A and B respectively and its output be Y.

Boolean Expression

$$Y = \overline{A + B}$$

Logic Symbol

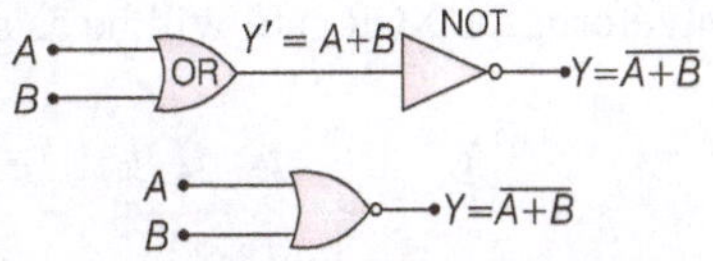

Truth Table

Input			Output
A	B	$Y' = A + B$	$Y = \overline{A + B}$
0	0	0	1
0	1	1	0
1	0	1	0
1	1	1	0

Input and Output Waveforms of NOR Gate

The output waveform for NOR gate will be as shown in figure.

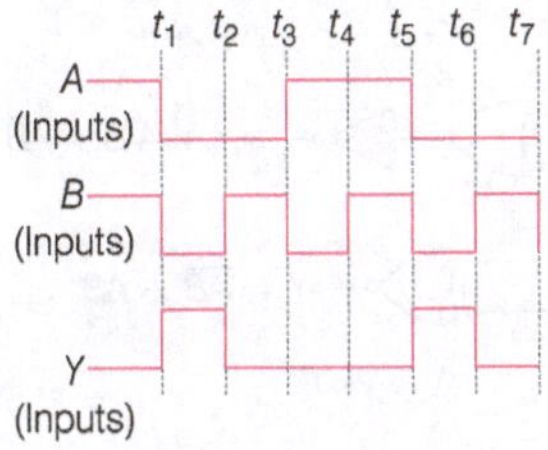

3. XOR Gate

It is also called the **exclusive OR function.** It is a function of two logical variables A and B which evaluates to 1, if one of two variables is 0 and the other is 1. The output is zero, if both the variables are 0 or 1.

Boolean Expression

$$Y = A \oplus B = A \text{ XOR } B \text{ or } Y = A \oplus B \text{ or } Y = \overline{A}B + A\overline{B}$$

Logic Symbol

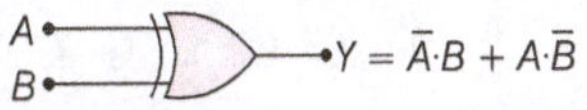

Truth Table

Input						Output
A	B	$\overline{A}$	$\overline{B}$	$A \cdot \overline{B}$	$\overline{A} \cdot B$	$A = A \cdot \overline{B} + \overline{A} \cdot B$
0	0	1	1	0	0	0
0	1	1	0	0	1	1
1	0	0	1	1	0	1
1	1	0	0	0	0	0

Input and Output Waveforms of XOR Gate

The output waveform for XOR gate will be as shown in Figure.

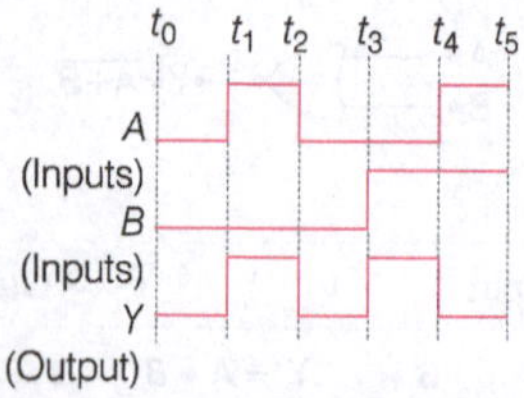

4. XNOR Gate

It is also called **exclusive NOR function**. It is a function of two logical variables A and B which evaluates to 0, if one of two variable is 0 and the other is 1. The output is one, if both the variables are 0 or 1.

Boolean Expression

$$Y = \overline{A \oplus B} = A \odot B \quad \text{or} \quad Y = \overline{A}\overline{B} + AB$$

Logic Symbol

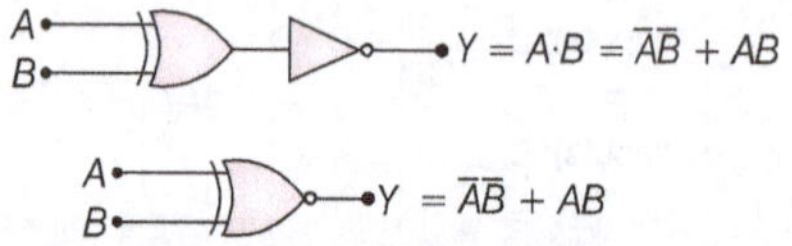

Truth Table

Input		Output
A	B	$Y = \overline{A}\overline{B} + AB$
0	0	1
0	1	0
1	0	0
1	1	1

Input and Output Waveforms of XNOR gate

The output waveform Y for XNOR gate is as shown in figure.

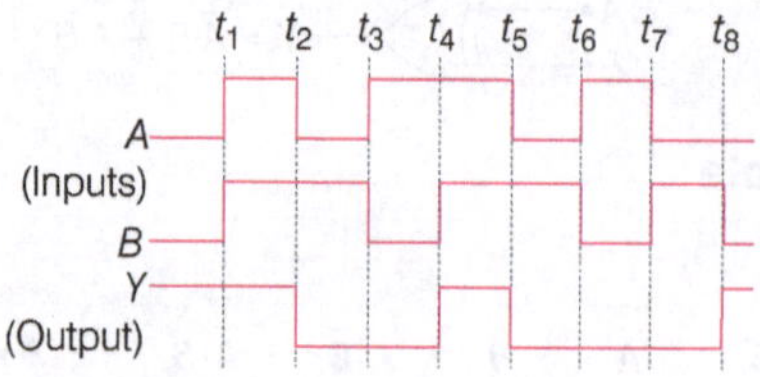

Mentor's Tip

- XOR gate and XNOR gate are known as **exclusive gates.**

NAND and NOR Gates as Digital Building Blocks

The repeated use of the OR, AND or the NOT gates alone cannot give a different gate. But the repeated use of the NAND or the NOR gates alone can give all basic gates like OR, AND and NOT gates. Hence, the NAND and the NOR gates are also called **universal gates.** In digital circuits, these gates serve as digital building blocks. Now, let us derive the basic logic gates one by one from NAND and NOR gates

Mentor's Tip

- Following two rules are very helpful in solving logics

$$\overline{\overline{A} + \overline{B}} = AB$$

$$\overline{\overline{A} \cdot \overline{B}} = A + B$$

NEET Close-up

Example Similar to PYQ Asked in NEET 2024, 2017 and 2015

The output Y of the given logic gate is similar to the output of an/a.

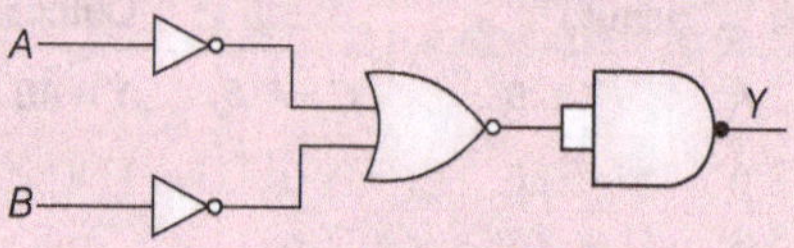

(a) NAND gate (b) NOR gate
(c) OR gate (d) AND gate

Sol. (a)

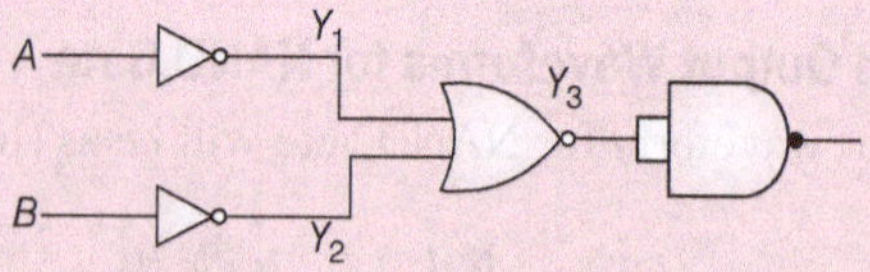

Here, $Y_1 = \overline{A}$ (NOT gate)

$Y_2 = \overline{B}$ (NOT gate)

$Y_3 = \overline{\overline{A} + \overline{B}} = AB$

$Y = \overline{Y_3 + Y_3} = \overline{Y_3} = \overline{AB}$

Hence, given circuit is equal to NAND gate.

Skill Builder

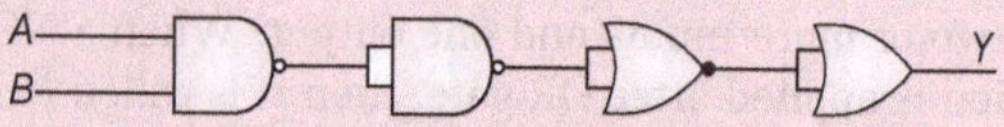

Identify equivalent logic gate of given circuit.
(a) AND gate (b) NAND gate
(c) NOR gate (d) OR gate

For more Practice Refer Q. No. 11, 20 of step up practice-3 and Q.No. 110, 116, 117 of Gearing up for NEET.

Example 24. *Name the equivalent gate that circuit represents. Write the truth table for the given circuit.*

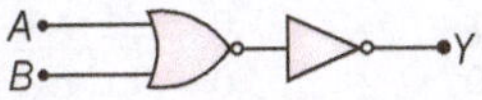

Sol. The given combination consists of NOR gate and NOT gate, so equivalent gate is OR gate.

Output, $Y = \overline{\overline{A + B}} = A + B$

Truth Table

A	B	Y = A + B
0	0	0
0	1	1
1	0	1
1	1	1

From the truth table, it is clear that the output is 1 only when atleast one of the inputs is at the high state (*i.e.* 1).

Example 25. *Let $X = A \cdot \overline{BC}$. Evaluate X for*

(i) $A = 1, B = 0, C = 1$,
(ii) $A = B = C = 1$
(iii) and $A = B = C = 0$.

Sol. (i) When $A = 1, B = 0$ and $C = 1$, then

$BC = 0$

$\therefore$ $\overline{BC} = 1$ or $A\overline{BC} = 1$

(ii) When $A = B = C = 1$,

then $BC = 1$ or $\overline{BC} = 0$

$\therefore$ $A\overline{BC} = 0$

(iii) When $A = B = C = 0$,

then $BC = 0$.

$\therefore$ $\overline{BC} = 1$ or $A\overline{BC} = 0$

Example 26. *Write the truth table for the logical function D = (A OR B) AND B.*

Sol. *A* OR *B* is a logical function, say it is equal to *X*, *i.e.*

$X = A \text{ OR } B = A + B$

Now, $D = X \text{ AND } B = X \cdot B$

The corresponding truth table is as under

A	B	X = A OR B	D = (A OR B) AND B
1	0	1	0
0	1	1	1
0	0	0	0
1	1	1	1

Mentor's TiP

The given function can also be written as $D = (A + B) \cdot B$.

Example 27. *Write down truth tables for*

(i) $X = \overline{A} \cdot \overline{B} + \overline{A} \cdot B$

(ii) $X = (A + \overline{B}) + \overline{A \cdot B}$

Sol. (i) The corresponding truth table is as under

A	B	$\overline{A}$	$\overline{B}$	$\overline{A} \cdot \overline{B}$	$\overline{A} \cdot B$	$X = \overline{A} \cdot \overline{B} + \overline{A} \cdot B$
0	0	1	1	1	0	1
0	1	1	0	0	1	1
1	0	0	1	0	0	0
1	1	0	0	0	0	0

(ii) The corresponding truth table is as under

A	B	$\overline{B}$	$A + \overline{B}$	$A \cdot B$	$\overline{A \cdot B}$	$X = (A + \overline{B}) + (\overline{A \cdot B})$
0	0	1	1	0	1	1
0	1	0	0	0	1	1
1	0	1	1	0	1	1
1	1	0	1	1	0	1

Example 28. *Let $Y = A\overline{BC} + B\overline{CA} + C\overline{AB}$. Find the output Y, if following inputs are given*

(i) $A = B = C = 0$ *(ii) $A = B = C = 1$*

(iii) $A = 1, B = 0, C = 1$

Sol.

A	B	C	$\overline{AB}$	$\overline{BC}$	$\overline{CA}$	$A\overline{BC}$	$B\overline{CA}$	$C\overline{AB}$	Y
0	0	0	1	1	1	0	0	0	0
1	1	1	0	0	0	0	0	0	0
1	0	1	1	1	0	1	0	1	1

(i) $Y = 0$ (ii) $Y = 0$ (iii) $Y = 1$

Example 29. *Write the truth table for the circuit given in figure.*

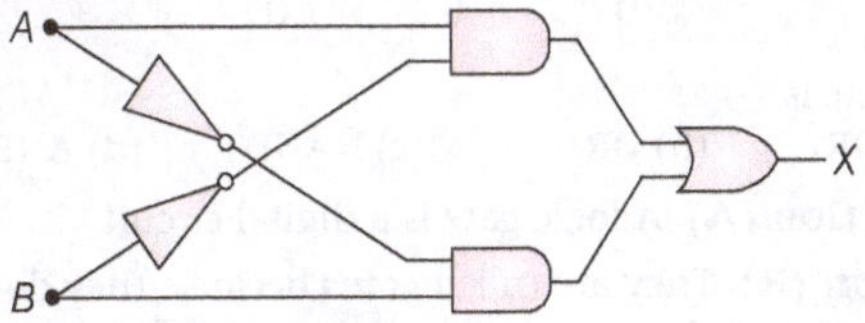

Sol. The circuit can be redrawn as

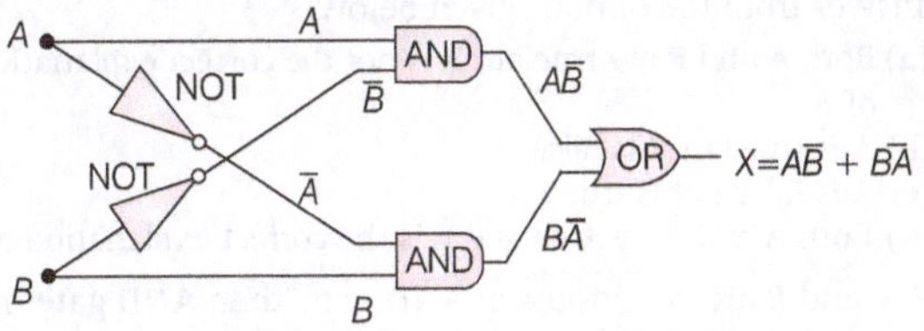

The corresponding truth table is shown below

A	B	$\overline{A}$	$\overline{B}$	$A\overline{B}$	$B\overline{A}$	$A\overline{B} + B\overline{A} = X$
0	0	1	1	0	0	0
0	1	1	0	0	1	1
1	0	0	1	1	0	1
1	1	0	0	0	0	0

Example 30. *Construct truth table for the function X of A and B as shown in the figure.*

(i)

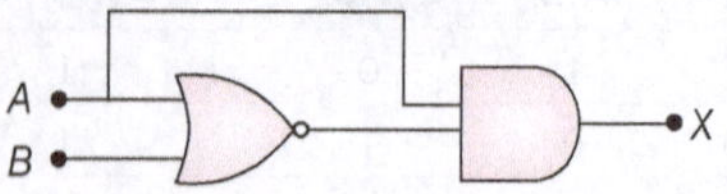

(ii)

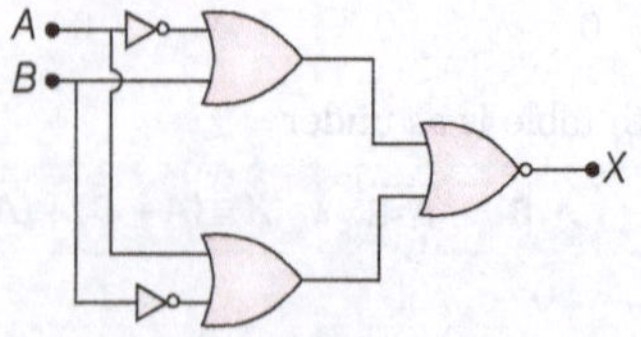

Sol. First write the boolean expression for the figure and then construct truth table.

(i)

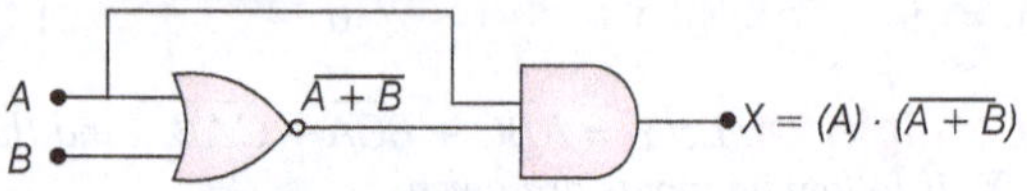

A	B	$\overline{A+B}$	$X = A \cdot (\overline{A+B})$
0	0	1	0
0	1	0	0
1	0	0	0
1	1	0	0

(ii)

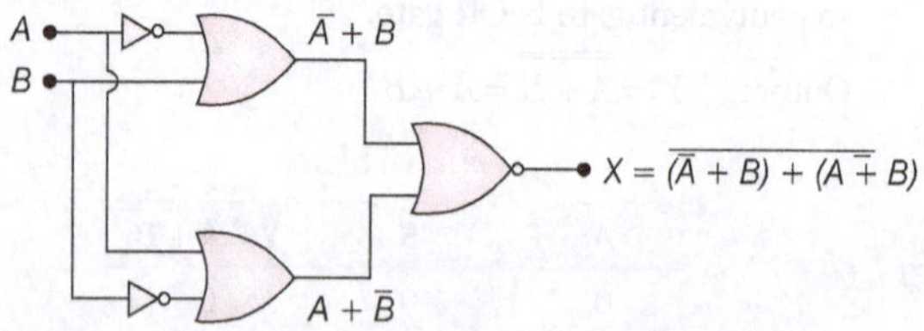

A	B	$\bar{A}$	$\bar{B}$	$\bar{A}+B$	$A+\bar{B}$	$X = \overline{(\bar{A}+B)+(A+\bar{B})}$
0	0	1	1	1	1	0
0	1	1	0	1	0	0
1	0	0	1	0	1	0
1	1	0	0	1	1	0

STEP UP Practice 3

1. A gate has the following truth table

P	Q	R
1	1	1
1	0	0
0	1	0
0	0	0

The gate is
(a) NOR (b) OR (c) NAND (d) AND

2. **Assertion (A)** A logic gate is a digital circuit.
Reason (R) They are called gates because they do not allow current through them,
In the light of the above statements, choose the correct answer from the options given below.
(a) Both A and R are true but R is not the correct explanation of A.
(b) A is true but R is false.
(c) A is false but is true.
(d) Both A and R are true and R is the correct explanation of A.

3. If A and B are two inputs in AND gate, then AND gate has an output of 0 when the value of A and B are
(a) $A = 0, B = 0$ (b) $A = 0, B = 1$
(c) $A = 1, B = 0$ (d) All are correct

4. The output of a NAND gate is 0,
(a) if both inputs are 0
(b) if one input is 0 and the other input is 1
(c) if both inputs are 1
(d) either if both inputs are 1 or if one of the inputs is 1 and the other 0

5. **Assertion (A)** NAND or NOR gates are universal gates.
Reason (R) A combination of NAND gates or a combination of NOR gates can be used to perform or implement any boolean function.
In the light of the above statements, choose the correct answer from the options given below.
(a) Both A and R are true but R is not the correct explanation of A.
(b) A is true but R is false.
(c) A is false but is true.
(d) Both A and R are true and R is the correct explanation of A.

6. The truth table given below is for

A	B	Y
0	0	1
0	1	1
1	0	1
1	1	0

(A and B are the inputs, Y is the output)
(a) NOR (b) AND (c) XOR (d) NAND

7. Any digital circuit can be realised by repetitive use of only
(a) NOT gates (b) OR gates
(c) AND gates (d) NOR gates

8. The logic gates having output 1 for the inputs of 1 and 0 are
(a) AND and OR (b) OR and NOR
(c) NAND and NOR (d) NAND and OR

9. If the two inputs of a NAND gate are shorted, the gate is equivalent to
(a) XOR (b) OR (c) NOR (d) NOT

10. Which of the following pair is incorrect about logic gates?

(a) OR gate $\rightarrow Y = A + B$

(b) AND gate $\rightarrow Y = A \cdot B$

(c) NOT gate $\rightarrow Y = \overline{A}$

(d) NOR gate $\rightarrow Y = \overline{A \cdot B}$

11. Which logic gate is represented by the following combination of logic gates?

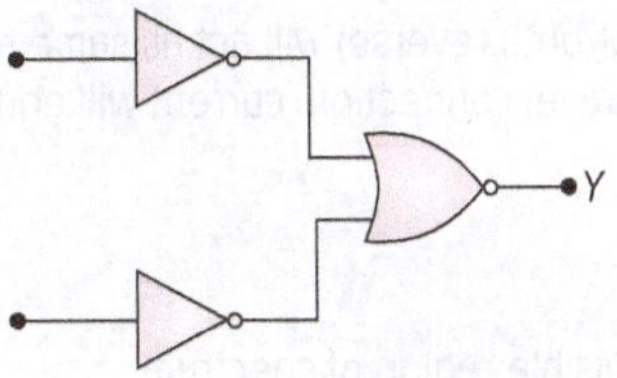

(a) OR (b) NAND
(c) AND (d) NOR

12. In the boolean algebra $(\overline{A} \cdot \overline{B}) \cdot A$ equals to

(a) $\overline{A + B}$ (b) A
(c) $\overline{A \cdot B}$ (d) $A + B$

13. In the given circuit as shown, the two input waveforms A and B are applied simultaneously. The resultant waveform Y is

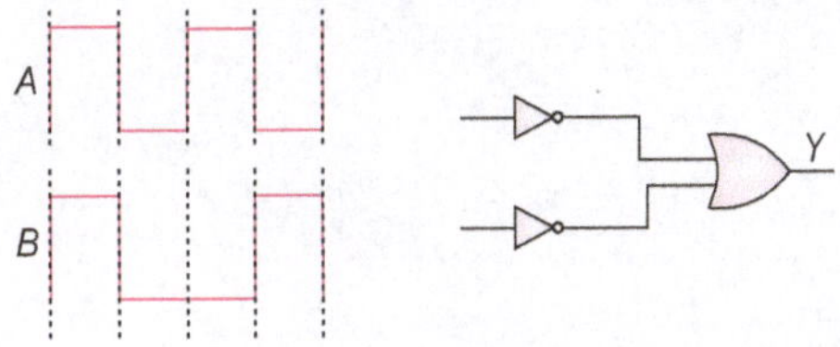

(a)  (b) 

(c) 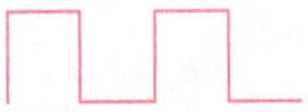 (d) 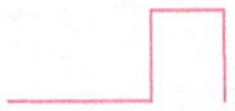

14. With reference to figure, which of the following is possible?

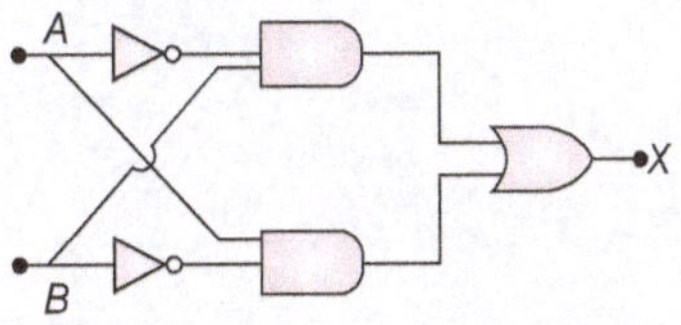

(a) $A = 0, B = 0, X = 1$ (b) $A = 0, B = 1, X = 0$
(c) $A = 1, B = 0, X = 0$ (d) $A = 1, B = 1, X = 0$

15. The truth table shown in figure is for

A	0	0	1	1
B	0	1	0	1
Y	1	0	0	1

(a) XOR (b) AND
(c) XNOR (d) OR

16. Assertion (A) A Logic gate can have one and only one output.

Reason (R) A boolean function like any other function can have a unique output.

In the light of the above statements, choose the correct answer from the options given below.

(a) Both A and R are true but R is not the correct explanation of A.
(b) A is true but R is false.
(c) A is false but is true.
(d) Both A and R are true and R is the correct explanation of A.

17. For the given combination of gates, if the logic states of inputs A, B, C are as follows $A = B = C = 0$ and $A = B = 1$, $C = 0$, then the logic states of output D are respectively.

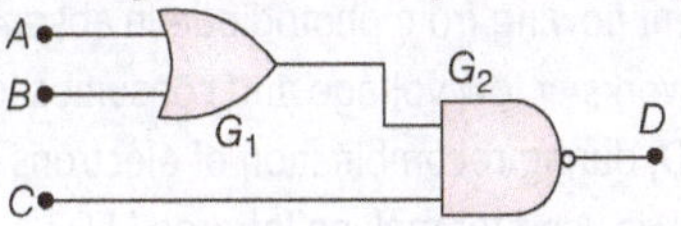

(a) 0, 0 (b) 0, 1 (c) 1, 0 (d) 1, 1

18. How many NAND gates are used to form an AND gate?

(a) 1 (b) 2 (c) 3 (d) 4

19. Assertion (A) A NAND gate is not obtained by using NOR gates only.

Reason (R) NOR and NAND gates are called universal gates.

In the light of the above statements, choose the correct answer from the options given below.

(a) Both A and R are true but R is not the correct explanation of A.
(b) A is true but R is false.
(c) A is false but is true.
(d) Both A and R are true and R is the correct explanation of A.

20. The figure shows two NAND gates followed by a NOR gate. The system is equivalent to which of the following logic gate?

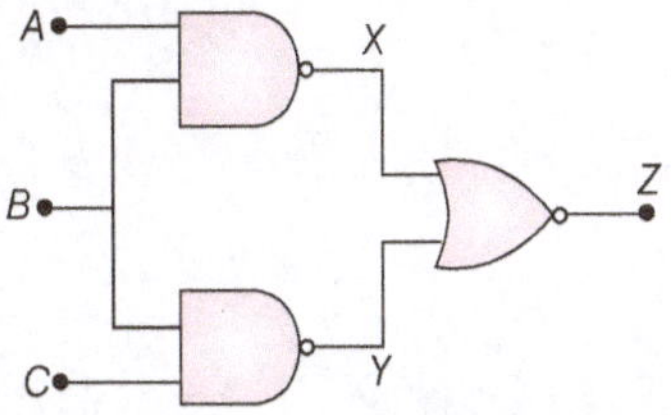

(a) OR (b) AND
(c) NAND (d) None of these

21. The diagram of a logic circuit is given below. The output F of the circuit is represented by

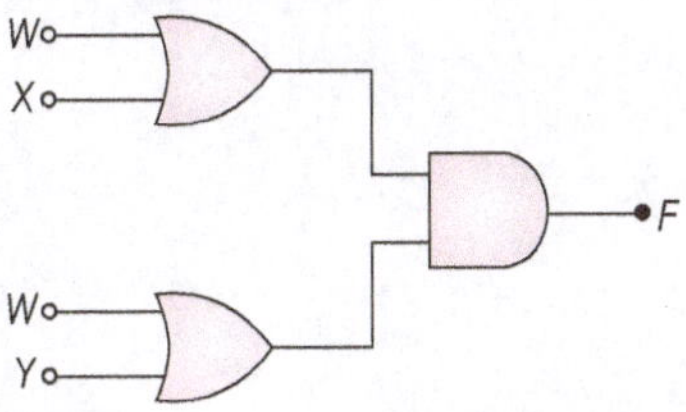

(a) $W \cdot (X + Y)$ (b) $W \cdot (X \cdot Y)$
(c) $W + (X \cdot Y)$ (d) $W + (X + Y)$

NEET Exclusive EXTRA BYTES

- Energy gap between conduction band and valence band is 5.5 eV for diamond, 1.1 eV for silicon and 0.7 eV for germanium.
- For low electric fields (less than 10^6 V/m), semiconductors follow Ohm's law.
- Impurity is mixed in semiconductor such low that it should not affect crystal structure of semiconductor material.
- Normal width of depletion layer in *p-n* junction is in order of 10^{-17} m.
- *p-n* junction is non-ohmic in nature.
- Two identical diodes connected in same type of biasing (either both forward or both reverse) will act as same resistance in a circuit. In such series connection, potential will equally get divided while in parallel connection, current will equally get divided.
- Current flowing from photodiode in absence of light is known as dark current.
- LED works at low voltage and consumes low power.
- In LED, during recombination of electrons and holes, energy is emitted in the visible region of spectrum.
- GaAsP is used for making infrared LED.
- Depletion layer of zener diode is thin in comparison to normal diode.
- NAND gate and NOR gate are known as universal gates as any logic can be performed using either of these gates.

GEARING UP FOR NEET

Single Correct Option

1. Number of electrons in the valence shell of a semiconductor is
(a) 1 (b) 2 (c) 3 (d) 4

2. Hole is *[NCERT Exemplar]*
(a) an anti-particle of electron
(b) a vacancy created when an electron leaves a covalent bond
(c) absence of free electrons
(d) an artificially created particle

3. A piece of copper and the other of germanium are cooled from the room temperature to 80 K, then which of the following would be a correct statement?
(a) Resistance of each increases.
(b) Resistance of each decreases.
(c) Resistance of copper increases, while that of germanium decreases.
(d) Resistance of copper decreases, while that of germanium increases.

4. A piece of semiconductor is connected in series in an electric circuit. On increasing the temperature, the current in the circuit will
(a) decrease (b) remain unchanged
(c) increase (d) stop flowing

5. E_g for silicon is 1.12 eV and that for germanium is 0.72 eV. Therefore, it can be concluded that
(a) more number of electron-hole pairs will be generated in silicon than in germanium at room temperature
(b) less number of electron-hole pairs will be generated in silicon than in germanium at room temperature
(c) equal number of electron-hole pairs will be generated in both at lower temperatures
(d) equal number of electron-hole pairs will be generated in both at higher temperatures

6. When the electrical conductivity of a semiconductor is due to the breaking of its covalent bonds, then the semiconductor is said to be
(a) donor (b) acceptor
(c) intrinsic (d) extrinsic

7. The majority charge carriers in p-type semiconductor are
(a) electrons (b) protons
(c) holes (d) neutrons

8. A p-type semiconductor can be obtained by adding
(a) arsenic to pure silicon
(b) gallium to pure silicon
(c) antimony to pure germanium
(d) phosphorus to pure germanium

9. p-type semiconductor is formed when
I. As impurity is mixed in Si
II. Al impurity is mixed in Si
III. B impurity is mixed in Ge
IV. P impurity is mixed in Ge
(a) Both I and III (b) Both I and IV
(c) Both II and III (d) Both II and IV

10. At room temperature, a p-type semiconductor has
(a) large number of holes and few electrons
(b) large number of free electrons and few holes
(c) equal number of free electrons and holes
(d) no electrons or holes

11. Which of the following statements is not true?
(a) The resistance of intrinsic semiconductor decreases with increase of temperature.
(b) Doping pure Si with trivalent impurities give p-type semiconductors.
(c) The majority carriers in n-type semiconductors are holes.
(d) A p-n junction can act as a semiconductor diode.

12. n-type semiconductor is formed
(a) when a germanium crystal is doped with an impurity containing three valence electrons
(b) from pure germanium
(c) from pure silicon
(d) when a germanium crystal are doped with an impurity containing five valence electrons

13. An n-type semiconductor is
(a) negatively charged (b) positively charged
(c) neutral
(d) negatively or positively charged depending upon the amount of impurity

14. Electrical conductivity of intrinsic and p-type semiconductor increases with increase in
(a) pressure (b) volume (c) density
(d) temperature

15. The valency of the impurity atom that is to be added to germanium crystal, so as to make it a n-type semiconductor, is
(a) 6 (b) 5 (c) 4 (d) 3

16. An n-type and a p-type silicon can be obtained by doping pure silicon with
(a) sodium and magnesium respectively
(b) phosphorus and boron respectively
(c) boron and phosphorus respectively
(d) indium and sodium respectively

17. The potential barrier for silicon diode is approximately
(a) 0.2 V (b) 0.6 V
(c) 1.1 V (d) 1.4 V

18. Serious drawback of the semiconductor device is that they
(a) cannot be used with high voltage
(b) pollute the environment
(c) are costly
(d) do not last for long time

19. Intrinsic semiconductor is electrically neutral. Extrinsic semiconductor having large number of current carriers would be
(a) positively charged
(b) negatively charged
(c) positively charged or negatively charged depending upon the type of impurity that has been added
(d) electrically neutral

20. The conductivity of a semiconductor increases with increase in temperature because *[NCERT Exemplar]*
(a) number density of free current carries increases
(b) relaxation time increases
(c) both number density of carries and relaxation time increase
(d) number density of carriers increases, relaxation time decreases but effect of decrease in relaxation time is much less than increase in number density

21. Temperature coefficient of resistance of semiconductor is
(a) zero (b) constant
(c) positive (d) negative

22. The temperature (T) dependence on resistivity (ρ) of a semiconductor is represented by

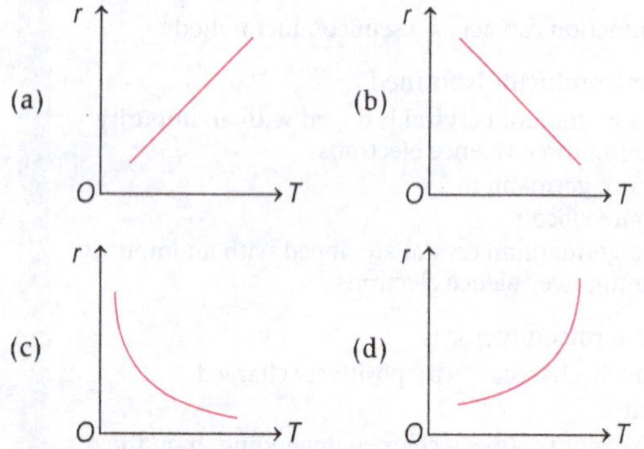

23. Mobilities of electrons and holes in a sample of intrinsic germanium at room temperature are 0.36 $m^2/V\text{-}s$ and 0.17 $m^2/V\text{-}s$. The electron and hole densities are each equal to 2.5×10^{19} m^{-3}. The electrical conductivity of germanium is
(a) 0.47 Sm^{-1}
(b) 5.18 Sm^{-1}
(c) 2.12 Sm^{-1}
(d) 1.09 Sm^{-1}

24. In a semiconductor, the concentration of electrons is 8×10^{14} / cm^3 and that of the holes is $5 \times 10^{12}/cm^3$. The semiconductor is
(a) *p*-type (b) *n*-type
(c) intrinsic (d) *p-n-p* type

25. A Si specimen is made into *p*-type semiconductor by doping on an average one indium atom per 6×10^7 silicon atoms. If the number density of atoms in Si be $6 \times 10^{28} m^{-3}$, then what is the indium atom per cm^3?
(a) 10^{12} (b) 10^{15} (c) 10^{18} (d) 10^{20}

26. A *p*-type semiconductor has acceptor level 57 meV above the valence band. The maximum wavelength of light required to create hole is
(a) 57 Å (b) 57×10^{-3} Å
(c) 217100 Å (d) 11.61×10^{-33} Å

27. If in a *p-n* junction, a square input signal of 10 V is applied as shown,

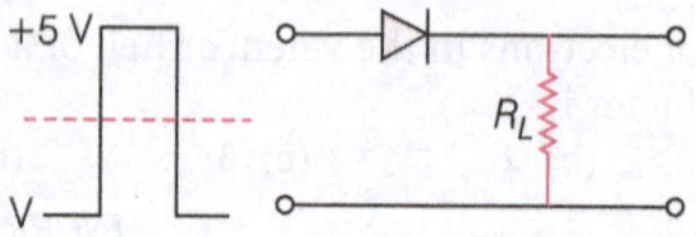

then the output across R_L will be

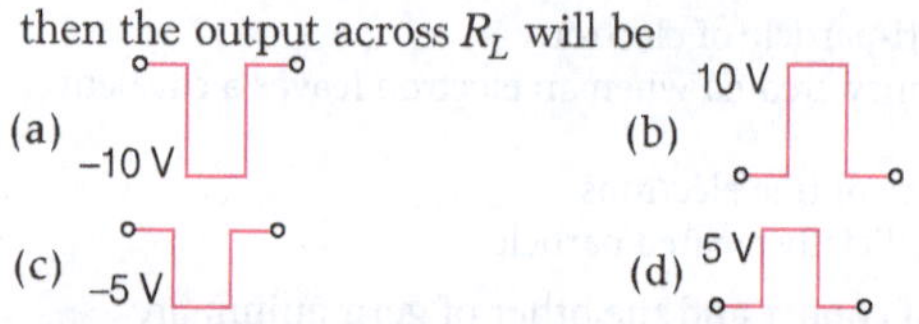

28. In a semiconducting material, the mobilities of electrons and holes are μ_e and μ_h, respectively. Which of the following is true?
(a) $\mu_e < \mu_h$ (b) $\mu_e = \mu_h$ (c) $\mu_e < 0, \mu_h > 0$ (d) $\mu_e > \mu_h$

29. The *p*-type semiconductor is
(a) positively charged
(b) negatively charged
(c) electrically neutral
(d) uncharged at 0 K or − 273 °C but charged at temperature higher than 0 K

30. The conductivity in the intrinsic semiconductor does not depend on
(a) band gap
(b) temperature
(c) fermi energy
(d) effective mass of charge carriers

31. In *n*-type semiconductor, electrons are majority charge carriers but it does not show any negative charge. The reason is
(a) electrons are stationary
(b) electrons neutralise with holes
(c) mobility of electrons is extremely small
(d) atom is electrically neutral

32. In *p*-type semiconductor, the acceptor level lies
(a) near the conduction band
(b) halfway between conduction and valence bands
(c) within conduction band
(d) near the valence band

33. Which one of the following statements is not correct in case of a semiconductor?
(a) Temperature coefficient of resistance is negative.
(b) Doping increases conductivity.
(c) At absolute zero temperature, it behaves like an insulator.
(d) Resistivity is in between that of a conductor and insulator.

34. In intrinsic semiconductor, at room temperature, number of electrons and holes are
(a) equal (b) zero
(c) unequal (d) infinite

35. If a small amount of antimony is added to germanium crystal,
(a) the antimony becomes an acceptor atom
(b) there will be more free electrons than holes in the semiconductor
(c) its resistance is increased
(d) it becomes a *p*-type semiconductor

36. A *p*-*n* junction has a thickness of the order of
(a) 1 cm (b) 1 mm
(c) 10^{-6} m (d) 10^{-12} cm

37. In comparison to half-wave rectifier, full wave rectifier gives lower
(a) efficiency (b) average DC
(c) average output voltage (d) None of these

38. Zener diode is used as
(a) half-wave rectifier (b) full wave rectifier
(c) AC voltage stabiliser (d) DC voltage stabiliser

39. When a forward bias is applied to *p*-*n* junction, then it
(a) raises the potential barrier
(b) reduces the majority carrier current to zero
(c) lowers the potential barrier
(d) None of the above

40. The drift current in a *p*-*n* junction is
(a) from the *n*-side to the *p*-side
(b) from the *p*-side to the *n*-side
(c) from the *n*-side to the *p*-side, if the junction is forward biased and in the opposite direction, if it is reverse biased
(d) from the *p*-side to the *n*-side, if the junction is forward biased and in the opposite direction, if it is reverse biased

41. The diffusion current in a *p*-*n* junction is
(a) from the *n*-side to the *p*-side
(b) from the *p*-side to the *n*-side
(c) from the *n*-side to the *p*-side, if the junction is forward biased and in the opposite direction, if it is reverse biased
(d) from the *p*-side to the *n*-side, if the junction is forward biased and in the opposite direction, if it is reverse biased

42. Diffusion current in a *p*-*n* junction is greater than the drift current in magnitude,
(a) if the junction is forward biased
(b) if the junction is reverse biased
(c) if the junction is unbiased
(d) None of the above

43. In the forward bias arrangement of a *p*-*n* junction diode, the
(a) *n*-end is connected to the positive terminal of the battery
(b) *p*-end is connected to the positive terminal of the battery
(c) direction of current is from *n*-end to *p*-end in the diode
(d) *p*-end is connected to the negative terminal of battery

44. Potential barrier developed in a junction diode opposes
(a) minority carrier in both regions only
(b) majority carrier only
(c) electrons in *n*-region
(d) holes in *p*-region

45. If n_e and v_d be the number of electrons and drift velocity in a semiconductor. When the temperature is increased,
(a) n_e increases and v_d decreases
(b) n_e decreases and v_d increases
(c) Both n_e and v_d increases
(d) Both n_e and v_d decreases

46. The dominant mechanisms for motion of charge carriers in forward and reverse biased silicon *p*-*n* junctions are
(a) drift in forward bias, diffusion in reverse bias
(b) diffusion in forward bias, drift in reverse bias
(c) diffusion in both forward and reverse bias
(d) drift in both forward and reverse bias

47. In *p*-*n* junction, avalanche current flows in circuit when biasing is
(a) forward (b) reverse
(c) zero (d) excess

48. In an unbiased *p*-*n* junction, holes diffuse from the *p*-region to *n*-region because
(a) free electrons in the *n*-region attract them
(b) they move across the junction by the potential difference
(c) hole concentration in *p*-region is more as compared to *n*-region
(d) All of the above

49. When the *p*-end of the *p*-*n* junction is connected to the negative terminal of the battery and the *n*-end to the positive terminal of the battery, then the *p*-*n* junction behaves like
(a) a conductor (b) an insulator
(c) a super conductor (d) a semiconductor

50. Select the correct statement.
(a) In a full wave rectifier, two diodes work alternately.
(b) In a full wave rectifier, two diodes work simultaneously.
(c) The efficiency of full wave and half-wave rectifiers is same.
(d) The full wave rectifier is bi-directional.

51. GaAs (with a band gap = 1.5 eV) as an LED can emit
(a) blue light (b) green light
(c) infrared rays (d) X-rays

52. If no external voltage is applied across *p*-*n* junction, then there would be
(a) no electric field across the junction
(b) an electric field pointing from *n*-type to *p*-type side across the junction
(c) an electric field pointing from *p*-type to *n*-type side across the junction
(d) a temporary electric field during formation of *p*-*n* junction that would subsequently disappear

53. When a diode is heavily doped, then
(a) the Zener voltage will be low
(b) the Avalanche voltage will be high
(c) the depletion region will be small
(d) the leakage current will be low

54. The electrical circuit used to get smooth DC output from a rectifier circuit is called
(a) oscillator (b) filter
(c) amplifier (d) logic gates

55. In given figure, V_0 is the potential barrier across a *p-n* junction, when no battery is connected across the junction *[NCERT Exemplar]*

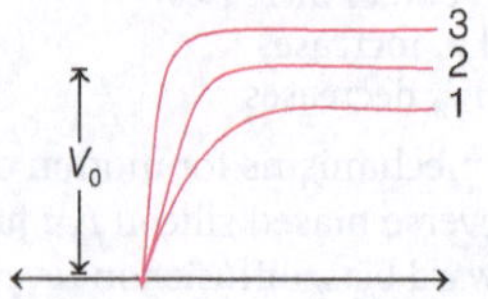

(a) 1 and 3 both correspond to forward bias of junction
(b) 3 corresponds to forward bias of junction and 1 corresponds to reverse bias of junction
(c) 1 corresponds to forward bias and 3 corresponds to reverse bias of junction
(d) 3 and 1 both correspond to reverse bias of junction

56. If a full wave rectifier circuit is operating in 50 Hz mains, then the fundamental frequency in the ripple will be
(a) 50 Hz (b) 70.7 Hz (c) 100 Hz (d) 25 Hz

57. With an AC input from 50 Hz power line, the ripple frequency is
(a) 50 Hz in the DC output of half-wave as well as full wave rectifier
(b) 100 Hz in the DC output of half-wave as well as full wave rectifier
(c) 50 Hz in the DC output of half-wave and 100 Hz in DC output of full wave rectifier
(d) 100 Hz in the DC output of half-wave and 50 Hz in the DC output of full wave rectifier

58. Under which of the following conditions, does an avalanche breakdown in a semiconductor diode occur?
(a) When potential barrier is reduced to zero
(b) When reverse bias exceeds a certain value
(c) When forward bias exceeds a certain value
(d) When forward current exceeds a certain value

59. The width of depletion region in a *p-n* junction diode is 500 nm and an intense electric field of $6 \times 10^5\ \text{Vm}^{-1}$ is also found to exist. The height of potential barrier is
(a) 0.30 V (b) 0.40 V (c) 3 V (d) 4 V

60. In figure given below, assuming the diodes to be ideal *[NCERT Exemplar]*

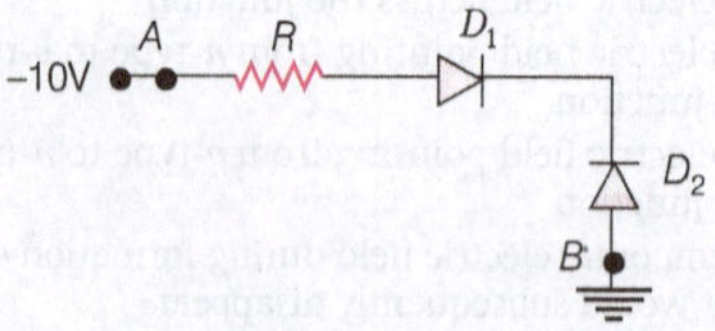

(a) D_1 is forward biased and D_2 is reverse biased and hence current flows from *A* to *B*
(b) D_2 is forward biased and D_1 is reverse biased and hence no current flows from *B* to *A* and *vice-versa*
(c) D_1 and D_2 are both forward biased and hence current flows from *A* to *B*
(d) D_1 and D_2 are both reverse biased and hence no current flows from *A* to *B* and *vice-versa*

61. A 220 V AC supply is connected between points *A* and *B* (figure). What will be the potential difference *V* across the capacitor? *[NCERT Exemplar]*

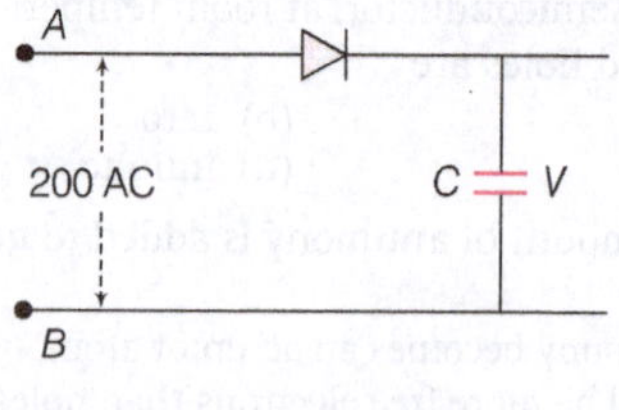

(a) 220V (b) 110 V (c) 0 (d) $220\sqrt{2}$V

62. In the diagram, the input is across the terminals *A* and *C* and the output is across *B* and *D*. Then, the output is

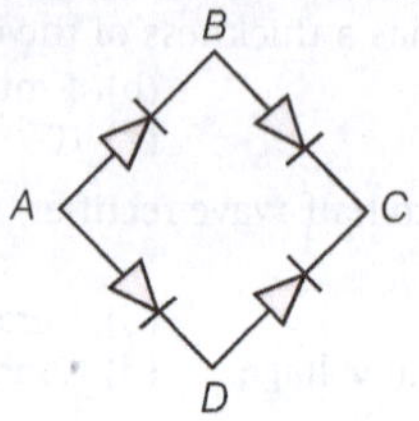

(a) zero (b) same as the input
(c) full wave rectifier (d) half wave rectifier

63. When forward bias is applied to a *p-n* junction, then what happens to the potential barrier V_B and the width of charge depleted region *x* ?
(a) V_B increases, *x* decreases (b) V_B decreases, *x* increases
(c) V_B increases, *x* increases (d) V_B decreases, *x* decreases

64. What is the current in the circuit shown below?

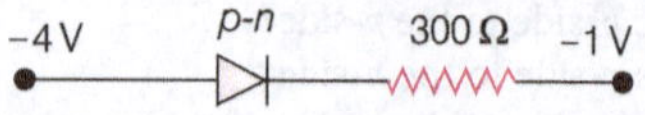

(a) Zero (b) 10^{-2} A (c) 1 A (d) 0.10 A

65. The diode shown in the circuit is a silicon diode. The potential difference between the points *A* and *B* will be

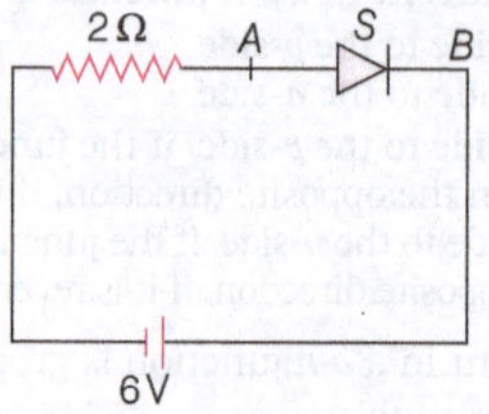

(a) 6 V (b) 0.6 V (c) 0.7 V (d) zero

66. The value of DC voltage in half-wave rectifier in converting AC voltage $V = 100\sin(314t)$ into DC is
(a) 100 V (b) 50 V (c) 30.3 V (d) 0 V

67. For the given circuit of *p-n* junction diode, which of the following statement is correct?

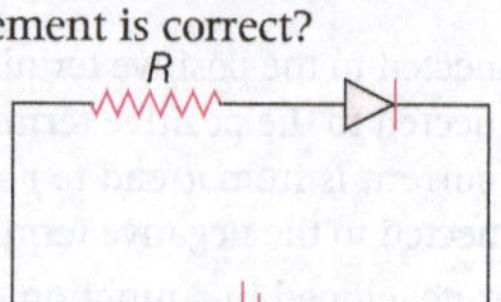

(a) In forward biasing, the voltage across *R* is *V*.
(b) In forward biasing, the voltage across *R* is 2*V*.
(c) In reverse biasing, the voltage across *R* is *V*.
(d) In reverse biasing, the voltage across *R* is 2*V*.

68. In the circuit given below, the value of the current is

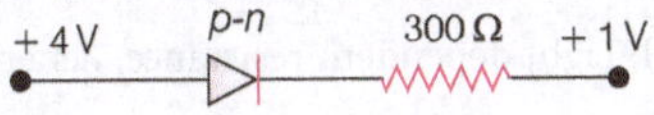

(a) zero (b) 10^{-2} A (c) 10^{2} A (d) 10^{-3} A

69. A potential barrier of 0.50 V exists across a *p-n* junction. If the depletion region is 5.0×10^{-7} m wide, then the intensity of the electric field in this region is

(a) 1×10^{6} Vm^{-1} (b) 1×10^{5} Vm^{-1}
(c) 2×10^{5} Vm^{-1} (d) 2×10^{6} Vm^{-1}

70. The output of the given circuit in figure given below, is *[NCERT Exemplar]*

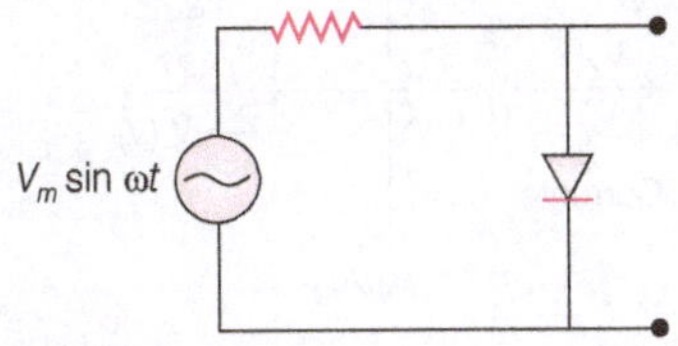

(a) would be zero at all times
(b) would be like a half wave rectifier with positive cycles in output
(c) would be like a half wave rectifier with negative cycles in output
(d) would be like that of a full wave rectifier

71. In the network shown,

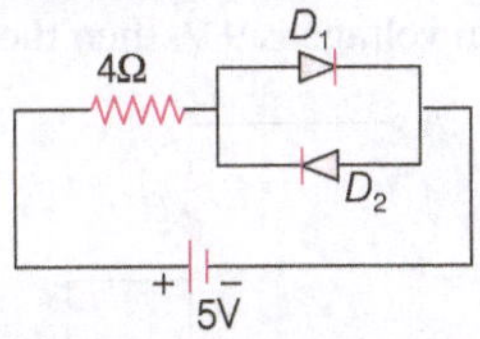

(a) the potential difference across D_2 is 5 V
(b) current through resistor equals 2.25 A
(c) current through diode D_1 is 1.25 A
(d) current through diode D_2 is 1.25 A

72. The current in the circuit will be

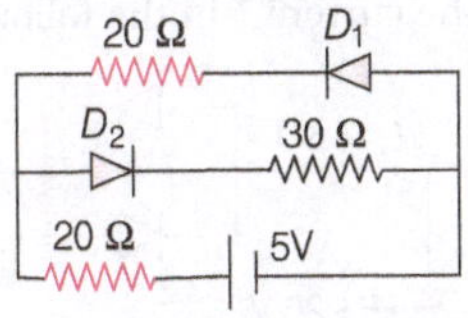

(a) (5/40) A (b) (5/50) A
(c) (5/10) A (d) (5/20) A

73. Which circuit will not show current in ammeter?

(a) 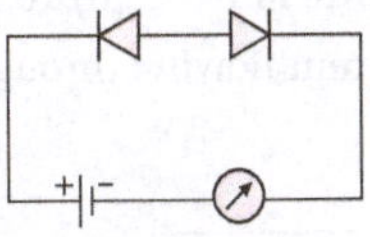 (b) 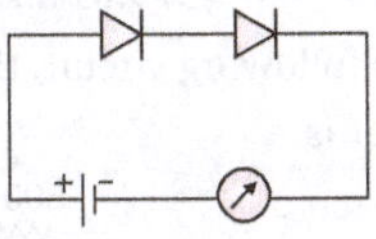

(c) 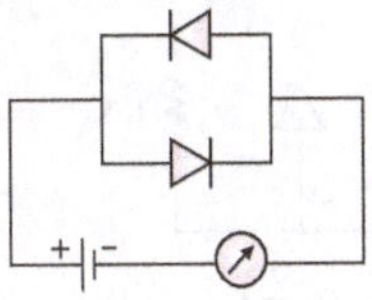 (d) 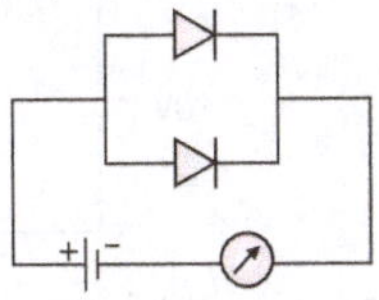

74. In the given figure, which of the diodes are forward biased?

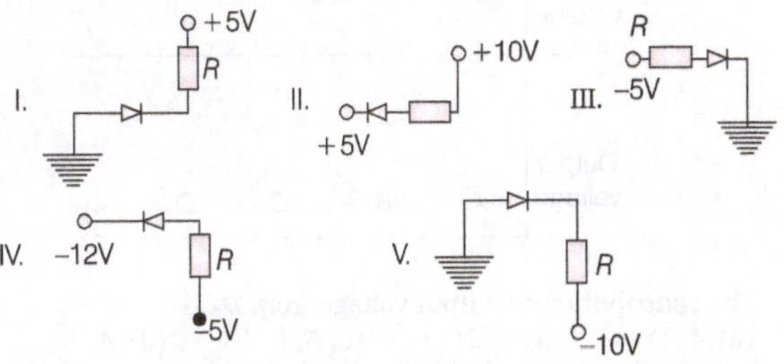

(a) I, II, III (b) II, IV, V (c) I, III, IV (d) II, III, IV

75. The equivalent resistance of the circuit across *AB* is given by

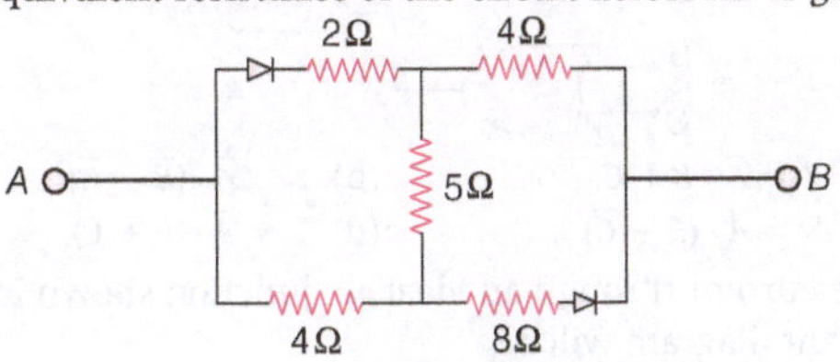

(a) 4Ω (b) 13Ω
(c) 4Ω or 13Ω (d) 4Ω or 0

76. In the circuit shown in figure given below, if the diode forward voltage drop is 0.3 V, the voltage difference between *A* and *B* is *[NCERT Exemplar]*

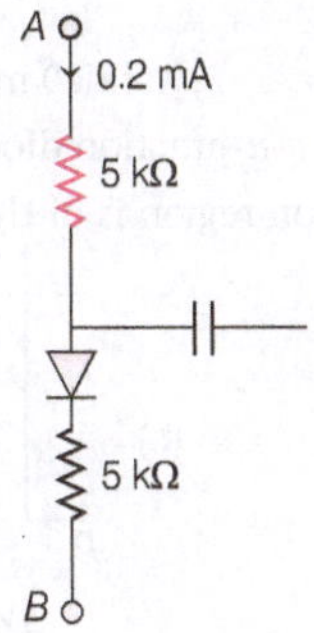

(a) 1.3 V (b) 2.3 V (c) 0 (d) 0.5 V

77. A Zener diode, having breakdown voltage equal to 15 V, is used in a voltage regulator circuit as shown in figure. The current through the diode is

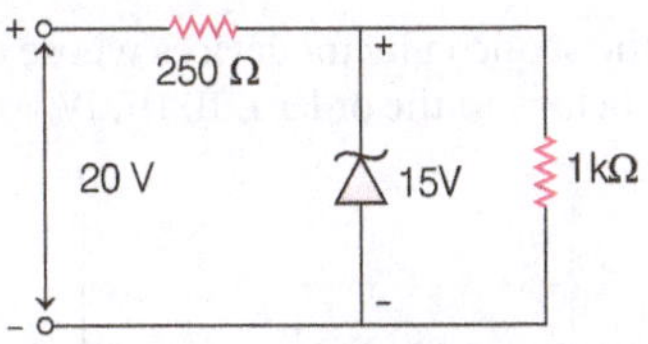

(a) 20 mA (b) 5 mA
(c) 10 mA (d) 15 mA

78. A full wave rectifier circuit along with the input and output voltages is shown in the figure

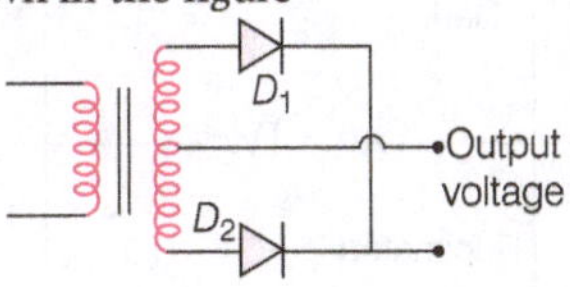

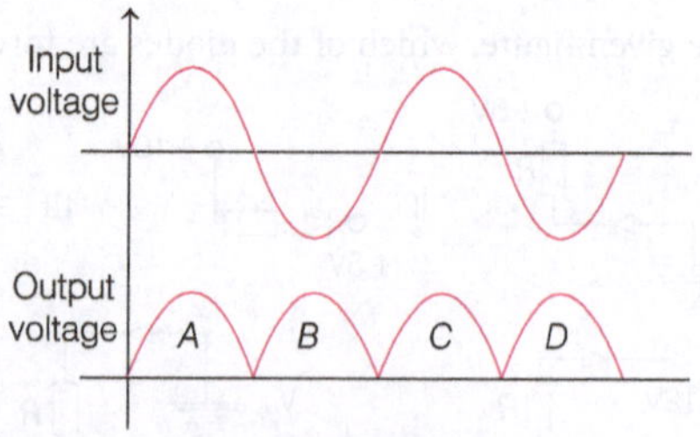

The contribution to output voltage from D_2 is

(a) A, C (b) B, D (c) B, C (d) A, D

79. The boolean expression for the circuit given in figure is

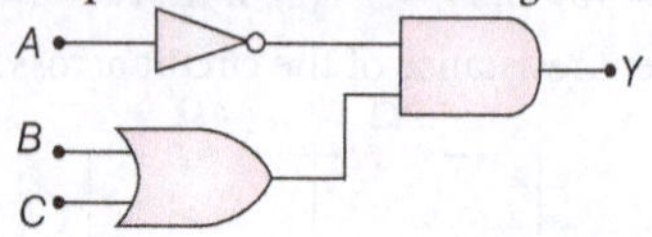

(a) $Y = \overline{A} \cdot B + C$ (b) $Y = \overline{A} \cdot (\overline{B} + \overline{C})$

(c) $Y = \overline{A} \cdot (B + \overline{C})$ (d) $Y = \overline{A} \cdot (B + C)$

80. The current through an ideal *p-n* junction shown in the circuit diagram will be

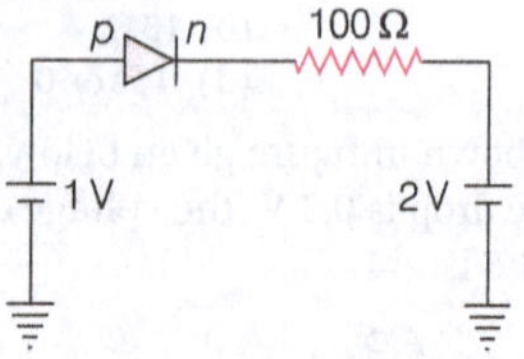

(a) zero (b) 1 mA (c) 10 mA (d) 30 mA

81. In a forwards biased *p-n*-junction diode, the potential barrier in the depletion region is of the form

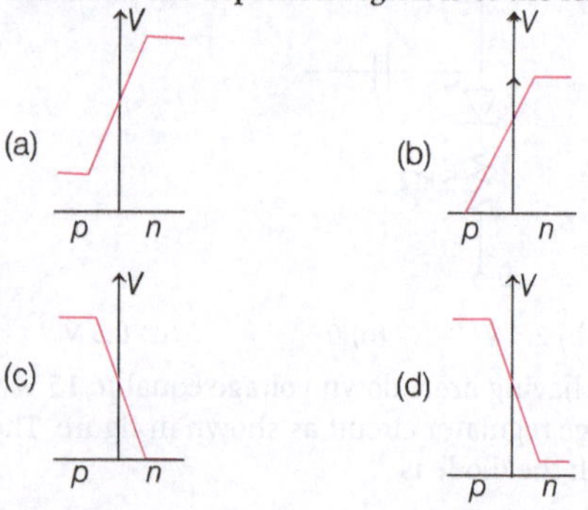

82. Identify the semiconductor devices whose characteristics are given below, in the order I, II, III, IV.

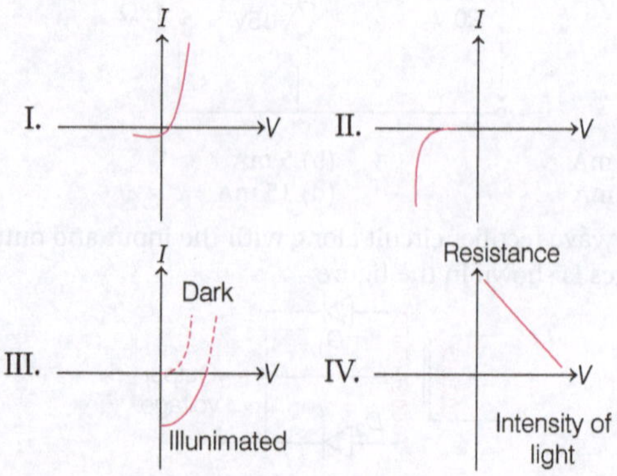

(a) Zener diode, Simple diode, Light dependent resistance, Solar cell

(b) Solar cell, Light dependent resistance, Zener diode, Simple diode

(c) Zener diode, Solar cell, Simple diode, Light dependent resistance

(d) Simple diode, Zener diode, Solar cell, Light dependent resistance

83. The graph given below represents the I -V characteristics of a Zener diode. Which part of the characteristics curve is most relevant for its operation as a voltage regulator?

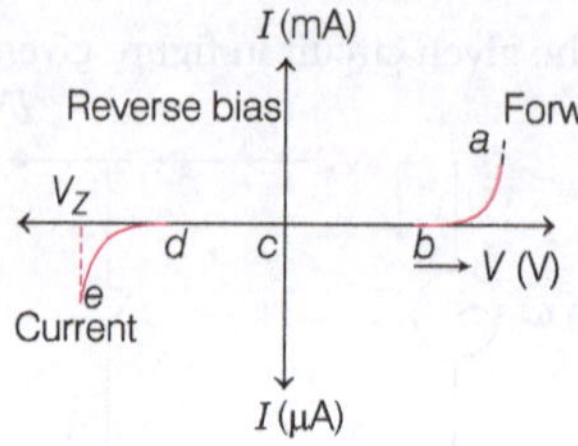

(a) *ab* (b) *bc* (c) *cd* (d) *de*

84. A diode having potential difference 0.5 V across its junction which does not depend on current, is connected in series with resistance of 20 Ω across source. If 0.1 A passes through resistance, then what is the voltage of the source?

(a) 1.5 V (b) 2.0 V (c) 2.5 V (d) 5 V

85. If the voltage between the terminals A and B is 17 V and Zener breakdown voltage is 9 V, then the potential across R is

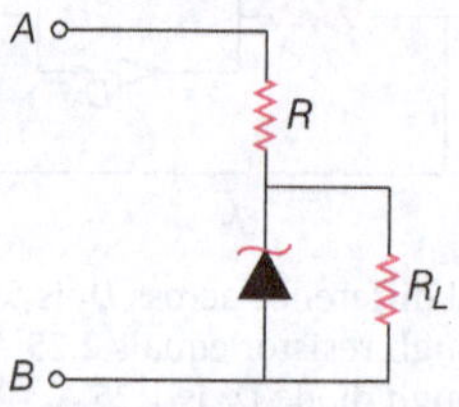

(a) 6 V (b) 8 V (c) 9 V (d) 17 V

86. Assuming the diodes to be of silicon with forward resistance zero, the current I in the following circuit is

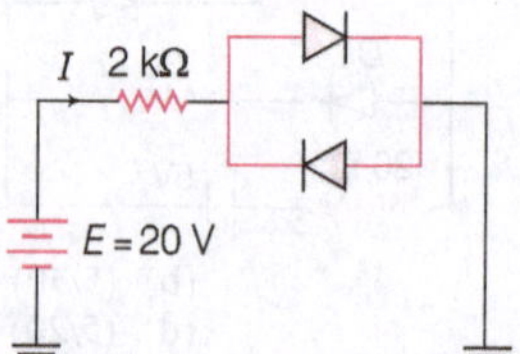

(a) zero (b) 9.65 mA (c) 10 mA (d) 10.36 mA

87. In the following circuit, the current flowing through 1 kΩ resistor is

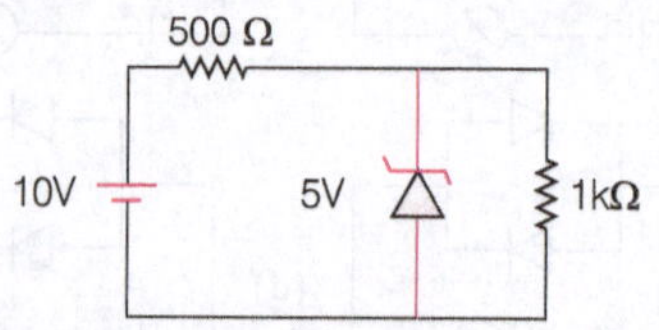

(a) zero (b) 5 mA (c) 10 mA (d) 15 mA

88. In the given circuit,

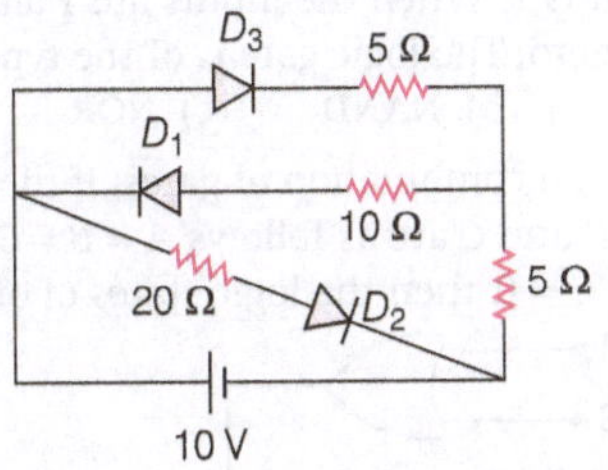

The current through the battery is

(a) 0.5 A (b) 1 A (c) 1.5 A (d) 2 A

89. Currents flowing in each of the circuits A and B respectively are

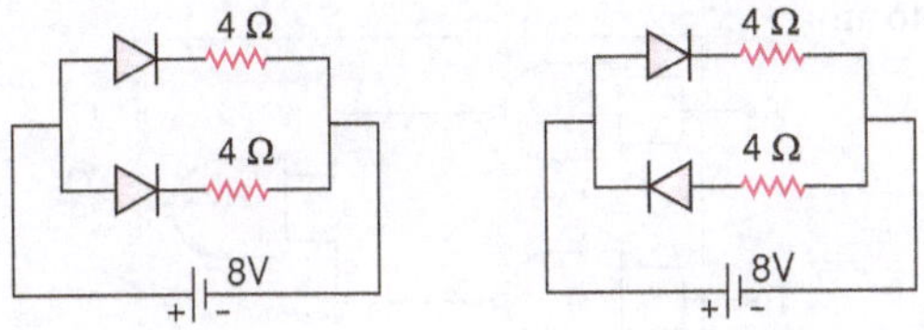

(Circuit A) (Circuit B)

(a) 1 A, 2 A (b) 2A, 1A
(c) 4 A, 2 A (d) 2 A, 4 A

90. An LED is constructed from a *p-n* junction based on a certain semi-conducting material whose energy gap is 1.9 eV, then the wavelength of the emitted light is

(a) 6.5×10^{-7} m (b) 2.9×10^{-9} m
(c) 9.1×10^{-5} m (d) 1.6×10^{-8} m

91. Assume that, each diode as shown in the figure has a forward bias resistance of 50 Ω and an infinite reverse bias resistance. The current through the resistance 150 Ω is

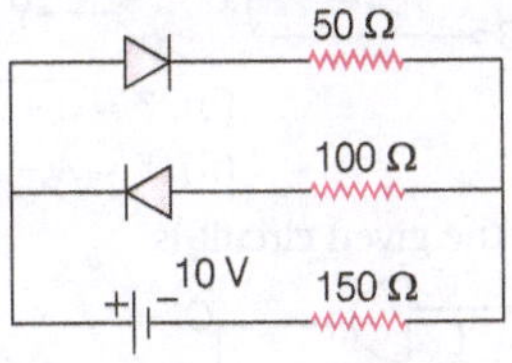

(a) 0.66 A (b) 0.05 A
(c) zero (d) 0.04 A

92. The given graph represents *V-I* characteristic for a semiconductor device.

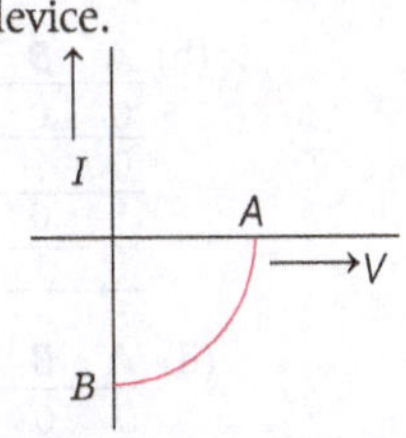

Which of the following statement is correct?

(a) It is *V-I* characteristic for solar cell, where point *A* represents open circuit voltage and point *B* short circuit current.
(b) It is for a solar cell and points *A* and *B* represent open circuit voltage and current, respectively.
(c) It is for a photodiode and points *A* and *B* represent open circuit voltage and current, respectively.
(d) It is for a LED and points *A* and *B* represents open circuit voltage and short circuit current, respectively.

93. In the circuit shown below, assume the diode to be ideal. When V_i increases from 2 V to 6 V, then the change in the current is (in mA)

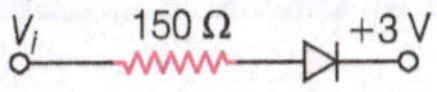

(a) zero (b) 20 (c) 80/3 (d) 40

94. The circuit has two oppositely connected ideal diodes in parallel as shown in figure. What is the current flowing in the circuit ?

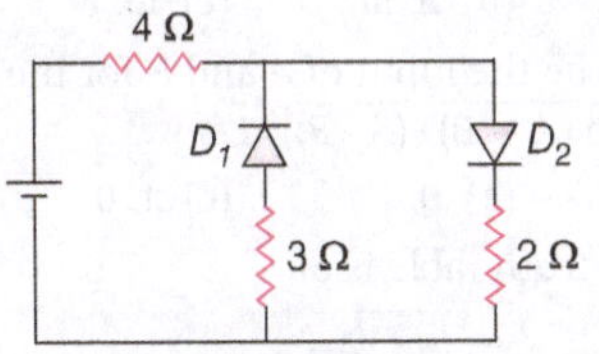

(a) 1.33 A (b) 1.71 A (c) 2.00 A (d) 2.31 A

95. Find the current in the circuit.

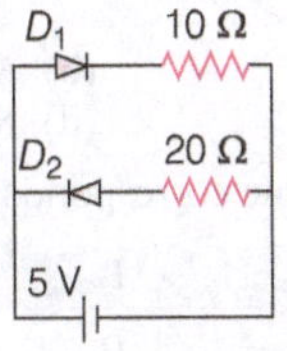

(a) 0.75 A (b) Zero (c) 0.25 A (d) 0.5 A

96. In the Boolean algebra, which of the following is not equal to *A*?

(a) $A \cdot A$ (b) $A + A$ (c) $\overline{A} \cdot A$ (d) $\overline{\overline{A} + \overline{A}}$

97. The given symbol represents

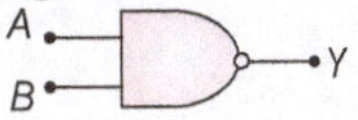

(a) NAND gate (b) OR gate
(c) AND gate (d) NOR gate

98. The boolean expression of NOR gate is

(a) $Y = A + B$ (b) $Y = \overline{A + B}$
(c) $Y = A \cdot B$ (d) $Y = \overline{A \cdot B}$

99. Which represents NAND gate?

(a) 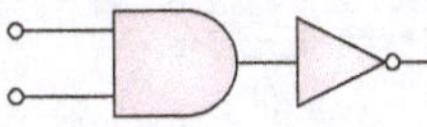 (b) 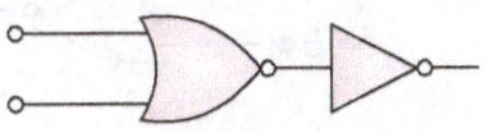

(c) 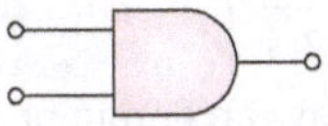 (d) 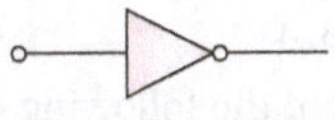

100. The following truth table corresponds to the logic gate

A	B	X
0	0	0
0	1	1
1	0	1
1	1	1

(a) NAND (b) OR (c) AND (d) XOR

101. Below we give four entries for the truth table of two point input OR gate. Which two are wrong?

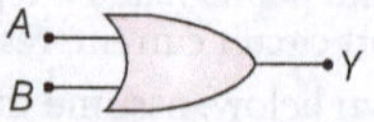

	A	B	Y
i	1	0	1
ii	1	1	0
iii	0	0	1
iv	0	1	1

(a) i, ii (b) ii, iii (c) iii, iv (d) iv, i

102. What will be the input of A and B for the boolean expression $(A + B) \cdot (A \cdot B) = 1$?

(a) 0, 0 (b) 0, 1 (c) 1, 0 (d) 1, 1

103. The given truth table is of

A	X
0	1
1	0

(a) OR gate (b) AND gate
(c) NOT gate (d) None of these

104. The below truth table corresponds to

A	B	Y
0	0	1
1	0	1
0	1	1
1	1	0

(a) NAND gate
(b) XOR gate
(c) OR gate
(d) NOR gate

105. Given below are four logic gate symbols (figure). Those for OR, NOR and NAND are respectively

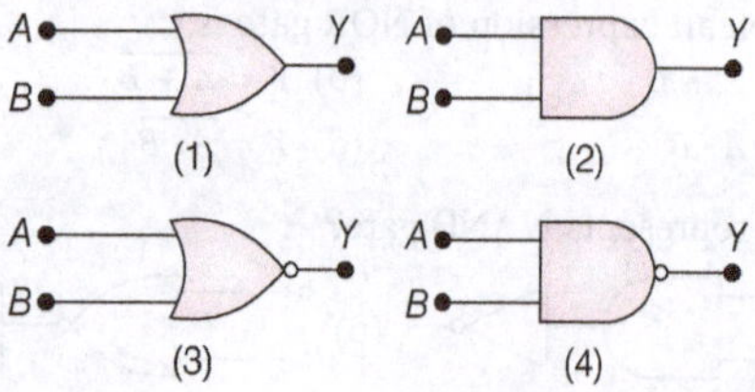

(a) 1, 4, 3 (b) 4, 1, 2
(c) 1, 3, 4 (d) 4, 2, 1

106. Which of the following gates will have an output of 1?

(a) 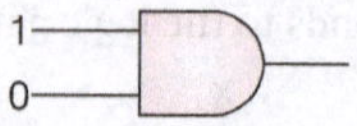

(b) 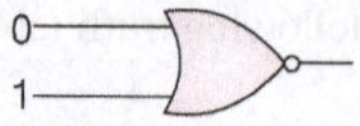

(c) 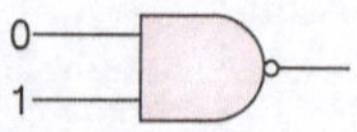

(d) 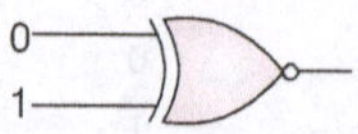

107. When the inputs of two input logic gates are 0 and 0, then the output is 1. When the inputs are 1 and 0, then the output is zero. The logic gate is of the type

(a) XOR (b) NAND (c) NOR (d) OR

108. For the given combination of gates, if the logic states of inputs A, B and C are as follows $A = B = C = 0$ and $A = B = 1, C = 0$, then the logic states of output D are

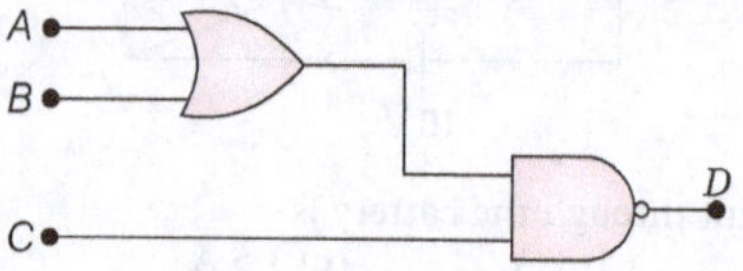

(a) 0, 0 (b) 0, 1 (c) 1,0 (d) 1, 1

109. The combination of NAND gates shown here are equivalent to an

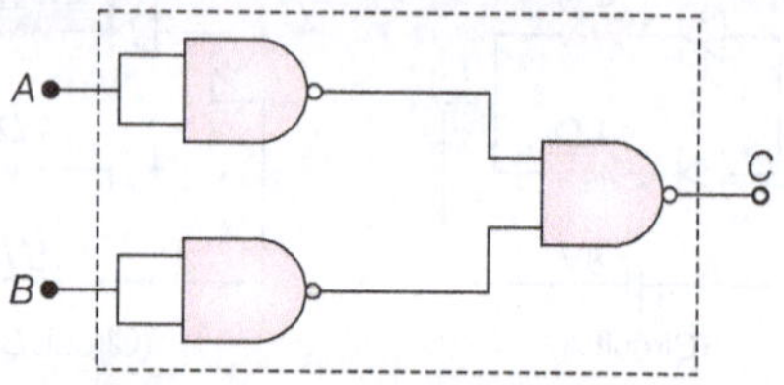

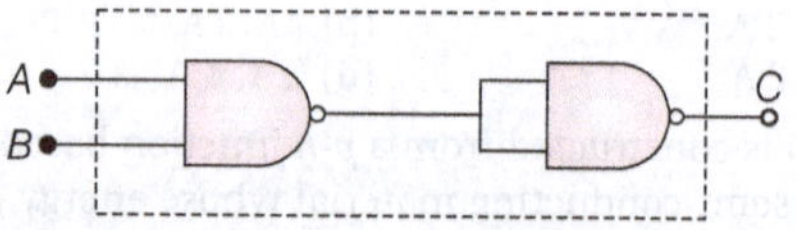

(a) OR gate and an AND gate, respectively
(b) AND gate and a NOT gate, respectively
(c) AND gate and an OR gate, respectively
(d) OR gate and a NOT gate, respectively

110. The boolean expression for the circuit given in the figure is

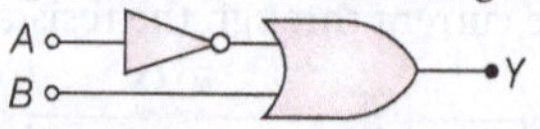

(a) $Y = A + \overline{B}$ (b) $Y = \overline{A + B}$
(c) $Y = \overline{A} + B$ (d) $Y = A + B$

111. Truth table for the given circuit is **[NCERT Exemplar]**

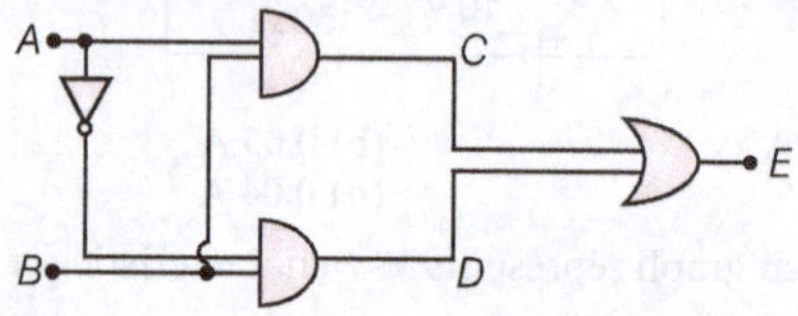

(a)

A	B	E
0	0	1
0	1	0
1	0	1
1	1	0

(b)

A	B	E
0	0	1
0	1	0
1	0	0
1	1	0

(c)

A	B	E
0	0	0
0	1	1
1	0	0
1	1	1

(d)

A	B	E
0	0	0
0	1	1
1	0	1
1	1	0

112. The logic circuit shown below has the input waveforms A and B as shown. Pick out the correct output waveform.

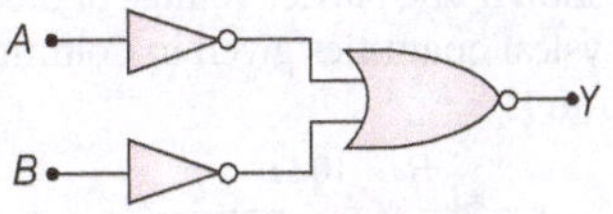

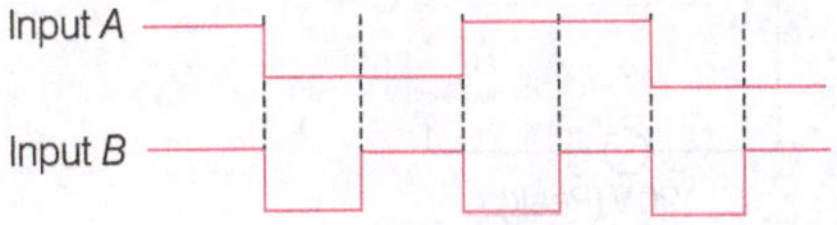

(a) 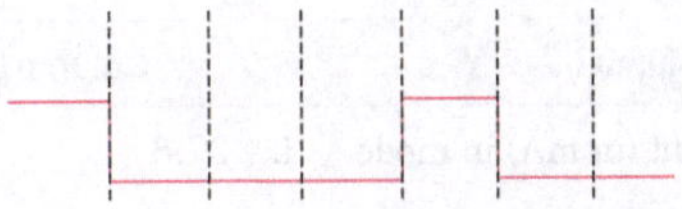

(b) 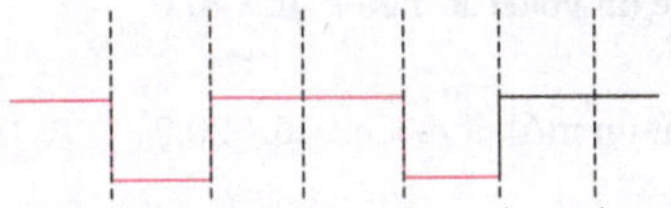

(c) 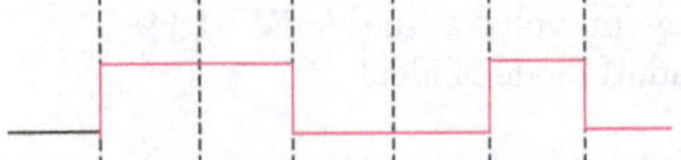

(d) 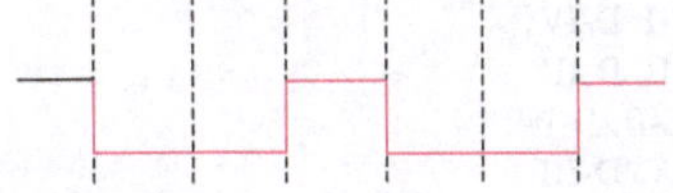

113. A researcher wants an alarm to sound when the temperature of air in his controlled research chamber rises above 40°C or falls below 20°C. The alarm can be triggered by the output of a

(a) NOT gate (b) AND gate
(c) NAND gate (d) OR gate

114 The combination of gates shown below yields is

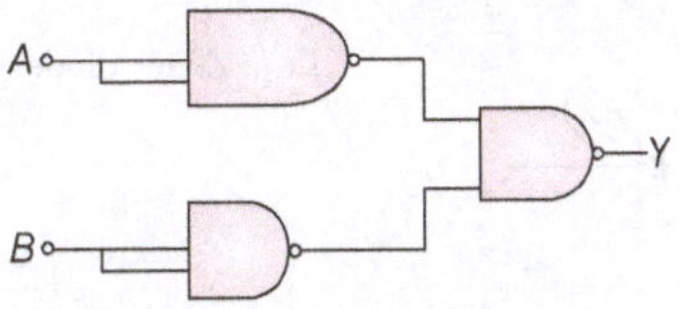

(a) NAND gate (b) NOR gate
(c) XOR gate (d) OR gate

115. The arrangement shown in figure performs the logic function of

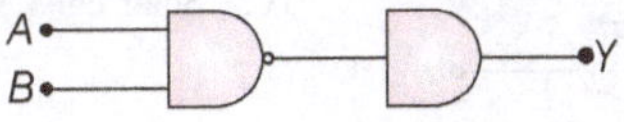

(a) AND gate (b) NAND gate
(c) OR gate (d) XOR gate

116. The equivalent circuit is

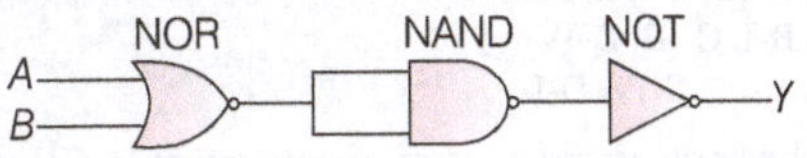

The circuit represents
(a) NAND gate
(b) OR gate
(c) AND gate
(d) NOR gate

117. The inputs to the digital circuit are as shown below. The output Y is

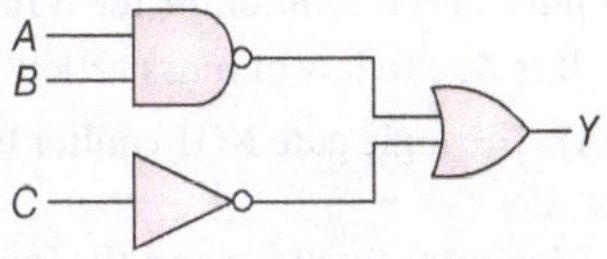

(a) $A + B + \overline{C}$ (b) $(A + B)\,\overline{C}$
(c) $\overline{A} + \overline{B} + \overline{C}$ (d) $\overline{A} + \overline{B} + C$

118 The following logic gate circuit in equivalent to an

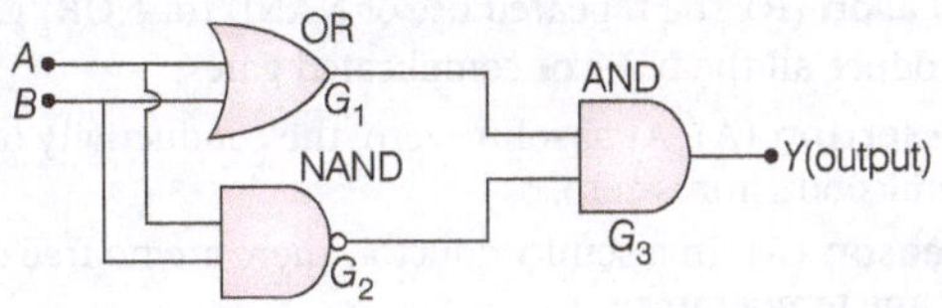

(a) NAND (b) OR
(c) XOR (d) NOT

119. Out of the following curves, which one represents a digital signal?

(a) 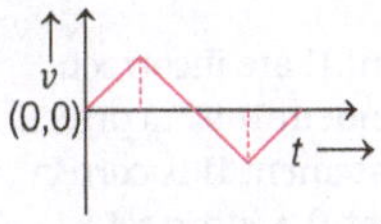

(b) 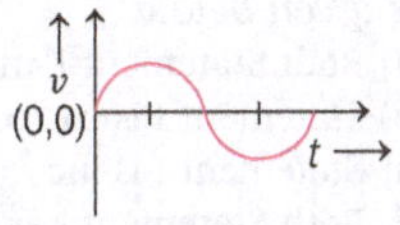

(c) 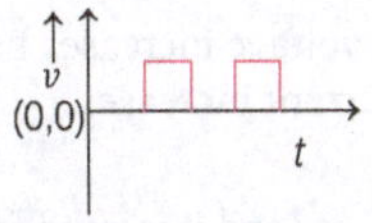

(d) 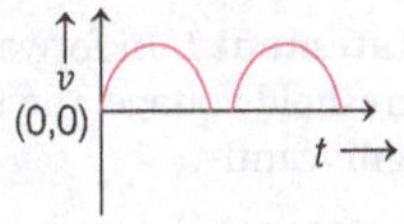

120. The figure shows a logic circuit with two inputs A and B and the output C. The voltage waveforms across A, B and C are as given. The logic circuit gate is

(a) OR gate
(b) NOR gate
(c) AND gate
(d) NAND gate

Assertion and Reason

Directions (Q. Nos. 1-5) *These questions consist of two statements each printed as Assertion (A) and Reason (R). While answering these questions, you are required to choose any one of the following four responses.*

(a) Both A and R are true but R is not the correct explanation of A.
(b) A is true but R is false.
(c) A is false but R is true.
(d) Both A and R are true and R is the correct explanation of A.

1. **Assertion** (A) If the temperature of a semiconductor is increased, then its resistance decreases.

   Reason (R) The energy gap between conduction band and valence band is very small.

2. **Assertion** (A) The number of conduction electrons in a *p*-type silicon semiconductor is less than the number of electrons in a pure silicon semiconductor at room temperature.

   Reason (R) It is due to law of mass action.

3. **Assertion** (A) The logic gate NOT cannot be built using diode.

   Reason (R) The output voltage and the input voltage of the diode have 180° phase difference.

4. **Assertion** (A) NAND or NOR gates are called digital building blocks.

   Reason (R) The repeated use of NAND (or NOR) gates can produce all the basic or complicated gates.

5. **Assertion** (A) At absolute zero, the conductivity of semiconductor is zero.

   Reason (R) In a semiconductor, there are no free electrons at any temperature.

Statement Type Questions

Directions (Q. Nos. 1-5) *These questions consist of two statements, choose the most appropriate answer from the options given below*

(a) Both Statement I and Statement II are incorrect.
(b) Statement I is correct but Statement II is incorrect.
(c) Statement I is incorrect but Statement II is correct.
(d) Both Statement I and Statement II are correct.

1. **Statement I** In forward bias as voltage increases beyond threshold voltage, the forward current increases significantly.

   Statement II Ohm's law states $V \propto I$ and it is valid for diode.

2. **Statement I** In equilibrium condition, *p*-side of a *p*-*n* junction is at positive potential.

   Statement II A *p*-type semiconductor contains more holes than electrons.

3. **Statement I** Silicon is preferred over germanium for making semiconductor devices.

   Statement II The energy band for germanium is more than the energy of silicon.

4. **Statement I** Ionisation energy of isolated pentavalent atom of phosphorus is very large, so in *n*-type semiconductor, there are no free charge carriers at room temperature.

   Statement II When current flows through a *p*-*n* junction diode, it becomes hot.

5. **Statement I** The conductivity of an intrinsic semiconductor depends on its temperature.

   Statement II The conductivity of an intrinsic semiconductor is slightly higher than that of a lightly doped *p*-type semiconductor.

Match the Columns

1. In the circuit shown, the barrier voltage of diode is 0.7 V. Match the physical quantities given in Column I to the results given in Column II.

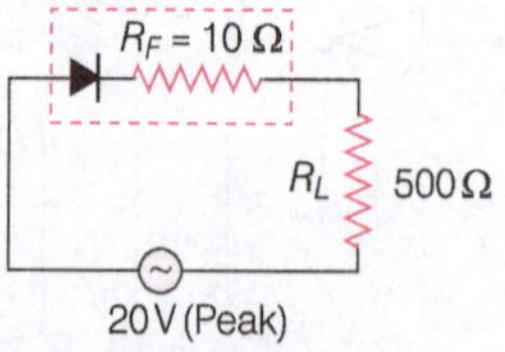

Column I	Column II
A. Peak current (in mA) in diode	I. 37.8
B. Peak voltage (in volts) at the ends of load	II. 40.0
C. Peak current (in mA), if diode is ideal	III. 20.2
D. Peak voltage (in volts) at the ends of load, if diode is ideal	IV. 18.9

Choose the correct answer from the options given below.
(a) A-III, B-II, C-I, D-IV
(b) A-I, B-IV, C-II, D-III
(c) A-IV, B-III, C-II, D-I
(d) A-II, B-I, C-IV, D-III

2. Match the symbol of diode given in Column I to the result given in Column II.

Column I	Column II
A. 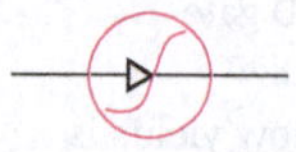	I. Light emitting diode
B. 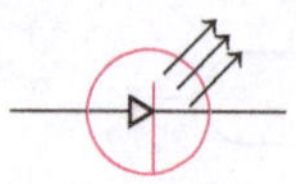	II. Zener diode
C. 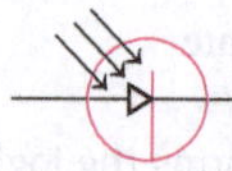	III. Photodiode
D. 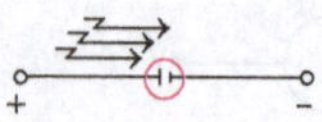	IV. Solar cells

Choose the correct answer from the options given below.
(a) A-I, B-III, C-IV, D-II
(b) A-II, B-III, C-I, D-IV
(c) A-II, B-I, C-III, D-IV
(d) A-II, B-III, C-IV, D-I

3. Match the boolean expression of gate given in Column I to the gate given in Column II.

Column I	Column II
A. $Y = A + B$	I. NAND gate
B. $Y = A \cdot B$	II. NOT gate
C. $Y = \overline{A}$	III. AND gate
D. $Y = \overline{A \cdot B}$	IV. OR gate

Choose the correct answer from the options given below.
(a) A-III, B-II, C-I, D-IV
(b) A-IV, B-III, C-II, D-I
(c) A-I, B-II, C-III, D-IV
(d) A-IV, B-III, C-II, D-I

4. Match the symbol of gate given in Column I to the gate given in Column II.

Column I	Column II
A. 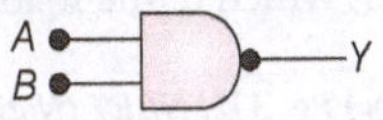	I. NOT
B. 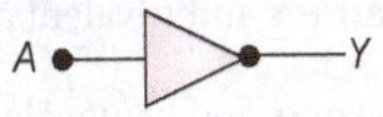	II. OR
C. 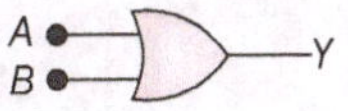	III. NAND
D. 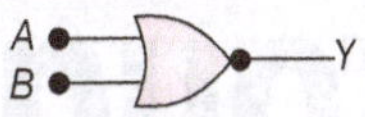	IV. NOR

Choose the correct answer from the options given below.
(a) A-III, B-I, C-II, D-IV
(b) A-IV, B-III, C-I, D-II
(c) A-II, B-IV, C-III, D-I
(d) A-I, B-II, C-IV, D-III

5. Match the Column I with Column II.

Column I	Column II
A. $\overline{A+B}$	I. $A + B$
B. $A + A \cdot B$	II. AB
C. $A(\overline{A} + B)$	III. A
D. $\overline{\overline{A} \cdot \overline{B}}$	IV. $\overline{A} \cdot \overline{B}$

Choose the correct answer from the options given below.
(a) A-II, B-I, C-III, D-IV
(b) A-II, B-III, C-I, D-IV
(c) A-IV, B-III, C-II, D-I
(d) A-IV, B-III, C-I, D-II

Final Check Through PYQs

Module-I Semiconductors and its Types

1. The electron concentration in an n-type semiconductor is the same as hole concentration in a p-type semiconductor. An external field (electric) is applied across each of them. Compare the currents in them. ***[NCERT (New) Pg. 331, NEET 2021]***

(a) Current in n-type = Current in p-type
(b) Current in p-type > Current in n-type
(c) Current in n-type > Current in p-type
(d) No current will flow in p-type, current will only flow in n-type

2. An intrinsic semiconductor is converted into n-type extrinsic semiconductor by doping it with ***[NCERT (New) Pg. 330, NEET (Oct.) 2020]***

(a) phosphorus
(b) aluminium
(c) silver
(d) germanium

3. The solids which have the negative temperature coefficient of resistance are

(a) insulators only ***[NCERT (New) Pg. 324, NEET (Sep.) 2020]***
(b) semiconductors only
(c) insulators and semiconductors
(d) metals

4. For a p-type semiconductor, which of the following statements is true? ***[NCERT (New) Pg. 331, NEET (National) 2019]***

(a) Holes are the majority carriers and trivalent atoms are the dopants.
(b) Holes are the majority carriers and pentavalent atoms are the dopants.
(c) Electrons are the majority carriers and pentavalent atoms are the dopants.
(d) Electrons are the majority carriers and trivalent atoms are the dopants.

Module-II Semiconductor Diode and Rectifiers

5. Consider the following statements A and B and identify the correct answer. ***[NCERT (Old) Pg. 489, NEET 2024]***

A. For a solar-cell, the I-V characteristics lies in the (IV) quadrant of the given graph.
B. In a reverse biased p-n junction diode, the current measured in (μA), is due to majority charge carriers.

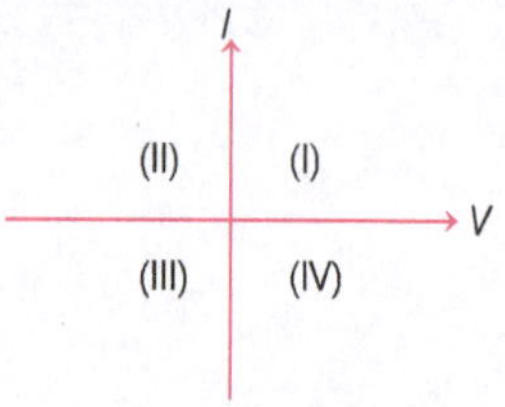

(a) A is correct but B is incorrect.
(b) A is incorrect but B is correct.
(c) Both A and B are correct.
(d) Both A and B are incorrect.

6. Choose the correct circuit which can achieve the bridge balance. ***[NCERT (New) Pg. 335, NEET 2024]***

(a)
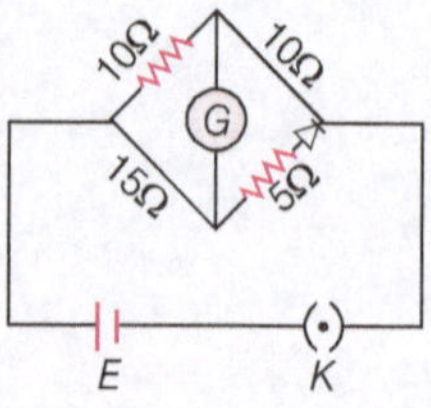

(b)
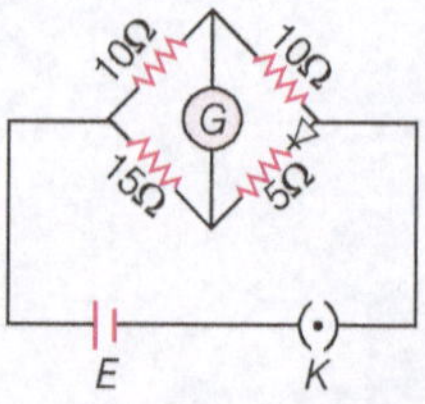

(c)
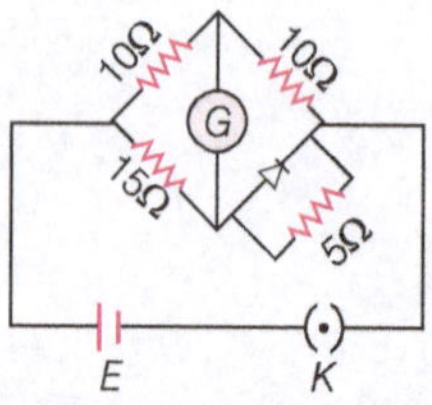

(d)
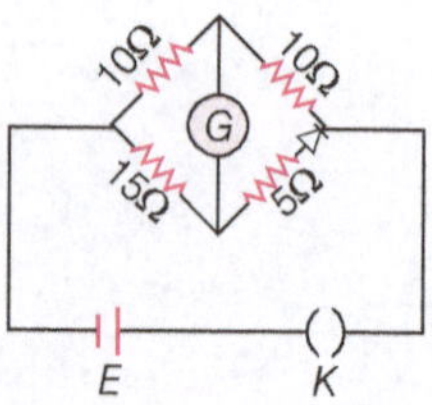

7. A full wave rectifier circuit consists of two p-n junction diodes, a centre-tapped transformer, capacitor and a load resistance. Which of these components remove the AC ripple from the rectified output? ***[NCERT (New) Pg. 335, NEET 2023]***

(a) p-n junction diodes
(b) Capacitor
(c) Load resistance
(d) A centre-tapped transformer

8. **Statement I** Photovoltaic devices can convert optical radiation into electricity.

Statement II Zener diode is designed to operate under reverse bias in breakdown region.

In the light of the above statements, choose the most appropriate answer from the options given below ***[NCERT (Old) Pg. 485, NEET 2023]***

(a) Both Statement I and Statement II are incorrect.
(b) Statement I is correct but Statement II is incorrect.
(c) Statement I is correct but Statement II is correct.
(d) Both Statement I and Statement II are correct.

9. In half-wave rectification, if the input frequency is 60 Hz, then the output frequency would be *[NCERT (New) Pg. 338, NEET 2022]*

(a) 30 Hz (b) 60 Hz
(c) 120 Hz (d) zero

10.

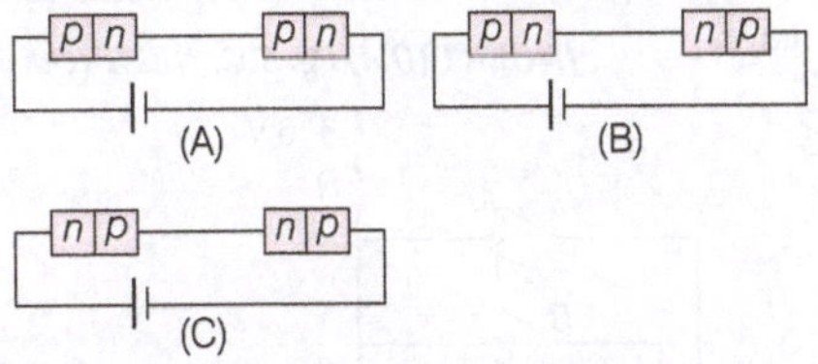

In the given circuits (A), (B) and (C), the potential drop across the two *p-n* junctions are equal, in *[NCERT (New) Pg. 334, NEET 2022]*

(a) circuit (B) only (b) circuit (C) only
(c) Both circuits (A) and (C) (d) circuit (A) only

11. Consider the following statements (A) and (B) and identify the correct answer. *[NCERT (Old) Pg. 485, NEET 2021]*

(A) A zener diode is connected in reverse bias, when used as a voltage regulator.
(B) The potential barrier of *p-n* junction lies between 0.1 V to 0.3 V.

(a) (A) and (B) both are correct.
(b) (A) and (B) both are incorrect.
(c) (A) is correct but (B) is incorrect.
(d) (A) is incorrect but (B) is correct.

12. Out of the following, which one is a forward biased diode? *[NCERT (New) Pg. 335, NEET (Oct.) 2020]*

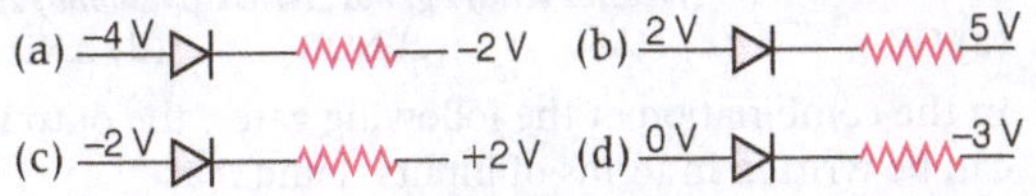

13. The increase in the width of the depletion region in a *p-n* junction diode is due to *[NCERT (New) Pg. 335, NEET (Sep.) 2020]*

(a) reverse bias only
(b) both forward bias and reverse bias
(c) increase in forward current
(d) forward bias only

14. An LED is constructed from a *p-n* junction diode using GaAsP. The energy gap is 1.9 eV. The wavelength of the light emitted will be equal to *[NCERT (Old) Pg. 488, NEET (Odisha) 2019]*

(a) 10.4×10^{-26} m (b) 654 nm
(c) 654 Å (d) 654×10^{-11} m

15. In a *p-n* junction diode, change in temperature due to heating *[NCERT (New) Pg. 335, NEET 2018]*

(a) does not affect resistance of *p-n* junction
(b) affects only forward resistance
(c) affects only reverse resistance
(d) affects the overall *V-I* characteristics of *p-n* junction

16. Which one of the following represents forward bias diode? *[NCERT (New) Pg. 335, NEET 2017]*

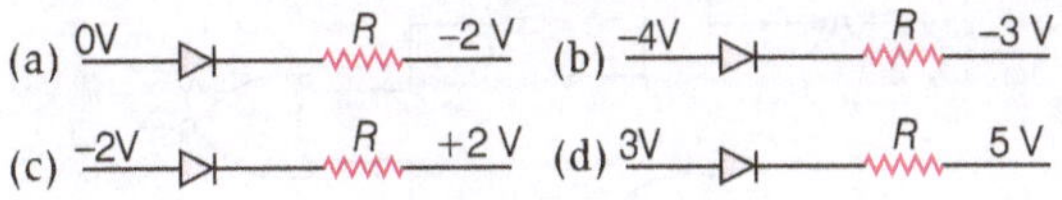

17. Consider the junction diode as ideal. The value of current flowing through *AB* is *[NCERT (New) Pg. 335, NEET 2016]*

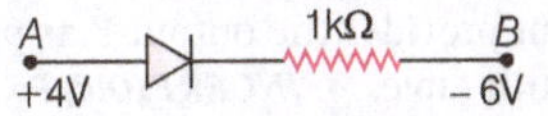

(a) 10^{-2} A (b) 10^{-1} A
(c) 10^{-3} A (d) 0

18. The given circuit has two ideal diodes connected as shown in the figure. The current flowing through the resistance R_1 will be *[NCERT (New) Pg. 335, NEET 2016]*

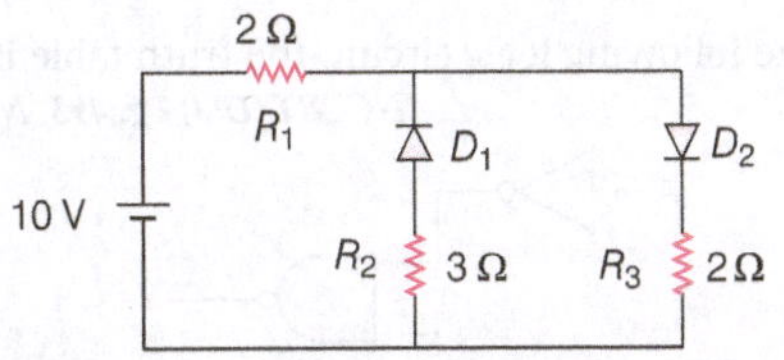

(a) 2.5 A (b) 10.0 A
(c) 1.43 A (d) 3.13 A

19. If in a *p-n* junction, a square input signal of 10 V is applied as shown *[NCERT (New) Pg. 335, AIPMT 2015]*

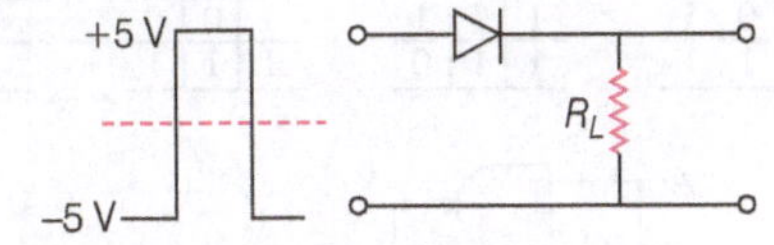

then the output across R_L will be

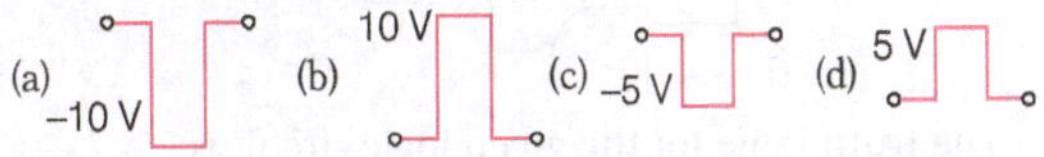

20. In the given figure, a diode *D* is connected to an external resistance $R = 100\,\Omega$ and an emf of 3.5V. If the barrier potential developed across the diode is 0.5 V, the current in the circuit will be *[NCERT (New) Pg. 335, AIPMT 2015]*

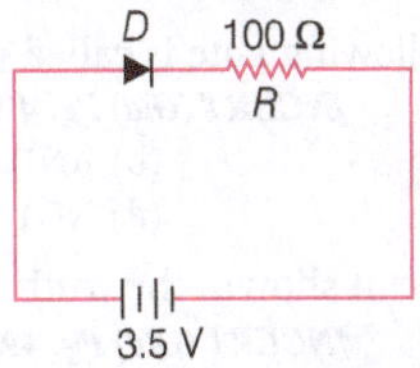

(a) 30 mA (b) 40 mA
(c) 20 mA (d) 35 mA

Module-III Logic Gates

21. The output Y of the given logic gate is similar to the output of an/a *[NCERT (Old) Pg. 493, NEET 2024]*

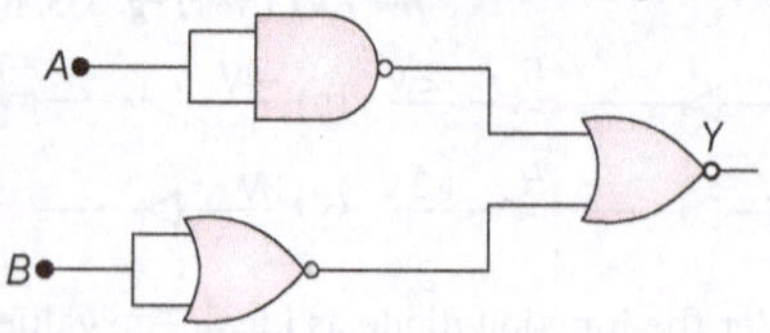

(a) NAND gate (b) NOR gate
(c) OR gate (d) AND gate

22. A logic circuit provides the output Y as per the following truth table. *[NCERT (Old) Pg. 493, NEET 2024]*

A	B	Y
0	0	1
0	1	0
1	0	1
1	1	0

The expression for the output Y is
(a) $A.B + \overline{A}$ (b) $A \cdot \overline{B} + \overline{A}$ (c) $\overline{B}$ (d) B

23. For the following logic circuit, the truth table is *[NCERT (Old) Pg. 493, NEET 2023]*

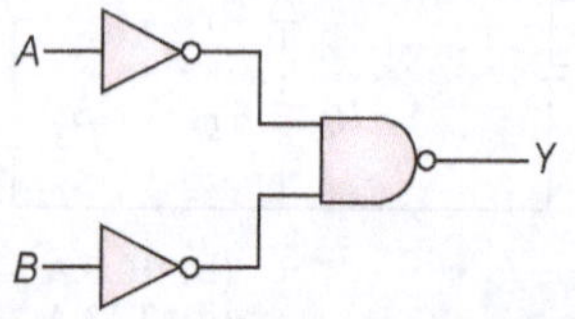

(a)

A	B	Y
0	0	0
0	1	1
1	0	1
1	1	1

(b)

A	B	Y
0	0	1
0	1	0
1	0	1
1	1	0

(c)

A	B	Y
0	0	0
0	1	0
1	0	0
1	1	1

(d)

A	B	Y
0	0	1
0	1	1
1	0	1
1	1	0

24.

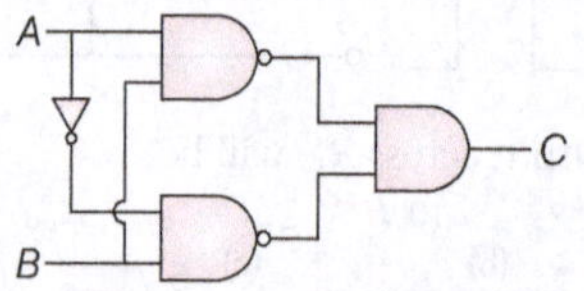

The truth table for the given logic circuit is *[NCERT (Old) Pg. 493, NEET 2022]*

(a)

A	B	C
0	0	1
0	1	0
1	0	0
1	1	1

(b)

A	B	C
0	0	1
0	1	0
1	0	1
1	1	0

(c)

A	B	C
0	0	0
0	1	1
1	0	0
1	1	1

(d)

A	B	C
0	0	1
0	1	1
1	0	1
1	1	0

25. Which of the following gate is called universal gate? *[NCERT (Old) Pg. 493, NEET (Oct.) 2020]*

(a) OR gate (b) AND gate
(c) NAND gate (d) NOT gate

26. For the logic circuit shown, the truth table is *[NCERT (Old) Pg. 493, NEET (Sep.) 2020]*

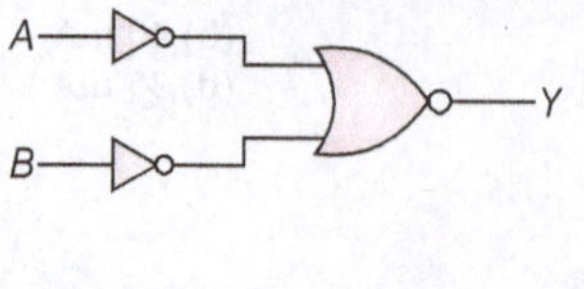

(a)

A	B	C
0	0	0
0	1	1
1	0	1
1	1	1

(b)

A	B	C
0	0	1
0	1	1
1	0	1
1	1	0

(c)

A	B	C
0	0	1
0	1	0
1	0	0
1	1	0

(d)

A	B	C
0	0	0
0	1	0
1	0	0
1	1	1

27. The circuit diagram shown here corresponds to the logic gate, *[NCERT (Old) Pg. 502, NEET (Odisha) 2019]*

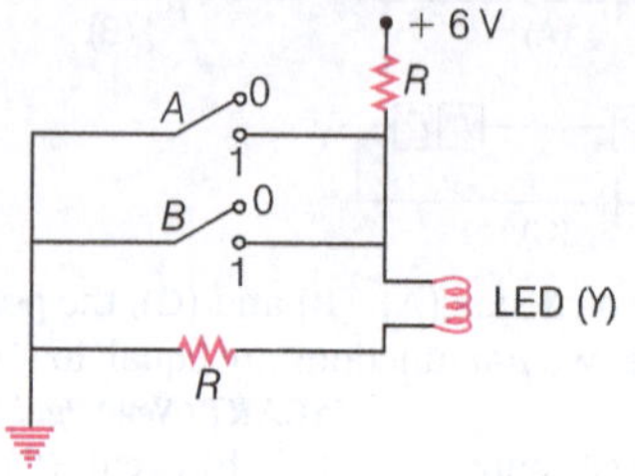

(a) NOR (b) AND
(c) OR (d) NAND

28.

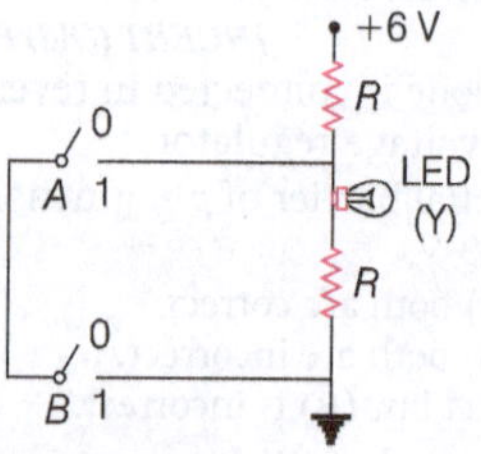

The correct boolean operation represented by the circuit diagram drawn is *[NCERT (Old) Pg. 502, NEET (National) 2019]*

(a) OR (b) NAND (c) NOR (d) AND

29. In the combination of the following gates, the output Y can be written in terms of inputs A and B as *[NCERT (Old) Pg. 493, NEET 2018]*

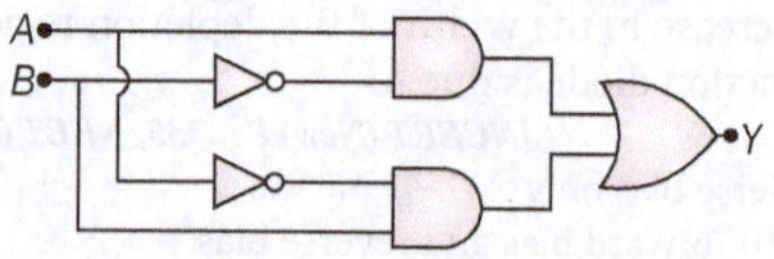

(a) $\overline{A \cdot B} + A \cdot B$
(b) $A \cdot \overline{B} + \overline{A} \cdot B$
(c) $\overline{A \cdot B}$
(d) $\overline{A + B}$

30. The given electrical network is equivalent to *[NCERT (Old) Pg. 493, NEET 2017]*

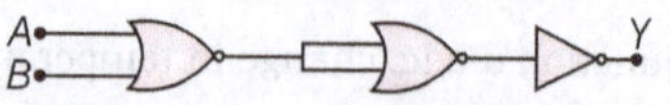

(a) AND gate (b) OR gate
(c) NOR gate (d) NOT gate

Final Check

31. To get output 1 for the following circuit, the correct choice for the input is *[NCERT (Old) Pg. 493, EET 2016]*

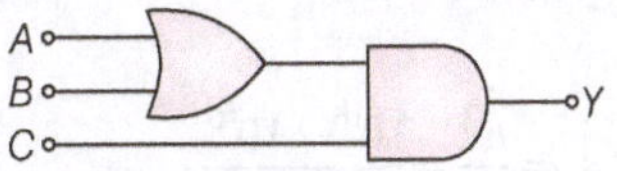

(a) $A = 1, B = 0, C = 0$
(b) $A = 1, B = 1, C = 0$
(c) $A = 1, B = 0, C = 1$
(d) $A = 0, B = 1, C = 0$

32. Which logic gate is represented by the following combination of logic gates? *[NCERT (Old) Pg. 493, AIPMT 2015]*

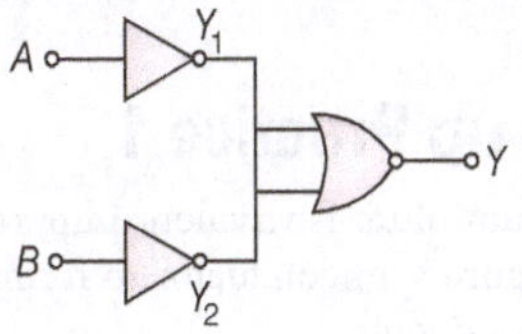

(a) OR (b) NAND (c) AND (d) NOR

Answers

Step up Practice 1

1 (a)	2 (a)	3 (b)	4 (d)	5 (d)	6 (c)	7 (c)	8 (b)	9 (d)	10 (b)
11 (c)	12 (b)	13 (c)	14 (d)	15 (a)	16 (c)	17 (c)	18 (c)		

Step up Practice 2

1 (c)	2 (b)	3 (a)	4 (b)	5 (c)	6 (a)	7 (b)	8 (d)	9 (a)	10 (d)
11 (b)	12 (b)	13 (d)	14 (b)	15 (d)	16 (b)	17 (a)	18 (a)	19 (d)	20 (c)
21 (d)									

Step up Practice 3

1 (d)	2 (b)	3 (d)	4 (c)	5 (d)	6 (d)	7 (d)	8 (d)	9 (d)	10 (d)
11 (c)	12 (b)	13 (a)	14 (d)	15 (c)	16 (a)	17 (d)	18 (b)	19 (c)	20 (b)
21 (c)									

Gearing up for NEET

1 (d)	2 (b)	3 (d)	4 (c)	5 (a)	6 (c)	7 (c)	8 (b)	9 (c)	10 (a)
11 (c)	12 (d)	13 (c)	14 (d)	15 (b)	16 (b)	17 (b)	18 (a)	19 (d)	20 (d)
21 (d)	22 (c)	23 (c)	24 (b)	25 (b)	26 (c)	27 (d)	28 (d)	29 (c)	30 (c)
31 (d)	32 (d)	33 (d)	34 (a)	35 (b)	36 (c)	37 (d)	38 (d)	39 (c)	40 (a)
41 (b)	42 (a)	43 (b)	44 (b)	45 (a)	46 (b)	47 (b)	48 (c)	49 (b)	50 (a)
51 (c)	52 (b)	53 (c)	54 (b)	55 (c)	56 (c)	57 (c)	58 (b)	59 (a)	60 (b)
61 (d)	62 (a)	63 (d)	64 (a)	65 (a)	66 (c)	67 (a)	68 (b)	69 (a)	70 (c)
71 (c)	72 (b)	73 (a)	74 (b)	75 (c)	76 (b)	77 (b)	78 (b)	79 (d)	80 (a)
81 (b)	82 (d)	83 (d)	84 (c)	85 (b)	86 (c)	87 (b)	88 (c)	89 (c)	90 (a)
91 (b)	92 (a)	93 (b)	94 (c)	95 (d)	96 (c)	97 (a)	98 (b)	99 (a)	100 (b)
101 (b)	102 (a)	103 (c)	104 (a)	105 (c)	106 (c)	107 (c)	108 (d)	109 (a)	110 (c)
111 (c)	112 (a)	113 (d)	114 (d)	115 (b)	116 (d)	117 (c)	118 (c)	119 (c)	120 (a)

Assertion and Reason

1 (d)	2 (d)	3 (b)	4 (d)	5 (b)

Statement Type Questions

1 (b)	2 (c)	3 (a)	4 (c)	5 (b)

Match the Columns

1 (b)	2 (c)	3 (d)	4 (a)	5 (c)

Final Check through PYQs : Module-I

1 (c)	2 (a)	3 (c)	4 (a)

Final Check through PYQs : Module-II

5 (a)	6 (a)	7 (b)	8 (d)	9 (b)	10 (c)	11 (c)	12 (d)	13 (a)	14 (b)
15 (d)	16 (a)	17 (a)	18 (a)	19 (d)	20 (a)				

Final Check through PYQs : Module-III

21 (d)	22 (c)	23 (a)	24 (b)	25 (c)	26 (d)	27 (a)	28 (b)	29 (b)	30 (c)
31 (c)	32 (c)								

Hints and Solutions

Step up Practice 1

1. (*a*) Aluminium is trivalent impurity which is doped with pure semiconductor to form *p*-type semiconductor.
2. (*a*) A hole is a vacancy left by an electron or a vacancy formed by an acceptor atom. Its own charge is zero (like charge on an atom). It behaves like a positive charge during conduction process.
3. (*b*) For *n*-type semiconducting material, number of free electrons is very large than number of holes, *i.e.* $n_e >> n_h$.
4. (*d*) Both A and R are true and R is the correct explanation of A.

   The ratio of the velocity to the applied field is called the mobility. Since, electron is lighter than holes, they move faster in applied field than holes.
5. (*d*) Copper, aluminium, iron are conductors, while germanium is semiconductor. Semiconductor have negative temperature coefficient.
6. (*c*) Phosphorus are pentavalent while indium is trivalent.
7. (*c*) In intrinsic semiconductors, the creation or liberation of one free electron by the thermal energy creates one hole simultaneously. Thus, in intrinsic semiconductors $n_e = n_h$.

   Hence, number of electron = number of hole.
8. (*b*) A is true as conductivity increases due to generation of more electron-hole pairs at elevated temperature.

   R is false as E_g is not affected by heating.
9. (*d*) We know that, in *p*-type semiconductors, holes are majority charge carriers and electrons are minority charge carriers.
10. (*b*) Temperature coefficient of resistance of metals are positive, while that of semiconductor is negative.
11. (*c*) Iron is a metal and silicon is a semiconductor.

    Resistivity of metal is directly proportional to its absolute temperature but resistivity of temperature is inversely proportional to its absolute temperature.
12. (*b*) As we know that,

    p-type → trivalent impurity doped, hence incorrect.

    n-type → pentavalent impurity, hence correct.

    Trivalent impurity → Arsenic, phosphorous, hence incorrect.

    Pentavalent impurity → Arsentic phosphorous, hence incorrect.
13. (*c*) We know that, $n_e n_h = n^2$

    or $$n_e = \frac{n^2}{n_h} = \frac{10^{16} \times 10^{16}}{4.5 \times 10^{22}} = \frac{10^{32}}{4.5 \times 10^{22}} \text{ m}^{-3}$$
14. (*d*) Ge + Trivalent → *p*-type semiconductor

    The valency of an impurity added to germanium to convert it into a *p*-type semiconductor is 3.
15. (*a*) Both A and R are true but R is not correct explanation of A.

    Rate of recombination is governed by laws of thermodynamics and at same temperature, both are equal.
16. (*c*) Number density of atoms in silicon specimen $= 5 \times 10^{28}$ atom/m^3 $= 5 \times 10^{22}$/cm^3

    Since one atom of indium is doped in 5×10^8 Si atom, so number of indium atoms doped per cm^3 silicon.

    $$n = \frac{5 \times 10^{22}}{5 \times 10^8} = 1 \times 10^{14} \text{ atom/cm}^3$$
17. (*c*) By using mass action law, $n_i^2 = n_e n_h$

    $$\Rightarrow \quad n_h = \frac{n_i^2}{n_e} = \frac{(10^{16})^2}{10^{21}} = 10^{11} \text{ per m}^3$$

    Hence, number of holes $= 10^{11}$ per m^3.
18. (*c*) A is false

    $E_g = \frac{1240\text{eV}}{\lambda(\text{nm})} = \frac{1240}{600} = 2.06$ eV as $\frac{hc}{\lambda}$ or hf is not greater than E_g in the given case.

    But, R is true.

Step up Practice 2

1. (*c*) When a large reverse voltage is applied across a *p-n* junction diode, a huge current flows in the reverse direction suddenly. This is called breakdown of *p-n* junction diode.
2. (*b*) At a particular reverse voltage in *p-n* junction avalanche breakdown occurs, hence a huge current flows in reverse direction known as avalanche current.
3. (*a*) Both Statement I and Statement II are incorrect.

   In a *p-n* junction with open ends, a depletion layer is created at the junction due to diffusion of majority carriers from one side to another and a constant electric field is set-up across the junction and therefore there is motion of charge carriers in *p-n* junction due to which depletion layer is created.

4. (*b*) The *p-n* junction is used to convert AC into DC (rectifier).

5. (*c*) When a light falls on the junction, new hole-electron pairs are created. Numbers of produced electron-hole pairs depend upon numbers of photons. So, photoemf or current is proportional to intensity of light.

6. (*a*) As, $-6\text{ V} < -3\text{V}$

i.e. p is at low potential than n.

$\therefore$Diode is reverse biased.

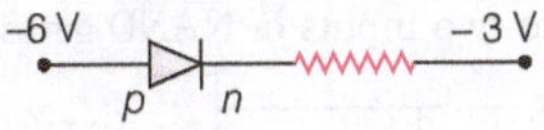

7. (*b*) Statement I is correct but Statement II is incorrect.

From the *V-I* characteristics of a junction diode, we see that it allows current to pass only when it is forward biased. So, if an alternating voltage is applied across a diode, the current flows only in that part of the cycle when the diode is forward biased.

8. (*d*) $\eta = \frac{\text{Output}}{\text{Input}} = \frac{I_{DC}}{I_{AC}}$

$$\eta = \frac{2I_0/\pi}{I_0/\sqrt{2}}$$

$$= \frac{2\sqrt{2}}{\pi} = 81.2\%$$

Hence, maximum efficiency of full wave rectifier is 81.2%.

9. (*a*) In an unbiased *p-n* junction, forward current is exactly equals to reverse current. So, net current across diode is zero.

10. (*d*) As we know,

$$I_{DC} = \frac{I_0}{\pi}, \quad V_{DC} = \frac{V_0}{\pi}, \quad I_0 = \frac{V_0}{r_f - R_L}$$

Hence, $V_{DC} = \frac{V_0}{\pi\left(1 + \frac{r_f}{R_L}\right)}$, is incorrect.

11. (*b*) Diode in upper branch is forward biased and in lower branch is reversed biased, so current through circuit $I = \frac{V}{R + r_d}$, here r_d = diode resistance in forward biasing = 0

$$\Rightarrow i = \frac{V}{R} = \frac{4}{10} = 0.4 \text{ A}$$

12. (*b*) Statement I is correct but Statement II is incorrect.

Due to diffusion of holes from the *p*-region to the *n*-region and of electrons from the *n*-region to the *p*-region and electric field is set up across the junction barrier. Once the depletion layer is formed, it is in equilibrium and becomes free of mobile charge carriers.

13. (*d*) The diode *D* will conduct for positive half cycle of AC supply because this is forward biased. For negative half cycle of AC supply, this is reverse biased and does not conduct. So, output would be half wave rectified and for half-wave rectified output.

$$V_{rms} = \frac{V_0}{2} = \frac{220\sqrt{2}}{2} = \frac{220}{\sqrt{2}} \text{ V}$$

Hence, voltage across the capacitor is $\frac{220}{\sqrt{2}}$ V.

14. (*b*) For the positive half cycle of input, the resulting network is shown below.

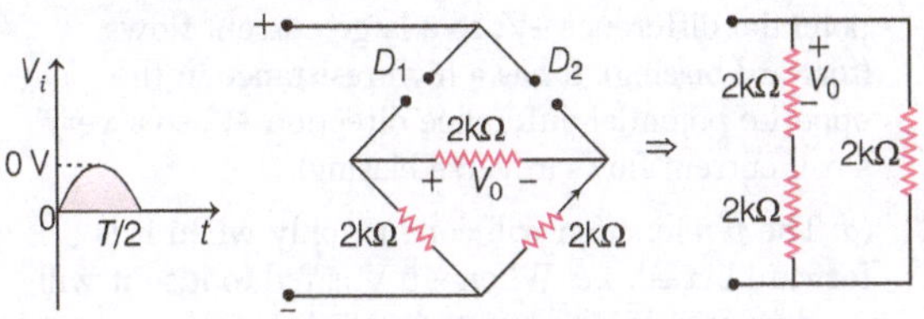

$$\Rightarrow (V_0)_{max} = \frac{1}{2}(V_i)_{max} = \frac{1}{2} \times 10 = 5 \text{ V}$$

Hence, the maximum output voltage V_0 is 5V.

15. (*d*) The electric field strength *versus* distance curve across the *p-n* junction is as follows

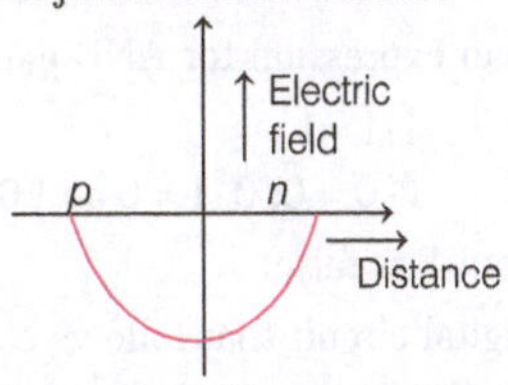

In the middle of the depletion layer of a reversed biased *p-n* junction, the electric field is maximum.

16. (*b*) Statement I is correct but Statement II is incorrect.

Due to diffusion of electrons, positive space-charge region on *n*-side of the junction and negative space charge region on *p*-side of the junction, an electric field directed from positive charge towards negative charge develops. Electric field is from *n*-side to *p*-side. Due to this field, an electron on *p*-side of the junction moves to *n*-side and a hole on *n*-side of the junction moves to *p*-side. The motion of charge carriers due to the electric field is called drift. Thus, a drift current, which is opposite in direction to the diffusion current starts. Concentration gradient is due to doping of sides. It is not affected by drift of charge carriers.

17. (*a*) If *p-n* junction diode is made from germanium or silicon, the energy released due to recombination of free electrons and holes is in the infrared region. However if the *p-n* junction diode is made from gallium arsenide or indium phosphide, then the energy released due to recombination of free electrons and holes is in the visible region.

18. (*a*) In forward biased *p-n* junction, external voltage decreases the potential barrier, so current is maximum. While in reversed biased *p-n* junction, external voltage increases the potential barrier, so the current is very small.

19. (*d*) Both Statement I and Statement II are correct.

A reverse bias on a *p-n* junction opposes the movement of the majority charge carriers thus stopping the diffusion current. It makes the free electrons and holes to drift across the junction. Therefore, a small current in μA flows even when the *p-n* junction is reverse biased. The drift current is due to the thermal excitations of the electrons and holes.

20. (*c*) *p-n* junction has low resistance in one direction of potential difference $+V$, so a large current flows (forward biasing). It has a high resistance in the opposite potential difference direction $-V$, so a very small current flows (reverse biasing).

21. (*d*) The *p-n* junction will conduct only when it is forward biased. *i.e.* When -5 V is fed to it,so it will conduct only for 3rd quarter part of signal shown and when it conducts potential drop 5 V will be across both the resistors, so output voltage across R is 2.5 V.

$\therefore \quad V_0 = -2.5$ V

Step up Practice 3

1. (*d*) The boolean expression for AND gate is $R = P \cdot Q$

$\Rightarrow \quad 1 \cdot 1 = 1$

$1 \cdot 0 = 0;\ 0 \cdot 1 = 0$ and $0 \cdot 0 = 0$

2. (*b*) A is true but R is false.

A gate is a digital circuit that follows certain logical relationship between the input and output voltages. Therefore, they are generally known as logic gates because they control the flow of information. The five common logic gates used are NOT, AND, OR, NAND and NOR.

3. (*d*) For AND gate, if output is 0, then one or both the inputs must be 0.

4. (*c*) If inputs are A and B, then output of NAND gate is $Y = \overline{AB}$.

If $A = B = 1$, then $Y = \overline{1 \cdot 1} = \overline{1} = 0$.

5. (*d*) Both A and R are true and R is the correct explanation of A.

Any boolean operation can be performed using either a combination of NOR gates or NAND gates.

6. (*d*) The given truth table is for NAND gate, since $Y = \overline{A \cdot B}$.

7. (*d*) Any digital circuit can be realised by repetitive use of NOR gate or NAND gate. NOR gate and NAND gate are called universal gates because by using these gates, we can realise other basic gates like OR, AND and NOT gates.

8. (*d*)

Input		Output			
		OR	AND	NOR	NAND
0	0	0	0	1	1
0	1	1	0	0	1
1	0	1	0	0	1
1	1	1	1	0	0

From the above truth tables, it is clear that the logic gates giving output 1 for the inputs 1 and 0 are NAND and OR gates.

9. (*d*) When the two inputs of NAND gates are shorted,

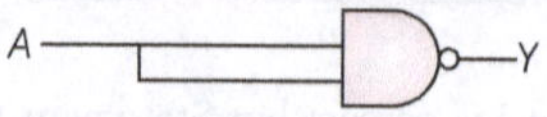

$Y = \overline{A} =$ which is equivalent to a NOT gate.

10. (*d*) As we know that,

NOR gate = NOT + OR

$= \overline{A + B}$, hence incorrect.

11. (*c*)

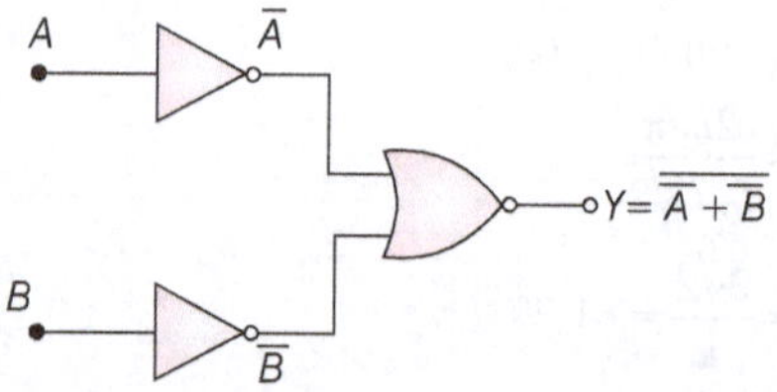

Hence, output $Y = \overline{\overline{A} + \overline{B}}$

According to de-Morgan's theorem,

$$Y = \overline{\overline{A} + \overline{B}} = \overline{\overline{A}} \cdot \overline{\overline{B}} = A \cdot B$$

This is the output equation of AND gate.

12. (*b*) $(\overline{\overline{A} \cdot \overline{B}}) \cdot A = (\overline{\overline{A}} + \overline{\overline{B}}) \cdot A = (A + B) \cdot A$

$= A \cdot A + AB + = A + AB = A(1 + B) = A$

Hence, $(\overline{\overline{A} + \overline{B}}) \cdot A = A$

13. (*a*) We consider (1 = high, 0 = low),

Input to A is in the sequence, 1, 0, 1, 0.

Input to B is in the sequence, 1, 0, 0, 1.

Sequence is inverted by NOT gate.

Thus inputs to OR gate becomes 0, 1, 0, 1 and 0, 1, 1, 0.

Since for OR gate, $0 + 1 = 1$. Hence, option (a) is correct.

14. (*d*) The output of both AND gates will be zero, so, OR gate does not respond.

Hence, $A = 1, B = 1, X = 0$.

15. (*c*) We know that,

for XNOR gate, $Y = \overline{A}\,\overline{B} + AB$

i.e. $\overline{0} \cdot \overline{0} + 0.0 = 1 \cdot 1 + 0 \cdot 0 = 1 + 0 = 1$

$\overline{0} \cdot \overline{1} + 0 \cdot 1 = 1 \cdot 0 + 0 \cdot 1 = 0 + 0 = 0$

$\bar{1}\cdot\bar{0}+1\cdot 0=0\cdot 1+1\cdot 0=0+0=0$

$\bar{1}\cdot\bar{1}+1\cdot .1=0\cdot 0+1\cdot 1=0+1=1$

Hence, the truth table shown here represents XNOR gate.

16. (*a*) Both A and R are true but R is not correct explanation of A.

The general nature of Boolean functions rather than specifically explaining logic gate has only one output.

17. (*d*) According to arrangement given in figure.

The output for the given combination,

$$D=\overline{(A+B)\cdot C}=\overline{(A+B)}+\overline{C}$$

If $A=B=C=0$,

then $D=\overline{(0+0)}+\overline{0}=\overline{0}+\overline{0}=1+1=1$

If $A=B=1, C=0$,

then $D=\overline{(1+1)}+\overline{0}=\overline{1}+\overline{0}=0+1=1$

Hence, the logic states of output D are 1, 1.

18. (*b*) If none of the AND gate's inputs are high, the output is low.

Two NAND gates are required as follows.

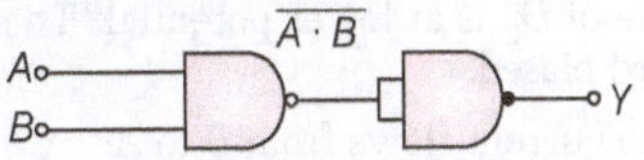

$$Y=\overline{\overline{A\cdot B}\cdot\overline{A\cdot B}}=A\cdot B$$

19. (*c*) A is false but R is true.

A NAND gate can be obtained by using NOR gates.

20. (*b*) $Z=\overline{\overline{(A\cdot B)}+\overline{(B\cdot C)}}$

$=(A\cdot B)\cdot(B\cdot C)=A\cdot B\cdot C$

Hence, the system is equivalent to AND gate.

21. (*c*) Output of upper OR gate $=W+X$

Output of lower OR gate $=W+Y$

Net output, $F=(W+X)(W+Y)$

$=WW+WY+XW+XY$ (Since, $WW=W$)

$=W(1+Y)+XW+XY$ (Since, $1+Y=1$)

$=W+XW+XY=W(1+X)+XY=W+XY$

Gearing up for NEET

2. (*b*) The concept of hole describes the lack of an electron at a position where one could exist in an atom or atomic lattice. If an electron is excited into a higher state, it leaves a hole in its old state.

Thus, hole can be defined as a vacancy created when an electron leaves a covalent bond.

3. (*d*) Resistance of conductor (Cu) decreases with decrease in temperature while that of semiconductor (Ge) increases with decrease in temperature.

4. (*c*) On increasing the temperature, the current in the circuit will increase because with rise in temperature, resistance of semiconductor decreases, hence overall resistance of the circuit decreases, which in turn increases the current in the circuit.

7. (*c*) The majority charge carriers in *p*-type semiconductor are holes, while electrons are minority charge carriers.

8. (*b*) *p*-type semiconductor can be made by doping a silicon atom in the crystal lattice with a gallium (a trivalent impurity).

9. (*c*) For making *p*-type semiconductor, we add trivalent impurity. So, B impurity is mixed in Ge and Al impurity is mixed in Si.

10. (*a*) At room temperature, a *p*-type semiconductor has large number of holes and few electrons, as holes are majority charge carriers.

15. (*b*) Pentavalent impurity atom is to be added to Ge crystal, so as to make a *n*-type semiconductor.

19. (*d*) Extrinsic semiconductors are also electrically neutral.

20. (*d*) The conductivity of a semiconductor increases with increase in temperature because the number density of current carriers increases. Here, due to high temperature, the relaxation time also decreases but effect of decrease in relaxation time is much less than increase in number density.

21. (*d*) Resistance of semiconductor decreases with increase in temperature. Hence, its temperature coefficient is negative.

22. (*c*) With the rise in temperature, resistivity of semiconductors decreases exponentially.

23. (*c*) The electrical conductivity of germanium,

$$\sigma=\frac{1}{\rho}=e(\mu_e n_e+\mu_h n_h)$$

$$=(1.6\times 10^{-19})[0.36+0.17](2.5\times 10^{19})$$

$$(\because n_e=n_h=2.5\times 10^{19}\ \text{m}^{-3})$$

$$=2.12\ \text{Sm}^{-1}$$

24. (*b*) As, $n_e >> n_h$

So, it is an *n*-type semiconductor.

25. (*b*) In 1 cm^3 of Si, there will be total $\frac{6\times 10^{28}}{10^6}$

$=6\times 10^{22}$ atoms

Per 6×10^7 silicon atoms, there is one indium atom. Therefore, total number of indium atoms will be

$$\frac{6\times 10^{22}}{6\times 10^7}=10^{15}$$

26. (*c*) $\lambda\ (\text{in Å})=\frac{12375}{E\ (\text{in eV})}=\frac{12375}{57\times 10^{-3}}\ \text{Å}\approx 217100\ \text{Å}$

27. (*d*) As the diode is forward biased, so it takes only positive value. Hence, option (d) is correct.

28. (*d*) The mobility of electron is greater than holes because electron require less energy to move.

29. (*c*) Each and every extrinsic semiconductor is electrically neutral whether it is *p*-type or *n*-type.

30. (*c*) The conductivity of the intrinsic semiconductor is independent of fermi energy. It depends upon band gap, temperature as well as effective mass of charge carriers.

31. (*d*) The *n*-type semiconductor region has (negative) electrons as majority charge carriers and an equal number of fixed positively charged donor ions. Again, the material as a whole is neutral. That is a reason, that atom is electrically neutral.

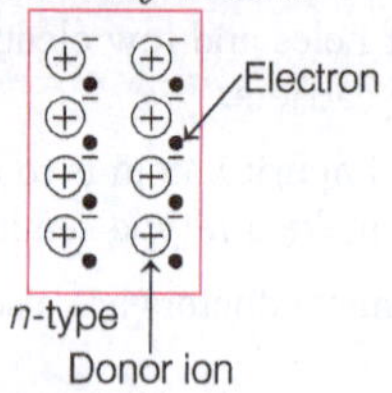

33. (*d*) Resistivity of a semiconductor is 10^{-5} -$10^{6}\Omega$-m while that of insulator is 10^{11}-$10^{19}\Omega$-m and conductor is 10^{-2} - $10^{-8}\Omega$-m.

34. (*a*) At room temperature, due to thermal vibrations, the few bonds of intrinsic semiconductor are broken and producing equal number of electrons and holes in the semiconductor.

35. (*b*) When a small amount of antimony is added to germanium crystal, the crystal becomes *n*-type semiconductor, because antimony is a pentavalent substrate and act as donor atom. So, there will be more free electrons than holes in the semiconductor.

43. (*b*) In the forward bias arrangement of a *p*-*n* junction diode, the *p*-end is connected to the positive terminal of the battery and *n*-end with negative terminal of battery.

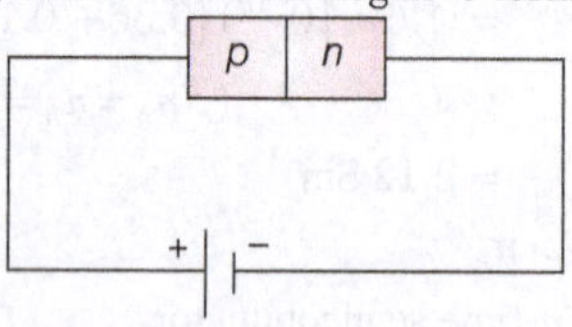

45. (*a*) As, $i = n_e A v_d$

So, $v_d = \dfrac{i}{n_e A}$

So, when temperature is increased, n_e increases and v_d decreases.

46. (*b*) In forward biasing, the diffusion current increases and drift current remains constant, so net current is due to diffusion. In reverse biasing diffusion is not possible, so net current (very small) is due to the drift.

47. (*b*) At a specific reverse voltage (breakdown voltage) in *p*-*n* junction, a huge current flows in reverse direction known as Avalanche current.

54. (*b*) From rectifier we get pulsating DC, which consists of AC ripple. To remove these unwanted ripples, we use filter circuits.

55. (*c*) When *p*-*n* junction is forward biased, it opposes the potential barrier at junction but when *p*-*n* junction is reverse biased, it supports the potential barrier at junction, resulting in increase in potential barrier across the junction.

56. (*c*) For full wave rectifier, the fundamental frequency in ripple is twice that of input frequency.

59. (*a*) Given, $E = 6 \times 10^5 \text{ Vm}^{-1}$

$$d = 500 \text{ nm}$$
$$= 500 \times 10^{-9} \text{m}$$

$\therefore$ Potential barrier, $V = Ed = (6 \times 10^5)(500 \times 10^{-9})$
$= 0.30$ V

60. (*b*) In the given circuit, *p*-side of *p*-*n* junction diode D_1 is connected to lower voltage and *n*-side of D_1 to higher voltage.

Thus D_1 is in reverse biased.

The *p* -side of *p*-*n* junction of D_2 is at higher potential and *n*-side of D_2 is at lower potential. Therefore, D_2 is in forward biased.

Hence, no current flows from *B* to *A*.

61. (*d*) As *p*-*n* junction conducts during positive half cycle only, the diode connected here will work in positive half cycle. Potential difference across C = peak voltage of the given AC voltage $= V_0 = V_{rms}\sqrt{2} = 220\sqrt{2}$ V.

62. (*a*) During the first half cycle when $V_A > V_C$, all the four diodes are forward biased. Hence, no current will flow through R_L. During second half cycle when $V_C > V_A$, all the four diodes are reverse biased. Again, no current will flow through R_L.

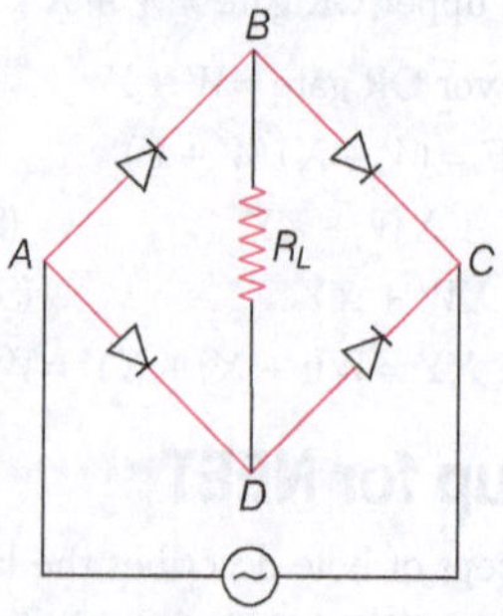

63. (*d*) In forward biasing, both potential barrier V_B and the width of charge depleted region *x* decreases.

64. (*a*) Here, diode is in reverse biased condition. In reverse biasing, it acts as open circuit, hence no current flows.

65. (*a*) In the given circuit, diode is in reverse biasing, so it acts as open circuit. Hence, potential difference between *A* and *B* is 6 V.

67. (*a*) In case of forward biasing, resistance of *p-n* junction diode is zero. So, whole voltage appears across the resistance.

68. (*b*) Diode is in forward biased condition. So, current flow $i = \frac{(4-1)}{300} = 10^{-2}$ A

69. (*a*) Intensity of electric field,

$$E = \frac{V}{d} = \frac{0.50}{5\times 10^{-7}} = 1.0\times 10^{6}\ \text{Vm}^{-1}$$

70. (*c*) Due to forward biasing during positive half cycle of input AC voltage, the resistance of *p-n* junction is low. The current in the circuit is maximum. In this situation, a maximum potential difference will appear across resistance connected in series of circuit. This result into zero output voltage across *p-n* junction.

Similarly during negative half cycle of AC voltage, the *p-n* junction is reverse biased. The resistance of *p-n* junction becomes high which will be more than resistance in series. That is why, there will be voltage across *p-n* junction with negative cycle in output.

71. (*c*) D_1 is forward biased and D_2 reverse biased. Therefore, current flows through the resistance and D_1 will be equal to $\frac{5}{4} = 1.25$ A

72. (*b*) D_1 is reverse biased, therefore no current will flow through 20 Ω resistance.

As, 30Ω and 20 Ω resistance are in series, so total current will be (5/50) A.

73. (*a*) First diode is in reverse biasing, it acts as open circuit, hence no current flows.

74. (*b*) For forward biasing, *p*-side is at higher potential and *n*-side is at lower potential, so diode in figures II, IV and V are forward biased.

75. (*c*) If $V_A > V_B$, then both the junction diodes are in forward biased and the given circuit diagram becomes a balanced Wheatstone bridge. The equivalent resistance in this case becomes 4 Ω.

If $V_A < V_B$, then the diodes are reverse biased. In that case, 4 Ω, 5 Ω and 4 Ω are in series, *i.e.* $R_{\text{net}} = 13\Omega$.

76. (*b*) Consider the figure given here, suppose the potential difference between *A* and *B* is *V*.

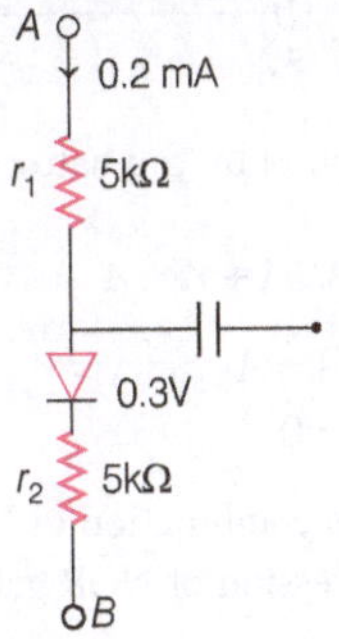

Then, $V - 0.3 = [(r_1 + r_2)10^3]\times(0.2\times 10^{-3})]$ $(\because V = ir)$

$$= [(5+5)\,10^3]\times(0.2\times 10^{-3})$$
$$= 10\times 10^3\times 0.2\times 10^{-3} = 2$$

$\Rightarrow$ $V = 2 + 0.3 = 2.3$ V

77. (*b*) Voltage across zener diode is constant,

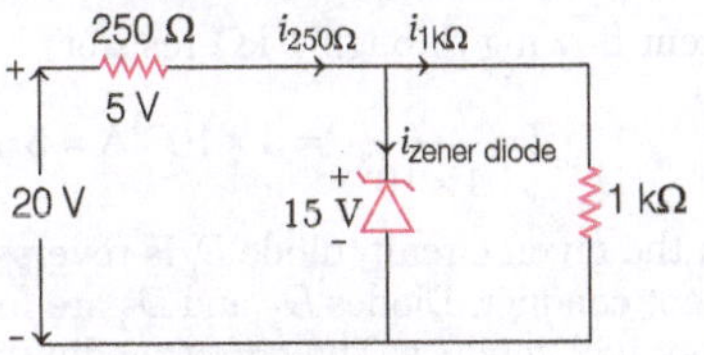

$$i_{1\text{k}\Omega} = \frac{15}{1\times 10^3} = 15\ \text{mA}$$

$$i_{250} = \frac{(20-15)}{250} = \frac{5}{250} = \frac{20}{1000} = 20\ \text{mA}$$

$\therefore$ $i_{\text{zener diode}} = (20 - 15) = 5$ mA

78. (*b*) In the positive half cycle of input AC signal, diode D_1 is in forward biased and D_2 is in reverse biased, so in the output voltage signal, *A* and *C* are due to diode D_1. In negative half cycle of input AC signal, diode D_2 is in forwards biased, hence it conducts, so output signals *B* and *D* are due to diode D_2.

80. (*a*) The diode is in reverse biasing, so no current flows through it.

81. (*b*) Potential across the *p-n* junction varies symmetrically linear, having *p* side negative and *n* side positive.

We know that in a forward biased *p-n* junction diode, the repulsion of holes and electrons takes place which decreases width of potential barrier by striking the combination of holes and electrons. We also know that the options (c) and (d) show the potential barrier in the reverse bias, whereas in options (a) and (b) show the potential barrier in forward bias. Moreover, the width of depletion layer in option (b) is less than shown in option (a). Thus, the option (b) is correct.

83. (*d*)

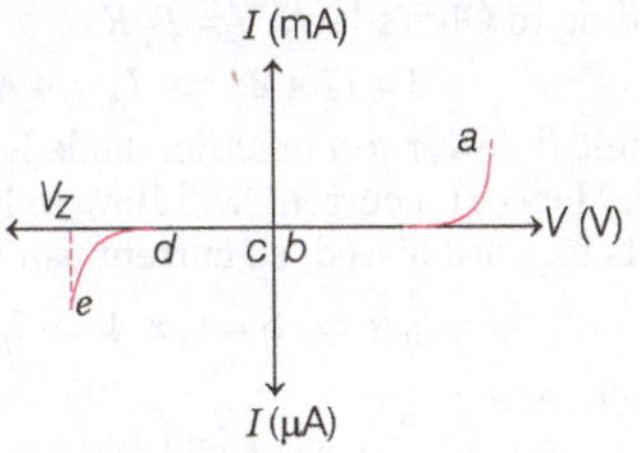

If the reverse bias voltage is greater than the V_Z, then there is breakdown condition. In breakdown region, *i.e.* $V_i > V_Z$ and for a long range of load (R_L), the voltage is constant.

84. (*c*) Voltage of the source,

$$V = V_D + iR = 0.5 + 0.1\times 20 = 2.5\ \text{V}$$

85. (*b*) The potential across,

$$R = 17\ \text{V} - 9\ \text{V} = 8\ \text{V}$$

86. (*c*) Total resistance in the circuit, $R = 2\,\text{k}\Omega$ and $E = 20\,\text{V}$

$\therefore$ Current, $I = \dfrac{E}{R} = \dfrac{20}{2000} = 10\,\text{mA}$

87. (*b*) In the given circuit, the Zener diode is used as a voltage regulating device. Hence, the voltage across $1\,\text{k}\Omega$ is 5 V.

Current flowing through $1\,\text{k}\Omega$ resistor,

$$I = \frac{5}{1\times 10^3} = 5\times 10^{-3}\,\text{A} = 5\,\text{mA}$$

88. (*c*) In the given circuit, diode D_1 is reverse biased, so it will not conduct. Diodes D_2 and D_3 are forward biased, so they will conduct. The corresponding equivalent circuit is as shown in the figure

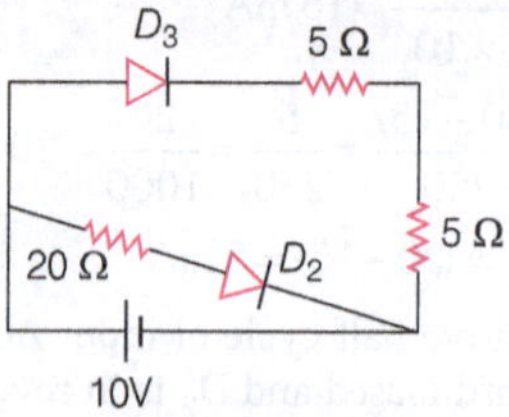

The equivalent resistance of the circuit is

$$R_{\text{eq}} = \frac{(5+5)\times 20}{(5+5)+20} = \frac{10\times 20}{10+20} = \frac{200}{30} = \frac{20}{3}\,\Omega$$

Current through the battery, $I = \dfrac{10}{\frac{20}{3}} = 1.5\,\text{A}$

89. (*c*) In circuit *A*, both the *p-n* junction diodes are in forward biased. Total resistance *R* is given by

$$\frac{1}{R} = \frac{1}{4} + \frac{1}{4}$$

$$\Rightarrow \frac{1}{R} = \frac{2}{4} \Rightarrow R = 2\,\Omega$$

According to Ohm's law, $V = I_A R$

$$\Rightarrow \quad 8 = I_A \times 2 \Rightarrow I_A = 4\,\text{A}$$

In circuit *B*, lower *p-n* junction diode is in reverse biased. Hence, no current will flow in it but upper diode is forward biased, so current can flow through it.

$$V = I_B R \Rightarrow 8 = I_B \times 4 \Rightarrow I_B = 2\,\text{A}$$

90. (*a*) Given, energy gap,

$E_g = 1.9\,\text{eV} = 1.9\times 1.6\times 10^{-19}\,\text{V}$

We know that, $E_g = \dfrac{hc}{\lambda} \Rightarrow \lambda = \dfrac{hc}{E_g}$

Wavelength of the emitted light,

$$\lambda = \frac{6.63\times 10^{-34}\times 3\times 10^{8}}{1.9\times 1.6\times 10^{-19}}$$

$$= 6.5\times 10^{-7}\,\text{m}$$

91. (*b*) The circuit is

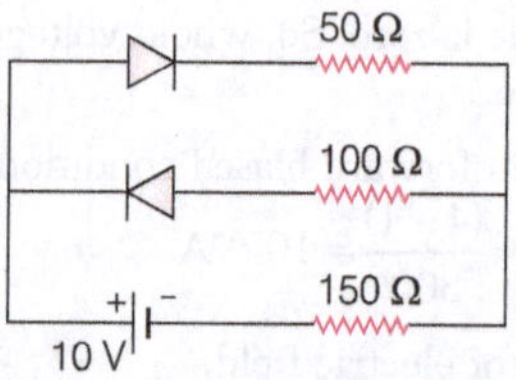

As the lower diode attached to $100\,\Omega$ resistance is in reverse biased, so it is non-conducting.

Now, the circuit can be redrawn as

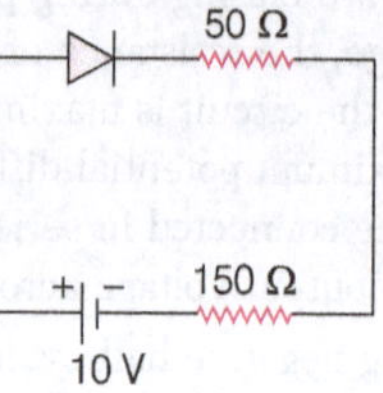

$\therefore$ Current through the circuit, $I = \dfrac{V}{R} = \dfrac{10}{200} = 0.05\text{A}$

92. (*a*) *V-I* characteristic of a solar cell is shown in the question, where *A* represents open circuit voltage and *B* shows short circuit current.

93. (*b*) Initial current, $I_{\text{in}} = 0$

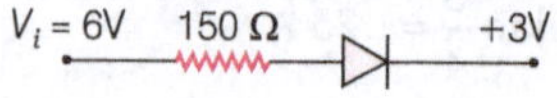

Final current, $I_f = \dfrac{(6-3)}{150} = 0.02\,\text{A}$

So, change in current, $\Delta I = I_f - I_{\text{in}} = 0.02 - 0$

$= 0.02\,\text{A} = 20\,\text{mA}$

94. (*c*) The diode D_1 is in reversed biased and D_2 is in forward biased. The resistance of D_1 in in becomes infinite and of D_2 is zero. Therefore, current in the circuit,

$$I = \frac{\text{emf}}{\text{total resistance}} = \frac{12}{4+2} = 2\,\text{A}$$

95. (*d*) Here in circuit D_1 is forward bias and D_2 is reverse bias, so current will flow only in diode D_1

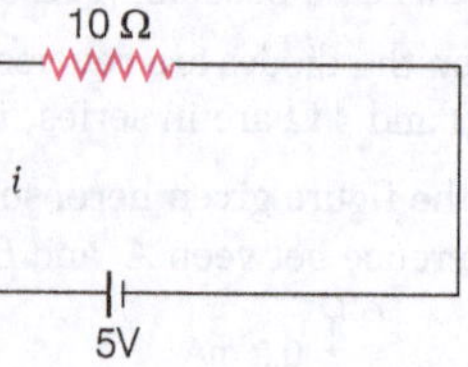

The current supplied by the battery, $i = \dfrac{5}{10} = 0.5\,\text{A}$

96. (*c*) Here, $A\cdot A = A,\ A + A = A$

and $\overline{A} + \overline{A} = \overline{A}\cdot\overline{A} = \overline{A}$

But $\overline{A}\cdot A = 0$

98. (*b*) A NOR gate is combination of NOT and OR gate. The boolean expression of NOR gate is $Y = \overline{A+B}$.

99. (a) In Fig. (a), first gate is AND gate and second gate is NOT gate. So, it is NAND gate.

102. (a) The given boolean expression can be written as

$$Y = \overline{(A+B)} \cdot \overline{(AB)}$$
$$= (\overline{A} \cdot \overline{B}) \cdot (\overline{A} + \overline{B}) = (\overline{A} \cdot \overline{A}) \cdot \overline{B} + \overline{A}(\overline{B} \cdot \overline{B})$$
$$= \overline{A} \cdot \overline{B} + \overline{A} \cdot \overline{B} = \overline{A} \cdot \overline{B}$$

So, the truth table is

A	B	Y
0	0	1
1	0	0
0	1	0
1	1	0

Hence, to get $Y = 1$, $A = 0$ and $B = 0$.

103. (c) In the truth table, output $X = \overline{A}$. So, this truth table is of NOT gate.

106. (c) For option (c), it is a NAND gate, its output $= \overline{0.1} = \overline{0} = 1$

108. (d) The output D for the given combination,

$$D = \overline{(A+B) \cdot C} = \overline{(A+B)} + \overline{C}$$

If $A = B = C = 0$, then

$$D = \overline{(0+0)} + \overline{0} = \overline{0} + \overline{0} = 1 + 1 = 1$$

If $A = B = 1$ and $C = 0$, then

$$D = \overline{(1+1)} + \overline{0} = \overline{1} + \overline{0} = 0 + 1 = 1$$

109. (a) For upper part,

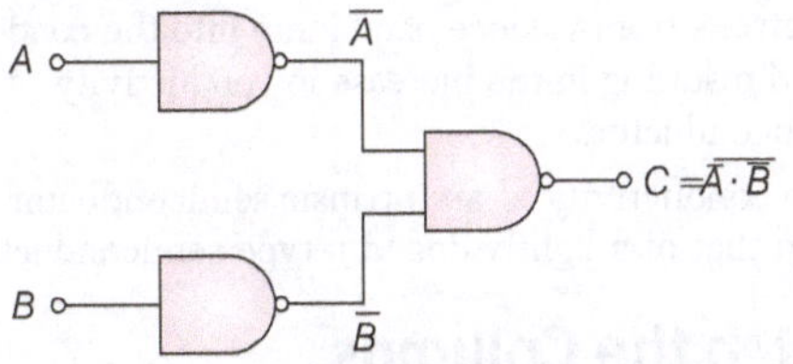

Here, $C = \overline{\overline{A} \cdot \overline{B}} = \overline{\overline{A}} + \overline{\overline{B}}$ (from de-Morgan's theorem)

$= A + B$

Here, output C is equivalent to OR gate.

For lower part,

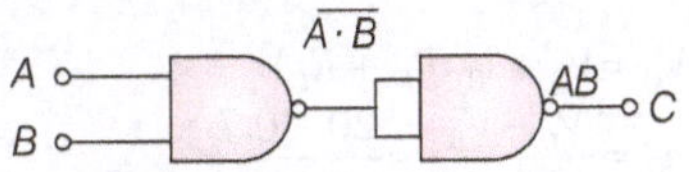

$$C = \overline{\overline{AB}} = AB$$

In this case, output C is equivalent to AND gate.

110. (c)

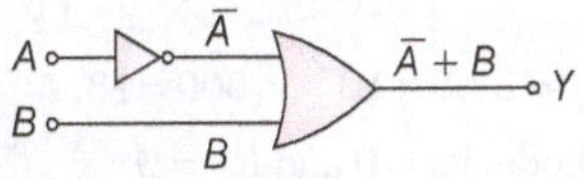

111. (c) Here, $C = A \cdot B$ and $D = \overline{A} \cdot B$

$$E = C + D = (A \cdot B) + (\overline{A} \cdot B)$$

Explanation The truth table of this arrangement of gates can be given by

A	B	$\overline{A}$	$C = A \cdot B$	$D = \overline{A} \cdot B$	$E = (C + D)$
0	0	1	0	0	0
0	1	1	0	1	1
1	0	0	0	0	0
1	1	0	1	0	1

112. (a) $Y = \overline{\overline{A} + \overline{B}} = A \cdot B$, *i.e.* it is a AND gate.

114. (d) The combination of three NAND gates are shown in the diagram

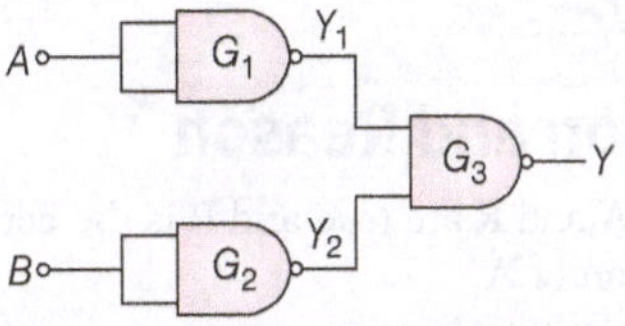

$Y_1 =$ Output due to NAND gate 1 $= \overline{A \cdot A} = \overline{A}$

$Y_2 =$ Output due to NAND gate 2 $= \overline{B \cdot B} = \overline{B}$

Output due to NAND gate 3

$$Y = \overline{Y_1 \cdot Y_2} = \overline{Y_1} + \overline{Y_2} = \overline{\overline{A}} + \overline{\overline{B}} = A + B$$

This is OR gate. Hence, the combination is equivalent to an OR gate.

115. (b) Given arrangement is

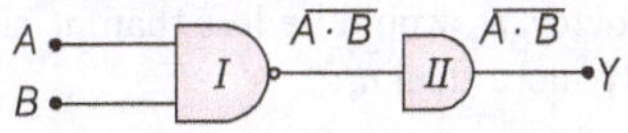

Gate I → NAND gate

Gate II → AND gate

Above arrangement represents NAND gate.

116. (d) Output of NOR gate, $Y' = \overline{A + B}$

Output of NAND gate,

$$Y'' = \overline{\overline{(A+B)} \cdot \overline{(A+B)}}$$
$$= (A+B) + (A+B) = A + B$$

Output of NOT gate, $Y''' = \overline{A + B}$

∴ The boolean expression is for NOR gate.

117. (c) The output of digital circuit can be given as $Y = \overline{AB} + \overline{C}$.

It will be same as $Y = \overline{A} + \overline{B} + \overline{C}$.

118. (c) The output of $G_1 = A + B$

Output of $G_2 = \overline{A \cdot B}$

and output of $G_3 = (A + B)(\overline{A \cdot B}) = A\overline{B} + B\overline{A}$

This output is same as the output of an XOR gate.

119. (c) A digital signal has only two values of voltage variation with time. Its value is either zero or maximum (1).

120. (a) From the given waveforms, the following truth table can be made

Input		Output
A	B	C
0	0	0
1	0	1
1	1	1
0	1	1

This truth table is similar to OR gate, so logic gate is OR gate.

Note The logic of the OR gate is, if any of the input is one, then output is one.

Assertion and Reason

1. (*d*) Both A and R are true and R is the correct explanation of A.

In semiconductors, the energy gap between conduction band and valence band is small (≈ 1 eV). Due to temperature rise, electron in the valence band gain thermal energy and may jump across the small energy gap, (to the conduction band). Thus, conductivity increases and hence resistance decreases.

2. (*d*) Both A and R are true and R is the correct explanation of A.

According to law of mass action, $n_i^2 = n_e n_h$. In intrinsic semiconductors, $n_i = n_e = n_h$ and for p-type semiconductor, n_e would be less than n_i, since n_h is necessarily more than n_i.

3. (*b*) A is true but R is false.

In diode, the output is in same phase with the input, therefore it cannot be used to built NOT gate.

4. (*d*) Both A and R are true and R is the correct explanation of A.

These gates are called digital building blocks because using these gates (either NAND or NOR), we can compile all other gates also (like OR, AND, NOT, XOR).

5. (*b*) A is true but R is false.

In a semiconductor, there are no free electrons at 0K. The number of free electrons increases with increase in temperature because with increase in temperature the electron get sufficient energy to cross forbidden band and reach conduction band. But total number of free electrons in a semiconductor is less than that in a conductor.

Statement Type Questions

1. (*b*) Statement I is correct but Statement II is incorrect.

In forward bias, forward current is obtained due to removal of barrier potential by externally applied potential. Ohm's law states $V \propto I$, not valid for diode.

2. (*c*) Statement I is incorrect and Statement II is correct.

The loss of electrons from the n-region and the gain of electrons by the p-region causes a difference of potential across the junction of the two regions. The polarity of this potential is such as to oppose further flow of carriers, so that a condition of equilibrium exists. Therefore potential at P-side is negative.

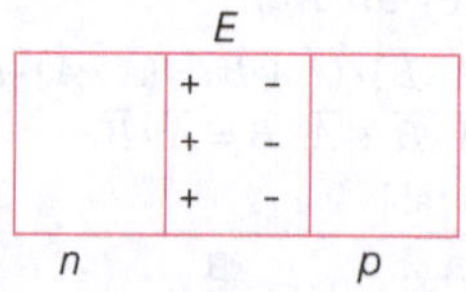

3. (*a*) Both Statement I and Statement II are incorrect.

The energy gap for germanium is less (0.72 eV) than the energy gap of silicon (1.1 eV). Therefore, germanium is preferred over silicon for making semiconductor device.

4. (*c*) Statement I is incorrect but Statement II is correct.

In a p-n junction or in a n-type semiconductor, phosphorus atoms are not isolated and there are enough free charge carriers in a semiconductor at room temperature.

Last or 5th electron of pentavalent phosphorus is rotating around an ion with net +1 unit charge. Energy of this electron is nearly $E = -\frac{13.6}{(\varepsilon_r)^2}$ eV.

ε_r for silicon is 12 so, $E = -0.1$ eV which is quite large and hence, this electron is not bounded to the core. So, ionisation is possible at room temperature.

5. (*b*) Statement I is correct but Statement II is incorrect.

As we increase the temperature, more number of electrons from valence band jump into the conductance band resulting in the increase in conductivity of intrinsic semiconductor.

The conductivity of an intrinsic semiconductor is less than that of a lightly doped p-type semiconductor.

Match the Columns

1. (*b*) Diode gets forward biased during positive half cycle of alternating source and current flows. Let the barrier voltage of diode is V_B and its forward resistance be R_F and load resistance be R_L, then peak voltage of applied signal,

$$V_0 = V_B + i_0 (R_F + R_L)$$

$$\therefore \quad i_0 = \frac{V_0 - V_B}{R_F + R_L} = \frac{20 - 0.7}{10 + 500}$$

$$= 37.8 \times 10^{-3} \text{ A} = 37.8 \text{ mA}$$

Peak voltage at the ends of the load R_L,

$$V_L = i_0 \times R_L = 37.8 \times 10^{-3} \times 500 = 18.9 \text{ V}$$

For ideal diode, $V_B = 0$ and $R_F = 0$

$$\therefore \quad i_0 = \frac{V_0}{R_L} = \frac{20}{500} = 0.04 \text{ A} = 40 \text{ mA}$$

and $\quad V_L = i_0 R_L = 0.04 \times 500 = 20 \text{ V}$

Hence, A-(I), B-(IV), C-(II), D-(III).

2. (*c*) Hence, A-(II), B-(I), C-(III), D-(IV).
3. (*d*) Hence, A-(IV), B-(III), C-(II), D-(I).
4. (*a*) Hence, A-(III), B-(I), C-(II), D-(IV).
5. (*c*) A. $\overline{(A+B)} = \overline{A} \cdot \overline{B}$ [By De-Morgan's theorem]

B. $A + (A \cdot B) = A(1 + B) = A$ [By Absorption laws]

C. $A(\overline{A} + B) = A\overline{A} + AB = AB$

D. $\overline{\overline{A} \cdot \overline{B}} = \overline{\overline{A}} + \overline{\overline{B}} = A + B$

Hence, A-(IV), B-(III), C-(II), D-(I).

Final Check Through PYQs

1. (*c*) Given, the electron concentration in *n*- type semiconductor is equal to the hole's concentration in *p*-type semiconductor.

   When electric field is applied across the semiconductor, the electrons and holes will move opposite to each other. The mobility of *n*-type semiconductor is greater than mobility of *p*-type semiconductor.

   So, the current in the *n*-type semiconductor is greater than current in the *p*-type semiconductor.
2. (*a*) When a pentavalent (phosphorous) impurities is doped with intrinsic semiconductor (Ge, Si), then *n* -type semiconductor is formed.
3. (*c*) Insulators and semiconductors are those solids, which have negative temperature coefficient of resistance.

   As, when temperature increases number of free electrons increases in both insulator and semiconductor.
5. (*a*) A is correct but B is incorrect.

   In reverse biased *p*-*n* junction, the current is due to minority charge carriers, which is very small and hence measured in terms of μA.
6. (*a*) For a diode to be active it must be forward biased. In options (b) and (d), diode is reverse biased.

   Hence, options (b) and (d) cannot achieve bridge balance.

   For option (a),

   Balance bridge condition is $\frac{10}{15} = \frac{10}{5+r}$

   If $r = 10\Omega$, bridge can be balanced.

   For option (c) : $\frac{10}{15} = \frac{10}{5 || r}$

   In this case, the resistance of 5Ω branch can only decrease.

   ∴ This circuit cannot achieve balance condition.
7. (*b*) When AC is converted into DC using a rectifier circuit, then converted DC is an unstable current that includes ripples.

   A capacitor is used to remove these ripples and maintain a constant voltage across load.
8. (*d*) Photovoltaic devices can convert optical radiation into electricity. The basic example of such device is solar photovoltaic system which converts solar energy directly into electrical energy.

   Zener diode is heavily doped *p*-*n* junction diode operating in reverse biased condition in breakdown region.
9. (*b*) In half wave rectification, input frequency,

   $f_{in} = 60$ Hz

   Since, frequency of output voltage obtained from the half- wave rectifier is same as frequency of input AC voltage.

   Hence, $f_{out} = 60$ Hz
10. (*c*) In the circuit diagram (A) and (C), both the *p*-*n* junction diodes are in same biasing conditions.

    So, both diodes offers equal resistances.

    Since, both diodes are in series, therefore equal potential will drop across the junction.
11. (*c*) Zener diode is a type of special *p*-*n* junction diode that operates in reverse bias. Thus, it is used as a voltage regulator. So, the statement (A) is correct.

    The potential barrier of *p*-*n* junction for silicon is 0.6-0.7 V and for germanium is 0.2-0.35 V. So, the statement (B) is incorrect.
12. (*d*) A *p*-*n* junction diode is in forward biased when *p*-side is connected with more positive potential than *n*-side.

    Since, $0V > -3V$.

    Hence in option (d), diode circuit is in forward biased.
13. (*a*) Under reverse bias condition, the holes of *p*-side are attracted towards the negative terminal of the battery and electrons of the *n*-side are attracted towards the positive terminal of the battery. This increases the width of the depletion layer.
14. (*b*) The energy of light of wavelength λ is given by

    $$E = h\nu = \frac{hc}{\lambda} \Rightarrow \lambda = \frac{hc}{E} \quad ...(i)$$

    Here, h = Planck's constant
    $= 6.63 \times 10^{-34}$ J-s

    c = speed of light $= 3 \times 10^8$ m/s

    E = energy gap $= 1.9$ eV
    $= 1.9 \times 1.6 \times 10^{-19}$ J

    Substituting the given values in Eq. (i), we get

    $$\Rightarrow \lambda = \frac{6.63 \times 10^{-34} \times 3 \times 10^8}{1.9 \times 1.6 \times 10^{-19}}$$

    $$= 6.54 \times 10^{-7} \text{ m} \approx 654 \text{ nm}$$

    Thus, the wavelength of light emitted from LED will be 654 nm.

15. (*d*) Due to increase in temperature because of heating, thermal collision between the electron and holes increases. Thus, net electron-hole pairs increase. This leads to increase in the current in diode and overall resistance of the diode changes.

This in turn changes both the forward biasing and the reverse biasing.

Thus, the overall *I-V* characteristics of *p-n* junction diode gets affected.

16. (*a*) In the forward biasing of *p-n* junction, *p*-side of junction diode is connected to higher potential and *n*-side of junction diode is connected to lower potential.

17. (*a*) Let us assume that current through the diode is *I*.

From the given condition

$$\because \quad I = \frac{V_A - V_B}{R} = \frac{4-(-6)}{1\,\text{k}\Omega} = \frac{10}{1\times 10^3}$$

$$= 10^{-2}\,\text{A}$$

18. (*a*) In the given circuit, the diode D_1 will be in reverse bias, so it will block the current and diode D_2 will be in forward bias, so it will pass the current,

$$i = \frac{V}{R_1 + R_3} = \frac{10}{2+2} = 2.5\,\text{A}$$

19. (*d*) As it is forward biased so it takes positive value. Hence, option (d) is correct.

20. (*a*) Given, external resistance $R = 100\,\Omega$ and an emf is 3.5 V.

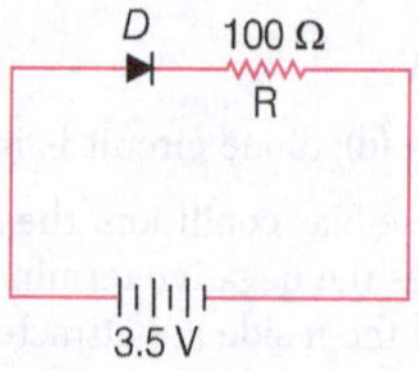

Potential barrier across the diode is 0.5 V.

Potential difference on $R = 3.5\text{ V} - 0.5\text{ V} = 3.0\text{ V}$

Current in circuit, $I = \frac{V}{R} = \frac{3}{100} = 0.03\text{ A} = 30\text{ mA}$

21. (*d*) The given combination of gates can be taken as

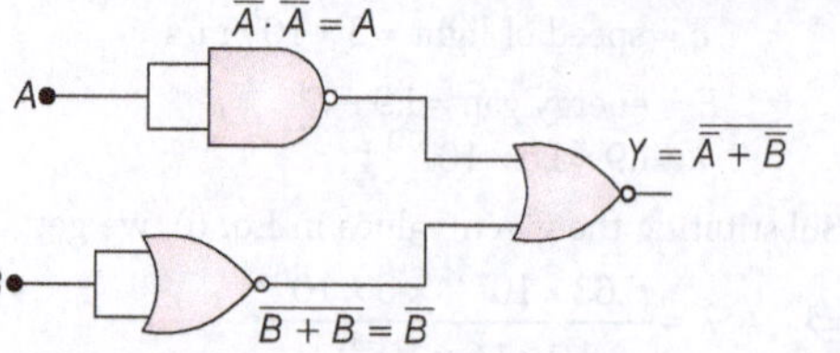

$$Y = \overline{\overline{A} + \overline{B}} = \overline{\overline{A}} \cdot \overline{\overline{B}} = A \cdot B$$

Hence, the output *Y* of the given logic gate is similar to AND gate.

22. (*c*) Output from the truth table

$$Y = \overline{AB} + \overline{AB}$$

$$\overline{B}\,(A + \overline{A})$$

$$Y = \overline{B}$$

So, correct option is (c).

23. (*a*) Output of the logic circuit is

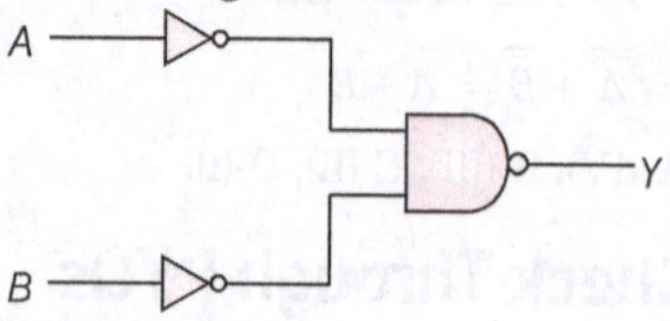

$$Y = \overline{\overline{A}\,\overline{B}} = \overline{\overline{A}} + \overline{\overline{B}} \qquad (\because \overline{xy} = \overline{x} + \overline{y})$$

$$= A + B \qquad (\because \overline{\overline{x}} = x)$$

$$= \text{output of OR gate}$$

Truth table is

A	B	Y = A + B
0	0	0
0	1	1
1	0	1
1	1	1

24. (*b*) The given logic circuit is represented as

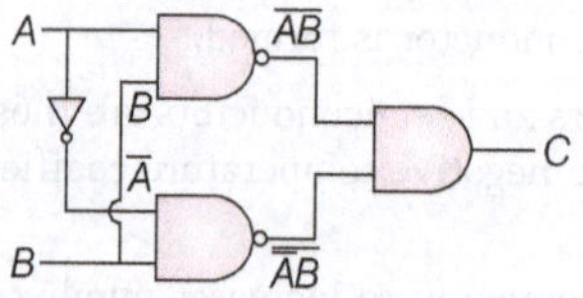

Output of logic circuit,

$$C = \overline{AB} \cdot \overline{\overline{A}B} = (\overline{A} + \overline{B}) \cdot (\overline{\overline{A}} + \overline{B})$$

$$= (\overline{A} + \overline{B}) \times (A + \overline{B})$$

$$= \overline{A}A + \overline{A}\,\overline{B} + \overline{B}A + \overline{B}\,\overline{B}$$

$$= 0 + \overline{A}\,\overline{B} + \overline{B}A + \overline{B} = \overline{A}\,\overline{B} + \overline{B}(A + 1)$$

$$= \overline{A}\,\overline{B} + \overline{B} = \overline{B}(\overline{A} + 1) = \overline{B}$$

Truth table is given as

A	B	C = $\overline{B}$
0	0	1
0	1	0
1	0	1
1	1	0

25. (*c*) NAND and NOR gate are called universal gate because all type of logic gates and boolean expressions can be realised with the help of NAND and NOR gate.

26. (*d*) Given, logic circuit is

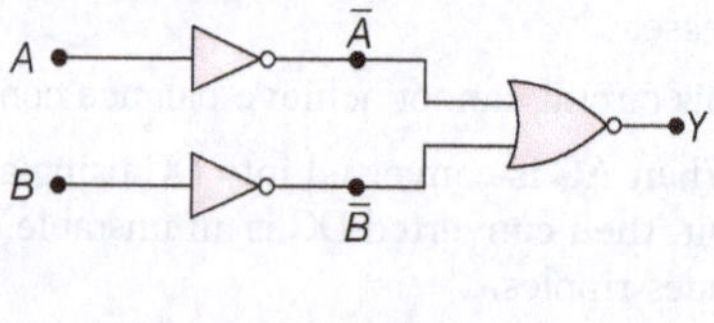

$$Y = \overline{\overline{A} + \overline{B}} = \overline{\overline{A}} \cdot \overline{\overline{B}}$$

[using de-Morgan's theorem, $\overline{x + y} = \overline{x} \cdot \overline{y}$]

$$= A \cdot B \qquad [\because \overline{\overline{x}} = x]$$

Truth table for above given logic circuit is

A	B	$\overline{A}$	$\overline{B}$	$Y = A \cdot B$
0	0	1	1	0
0	1	1	0	0
1	0	0	1	0
1	1	0	0	1

$\Rightarrow$

A	B	Y
0	0	0
0	1	0
1	0	0
1	1	1

Hence, correct option is (d).

27. (*a*) From the circuit diagram given below, it can be seen that the current will flow to ground if any of the switch is closed. Also, the LED will only glow when current flows through it.

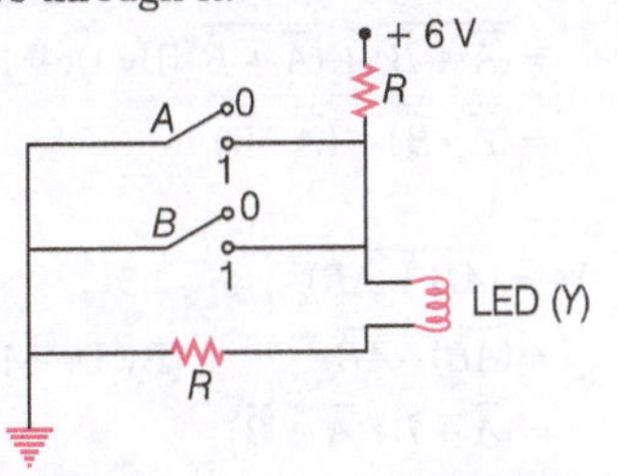

Thus, the truth table for the circuit diagram can be formed as circuit diagram in given solution.

A	B	Y
0	0	1
0	1	0
1	0	0
1	1	0

The output (Y) is equivalent to that of NOR gate.

28. (*b*) The LED will glow when the current flows through it, i.e. when the voltage across it is high. The truth table can be formed from this

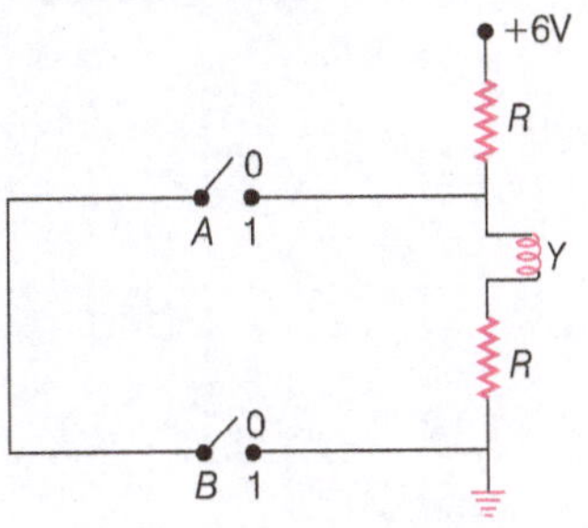

A	B	Y
0	0	1
0	1	1
1	0	1
1	1	0

The output Y is same as that come from NAND gate.

29. (*b*) According to the question, the figure of combination of gates in terms of inputs and outputs can be given as

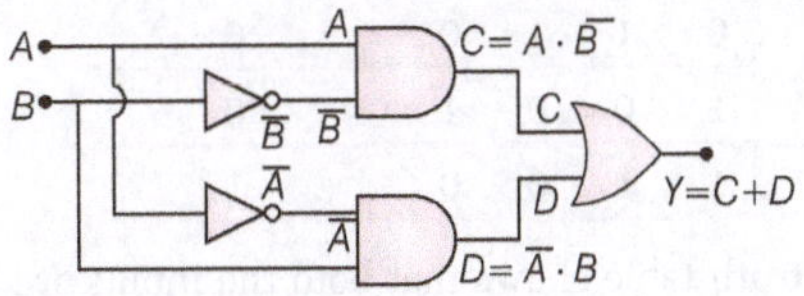

Thus,

$$Y = A \cdot \overline{B} + \overline{A} \cdot B$$

30. (*c*) Truth table for given network is

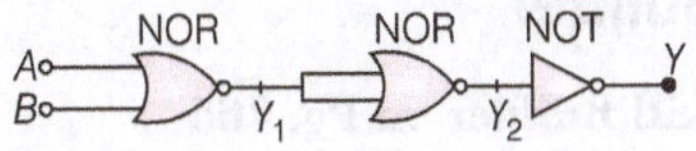

A	B	Y_1	Y_2	Y
0	0	1	0	1
1	0	0	1	0
0	1	0	1	0
1	1	0	1	0

Output Y of network matches with that of NOR gate.

31. (*c*) Consider the given figure in question,

The resultant boolean expression of the above logic circuit will be

$$Y = (A + B) \cdot C$$

Now, let us try with inputs A, B and C given in the options and lets see, which one of them will give output 1 at Y.

If $A = 0, B = 0, C = 0$

$\Rightarrow$ $Y = (0 + 0) \cdot 0$

$\Rightarrow$ $Y = 0$

If $A = 1, B = 1, C = 0$

$\Rightarrow$ $Y = (1 + 1) \cdot 0$

$\Rightarrow$ $Y = 1 \cdot 0$

$\Rightarrow$ $Y = 0$

If $A = 1, B = 0, C = 1$

$\Rightarrow$ $Y = (1 + 0) \cdot 1$

$\Rightarrow$ $Y = 1 \cdot 1$

$\Rightarrow$ $Y = 1$

If $A = 0, B = 1, C = 0$

$\Rightarrow$ $Y = (0 + 1) \cdot 0$

$\Rightarrow$ $Y = 1 \cdot 0$

$\Rightarrow$ $Y = 0$

So, we have seen that among the given options, only option (c) is the correct choice, *i.e.*

Output $Y = 1$ only when inputs

$$A = 1, B = 0 \text{ and } C = 1$$

32. (*c*) The truth table for the given circuit is

A	B	Y_1	Y_2	$Y = \overline{Y_1 + Y_2}$
0	0	1	1	0
0	1	1	0	0
1	0	0	1	0
1	1	0	0	1

The truth table shows that both the inputs are high, then we are getting high value of output otherwise zero.

Hence, the combination represents AND gate.

Skill Builder

Sol. of Skill Builder on Pg. 765

(*b*) For the forward biasing, *p*-part of diode must be at higher potential than *n*-part of diode.

Sol. of Skill Builder on Pg. 766

(*a*) For diode to be active, it must be forward biased. In options (b), (c) and (d), diodes are reverse biased.

Hence, options (b), (c) and (d) cannot achieve bridge balance.

For option (a),

balance bridge condition is $\frac{5}{2} = \frac{15}{5 + r_d}$.

If $r_d = 1\,\Omega$, bridge can be balanced.

Sol. of Skill Builder on Pg. 778

(*c*) Here, the two switches can be operated in different combinations.

Switch *A*	Switch *B*	Bulb	A	B	Y
OFF	OFF	ON	0	0	1
OFF	ON	ON	0	1	1
ON	OFF	OFF	1	0	0
ON	ON	OFF	1	1	0

From above table we can conclude that switch *B* doesn't effect the circuit but *A* does, when switch *A* is 'ON', then current will flow to ground and bulb will not glow. The bulb will only glow when current will pass through it.

Hence, $Y = \overline{A}$

It will behave like NOT gate for switch '*A*'.

Sol. of Skill Builder on Pg. 780

(*b*)

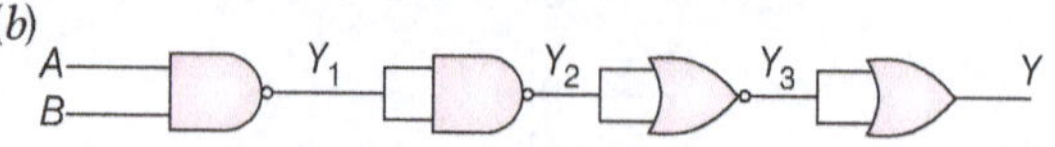

Here, $Y_1 = \overline{(A \cdot B)}$ [NAND gate]

$= (\overline{A} + \overline{B})$ [De-Morgon's theorem]

$Y_2 = \overline{(\overline{A} + \overline{B}) \cdot (\overline{A} + \overline{B})}$ [NAND gate]

$= \overline{(\overline{A} + \overline{B})} + \overline{(\overline{A} + \overline{B})}$ [By De-Morgan's theorem]

$= (\overline{\overline{A}} \cdot \overline{\overline{B}}) + (\overline{\overline{A}} \cdot \overline{\overline{B}})$

$= AB$

$Y_3 = \overline{(AB + AB)}$ [NOR gate]

$= (\overline{AB}) \cdot (\overline{AB})$ [By De-Morgan's theorem]

$= (\overline{A} + \overline{B})(\overline{A} + \overline{B})$

$= (\overline{A} + \overline{B})$

$Y = (\overline{A} + \overline{B})(\overline{A} + \overline{B})$ [OR gate]

$= (\overline{A} + \overline{B})$

$= \overline{(A \cdot B)}$

Hence, given circuit is equal to NAND gate.

For deeper insight
Scan the QR Code

Chapter 16

Experimental Skills

Learning Objectives

Module-I

- Experiment-1
- Experiment-2
- Experiment-3
- Experiment-4

Module-II

- Experiment-5
- Experiment-6
- Experiment-7
- Experiment-8
- Experiment-9

Module-III

- Experiment-10
- Experiment-11
- Experiment-12

Module-IV

- Experiment-13
- Experiment-14
- Experiment-15
- Experiment-16
- Experiment-17

Chapter Overview with
NEET Connection

This chapter provides better understanding of all other chapters of class 11th and 12th by providing experimental exposure of concepts. Having good grasp of this chapter can help us to understand the other chapter very easily.

Special format questions from each of the experiment can be easily framed on the following topics

- Conceptual information of components
- Experimental data based questions

For better understanding of this chapter

- Concerned theoritical chapter must be revisited.
- Basic exposure to components of different experiments in Physics laboratory will be very helpful.

Introduction

A practical physics course should enable us to do experiments on the fundamental laws and principles, and gain experience of using a variety of measuring instruments. Practical work improves basic learning skill. To enhance focus of students on experiments of Physics, experimental skills chapter is introduced with additional purpose to enhance experiments related problems solving abilities.

In this chapter, we will study about seventeen experiments which as listed in NTA's NEET-UG syllabus and describes concepts, formulae, important results of experiments followed by few practice questions.

Module 1

Experiments Related to Vernier Caliper, Screw Gauge, Simple Pendulum and Meter Scale

EXPERIMENT-1

Vernier Caliper

To measure internal and external diameter and depth of vessel.

Summary

The least count of vernier caliper = $M - V$ ...(i)

where, M = the distance between two consecutive divisions on the main scale.

V = The distance between two consecutive divisions on the vernier scale.

The length of x divisions on vernier scale = The length of y divisions on the main scale.

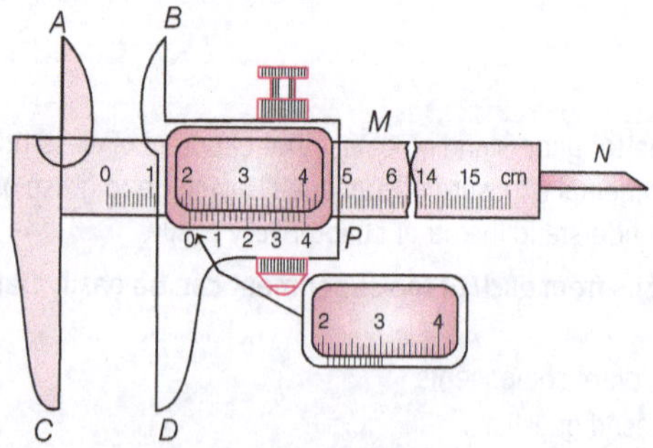

Therefore, $xV = yM$

$$V = \frac{y}{x}M$$

From Eq. (i), the LC of vernier caliper

$$= M - \left(\frac{yM}{x}\right) = M\left(\frac{x-y}{x}\right)$$

If $x - y = 1$, then least count

$$= \frac{M}{x} = \frac{\text{1 Main scale division}}{\text{Number of division in vernier scale}}$$

Zero Error

When the jaws are made to touch each other, the zero mark of the main scale and vernier scale may not be in the straight line. Reading in this case is known as zero error.

- When zero of vernier scale is on right of zero of main scale, then zero error is positive.
- When zero of vernier scale is on left of zero of main scale, then zero error is negative.
- Zero error = Vernier scale reading with closed jaws × least count
- Corrected reading = Observed reading − Zero error

NEET Close-up

Example Similar to PYQ Asked in NEET 2024

Each part of the main scale of vernier caliper is divided into 40 equal parts. If the 20th vernier scale division coincides with 19th main scale division, then the value of vernier constant (in cm) is

(a) 4.25×10^{-3} (b) 6.25×10^{-2}
(c) 2.25×10^{-4} (d) 1.25×10^{-3}

Sol. (*d*) 1 cm is divided into 40 equal parts.

$\therefore$ $1 \text{ MSD} = \frac{1}{40} \text{ cm}$

$\because$ $20 \text{ VSD} = 19 \text{ MSD}$

$\therefore$ $1 \text{ VSD} = \frac{19}{20} \text{ MSD}$

Then, least count $= 1 \text{ MSD} - 1 \text{ VSD}$

$$= 1 \text{ MSD} - \frac{19}{20} \text{ MSD} = \frac{1}{20} \text{ MSD} = \frac{1}{20} \times \frac{1}{40} = \frac{1}{800} \text{ cm} = 1.25 \times 10^{-3} \text{ cm}$$

Skill Builder

Each part of the main scale division of a vernier calipers is divided into 20 equal parts.

If the 10th vernier scale division coincides with 9th main scale division, then the value of vernier constant (in cm) is

(a) 5×10^{-3} (b) 4×10^{-3}
(c) 2×10^{-3} (d) 3.25×10^{-3}

For more Practice Refer Q. No. 7 of step up practice 1.

EXPERIMENT-2

Micrometer screw gauge

To measure thickness/ diameter of thin sheet/wire.

Summary

Least count of screw gauge

$$= \frac{\text{Pitch}}{\text{Total number of divisions on circular scale}}$$

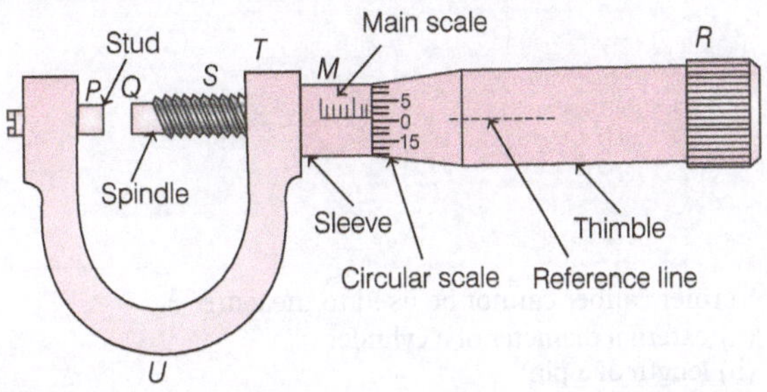

Concept ladder

- A normal screw gauge has 1MSD = 1 mm and 100 divisions in circular scale. (LC = 0.01 mm)
- Pitch = Change in MS (Main Scale) in one complete rotation of CS (Circular Scale).
- Final (observed) value = Main scale reading + Circular deflection × Least count

Zero Error

In case of **positive zero error**, zero of CS (Circular Scale) is below the reference line.

$$ZE = n \times LC \qquad (n = \text{circular deflection})$$

Corrected reading = Observed reading – Zero error

In case of **negative zero error**, zero of CS (circular scale) is above the reference line.

$$ZE = (n - 100) \times LC$$

EXPERIMENT-3

Simple pendulum

Dissipation of energy by plotting graph between the square of amplitude and time

Summary

- Restoring force (SHM), $F = -kx$
- Damping force (drag force), $F = -bv$

Equation of damped motion,

$$\frac{md^2x}{dt^2} + b\frac{dx}{dt} + kx = 0$$

Solution of above equation,

$$x = A_0 e^{-bt/2m} \cos(\omega' t + \phi)$$

$$\text{where, } \omega' = \sqrt{\frac{k}{m} - \frac{b^2}{4m^2}}$$

x versus t graph

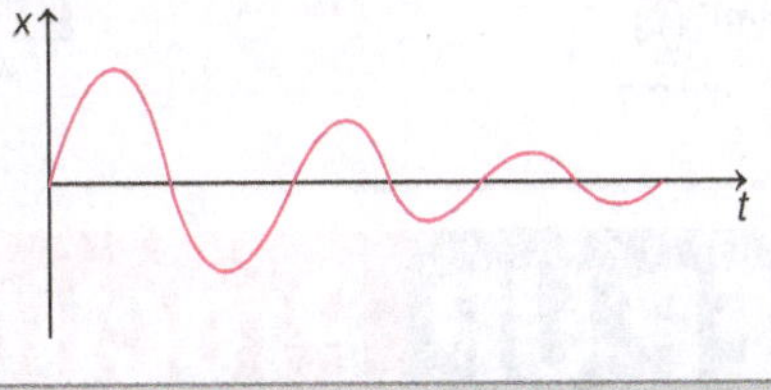

Damped Oscillation

1. (Amplitude)^2 $\quad A^2 = A_0^2 e^{-bt/m}$

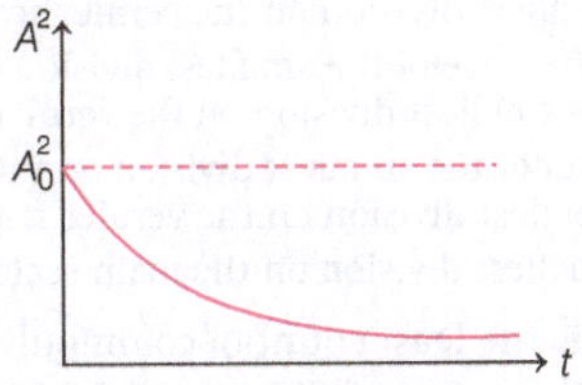

2. Total energy

$$E = \frac{1}{2}kA^2 = \frac{1}{2}k\left[A_0 e^{\frac{-bt}{2m}}\right]^2$$

$$E = \left(\frac{1}{2}kA_0^2\right)e^{-bt/m} = E_0 e^{-bt/m}$$

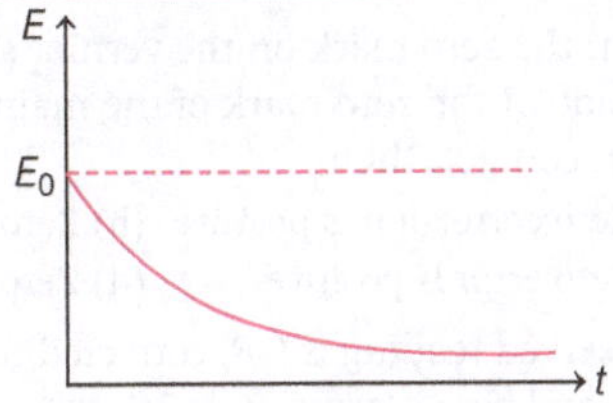

Concept ladder

- Graph of (amplitude)^2 *versus* time is same as energy-time graph.
- All three graphs (amplitud *versus* time, energy *versus* time and (amplitude)^2 *versus* time decay exponentially with time.

EXPERIMENT-4

Meter Scale

Mass of given object by the principle of moments.

Summary

A meter rod is supported at its centre of gravity on a wedge as shown.

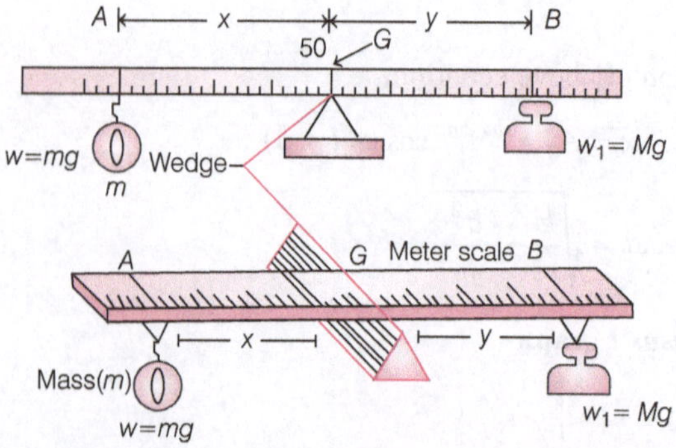

As unknown mass m is suspended from the left arm at a distance x and known as **standard mass.** M is suspended from the right arm at a distance y. The distances are measured from the knife edge.

For equilibrium, the moments of forces about the fulcrum of knife edge is equal, so we have

$$mg \times x = Mg \times y$$

$$\Rightarrow \quad m = M\left(\frac{y}{x}\right)$$

STEP UP Practice 1

1. What is the least count of the vernier caliper?
   (a) Smallest division on the vernier scale.
   (b) Difference of the smallest division on the main scale and the smallest division on the vernier scale.
   (c) Sum of the smallest division on the main scale and the smallest division on the vernier scale.
   (d) Smallest division on the main scale.

2. What is the least count of commonly available vernier?
   (a) 0.01 cm (b) 0.001 cm (c) 0.0001 cm (d) 0.1 cm

3. When the zero mark on the vernier scale lies towards the right side of the zero mark of the main scale, the jaws are in contact, then what will be the zero error?
   (a) Zero error is positive (b) Zero error is negative
   (c) Zero correction is positive (d) Zero error does not exist

4. When the zero mark on the vernier scale lies towards the left side of the zero mark of the main scale, when the jaws are in contact, then
   (a) Zero correction is positive (b) Zero correction is negative
   (c) Zero error is positive (d) Zero error does not exist

5. If observed reading is OR, corrected reading is CR, zero error is ZE and zero correction is ZC, then what will be the possibility?
   (a) CR = OR + ZC and ZE = CR − OR
   (b) CR = OR + ZE and ZC = CR − OR
   (c) CR = OR − ZC and SE = OR − CR
   (d) CR = OR − ZE and ZC = CR − OR

6. When the jaws of a standard vernier are together, zero of main scale is not coinciding with zero of vernier scale. If 4th division of vernier scale meets exactly with 4th division of main scale, zero error is;
   (a) − 0.04 mm (b) − 0.4 mm
   (c) + 0.4 mm (d) + 0.04 mm

7. In an unusual vernier, 10 vernier scale divisions, coincide with 8 main scale divisions, then what is the least count of the vernier? (1 MSD = 1 mm)
   (a) 0.1 mm (b) 0.2 mm
   (c) 0.8 mm (d) $\frac{1}{8}$ mm

8. Vernier caliper cannot be used to measure
   (a) external diameter of a cylinder
   (b) length of a pin
   (c) diameter of hair
   (d) internal diameter of a cylinder

9. One main scale division of vernier caliper is of 0.5 mm and its least count is to be 0.005 cm. The number of vernier divisions is
   (a) 10 (b) 20 (c) 30 (d) 40

10. **Assertion** (A) A vernier caliper has a positive error of 0.5 mm, then the correction is − 0.5 mm.
    Reason (R) In case of positive zero error, measured length is greater than the actual length.
    In the light of the above statements, choose the correct answer from the options given below.
    (a) Both A and R are true but R is not the correct explanation of A.
    (b) A is true but R is false.
    (c) A is false but R is true.
    (d) Both A and R are true and R is the correct explanation of A.

11. When the edge of circular scale lies to the left of 0 mark on the main scale, when the stud and spindle touch each other. Then, what will be the zero error?
    (a) Zero error is negative (b) Zero error is positive
    (c) Zero error does not exist (d) Zero correction is negative

12. When the edge of the circular scale lies to the right of the 0 mark on the main scale, when the stud and the spindle touch each other. Then
    (a) Zero correction is negative
    (b) Zero error is negative
    (c) Zero error does not exist
    (d) Zero correction is positive

13. When the screw and stud touch each other, zero of the circular scale is above reference line and the 96th division of the circular scale coincides with the reference line of main scale, then what is the value of zero error?
    (a) + 0.96 mm (b) − 0.96 mm
    (c) + 0.04 mm (d) − 0.04 mm

14. When the screw and stud touch each other, the edge of certain screw gauge is to the right of the 0 mark on the main scale and 5th division of the circular scale coincides with the line of graduation, then what is the value of zero error?

(a) + 0.95 mm (b) – 0.95 mm
(c) + 0.05 mm (d) – 0.05 mm

15. Screw gauge A has a pitch of 1 mm and 50 divisions on its circular scale and screw gauge B has a pitch of 0.5 mm and 100 divisions on its circular scale. If (L × C) is least count, then which possibility is true?

(a) $2(LC)_A = (LC)_B$ (b) $(LC)_A = 4(LC)_B$
(c) $(LC)_A = (LC)_B$ (d) $(LC)_A = 2(LC)_B$

16. The screw gauge shown has a zero error of – 0.02 mm and 100 divisions on the circular scale. What is the diameter of wire?

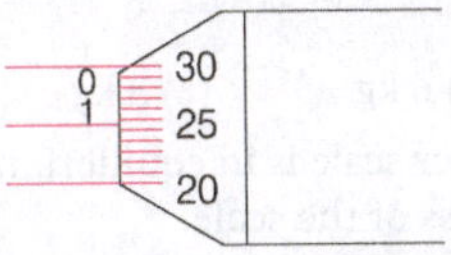

(a) 0.28 mm (b) 0.22 mm
(c) 0.24 mm (d) 0.26 mm

17. Match the Column I and Column II.

Column I	Column II
(a) A	(p) Main scale
(b) B	(q) circular scale
(c) C	(r) stud
(d) D	(s) spindle
(e) E	(t) Ratchet
(f) F	(u) Thimble
(g) G	(v) Screen

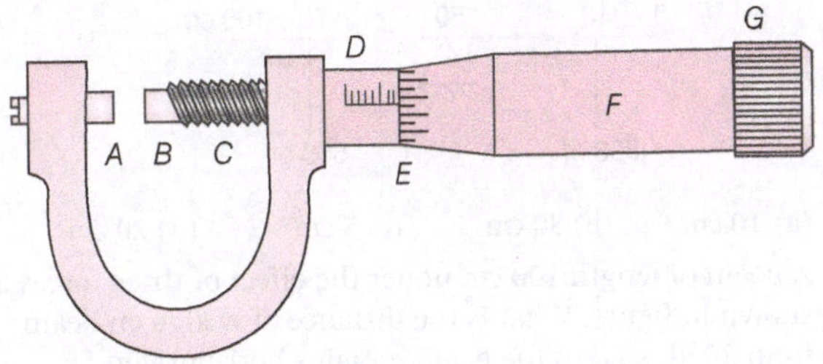

(a) a → r, b → s, c → v, d → p, e → q, f → u, g → t
(b) a → u, b → I, c → v, d → p, e → q, f → r, g → s
(c) a → v, b → p, c → r, d → s, e → t, f → q, g → u
(d) a → p, b → q, c → u, d → t, e → r, f → s, g → v

18. For the pitch of a screw 0.1 cm and 200 divisions on circular scale, then least count will be

(a) 0.5 mm (b) 0.05 mm
(c) 0.005 mm (d) 0.0005 mm

19. The screw gauge has least count of 0.005 mm and its circular scale is divided into 100 equal divisions. What is the distance between two consecutive threads of its screw?

(a) 0.5 mm (b) 0.05 mm
(c) 0.01 mm (d) 0.1 mm

20. A screw gauge with a pitch of 0.5 mm and a circular scale with 50 divisions is used to measure the thickness of a thin sheet of aluminium. Before starting the measurement, it is found that when the anvil and screw are in contact with each other, the 45th division coincides with the main scale line and that the zero of the main scale is not visible. What is the thickness of the sheet, if the main scale reading is zero and the 25th division coincides with the main scale line?

(a) 0.50 mm (b) 0.45 mm (c) 0.20 mm (d) 0.50 mm

21. If the time period of undamped oscillation is T and that of damped oscillation is T', then what is the relation between T and T'

(a) $T' < T$
(b) Nothing can be said, unless the drag force constant is known
(c) $T' = T$
(d) $T' > T$

22. The energy dissipated in a damped oscillation

(a) decays exponentially
(b) decays curve will depend on the drag constant
(c) decays linearly
(d) decays following a sine curve with diminishing amplitude.

23. What is the equation for a damped oscillator, where k and b are constants and x is displacement?

(a) $\frac{md^2x}{dt^2} + kx + \frac{bdx}{dt} = 0$ (b) $\frac{md^2x}{dt^2} xkx = \frac{bdx}{dt}$
(c) $m\frac{d^2x}{dt^2} + kx + \frac{bdx}{dt}$ (d) $\frac{md^2x}{dt^2} + kx = b\frac{dx}{dt}$

24. Which of the following change with time when damping is considered for an SHM?

(i) Time period (ii) Angular frequency
(iii) Amplitude (iv) Energy
(a) (i) and (ii) (b) (iii) and (iv)
(c) (ii) and (iii) (d) All of these

25. Which of the following represent the correct graph for the square of amplitude with time for a damped SHM?

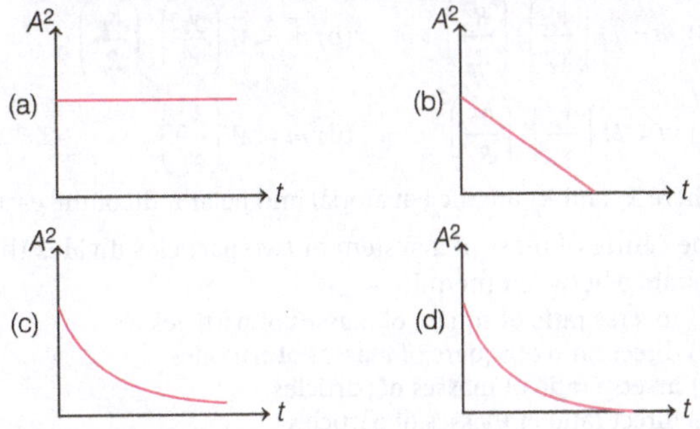

26. Which of the following represent the correct graph for energy with time for a damped SHM?

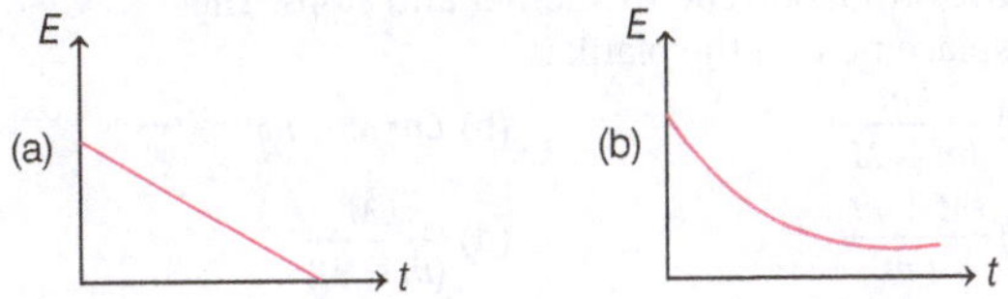

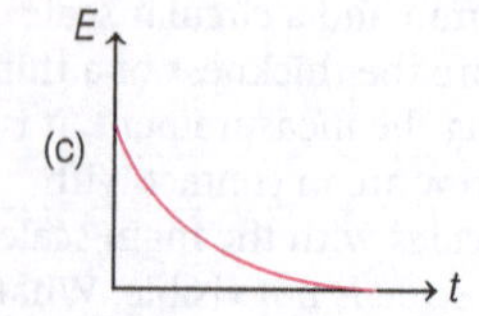

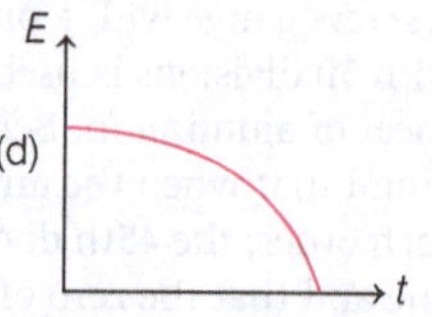

27. The amplitude of a damped SHM becomes half in 1 min and $\frac{1}{x}$ times in 3 min. Then, the value of x will be

(a) 16 (b) 4 (c) 8 (d) 6

28. In a damped oscillation, the amplitude after 50 oscillations is $0.8\,a_0$, where a_0 is the initial amplitude, then amplitude after 150 oscillations is

(a) $0.28\,a_0$ (b) $0.512\,a_0$ (c) zero (d) a_0

29. In the experiment of simple pendulum we keep $\theta < 5°$, so as ensure

(a) mass m does not interfere in the time period
(b) g remains constant
(c) the air drag is not too much
(d) $\sin\theta \cong \theta$ where by motion becomes simple harmonic

30. When the moment of force is maximum, then what is the angle between force and position vector of the force?

(a) 90° (b) 0° (c) 30° (d) 45°

31. In the scale and wedge experiment, m situated at x from the wedge and M is situated at y from wedge at equilibrium. Now, if $m < M$, then what is the relation between x and y?

(a) $x = y$
(b) $x < y$
(c) $x > y$
(d) Nothing can be said about $-x$ and y unless values of m and M one know.

32. When the "wedge and scale" experiment is performed at the equator, we get $m = M\left(\frac{y_e}{x_e}\right)$. If the same experiment is performed at the poles, then what is the right equation?

(a) $m = M\left(\frac{y_e}{x_e}\right)\cdot\left(\frac{R_e}{R_p}\right)$ (b) $m = M\left(\frac{y_e}{x_e}\right)\cdot\left(\frac{R_p}{R_e}\right)$

(c) $m = M\left(\frac{y_e}{x_e}\right)\cdot\left(\frac{R_p}{R_e}\right)^2$ (d) $m = M\left(\frac{y_e}{x_e}\right)$

where R_e and R_p are the equatorial and polar radii of the earth.

33. The centre of mass of a system of two particles divides the distance between them in

(a) inverse ratio of square of masses of particles
(b) direct ratio of square of masses of particles
(c) inverse ratio of masses of particles
(d) direct ratio of masses of particles

34. A person of mass m is standing on one end of a plank of mass M and length L and floating in water. The person moves from one end to another and stops. The displacement of the plank is

(a) $\frac{Lm}{(m+M)}$ (b) $Lm(M+m)$

(c) $\frac{(M+m)}{Lm}$ (d) $\frac{LM}{(m+M)}$

35. Two particles of masses 5 kg of 10 kg respectively, are attached to the two ends of a rigid rod of length 1m with negligible mass.

The centre of mass of the system from the 5 kg particle is nearly at a distance of

(a) 80 cm (b) 33 cm
(c) 50 cm (d) 67 cm

36. In an experiment with a meter scale an unknown mass m is balanced by two known masses of 16 kg and 4 kg as shown in figure. Find m.

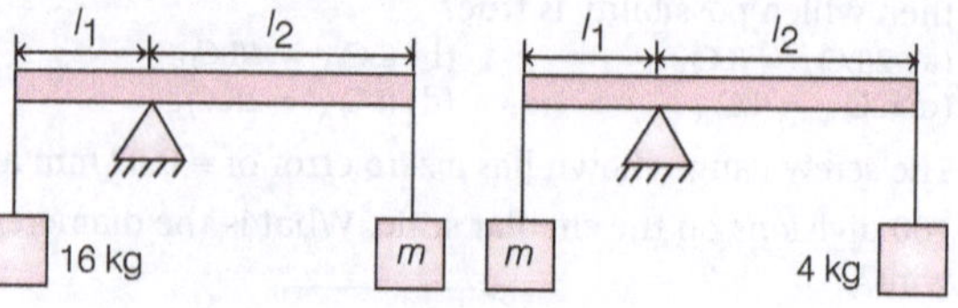

(a) 10 kg (b) 6 kg (c) 8 kg (d) 12 kg

37. If a uniform meter scale is in equilibrium position, then calculate the mass of the scale.

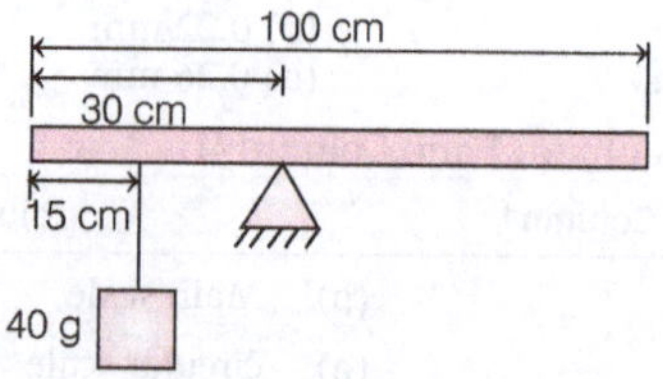

(a) 20 g (b) 30 g (c) 40 g (d) 10 g

38. Figure shows a uniform meter scale weighing 200 gf, pivoted at its centre. Two weight 300 gf and 500 gf are suspended from the ruler as shown in the figure. The distance from mid-point where a 200 gf should be suspended to balance the meter scale is

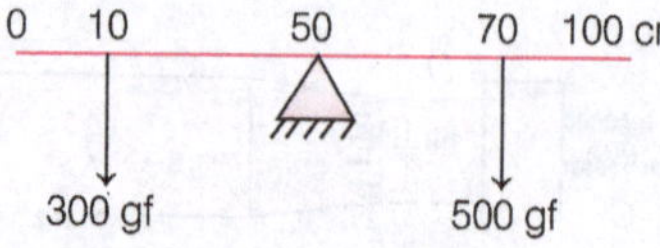

(a) 10 cm (b) 30 cm (c) 5 cm (d) 20 cm

39. A beam of length 100 cm under the effect of three forces as shown in figure. What is the distance of wedge on beam from 80 gf, so that the beam remains horizontal in equilibrium?

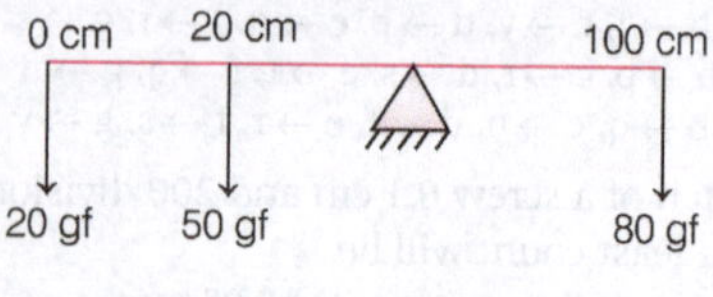

(a) 30 cm (b) 35 cm
(c) 40 cm (d) 50 cm

40. A uniform meter scale is balanced at 60 cm mark, when weight of 5 gf and 40 gf are suspended at 10 cm and 80 cm mark, respectively. Calculate the weight of the meter scale.

(a) 65 gf (b) 60 gf
(c) 75 gf (d) 55 gf

Module 2

Experiments Related to Young's Modulus, Surface Tension of Liquid by Capillary, Viscosity, Resonance Tube and Specific Heat Capacity

EXPERIMENT-5

To determine the Young's modulus of elasticity of the material of a metallic wire.

Summary

Where a wire of length L is stratched by a force F. Its cross-section is A and it extends by 1.

Young's modulus, $Y = \frac{FL}{Al} = \frac{mgL}{\pi r^2 l}$

where, r is radius of wire.

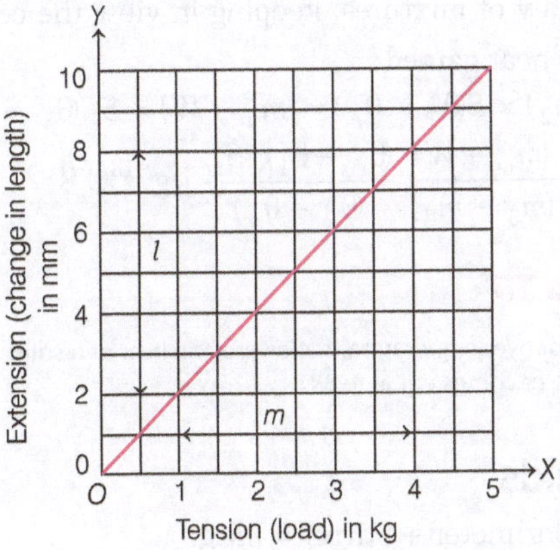

Clearly $l \propto F$ or extension is proportional to the tension

EXPERIMENT-6

To determine the surface tension of liquid by capillary rise method and effect of detergents.

Summary

Weight of meniscus $= \left(\frac{\pi r^3}{3}\right) \rho g$, if r is small

where, ρ is the density of liquid and r is the radius of capillary.

Surface tension, $T = \frac{rh\rho g}{2\cos\theta}$

$T \propto rh$(ρ, θ and g are constants)

for clean glass capillary and pure water $\theta \approx 0°$

where, ρ = density

h = height of liquid and

θ = angle of contact

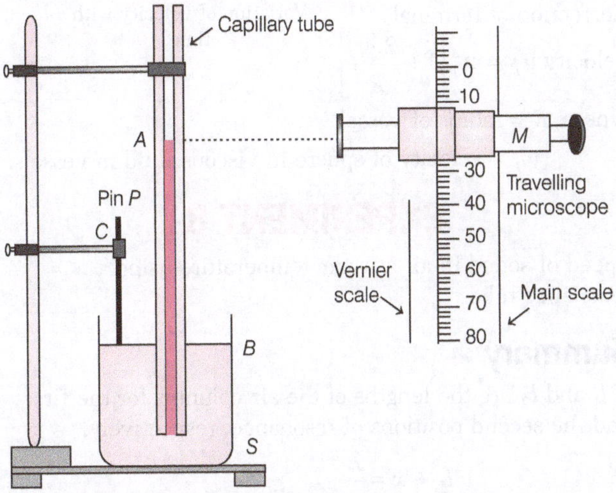

To determine the surface tension of liquid by capillary rise method

If correction is applied, then formula will be

$$T = \frac{r\rho g\left[h + \frac{r}{3}\right]}{2\cos\theta}$$

for water

$$T = \frac{h\rho g r}{2}$$

EXPERIMENT-7

Coefficient of viscosity of a given viscous liquid by measuring terminal velocity of a given spherical body.

Summary

Stoke's force, $F = 6\pi\eta r v$

where,

η = coefficient of viscosity,

r = radius of sphere and

v = velocity of sphere

$$\eta = \frac{2}{9} r^2 g \left(\frac{\rho - \sigma}{v_T}\right)$$

$$\Rightarrow \quad v_T = \frac{2}{9}\frac{r^2 g(\rho - \sigma)}{\eta}$$

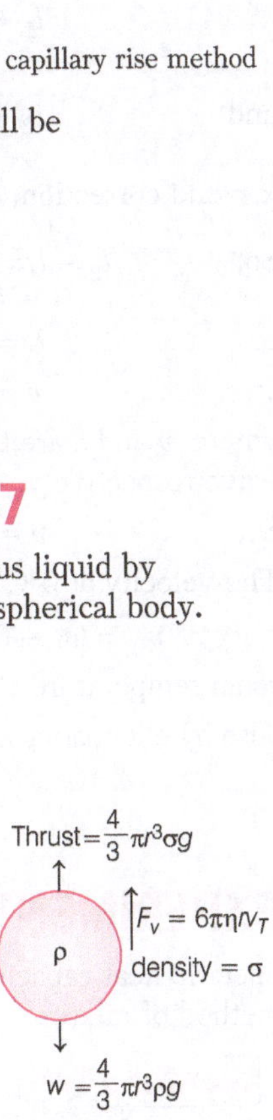

where,

η = viscosity of liquid

r = radius of sphere

ρ = density of sphere

σ = density of liquid

v_T = terminal velocity

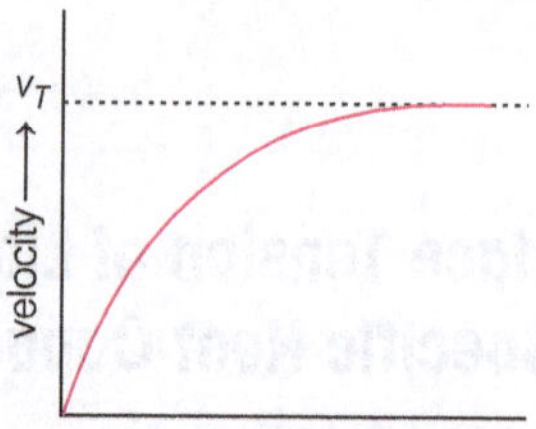

Variation of velocity with time

Correction of terminal velocity $v_T = v_0\left[1+\frac{2.4r}{R}\right]$

where, R = radius of vessel

v_0 = velocity of sphere in viscous fluid in vessels.

EXPERIMENT-8

Speed of sound in air at room temperature using a resonance tube.

Summary

If l_1 and l_2 are the lengths of the air columns for the first and the second positions of resonance, respectively.

$$l_1 + x = \frac{\lambda}{4} \quad \text{...(i)}$$

and

$$l_2 + x = \frac{3\lambda}{4} \quad \text{...(ii)}$$

x = end correction, λ = wavelength of the sound wave.

So, $$l_2 - l_1 = \frac{\lambda}{2}$$

or $$\lambda = 2(l_2 - l_1)$$

$\because$ $$v = n\lambda$$

where, v and n are the velocity and frequency of the sound wave respectively.

So, $$v = 2n(l_2 - l_1)$$

The velocity at 0°C is given by

$v_0 = (v_t - 0.61 \times t)$ in ms^{-1} where, v_t is velocity at room temperature t°C.

Also by eliminating λ from Eqs. (i) and (ii), the end correction.

$$x = \frac{l_2 - 3l_1}{2}$$

EXPERIMENT-9

Specific heat capacity of a given (i) solid and (ii) liquid by method of mixture.

Mentor's TiP

- In resonant tube (organ pipe) open at both ends, both odd and even harmonics are present.

Summary

Law of mixtures i.e., **Heat gained by cold substance = Heat loss by hot substance**

(Assuming no heat loss to the atmosphere)

For Solids

Mass of calorimeter + Stirrer + Lid = m_1 g.

Mass of calorimeter + Lid + Cold water = m_2 g.

Temperature of cold water in calorimeter = θ_1 °C.

Steady temperature of solid in hypsometer by thermometer $B = \theta_2$ °C.

Final, *i.e.* equilibrium temperature of the mixture θ_e °C.

Mass of calorimeter + Stirrer + Liq. + water + Solid = m_3 g.

Water equivalent of calorimeter + stirrer, $W = m$ (mass of calorimeter) $\times \frac{S_C}{S_W}$

Applying law of mixtures, keeping in view the conditions, heat lost = heat gained

$$(m_3 - m_2) \times S(\theta_2 - \theta_e) = (m_w + W) \times S_w(\theta_e - \theta_1)$$

$$\therefore \quad S = \frac{(m_w + W)}{(m_3 - m_2)} \frac{(\theta_e - \theta_1)\cdot S_w}{(\theta_2 - \theta_e)} \text{ J/g}^{-1}{}^\circ\text{C}^{-1}$$

Mentor's TiP

- At the debye temperature, molar specific heat of a solid at constant volume becomes equal to 3*R*.

For Liquids

Mass of calorimeter + Stirrer = m_1 g.

Mass of calorimeter + Stirrer + Oil = m_2 g.

Temperature of oil in the calorimeter = θ_1 °C.

Mass of the cylindrical piece tied to thread = m_3 g

Temperature of boiling water in the beaker, *i.e.*, temperature of metal piece $\theta_2 = 100$ °C.

Steady equilibrium temperature of mixture = 0_e° C.

Water equivalent of calorimeter,

$$W = \text{Mass} \times \frac{\text{Specific heat of material of calorimeter}}{\text{Specific heat of water}}$$

Mass of oil, $m = m_2 \times 0.095$ (for copper calorimeter)

Applying law of mixtures

$$(\theta_e - \theta_1)(W + mS_t) = m_3 \times S \times (100 - \theta_e)$$

Specific heat of liquid,

$$S_l = \frac{m_3 \cdot S(100 - \theta_e)}{m(\theta_e - \theta_1)} - \frac{W}{m} (\text{J g}^{-1}{}^\circ\text{C}^{-1})$$

STEP UP Practice 2

1. Two rods of different materials having coefficients of thermal expansions α_1, α_2 and Young's moduli Y_1, Y_2 respectively, are fixed between two rigid walls. The rods are heated such that they undergo the same increase in temperature. There is no bending of the rod, if $\alpha_1 : \alpha_2 = 2:3$ the thermal stresses developed in the rod are equal provided $Y_1 : Y_2$ equals.
(a) 3 : 2
(b) 2 : 3
(c) 4 : 9
(d) 1 : 1

2. A uniform rod of length L and density ρ is being pulled along a smooth floor with a horizontal acceleration α. What is the magnitude of the stress at the transverse cross-section through the mid-point of the rod?
(a) $\frac{1}{3}L\rho\alpha$
(b) $L\rho\alpha$
(c) $\frac{2}{3}L\rho\alpha$
(d) $\frac{L\rho\alpha}{2}$

3. A solid cylindrical steel column is 4 m long and 9 cm in diameter. ($Y_{steel} = 1.9 \times 10^{11}$ Nm^{-2}). The decrease in length of the column, while carrying a load of 80000 kg is
(a) 3.2 mm
(b) 1.8 mm
(c) 4.4 mm
(d) 2.6 mm

4. In the Searle's experiment following four wires are made of the same material. Which of these will have the largest extension when the same tension is applied?
(a) Length = 300 cm, diameter = 3 mm
(b) Length = 50 cm, diameter = 0.5 mm
(c) Length = 100 cm, diameter = 1 mm
(d) Length = 200 cm, diameter = 2 mm

5. Copper of fixed volume V is drawn into wire of length l. When this wire is subjected to a constant force F, the extension produced in the wire is Δl. Which of the following graphs is a straight line?
(a) Δl versus $\frac{1}{l}$
(b) Δl versus l^2
(c) Δl versus $\frac{1}{l^2}$
(d) Δl versus l

6. In determination of Young's modulus of elasticity of wire, a force is applied and extension is recorded. Initial length of wire is 1m. The curve between extension and stress is depicted, then Young's modulus of wire will be

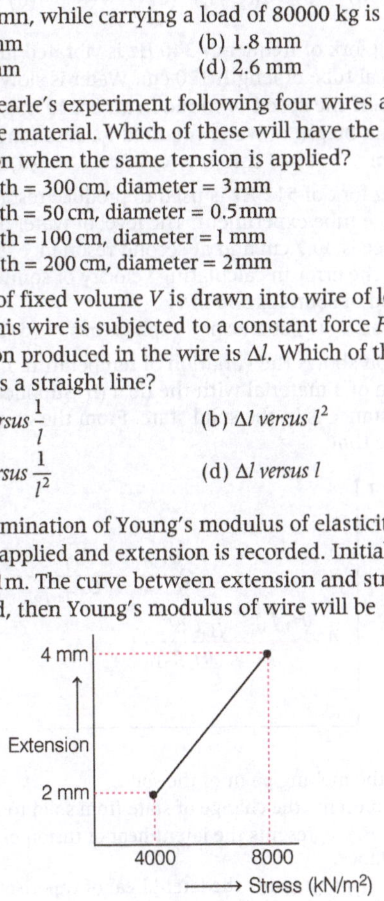

(a) 2×10^9 N/m^2
(b) 1×10^9 N/m^2
(c) 2×10^{10} N/m^2
(d) 1×10^{10} N/m^2

7. The maximum load a test wire in Searle's experiment can withstand without breaking, when its length is reduced to half of its original length, will
(a) be double.
(b) be half.
(c) be four times.
(d) remain same.

8. Overall changes in volume and radii of a uniform cylindrical steel wire are 0.2% and 0.002% respectively, when subjected to some suitable force. Longitudinal tensile stress acting on the wire is ($Y = 2.0 \times 10^{11}$ N/m^2)
(a) 3.2×10^9 Nm^{-2}
(b) 3.2×10^7 Nm^{-2}
(c) 3.6×10^9 Nm^{-2}
(d) 3.9×10^8 Nm^{-2}

9. The Young's modulus of a wire of length L and radius r is Y newton per square metre. If the length is reduced to $\frac{L}{2}$ and radius of $\frac{r}{2}$, its Young's modulus will be
(a) $\frac{Y}{2}$
(b) Y
(c) $2Y$
(d) $4Y$

10. The Young's modulus of the material of a wire is equal to the
(a) stress required to increase its length four times
(b) stress required to produce unit strain
(c) strain produced in it
(d) half the strain produced in it

11. If the temperature of a wire is doubled, then the Young's modulus of elasticity will
(a) also double.
(b) become four times.
(c) remain same.
(d) decrease.

12. To what height can mercury be filled in a vessel without any leakage, if there is a pin hole of diameter 0.1 mm at the bottom of the vessel? (Density of mercury $= 1.36 \times 10^4$ kg m^{-3}, surface tension of mercury $= 550 \times 10^{-3}$ Nm^{-1} and angle of contact with the vessel for mercury = 0°)
(a) 16.5 cm
(b) 18.5 cm
(c) 20 cm
(d) 12.5 cm

13. A spherical soap bubble of radius 2 cm attached to the outside of a spherical bubble of radius 4 cm. Then, what is the radius of the common surface?
(a) 3.5 cm
(b) 4 cm
(c) 4.5
(d) 3 cm

14. By how much depth will the surface of a liquid be depressed in a glass tube of radius 0.2 mm if the angle of contact of the liquid is 135° and the surface tension is 0.547 Nm^{-1}? (Density of the liquid is 1.28×10^4 kg m^{-3})
(a) 3 cm
(b) 4 cm
(c) 5 cm
(d) 2 cm

15. Complete the sentence

If the height of a capillary is smaller than the height to which water should rise, then ....

(a) water stops gets depressed in the capillary below the water surface.
(b) water rises up to the height of the capillary and meniscus becomes less concave.
(c) water does not rise in such a capillary at all.
(d) water states flowing out like a fountain.

16. Water rise in a capillary upto an extension height such that upward force of surface tension balances the force of 75×10^{-4} N due to weight of water. If surface tension of water is 6×10^{-2} N/m. The internal circumference of the capillary must be

(a) 12.5×10^{-2} m (b) 6.5×10^{-2} m
(c) 0.5×10^{-2} m (d) 1.25×10^{-2} m

17. Internal radius of a capillary tube is $\frac{1}{14}$ cm and surface tension of water is 70 dyne/cm, if angle of contact is zero, then water will rise up in the tube up to height ($g = 980$ cm/s^2)

(a) 4 cm (b) 2 cm (c) 14 cm (d) 18 cm

18. The wettability of a surface by a liquid depends primarily on

(a) angle of contact between the surface and the liquid
(b) viscosity
(c) surface tension
(d) density

19. Water rises to height h in capillary tube, if the length of capillary tube above the surface of water is made less than h, then

(a) water does not rise at all.
(b) water rises upto the tip of capillary tube and then starts overflowing like a fountain.
(c) water rises upto the top of capillary tube and stays there without overflowing.
(d) water rises upto a point a little below the top and stays there.

20. Three liquids of densities ρ_1, ρ_2 and ρ_3 (with $\rho_1 > \rho_2 > \rho_3$), having the same value of surface tension T, rise to the same height in three identical capillaries. The angles of contact θ_1, θ_2 and θ_3 obey.

(a) $\frac{\pi}{2} < \theta_1 < \theta_2 < \theta_3 < \pi$ (b) $\pi > \theta_1 > \theta_2 > \theta_3 > \frac{\pi}{2}$
(c) $\frac{\pi}{2} > \theta_1 > \theta_2 > \theta_3 \geq 0$ (d) $0 \leq \theta_1 < \theta_2 < \theta_3 < \frac{\pi}{2}$

21. **Statement I** Viscosity of liquids decreases with decrease in temperature.

Statement II Surface tension of a liquid decreases with increase in temperature.

In the light of the above statement, choose the most appropriate answer from the options given below

(a) Both Statement I and Statement II are incorrect.
(b) Statement I is correct but Statement II is incorrect.
(c) Statement I is incorrect but Statement II is correct.
(d) Both Statement I and Statement II are correct.

22. A tube closed at one end and containing air produces, when excited, the fundamental note of frequency 512 Hz. If the tube is open at both ends, the fundamental frequency that can be excited is (in Hz)

(a) 1024 (b) 512 (c) 256 (d) 128

23. An air column in pipe, which is closed at one end will be in resonance with a vibrating tuning fork of frequency 264 Hz if the length of the column (in cm) is [$v = 330$ m/s]

(a) 31.25 (b) 62.50 (c) 110 (d) 125

24. Velocity of sound in air is 320 m/s. A pipe closed at one end has a length of 1 m neglecting end corrections, the air column in the pipe can resonant for sound of frequency.

(1) 80 Hz (2) 240 Hz (3) 500 Hz (4) 400 Hz
(a) 1 (b) 1, 2 (c) 1, 2, and 4 (d) 1, 4

25. In a long cylindrical tube, the water level is adjusted and the air column above it is made to vibrate in unison with a vibrating tuning fork kept at the open end. Maximum sound is heard when the air column lengths are equal to

(a) $\frac{\lambda}{4}, \frac{\lambda}{2}, \frac{3\lambda}{4}$ (b) $\frac{\lambda}{2}, \lambda, \frac{3\lambda}{2}$ (c) $\frac{\lambda}{2}, \frac{3\lambda}{2}, \frac{5\lambda}{2}$ (d) $\frac{\lambda}{4}, \frac{3\lambda}{4}, \frac{5\lambda}{4}$

26. If l_1 and l_2 are the lengths of air column for the first and second resonance when a tuning fork of frequency n is sounded on a resonance tube, then the distance of the displacement anti-node from the top end of the resonance tube is

(a) $2(l_2 - l_1)$ (b) $\frac{1}{2}2(l_2 - l_1)$ (c) $\frac{l_2 - 3l_1}{2}$ (d) $\frac{l_2 - l_1}{2}$

27. A tuning fork of frequency 340 Hz is vibrated just above a cylindrical tube of length 120 cm. Water is slowly poured in the tube. If the speed of sound in air is 340 m/s, then the minimum height of water required for resonance is

(a) 25 cm (b) 45 cm (c) 75 cm (d) 95 cm

28. A tuning fork of 512 Hz is used to produce resonance in a resonance tube experiment. The level of water at first resonance is 30.7 cm and at second resonance is 63.2 cm. What is the error in calculating velocity of sound? Assume the speed of sound is 330 m/s.

(a) 58 cm/s (b) 204.1 cm/s (c) 280 cm/s (d) 110 cm/s

29. The graph shows the variation of temperature T of one kilogram of a material with the heat (H) supplied to it, at O, the substance is in the solid state. From the graph, we can conclude that.

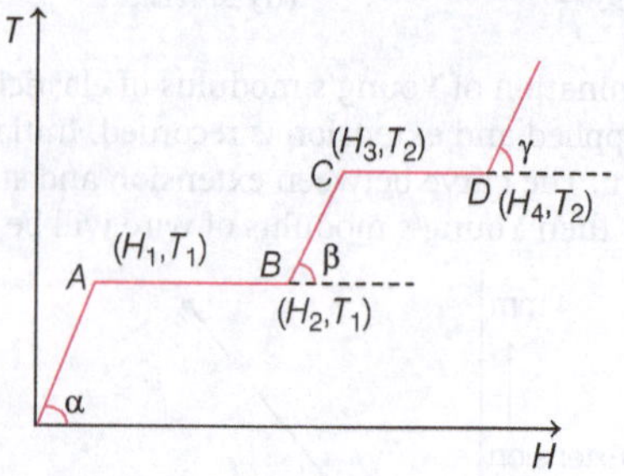

(a) T_2 is the melting point of the solid.
(b) BC represents the change of state from solid to liquid.
(c) $(H_2 - H_1)$ represents the latent heat of fusion of the substance.
(d) $(H_3 - H_1)$ represents the latent heat of vaporisation of the liquid

30. A block of ice at –10°C is slowly heated and converted to steam at 100°C. Which of the following curves represents the phenomenon qualitatively ?

(a)

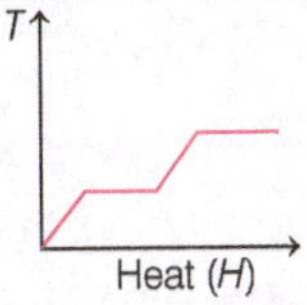

(b)

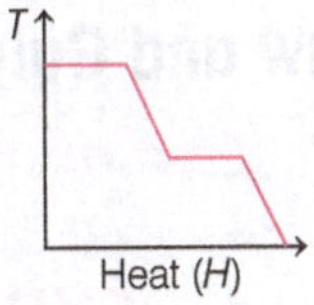

(c)

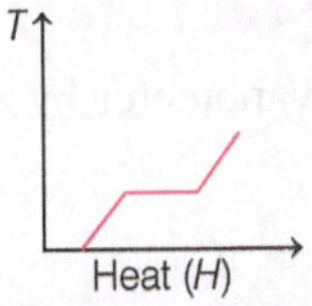

(d)

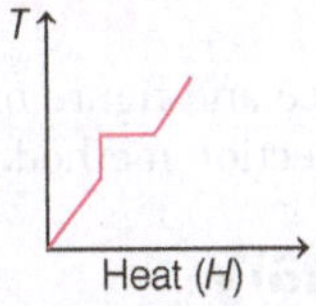

31. Which of the substances *A*, *B* or *C* has the highest specific heat in the temperature *versus* time graph is shown ?

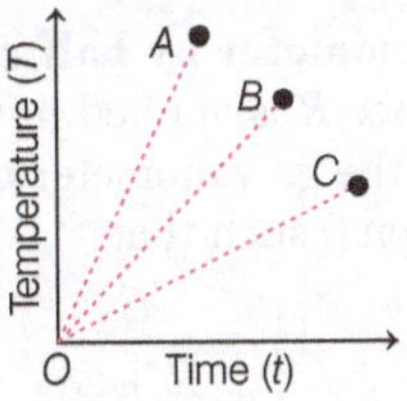

(a) *A*
(b) *B*
(c) *C*
(d) All have equal specific heat

32. Equal amount of heat energy is transferred into equal mass of ethyl alcohol and water sample. The rise in temperature of water sample is 25°C.
The temperature rise of ethyl alcohol will be
(Specific heat of ethyl alcohol is one half of the specific heat of water)
(a) 12.5°C
(b) 25°C
(c) 50°C
(d) It depends on the rate of energy transfer.

33. A block of mass 2.4 kg is heated to temperature of 500°C and placed on a large ice block. What is the maximum amount of ice that can melt (approx)? (Specific heat for the block = 0.1 cal/g°C.)
(a) 1 kg (b) 1.5 kg (c) 2 kg (d) 2.5 kg

34. 10 g of ice at 0°C is kept in a calorimeter of water equivalent 10 g. How much heat should be supplied to the apparatus to evaporate the water thus formed? (Neglect loss of heat)
(a) 6200 cal (b) 7200 cal
(c) 13600 cal (d) 8200 cal

35. 1 kg of ice of 0°C is mixed with 1 kg of steam at 100°C. What will be the composition of the system when thermal equilibrium is reached? Latent heat of fusion of ice $= 3.36 \times 10^5$ J/kg and latent heat of vaporisation of water $= 2.26 \times 10^6$ J/kg.
(a) 2000 g water
(b) 665 g steam and 1335 g water
(c) 665 g ice and 1335 g water
(d) 2000 g steam

36. A copper ball of mass 100 g is at a temperature *T*. It is dropped in a copper calorimeter of mass 100 g, filled with 170 g of water at room temperature. Subsequently, the temperature of the system is found to be 75°C. *T* is given by (Given, room temperature = 30° C, specific heat of copper = 0.1 cal/g°C)
(a) 1250°C (b) 825°C
(c) 800°C (d) 885°C

37. The amount of heat required in converting 1 g ice at –10°C into steam at 100°C will be
(a) 3030 J (b) 6065 J
(c) 721 J (d) 616 J

38. 2 kg ice at –20°C is mixed with 5 kg water at 20°C. Then, final amount of water in the mixture would be,
(Given, specific heat of ice = 0.5 cal/g°C,
specific heat of water = 1 cal/g°C,
latent heat of fusion for ice = 80 cal/g.)
(a) 6 kg (b) 5 kg
(c) 4 kg (d) 2 kg

39. 420 J of energy supplied to 10 g of water will raise its temperature by nearly
(a) 1°C (b) 4.2°C
(c) 10°C (d) 42°C

40. Two liquids are at temperatures 20°C and 40°C. When same mass of both of them is mixed the temperature of mixture is 32°C. What is ratio of their specific heat ?
(a) 1/3 (b) 2/3
(c) 1/5 (d) 2/5

Module 3

Experiments Related to Meter Bridge, Ohm's Law and Galvanometer

EXPERIMENT-10

To find resistivity of the material of a given wire using meter bridge.

Summary

According to Wheatstone bridge principle, at the null point.

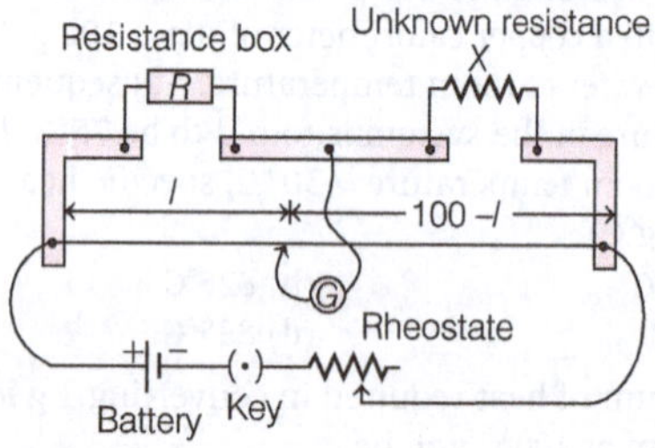

$$\frac{R}{X}=\frac{\lambda l}{\lambda(100-l)} \Rightarrow X=\frac{R}{l}(100-l)$$

$$\text{Resistivity}=\frac{XA}{l}$$

where, λ = resistance per cm

A = cross-section area

X = resistance

l = length of resistor

$$\rho=\frac{X\cdot\pi D^2}{4l}$$

where, D = diameter of resistor

EXPERIMENT-11

To find resistance of a given wire using Ohm's law.

Summary

Ohm's law $I \propto V$ or $V \propto I$ (provided physical conditions remains same)

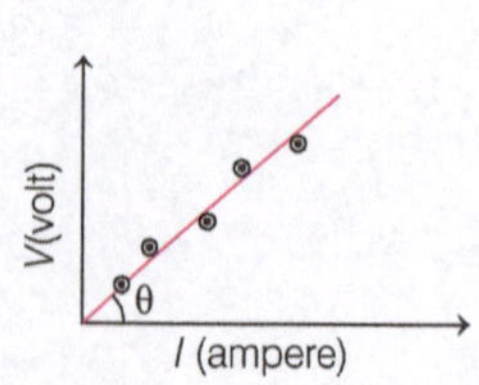

$$R=\frac{V}{I}$$

If the current is steady for different voltage across to resistor R, the graph nature of $V \rightarrow I$ is straight line with positive slope. (*i.e.* Temperature of resistor is constant)

Slope of graph $V \rightarrow I$ gives values of resistor.

EXPERIMENT-12

Resistance and figure of merit of a galvanometer by half-deflection method.

Summary

Galvanometer constant, $K=\left(\frac{c}{NAB}\right)$

Resistance of galvanometer by half deflection method

When a high resistance R is applied in the circuit with K_1 closed and K_2 open, the galvanometer draws a current I_g and shows a deflection θ such that

$$I_g=\frac{E}{R+G} \qquad \text{...(i)}$$

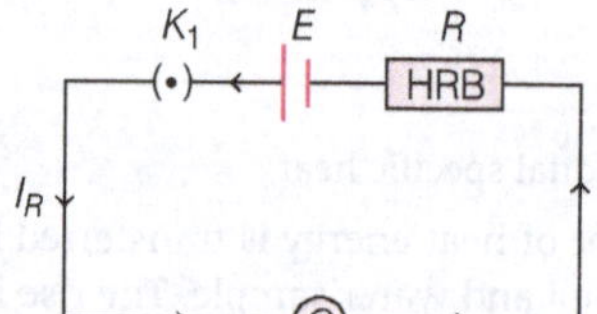

where, E is emf of the battery and G is resistance of the galvanometer.

Now, K_2 is closed. Adjust the resistance, in LRB such that galvanometer deflection becomes equal to $\frac{\theta}{2}$.

Now, the galvanometer draw the current.

$$I'_g=\frac{IS}{G+S}=\frac{ES}{R(G+S)+GS} \qquad \left(\text{where, } I=\frac{E}{R+\frac{GS}{S}}\right)$$

Also $I'_g=\frac{1}{2}I_g$

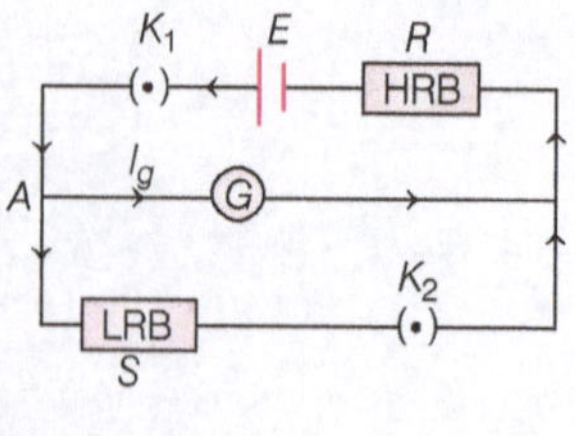

$$\therefore \quad \frac{ES}{R(G+S)\;GS}=\frac{1}{2}\cdot\frac{E}{R+G}$$

gives, $G = \frac{RS}{R - S}$

where,

G = resistance of galvanometer coil,

R = series resistance and

θ = deflection in galvanometer

- Galvanometer resistance, $G = \frac{RS}{R - S}$

  where, S = resistance of shunt

- Shunt

$$S = \frac{I_g \cdot G}{(I - I_g)} = \frac{G}{n - 1} \text{ where, }$$

$$n = \frac{I}{I_g}$$

Value of high series resistance,

$$R_S = \frac{V}{I} - G = [(n-1)G] \text{ where, } n = \frac{V}{V_g}$$

$$\text{Figure of merit} = \frac{C}{NAB}$$

Current sensitivity of galvanometer,

$$S_i = \frac{\theta}{i} = \frac{NAB}{C}$$

Voltage sensitivity of galvanometer

$$S_V = \frac{\theta}{V} = \frac{NAB}{CR}$$

Mentor's TIP

- The linear relationship between current (I) and angle of twist (α) makes the moving coil galvanometer useful for current measurement and detection.

STEP UP Practice 3

1. Which of the following statement(s) is/are true regarding null point in finding resistance of unknown wire using meter bridge.

(i) At null point, current through galvanometer is zero.

(ii) At null point, condition is balanced Wheatstone bridge.

(iii) Deflection of galvanometer in same direction, either side of null point.

(a) (i) only (b) (i) and (iii)
(c) (i) and (ii) (d) All of these

2. Wheatstone bridge is an arrangement of .... resistors used for accurate measurement of resistance.

(a) three (b) six
(c) five (d) four

3. The resistivity of the material depends on

(a) length of the wire (b) diameter of the wire
(c) density of the wire (d) material of the wire

4. A thin uniform wire AB of length 1 m, an unknown resistance X and a resistance of 12 Ω are connected by thick conducting strips as shown in figure. A battery and a galvanometer (with a sliding jockey connected to it) are also available. In the following diagram, connections are given to measure the unknown resistance X using the principle of Wheatstone bridge. The appropriate connection are

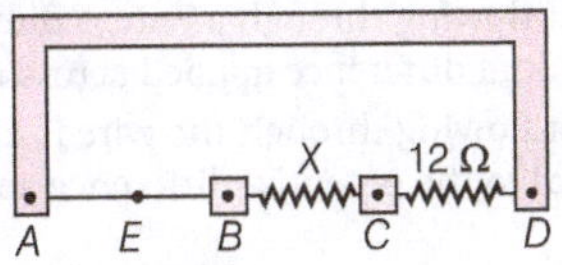

(E is the balance point for Wheatstone bridge)

(a) battery across EB and galvanometer across BC
(b) battery across EC and galvanometer across BD
(c) battery across BD and galvanometer across EC
(d) battery across BC and galvanometer across CD

5. In meter bridge experiment, a thin uniform wire AB of length 1 m and unknown resistance X and a resistance of 12 Ω are connected.

In the above question, after appropriate connection are made, it is found that no deflection takes places in the galvanometer where the sliding jockey touches the wire at a distance of 60 cm from A. What is the value of the resistance X?

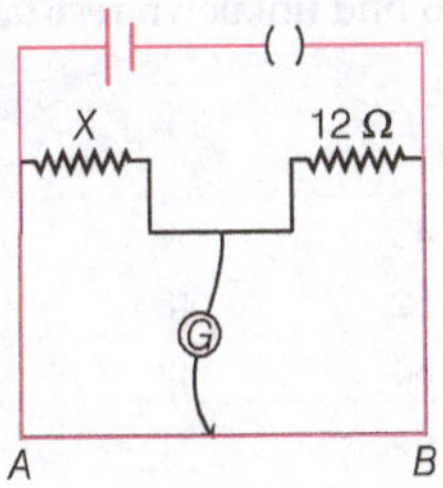

(a) 18 Ω (b) 6 Ω
(c) 16 Ω (d) 4 Ω

6. In a simple meter bridge circuit, the both gaps are bridge by coils P and Q having the smaller resistance. A balance is obtained when the jockey key makes contact at a point of the bridge wire 40 cm from the P end. On shunting the coil Q with a resistance of 50 Ω the balance point is moved through 10 cm. What are the resistances of P and Q?

(a) $\frac{100}{3}\Omega, \frac{100}{2}\Omega$ respectively
(b) $\frac{50}{3}\Omega, \frac{50}{2}\Omega$ respectively
(c) $\frac{25}{3}\Omega, \frac{25}{2}\Omega$ respectively
(d) $\frac{75}{3}\Omega, \frac{75}{2}\Omega$ respectively

7. Resistance in the two gaps of a meter bridge are 10 ohms and 30 ohms, respectively. If the resistances are interchanged, the balance point shifts by
(a) 33.3 cm (b) 66.67 cm (c) 25 cm (d) 50 cm

8. An unknown resistance R_1 is connected in series with a resistance of 10Ω. This combination is connected to one gap of a meter bridge while a resistance R_2 is connected in the other gap. The balance point is at 50 cm. Now, when the 10Ω resistance is removed the balance point shifts to 40 cm. The value of R_1 is (in ohms)
(a) 20 (b) 10 (c) 60 (d) 40

9. The meter bridge shown in a balanced position with $\frac{P}{Q} = \frac{l_1}{l_2}$.

If we now interchange the positions of galvanometer and cell, will the bridge work? If yes, what will be balance condition?

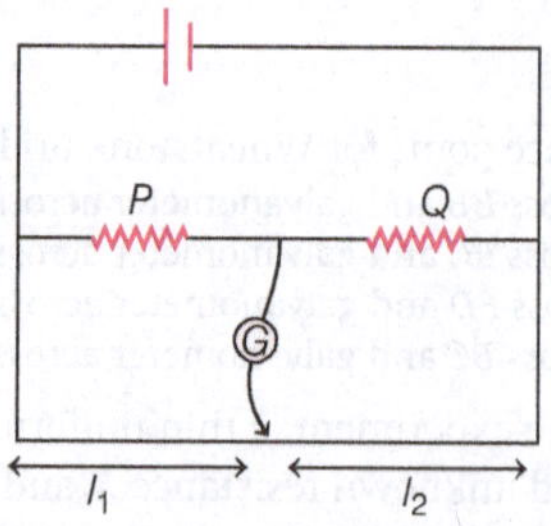

(a) Yes, $\frac{P}{Q} = \frac{l_2 - l_1}{l_2 + l_1}$ (b) No, no null point
(c) Yes, $\frac{P}{Q} = \frac{l_2}{l_1}$ (d) Yes, $\frac{P}{Q} = \frac{l_1}{l_2}$

10. A student obtained following observations in an experiment of meter bridge to find unknown resistance of given wire.

S. No.	R	l	100 − l	$S = \left(\frac{100 - l}{l}\right)R$
1	2 Ω	43	57	2.65
2	3 Ω	52	48	2.77
3	4 Ω	58	42	2.89
4	5 Ω	69	31	2.25

The most accurate value of unknown resistance will be
(a) 2.65 Ω (b) 2.77 Ω (c) 2.89 Ω (d) 2.25 Ω

11. In a meter bridge experiment null point is obtained at 20 cm from one end of the wire when resistance X is balanced against another resistance Y. If $X < Y$, then where will be the new position of the null point from the same end, if one decide to balance a resistance of $4X$ against Y?
(a) 50 cm (b) 80 cm (c) 40 cm (d) 70 cm

12. A meter bridge is set-up as shown, to determine an unknown resistance X using a standard 10 ohm resistor. The galvanometer shows null point when tapping-key is at 52 cm mark. The end corrections are 1 cm and 2 cm respectively, for the ends A and B. The determined value of ' X is

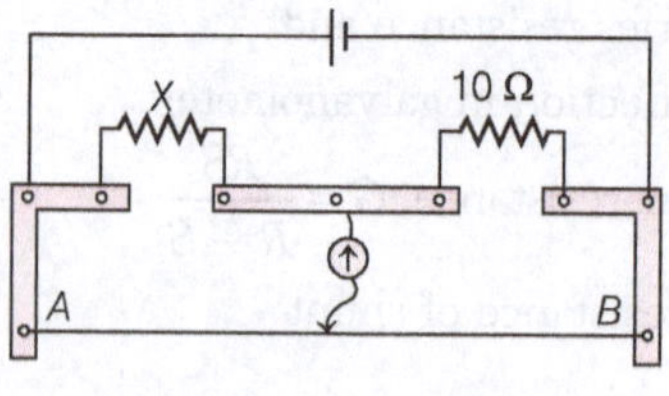

(a) 10.2 Ω (b) 10.6 Ω (c) 10.8 Ω (d) 11.1 Ω

13. **Assertion** (A) Meter bridge wire is made up of manganin.
Reason (R) The temperature of coefficient of resistance is very small for manganin.
In the light of the above statements, choose the correct answer from the options given below
(a) Both A and R are true but R is not the correct explanation of A.
(b) A is true but R is false.
(c) A is false but R is true.
(d) Both A and R are true and R is the correct explanation of A.

14. The point to be kept in mind of verification of Ohm's law is
(a) ammeter and voltmeter should be connected in series
(b) ammeter should be connected in series and voltmeter in parallel
(c) ammeter should be connected in parallel and voltmeter in series
(d) More the one of the above

15. From the given V-I graph for three resistors R_1, R_2 and R_3 it may be concluded that

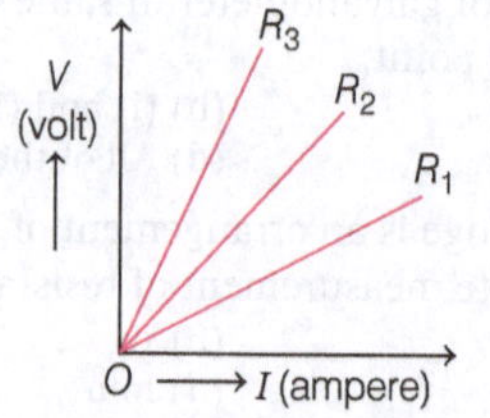

(a) $R_1 > R_2 > R_3$ (b) $R_1 < R_2 < R_3$
(c) $R_1 = R_2 = R_3$ (d) None of these

16. In an electric circuit, current becomes half when resistance is
(a) removed (b) doubled
(c) halved (d) None of these

17. According to Ohm's Law, which of the following is true?
(a) The current flowing through a wire is inversely proportional to its length.
(b) The current flowing through a wire is directly proportional to its resistance.
(c) The current flowing through a wire is directly proportional to the potential difference applied across its ends.
(d) The current flowing through the wire is inversely proportional to the potential difference applied across its ends.

18. Choose the correct statement regarding Ohm's law.
(a) It is valid for any circumstances, *i.e.* independent of temperature.
(b) Ohm's law is valid for all conducting materials.
(c) The temperature must be constant for validation of this law
(d) All are wrong.

19. The electric resistance of a certain wire of iron is R. If its length and radius both are doubled, then
(a) the resistance will be halved and the specific resistance will remain unchanged.
(b) the resistance will be halved and the specific resistance will be doubled.
(c) the resistance and the specific resistance will both remain unchanged.
(d) the resistance will be doubled and the specific resistance will be halved.

20. When a piece of aluminium wire of finite length is drawn to reduce its diameter to half its original value, its resistance will become
(a) two times (b) four times
(c) eight times (d) sixteen times

21. As the temperature of a metallic resistor is increased, the product of resistivity and conductivity,
(a) increases
(b) decreases
(c) may increase or decrease
(d) remains constant

22. The length of a given cylindrical wire is increased by 100%. Due to the consequent decrease in diameter the change in the resistance of the wire will be
(a) 300% (b) 200%
(c) 100% (d) 50%

23. The current voltage graph for a given metallic conductor at two different temperatures T_1 and T_2 are as shown in the figure. Then,

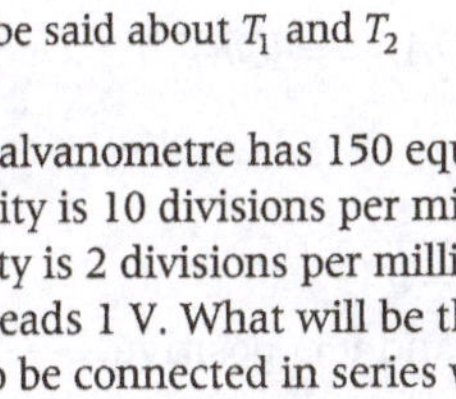

(a) $T_1 > T_2$
(b) $T_1 = T_2$
(c) nothing can be said about T_1 and T_2
(d) $T_1 < T_2$

24. A moving coil galvanometre has 150 equal divisions. Its current sensitivity is 10 divisions per milliampere and voltage senstivity is 2 divisions per millivolt. In order that each divisions reads 1 V. What will be the resistance in ohms needed to be connected in series with the coil?
(a) 10^3 (b) 99995
(c) 9995 (d) 10^5

25. A galvanometre of resistance 200 Ω gives full scale deflection for a current of 10^{-3} A. To convert it into an ammetre capable of measuring upto 1 A. What resistance should be connected in parallel with it?
(a) $2\times10^{-1}\,\Omega$ (b) 2Ω
(c) $2\times10^{-3}\,\Omega$ (d) $2\times10^{-6}\,\Omega$

26. A galvanometre with resistance 100 Ω is converted into an ammetre with a resistance of 0.1. The galvanometre shows full scale deflection with current of 100 μA. Then, what will be the minimum current in the circuit for all scale deflection of galvanometre?
(a) 0.1001 mA (b) 100.1 mA
(c) 1000.1 mA (d) 1.001 mA

27. The range of a galvanometre of resistance G ohm is V volt. The resistance required to be connected in series with it in order to convert it into voltmetre of range nv volt will be
(a) $\frac{G}{n}$ (b) nG
(c) $(n-1)G$ (d) $\frac{G}{(n-1)}$

28. The scale of a galvanometre of resistance 100 Ω contains 25 divisions. It gives a deflection of I division on passing a current 4×10^{-4} A. The resistance in ohm to be added to it. So that, it may become a voltmetre of range 2.5 V is
(a) 250 (b) 300 (c) 150 (d) 100

29. A galvanometre of resistance 200 Ω gives full scale deflection with 15 milliampere current. In order to convert it into a 15 V range voltmetre. What is the value of resistance connected in series?
(a) 1000 Ω (b) 800 Ω
(c) 2500 Ω (d) 1500 Ω

30. What is the relation between figure of merit (k) and current sensitivity (S_I)?
(a) $S_I = k^{-1}$ (b) $S_I = \frac{k}{2}$
(c) $S_I = kV$ (d) $S_I = (k)I$

31. One micrometre has a resistance of 100 Ω and a full scale range of 50 μ A. It can be used as a voltmetre or as a higher range ammetre provided a resistance is added to it. Pick the correct range and resistance combination (s).
(a) 5 mA range with 2 Ω resistance in parallel
(b) 10 mA range with 1 Ω resistance in parallel
(c) 10 V range with 200 kΩ resistance in series
(d) 50 mV range with 10 kΩ resistance in series

32. Current sensitivity of a moving coil galvanometre is 5 div/mA and its voltage sensitivity (angular deflection per unit voltage applied) is 20 div/V.
The resistance of the galvanometre is
(a) 40 Ω (b) 25 Ω
(c) 250 Ω (d) 500 Ω

Module 4

Experiments Related to Mirror & Lens, Prism, Travelling Microscope, p-n Junction Diode and Zener Diode

EXPERIMENT-13

Focal length of (i) Concave mirror (ii) Convex mirror and (iii) Convex lens

Summary

(i) Concave Mirror

Formula for focal length, $f = \dfrac{uv}{u+v}$

Here, u = distance of object from pole of mirror and
v = distance of image from pole of mirror.

- We use **optical bench** for these three experiments.
- u and v both are negative for concave mirror.

Graphs

(a) Graph between u and v

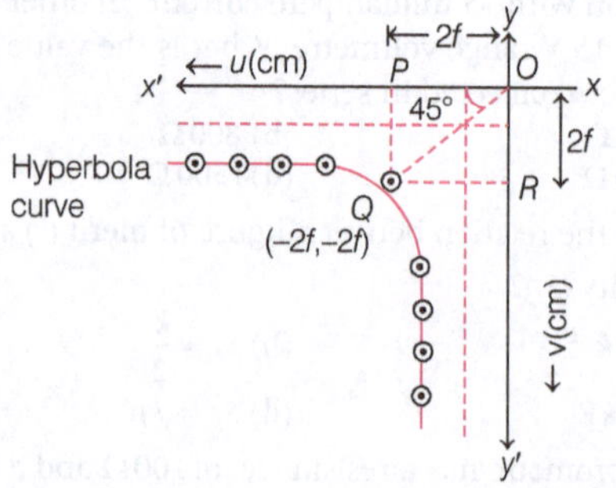

In this graph, focal length, $f = \dfrac{OP}{2} = \dfrac{OR}{2}$

(b) Graph between $\dfrac{1}{u}$ and $\dfrac{1}{v}$

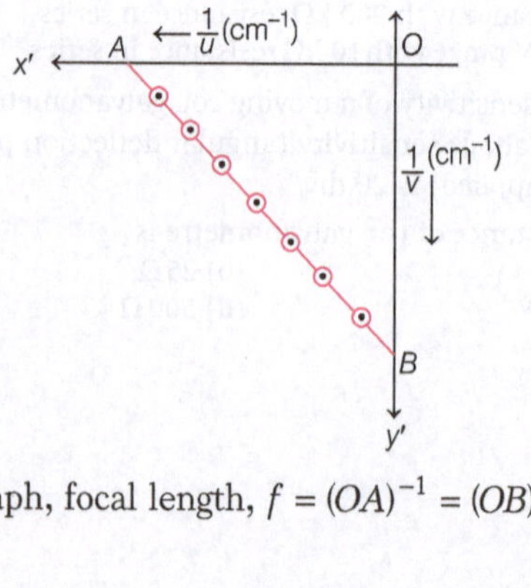

In this graph, focal length, $f = (OA)^{-1} = (OB)^{-1}$

(ii) Convex Mirror

Formula for focal length, $f = \dfrac{uv}{u+v}$

Here, u is negative and v is positive

Graphs

(a) Graph between u and v

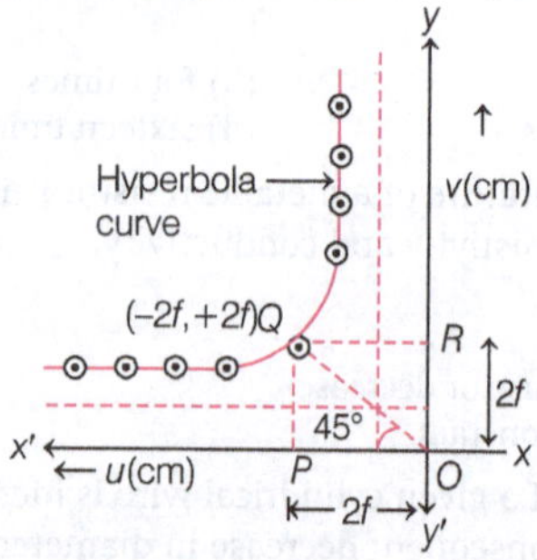

In this graph, focal length, $f = \dfrac{OP}{2} = \dfrac{OR}{2}$

(b) Graph between $\dfrac{1}{u}$ and $\dfrac{1}{v}$

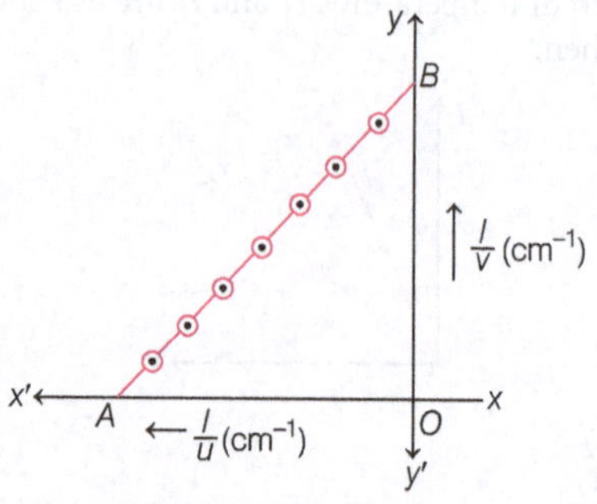

In this graph, $f = (OA)^{-1} = (OB)^{-1}$

(iii) Convex Lens

Focal length, $f = \dfrac{uv}{u-v}$

Here, u is negative and v is positive.

Graphs between u and v, $\dfrac{1}{u}$ and $\dfrac{1}{v}$ are similar to that of concave mirror.

> **Concept ladder**
> Bench error (of optical bench) is given by
> Bench error = Actual distance − Observed distance

EXPERIMENT-14

Plot of angle of the deviation *versus* angle of incidence for a triangular prism.

Summary

Deviation of ray through prism is shown below.

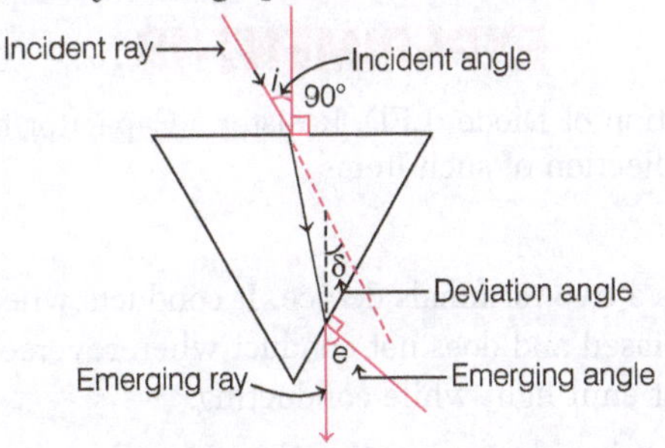

This experiment is performed for different incident angles (30° to 60°, in increments of 5°)

Graph between i and δ

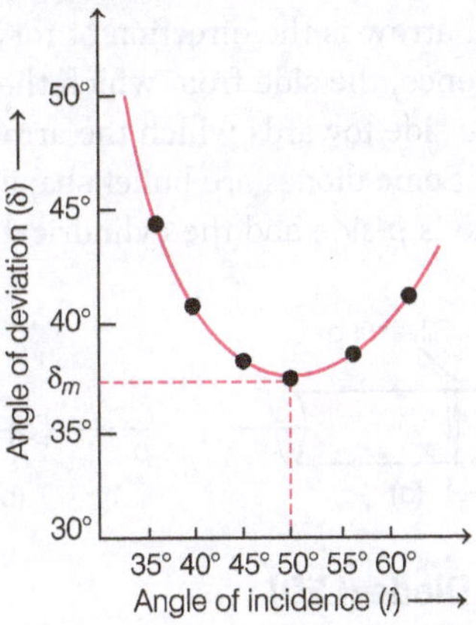

Here, δ_m is known as **angle of minimum deviation.**

> **Concept ladder**
>
> - Refractive Index of prism is given by $\mu = \dfrac{\sin\left(\dfrac{A+\delta_m}{2}\right)}{\sin\left(\dfrac{A}{2}\right)}$
> - In case of minimum deviation, $i = e$ and angle of refraction, $r = \dfrac{A}{2}$

EXPERIMENT-15

Refractive index of a glass slab using a travelling microscope.

Summary

Formula $\mu = \dfrac{\text{Real depth (thickness)}}{\text{Apparent depth (thickness)}}$

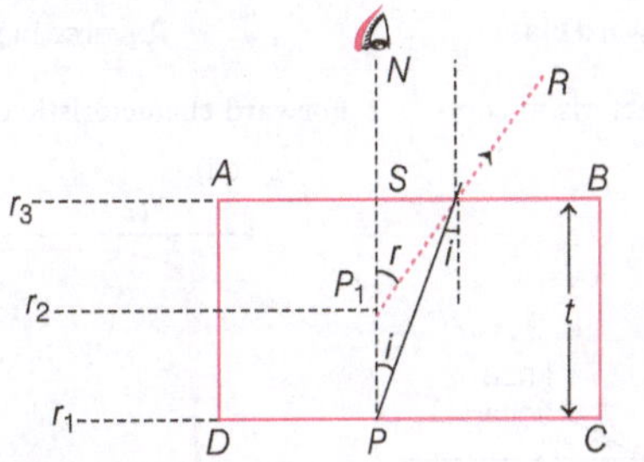

Refractive index (in this case)

$$\mu = \frac{r_3 - r_1}{r_2 - r_1}$$

EXPERIMENT 16

Characteristic curves of a *p-n* junction diode in forward and reverse bias.

Summary

Circuit diagram

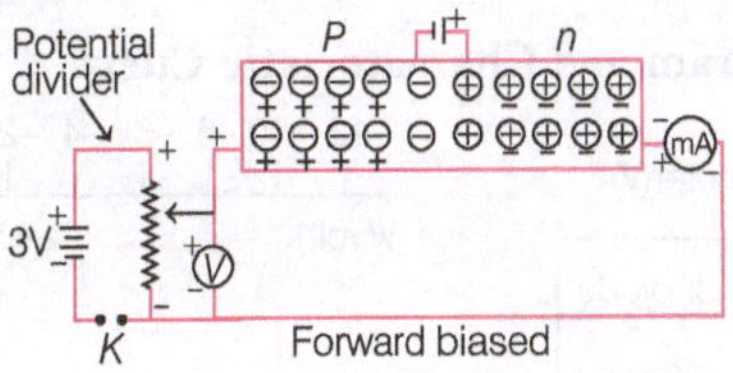

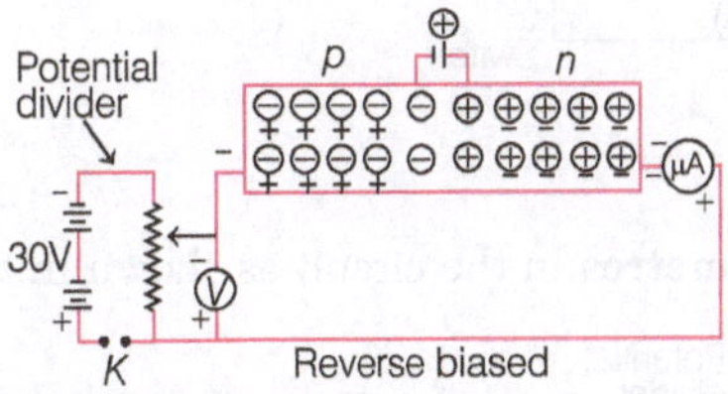

Forward bias	Reverse bias
p → positive n → negative 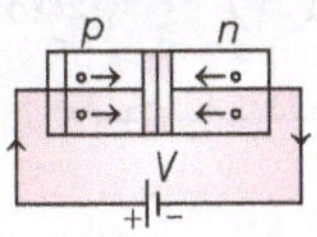	p → negative n → positive 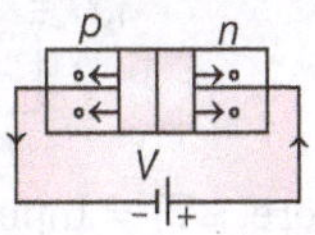
Potential barrier reduces.	Potential barrier increases.
Width of depletion layer decreases.	Width of depletion layer increases.
p-n junction provides very small resistance.	*p-n* junction provides high resistance.
Order of forward current is milliampere.	Order of current is micro- ampere (Ge) or nanoampere (Si).
Current flows mainly due to majority charge carrier.	Current flows mainly due to minority charge carrier.

Forward bias	Reverse bias
Forward characteristic curve	Forward characteristic curve
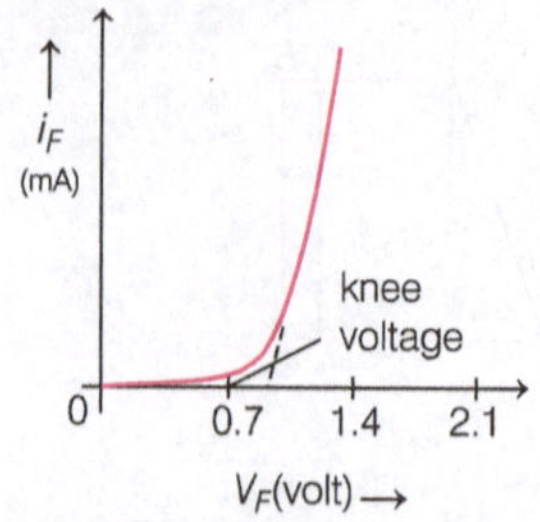	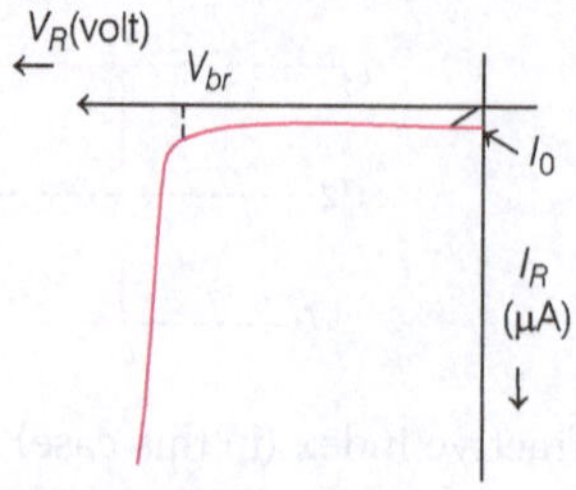
Forward resistance $R_f = \dfrac{\Delta V_f}{\Delta I_f} \approx 100\,\Omega$	Reverse resistance $R_B = \dfrac{\Delta V_B}{\Delta I_B} \approx 10^6\,\Omega$

EXPERIMENT-17

Characteristics curve of a zener diode and finding reverse breakdown voltage.

Summary

Circuit Diagram and **Characteristic Curve.**

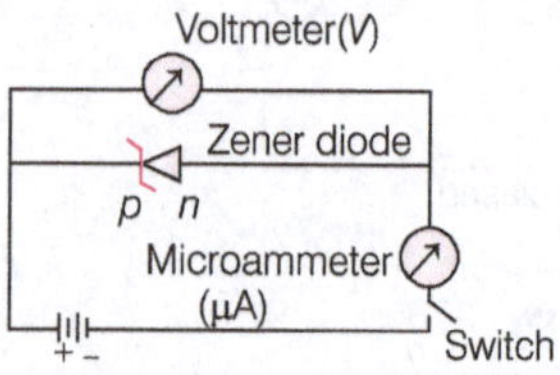

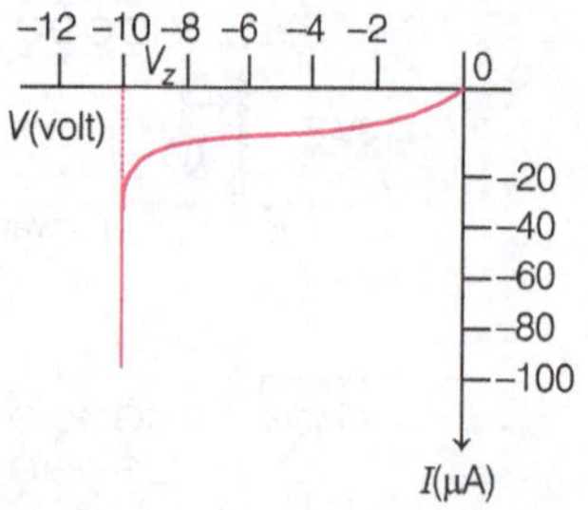

Circuit parametres In the circuit as shown in the figure above.

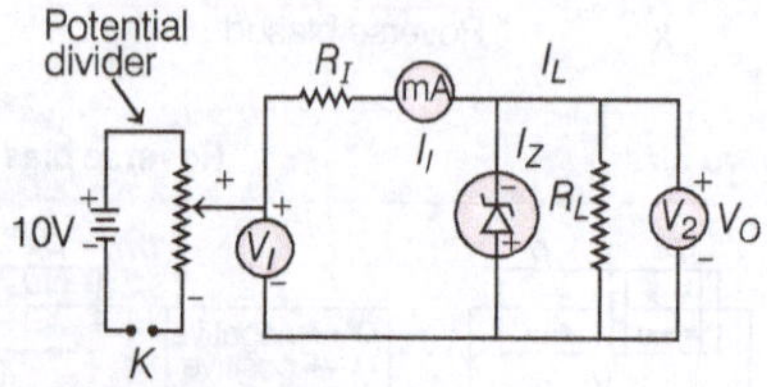

where, V_I = Input voltage

V_O = Output voltage

R_I = Input resistance

R_L = Load resistance

I_I = Input current

I_Z = Zener diode current and

I_L = Load current

Relations

$$I_L = I_I - I_z \quad \text{...(i)}$$

$$V_O = V_I - R_I I_I \quad \text{...(ii)}$$

$$V_0 = I_L R_L$$

Initially as V_1 is increased, I_I increases a little, then V_O increases.

At breakdown, increase of V_I, increases I_I by large amount, so that $V_O = V_I - R_I I_I$ becomes constant.

This constant value of V_O which is the reverse breakdown voltage is called **zener voltage.**

EXPERIMENT-18

Identification of Diode, LED, Resistor a Capacitor from a Mixed Collection of such Items

Diode

A diode is a two terminals device. It conducts when forward biased and does not conduct when reverse biased. It does not emit light while conducting.

In some semiconductor junction diodes, a silver ring is shown on one of its end. This end of the diode is *n*-side and the other end is *p*-side [Fig. (a)]. In some diodes, the symbol of the diode is painted on the body of the diode. The direction of arrow is the direction of forward bias current flow. Hence, the side from which the arrow starts is *p*-side and the side towards which the arrow ends is *n*-side [Fig. (b)]. Some diodes are bullet shaped in which case the flat side is *p*-side and the cylindrical side is *n*-side.

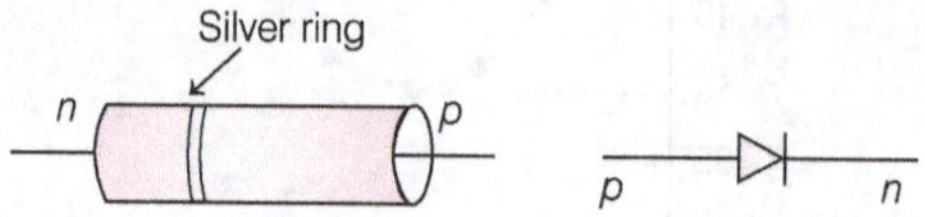

(a) (b)

Light Emitting Diode (LED)

An LED (Light Emitting Diode) is also a two terminals device. It conducts when forward biased and does not conduct when reverse biased. It emits light while conducting.

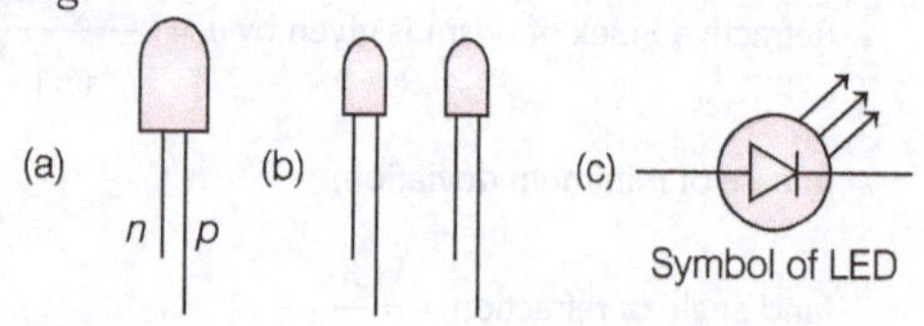

Semiconductor ased for LED is such that $E_g = h\nu = \dfrac{hc}{\lambda}$

If the deflection is accompanied with emission of light, in one direction and a much less or zero deflection in the other direction the component is an LED.

Resistor

A resistor is a two terminals device. it conducts equally in both directions.

Look for colour bands, if it has a typical set of three colour bands followed by a silver or gold band, the component is a resistor.

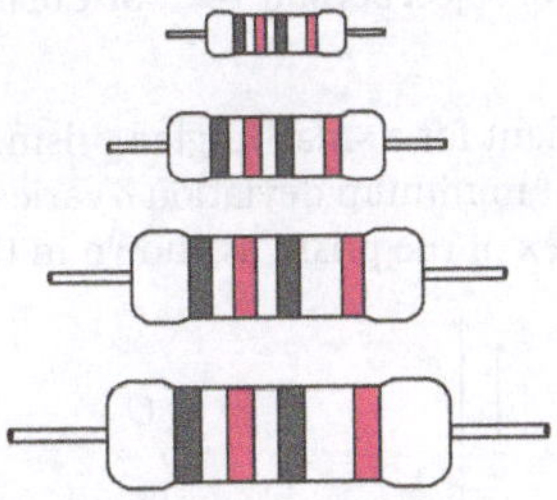

Capacitor

Capacitor is a device that store electrical charge. A capacitor blocks the passage of DC while it allows AC to flow through it.

There are many types of capacitor having different types of dielectrics in general use. These are

(i) Air capacitor (variable gang capacitors)
(ii) Mica capacitor (low capacitance)
(iii) Ceramic capacitor (very low capacitance)
(iv) Paper capacitor (low capacitance)
(v) Plastic capacitor
(vi) Electrolytic capacitor (medium capacitance)
(vii) Oil filled capacitor (high capacitance)

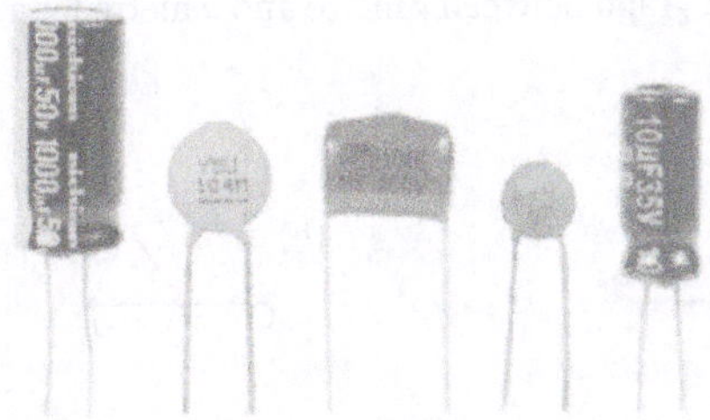

A capacitor is a two terminal device. It does not conduct but stores some charge when DC voltage is applied. If the multimeter does not show any deflection on connecting its terminals either way to the component, it is a capacitor. But if capacitance of capacitor is large, multimeter may show a momentary deflection.

Summary Table

Possible current flow	Device
Unidirectional emits no light	Diode
Unidirectional emits light	LED
Both directions (steady)	Resistor
Initially very high which eventually decays to zero	Capacitor

STEP UP Practice 4

1. Which of the following graph is the magnification of a real image against the distance from the focus of a concave mirror?

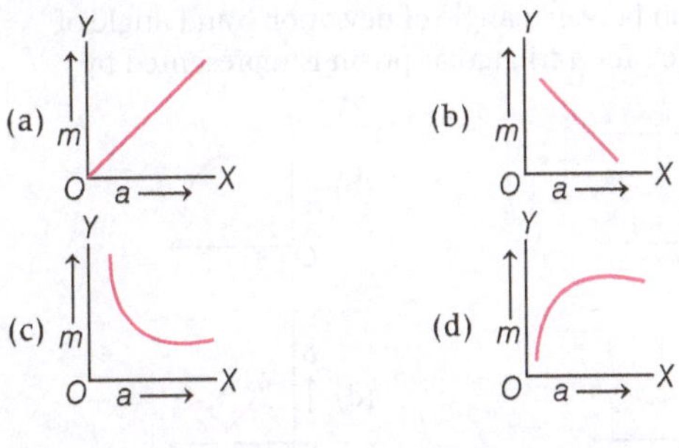

2. A student gets a graph u *versus* v for a mirror. Point plotted above the point P on the curve are for values of v

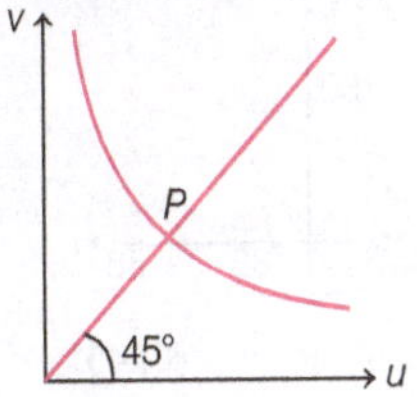

(a) smaller than f
(b) smaller than $2f$
(c) larger than $2f$
(d) larger than f

3. In an optics experiment, with the position of the object fixed, a student varies the position of a convex lens and for each position, the screen is adjusted to get a clear image of the object. A graph between the object distance u and the image distance v, from the lens, is plotted using the same scale for the two axes. A straight line passing through the origin and making an angle of 45° with the X-axis meets the experimental curve at P. The coordinates of P will be

(a) $(2f, 2f)$ (b) $\left(\frac{f}{2}, \frac{f}{2}\right)$ (c) (f, f) (d) $(4f, 4f)$

4. In the figure shown, the image of a real object is formed at point I. AB is the principal axis of the mirror. The mirror must be

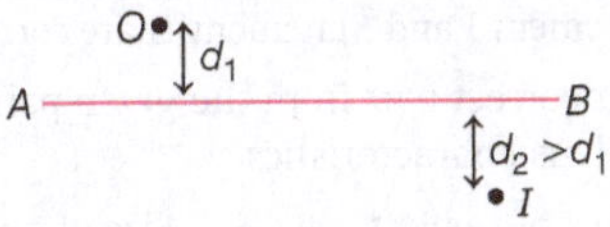

(a) concave and placed towards right of I
(b) concave and placed towards left of I
(c) convex and placed towards right of I
(d) convex and placed towards left of I

5. Select a graph between v metre and u metre for a concave mirror.

(a) 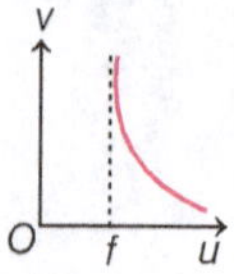

(b) 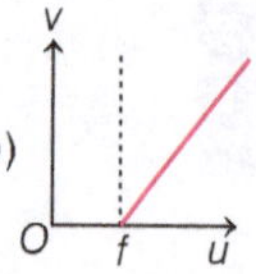

(c) 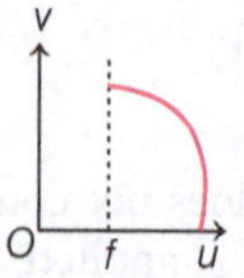

(d) 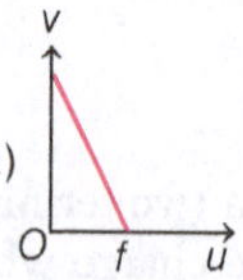

6. In the displacement method, a convex lens is placed in between an object and a screen. If the magnification in the two positions are m_1 and m_2, ($m_1 > m_2$), the distance between the two positions of the lens is x, the focal length of the lens is

(a) $\frac{x}{m_1 + m_2}$ (b) $\frac{x}{m_1 - m_2}$ (c) $\frac{x}{(m_1 + m_2)^2}$ (d) $\frac{x}{(m_1 - m_2)^2}$

7. For practical use, which colour we take for the refractive index of a material of lens and glass slab?

(a) Red (b) Blue
(c) Yellow (d) Green

8. An object is placed 25 cm from the surface of a convex mirror and a plane mirror is set, so that the image formed by the two mirror lie adjacent to each other is same plane (no parallax). The plane mirror is placed at 20 cm from the object. What is the radius of curvature of convex mirror?

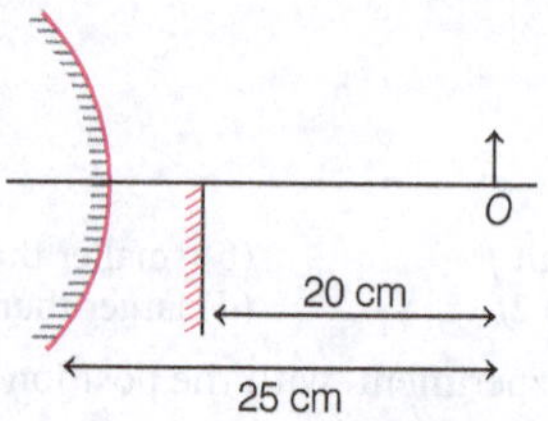

(a) 50 cm (b) 75 cm
(c)90 cm (d) 60 cm

9. **Statement I** When a concave mirror is held under water its focal length will increase.

Statement II The focal length of a concave mirror is independent of the medium in which it is placed.

In the light of the above statements, choose the most appropriate answer from the options given below.

(a) Both Statement I and Statement II are incorrect.
(b) Statement I is correct but Statement II is incorrect.
(c) Statement I is incorrect but Statement II is correct.
(d) Both Statement I and Statement II are correct.

10. Choose the incorrect pair from the given pair by considering the concave lens characteristics.

(a) Position of object at infinity → Size of image is extremely diminished
(b) Position of object at $2f_1$ → Size of image is same as object
(c) Position of object at f_1 → Size of image is highly magnified
(d) Position of object beyond $2f_1$ → Size of image is magnified

11. In an experiment for a small angled prism, angle of prism A, the angle of minimum deviation δ varies with the refractive index of the prism as shown in the graph.

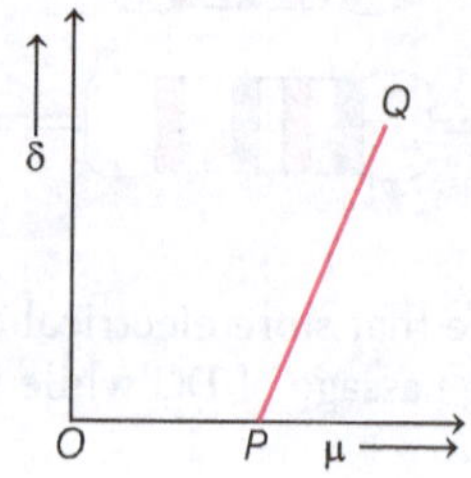

(a) Point P corresponds to $\mu = 1$
(b) Slope of the line, $PQ = \frac{A}{2}$
(c) Slope $= 2A$
(d) None of the above statement is true

12. A given ray of light suffers minimum deviation in an equilateral prism P. If refractive index increases slightly then the ray will suffer

(a) greater deviation
(b) no deviation
(c) same deviation as before
(d) lesser deviation

13. When a ray of light is refracted by a prism such that the angle of deviation is minimum, then

(a) the angle of emergence is equal to the angle of incidence
(b) the angle of emergence is greater than the angle of incidence
(c) the angle of emergence is smaller than the angle of incidence
(d) the sum of the angle of incidence and the angle of emergence is equal to 90°

14. The graph between angle of deviation δ and angle of incidence i for a triangular prism is represented by

(a) 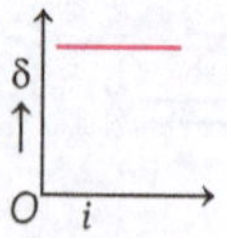

(b) 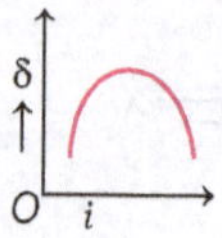

(c) 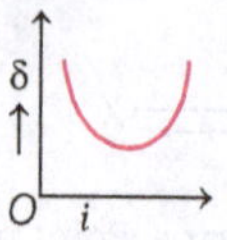

(d) 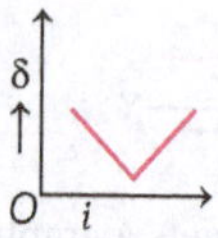

15. From the graph, (between δ and i) prism angle is

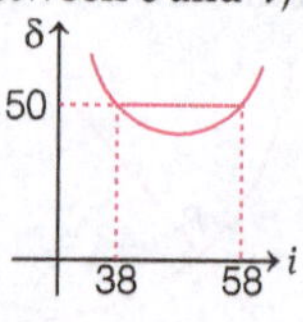

(a) 47° (b) 46° (c) 45° (d) 60°

16. If a ray is passing through a broken prism, find angular deviation for the ray

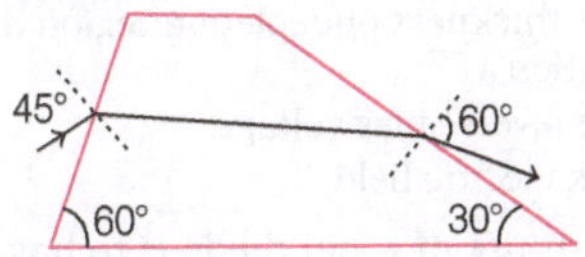

(a) 105° (b) 30° (c) 60° (d) 15°

17. Light travels through a glass plate of thickness t and having refractive index μ. If c be the velocity of light in vacuum, the time taken by the light to travel this thickness of glass is

(a) $\frac{t}{\mu c}$ (b) $t\mu c$ (c) $\frac{\mu t}{c}$ (d) $\frac{tc}{\mu}$

18. A vessel of depth t is half filled with oil of refractive index μ_1 and the other half is filled with water (refractive index μ_2). The apparent depth of the vessel when viewed from above is

(a) $\frac{t(\mu_1 + \mu_2)}{2\mu_1 \mu_2}$ (b) $\frac{t(\mu_1 - \mu_2)}{2\mu_1 \mu_2}$

(c) $\frac{2t(\mu_1 + \mu_2)}{\mu_1 \mu_2}$ (d) $\frac{2(\mu_1 - \mu_2)}{\mu_1 \mu_2}$

19. An experiment is performed to find the refractive index of glass using a travelling microscope. In this experiment distances are measured by
(a) a standard laboratory scale
(b) a metre scale provided on the microscope
(c) a screw gauge provided on the microscope
(d) a vernier scale provided on the microscope

20. A microscope is focussed on a mark on a piece of paper and then a slab of glass of thickness 3 cm and refractive index 1.5 is placed over the mark. How should the microscope be moved to get the mark in focus again
(a) 1 cm upward (b) 4.5 cm downward
(c) 1 cm downward (d) 2 cm upward

21. A travelling microscope is focused on a mark on a piece of paper and the scale reading is A. A rectangular block of glass is placed on the paper and the microscope is raised and focused the mark on the paper, then microscope reading is B. A layer of lycopodium power is sprinted on the block of glass. The reading now is C. The refractive index of the material of the block is

(a) $\frac{C-B}{C-A}$ (b) $\frac{C-A}{C-B}$ (c) $\frac{C-A}{B-A}$ (d) $\frac{C}{C-A}$

22. In a semiconductor diode, the barrier potential offers opposition to only
(a) majority carriers in both regions
(b) minority carriers in both regions
(c) free electrons in n region
(d) holes in the p region

23. When a p-n junction diode is reverse biased
(a) electrons and holes are attracted towards each other and move towards the depletion region.
(b) electrons and holes move away from the junction depletion region.
(c) height of the potential barriers decreases.
(d) no change in the current takes place.

24. The reverse biasing in junction diode
(a) decreases the potential barrier
(b) increases the potential barrier
(c) increases the number of minority charge carriers
(d) increases the number of majority charge carriers

25. When a p-n junction diode is in forward biased condition, the flow of current is mainly due to
(a) the drift of electrons
(b) the diffusion of electrons
(c) both by drift and diffusion of electrons
(d) None of the above

26. The V-I characteristic for a p-n junction diode is plotted as shown in the figure. From the plot we can conclude that [$V_b \to$ breakdown voltage, $V_k \to$ knee voltage]

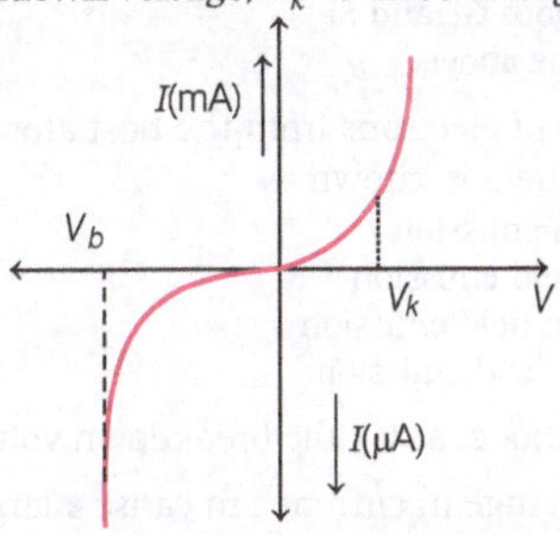

(a) the forward bias resistance of diode is very high, almost infinity for small values of V and after a certain value it becomes very low.
(b) the reverse bias resistance of diode is very high in the beginning up to breakdown voltage is not achieved.
(c) both forward and reverse bias resistances are same for all voltages.
(d) Both (a) and (b)

27. Pick out the incorrect statement.
The reverse current in an ideal p-n junction diode
(a) can be minimum and constant before breakdown voltage.
(b) remains constant even after the breakdown voltage.
(c) becomes infinity at breakdown.
(d) reverse current is controlled by external resistance.

28. **Statement I** A p-n junction with reverse bias can be used as a photodiode to measure light intensity.
Statement II In a reverse bias condition the current is small but is more sensitive to changes in incident light intensity.
In the light of the above statements, choose the most appropriate answer from the options given below.
(a) Both Statement I and Statement II are incorrect.
(b) Statement I is correct but Statement II is incorrect.
(c) Statement I is incorrect but Statement II is correct.
(d) Both Statement I and Statement II are correct.

29. Choose in incorrect pair from the following pair by considering forward bias p-n junction diode.

(a)	Potential barrier	→	reduces
(b)	Width of depletion layer	→	decreases
(c)	p-n junction provided resistance	→	very small
(d)	Order of forward current	→	in ampere

30. Avalanche breakdown in a semiconductor diode happens when
(a) forward current exceeds a certain value
(b) reverse bias exceeds a certain value
(c) forward bias exceeds a certain value
(d) the potential barrier is reduced to zero

31. What constitutes the reverse current?
(a) Holes in p-type and free electrons in n-type
(b) Free electrons in p-type and holes in n-type
(c) Holes in both p-type and n-type
(d) Free electrons in both p-type and n-type

32. For the same density of impurity atoms knee voltage is
(a) higher for silicon than for germanium
(b) higher for Ge than for Si
(c) same for both Ge and Si
(d) None of the above

33. The emission of electrons from the host atoms due to the high electric field is known as
(a) zener field emission
(b) internal field emission
(c) breakdown field emission
(d) avalanche field emission

34. In the zener diode, at V_Z, the breakdown voltage
(a) a small change in current can cause a large change in the voltage.
(b) a small change in current causes a small change in the voltage.
(c) a large change in current produces an insignificant change in the voltage.
(d) a large change in voltage produces an insignificant change in the current.

35. The breakdown in a reverse biased p-n junction diode is more likely to occur due to
(i) large velocity of the minority charge carriers if the doping concentration is small.
(ii) large velocity of the minority charge carriers if the doping concentration is large.
(iii) strong electric field in a depletion region if the doping concentration is small.
(iv) strong electric field in the depletion region if the doping concentration is large.
(a) (i) and (ii) (b) (ii) and (iii)
(c) (i) and (iii) (d) (i) and (iv)

36. Zener diode is a p-n junction which has
(a) p-end heavily doped, n-end lightly doped.
(b) n-end heavily doped, p-end lightly doped.
(c) both p and n-ends heavily doped.
(d) both p and n-ends lightly doped.

37. Zener diode has both p and n-ends heavily doped, so that
(a) it has small thickness of depletion region
(b) it has large thickness of depletion region due to large recombination
(c) it has large reverse bias voltage
(d) it has weak electric field

38. Most important use of zener diode is to have
(a) constant voltage across applied load
(b) any desired current at constant voltage
(c) a p-n junction working under constant regulated voltage conditions
(d) a p-n junction to operate at high voltage

39. In given figure when input voltage increases,

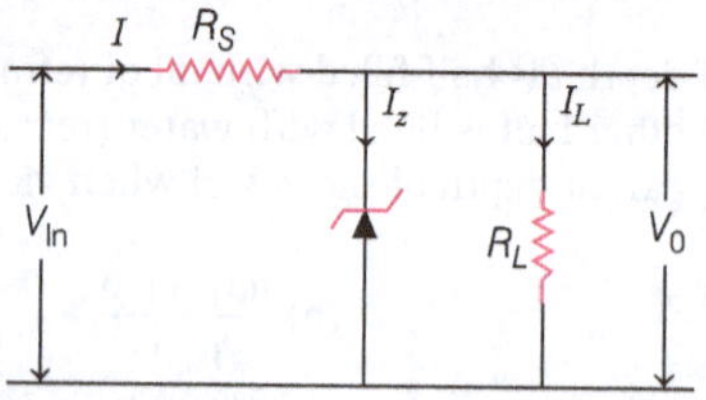

(a) the current through R_S, R_L and zener increases.
(b) the current through R_S increases, zener increases but through R_L remains constant.
(c) the current through R_S increases, through zener decreases, R_L increases.
(d) the current through R_S increases, through zener remains constant but R_L increases.

40. In some seimconductor junction, a silver ring is shown an one of its end. This end of the diode is
(a) n-side (b) p-side
(c) base-side (d) Data is not sufficient

41. Light emitting diode conducts when it is in
(a) forward biased
(b) reverse biased
(c) stable condition
(d) None of the above

42. Electrical item which allow flow of electric current in both direction.
(a) LED (b) Diode
(c) Resistor (d) None of these

43. From the given symbol, choose the symbol of diode.

(a) 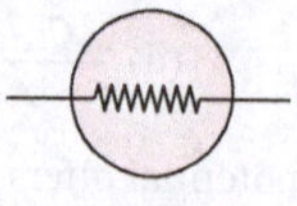 (b) 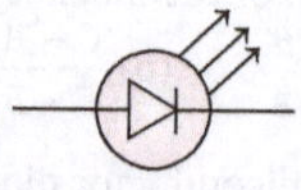

(c) 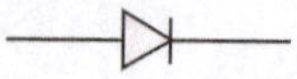 (d) 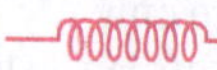

GEARING UP FOR NEET

Single Correct Option

1. On measuring the diameter of a spherical body using vernier caliper, main scale reading = 1.3 cm, 5th vernier scale division is coinciding with any main scale division and zero error is – 0.03 cm, what will be corrected reading?
(a) 1.38 cm (b) 1.32 cm
(c) 1.35 cm (d) –1.38 cm

2. You are given two different vernier calipers A and B having 10 divisions on vernier scale that coincide with 9 divisions on the main scale each. If 1 cm of main scale A is divided into 10 parts and that of B in 20 parts, then least count of A and B are
(a) 0.001 cm and 0.005 cm
(b) 0.01 cm and 0.05 cm
(c) 0.01 cm and 0.005 cm
(d) 0.01 cm and 0.001 cm

3. One main scale division of a vernier caliper is a cm and nth division of the vernier scale coincide with $(n-1)$th division of the main scale. The least count of the caliper (in mm) is
(a) $\frac{10na}{(n-1)}$ (b) $\frac{10a}{(n-1)}$
(c) $\left(\frac{n-1}{10n}\right)a$ (d) $\frac{10a}{n}$

4. A student constructed a vernier caliper as shown. He used two identical inclines and tried to measure the length of line PQ. For this instrument determine the least count.

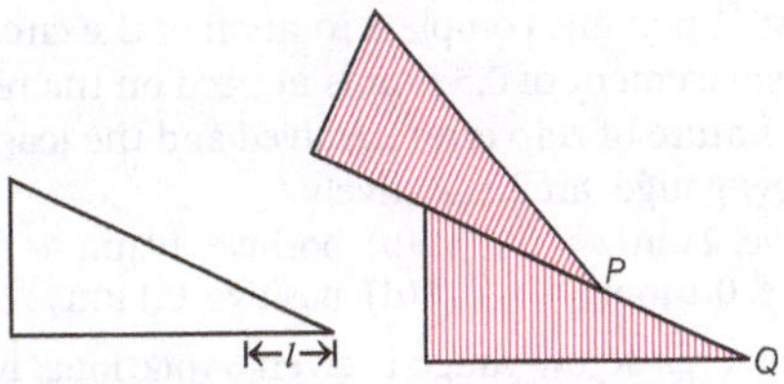

(a) $\frac{l(1-\cos\theta)}{\cos\theta}$ unit (b) $\frac{l}{\cos\theta}$ unit
(c) $l(1-\cos\theta)$ unit (d) $\frac{1-\cos\theta}{l}$ unit

5. For the following diagram [used to measure the length of a small metal piece by using vernier caliper], determine the length of the metal piece. [Least count of the vernier caliper is 0.1 mm]

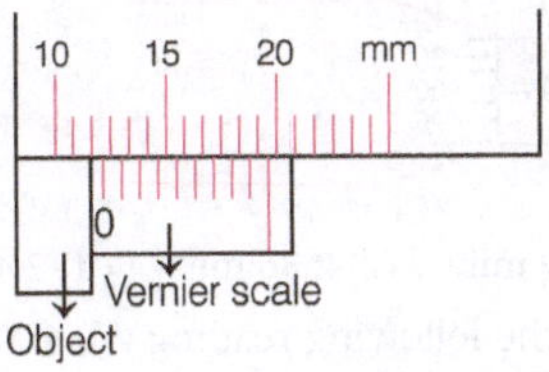

(a) 18 mm (b) 15.7 mm
(c) 12.6 mm (d) None of these

6. A spectrometer gives the following reading when used to measure the angle of a prism.
Main scale reading – 58.5 degree
Vernier scale reading – 09 divisions
Given that 1 division on main scale corresponds to 0.5 degree. Total divisions on the vernier scale is 30 and match with 29 divisions of the main scale. The angle of the prism from the above data is
(a) 58.59° (b) 58.77° (c) 58.65° (d) 59°

7. In an experiment the angles are required to be measured using an instrument. 29 divisions of the main scale exactly coincide with the 30 divisions of the vernier scale. If the smallest division of the main scale is half a degree (*i.e.* 0.5°), then the least count of the instrument is
(a) one minute (b) half minute
(c) one degree (d) half degree

8. N divisions on the main scale of a vernier caliper coincides with $(N+1)$ divisions on the vernier scale. If each division on the main scale is of a unit, the least count of instrument is
(a) $\frac{a}{N+1}$ (b) $\frac{a}{N-1}$
(c) $\frac{N+1}{a}$ (d) $\frac{N-1}{a}$

9. The edge of a cube is measured using a vernier caliper (9 divisions of the main scale is equal to 10 divisions of vernier scale and 1 main scale division is 1 mm). The main scale division reading is 10 and 1 division of vernier scale was found to be coinciding with the main scale. The mass of the cube is 2.736 g. What will be the density in $\frac{g}{cm^3}$ upto correct (significant figures)?
(a) $2.66\times10^{-3}\ \frac{g}{cm^3}$ (b) $2.66\times10^{3}\ \frac{g}{cm^3}$
(c) $2.66\ \frac{g}{cm^3}$ (d) $2.66\times10^{-6}\ \frac{g}{cm^3}$

10. The incorrect statement is
(a) The least count of screw gauge depends only on the number of circular scale divisions.
(b) In a positive zero error, the zero of circular scale lies below the reference line.
(c) In a positive zero error, the zero of the main scale is visible.
(d) The screw gauge with a pitch of 0.5 mm is more precise than the instruments with a pitch of 1 mm if both have the same number of circular divisions.

11. What is the reading of micrometer screw gauge shown in figure (no. of divisions on circular scale is 50)

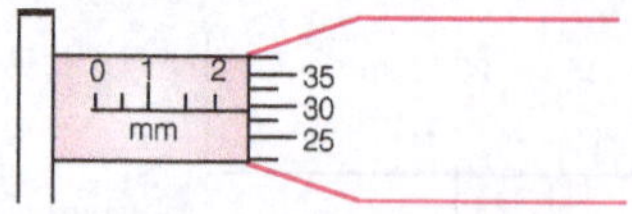

(a) 2.30 mm (b) 2.29 mm (c) 2.36 mm (d) 2.41 mm

12. A screw gauge gives the following reading when used to measure the diameter of a wire.
Main scale reading – 0 mm.
Circular scale reading–52 divisions
Given that, 1 mm on main scale corresponds to 100 divisions of the circular scale.
The diameter of wire from the above date is
(a) 0.026 cm (b) 0.005 cm (c) 0.52 cm (d) 0.052 cm

13. The circular divisions of shown screw gauge are 50. It moves 0.5 mm on main scale in one rotation. The diameter of the ball is

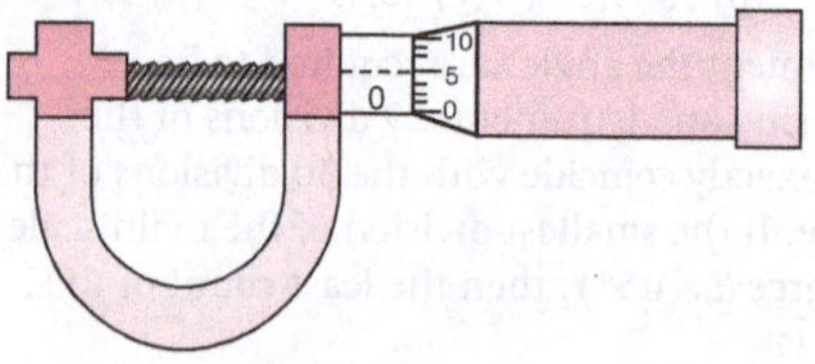

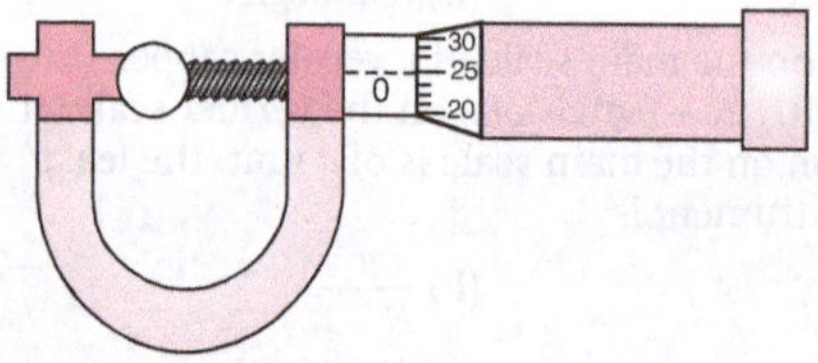

(a) 2.25 mm (b) 2.20 mm (c) 1.20 mm (d) 1.25 mm

14. The pitch and the number of divisions, on the circular scale, for a given screw gauge are 0.5 mm and 100 respectively. When the screw gauge is fully tightened without any object, the zero of its circular scale lies 3 divisions below the mean line.
The readings of the main scale and the circular scale, for a thin sheet, are 5.5 mm and 48 mm respectively, the thickness of this sheet is
(a) 5.755 m (b) 5.725 mm
(c) 5.740 m (d) 5.950 mm

15. The least count of the main scale of a screw gauge is 1 mm. The minimum number of divisions on its circular scale required to measure 5μm diameter of wire is
(a) 50 (b) 100 (c) 200 (d) 500

16. Using screw gauge of pitch 0.1 cm and 50 divisions on its circular scale, the thickness of an object is measured. It should correctly be recorded as
(a) 2.123 cm (b) 2.125 cm (c) 2.121 cm (d) 2.124 cm

17. A screw gauge of pitch 0.5 mm is used to measure the diameter of uniform wire of length 6.8 cm, the main scale reading is 1.5 mm and circular scale reading is 7. The calculated curved surface area of wire to appropriate significant figures is [Screw gauge has 50 divisions on the circular scale]
(a) 6.8 cm^2 (b) 3.4 cm^2 (c) 3.9 cm^2 (d) 2.4 cm^2

18. If the amplitude of a SHM becomes $\frac{1}{27}$ times in 6 min and the amplitude becomes $\frac{1}{n}$ times in first 4 min. The value of n would be
(a) 4 (b) 8 (c) 6 (d) 9

19. On measuring diameter of a wire with help of screw gauge, main scale reading is 1 mm and 6th division of circular scale lying over reference line. On measuring zero error, it is found that zero of circular scale has advanced from reference line by 3 divisions on circular scale, then corrected diameter is
(a) 1.09 mm (b) 1.06 mm
(c) 1.03 mm (d) 1.60 mm

20. On measuring the thickness of a given sheet using screw gauge, observed readings are

S. No.	LSR (mm)	Circular scale division coinciding
1.	1	4
2.	1	6
3.	1	8

If zero error is + 0.06 mm, then corrected thickness of the sheet (in cm) is
(a) 0.1 (b) 1.0 (c) 0.01 (d) 0.11

21. A screw gauge has 50 divisions on its circular scale. The circular scale is 4 units ahead of the pitch scale marking, prior to use. Upon one complete rotation of the circular scale, a displacement of 0.5 mm is noticed on the pitch scale. The nature of zero error involved and the least count of the screw gauge, are respectively
(a) negative, 2 μm (b) positive, 10 μm
(c) positive, 0.1 mm (d) positive, 0.1 μm

22. If the screw on a screw gauge is given 6 rotations, it moves by 3 mm on the main scale. If there are 50 divisions on the circular scale, the least count of the screw gauge is
(a) 0.001 cm (b) 0.01 cm (c) 0.02 cm (d) 0.001 cm

23. A screw gauge gives the following reading when used to measure the diameter of a wire.
Main scale reading – 0 mm
Circular scale reading – 52 divisions

Given that 1 mm on main scale corresponds to 100 divisions of the circular scale.
The diameter of wire from the above data is
(a) 0.052 cm (b) 0.026 cm (c) 0.005 cm (d) 0.52 cm

24. For a simple pendulum, when a graph is plotted between displacement d, KE $= \frac{1}{2} mv^2$ and PE $= mgh$, taking d along X-axis and $\frac{1}{2} mv^2$ and mgh along Y-axis, the graph comes as

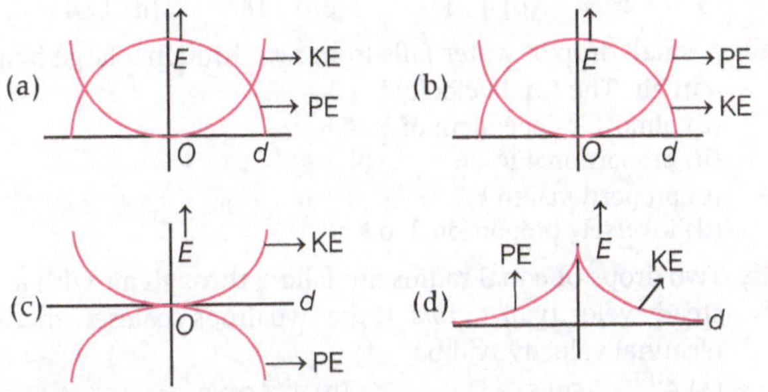

25. A simple pendulum is being used to determine the value of gravitational acceleration g at a certain place. The length of the pendulum is 25.0 cm and a stop watch with 1s resolution measures the time taken for 40 oscillations to be 50 s. The accuracy in g is
(a) 2.40% (b) 5.40% (c) 4.40% (d) 3.40%

26. If m and M are the masses of two bodies that are tied at two ends of a metre scale that is balanced on a sharp edge of a heavy broad wedge. If $M = 20$ g, its distance from centre = 30 cm and distance of mass m from centre is 25 cm when metre scale is balanced, then m is
(a) 23 g (b) 24 g (c) 25 g (d) 26 g

27. If two masses M and m are tied to two ends of a metre scale. If a balanced point is obtained at point P and if $M > m$, then

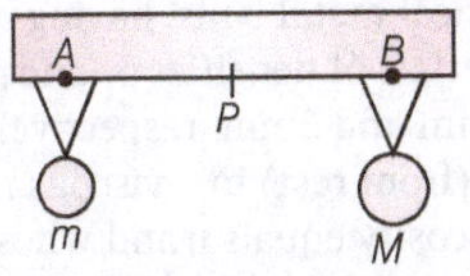

(a) $PA = PB$ (b) $PA > PB$ (c) $PB > PA$ (d) $PA = 3PB$

28. In measurement of mass of a given object by the principle of moments, the metre scale is hung from its mid-point. A known weight of mass 2 kg is hung at one end of metre scale and unknown weight of mass m kg is hung at 20 cm from the centre on other side. The value of m is
(a) 2 kg (b) 5 kg (c) 2.5 kg (d) 0.8 kg

29. In the above question mass of scale is 1 kg and instead of mid-point it is hung at 60 cm from the end where known mass of 2 kg has hung. A mass of 5 kg has to hung at a distance of x cm from pivot to carry out the experiment, then value of x is
(a) 20 cm (b) 10 cm (c) 26 cm (d) 5 cm

30. Two wires A and B have same lengths and made of the same material but A is thicker than B. Both are subjected to the same extending load. Which will extend more?
(a) A (b) B
(c) Same extension (d) Can't predict

31. In experiment for measuring surface tension by capillary rise method, readings for positions A, B, C and D for internal diameter of capillary tube are given as under. Mean internal radius of capillary is

A (cm) = 1.006
B (cm) = 1.009
C (cm) = 1.004
D (cm) = 1.009

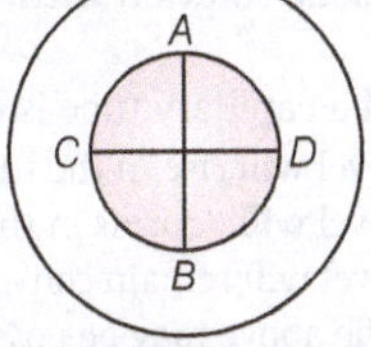

(a) 0.002 cm (b) 0.003 cm (c) 0.004 cm (d) 0.005 cm

32. When a glass capillary tube of radius 0.015 cm is dipped in water, the water rises to a height of 15 cm within it. Assuming contact angle between water and glass to be 0°, the surface tension of water is
$[\rho_{water} = 1000 \text{ kg m}^{-3}, g = 9.81 \text{ ms}^{-2}]$
(a) 0.11 Nm^{-1} (b) 0.7 Nm^{-1}
(c) 0.072 Nm^{-1} (d) None of these

33. While measuring surface tension of water using capillary rise method, height of the lower meniscus from free surface of water is 3 cm while inner radius of capillary tube is found to be 0.5 cm. Then, compute surface tension of water using this data. [Take, contact angle between glass and water as 0° and $g = 9.81 \text{ms}^{-2}$]
(a) 0.72 Nm^{-1} (b) 0.77 Nm^{-1}
(c) 1.67 Nm^{-1} (d) None of these

34. While performing experiment to measure surface tension of water using capillary rise method, the necessary precautions to be taken is
(1) both capillary tube and water should be free from contamination.
(2) capillary tube should be clean while water may contain some dirt or grease.
(3) temperature of water should be observed while performing experiment.
(4) internal diameter of capillary should be measured in two mutually perpendicular direction.
(a) (1), (3) (b) (2), (4)
(c) (2), (3) (d) (3), (4)

35. While measuring the surface tension of water, by capillary rise method, which of the following precaution is/are necessary.
(1) Capillary tube and water must be clean and free from contamination/grease
(2) Capillary tube should be set vertical and the temperature of the water should be noted
(3) Travelling microscope should be moved in lower direction only avoid back lash error
(4) Internal diameter of capillary tube should be measured in two mutually perpendicular directions
(a) 2 and 3 (b) 2
(c) 3 and 4 (d) 1, 2, 3 and 4

36. Choose the incorrect statement among the following.
(a) Capillary action is due to both cohesion and adhesion.
(b) Falling raindrop becomes a spherical due to cohesion and surface tension.
(c) Surface tension is due to cohesion between atoms at the free surface.
(d) Mixing soap solution with water, increases its surface tension.

37. If an end of a capillary tube is dipped into a liquid, then
(a) liquid level will rise in the tube
(b) liquid level will depress in the tube
(c) liquid level will remain constant as surrounding liquid
(d) any of the above may be possible

38. Choose the incorrect statement from the following.
(a) Small droplets of a liquid are spherical due to the surface tension.
(b) Oil rises through the wick due to capillarity.
(c) In drinking liquids through a straw, we use of phenomenon of capillarity.
(d) None of the above

39. liquid reaches an equilibrium as shown, in a capillary tube of internal radius r. If the surface tension of the liquid is T, the angle of contact θ and density of liquid ρ, then the pressure difference between P and Q is

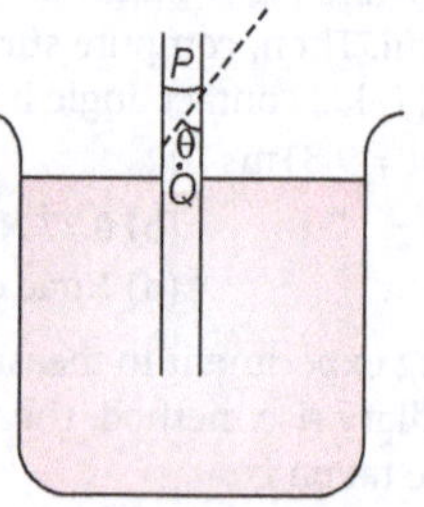

(a) $\left(\frac{2T}{r}\right)\cos\theta$ (b) $\frac{T}{r\cos\theta}$
(c) $\frac{2T}{r\cos\theta}$ (d) $\left(\frac{4T}{r}\right)\cos\theta$

40. The velocity of falling rain drop attain limiting value because of
(a) surface tension
(b) upthrust due to air
(c) viscous force exerted by air
(d) None of the above

41. A glass capillary tube is lowered vertically into liquid in a vessel. Now, choose the incorrect pair from the below pair.
(a) For concave meniscus → Contact angle is less than 90°
(b) For convex meniscus → Contact angle is equal to 90°
(c) For concave meniscus → Liquid in capillary tube ascends.
(d) For convex meniscus → Liquid in capillary tube descends.

42. A body of density D_1 and mass M is moving downward with uniform velocity in glycerine of density D_2. What is the viscous force acting on it
(a) $Mg\left(1-\frac{D_2}{D_1}\right)$ (b) $Mg\left(1-\frac{D_1}{D_2}\right)$
(c) $Mg\,D_1$ (d) $Mg\,D_2$

43. Two small spheres of radii r and $4r$ fall through a viscous liquid with the same terminal velocity. The ratio of the viscous forces acting on them is
(a) 1 : 2 (b) 4 : 1 (c) 1 : 16 (d) 1 : 4

44. A small drop of water falls from rest through a large height h in air. The final velocity is
(a) almost independent of h
(b) proportional to $\sqrt{h}$
(c) proportional to h
(d) inversely proportional to h

45. Two drops of equal radius are falling through air with a steady velocity of 1 cm/s. If the two drops coalesce, then its terminal velocity will be
(a) $4^{1/3} \times 5$ cm/s (b) $4^{1/3}$ cm/s
(c) $5^{1/3} \times 4$ cm/s (d) $4^{2/3} \times 5$ cm/s

46. Two rain drops falling through air have radii in the ratio 3 : 2. They will have terminal velocity in the ratio
(a) 4 : 1 (b) 9 : 4 (c) 2 : 1 (d) 4 : 9

47. A sphere of mass M and radius R is falling in a viscous fluid. The square of the terminal velocity attained by the falling object will be proportional to
(a) MR^2 (b) M/R (c) M^2/R^2 (d) M/R^2

48. A small sphere of radius r falls from rest in a viscous liquid. As a result, heat is produced due to viscous force. The rate of production of heat when the sphere attains its terminal velocity, is proportional to
(a) r^3 (b) r^2 (c) r^5 (d) r^4

49. Two small spherical metal balls, having equal masses, are made from materials of densities ρ_1 and $\rho_2 (\rho_1 = 8\rho_2)$ and have radii of 1 mm and 2mm, respectively. They are made to fall vertically (from rest) in a viscous medium whose coefficient of viscosity equals η and whose density is $0.1\,\rho_2$. The ratio of their terminal velocities would be
(a) $\frac{79}{72}$ (b) $\frac{19}{36}$ (c) $\frac{39}{72}$ (d) $\frac{79}{36}$

50. The velocity of a small ball of mass M and density d, when dropped in a container filled with glycerine becomes constant after some time. If the density of glycerine is $\frac{d}{2}$, then the viscous force acting on the ball will be
(a) $\frac{Mg}{2}$ (b) Mg (c) $\frac{3}{2}Mg$ (d) $2Mg$

51. The correct statement about the variation of viscosity of fluid with increase in temperature is
(a) viscosity of both liquids and gases increases.
(b) viscosity of liquids increases.
(c) viscosity of liquids decreases.
(d) viscosity of gases decreases.

52. The terminal velocity of a copper ball of radius 5 mm falling through a tank of oil at room temperature is 10 cm s^{-1}. If the viscosity of oil at room temperature is 0.9 kg m^{-1} s^{-1}, the viscous drag force is
(a) 8.48×10^{-3} N (b) 8.48×10^{-5} N
(c) 4.23×10^{-3} N (d) 4.23×10^{-6} N

53. If the terminal velocity of a sphere of gold (density = 19.5 kg/m^3) is 0.8 m/s in a viscous liquid (density = 1.5 kg/m^3), find the terminal speed of a sphere of silver (density = 10.5 kg/m^3) of the same size in the same liquid
(a) 0.4 m/s (b) 0.133 m/s (c) 0.1 m/s (d) 0.2 m/s

54. A small ball of mass m and radius r is falling under gravity through a viscous liquid of coefficient of viscosity η. If g is the acceleration due to gravity, then the terminal velocity of the ball is proportional to
(a) $\frac{mg\eta}{r}$ (b) $mg\eta r$ (c) $\frac{mgr}{\eta}$ (d) $\frac{mg}{r\eta}$

55. The graph AB shown in figure is a plot of temperature of body in degree celsius and degree fahrenheit, then......

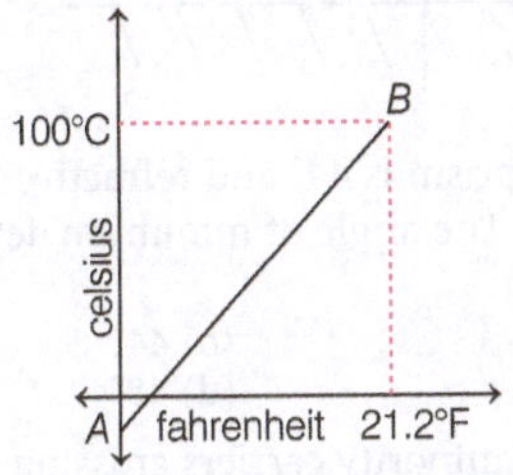

(a) slope line AB is $\frac{9}{5}$ (b) slope line AB is $\frac{5}{9}$
(c) slope line AB is $\frac{1}{9}$ (d) slope line AB is $\frac{3}{9}$

56. In an experiment for determining coefficient of viscosity, one lead shot A is having radius r_1 and the other B is having $\frac{r_1}{2}$. Which one will fall fast?
(a) A (b) B
(c) Both with same speed (d) Can't say

57. A wide jar is filled with water, in which a steel ball of radius 0.25 cm has been dropped to measure the viscosity of water by using terminal velocity concept.
(a) This method is appropriate
(b) This method is not appropriate
(c) If we take a jar of length 2 m, it will work
(d) None of the above

58. A wide jar is filled with glycerine having specific gravity 1.26, in this jar, a steel ball of radius 0.25 cm has been dropped. After some time it has been observed that ball is taking equal interval of time (1.8 s) to cover equal successive distances, of 20 cm.
[Take, $\rho_{steel} = 7.8 \times 10^3$ kg -m^3, $g = 9.81$ ms^{-2}]. The viscosity of glycerine (in N-sm^{-2}) is
(a) 0.802 (b) 1.67
(c) 0.76 (d) 0.963

59. While measuring viscosity of caster oil using terminal velocity concept the following observation table has been taken by a student.
Which one is the first correct reading which he should consider for the computation of terminal velocity?

S.No.	Distance	Time
1.	20 cm	1 s
2.	20 cm	1.4 s
3.	20 cm	1.8 s
4.	20 cm	1.81 s
5.	20 cm	1.82 s

(a) 1 (b) 2 (c) 3 (d) 4

60. In the experiment of measuring speed of sound by resonance tube, it is observed that for tuning fork of frequency $\nu = 480$ Hz, length of air column $l_1 = 30$ cm, $l_2 = 70$ cm, then v_1 is equal to
(a) 338 ms^{-1} (b) 379 ms^{-1}
(c) 384 ms^{-1} (d) 332 ms^{-1}

61. A heating curve has been plotted for a solid object as shown in the figure. If the mass of the object is 200 g, then latent heat of vaporisation for the material of the objects, is (Power supplied to the object is constant and equal to 1 kW)

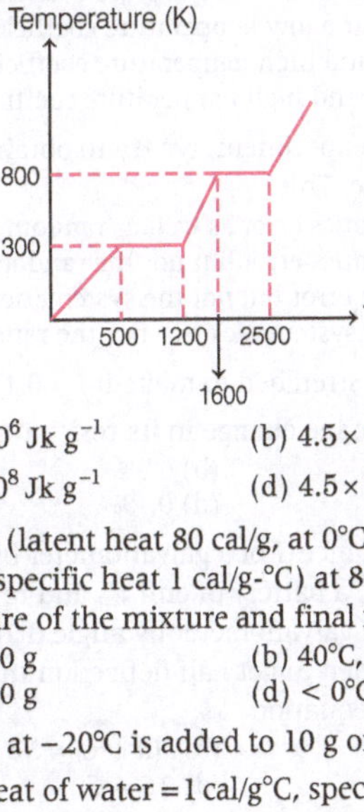

(a) 4.5×10^6 Jk g^{-1} (b) 4.5×10^6 cal g^{-1}
(c) 4.5×10^8 Jk g^{-1} (d) 4.5×10^4 cal g^{-1}

62. 50 g of ice (latent heat 80 cal/g, at 0°C) is mixed with 50 g of water (specific heat 1 cal/g-°C) at 80°C. The final temperature of the mixture and final mass of water will be
(a) 0°C, 100 g (b) 40°C, 100 g
(c) 80°C, 50 g (d) < 0°C, 0g

63. 10 g of ice at −20°C is added to 10 g of water at 50°C. Specific heat of water = 1 cal/g°C, specific heat of ice = 0.5 cal/g°-C specific heat of ice = 0.5 cal/g°C. Latent heat of ice = 80 cal/g, the amount of ice in the mixture at the resulting temperature is
(a) 10 g (b) 5 g (c) 0 g (d) 20 g

64. 19 g of water at 30°C and 5 g of ice at −20°C are mixed together in a calorimeter. What is the final temperature of the mixture? Given, specific heat of ice = 0.5 cal g^{-1} $(°C)^{-1}$ and latent heat of fusion of ice = 80 cal g^{-1}.
(a) 0°C (b) −5°C (c) 5°C (d) 10°C

65. 5 g of steam at 100°C is passed into 6 g of ice at 0°C. If the latent heats of steam and ice in cal per g are 540 and 80 respectively, then the final temperature is
(a) 0°C (b) 100°c
(c) 50°C (d) 30°C

66. In the measurement of resistance of a wire using Ohm's law, the plot between V and I is drawn as shown.

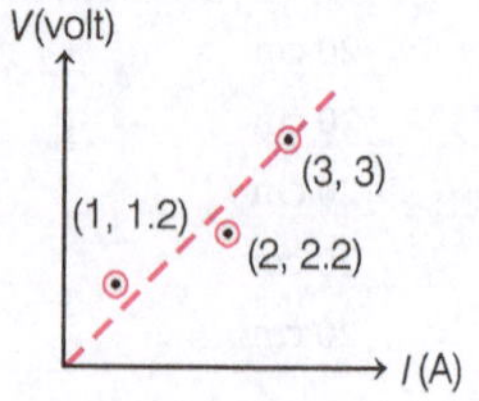

The resistance of the wire is
(a) 0.833 Ω (b) 0.9 Ω
(c) 1 Ω (d) None of these

67. In the experiment of Ohm's law, a potential difference of 5.0 V is applied across the end of a conductor of length 10.0 cm and diameter of 5.00 mm. The measured current in the conductor is 2.00 A. The maximum permissible percentage error in the resistivity of the conductor is
(a) 3.9 (b) 8.4
(c) 7.5 (d) 3.0

68. In a meter bridge set up, which of the following should be the properties of the one metre long wire?
(a) High resistivity and low temperature coefficient
(b) Low resistivity and low temperature coefficient
(c) Low resistivity and high temperature coefficient
(d) High resistivity and high temperature coefficient

69. In a meter bridge experiment, we try to obtain the null point at the middle. This
(a) reduces systematics error as well as random error.
(b) reduces systematics error but not the random error.
(c) reduces random error but not the systematic error.
(d) reduces neither systematic error nor the random error.

70. If a copper wire is stretched to make it $l = 0.1\%$ longer, then what is the percentage change in its resistance?
(a) 0.2% (b) 0.3%
(c) 0.4% (d) 0.1%

71. To know the resistance G of a galvanometer by half deflection method, a battery of emf V_E and resistance R is used to deflect the galvanometer by angle θ. If a shunt of resistance S is needed to get half deflection then, G, R and S are related by the equation
(a) $2S(R+G) = RG$ (b) $S(R+G) = RG$
(c) $2G = S$ (d) $2S = G$

72. Monochromatic light of wavelength λ_1 travelling in a medium of refractive index n_1 enters a denser medium of refractive index n_2. The wavelength in the second medium is
(a) $\lambda_1\left(\frac{n_1}{n_2}\right)$ (b) $\lambda_1\left(\frac{n_2}{n_1}\right)$
(c) $\frac{\lambda_1(n_2-n_1)}{n_2}$ (d) $\frac{\lambda_1(n_2-n_1)}{n_1}$

73. There are certain material developed in laboratories which have a negative refractive index figure.
A ray incident from air (medium 1) into such a medium (medium 2) shall follow a path given by

(a)
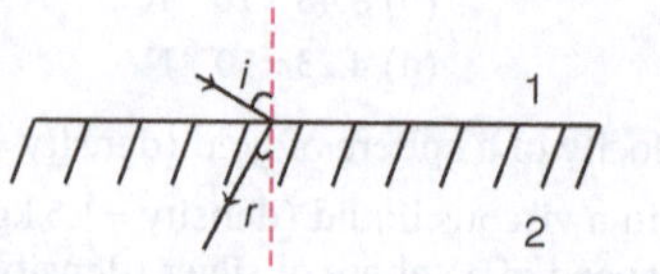

(b)
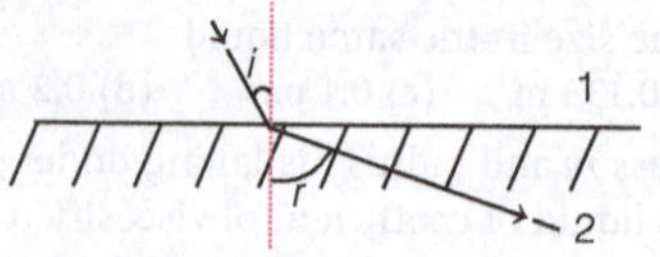

(c)
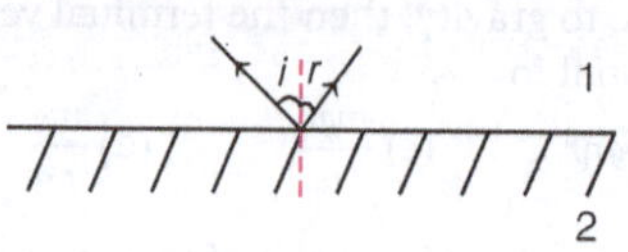

(d)
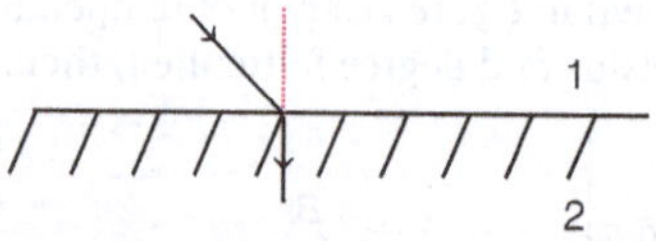

74. The angle of a prism is 44° and refractive index of its material is 1.5. The angle of minimum deviation for this prism is
(a) 22° (b) 44°
(c) 36° (d) 48°

75. The number of minority carriers crossing the junction of a diode depends primarily on the
(a) concentration of doping impurities
(b) magnitude of potential barrier
(c) magnitude of the forward bias barrier
(d) rate of thermal generation of electron-hole pair

76. The electrical resistance of depletion layer is large because
(a) it has no charge carriers
(b) it has large number of charge carriers
(c) it contains electrons as charge carriers
(d) it has holes as charge carriers

77. The readings corresponding to zener diode are given below in the table. From given table, determine the reverse breakdown voltage of the zener diode.

Forward bias		Reverse bias	
V (volt)	I (mA)	V (volt)	I (μA)
0.5	5	0.5	2.0
0.7	20	1.0	2.0
0.8	40	3.0	2.0
1.0	250	5.0	2.0
		5.5	100.0
		5.5	120.0

(a) It is lying between 1.0 V to 5.0 V
(b) 1.0 V
(c) Approx. 5.3 V
(d) None of the above

78. The zener diode normally operates under reverse bias condition, the major use of this fact is in the applications where we require
(a) large value of current
(b) a constant voltage
(c) a current that is increasing without any change in applied voltage
(d) All of the above

79. A zener diode is operating in its normal region *i.e.*, the breakdown region for which the circuit diagram is as shown in the figure.

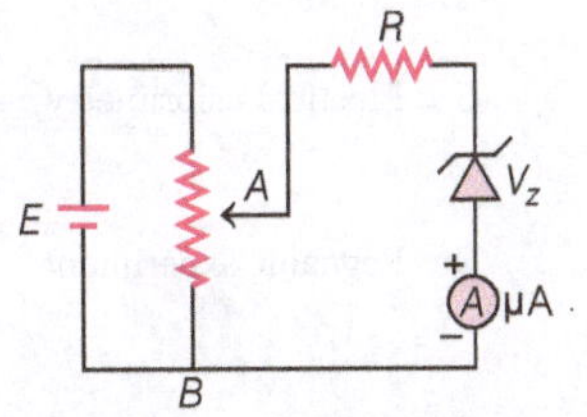

Here, take $V_Z = 7$ V and $R = 10\ k\Omega$. For potential difference equal to 8 V across *AB*, what is the current through microammeter?
(a) 1000 μA (b) 1 mA (c) 10 μA (d) 100 μA

80. The forward bias characteristics of two diodes D_1 and D_2 are shown, the knee voltages for D_1 and D_2 are respectively (approx.)

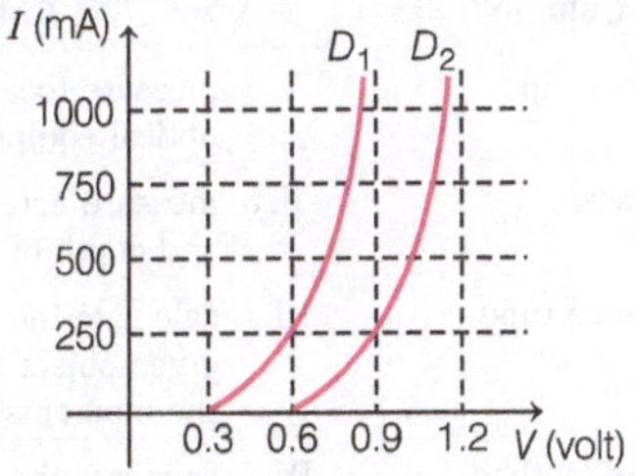

(a) 0.4 V and 0.7 V
(b) 0.6 V and 0.9 V
(c) 0.6 V and 0.8 V
(d) 0.4 V and 0.9 V

Assertion and Reason

Directions (Q. Nos. 1-5) *These questions consist of two statements each printed as Assertion (A) and Reason (R). While answering these questions you are required to choose any one of the following four responses.*
(a) Both A and R are true but R is not the correct explanation of A.
(b) A is true but R is false.
(c) A is false but R is true.
(d) Both A and R are true and R is the correct explanation of A.

1. Assertion (A) In meter bridge experiment a high resistance is connected in series with the galvanometer.
Reason (R) As resistance increases, current through the circuit increases.

2. Assertion (A) If we perform an experiment in our laboratory today and repeat the same experiment on the same object under identical conditions after a year, the result are found to be the different.
Reason (R) The law of nature do not change with time.

3. Assertion (A) Meter bridge does not give accurate readings.
Reason (R) End error cannot be fully eradicated.

4. Assertion (A) In forward biasing electrons from valance band are excited to conduction band.
Reason (R) In forward biasing, electrons on *n*-side diffuses into *p*-side.

5. Assertion (A) A zenner diode is a *p-n* junction with heavy doping.
Reason (R) Heavy doping results in low breakdown voltage.

Statement Type Questions

Directions (Q. Nos. 1-7) *These questions consist of two statements, choose the most appropriate answer from the options given below.*
(a) Both Statement I and Statement II are incorrect.
(b) Statement I is correct but Statement II is incorrect.
(c) Statement I is incorrect but Statement II is correct.
(d) Both Statement I and Statement II are correct.

1. Statement I If a meter scale has 1000 divisions, its least count is 1 mm.
Statement II Least count is the least value of measurement that an instrument can give us.

2. Statement I In meter bridge experiment, if diameter of meter bridge wire is increased, then balancing length does not change.
Statement II Meter bridge experiment is useful to measure the value of unknown resistance.

3. Statement I In the measurement of specific heat of a liquid using calorimeter, while performing the experiment we keep the value of current constant by adjusting rheostat.
Statement II Charging current damages the coil of heater.

4. Statement I In Searle's experiment after every step of loading, we wait for 2 min or 3 min before taking reading.
Statement II Young's modulus of elasticity $= \dfrac{\text{Stress}}{\text{Strain}}$.

5. Statement I If we use tuning fork of smaller frequency, then we require a large tube in resonance column method.
Statement II In resonance column method, $v = 2f(l_2 - l_1)$
Here, v = velocity of sound in air,
f = frequency of tuning fork,
l_1 = first resonance length of air column,
l_2 = second resonance length of air column.

6. Statement I In a experiment, increasing the voltage across a resistor in a circuit will increase the current flowing through it.
Statement II According to Ohm's law, current is directly proportional to voltage when resistance is constant.

7. **Statement I** When colour of light changes, the focal length of thin lens change but that of spherical mirror does not change.

Statement II Refractive index of material depends on wavelength of light while reflection of light does not depend on wavelength of light.

Match the Columns

1. Match the following columns.

Column I		Column II
A. The difference between one main scale division and one vernier scale division, used to measure with high precision.	I.	Main scale
B. The part of the vernier caliper that provides the primary reading. Usually in millimeters or centimeters.	II.	Vernier scale
C. A correction needed when the zero mark of the vernier scale does not coincide with the zero mark of the main scale when the jaws are closed.	III.	Zero error
D. The part of the vernier caliper that provides the additional decimal places to the main scale reading.	IV.	Least count

Choose the correct answer from the options given below.

(a) A-II, B-I, C-IV, D-III
(b) A-IV, B-I, C-III, D-II
(c) A-III, B-IV, C-II, D-I
(d) A-I, B-IV, C-I, D-II

2. Match the following columns.

Column I		Column II
A. Meter bridge	I.	A instrument used to detect and measure small electric currents.
B. Galvanometer	II.	A practical method used to determine the unknown resistance by balancing two legs of a bridge circuit.
C. Electical calorimetry	III.	A experimental setup used to measure the specific capacity of substances.
D. Regnault experiment	IV.	A method used to measure the electrical equivalent of heat by determining the amount of heat produced by an electric current.

Choose the correct answer from the options given below.

(a) A-II, B-I, C-IV, D-III
(b) A-I, B-II, C-III, D-IV
(c) A-III, B-I, C-II, D-IV
(d) A-I, B-IV, C-III, D-II

3. Match the Columns I with column II.

Column I		Column II
A. Vernier caliper	I.	measure focal length of the optical equipment
B. Meter scale	II.	measure external, internal and depth of vessel
C. Resonance tube	III.	calculate the mass of the given object by principle of the moments
D. Parallax method	IV.	calculate the speed of sound in air at room temperature

Choose the correct answer from the options given below.

(a) A-II, B-III, C-IV, D-I
(b) A-I, B-II, C-III, D-IV
(c) A-III, B-I, C-IV, D-II
(d) A-IV, B-I, C-II, D-III

Answers

Step up Practice 1

1 (b)	2 (a)	3 (a)	4 (a)	5 (d)	6 (c)	7 (b)	8 (c)	9 (a)	10 (d)
11 (a)	12 (a)	13 (d)	14 (c)	15 (b)	16 (d)	17 (a)	18 (c)	19 (a)	20 (c)
21 (d)	22 (a)	23 (a)	24 (b)	25 (c)	26 (b)	27 (c)	28 (b)	29 (d)	30 (a)
31 (c)	32 (d)	33 (c)	34 (a)	35 (d)	36 (c)	37 (b)	38 (a)	39 (c)	40 (d)

Step up Practice 2

1 (a)	2 (d)	3 (d)	4 (b)	5 (b)	6 (a)	7 (d)	8 (d)	9 (b)	10 (b)
11 (d)	12 (a)	13 (b)	14 (a)	15 (b)	16 (a)	17 (b)	18 (a)	19 (c)	20 (d)
21 (c)	22 (a)	23 (a)	24 (c)	25 (d)	26 (c)	27 (b)	28 (c)	29 (c)	30 (a)
31 (c)	32 (c)	33 (b)	34 (d)	35 (b)	36 (d)	37 (a)	38 (a)	39 (c)	40 (b)

Step up Practice 3

1 (c)	2 (d)	3 (d)	4 (c)	5 (a)	6 (b)	7 (d)	8 (a)	9 (d)	10 (b)
11 (a)	12 (b)	13 (d)	14 (b)	15 (b)	16 (b)	17 (c)	18 (c)	19 (a)	20 (d)
21 (d)	22 (a)	23 (d)	24 (c)	25 (a)	26 (b)	27 (c)	28 (c)	29 (b)	30 (a)
31 (c)	32 (c)								

Step up Practice 4

1 (c)	2 (c)	3 (a)	4 (a)	5 (a)	6 (b)	7 (c)	8 (b)	9 (c)	10 (d)
11 (a)	12 (a)	13 (a)	14 (c)	15 (b)	16 (d)	17 (c)	18 (a)	19 (d)	20 (a)
21 (b)	22 (b)	23 (b)	24 (b)	25 (b)	26 (d)	27 (b)	28 (d)	29 (d)	30 (b)
31 (b)	32 (d)	33 (b)	34 (c)	35 (d)	36 (c)	37 (a)	38 (a)	39 (b)	40 (a)
41 (a)	42 (c)	43 (c)							

Gearing up for NEET

1 (a)	2 (c)	3 (d)	4 (a)	5 (c)	6 (c)	7 (a)	8 (a)	9 (c)	10 (a)
11 (a)	12 (d)	13 (c)	14 (b)	15 (c)	16 (d)	17 (b)	18 (d)	19 (a)	20 (a)
21 (b)	22 (a)	23 (a)	24 (b)	25 (c)	26 (b)	27 (b)	28 (b)	29 (c)	30 (b)
31 (a)	32 (a)	33 (b)	34 (c)	35 (d)	36 (d)	37 (d)	38 (c)	39 (a)	40 (c)
41 (b)	42 (a)	43 (d)	44 (a)	45 (b)	46 (b)	47 (c)	48 (c)	49 (d)	50 (a)
51 (c)	52 (a)	53 (a)	54 (d)	55 (b)	56 (a)	57 (b)	58 (a)	59 (c)	60 (c)
61 (a)	62 (a)	63 (b)	64 (c)	65 (b)	66 (c)	67 (a)	68 (a)	69 (a)	70 (a)
71 (b)	72 (a)	73 (a)	74 (a)	75 (d)	76 (a)	77 (c)	78 (b)	79 (d)	80 (a)

Assertion and Reason

1 (b)	2 (c)	3 (d)	4 (c)	5 (d)

Statement Type Questions

1 (d)	2 (d)	3 (b)	4 (d)	5 (d)	6 (d)	7 (d)

Match the Columns

1 (b)	2 (a)	3 (a)

Hints and Solutions

Step up Practice 1

1. (*b*) $LC = 1M - 1V$

2. (*a*) $\text{Least count} = \dfrac{1\text{ MSD}}{\text{No. of div. in CS}} = \dfrac{1\text{ mm}}{10}$
$= 0.1\text{ mm} = 0.01\text{ cm}$

3. (*a*) Here, zero error is positive and zero correction is negative.

4. (*a*) ZE = negative ZC = positive

5. (*d*) CR = OR − ZE and ZC = CR − OR

6. (*c*) We have the situation given shown.

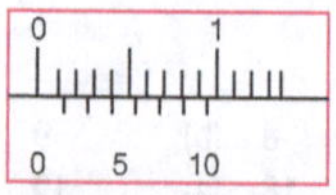

Positive zero error

Clearly zero error is positive and zero error
$e = +4\text{ VSD} = +(4 \times 0.1\text{ mm})$
$= 0.4\text{ mm}$

7. (*b*) Given, 10 VSD = 8 MSD

So, $1\text{ VSD} = \dfrac{8}{10}\text{ MSD}$
$LC = 1\text{ MSD} - 1\text{ VSD}$
$= 1\text{ MSD} - \dfrac{8}{10}\text{ MSD}$
$= \dfrac{2}{10} \times \text{MSD}$
$LC = 0.2\text{ mm}$

8. (*c*) Vernier caliper cannot measure diametre of range of micron.

9. (*a*) $\text{Least count} = \dfrac{1\text{ MSD}}{\text{No. of div. in VS}}$
$\Rightarrow \quad 0.05\text{ mm} = \dfrac{0.5\text{ mm}}{\text{No. of Div. in VS}}$
$\text{No. of div. in VS} = \dfrac{0.5}{0.05} = 10$

10. (*d*) Both A and R are true and R is the correct explanation of A.
When the zero error of a caliper is positive, it will be subtracted from the measured value because the positive zero error gives the extra measured value. So, the measured value is greater than of actual value.

11. (*a*) Zero error is negative here.

12. (*a*) Here, zero error is positive, so zero correction is negative.

13. (*d*) Here, the zero error is negative.
$Z = (96 - 100) \times LC = -4 \times 0.01\text{ mm} = -0.04\text{ mm}$

14. (*c*) Here, the zero error is positive.
$Z = 5 \times LC = 5 \times 0.01\text{ mm} = +0.05\text{ mm}$

15. (*b*) $\text{Least count} = \dfrac{\text{Pitch}}{\text{No. of divisions on circular scale}}$
$(LC)_A = \dfrac{1\text{mm}}{50\text{ division}} = 0.02\text{ mm/division}$
$(LC)_B = 0.005\text{ mm/division}$
$\dfrac{(LC)_A}{(LC)_B} = \dfrac{0.02}{0.005} = 4$
$(LC)_A = 4\,(LC)_B$

16. (*d*) The observed reading is 0.24 mm.
The correct reading = Observe reading − Zero error.
$= 0.24\text{ mm} - (-0.02\text{ mm}) = 0.26\text{ mm}$

18. (*c*) $LC = \dfrac{0.1\text{cm}}{200} = \dfrac{1\text{mm}}{200} = 0.005\text{ mm}$

19. (*a*) Distance between consecutive threads = Pitch
$LC = 0.005\text{ mm} = \dfrac{\text{Pitch}}{100}$
$\Rightarrow \quad \text{Pitch} = 0.5\text{ mm}$

20. (*c*) $LC = \dfrac{0.5\text{mm}}{50} = 0.01\text{ mm}$
$ZE = -(50 - 45) \times 0.01\text{ mm} = -0.05\text{ mm}$
$MSR = 0$
$CSR = 25 \times 0.01\text{ mm} = 0.25\text{ mm}$
$\text{Corrected reading} = [0 + 0.25 - (0.05)] = 0.2\text{ mm}$

21. (*d*) $T \propto \dfrac{1}{\omega},\ \omega = \sqrt{\dfrac{k}{m}} \Rightarrow T = 2\pi\sqrt{\dfrac{m}{k}}$
where, $T' \propto \dfrac{1}{\omega'}$
$\omega = \sqrt{\dfrac{k}{m} - \dfrac{b^2}{4m^2}}$ as $\omega' < \omega \Rightarrow T' > T$

22. (*a*) $E = E_0 e^{-\lambda t}$

23. (*a*) $F = -kx - bv \Rightarrow m\dfrac{d^2x}{dt^2} + \dfrac{bdx}{dt} + kx = 0$

24. (*b*) Amplitude and energy decrease exponentially.

25. (*c*) $A^2 = A_0^2 e^{\frac{-bt}{m}}$

26. (*b*) $E = E_0 e^{\frac{-bt}{m}}$

27. (c) As, $A = A_0 e^{-\alpha t}$

$$\Rightarrow \frac{A_0}{2} = A_0 e^{-\alpha} \quad \text{... (i)}$$

and $$\frac{A_0}{x} = A_0 e^{-\alpha \cdot 3} \quad \text{... (ii)}$$

From Eqs. (i) and (ii), we get

$$\frac{1}{x} = \left(\frac{1}{2}\right)^3 = \frac{1}{8} \quad \therefore \quad x = 8$$

28. (b) $a = a_0 e^{-\alpha t}$

$$0.8 a_0 = a_0 e^{-50\alpha T} \Rightarrow 0.8 = e^{50\alpha T}$$

$$a = a_0 e^{-150\alpha T}$$

$$a = a_0 e^{-150\alpha T} = a_0 \left(\frac{0.8 a_0}{a_0}\right)^3 = 0.512 a_0$$

29. (d) In the experiment of simple pendulum, we keep $\theta <$ 5° i.e. angular displacement very small, so that motion becomes SHM because as θ very small.

$$\therefore \quad \sin\theta = \theta$$

$$F = -mg \sin\theta = -mg\,\theta$$

$$\Rightarrow \quad F = -\left(\frac{mg}{l}\right) \cdot x \quad \text{or} \quad F \propto -x$$

30. (a) $\tau = Fr \sin\theta$

$(\sin\theta)_{max} = 1$ for $\theta = 90°$

31. (c) $m = M\left(\frac{y}{x}\right)$

32. (d) When we take moments of force at equilibrium, the terms of g cancel on both sides.

$$mg \cdot x_e = Mg \cdot y_e$$

$$m = M \cdot \left(\frac{y_e}{x_e}\right)$$

The mass is independent of the gravity at that point, so mass at the poles will be same as mass at the equator.

33. (c) $\because m_1 r_1 = m_2 r_2$

$$\frac{r_1}{r_2} = \frac{m_2}{m_1} \Rightarrow r \propto \frac{1}{m}$$

34. (a) Let plank shifted by x, then $\Delta x_{CM} = 0$, as there is no external force on the system.

$$m(L - x_{plank}) - Mx_{plank} = 0$$

$$x_{plank} = \frac{mL}{M + m}$$

35. (d)

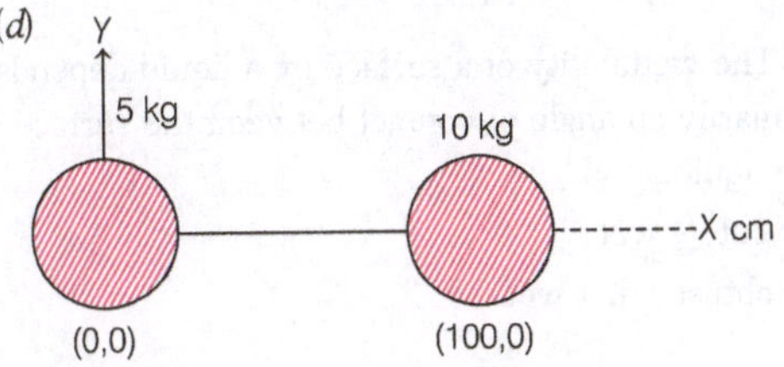

Centre of mass of the system from the 5 kg particle

$$X_{CM} = \frac{m_1 x_1 + m_2 x_2}{m_1 + m_2} = \frac{5 \times 0 + 100 \times 10}{m_1 + m_2} = \frac{200}{3}$$

$$= 66.66 \text{ cm}$$

$$X_{CM} = 67 \text{ cm}$$

36. (c) According to questions,

$$16 l_1 = m l_2 \quad \text{...(i)}$$

$$m l_1 = 4 l_2 \quad \text{...(ii)}$$

Dividing Eq. (i) by Eq. (ii), we get

$$\frac{16}{m} = \frac{m}{4}$$

$$\Rightarrow \quad m^2 = 64 \Rightarrow m = 8 \text{ kg}$$

37. (b) $$m l_1 = m_2 l_2$$

$$m \times 20 = 40 \times 15 \Rightarrow m = 30 \text{ g}$$

38. (a) $\tau_R = (300 \times 40) - (500 \times 20) = m_1 r_1 - m_2 r_2$

$= 2000$ gf cm

Let 100 gf be suspended at x distance at right hand side.

In balanced condition

$$\tau_R' = m_1' r'_1 = m_2 r_2' = 0$$

$$12000 - 10000 - 200x = 0$$

$$x = 10 \text{ cm}$$

39. (c)

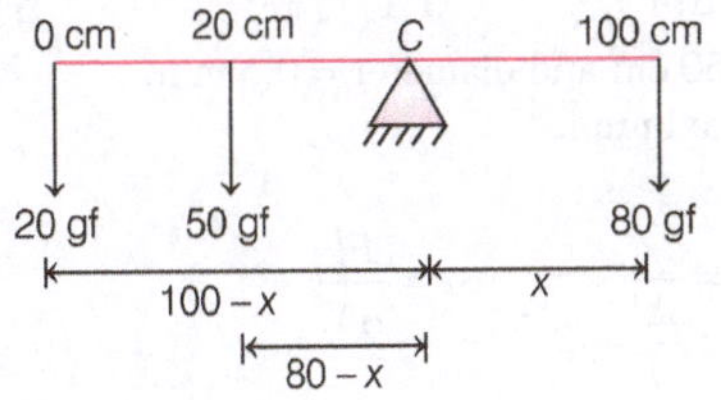

In equilibrium at C

$$80x = 20(100 - x) + 50(80 - x)$$

$$x = 40 \text{ cm}$$

40. (d) $(5 \times 50) + w \times 10 = 20 \times 40$

$$250 + 10w = 800$$

$$10w = 550$$

$$w = \frac{550}{10}$$

$$w = 55 \text{ gf}$$

Step up Practice 2

1. (a) $Y = \frac{FL}{A\Delta L}, \quad \frac{\Delta L}{L} = \alpha\,\Delta T$

$$F = \frac{YA\Delta L}{L} = YA\alpha\,\Delta T$$

$$Y_1 A \alpha_1 \Delta T = Y_2 A \alpha_2 \Delta T$$

$$\frac{\alpha_1}{\alpha_2} = \frac{Y_2}{Y_1} \Rightarrow \frac{Y_1}{Y_2} = \frac{3}{2}$$

2. (*d*) $F = M\alpha = (LA\rho)\alpha$

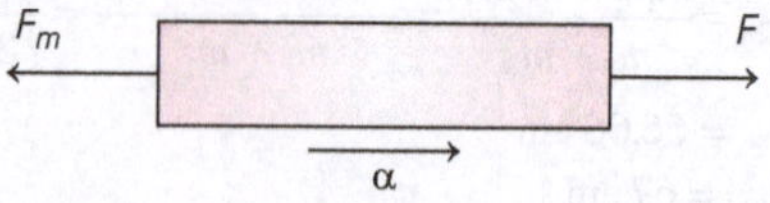

$$F - F_m = \left(\frac{LA\rho}{2}\right)\alpha \Rightarrow F_m = \left(\frac{LA\rho}{2}\right)\alpha$$

Stress at mid-point $= \frac{F_m}{A} = \left(\frac{L\rho\alpha}{2}\right)$

3. (*d*) $y = \frac{FL}{Al}$ ...(i)

$L = 4$ m

$A = \frac{\pi d^2}{4} = \frac{\pi}{4} \times (9 \times 10^{-2})^2$

$A = 63.61 \times 10^{-4}\ \text{m}^2$

$\gamma = 1.9 \times 10^{11}\ \text{N/m}^2$

$F = mg = 80000 \times 10 = 8 \times 10^5$ N

Now, from Eq. (i),

$$l = \frac{8 \times 10^5 \times 4}{1.9 \times 10^{11} \times 63.61 \times 10^{-4}}$$

$l = 2.6$ mm

4. (*b*) $Y = \frac{F/A}{\Delta l/l} \Rightarrow \Delta l = \frac{Fl}{YA} = \frac{Fl}{Y\pi r^2} \Rightarrow \Delta l \propto \frac{l}{r^2}$

for $l = 50$ cm and diameter $= 0.5$ mm, Δl is maximum.

5. (*b*) $\because Y = \frac{\frac{F}{A}}{\frac{\Delta l}{l}} \Rightarrow \Delta l = \frac{Fl}{AY}$

But $V = Al$, so $A = \frac{V}{l}$ (V = volume)

$\therefore\ \Delta l = \frac{Fl^2}{VY}$

So, $\Delta l \propto l^2$

6. (*a*) $Y = \frac{\text{Stress}}{\text{Strain}} = \frac{\text{Stress}}{\text{Extension / Initial length}}$

$= \frac{4000 \times 10^3}{2 \times 10^{-3}/1} = 2 \times 10^9\ \text{N/m}^2$

7. (*d*) Stress same

Maximum stress remains same.

8. (*d*) $V = \pi r^2 l \Rightarrow \frac{\Delta V}{V} = 2\frac{\Delta r}{r} + \frac{\Delta l}{l}$

$\frac{\Delta l}{l} = 0.2\% - 2 \times 0.002\% = 0.2\% - 0.004\% = 0.196\%$

$\therefore$Stress $= Y\frac{\Delta l}{l} = 2 \times 10^{11} \times 0.196 \times 10^{-2}$

$= 0.392 \times 10^9$

$= 3.9 \times 10^8\ \text{N/m}^2$

9. (*b*) Young's modulus of elasticity is independent from length and radius of wire.

10. (*b*) $Y = \frac{\text{Stress}}{\text{Strain}}$

if strain = 1, then Y = stress

11. (*d*) As, $Y = \frac{FL}{A\Delta L}$, when $T\uparrow, \Delta L\uparrow \Rightarrow Y\downarrow$

The temperature of a wire is doubled the Young's modulus of elasticity will decrease.

12. (*a*) Mercury will start leaking when $\rho gh = 2\frac{T}{r}$

$$h_{\min} = \frac{2T}{\rho gr} = \frac{4T}{\rho gd} = \frac{4 \times 550 \times 10^{-3} \times 10^4}{9.8 \times 1 \times 13.6 \times 10^3}$$

$= 0.165$ m $= 16.5$ cm

13. (*b*) $p_2 - p_1 = 4T\left(\frac{1}{r_2} - \frac{1}{r_1}\right) = \frac{4T}{r}$

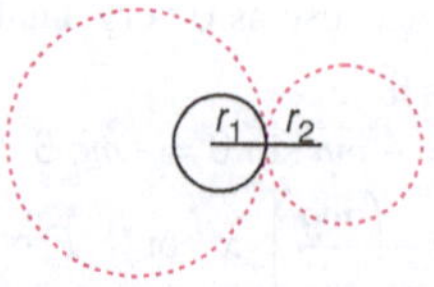

$\frac{1}{r} = \frac{1}{r_2} - \frac{1}{r_1} = \frac{1}{2} - \frac{1}{4} = \frac{1}{4} \Rightarrow r = 4$ cm

14. (*a*) $h = \frac{2T\cos\theta}{\rho gr} = -0.029$ m

≈ 0.03 m or 3 cm

15. (*b*) $T = \frac{h\rho gr}{2\cos\theta}$

If h is not sufficient, then θ changes to balance the surface tension.

16. (*a*) At equilibrium force due to surface tension

= Weight of liquid rise

$(2\pi)T\cos\theta_c = mg$

$\therefore\ 2\pi rT$ = weight

$\Rightarrow\ 2\pi r = \frac{\text{weight}}{T}$

$= \frac{75 \times 10^{-4}}{6 \times 10^{-2}} = 12.5 \times 10^{-2}$ m

17. (*b*) $h = \frac{2T\cos\theta}{r\rho g} = \frac{2 \times 70 \times 1}{\frac{1}{14} \times 1 \times 980} = 2$ cm

18. (*a*) The wettability of a surface by a liquid depends primarily on angle of contact between the surface and the liquid.

(I) acute - wet

(II) obtuse - not wet

19. (c) Water will rise upto the top level but will not overflow. Radius of curvature R' increases in such a way that final height h' is reduced and given by

$h' = \frac{hR}{R'}$ (it is in accordance with Zurin's law)

20. (d) $h = \frac{2T \cos\theta}{\rho g r}$

As r, h, T are same, $\frac{\cos\theta}{\rho} = \text{constant}$

$$\therefore \quad \frac{\cos\theta_1}{\rho_1} = \frac{\cos\theta_2}{\rho_2} = \frac{\cos\theta_3}{\rho_3}$$

As $\rho_1 > \rho_2 > \rho_3$

$\therefore \cos\theta_1 > \cos\theta_2 > \cos\theta_3 \Rightarrow \theta_1 < \theta_2 < \theta_3$

As, water rises, so θ must be acute

So, $0 \le \theta_1 < \theta_2 < \theta_3 < \frac{\pi}{2}$

21. (c) For liquids

$T\downarrow, \eta\uparrow$

and for surface tension

$T\uparrow$, ST$\downarrow$

So, statement I is incorrect and statement II is correct.

22. (a) For closed pipe

$$n = \frac{v}{4l} = 512 \text{ Hz}$$

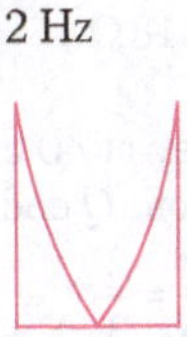

For open pipe

$$n = \frac{v}{2l} = 1024$$

$$n = 1024 \text{ Hz}$$

23. (a) $n = \frac{v}{4l}$

$$n = 264 \text{ Hz}$$

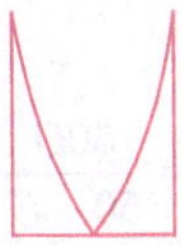

$$v = 330 \text{ m/s}$$

Then, $\quad l = 31.25$ cm

24. (c) Fundamental frequency

$$n = \frac{v}{4l}$$

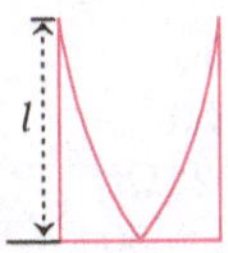

$$v = 320 \text{ m/s}$$

$$l = 1 \text{ m}, n = 80 \text{ Hz}$$

For closed pipe

$n_1 : n_2 : n_3 = \ldots\ldots = 1:3:5:\ldots\ldots$

Frequency 80Hz, 240Hz, 400Hz, ...

25. (d) $L = (2n-1)\frac{\lambda}{4}$

$$= \frac{\lambda}{4}, \frac{3\lambda}{4}, \frac{5\lambda}{4}, \ldots\ldots\ldots\ldots \quad \text{(where, } n = 1, 2, 3\text{)}$$

26. (c) $L = (2n-1)\frac{\lambda}{4}$

$$\Rightarrow \quad l_1 = \frac{\lambda}{4} \quad \ldots\text{(i)}$$

$$\Rightarrow \quad l_2 = \frac{3\lambda}{4} \quad \ldots\text{(ii)}$$

Distance of displacement anti-node from top.

$$= \frac{l_2 - 3l_1}{2}$$

27. (b) $v = f\lambda$

$$\lambda = \frac{340}{340} = 1 \text{ m}$$

$$x = 1.2 - \frac{3\lambda}{4}$$

$$= 1.2 - 0.75$$

$$x = 0.45 \text{ m or } 45 \text{ cm}$$

28. (c) $\frac{\lambda}{2} = (63.2 - 30.7)$ cm or $\lambda = 0.65$ m

$\therefore$ Speed of sound observed, $v_O = f\lambda$

$$= 512 \times 0.65 = 332.8 \text{ m/s}$$

So, $\quad \text{error} = 332.8 - 330$

$$= 2.8 \text{ m/s} = 280 \text{ cm/s}$$

29. (c) Since, in the region AB temperature is constant therefore at this temperature phase of the material changes from solid to liquid and $(H_2 - H_1)$ heat will be absorb by the material. This heat is known as the heat of melting of the solid. Similarity in the region CD temperature is constant therefore at this temperature phase of the material changes from liquid to gas and $(H_4 - H_3)$ heat will be absorbed by the material. This heat as known as the heat of vaporisation of the liquid.

30. (a) Initially on heating temperature rises from $-10°$C to 0°C. Then, ice melts and temperature does not rise. After the whole ice has melted, temperature begins to rise until it reaches 100°C. Then, it becomes constant, as at the boiling point will not rise.

31. (c) If we draw a line parallel to the time axis, then it cuts the given graph at three different points. Corresponding points on the times axis shows that

$$t_C > t_B > t_A \Rightarrow C_C > C_B > C_A$$

32. (c) $\Delta Q = ms_1\Delta T_1 = ms_2\Delta T_2$

$$ms(25) = m\frac{s}{2}(\Delta T)$$

$$\Delta T = 50°\text{C}$$

33. (b) $m_{ice}L_f = m_b S_b \Delta T$

$m_{ice}(80) = (2400)(0.1)(500-0)$

$m_{ice} = 1500\text{ g} = 1.5\text{ kg}$

34. (d) $Q = m_i L_f + m_w S_w(\Delta T) + m_w L_w + m_a s_a(\Delta T)$

from water equivalent concept

$m_a s_a = m_w s_w$

$Q = 10\times 80 + 10\times 1\times 100 + 10\times 540 + 10\times 1\times 100$

$= 8200\text{ cal}$

35. (b) Heat released by the steam when it converts to water at 100°C $= 1\times 2.26\times 10^6 = 226\text{ kJ}$

Heat given to ice to convert in water at 0°C

$= 1\times 3.36\times 10^5 = 336\text{ kJ}$

Heat given to rise temperature 0° to 100°C

$= 1\times 4.2\times 10^3\times 100 = 420\text{ kJ}$

Total heat required $= 420 + 336 = 756\text{ kg}$

$= 756000\text{ g}$

Let m mass of system is converted into water at 100°C by giving out this much amount of heat.

Then, $m\times 2.26\times 10^6 = \dfrac{756000}{2.26\times 10^6}$

$\Rightarrow \quad m = 0.335\text{ kg}$

Therefore, at equilibrium, the steam will be

$= 1 - 0.335 = 0.665\text{ kg}$

and water will be $1 + 0.335 = 1.335\text{ kg}$

The temperature of both will be 100°C.

Thus, the final composition of the system,

water $= 1335\text{ g}$, steam $= 665\text{ g}$

36. (d) Heat given = Heat taken

$(100)(0.1)(T-75) = (100)(0.1)(45) + (170)(45)$

$10(T-75) = 450 + 7650 = 8100$

$T - 75 = 810$

$T = 885°\text{ C}$

37. (a) $Q = ms_{ice}\ \Delta T = mL_F + ms_{water}\Delta T + mL_v$

$= (1)(0.5)(10) + (1)(80) + (1)(1)(100) + (1)(540)$

$= 5 + 80 + 100 = 540 = 725\text{ cal}$

or $725\times 4.18 = 3030\text{ J}$

38. (a) 2 kg ice at −20°C + 5 kg water at 20°C

$Q_{gain} = Q_{lost}$

$2\times \frac{1}{2}\times 20 + M\times 80 = 5\times 1\times 20$

(M = amount of ice melted)

$M = 1\text{ kg}$

Water $= 5 + 1 = 6\text{ kg}$

39. (c) $\Delta Q = msd\theta$

$420\text{ J} = 10g\times 4.2\times d\theta$

$d\theta = 10°\text{ C}$

40. (b) Let specific heat of liquids be s_1 and s_2 respectively, so heat gain by 1st = heat loss by 2nd

$ms_1(32-200) = ms_2(40-32)$

$\Rightarrow \quad \dfrac{s_1}{s_2} = \dfrac{8}{12} = \dfrac{2}{3}$

Step up Practice 3

1. (c) At null point, deflection through galvanometer is zero, also deflection in galvanometer in opposite direction, either side of null point.

2. (d) Wheatstone bridge is combination of four resistors.

3. (d) Resistivity of material is property of that material only. It does not depend on geometry of material.

4. (c)

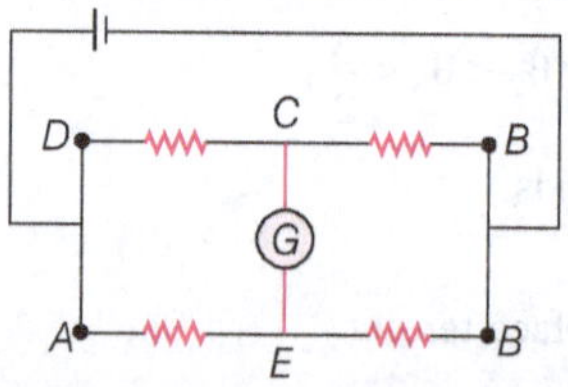

Battery connected across BD and galvanometer connected across EC

5. (a) $\dfrac{X}{60} = \dfrac{12}{40} \Rightarrow X = 18\Omega$

6. (b) Initially, jockey key at 40 cm from P end i.e. $(100-40) = 60$ cm from Q end.

$\therefore \quad \dfrac{P}{Q} = \dfrac{40}{60} = \dfrac{2}{3}$

$\dfrac{P}{Q} = \dfrac{2}{3}$ ...(i)

Now, Q is shunted with 50Ω.

$\therefore$ New resistance, $Q' = \left[\dfrac{50Q}{50+Q}\right]$ and new balance point is moved by 10 cm.

Hence, $\dfrac{P}{Q'} = \dfrac{50}{50} = 1$

$\therefore \quad P = Q'$ i.e. $P = \dfrac{50Q}{50+Q}$

$\therefore \quad \dfrac{P}{Q} = \dfrac{50}{50+Q}$

From Eq. (i),

$\dfrac{2}{3} = \dfrac{50}{50+Q}$

$\therefore \quad 100 + 2Q = 5Q$

$2Q = 50$

$Q = 25\Omega$

and $P = \dfrac{2}{3}Q = \dfrac{2}{3}\times 25 = \dfrac{50}{3}\Omega$

7. (d) Initially

$$\frac{R_1}{R_2} = \frac{x}{(1-x)} = \frac{10}{30} \Rightarrow x = 25 \text{ cm}$$

Finally after interchange

$$\frac{y}{1-y} = \frac{30}{10} \Rightarrow y = 75 \text{ cm}$$

shifting = 50 cm

8. (a) $\frac{R_1 + 10}{R_2} = \frac{50}{50} = 1 \Rightarrow R_1 + 10 = R_2$ ...(i)

$$\frac{R_1}{R_2} = \frac{40}{60} \Rightarrow 3R_1 = 2R_2 \quad \text{...(ii)}$$

From Eqs. (i) and (ii), we get

$$R_1 + 10 = \frac{3}{2}R_1 \Rightarrow R_1 = 20\,\Omega$$

9. (d) Interchanging cell and galvanometer do not effect balance condition.

10. (b) Average value of 1st three measurement is 2.77 Ω. So, this can be taken as true value.

11. (a) $\frac{X}{20} = \frac{Y}{80}$ ...(i)

$$\frac{4X}{l} = \frac{Y}{100-l} \quad \text{...(ii)}$$

$$\Rightarrow l = 100 - l \Rightarrow l = 50 \text{ cm}$$

12. (b) $\frac{X}{52+1} = \frac{10}{48+2} \Rightarrow X = 10.6\,\Omega$

13. (d) Both A and R are true and R is the correct explanation of A.

The bridge wire is made up of manganin because it have large resistivity.

The temperature coefficient of manganin is very small. Thats why its resistivity is nearly constant over large value of temperature which is exactly required for bridge wire.

14. (b) Ammeter should be connected in series and voltmeter should be connected in parallel.

15. (b)

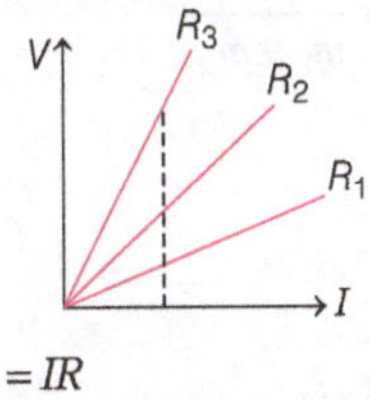

$\because \quad V = IR$

For I = constant $\Rightarrow V \propto R$

Clearly, $R_3 > R_2 > R_1$

16. (b) $V = iR$

$\Rightarrow R$ = Double = Current will reduce to half.

17. (c) $V = IR$

$$I \propto V$$

18. (c) For the validation of Ohm's law temperature must be kept constant.

19. (a) Material same ⇒ ρ unchanged

$$R = \frac{\rho l}{A} = \frac{\rho l}{\pi a^2} \Rightarrow R \propto \frac{l}{a^2}$$

Therefore, $R' \propto \frac{2l}{(2a)^2} \Rightarrow R' = \frac{R}{2}$

20. (d)

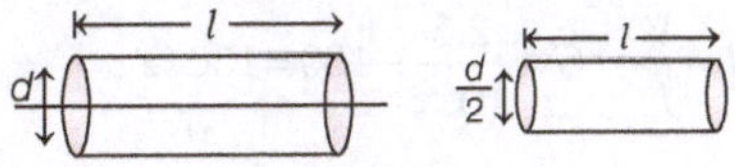

Initial volume = Final volume

$$\frac{\pi d^2 l}{4} = \frac{\pi d^2 L}{16} \Rightarrow L = 4l \qquad A_f = \frac{A_i}{4}$$

$$R_i = \frac{\rho l}{A_i} \qquad R_f = \rho\left(\frac{4l}{\frac{A_i}{4}}\right) = 16R_i$$

21. (d) $\rho = \frac{1}{\sigma} \Rightarrow \rho \times \sigma = \text{constant}$

22. (a) Volume remains same ⇒ $Al = A'(2L)$

$$A' = \frac{A}{2}, R_i = \frac{\rho L}{A}$$

$$R_f = \frac{\rho(2L)}{(A/2)} = 4R_i$$

$$\text{Percentage change} = \frac{4R_i - R_i}{R_i} \times 100 = 300\%$$

23. (d) For I-V curve

$$\text{slope} = \frac{I}{V} = \frac{1}{R}$$

$$R = \frac{1}{\text{slope}}$$

$\because \quad R_2 > R_1$

$\therefore \quad T_2 > T_1$

24. (c) $I_g = \frac{V}{(R+G)}, \frac{V_{max}}{I_{max}} = 5\Omega$

$$\frac{V}{I_g} = 10^4 \Rightarrow R = 10000 - 5 = 9995\,\Omega$$

25. (a) $S = \left(\frac{I_g}{I - I_g}\right)G \Rightarrow S = \left(\frac{10^{-3}}{1 - 10^{-3}}\right) \times 200$

$$\Rightarrow S = 0.2\,\Omega$$

26. (b) $I_g \times G = (I - I_g)S$

$$\Rightarrow I = 1001 \times 100 \times 10^{-6} = 100.1 \text{ mA}$$

27. (c) Given, the voltmeter of resistance G gives the full scale deflection for potential difference V.

$$\therefore \quad I_g = \frac{V}{G}$$

Voltage across voltmeter and resistance is

$$V' = I_g(R+G)$$

Here, $V' = nV$, $I_g = \dfrac{V}{G}$

$$nV = \frac{V}{G}(R+G)$$

$$\therefore \quad R = nG - G = (n-1)G$$

28. (c) For full scale deflection, $I_g = nk = 10^{-2}\text{A}$

Now, $R = \dfrac{V}{I_g} - G = \dfrac{2.5}{10^{-2}} - 100 = 150\,\Omega$

29. (b) $R = \left(\dfrac{V}{I_g}\right) - G = \dfrac{15}{15\times10^{-3}} - 200 = 800\,\Omega$

30. (a) $S_I = \dfrac{1}{k}$

31. (c) This is only possible, if we take $V = 10r$

$$V = I_g(G+R)$$

$$R = \frac{V}{I_g} - G$$

$$R = \frac{10}{50\times10^{-6}} - 100$$

$$R \approx 200\,\text{k}\Omega$$

32. (c) $\dfrac{\theta}{i} = \dfrac{50}{10^{-3}} = 5000,\ \dfrac{\theta}{V} = 20$

$$\Rightarrow \frac{\theta/i}{\theta/V} = \frac{5000}{20} = 250 \Rightarrow \frac{V}{i} = R = 250\,\Omega$$

Step up Practice 4

1. (c) Magnification, $m = \dfrac{f}{u-f} = \dfrac{f}{a}$

Clearly graph between f and a must be rectangular hyperbola.

2. (c) Points above the P have $v > 2f$ while points below the P have $u > 2f$.

3. (a)

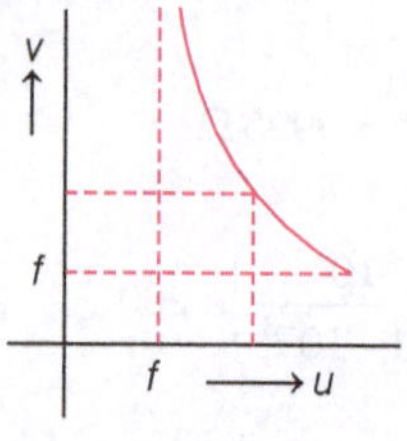

From u-v graph

Slope $= \tan 45° = \dfrac{v}{u} \Rightarrow v = u$

$$\Rightarrow \frac{1}{f} = \frac{1}{v} - \frac{1}{u} \Rightarrow \frac{1}{f} = \frac{1}{v} - \frac{1}{-v}$$

$$\Rightarrow \quad v = 2f = 4 \Rightarrow P = 2f,\ 2f$$

4. (a) Concave mirror formed real and inverted image. The image formed by a concave mirror is real only, if the image and object lie on the same side, which is left according to convention of the mirror.

So, option (a) is correct.

5. (a) $\dfrac{1}{v} + \dfrac{1}{u} = \dfrac{1}{f} \Rightarrow \dfrac{1}{v} = \dfrac{1}{f} - \dfrac{1}{u} \Rightarrow v = \dfrac{fu}{u-f}$

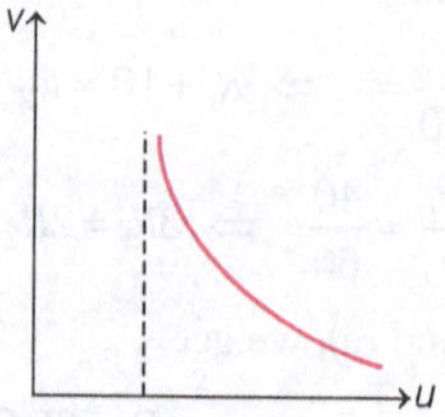

6. (b)

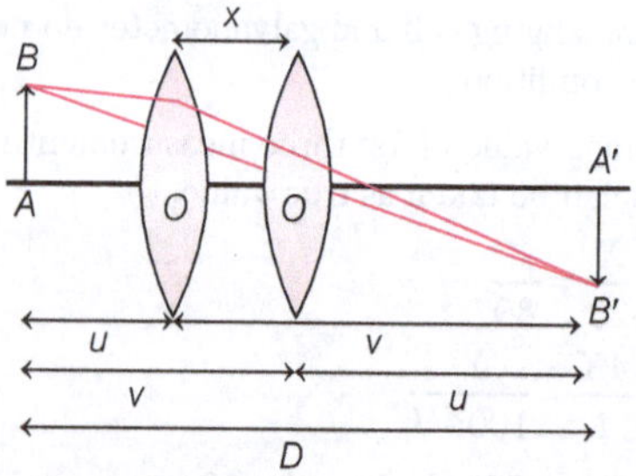

$m_1 = \dfrac{v}{u}$, $m_2 = \dfrac{u}{v}$ (v and u interchange value between the object and screen)

$$m_1 - m_2 = \frac{v}{u} - \frac{u}{v}$$

$$m_1 - m_2 = \frac{v^2 - u^2}{uv} = \frac{(v-u)(v+u)}{uv}$$

Now, $\quad v - u = x,\ \dfrac{1}{f} = \dfrac{1}{v} - \dfrac{1}{(-v)}$

$$\frac{1}{f} = \frac{u+v}{uv}$$

$$\therefore \quad m_1 - m_2 = \frac{x}{f}$$

$$\Rightarrow \quad f = \frac{x}{m_1 - m_2}$$

8. (b) $\dfrac{1}{v} + \dfrac{1}{u} = \dfrac{1}{f}$

By solving $f = \dfrac{75}{2}$,

$$\Rightarrow \quad R = 75 \text{ cm}$$

9. (c) Statement I is incorrect but Statement II is correct.

Focal length is the property of mirror and is independent of the medium in which it is placed.

10. (d) If position of object beyond $2f_1$, then size of image is diminished.

11. (a) $\mu = \dfrac{\sin\left(\dfrac{A+\delta_m}{2}\right)}{\sin\left(\dfrac{A}{2}\right)}$

At point P, $\delta_m = 0$

$\Rightarrow \quad \mu = \dfrac{\sin A/2}{\sin A/2} = 1$

12. (a) $\mu = \dfrac{\sin\left(\dfrac{A+\delta_m}{2}\right)}{\sin\left(\dfrac{A}{2}\right)}$

When μ is increased δ_m will also increase, hence the deviation will also increase.

13. (a) When light rays deviation by prism is minimum, then angle of incident and emergence are equal.

15. (b) $\angle i = 38°$, $\angle e = 58°$, $\delta = 50°$

$\because \delta = i + e - A \Rightarrow A = 46°$

16. (d) $\angle A = 90°$, $\angle i = 45°$, $\angle e = 60°$

$\because \delta = i + e - A = 15°$

17. (c) $\mu = \dfrac{\text{Velocity of light in vacuum}}{\text{Velocity of light in glass plate}} = \dfrac{c}{c'}$

or $c' = \dfrac{c}{\mu}$

Time taken $= \dfrac{\text{Distance}}{\text{Velocity}} = \dfrac{t}{(c/\mu)} = \dfrac{\mu t}{c}$

18. (a) Then, apparent depth is given by

$$I' = \frac{t_1}{\mu_1} + \frac{t_2}{\mu_2}$$
$$= \frac{(t/2)}{\mu_1} + \frac{(t/2)}{\mu_2} = \frac{t(\mu_1 + \mu_2)}{2\mu_1\mu_2}$$

20. (a) Movement of microscope = Normal shift

$$= \left(1 - \frac{1}{u}\right)t = \left(1 - \frac{1}{1.5}\right)3 = 1 \text{ cm}$$

21. (b) $\mu = \dfrac{\text{real depth}}{\text{apparent depth}} = \dfrac{C-A}{C-B}$

28. (d) Both Statement I and Statement II are correct.

A photodiode is a semiconductor device that converts light into current. The current is generated when photons are absorbed in the photodiode. For this purpose, a p-n junction diode is reversed biased.

29. (d) Order of forward current is milliampere.

39. (b) Since, voltage across zener diode (and hence R_S) is regulated, so current through $R_L\left(\dfrac{V}{R_L}\right)$ will remain unchanged.

Gearing up for NEET

1. (a) As, TR = MSR + $n \times$ LC

$= 1.3 + 5 \times 0.01$

$= 1.35$ cm

Zero error $= -0.03$ cm

Zero correction $= +0.03$ cm

Corrected reading $= 1.35 + 0.03 = 1.38$ cm

2. (c) Least count of $A = \dfrac{(1/10)}{10} = 0.01$ cm

Least count of $B = \dfrac{(1/20)}{10} = 0.005$ cm

3. (d) $(n-1)a = n(a')$

$$a' = \frac{(n-1)a}{n}$$

$\therefore \quad$ LC = 1 MSD − 1 VSD

$= (a - a')$ cm

$= a - \dfrac{(n-1)a}{n} = \dfrac{na - na + a}{n} = \dfrac{a}{n}$ cm

$= \left(\dfrac{10a}{n}\right)$ mm

4. (a) Let θ be the angle of incline. Here, the incline kept horizontally is working as main scale while the other incline kept on horizontally placed incline is treated as vernier scale.

From the given figure, it is clear that,

1 MSD $= \dfrac{l}{\cos\theta}$ unit and 1 VSD $= l$ unit,

So, LC of instrument, LC = 1 MSD − 1 VSD

$$= \left(\frac{l}{\cos\theta} - l\right) = \frac{l(1-\cos\theta)}{\cos\theta} \text{ unit}$$

5. (c) As, 6th VSD is coinciding with one of the MSD, so reading of the vernier caliper is

$12 + 6 \times 0.1 = 12.6$ mm

6. (c) 1 Vernier scale division $= \dfrac{29}{30}$ Main scale division

$\Rightarrow \quad 1 \text{ VSD} = \dfrac{29}{30} \times 0.5° = \left(\dfrac{29}{60}\right)^\circ$

$\therefore$ The least count = 1 MSD − 1 VSD

$$= \left(\frac{1}{2}\right)^\circ - \left(\frac{29}{60}\right)^\circ = \left(\frac{1}{60}\right)^\circ$$

So, reading = main scale reading + vernier scale reading

$= \text{MSR} + n \times \text{LC}$

$= 58.5° + 9 \times \left(\dfrac{1}{60}\right)^\circ = 58.65°$

7. (a) As, least count

$= \dfrac{\text{value of main scale division}}{\text{number of divisions on vernier scale}}$

$= \dfrac{1}{30}\text{ MSD} = \dfrac{1}{30} \times \dfrac{1°}{2} = \dfrac{1°}{60} = 1$ min

8. (a) $(N+1)\text{VSD} = N\ \text{MSD}$

$$1\ \text{VSD} = \frac{N}{N+1}\text{MSD}$$

least count = 1 MSD − 1 VSD

$$= 1\ \text{MSD} - \frac{N}{N+1}\text{MSD}$$

$$= \frac{1}{N+1}\text{MSD}$$

$$\text{LC} = \frac{a}{N+1}$$

9. (c) 1 MSD = 1 mm

9 MSD = 10 VSD

∴ Least count, LC = 1MSD − 1VSD

$$= 1\ \text{mm} - \frac{9}{10}\ \text{mm}$$

$$= \frac{1}{10}\ \text{mm}$$

Measure reading of edge = MSR + VSR(LC)

$$= 10 + 1\frac{1}{10} = 10.1\ \text{mm}$$

Volume of cube, $V = (1.01)^3\ \text{cm}^3 = 1.03\ \text{cm}^3$

[After rounding off upto 3 significant digits, as edge length is measured upto 3 significant digits]

$$\text{Density of cube} = \frac{2.736}{1.03} = 2.6563\frac{\text{g}}{\text{cm}^3} = 2.66\frac{\text{g}}{\text{cm}^3}$$

(After rounding off to 3 significant digits)

10. (a) Least count depends on main scale and circular scale.

11. (a) MSR = 2 mm, CSR = 30 × 0.01 mm = 0.30 mm

Reading = 2 mm + 0.30 mm = 2.30 mm

12. (d) MSR = 0 mm, CSR = 52 div,

$$\text{LC} = \frac{1}{100} = 0.01\ \text{mm}$$

Diametre = (0 + 52 × 0.01) mm = 0.052 cm

13. (c) Pitch = 0.5 mm, $\text{LC} = \frac{0.5\ \text{mm}}{50} = 0.01\ \text{mm}$

ZE = (+ 5 × 0.01 mm) = + 0.05 mm

During measurement MSR = 2 × 0.5 mm = 1 mm

CSR = 25 × 0.01 mm = 0.25 mm

Corrected reading = 1 mm + 0.25 mm − 0.05 mm

= 1.20 mm

14. (b) Pitch = 0.5 mm, $\text{LC} = \frac{0.5\ \text{mm}}{100} = 0.005\ \text{mm}$

ZE = + *ve*; ZE = (+3 × 0.005) = + 0.015 mm

During measurement MSR = 5.5 mm

CSR = 48 × 0.005 mm = 0.240 mm

Corrected reading = (5.5 + 0.240 − 0.015)

= 5.725 mm

15. (c) $\text{LC} = (5\times10^{-6})\times10^3\ \text{mm} = \frac{1\ \text{mm}}{\text{No. of CSD}}$

$$\Rightarrow \text{No. of CSD} = \frac{1}{5\times10^{-3}} = 200$$

16. (d) $\text{LC} = \frac{0.1\text{cm}}{50} = 0.002\ \text{cm}$

Measurement should be integer multiple of least count.

17. (b) LC = 0.01 mm, l = 6.8 cm

Diametre = (1.5 + 7 × 0.01) = 1.57 mm

= 0.157 cm

$$\text{SA} = (\pi dl) = (3.141)(0.157)(6.8) = 3.4\ \text{cm}^2$$

18. (d) In 2 min, $A = \frac{A_0}{3}$

$$\Rightarrow \text{In 4 min, } A = \frac{A_0}{3^2} = \frac{A_0}{9}$$

19. (a) Observed reading = 1 mm + 6 × 0.01 mm

= 1.06 mm

Zero error = − 0.03 mm

Zero correction = + 0.03 mm

Corrected reading = 1.06 + 0.03 = 1.09 mm

20. (a) Corrected thickness of the sheet

$$= \frac{(1.04-0.06)+(1.06-0.06)+(1.08-0.06)}{3}$$

$$= \frac{0.98+1+1.02}{3}$$

$$= \frac{3}{3}\text{mm} = 0.10\ \text{cm}$$

21. (b) Given that, number of divisions on circular scale = 50

Pitch = 0.5 mm = 5×10^{-4} m

Least count of screw gauge

$$= \frac{\text{Pitch}}{\text{Number of divisions on circular scale}}$$

$$= \frac{5\times10^{-4}}{50} = 1\times10^{-5}\ \text{m} = 10\ \mu\text{m}$$

Since, circular scale is 4 units ahead of the pitch scale marking which means screw gauge has positive zero error.

22. (a) Pitch of screw of a screw gauge

$$= \frac{\text{Distance moved by screw}}{\text{Number of rotations}}$$

$$= \frac{3\ \text{mm}}{6} = 0.5\ \text{mm}$$

and least count of screw gauge

$$= \frac{\text{pitch}}{\text{number of circular scale divisions}}$$

$$= \frac{0.5\ \text{mm}}{50} = 0.01\ \text{mm} = 0.001\ \text{cm}$$

23. (a) Diametre of wire,

$$d = \text{MSR} + \text{CSR} \times \text{LC}$$

$$= 0 + 52 \times \frac{1}{100} = 0.52 \text{ mm} = 0.052 \text{ cm}$$

24. (b) For a simple pendulum, KE is maximum at mean position and PE is maximum at extreme position. Therefore, curve (b) is correct.

25. (c) Given, length of pendulum, $l = 25.0$ cm. So, there is an uncertainty of 0.1 cm in measurement of length. Resolution of stop watch is 1s, so uncertainty in measurement of time is 1s.

Now using, $T = 2\pi\sqrt{\frac{l}{g}}$ or $g = \frac{4\pi^2 l}{T^2}$

We have, $\frac{\Delta g}{g} = \frac{\Delta l}{l} + \frac{2\Delta T}{T}$

$$\Rightarrow \frac{\Delta g}{g} \times 100\% = \left(\frac{\Delta l}{l} + \frac{2\Delta T}{T}\right) \times 100\%$$

Accuracy in measurement of g is

$$\frac{\Delta g}{g} \times 100\% = \left(\frac{01}{25} + \frac{2 \times 1}{50}\right) \times 100\%$$

$$= (0.004 + 0.04) \times 100\,\% = 4.40\%$$

26. (b) As, $ma = MA$ [principle of moments]

$$\Rightarrow m \times 25 = 20 \times 30$$

$$m = \frac{20 \times 30}{25} = 24 \text{ g}$$

27. (b) In equilibrium, $m \times PA = M \times PB$

$$\frac{PA}{PB} = \frac{M}{m} > 1$$

$$\therefore PA > PB$$

28. (b) Taking moments about the point O.

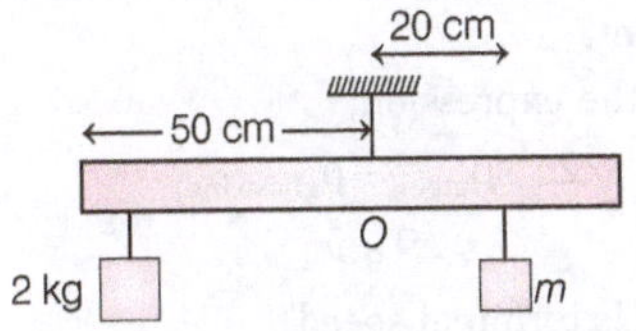

$$2g \times 0.5 = mg \times 0.2$$

$$\Rightarrow m = 5 \text{ kg}$$

29. (c) Taking torque about hanging point.

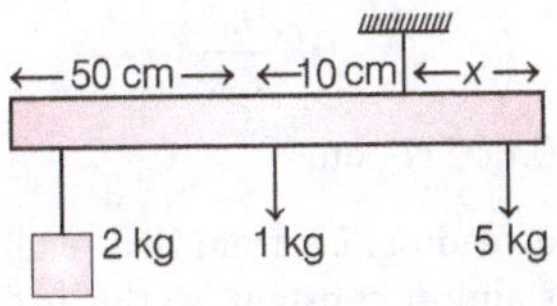

$$2g \times 60 + 1g \times 10 = mg \times x$$

$$\Rightarrow x = \frac{2 \times 60 + 1 \times 10}{5} = 26 \text{ cm}$$

30. (b) As, Young's modulus, $Y = \frac{F \cdot l}{A\Delta l} \Rightarrow \Delta l = \frac{F \cdot l}{YA}$

$$\Rightarrow \Delta l \propto \frac{1}{A}$$

$$\therefore \frac{\Delta l_A}{\Delta l_B} = \frac{A_B}{A_A}$$

As, $A_A > A_B \therefore \Delta l_B > \Delta l_A$

31. (a) Here, $AB = 1.009 - 1.006 = 0.003$ cm

and $CD = 1.009 - 1.004 = 0.005$ cm

$$\therefore d = \frac{AB + CD}{2} = \frac{0.008}{2} = 0.004 \text{ cm}$$

$$r = d/2 = 0.002 \text{ cm}$$

32. (a) For the liquid of meniscus, $2\pi r \times T \cos\theta = \pi r^2 h\rho g$

$$\Rightarrow T = \frac{rh\rho g}{2}$$

$$= \frac{0.015 \times 10^{-2} \times 15 \times 10^{-2} \times 1000 \times 9.81}{2}$$

$$= 0.11 \text{ Nm}^{-1}$$

33. (b) As, $T = \frac{r\left(h + \frac{r}{3}\right)\rho g}{2\cos\theta}$

$$= \frac{0.5 \times 10^{-2}\left(3 + \frac{0.5}{3}\right) \times 10^{-2} \times 10^3 \times 9.81}{2}$$

$$= 0.77 \text{ Nm}^{-1}$$

39. (a) $\Delta p = \frac{2T}{R}$

$$R = \frac{r}{\cos\theta} \Rightarrow \Delta p = \frac{2T}{r}\cos\theta$$

40. (c) The velocity of falling rain drop attain limiting value because viscous force exerted by air.

41. (b) For convex meniscus contact angle is greater 90°.

42. (a) $F_v = Mg - F_{\text{Th}}$

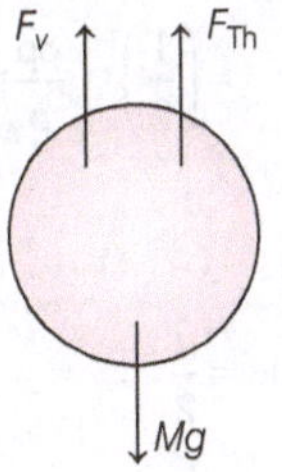

$$= Mg\left(1 - \frac{F_{\text{Th}}}{Mg}\right) = Mg\left(1 - \frac{D_2}{D_1}\right)$$

43. (d) $F_v = 6\pi\eta r v_T$

For same fluid and terminal velocity

$$F_v \propto r \Rightarrow \frac{F_{v_1}}{F_{v_2}} = \frac{1}{4}$$

44. (a) Final velocity is terminal velocity which is independent from h

$$v_T = \frac{2r^2}{9}\frac{(\rho - \sigma)}{\eta}g$$

45. (b) $v_r \propto r^2$

$$\therefore \frac{v'_T}{v_T} = \left(\frac{R}{r}\right)^2 \text{ or } v'_T = \left(\frac{R}{r}\right)^2 v_T \quad \text{...(i)}$$

when 2 droplets of radius r coalesce to form a big drop of radius R, then

$$\frac{4}{3}\pi R^3 = 2 \times \frac{4}{3}\pi r^3 \Rightarrow \frac{R}{r} = 2^{1/3} \quad \text{...(ii)}$$

From Eqs. (i) and (ii)

$v'_T = (2^{1/3})^2 \times 1 = 4^{1/3}$ cm/s

46. (b) $v_T \propto r^2 \Rightarrow \frac{v_{T_1}}{v_{T_2}} = \left(\frac{r_1}{r_2}\right)^2 = \left(\frac{3}{2}\right)^2 = 9:4$

47. (c) $v_T \propto R^2$ and $M \propto R^3 \Rightarrow v_T^2 \propto \frac{M^2}{R^2}$

48. (c) Rate of heat produced

$$\frac{dQ}{dt} = F_v \times v_T$$

$$= 6\,\pi\eta r v_T \times v_T$$

$$\therefore \frac{d\theta}{dt} \propto r v_T^2 \propto r^5 \quad \left(\text{as } v_T = \frac{2r^2}{9\eta}(\rho - \sigma)g\right)$$

49. (d)

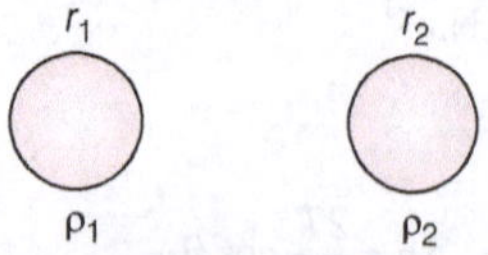

$$v_T = \frac{2r^2(\sigma - \rho)g}{9\eta}$$

$$\frac{v_1}{v_2} = \left(\frac{r_1}{r_2}\right)^2 \frac{(\sigma_1 - \rho)}{(\sigma_2 - \rho)}$$

$$= \left(\frac{1}{2}\right)^2 \left(\frac{8\rho_2 - 0.1\rho_2}{\rho_2 - 0.1\rho_2}\right) = \frac{79}{36}$$

50. (a) Mass $= M$

Density of ball $= d$

Density of glycerine $= \frac{d}{2}$

$$F_B = V_S \rho g = V\frac{d}{2}g$$

$$F_g = Mg = Vdg$$

For constant velocity, $F_{net} = 0$

$$\therefore F_B + F_v = Mg$$

$$F_v = Mg - F_B = Vdg - \frac{Vdg}{2} = \frac{Vdg}{2} = \frac{Mg}{2}$$

51. (c) Viscosity of liquid decreases with increase of temperature.

52. (a) $F = 6\pi\eta r v$

$$= 6 \times 3.14 \times 0.9 \times 5 \times 10^{-3} \times 10 \times 10^{-2}$$

$$= 847.8 \times 10^{-5}\text{ N}$$

$$= 8.48 \times 10^{-3}\text{ N}$$

53. (a) $v_T = \frac{2r^2}{9}\frac{(\rho - \sigma)}{\eta}g$

For same size and same liquid

$$v_T \propto \rho_b - \rho_l$$

$$\therefore \frac{(v_T)_{silver}}{(v_T)_{gold}} = \frac{\rho_{silver} - \rho_{liq}}{\rho_{gold} - \rho_{liq}}$$

$$\therefore (v_T)_{silver} = \left(\frac{10.5 - 1.5}{19.5 - 1.5}\right) \times 0.8 = 0.4\text{ m/s}$$

54. (d) $v_T = \frac{2r^2}{9}\frac{(\rho_B - \sigma_L)}{\eta}g, \; v_T \propto \frac{r^2 g}{\eta}$

but $m \propto r^3 \Rightarrow \frac{m}{r} \propto r^2 \Rightarrow v_T \propto \frac{mg}{\eta r}$

55. (b) $\frac{C}{5} = \frac{F - 32}{9} \Rightarrow C = \frac{5}{9}F - \frac{160}{9}$

Equating above equation with standard equation of line.

$y = mx + c$, we get slope of the line AB in $m = \frac{5}{9}$

56. (a) For lead shot, $v_T \propto r^2$

Hence, A will fall faster.

57. (b) As, water is having low viscosity, the terminal velocity will not be acquired by steel ball very soon, so to serve the purpose a very long jar of approximately 1000 m, is needed which is not suitable to perform the experiment.

58. (a) From the expression,

$$\eta = \frac{2r^2(\rho_{steel} - \rho_{glycerine})}{9 \times v} \times g$$

where, v is terminal speed.

Here, $v = \frac{0.2}{1.8}\text{ ms}^{-1}$

$$\therefore \eta = \frac{2 \times (0.25 \times 10^{-2})^2 \times (7.8 - 1.26) \times 10^3 \times 9.81}{9 \times \frac{0.2}{1.8}}$$

$$= 0.802\text{ N-sm}^{-2}$$

59. (c) After 2nd reading, *i.e.* from 3rd reading the velocity of the ball is almost constant, so this is the first correct reading which shows that terminal speed has been acquired by ball.

60. (c) $v = 2\nu(l_2 - l_1)$

$= 2 \times 480 \times \frac{(70-30)}{100}$ (Convert cm in m)

$= 2 \times 480 \frac{40}{100} = 384\ \text{ms}^{-1}$

61. (a) As, $\int_{1600}^{2500} P dt = mL_v$

where, P = power developed,

m = mass

and L_v = latent heat of vaporisation.

$\Rightarrow 10^3 \times 900 = 0.2 \times L_v$

($\because$ time duration is 1600 s to 2500 s)

$\Rightarrow L_v = 4.5 \times 10^6\ \text{Jkg}^{-1}$

62. (a)

Available heat	Required heat
50g water (80°C)	50g ice (0°C)
$ms\Delta\theta \downarrow$ = 4000 cal	$mL \downarrow$ = 4000 cal
50g water (0°C)	50g water (50°C)

Therefore, final temperature will be 0°C

Also all ice will melt and final amount of water = 50 + 50 = 100 g

63. (b) **Available heat**

10 g water at 50°C

$ms\Delta\theta \downarrow = 10 \times 1 \times 50 = 500$ cal

10 g water at 0°C

Required heat

10 g ice −20°C

$ms\Delta\theta \downarrow = 10 \times 0.5 \times 20 = 100$ cal

10 g water 0°C

$ms\Delta\theta \downarrow = 10 \times 80 = 800$ cal

10 g water 0°C

$\therefore$ Final temperature = 0°C

So, heat utilised to melt the ice is 400 cal

Mass of ice melted $= \frac{400}{80} = 5$ g

$\therefore$ Final amount of ice in mixture = 10 − 5 = 5 g

64. (c) **Available heat**

19 g water at 30°C

$ms\Delta\theta \downarrow = 19 \times 1 \times 30 = 570$ cal

19 g water at 0°C

Required heat

5 g ice at −20°C

$ms\Delta\theta \downarrow = 5 \times 0.5 \times 20 = 50$ cal

5 g ice at 0°C

$mL \downarrow = 5 \times 80 = 400$ cal

5 g water at 0°C

As available heat is more than required heat so, $\theta_f \neq 0°C$

$\Rightarrow \theta_f = \frac{\text{Excess heat}}{\text{total mass}} = \frac{570 - 450}{19 + 5} = \frac{120}{24} = 5°C$

65. (b) **Available heat**

5 g steam at 100°C

$mL \downarrow = 5 \times 540 = 2700$ cal

5 g water at 100°C

Required heat

6 g ice at 0°C

$mL \downarrow = 6 \times 80 = 480$ cal

6 g water at 0°C

$ms\Delta\theta \downarrow = 6 \times 1 \times 100 = 600$ cal

6 g water at 100°C

As available heat is more than required heat

So, final temperature = 100°C

66. (c) We know that, V-I curve for a linear device is a straight line passing through origin. Due to some errors/carelessness on the part of experiment all points may not come on the same line. In this situation, we draw the most appropriate curve.

From the diagram, $R = \frac{3}{3} = 1\,\Omega$.

67. (a) $R = \frac{\rho l}{A} = \frac{V}{I}$

$\rho = \frac{AV}{Il} = \frac{\pi d^2 V}{4Il}$ $\left(A = \frac{\pi d^2}{4}\right)$

$\therefore \frac{\Delta\rho}{\rho} = \frac{2\Delta d}{d} + \frac{\Delta V}{V} + \frac{\Delta I}{I} + \frac{\Delta l}{l}$

$\frac{\Delta\rho}{\rho} = 2\left(\frac{0.01}{5.00}\right) + \frac{0.1}{5.0} + \frac{0.01}{2.00} + \frac{0.1}{10.0}$

$\frac{\Delta\rho}{\rho} = 0.004 + 0.02 + 0.005 + 0.01$

$\frac{\Delta\rho}{\rho} = 0.039$

Percentage error $= \frac{\Delta\rho}{\rho} \times 100 = 0.039 \times 100 = 3.90\%$

68. (a) Wire of meter bridge should have high resistivity and low temperature coefficient.

69. (a) To reduces systematic error as well as random error.

70. (a) $R \propto l^2$

$\Rightarrow \frac{\Delta R}{R} = \frac{2\Delta l}{l} = 0.2\%$

71. (b) $i_1 = \frac{E}{R + G}$, $i_2 = \frac{E}{R + \frac{GS}{G+S}} = \frac{E(G+S)}{RG + RS + GS}$

$\frac{i_1}{2} G = \left(i_2 - \frac{i_1}{2}\right) S$

$$\frac{i}{2}(G+S)=\frac{E(G+S)}{RG+RS+GS}\cdot S$$

$$\frac{1}{2(R+G)}=\frac{S}{RG+RS+GS}$$

$$2RS+2SG=RG+RS+GS$$

$$RS+GS=RG$$

$$S(R+G)=RG$$

72. (a) $\lambda_a=\frac{c}{\nu}$ or $\lambda_m=\frac{v}{\nu}=\frac{c}{\mu_m\nu}$

$\therefore \lambda_1=\frac{c}{n_1\nu}$ and $\lambda_2=\frac{c}{n_2\nu}$ or $\lambda_1 n_1=\lambda_2 n_2$ and $\lambda_2=\lambda_1\frac{n_1}{n_2}$

73. (a) The negative refractive index or metamaterials are those in which incident ray from air (Medium 1) to them refract or bend differently to that of positive refractive index medium.

74. (a) $\delta_{min}=(\mu-1)A$

$=(1.5-1)44°=22°$

77. (c) Current changes by large amount when we change reverse bias voltage from 5 V to 5.5 V, so reverse breakdown voltage is some where there only and there after current increases even though no change in voltage occurs.

78. (b) The circuit used for working zener diode is shown. Once the diode attains the breakdown voltage, then there is no change in voltage across the diode even if we change the current in circuit by changing the position of rheostat and that is why the voltage across zener diode is constant.

79. (d) Write KVL equation, $-V_{BA}+IR+V_Z=0$

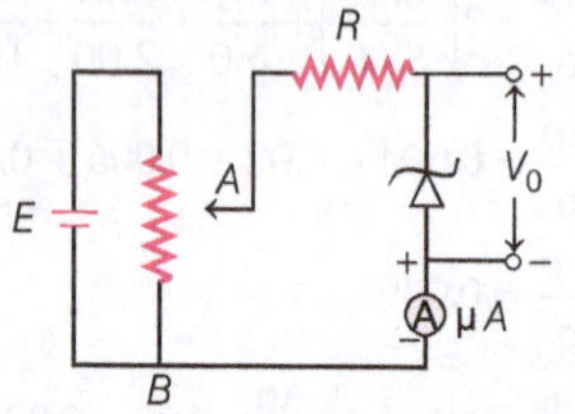

[As diode is operating in breakdown region]

$\Rightarrow \quad IR=V_{BA}-V_Z=8-7$

or, $\quad I=\frac{1\text{V}}{10\,\text{k}\Omega}=100\,\mu\text{A}$

80. (a) The forward voltage when current in circuit starts increasing abruptly, is the knee voltage.

Assertion and Reason

1. (b) A is true but R is false.

The purpose of connecting the high resistance in series with galvanometer is to protect the galvanometer from the high current. i.e., high current flow through the galvanometer damage its coil.

2. (c) A is false but R is true.

Laws of nature like law of conservation of energy do not change with time. So, experiment result does not change with time under identical conditions.

3. (d) By changing position of resistance box and unknown resistance and taking average of both values, end error can be minimised but it cannot be fully eradicated.

4. (c) In forward biasing electrons of n-side (from conduction band) combines with holes of p-side (in valance band).

So electrons move from higher energy levels to lower levels.

5. (d) Heavy doping results in a narrow depletion zone with high junction field and low breakdown voltages.

Statement Type Questions

1. (d) Both Statement I and Statement II are correct.

$$\text{Least count}=\frac{1\text{m}}{1000}=\frac{1000\text{ mm}}{1000}=1\text{ mm}$$

2. (d) Both Statement I and Statement II are correct.

In meter bridge, unknown resistance is function of length of metre bridge.

3. (b) Statement I is correct but Statement II is incorrect.

Charging current does not damage the coil of heater.

4. (d) Both Statement I and Statement II are correct.

Wire takes some time to acquire the actual extension.

According to Hooke's law

$$\text{Young's modulus of elasticity}=\frac{\text{Stress}}{\text{Strain}}$$

5. (d) Both Statement I and Statement II are correct.

$$\because \quad v=2f(l_2-l_1)$$

$$l_2-l_1=\frac{v}{2f}$$

If means lower frequency of tuning fork gives two resonance positions for relatively long length of air column.

So, large tube is required to obtain the two resonance positions.

6. (d) Both Statement I and Statement II are correct.

As per Ohm's law, $V=IR$, if voltage increases and resistance remains constant, current will increase.

7. (d) Both statement I and Statement II are correct.

$$\because \quad \frac{1}{f}=(\mu-1)\left(\frac{1}{R_1}-\frac{1}{R_2}\right)$$

and $\quad \mu\propto\frac{1}{\lambda}$

Match the Columns

1. (*b*) A-IV, B-I, C-III, D-II
2. (*a*) A-II, B-I, C-IV, D-III
3. (*a*) A-II, B-III, C-IV, D-I

Skil Builder

■ Sol. of Skill Builder on Pg. 814

(*a*) Here, 1 cm is divided in 20 equal parts.

$$\therefore \quad 1 \text{ MSD} = \frac{1}{20} \text{ cm}$$

Since, $10 \text{ VSD} = 9 \text{ MSD}$

$$\therefore \quad 1 \text{ VSD} = \frac{9}{10} \text{ MSD}$$

$$\text{Least Count} = 1 \text{ MSD} - 1 \text{ VSD}$$
$$= 1 \text{ MSD} - \frac{9}{10} \text{ MSD}$$
$$= \frac{1}{10} \text{ MSD}$$
$$= \frac{1}{10} \times \frac{1}{20}$$
$$= 5 \times 10^{-3} \text{cm}$$

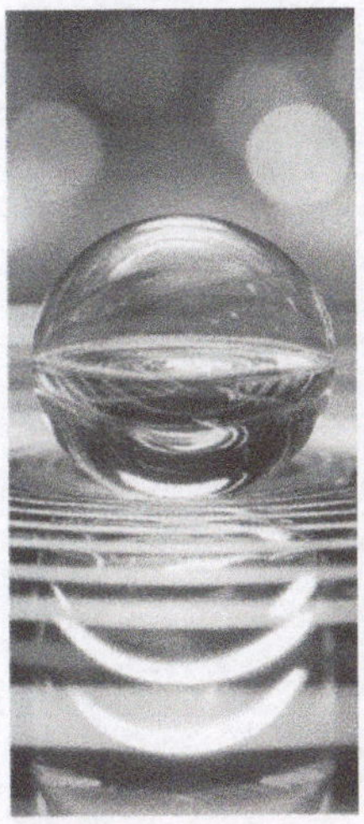

Practice Tests (1-3)

Class 12th (Syllabus Only)

Practice Test 01

Important Instructions

- The test of 1 hour duration and contains 50 Multiple Choice Questions (four options with a single correct answer) from Physics.
- There are 50 questions in each subject, divided into **two Sections** : Section A and Section B.
  (a) **Section A** contains 35 questions in each subject and all questions are compulsory.
  (b) **Section B** contains 15 questions from each subject out of which 10 questions are to be attempted.
- Each question carries 4 marks. For each correct response, the candidate will get 4 marks. For each incorrect response, one mark will be deducted from the total score.

Section-A (Q. No. 1 to 35)

1. An electron travels with velocity $\mathbf{v} = 60\,\hat{\mathbf{i}}$ m/s through a point in space, where $\mathbf{B} = 0.1\,\hat{\mathbf{j}}$ T. The force on the electron at this point is $\mathbf{F} = (9.6 \times 10^{-19}\,\hat{\mathbf{i}} - 9.6 \times 10^{-19}\hat{\mathbf{k}})$ N. The electric field $\mathbf{E}$ will be

(a) $-6\,\hat{\mathbf{i}}$ N/C (b) $(6\hat{\mathbf{i}} - 12\hat{\mathbf{k}})$ N/C
(c) $(-12\hat{\mathbf{i}} + 6\hat{\mathbf{k}})$ N/C (d) $(-6\hat{\mathbf{i}} - 6\hat{\mathbf{j}} + 6\hat{\mathbf{k}})$ N/C

2. In the circuit shown below, the diode has 20Ω forward bias resistance. When V_i increases from 8 V to 12 V, the change in the current will be

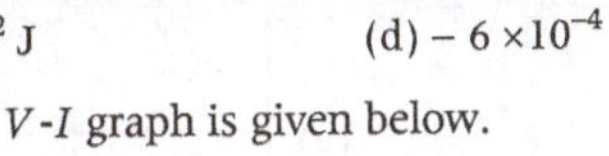

(a) 9 mA (b) 50 mA
(c) 47 mA (d) 40 mA

3. A short bar magnet of magnetic moment of 0.15 J/T is placed in a uniform magnetic field of 0.4 T. The potential energy of the magnet in unstable equilibrium is

(a) 6×10^{-4} J (b) -6×10^{-2} J
(c) 6×10^{-2} J (d) -6×10^{-4} J

4. For a cell, V-I graph is given below.

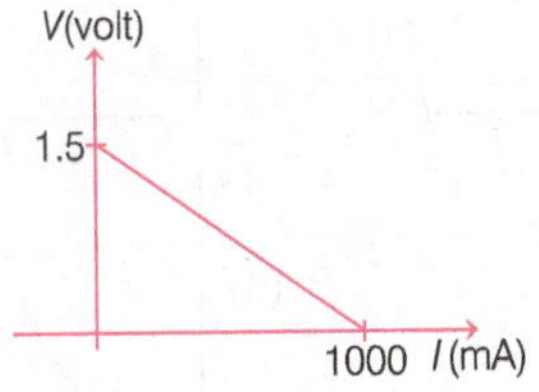

Which of the following options gives correct value of emf of cell and its internal resistance?

(a) 1.5 V, 1.0Ω (b) 1.5 V, 2.0Ω
(c) 1.0 V, 1.5Ω (d) 1.5 V, 1.5Ω

5. Two coaxial solenoids are made by winding thin insulated wire over a pipe of cross-sectional area $A = 10\,\text{cm}^2$ and length = 20 cm. If one of the solenoids has 500 turns and the other 300 turns, then their mutual inductance is ($\mu_0 = 4\pi \times 10^{-7}\,\text{TmA}^{-1}$)

(a) $2.4\pi \times 10^{-5}$H (b) $3.0\pi \times 10^{-4}$H
(c) $4.8\pi \times 10^{-5}$H (d) $2.4\pi \times 10^{-4}$H

6. Focal length of a convex lens of refractive index 1.5 is 20 cm. Focal length of the lens when immersed in a liquid of refractive index of 1.25 will be

(a) 8 cm (b) 25 cm (c) 75 cm (d) 50 cm

7. **Statement I** Infrared wave is absorbed by the ozone layer of the atmosphere.

Statement II During the propagation of EM waves in a medium, the electric energy density is equal to magnetic energy density.

In the light of the above statements, choose the most appropriate answer from the options given below.

(a) Both Statement I and Statement II are incorrect.
(b) Statement I is correct and Statement II is incorrect.
(c) Statement I is incorrect and Statement II is correct.
(d) Both Statement I and Statement II are correct.

8. A point charge $q = 6\mu$C is moving with velocity $\mathbf{v} = 5 \times 10^4\,\hat{\mathbf{i}}\,\text{ms}^{-1}$. Magnitude of magnetic field at origin (in T) when charge reaches at point P(3m, 4m, 0) will be

(a) $9.6 \times 10^{-1}\,\hat{\mathbf{k}}$ (b) $24 \times 10^{-8}\,\hat{\mathbf{k}}$
(c) $9.6 \times 10^{-10}\,\hat{\mathbf{j}}$ (d) zero

9. What should be the value of distance d, so that final image is formed on the object itself?

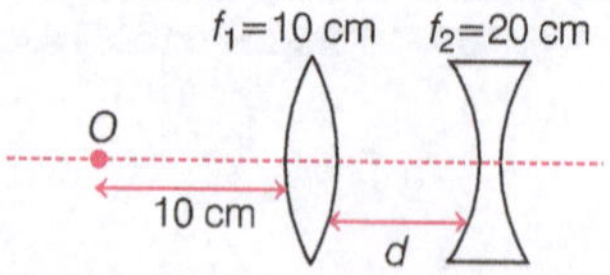

(a) 5 cm (b) 10 cm
(c) 20 cm (d) None of these

10. The ratio of minimum wavelengths of Balmer and Paschen series of hydrogen atom will be
(a) 1 : 4 (b) 4 : 9 (c) 9 : 4 (d) 4 : 1

11. If an electron in $n = 4$ orbit of hydrogen atom jumps down to $n = 3$ orbit, the amount of energy released and the wavelength of radiation emitted are
(a) 0.66 eV, 1.88×10^{-6} m (b) 1.89 eV, 1.98×10^{-7} m
(c) 0.29 eV, 1.78×10^{-5} m (d) 0.98 eV, 0.93×10^{-6} m

12. If the frequency of incident photon on metal surface is doubled, then stopping potential will become
(a) doubled (b) less than double
(c) more than double (d) less than existing value

13. In an L-R series circuit, resistance is R and inductive reactance $X_L = 3R$. When a capacitor is added in a circuit such that $X_C = 2R$.
The ratio of initial and final power factors of circuit is
(a) $\sqrt{3}$ (b) $\sqrt{5}$ (c) $1/\sqrt{3}$ (d) $\frac{1}{\sqrt{2}}$

14. Infinite long wire have a linear charge density of 0.2 C/m. Find the electric field intensity at a distance of 2 m from wire.
(a) 1.8×10^9 V/m (b) 0.9×10^9 V/m
(c) 27×10^9 V/m (d) 0.3×10^5 V/m

15. I. The total current i is the sum of the conduction current denoted by i_c and the displacement current denoted by $i_d = \varepsilon_0 \, (d\phi_E / dt)$.
II. Outside the capacitor plates, we have only conduction current $i_c = i$ and displacement current, $i_d \neq 0$.
III. Inside the capacitor, there is no conduction current, i.e. $i_c = 0$ and there is only displacement current, so that $i_d = i$.
Which of the above statement(s) is/are correct?
(a) Both I and III (b) Both II and III
(c) Both I and II (d) I, II and III

16. A 27 mW laser beam has an area of cross-section of 20 mm^2. Magnitude of maximum electric field in laser is (Take, $\varepsilon_0 = 9 \times 10^{-12}$ SI unit and $c = 3 \times 10^8$ m/s)
(a) 1 kV/m (b) 0.7 kV/m
(c) 2 kV/m (d) 1.4 kV/m

17. A source of 6.6 kW produces 10^{20} photons per second, then emitted wave
(a) radio wave is (b) microwave
(c) X-rays (d) infrared rays

18. A hydrogen atom emits a photon as its electron jumps from $n = 5$ to $n = 1$ state. Recoil speed of hydrogen atom will be
(a) 7.7 km/s (b) 2.19 km/s
(c) 3.5 km/s (d) 4.34 km/s

19. A measurement taken from an instrument having lower least count increases which of these?
(a) Accuracy of measurement
(b) Precision of measurement
(c) Significant digits in measurement
(d) Value of measured quantity

20. In an AC circuit, the instantaneous voltage and current are given by $V = 100\sin(100\pi t)$ V and $i = 20\cos\left(100\pi t - \frac{\pi}{6}\right)$ A. In one cycle of AC, the average power consumed by the circuit and wattless current are, respectively
(a) 500 W, $5\sqrt{6}$ A (b) $500\sqrt{3}$ W, $10\sqrt{2}$ A
(c) 1000 W, $5\sqrt{2}$ A (d) $1000\sqrt{3}$ W, 0 A

21. Which of the following is not a characteristic of diamagnetic materials?
(a) The diamagnetic materials are repelled by a magnetic field.
(b) Susceptibility of diamagnetic materials is inversely proportional to the absolute temperature.
(c) Magnetic susceptibility of diamagnetic material is small and negative.
(d) Diamagnetic material moves from a region of strong magnetic field to weak magnetic field.

22. A battery of emf 12 V and internal resistance 0.3Ω is connected across a variable resistance R. The value of R for which the power delivered in it is maximum
(a) 0.3Ω (b) 0.5Ω (c) 1.0Ω (d) 0.25Ω

23. An inductor 30 mH, a capacitor 50 μF and a resistance 60Ω are connected in series across a source of emf $V = 12\sin 314t$. The power loss in the circuit is,
(a) 0.8W (b) 1.1W (c) 1.5W (d) 0.6W

24. A straight wire carrying a current of 12 A is bent into a semi-circular loop of radius 2.0 cm. What will be magnetic field at the centre of the semi-circular loop?

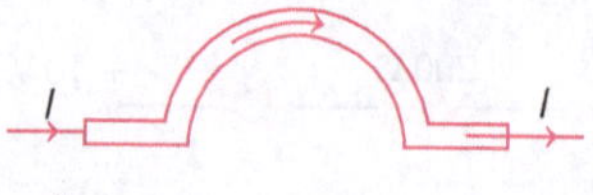

(a) $\mathbf{B} = 1.9 \times 10^{-4}$ T, ⊙ (b) $\mathbf{B} = 1.9 \times 10^{4}$ T, ⊙
(c) $\mathbf{B} = 1.9 \times 10^{-4}$ T, ⊗ (d) $\mathbf{B} = 1.9 \times 10^{4}$ T, ⊗

25. If an uncharged capacitor is being charged by a constant current, then which graph represents correct variation in change in voltage across the capacitor with time t?

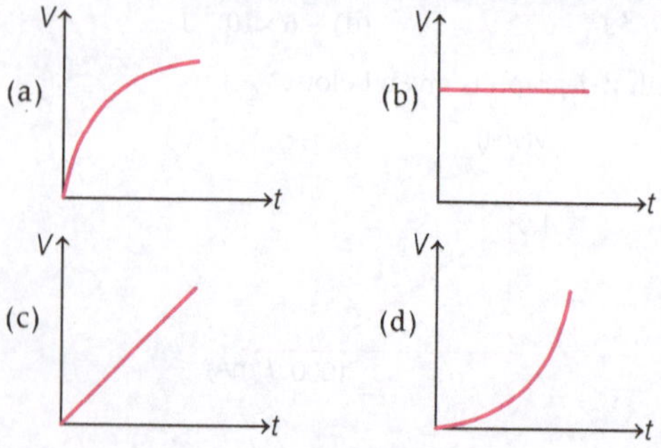

26. In an AC circuit, the current flowing is $I = 12\sin(100t - \pi/2)$ A and the potential difference is $V = 220\sin(100t)$ V. The power consumption is
(a) 1000 W (b) 400 W (c) 600 W (d) 0 W

27. A nucleus (mass number = 184) initially at rest emits an α-particle. Q-value of reaction is 5.5 MeV. Kinetic energy of emitted α-particle is
(a) 5 MeV (b) 5.5 MeV (c) 0.12 MeV (d) 5.38 MeV

28. A metal surface is illuminated with photons of energies $E_1 = 4$ eV and $E_2 = 2.5$ eV respectively. The ratio of maximum speeds of the photoelectrons in two cases is 2. Work function of metal surface will be
(a) 2.5 eV (b) 5 eV (c) 4 eV (d) 2 eV

29. **Assertion** (A) A pure semiconductor has negative temperature coefficient of resistance.

Reason (R) In a semiconductor on raising the temperature, more charge carriers are released, conductor conductance increases and resistance decreases.

In the light of the above statements, choose the most appropriate answer from the options given below.
(a) Both A and R are true and R is the correct explanation of A.
(b) Both A and R are true but R is not the correct explanation of A.
(c) A is true but R is false.
(d) A is false but R is also false.

30. I. Electric field, electric displacement and electric polarisation are related by the relation as $D = \varepsilon_0 E - P$.
II. Electric field vector **E**, electric displacement vector **D** and electric polarisation vector **P** are mutually perpendicular to each other.
III. Electric field vector **E**, electric displacement vector **D** and electric polarisation vector **P** are mutually parallel to each other.

Which of the following statement(s) is/are correct?
(a) Only I (b) Both II and III
(c) Both I and III (d) Only III

31. The electric field lines due to positive charge has been shown in the following figure. If a small negative charge is released at point B, then the difference of potential energy of negative charge between the points B and A is

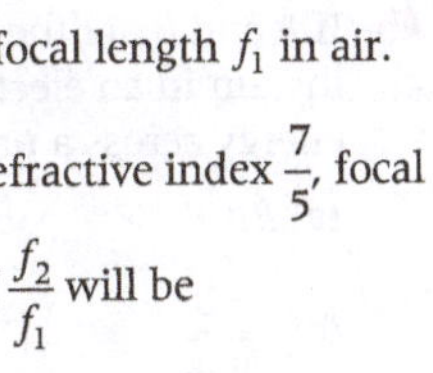

(a) positive (b) negative
(c) zero (d) either positive or negative

32. A thin lens made of glass $\left(n_g = \dfrac{3}{2}\right)$ of focal length f_1 in air. This lens when dipped in a liquid of refractive index $\dfrac{7}{5}$, focal length of lens will become f_2. Ratio of $\dfrac{f_2}{f_1}$ will be
(a) 1 (b) 5
(c) 7 (d) 9

33. A generator produces a voltage that is given by $V = 240\sin 120t$, where t is in seconds. The frequency and rms voltage are
(a) 60 Hz and 240 V (b) 19 Hz and 120 V
(c) 19 Hz and 170 V (d) 754 Hz and 70 V

34. Two non-ideal batteries are connected in parallel. Consider the following statements.

Statement I The equivalent emf is smaller than either of the two emf's.

Statement II The equivalent internal resistance is smaller than either of the two internal resistances.

In light of above statements choose the most appropriate answer from the options given below.
(a) Both Statement I and Statement II are incorrect.
(b) Statement I is correct but Statement II is incorrect.
(c) Statement I is incorrect but Statement II is correct.
(d) Both Statement I and Statement II are correct.

35. I. Dots and arrows indicates that both polarisations are present in the incident and refracted waves.
II. The reflected light is not linearly polarised.
III. Transmitted intensity will be zero when the axis of the analyser is in the plane of the figure, i.e. the plane of incidence.

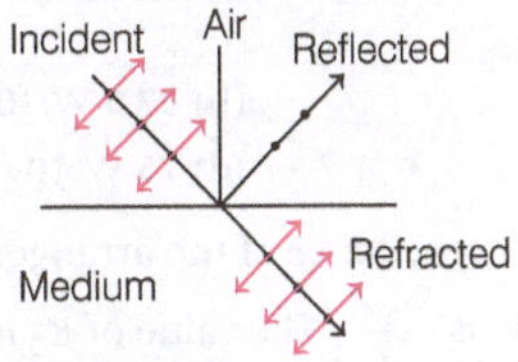

Which of the following statement(s) is/are correct with reference to the figure given?
(a) Only I (b) Only II
(c) Both I and III (d) Both I and II

Section-B (Q. No. 36 to 50)

36. Identify the correct output signal Y in the given combination of gates for the given inputs A and B shown in the figure.

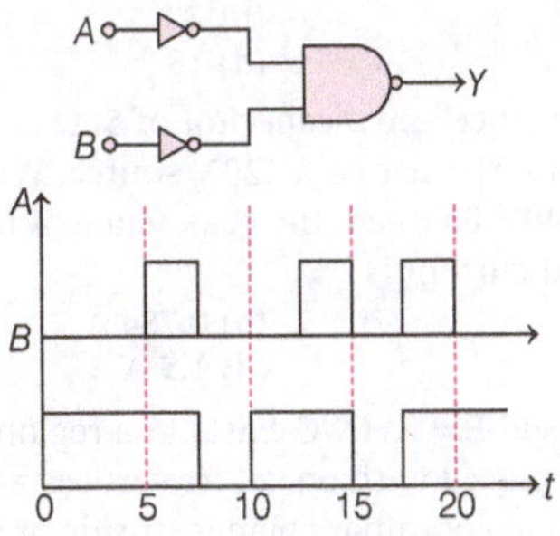

(a)

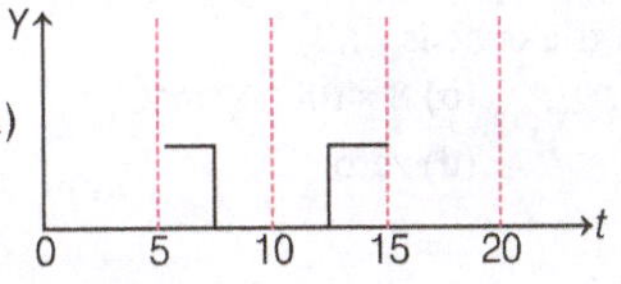

(b)

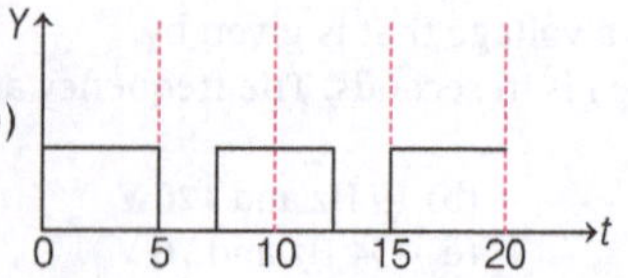

(c)

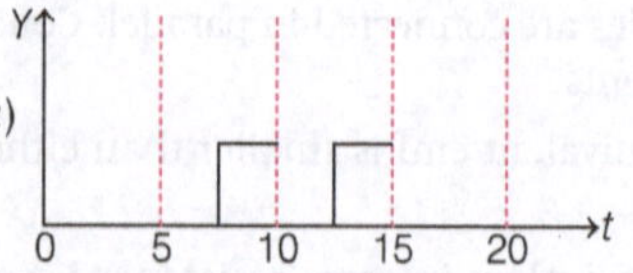

(d)

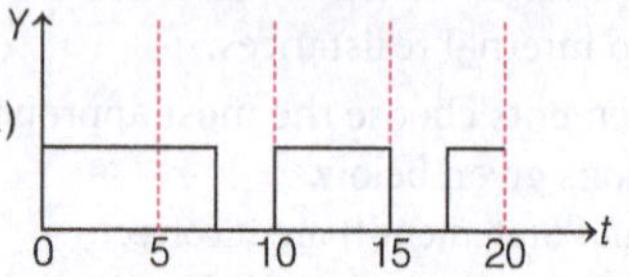

37. In YDSE, monochromatic light falls on a screen 1.80 m from two slits separated by 2.08 mm. The first and second order bright fringes are separated by 0.553 mm. The wavelength of light used is

(a) 520 nm (b) 639 nm (c) 715 nm (d) None of these

38. A resistance of $10\,\Omega$ draws power 150 W when connected to an AC source. If an inductor is now placed in series with the resistance, such that the impedance of the circuit becomes $20\,\Omega$, the power drawn and inductive reactance are respectively.

(a) 37.5 W, $10\,\Omega$ (b) 37.5 W, $10\sqrt{3}\,\Omega$

(c) 75 W, $10\,\Omega$ (d) 75 W, $10\sqrt{3}\,\Omega$

39. The equivalent capacitance of the arrangement shown in the figure below is $\frac{3\varepsilon_0 A}{d}$. The value of K_3 is

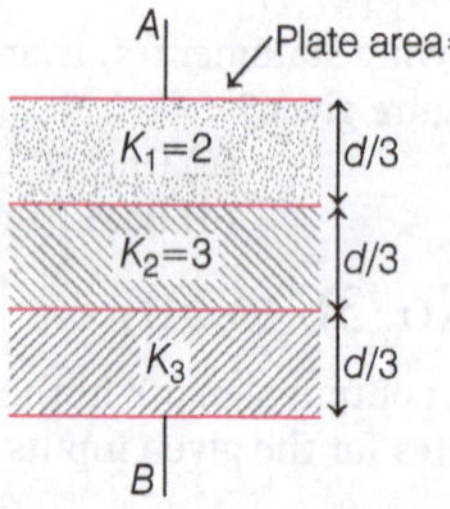

(a) 1 (b) 2

(c) 3 (d) 18

40. A $150\,\Omega$ resistance and a capacitor of 50Ω reactance are connected in series across a 220 V source. When the capacitor is 40% charged, the peak value of the displacement current is

(a) 2.2 A (b) 0.784 A

(c) $11\sqrt{2}$ A (d) 1.5 A

41. An electric field $\mathbf{E} = 2x\hat{\mathbf{i}}$ N/C exists in a region. A cubical metal box is placed with one of its vertices at origin and sides parallel to coordinate planes. If side of cube is 2 cm, then net flux through the cube is

(a) 4×10^{-2} Nm^{2}C^{-1} (b) 8×10^{-2} Nm^{2}C^{-1}

(c) 0.5×10^{-2} Nm^{2}C^{-1} (d) zero

42. A charge passing through a resistor is varying with time as shown in the figure. The amount of heat generated H in time t as a function of time is best represented by

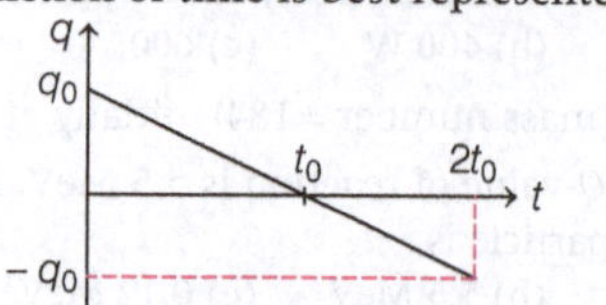

(a)

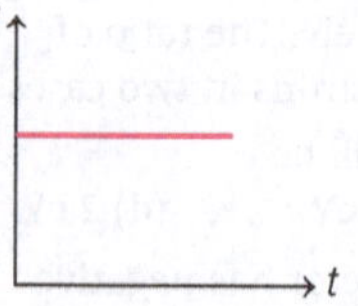

(b)

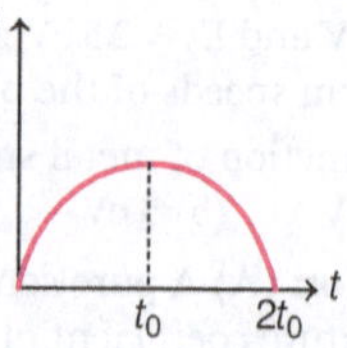

(c)

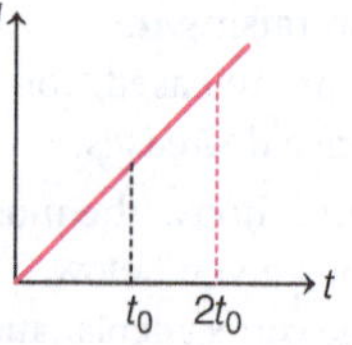

(d)

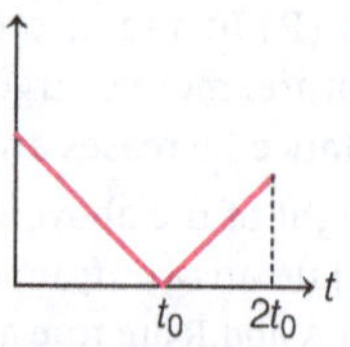

43. An electric dipole with dipole moment $\mathbf{p} = (3\hat{\mathbf{i}} + 4\hat{\mathbf{j}})\times10^{-30}$ C-m is placed in an electric field $\mathbf{E} = 4000\,\hat{\mathbf{i}}$ N/C. The dipole is rotated very slowly until its electric dipole moment becomes $(-4\,\hat{\mathbf{i}} + 3\hat{\mathbf{j}})\times10^{-30}$ C-m. The work done by external torque is equal to

(a) -4×10^{-28} J (b) 4×10^{-28} J

(c) 2.8×10^{-26} J (d) -2.8×10^{-26} J

44. In the circuit shown in the adjoining figure, the current between B and D is zero, the unknown resistance is of

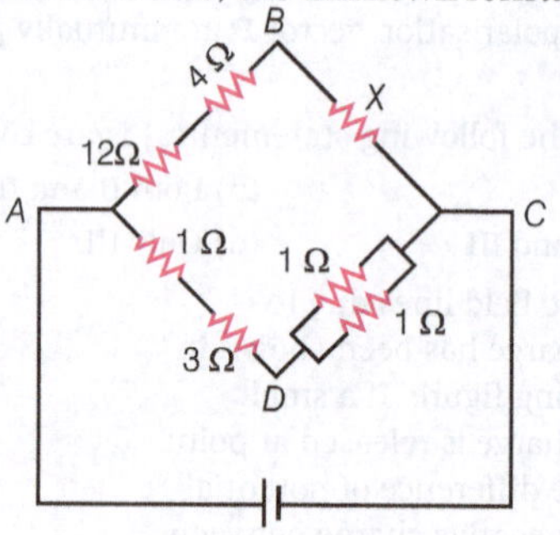

(a) 4Ω

(b) 2Ω

(c) 3Ω

(d) emf of a cell is required to find the value of X

45. If E and B are the electric field and magnetic field at any instant in an electromagnetic wave, then rate of flow of energy across a unit area at any instant is given as

(a) EB (b) $\frac{EB}{\mu_0}$

(c) $\frac{EB}{\sqrt{\mu_0\varepsilon_0}}$ (d) $\frac{EB}{c^2}$

46. The minimum radial distance between first orbit and second orbit in He^+ ion, if the de-Broglie wavelength of an electron in first orbit is λ, will be

(a) 2λ (b) $\frac{2\lambda}{\pi}$ (c) $\frac{\lambda}{2\pi}$ (d) $\frac{\lambda}{4\pi}$

47. A charge q is enclosed by an imaginary Gaussian surface. If the radius of Gaussian surface is increasing at a rate $\frac{dr}{dt} = \alpha$, then flux linked with surface is

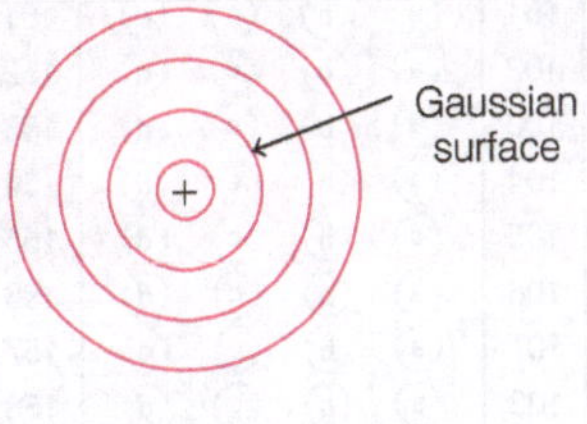

(a) increasing at a rate, $\frac{d\phi}{dt} = \alpha$

(b) decreasing at a rate, $\frac{d\phi}{dt} = -\alpha$

(c) decreasing at a rate, $\frac{d\phi}{dt} = \frac{1}{k}$

(d) $\frac{q}{\varepsilon_0}$

48. Two light waves having same wavelength of 550 nm are travelling through vacuum are in phase initially.

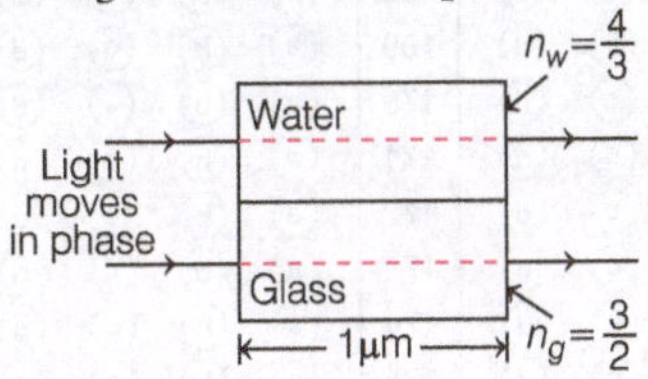

They pass through 1 μm blocks of water and glass, respectively as shown above. Phase difference between waves as they emerge out is

(a) 0.4 π rad

(b) 0.5 π rad

(c) 0.7 π rad

(d) 0.6 π rad

49. A germanium crystal is doped with arsenic atoms and indium atoms simultaneously. Number of arsenic atoms used $= 5 \times 10^{22}$ per m^3 and number of indium atoms used $= 5 \times 10^{20}$ per m^3, then resulting crystal is a/an

(a) *p-n* junction

(b) *p*-type semiconductor

(c) *n*-type semiconductor

(d) Depends on number of germanium atoms in given sample.

50. A thin equiconvex lens of glass has radii of curvature of each surface 30 cm. The lens has different medium on its left and right side of refractive indices 1.2 and 1.6, respectively. If the refractive index of the glass is 1.5, then focal length of this lens for parallel beam incident from left is

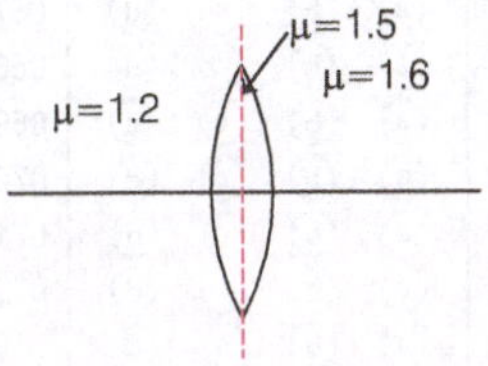

(a) 30 cm (b) 60 cm (c) 120 cm (d) 240 cm

Answer key

Section A

1 (a)	2 (a)	3 (c)	4 (d)	5 (b)	6 (a)	7 (c)	8 (b)	9 (b)	10 (b)
11 (a)	12 (c)	13 (d)	14 (a)	15 (a)	16 (a)	17 (c)	18 (a)	19 (b)	20 (a)
21 (b)	22 (a)	23 (b)	24 (a)	25 (c)	26 (d)	27 (d)	28 (d)	29 (a)	30 (d)
31 (a)	32 (c)	33 (c)	34 (d)	35 (c)					

Section B

36 (d)	37 (b)	38 (b)	39 (b)	40 (b)	41 (d)	42 (c)	43 (c)	44 (b)	45 (b)
46 (c)	47 (d)	48 (d)	49 (c)	50 (d)					

Scan this QR Code for Detailed Solutions

ANSWER SHEET

Instructions for filling the sheet
1. Use only blue/ black ball pen to fill the circle.
2. Use of pencil is strictly prohibited.
3. Circle should be darkened completely and properly.

SECTION-A Attempt all 35 Questions in each subject

Q.No	Response	Q.No	Response	Q.No	Response	Q.No	Response
001	a b c d	051	a b c d	101	a b c d	151	a b c d
002	a b c d	052	a b c d	102	a b c d	152	a b c d
003	a b c d	053	a b c d	103	a b c d	153	a b c d
004	a b c d	054	a b c d	104	a b c d	154	a b c d
005	a b c d	055	a b c d	105	a b c d	155	a b c d
006	a b c d	056	a b c d	106	a b c d	156	a b c d
007	a b c d	057	a b c d	107	a b c d	157	a b c d
008	a b c d	058	a b c d	108	a b c d	158	a b c d
009	a b c d	059	a b c d	109	a b c d	159	a b c d
010	a b c d	060	a b c d	110	a b c d	160	a b c d
011	a b c d	061	a b c d	111	a b c d	161	a b c d
012	a b c d	062	a b c d	112	a b c d	162	a b c d
013	a b c d	063	a b c d	113	a b c d	163	a b c d
014	a b c d	064	a b c d	114	a b c d	164	a b c d
015	a b c d	065	a b c d	115	a b c d	165	a b c d
016	a b c d	066	a b c d	116	a b c d	166	a b c d
017	a b c d	067	a b c d	117	a b c d	167	a b c d
018	a b c d	068	a b c d	118	a b c d	168	a b c d
019	a b c d	069	a b c d	119	a b c d	169	a b c d
020	a b c d	070	a b c d	120	a b c d	170	a b c d
021	a b c d	071	a b c d	121	a b c d	171	a b c d
022	a b c d	072	a b c d	122	a b c d	172	a b c d
023	a b c d	073	a b c d	123	a b c d	173	a b c d
024	a b c d	074	a b c d	124	a b c d	174	a b c d
025	a b c d	075	a b c d	125	a b c d	175	a b c d
026	a b c d	076	a b c d	126	a b c d	176	a b c d
027	a b c d	077	a b c d	127	a b c d	177	a b c d
028	a b c d	078	a b c d	128	a b c d	178	a b c d
029	a b c d	079	a b c d	129	a b c d	179	a b c d
030	a b c d	080	a b c d	130	a b c d	180	a b c d
031	a b c d	081	a b c d	131	a b c d	181	a b c d
032	a b c d	082	a b c d	132	a b c d	182	a b c d
033	a b c d	083	a b c d	133	a b c d	183	a b c d
034	a b c d	084	a b c d	134	a b c d	184	a b c d
035	a b c d	085	a b c d	135	a b c d	185	a b c d

SECTION-B Attempt any 10 Questions in each subject

Q.No	Response	Q.No	Response	Q.No	Response	Q.No	Response
036	a b c d	086	a b c d	136	a b c d	186	a b c d
037	a b c d	087	a b c d	137	a b c d	187	a b c d
038	a b c d	088	a b c d	138	a b c d	188	a b c d
039	a b c d	089	a b c d	139	a b c d	189	a b c d
040	a b c d	090	a b c d	140	a b c d	190	a b c d
041	a b c d	091	a b c d	141	a b c d	191	a b c d
042	a b c d	092	a b c d	142	a b c d	192	a b c d
043	a b c d	093	a b c d	143	a b c d	193	a b c d
044	a b c d	094	a b c d	144	a b c d	194	a b c d
045	a b c d	095	a b c d	145	a b c d	195	a b c d
046	a b c d	096	a b c d	146	a b c d	196	a b c d
047	a b c d	097	a b c d	147	a b c d	197	a b c d
048	a b c d	098	a b c d	148	a b c d	198	a b c d
049	a b c d	099	a b c d	149	a b c d	199	a b c d
050	a b c d	100	a b c d	150	a b c d	200	a b c d

Complete Syllabus (11th & 12th)

Practice Test 02

Important Instructions

- The test of 1 hour duration and contains 50 Multiple Choice Questions (four options with a single correct answer) from Physics.
- There are 50 questions in each subject, divided into **two Sections** : Section A and Section B.
  (a) **Section A** contains 35 questions in each subject and all questions are compulsory.
  (b) **Section B** contains 15 questions from each subject out of which 10 questions are to be attempted.
- Each question carries 4 marks. For each correct response, the candidate will get 4 marks. For each incorrect response, one mark will be deducted from the total score.

Section-A (Q. No. 1 to 35)

1. A uniform rod of mass 1.5 kg is hanged with one end attached to ceiling. The rod is 60 cm long and have 100 cm^2 area of cross-section. If the Young's modulus of the rod is $1.2 \times 10^{11} N/m^2$, then elongation of the rod due to its weight is
(a) 3.67×10^{-9}m (b) 7.35×10^{-11} m
(c) 1.47×10^{-10}m (d) 7.35×10^{-9}m

2. A pipe, 30 cm long is open at both ends, harmonic mode of the pipe which resonates at 1.65 kHz source is (speed of sound is 330 ms^{-1})
(a) third (b) fourth
(c) first (d) second

3. Two persons *A* and *B* perform same amount of work in moving a body through same distance *d* with application of forces acting at angles 45° and 60°, respectively with the direction of displacement. The ratio of force applied by person *A* to the force applied by person *B* is
(a) 1 : 1 (b) $1 : \sqrt{2}$
(c) $\sqrt{2} : 1$ (d) $\sqrt{3} : 2$

4. Consider the situation shown below.

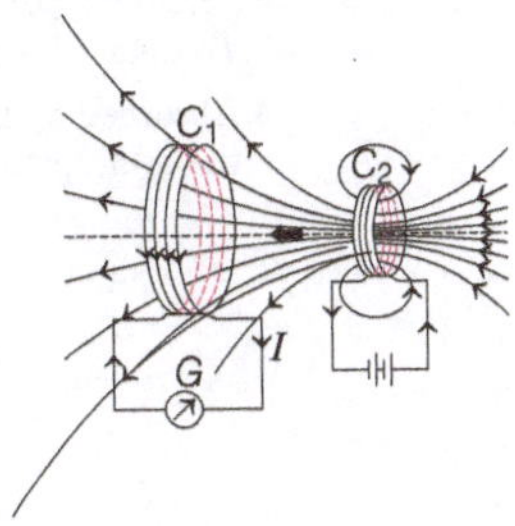

I. Because of change in current in C_2, emf is induced in C_1.
II. The steady current in the coil C_2 produces a steady magnetic field.
III. If coil C_2 is moved towards the coil C_1, the galvanometer shows a deflection. This indicates that electric current is induced in coil C_1.
Which of the above statements are correct for the figure shown?
(a) Only I
(b) Both II and III
(c) Both I and III
(d) I, II and III

5. Force acting on a particle is 5 N. If unit of length and time are doubled and unit of mass is halved, then the numerical value of the force in the new unit will be
(a) 4 times (b) 2 times
(c) 1/4 times (d) 1/2 times

6. The points *A* and *B* are situated perpendicular to the axis of 2 cm long bar magnet at large distances *x* and 3 *x* from the centre on opposite sides. The ratio of magnetic fields at *A* and *B* will be approximately equal to
(a) 27 : 1 (b) 1 : 27
(c) 9 : 1 (d) 1 : 9

7. **Assertion** (A) Photosensitivity of metal is high, if its work function is small.
Reason (R) Work function = hf_0, where f_0 is the threshold frequency.
In the light of above statements, choose the most appropriate answer from the options given below.

(a) Both A and R are true and R is the correct explanation of A.
(b) Both A and R are true but R is not the correct explanation of A.
(c) A is true but R is false.
(d) A is false but R is true.

8. **Statement I** The resistance of *p-n* junction diode decreases when forward biased and increases when reverse biased.

Statement II In forward biased, the potential barrier is supported by the battery and in reverse biased, potential barrier is opposed by battery.

In light of above statements, choose the most appropriate answer from the options given below.
(a) Both Statement I and Statement II are incorrect.
(b) Statement I is correct and Statement II is incorrect.
(c) Statement I is incorrect and Statement II is correct.
(d) Both Statement I and Statement II are correct.

9. The heat given to a body to raise its temperature is given by $Q = ms\Delta\theta$, where Q = heat given, m = mass of body, s = specific heat and $\Delta\theta$ = change in temperature.
The dimensional formula of specific heat is
(a) $[M^1L^2T^{-2}K^{-1}]$ (b) $[M^0L^2T^{-2}K^0]$
(c) $[M^0L^1T^{-2}K^{-2}]$ (d) $[M^0L^2T^{-2}K^{-1}]$

10. The displacement-time graph of a moving particle is shown below.

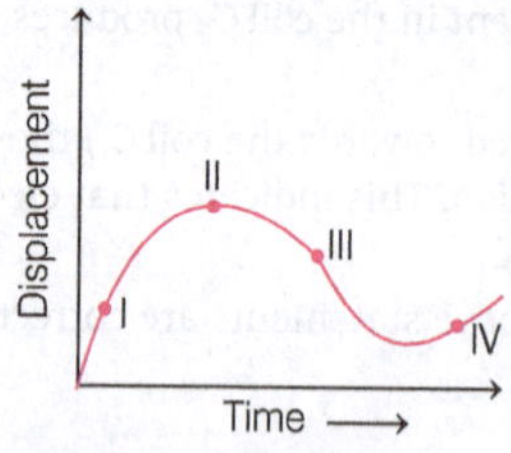

The instantaneous velocity of the particle is negative at the point
(a) IV (b) I (c) II (d) III

11. The straight wire *AB* carries a current *I*. The ends of the wire subtend angles θ_1 and θ_2 at the point *P* as shown in figure. The magnetic field at the point *P* is

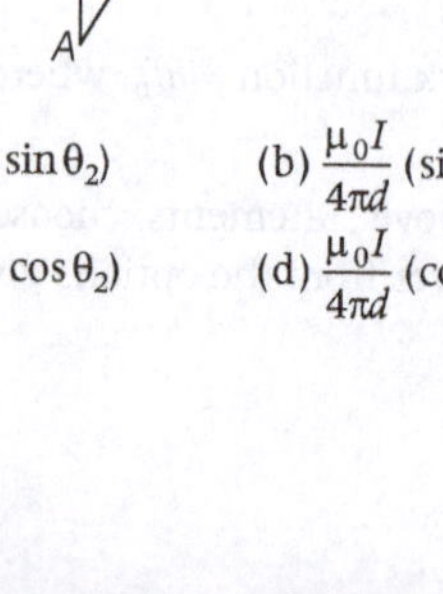

(a) $\frac{\mu_0 I}{4\pi d}(\sin\theta_1 - \sin\theta_2)$ (b) $\frac{\mu_0 I}{4\pi d}(\sin\theta_1 + \sin\theta_2)$
(c) $\frac{\mu_0 I}{4\pi d}(\cos\theta_1 - \cos\theta_2)$ (d) $\frac{\mu_0 I}{4\pi d}(\cos\theta_1 + \cos\theta_2)$

12. A mass of 50 kg is placed at the centre of uniform spherical shell of mass 100 kg and radius 50 m. The gravitational potential at a point 25 m from the centre will be
(a) $4G$ J/kg (b) $-4G$ J/kg
(c) $3G$ J/kg (d) $-5G$ J/kg

13. A particle is moving along the curved path with acceleration $-5\hat{j}$ m/s^2. At an instant, its velocity is $(8\hat{i} - 6\hat{j})$ m/s^2. The tangential acceleration vector at this instant is given by
(a) $(24\hat{i} - 18\hat{j})$ m/s^2 (b) $(26\hat{i} + 18\hat{j})$ m/s^2
(c) $(-24\hat{i} + 18\hat{j})$ m/s^2 (d) $(-26\hat{i} - 18\hat{j})$ m/s^2

14. A series *R-L-C* circuit is subjected to an AC source of voltage 220 V and 50 Hz frequency. The circuit contains a resistor $R = 10\ k\Omega$, an inductor of inductance 2.5 H and an unknown capacitor. What value of capacitance should be taken, so that power consumption in circuit can be maximum?
(a) 4 μF (b) 40 μF (c) 25μF (d) 400 μF

15. A 5.80 μF parallel plate air capacitor has a plate separation of 5 mm and is charged to a potential difference of 400 V. The energy density in the region between the plates is
(a) 2.83×10^{-2} J/m^3 (b) 2.83 J/m^3
(c) 2.83×10^{-4} J/m^3 (d) 2.83×10^{6} J/m^3

16. The volume occupied by the molecules contained in 3.6 kg water at STP, if the intermolecular force vanish away is
(a) 2.8 m^3 (b) 8.3 m^3
(c) 5.44 m^3 (d) 6.0 m^3

17. In photoelectric experiment, a light of wavelength 480 nm is incident on a metal surface of work function 1.67 eV, then photoelectrons are emitted. A fastest photoelectron combines with an excited He^{+2} ion in its third excited state to form He^{+} ion. What is energy of photon emitted by de-excitation of He^{+} ion?
(a) 4.5 eV (b) 4.3 eV
(c) 6.9 eV (d) 0.9 eV

18. A sphere encloses an electric dipole with charges $\pm 2.5 \times 10^{-6}$C. What is the total electric flux across the sphere?
(a) 6×10^{-5} Nm^2/C (b) -2.5×10^{-6} Nm^2/C
(c) 0 (d) 2.5×10^{-6} Nm^2/C

19. Match List I (Electromagnetic wave type) with List II (its association/application).

	List I	List II
A.	Infrared waves	1. To treat muscular strain
B.	Radiowaves	2. For broadcasting
C.	X-rays	3. To detect fracture of bones
D.	Ultraviolet	4. Absorbed by the ozone layer of the atmosphere

Codes

	A	B	C	D
(a)	4	3	2	1
(b)	1	2	4	3
(c)	3	2	1	4
(d)	1	2	3	4

20. The displacement time equations of two particles A and B executing SHM are given as

$$x_A = 4\sin\left(\omega t + \frac{\pi}{4}\right) + 3\cos\left(\omega t - \frac{\pi}{4}\right) \text{ m}$$

$$x_B = 5\sqrt{2}(\sin 2\pi t + \cos 2\pi t) \text{ m}$$

The ratio of amplitudes of particles A and B is

(a) 1 (b) $\frac{1}{2}$

(c) $\frac{1}{\sqrt{3}}$ (d) $\frac{7}{10}$

21. Consider arrangement given below

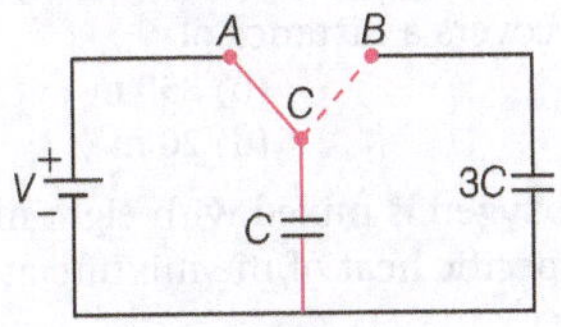

When C and A are in contact, charge on capacitor of capacity C is q. Energy dissipated when C is connected to B will be

(a) $\frac{3}{4}\frac{q^2}{C}$ (b) $\frac{5}{8}\frac{q^2}{C}$ (c) $\frac{1}{8}\frac{q^2}{C}$ (d) $\frac{3}{8}\frac{q^2}{C}$

22. **Statement I** The net work done by a conservative force on an object moving along a close loop is always non-zero.

Statement II For a charged particle moving from point P to point Q, the net work done by electric field on the particle is independent of path.

In the light of above statements, choose the most appropriate answer from the options given below.

(a) Both Statement I and Statement II are incorrect.

(b) Statement I is correct and Statement II is incorrect.

(c) Statement I is incorrect and Statement II is correct.

(d) Both Statement I and Statement II are correct.

23. Magnetic field in a region is changing at a constant rate. As a result, an induced electric field appears in the region which give rise to an emf. Induced electric field lines are

(a) open curves

(b) closed loops

(c) can be open or closed depending on magnetic field

(d) no field lines are produced

24. In context of diamagnetic material, the correct graphs for intensity of magnetisation *versus* magnetic field strength and susceptibility *versus* temperature are

(a) 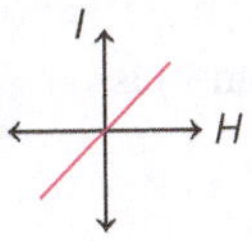

(b) 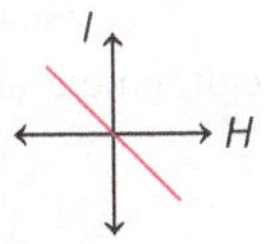

(c) 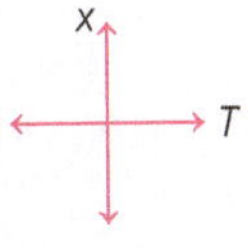

(d) 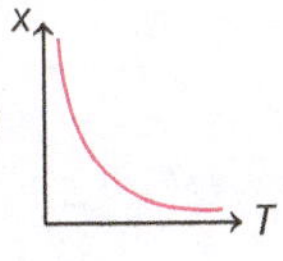

25. In a He^+ ion, if potential energy of electron in ground state is assumed to be zero, then its energy in first excited state is equal to

(a) 13.6 eV (b) 27.2 eV

(c) 54.4 eV (d) 95.2 eV

26. An unknown resistance R is connected to left gap of a meter bridge and another unknown resistance S is connected to right gap, such that the balance point from left end is at 30 cm. If a resistance of $2\,\Omega$ is connected in parallel with S, the null point occurs at 40 cm. The value of S is

(a) $1.1\,\Omega$ (b) 2Ω (c) 3.2Ω (d) 4Ω

27. I. The resistance R of a conductor depends on its length l and cross-sectional area A through the relation $R = \frac{\rho A}{l}$.

II. Metals have low resistivity in the range of $10^{-8}\,\Omega$-m to $10^{-6}\Omega$-m.

III. In most substances, the carriers of current are electrons, while in some cases,e.g. in ionic crystals and electrolytic liquids, positive and negative ions.

Which of the following statement(s) is/are correct?

(a) Only I (b) Both II and III

(c) Both I and II (d) Both I and III

28. A particle is projected with initial speed of 30 m/s making an angle 60° with horizontal. The velocity of particle when its velocity makes angle of 30° with horizontal is

(a) 10 m/s

(b) $10\sqrt{2}$ m/s

(c) $10\sqrt{3}$ m/s

(d) 20 m/s

29. Which of the following transitions of He^+ ion will give rise to spectral line which has same wavelength as the spectral line in hydrogen atom?

(a) $n = 4$ to $n = 2$

(b) $n = 6$ to $n = 5$

(c) $n = 6$ to $n = 3$

(d) None of the above

30. A 0.124 m long pencil is oriented perpendicular to the principal axis of a concave spherical mirror that has a radius of curvature of 0.3 m. If the pencil is 0.018 m from the mirror, then height of image is

(a) 2.13 cm (b) 16.5 cm

(c) 9.3 cm (d) 1.6 cm

31. Inside a solenoid of radius 0.5 m, magnetic field is changing at a rate of 50×10^{-6} T/s. Acceleration of an electron placed at a distance of 0.3 m from axis of solenoid will be

(a) 23×10^6 ms^{-2} (b) 2.6×10^6 m/s^2

(c) 1.3×10^9 ms^{-2} (d) 2.6×10^9 m/s^2

32. A particle is executing SHM on a straight line starting from its mean position. It passes through the mean position at successive intervals 1.5 s and 3 s with a speed of 1.57 m/s. The amplitude of the motion is

(a) 0.5 m (b) 0.75 m

(c) 1 m (d) 1.5 m

33. A rectangular block of glass is placed on a printed page lying on a horizontal surface. The minimum value of the refractive index of glass for which the letters on the page are not visible from any of the vertical faces of the block is

(a) 2 (b) $\sqrt{3}$ (c) $\sqrt{2}$ (d) 4/3

34. Two diodes of silicon and germanium are connected in series as shown below. The current flowing through the circuit will be around

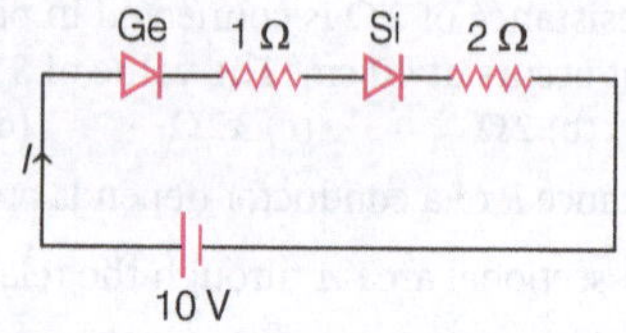

(a) 0 (b) 3 A
(c) 4 A (d) 3.5 A

35. A car turns on a banked road of radius 300 m. If the coefficient of friction between the tyres and the road is 0.3, then maximum speed of the car on the turn is (Take, $g = 10 \text{ m/s}^2$)

(a) 10 m/s (b) 30 m/s
(c) 40 m/s (d) 50 m/s

Section-B (Q. No. 36 to 50)

36. The graph between angle of deviation δ and angle of incidence i for a triangular prism is represented by

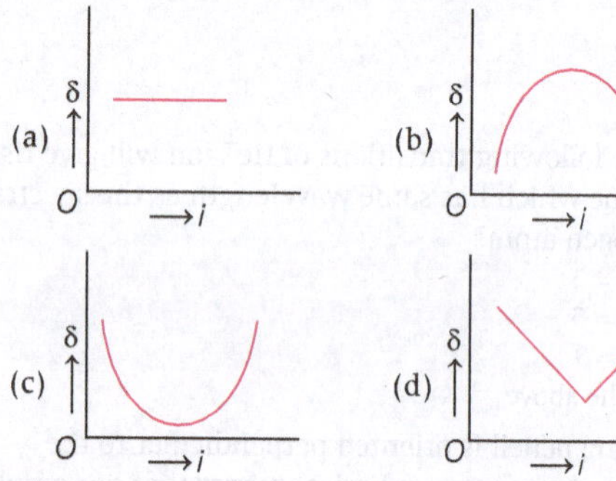

37. Side of a cube measured using a vernier caliper is $L = (30.0 \pm 0.1)$ mm. Percentage uncertainty in volume is about

(a) 0.1% (b) 0.3%
(c) 1% (d) 3%

38. A system consisting of two masses connected by a massless rod lies along the X-axis. A 0.4 kg mass is at a distance $x = 2$ m while a 0.6 kg mass is at a distance $x = 7$ m. The x-coordinate of the centre of mass is

(a) 5 m (b) 3.5 m
(c) 4.5 m (d) 4 m

39. In the following circuit diagram, potential difference across 4 μF capacitor is

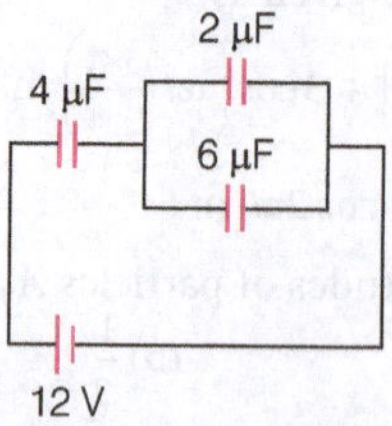

(a) 19 V (b) 14 V
(c) 16 V (d) 8 V

40. If a car at rest accelerates uniformly to a speed of 72 km/h in 25s, then it covers a distance of

(a) 450 m (b) 250 m
(c) 800 m (d) 20 m

41. Two moles of oxygen is mixed with eight mole of helium. The effective specific heat of the mixture at constant volume will be

(a) 2.5 R (b) 1.7 R
(c) 1.4 R (d) 1.8 R

42. A rectangular film of liquid is extended from 4 cm × 2 cm to 5 cm × 4 cm. If the work done is 6×10^{-4} J, then the value of the surface tension of the liquid is

(a) 0.25 N/m (b) 0.50 N/m
(c) 0.75 N/m (d) 1.25 N/m

43. A conducting wire is stretched by applying a deforming force, so that its diameter decreases to 40% of original value. The percentage change in its resistance will be

(a) 0.9% (b) 0.12%
(c) 1.6% (d) 0.5%

44. In Young's double slit experiment, if the distance between the slits and screen is increased to double and distance between the slits is decreased to half, then fringe width is

(a) increased to four times
(b) decreased to one-third
(c) decreased to half
(d) decreased to one-fourth

45.

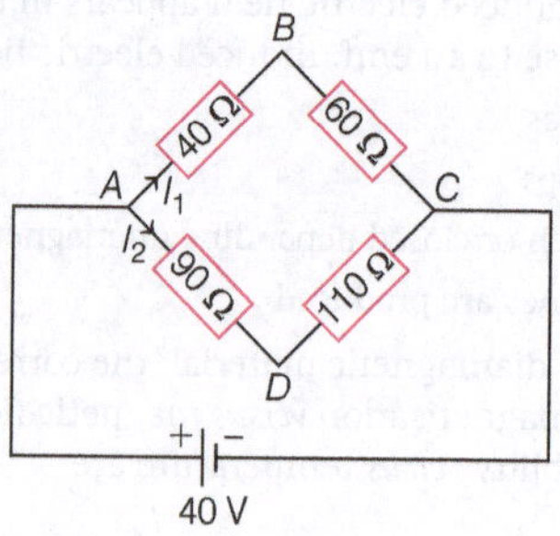

In above circuit, potential drop $V_B - V_D$ (in V) is

(a) 0 (b) 2
(c) 3 (d) 4

46. I. The reflected ray goes through the focus of the mirror, when it is incident parallel to the principal axis.

II. The reflected ray is perpendicular to the principal axis when incident ray passes through the focus of the concave mirror or appear to pass through the focus of a convex mirror.

III. For the ray incident at any angle at the pole, the reflected ray follows laws of reflection.

Which of the following statement is incorrect?

(a) Only I
(b) Both I and II
(c) Only II
(d) Both I and III

47. A proton and an α-particle, both are accelerated from rest with same energy. The ratio of de-Broglie wavelength of α-particle to that of proton is

(a) 1 : 4 (b) 4 : 1
(c) 1 : 2 (d) 2 : 1

48 The binding energy of ${}_1^2H$ is 1.15 MeV per nucleon, an alpha particle ${}_2^4He$ has a binding energy of 7.1 MeV per nucleon. The Q-value of the following reaction is

$${}_1^2H + {}_1^2H \rightarrow {}_2^4He + Q$$

(a) 5.95 MeV (b) 23.8 MeV
(c) 26.1 MeV (d) 28.9 MeV

49. A cylinder contains 3 moles of oxygen and 1 mole of argon gas at room temperature of 27°C. Total internal energy of the system is

(a) $3600R$ (b) $5500R$
(c) $2700R$ (d) $3200R$

50. In a certain process $pV^n =$ constant, the heat Q given to a monoatomic gas leads to a change in internal energy of a gas which is equal to $\frac{Q}{4}$. The value of n is

(a) $\frac{7}{9}$ (b) 2 (c) $\frac{3}{5}$ (d) $\frac{6}{7}$

Answer key

Section A

1 (a)	2 (a)	3 (b)	4 (d)	5 (a)	6 (a)	7 (b)	8 (b)	9 (d)	10 (d)
11 (a)	12 (b)	13 (a)	14 (a)	15 (c)	16 (c)	17 (b)	18 (c)	19 (d)	20 (d)
21 (d)	22 (c)	23 (a)	24 (b)	25 (d)	26 (a)	27 (b)	28 (c)	29 (a)	30 (b)
31 (a)	32 (b)	33 (c)	34 (b)	35 (b)					

Section B

36 (c)	37 (c)	38 (a)	39 (d)	40 (b)	41 (b)	42 (a)	43 (c)	44 (a)	45 (b)
46 (c)	47 (c)	48 (b)	49 (c)	50 (a)					

Scan this QR Code for Detailed Solutions

ANSWER SHEET

Instructions for filling the sheet
1. Use only blue/ black ball pen to fill the circle.
2. Use of pencil is strictly prohibited.
3. Circle should be darkened completely and properly.

SECTION-A Attempt all 35 Questions in each subject

Q.No	Response	Q.No	Response	Q.No	Response	Q.No	Response
001	a b c d	051	a b c d	101	a b c d	151	a b c d
002	a b c d	052	a b c d	102	a b c d	152	a b c d
003	a b c d	053	a b c d	103	a b c d	153	a b c d
004	a b c d	054	a b c d	104	a b c d	154	a b c d
005	a b c d	055	a b c d	105	a b c d	155	a b c d
006	a b c d	056	a b c d	106	a b c d	156	a b c d
007	a b c d	057	a b c d	107	a b c d	157	a b c d
008	a b c d	058	a b c d	108	a b c d	158	a b c d
009	a b c d	059	a b c d	109	a b c d	159	a b c d
010	a b c d	060	a b c d	110	a b c d	160	a b c d
011	a b c d	061	a b c d	111	a b c d	161	a b c d
012	a b c d	062	a b c d	112	a b c d	162	a b c d
013	a b c d	063	a b c d	113	a b c d	163	a b c d
014	a b c d	064	a b c d	114	a b c d	164	a b c d
015	a b c d	065	a b c d	115	a b c d	165	a b c d
016	a b c d	066	a b c d	116	a b c d	166	a b c d
017	a b c d	067	a b c d	117	a b c d	167	a b c d
018	a b c d	068	a b c d	118	a b c d	168	a b c d
019	a b c d	069	a b c d	119	a b c d	169	a b c d
020	a b c d	070	a b c d	120	a b c d	170	a b c d
021	a b c d	071	a b c d	121	a b c d	171	a b c d
022	a b c d	072	a b c d	122	a b c d	172	a b c d
023	a b c d	073	a b c d	123	a b c d	173	a b c d
024	a b c d	074	a b c d	124	a b c d	174	a b c d
025	a b c d	075	a b c d	125	a b c d	175	a b c d
026	a b c d	076	a b c d	126	a b c d	176	a b c d
027	a b c d	077	a b c d	127	a b c d	177	a b c d
028	a b c d	078	a b c d	128	a b c d	178	a b c d
029	a b c d	079	a b c d	129	a b c d	179	a b c d
030	a b c d	080	a b c d	130	a b c d	180	a b c d
031	a b c d	081	a b c d	131	a b c d	181	a b c d
032	a b c d	082	a b c d	132	a b c d	182	a b c d
033	a b c d	083	a b c d	133	a b c d	183	a b c d
034	a b c d	084	a b c d	134	a b c d	184	a b c d
035	a b c d	085	a b c d	135	a b c d	185	a b c d

SECTION-B Attempt any 10 Questions in each subject

Q.No	Response	Q.No	Response	Q.No	Response	Q.No	Response
036	a b c d	086	a b c d	136	a b c d	186	a b c d
037	a b c d	087	a b c d	137	a b c d	187	a b c d
038	a b c d	088	a b c d	138	a b c d	188	a b c d
039	a b c d	089	a b c d	139	a b c d	189	a b c d
040	a b c d	090	a b c d	140	a b c d	190	a b c d
041	a b c d	091	a b c d	141	a b c d	191	a b c d
042	a b c d	092	a b c d	142	a b c d	192	a b c d
043	a b c d	093	a b c d	143	a b c d	193	a b c d
044	a b c d	094	a b c d	144	a b c d	194	a b c d
045	a b c d	095	a b c d	145	a b c d	195	a b c d
046	a b c d	096	a b c d	146	a b c d	196	a b c d
047	a b c d	097	a b c d	147	a b c d	197	a b c d
048	a b c d	098	a b c d	148	a b c d	198	a b c d
049	a b c d	099	a b c d	149	a b c d	199	a b c d
050	a b c d	100	a b c d	150	a b c d	200	a b c d

Complete Syllabus (11th & 12th)

Practice Test 03

Important Instructions

- The test of 1 hour duration and contains 50 Multiple Choice Questions (four options with a single correct answer) from Physics.
- There are 50 questions in each subject, divided into **two Sections** : Section A and Section B.
  (a) **Section A** contains 35 questions in each subject and all questions are compulsory.
  (b) **Section B** contains 15 questions from each subject out of which 10 questions are to be attempted.
- Each question carries 4 marks. For each correct response, the candidate will get 4 marks. For each incorrect response, one mark will be deducted from the total score.

Section-A (Q. No. 1 to 35)

1. Young's double slit experiment is performed in a medium of refractive index of 1.33. The maximum intensity is I_0. The intensity at a point on the screen, where path difference between the light coming out from slits is $\frac{\lambda}{4}$, is

(a) 0 (b) $\frac{I_0}{2}$ (c) $\frac{3I_0}{8}$ (d) $\frac{2I_0}{3}$

2. A particle moves in a straight line with a constant acceleration. It changes its velocity from 15 m/s to 25 m/s while passing through a distance 150 m in t s. The value of t is

(a) 9 (b) 8.5 (c) 7.5 (d) 10

3. If a equiconvex lens is made of number of layers of different refractive indices for a given wavelength as shown in the figure, then number of images formed for an object kept in front is

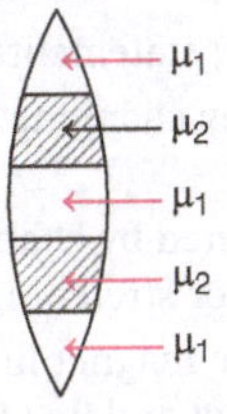

(a) only 1 (b) 2 (c) 2.5 (d) 5

4. Calculate the radius of the second Bohr's orbit of electron of hydrogen atom.

(a) 3.68Å (b) 2.12Å
(c) 4.77Å (d) 2.68Å

5. The period of revolution of a planet A around the sun is 27 times that of B. The distance of A from the sun is how many times greater than that of B from the sun ?

(a) 4 (b) 6 (c) 9 (d) 12

6. The output of the given arrangement of logic gates for $A = 0, B = 1$ and $A = 1, B = 1$ will be

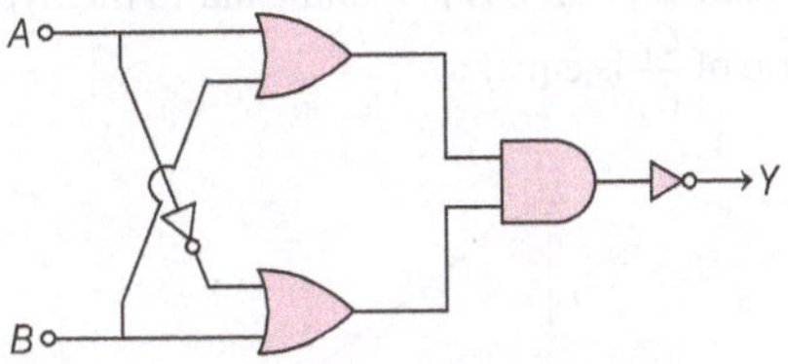

(a) (0, 0) (b) (0, 1)
(c) (1,1) (d) (1, 0)

7. Which of these graphs correctly shows change of kinetic energy K of a small steel ball in a deep water lake?

(a)
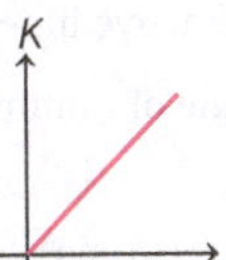

(b)
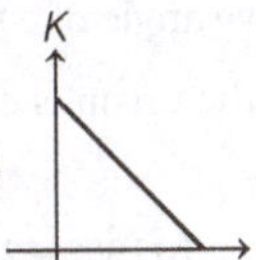

(c)
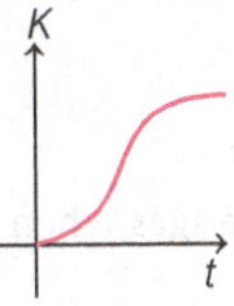

(d)
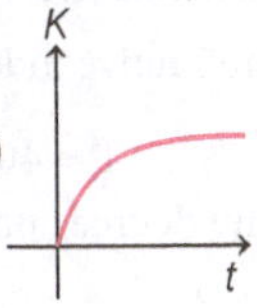

8. A solid sphere of mass M is rolling with a velocity v on a smooth horizontal surface and strikes a massless spring of force constant k attached to a massless smooth platform, then the maximum compression of spring is

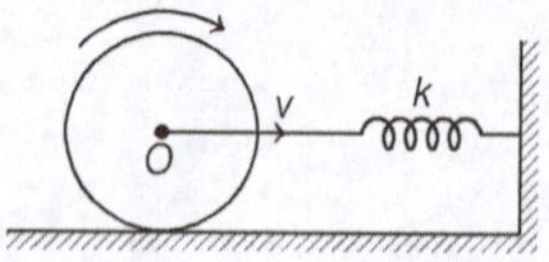

(a) $v\sqrt{\frac{7M}{5k}}$ (b) $v\sqrt{\frac{2M}{3k}}$ (c) $v\sqrt{\frac{M}{5k}}$ (d) $v\sqrt{\frac{5M}{3k}}$

9. **Assertion** (A) Specific heat capacity and molar specific heat capacity both have same units.

Reason (R) Specific heat capacity and molar specific heat capacity both do not depend on mass.

In the light of above statements choose the most appropriate answer from the options given below.

(a) Both A and R are true and R is the correct explanation of A.
(b) Both A and R are true but R is not the correct explanation of A.
(c) A is true but R is false.
(d) A is false but R is true.

10. In a plane electromagnetic wave, the electric field oscillate sinusoidally at a frequency of 2×10^{10} Hz and amplitude 48 V/m. The wavelength of the wave is

(a) 24×10^{-10} m (b) 1.5×10^{-2} m
(c) 4.16×10^{8} m (d) 3×10^{8} m

11. Two point charges Q_1 and Q_2 are placed on two vertices of a right angle triangle as shown in figure. The resultant electric field at point O is perpendicular to the hypotenuse, then ratio of $\frac{Q_1}{Q_2}$ is equal to

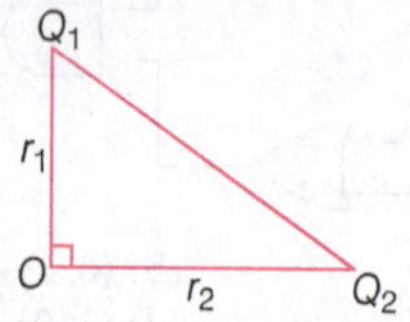

(a) $\frac{r_1}{r_2}$ (b) $\frac{r_2}{r_1}$ (c) $\frac{r_1^2}{r_2^2}$ (d) $\frac{r_2^3}{r_1^3}$

12. The refractive angle of a prism is A. If refractive index of material of the prism is $\cot\left(\frac{A}{2}\right)$, then angle of minimum deviation is

(a) $180° - A$ (b) $180° - 2A$ (c) $2A$ (d) $90° - A$

13. Electric field associated with an electromagnetic wave in a medium of refractive index $\frac{3}{2}$ is

$$E = 40\cos(kz - 6 \times 10^8 t)$$

By how many degrees phase of wave changes when it travels $\left(\frac{\pi}{2}\right)$ m?

(a) 90° (b) 180° (c) 270° (d) 360°

14. A coil of area 10 cm² and 10 turns is in magnetic field directed perpendicular to the plane and changing at a rate of 10^8 G/s. The resistance of coil is 20 Ω. The current in the coil will be

(a) 0.5 A (b) 5×10^{-3} A
(c) 0.05 A (d) 5 A

15. Four different configurations of charges has been shown in the figure. The increasing order of electrostatics potential energies of the given system of charges is

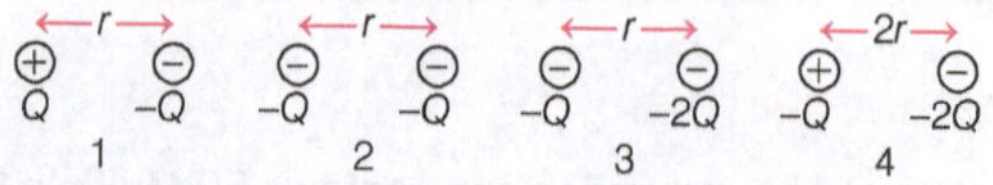

(a) $U_1 = U_4 < U_2 < U_3$ (b) $U_2 = U_4 < U_3 < U_1$
(c) $U_2 = U_3 < U_1 < U_4$ (d) $U_3 < U_1 < U_2 < U_4$

16. **Statement I** In a nuclear reactor, heavy water or graphite can be used as moderator.

Statement II When a light object collides with a heavy object, nearly whole of kinetic energy is given to heavier object.

In light of above statements choose the most appropriate answer from the options given below

(a) Both Statement I and Statement II are incorrect.
(b) Statement I is correct and Statement II is incorrect.
(c) Statement I is incorrect and Statement II is correct.
(d) Both Statement I and Statement II are correct.

17. A rectangular film of liquid is extended from 16 cm² to 40 cm². If the work done is 5×10^{-4} J. The value of the surface tension of liquid is

(a) 0.1 N/m (b) 0.2 N/m (c) 0.3 N/m (d) 0.5 N/m

18. The graph between current I and voltage V has been shown in figure given below, so which portion of the graph shows the negative dynamic resistance?

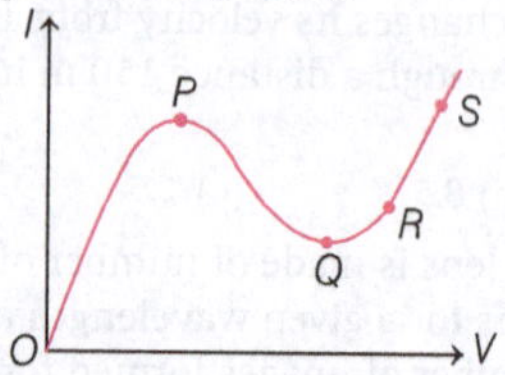

(a) OP (b) PQ (c) QS (d) RS

19. Which of the following statement(s) is/are incorrect ?

I. Flux can be varied by changing any one or more of the terms B, A and θ.
II. Flux can also be altered by changing the shape of a coil (i.e. by shrinking it or stretching it) in a magnetic field.
III. A gentle push on the magnet in magnetic field initiates the motion in magnet and its kinetic energy continuously increases without expanding any energy.
IV. When a bar magnet experiences a repulsive force due to the induced current, a person has to do work in moving the magnet. The energy spent by the person is dissipated by joule heating produced by the induced current.

(a) Only I (b) Both II and III
(c) Only III (d) I, II, III

20. Which of the following equations can be derived using method of dimensional analysis?
(a) $N = N_0 \cdot e^{-\lambda t}$
(b) $y = A\sin(\omega t + kx)$
(c) $E = \frac{1}{2}mv^2 + \frac{1}{2}I\omega^2$
(d) None of these

21. The equation of a transverse wave propagating in a string is given by $y = 0.02\sin(x + 30t)$, where x and y are in metres and t is in second. If linear density of the string is 1.3×10^{-4} kg/m, then the tension in the string is
(a) 0.12 N
(b) 1.2 N
(c) 12 N
(d) 120 N

22. The bottom end of a cubical block of side 5×10^{-2} m is fixed. A force of 10^5N tangential to the top face displaces it by 1.2×10^{-4} m. The rigidity modulus is
(a) 6×10^{-10} Nm^{-2}
(b) 6×10^{-9} Nm^{-2}
(c) 1.67×10^{10} Nm^{-2}
(d) 10^{11} Nm^{-2}

23. A large glass surface is 2 mm thick. The outside temperature is – 20°C and the inside temperature is 25°C. If the thermal conductivity of glass is 0.8 W/m-K, then the temperature at the mid-point of the window is
(a) 0 °C
(b) 2.5 °C
(c) – 25°C
(d) 22.5 °C

24. In a Young's double slit experiment, if there is no initial phase difference between the light from the two slits. The point on the screen corresponding to the 8th minimum has path difference
(a) 4λ
(b) $\frac{9}{2}\lambda$
(c) $\frac{15}{2}\lambda$
(d) 8λ

25. If the earth shrinks to n times of its radius without changing its mass, then duration of the day will be
(a) nT
(b) $\frac{T}{n}$
(c) n^2T
(d) $\frac{T}{n^2}$

(where, T = duration of day before shrinking)

26. A particle moves in a straight line, its angular momentum with respect to a choosen origin is
(a) a constant
(b) keeps on increasing with time
(c) first increases then decreases
(d) keeps on decreasing

27. A water drop in air refracts the light rays as

(a)
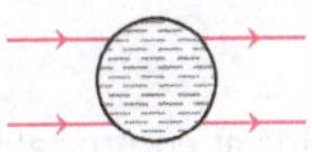

(b)
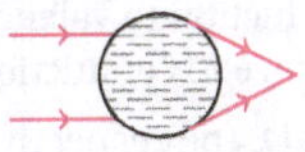

(c)
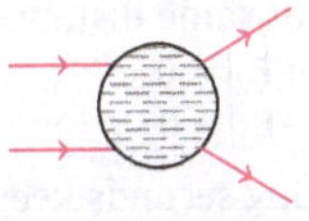

(d)
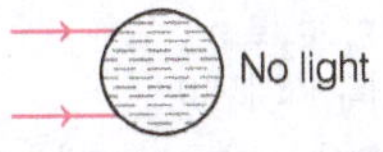

28. Two balls of masses m_1 and m_2 are moving with velocities $v_1\hat{i}$ and $v_2\hat{i}$ undergoes a collinear collision. After collision, velocities of m_1 and m_2 are $v_3\hat{i}$ and $v_4\hat{i}$ respectively. If $m_2 = 0.5m_1$ and $v_3 = 0.5v_1$, then value of v_1 is
(a) $v_4 + v_2$
(b) $v_4 - \frac{v_2}{4}$
(c) $v_4 - \frac{v_2}{2}$
(d) $v_4 - v_2$

29. The p-V graph of three different gases A, B and C during adiabatic expansion has been plotted. The gases A, B and C can be respectively,

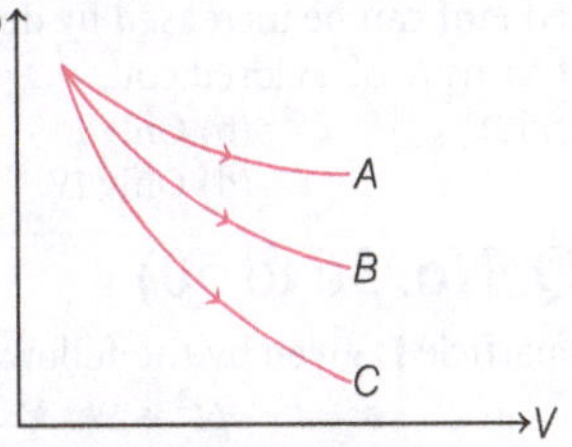

(a) monoatomic, diatomic, polyatomic
(b) polyatomic, diatomic, monoatomic
(c) diatomic, triatomic (linear), triatomic (non-linear)
(d) monoatomic, triatomic (linear), triatomic (non-linear)

30. A boy riding a bike with a speed of 5 m/s towards east direction observes raindrops falling vertically downwards. On increasing the speed of 15 m/s, rain appears to fall making an angle at 45° of the vertical. The magnitude of velocity of rain w.r.t. ground is
(a) 5 m/s
(b) $5\sqrt{5}$ m/s
(c) 25 m/s
(d) 10 m/s

31. A 50 Hz, 10 V source is connected to a resistance of 40Ω, an inductance of 191 mH and a capacitance of 106 μF in series. The time in which the resistor having heat capacity 6 J/°C gets heated by 80°C is
(a) 4 s
(b) 6 s
(c) 12 s
(d) 480 s

32. Dimensional formula $[ML^{-1}T^{-2}]$ does not represent the physical quantity.
(a) Young's modulus of elasticity
(b) Stress
(c) Strain
(d) Pressure

33. A particle is projected from ground at an angle θ with the vertical such that its horizontal range R is related to its time of flight T as $R = 10\frac{\sqrt{3}}{2}T^2$. The value of projection angle θ is
(Take, $g = 10\,\text{m/s}^2$)
(a) 30°
(b) 45°
(c) 60°
(d) None of these

34. A DC battery of 2 V emf and internal resistance 1 Ω are connected through the external load. Current of 1 A is flowing through the external load. If this type of battery is connected twice in series, then the value of current through same load is
(a) 1.33 A
(b) 2.7 A
(c) 0.67 A
(d) 1.11 A

35. Which of the following statement(s) is/are incorrect ?
I. The phenomenon in which electric current is generated by varying magnetic field is appropriately called electromagnetic induction.

II. If the magnetic field has different magnitudes and directions at various parts of a surface, then the magnetic flux through the surface is, $\phi_B = \sum \mathbf{B}_i d\mathbf{A}_i$

III. An emf is induced in a coil when magnetic flux through the coil changes with time, whose magnitude is equal to the time rate of change of magnetic flux through the circuit.

IV. The induced emf can be increased by decreasing the number of turns N of a closed coil.

(a) Both III and IV
(b) Only I
(c) I, II, III
(d) Only IV

Section-B (Q. No. 36 to 50)

36. Position of a particle is given by the following equation,

$$x = t^3 - 6t^2 + 9t$$

Ratio of distance and displacement of body in first five second will be

(a) 1
(b) 2
(c) $\frac{3}{7}$
(d) $\frac{7}{5}$

37. An EM wave of wavelength λ is incident on a photosensitive surface of negligible work function. If the photoelectrons emitted from the surface have the de-Broglie wavelength λ_0, then λ is equal to

(a) $\lambda_0\sqrt{\frac{2mc}{h}}$
(b) $\lambda_0^2\left(\frac{2mc}{h}\right)$
(c) $\sqrt{\lambda_0 \frac{h}{2mc}}$
(d) $\lambda_0\left(\frac{2mc}{h}\right)^2$

38. Four moles of an ideal gas is taken through the process ABC as shown in the following figure. The total work done by the gas is

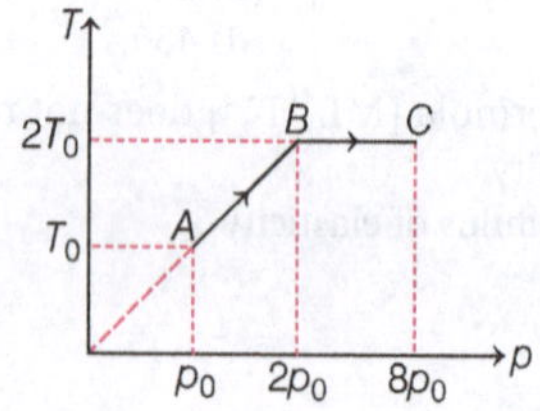

(a) $8RT_0 \ln 2$
(b) $-8RT_0 \ln 2$
(c) $16RT_0 \ln 2$
(d) $-16RT_0 \ln 2$

39. I. The reflected ray goes through the focus of the mirror, when it is incident parallel to the principal axis.

II. The reflected ray is perpendicular to the principal axis when incident ray passes through the focus of the concave mirror or appear to pass through the focus of a convex mirror.

III. For the ray incident at any angle at the pole, the reflected ray follows laws of reflection.

Which of the following statement is incorrect?

(a) Only I
(b) Both I and II
(c) Only II
(d) Both I and III

40. Match the quantities in Column I with their orders in Column II and choose the correct answer from the options given below.

	Column I		Column II
A	Drift velocity of electron in a metallic conductor	P	10^{-4}
B	Speed of electron in an atomic orbit	Q	10^{-3}
C	Resistivity of metals	R	10^{-8}
D	Temperature coefficient of resistivity of metals	S	10^{6}

(a) $A \rightarrow P, B \rightarrow S, C \rightarrow R, D \rightarrow Q$
(b) $A \rightarrow Q, B \rightarrow P, C \rightarrow R, D \rightarrow S$
(c) $A \rightarrow R, B \rightarrow Q, C \rightarrow P, D \rightarrow S$
(c) $A \rightarrow P, B \rightarrow R, C \rightarrow Q, D \rightarrow S$

41. The electric potential V is given as a function of distance as $V = (10x^2 + 5x + 2)$ V, where x is in metre. The difference of electrostatic potential energy of a charge $+2\,\mu C$ at $x = 1$ m and $x = 2$ m is

(a) $7\mu J$
(b) $3.5\,\mu J$
(c) $70\,\mu J$
(d) $35\,\mu J$

42. Which among the following graphs shows the correct variation of photoelectric current with intensity of light for a given frequency?

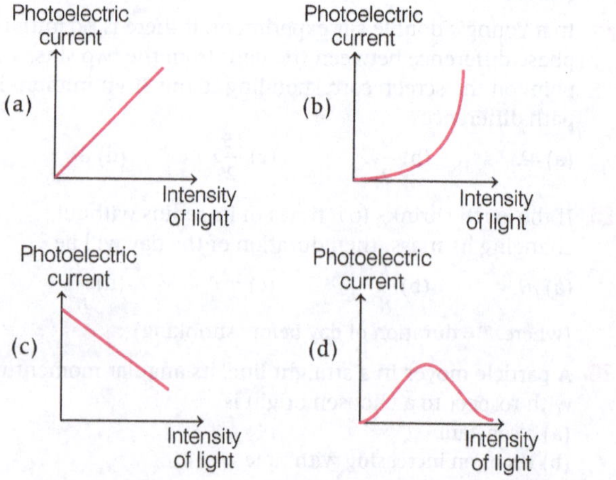

43. In an LED, electrons move from

(a) lower level to higher in conduction band
(b) lower level to higher in valence band
(c) conduction to valence band
(d) valence to conduction band

44. If $\mathbf{E}_1$ and $\mathbf{E}_2$ be respective electric fields at equitorial position and axial position of electric dipole at same distance, then

(a) $\mathbf{E}_1 \cdot \mathbf{E}_2 = 0$
(b) $|\mathbf{E}_1 + \mathbf{E}_2| = 0$
(c) $|\mathbf{E}_1 \times \mathbf{E}_2| = 0$
(d) $|\mathbf{E}_1 - \mathbf{E}_2| = 0$

45. A clock with a metal pendulum beating seconds keeps correct time at 0°C. If it loses 14.5 s a day at 25°C, the coefficient of linear expansion of metal pendulum is

(a) 1.34×10^{-5}/°C
(b) 234×10^{-5}/°C
(c) 7.24×10^{8}/°C
(d) 7.24×10^{-8}/°C

46. An electron is travelling horizontally towards east. A magnetic field in vertically downward direction exerts a force on the electron along

(a) east (b) west
(c) north (d) south

47. A transformer with efficiency of 90% works at 10 kW and 2000 V. If the secondary voltage is 100 V, then the primary and secondary currents are, respectively

(a) 5 A, 90 A (b) 4.5 A, 100 A
(c) 5 A, 50 A (d) 10 A, 45 A

48. The graph between intensity of magnetisation I and magnetic field strength H is for an unknown substance is found as shown in the figure, then the substance is

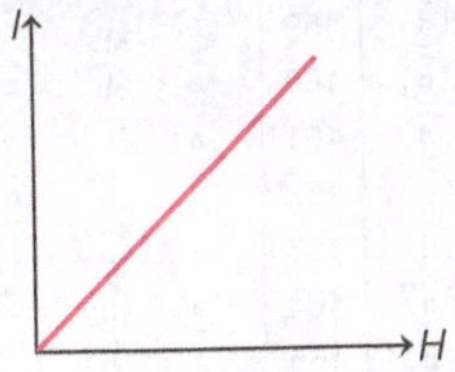

(a) diamagnetic (b) paramagnetic
(c) Both (a) and (b) (d) ferromagnetic

49. A dipole is placed parallel to an electric field. Let W is work done in rotating the dipole by 60°, then work done in rotating dipole by 180° will be

(a) $2W$ (b) $3W$
(c) $4W$ (d) $0.5W$

50. In the circuit shown below, diode has potential barrier of 0.5 V across it. A current greater than 10 mA produces large amount of heat and damages diode. If diode is to be operated at 5 mA, the required series resistance R is (the internal resistance of battery)

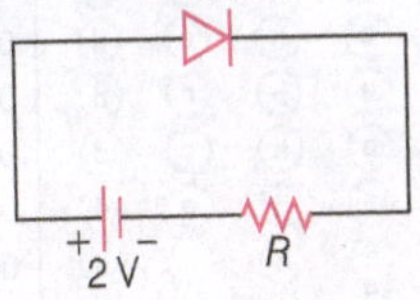

(a) 300 Ω (b) 300 kΩ
(c) 200 kΩ (d) 3 kΩ

Answer key

Section A

1 (b)	2 (c)	3 (b)	4 (b)	5 (c)	6 (a)	7 (d)	8 (a)	9 (d)	10 (b)
11 (a)	12 (b)	13 (c)	14 (d)	15 (a)	16 (b)	17 (a)	18 (b)	19 (c)	20 (d)
21 (a)	22 (c)	23 (b)	24 (c)	25 (d)	26 (a)	27 (b)	28 (d)	29 (b)	30 (b)
31 (b)	32 (c)	33 (a)	34 (a)	35 (d)					

Section B

36 (d)	37 (b)	38 (d)	39 (c)	40 (a)	41 (c)	42 (a)	43 (c)	44 (c)	45 (a)
46 (d)	47 (a)	48 (b)	49 (c)	50 (a)					

Scan this QR Code for Detailed Solutions

ANSWER SHEET

Instructions for filling the sheet
1. Use only blue/ black ball pen to fill the circle.
2. Use of pencil is strictly prohibited.
3. Circle should be darkened completely and properly.

SECTION-A Attempt all 35 Questions in each subject

Q.No	Response	Q.No	Response	Q.No	Response	Q.No	Response
001	a b c d	051	a b c d	101	a b c d	151	a b c d
002	a b c d	052	a b c d	102	a b c d	152	a b c d
003	a b c d	053	a b c d	103	a b c d	153	a b c d
004	a b c d	054	a b c d	104	a b c d	154	a b c d
005	a b c d	055	a b c d	105	a b c d	155	a b c d
006	a b c d	056	a b c d	106	a b c d	156	a b c d
007	a b c d	057	a b c d	107	a b c d	157	a b c d
008	a b c d	058	a b c d	108	a b c d	158	a b c d
009	a b c d	059	a b c d	109	a b c d	159	a b c d
010	a b c d	060	a b c d	110	a b c d	160	a b c d
011	a b c d	061	a b c d	111	a b c d	161	a b c d
012	a b c d	062	a b c d	112	a b c d	162	a b c d
013	a b c d	063	a b c d	113	a b c d	163	a b c d
014	a b c d	064	a b c d	114	a b c d	164	a b c d
015	a b c d	065	a b c d	115	a b c d	165	a b c d
016	a b c d	066	a b c d	116	a b c d	166	a b c d
017	a b c d	067	a b c d	117	a b c d	167	a b c d
018	a b c d	068	a b c d	118	a b c d	168	a b c d
019	a b c d	069	a b c d	119	a b c d	169	a b c d
020	a b c d	070	a b c d	120	a b c d	170	a b c d
021	a b c d	071	a b c d	121	a b c d	171	a b c d
022	a b c d	072	a b c d	122	a b c d	172	a b c d
023	a b c d	073	a b c d	123	a b c d	173	a b c d
024	a b c d	074	a b c d	124	a b c d	174	a b c d
025	a b c d	075	a b c d	125	a b c d	175	a b c d
026	a b c d	076	a b c d	126	a b c d	176	a b c d
027	a b c d	077	a b c d	127	a b c d	177	a b c d
028	a b c d	078	a b c d	128	a b c d	178	a b c d
029	a b c d	079	a b c d	129	a b c d	179	a b c d
030	a b c d	080	a b c d	130	a b c d	180	a b c d
031	a b c d	081	a b c d	131	a b c d	181	a b c d
032	a b c d	082	a b c d	132	a b c d	182	a b c d
033	a b c d	083	a b c d	133	a b c d	183	a b c d
034	a b c d	084	a b c d	134	a b c d	184	a b c d
035	a b c d	085	a b c d	135	a b c d	185	a b c d

SECTION-B Attempt any 10 Questions in each subject

Q.No	Response	Q.No	Response	Q.No	Response	Q.No	Response
036	a b c d	086	a b c d	136	a b c d	186	a b c d
037	a b c d	087	a b c d	137	a b c d	187	a b c d
038	a b c d	088	a b c d	138	a b c d	188	a b c d
039	a b c d	089	a b c d	139	a b c d	189	a b c d
040	a b c d	090	a b c d	140	a b c d	190	a b c d
041	a b c d	091	a b c d	141	a b c d	191	a b c d
042	a b c d	092	a b c d	142	a b c d	192	a b c d
043	a b c d	093	a b c d	143	a b c d	193	a b c d
044	a b c d	094	a b c d	144	a b c d	194	a b c d
045	a b c d	095	a b c d	145	a b c d	195	a b c d
046	a b c d	096	a b c d	146	a b c d	196	a b c d
047	a b c d	097	a b c d	147	a b c d	197	a b c d
048	a b c d	098	a b c d	148	a b c d	198	a b c d
049	a b c d	099	a b c d	149	a b c d	199	a b c d
050	a b c d	100	a b c d	150	a b c d	200	a b c d